Mosby's
DRUG
REFERENCE *for*
HEALTH
PROFESSIONS

Second Edition

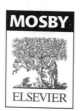

MOSBY

ELSEVIER

MOSBY
ELSEVIER

11830 Westline Industrial Drive
St. Louis, Missouri 63146

MOSBY'S DRUG REFERENCE FOR
HEALTH PROFESSIONS

ISBN: 978-0-323-06362-3

Notice

Knowledge and best practice in this field are constantly changing. As new research and experience broaden our knowledge, changes in practice, treatment and drug therapy may become necessary or appropriate. Readers are advised to check the most current information provided (i) on procedures featured or (ii) by the manufacturer of each product to be administered, to verify the recommended dose or formula, the method and duration of administration, and contraindications. It is the responsibility of the practitioner, relying on their own experience and knowledge of the patient, to make diagnoses, to determine dosages and the best treatment for each individual patient, and to take all appropriate safety precautions. To the fullest extent of the law, neither the Publisher nor the Editors assume any liability for any injury and/or damage to persons or property arising out of or related to any use of the material contained in this book.

ISBN: 978-0-323-06362-3

Vice President and Publisher: Linda Duncan
Senior Editor: Kellie White
Senior Developmental Editor: Jennifer Watrous
Publishing Services Manager: Pat Joiner-Myers
Project Manager: Srikumar Narayanan
Designer: Kimberly Denando

Printed in the United States of America

Last digit is the print number: 9 8 7 6 5 4 3

Working together to grow
libraries in developing countries
www.elsevier.com | www.bookaid.org | www.sabre.org

ELSEVIER   BOOK AID International   Sabre Foundation

CONSULTANTS

MaryAnne Hochadel,
PharmD, BCPS
Editor Emeritus
ELSEVIER/Gold Standard
Tampa, Florida

John J. Smith, EdD
AVP, Curriculum
Corinthian Colleges, Inc.
Santa Ana, California

Stephanie Schroeder, PharmD
ELSEVIER/Gold Standard
Wichita, Kansas

CONTRIBUTORS

Deborah A. DeLuca, MS ChE, JD
Assistant Professor
Health Professions Leadership
Seton Hall University School of
 Health and Medical Sciences
South Orange, New Jersey

Julie Karpinski, PharmD, BCPS
Assistant Director, Drug Information
 Center
Assistant Professor, Pharmacy
 Practice
Southern Illinois University
 Edwardsville
Edwardsville, Illinois

Kristi Kelley, PharmD, BCPS, CDE
Associate Clinical Professor
Department of Pharmacy Practice
Auburn University Harrison School
 of Pharmacy
Birmingham, Alabama

Terri L. Levien, PharmD
Clinical Associate Professor
Pharmacotherapy Department
College of Pharmacy
Washington State University
 Spokane
Spokane, Washington

Erin M. Timpe, PharmD, BCPS
Director, Drug Information Center
Assistant Professor, Pharmacy
 Practice
School of Pharmacy
Southern Illinois University
 Edwardsville
Edwardsville, Illinois

REVIEWERS

Susan G. Salvo, BEd, LMT, NTS, CI, NCTMB
Co-Director and Instructor
Louisiana Institute of Massage Therapy
Lake Charles, Louisiana

Erica Seamon, PharmD
Natural Standard Research Collaboration
Cambridge, Massachusetts

Catherine E. Ulbricht, PharmD
Natural Standard Research Collaboration
Cambridge, Massachusetts
www.naturalstandard.com
Department of Pharmacy
Massachusetts General Hospital
Boston, Massachusetts

Health care professionals face many challenges in today's environment, not the least of which is familiarity with the large number of medications available. New medications are being introduced, and new applications, dosage forms, and different routes of administration for existing medications are increasing at a rapid rate. This voluminous amount of drug information must be quickly integrated into the patient care environment. *Mosby's Drug Reference for Health Professions* is designed as an easy-to-use source of the current drug information needed by the busy health care provider.

This guide contains:

1. Practice-oriented precautions and considerations. Every drug entry provides extensive, practice-oriented precautions and considerations, putting essential drug facts directly into the context of your care.
2. Vital lifespan considerations. Throughout its pages, the book highlights key points related to drug therapy in pregnant, breast-feeding, pediatric, and elderly patients.
3. Informative appendices. Five ready-reference appendices give you easy access to additional vital drug-related information, such as the English-Spanish Drug Phrase Translator and Normal Laboratory Values for a quick reference when working with clients and patients.
4. Prioritized side effects. Drug entries rank side effects by frequency of occurrence, from most common to least common. Entries also include the percentage of frequency, when known. This information helps you focus your

care by knowing which effects to monitor more closely.
5. Highlights on serious adverse reactions. The book calls attention to dangerous or life-threatening reactions so that you can identify them easily and act on them promptly.
6. Alert icons. Alert icons are used to spotlight critical health professions considerations that require special attention.

A detailed guide to *Mosby's Drug Reference for Health Professions:*

Essential drug information in a user-friendly format. The bulk of the handbook contains an alphabetical listing of drug entries by generic name. Drug entries include the following:

Generic and Brand Names. Drug entries begin with the generic drug name, followed by its pronunciation and U.S. and Canadian brand names.

Classification. Each entry highlights this important information for easy identification.

Category and schedule. This section lists the drug's pregnancy risk category and, when appropriate, its controlled substance schedule or over-the-counter (OTC) status.

Mechanism of action. This section clearly and concisely details the drug's mechanism of action and therapeutic effects.

Pharmacokinetics. This heading, outlines the drug's route, onset, peak, and duration, when known. This information is followed by a discussion of the drug's absorption, distribution, metabolism, excretion, and half-life.

Availability. This section identifies the forms that the drug comes in, such as tablets, sustained-release capsules, or an injectable solution. Available doses and concentrations are also listed.

Indications and dosages. Here, you'll find the approved indications and routes, along with the dosage information for all age groups and populations, including adults, elderly patients, children, neonates, and those with pre-existing conditions such as liver or kidney disease.

Contraindications. Entries list the most common conditions in which use of the generic drug is contraindicated and should not be used.

Interactions. For drugs, herbal supplements, and food, this section supplies vital information about interactions with the topic drug.

Diagnostic test effects. Under this heading, you'll see a brief description of the drug's effects on laboratory and diagnostic test results, such as liver enzyme levels and electrocardiogram tracings, when known.

IV incompatibilities and IV compatibilities. These twin sections let you know which IV drugs can and cannot be given with the featured drug. These listings are not meant to be inclusive, but rather are exemplary of common incompatibilities and compatibilities.

Side effects. Unlike other handbooks that mix common, deadly effects with rare, minor ones in a long, undifferentiated list, this book ranks side effects by frequency of occurrence by indicating: expected, frequent, occasional, and rare. Within each frequency, effects are listed by highest to lowest percentage of occurrence, when known.

Serious reactions. Because serious reactions are life-threatening responses that require prompt intervention, this section highlights them, apart from other side effects, for easy identification.

Precautions and considerations. Using a practice-oriented format and written specifically for health professions, this section presents precautions and considerations for each drug entry.

Mosby's Drug Reference for Health Professions is an easy-to-use source of the current drug information for a wide spectrum of health care providers. When it comes to providing quality patient care, you'll need no other drug reference.

CONTENTS

Contributors, iii

Reviewers, iv

Introduction, vi

A to Z Drug Entries, 1

Appendices
- A General Anesthetics, 1647
- B English-to-Spanish Drug Phrases Translator, 1648
- C FDA Pregnancy Categories, 1666
- D Normal Laboratory Values, 1667
- E Error-Prone Drug Name Abbreviations, 1670

Glossary, 1673

Index, 1691

Abacavir
ah-bah´-cah-veer
(Ziagen)

CATEGORY AND SCHEDULE
Pregnancy Risk Category: C

Classification: Antiretroviral, nucleoside analog

MECHANISM OF ACTION
An antiretroviral that inhibits the activity of HIV-1 reverse transcriptase by competing with the natural substrate deoxyguanosine-5´-triphosphate (dGTP) and by its incorporation into viral DNA. *Therapeutic Effect:* Inhibits viral DNA growth.

PHARMACOKINETICS
Rapidly and extensively absorbed after PO administration. Protein binding: 50%. Widely distributed, including to CSF and erythrocytes. Metabolized in the liver to inactive metabolites. Excreted primarily in urine. Unknown whether removed by hemodialysis. *Half-life: 1.5 h.*

AVAILABILITY
Tablets: 300 mg.
Oral Solution: 20 mg/mL.

INDICATIONS AND DOSAGES
▶ **HIV infection (in combination with other antiretrovirals)**
PO
Adults. 300 mg twice a day or 600 mg once daily.
Children (3 mo–16 yr). 8 mg/kg twice a day. Maximum: 300 mg twice a day.
▶ **Dosage in hepatic impairment**
Mild impairment
Adults: 200 mg twice a day.

Moderate to Severe Impairment
Not recommended.

CONTRAINDICATIONS
Hypersensitivity to abacavir or its components.
Moderate to severe hepatic impairment.

INTERACTIONS
Drug
Ethanol: Increased abacavir levels.
Methadone: Methadone levels may be increased.
Herbal
None known.
Food
None known.

SIDE EFFECTS
Frequent
Adults: Nausea, nausea with vomiting, diarrhea, decreased appetite.
Children: Nausea with vomiting, fever, headache, diarrhea, rash.
Occasional
Adults: Insomnia.
Children: Decreased appetite.

SERIOUS REACTIONS
• A hypersensitivity reaction may be life threatening. Signs and symptoms include fever, rash, fatigue, intractable nausea and vomiting, severe diarrhea, abdominal pain, cough, pharyngitis, and dyspnea.
• Life-threatening hypotension may occur.
• Lactic acidosis and severe hepatomegaly may occur.

PRECAUTIONS & CONSIDERATIONS
Serious and sometimes fatal hypersensitivity reactions have been associated with abacavir therapy. Hypersensitivity reactions to abacavir may be characterized

by constitutional symptoms such as achiness, fatigue, or generalized malaise; fever; GI symptoms including abdominal pain, diarrhea, nausea, or vomiting; rash; and respiratory symptoms including cough, dyspnea, or pharyngitis. Abacavir therapy should be discontinued if hypersensitivity is suspected. Abacavir therapy should never be restarted following a hypersensitivity reaction. *A Medication Guide* and warning card that provide information about recognition of hypersensitivity reactions should be dispensed with each new prescription and refill. Screen all patients before initiation of abacavir therapy for the presence of the *HLA-B*5701* allele. Patients showing a positive result should have an abacavir allergy recorded and should **NOT** receive the medication. Patients taking abacavir appear to be at greater risk of having a myocardial infarction than are patients receiving other nucleoside reverse transcriptase inhibitors. Risk of myocardial infarction appears greatest with recent use and in patients with other heart disease risk factors. Lactic acidosis and severe hepatomegaly with steatosis, including fatal cases, have been reported with the use of nucleoside analogs alone or in combination, including abacavir and other antiretrovirals. Fat redistribution has also been observed in patients receiving antiretroviral therapy.

Storage
Store abacavir tablets and solution at room temperature. Abacavir solution may also be stored in the refrigerator, but it should be protected from freezing.

Administration
Abacavir may be taken with or without food. Abacavir should always be used in combination with other antiretroviral agents.

Abarelix
a-ba-rel′iks
(Plenaxis)

CATEGORY AND SCHEDULE
Pregnancy Risk Category: X

Classification: Antineoplastics, hormones/hormone modifiers, gonadotropin-releasing hormone (GnRH) analogs.

MECHANISM OF ACTION
A luteinizing hormone-releasing hormone (LHRH) antagonist that inhibits gonadotropin and androgen production by blocking GnRH receptors in the pituitary. *Therapeutic Effect:* Suppresses luteinizing hormone, follicle stimulating hormone secretion, reducing the secretion of testosterone by the testes.

PHARMACOKINETICS
Slowly absorbed following IM administration. Distributed extensively. Protein binding: 96%-99%. *Half-life:* 13.2 days.

AVAILABILITY
Powder for Injection: 113 mg kit containing 10 mL 0.9% NaCl, 18-gauge needle, 22-gauge needle.

INDICATIONS AND DOSAGES
▶ **Prostate cancer:** Palliative treatment of advanced prostate cancer when LHRH agonist therapy is not appropriate.

IM

Adults, Elderly. 100 mg on days 1, 15, 29, and every 4 wks thereafter. Treatment failure can be detected by obtaining serum testosterone concentration before abarelix administration, beginning day 29 and every 8 wks thereafter.

CONTRAINDICATIONS

Known hypersensitivity to any of the product ingredients.

This drug should not be used in women and children.

INTERACTIONS

Drug

None known.

Herbal

None known.

Food

None known.

DIAGNOSTIC TEST EFFECTS

May increase serum transaminase, serum SGOT (AST), SGPT (ALT), and serum triglyceride levels. May slightly decrease blood hemoglobin concentrations. May decrease bone mineral density.

SIDE EFFECTS

Frequent (30%-79%)

Hot flashes, sleep disturbances, breast enlargement.

Occasional (11%-20%)

Breast pain, nipple tenderness, back pain, constipation, peripheral edema, dizziness, upper respiratory tract infection, diarrhea.

Rare (10%)

Fatigue, nausea, dysuria, micturition frequency, urinary retention, urinary tract infection.

SERIOUS REACTIONS

• Immediate-onset systemic allergic reaction characterized by hypotension, urticaria, pruritus, periorbital and/or circumoral edema, shortness of breath, wheezing, and syncope may occur.

• Prolongation of the QT interval may occur; tightening of throat, tongue swelling, wheezing, shortness of breath, and low blood pressure occur rarely.

PRECAUTIONS & CONSIDERATIONS

May be prescribed only by clinicians who have enrolled in the Plenaxis PLUS limited distribution program. Caution is warranted in patients with prolonged QT interval or who weigh more than 225 lb (103 kg). Be aware that this drug is not for use in women or children. Be aware that there are no age-related precautions noted in the elderly.

Potential side effects, including hot flashes, sleep disturbances, breast enlargement, and nipple tenderness, may occur. Notify the physician if rash, hives, itching, tingling, or flushing develops; the skin reaction may occur immediately after injection or several days later. Immediate-onset systemic allergic reactions (urticaria, pruritus, hypotension, syncope) can occur after any dose, including the first dose. Patients should be observed for at least 30 min after each dose. Serum testosterone concentration should be measured before administration beginning on day 29 and every 8 wks thereafter. Serum PSA and serum transaminase levels should be periodically monitored.

Storage

Store at room temperature.

Administration

Shake abarelix vial gently before reconstituting. Withdraw 2.2 mL of 0.9% NaCl using an 18-gauge needle and a 3-mL syringe. Insert the needle into the abarelix vial and inject the diluent quickly.

Shake immediately for 15 s. Allow vial to stand for 2 min. Tap the vial to reduce foaming, and swirl the vial. Shake the vial again for 15 s, and allow it to stand again for 2 min. Insert 18-gauge needle, invert the vial, and draw up some of the suspension into the syringe. Without removing the needle from the vial, reinject it at any remaining solids in the vial. Repeat this process until all solids are dispersed. Swirl the vial before withdrawal, then withdraw the entire contents, about 2.2 mL. Reconstitution will provide a concentration of 50 mg/mL and should be used within 1 h of reconstitution. Exchange the 18-gauge needle with the 22-gauge needle and give entire suspension IM into the dorsogluteal or vetrogluteal region of the buttock. Monitor the patient for 30 min. The cumulative risk for allergic reaction increases with each injection.

Abciximab
ab-six′ih-mab
(c7E3 Fab, ReoPro)

CATEGORY AND SCHEDULE
Pregnancy Risk Category: C

Classification: Monoclonal antibodies, platelet inhibitors, recombinant DNA origin

MECHANISM OF ACTION
A glycoprotein IIb/IIIa receptor inhibitor that rapidly inhibits platelet aggregation by preventing the binding of fibrinogen to GP IIb/IIIa receptor sites on platelets. *Therapeutic Effect:* Prevents closure of treated coronary arteries. Prevents acute cardiac ischemic complications.

PHARMACOKINETICS
Rapidly cleared from plasma. Initial-phase half-life is < 10 min; second-phase half-life is 30 min. Platelet function generally returns within 48 h.

AVAILABILITY
Injection: 2 mg/mL (5-mL vial).

INDICATIONS AND DOSAGES
▸ **Percutaneous coronary intervention (PCI)**
IV BOLUS
Adults. 0.25 mg/kg 10-60 min before angioplasty or atherectomy, then 12-h IV infusion of 0.125 mcg/kg/min. Maximum: 10 mcg/min.
▸ **PCI (Unstable angina)**
IV BOLUS
Adults. 0.25 mg/kg, followed by 18- to 24-h infusion of 10 mcg/min, ending 1 h after procedure.

CONTRAINDICATIONS
Active internal bleeding, arteriovenous malformation or aneurysm, bleeding diathesis, history of cerebrovascular accident (CVA) within the past 2 yr or CVA with residual neurologic defect, hypersensitivity to any product component or to murine proteins, oral anticoagulant use within the past 7 days unless PT is < 1.2 times control, history of vasculitis, intracranial neoplasm, prior IV dextran use before or during PTCA, recent surgery or trauma (within the past 6 wks), recent (within the past 6 wks or less) GI or genitourinary bleeding,

thrombocytopenia ($\leq 100,000$ cells/μL), and severe uncontrolled hypertension.

INTERACTIONS
Drug
Anticoagulants, including heparin: May increase risk of hemorrhage.
Platelet aggregation inhibitors (such as aspirin, dextran, thrombolytic agents): May increase risk of bleeding.
Herbal
None known.
Food
None known.

DIAGNOSTIC TEST EFFECTS
Increases activated clotting time (ACT), aPTT, and PT. Decreases platelet count.

Ⓓ IV INCOMPATIBILITIES
Administer in separate line; no other medication should be added to infusion solution.

SIDE EFFECTS
Frequent
Nausea (16%), hypotension (12%), back pain (17%), chest pain (11%).
Occasional (9%)
Vomiting, minor bleeding, headache.
Rare (3%)
Bradycardia, confusion, dizziness, pain, peripheral edema, thrombocytopenia, urinary tract infection.

SERIOUS REACTIONS
• Major bleeding complications may occur. If complications occur, stop the infusion immediately.
• Hypersensitivity reaction may occur.
• Atrial fibrillation or flutter, pulmonary edema, and complete atrioventricular block occur occasionally.

PRECAUTIONS & CONSIDERATIONS
Caution is warranted with persons who weigh < 75 kg, those who are over age 65, those who have a history of GI disease, and those who are receiving aspirin, heparin, or thrombolytics. Also use abciximab cautiously in those who have had a PTCA within 12 h of the onset of signs and symptoms of acute myocardial infarction, who have had a prolonged PTCA ($\geq$70 min), or who have had a failed PTCA because they are at increased risk for bleeding. It is unknown whether abciximab is distributed in breast milk. Safety and efficacy have not been established in children. There is an increased risk of bleeding in elderly patients. An electric razor and soft toothbrush should be used to prevent bleeding.

Notify the physician of signs of bleeding, including black or red stool, coffee-ground emesis, red or dark urine, or red-speckled mucus from cough. Assess for preexisting blood abnormalities, aPTT, platelet count, and PT before abciximab infusion, 2-4 h after treatment, and 24 h after treatment or before discharge, whichever is first. Signs and symptoms of hemorrhage, including a decrease in BP, increase in pulse rate, abdominal or back pain, and severe headache, should be monitored. Laboratory test results, including ACT, aPTT, platelet count, and PT, should also be assessed. Females' menstrual discharge should be determined and monitored for increase.
Storage
Store vials in refrigerator. Do not freeze.
Administration
Solution for injection normally appears clear and colorless. Do not shake. Discard any unused portion or

any preparation that contains opaque particles. Avoid IM injections and venipunctures; also avoid using indwelling urinary catheters and nasogastric tubes. Expect to discontinue heparin 4 h before the arterial sheath is removed. Stop abciximab and heparin infusion if serious bleeding uncontrolled by pressure occurs.

For bolus injection and continuous infusion, use an in-line sterile, nonpyrogenic, low protein-binding 0.2- or 0.22-µm filter. The continuous infusion may be filtered either during drug preparation or at the time of administration. The bolus dose may be given undiluted. Withdraw the desired dose and dilute in 250 mL of 0.9% NaCl or D5W (for example, 10 mg in 250 mL equals a concentration of 40 mcg/mL). Give in separate IV line; do not add other medications to infusion. While femoral artery sheath is in position, maintain patient on complete bed rest with the head of bed elevated at 30 degrees. Maintain the affected limb in straight position. After the sheath has been removed, apply femoral pressure for 30 min, either manually or mechanically; then apply a pressure dressing. Bed rest should be maintained for 6-8 h after the sheath is removed or the drug is discontinued, whichever is later.

Absorbable Gelatin Sponge
(Gelfoam)

CATEGORY AND SCHEDULE
Hemostatic
Hemostatic, purified gelatin sponge

MECHANISM OF ACTION
Absorbs blood, provides area for clot formation.

PHARMACOKINETICS
Implant: Absorbed in 4-6 wks.

AVAILABILITY
Sponges, packs, prostatectomy cones.

INDICATIONS AND DOSAGES
▸ **Surgical hemostatic adjunct**
Adult. Can be applied dry or moistened with normal saline solution; blot on sterile gauze to remove excess solution, shape to fit with light finger compression; hold pressure until hemostasis results. Apply to bleeding surfaces. Material may be cut to appropriate size or secured in extraction sites with sutures.

SIDE EFFECTS
• Infection, abscess formation.

CONTRAINDICATIONS
Not for use in closure of skin incisions.
Control of postpartum bleeding or menorrhagia.
Should not be placed in intravascular compartments.
Hypersensitivity to porcine collagen infection.
Caution
Avoid use in presence of infection; potential nidus of infection. Do not resterilize product.

INTERACTIONS
None known.

DIAGNOSTIC TEST EFFECTS
None known.

SERIOUS REACTIONS
• Abscesses.

Use only the minimum amount required; once hemostasis is achieved, excess material should be removed. Remove after use in laminectomy or in foramina of bone to avoid nerve damage as material swells.

Storage
Store at room temperature. Opened, unused packages should be discarded.

Administration
Sterile technique should always be used. Sponge should be cut to the minimum size required. May be applied dry or saturated with saline solution. When applied dry, the sponge should be manually compressed before application to the bleeding site. When used with saline, the sponge should be soaked in the solution, then withdrawn, squeezed between gloved fingers to expel air bubbles, replaced in saline, and kept there until needed. Sponges can be used wet or blotted to dampness on gauze before application to the bleeding site.

Acamprosate
ah-cam′pro-sate
(Campral)

CATEGORY AND SCHEDULE
Pregnancy Risk Category: C

Classification: Alcohol-abuse deterrent

MECHANISM OF ACTION
Actual mechanism unknown; may facilitate balance between GABA and glutamate neurotransmitter systems in the CNS to decrease alcohol craving.

PHARMACOKINETICS
Partially absorbed from the GI tract. Steady-state levels reached within 5 days of dosing; Protein binding negligible. *Half-life:* 20-33 h. Does not undergo metabolism; excreted unchanged in urine.

AVAILABILITY
Tablets, Enteric-Coated: 333 mg.

INDICATIONS AND DOSAGES
▸ **Maintenance of alcohol abstinence in alcohol-dependent patients who are abstinent at initiation of treatment**
PO
Adults, Elderly: 666 mg 3 times a day with or without food.
▸ **Dosage in renal impairment**
For patients with creatinine clearance of 30-49 mL/min, dosage is decreased to 333 mg 3 times a day.

CONTRAINDICATIONS
Hypersensitivity.
Severe renal impairment (creatinine clearance of ≤ 30 mL/min).

INTERACTIONS
Drug
Antidepressants: May cause weight gain or loss.
Naltrexone: May increase acamprosate blood concentration.
Herbal
None known.
Food
None known.

DIAGNOSTIC TEST EFFECTS
None known.

SIDE EFFECTS
Frequent (17%)
Diarrhea.
Occasional (4%-6%)
Insomnia, asthenia, fatigue, anxiety, flatulence, nausea, depression, pruritus.

Rare (1%-3%)
Dizziness, anorexia, paraesthesia, diaphoresis, dry mouth.

SERIOUS REACTIONS
• Suicidal ideation/suicide attempts.

PRECAUTIONS & CONSIDERATIONS

It is unknown whether acamprosate is distributed in breast milk. The safety and efficacy of acamprosate have not been established in children. Age-related renal impairment may require a dosage adjustment in elderly patients. Be aware that acamprosate does not eliminate or diminish withdrawal symptoms. Acamprosate helps maintain abstinence only when used as part of a treatment program that includes counseling and support. Avoid tasks that require mental alertness or motor skills until response to the drug has been established.

Dizziness may occur. BUN and serum creatinine levels should be obtained before beginning treatment. Know that acamprosate use is contraindicated with severe renal impairment (creatinine clearance of ≤30 mL/min). Pattern of daily bowel activity should be assessed during therapy.

Storage

Store at room temperature.

Administration

! Expect to decrease the dosage with moderate renal impairment (creatinine clearance of 30-50 mL/min).

Do not crush or break enteric-coated tablets. Take acamprosate without regard to food. However, persons who regularly eat three meals a day may be more compliant with the drug regimen if instructed to take acamprosate with food.

Acarbose
a-car'bose
(α-amylase inhibitor, α-glucosidase inhibitor, antidiabetic, hypoglycemic)
(Glucobay [AUS], Prandase [CAN], Precose)
Do not confuse Precose with PreCare.

CATEGORY AND SCHEDULE
Pregnancy Risk Category: B

Classification: α-glucosidase inhibitors, oral antidiabetic agents

MECHANISM OF ACTION
An α-glucosidase inhibitor that delays glucose absorption and digestion of carbohydrates, resulting in a smaller rise in blood glucose concentration after meals. *Therapeutic Effect:* Lowers postprandial hyperglycemia.

PHARMACOKINETICS
PO
Limited oral absorption, absorbed dose excreted in urine, metabolized in the GI tract and major portion of dose excreted in feces; systemic exposure increased sixfold in subjects with severe renal impairment.

AVAILABILITY
Tablets: 25 mg, 50 mg, 100 mg.

INDICATIONS AND DOSAGES
▶ Diabetes Mellitus
Use as single drug or in combination with insulin or oral hypoglycemics (sulfonylureas, metformin) in type 2 diabetes (non-insulin-dependent diabetes mellitus [NIDDM]) when diet

control is ineffective in controlling blood glucose levels.
PO
Adults, Elderly. Initially, 25 mg 3 times a day with first bite of each main meal. Increase at 4- to 8-wks intervals. Maximum: For patients weighing more than 60 kg, 100 mg 3 times a day; for patients weighing 60 kg or less, 50 mg 3 times a day.

CONTRAINDICATIONS

Chronic intestinal diseases associated with marked disorders of digestion or absorption, cirrhosis, colonic ulceration, conditions that may deteriorate as a result of increased gas formation in the intestine, diabetic ketoacidosis, hypersensitivity to acarbose, inflammatory bowel disease, partial intestinal obstruction or predisposition to intestinal obstruction, significant renal dysfunction (serum creatinine level ≥2 mg/dL).

INTERACTIONS
Drug
Digestive enzymes, intestinal absorbents (such as charcoal): Reduces effects of acarbose; avoid concomitant use.
Digoxin: May affect bioavailability of oral digoxin, and dose adjustment may be needed.
Herbal
None known.
Food
None known.

DIAGNOSTIC TEST EFFECTS
May increase AST(SGOT) and ALT levels.

SIDE EFFECTS
Side effects diminish in frequency and intensity over time.

Frequent
Transient GI disturbances: flatulence (77%), diarrhea (33%), abdominal pain (21%).

SERIOUS REACTIONS
• Elevated liver transaminases may occur. May cause jaundice.

PRECAUTIONS & CONSIDERATIONS
Caution is warranted with fever or infection and in those who have had surgery or trauma because these states may cause loss of glycemic control. Acarbose use is not recommended during pregnancy. It is unknown if acarbose is distributed in breast milk. Safety and efficacy have not been established in children. Hypoglycemia may be difficult to recognize in the elderly. Avoid alcoholic beverages.

Food intake and blood glucose should be monitored before and during therapy. Glycosylated hemoglobin and AST (SGOT) levels should also be assessed. Consult the physician when glucose demands are altered (such as with fever, heavy physical activity, infection, stress, trauma). Exercise, good personal hygiene (including foot care), not smoking, and weight control are essential parts of therapy. Patients should be advised to have oral glucose (dextrose) available to treat hypoglycemia if also treated with a sulfonylurea or insulin, since acarbose delays/inhibits breakdown of table sugar making it ineffective for the rapid treatment of hypoglycemia.
Storage
Do not store above 25° C (77° F). Protect from moisture. Keep container tightly closed.
Administration
Take acarbose with the first bite of each main meal. Do not skip or delay meals.

Acebutolol

a-se-byoo'toe-lole
(Monitan [CAN], Novo-Acebutolol
[CAN], Rhotral [CAN], Sectral)
**Do not confuse with Factrel or
Septra.**

CATEGORY AND SCHEDULE

Pregnancy Risk Category: B (D if
used in second or third trimester)

Classification: Antiadrenergics,
β-blocking antihypertensives,
antiarrhythmics, class II

MECHANISM OF ACTION

A β_1-adrenergic blocker that
competitively blocks β_1-adrenergic
receptors in cardiac tissue.
Reduces the rate of spontaneous
firing of the sinus pacemaker
and delays AV conduction.
Therapeutic Effect: Slows heart rate,
decreases cardiac output, decreases
BP, and exhibits antiarrhythmic
activity.

PHARMACOKINETICS

Route	Onset	Peak	Duration
PO (hypo-tensive)	1-1.5 h	2-8 h	24 h

Well absorbed from the GI
tract. Protein binding: 26%.
Undergoes extensive first-pass
liver metabolism to active
metabolite. Eliminated via bile,
secreted into GI tract via intestine,
and excreted in urine. Removed
by hemodialysis. *Half-life:* 3-4 h;
metabolite, 8-13 h.

AVAILABILITY

Capsules: 200 mg, 400 mg.

INDICATIONS AND DOSAGES
▸ **Mild to moderate hypertension**
PO
Adults. Initially, 400 mg/day in
1 or 2 divided doses. Range: Up to
1200 mg/day in 2 divided doses.
Maintenance: 400-800 mg/day.
▸ **Ventricular arrhythmias**
PO
Adults. Initially, 200 mg q12h.
Increase gradually to 600-1200
mg/day in 2 divided doses.
Elderly. Initially, 200-400 mg/day.
Maximum: 800 mg/day.
▸ **Dosage in Renal Impairment**
Dosage is modified based on
creatinine clearance.

Creatinine % Clearance (mL/min)	Usual Dosage
25-49	Reduce dose by 50%
< 25	Reduce dose by 75%

OFF-LABEL USES

Treatment of chronic angina pectoris,
myocardial infarction.

CONTRAINDICATIONS

Cardiogenic shock, heart block
greater than first degree, overt heart
failure, severe bradycardia.

INTERACTIONS
Drug
Diuretics, other antihypertensives:
May increase hypotensive effect of
acebutolol.
Sympathomimetics, xanthines:
May mutually inhibit effects of
acebutolol; increased dosages of
β-agonist bronchodilators may be
necessary.
Antidiabetic agents: May
mask symptoms of hypoglycemia
and prolong hypoglycemic
effect of insulin and oral
hypoglycemics.

α-adrenergic agonists: Increased risk of hypertensive reaction.
Herbal
None known.
Food
None known.

DIAGNOSTIC TEST EFFECTS

May increase antinuclear antibody titer and serum alkaline phosphatase, serum bilirubin, BUN, serum creatinine, HDL, lipoproteins, serum potassium, AST (SGOT), ALT (SGPT), triglyceride, and uric acid levels.

SIDE EFFECTS

Frequent
Hypotension manifested as dizziness, nausea, diaphoresis, headache, cold extremities, fatigue, constipation, or diarrhea.
Occasional
Insomnia, urinary frequency, impotence or decreased libido.
Rare
Rash, arthralgia, myalgia, confusion (especially in elderly patients), altered taste.

SERIOUS REACTIONS

• Overdose may produce profound bradycardia and hypotension.
• Abrupt withdrawal may result in diaphoresis, palpitations, headache, and tremors.
• Acebutolol administration may precipitate CHF or MI in patients with heart disease; thyroid storm in those with thyrotoxicosis; or peripheral ischemia in those with existing peripheral vascular disease.
• Hypoglycemia may occur in patients with previously controlled diabetes.
• Signs of thrombocytopenia, such as unusual bleeding or bruising, occur rarely.

PRECAUTIONS & CONSIDERATIONS

Caution is warranted with bronchospastic disease, diabetes, hyperthyroidism, impaired renal or hepatic function, inadequate cardiac function, and peripheral vascular disease. Acebutolol readily crosses the placenta and is distributed in breast milk. Acebutolol use should be avoided in pregnant women after the first trimester because it may result in low-birth-weight infants. The drug may also produce apnea, bradycardia, hypoglycemia, or hypothermia during childbirth. No age-related precautions have been noted in children, and dosages have not been established. Use cautiously in elderly patients, who may have age-related peripheral vascular disease. Be aware that salt and alcohol intake should be restricted. Nasal decongestants or OTC cold preparations (stimulants) should not be used without physician approval.

Notify the physician of excessive fatigue, headache, prolonged dizziness, shortness of breath, or weight gain. BP for hypotension; respiratory status for shortness of breath; pattern of daily bowel activity and stool consistency; ECG for arrhythmias; and pulse for quality, rate, and rhythm should be monitored during treatment. If pulse rate is 60 beats/min or lower or systolic BP is < 90 mm Hg, withhold the medication and contact the physician. Signs and symptoms of CHF, such as decreased urine output, distended neck veins, dyspnea (particularly on exertion or lying down), night cough, peripheral edema, and weight gain should also be assessed.
Storage
Store at room temperature.

Administration
Acebutolol may be taken without regard to meals. Do not abruptly discontinue the drug.

Acetaminophen
ah-seet′ah-min-oh-fen
(Abenol [CAN], Apo-Acetaminophen [CAN], Atasol [CAN], Dymadon [AUS], Feverall, Panadol [AUS], Panamax [AUS], Paralgin [AUS], Setamol [AUS], Tempra, Tylenol)
Do not confuse with Fiorinal, Hycodan, Indocin, Percodan, or Tuinal.

CATEGORY AND SCHEDULE
Pregnancy Risk Category: B
OTC

Classification: Analgesics, nonnarcotic, antipyretics

MECHANISM OF ACTION
A central analgesic whose exact mechanism is unknown but appears to inhibit prostaglandin synthesis in the CNS and, to a lesser extent, block pain impulses through peripheral action. Acetaminophen acts centrally on the hypothalamic heat-regulating center, producing peripheral vasodilation (heat loss, skin erythema, sweating). *Therapeutic Effect:* Results in antipyresis. Produces analgesic effect.

PHARMACOKINETICS

Route	Onset	Peak	Duration
PO	15-30 min	1-1.5 h	4-6 h

Rapidly, completely absorbed from GI tract; rectal absorption variable. Protein binding: 20%-50%. Widely distributed to most body tissues. Metabolized in liver; excreted in urine. Removed by hemodialysis. *Half-life:* 1-4 h (half-life is increased in those with liver disease, elderly, neonates; decreased in children).

AVAILABILITY
Caplet (Genapap, Tylenol): 500 mg.
Caplet, Extended Release (Mapap, Tylenol Arthritis Pain): 650 mg.
Capsule (Mapap): 500 mg.
Elixir: 160 mg/5 mL.
Liquid, Oral: 160 mg/5 mL, (*Tylenol Extra Strength*): 500 mg/15 mL.
Solution, Oral Drops (Genapap Infant): 80 mg/0.8 mL.
Suppository, Rectal (Feverall): 80 mg, (*Acephen, Feverall*): 120 mg, 325 mg, 650 mg.
Suspension, Oral (Tylenol): 160 mg/5 mL.
Tablet (Genapap, Mapap, Tylenol): 325 mg, 500 mg.
Tablet, Chewable (Genapap, Mapap, Tylenol): 80 mg, 160 mg, 500 mg.
Tablet, Disintegrating/Dispersible (Quick Melts, Tylenol): 80 mg, 160 mg.

INDICATIONS AND DOSAGES
▸ **Analgesia and antipyresis**
PO
Adults, Elderly. 325-650 mg q4-6h or 1 g 3-4 times/day. Maximum: 4 g/day.
Children. 10-15 mg/kg/dose q4-6h as needed. Maximum: 5 doses/24 h.
Neonates. 10-15 mg/kg/dose q6-8h as needed.
Rectal
Adults. 650 mg q4-6h. Maximum: 6 doses/24 h.
Children. 10-20 mg/kg/dose q4-6h as needed. Maximum: no more than 6 doses/24 h.

Neonates. 10-15 mg/kg/dose q6-8h as needed.

▸ **Dosage in renal impairment**

Creatinine Clearance (mL/min)	Frequency
10-50	q6h
< 10	q8h

CONTRAINDICATIONS
Active alcoholism, liver disease, or viral hepatitis, all of which increase the risk of hepatotoxicity.

INTERACTIONS
Drug
Alcohol (chronic use), hepatotoxic medications (e.g., phenytoin), liver-enzyme inducers (e.g., cimetidine): May increase risk of hepatotoxicity with prolonged high dose or single toxic dose.
Warfarin: May increase the risk of bleeding with regular use.
Herbal
Chaparral: Potential additive hepatotoxicity; avoid concomitant use.
Comfrey: Potential additive hepatotoxicity; avoid concomitant use.

DIAGNOSTIC TEST EFFECTS
May increase serum bilirubin, PT (may indicate hepatotoxicity), SGOT (AST), and SGPT (ALT). Therapeutic serum level: 10-30 mcg/mL; toxic serum level: > 200 mcg/mL. Must use nomogram to determine risk of toxicity.

SIDE EFFECTS
Rare
Hypersensitivity reaction.

SERIOUS REACTIONS
Hepatotoxicity
• Acetaminophen toxicity is the primary serious reaction.

• Early signs and symptoms of acetaminophen toxicity include anorexia, nausea, diaphoresis, and generalized weakness within the first 12 to 24 h.
• Later signs of acetaminophen toxicity include vomiting, right upper quadrant tenderness, and elevated liver function tests within 48-72 h after ingestion.
• The antidote to acute acetaminophen toxicity is acetylcysteine (Mucomyst), and it should be administered as soon as possible following toxic dose.

PRECAUTIONS & CONSIDERATIONS
Caution is warranted with liver disease, G6PD deficiency, phenylketonuria, sensitivity to acetaminophen, and severe impaired renal function. Adult dose should not exceed 4 g per day. Chronic alcoholics should limit intake to 2 g or less per day. Acetaminophen crosses the placenta and is distributed in breast milk. Acetaminophen is routinely used in all stages of pregnancy and appears safe for short-term use. There are no age-related precautions noted in children or in elderly patients. Be aware that children may receive repeat doses 4-5 times a day to a maximum of 5 doses in 24 h. Withhold the drug and contact the physician if respirations are 12/ min or lower (20/min or lower in children).

Consult with the physician before using acetaminophen in children under 2 yr of age; oral use for more than 5 days in children, more than 10 days in adults, or fever lasting more than 3 days. Severe or recurrent pain or high, continuous fever, which may indicate a serious illness, should be monitored. Be aware that the therapeutic serum level is

10-30 mcg/mL and a toxic serum level is > 200 mcg/mL.

Storage
Store at room temperature. Avoid high heat, excessive humidity, and freezing.

Administration
Take oral acetaminophen without regard to meals. Tablets may be crushed.

For rectal use, moisten suppository with cold water before inserting well up into the rectum.

Acetazolamide
ah-seat-ah-zole-ah-myd
(Apo-Acetazolamide [CAN], Diamox, Diamox Sequels)
Do not confuse with acetohexamide.

CATEGORY AND SCHEDULE
Pregnancy Risk Category: C

Classification: Diuretic, Anticonvulsant, Carbonic anhydrase inhibitors

MECHANISM OF ACTION
A carbonic anhydrase inhibitor that reduces formation of hydrogen and bicarbonate ions from carbon dioxide and water by inhibiting, in proximal renal tubule, the enzyme carbonic anhydrase, thereby promoting renal excretion of sodium, potassium, bicarbonate, water. *Ocular:* Reduces rate of aqueous humor formation, lowers intraocular pressure.
Therapeutic Effect: Produces anticonvulsant activity; by retarding neuronal conduction in the brain; produces a diuretic effect generally.

PHARMACOKINETICS
SR: Absorption 3-6 h; onset 2 h; peak activity attained 3-6 h; duration 18-24 h.

IR: Absorption 1-4 h; onset 1-1.5 h; peak activity attained 1-4 h; duration 8-12 h.
IV: Onset 2 min; Peak activity attained 15 min; duration 4-5 h.
Excreted unchanged in urine. Removed by hemodialysis. *Half-life:* 2.4-5.8 h.

AVAILABILITY
Capsules, sustained release: 500 mg (Diamox Sequels).
Powder for reconstitution: lyophilized 500 mg.
Tablets: 125 mg, 250 mg (Diamox).

INDICATIONS AND DOSAGES
▸ **Chronic simple (open-angle) glaucoma**
PO
Adults. 250 mg 1-4 times/day, not to exceed 1 g/day. *Extended-Release:* 500 mg 1-2 times/day usually given in morning and evening, not to exceed 1 g/day.
▸ **Secondary glaucoma, preop treatment of closed-angle glaucoma (short term)**
PO
Adults. 250 mg q 4h or 250 mg twice a day.
▸ **Acute Glaucoma**
IV
Adults: PO: Initially 500 mg; then increase to 125-250 mg q 4h.
Adults: IV: Use for rapid relief of increased intraocular pressure. Direct IV administration is preferred.
▸ **Drug-induced edema**
PO/IV
Adults. 250-375 mg daily for 1-2 days, alternating with a day of rest.
▸ **Epilepsy**
ORAL
Adults: Optimum range is 375-1000 mg/day in 1-4 divided doses, unless given with another anticonvulsant therapy where initial dosage should be 250 mg/day.

▸ **Acute mountain sickness**
PO
Adults. 500-1000 mg/day in divided doses using tablets or sustained release capsules. If possible, begin 24-48 h before ascent; continue at least 48 h at high altitude.

▸ **Diuresis in CHF**
Adults. PO/IV: Initially 250-375 mg (5 mg/kg) every morning, then given on alternate days or for 2 days alternating with 1 day of rest. Use lowest effective dosage.

▸ **Dosage in renal impairment**

Creatinine Clearance (mL/min)	Dosage Interval
10-50	q12h
Less than 10	Avoid use

CONTRAINDICATIONS
Hypersensitivity to other sulfonamides; severe renal disease, hepatic cirrhosis, decreased sodium or potassium serum levels, adrenal insufficiency, hypochloremic acidosis, severe pulmonary obstruction with increased risk of acidosis, hypersensitivity to acetazolamide, to any component of the formulation, or to sulfonamides. Long-term use is contraindicated in patients with chronic noncongestive angle-closure glaucoma.

INTERACTIONS
Drug (not limited to the following)
Phenytoin: May increase serum concentrations of phenytoin.
Primidone: May decrease serum concentrations of primidone.
Quinidine: May decrease urinary excretion of quinidine and increase effects.
Salicylates: May increase risk of acetazolamide accumulation and toxicity including CNS depression and metabolic acidosis.
Herbal and Food
None known.

DIAGNOSTIC TEST EFFECTS
May increase ammonia, bilirubin, glucose, chloride, uric acid, calcium. May decrease bicarbonate, potassium. May cause false-positive results for urinary protein with Albustix®, Labstix®, Albutest®, Bumintest®; interferes with HPLC theophylline assay and serum uric acid levels.

ⓘ IV INCOMPATIBILITIES
No drug incompatibilities reported.

ⓘ IV COMPATIBILITIES
Cimetidine (Tagament), procaine, ranitidine (Zantac).

SIDE EFFECTS
Frequent
Drowsiness, dizziness; confusion, sensory disturbances including parathesia and loss of appetite; convulsions; transient myopia; unusually tired/weak, diarrhea, increased urination/frequency, decreased appetite/weight, altered taste (metallic), nausea, vomiting, numbness or tingling in extremities, lips, mouth.
Occasional
Depression, drowsiness, taste alterations; skin rash; uticaria.
Rare
Headache, photosensitivity, confusion, tinnitus, severe muscle weakness, loss of taste, bruising; transient myopia; hearing disturbances.
Other
Flaccid paralysis; fever; flank or loin pain; severe adverse reactions otherwise associated with sulfonamides; Stevens–Johnson

syndrome; toxic epidermal necrolysis and photosensitivity.

SERIOUS REACTIONS
• Long-term therapy may result in acidotic state.
• Nephrotoxicity/hepatotoxicity occurs occasionally, manifested as dark urine/stools, pain in lower back, jaundice, dysuria, crystalluria, renal colic/calculi.
• Bone marrow depression may be manifested as aplastic anemia, thrombocytopenia, thrombocytopenic purpura, leukopenia, agranulocytosis, hemolytic anemia.

PRECAUTIONS & CONSIDERATIONS
Advise patient to stop taking acetazolamide immediately and to contact their healthcare provider if any of the following symptoms occur: sore throat, unexplained fever, pallor, purpura, hematuria, unusual bleeding or bruising; blood in urine; tingling or tremors in hands or feet; hearing changes; flank or loin pain.

Caution is warranted in patients being treated for glaucoma; intraocular pressures should be measured and documented in the patient's record before starting therapy and periodically during therapy. When the patient is using acetazolamide to prevent symptoms from high altitude sickness, adivse patient that if rapid ascent causes high altitude sickness, rapid descent is necessary.

It is unknown if acetazolamide crosses the placenta or is distributed in the breast milk. Safety and efficacy has not been established in children. Acetazolamide may cause drowsiness. Avoid alcohol and performing tasks that require mental alertness or motor skills. Patient should avoid unnecessary exposure to sunlight and artificial tanning.

Storage
Reconstituted solution for injection may be stored up to 12 h at room temperature and for 3 days under refrigeration.
Administration
IM administration is not recommended because of pain secondary to the alkaline pH. Standard diluent is 500 mg/50 mL D5W. Minimum volume is 50 mL D5W. Reconstitute with at least 5 mL of sterile water to provide a solution containing not more than 100 mg/ml. Further dilute in 50 mL of either D5W or 0.9% NaCl for IV infusion administration. Recommended rate of administration is 100-500 mg/min for IV push and 4-8 h for IV infusions. Maximum concentration is 100 mg/mL. Maximum rate of IV infusion is 500 mg/mL. Do not administer if particulate matter, cloudiness or discoloration is noted.

Give oral acetazolamide with food. Do not crush, chew, or swallow contents of long-acting capsule. Capsules may be opened and sprinkled on soft food.

Acetic Acid
a-cee′tik as′id
(Acetasol; Acidic Vaginal Jelly; Acid Jelly; Aci-Jel; Borofair; Fem pH; Relagard; Vasotate; Vosol; Aquaear [AUS])
Do not confuse with salicylic acid.

Classification: Anti-infectives, otics

MECHANISM OF ACTION
The mechanism by which acetic acid exerts its antibacterial and antifungal actions is unknown.

Therapeutic Effect: Antibacterial and antifungal.

PHARMACOKINETICS
Unknown.

AVAILABILITY
Solution (Irrigation): 0.25%.
Solution (Otic): 2%.
Gel (Vaginal): 0.92%.
Solution (Compounding): 36%.

INDICATIONS AND DOSAGES
▶ **Superficial infections of the external auditory canal**
TOPICAL
Adults, Elderly, Children. Carefully remove all cerumen and debris to allow acetic acid to contact infected surfaces directly. To promote continuous contact, insert a wick saturated with acetic acid into the ear canal; the wick may also be saturated after insertion. Instruct the patient to keep the wick in for at least 24 h and to keep it moist by adding 3-5 drops of acetic acid every 4-6 h. The wick may be removed after 24 h, but the patient should continue to instill 5 drops of acetic acid 3 or 4 times daily thereafter, for as long as indicated. Dosing should be tapered gradually after apparent response to avoid relapse.
▶ **Bladder irrigation**
For continuous irrigation of the urinary bladder with 0.25% irrigation, the rate approximates urine flow rates or 500-1500 mL/24 h; for periodic irrigation of an indwelling catheter to maintain patency, about 50 mL of 0.25% irrigation is required.

CONTRAINDICATIONS
Hypersensitivity to acetic acid or any of the ingredients. Perforated tympanic membrane is frequently considered a contraindication to the use of any medication in the external ear canal.

DIAGNOSTIC TEST EFFECTS
None known.

SIDE EFFECTS
Occasional
Stinging or burning.
Rare
Local irritation, superinfection, hematuria.

SERIOUS REACTIONS
• Superinfection with prolonged use.
! Discontinue promptly if sensitization or irritation occurs.

PRECAUTIONS & CONSIDERATIONS
Acidosis may occur with systemic absorption of irrigation solution. It is unknown whether acetic acid crosses the placenta or is distributed into breast milk. No age-related precautions have been noted in children or the elderly. Discontinue otic solution if sensitization or irritation occurs.

Transient burning or stinging may be noted when otic solution is first instilled into acutely inflamed ear.
Administration
Insert saturated wick of cotton into the ear canal and leave for at least 24 h, keeping moist by adding 3-5 drops every 4-6 h. For maintenance, instill drops as long as indicated.

To restore and maintain vaginal acidity, use 1 applicatorful intravaginally in the morning and evening and determine the duration of treatment based on the individual's response.

Acetylcysteine

a-see-til-sis'tay-een
(Acetadote, Mucomyst, Parvolex
[CAN])
**Do not confuse acetylcysteine
with acetylcholine.**

CATEGORY AND SCHEDULE

Pregnancy Risk Category: B

Classification: Antidotes,
mucolytics

MECHANISM OF ACTION

An intratracheal respiratory inhalant
that splits the linkage of mucoproteins,
reducing the viscosity of pulmonary
secretions. Protects against
acetaminophen-induced hepatotoxicity
by maintaining or restoring
glutathione levels or by acting as an
alternate substrate for conjugation
with, and thus detoxification of,
the toxic acetaminophen reactive
metabolite. *Therapeutic Effect:*
Facilitates the removal of pulmonary
secretions by coughing, postural
drainage, mechanical means. Protects
against acetaminophen overdose-
induced hepatotoxicity.

PHARMACOKINETICS

Low oral bioavailability, *Half-life:*
11 h (newborns), 5.6 h (adults).

AVAILABILITY

Injection (Acetadote): 20%
(200 mg/mL).
Inhalation Solution (Mucomyst): 10%
(100 mg/mL), 20% (200 mg/mL).

INDICATIONS AND DOSAGES
▸ **Adjunctive treatment of viscid
mucus secretions from chronic
bronchopulmonary disease and for
pulmonary complications of cystic
fibrosis**

Nebulization
Adults, Elderly, Children. 3-5 mL
(20% solution) 3-4 times a day or
6-10 mL (10% solution) 3-4 times a
day. Range: 1-10 mL (20% solution)
q2-6h or 2-20 mL (10% solution)
q2-6h.
Infants. 1-2 mL (20%) or 2-4 mL
(10%) 3-4 times a day.
▸ **Treatment of viscid mucus
secretions in patients with a
tracheostomy**
INTRATRACHEAL
Adults, Children. 1-2 mL of 10%
or 20% solution instilled into
tracheostomy q1-4h.
▸ **Acetaminophen overdose**
PO (ORAL SOLUTION 5%)
Adults, Elderly, Children. Loading
dose of 140 mg/kg, followed in 4 h
by maintenance dose of 70 mg/kg
q4h for 17 additional doses (unless
acetaminophen assay reveals
nontoxic level). Repeat dose
if emesis occurs within 1 h of
administration.
IV (ACETADOTE)
Adults, Elderly, Children. 150 mg/kg
infused over 60 min, then
50 mg/kg infused over 4 h, then
100 mg/kg infused over 16 h.
▸ **Prevention of renal damage from
dyes used during certain diagnostic
tests**
PO (ORAL SOLUTION 5%)
Adults, Elderly. 600-1200 mg twice
a day for 4 doses starting the day
before the procedure.

OFF-LABEL USES (PO)

Prevention of renal damage from
dyes given during certain diagnostic
tests (such as CT scans).

CONTRAINDICATIONS

None known.

DIAGNOSTIC TEST EFFECTS

None known.

SIDE EFFECTS
Frequent
Inhalation: Stickiness on face, transient unpleasant odor.
Occasional
Inhalation: Increased bronchial secretions, throat irritation, nausea, vomiting, rhinorrhea.
IV: Nausea, vomiting, flushing, pruritus, rash, tachycardia.
Rare
Inhalation: Rash.
Oral: Facial edema, bronchospasm, wheezing.

SERIOUS REACTIONS
• Large doses may produce severe nausea and vomiting.

PRECAUTIONS & CONSIDERATIONS
Caution is warranted with bronchial asthma and in elderly or debilitated patients with severe respiratory insufficiency. Maintain adequate hydration. A disagreeable color may emanate from the solution during initial administration, but it disappears quickly.

If bronchospasm occurs, discontinue treatment; notify the physician. A bronchodilator may be needed. Assess respiratory rate, depth, rhythm, and type (such as abdominal or thoracic) and color, consistency, and amount of sputum.
Storage
Injectable solution: Store at room temperature. Following reconstitution with D5W, solution is stable for 24 h at room temperature. A color change may occur in opened vials (light purple) but does not affect the safety or efficacy.

Inhalation solution: Store at room temperature; once opened, store under refrigeration and use within 96 h. Use diluted solutions within 1 h. A color change may occur in opened vials (light purple) but does not affect the safety or efficacy.

Administration
To create the oral solution, dilute 20% solution with water or soft drinks to create a 5% concentration. Use within 1 h. When administering the solution by nebulizer, avoid using equipment that contains copper, iron, or rubber because the drug will react with these materials on contact.

For adults ≥ 40 kg: For IV use, give 3 infusions of different strengths: first dose (150 mg/kg) in 200 mL D5W and infused over 15 min, second dose (50 mg/kg) in 500 mL D5W and infused over 4 h, third dose (100 mg/kg) in 1000 mL D5W and infused over 16 h.

For children and adults < 40 kg; Dilutions are adjusted. Consult prescribing information. For inhalation, may administer either undiluted or diluted with 0.9% NaCl.

Acitretin
a-si-tre′tin
(Soriatane)

CATEGORY AND SCHEDULE
Pregnancy Risk Category: X

Classification: Antipsoriatics, dermatologics, systemic retinoids

MECHANISM OF ACTION
A second-generation retinoid that adjusts factors influencing epidermal proliferation, RNA/DNA synthesis, controls glycoprotein, and governs immune response. *Therapeutic Effect:* Regulates keratinocyte growth and differentiation.

PHARMACOKINETICS
Well absorbed from the GI tract. Food increases the rate of absorption.

Protein binding: > 99%. Metabolized in liver. Excreted in bile and urine. Not removed by hemodialysis.
Half-life: 49 h.
With alcohol consumption, acitretin is converted to etretinate, which has a half-life of 120 days.

AVAILABILITY
Capsules: 10 mg, 25 mg (Soriatane).

INDICATIONS AND DOSAGES
▸ **Psoriasis**
PO
Adults, Elderly. 25-50 mg/day as a single dose with main meal. May increase to 75 mg/day if necessary and dose tolerated. Maintenance: 25-50 mg/day after the initial response is noted. Continue until lesions have resolved.

OFF-LABEL USES
Treatment of nonpsoriatic dermatoses, keratinization disorders, Darier's disease, palmoplantar keratoses, lichen planus; children with lamellar ichthyosis, nonbullous and bullous ichthyosiform erythroderma, Sjögren-Larsson syndrome; should be prescribed only by physicians knowledgeable in the use of systemic retinoids.

CONTRAINDICATIONS
Pregnancy or those who intend to become pregnant within 3 yr following discontinuation of therapy, severely impaired liver or kidney function, chronic abnormal elevated lipid levels, concomitant use of methotrexate or tetracyclines, ingestion of alcohol (in females of reproductive potential), hypersensitivity to acitretin, etretinate, or other retinoids, sensitivity to parabens (used as preservative in gelatin capsule).

INTERACTIONS
Drug
Alcohol: May prevent elimination of acitretin by conversion of drug to etiretinate. Females must *not* drink alcohol for 2 mo after treatment with acitretin.
"Minipill" oral contraceptive: May interfere with contraceptive effect.
Methotrexate: May increase risk of hepatotoxicity.
Tetracyclines: May increase risk of increased intracranial pressure.
Vitamin A: May increase risk of vitamin A toxicity.
Herbal
St. John's wort: May increase risk of unplanned pregnancy as a result of lessening of effects of hormonal contraceptives.
Sulfonylureas: May potentiate blood glucose lowering.
Phenytoin: May increase phenytoin free levels via decreased protien binding.
Food
None known.

DIAGNOSTIC TEST EFFECTS
May increase triglycerides, SGOT (AST), SGPT (ALT). May decrease HDL (high density lipoprotein). May alter blood glucose control.

SIDE EFFECTS
Frequent
Lip inflammation, alopecia, skin peeling, shakiness, dry eyes, rash, hyperesthesia, paresthesia, sticky skin, dry mouth, epistaxis, dryness/thickening of conjunctiva.
Occasional
Eye irritation, brow and lash loss, sweating, chills, sensation of cold, flushing, edema, blurred vision, diarrhea, nausea, thirst.

SERIOUS REACTIONS
• Benign intracranial hypertension (pseudotumor cerebri) occurs rarely.

PRECAUTIONS & CONSIDERATIONS
Caution is warranted with impaired hepatic or renal function and in those with elevated cholesterol/triglycerides. Triglycerides should be monitored at 1- to 2-wks intervals until response to drug is established. Safety and efficacy have not been established in children. Be aware that acitretin should be avoided in elderly patients with renal impairment. Decreased tolerance to contact lenses may develop. Follow a cholesterol-free diet for best results. Depression and other psychiatric symptoms such as aggression or thoughts of self-harm have occurred during therapy with systemic retinoids, including acitretin. Photosensitivity may occur.

Be aware that acitretin is contraindicated in pregnant women. Women should not take acitretin if pregnant or planning to become pregnant within the next 3 yr. Two pregnancy tests with negative results must be obtained before starting treatment. Two forms of birth control must be used for 1 mo before beginning with acitretin, during treatment, and 3 yr after treatment. Acitretin has teratogenic effects. An agreement/informed consent must be signed before treatment begins. Patients should not donate blood during and for at least 3 yr after completing acitretin therapy so that women of childbearing potential do not receive blood from patients receiving acetretin.

Storage
Store at room temperature.
Administration
Give with main meal of the day or milk.

Acyclovir
ay-sye'kloe-ver
(Aciclovir-BC IV [AUS], Acihexal [AUS], Acyclo-V [AUS], Avirax [CAN], Lovir [AUS], Zovirax, Zyclir [AUS])
Do not confuse with Zostrix, Zyvox.

CATEGORY AND SCHEDULE
Pregnancy Risk Category: B

Classification: Antivirals

MECHANISM OF ACTION
A synthetic nucleoside that converts to acyclovir triphosphate, becoming part of the DNA chain. *Therapeutic Effect:* Interferes with DNA synthesis and viral replication. Virustatic.

PHARMACOKINETICS
Poorly absorbed from the GI tract; minimal absorption following topical application. Protein binding: 9%-36%. Widely distributed. Partially metabolized in liver. Excreted primarily in urine. Removed by hemodialysis. *Half-life:* 2.5 h (increased in impaired renal function).

AVAILABILITY
Capsules: 200 mg.
Tablets: 400 mg, 800 mg.
Injection, (lyophylized powder for reconstitution): 50 mg/mL once reconstituted.
Oral Suspension: 200 mg/5 mL.
Injection, Solution: 25 mg/mL.
Cream: 5%.
Ointment: 5%/50 mg.

INDICATIONS AND DOSAGES
▸ **Genital herpes (initial episode)**
IV
Adults, Elderly, Children 12 yr and older. 5 mg/kg q8h for 5 days.

PO
Adults, Elderly, Children 12 yr and older. 200 mg q4h 5 times a day.
TOPICAL (OINTMENT)
Cover all lesions every 3 h, 6 times a day for 7 days. Begin as soon as signs and symptoms appear.

▸ **Genital herpes (recurrent)**
Less than 6 episodes per year:
PO
Adults, Elderly, Children 12 yr and older. 200 mg q4h 5 times a day for 5 days.
6 episodes or more per year:
PO
Adults, Elderly, Children 12 yr and older. 400 mg 2 times a day or 200 mg 3-5 times a day for up to 12 mo.

▸ **Herpes labialis (cold sores), recurrent**
TOPICAL CREAM
Adults, Children 12 yr and older. Apply 5 times per day for 4 days (i.e., during the prodrome or when lesions appear).

▸ **Herpes simplex mucocutaneous**
IV
Adults, Elderly, Children 12 yr and older. 5 mg/kg/dose q8h for 7 days.
Children younger than 12 yr. 10 mg/kg q8h for 7 days.

▸ **Herpes simplex neonatal**
IV
Children younger than 4 mo. 10 mg/kg q8h for 10 days.

▸ **Herpes simplex encephalitis**
IV
Adults, Elderly, Children 12 yr and older. 10 mg/kg q8h for 10 days.
Children 3 mo to younger than 12 yr. 20 mg/kg q8h for 10 days.

▸ **Herpes zoster (caused by varicella)**
IV
Adults, Elderly, Children 12 yr and older. 10 mg/kg q8h for 7 days.
Children younger than 12 yr. 20 mg/kg q8h for 7 days.

▸ **Herpes zoster (shingles)**
PO
Adults, Elderly, Children 12 yr and older. 800 mg q4h 5 times a day for 7-10 days.

▸ **Varicella (chickenpox)**
PO
Adults, Elderly, Children older than 12 yr or children 2-12 yr, weighing 40 kg or more. 800 mg 4 times a day for 5 days.
Children 2-12 yr, weighing < 40 kg. 20 mg/kg 4 times a day for 5 days. Maximum: 800 mg/dose.

▸ **Dosage in renal impairment**
Dosage and frequency are modified based on severity of infection and degree of renal impairment.
PO
If normal dose is 800 mg 5 times/day, decrease to 800 mg q12h. If normal dose is 200 mg 5 times/day or 400 mg q12h, decrease dose to 200 mg q12h.
IV

Creatinine Clearance (mL/min)	Dosage %	Dosage Interval
> 50	100	8 h
25-50	100	12 h
10-25	100	24 h
< 10	50	24 h

OFF-LABEL USES
Treatment of herpes simplex ocular infections, infectious mononucleosis.

CONTRAINDICATIONS
Hypersensitivity to acyclovir or valacyclovir; use in neonates when acyclovir is reconstituted with bacteriostatic water containing benzyl alcohol.

INTERACTIONS
Drug
Nephrotoxic medications (such as aminoglycosides): May increase the nephrotoxicity of acyclovir.

Probenecid: May increase acyclovir half-life.

DIAGNOSTIC TEST EFFECTS
May increase BUN and serum creatinine concentrations.

🚱 IV INCOMPATIBILITIES
In general, do not mix any other drugs in an acyclovir syringe. Acyclovir has as many incompatibilities as compatibilities. Caution should be used with *any* administration at a Y-site. Aztreonam (Azactam), cefepime (Maxipime), diltiazem (Cardizem), dobutamine (Dobutrex), dopamine (Intropin), levofloxacin (Levaquin), meropenem (Merrem IV), ondansetron (Zofran), piperacillin, and tazobactam (Zosyn); blood products and protein-containing solutions.

🚱 IV COMPATIBILITIES
Allopurinol (Alloprim), amikacin (Amikin), ampicillin, cefazolin (Ancef), cefotaxime (Claforan), ceftazidime (Fortaz), ceftriaxone (Rocephin), cimetidine (Tagamet), clindamycin (Cleocin), famotidine (Pepcid), fluconazole (Diflucan), gentamicin, heparin, hydromorphone (Dilaudid), imipenem (Primaxin), lorazepam (Ativan), magnesium sulfate, methylprednisolone (Solu-Medrol), metoclopramide (Reglan), metronidazole (Flagyl), morphine, multivitamins, potassium chloride, propofol (Diprivan), ranitidine (Zantac), vancomycin.

SIDE EFFECTS
Frequent
Parenteral (7%-9%): Phlebitis or inflammation at IV site, nausea, vomiting.
Topical ointment (28%): Burning, stinging.

Occasional
Parenteral (3%): Pruritus, rash, urticaria.
Oral (6%-12%): Malaise, nausea.
Topical ointment (4%): Pruritus.
Rare
Oral (1%-3%): Vomiting, rash, diarrhea, headache.
Parenteral (1%-2%): Confusion, hallucinations, seizures, tremors.
Topical (< 1%): Rash.

SERIOUS REACTIONS
• Rapid parenteral administration, excessively high doses, or fluid and electrolyte imbalance may produce renal failure exhibited by such signs and symptoms as abdominal pain, decreased urination, decreased appetite, increased thirst, nausea, and vomiting.
• Extravasation may cause tissue necrosis.

PRECAUTIONS & CONSIDERATIONS
Caution is warranted with concurrent use of nephrotoxic agents, dehydration, fluid and electrolyte imbalance, neurologic abnormalities, or renal or hepatic impairment. Acyclovir crosses the placenta and is distributed in breast milk. Be aware that safety and efficacy have not been established in children < 2 yr of age or < 1 yr of age for IV use. In the elderly, age-related renal impairment may require dosage adjustment. Analgesics and comfort measures should be provided, especially to elderly patients. Females should have a Pap smear at least annually because of the increased risk of cervical cancer in women with genital herpes. Avoid touching lesions with fingers to prevent spreading infection to new sites.

History of allergies, particularly to acyclovir, should be obtained before treatment. Herpes simplex lesions should be assessed before treatment to compare baseline with treatment effect. IV site should be assessed for signs and symptoms of phlebitis, including heat, pain, or red streaking over the vein. Cutaneous lesions should be evaluated for signs of effective drug treatment. Adequate ventilation as well as hydration should be maintained. Appropriate isolation precautions should be maintained in persons with chickenpox and disseminated herpes zoster.

Storage

Store capsules, tablets, cream, ointment, suspension at room temperature. Store vials at room temperature. Solutions of 50 mg/mL will remain stable for 12 h at room temperature; may form precipitate when refrigerated. Potency not affected by precipitate and redissolution. IV infusion (piggyback) is stable for 24 h at room temperature. Yellow discoloration does not affect potency.

Administration

Oral: Shake suspension well before administration. Take without regard to food.

Topical: Use finger cot or rubber glove to prevent autoinoculation to apply topical acyclovir. Avoid eye contact.

IV: Add 10 mL sterile water for injection to each 500-mg vial (50 mg/mL). Do not use bacteriostatic water for injection containing benzyl alcohol or parabens because this will cause a precipitate to form. Shake well until solution is clear. Further dilute with at least 100 mL D5W or 0.9% NaCl. Final concentration should be ≤ 7 mg/mL.

Infuse over at least 1 h because renal tubular damage may occur with too rapid administration. Maintain adequate hydration during infusion and for 2 h following IV administration. Use syringe pump for neonatal administration.

Adalimumab
Ah-dah-lim'-you-mab
(Humira)
Do not confuse with Humulin

CATEGORY AND SCHEDULE
Pregnancy Risk Category: B

Classification: Disease-modifying antirheumatic drugs, immunomodulators, monoclonal antibodies, tumor necrosis factor (TNF) modulators.

MECHANISM OF ACTION
A monoclonal antibody that binds specifically to TNF-α, blocking its interaction with cell surface TNF receptors. *Therapeutic Effect:* Reduces inflammation, tenderness, and swelling of joints; slows or prevents progressive destruction of joints in rheumatoid arthritis.

PHARMACOKINETICS
Time to peak serum concentration 131 h. *Half-life:* 10-20 days.

AVAILABILITY
Pediatric Injection: 20 mg/0.4 mL in prefilled syringes.
Injection: 40 mg/0.8 mL in prefilled syringes or prefilled pens.

INDICATIONS AND DOSAGES
▸ **Ankylosing Spondylitis**
SC
Adults. 40 mg every other week.
▸ **Crohn disease**
SC
Adults. 160 mg initially on day 1 (given as four 40-mg injections in 1 day or as two 40-mg injections per day for 2 consecutive days), followed by 80 mg 2 wks later (day 15). Two weeks later (day 29), begin a maintenance dosage of 40 mg every other week.

> ‣ **Juvenile idiopathic arthritis**
SC
Children 4-17 yr of age. Weight-based dosing. For patients weighing 15 kg (33 lb) to < 30 kg (66 lb), the dose is 20 mg every other week. For patients weighing 30 kg (66 lbs) or more, the dose is 40 mg every other week.
> ‣ **Plaque psoriasis**
SC
Adults. 80 mg initial dose (given as two 40-mg injections on day 1), followed by 40 mg every other week starting 1 wk after the initial dose.
> ‣ **Psoriatic arthritis**
SC
40 mg every other week.
> ‣ **Rheumatoid arthritis**
SC
Adults, Elderly. 40 mg every other week. Dose may be increased to 40 mg/wk in those not taking methotrexate.

CONTRAINDICATIONS
Active infections.

INTERACTIONS
Drug
Abatacept: Concomitant use not recommended. Increased risk of serious infections with combined use.
Anakinra: Concomitant use not recommended. Increased risk of serious infections with combined use.
Methotrexate: Reduces the absorption of adalimumab by 29%-40%, but dosage adjustment is unnecessary if given concurrently.
Rilonacept: Concomitant use not recommended. Increased risk of serious infections with combined use.
Vaccines, live: Use not recommended. Altered immune response. Increased risk of secondary transmission of infection from vaccine.

DIAGNOSTIC TEST EFFECTS
May increase levels of blood cholesterol, other lipids, liver aminotransferases, creatine phosphokinase, and serum alkaline phosphatase.

SIDE EFFECTS
Frequent (20%)
Injection site reactions: erythema, pruritus, pain, and swelling.
Occasional (9%-12%)
Headache, rash, sinusitis, nausea.
Rare (5%-7%)
Abdominal or back pain, hypertension.

SERIOUS REACTIONS
• Rare reactions include hypersensitivity reactions, malignancies, neurologic events, respiratory tract infections, bronchitis, UTIs, and more serious infections (such as pneumonia, tuberculosis, cellulitus, pyelonephritis, and septic arthritis).

PRECAUTIONS & CONSIDERATIONS
Serious infections, sepsis, tuberculosis, and opportunistic infections have occurred during therapy with TNF blockers, including adalimumab. Patients should be screened for active or recent infection, tuberculosis risk factors, and latent tuberculosis infection before initiating therapy. Closely monitor patients developing infection during therapy. Use of adalimumab may increase the risk of reactivation of hepatitis B virus in patients who are chronic carriers of the virus. Caution is warranted with cardiovascular disease, demyelinating disorders, history of sensitivity to monoclonal antibodies, preexisting or recent onset of CNS disturbances, in elderly patients, and in pregnant women. It is unknown whether adalimumab is excreted in breast milk. The safety and efficacy of

adalimumab have not been established in children younger than 4 yr of age. Cautious use in the elderly is necessary because they are at increased risk for serious infection and malignancy. Avoid receiving live vaccines during adalimumab treatment. Syringe needle cover contains latex; avoid contact if sensitive to latex.

Laboratory values, particularly serum alkaline phosphatase levels, should be monitored before and during therapy. Therapeutic response, such as improved grip strength, increased joint mobility, reduced joint tenderness, and relief of pain, stiffness, and swelling, should also be assessed.

Storage

Refrigerate adalimumab. Do not freeze. Protect from light; store in original carton until administration.

Administration

For subcutaneous use, rotate injection sites. Administer each injection at least 1 inch from previous site. Never inject drug into bruised, hard, red, or tender areas. Discard any unused portion. Injection site reactions generally occur in the first month of treatment and decrease with continued therapy. Do not inject within 2 in of the navel.

Adapalene
a-dap′ah-leen
(Differin)

CATEGORY AND SCHEDULE
Pregnancy Risk category: C

Classification: Dermatologics, retinoids

MECHANISM OF ACTION
Binds to retinoic acid receptors in cell nuclei modulating cell differentiation, keratinization. Possesses anti-inflammatory properties. *Therapeutic Effect:* Normalizes differentiation of follicular epithelial cells.

PHARMACOKINETICS
Absorption through the skin is low. Trace amount found in plasma following topical application. Excreted primarily by biliary route.

AVAILABILITY
Gel: 0.1%, 0.3%.
Cream: 0.1%.

INDICATIONS AND DOSAGES
▸ **Acne vulgaris**
TOPICAL
Adults, Elderly, Children > 12 yr.
Apply to affected area once daily at bedtime after washing.

CONTRAINDICATIONS
Hypersensitivity to adapalene, vitamin A, or any one of its components. Do not use if patient has current sunburn. Wait until fully recovered.

INTERACTIONS
Drug
Quinolones (particularly sparfloxacin), phenothiazines, sulfonamides, sulfonylureas, tetracyclines, thiazide diuretics: Adapalene may increase the effects of these photosensitizing agents.
Benzoyl peroxide, salicylic acid, sulfur, resorcinol, alcohol: Additive local irritation when used with adapalene.

DIAGNOSTIC TEST EFFECTS
None known.

SIDE EFFECTS
Frequent
Erythema, scaling, dryness, pruritus, burning (likely to occur first 2-4 wks, lessens with continued use).

Occasional
Skin irritation, stinging, sunburn, acne flares, erythema, photosensitivity, xerosis.

SERIOUS REACTIONS
• Concurrent use of other potential irritating topical products (soaps, cleansers, aftershave, cosmetics) may produce severe topical irritation.

PRECAUTIONS & CONSIDERATIONS
Caution is warranted for patients with eczema and seborrheic dermatitis. Adapalene has not been studied in pregnant women. It is unknown whether adapalene enters the breast milk. Safety and efficacy have not been established in children younger than 12 yr or in elderly patients.

A burning sensation, stinging, dryness, itching, or redness of the skin may occur, especially during the first month of use. Other skin products such as hair-removal products, shaving creams with a large amount of alcohol, other acne medications, and certain soaps and cleansers may irritate the skin while using adapalene. Minimize sun exposure.
Storage
Store at room temperature.
Administration
Apply a small amount as a thin film once a day, at least 1 h before bedtime. Apply the medicine to dry, clean areas affected by acne. Rub in gently and well. Avoid contact with eyes, lips, angles of the nose, and mucous membranes. Do not apply to cuts, abrasions, eczematous skin, or sunburned skin.

Adefovir dipivoxil
ah-deh'foh-veer
(Hepsera)

CATEGORY AND SCHEDULE
Pregnancy Risk Category: C

Classification: Antiretroviral, nucleoside reverse transcriptase inhibitor

MECHANISM OF ACTION
An antiviral that inhibits the enzyme DNA polymerase, causing DNA chain termination after its incorporation into viral DNA. *Therapeutic Effect:* Prevents cell replication of viral DNA.

PHARMACOKINETICS
Prodrug converted to adefovir. Excreted in urine. *Half-life:* 7 h (increased in impaired renal function).

AVAILABILITY
Tablets: 10 mg.

INDICATIONS AND DOSAGES
▶ **Chronic hepatitis B in patients with normal renal function**
PO
Adults, Elderly. 10 mg once a day.
▶ **Chronic hepatitis B in patients with impaired renal function (adults)**
Adults, Elderly with creatinine clearance 20-49 mL/min. 10 mg q48h.
Adults, Elderly with creatinine clearance 10-19 mL/min. 10 mg q72h.
Adults, Elderly on hemodialysis. 10 mg every 7 days following dialysis.

CONTRAINDICATIONS
Hypersensitivity.

INTERACTIONS
Drug
Ibuprofen: Increases adefovir bioavailability and plasma concentration.
Metformin: Adefovir may compete for renal elimination. May increase risk of lactic acidosis.
Nephrotic drugs: Watch for increased risk of renal effects.

DIAGNOSTIC TEST EFFECTS
May increase serum amylase, serum creatinine, AST (SGOT) and ALT (SGPT) levels.

SIDE EFFECTS
Frequent (13%)
Asthenia.
Occasional (4%-9%)
Headache, abdominal pain, nausea, flatulence.
Rare (3%)
Diarrhea, dyspepsia.

SERIOUS REACTIONS
• Nephrotoxicity (characterized by increased serum creatinine and decreased serum phosphorus levels) is a treatment-limiting toxicity of adefovir therapy.
• Lactic acidosis and severe hepatomegaly occur rarely, particularly in those who are overweight, in combination with other antiretrovirals, or in female patients.

PRECAUTIONS & CONSIDERATIONS
Caution is warranted with impaired renal function and known risk factors for liver disease and in elderly patients. Baseline renal function laboratory values should be obtained before therapy begins and routinely thereafter. Adjust adefovir dosage with preexisting renal insufficiency. Blood specimen should be obtained for HIV antibody testing before therapy begins because unrecognized or untreated HIV infection may result in an emergence of HIV resistance.
! Notify the physician immediately if unusual muscle pain, stomach pain with nausea and vomiting, cold feeling in arms and legs, or dizziness occurs. These signs and symptoms may signal the onset of lactic acidosis. Continue to take adefovir as prescribed because there is a risk for developing a worse or very serious hepatitis if the drug is stopped. Notify physician if yellow skin color or yellowing of the whites of the eyes or other unusual signs or symptoms occur. Reliable forms of contraception should be used.
Storage
Store at room temperature.
Administration
Give adefovir without regard to food.

Adenosine
ah-den′oh-seen
(Adenocard, Adenocor [AUS], Adenoscan)

CATEGORY AND SCHEDULE
Pregnancy Risk Category: C

Classification: Antiarrhythmics, diagnostics, nonradioactive

MECHANISM OF ACTION
A cardiac agent that slows impulse formation in the SA node and conduction time through the AV node. Adenosine also acts as a diagnostic aid in myocardial perfusion imaging or stress echocardiography. *Therapeutic Effect:* Depresses left ventricular function and restores normal sinus rhythm.

PHARMACOKINETICS
Rapidly cleared from blood after IV administration, metabolized to cyclic AMP and inosine primarily by red blood cells and vascular endothelial cells. *AMP half-life:* < 10 s.

AVAILABILITY
Injection (Adenocard): 3 mg/mL in 2-mL, 4-mL syringes.
Injection (Adenoscan): 3 mg/mL in 20-mL, 30-mL vials.

INDICATIONS AND DOSAGES
▸ **Paroxysmal supraventricular tachycardia (PSVT)**
RAPID IV BOLUS
Adults, Elderly. Initially, 6 mg given over 1-2 s. If first dose does not convert within 1-2 min, give 12 mg; may repeat 12-mg dose in 1-2 min if no response has occurred.
Children. Initially 0.1 mg/kg (maximum: 6 mg). If ineffective, may give 0.2 mg/kg (maximum: 12 mg).
▸ **Diagnostic testing**
IV INFUSION
Adults. 140 mcg/kg/min for 6 min.

CONTRAINDICATIONS
Atrial fibrillation or flutter, second- or third-degree AV block or sick sinus syndrome (except with functioning pacemaker), ventricular tachycardia.

INTERACTIONS
Drug
Carbamazepine: May increase degree of heart block caused by adenosine.
Dipyridamole: May increase effect of adenosine.
Methylxanthines (e.g., caffeine, theophylline): May decrease the effect of adenosine.

Food
Caffeine: May decrease effect of adenosine. Avoid dietary caffeine 12-24 h before adenosine stress testing.

DIAGNOSTIC TEST EFFECTS
None known.

⊘ IV INCOMPATIBILITIES
Any drug or solution other than 0.9% NaCl or D5W.

SIDE EFFECTS
Frequent (12%-18%)
Facial flushing, dyspnea.
Occasional (2%-7%)
Headache, nausea, light-headedness, chest pressure.
Rare (≤1%)
Numbness or tingling in arms; dizziness; diaphoresis; hypotension; palpitations; chest, jaw, or neck pain.

SERIOUS REACTIONS
• May produce short-lasting heart block.

PRECAUTIONS & CONSIDERATIONS
Caution is warranted with arrhythmias at the time of conversion, asthma, heart block, and hepatic and renal failure. Additional caution is advised in elderly patients who may be at increased risk for severe bradycardia or AV block.

Facial flushing, headache, and nausea may occur, but these symptoms will resolve. Notify the physician if chest pain, pounding, or palpitations or difficultly breathing or shortness of breath occurs. Before administering adenosine, the arrhythmia should be identified on a 12-lead EKG. Heart rate and rhythm on a continuous cardiac monitor and the apical pulse rate, rhythm, and quality should be assessed. BP, respirations, intake and output, and electrolytes should also be monitored.

Storage
Solution may be stored at room temperature and normally appears clear. Crystallization occurs if solution is refrigerated. If crystallization occurs, dissolve crystals by warming to room temperature. Discard unused portion.

Administration
Administer undiluted very rapidly, over 1-2 s, directly into vein, or if using an IV line, use the port closest to the insertion site. If the IV line is infusing fluid other than 0.9% NaCl, flush the line first before administering adenosine. Follow the rapid bolus injection with a rapid 0.9% NaCl flush.

IV infusion (diagnostic use): Administer undiluted using a syringe pump or volumetric infusion pump.

Agalsidase-β
a-gal′si-daze
(Fabrazyme)

CATEGORY AND SCHEDULE
Pregnancy Risk Category: B

Classification: Enzymes, metabolic

MECHANISM OF ACTION
An enzyme that treats Fabry disease, an X-linked genetic disorder, by catalyzing the hydrolysis of glycosphingolipids, reducing their accumulation in the kidneys' capillary endothelium and other body tissues. *Therapeutic Effect:* Provides an exogenous source of α-galactosidase A, an enzyme, missing in those with Fabry disease.

PHARMACOKINETICS
Nonlinear pharmacokinetics. *Half-life:* 45-102 min, dose-dependent.

AVAILABILITY
Powder for Injection: 5 mg, 35 mg (5 mg/mL when reconstituted).

INDICATIONS AND DOSAGES
▶ **Fabry disease**
IV
Adults, Elderly. 1 mg/kg q2wk. Give no more than 0.25 mg/min (15 mg/h). May slow infusion rate if infusion-related reaction occurs. If no reaction occurs, infusion rate may be increased in increments of 0.05-0.08 mg/min (3-5 mg/h).

CONTRAINDICATIONS
None known.

DIAGNOSTIC TEST EFFECTS
None known.

⊘ IV INCOMPATIBILITIES
Do not mix any other medications with agalsidase-β.

SIDE EFFECTS
Expected (45%-52%)
Infusion reactions (rigors, fever, headache).
Frequent (21%-38%)
Rhinitis, nausea, anxiety, pharyngitis, edema, skeletal pain.
Occasional (14%-17%)
Temperature change sensation, hypotension, pallor, paresthesia, pruritus, urticaria, bronchitis.
Rare (7%-10%)
Depression, arthralgia, dyspepsia, laryngitis, sinusitis.

SERIOUS REACTIONS
• Serious infusion reactions, such as tachycardia, hypertension, throat tightness, chest pain, dyspnea, vomiting, lip edema, and rash, occur frequently.

• Other serious reactions include bradycardia, arrhythmias, vertigo, nephrotic syndrome, CVA, and cardiac arrest.

PRECAUTIONS & CONSIDERATIONS

Caution is warranted with fever, compromised cardiac function, moderate to severe hypertension, and renal impairment.

Storage

Store vials in the refrigerator. Allow them to reach room temperature before reconstitution, which takes about 30 min. The reconstituted and diluted solution should be used immediately; if this is not possible, the solution may be stored in the refrigerator for 24 h.

Administration

Pretreatment antipyretics should be administered. Reconstitute each 37-mg vial by slowly injecting 7.2 mL of sterile water for injection. Roll and tilt gently. Do not shake or agitate. Before adding the reconstituted solution to 500 mL 0.9% NaCl, remove an equal volume from the 500-mL infusion bag, and then add the agalsidase-β to the 500-mL 0.9% NaCl infusion bag. Administer at a rate of no more than 0.25 mg/min (15 mg/h). Expect to decrease the infusion rate if an infusion reaction occurs. If no reaction occurs, the infusion rate may be increased in increments of 0.05-0.08 mg/min (3-5 mg/h). Plan to decrease the infusion rate or temporarily stop the infusion if a reaction occurs. As prescribed, give additional antipyretics, antihistamines, or steroids to alleviate these symptoms. Patients with compromised cardiac function should be closely monitored because they are at increased risk for ≤ severe complications from infusion reactions.

Albendazole
all-ben´dah-zole
(Albenza)

CATEGORY AND SCHEDULE

Pregnancy Risk Category: C

Classification: Anthelmintic, systemic

MECHANISM OF ACTION

A benzimidazole carbamate anthelmintic that degrades parasite cytoplasmic microtubules, irreversibly blocks cholinesterase secretion and glucose uptake in helminth and larvae (depletes glycogen, decreases ATP production, depletes energy). Vermicidal. *Therapeutic Effect:* Immobilizes and kills worms.

PHARMACOKINETICS

Poorly and variable absorbed GI tract. Widely distributed, cyst fluid, including CSF. Protein binding: 70%. Extensively metabolized in liver. Primarily excreted in bile. Not removed by hemodialysis. *Half-life:* 8-12 h (prolonged in impaired heptatic function).

AVAILABILITY

Tablets: 200 mg (Albenza).

INDICATIONS AND DOSAGES
▸ **Neurocysticercosis**
PO
Adults, Elderly weighing ≥ 60 kg. 400 mg 2 times/day. Give for 8 to 30 days.
Adults, Elderly weighing < 60 kg. 15 mg/kg/day, given in two divided doses (maximum 800 mg/day). Give for 8 to 30 days. Rest 14 days, repeat cycle 3 times.

▸ **Cystic hydatid**
PO
Adults, Elderly weighing ≤ 60 kg. 400 mg
2 times/day for 28 days, rest 14 days,
repeat 3 times.
Adults, Elderly weighing < 60 kg.
15 mg/kg/day given in two divided
doses (maximum 800 mg/day).

OFF-LABEL USES
Giardiasis, microsporidiosis,
taeniasis, gnathostomiasis, liver
flukes, trichuriasis.

CONTRAINDICATIONS
Hypersensitivity to albendazole,
benzimidazoles, or any component of
the formulation.

INTERACTIONS
Drug
**Cimetidine, dexamethasone,
praziquantel:** May increase
albendazole concentration.
Theophylline: May increase risk of
theophylline toxicity.
Herbal
Ginseng: May increase intestinal
elimination.
Food
Grapefruit juice: May increase risk
of albendazole adverse effects.

DIAGNOSTIC TEST EFFECTS
May decrease total white blood cell
(WBC) count. Monitor liver function
tests.

SIDE EFFECTS
Frequent
Neurocysticercosis: Nausea,
vomiting, headache.
Hydatid: Abnormal liver function
tests, abdominal pain, nausea,
vomiting.
Occasional
Neurocysticercosis: Increased
intracranial pressure, meningeal
signs.

Hydatid: Headache, dizziness,
alopecia, fever.

SERIOUS REACTIONS
• Granulocytopenia or pancytopenia
occurs rarely.
• In the presence of cysticercosis,
drug may produce retinal damage in
presence of retinal lesions.
• Hepatoxicity is rare.

PRECAUTIONS & CONSIDERATIONS
Caution is warranted in patients
with liver impairment or biliary
obstruction; hypersensitivity to other
triazoles, such as itraconazole or
terconazole; or hypersensitivity to
imidazoles, such as butoconazole
and ketoconazole. It is unknown
whether albendazole is excreted in
breast milk. Safety and efficacy data
are limited for children, particularly
children younger than 6 yr.
Therefore, expect to use the smallest
dose necessary to achieve optimal
results. There are no age-related
precautions noted in elderly patients.
Fecal specimens should be obtained
3 wks after treatment. Patients
being treated for neurocysticercosis
should receive corticosteroid and
anticonvulsant therapy, as indicated.
    If fever, chills, sore throat, unusual
bleeding or bruising, rash, or hives
occurs, notify the physician. All
patients should have monitoring of
blood cell counts and transaminases
before therapy and every 2 wks
during therapy. Patients should
be advised to avoid becoming
pregnancy while on therapy and
for 1 mo after completing therapy.
Therapy should be initiated after
a negative pregnancy test. Use in
pregnancy only if no alternative
therapy is appropriate.
Administration
Take albendazole with meals. Fatty
meals are preferred. For young

children, the tablets should be crushed or chewed and swallowed with a drink of water.

Albumin, Human

al-byew′min
(Albumex [AUS], Albuminar, Albutein, Buminate, Plasbumin)
Do not confuse with albuterol.

CATEGORY AND SCHEDULE

Pregnancy Risk Category: C

Classification: Plasma expanders

MECHANISM OF ACTION

A plasma protein fraction that acts as a blood volume expander. *Therapeutic Effect:* Provides temporary increase in blood volume; reduces hemoconcentration and blood viscosity.

PHARMACOKINETICS

Distributed throughout extracellular fluid. *Half-life:* 15-20 days.

AVAILABILITY

Injection: 5%, 20%, 25%.

INDICATIONS AND DOSAGES
▸ **Hypovolemia**
IV
Adults, Elderly. Initially, 25 g; may repeat in 15-30 min. Maximum: 250 g within 48 h.
Children. 0.5-1 g/kg/dose (10-20 mL/kg/dose of 5% albumin). Maximum: 6 g/kg/day.
▸ **Hypoproteinemia**
IV
Adults, Elderly. 25 g IV. May repeat in 15-30 min. Maximum: 250 g in 48 h.

Children. 0.5-1 g/kg/dose (10-20 mL/kg/dose of 5% albumin). Repeat in 1-2 days.
▸ **Burns**
IV
Adults, Elderly, Children. Initially, give large volumes of crystalloid infusion to maintain plasma volume. After 24 h, give 25 g, then adjust dosage to maintain plasma albumin concentration of 2-2.5 g/100 mL.
▸ **Cardiopulmonary bypass**
IV
Adults, Elderly. 5% or 25% albumin with crystalloid to maintain plasma albumin concentration of 2.5 g/100 mL.
▸ **Acute nephrosis, nephrotic syndrome**
IV
Adults, Elderly. 25 g of 25% injection, with diuretic once a day for 7-10 days.
▸ **Hemodialysis**
IV
Adults, Elderly. 100 mL (25 g) of 25% albumin.
▸ **Hyperbilirubinemia, erythroblastosis fetalis**
IV
Infants. 1 g/kg 1-2 h before transfusion.

CONTRAINDICATIONS

Heart failure, history of allergic reaction to albumin level, hypervolemia, normal serum albumin, pulmonary edema, severe anemia.

DIAGNOSTIC TEST EFFECTS

May increase serum alkaline phosphatase concentration.

🚫 IV INCOMPATIBILITIES

Midazolam (Versed), vancomycin (Vancocin), verapamil (Isoptin), protein hydrolysates, amino acid solutions, alcohol-containing solutions.

IV COMPATIBILITIES

Diltiazem (Cardizem), lorazepam (Ativan), whole blood, plasma, 0.9% NaCl, D5W, sodium lactate.

SIDE EFFECTS

Rare

High dose in repeated therapy: altered vital signs, chills, fever, increased salivation, nausea, vomiting, urticaria, tachycardia.

SERIOUS REACTIONS

- Fluid overload may occur, marked by increased BP and distended neck veins. Neurologic changes that may occur include headache, weakness, blurred vision, behavioral changes, incoordination, and isolated muscle twitching. Pulmonary edema may also occur, evidenced by rapid breathing, rales, wheezing, and coughing.

PRECAUTIONS & CONSIDERATIONS

Caution is warranted with hepatic or renal impairment, hypertension, normal serum albumin level, poor heart function, and pulmonary disease. It is unknown whether albumin crosses the placenta or is distributed in breast milk. No age-related precautions have been noted in children or in elderly patients.

Notify the physician of difficulty breathing, itching, or rash. BP for hypertension or hypotension, intake and output, and skin for flushing and urticaria should be monitored. Signs and symptoms of fluid overload and pulmonary edema should be assessed frequently.

Storage

Store at room temperature. Albumin normally appears as a clear, brownish, odorless, and moderately viscous fluid. Do not use if the solution has been frozen, appears turbid, or contains sediment or if the vial has been open 4 h or longer.

Administration

! Dosage is based on the condition; duration of administration is based on the response. Make a 5% solution from 25% solution by adding 1 volume 25% solution to 4 volumes 0.9% NaCl (preferred) or D5W. Do not use sterile water for injection because life-threatening acute renal failure and hemolysis can occur. Give by IV infusion. Rate varies depending on therapeutic use, blood volume, and concentration of the solute. Give 5% solution at 5-10 mL/min. Give 25% at a usual rate of 2-3 mL/min. A slower rate (1 mL/min) is recommended in patients with normal blood volume. Administer 5% solution undiluted; administer 25% solution undiluted or diluted with 0.9% NaCl (preferred) or D5W. May give without regard to patient's blood group or Rh factor.

Albuterol

al-byoo′ter-ole
(AccuNeb, Airomir [AUS], Asmol CFC-Free [AUS], Epaq Inhaler [AUS], Novosalmol [CAN], Proventil, Proventil Repetabs, Respax [AUS], Ventolin, Ventolin CFC-Free [AUS], Volmax, VoSpire ER)
Do not confuse albuterol with Albutein or atenolol, or Proventil with Prinivil. Also known as salbutamol.

CATEGORY AND SCHEDULE

Pregnancy Risk Category: C

Classification: Adrenergic β_2 agonist, bronchodilator

MECHANISM OF ACTION

A sympathomimetic that stimulates β_2-adrenergic receptors in the lungs, resulting in relaxation of bronchial smooth muscle. *Therapeutic Effect:* Relieves bronchospasm and reduces airway resistance.

PHARMACOKINETICS

Route	Onset (min)	Peak (h)	Duration (h)
PO	15-30	2-3	4-6
PO (extended-release)	30	2-4	12
Inhalation	5-15	0.5-2	2-5

Rapidly, well absorbed from the GI tract; gradually absorbed from the bronchi after inhalation. Metabolized in the liver. Primarily excreted in urine. *Half-life:* 2.7-5 h (PO); 3.8 h (inhalation).

AVAILABILITY

Syrup: 2 mg/5 mL.
Tablet: 2 mg, 4 mg.
Tablets (Extended-Release [Volmax, VoSpire ER]): 4 mg, 8 mg.
Inhalation (Aerosol [Proventil, Ventolin]): 90 mcg/spray.
Inhalation (Solution [AccuNeb]): 0.75 mg/3 mL, 1.5 mg/3 mL.
Inhalation (Solution [Proventil]): 0.083%, 0.5%.

INDICATIONS AND DOSAGES
▶ **Bronchospasm**
PO
Adults, Children older than 12 yr. 2-4 mg 3-4 times a day. Maximum: 8 mg 4 times/day.
Elderly. 2 mg 3-4 times a day. Maximum: 8 mg 4 times a day.
Children 6-12 yr. 2 mg 3-4 times a day. Maximum: 24 mg/day.
PO (EXTENDED-RELEASE)
Adults, Children older than 12 yr. 4-8 mg q12h.
Children 6-12 yr. 4 mg q12h.
INHALATION
Adults, Elderly, Children older than 12 yr. 1-2 puffs by metered dose inhaler q4-6h as needed.

Children 4-12 yr. 1-2 puffs 4 times a day.
NEBULIZATION
Adults, Elderly, Children older than 12 yr. 2.5 mg 3-4 times a day.
Children 2-12 yr. 0.63-1.25 mg 3-4 times a day.
▶ **Exercise-induced bronchospasm**
INHALATION
Adults, Elderly, Children 4 yr and older. 2 puffs 15-30 min before exercise.

OFF-LABEL USES
Acute treatment of hyperkalemia.

CONTRAINDICATIONS
History of hypersensitivity to sympathomimetics.

INTERACTIONS
Drug
β-blockers: Antagonize effects of albuterol.
Digoxin: May increase the risk of arrhythmias.
Diuretics: Hypokalemia associated with diuretic may worsen with albuterol. Monitor potassium levels.
MAOIs, tricyclic antidepressants: May potentiate cardiovascular effects.
Food
Caffeine: Limit use of caffeine, increased CNS stimulation.

DIAGNOSTIC TEST EFFECTS
May increase blood glucose level. May decrease serum potassium level.

SIDE EFFECTS
Frequent
Headache (27%); nausea (15%); restlessness, nervousness, tremors (20%); dizziness (< 7%); throat dryness and irritation, pharyngitis (< 6%); BP changes, including hypertension (3%-5%); heartburn, transient wheezing (< 5%).

Occasional (2%-3%)
Insomnia, asthenia, altered taste.
Inhalation: Dry, irritated mouth or
throat; cough; bronchial irritation.
Rare
Somnolence, diarrhea, dry mouth,
flushing, diaphoresis, anorexia.

SERIOUS REACTIONS

• Excessive sympathomimetic
stimulation may produce palpitations,
extrasystole, tachycardia, chest pain,
a slight increase in BP followed
by a substantial decrease, chills,
diaphoresis, and blanching of skin.
• Too-frequent or excessive use may
lead to decreased bronchodilating
effectiveness and severe, paradoxical
bronchoconstriction.

PRECAUTIONS & CONSIDERATIONS
Caution is warranted in patients
with cardiovascular disease, diabetes
mellitus, hypertension, glaucoma,
seizure disorders, and hyperthyroidism.
Albuterol appears to cross the placenta;
it is unknown whether albuterol is
distributed in breast milk. Albuterol
may inhibit uterine contractility. The
safety and efficacy of this drug have
not been established in children < 2 yr
of age (syrup, nebulizer solution),
< 4 yr of age (inhaler), or < 6 yr of
age (tablets). Elderly patients may be
more prone to tremors and tachycardia
because of increased sensitivity to
sympathomimetics. Drink plenty
of fluids to decrease the thickness
of lung secretions. Avoid excessive
use of caffeinated products, such as
chocolate, cocoa, cola, coffee, and tea.
Pulse rate and quality, 12-lead
ECG, respiratory rate, depth, rhythm
and type, ABG, and serum potassium
levels should be monitored.
Storage
Store at room temperature. Use
nebulization solution within 1 wk of
opening foil pouch.

Administration
Do not crush or break extended-
release tablets. Take albuterol
without regard to food.
For inhalation, shake the
container well before inhalation.
Prime before first use or if inhaler
has not been used for 2 wks. Wait
2 min before inhaling the second
dose to allow for deeper bronchial
penetration. Rinse mouth with water
immediately after inhalation to
prevent mouth and throat dryness.
Take no more than 2 inhalations
at any one time because excessive
use may decrease the drug's
effectiveness or produce paradoxical
bronchoconstriction.
For nebulizer use, dilute 0.5 mL
of 0.5% solution to a final volume
of 3 mL with 0.9% NaCl to provide
2.5 mg. Administer over 5-15 min.
The nebulizer should be used with
compressed air or oxygen (O_2) at a
rate of 6-10 L/min.
Note: The 0.083% nebulization
solution requires no dilution before
nebulizer administration.

Alclometasone
al-kloe-met´a-sone
(Aclovate)
Do not confuse with Accolate.

CATEGORY AND SCHEDULE
Pregnancy Risk Category: C

Classification: Corticosteroids,
topical, dermatologics

MECHANISM OF ACTION
Topical corticosteroids exhibit
anti-inflammatory, antipruritic,
and vasoconstrictive properties.
Clinically, these actions correspond
to decreased edema, erythema,

pruritus, plaque formation, and scaling of the affected skin.
Low- to medium-potency topical corticosteroid.

PHARMACOKINETICS

Approximately 3% is absorbed during an 8-h period. Metabolized in the liver. Excreted in the urine.

AVAILABILITY

Cream, as Dipropionate: 0.05% (Aclovate).
Ointment, as Diproprionate: 0.05% (Aclovate).

INDICATIONS AND DOSAGES

▶ **Corticosteroid-responsive dermatoses: atopic dermatitis, contact dermatitis, dermatitis, discoid lupus erythematosus, eczema, exfoliative dermatitis, granuloma annulare, lichen planus, lichen simplex, polymorphous light eruption, pruritus, psoriasis, Rhus dermatitis, seborrheic dermatitis, xerosis**
TOPICAL
Adults, Elderly, Children 1 yr and older. Apply a thin film to the affected area 2-3 times a day.

CONTRAINDICATIONS

Hypersensitivity to alclometasone, other corticosteroids, or any of its components.

DIAGNOSTIC TEST EFFECTS

None known.

SIDE EFFECTS

Frequent
Burning, erythema, maculopapular rash, pruritus, skin irritation, xerosis.
Occasional
Acneiform rash, contact dermatitis, folliculitis, glycosuria, growth inhibition, headache, hyperglycemia, infection, miliaria, papilledema, skin atrophy, skin hypopigmentation, skin ulcer, striae, telangiectasia.
Rare
Adrenocortical insufficiency, increased intracranial pressure, pseudotumor cerebri, impaired wound healing, Cushing syndrome, HPA suppression, skin ulcers, tolerance, withdrawal, visual impairment, ocular hypertension, cataracts.

PRECAUTIONS & CONSIDERATIONS

Caution is warranted with pregnancy. It is unknown whether alclometasone is distributed in breast milk. Alclometasone should not be used for diaper dermatitis. Children are more susceptible to HPA axis suppression than adults. There are no age-related precautions noted for elderly patients. Avoid use on herpetic lesions; avoid use as monotherapy on sites with bacterial or fungal infections.

The most common side effect is transient mild skin irritation consisting of burning, pruritus, or erythema.
Storage
Store at room temperature.
Administration
Do not use occlusive dressings unless directed by physician. Apply a thin film topically to affected area 2-3 times daily. Massage gently until medication disappears.

Aldesleukin

Al-des-lew´-kin
(Interleukin-2, IL-2, Proleukin)
Do not confuse interleukin-2 with interferon 2.

CATEGORY AND SCHEDULE

Pregnancy Risk Category: C

Classification: Antineoplastics, biologic response modifier

MECHANISM OF ACTION
A biological response modifier that acts like human recombinant interleukin-2, promoting proliferation, differentiation, and recruitment of T and B cells, lymphokine-activated and natural cells, and thymocytes. *Therapeutic Effect:* Enhances cytolytic activity in lymphocytes.

PHARMACOKINETICS
Primarily distributed into plasma, lymphocytes, lungs, liver, kidney, and spleen. Metabolized to amino acids in the cell lining the kidneys. *Half-life:* 85 min.

AVAILABILITY
Powder for Injection, 22 million units (1.3 mg).

INDICATIONS AND DOSAGES
▸ **Metastatic melanoma, metastatic renal cell carcinoma**
IV
Adults. 600,000 units/kg q8h for 14 doses; followed by 9 days of rest, then another 14 doses for a total of 28 doses per course. Course may be repeated after rest period of at least 7 wks from date of hospital discharge.

OFF-LABEL USES
Treatment of colorectal cancer, Kaposi sarcoma, non-Hodgkin lymphoma.

CONTRAINDICATIONS
Abnormal pulmonary function or thallium stress test results, organ allografts, retreatment in those who experience any of the following toxicities: bowel ischemia or perforation, coma, or toxic psychosis lasting longer than 48 h, GI bleeding requiring surgery, intubation lasting more than 72 h, pericardial tamponade, renal dysfunction requiring dialysis for longer than 72 h, repetitive or difficult-to-control

seizures; angina, MI, recurrent chest pain with ECG changes, sustained ventricular tachycardia, uncontrolled or unresponsive cardiac rhythm disturbances.

INTERACTIONS
Drug
Antihypertensives: May increase hypotensive effect.
Cardiotoxic, hepatotoxic, myelotoxic, or nephrotoxic medications: May increase the risk of toxicity.
Glucocorticoids: May decrease the effects of aldesleukin.
Interferon-α: May increase the risk of myocardial injury, including myocardial infarction, myocarditis, ventricular hypokinesia, and severe rhabdomyolysis.
Iodinated contrast media: Administration subsequent to aldesleukin associated with acute, atypical adverse reactions within hours of contrast media.
Herbal
None known.
Food
None known.

DIAGNOSTIC TEST EFFECTS
May increase BUN and serum alkaline phosphatase, bilirubin, creatinine, AST (SGOT), and ALT (SGPT) levels. May decrease serum calcium, magnesium, phosphorus, potassium, and sodium levels.

ⓘ IV INCOMPATIBILITIES
Ganciclovir (Cytovene), lorazepam (Ativan), pentamidine (Pentam), prochlorperazine (Compazine), promethazine (Phenergan).

ⓘ IV COMPATIBILITIES
Calcium gluconate, dopamine (Intropin), heparin, magnesium, potassium.

SIDE EFFECTS/ADVERSE REACTIONS

Side effects are generally self-limiting and reversible within 2-3 days after discontinuing therapy.

Frequent (48%-89%)
Fever, chills, nausea, vomiting, hypotension, diarrhea, oliguria or anuria, mental status changes, irritability, confusion, depression, sinus tachycardia, pain (abdominal, chest, back), fatigue, dyspnea, pruritus.

Occasional (17%-47%)
Edema, erythema, rash, stomatitis, anorexia, weight gain, infection (urinary tract infection, injection site, catheter tip), dizziness.

Rare (4%-15%)
Dry skin, sensory disorders (vision, speech, taste), dermatitis, headache, arthralgia, myalgia, weight loss, hematuria, conjunctivitis, proteinuria.

SERIOUS REACTIONS

• Anemia, thrombocytopenia, and leukopenia occur commonly.
• GI bleeding and pulmonary edema occur occasionally.
• Capillary leak syndrome results in hypotension (systolic pressure < 90 mm Hg or a 20-mm Hg drop from baseline systolic pressure), extravasation of plasma proteins and fluid into extravascular space, and loss of vascular tone. It may result in cardiac arrhythmias, angina, MI, and respiratory insufficiency.
• Other rare reactions include fatal malignant hyperthermia, cardiac arrest, CVA, pulmonary emboli, bowel perforation, gangrene, and severe depression leading to suicide.

PRECAUTIONS & CONSIDERATIONS

Extreme caution should be used in patients with a history of cardiac or pulmonary disease even if they have normal thallium stress and pulmonary function test results. Also use the drug cautiously with fixed requirements for large volumes of fluid (such as those with hypercalcemia) or a history of seizures. Aldesleukin use should be avoided in patients of either sex who do not practice effective contraception. The safety and efficacy of aldesleukin have not been established in children. Elderly patients may require cautious use of the drug because of age-related renal impairment. They are also less able to tolerate drug-related toxicities.

Notify the physician of difficulty urinating, black tarry stools, pinpoint red spots on skin, bruising, fever, signs of local infection, sore throat, or unusual bleeding from any site. Treat persons with bacterial infection and those with indwelling central lines with antibiotic therapy before beginning aldesleukin therapy. A negative CT scan must be obtained before beginning therapy. Immediately report any symptoms of depression or suicidal ideation. CBC, electrolytes, liver and renal function, amylase concentration, BP, mental status, intake and output, extravascular fluid accumulation, platelet count, pulse oximetry values, and weight should be assessed.

Consider the use of medications to reduce aldesleukin side effects: NSAIDs/antipyretics starting before first dose to reduce fever, meperidine to control rigors associated with fever, H2 antagonists/PPIs to reduce gastrointestinal (GI) bleeding/irritation, antiemetics and antidiarrheals, hydroxyzine or diphenhydramine for pruritic rashes, and antibiotic prophylaxis.

Storage
Refrigerate—do not freeze—unopened vials. The reconstituted

solution is stable for 48 h at room temperature or refrigerated (refrigerated is preferred).

Administration

! Withhold the drug in patients who exhibit moderate to severe lethargy or somnolence because continued administration may result in coma. Restrict aldesleukin therapy to patients with normal cardiac and pulmonary function as determined by thallium stress testing and pulmonary function testing. Dosage is individualized based on clinical response and tolerance of the drug's adverse effects. Aldesleukin should be administered only in a hospital setting with availability of an intensive care facility and specialists skilled in cardiopulmonary or intensive care medicine.

For IV use, reconstitute the 22-million-unit vial with 1.2 mL sterile water for injection to provide a concentration of 18 million units/mL. Do not use bacteriostatic water for injection or 0.9% NaCl. During reconstitution, direct the diluent at the side of the vial. Swirl the content gently; do not shake to avoid foaming. Further dilute the dose in 50 mL D5W and infuse over 15 min. Do not use an in-line filter. Warm the solution to room temperature before infusion. Closely monitor the patient for a drop in mean arterial BP, a sign of capillary leak syndrome. Continued treatment may result in edema, pleural effusion, mental status changes, and significant hypotension (systolic pressure < 90 mm Hg or a 20 mm Hg drop from baseline systolic pressure).

Alefacept

ale´fah-cept
(Amevive)

CATEGORY AND SCHEDULE

Pregnancy Risk Category: B

Classification:
Immunosuppressives

MECHANISM OF ACTION

An immunologic agent that interferes with the activation of T lymphocytes by binding to the lymphocyte antigen, thus reducing the number of circulating T lymphocytes. *Therapeutic Effect:* Prevents T cells from becoming overactive, which may help reduce symptoms of chronic plaque psoriasis.

PHARMACOKINETICS

Bioavailability 63% with IM administration, *Half-life:* 270 h.

AVAILABILITY

Powder for Injection: 15 mg. Alefacept is distributed to physicians' offices and specialty pharmacies, with administration intended in the physician's office.

INDICATIONS AND DOSAGES
▸ **Plaque psoriasis**
IV
Adults, Elderly. 7.5 mg once weekly for 12 wks. Retreatment for one additional cycle acceptable after 12 wks of rest.
IM
Adults, Elderly. 15 mg once weekly for 12 wks. Retreatment for one additional cycle acceptable after 12 wks of rest.

CONTRAINDICATIONS

HIV infection, history of systemic malignancy, concurrent use of immunosuppressive agents or phototherapy, active serious infection or sepsis.

Hypersensitivity to drug or hamster proteins.

INTERACTIONS
Drug
Live virus vaccines: avoid concurrent use.

DIAGNOSTIC TEST EFFECTS
Decreases serum T-lymphocyte levels. May increase serum AST (SGOT) and ALT (SGPT) levels.

ⓘ IV INCOMPATIBILITIES
Do not mix alefacept with any other medications. Do not reconstitute it with any diluent other than that supplied by the manufacturer.

SIDE EFFECTS
Frequent (16%)
Injection site pain and inflammation (with IM administration).
Occasional (5%)
Chills.
Rare (2% or less)
Pharyngitis, dizziness, cough, nausea, myalgia.

SERIOUS REACTIONS
• Rare reactions include hypersensitivity reactions, infusion reactions, liver injury, lymphopenia, malignancies, and serious infections requiring hospitalization (such as abscess, pneumonia, and postoperative wound infection).
• Coronary artery problems or disorder and MI occur in fewer than 1% of patients.

PRECAUTIONS & CONSIDERATIONS

Caution is warranted in patients with chronic infections, history of recurrent infections, high risk for malignancy, and in elderly patients.

It is unknown whether alefacept crosses the placenta or is distributed in breast milk. The safety and efficacy of this drug have not been established in children. Cautious use is necessary in elderly patients because they are at increased risk for infections and certain malignancies. Avoid contact with infected individuals and situations that might increase the risk for infection.

Notify the physician of any signs of infection or malignancy. CD4+ T-lymphocyte counts should be monitored before and weekly during the 12-wks treatment period. Withhold the dose if the CD4+ count is < 250 cells/μL. Discontinue treatment if the count remains below 250 cells/μL.

Storage
Store unopened vials in the refrigerator protected from light. Do not freeze. Use the drug immediately after reconstitution or within 4 h if refrigerated. Discard unused portion within 4 h of reconstitution.

Administration
! The patient may be retreated for an additional 12 wks, as prescribed, if at least 12 wks have elapsed since the previous course of therapy and the patient's CD4+ T-lymphocyte count is within normal limits. For both IV and IM administration, withdraw 0.6 mL of the supplied diluent and, with the needle pointed at the sidewall of the vial, slowly inject the diluent into the vial of alefacept. Swirl the vial gently to dissolve the contents; do not shake or vigorously agitate the vial to avoid excessive foaming. The reconstituted solution should be clear and colorless to slightly yellow. Do not use if it becomes discolored or cloudy or contains undissolved material. Note: IV and IM dosages differ.

For IV use, reconstitute the 7.5-mg vial with 0.6 mL of the supplied diluent (sterile water for injection); final concentration is 7.5 mg/0.5 mL. Prepare two syringes with 3 mL 0.9% NaCl for a pre- and post-administration flush. Prime the winged infusion set with 3 mL 0.9% NaCl and insert the set into the vein. Attach the drug-filled syringe to the infusion set, and administer the solution over no more than 5 s. Flush the infusion set with 3 mL 0.9% NaCl.

For IM use, reconstitute 15-mg vial with 0.6 mL of the supplied diluent (sterile water for injection); final concentration is 15 mg/0.5 mL. Inject the full 0.5 mL of solution. Use a different IM site for each new IM injection at least 1 inch from an old site, avoiding tender, bruised, red, or hard areas.

Alemtuzumab
Al-em-two'-zoo-mab
(Campath)

CATEGORY AND SCHEDULE
Pregnancy Risk Category: C

Classification: Antineoplastics

MECHANISM OF ACTION
Binds to CD52, a cell surface glycoprotein, found on the surface of all B and T lymphocytes, most monocytes, macrophages, natural killer cells, and granulocytes.
Therapeutic Effect: Produces cytotoxicity, reducing tumor size.

PHARMACOKINETICS
Half-life: 11 h after the first dose and 6 days after the last dose. Peak

and trough levels rise during first few weeks of therapy and approach steady state by about wks 6.

AVAILABILITY
Solution for Injection: 30 mg/3 mL.

INDICATIONS AND DOSAGES
▸ **B-cell chronic lymphocytic leukemia in patients who have been treated with alkylating agents and failed fludarabine therapy**
IV
Adults, Elderly. Initially, 3 mg/day as a 2-h infusion. When the 3-mg daily dose is tolerated (with only low-grade or no infusion-related toxicities), increase daily dose to 10 mg. When the 10 mg/day dose is tolerated, maintenance dose may be initiated.
Maintenance: 30 mg/day 3 times/wk on alternate days (such as Monday, Wednesday, and Friday or Tuesday, Thursday, and Saturday) for up to 12 wks. The increase to 30 mg/day is usually achieved in 3-7 days.

CONTRAINDICATIONS
Active systemic infections, history of hypersensitivity or anaphylactic reaction to the drug, or hamster proteins.

INTERACTIONS
Drug
Live virus vaccines: May potentiate viral replication, increase side effects, and decrease the patient's antibody response to the vaccine.
Herbal
None known.
Food
None known.

DIAGNOSTIC TEST EFFECTS
May decrease hemoglobin level, platelet count, and WBC count.

🕥 IV INCOMPATIBILITIES
Do not mix alemtuzumab with any other medications.

SIDE EFFECTS
Frequent
Rigors (86%-89%), tremors (86%), fever (85%), nausea (54%), vomiting (41%), rash (40%), fatigue (34%), hypotension (32%), urticaria (30%), pruritus (14%-24%), skeletal pain, headache (24%), diarrhea (22%), anorexia (20%).
Occasional (< 10%)
Myalgia, dizziness, abdominal pain, throat irritation, vomiting, neutropenia, rhinitis, bronchospasm, urticaria.

SERIOUS REACTIONS
• Neutropenia occurs in 85% of patients, anemia occurs in 80% of patients, and thrombocytopenia occurs in 72% of patients.
• A rash occurs in 40% of patients.
• Respiratory toxicity, manifested as dyspnea, cough, bronchitis, pneumonitis, and pneumonia, occurs in 16%-26% of patients.

PRECAUTIONS & CONSIDERATIONS
Alemtuzumab has the potential to cause depletion of B- and T-lymphocytes in the fetus. Effective contraception is recommended during and for 6 mo after treatment for women of childbearing potential and men of reproductive potential. Discontinue breastfeeding during treatment and for at least 3 mo after the last dose. The safety and efficacy of alemtuzumab have not been established in children. No age-related precautions have been noted in the elderly. Vaccinations and contact with anyone who has recently received a live-virus vaccine should be avoided. Crowds and those with known infection should also be avoided.

Infusion-related reactions, including chills, fever, hypotension, and rigors, should be monitored which usually occur 30 min to 2 h after starting the first infusion; these reactions may resolve by slowing the drip rate. Signs and symptoms for hematologic toxicity, including excessive fatigue or weakness, ecchymosis, fever, signs of local infection, sore throat, or unusual bleeding from any site, should be assessed. CBC should be monitored frequently during and after therapy to assess for anemia, neutropenia, and thrombocytopenia. Prophylactic therapy against PCP pneumonia and herpes viral infections is recommended upon initiation of therapy and for at least 2 mo following the last dose or until CD4+ counts are ≥200 cells/µL (whichever is later).
Storage
Refrigerate ampules before dilution. Do not freeze them. Use the solution within 8 h after dilution. The diluted solution may be stored at room temperature or refrigerated. Discard the solution if it becomes discolored or contains particulate matter.
Administration
! Expect to pretreat with 650 mg of acetaminophen and 50 mg of diphenhydramine before each infusion to prevent infusion-related side effects.

Withdraw the needed amount from the vial into a syringe. Inject it into 100-mL 0.9% NaCl or D5W. Gently invert the bag to mix the contents; do not shake it. Give the 100-mL solution as a 2-h IV infusion. Do not give alemtuzumab by IV push or bolus.

Alendronate
ah-len´dro-nate
(Fosamax)
Do not confuse Fosamax with Flomax.

CATEGORY AND SCHEDULE
Pregnancy Risk Category: C

Classification: Bisphosphonates

MECHANISM OF ACTION
A bisphosphonate that inhibits normal and abnormal bone resorption, without retarding mineralization. *Therapeutic Effect:* Leads to significantly increased bone mineral density; reverses the progression of osteoporosis.

PHARMACOKINETICS
Poorly absorbed after oral administration; oral bioavailability < 1%. Protein binding: 78%. After oral administration, rapidly taken into bone, with uptake greatest at sites of active bone turnover. Excreted in urine. *Terminal half-life:* > 10 yr (reflects release from skeleton as bone is resorbed).

AVAILABILITY
Tablets: 5 mg, 10 mg, 35 mg, 40 mg, 70 mg.
Oral Solution: 70 mg/75 mL.

INDICATIONS AND DOSAGES
▸ **Osteoporosis (in men)**
PO
Adults, Elderly. 10 mg once a day in the morning.
▸ **Glucocorticoid-induced osteoporosis**
PO
Adults, Elderly. 5 mg once a day in the morning.

Postmenopausal women not receiving estrogen. 10 mg once a day in the morning.
▸ **Postmenopausal osteoporosis**
PO (TREATMENT)
Adults, Elderly. 10 mg once a day in the morning or 70 mg once weekly.
PO (PREVENTION)
Adults, Elderly. 5 mg once a day in the morning or 35 mg once weekly.
▸ **Paget disease**
PO
Adults, Elderly. 40 mg once a day in the morning for 6 mo; reevaluate before treatment.

CONTRAINDICATIONS
Abnormalities of the esophagus that delay esophageal emptying, such as stricture or achalasia; hypocalcemia; inability to stand or sit upright for at least 30 min; renal impairment (CrCl < 35 mL/min); sensitivity to alendronate or phosphonates; patients with aspiration risk.

INTERACTIONS
Drug
Aspirin: May increase GI disturbances.
IV ranitidine: May double the bioavailability of alendronate.
Herbal
None known.
Food
Beverages other than plain water, dietary supplements, food: May interfere with absorption of alendronate.

DIAGNOSTIC TEST EFFECTS
Reduces serum calcium and serum phosphate concentrations. Significantly decreases serum alkaline phosphatase level in patients with Paget disease.

SIDE EFFECTS
Frequent (7%-8%)
Back pain, abdominal pain.

Occasional (2%-3%)
Nausea, abdominal distension,
constipation, diarrhea,
flatulence.
Rare (< 2%)
Rash.

SERIOUS REACTIONS

• Overdose causes hypocalcemia,
hypophosphatemia, and significant
GI disturbances.
• Esophageal irritation occurs if
alendronate is not given with 6-8
oz of plain water or if the patient
lies down within 30 min of drug
administration.
• Severe and occasionally debilitating
bone, joint, or muscle pain.
• Osteonecrosis of the jaw.

PRECAUTIONS & CONSIDERATIONS

Caution is warranted with
hypocalcemia or vitamin D
deficiency and in patients with
GI disease, including dysphagia,
frequent heartburn, GI reflux
disease, hiatal hernia, and
ulcers. Alendronate may cause
decreased maternal weight gain
and incomplete fetal ossification
and delay delivery. It is unknown
whether alendronate is excreted in
breast milk. Do not give to women
who are breastfeeding. Safety and
efficacy of alendronate have not
been established in children. No
age-related precautions have been
noted for elderly patients.

Consider beginning weight-
bearing exercises and modifying
behavioral factors, such as reducing
alcohol consumption and stopping
cigarette smoking. Plan to correct
hypocalcemia and vitamin D
deficiency, if present, before
starting alendronate therapy. Serum
electrolytes, including serum alkaline
phosphatase and serum calcium
levels, should be monitored.

Administration
❗ Give at least 30 min before the
first food, beverage, or medication
of the day.

Expected benefits occur only when
alendronate is taken with a full
glass (6-8 oz) of plain water first
thing in the morning and at least
30 min before the first food,
beverage, or medication of the day.
Taking alendronate with beverages
other than plain water, including
mineral water, orange juice, and
coffee, significantly reduces
absorption of the medication.
❗ Do not lie down for at least 30
min after taking the medication.
Remaining upright helps the drug
move quickly to the stomach and
reduces the risk of esophageal
irritation.

Alfuzosin
al-few-zoe'sin
(Uroxatral)

CATEGORY AND SCHEDULE
Pregnancy Risk Category: B;
however, this drug is not indicated
for use in women.

Classification: Antiadrenergics,
α-blocking, peripheral

MECHANISM OF ACTION
An α-1 antagonist that targets
receptors around bladder neck
and prostate capsule. *Therapeutic
Effect:* Relaxes smooth muscle and
improves urinary flow and symptoms
of prostatic hyperplasia.

PHARMACOKINETICS
Bioavailability 49% following
meal; reduced 50% in fasting
state. Peak levels reached in 8 h.

Protein binding: 90%. Extensively metabolized in the liver. Primarily excreted in urine. *Half-life:* 3-9 h.

AVAILABILITY
Tablets (Extended-Release): 10 mg.

INDICATIONS AND DOSAGES
▸ **Benign prostatic hyperplasia**
PO
Adult men. 10 mg once a day, approximately 30 min after same meal each day.

CONTRAINDICATIONS
History of hypersensitivity to alfuzosin; moderate to severe hepatic insufficiency (Child Pugh Class B and C); potent CYP3A4 inhibitors (itraconazole, ketoconazole, ritonavir).

INTERACTIONS
Drug
Antihypertensive agents, nitrates: Increased potential for hypotension.
Cimetidine: May increase alfuzosin blood concentration.
CYP3A4 inducers: May reduce alfuzosin levels, decrease effect.
CYP3A4 inhibitors: May increase alfuzosin levels and increase side effects; potent inhibitors (e.g., itraconazole, ketoconazole, ritonavir) are contraindicated.
Other α-blockers, such as doxazosin, prazosin, tamsulosin, and terazosin: May increase the α-blockade effects of both drugs.
Herbal
None known.
Food
Food increases extent of absorption.

DIAGNOSTIC TEST EFFECTS
None known.

SIDE EFFECTS
Frequent (6%-7%)
Dizziness, headache, malaise.
Occasional (4%)
Dry mouth.
Rare (2%-3%)
Nausea, dyspepsia (such as heartburn and epigastric discomfort), diarrhea, orthostatic hypotension, tachycardia, drowsiness.

SERIOUS REACTIONS
• Ischemia-related chest pain may occur rarely.

PRECAUTIONS & CONSIDERATIONS
Caution is warranted for patients with coronary artery disease, hepatic impairment, known history of QT-interval prolongation, orthostatic hypotension, severe renal impairment, or under general anesthesia. Alfuzosin is not indicated for use in women and children. No age-related precautions have been noted for elderly patients.

Dizziness and lightheadedness may occur. Tasks that require mental alertness or motor skills should be avoided until response to the drug is established. Notify the physician if headache occurs.
Administration
Take after the same meal each day. The extended-release tablet should not be crushed or chewed.

Aliskiren
a-lis-kye-ren
(Tekturna)

CATEGORY AND SCHEDULE
Pregnacy Risk Category: C (first trimester) and D (second and third trimesters)

Classification: Antihypertensive. Renin inhibitor.

MECHANISM OF ACTION
A direct renin inhibitor that decreases plasma renin activity and inhibits the conversion of angiotensinogen to angiotensin I. *Therapeutic Effect:* reduced blood pressure.

PHARMACOKINETICS
Poorly absorbed; oral bioavailability 2.5%; high-fat meal reduced extent of absorption 71%. Metabolized by CYP3A4. *Half-life:* 24 h.

AVAILABILITY
Tablets: 150 mg, 300 mg.

INDICATIONS AND DOSAGES
▸ **Hypertension**
PO
Adults. 150 mg once daily, may increase to 300 mg once daily after 2 wks. Take consistently with regard to meals.

CONTRAINDICATIONS
None.

INTERACTIONS
Drug
Cyclosporine: May increase aliskiren concentrations; concomitant use not recommended.
Furosemide: May reduce furosemide concentrations, reducing furosemide activity.
Potassium-sparing diuretics, potassium supplements, salt substitutes containing potassium, or other drugs that increase potassium: Caution is advised.
Herbal
None known.
Food
High-fat meal reduces the extent of absorption; aliskiren should be administered consistently with regard to meals.

DIAGNOSTIC TEST EFFECTS
May increase serum creatinine and BUN, serum potassium, serum uric acid, and creatine kinase; may reduce hemoglobin and hematocrit.

SIDE EFFECTS
Occasional (> 2%)
Diarrhea.
Rare (< 2%)
Abdominal pain, angioedema, cough, dyspepsia, edema, GI reflux, gout, hypotension, rash, renal stones.

SERIOUS REACTIONS
• Angioedema, seizures.

PRECAUTIONS & CONSIDERATIONS
Use in pregnancy can cause injury and death to the developing fetus. Discontinue as soon as possible if pregnancy occurs. Safety and effectiveness have not been established in pediatric patients. No age-related cautions precautions noted in elderly patients. Use with caution in patients with severe renal impairment.
Storage
Store at room temperature; protect from moisture.
Administration
Take consistently with regard to meals. Antihypertensive effect at a given dose generally observed by 2 wks. May be taken with other anti-hypertensives. Doses above 300 mg did not result in additional blood pressure lowering but were associated with increased incidence of diarrhea.

Alitretinoin
ah-lee-tret´-ih-noyn
(Panretin)

CATEGORY AND SCHEDULE
Pregnancy Risk Category: D

Classification: Topical retinoid

MECHANISM OF ACTION

Binds to and activates all known retinoid receptors. Once activated, receptors act as transcription factors, regulating genes that control cellular differentiation and proliferation. *Therapeutic Effect:* Inhibits growth of Kaposi sarcoma (KS) cells.

PHARMACOKINETICS

Minimally absorbed following topical administration; plasma concentrations not detectable.

AVAILABILITY

Gel: 0.1%.

INDICATIONS AND DOSAGES
▸ KS skin lesions
TOPICAL
Adults. Initially, apply twice a day to lesions. May increase to 3 or 4 times a day.

CONTRAINDICATIONS

Hypersensitivity to retinoids or alitretinoin ingredients; when systemic therapy is required (more than 10 new KS lesions in the previous month, symptomatic pulmonary KS, symptomatic visceral involvement, symptomatic lymphedema).

INTERACTIONS
Drug
DEET insect repellant: A litretinoin increases DEET systemic absorption; do not use DEET products.

DIAGNOSTIC TEST EFFECTS

None known.

SIDE EFFECTS
Frequent (3%-77%)
Rash (erythema, scaling, irritation, redness, dermatitis), itching, exfoliative dermatitis (flaking, peeling, desquamation, exfoliation),

stinging, tingling, edema, skin disorders (scabbing, crusting, drainage).

SERIOUS REACTIONS

• Severe local skin reaction (intense erythema, edema, vesiculation) may limit treatment.

PRECAUTIONS & CONSIDERATIONS

Avoid pregnancy, and discontinue breastfeeding when used. Safety and efficacy are unknown for children and patients older than 65 yr, do not use products containing DEET. May cause photosensitivity; minimize exposure of treated areas to sunlight and sunlamps.
Storage
Store at room temperature.
Administration
Apply sufficient gel to cover the lesion with a generous coating. Allow gel to dry for 3-5 min before covering with clothing. Do not cover with occlusive dressings. Avoid bathing, showering, and swimming for 3 h after application. Because unaffected skin may become irritated, avoid application of the gel to healthy skin surrounding the lesions. In addition, do not apply the gel on or near mucosal surfaces of the body. If application site toxicity occurs, the application frequency can be reduced. If severe irritation occurs, application of drug can be discontinued for a few days until the symptoms subside.

A response of KS lesions may be seen as soon as 2 wks after initiation of therapy, but most patients require longer application. With continued application, further benefit may be attained. Some patients have required more than 14 wks to respond. Continue alitretinoin gel as long as the patient is benefitting.

Allopurinol
al-oh-pure′ih-nole
(Allohexal [AUS], Allosig [AUS],
Aloprim, Apo-Allopurinol [CAN],
Capurate [AUS], Progout [AUS],
Purinol [CAN], Zyloprim)
**Do not confuse Zyloprim with
ZORprin.**

CATEGORY AND SCHEDULE
Pregnancy Risk Category: C

Classification: Antigout
agents, purine analogs,
antihyperuricemic

MECHANISM OF ACTION
A xanthine oxidase inhibitor that
decreases uric acid production by
inhibiting xanthine oxidase, an
enzyme. *Therapeutic Effect:* Reduces
uric acid concentrations in both
serum and urine.

PHARMACOKINETICS

Route	Onset	Peak	Duration
PO/IV	2-3 days	1-3 wks	1-2 wks

Well absorbed from the GI tract.
Widely distributed. Metabolized
in the liver to active metabolite.
Excreted primarily in urine.
Removed by hemodialysis. *Half-life:*
1-3 h; metabolite, 12-30 h.

AVAILABILITY
Tablets (Zyloprim): 100 mg, 300 mg.
Powder for Injection (Aloprim):
500 mg.

INDICATIONS AND DOSAGES
▸ **For primary or secondary gout (tophi,
arthritis, uric acid, lithiasis, etc.)**
PO
*Adults, Children older than
10 yr.* Initially, 100 mg/day; may
increase by 100 mg/day at weekly
intervals. Maximum: 800 mg/day.
Maintenance: 100-200 mg 2-3 times
a day or 300 mg/day.
▸ **To prevent uric acid nephropathy
during chemotherapy**
PO
Adults. Initially, 600-800 mg/day,
given in divided doses, starting
2-3 days before initiation of
chemotherapy or radiation therapy.
Children 6-10 yr. 100 mg 3 times a
day or 300 mg once a day. Reassess
at 48 h.
Children < 6 yr. 50 mg 3 times a day.
IV
Adults. 200-400 mg/m^2/day
beginning 24-48 h before initiation
of chemotherapy.
Children. 200 mg/m^2/day. Maximum:
600 mg/day.
▸ **Recurrent calcium oxalate calculi**
PO
Adults. 200-300 mg/day.
Elderly. Initially, 100 mg/day,
gradually increased until optimal uric
acid level is reached.
▸ **Dosage in renal impairment**
Dosage is modified based on
creatinine clearance.

Creatinine Clearance (mL/min)	Dosage Adjustment
10-20	200 mg/day
3-9	100 mg/day
< 3	100 mg at extended intervals

CONTRAINDICATIONS
Asymptomatic hyperuricemia, history
of severe hypersensitivity reactions to
allopurinol.

INTERACTIONS
Drug
ACE inhibitors: May increase risk
of hypersensitivity reactions.

Amoxicillin, ampicillin: May increase incidence of rash.
Azathioprine, mercaptopurine: May increase therapeutic effect and toxicity of azathioprine and mercaptopurine.
Cyclophosphamide: May increase cyclophosphamide myelosuppressive effect, increasing risk of bleeding and infection.
Oral anticoagulants: May increase anticoagulant effect of coumarins.
Thiazide diuretics: May decrease renal elimination of allopurinol. Monitor need for dose adjustment.
Herbal
None known.
Food
None known.

DIAGNOSTIC TEST EFFECTS

May increase BUN, serum creatinine, serum alkaline phosphatase, AST (SGOT), and ALT (SGPT) levels.

⊘ IV INCOMPATIBILITIES

Amikacin (Amikin), amphotericin B, carmustine (BiCNU), cefotaxime (Claforan), chlorpromazine (Thorazine), cimetidine (Tagamet), clindamycin (Cleocin), cytarabine (Ara-C), dacarbazine (DTIC), daunorubicin, diphenhydramine (Benadryl), doxorubicin (Adriamycin), doxycycline (Vibramycin), droperidol (Inapsine), floxuridine, fludarabine (Fludara), gentamicin (Garamycin), haloperidol (Haldol), hydroxyzine (Vistaril), idarubicin (Idamycin), imipenem-cilastatin (Primaxin), mechlorethamine, meperidine (Demerol), methylprednisolone (Solu-Medrol), metoclopramide (Reglan), minocycline, nalbuphine, netilmicin, ondansetron (Zofran), prochlorperazine (Compazine), promethazine (Phenergan), sodium bicarbonate, streptozocin (Zanosar), tobramycin (Nebcin), vinorelbine (Navelbine).

⊌ IV COMPATIBILITIES

Bumetanide (Bumex), calcium gluconate, furosemide (Lasix), heparin, hydromorphone (Dilaudid), lorazepam (Ativan), morphine, potassium chloride.

SIDE EFFECTS

Occasional
Oral: Somnolence, unusual hair loss.
IV: Rash, nausea, vomiting.
Rare
Diarrhea, headache.

SERIOUS REACTIONS

! Pruritic maculopapular rash possibly accompanied by malaise, fever, chills, joint pain, nausea, and vomiting should be considered a toxic reaction.
• Severe hypersensitivity may follow appearance of rash.
• Bone marrow depression, hepatic toxicity, peripheral neuritis, and acute renal failure occur rarely.

PRECAUTIONS & CONSIDERATIONS

Caution is warranted with CHF, diabetes mellitus, hypertension, and impaired renal or hepatic function. It is unknown whether allopurinol crosses the placenta. Allopurinol is excreted in breast milk; use with caution in nursing women. No age-related precautions have been noted in children or in elderly patients. The drug should be discontinued if rash or other evidence of allergic reaction appears. Avoid tasks that require mental alertness or motor skills until response to the drug has been established.

High fluid intake (3000 mL/day) should be encouraged; intake and output should be monitored; output should be at least 2000 mL/day, urine for cloudiness and unusual color and odor, CBC, hepatic enzyme test results, and serum uric acid levels should also be assessed. Signs and symptoms of a therapeutic response, including improved joint range of motion and reduced redness, swelling, and tenderness, should be evaluated.

Storage

Store unreconstituted vials at room temperature. Store reconstituted solution at room temperature; give within 10 h. Do not refrigerate reconstituted or diluted solutions. Do not use if precipitate forms or solution is discolored.

Administration

May take with or immediately after meals or milk. Drink enough fluid daily to maintain a urine output of 2 L/day, if possible. Administer dosages > 300 mg/day in divided doses. It may take 1 wk or longer for the full therapeutic effect of the drug to be evident.

For IV use, reconstitute 500-mg vial with 25 mL sterile water for injection, which produces a clear, almost colorless solution (concentration of 20 mg/mL). Further dilute with 0.9% NaCl or D5W (19 mL of added diluent yields 1 mg/mL, 9 mL yields 2 mg/mL, and 2.3 mL yields a maximum concentration of 6 mg/mL). Infuse over 30-60 min.

Almotriptan
al-moe-trip'tan
(Axert)
Do not confuse Axert with Antivert.

CATEGORY AND SCHEDULE
Pregnancy Risk Category: C

Classification: Selective serotonin receptor agonists, antimigraine agents

MECHANISM OF ACTION
A serotonin receptor agonist that binds selectively to vascular receptors, producing a vasoconstrictive effect on cranial blood vessels. *Therapeutic Effect:* Produces relief of migraine headache.

PHARMACOKINETICS
Well absorbed after PO administration; bioavailability 70%. Metabolized by MAO type A and CYP3A4 and 2D6, excreted in urine (40% as unchanged drug). *Half-life:* 3-4 h.

AVAILABILITY
Tablets: 6.5 mg, 12.5 mg.

INDICATIONS AND DOSAGES
▸ **Migraine headache**
PO
Adults, Elderly. 6.25-12.5 mg. If headache improves but then returns, dose may be repeated after 2 h. Maximum: 2 doses/24 h.
▸ **Dosage in hepatic or renal impairment (CrCl < 10 mL/min)**
Adult, Elderly. Recommended initial dose is 6.25 mg and maximum daily dose is 12.5 mg.

CONTRAINDICATIONS
Arrhythmias associated with conduction disorders, hemiplegic or basilar migraine, ischemic heart disease (including angina pectoris, history of MI, silent ischemia, and Prinzmetal's angina), uncontrolled hypertension, use within 24 h of ergotamine-containing preparation or another serotonin receptor agonist; use within 14 days of MAOIs, Wolff-Parkinson-White syndrome.

INTERACTIONS
Drug
Ergotamine-containing medications: May produce a

vasospastic reaction. Do not use triptan within 24 hr of ergot drug.

Erythromycin, itraconazole, ketoconazole, ritonavir: May increase the almotriptan plasma level.

MAOIs: Do not take within 2 wks of MAOI treatment.

SSRIs/SNRIs (citalopram, desvenlafaxine, duloxetine, escitalopram, fluoxetine, fluvoxamine, paroxetine, sertraline, venlafaxine): May produce weakness, hyperreflexia, and incoordination; serotonin syndrome.

DIAGNOSTIC TEST EFFECTS
None known.

SIDE EFFECTS
Frequent (> 1%)
Nausea, dry mouth, paresthesia, flushing.
Occasional (< 1%)
Changes in temperature sensation, asthenia, dizziness, chest pain, neck pain, back pain.

SERIOUS REACTIONS
• Excessive dosage may produce tremor, red extremities, reduced respirations, cyanosis, seizures, chest pain, and serotonin syndrome.
• Serious arrhythmias occur rarely, particularly in patients with hypertension or diabetes, obese patients, smokers, and those with a strong family history of coronary artery disease.
• Hypertensive crisis.

PRECAUTIONS & CONSIDERATIONS
Caution is warranted with controlled hypertension, a history of CVA, mild to moderate hepatic or renal impairment, and cardiovascular risk factors. It is unknown whether

almotriptan is distributed in breast milk. The safety and efficacy of almotriptan have not been established in children younger than 12 yr. No age-related precautions have been noted in elderly patients. Tasks that require mental alertness or motor skills should be avoided.

Notify the physician immediately if palpitations, pain or tightness in the chest or throat, or pain or weakness in the extremities occurs. Migraines and associated symptoms, including nausea and vomiting, photophobia, and phonophobia (sound sensitivity), should be assessed before and during treatment.

Alosetron
a-low-seh-tron
(Lotronex)
Do not confuse Lotronex with Lovenox

CATEGORY AND SCHEDULE
Pregnancy Risk Category: B

Classification: Selective serotonin receptor antagonist, neuroenteric modulator

MECHANISM OF ACTION
A serotonin (5-HT$_3$) receptor antagonist that mediates abdominal pain, bloating, nausea, vomiting, peristalsis, and secretory reflexes. *Therapeutic Effect:* Alleviates diarrhea, reduces gastric pain.

PHARMACOKINETICS
Rapidly absorbed after PO administration. Extensively metabolized in liver. Excreted primarily in urine and, to a lesser extent, in feces. *Half-life:* 1.5 h.

AVAILABILITY
Tablets: 0.5 mg, 1 mg.

INDICATIONS AND DOSAGES
▶ **Irritable bowel syndrome (IBS), diarrhea predominant**
PO
Adult women. 0.5 mg twice a day. If, after 4 wks the 0.5-mg twice daily dose is well tolerated but does not adequately control IBS symptoms, the dose can be increased up to 1 mg twice a day. Maximum: 2 mg/day.

CONTRAINDICATIONS
Constipation; concomitant fluvoxamine; diverticulitis (active or history of); GI bleeding, obstruction, or perforation; history of ischemic colitis, ulcerative colitis, or Crohn disease; history of severe or chronic constipation or sequelae from constipation; severe hepatic impairment; thrombophlebitis; unable to understand or comply with required patient-physician agreement.

INTERACTIONS
Drug
Apomorphine: May enhance hypotensive effect of apomorphine; contraindicated.
Fluvoxamine: Substantially increases alosetron concentrations; contraindicated.
CYP1A2 inhibitors: May increase levels and effects of alosetron; use with caution.
CYP3A4 inhibitors: May increase levels and effects of alosetron; use with caution.
Hydralazine, isoniazid, procainamide: May alter the effects of these drugs.
Food
All foods: May decrease the absorption or delay the peak blood concentration of alosetron.

DIAGNOSTIC TEST EFFECTS
May increase serum alkaline phosphatase, bilirubin, ALT (SGPT), and AST (SGOT) levels.

SIDE EFFECTS
Frequent (29%)
Constipation.
Occasional (2%-10%)
Nausea, GI or abdominal discomfort or pain, abdominal distension, hemorrhoids, regurgitation and reflux.
Rare (< 1%)
Sedation, abnormal dreams, anxiety, hypertension, clinical depression.

SERIOUS REACTIONS
• Acute ischemic colitis and serious complications of constipation have resulted in the rare need for blood transfusions and surgery or have caused death.

PRECAUTIONS & CONSIDERATIONS
Caution is warranted with hepatic function impairment. Be aware alosetron is indicated for use in women only. The safety and efficacy of this drug have not been established in men. It is unknown whether alosetron is excreted in breast milk. The safety and efficacy of alosetron have not been established in children. Caution is advised for elderly patients, who may be at greater risk for complications of constipation.

Urgency and diarrhea may be reduced within 1 wk of treatment, but the drug's full therapeutic effects may not occur for up to 4 wks. Persistent constipation may require interruption of treatment or drug management. Notify the physician or nurse if bloody diarrhea, severe constipation, or a sudden worsening of stomach pain occurs. Therapy should be discontinued immediately in patients developing constipation or symptoms of ischemic colitis; therapy should not be resumed in patients developing ischemic colitis. Pattern of daily bowel activity and stool consistency should be monitored. Adequate hydration should be maintained.

Only physicians enrolled in the manufacturer's prescribing program may prescribe alosetron. Program stickers must be affixed to all prescriptions. A Med Guide must be distributed with alosetron each time an outpatient prescription or refill is dispensed.

Storage
Store at room temperature.
Protect from light and moisture.

Administration
Take alosetron without regard to food. Therapy should be discontinued in patients without an adequate response after 4 wks of treatment at a dose of 1 mg twice daily.

Alprazolam
al-pray'zoe-lam
(Apo-Alpraz [CAN], Kalma [AUS], Novo-Alprazol [CAN], Xanax, Xanax XR)

Do not confuse alprazolam with lorazepam, or Xanax with Tenex or Zantac.

CATEGORY AND SCHEDULE
Pregnancy Risk Category: D
Controlled Substance: Schedule IV

Classification: Anxiolytics, benzodiazepines, sedatives/hypnotics

MECHANISM OF ACTION
A benzodiazepine that enhances the action of the inhibitory neurotransmitter γ-aminobutyric acid in the brain. *Therapeutic Effect:* Produces anxiolytic effect from its CNS depressant action.

PHARMACOKINETICS
Well absorbed from GI tract. Protein binding: 80%. Metabolized in the liver primarily by CYP3A4. Primarily excreted in urine. Minimal removal by hemodialysis. *Half-life:* 11-16 h.

AVAILABILITY
Oral Solution: 1 mg/mL.
Tablets: 0.25 mg, 0.5 mg, 1 mg, 2 mg.
Tablets (Extended-Release): 0.5 mg, 1 mg, 2 mg, 3 mg.
Tablets (Orally Disintegrating): 0.25 mg, 0.5 mg, 1 mg, 2 mg.

INDICATIONS AND DOSAGES
▸ **Anxiety disorders**
PO
Adults (immediate release). Initially, 0.25-0.5 mg 3 times a day. May titrate q3-4 days. Maximum: 4 mg/day in divided doses.
Elderly, Debilitated Patients. Patients with hepatic disease or low serum albumin. Initially, 0.25 mg 2-3 times a day. Gradually increase to optimum therapeutic response.
PO (ORALLY DISINTEGRATING)
Adults. 0.25-0.5 mg 3 times a day. Maximum: 4 mg/day in divided doses.
▸ **Anxiety with depression**
PO
Adults. 2.5-3 mg/day in divided doses.
▸ **Panic disorder**
PO, IMMEDIATE RELEASE
Adults. Initially, 0.5 mg 3 times a day. May increase at 3- to 4-day intervals. Range: 5-6 mg/day.
Elderly. Initially, 0.125-0.25 mg 2 times a day; may increase in 0.125-mg increments until desired effect attained.
PO, EXTENDED RELEASE
Alert to switch from immediate-release to extended-release form, give total daily dose (immediate release) as a single daily dose of extended-release form.

Adults. Initially, 0.5-1 mg once a day. May titrate at 3- to 4-day intervals. Range: 3-6 mg/day.
Elderly. Initially, 0.5 mg once a day.
PO, ORALLY DISINTEGRATING
Adults. Initially, 0.5 mg 3 times a day. May increase at 3- to 4-day intervals. Range: 5-6 mg/day.

CONTRAINDICATIONS

Acute alcohol intoxication with depressed vital signs, acute angle-closure glaucoma, concurrent use of itraconazole or ketoconazole, myasthenia gravis, severe COPD.

INTERACTIONS

Drug
Alcohol, other CNS depressants: Potentiate effects of alprazolam and may increase sedation.
CYP3A4 inhibitors, cimetidine, erythromycin, fluvoxamine, nefazodone, oral contraceptives, propoxyphene: May inhibit metabolism and increase serum concentrations of alprazolam; use with caution.
CYP3A4 inducers, carbamazepine: May induce metabolism and decrease serum concentration of alprazolam.
Itraconazole, ketoconazole: Increase alprazolam serum concentration; contraindicated.
Herbal
Gotu kola, kava kava, valerian: May increase CNS depressant effect of alprazolam.
St. John's wort: Increases alprazolam clearance; decreases alprazolam half-life from 12 h to 6 h.
Food
Grapefruit, grapefruit juice: May inhibit alprazolam's metabolism.
High-fat meal: May alter the rate, but not extent, of absorption.

DIAGNOSTIC TEST EFFECTS

None known.

SIDE EFFECTS

Frequent (> 10%)
Ataxia; lightheadedness; somnolence; depression, headache, memory impairment, dry mouth, slurred speech (particularly in elderly or debilitated patients), constipation, diarrhea.
Occasional
Confusion, blurred vision, confusion, hypotension, nausea.
Rare
Behavioral problems such as anger, impaired memory, paradoxical reactions such as insomnia, nervousness, or irritability.

SERIOUS REACTIONS

• Abrupt or too rapid withdrawal may result in pronounced restlessness, irritability, insomnia, hand tremors, abdominal and muscle cramps, diaphoresis, vomiting, and seizures.
• Overdose results in somnolence, confusion, diminished reflexes, and coma.
• Blood dyscrasias have been reported rarely.

PRECAUTIONS & CONSIDERATIONS

Caution is warranted with impaired renal or hepatic function. Dizziness and drowsiness may occur. Change positions slowly from recumbent, to sitting, before standing to prevent dizziness. Alcohol, tasks that require mental alertness or motor skills, and smoking should also be avoided. Women on long-term therapy should use effective contraception during therapy and notify the physician immediately if they become or may be pregnant. Breastfeeding is not recommended.
Storage
Store at room temperature. Keep tightly closed.

Administration

Take alprazolam without regard to food. Crush tablets as needed. Mix concentrated oral solution with liquids or semisolid foods (e.g., water, juice, soda or soda-like beverages, applesauce, pudding). Use the calibrated dropper to measure doses. Handle orally disintegrating tablets with dry hands. If only half an orally disintegrating tablet is used, the other half should be discarded because it might not remain stable.

Take extended-release once a day; swallow tablets whole and do not break, chew, or crush tablets.

Alprostadil

al-pros´ta-dil
(Caverject, Caverject Impulse, Edex, Muse, Prostin VR Pediatric)

CATEGORY AND SCHEDULE

Pregnancy Risk Category: X/C

Classification: Naturally occurring prostaglandin (E1, PGE1)

MECHANISM OF ACTION

A prostaglandin that directly affects vascular and ductus arteriosus smooth muscle and relaxes trabecular smooth muscle. *Therapeutic Effect:* Causes vasodilation; dilates cavernosal arteries, allowing blood flow to and entrapment in the lacunar spaces of the penis.

PHARMACOKINETICS

Rapidly metabolized and cleared from the body by urinary excretion. *Half-life:* 5-10 min.

AVAILABILITY

Injection (Prostin VR Pediatric): 500 mcg/mL.
Injection, Aqueous (Caverject): 10 mcg/mL, 20 mcg/mL, 40 mcg/mL.
Powder for Injection (Caverject, Edex): 5 mcg, 10 mcg, 20 mcg, 40 mcg.
Powder for Injection (Caverject Impulse): 10 mcg, 20 mcg.
Urethral Pellet (Muse): 125 mcg, 250 mcg, 500 mcg, 1000 mcg.

INDICATIONS AND DOSAGES
▸ **Maintain patency of ductus arteriosus**
IV INFUSION
Neonates. Initially, 0.05-0.1 mcg/kg/min. Maintenance: 0.01-0.4 mcg/kg/min. Use lowest possible dose that maintains response. Maximum: 0.4 mcg/kg/min.
▸ **Impotence**
PELLET (MUSE)
Adult. Initial dose 125-250 mcg, maintenance dose individualized. Maximum: 2 systems per 24 h.
INTRACAVERNOSAL (CAVERJECT)
Adults. Dosage is individualized. Initial dose titrated in physician's office.

CONTRAINDICATIONS

Conditions predisposing to priapism (sickle cell anemia, multiple myeloma, leukemia); anatomic deformation of penis, penile implants, hyaline membrane disease, neonatal respiratory distress syndrome.

INTERACTIONS

Drug
Anticoagulants, including heparin, thrombolytics: May increase the risk of bleeding.
Sympathomimetics: May decrease the effect of alprostadil.
Vasodilators: May increase risk of hypotension.
Herbal
None known.
Food
None known.

DIAGNOSTIC TEST EFFECTS

May increase blood bilirubin levels. May decrease glucose, serum calcium, and serum potassium levels.

⚗ IV INCOMPATIBILITIES

Do not mix with any other drugs.

SIDE EFFECTS

Frequent

Intracavernosal (1%-4%): Penile pain (37%), prolonged erection, hypertension, localized pain, penile fibrosis, injection site hematoma or ecchymosis, headache, respiratory infection, flu-like symptoms.

Intraurethral (3%): Penile pain (36%), urethral pain or burning, testicular pain, urethral bleeding, headache, dizziness, respiratory infection, flulike symptoms.

Systemic (> 1%): Fever, seizures, flushing, bradycardia, hypotension, tachycardia, apnea, diarrhea, sepsis.

Occasional

Intracavernosal (< 1%): Hypotension, pelvic pain, back pain, dizziness, cough, nasal congestion.

Intraurethral (< 3%): Fainting, sinusitis, back and pelvic pain.

Systemic (< 1%): Anxiety, lethargy, myalgia, arrhythmias, respiratory depression, anemia, bleeding, thrombocytopenia, hematuria.

SERIOUS REACTIONS

• Systemic overdose is manifested as apnea, flushing of the face and arms, and bradycardia.

• Cardiac arrest and sepsis occur rarely.

PRECAUTIONS & CONSIDERATIONS

Caution is warranted with coagulation defects, polycythemia, severe hepatic disease, and thrombocythemia. Be aware that erection should occur within 2-5 min of administration. Notify the physician if erection lasts for longer than 4 h or becomes painful. Alprostadil should not be used if sexual partner is pregnant unless a condom barrier is being used.

Use with caution in neonates with bleeding tendencies. Arterial pressure by auscultation, Doppler transducer, or umbilical artery catheter should be monitored with ductus arteriosus. Infusion rate should be decreased immediately if a significant decrease in arterial pressure occurs. Continuous cardiac monitoring should be performed. Heart sounds, femoral pulse (to monitor lower extremity circulation), and respiratory status should be assessed. In addition, signs and symptoms of hypotension should be monitored and BP, ABG values, and temperature should be assessed. Apnea usually appears during the first hour of infusion. If apnea or bradycardia occurs, infusion should be discontinued immediately and the physician should be notified.

Storage

Store aqueous injection (Caverject) in the freezer until dispensed; once dispensed store in freezer up to 3 mo. May be kept in refrigerator for up to 7 days; once refrigerated, it must be used within 7 days or discarded; do not refreeze. Once the ampule is removed from the foil wrapper, it must be used immediately after allowing to warm to room temperature or discarded. Open ampules of alprostadil injection must be used immediately. Alprostadil lyophilized powder (Caverject) should be stored in a refrigerator until dispensed. Once dispensed it can be stored at room temperature for up to 3 mo. Reconstitued solution should be used within 24 h when stored at room temperature. Do not refrigerate or freeze reconstituted solution. Alprostadil dual-chamber system (Caverject Impulse) and cartridges (Edex) should be stored at room temperature. Refrigerate Muse pellet unless used within 14 days. Store the pediatric parenteral form in refrigerator. Dilute drug before administration. Prepare fresh dose every 24 h and discard unused portions.

Administration
! Doses > 40 mcg (Edex) or 60 mcg (Caverject) are not recommended.
! *Pediatric injection:* Give by continuous IV infusion or through umbilical artery catheter placed at ductal opening. Prepare continuous IV infusion by diluting 1 mL of alprostadil containing 500 mcg, with D5W or 0.9% NaCl to yield a solution containing 2-20 mcg/mL. Diluting volumes can range from 25 to 250 mL, depending on the patient and the available infusion device. Infuse the lowest possible dose over the shortest possible time. Decrease the infusion rate immediately if a significant decrease in arterial pressure is noted via auscultation, Doppler transducer, or umbilical artery catheter. Discontinue the infusion immediately if signs and symptoms of overdose, such as apnea and bradycardia, occur.

Alteplase
al'-te-plase
(Actilyse, Activase [AUS], Activase Cathflo)
Do not confuse alteplase or Activase with Altace.

CATEGORY AND SCHEDULE
Pregnancy Risk Category: C

Classification: Thrombolytics, tissue plasminogen activator

MECHANISM OF ACTION
A tissue plasminogen activator that acts as a thrombolytic by binding to the fibrin in a thrombus and converting entrapped plasminogen to plasmin. This process initiates fibrinolysis. *Therapeutic Effect:* Degrades fibrin clots, fibrinogen, and other plasma proteins.

PHARMACOKINETICS
Rapidly metabolized in the liver. Primarily excreted in urine. Approximately 80% present in plasma cleared within 10 min.

AVAILABILITY
Powder for Injection (Activase Cathflo): 2 mg.
Powder for Injection (Activase): 50 mg, 100 mg.

INDICATIONS AND DOSAGES
▸ **Acute MI**
IV INFUSION
Adults weighing > 67 kg. 100 mg over 90 min, starting with 15-mg bolus over 1-2 min, then 50 mg over 30 min, then 35 mg over 60 min. Or a 3-h infusion, giving 60 mg over first h (6-10 mg as bolus over 1-2 min), 20 mg over second hour, and 20 mg over third hour.
Adults weighing 67 kg or less. 100 mg over 90 min, starting with

15-mg bolus, then 0.75 mg/kg over 30 min (maximum: 50 mg), then 0.5 mg/kg over 60 min (maximum: 35 mg). Or 3-h infusion of 1.25 mg/kg giving 60% of dose over first hour (6%-10% as 1- to 2-min bolus), 20% over second hour, and 20% over third hour.

▸ **Acute pulmonary emboli**
IV INFUSION
Adults. 100 mg over 2 h. Institute or reinstitute heparin near end or immediately after infusion when aPTT or thrombin time (TT) returns to twice normal or less.

▸ **Acute ischemic stroke**
IV INFUSION
Adults. 0.9 mg/kg over 60 min (10% total dose as initial IV bolus over 1 min).

▸ **Central venous catheter clearance**
IV
Adults, Elderly, Children (weighing 30 kg or more). 2 mg; may repeat after 2 h if catheter function not restored.
Children weighing 10 kg - 30 kg. Instill 110% of the internal lumen volume of the catheter, not to exceed 2 mg in 2 mL. May repeat after 2 h if catheter function is not restored.

OFF-LABEL USES
Coronary thrombolysis, to decrease ischemic events in unstable angina.

CONTRAINDICATIONS
Active internal bleeding, AV malformation or aneurysm, bleeding diathesis, intracranial neoplasm, intracranial or intraspinal surgery or trauma, recent (within past 2 mo) cerebrovascular accident, severe uncontrolled hypertension; additional contraindication in acute stroke includes evidence of intracranial hemorrhage on pretreatment evaluation, suspicion of subarachnoid hemorrhage, history of intracranial hemorrhage, seizure at onset of stroke.

INTERACTIONS
Drug
Anticoagulants, including cefotetan, heparin, plicamycin, valproic acid: May increase risk of hemorrhage.
Nitroglycerin: May decrease alteplase concentrations, thereby reducing alteplase effect.
Platelet aggregation inhibitors, including aspirin, NSAIDs, ticlopidine: May increase the risk of bleeding.
Herbal
Cat's claw, dong quai, evening primrose, feverfew, red clover, horse chestnut, garlic, green tea, ginseng, ginkgo: Can have antiplatelet activity, may increase risk of bleeding.
Food
None known.

DIAGNOSTIC TEST EFFECTS
Decreases plasminogen and fibrinogen levels during infusion, which decreases clotting time (and confirms the presence of lysis). Decreases hemoglobin and hematocrit levels.

⊘ IV INCOMPATIBILITIES
Do not add other medications to the container of alteplase solution or administer other medications through the same IV line. Incompatible with dobutamine, dopamine, heparin, nitroglycerin.

⊜ IV COMPATIBILITIES
Lidocaine, metoprolol (Lopressor), morphine, propranolol (Inderal).

SIDE EFFECTS
Frequent
Superficial bleeding at puncture sites, decreased BP.
Occasional
Allergic reaction, such as rash or wheezing; bruising.

SERIOUS REACTIONS
• Severe internal hemorrhage may occur.
• Lysis of coronary thrombi may produce atrial or ventricular arrhythmias or stroke.

PRECAUTIONS & CONSIDERATIONS
Caution is warranted with recent (within past 10 days) major surgery or GI bleeding, organ biopsy, trauma, cerebrovascular disease, cardiopulmonary resuscitation, diabetic retinopathy, endocarditis, left heart thrombus, occluded AV cannula at infected site, severe hepatic or renal disease, thrombophlebitis, in elderly patients, and in pregnant women or within the first 10 postpartum days. Alteplase is used only when the benefit to the mother outweighs the risk to a fetus. Also, it is unknown whether alteplase crosses the placenta or is distributed in breast milk. Safety and efficacy have not been established in children (Activase) or in children < 2 yr or weighing < 10 kg (Activase Cathflo). In elderly patients, there is an increased risk of bleeding. Patients must be carefully selected and monitored. An electric razor and a soft toothbrush should be used to reduce the risk of bleeding.

Immediately report signs of bleeding, such as oozing from cuts or gums. Serum creatine kinase (CK), CK-MB concentrations, 12-lead ECG, electrolyte levels, hematocrit, platelet count, TT, aPTT, PT, and fibrinogen levels should be evaluated before therapy starts. BP and pulse and respiration rates should be checked every 15 min until stable; then check hourly. Continuous cardiac monitoring should be performed.

Storage
Store 50-mg and 100-mg vials at room temperature or in refrigerator. Solution is stable for 8 h after reconstitution. Discard unused portion. Store 2-mg vials in refrigerator.

Administration
Reconstitute immediately before use with sterile water for injection. Reconstitute 100-mg vial with 100 mL sterile water for injection (50-mg vial with 50 mL sterile water for injection) without preservative to provide a concentration of 1 mg/mL. May dilute further with equal volume of D5W or 0.9% NaCl to provide a concentration of 0.5 mg/mL. Gently swirl or slowly invert vial; avoid excessive agitation. After reconstitution, solution normally appears colorless to pale yellow. Give by IV infusion via infusion pump. (See individual dosages above.) If minor bleeding occurs at puncture site, apply pressure for 30 s; if unrelieved, apply a pressure dressing. If uncontrolled hemorrhage occurs, discontinue the infusion immediately. Slowing the rate of infusion may worsen the hemorrhage. Avoid undue pressure when injecting the drug into the catheter because the catheter can rupture or expel a clot into circulation.

Aluminum Chloride Hexahydrate
a-loo′mi-num klor′ide heks-a-hye′drate
(Drysol, Xerac AC)
(powder, solution)

CATEGORY AND SCHEDULE
Pregnancy Risk Category: C

Classification:
Antiperspirants

MECHANISM OF ACTION

Aluminum salts cause an obstruction of the distal sweat gland. This obstruction causes metal ions to precipitate with mucopolysaccharides, damaging epithelial cells along the lumen of the duct and forming a plug to block sweat output. *Therapeutic Effect:* Results in decreased secretion of the sweat glands.

PHARMACOKINETICS

Not known.

AVAILABILITY

Topical Solution: 6.25% (Xerac AC), 12% (Certain Dri), 20% (Drysol, Hypercare).

INDICATIONS AND DOSAGES

▶ **Antiperspirant**
TOPICAL
Adults, Elderly, Children 12 yr and older. Apply to each underarm once a day at bedtime.
▶ **Hyperhidrosis**
TOPICAL
Adults, Elderly, Children 12 yr and older. Apply to affected areas once a day, at bedtime.

CONTRAINDICATIONS

Hypersensitivity to aluminum chloride or any one of its components.

INTERACTIONS

Drug
None known.
Herbal
None known.
Food
None known.

DIAGNOSTIC TEST EFFECTS

None known.

🜨 IV INCOMPATIBILITIES

None known.

🜨 IV COMPATIBILITIES

None known.

SIDE EFFECTS

Frequent
Itching, burning, tingling sensation.
Occasional
Rash.

SERIOUS REACTIONS

• Hypersensitivity reaction, such as rash, may occur.

PRECAUTIONS & CONSIDERATIONS

It is unknown whether aluminum chloride hexahydrate crosses the placenta or is distributed in breast milk. Deodorants or antiperspirants should be avoided during treatment. It may be harmful to cotton fibers and certain metals.

Skin may become irritated during use. Aluminum chloride hexahydrate should not be applied to broken, irritated, or recently shaved skin.

Administration
Aluminum chloride hexahydrate is for external use only. It should be applied to dry skin. The treated area should be covered with a sheet of plastic wrap held in place with a snug t-shirt to avoid aluminum chloride hexahydrate rubbing off at night. The next morning, discard the plastic wrap if used and wash the skin with a mild soap. Excessive sweating may be stopped after 2 or more treatments; thereafter, apply 1-2 times/wk or as needed.

Aluminum Hydroxide

a-loo'mi-num hye-drox'ide
(Alternagel, Alu-Tab, Amphojel
[CAN], Basaljel [CAN])

CATEGORY AND SCHEDULE

Pregnancy Risk Category: C
(Considered safe except for
chronic, high-dose use).
OTC

Classification: Gastrointestinals,
vitamins/minerals

MECHANISM OF ACTION

An antacid that reduces gastric
acid by binding with phosphate in
the intestine and is then excreted
as aluminum carbonate in feces;
decreased serum phosphate levels
may result in increased absorption
of calcium. The drug also has
astringent and adsorbent properties.
Therapeutic Effect: Neutralizes
or increases gastric pH; reduces
phosphate levels in urine, preventing
formation of phosphate urinary
calculi; reduces the serum phosphate
level; decreases the fluidity of
stools.

AVAILABILITY

Capsules: 400 mg (Alu-Cap),
500 mg (Dialume).
Liquid: 600 mg/5 mg (ALternagel).
Suspension: 320 mg/5 mL
(Amphojel), 450 mg/5 mL,
675 mg/5 mL.
Tablets: 300 mg (Amphojel),
500 mg (Alu-Tab), 600 mg (Amphojel).

INDICATIONS AND DOSAGES
▸ Antacid
PO
Adults, Elderly. 500-1500 mg 3-6
times daily, between meals and at
bedtime.

▸ Hyperphosphatemia
PO
Adults, Elderly. Initially, 300-600 mg
3 times a day with meals.
Children. 50-150 mg/kg/day in
divided doses q4-6h.

CONTRAINDICATIONS

Children age 6 yr or younger,
intestinal obstruction.

INTERACTIONS

Drug
**Bisphosphonates, iron preparations,
isoniazid, ketoconazole, phenytoin,
quinolones, tetracyclines,
alumimun hydroxide:** May decrease
absorption of this drug.
Methenamine: May decrease effects
of the methenamine.
Salicylate: May increase salicylate
excretion.
Herbal
None known.
Food
None known.

DIAGNOSTIC TEST EFFECTS

May increase the serum gastrin
level and systemic and urinary pH.
May decrease the serum phosphate
level.

SIDE EFFECTS

Frequent
Chalky taste, mild constipation,
abdominal cramps.
Occasional
Nausea, vomiting, speckling
or whitish discoloration of
stools.

SERIOUS REACTIONS

• Prolonged constipation may result
in intestinal obstruction.
• Excessive or chronic use may
produce hypophosphatemia
manifested as anorexia, malaise,
muscle weakness, or bone pain,

which may result in osteomalacia and osteoporosis.
• Prolonged use may produce urinary calculi.

PRECAUTIONS & CONSIDERATIONS
Caution is warranted with Alzheimer disease, chronic diarrhea, cirrhosis, constipation, dehydration, edema, fecal impaction, fluid restrictions, gastric outlet obstruction, GI or rectal bleeding, heart failure, impaired renal function, low sodium diets, symptoms of appendicitis, and in elderly patients. Aluminum hydroxide is contraindicated for children 6 yr or younger. Elderly patients may be at increased risk of constipation and fecal impaction.

Stool discoloration may occur but will resolve when the drug is discontinued. Adequate hydration should be maintained. Pattern of daily bowel activity and stool consistency and serum aluminum, calcium, phosphate, and uric acid levels should be monitored.
Administration
Take aluminum hydroxide 1-3 h after meals and at bedtime when used as an antacid. Expect the dosage to be individualized based on the antacid's neutralizing capacity. Thoroughly chew chewable tablets (combination forms) before swallowing, and then drink a glass of water or milk. Shake the suspension well before use. Do not take other oral drugs within 1-2 h of antacid administration.

Aluminum Salts
a-loo´mi-num
Aluminum acetate and acetic acid (Otic Domeboro); aluminum hydroxide and magnesium carbonate (Gaviscon Extra Strength, Gaviscon Liquid); aluminum hydroxide and magnesium hydroxide (Diovol [CAN], Diovol EX [CAN], Gelusil [CAN], Gelusil Extra Strength [CAN], Maalox, Maalox TC, Mylanta [CAN], Univol [CAN]); aluminum hydroxide and magnesium trisillicate (Gaviscon); aluminum hydroxide, magnesium hydroxide, and simethicone (Diovol Plus [CAN], Maalox Fast Release Liquid, Maalox Max, Mylanta Double Strength [CAN], Mylanta Extra Strength [CAN], Mylanta Extra Strength Liquid, Mylanta Liquid, Mylanta Regular Strength [CAN]); aluminum sulfate and calcium acetate (Bluboro, Domeboro, Pedi-Boro)

CATEGORY AND SCHEDULE
Pregnancy Risk Category: C

Classification: Antacid

MECHANISM OF ACTION
An antacid that reduces gastric acid by binding with phosphate in the intestine and then is excreted as aluminum carbonate in feces. Aluminum carbonate may increase the absorption of calcium because of decreased serum phosphate levels. The drug also has astringent and adsorbent properties. *Therapeutic Effect:* Neutralizes or increases gastric pH; reduces phosphates in urine, preventing formation of

phosphate urinary stones; reduces serum phosphate levels; decreases fluidity of stools.

PHARMACOKINETICS
Varies in each formulation.

AVAILABILITY
Aluminum Acetate and Acetic Acid
(Otic Domeboro)
Otic Solution: 2% acetic acid and aluminum acetate (Otic Domeboro).
Aluminum Hydroxide and Magnesium Carbonate
Liquid: 31.7 mg aluminum hydroxide and 119.3 mg magnesium carbonate/5 mL (Gaviscon Liquid), 84.6 mg aluminum hydroxide and 79.1 mg magnesium carbonate/5 mL (Gaviscon Extra Strength).
Tablets, Chewable: 160 mg aluminum hydroxide and 1.5 mg magnesium carbonate (Gaviscon Extra Strength Relief).
Aluminum Hydroxide and Magnesium Hydroxide
Suspension: 225 mg aluminum hydroxide and 200 mg magnesium hydroxide/5 mL (Maalox).
Suspension: 600 mg aluminum hydroxide and 300 mg magnesium hydroxide/5 mL (Maalox TC).
Aluminum Hydroxide and Magnesium Trisilicate
Tablets, Chewable: 80 mg aluminum hydroxide and 20 mg magnesium hydroxide (Gaviscon).
Aluminum Hydroxide, Magnesium Hydroxide, and Simethicone
Liquid: 200 mg aluminum hydroxide, 200 mg magnesium hydroxide, and 20 mg simethicone/5 mL (Mylanta), 400 mg aluminum hydroxide, 400 mg magnesium hydroxide, and 40 mg simethicone/5 mL (Maalox Max), 500 mg aluminum hydroxide, 450 mg magnesium hydroxide, and 20 mg simethicone/5 mL (Maalox Fast Release), 400 mg aluminum hydroxide, 400 mg magnesium hydroxide, and 40 mg simethicone/5 mL (Mylanta Extra Strength).
Aluminum Sulfate and Calcium Acetate
Powder, for Topical Solution: packets (Bluboro, Domeboro, Pedi-Boro).
Tablets, Effervescent, for Topical Solution: Effervescent tablets (Domeboro).

INDICATIONS AND DOSAGES
Aluminum Acetate and Acetic Acid
▸ **Superficial infections of the external auditory canal**
OTIC
Adults, Elderly. Instill 4-6 drops in ear(s) q2-3h.
Aluminum Hydroxide and Magnesium Carbonate
▸ **Antacid**
PO
Adults, Elderly. 15-30 mL 4 times/day of the liquid; chew 2-4 tablets 4 times/day.
Aluminum Hydroxide and Magnesium Hydroxide
▸ **Antacid**
PO
Adults, Elderly. 5-10 mL 4-6 times/day.
Aluminum Hydroxide and Magnesium Trisilicate

▸**Antacid**
PO
Adults, Elderly. Chew 2-4 tablets
4 times/day or as directed.
**Aluminum Hydroxide, Magnesium
Hydroxide, and Simethicone**
▸**Antacid (with flatulence)**
PO
Adults, Elderly. 10-20 mL or
2-4 tablets 4-6 times/day.
**Aluminum Sulfate and Calcium
Acetate**
▸**Inflammatory skin conditions with
weeping that occurs in dermatitis**
TOPICAL
Adults, Elderly. Soak affected
area in solution 2-4 times/day
for 15-30 min or apply wet
dressing soaked in solution 2-4
times/day for 30-min treatment
periods. Domeboro: Saturate
dressing and apply to affected
area and saturate every 15-30
min; or soak for 15-30 min
3 times/day.

CONTRAINDICATIONS
Children age 6 yr or younger,
intestinal obstruction,
hypersensitivity to aluminum
or any component of the
formulation.

INTERACTIONS
Drug
**Bisphosphonates, iron
preparations, isoniazid,
ketoconazole, phenytoin,
quinolones, tetracyclines,
aluminum hydroxide:** May
decrease absorption.
Methenamine: May decrease effects
of methenamine.
Salicylate: May increase salicylate
excretion.
Herbal
None known.

Food
None known.

DIAGNOSTIC TEST EFFECTS
May increase serum gastrin levels
and systemic and urinary pH.
May decrease serum phosphate
levels.

SIDE EFFECTS
Frequent
PO: Chalky taste, mild constipation,
stomach cramps, diarrhea.
Topical: Burning, itching.
Occasional
PO: Nausea, vomiting, speckling
or whitish discoloration of
stools
Otic: Burning or stinging in
ear.
Topical: New or continued redness,
skin dryness.
Rare
PO: Hypermagnesemia,
hypophosphatemia, osteomalacia.
Otic: Skin rash, redness, swelling, or
pain in the ear.

SERIOUS REACTIONS
• Prolonged constipation may result
in intestinal obstruction.
• Excessive or chronic use may
produce hypophosphatemia
manifested as anorexia, malaise,
muscle weakness, or bone pain and
resulting in osteomalacia and
osteoporosis.
• Prolonged use may produce urinary
calculi.

PRECAUTIONS & CONSIDERATIONS
Caution is warranted with Alzheimer
disease, chronic diarrhea, cirrhosis,
constipation, dehydration, edema,
fecal impaction, fluid restrictions,
gastric outlet obstruction, GI or
rectal bleeding, heart failure,

impaired renal function, low sodium diets, symptoms of appendicitis, and in elderly patients. Aluminum hydroxide is contraindicated for children 6 yr or younger. Elderly patients may be at increased risk of constipation and fecal impaction.

Administration

Administer 1-3 h after meals when used as an antacid. Expect the dosage to be individualized based on the neutralizing capacity of the antacid.

For chewable tablets, thoroughly chew tablets before swallowing and then drink a glass of water or milk.

If administering a suspension, shake well before use.

For otic solution, insert saturated wick and keep moist for 24 h.

For topical preparation, rewet dressings with solution every few minutes to keep it moist. Do not cover with plastic.

Amantadine Hydrochloride

a-man′ta-deen hi-droh-klor′ide
(Endantadine [CAN], PMS-Amantadine [CAN], Symmetrel)

CATEGORY AND SCHEDULE
Pregnancy Risk Category: C

Classification: Antiparkinson agents, antivirals

MECHANISM OF ACTION
A dopaminergic agonist that blocks the uncoating of influenza A virus, preventing penetration into the host and inhibiting M2 protein in the assembly of progeny virions. Amantadine also blocks the reuptake of dopamine into presynaptic neurons and causes direct stimulation of postsynaptic receptors. *Therapeutic Effect:* Antiviral and antiparkinsonian activity.

PHARMACOKINETICS
Rapidly and completely absorbed from the GI tract. Protein binding: 67%. Widely distributed. Primarily excreted in urine. Minimally removed by hemodialysis. *Half-life:* 16 h (increased in the elderly and in impaired renal function).

AVAILABILITY
Capsule: 100 mg.
Syrup: 50 mg/5 mL.
Tablets: 100 mg.

INDICATIONS AND DOSAGES
▸ **Prevention and symptomatic treatment of respiratory illness due to influenza A virus**
ALERT! Due to increased resistance, the CDC recommends that amantadine no longer be used for treatment or prophylaxis of

influenza A in the United States until susceptibility is re-established.

PO

Adults older than 64 yr. 100 mg/day.
Adults and children 13-64 yr.
200 mg/day or 100 mg twice a day.
Children 10-12 yr. 5 mg/kg/day up to 200 mg/day in two divided doses.
Children 1-9 yr. 5 mg/kg/day in two divided doses (up to 150 mg/day).

▸ **Parkinson's disease, extrapyramidal symptoms**

PO

Adults, Elderly. 100 mg twice a day.
May increase up to 300 mg/day in divided doses.

▸ **Dosage in renal impairment**

Dose and frequency are modified based on creatinine clearance.

Creatinine Clearance (mL/min)	Dosage
30-50	200 mg first day; 100 mg/day thereafter
15-29	200 mg first day; 100 mg on alternate days
< 15	200 mg every 7 days

CONTRAINDICATIONS

Hypersensitivity to amantadine, rimantadine, or any product ingredients.

INTERACTIONS

Drug

Alcohol: May increase CNS effects, including dizziness, confusion, light-headedness, and orthostatic hypotension.
Anticholinergics, antihistamines, phenothiazine, tricyclic antidepressants: May increase anticholinergic effects of amantadine.
Hydrochlorothiazide, triamterene: May increase amantadine blood concentration and risk for toxicity.

Live attenuated influenza vaccine: Avoid use of vaccine within 2 wks before or 48 h after amantadine; may reduce vaccine response.
Herbal
None known.
Food
None known.

DIAGNOSTIC TEST EFFECTS

None known.

SIDE EFFECTS

Frequent (5%-10%)
Nausea, dizziness, poor concentration, insomnia, nervousness.
Occasional (1%-5%)
Orthostatic hypotension, anorexia, headache, livedo reticularis (reddish blue, netlike blotching of skin), blurred vision, urine retention, dry mouth or nose, depression, anxiety and irritability, hallucinations, somnolence, abnormal dreams, agitation.
Rare
Vomiting, irritation or swelling of eyes, rash, visual disturbances.

SERIOUS REACTIONS

• CHF, leukopenia, and neutropenia occur rarely.
• Hyperexcitability, seizures, and ventricular arrhythmias may occur.
• Neuroleptic malignant syndrome has occurred upon rapid dose reduction or withdrawal.
• Suicide, suicidal ideation or attempt.

PRECAUTIONS & CONSIDERATIONS

Caution is warranted with cerebrovascular disease, CHF, history of seizures, liver disease, orthostatic hypotension, peripheral edema, psychosis, recurrent eczematoid dermatitis, renal dysfunction, and those receiving CNS stimulants. Avoid use in patients with untreated angle-closure glaucoma. There have been reports of suicidal ideation and suicide attempts in patients with and without a history of psychiatric illness. May exacerbate psychiatric symptoms in patients with a history of psychiatric illness. Teratogenic effects observed in animal studies and impaired fertility observed in animal studies and humans. It is distributed into breast milk; use is not recommended in breastfeeding. There are no safety or efficacy data in children < 1 yr of age. Elderly patients may exhibit increased sensitivity to amantadine's anticholinergic effects. In elderly patients, age-related decreased renal function may require dosage adjustment. Avoid alcohol and taking any medications, including over-the-counter (OTC) drugs without first consulting the physician.

Skin should be monitored for peripheral edema, blotching, or rash, Dizziness should be monitored. Food tolerance and episodes of nausea and vomiting should be evaluated. If new symptoms, especially blurred vision, dizziness, nausea or vomiting, and skin blotching or rash occurs, notify the physician. Get up slowly from a sitting or lying position. Do not drive, use machinery, or engage in other activities that require mental acuity if dizziness or blurred vision occurs.

Administration
! Give as a single or in 2 divided doses. Use of 2 divided doses may reduce CNS side effects. May take without regard to food. Administer nighttime dose several hours before bedtime to prevent insomnia. Continue therapy for the full length of treatment and evenly space drug doses around the clock.

Ambenonium
am-be-noe´nee-um
(Mytelase)

CATEGORY AND SCHEDULE
Pregnancy Risk Category: C

Classification: Cholinesterase inhibitors

MECHANISM OF ACTION
A cholinesterase inhibitor that enhances and prolongs cholinergic function by increasing the concentration of acetylcholine through inhibition of the hydrolysis of acetylcholine. *Therapeutic Effect:* Increases muscle strength in myasthenia gravis.

PHARMACOKINETICS
Poorly absorbed after PO administration. Onset of action observed within 20-30 min.

AVAILABILITY
Tablets: 10 mg (Mytelase).

INDICATIONS AND DOSAGES
▸ **Myasthenia gravis**
PO
Adults. 5-25 mg 3 or 4 times a day. If well tolerated, after 1 or 2 days, may increase to 50-75 mg 3 times a day if needed. Maximum: 5-200 mg/day in divided doses.

CONTRAINDICATIONS
Not recommended in patients receiving routine administration of atropine or other belladonna derivatives. Not recommended in patients receiving mecamylamine.

INTERACTIONS
Drug
Atropine: Suppresses GI side effects; may mask the

symptoms of ambenonium overdose.
Herbal
None known.
Food
None known.

DIAGNOSTIC TEST EFFECTS
None known.

SIDE EFFECTS
Frequent
Abdominal pain, diarrhea, increased salivation, miosis, sweating, and vomiting.
Occasional
Anxiety, blurred vision, and urinary urgency.
Rare
Trembling, difficulty moving or controlling movement of the tongue, neck, or arms.

SERIOUS REACTIONS
• Overdosage may result in cholinergic crisis, characterized by severe nausea, vomiting, diarrhea, increased salivation, diaphoresis, bradycardia, hypotension, flushed skin, stomach pain, respiratory depression, seizures, and paralysis of muscles.
• Increasing muscle weakness of myasthenia gravis may occur. Antidote: 0.5-1 IV atropine sulfate with other supportive treatment.

PRECAUTIONS & CONSIDERATIONS
Caution is warranted in patients with asthma, bladder outflow obstruction, bradycardia, COPD, recent coronary occlusion, vagotonia, hyperthyroidism, cardiac arrhythmias, Parkinson disease, and a history of peptic ulcer disease. It is unknown whether ambenonium crosses the placenta or is excreted in breast milk. Safety and efficacy of ambenonium have not been established in children.

Anticholinergic insensitivity may develop; reduce or withhold ambenonium until the patient becomes sensitive again. Cholinergic reaction, such as diaphoresis, dizziness, excessive salivation, feeling of facial warmth, GI cramping or discomfort, lacrimation, pallor, trembling or difficulty moving or controlling movement of the tongue, neck, or arms, and urinary urgency should be reported.
Administration
Ambenonium should be given after food in divided doses at the same times each day.

Ambrisentan
am-bri-sen´tan
(Letairis)

CATEGORY AND SCHEDULE
Pregnancy Risk Category: X

Classification: Endothelin antagonist, vasodilator

MECHANISM OF ACTION
Endothelin receptor antagonist with greater selectivity for the endothelin A receptor than the endothelin B receptor. Stimulation of endothelin receptors is associated with vasoconstriction. Endothelin levels are increased in pulmonary arterial hypertension and correlate with increased mean right arterial pressure and disease severity.
Therapeutic Effect: symptomatic improvement in pulmonary artery hypertension and reduced rate of clinical worsening.

PHARMACOKINETICS
Rapidly absorbed; peak concentrations reached within 2 h. Highly plasma protein

bound: 99%. Nonrenal
elimination. *Half-life:* 9 h.

AVAILABILITY

Tablets: 5 mg, 10 mg.

INDICATIONS AND DOSAGES
▸ **Pulmonary Arterial Hypertension**
PO
Adult. Initiate at 5 mg once daily,
consider increasing to 10 mg once
daily if 5 mg tolerated.

CONTRAINDICATIONS

Pregnancy.

INTERACTIONS
Drug
Cyclosporine: May increase
ambrisentan concentrations and
effects; use with caution.
**CYP3A4 potent inhibitors (e.g.,
itraconazole, ketoconazole):** May
increase ambrisentan concentrations
and effects; use with caution.
**CYP2C19 potent inhibitors
(e.g., omeprazole):** May increase
ambrisentan concentrations and
effects; use with caution.
Herbal
St. John's wort: may reduce
abrisentan concentrations and
effects; avoid concomitant use.
Food
Grapefruit juice: may increase
ambrisentan concentrations and effects.

DIAGNOSTIC TEST EFFECTS

Decreased hemoglobin, increased
liver aminotransferases (ALT, AST).

SIDE EFFECTS
Frequent (> 10%)
Peripheral edema, headache.
Occasional (1%-10%)
Nasal congestion, sinusitis, flushing,
palpitations, abdominal pain,
constipation, decreased hemoglobin,
increased hepatic transaminases,
dyspnea.

SERIOUS REACTIONS
• Serious liver injury, fluid retention
with decompensated heart failure.

PRECAUTIONS & CONSIDERATIONS
Ambrisentan is only available through
a restricted distribution system
because of the risks of serious liver
toxicity and birth defects. The name
of the program is Letairis Education
and Access Program (LEAP). A Med
Guide must be dispensed with every
prescription and refill.

Treat women of childbearing
potential only after a negative
pregnancy test. Women of
childbearing potential must use two
reliable methods of contraception.
Monthly pregnancy tests are
required. It is not known whether
ambrisentan is distributed in
breast milk; breastfeeding is not
recommended.

Ambrisentan is not recommended
in patients with moderate or
severe hepatic impairment. Liver
aminotransferases should be
monitored monthly; discontinue
therapy if elevated to 5 times the
upper limit of normal or if elevations
are accompanied by increases in
bilirubin or signs or symptoms of
liver dysfunction.

Monitor hemoglobin at initiation,
1 mo after initiation, and periodically
thereafter; reductions in hemoglobin
levels have been observed within the
first few weeks of therapy.

Safety and efficacy have not been
established in pediatric patients.
Peripheral edema occurs more
frequently in elderly patients.
Storage
Store at room temperature in the
original blister packaging.
Administration
May be taken with or without food.
Tablets should not be split, crushed,
or chewed. Take at about the same
time each day.

Amcinonide
am-sin'oh-nide
(Cyclocort)

CATEGORY AND SCHEDULE
Pregnancy Risk Category: C

Classification: Anti-
inflammatory, steroidal, topical

MECHANISM OF ACTION
Topical corticosteroids have anti-
inflammatory, antipruritic, and
vasoconstrictive properties. The exact
mechanism of the anti-inflammatory
process is unclear. Amcinonide is
categorized as a high-potency topical
corticosteroid. *Therapeutic Effect:*
Reduces or prevents tissue response
to inflammatory process. High-
potency fluorinated corticosteroid.

PHARMACOKINETICS
Well absorbed systemically. Large
variation in absorption among sites:
forearm 1%, scalp 4%, forehead 7%,
scrotum 36%. Greatest penetration
occurs at groin, axillae, and face.
Protein binding in varying degrees.
Metabolized in liver. Primarily
excreted in urine.

AVAILABILITY
Cream: 0.1% (Cyclocort).
Ointment: 0.1% (Cyclocort).

INDICATIONS AND DOSAGES
▸ **Corticosteroid-responsive
dermatoses**
TOPICAL
Adults, Elderly. Apply sparingly 2-3
times/day.

CONTRAINDICATIONS
History of hypersensitivity to
amcinonide or other corticosteroids;
use on face, groin, or axilla.

INTERACTIONS
Drug
None known.
Herbal
None known.
Food
None known.

DIAGNOSTIC TEST EFFECTS
Urinary free cortisol test and ACTH
stimulation test can be used to
evaluate HPA axis suppression.

SIDE EFFECTS
Frequent
Itching, redness, irritation, burning.
Occasional
Dryness, folliculitis, hypertrichosis,
acneiform eruptions, hypopigmentation,
perioral dermatitis.
Rare
Allergic contact dermatitis,
maceration of the skin, secondary
infection, skin atrophy.
Systemic: Absorption more likely
with occlusive dressings or extensive
application in young children.

SERIOUS REACTIONS
• The serious reactions of
long-term therapy and the
addition of occlusive dressings are
reversible hypothalamic-pituitary-
adrenal (HPA) axis suppression,
manifestations of Cushing syndrome,
hyperglycemia, and glucosuria.
• Abruptly withdrawing the drug
after long-term therapy may require
supplemental systemic corticosteroids.

PRECAUTIONS & CONSIDERATIONS
Caution is necessary when using
amcinonide over large surface areas,
prolonged use, and the addition
of occlusive dressings. Long-term
therapy and the addition of occlusive
dressings can lead to reversible
hypothalamic-pituitary-adrenal
(HPA) axis suppression,

manifestations of Cushing syndrome, hyperglycemia, and glucosuria. Children may absorb larger amounts and may be more susceptible to toxicity. It is unknown whether amcinonide is distributed in breast milk.

Signs of a rash in addition to fever and sore throat should be reported. Sunlight should be avoided.

Administration
Amcinonide should be applied sparingly to the skin and rubbed gently into affected area. Apply after bath or shower for best absorption, and do not cover the area with any coverings, plastic pants, or tight diapers unless instructed. Occlusive dressings may be used in the management of psoriasis or recalcitrant conditions. Avoid contact with eyes.

Amifostine
am-ih-fos´-teen
(Ethyol)
Do not confuse Ethyol with ethanol.

CATEGORY AND SCHEDULE
Pregnancy Risk Category: C

Classification: Cytoprotective, radioprotective

MECHANISM OF ACTION
An antineoplastic adjunct and cytoprotective agent that is converted to an active metabolite by alkaline phosphatase in tissues. The active metabolite binds to and detoxifies metabolites of cisplatin. These actions occur more readily in normal tissues than in tumor tissue. *Therapeutic Effect:* Reduces the toxic effect of the chemotherapeutic agent cisplatin.

PHARMACOKINETICS
Rapidly cleared from plasma. Converted in tissue to active free thiol metabolite. Tissue uptake highest in bone marrow, skin, GI mucosa, salivary glands. *Half-life:* distribution half-life < 1 min; elimination half-life 8 min. Less than 10% remains in plasma 6 min after drug administration.

AVAILABILITY
Lyophilized Powder for Injection: 500 mg.

INDICATIONS AND DOSAGES
▸ **To reduce cumulative renal toxicity from repeated administration of cisplatin in patients with advanced ovarian cancer**
IV
Adults. 910 mg/m^2 once a day as 15-min infusion, beginning 30 min before chemotherapy. A 15-min infusion is better tolerated than extended infusions. If the full dose cannot be administered, dose for subsequent cycles should be 740 mg/m^2.
▸ **Treatment of postoperative radiation-induced xerostomia in patients with head and neck cancer**
IV
Adults. 200 mg/m^2 once a day as 3-min infusion, starting 15-30 min before radiation therapy.

CONTRAINDICATIONS
Sensitivity to aminothiol compounds or mannitol.

INTERACTIONS
Drugs
Antihypertensives: Increased risk of hypotension; interrupt antihypertensive therapy for at least 24 h before amifostine administration.

DIAGNOSTIC TEST EFFECTS
May lower serum calcium levels with multiple doses.

🖐 IV INCOMPATIBILITIES
Do not mix with any other drugs or solutions except those with established compatibility.

🖐 IV COMPATIBILITIES
Compatibility only established with 0.9% sodium chloride and sodium chloride with other additives.

SIDE EFFECTS
Frequent (> 10%)
Transient reduction in BP (usually starts 14 min into infusion, lasts about 6 min and returns to normal in 5–15 min); severe nausea, vomiting.
Occasional
Flushing or feeling of warmth or chills or feeling of coldness; dizziness, hiccups, sneezing, somnolence.
Rare
Clinically relevant hypocalcemia, mild rash.

SERIOUS REACTIONS
• A pronounced drop in BP may require temporary cessation of amifostine and fluid resuscitation.
• Serious cutaneous reactions, including erythema multiforme, Stevens-Johnson syndrome, toxic epidermal necrolysis, toxoderma, and exfoliative dermatitis.
• Anaphylaxis, arrhythmias, seizures, syncope.

PRECAUTIONS & CONSIDERATIONS
Patients should be well hydrated. Monitor BP frequently during infusion and as clinically indicated following completion of infusion. Safety not established in patients with cardiovascular disease, in elderly patients, in lactating women, or in children. Antiemetic medications should be administered before and in conjunction with amifostine. Interrupt antihypertensive therapy 24 h preceding amifostine administration. Should not be used in cancers in which chemotherapy or radiation could produce cure except in a clinical trial.

Patients should be closely assessed for cutaneous reactions before each dose. Therapy should be permanently discontinued for serious or severe cutaneous reactions or cutaneous reactions associated with fever or other constitutional symptoms.
Storage
Store unreconstituted vials at room temperature. Reconstituted solution is stable for up to 5 h at room temperature or up to 24 h in the refrigerator. The infusion solution prepared in polyvinylchloride bags at concentrations of 5-40 mg/mL is stable for up to 5 h at room temperature or 24 h in the refrigerator.
Administration
Reconstitute each vial with 9.7 mL normal saline. Before chemotherapy, amifostine should be administered as a 15-min infusion. Before radiation therapy, amifostine should be administered as a 3-min infusion.

Amikacin
am-i-kay´sin
(Amikin)
Do not confuse with Amicar.

CATEGORY AND SCHEDULE
Pregnancy Risk Category: C

Classification: Antibiotics, aminoglycosides

MECHANISM OF ACTION
An aminoglycoside antibiotic that irreversibly binds to protein on bacterial ribosomes. *Therapeutic Effect:* Interferes with protein synthesis of susceptible bacterial microorganisms.

PHARMACOKINETICS
Rapid, complete absorption after IM administration. Protein binding: 0%-10%. Widely distributed (does not cross the blood-brain barrier, low concentrations in CSF). Excreted unchanged in urine. Removed by hemodialysis. *Half-life:* 2-4 h (increased in impaired renal function and neonates; decreased in cystic fibrosis and burn or febrile patients).

AVAILABILITY
Injection. 50 mg/mL, 250 mg/mL.

INDICATIONS AND DOSAGES
▸ **Uncomplicated urinary tract infections**
IV, IM
Adults, Elderly. 250 mg q12h.
▸ **Moderate to severe infections**
IV, IM
Adults, Elderly. 15 mg/kg/day in divided doses q8-12h. Maximum 1.5 g/day.
Children, Infants. 15 mg/kg/day in divided doses q8h.
Neonates. 10 mg/kg loading dose, followed by 7.5 mg/kg q12h.
▸ **Dosage in renal impairment**
Dosage and frequency are modified based on the degree of renal impairment and serum drug concentration. After a loading dose of 5-7.5 mg/kg, the maintenance dose and frequency are based on serum creatinine levels and creatinine clearance.

CONTRAINDICATIONS
Hypersensitivity to amikacin, other aminoglycosides (cross-sensitivity), or their components.

INTERACTIONS
Drug
Loop diuretics: May increase the risk of ototoxicity because both agents have the potential to cause ototoxicity and potent diuretics may alter amikacin concentrations.
Nephrotoxic medications, other aminoglycosides, ototoxic medications: May increase the risk of nephrotoxicity or ototoxicity.
Neuromuscular blockers: May enhance neuromuscular blockade.

DIAGNOSTIC TEST EFFECTS
May increase serum bilirubin, BUN, serum creatinine, serum LDH, SGOT (AST), and SGPT (ALT) levels. May decrease serum calcium, magnesium, potassium, and sodium concentrations. Therapeutic peak serum level is 15-35 mcg/mL, and therapeutic trough is < 4-8 mcg/mL, depending on infection severity and site of infection. Toxic peak concentration is > 35 mcg/mL and toxic trough serum level is > 10 mcg/mL.

🚫 IV INCOMPATIBILITIES
Amphotericin, ampicillin, cefazolin (Ancef), heparin, propofol (Diprivan).

🙼 IV COMPATIBILITIES
Amiodarone (Cordarone), aztreonam (Azactam), calcium gluconate, cefepime (Maxipime), cimetidine (Tagamet), ciprofloxacin (Cipro), clindamycin (Cleocin), diltiazem (Cardizem), enalapril (Vasotec), esmolol (BreviBloc), fluconazole (Diflucan), furosemide (Lasix), levofloxacin (Levaquin), lorazepam (Ativan), magnesium sulfate,

midazolam (Versed), morphine, ondansetron (Zofran), potassium chloride, ranitidine (Zantac), vancomycin.

SIDE EFFECTS
Frequent
IM: Pain, induration.
IV: Phlebitis, thrombophlebitis.
Occasional
Hypersensitivity reactions (rash, fever, urticaria, pruritus).
Rare
Neuromuscular blockade (difficulty breathing, drowsiness, weakness).

SERIOUS REACTIONS
• Serious reactions may include nephrotoxicity (as evidenced by increased thirst, decreased appetite, nausea, vomiting, increased BUN and serum creatinine levels, and decreased creatinine clearance); neurotoxicity (manifested as muscle twitching, visual disturbances, seizures, and tingling); and ototoxicity (as evidenced by tinnitus, dizziness, and loss of hearing).

PRECAUTIONS & CONSIDERATIONS
Caution is warranted with patients with 8th cranial nerve (vestibulocochlear nerve) impairment, decreased renal function, myasthenia gravis, and Parkinson disease. Amikacin readily crosses the placenta, and small amounts are distributed in breast milk. It may produce fetal nephrotoxicity. Neonates and premature infants may be more susceptible to amikacin toxicity because of their immature renal function. Elderly patients are at increased risk for amikacin toxicity because of age-related renal impairment as well as an increased risk for hearing loss. Signs and symptoms of superinfection, particularly changes in the oral mucosa, diarrhea, and genital or anal pruritus, should be monitored. Safety for treatment periods exceeding 14 days have not been established.

Determine the history of allergies, especially to aminoglycosides and sulfites. Expect to correct dehydration before beginning aminoglycoside therapy. Establish the baseline hearing acuity before beginning therapy. Obtain a specimen for culture and sensitivity testing before giving the first dose. Therapy may begin before test results are known. Urinalysis results to detect casts, RBCs, WBCs, and decreased specific gravity should be monitored. Expect to monitor peak and trough serum amikacin levels. Be alert for ototoxic and neurotoxic side effects.

Storage
Store vials at room temperature. Solutions normally appear clear but may become pale yellow; the yellow color does not affect the drug's potency. Discard the solution if a precipitate forms or dark discoloration occurs. Intermittent IV infusion (piggyback) is stable for 24 h at room temperature.

Administration
For intermittent IV infusion (piggyback), dilute each 500 mg with 100 mL of 0.9% NaCl or D5W. Infuse over 30-60 min for adults and older children. Dilution volumes for younger children and infants must be individualized. Infuse over 60-120 min for infants and young children.

For IM injection, administer slowly to minimize patient discomfort. Injections administered into the gluteus maximus are less painful than those given in the lateral aspect of the thigh.

Amiloride Hydrochloride

a-mill′oh-ride hi-droh-klor′-ide
(Kaluril [AUS], Midamor)
Do not confuse with amiodarone or amlodipine.

CATEGORY AND SCHEDULE

Pregnancy Risk Category:
B (D if used in pregnancy-induced hypertension)

Classification: Diuretics, potassium sparing

MECHANISM OF ACTION

A guanidine derivative that acts as a potassium-sparing diuretic, antihypertensive, and antihypokalemic by directly interfering with sodium reabsorption in the distal tubule. *Therapeutic Effect:* Increases sodium and water excretion and decreases potassium excretion.

PHARMACOKINETICS

Route	Onset	Peak	Duration
PO	2 h	6-10 h	24 h

Incompletely absorbed from GI tract. Protein binding: Minimal. Primarily excreted in urine; partially eliminated in feces. *Half-life:* 6-9 h.

AVAILABILITY

Tablets: 5 mg.

INDICATIONS AND DOSAGES

▸**To treat of hypertension and congestive heart failure and to counteract potassium loss induced by other diuretics**
PO
Adults. 5-10 mg/day up to 20 mg.

Elderly. Initially, 5 mg/day or every other day.

▸**Dosage in renal impairment**

Creatinine Clearance (mL/min)	Dosage
10-50	50% of normal
< 10	Avoid use

OFF-LABEL USES

Liver cirrhosis and nephrotic syndrome.

CONTRAINDICATIONS

Acute or chronic renal insufficiency, anuria, diabetic nephropathy, patients on other potassium-sparing diuretics, serum potassium > 5.5 mEq/L.

INTERACTIONS

Drug
ACE inhibitors, including captopril, and potassium-sparing diuretics: May increase potassium levels.
Anticoagulants, including heparin: May decrease effect of anticoagulants, including heparin.
Drospirenone: May increase potassium levels.
Lithium: May decrease lithium clearance and increase risk of lithium toxicity.
NSAIDs: May decrease antihypertensive effect.
Herbal
None known.
Food
None known.

DIAGNOSTIC TEST EFFECTS

May increase BUN, calcium excretion, and glucose, serum creatinine, serum magnesium, serum potassium, and uric acid levels. May decrease serum sodium levels.

SIDE EFFECTS
Frequent (3%-8%)
Headache, nausea, diarrhea,
vomiting, decreased appetite.
Occasional (1%-3%)
Dizziness, constipation, abdominal
pain, weakness, fatigue, cough,
impotence, hyperkalemia.
Rare (< 1%)
Tremors, vertigo, confusion,
nervousness, insomnia, thirst,
dry mouth, heartburn, shortness
of breath, increased urination,
hypotension, rash.

SERIOUS REACTIONS
• Severe hyperkalemia may produce
irritability, anxiety, a feeling of
heaviness in the legs, paresthesia of
hands, face, and lips, hypotension,
bradycardia, tented T waves,
widening of QRS, and ST depression.

PRECAUTIONS & CONSIDERATIONS
Caution is warranted with
cardiopulmonary disease, diabetes
mellitus, or liver insufficiency,
BUN > 30 mg/dL or serum creatinine
> 1.5 mg/dL, and in elderly and
debilitated patients. Be aware that
it is unknown whether amiloride
crosses the placenta or is distributed in
breast milk. There are no age-related
precautions noted in children. In
elderly patients, age-related decreased
renal function increases the risk of
hyperkalemia and may require caution.
Incidence of hyperkalemia is increased
when administered without a kaliuretic
diuretic. Be aware a high-potassium
diet and potassium supplements can
be dangerous, especially with liver or
kidney problems.
　Notify the physician of signs and
symptoms of hyperkalemia: confusion;
difficulty breathing; irregular
heartbeat; nervousness; numbness
of the hands, feet, or lips; unusual
tiredness; and weakness in the legs.

BP, vital signs, electrolytes, intake and
output, weight, and potassium levels
should be monitored before and during
treatment. A baseline 12-lead ECG
should also be obtained.
Administration
Take with food. Therapeutic effect of
the drug takes several days to begin
and can last for several days after the
drug is discontinued.

Aminocaproic Acid
a-mee-noe-ka-proe´ik
(Amicar)
**Do not confuse Amicar with
amikacin or Amikin.**

CATEGORY AND SCHEDULE
Pregnancy Risk Category: C

Classification: Hemostatic

MECHANISM OF ACTION
A systemic hemostatic that acts as an
antifibrinolytic and antihemorrhagic by
inhibiting the activation of plasminogen
activator substances. *Therapeutic
Effect:* Prevents fibrinolysis.

PHARMACOKINETICS
Mean peak concentration reached
within 1-2 h. Primarily excreted
unchanged in the urine (65%).
Half-life: 2 h.

AVAILABILITY
Syrup: 250 mg/mL.
Tablets: 500 mg, 1000 mg.
Injection: 250 mg/mL.

INDICATIONS AND DOSAGES
▸ **Acute bleeding**
PO, IV INFUSION
Adults, Elderly. 4-5 g over first
hour; then 1-1.25 g/h. Continue for

8 h or until bleeding is controlled.
Maximum: 30 g/24 h.
Children. 3 g/m^2 over first hour; then
1 g/m^2/h. Maximum: 18 g/m^2/24 h.

OFF-LABEL USES
Prevention of recurrence of
subarachnoid hemorrhage,
prevention of hemorrhage in
hemophiliacs following dental
surgery.

CONTRAINDICATIONS
Evidence of active intravascular
clotting process, disseminated
intravascular coagulation without
concurrent heparin therapy,
hematuria of upper urinary
tract origin (unless benefit
outweighs risk); newborns
(parenteral form).

INTERACTIONS
Drug
Oral contraceptives, estrogens:
May increase clotting factors leading
to a hypercoaguable state.

DIAGNOSTIC TEST EFFECTS
May elevate serum potassium level.

ⓘ IV INCOMPATIBILITIES
Sodium lactate. Do not mix with
other medications.

SIDE EFFECTS
Occasional
Nausea, diarrhea, cramps, decreased
urination, decreased BP, dizziness,
headache, muscle fatigue and
weakness, myopathy, bloodshot eyes.

SERIOUS REACTIONS
• Too rapid IV administration
produces tinnitus, rash, arrhythmias,
unusual fatigue, and weakness.
• Rarely, a grand mal seizure occurs,
generally preceded by weakness,
dizziness, and headache.

PRECAUTIONS & CONSIDERATIONS
Caution is warranted with
hyperfibrinolysis and impaired
cardiac, hepatic, or renal function. No
information is available concerning
the distribution of aminocaproic
acid in breast milk. There is no
documented evidence of age-related
problems in children; however,
injectable contains benzyl alcohol
and is not recommended for use
in newborns. Although no elderly-
related problems have been noted,
cautious use is advised because of the
risk of age-related renal impairment,
which may require dosage reduction.
Women may experience an increase
in menstrual flow.
    Notify the physician of red or dark
urine, muscular pain or weakness,
abdominal or back pain, gingival
bleeding, black or red stool, coffee-
ground vomitus, or blood-tinged
mucus from cough. BP, heart rate
and rhythm, and pulse rate, serum
creatine kinase, and AST (SGOT)
levels should be monitored.
Storage
Store tablets and solution at room
temperature; keep tightly closed.
Do not freeze solution.
    Store injection at room
temperature.
Caution
Use only for gingival bleeding. Most
treatment during dental surgery
requires oral treatment.
Administration
! Expect to administer a reduced
dose if the patient has cardiac, renal,
or hepatic impairment. The syrup
may be given as an oral rinse for the
control of bleeding during dental and
oral surgery in hemophilic patients.
    For IV use, dilute each 1 g in
up to 50 mL 0.9% NaCl, D5W,
Ringer's solution, or sterile water
for injection. Do not use sterile
water for injection in those with

subarachnoid hemorrhage. Do not give by direct injection. Give only by IV infusion. Infuse 5 g or less over the first hour in 250 mL of solution. Give each succeeding 1 g over 1 h in 50-100 mL of solution. Monitor for hypotension during the infusion. Be aware that rapid infusion may produce arrhythmias, including bradycardia.

Aminophylline
am-in-off'i-lin
(Phyllocontin)
Do not confuse aminophylline with amitriptyline or ampicillin.

CATEGORY AND SCHEDULE
Pregnancy Risk Category: C

Classification: Bronchodilators, xanthine derivatives

MECHANISM OF ACTION
A xanthine derivative that acts as a bronchodilator by directly relaxing smooth muscle of the bronchial airways and pulmonary blood vessels. *Therapeutic Effect:* Relieves bronchospasm and increases vital capacity.

PHARMACOKINETICS
Aminophylline is rapidly converted to theophylline. See theophylline monograph.

AVAILABILITY
Tablets: 100 mg, 200 mg.
Injection (aminophylline): 25 mg/mL.

INDICATIONS AND DOSAGES
Note that aminophylline dose equals theophylline dose divided by 0.8. Doses should be calculated based on ideal body weight.

Theophylline is usually preferred for oral dosages.

▸ **Chronic bronchospasm**
PO
Adults, Elderly, Children weighing more than 45 kg. Aminophylline 380 mg/day divided every 6-8 h, after 3 days if tolerated may increase to aminophylline 507 mg/day divided every 6-8 h, and after 3 additional days if tolerated and increased dose is necessary may increase to aminophylline 760 mg/day divided every 6-8 h. Maximum dose is theophylline 400 mg/day in adults with risk factors for reduced clearance or when concentration monitoring is not feasible.

▸ **Acute bronchospasm in patients not currently taking theophylline**
PO
Adults, children older than 1 yr. Initially, loading dose of aminophylline 6.25 mg/kg, then maintenance dosage of oral theophylline based on patient group (shown below).

Patient Group	Maintenance Theophylline Dosage*
Healthy, nonsmoking adults	3 mg/kg q8h
Elderly patients, patients with cor pulmonale	2 mg/kg q8h
Patients with CHF or hepatic disease	1-2 mg/kg q12h
Children 9-16 yr, young adult smokers	3 mg/kg q6h
Children 1-8 yr	4 mg/kg q6h

*Convert dose to aminophylline equivalent if using aminophylline.

IV INFUSION
Adults, Children older than 1 yr. Initially, loading dose of 6 mg/kg (aminophylline); maintenance dosage of aminophylline based on patient group (shown next).

Patient Group	Maintenance Aminophylline Dosage
Healthy, nonsmoking adults	0.7 mg/kg/h
Elderly patients, patients with cor pulmonale, CHF, or hepatic impairment	0.25 mg/kg/h
Children 13-16 yr	0.7 mg/kg/h
Children 9-12 yr, young adult smokers	0.9 mg/kg/h
Children 1-8 yr	1-1.2 mg/kg/h
Children 6 mo to 1 yr	0.6-0.7 mg/kg/h
Children 6 wks to 6 mo	0.5 mg/kg/h
Neonates	5 mg/kg q12h

▸ **Acute bronchospasm in patients currently taking theophylline**
PO, IV
Adults, children older than 1 yr.
Obtain serum theophylline level. If not possible and patient is in respiratory distress and not experiencing toxic effects, may give theophylline 2.5 mg/kg dose. Maintenance: Dosage based on peak serum theophylline concentration, clinical condition, and presence of toxicity.

CONTRAINDICATIONS
History of hypersensitivity to caffeine or xanthine.

INTERACTIONS
Drug
β-blockers: May decrease the effects of aminophylline.
Cimetidine, ciprofloxacin, erythromycin, fluvoxamine, norfloxacin, tacrine: May increase theophylline blood concentration and risk of aminophylline toxicity.
Phenytoin, primidone, rifampin: May increase theophylline metabolism.

Smoking: May decrease theophylline blood concentration.
Food
Charcoal-broiled foods; high-protein, low-carbohydrate diet: May decrease the theophylline blood level.

DIAGNOSTIC TEST EFFECTS
None known. Measure serum theophylline level to guide all dosage adjustments.

ⓓ IV INCOMPATIBILITIES
Amiodarone (Cordarone), ciprofloxacin (Cipro), dobutamine (Dobutrex), epinephrine, hydroxyzine, magnesium sulfate, norepinephrine, ondansetron (Zofran).

ⓓ IV COMPATIBILITIES
Aztreonam (Azactam), ceftazidime (Fortaz), dopamine, fluconazole (Diflucan), heparin, morphine, potassium chloride.

SIDE EFFECTS
Frequent
Altered smell (during IV administration), restlessness, tachycardia, tremor.
Occasional
Heartburn, vomiting, headache, mild diuresis, insomnia, nausea.

SERIOUS REACTIONS
• Too-rapid IV administration may produce marked hypotension with accompanying faintness, light-headedness, palpitations, tachycardia, hyperventilation, nausea, vomiting, angina-like pain, seizures, ventricular fibrillation, and cardiac standstill.

PRECAUTIONS & CONSIDERATIONS
Caution is warranted with diabetes mellitus; glaucoma; hypertension; hyperthyroidism; cardiac, renal, or hepatic impairment; peptic

ulcer disease; and seizure disorder. Aminophylline crosses the placenta and small amounts of the drug may be distributed in breast milk and cause irritability in the breastfeeding infant. Use the drug cautiously in children < 1 yr. Drink plenty of fluids to decrease the thickness of lung secretions. Avoid excessive use of caffeinated products, such as chocolate, cocoa, cola, coffee, and tea. Smoking, charcoal-broiled foods, and a high-protein, low-carbohydrate diet may decrease the theophylline level.

Pulse rate and quality; respiratory rate, depth, rhythm, and type; ABG levels; and serum potassium levels should be monitored. Peak serum concentration should be obtained 1 h after an IV dose, 1-2 h after an immediate-release dose, and 3-8 h after a sustained-release dose. Serum trough level should be obtained just before the next dose. Lips and fingernails should be assessed for signs of hypoxemia, such as a blue or gray color in light-skinned patients and a gray color in dark-skinned patients.

Storage

Store injection vials at room temperature. Do not use if crystals are present.

Store tablets and oral solution at room temperature.

Protect from light and moisture.

Administration

Take oral aminophylline with food to avoid GI distress.

Discard the solution for injection if it contains a precipitate. For IV use, give loading dose diluted in 100-200 mL of D5W or 0.9% NaCl. Prepare maintenance dose in larger-volume parenteral infusion. Usual concentration for maintenance infusion is 1 mg/mL. Do not exceed a flow rate of 25 mg/min for either piggyback or infusion. Administer loading dose over 20-30 min. Use an infusion pump or microdrip to regulate IV administration.

Aminosalicylic Acid
a-mee-noe-sal-i-sil-ik as-id
(Nemasol [CAN], Paser)

CATEGORY AND SCHEDULE
Pregnancy Risk Category: C

Classification: Antitubercular anti-infective

MECHANISM OF ACTION
An antitubercular agent active against *M. tuberculosis.* Thought to exhibit competitive antagonism of folic acid synthesis. *Therapeutic Effect:* Bacteriostatic activity in susceptible microorganisms.

PHARMACOKINETICS
Readily absorbed from the GI tract. Protein binding: 50%-60%. Widely distributed (including CSF). Metabolized in liver. Primarily excreted in urine. Removed by hemodialysis. *Half-life:* 1.1-1.62 h.

AVAILABILITY
Packet Granules: 4 g/packet granules (Paser).
Tablets, Enteric-Coated: 7.7 grains (Paser).
Tablets, Sustained-Release: 500 mg (Paser).

INDICATIONS AND DOSAGES
▸ **Tuberculosis**
PO
Adults, Elderly. 4 g in divided doses 3 times/day.

Children. 150 mg/kg/day in divided doses 3 times/day. Maximum: 12 g/day.

OFF-LABEL USES
Crohn disease, hyperlipidemia, ulcerative colitis.

CONTRAINDICATIONS
End-stage renal disease, hypersensitivity to aminosalicylic acid products.

INTERACTIONS
Drug
Cyanocobalamin: May decrease cyanocobalamin absorption.
Digoxin: May decrease digoxin absorption.
Isoniazid: May increase isoniazid serum levels.

DIAGNOSTIC TEST EFFECTS
May alter bilirubin levels in urinalysis.

SIDE EFFECTS
Occasional
Abdominal pain, diarrhea, nausea, vomiting.
Rare
Hypersensitivity reactions, hepatotoxicity, thrombocytopenia.

SERIOUS REACTIONS
• Liver toxicity and hepatitis, blood dyscrasias occur rarely.
• Agranulocytosis, methemoglobinemia, thrombocytopenia have been reported.

PRECAUTIONS & CONSIDERATIONS
Precaution is necessary with liver insufficiency, peptic ulcer disease, impaired renal function, and congestive heart failure. It is unknown whether aminosalicylic acid crosses the placenta or is excreted in breast milk. There are no age-related precautions noted in children or in elderly patients. Be aware that skeleton of the granules may appear in the stool.

Liver function should be monitored during therapy. Symptoms of hepatitis as evidenced by anorexia, dark urine, fatigue, jaundice, nausea, vomiting, and weakness should be assessed. If hepatitis is suspected, withhold the drug and notify the physician promptly.
Storage
Store in refrigerator or freezer.
Administration
May sprinkle granules on acidic food such as applesauce or yogurt or mix with acidic drink such as tomato, orange, grapefruit, grape, cranberry, or apple juice or fruit punch. Granules must be swirled in drink since they will not dissolve. Care must be taken to maintain the enteric coating; in the presence of gastric acid, unprotected aminosalicylic acid is converted to a known hepatotoxin. Discard medication if the package is swollen or the granules are dark brown or purple.

Amiodarone
a-mee′oh-da-rone
(Aratac [AUS], Cordarone, Cordarone X [AUS], Pacerone)
Do not confuse amiodarone with amiloride or Cordarone with Cardura.

CATEGORY AND SCHEDULE
Pregnancy Risk Category: D

Classification: Antiarrhythmics, class III

MECHANISM OF ACTION
A cardiac agent that prolongs duration of myocardial cell action potential and refractory period

by acting directly on all cardiac tissue. Decreases AV and sinus node function. *Therapeutic Effect:* Suppresses arrhythmias.

PHARMACOKINETICS

Route	Onset	Steady State	Duration
PO	3 days to 3 wks	1 wk to 5 mo	7-50 days after discontinuation

Slowly, variably absorbed from GI tract; oral bioavailability is 35%-65%. Protein binding: 96%. Extensively metabolized by CYP3A4 and CYP2C8 to active metabolite. Excreted via bile; not removed by hemodialysis. *Half-life:* 26-107 days; metabolite, 61 days.

AVAILABILITY

Tablets (Cordarone): 200 mg.
Tablets (Pacerone): 100 mg, 200 mg, 400 mg.
Injection (Cordarone): 50 mg/mL.

INDICATIONS AND DOSAGES
▸ **Life-threatening recurrent ventricular fibrillation or hemodynamically unstable ventricular tachycardia**
PO
Adults, Elderly. Initially, load with (unless patient has been on IV treatment) 800-1600 mg/day in 2-4 divided doses for 1-3 wks. After arrhythmia is controlled or side effects occur, reduce to 600-800 mg/day for about 4 wks. Maintenance: 200-600 mg/day with a usual maintenance dose of 400 mg/day.
IV INFUSION
Adults. Initially, 150 mg over 10 min, then 360 mg over 6 h; then 540 mg over 18 h. May continue at 0.5 mg/min for up to 2-3 wks regardless of age or renal or left ventricular function.

OFF-LABEL USES
Treatment and prevention of supraventricular arrhythmias and symptomatic atrial flutter refractory to conventional treatment.

CONTRAINDICATIONS
Bradycardia-induced syncope (except in the presence of a pacemaker), cardiogenic shock, second- and third-degree AV block, severe hepatic disease, severe sinus-node dysfunction; hypersensitivity to amiodarone or its components, including iodine.

INTERACTIONS
Drug
Antiarrhythmics: May increase cardiac effects.
Azole antifungals, fluoroquinolones, macrolides, ranolazine, thioridazine, vardenafil, ziprasidone: Risk of cardiac arrhythmias, including torsades de pointes, may be increased.
β-blockers, oral anticoagulants: May increase effect of β-blockers and oral anticoagulants.
Cyclosporine: Increased cyclosporine concentrations.
Digoxin, phenytoin: May increase drug concentration and risk of toxicity of digoxin and phenytoin.
Protease inhibitors: Increased amiodarone concentrations/toxicity; ritonavir and nelfinavir are contraindicated with amiodarone.
Simvastatin: May increase risk of myopathy/rhabdomyolysis.
Warfarin: Increased anticoagulant effect; closely monitor International Normalized Ratio.
Herbal
St. John's wort: May reduce amiodarone concentrations.

Food
All foods: Food increases the rate and extent of absorption. Dose consistently with regard to meals.
Grapefruit juice: Increased amiodarone concentrations; avoid grapefruit juice.

DIAGNOSTIC TEST EFFECTS
May increase antinuclear antibody titers and AST (SGOT), ALT (SGPT), and serum alkaline phosphatase levels. May cause changes in ECG and thyroid function test results. Therapeutic serum level is 0.5-2.5 mcg/mL but not well correlated with efficacy as a result of long half-life of drug.

ⓘ IV INCOMPATIBILITIES
Aminophylline (theophylline), cefamandole, cefazolin (Ancef), heparin, mezlocillin, sodium bicarbonate.

ⓘ IV COMPATIBILITIES
Dobutamine (Dobutrex), dopamine (Intropin), furosemide (Lasix), insulin (regular), labetalol (Normodyne), lidocaine, midazolam (Versed), morphine, nitroglycerin, norepinephrine (Levophed), phenylephrine (Neo-Synephrine), potassium chloride, vancomycin.

SIDE EFFECTS
Expected
Corneal microdeposits are noted in almost all patients treated for more than 6 mo (can lead to blurry vision).
Frequent (> 3%)
Parenteral: Hypotension, nausea, fever, bradycardia.
Oral: Constipation, headache, decreased appetite, nausea, vomiting, paresthesias, photosensitivity, muscular incoordination, hypothyroidism, malaise, fatigue, tremor, abnormal liver function tests.

Occasional (< 3%)
Oral: Bitter or metallic taste, decreased libido, dizziness, facial flushing, blue-gray coloring of skin (face, arms, and neck), blurred vision, bradycardia, asymptomatic corneal deposits, hyperthyroidism.
Rare (< 1%)
Oral: Rash, vision loss, blindness, peripheral neuropathy.

SERIOUS REACTIONS
• Serious, potentially fatal pulmonary toxicity (alveolitis, pulmonary fibrosis, pneumonitis, acute respiratory distress syndrome) may begin with progressive dyspnea and cough with crackles, decreased breath sounds, pleurisy, CHF, or hepatotoxicity.
• Amiodarone may worsen existing arrhythmias or produce new arrhythmias (called proarrhythmias).

PRECAUTIONS & CONSIDERATIONS
A Med Guide must be dispensed with every prescription and refill.
   Caution is warranted with thyroid disease. Amiodarone crosses the placenta and is distributed in breast milk; it adversely affects fetal development. Safety and efficacy of amiodarone have not been established in children. Elderly patients may be more sensitive to amiodarone's effects on thyroid function and may experience increased incidence of ataxia or other neurotoxic effects. Amiodaron may cause photosensitivity; wear sunscreen and sun-protective clothing.
! Signs and symptoms of pulmonary toxicity, including progressively worsening cough and dyspnea, should be assessed. Dosage should be discontinued or reduced if toxicity occurs.
   Chest x-ray, ECG, pulmonary function tests, liver enzyme tests, AST, ALT, and serum alkaline phosphatase level should be obtained at baseline

and during therapy. Apical pulse and BP should be assessed immediately before giving amiodarone. Withhold the medication and notify the physician if the pulse rate is 60 beats/min or lower or the systolic BP is < 90 mm Hg. Pulse rate for bradycardia, an irregular rhythm, and quality should be monitored. ECG for changes such as widening of the QRS complex and prolonged PR and QT intervals should be assessed; notify the physician of significant interval changes. Signs and symptoms of hyperthyroidism, such as difficulty breathing, bulging eyes (exophthalmos), eyelid edema, frequent urination, hot and dry skin, and weight loss, and signs and symptoms of hypothyroidism, such as cool and pale skin, lethargy, night cramps, periorbital edema, and pudgy hands and feet should also be monitored.

Storage

Store unopened vials at room temperature. Protect from light.
Store tablets at room temperature.

Administration

For oral use, take with meals to reduce GI distress. Dose consistently with regard to meals. Tablets may be crushed if necessary.

! Solution concentrations > 3 mg/mL can cause peripheral vein phlebitis. For IV administration, use glass or polyolefin containers for dilution. Avoid evacuated glass containers. Dilute the loading dose of 150 mg in 100 mL D5W to yield a solution of 1.5 mg/mL. Dilute the maintenance dose of 900 mg in 500 mL D5W to yield a solution of 1.8 mg/mL. Avoid solution with a concentration exceeding 2 mg/mL unless a central venous catheter is used. Administer with a volumetric infusion pump. When possible, administer through central venous catheter used only for amiodarone. Use an in-line filter.

Amitriptyline
a-mee-trip′ti-leen
(Apo-Amitriptyline [CAN], Elavil, Endep [AUS], Levate [CAN], Novo-Triptyn [CAN], Tryptanol [AUS])
Do not confuse amitriptyline with aminophylline or nortriptyline, or Elavil with Equanil or Mellaril.

CATEGORY AND SCHEDULE
Pregnancy Risk Category: C

Classification: Antidepressants, tricyclic

MECHANISM OF ACTION
A tricyclic antidepressant that blocks the reuptake of neurotransmitters, including norepinephrine and serotonin, at presynaptic membranes, thus increasing their availability at postsynaptic receptor sites. Also has strong anticholinergic activity. *Therapeutic Effect:* Relieves depression.

PHARMACOKINETICS
Rapidly and well absorbed from the GI tract. Protein binding: 90%. Undergoes first-pass metabolism in the liver. Primarily excreted in urine. Minimal removal by hemodialysis. *Half-life:* 10-26 h.

AVAILABILITY
Tablets: 10 mg, 25 mg, 50 mg, 75 mg, 100 mg, 150 mg.

INDICATIONS AND DOSAGES
▸ **Depression**
PO
Adults. Initially, 25-75 mg/day as a single dose at bedtime or in divided

doses. May gradually increase up to 300 mg/day. Titrate to lowest effective dosage.
Elderly. Initially, 10-25 mg at bedtime. May increase by 10-25 mg at weekly intervals. Range: 25-150 mg/day.
▸ **Neuropathic pain**
PO
Adults, Elderly. Range of 10-150 mg at bedtime. Follow titration schedule as for depression.

OFF-LABEL USES

Relief of neuropathic pain, such as that experienced by patients with diabetic neuropathy or postherpetic neuralgia; treatment of bulimia nervosa.

CONTRAINDICATIONS

Acute recovery period after MI; use within 14 days of MAOIs, hypersensitivity.

INTERACTIONS

Drug
Antithyroid agents: May increase the risk of agranulocytosis.
Cimetidine, valproic acid: May increase amitriptyline blood concentration and risk of toxicity.
Clonidine, guanadrel: May decrease the effects of these drugs.
CNS depressants (including alcohol, anticonvulsants, barbiturates, phenothiazines, and sedative-hypnotics): May increase CNS and respiratory depression and the hypotensive effects of amitriptyline.
CYP2D6 inhibitors: May increase amitriptyline blood concentrations and risk of toxicity.
MAOIs: May increase the risk of neuroleptic malignant syndrome, seizures, hypertensive crisis, and hyperpyresis. Contraindicated for concomitant use. Make sure at least

14 days elapse between the use of MAOIs and amitriptyline.
Phenothiazines: May increase the sedative and anticholinergic effects of amitriptyline.
Sympathomimetics: May increase the risk of cardiac effects.
Herbal
St. John's wort: May decrease amitriptyline concentration.

DIAGNOSTIC TEST EFFECTS

May alter blood glucose levels and ECG readings. Therapeutic serum drug level is 120-250 ng/mL; toxic serum drug level is > 500 ng/mL.

SIDE EFFECTS

Frequent
Dizziness, somnolence, dry mouth, orthostatic hypotension, headache, increased appetite, weight gain, nausea, unusual fatigue, unpleasant taste.
Occasional
Blurred vision, confusion, constipation, hallucinations, delayed micturition, eye pain, arrhythmias, fine muscle tremors, parkinsonian syndrome, anxiety, diarrhea, diaphoresis, heartburn, insomnia.
Rare
Hypersensitivity, alopecia, tinnitus, breast enlargement, photosensitivity.

SERIOUS REACTIONS

• Overdose may produce confusion, seizures, severe somnolence, arrhythmias, fever, hallucinations, agitation, dyspnea, vomiting, and unusual fatigue or weakness.
• Abrupt discontinuation after prolonged therapy may produce headache, malaise, nausea, vomiting, and vivid dreams.

• Blood dyscrasias and cholestatic jaundice occur rarely.

PRECAUTIONS & CONSIDERATIONS

Caution is warranted with cardiovascular disease, diabetes mellitus, angle-closure glaucoma, hiatal hernia, history of seizures, history of urine retention or urinary obstruction, hyperthyroidism, increased intraocular pressure, hepatic or renal disease, benign prostatic hyperplasia, and schizophrenia. Amitriptyline crosses the placenta and is minimally distributed in breast milk. Children are more sensitive to an acute overdose and are at increased risk for amitriptyline toxicity. In addition, antidepressants have been associated with an increased risk of suicidal thinking and behavior in children, adolescents, and young adults with major depressive disorder and other psychiatric disorders. Elderly patients are more sensitive to the drug's anticholinergic effects and are at increased risk for amitriptyline toxicity.

Anticholinergic, sedative, and hypotensive effects may occur, but tolerance usually develops to these effects. Because dizziness may occur, change positions slowly, and avoid alcohol and tasks that require alertness or motor skills. CBC and blood chemistry profile should be obtained before and periodically during therapy, especially with long-term use. BP and pulse rate should be monitored to detect for arrhythmias and hypotension.

Administration

A Med Guide should be dispensed with every prescription and refill.

Take oral amitriptyline tablets with food or milk if GI distress occurs. Do not abruptly discontinue the drug. Full therapeutic effect may be noted in 2-4 wks.

Bedtime once-daily administration may increase compliance and limit side effects.

Amlexanox
am-lecks-ah-knocks
(Aphthasol)
Do not confuse with Ambesol.

CATEGORY AND SCHEDULE
Pregnancy Risk Category: B

Classification: Topical anti-inflammatory

MECHANISM OF ACTION

A mouth agent that has antiallergic and anti-inflammatory properties. Appears to inhibit formation and/or release of inflammatory mediators (e.g., histamine) from mast cells, neutrophils, and mononuclear cells. *Therapeutic Effect:* Alleviates signs and symptoms of aphthous ulcers.

PHARMACOKINETICS

After topical application, most systemic absorption occurs from the GI tract. Metabolized to inactive metabolite. Excreted in urine. *Half-life:* 3.5 h.

AVAILABILITY

Paste: 5% (Aphthasol).

INDICATIONS AND DOSAGES
▸ **Aphthous ulcers**
TOPICAL
Adults, Elderly. Administer ¼ inch directly to ulcers 4 times/day (after meals and at bedtime) following oral hygiene.

CONTRAINDICATIONS
Hypersensitivity to amlexanox or any component of the formulation.

INTERACTIONS
Drug
None known.
Herbal
None known.
Food
None known.

DIAGNOSTIC TEST EFFECTS
None known.

SIDE EFFECTS
Occasional (1%-2%)
Stinging, burning at administration site, transient pain.
Rare (< 1%)
Contact mucositis, rash, nausea, diarrhea.

SERIOUS REACTIONS
• Ingestion of a full tube could result in nausea, vomiting, and diarrhea.

PRECAUTIONS & CONSIDERATIONS
Be aware that amlexanox should be discontinued if rash or contact mucositis develops. It is unknown whether amlexanox crosses the placenta or is distributed in breast milk. There are no age-related precautions noted in children or the elderly.
Storage
Store at room temperature.
Administration
Apply as soon as possible after noticing symptoms. Apply directly on ulcers following oral hygiene, after meals, and at bedtime. Dry ulcer before applying by gently patting with a soft, clean cloth. Continue use until ulcer heals.

Amlodipine
am-low′di-peen
(Norvasc)
Do not confuse amlodipine with amiloride, or Norvasc with Navane or Vascor.

CATEGORY AND SCHEDULE
Pregnancy Risk Category: C

Classification: Calcium channel blockers

MECHANISM OF ACTION
A calcium channel blocker that inhibits calcium movement across cardiac and vascular smooth-muscle cell membranes. *Therapeutic Effect:* Relieves angina by dilating coronary arteries, peripheral arteries, and arterioles. Decreases total peripheral vascular resistance and BP by vasodilation.

PHARMACOKINETICS

Route	Onset	Peak	Duration
PO	0.5-1 h	6-12 h	24 h

Slowly absorbed from the GI tract. Protein binding: 93%. Undergoes first-pass metabolism in the liver. Excreted primarily in urine. Not removed by hemodialysis.
Half-life: 30-50 h (increased in elderly patients and in those with liver cirrhosis).

AVAILABILITY
Tablets: 2.5 mg, 5 mg, 10 mg.

INDICATIONS AND DOSAGES
▸ **Hypertension**
PO
Adults. Initially, 5 mg/day as a single dose. Maximum: 10 mg/day.

Elderly and Debilitated Patients.
Initially, 2.5 mg/day as a single dose.
Titrate to 5 mg/day if needed.
Children 6-17 yr. 2.5-5 mg/day as a single dose.
▸ **Angina (chronic stable or vasospastic)**
PO
Adults. 5-10 mg/day as a single dose.
Elderly. 5 mg/day as a single dose.
Maximum: 10 mg.
▸ **Dosage in hepatic impairment**
For adults and elderly patients, give 2.5 mg/day for hypertension; 5 mg/day for angina.

CONTRAINDICATIONS
Severe hypotension.

INTERACTIONS
Drug
None known.
Herbal
St. John's wort: May decrease amlodipine levels.

DIAGNOSTIC TEST EFFECTS
None known.

SIDE EFFECTS
Frequent (> 5%)
Peripheral edema, headache, flushing.
Occasional (< 5%)
Dizziness, palpitations, nausea, unusual fatigue or weakness (asthenia).
Rare (< 1%)
Chest pain, bradycardia, orthostatic hypotension.

SERIOUS REACTIONS
• Overdose may produce excessive peripheral vasodilation and marked hypotension with reflex tachycardia.

PRECAUTIONS & CONSIDERATIONS
Caution is warranted with aortic stenosis, CHF, and impaired hepatic function. Expect to adjust dosage in hepatic impairment. It is unknown whether amlodipine crosses the placenta or is distributed in breast milk. The safety and efficacy of amlodipine have not been established in children younger than 6 yr of age. Elderly patients are more sensitive to amlodipine's hypotensive effects, and its half-life may be increased in these patients. Tasks that require alertness and motor skills should be avoided until drug effects are known.

Asthenia or headache may occur. Apical pulse, BP, and renal and hepatic function test results should be monitored before and during therapy. Skin should be assessed for flushing and peripheral edema, especially behind the medial malleolus and the sacral area.
Administration
! Expect to increase amlodipine dosage slowly over 7-14 days based on response. Amlodipine may be taken without regard to food. Do not abruptly discontinue amlodipine.

Ammonium Lactate
ah-moe′nee-um lack′tate
(Amlactin, Lac-Hydrin, Lac-Hydrin Five, LAClotion)

CATEGORY AND SCHEDULE
Pregnancy Risk Category: C

Classification: Dermatologics

MECHANISM OF ACTION
Lactic acid is an α-hydroxy acid that influences hydration, decreases corneocyte cohesion, reduces excessive epidermal keratinization in hyperkeratotic conditions, and induces synthesis of mucopolysaccharides

and collagen in photodamaged skin. The exact mechanism is not known. *Therapeutic Effect:* Increases hydration of the skin.

PHARMACOKINETICS
Not known.

AVAILABILITY
Cream: 12% (Amlactin).
Lotion: 5% (Lac-Hydrin Five), 12% (Amlactin, Lac-Hydrin. LAClotion).

INDICATIONS AND DOSAGES
▸ **Treatment of ichthyosis vulgaris and xerosis**
PO
Adults, Elderly, Children. Apply sparingly and rub into area thoroughly twice daily.

CONTRAINDICATIONS
Hypersensitivity to ammonium lactate.

INTERACTIONS
Drug
Calcipotriene: May decrease the effects of calcipotriene.

DIAGNOSTIC TEST EFFECTS
None known.

SIDE EFFECTS
Occasional (2%-15%)
Burning, stinging, rash, itching, dry skin.

PRECAUTIONS & CONSIDERATIONS
Ammonium lactate should not be used on broken skin or in areas of infection, and do not apply to the face, inguinal areas, or abraded skin. It is not known whether ammonium lactate is distributed in breast milk. Safety and efficacy have not been established in children younger than 2 yr of age. May be sensitive to sunlight (UV) exposure.

Administration
Gently cleanse area before application. Shake lotion well before application. Use occlusive dressings only as ordered. Apply sparingly and rub into area thoroughly. Avoid contact with the eyes and mucous membranes.

Amobarbital
am-oh-bar´bi-tal
(Amytal Sodium, Neur-Amyl [AUS])

CATEGORY AND SCHEDULE
Pregnancy Risk Category: D
Controlled substance: Schedule II

Classification: Barbiturates, preanesthetics, sedatives/hypnotics

MECHANISM OF ACTION
A barbiturate that depresses the sensory cortex, decreases motor activity, and alters cerebellar function. *Therapeutic Effect:* Produces drowsiness, sedation, and hypnosis.

PHARMACOKINETICS
Protein binding: 60%. Metabolized in liver primarily by the hepatic microsomal enzyme system. Primarily excreted in urine. *Half-life:* 16-40 h.

AVAILABILITY
Powder for Injection: 500 mg (Amytal Sodium).

INDICATIONS AND DOSAGES
▸ **Preanesthetic sedative**
IM/IV
Adults, Children 6 yr and older. 65-200 mg single dose. Alternatively,

use a weight-based dose:
3-5 mg/kg/dose.
▶ **Short-term treatment of insomnia**
IM/IV
Adults. 65-200 mg at bedtime.
Maximum: 500 mg.
Elderly. Not recommended.
Children older than 6 yr.
2-3 mg/kg/dose at bedtime.

OFF-LABEL USES
Refractory seizures.

CONTRAINDICATIONS
History of manifest or latent
porphyria, marked liver dysfunction,
marked respiratory disease in which
dyspnea or obstruction is evident,
and hypersensitivity to amobarbital
products.

INTERACTIONS
Drug
Anticoagulants, steroids: May
decrease the effects of anticoagulants
and steroids.
**Anticonvulsants, barbiturates,
benzodiazepines, valproic acid:**
May increase the metabolism
of anticonvulsants, barbiturates,
benzodiazepines, and valproic
acid.
CNS depressants: May increase
respiratory depression and
hypotension.
**Corticosteroids, doxycycline,
griseofulvin:** May decrease
the effect of corticosteroids,
doxycycline, and griseofulvin.
MAOIs: May cause convulsions and
hypertensive crises.
Herbal
Valerian: May increase CNS
depression.
St. John's wort: May decrease the
effects of amobarbital sodium.
Food
Ethanol: May increase CNS
depression.

All foods: Food may decrease the
rate of absorption.

DIAGNOSTIC TEST EFFECTS
May falsely elevate phenobarbital
levels when measured with EMIT(R)
system.

Ⓥ IV INCOMPATIBILITIES
Anileridine [can], atracurium
(Tracrium), cefazolin (Ancef),
cephalothin (Ceporacin [can]),
chlorpromazine (Thorazine),
cimetidine (Tagamet), clindamycin
(Cleocin), codeine, dimenhydrinate
(Dramamine), diphenhydramine
(Benadryl), droperidol (Inapsine),
hydrocortisone, hydroxyzine (Atarax,
Vistaril), insulin, isoproterenol
(Isuprel), levorphanol
(Levo-Dromaron), meperidine
(Demerol), metaraminol
(Aramine), methadone (Dolophine,
Methadose), methyldopa (Aldomet),
methylphenidate (Concerta, Ritalin),
morphine (Avinza, Kadian, Roxanol),
norepinephrine (Levophed),
oxytetracycline (Terramycin),
pancuronium (Pavulon), penicillin
G (Bicillin), pentazocine (Talwin),
phytonadione (AquaMEPHYTON,
Mephyton), procaine (Novocain),
prochlorperazine (Compazine),
propiomazine (Largon),
streptomycin, succinylcholine
(Anectine), tetracycline (Sumycin),
vancomycin (Vancocin).

🝱 IV COMPATIBILITIES
Amikacin, aminophylline, sodium
bicarbonate.

SIDE EFFECTS
Frequent
Somnolence, headache, confusion,
dizziness.
Occasional
Nausea, vomiting, visual
abnormalities, such as spots before

eyes, difficulty focusing, blurred vision, dry mouth or pharynx, tongue irritation, water retention, increased sweating, constipation, or diarrhea.

SERIOUS REACTIONS
• Overdosage results in severe respiratory depression, skeletal muscle flaccidity, bronchospasm, cardiovascular disturbances, such as congestive heart failure (CHF), hypotension or hypertension, arrhythmias, cold and clammy skin, cyanosis, and coma.
• Tolerance may occur with repeated use.
• Extravasation may cause local tissue damage.

PRECAUTIONS & CONSIDERATIONS
Caution is necessary in patients with impaired cardiac, liver, or renal function. Amobarbital crosses the placenta and is distributed in breast milk. Teratogenic effects have been reported after first-trimester exposure; withdrawal reactions have been observed in infants following third-trimester exposure. Behavioral changes are more likely to occur in children and elderly patients. BP for hypotension, level of sedation, and pulse for bradycardia as well as respiratory rate and rhythm should be monitored. Change positions slowly to avoid orthostatic hypotension. Tasks that require mental alertness or motor skills should be avoided.
Storage
Store at room temperature.
Administration
IM: Administer deeply into a large muscle. Do not use more than 5 mL at any single site (may cause tissue damage). Maximum: 500 mg.
IV: Use only when IM administration is not feasible.

Administer by slow IV injection. Each 125 mg must be diluted with a maximum of 1.25 mL of sterile water for injection to make a 10% solution. Do not use solution that has not become clear within 5 min of addition of diluent. Vial should not be left opened for more than 30 min until it is injected. Administer IV only when IM not feasible. The rate of IV injection should not exceed 50 mg/min in adults to prevent sudden respiratory depression, apnea, and hypotension.

Amoxapine
a-moks-a-peen
(Ascendin)
Do not confuse with atomoxetine or atropine.

CATEGORY AND SCHEDULE
Pregnancy Risk Category: C

Classification: Antidepressants, tricyclic

MECHANISM OF ACTION
A tricyclic antidepressant that blocks the reuptake of neurotransmitters, such as norepinephrine and serotonin, at CNS presynaptic membranes, increasing their availability at postsynaptic receptor sites. The metabolite 7-OH-amoxapine has significant dopamine receptor blocking activity similar to that of haloperidol. *Therapeutic Effect:* Produces antidepressant effects.

PHARMACOKINETICS
Rapidly, well absorbed from the GI tract. Protein binding: 90%. Metabolized in liver. Excreted in urine and feces. *Half-life:* 8 h.

AVAILABILITY
Tablets: 25 mg, 50 mg, 100 mg, 150 mg (Ascendin).

INDICATIONS AND DOSAGES
▸ **Depression**
PO
Adults. 50 mg 2-3 times/day. May increase to 100 mg 2-3 times/day. Maximum: 300 mg/day (outpatient); higher doses have been used rarely (inpatient).
Elderly. Initially, 25 mg at bedtime. May increase by 25 mg/day q3-7 days.

CONTRAINDICATIONS
Acute recovery period following myocardial infarction (MI), within 14 days of MAOI ingestion, hypersensitivity to dibenzoxazepine compounds.

INTERACTIONS
Drug
Alcohol, CNS depressants: May increase CNS and respiratory depression and amoxapine's hypotensive effects.
Antithyroid agents: May increase risk of agranulocytosis.
Cimetidine: May increase amoxapine blood concentration and risk of toxicity.
Clonidine, guanadrel: May decrease the effects of clonidine and guanadrel.
Estrogens, SSRIs: May increase risk of amoxapine toxicity.
Fluoroquinolones, sympathomimetics: May increase cardiac effects.
MAOIs: May increase the risk of convulsions, hyperpyresis, and hypertensive crisis. Contraindicated.

Nefopam: May increase risk of seizures.
Phenothiazines: May increase the anticholinergic and sedative effects of clomipramine.
Herbal
St. John's wort: May increase risk of serotonin syndrome.
Food
None known.

DIAGNOSTIC TEST EFFECTS
May increase serum glucose levels.

SIDE EFFECTS
Frequent
Drowsiness, fatigue, xerostomia, constipation, weight gain.
Occasional
Nausea, dizziness, headache, confusion, nervousness, restlessness, insomnia, edema, tremor, blurred vision, aggressiveness, muscle weakness.
Rare
Paradoxical reactions (agitation, restlessness, nightmares, insomnia, extrapyramidal symptoms, particularly fine hand tremor), laryngitis, seizures.

SERIOUS REACTIONS
• High dosage may produce cardiovascular effects, including severe postural hypotension, dizziness, tachycardia, palpitations, arrhythmias, and seizures. High dosage may also result in altered temperature regulation, such as hyperpyrexia or hypothermia.
• Abrupt withdrawal from prolonged therapy may produce headache, malaise, nausea, vomiting, and vivid dreams.
• Extrapyramidal reactions, neuroleptic malignant syndrome, and tardive dyskinesia may occur as a result of the dopamine receptor blocking activity of the metabolite.

PRECAUTIONS & CONSIDERATIONS

Caution is warranted with cardiac conduction disturbances, cardiovascular disease, hyperthyroidism, seizure disorders, and urinary retention and in persons taking thyroid replacement therapy. Be aware that amoxapine is distributed in breast milk. Safety and effectiveness have not been established in children. Antidepressants have been associated with an increased risk of suicidal thinking and behavior in children, adolescents, and young adults with major depressive disorder and other psychiatric disorders.

Expect to use lower dosages in elderly patients. Higher dosages are not tolerated well and increase the risk of toxicity in elderly patients. Blurred vision, drowsiness, constipation, and dry mouth may occur during therapy. Change positions slowly to avoid postural hypotension. Avoid alcohol and tasks that require mental alertness or motor skills. Tolerance usually develops to amoxapine's anticholinergic effects, postural hypotension, and sedative effects. The risk of tardive dyskinesia must be considered when contemplating chronic use.

Storage

Store at room temperature.

Administration

Once dose is established, may be taken as a single dose usually at bedtime, usually without food. May be taken with food to improve GI tolerability. Doses > 300 mg/day should be taken in divided doses.

Amoxicillin
a-mox′i-sill-in
(Alphamax [AUS], Amohexal [AUS], Amoxil, Apo-Amoxi [CAN], Cilamox [AUS], Clamoxyl [AUS], DisperMox, Fisamox [AUS], Moxamox [AUS], Moxacin [AUS], Moxatag, Novamoxin [CAN], Polymox, Trimox, Wymox)
Do not confuse amoxicillin with amoxapine, Diamox, Trimox, or Tylox.

CATEGORY AND SCHEDULE
Pregnancy Risk Category: B

Classification: Antibiotics, penicillins

MECHANISM OF ACTION
A penicillin that inhibits bacterial cell wall synthesis. *Therapeutic Effect:* Bactericidal in susceptible microorganisms.

PHARMACOKINETICS
Well absorbed from the GI tract. Protein binding: 20%. Partially metabolized in the liver. Primarily excreted in urine. Removed by hemodialysis. *Half-life:* 1-1.3 h (increased in impaired renal function).

AVAILABILITY
Capsules (Amoxil, Moxillin, Trimox): 250 mg, 500 mg.
Powder for Suspension, Oral Drops (Amoxil): 50 mg/mL.
Powder for Oral Suspension: 125 mg/5 mL, 200 mg/5 mL, 250 mg/5 mL, 400 mg/5 mL.
Tablets (Amoxil): 500 mg, 875 mg.
Tablets, Chewable (Amoxil): 125 mg, 200 mg, 250 mg, 400 mg.
Tablets for Oral Suspension (DisperMox): 200 mg, 400 mg.

*Tablets, Extended-Release
(Moxatag):* 775 mg.

INDICATIONS AND DOSAGES
▸ **Ear, nose, throat, genitourinary,
skin, and skin-structure infections**
PO
*Adults, Elderly, Children weighing
more than 40 kg.* 250-500 mg q8h or
500-875 mg (tablets) twice a day.
Adults, Children 12 yr of age and older.
775 mg once daily (tonsillitis/pharyngitis
due to *Streptococcus pyogenes*).
Children weighing < 40 kg. 20-45
mg/kg/day in divided doses q8-12h.
▸ **Lower respiratory tract infections**
PO
*Adults, Elderly, Children weighing
more than 40 kg.* 500 mg q8h or 875
mg (tablets) twice a day.
Children weighing < 40 kg.
40 mg/kg/day in divided doses q8h or
45 mg/kg/day in divided doses q12h.
▸ **Acute, uncomplicated gonorrhea**
PO
Adults. 3 g one time with 1 g
probenecid. Follow with tetracycline
or erythromycin therapy.
*Prepubertal children 2 yr and
older.* 50 mg/kg plus probenecid
25 mg/kg as a single dose. Do not
use in children < 2 yr old.
▸ **Acute otitis media**
PO
Children. 80-90 mg/kg/day in
divided doses q12h.
▸ ***Helicobacter pylori* infection**
PO
Adults, Elderly. 1 g two or
three times/day for 14 days (in
combination with other antibiotics).
▸ **Prevention of endocarditis**
PO
Adults, Elderly. 2 g 1 h before
procedure.
Children. 50 mg/kg 1 h before
procedure.
▸ **Usual neonatal and young infant
dosage**

*Children younger than 3 mo,
Neonates.* 20-30 mg/kg/day in
divided doses q12h.
▸ **Dosage in renal impairment (adults)**
Dosage interval is modified based on
creatinine clearance.
Creatinine clearance 10-30 mL/min.
250-500 mg q12h.
Creatinine clearance < 10 mL/min.
250-500 mg q24h.

OFF-LABEL USES
Treatment of Lyme disease and
typhoid fever.

CONTRAINDICATIONS
Hypersensitivity to any penicillin.

INTERACTIONS
Drug
Allopurinol: May increase incidence
of rash.
Oral contraceptives: May
decrease effectiveness of oral
contraceptives.
Probenecid: Increase amoxicillin
blood concentration.

DIAGNOSTIC TEST EFFECTS
May increase BUN and serum LDH,
bilirubin, creatinine, AST (SGOT),
and ALT (SGPT) levels. May cause a
positive Coombs' test.

SIDE EFFECTS
Frequent
GI disturbances (mild diarrhea,
nausea, or vomiting), headache, oral
or vaginal candidiasis.
Occasional
Generalized rash, urticaria,

SERIOUS REACTIONS
• Antibiotic-associated colitis and
other superinfections may result from
altered bacterial balance.
• Severe hypersensitivity reactions,
including anaphylaxis and acute
interstitial nephritis, occur rarely.

PRECAUTIONS & CONSIDERATIONS

Caution is warranted with antibiotic-associated colitis or a history of allergies, especially to cephalosporins. Amoxicillin crosses the placenta, appears in cord blood and amniotic fluid, and is distributed in breast milk in low concentrations. Amoxicillin administration may lead to allergic sensitization, candidiasis, diarrhea, and skin rash in infants. Immature renal function in neonates and young infants may delay renal excretion of amoxicillin. Age-related renal impairment may require dosage adjustment in elderly patients.

History of allergies, especially to cephalosporins or penicillins, should be determined before giving the drug. Withhold amoxicillin and promptly notify the physician if rash or diarrhea occurs. A high percentage of patients with infectious mononucleosis have developed rash during amoxicillin therapy. Severe diarrhea with abdominal pain, blood or mucus in stool, and fever may indicate antibiotic-associated colitis. Signs and symptoms of superinfection, including anal or genital pruritus, black hairy tongue, diarrhea, increased fever, sore throat, ulceration or changes of oral mucosa, and vomiting, should be monitored.

Storage
Store capsules or tablets at room temperature. After reconstitution, the oral suspension is stable for 14 days either at room temperature or refrigerated. Refrigeration is preferred.

Administration
Chew or crush chewable tablets thoroughly before swallowing. Take amoxicillin capsules, tablets, chewable tablets, and suspension without regard to food; extended-release tablets should be taken within 1 h of finishing a meal. Take evenly around the clock and continue for the full course of treatment. Suspension may be mixed with formula, milk, fruit juice, ginger ale, or cold drinks; administered immediately after mixing. Consume the entire dose.

Amoxicillin/ Clavulanate

a-mox´i-sill-in clav-u-lan´ate
(Augmentin, Augmentin ES 600, Augmentin XR, Ausclav [AUS], Ausclav Duo Forte [AUS], Ausclav Duo 400 [AUS], Clamoxyl [AUS], Clamoxyl Duo 400 [AUS], Clamoxyl Duo Forte [AUS], Clavulin [CAN], Clavulin Duo Forte [AUS])
Do not confuse with amoxapine.

CATEGORY AND SCHEDULE
Pregnancy Risk Category: B

Classification: aminopenicillin with a β-lactamase inhibitor

MECHANISM OF ACTION
Amoxicillin inhibits bacterial cell wall synthesis, while clavulanate inhibits bacterial β-lactamase. *Therapeutic Effect:* Amoxicillin is bactericidal in susceptible microorganisms. Clavulanate protects amoxicillin from enzymatic degradation.

PHARMACOKINETICS
Well absorbed from the GI tract. Protein binding: 20%. Partially metabolized in the liver. Primarily excreted in urine. Removed by hemodialysis. *Half-life:* 1-1.3 h (increased in impaired renal function).

AVAILABILITY

Powder for Oral Suspension:
125 mg/31.25 mg per 5 mL,
200 mg/28.5 mg per 5 mL,
250 mg/62.5 mg per 5 mL,
400 mg/57 mg per 5 mL,
600 mg/42.9 mg per 5 mL.
Tablets: 250 mg/125 mg, 500 mg/
125 mg, 875 mg/125 mg.
Tablets (Extended-Release):
1000 mg/62.5 mg.
Tablets (Chewable): 200 mg/28.5 mg,
250 mg/62.5 mg, 400 mg/57 mg.

INDICATIONS AND DOSAGES

Note: Weight-based dosing is based
on amoxicillin component.
▸ **Mild to moderate infections**
PO
*Adults, Elderly, Children weighing
more than 40 kg.* 250 mg q8h or
500 mg q12h.
Children weighing < 40 kg. 20 mg/
kg/day in divided doses q8h or
25 mg/kg/day in divided doses q12h.
▸ **Respiratory tract and other severe
infections**
PO
*Adults, Elderly, Children weighing
more than 40 kg.* 500 mg q8h or
875 mg q12h.
Children weighing < 40 kg. 40 mg/
kg/day in divided doses q8h or
45 mg/kg/day in divided doses q12h.
▸ **Otitis media**
PO
Children. 90 mg/kg/day in divided
doses q12h for 10 days.
▸ **Sinusitis, lower respiratory tract
infections**
PO
Children. 40 mg/kg/day in divided
doses q8h or 45 mg/kg/day in
divided doses q12h.
▸ **Usual neonate dosage**
PO
*Neonates, Children younger than
3 mo.* 30 mg/kg/day in divided doses
q12h.

▸ **Dosage in renal impairment**
Dosage and frequency are modified
based on creatinine clearance. Adults:
Creatinine clearance 10-30 mL/min:
250-500 mg q12h.
Creatinine clearance < 10 mL/min:
250-500 mg q24h.

OFF-LABEL USES

Treatment of bronchitis and
chancroid.

CONTRAINDICATIONS

Hypersensitivity to any penicillins,
history of cholestatic jaundice/
hepatic function impairment
associated with amoxicillin/
clavulanate; extended-release
formulation also contraindicated
in severe renal impairment (CrCl
< 30 mL/min) and in hemodialysis
patients.

INTERACTIONS

Drug
Allopurinol: May increase incidence
of rash.
Oral contraceptives: May decrease
effects of oral contraceptives.
Probenecid: May increase amoxicillin
and clavulanate blood concentration.

DIAGNOSTIC TEST EFFECTS

May increase serum AST (SGOT)
and ALT (SGPT) levels. May cause a
positive Coombs' test.

SIDE EFFECTS

Frequent
GI disturbances (mild diarrhea,
nausea, vomiting), headache, oral or
vaginal candidiasis.
Occasional
Generalized rash, urticaria.

SERIOUS REACTIONS

• Antibiotic-associated colitis and
other superinfections may result from
altered bacterial balance.

• Severe hypersensitivity reactions, including anaphylaxis and acute interstitial nephritis, occur rarely.
• Hepatotoxicity (rare).

PRECAUTIONS & CONSIDERATIONS
Caution is warranted with antibiotic-associated colitis or a history of allergies, especially to cephalosporins. Amoxicillin and clavulanate cross the placenta, appear in cord blood and amniotic fluid, and are distributed in breast milk in low concentrations. Amoxicillin and clavulanate may lead to allergic sensitization, candidiasis, diarrhea, and skin rash in infants. Immature renal function in neonates and young infants may delay renal excretion of amoxicillin and clavulanate. Age-related renal impairment may require dosage adjustment in elderly patients.

History of allergies, especially to cephalosporins or penicillins, should be determined before giving the drug. Withhold and promptly notify the physician if rash or diarrhea occurs. Severe diarrhea with abdominal pain, blood or mucus in stool, and fever may indicate antibiotic-associated colitis. Signs and symptoms of superinfection, including anal or genital pruritus, black hairy tongue, diarrhea, increased fever, sore throat, ulceration or changes of oral mucosa, and vomiting, should be monitored.

Storage
Store capsules or tablets at room temperature. After reconstitution, the oral suspension is stable for 10 days refrigerated.

Administration
! Drug dosage is expressed in terms of amoxicillin. Dosage forms cannot be interchanged based on amoxicillin component alone; must also consider clavulanate content.

May be taken without regard to meals; however, absorption is enhanced and tolerability improved when taken at the start of a meal. Chew or crush chewable tablets thoroughly before swallowing. Space doses evenly around the clock and continue for the full course of treatment.

Amphetamine; Dextroamphetamine
am-fet'ah-meen
(Adderall, Adderall XR)

CATEGORY AND SCHEDULE
Pregnancy Risk Category: C
Controlled substance: Schedule II

Classification: Adrenergic agonists, amphetamines, anorexiants, stimulants, central nervous system

MECHANISM OF ACTION
A sympathomimetic amine that produces CNS and respiratory stimulation, mydriasis, bronchodilation, a pressor response, and contraction of the urinary sphincter. Directly affects α and β receptor sites in peripheral system. Enhances release of norepinephrine by blocking reuptake, inhibiting monoamine oxidase. *Therapeutic Effect:* Increases motor activity, mental alertness; decreases drowsiness, fatigue. Mechanism in attention-deficit hyperactivity disorder (ADHD) is not known.

PHARMACOKINETICS
Well absorbed from the GI tract. Protein binding: 20%. Widely distributed (including CSF).

Metabolized in liver. Excreted in urine. Unknown if removed by hemodialysis. *Half-life:* 9-14 h.

AVAILABILITY

Adderall XR Capsules (Extended-Release): 5-mg, 10-mg, 15-mg, 20-mg, 25-mg, and 30-mg tablets.
Tablets: 5 mg, 7.5 mg, 10 mg, 12.5 mg, 15 mg, 20 mg, 30 mg.

INDICATIONS AND DOSAGES
▸ **ADHD**
PO
Adults. 5-20 mg 1-3 times/day.
Adults, Children older than 12 yr. Initially, 5 mg twice a day. Increase by 10 mg at weekly intervals until therapeutic response achieved. Usual maximum: 60 mg/day.
Children 6-12 yr. Initially, 5 mg twice a day. Increase by 5 mg/day at weekly intervals until therapeutic response achieved. Usual maximum: 40 mg/day.
Children 3-6 yr. Initially, 5 mg once or twice a day. Increase by 5 mg/day at weekly intervals until therapeutic response achieved.
▸ **Narcolepsy**
PO
Adults. 5-20 mg 1-3 times/day.
Children older than 12 yr. Initially, 5 mg twice a day. Increase by 10 mg at weekly intervals until therapeutic response achieved. Usual maximum: 60 mg/day.
Children 6-12 yr. Initially, 5 mg once or twice a day. Increase by 5 mg/day at weekly intervals until therapeutic response achieved. Usual maximum: 60 mg/day.
▸ **Extended-release tablets**
Adults. Usual 5-20 mg once daily. Maximum: 30 mg/day.
Children 6 yr and older. Initially, 5-10 mg once daily. Increase by 5 or 10 mg weekly to effective dose. Maximum: 30 mg/day.

Children < 6 yr. Do not use extended release.

OFF-LABEL USES
Depression, obsessive-compulsive disorder.

CONTRAINDICATIONS
Advanced arteriosclerosis, agitated states, glaucoma, history of drug abuse, history of hypersensitivity to sympathomimetic amines, hyperthyroidism, moderate to severe hypertension, symptomatic cardiovascular disease, within 14 days following discontinuation of an MAOI.

INTERACTIONS
Drug
β-blockers: May increase risk of bradycardia, heart block, and hypertension.
CNS stimulants: May increase the effects of amphetamine.
Digoxin: May increase the risk of arrhythmias with this drug.
MAOIs: May prolong and intensify the effects of amphetamine. Contraindicated.
Meperidine: May increase the risk of hypotension, respiratory depression, seizures, and vascular collapse.
Tricyclic antidepressants: May increase cardiovascular effects.

DIAGNOSTIC TEST EFFECTS
May increase plasma corticosteroid concentrations.

SIDE EFFECTS
Frequent
Irregular pulse, increased motor activity, talkativeness, nervousness, mild euphoria, insomnia.
Occasional
Headache, chills, dry mouth, GI distress, worsening depression in

patients who are clinically depressed, tachycardia, palpitations, chest pain.

SERIOUS REACTIONS
• Overdose may produce skin pallor or flushing, arrhythmias, and psychosis.
• Abrupt withdrawal following prolonged administration of high dosage may produce lethargy (may last for weeks).
• Prolonged administration to children with ADHD may produce a temporary suppression of normal weight and height patterns.

PRECAUTIONS & CONSIDERATIONS
Med Guide is required with each prescription and refill. Precaution is necessary with acute stress reaction, emotional instability, history of drug dependence, hypertension, seizures, and in elderly and debilitated patients and those who are tartrazine-sensitive. Amphetamine crosses the placenta and is distributed in breast milk. Use in pregnancy may be associated with teratogenic effects, premature delivery, low birthweight, and infant withdrawal symptoms. Children may be more susceptible to develop abdominal pain, anorexia, decreased weight, and insomnia. A thorough cardiovascular assessment is recommended before initiation of therapy in pediatric patients; assessment should include medical history, family history, and physical examination with consideration of ECG testing. There are no age-related precautions noted for elderly patients.

Decreased appetite, dizziness, dry mouth, or pronounced nervousness may be experienced. Tasks that require mental alertness or motor skills should be avoided until the effects of the drug are determined.

Storage
Store at room temperature.
  Protect from light.
  Keep tightly closed.
Administration
Do not take in afternoon or evening because the drug can cause insomnia.
  The first dose is given on awakening.
  Do not crush, chew, or cut XR form.
  XR form may be opened and sprinkled on 1 tsp of applesauce; entire dose is swallowed immediately.

Amphotericin B/ Amphotericin B Cholesteryl/ Amphotericin B Lipid Complex/ Liposomal Amphotericin B
am-foe-ter′i-sin bee
(Abelcet, AmBisome, Amphocin, Amphotec, Fungizone)

CATEGORY AND SCHEDULE
Pregnancy Risk Category: B

Classification: Antifungals

MECHANISM OF ACTION
An antifungal and antiprotozoal that is generally fungistatic but may become fungicidal with high dosages or very susceptible microorganisms. This drug binds to sterols in the fungal cell membrane. Lipid-based formulations deliver higher drug concentrations to sites of infection and reduced levels in normal tissues. *Therapeutic Effect:* Increases fungal cell-membrane permeability, allowing loss of potassium and other cellular components. Fungicidal.

PHARMACOKINETICS

Protein binding: 90%. Widely distributed. Metabolic fate unknown. Excreted slowly over weeks to months by the kidneys. Approximately 40% of a given dose is excreted in the first 7 days. Minimal removal by hemodialysis. Amphotec and Abelcet are not dialyzable. *Half-life:* amphotericin B desoxycholate, 24 h (increased in neonates and children); Amphotec, 26-28 h; Abelcet, 7.2 days; AmBisome, 100-153 h.

AVAILABILITY

Injection, Powder for Reconstitution: (Amphotec): 50 mg, 100 mg.
Injection, Powder for Reconstitution (AmBisome, Amphocin, amphotericin B desoxycholate): 50 mg.
Injection, Suspension (Abelcet): 5 mg/mL.

INDICATIONS AND DOSAGES
▸ **Cryptococcosis; blastomycosis; systemic candidiasis; disseminated forms of moniliasis, coccidioidomycosis, and histoplasmosis; zygomycosis; sporotrichosis; aspergillosis**
IV INFUSION (AMPHOTERICIN B DESOXYCHOLATE)
Adults, Elderly. Dosage based on patient tolerance and severity of infection. Initially, 1-mg test dose is given over 20-30 min. If test dose is tolerated, 5-mg dose may be given the same day. Subsequently, dosage is increased by 5 mg q12-24h until desired daily dose is reached. Alternatively, if test dose is tolerated, 0.25 mg/kg is given on same day and 0.5 mg/kg on second day; then dosage is increased until desired daily dose is reached. Total daily dose: 1 mg/kg/day up to 1.5 mg/kg every other day. Maximum: 1.5 mg/kg/day.
Children. Test dose of 0.1 mg/kg/dose (maximum 1 mg) is infused over 20-60 min. If test dose is tolerated, initial dose of 0.4 mg/kg may be given on same day; dosage is then increased in 0.25-mg/kg increments as needed. Maintenance dose: 0.25-1 mg/kg/day.
▸ **Invasive fungal infections unresponsive to or intolerant of amphotericin B.**
IV INFUSION (ABELCET)
Adults, Children. 5 mg/kg at rate of 2.5 mg/kg/h.
▸ **Empiric treatment of fungal infections in patients with febrile neutropenia; aspergillosis, candidiasis, or cryptococcosis in patients with renal impairment and those who have experienced toxicity or treatment failure with amphotericin B desoxycholate**
IV INFUSION (AMBISOME)
Adults, Children. 3-5 mg/kg over 1 h.
▸ **Invasive aspergillosis in patients with renal impairment and those who have experienced toxicity or treatment failure with amphotericin B desoxycholate**
IV INFUSION (AMPHOTEC)
Adults, Children. 3-4 mg/kg over 2-4 h.

CONTRAINDICATIONS
Hypersensitivity to amphotericin B.

INTERACTIONS
Drug
Bone marrow depressants: May increase the risk of anemia.
Digoxin: May increase the risk of digoxin toxicity from hypokalemia.
Nephrotoxic medications: May increase the risk of nephrotoxicity.
Steroids: May cause severe hypokalemia.

DIAGNOSTIC TEST EFFECTS
May increase BUN, serum alkaline phosphatase, serum creatinine, serum SGOT (AST), and SGPT (ALT)

levels. May decrease serum calcium, magnesium, and potassium levels.

ⓘ IV INCOMPATIBILITIES

Abelcet, AmBisome, Amphotec: Do not mix with any other drug, diluent, or solution. Amphotericin B desoxycholate: Allopurinol (Aloprim), amifostine (Ethyol), aztreonam (Azactam), calcium gluconate, cefepime (Maxipime), cimetidine (Tagamet), ciprofloxacin (Cipro), docetaxel (Taxotere), dopamine (Intropin), doxorubicin (Adriamycin), enalapril (Vasotec), etoposide (VP-16), filgrastim (Neupogen), fluconazole (Diflucan), fludarabine (Fludara), foscarnet (Foscavir), gemcitabine (Gemzar), magnesium sulfate, meropenem (Merrem IV), ondansetron (Zofran), paclitaxel (Taxol), piperacillin and tazobactam (Zosyn), potassium chloride, propofol (Diprivan), vinorelbine (Navelbine).

ⓘ IV COMPATIBILITIES

Do not mix with other medications or electrolytes or preservatives.

SIDE EFFECTS

Frequent (> 10%)
Abelcet: Chills, fever, increased serum creatinine level, multiple organ failure.
AmBisome: Hypokalemia, hypomagnesemia, hyperglycemia, hypocalcemia, edema, abdominal pain, back pain, chills, chest pain, hypotension, diarrhea, nausea, vomiting, headache, fever, rigors, insomnia, dyspnea, epistaxis, increased hepatic or renal function test results.
Amphotec: Chills, fever, hypotension, tachycardia, increased serum creatinine level, hypokalemia, bilirubinemia.
Amphotericin B desoxycholate: Fever, chills, headache, anemia,

hypokalemia, hypomagnesemia, anorexia, malaise, generalized pain, nephrotoxicity.

SERIOUS REACTIONS

• Cardiovascular toxicity (as evidenced by hypotension, ventricular fibrillation, and anaphylaxis) occurs rarely.
• Altered vision and hearing, seizures, hepatic failure, coagulation defects, multiple organ failure, and sepsis may be noted.

PRECAUTIONS & CONSIDERATIONS

Caution is warranted with renal impairment and in combination with antineoplastic therapy. Drug is prescribed only for progressive, potentially fatal fungal infection. Keep in mind that conventional amphotericin, amphotericin B desoxycholate, is more nephrotoxic than the alternative formulations of amphotericin B, including Albecet, AmBisome, and Amphotec. Amphotericin B crosses the placenta, and it is unknown whether amphotericin B is distributed in breast milk. There are no age-related precautions noted in children or in elderly patients.

History of allergies, especially to amphotericin B and sulfites, should be determined before giving the drug. Be aware that other nephrotoxic medications should be avoided, if possible. Antiemetics, antihistamines, antipyretics, or small doses of corticosteroids may be given before or during amphotericin administration to help control adverse reactions.

BP, pulse, respirations, and temperature should be monitored twice every 15 min, then every 30 min for the initial 4 h of the infusion to assess for adverse reactions. Adverse reactions include abdominal pain, anorexia, chills, fever, nausea, shaking, and vomiting. If signs and symptoms of adverse reactions occur, slow the infusion and give prescribed drugs to provide symptomatic relief. For a severe reaction or for patients without orders for symptomatic relief, stop the infusion and notify the physician.

Storage

Refrigerate Albecet as unreconstituted solution. Albecet reconstituted solution is stable for 48 h if refrigerated and 6 h at room temperature.

Refrigerate AmBisome as unreconstituted solution. AmBisome reconstituted solution of 4 mg/mL is stable for 24 h. AmBisome reconstituted solution concentration of 1-2 mg/mL is stable for 6 h.

Store Amphotec as unreconstituted solution at room temperature. Amphotec reconstituted solution and diluted for infusion are stable for 24 h if refrigerated.

Refrigerate Fungizone as unreconstituted solution. Fungizone reconstituted solution is stable for 24 h at room temperature or 7 days if refrigerated. Diluted solution ≤ 0.1 mg/mL should be used promptly. Do not use the solution if it is cloudy or contains a precipitate. Protect from light.

Administration

To prevent inadvertent overdose with amphotericin B, verify product name and dosage if dose exceeds 1.5 mg/kg. Amphotericin products are not interchangeable. For IV use, observe strict aseptic technique because no bacteriostatic agent or preservative is present.

Shake Abelcet 20-mL (100-mg) vial gently until contents are dissolved. Withdraw required Abelcet dose using a 5-μm filter needle supplied by manufacturer. Inject Abelcet dose into D5W; 4 mL D5W is required for each 1 mL (5 mg) to final concentration of 1 mg/mL. Double concentration for pediatric and fluid-restricted patients (2 mg/mL). Infuse Abelcet over 2 h by slow IV infusion. Shake the contents if the infusion is > 2 h. Reconstitute each 50-mg AmBisome vial with 12 mL sterile water for injection to provide concentration of 4 mg/mL. Shake AmBisome vial vigorously for 30 s. Then withdraw the required AmBisome dose and empty the syringe contents through a 5-μm filter into an infusion of D5W to provide final concentration of 1-2 mg/mL. Infuse AmBisome over 1-2 h by slow IV infusion.

Add 10 mL sterile water for injection to each 50-mg Amphotec vial to provide a concentration of 5 mg/mL. Shake the Amphotec vial gently. Further dilute Amphotec vial only with D5W using specific amount recommended by manufacturer to provide concentration of 0.16-0.83 mg/mL. Infuse Amphotec over 2-4 h by slow IV infusion.

Rapidly inject 10 mL Sterile Water for Injection to each 50-mg amphotericin B desoxycholate vial to provide concentration of 5 mg/mL. Immediately shake amphotericin B desoxycholate vial until the solution is clear. Further dilute each 1 mg amphotericin B desoxycholate in at least 10 mL D5W to provide a concentration of 0.1 mg/mL. Be aware that the potential for thrombophlebitis may be less with the use of pediatric scalp vein needles or by adding dilute heparin solution, as prescribed. Infuse conventional amphotericin over 2-6 h by slow IV infusion.

Ampicillin Sodium
am-pi-sill'in soe'dee-um
(Alphacin [AUS], Apo-Ampi [CAN],
Novo-Ampicillin [CAN], Nu-Ampi
[CAN], Principen)
**Do not confuse ampicillin with
aminophylline, Imipenem, or
Unipen.**

CATEGORY AND SCHEDULE
Pregnancy Risk Category: B

Classification: aminopenicillin

MECHANISM OF ACTION
A penicillin that inhibits cell wall
synthesis in susceptible microorganisms.
Therapeutic Effect: Bactericidal.

PHARMACOKINETICS
Moderately absorbed from the GI
tract. Protein binding: 28%. Widely
distributed. Partially metabolized in
the liver. Primarily excreted in urine.
Removed by hemodialysis. *Half-life:*
1-1.5 h (increased in impaired renal
function).

AVAILABILITY
Capsules: 250 mg, 500 mg.
Powder for Oral Suspension:
125 mg/5 mL, 250 mg/5 mL,
Powder for Injection: 250 mg,
500 mg, 1 g, 2 g.

INDICATIONS AND DOSAGES
▶ **Respiratory tract, skin, and
skin-structure infections**
PO
*Adults, Elderly, Children weighing
more than 40 kg.* 250-1000 mg q6h.
Children weighing < 20 kg.
50-100 mg/kg/day in divided doses
q6h.
IV, IM
*Adults, Elderly, Children weighing
more than 40 kg.* 500-1000 mg q6h.

Children weighing < 40 kg. 25-50
mg/kg/day in divided doses q6h.
▶ **Bacterial meningitis, septicemia**
IV, IM
Adults, Elderly. 2 g q4h or 3 g q6h.
Children. 100-200 mg/kg/day in
divided doses q3-4h.
▶ **Uncomplicated gonococcal
infections**
PO
Adults. 3.5 g one time with 1 g
probenecid.
▶ **Perioperative prophylaxis**
IV, IM
Adults, Elderly. 2 g 30 min before
procedure. May repeat in 8 h.
Children. 50 mg/kg 30 min before
procedure. May repeat in 8 h.
▶ **Usual neonatal dosage**
Neonates 7-28 days old. 75 mg/kg/
day in divided doses q8h up to 200
mg/kg/day in divided doses q6h.
Neonates 0-7 days old. 50 mg/kg/day
in divided doses q12h up to 150
mg/kg/day in divided doses q8h.
▶ **Dosage in renal impairment (adults)**

Creatinine Clearance (mL/min)	% of Normal Dosage
10-30	Give q6-12h
< 10	Give q12h

CONTRAINDICATIONS
Hypersensitivity to any penicillin.

INTERACTIONS
Drug
Allopurinol: May increase incidence
of rash.
Oral contraceptives: May decrease
effectiveness of oral contraceptives.
Probenecid: May increase
ampicillin blood concentration.
Herbal
None known.
Food
None known.

DIAGNOSTIC TEST EFFECTS
May increase AST (SGOT) and ALT (SGPT) levels. May cause a positive Coombs' test.

⑦ IV INCOMPATIBILITIES
Amikacin (Amikin), diltiazem (Cardizem), gentamicin, midazolam (Versed).

🍶 IV COMPATIBILITIES
Calcium gluconate, cefepime (Maxipime), dopamine (Intropin), famotidine (Pepcid), furosemide (Lasix), heparin, hydromorphone (Dilaudid), insulin (regular), levofloxacin (Levaquin), magnesium sulfate, morphine, multivitamins, potassium chloride, propofol (Diprivan).

SIDE EFFECTS
Frequent
Pain at IM injection site, GI disturbances (mild diarrhea, nausea, vomiting), oral or vaginal candidiasis.
Occasional
Generalized rash, urticaria, phlebitis or thrombophlebitis (with IV administration), headache.
Rare
Dizziness, seizures (especially with IV therapy).

SERIOUS REACTIONS
• Antibiotic-associated colitis and other superinfections may result from altered bacterial balance.
• Severe hypersensitivity reactions, including anaphylaxis and acute interstitial nephritis, occur rarely.

PRECAUTIONS & CONSIDERATIONS
Caution is warranted with antibiotic-associated colitis or a history of allergies, especially to cephalosporins. Ampicillin readily crosses the placenta, appears in cord blood and amniotic fluid, and is distributed in breast milk in low concentrations. Ampicillin may lead to allergic sensitization, candidiasis, diarrhea, and skin rash in infants. Immature renal function in neonates and young infants may delay renal excretion of ampicillin. Keep in mind that high dosages may be needed for neonatal meningitis. Age-related renal impairment may require dosage adjustment for elderly patients.

History of allergies, especially to cephalosporins or penicillins, should be determined before giving the drug. Withhold and promptly notify the physician if rash or diarrhea occurs. A high incidence of rash has been observed in patients with infectious mononucleosis treated with ampicillin. Severe diarrhea with abdominal pain, blood or mucus in stool, and fever may indicate antibiotic-associated colitis. Signs and symptoms of superinfection, including anal or genital pruritus, black hairy tongue, diarrhea, increased fever, sore throat, ulceration or changes in oral mucosa, and vomiting, should be monitored. Intake and output, renal function tests, urinalysis, and the injection sites should be assessed.
Storage
Store capsules at room temperature. After reconstitution, the oral solution is stable for 7 days at room temperature or 14 days if refrigerated. Refrigeration is preferred. An IV solution diluted with 0.9% NaCl is stable for 2-8 h at room temperature or 3 days if refrigerated. An IV solution diluted with D5W is stable for 2 h at room temperature or 3 h if refrigerated. Discard the IV solution if a precipitate forms. The reconstituted solution for IM injection is stable for 1 h.
Administration
Give oral forms 1 h before or 2 h after meals for maximum absorption. Shake oral solution well before use.

For IV injection, dilute each 250- or 500-mg vial with 5 mL sterile water for injection and each 1- or 2-g vial with 10 mL. For intermittent IV infusion (piggyback), further dilute with 50-100 mL 0.9% NaCl or D5W. Administer each 125-, 250-, or 500-mg dose over 3-5 min and each 1- to 2-g dose over 10-15 min. Infuse intermittent IV infusion (piggyback) over 20-30 min. Because of the potential for hypersensitivity and anaphylaxis, start the initial dose at a few drops per minute, increase the dosage slowly to the prescribed rate, and stay with the patient for the first 10-15 min. Then assess every 10 min during the infusion for signs and symptoms of hypersensitivity or anaphylaxis. Expect to switch to the oral route as soon as possible.

For IM use, reconstitute each vial with sterile water for injection or bacteriostatic water for injection. Consult individual ampicillin vials or package insert for specific volumes of diluent. Inject the drug deep into a large muscle mass.

Ampicillin/ Sulbactam
am'pi-sill-in/sul-bac'tam
(Unasyn)

CATEGORY AND SCHEDULE
Pregnancy Risk Category: B

Classification: Aminopenicillin

MECHANISM OF ACTION
Ampicillin inhibits bacterial cell wall synthesis, whereas sulbactam inhibits bacterial β-lactamase. *Therapeutic Effect:* Ampicillin is bactericidal in susceptible microorganisms. Sulbactam protects ampicillin from enzymatic degradation.

PHARMACOKINETICS
Protein binding: 28%-38%. Widely distributed. Partially metabolized in the liver. Primarily excreted in urine. Removed by hemodialysis. *Half-life:* 1 h (increased in impaired renal function).

AVAILABILITY
Powder for Injection: 1.5 g (ampicillin 1 g/sulbactam 500 g), 3 g (ampicillin 2 g/sulbactam 1 g).

INDICATIONS AND DOSAGES
▸ **Skin/skin-structure, intra-abdominal, and gynecologic infections**
IV, IM
Adults, Elderly, Children > 40 kg.
1.5 g (1 g ampicillin/500 mg sulbactam) to 3 g (2 g ampicillin/1 g sulbactam) q6h.
Children 1-12 yr and < 40 kg. 150-300 mg/kg/day in divided doses q6h.
▸ **Dosage in renal impairment**
Dosage and frequency are modified based on creatinine clearance and the severity of the infection.

Creatinine Clearance (mL/min)	Adult Dosage
> 30	1.5-3 g q6-8h
15-29	1.5-3 g q12h
5-14	1.5-3 g q24h
< 5	Not recommended

CONTRAINDICATIONS
Hypersensitivity to any penicillin.

INTERACTIONS
Drug
Allopurinol: May increase incidence of rash.

Oral contraceptives: May decrease effectiveness of oral contraceptives.
Probenecid: May increase ampicillin blood concentration.
Herbal
None known.
Food
None known.

DIAGNOSTIC TEST EFFECTS

May increase serum LDH, alkaline phosphatase, creatinine, AST (SGOT), and ALT (SGPT) levels. May cause a positive Coombs' test.

⚕ IV INCOMPATIBILITIES

Acyclovir, diltiazem (Cardizem), idarubicin (Idamycin), ondansetron (Zofran), sargramostim (Leukine).

SIDE EFFECTS

Frequent
Diarrhea and rash (most common), urticaria, pain at IM injection site, thrombophlebitis with IV administration, oral or vaginal candidiasis.
Occasional
Nausea, vomiting, headache, malaise, urine retention.

SERIOUS REACTIONS

• Severe hypersensitivity reactions, including anaphylaxis, acute interstitial nephritis, and blood dyscrasias, may occur.
• Antibiotic-associated colitis and other superinfections may result from altered bacterial balance.
• Overdose may produce seizures.

PRECAUTIONS & CONSIDERATIONS

Caution is warranted with antibiotic-associated colitis or a history of allergies, especially to cephalosporins. Ampicillin and sulbactam readily cross the placenta, appear in cord blood and amniotic fluid, and are distributed in breast milk in low concentrations. Ampicillin and sulbactam may lead to allergic sensitization, candidiasis, diarrhea, and skin rash in infants. The safety and efficacy of ampicillin and sulbactam have not been established in children younger than 1 yr. Age-related renal impairment may require dosage adjustment in elderly patients.

History of allergies, especially to cephalosporins or penicillins, should be determined before giving the drug. Withhold and promptly notify the physician if rash or diarrhea occurs. A high incidence of rash has been observed in patients with infectious mononucleosis treated with ampicillin. Severe diarrhea with abdominal pain, blood or mucus in stool, and fever may indicate antibiotic-associated colitis. Signs and symptoms of superinfection, including anal or genital pruritus, black hairy tongue, diarrhea, increased fever, sore throat, ulceration or changes of oral mucosa, and vomiting, should be monitored. Intake and output, renal function tests, urinalysis, and the injection sites should be assessed.
Storage
Store at room temperature prior to reconstitution. When reconstituted with 0.9% NaCl, the IV solution is stable for 8 h at room temperature or 48 h if refrigerated. Stability may differ with other diluents. Discard the IV solution if a precipitate forms.
Administration
For IV injection, dilute with 10-20 mL sterile water for injection. For intermittent IV infusion (piggyback), further dilute with 50-100 mL D5W or 0.9% NaCl. Administer IV injection slowly, over 10-15 min. Administer intermittent IV infusion (piggyback) over 15-30 min. Because of the potential for hypersensitivity and anaphylaxis, start the initial dose at a few drops

per minute and then increase the dose slowly to the ordered rate. Stay with the patient for the first 10-15 min; then check every 10 min during the infusion for signs and symptoms of hypersensitivity or anaphylaxis. Expect to switch to an oral antibiotic as soon as possible.

For IM use, reconstitute each 1.5-g vial with 3.2 mL or each 3-g vial with 6.4 mL of sterile water for injection to provide a concentration of 250 mg ampicillin/125 mg sulbactam per milliliter. Administer the injection deep into a large muscle mass within 1 h of preparation.

Amyl Nitrite
am′il nye′-trite
(Amyl Nitrite)
Do not confuse with Nicobid, Nicoderm, Nilstat, nitroprusside, Nitrates, Nizoral, or Nystatin.

CATEGORY AND SCHEDULE
Pregnancy Risk Category: C

Classification: Antianginal; nitrates, vasodilators

MECHANISM OF ACTION
A nitrite vasodilator that relaxes smooth muscles. Reduces afterload and improves vascular supply to the myocardium. *Therapeutic Effect:* Dilates coronary arteries, improves blood flow to ischemic areas within myocardium. Following inhalation, systemic vasodilation occurs.

PHARMACOKINETICS
The vapors are absorbed rapidly through the pulmonary alveoli and metabolized rapidly. Partially excreted in the urine.

AVAILABILITY
Inhalation: 0.3 mL glass ampule (amyl nitrite).

INDICATIONS AND DOSAGES
▸ **Acute relief of angina pectoris**
NASAL INHALATION
Adults, Elderly. Place crushed capsule to nostrils for 0.18-0.3 mL inhalation of vapors. Repeat at 5- to 10-min intervals. No more than 3 doses in 30-min period. Call emergency if pain is not relieved after one dose, even though repeat dose will be given.

OFF-LABEL USES
Cyanide toxicity.

CONTRAINDICATIONS
Closed-angle glaucoma, cerebral hemorrhage or recent head injury, postural hypotension, hypersensitivity to nitrates.

INTERACTIONS
Drug
Sildenafil: May increase hypotensive effects. Contraindicated.
Herbal
None known.
Food
Ethanol: May increase hypotensive effects.

DIAGNOSTIC TEST EFFECTS
None known.

SIDE EFFECTS
Frequent
Headache (may be severe) occurs mostly in early therapy, diminishes rapidly in intensity, usually disappears during continued treatment; transient flushing of face and neck; dizziness (especially if patient is standing immobile or is in a warm environment); weakness; postural hypotension.

Occasional
Nausea, rash, vomiting.
Rare
Involuntary passage of urine and feces, restlessness, weakness.

SERIOUS REACTIONS
• Large doses may produce hemolytic anemia or methemoglobinemia.
• Severe postural hypotension manifested by fainting, pulselessness, cold or clammy skin, and profuse sweating may occur.
• Tolerance may occur with repeated, prolonged therapy.
• High dose tends to produce severe headache.

PRECAUTIONS & CONSIDERATIONS
Caution is warranted in patients with acute MI, blood volume depletion from diuretic therapy, glaucoma (contraindicated in closed-angle glaucoma), liver or renal disease, severe anemia, and systolic BP < 90 mm Hg. Test for apical pulse and blood pressure before amyl nitrite is administered and periodically after dose. Facial or neck flushing should be reported.

It is unknown whether amyl nitrite crosses the placenta or is distributed in breast milk. Safety and efficacy of amyl nitrite have not been established in children. Elderly patients are more susceptible to the hypotensive effects of amyl nitrite, and age-related renal impairment may require cautious use.
Storage
Store at room temperature and protect from light. Keep the drug container away from heat and moisture.
Administration
Capsules for inhalation should be used at the first sign of angina. Wrap ampule in woven sterile gauze. Crush amyl nitrite capsule with fingers and hold to the nostrils for inhalation of vapors. Wave under the nose; patient should inhale 1-6 times. May repeat in 3-5 min.

Anagrelide
ah-na′greh-lide
(Agrylin)

CATEGORY AND SCHEDULE
Pregnancy Risk Category: C

Classification: Platelet count-reducing agent

MECHANISM OF ACTION
A hematologic agent that reduces platelet production and prevents platelet shape changes caused by platelet-aggregating agents. *Therapeutic Effect:* Inhibits platelet aggregation.

PHARMACOKINETICS
After oral administration, plasma concentration peaks within 1 h. Extensively metabolized. Primarily excreted in urine. *Half-life:* 1.3 h.

AVAILABILITY
Capsules: 0.5 mg, 1 mg.

INDICATIONS AND DOSAGES
▸ **Thrombocythemia secondary to myeloproliferative disorders**
PO
Adults, Elderly. Initially, 0.5 mg 4 times a day or 1 mg twice a day. Adjust to lowest effective dosage, increasing by up to 0.5 mg/day or less in any 1 wk. Maximum: 10 mg/day or 2.5 mg/dose.
Children. Initially 0.5 mg/day. Adjust to lowest effective dose, increasing by up to 0.5 mg/day or less in any

1 wk. Maximum: 10 mg/day or 2.5 mg/dose.
Dose in hepatic impairment. Initially 0.5 mg/day. Adjust to lowest effective dose, increasing by up to 0.5 mg/day or less in any 1 wk.

CONTRAINDICATIONS
Severe hepatic impairment.

INTERACTIONS
Drug
None known.
Herbal
None known.
Food
None known.

DIAGNOSTIC TEST EFFECTS
May increase hepatic enzyme levels (rare).

SIDE EFFECTS
Frequent (≥5%)
Headache, palpitations, diarrhea, abdominal pain, nausea, flatulence, bloating, asthenia, pain, dizziness.
Occasional (< 5%)
Tachycardia, chest pain, vomiting, paresthesia, peripheral edema, anorexia, dyspepsia, rash.
Rare
Confusion, insomnia.

SERIOUS REACTIONS
• Angina, heart failure, and arrhythmias occur rarely.

PRECAUTIONS & CONSIDERATIONS
Caution is warranted with cardiac disease and hepatic or renal impairment. It is unknown whether anagrelide crosses the placenta or is distributed in breast milk. Anagrelide may cause fetal harm; it is not recommended in pregnant women. Strongly urge women to use contraceptives while taking anagrelide. Age-related precautions

have not been observed in pediatric patients. Use anagrelide cautiously in elderly patients, who may have age-related cardiac disease and decreased renal and hepatic function.

Hemoglobin, hematocrit, and platelet and WBC counts should be obtained before treatment, every 2 days during the first week of treatment, and weekly thereafter until therapeutic range is achieved. Skin should be monitored for bruises or petechiae, and catheter and needle sites should be inspected for bleeding. Persons with suspected heart disease should be assessed for tachycardia, palpitations, and signs and symptoms of CHF, such as dypsnea.
Storage
Store at room temperature. Protect from light.
Administration
Take without regard to food. Platelet count should respond within 7-14 days of beginning therapy.

Anakinra
an-a-kin′ra
(Kineret)
Do not confuse with amikacin.

CATEGORY AND SCHEDULE
Pregnancy Risk Category: B

Classification: Disease modifying antirheumatic drugs, interleukin-receptor antagonists

MECHANISM OF ACTION
An interleukin-1 (IL-1) receptor antagonist that blocks the binding of IL-1, a protein that is a major mediator of joint disease and is present in excess amounts in patients with rheumatoid arthritis.
Therapeutic Effect: Inhibits the inflammatory response.

PHARMACOKINETICS

No accumulation of anakinra in tissues or organs was observed after daily subcutaneous doses. Excreted in urine. *Half-life:* 4-6 h.

AVAILABILITY

Solution: 100-mg syringe.

INDICATIONS AND DOSAGES

▶ **Rheumatoid arthritis**
SC
Adults, Elderly. 100 mg/day, given at same time each day.
▶ **Renal impairment**
Creatinine clearance < 30 mL/min: Consider decreasing the dose to q48h (every other day).

CONTRAINDICATIONS

Known hypersensitivity to *Escherichia coli*–derived proteins, serious infection.

INTERACTIONS

Drug
Live-virus vaccines: Avoid because of potential risk of infection.

DIAGNOSTIC TEST EFFECTS

May decrease WBC, platelet, and absolute neutrophil counts.

SIDE EFFECTS

Frequent (> 10%)
Injection site ecchymosis, erythema, and inflammation; infection; headache.
Occasional
Nausea, diarrhea, abdominal pain, neutropenia.

SERIOUS REACTIONS

• Infections, including upper respiratory tract infection, sinusitis, flu-like symptoms, and cellulitis, have been noted.
• Neutropenia may occur, particularly when anakinra is used in combination with tumor necrosis factor-blocking agents.

PRECAUTIONS & CONSIDERATIONS

Caution is warranted with asthma and renal impairment. Asthmatics are at increased risk for serious infection, and those with renal impairment are at increased risk for a toxic reaction. It is unknown whether anakinra is distributed in breast milk. The safety and efficacy of anakinra have not been established in children. Use anakinra cautiously in elderly patients, who may experience age-related renal impairment. Avoid contact with infected individuals and situations that might increase risk for infection.

Neutrophil count should be monitored before therapy begins, monthly for 3 mo during therapy, and then quarterly for up to 1 yr. Evaluate for inflammatory reactions, especially during the first 4 wks of therapy. Inflammation is uncommon after the first month of therapy.
Storage
Keep the drug refrigerated. Do not freeze or shake it. Protect from light.
Administration
Do not use the drug if it becomes discolored or contains particles. Give the drug by subcutaneous injection.

Anastrozole
(Arimidex)
Do not confuse Arimidex with Imitrex.

CATEGORY AND SCHEDULE
Pregnancy Risk Category: D

Classification: Antineoplastics, aromatase inhibitors, hormones/hormone modifiers

MECHANISM OF ACTION
Decreases the circulating estrogen level by inhibiting aromatase, the enzyme that catalyzes the final step in estrogen production. *Therapeutic Effect:* Inhibits the growth of breast cancers that are stimulated by estrogens.

PHARMACOKINETICS
Well absorbed into systemic circulation (absorption not affected by food). Protein binding: 40%. Extensively metabolized in the liver. Eliminated by biliary system and, to a lesser extent, kidneys. *Mean half-life:* 50 h in postmenopausal women. Steady-state plasma levels reached in about 7 days.

AVAILABILITY
Tablets: 1 mg.

INDICATIONS AND DOSAGES
▸ **Breast cancer**
PO
Adults, Elderly. 1 mg once a day.

CONTRAINDICATIONS
Pregnancy.

INTERACTIONS
Drug
Estrogen-containing products: May reduce anastrozole therapeutic effect.
Tamoxifen: May reduce anastrozole concentrations.
Herbal
Black cohosh, hops, licorice, red clover, thyme, and dong quai: Avoid herbals with potential estrogenic activity.
Food
None known.

DIAGNOSTIC TEST EFFECTS
May elevate serum GGT level in patients with liver metastasis. May increase serum LDL, serum alkaline phosphate, AST (SGOT), ALT (SGPT), and total cholesterol levels. May reduce bone mineral density.

SIDE EFFECTS
Frequent (8%-16%)
Asthenia, nausea, headache, hot flashes, back pain, vomiting, cough, diarrhea.
Occasional (4%-6%)
Constipation, abdominal pain, anorexia, bone pain, pharyngitis, dizziness, rash, dry mouth, peripheral edema, pelvic pain, depression, chest pain, paresthesia.
Rare (1%-2%)
Weight gain, diaphoresis, persistent vaginal bleeding.

SERIOUS REACTIONS
• Thrombophlebitis, and thromboembolism occur rarely.

PRECAUTIONS & CONSIDERATIONS
Anastrozole is indicated only for postmenopausal women. Women who are or may be pregnant should not use anastrozole because the drug crosses the placenta and may cause fetal harm. Pregnancy should be excluded before therapy begins. It is unknown whether anastrozole is excreted in breast milk. The safety and efficacy of anastrozole have not been established in children. No age-related precautions have been noted in elderly patients.

Potential side effects, including dizziness and weakness, may occur. Notify the physician if asthenia, hot flashes, and nausea become unmanageable. If diarrhea occurs, an antidiarrheal should be given; if nausea or vomiting occurs, an antiemetic should be prescribed.
Storage
Store at room temperature.

Administration
Take oral anastrozole without regard to food.

Anidulafungin
ann-id-yoo-la-fun´-jin
(Eraxis)

CATEGORY AND SCHEDULE
Pregnancy Risk Category: C

Classification: Antifungal, echinocandins

MECHANISM OF ACTION
An antifungal that inhibits the synthesis of 1,3-β-D-glucan, an essential component of the fungal cell wall. *Therapeutic Effect:* Fungicidal.

PHARMACOKENETICS
Protein binding: 84%. Metabolism in the liver has not been observed. Approximately 30% eliminated in feces; < 1% excreted in the urine. *Half-life: 26.5 h.*

AVAILABILITY
Lyophilized Powder for Injection: 50 mg, 100 mg.

INDICATIONS AND DOSAGES
▸ **Candidemia**
IV
Adults. 200 mg loading dose on day 1, followed by 100 mg daily thereafter. Continue for at least 14 days after the last positive culture.
▸ **Esophageal candidiasis**
IV
Adults. 100 mg loading dose on day 1, followed by 50 mg daily for a minimum of 14 days and for at least 7 days following resolution of symptoms.

Children. Safety and efficacy have not been established.

CONTRAINDICATIONS
Hypersensitivity to anidulafungin or its components.

INTERACTIONS
Drug
Cyclosporine: May increase anidulafungin concentrations, but no dose adjustment needed.

DIAGNOSTIC TEST EFFECTS
Increased liver function test values.

ⓘ IV INCOMPATIBILITIES
Do not confuse with other medications.

SIDE EFFECTS
Occasional (2%-10%)
Diarrhea, hypokalemia, abnormal liver function.
Rare (< 2%)
Rash, urticaria, flushing, pruritus, dyspnea, hypotension, deep vein thrombosis.

SERIOUS REACTIONS
• Histamine-mediated symptoms, including rash, urticaria, flushing, pruritus, dyspnea, and hypotension, have been reported.

PRECAUTIONS & CONSIDERATIONS
Caution in patients with preexisting hepatic impairment and neutropenia. Abnormal liver function test results have been observed in patients treated with anidulafungin. Clinical hepatic abnormalities have been observed in patients with preexisting hepatic impairment or concomitant medical conditions. Teratogenic effects observed in animal studies; use in pregnancy only if clearly needed. Use with

caution in breastfeeding. Safety and effectiveness have not been established in pediatric patients.
Storage
Store unreconstituted vials, reconstituted solution, and diluted solution at room temperature. Reconstituted solution must be administered within 24 h.
Administration
Reconstitute with supplied diluent (20% [wt/wt] dehydrated alcohol in water for injection) and further dilute with D5W or NS. Final concentrations are 0.36 mg/mL or 0.43 mg/mL. Rate of infusion should not exceed 1.1 mg/min.

Anthralin
anth-rah′lin
(A-Fil, Anthra-Derm, Anthra-forte [CAN], Anthranol [CAN], Anthrascalp [CAN], Dithrocream [AUS], Drithocreme, Dritho-Scalp, Micanol, Psoriatec)
Do not confuse with Antagon, Antabuse, or Andriol.

CATEGORY AND SCHEDULE
Pregnancy Risk Category: C

Classification: Antipsoriatic

MECHANISM OF ACTION
A topical agent that binds DNA, inhibiting synthesis of nucleic protein, and reduces mitotic activity.

PHARMACOKINETICS
Poorly absorbed systemically but excellent epidermal absorption. Auto-oxidized to inactive metabolites—danthrone and dianthrone. Rapid urinary excretion, so significant levels do not accumulate in the blood or other tissues.
Half-life: 6 h.

AVAILABILITY
Cream: 0.5% (Dritho-Scalp), 1% (Anthralin, Psoriatec).

INDICATIONS AND DOSAGES
▸ **Psoriasis**
TOPICAL
Adults, Elderly. Apply in a thin layer to affected areas once daily. Application time may be gradually increased from 5-10 min to 20-30 min.

OFF-LABEL USES
Inflammatory linear verrucous epidermal nevus.

CONTRAINDICATIONS
Acute psoriasis where inflammation is present, erythroderma, hypersensitivity to anthralin.

INTERACTIONS
Drug
Topical corticosteroids: Because psoriasis may worsen upon discontinuation of long-term topical corticosteroid therapy, allow 1 wk between discontinuation of corticosteroid therapy and initiation of anthralin therapy.
Herbal
None known.
Food
None known.

SIDE EFFECTS
Frequent
Irritation.
Rare
Neutrophilia, proteinuria, staining of the skin or fingernails.

SERIOUS REACTIONS
• Hypersensitivity reaction, such as burning, erythema, and dermatitis, may occur.

PRECAUTIONS & CONSIDERATIONS
Caution should be used in renal disease. Patch test should be obtained to rule out the possibility of allergy versus an irritation reaction. It is unknown whether anthralin crosses the placenta and is detected in breast milk. Safety and effectiveness have not been determined for use in children. Severe irritation or edema should be reported.

Administration
For external use only. Apply only to the skin affected with psoriasis. Do not apply to face or genitalia areas. For skin application, apply sparingly only to psoriatic lesions and rub gently and carefully into the skin until absorbed. For scalp application, comb hair to remove scalar debris, wet hair, and, after suitably parting, rub cream well into the lesions, taking care to prevent the cream from spreading onto the forehead or neck. Wash hands thoroughly after using because anthralin may stain skin, hair, and fabric. After prescribed time, rinse area where applied with cool or lukewarm water only. Avoid hot water and soap or shampoo as they could cause product to stain or irritate. Following anthralin removal, the area can be cleaned with usual soap or shampoo.

Antihemophilic Factor (Factor VIII, AHF)
(Advate, Alphanate, Helixate FS, Hemofil M, Humanate P, Hyate C, Koate DVI, Kogenate FS, Monarc M, Monoclate-P, Recombinate, ReFacto, Xyntha)
Do not confuse with Alfenta.

CATEGORY AND SCHEDULE
Pregnancy Risk Category: C

Classification: Antihemophilic agents, blood clotting factors

MECHANISM OF ACTION
An antihemophilic agent that assists in conversion of prothrombin to thrombin, essential for blood coagulation. Replaces missing clotting factor. *Therapeutic Effect:* Produces hemostasis; corrects or prevents bleeding episodes.

AVAILABILITY
Injection: Actual number of AHF units is listed on each vial and varies from brand to brand.

INDICATIONS AND DOSAGES
▶ **Treatment and prevention of bleeding in patients with hemophilia A factor VIII deficiency, hypofibrinogenemia, von Willebrand disease**
IV
Adults, Elderly, Children. Dosage is highly individualized and is based on patient's weight, severity of bleeding, and coagulation studies.

OFF-LABEL USES
Treatment of disseminated intravascular coagulation.

CONTRAINDICATIONS

Hypersensitivity to mouse, hamster, or bovine protein, or to porcine or murine factor, depending on product source.

INTERACTIONS

Drug
None known.
Herbal
None known.
Food
None known.

DIAGNOSTIC TEST EFFECTS

None known.

ⓦ IV INCOMPATIBILITIES

Do not mix with other IV solutions or medications.

SIDE EFFECTS

Occasional
Allergic reaction, including fever, chills, urticaria, wheezing, hypotension, nausea, feeling of chest tightness; stinging at injection site; dizziness; dry mouth; headache; altered taste.

SERIOUS REACTIONS

• There is a risk of transmitting viral hepatitis and other viral illnesses with product derived from pooled human plasma.
• Intravascular hemolysis may occur if large or frequent doses are used with blood group A, B, or AB.

PRECAUTIONS & CONSIDERATIONS

Caution is warranted with hepatic disease and in those with blood type A, B, or AB. If large doses are given with these blood types, expect to monitor Hct and direct Coombs' test to check for hemolytic anemia. If hemolytic anemia occurs, expect to give transfusions with type O blood. Avoid overinflating cuff when monitoring BP. Take BP manually, avoiding automatic BP cuffs. Electric razor and soft toothbrush should be used to prevent bleeding.

Notify the physician of abdominal or back pain, gingival bleeding, black or red stool, coffee-ground emesis, dark or red urine, or red-speckled mucus from cough. IV site should be monitored for oozing. Vital signs should also be monitored throughout therapy.

Administration
For IV use, refer to individual vials for specific storage requirements. Warm concentrate and diluent to room temperature. Gently agitate or rotate to dissolve. Do not shake vigorously. Complete dissolution may take 5-10 min. Filter before administering. Use plastic syringes. A controlled infusion device is often used. Administer IV at a rate of approximately 2 mL/min. Can give up to 10 mL/min.

Apomorphine
aye-poe-more'feen
(Apokyn)

CATEGORY AND SCHEDULE
Pregnancy Risk Category: C

Classification: Antiparkinson agents, dopaminergics

MECHANISM OF ACTION

An antiparkinson agent that stimulates postsynaptic dopamine receptors in the brain. *Therapeutic Effect:* Relieves signs and symptoms of Parkinson disease and improves motor function.

PHARMACOKINETICS

Rapidly absorbed after subcutaneous administration.

Protein binding: 99.9%. Widely distributed. Rapidly eliminated from plasma. Not detected in urine or secretions. *Half-life:* 41-45 min.

AVAILABILITY

Injection: 10 mg/mL in cartridges to be used with injection pen.

INDICATIONS AND DOSAGES

▸ **Acute, intermittent treatment of hypomobility ('off' episodes) associated with advanced Parkinson disease**

SC

Adults, Elderly. Initially, 0.2 mL (2 mg) used "as needed" to treat an acute "off" episode; may be increased in 0.1-mL (1-mg) increments every few days. Maximum: 0.6 mL (6 mg). For Parkinson disease, apomorphine is dosed from 0.2 mL (2 mg) to 0.6 mL (6 mg) subcutaneously as needed and titrated upward in 0.1 mL (1 mg) increments every few days if necessary. Initial doses are determined by administering test doses in-clinic where a medical professional can closely monitor BP pre-dose and at 20, 40, and 60 min post dose. No more than 1 dose per "off" episode should be administered. Doses > 0.6 mL (6 mg), total daily doses > 2 mL (20 mg), and dosing more than 5 times per day are not recommended. Rotate injection sites.

▸ **Dose in renal impairment.**

Test dose and startng dose should be reduced to 0.1 mL (1 mg).

CONTRAINDICATIONS

Concurrent use of alosetron, dolasetron, granisetron, ondansetron, or palonosetron; hypersensitivity to apomorphine or any of the product ingredients (sodium metabisulfite); IV administration.

INTERACTIONS

Drug

Alosetron, dolasetron, granisetron, ondansetron, palonosetron: May produce profound hypotension and loss of consciousness. Contraindicated.

Butyrophenones, metoclopramide, phenothiazines, thioxanthenes: Decrease the effectiveness of apomorphine.

CNS depressants: May increase CNS depressant effects.

Antihypertensives, vasodilators: Increased risk of hypotension and adverse events.

Drugs that prolong QT interval: Increased risk of QT interval prolongation and torsades de pointes. Apomorphine should be given with an antinauseant but not a serotonin 5-HT3 antagonist. Trimethobenzamide is recommended at a dose of 300 mg 3 times daily started 3 days before the initial dose of apomorphine and continued for at least the first 2 mo of therapy to combat nausea.

Food

Alcohol: Can worsen side effects; avoid.

DIAGNOSTIC TEST EFFECTS

May increase serum alkaline phosphatase level.

SIDE EFFECTS

Occasional (3%-4%)

Injection site discomfort, arthralgia, somnolence, hypersalivation, pallor, yawning, headache, dizziness, diaphoresis, vomiting, orthostatic hypotension, dyskinesia or worsening dyskinesia.

Rare (< 2%)

Psychosis, stomatitis, altered taste, hallucinations.

SERIOUS REACTIONS

• Respiratory depression or CNS stimulation (characterized by

tachypnea, bradycardia, or persistent vomiting) may occur.
• Apomorphine use may cause or exacerbate preexisting dyskinesia.
• Cardiovascular events.
• Falls.
• Priapism.

PRECAUTIONS & CONSIDERATIONS

Caution is warranted with asthma, cardiac decompensation, cardiovascular or cerebrovascular disease, concomitant use of alcohol, antihypertensives or vasodilators, hypotension, sleep disorders, and renal impairment. Caution should also be used in persons prone to nausea and vomiting and those susceptible to QT/QTc prolongation, such as persons with hypokalemia, hypomagnesemia, bradycardia, genetic predisposition or concomitant use of drugs that prolong the QTc interval. It is unknown whether apomorphine is distributed in breast milk. The safety and efficacy of apomorphine have not been established in children. Elderly patients are more likely to develop hallucinations and confusion and to experience falls, cardiovacular events, and respiratory disorders.

Nausea, vomiting, headache, hallucinations, somnolence, sedation, dizziness, bradycardia, and hypotension may occur. Chronic subcutaneous administration produces painful nodules. Rarely, syncope has occurred during use of sublingual apomorphine. Prolonged QT intervals have been reported with apomorphine.

Storage
Store at room temperature.
Administration
! Do not use intravenously.
The manufacturer recommends expressing the dose of apomorphine

in milliliters (mL) not milligrams (mg) to avoid confusion.

Apomorphine is administered subcutaneously via use of a multidose-containing dosing pen. Follow directions carefully for use of the dosing pen.

Apraclonidine Hydrochloride

ap-ra-kloe´-ni-deen hi-droh-klor´-ide
(Iopidine)
Do not confuse with Cetapred, clomiphene, Klonopin, or quinidine.

CATEGORY AND SCHEDULE

Pregnancy Risk Category: C

Classification: Selective α_2-adrenergic agonist

MECHANISM OF ACTION

An ocular α-adrenergic agent that is relatively selective for α_2 receptor agonist. *Therapeutic Effect:* Reduces intraocular pressure.

PHARMACOKINETICS

Onset of action occurs within 1 h. The duration of a single dose is about 12 h. *Half-life:* 8 h.

AVAILABILITY

Ophthalmic Solution: 0.5%, 1%.

INDICATIONS AND DOSAGES

▸ **Glaucoma**
OPHTHALMIC
Adults, Elderly. Instill 1 drop of 0.5% solution to affected eye(s) 3 times a day.

▸ **Intraocular hypertension post laser surgery**
OPHTHALMIC
Adults, Elderly. Instill 1 drop of 1% solution in operative eye(s) 1 h before surgery and 1 drop postoperatively.

CONTRAINDICATIONS
Hypersensitivity to apraclonidine or clonidine or any component of the formulation; MAO inhibitor therapy.

DRUG INTERACTIONS
Drugs
MAO inhibitors: concomitant use contraindicated.

DIAGNOSTIC TEST EFFECTS
None known.

SIDE EFFECTS/ADVERSE REACTIONS
Frequent (5%-15%)
Eye discomfort, hyperemia, pruritus, dry mouth.
Occasional (1%-5%)
Headache, constipation, dizziness, somnolence, conjunctivitis, changes in visual acuity, mydriasis, ocular inflammation.
Rare
Nasal decongestion.

SERIOUS REACTIONS
• Allergic reaction occurs rarely.
• Peripheral edema and arrhythmias have been reported.

PRECAUTIONS & CONSIDERATIONS
Tachyphylaxis frequently develops. Use with caution in patients with impaired renal or liver function, depression, cardiovascular disease, cerebrovascular disease, Raynaud disease, or thromboangiitis obliterans and in patients receiving concomitant cardiovascular drugs. Safety and effectiveness have not been established in pediatric patients. No unique precautions have been identified in elderly patients.
Storage
Store at room temperature.
Administration
Wait 5 min between instillation of other ophthalmic agents. Use nasolacrimal occlusion to reduce systemic exposure.

Aprepitant
ap-re′pi-tant
(Emend)

CATEGORY AND SCHEDULE
Pregnancy Risk Category: B

Classification: Antiemetics/anti-vertigo, substance P antagonists

MECHANISM OF ACTION
A selective human substance P and neurokinin-1 (NK1) receptor antagonist that inhibits chemotherapy-induced nausea and vomiting centrally in the chemoreceptor trigger zone.
Therapeutic Effect: Prevents the acute and delayed phases of chemotherapy-induced emesis, including vomiting caused by high-dose cisplatin.

PHARMACOKINETICS
Crosses the blood-brain barrier. Extensively metabolized in the liver. Eliminated primarily by liver metabolism (not excreted renally). *Half-life:* 9-13 h.

AVAILABILITY
Capsules: 80 mg, 125 mg.

INDICATIONS AND DOSAGES
▸ **Prevention of chemotherapy-induced nausea and vomiting**

PO
Adults, Elderly. 125 mg 1 h before chemotherapy on day 1 and 80 mg once a day in the morning on days 2 and 3. Given as part of regimens that include a steroid and an 5-HT3 antagonist.
▸ **Prevention of postoperative nausea and vomiting**
PO
Adults, Elderly. 40 mg within 3 h before induction of anesthesia.

CONTRAINDICATIONS
Hypersensitivity, concurrent use of pimozide (Orap), cisapride.

INTERACTIONS
Drug
Alprazolam, docetaxel, etoposide, ifosfamide, imatinib, irinotecan, midazolam, paclitaxel, triazolam, vinblastine, vincristine, vinorelbine: May increase the plasma concentrations of these drugs.
Antifungals, clarithromycin, diltiazem, nefazodone, nelfinavir, ritonavir: Increase aprepitant plasma concentration.
Carbamazepine, phenytoin, rifampin: Decrease aprepitant plasma concentration.
Contraceptives: May decrease the effectiveness of estrogen or progestin contraceptives.
Corticosteroids: Increase levels of systemic corticosteroids. If the patient is also receiving a steroid, expect to reduce the IV steroid dose by 25% and the oral dose by 50%.
Paroxetine: May decrease the effectiveness of either drug.
Steroids: Increase the blood levels and effects of steroids.
Warfarin: May decrease the effectiveness of warfarin.
Herbal
St. John's wort: May decrease aprepitant levels.

Food
Grapefruit juice: may increase aprepitant concentrations.

DIAGNOSTIC TEST EFFECTS
May increase BUN level and serum creatinine, AST (SGOT), and ALT (SGPT) levels. May produce proteinuria.

SIDE EFFECTS
Frequent (10%-17%)
Fatigue, nausea, hiccups, diarrhea, constipation, anorexia.
Occasional (4%-8%)
Headache, vomiting, dizziness, dehydration, heartburn.
Rare (≤3%)
Abdominal pain, epigastric discomfort, gastritis, tinnitus, insomnia.

SERIOUS REACTIONS
• Neutropenia and mucous membrane disorders occur rarely.

PRECAUTIONS & CONSIDERATIONS
Caution in hepatic impairment. It is unknown whether aprepitant crosses the placenta or is distributed in breast milk. The safety and efficacy of aprepitant have not been established in children. No age-related precautions have been noted in elderly patients.
   Nausea and vomiting should be relieved shortly after drug administration. Notify the physician if headache or persistent vomiting occurs. Pattern of daily bowel activity and stool consistency should be assessed.
Storage
Store at room temperature in original package.
Administration
As prescribed, aprepitant is given with corticosteroids and a serotonin (5 HT3) antagonist.
   Take aprepitant orally without regard to food.

Arformoterol Tartrate

ar-for-moe´-ter-ole tar´-trate
(Brovana)

CATEGORY AND SCHEDULE
Pregnancy Risk Category: C
β_2 agonist

MECHANISM OF ACTION
A long-acting β_2 agonist that
stimulates adrenergic receptors in
bronchial smooth muscle, causing
relaxation of smooth muscle.
Therapeutic Effect: Produces
bronchodilation.

PHARMACOKENETICS
Primarily absorbed by the
pulmonary system following
inhalation. Protein binding: 52%-65%.
Primarily metabolized by
glucuronidation. Primarily excreted
in urine; partial elimination in feces.
Half-life: 26 h.

AVAILABILITY
Solution for Nebulization: 15 mcg/
2 mL.

INDICATIONS AND DOSAGES
▸ COPD
ORAL INHALATION
Adults. 15 mcg (2 mL) twice a day
by nebulization.
Children. Safety and efficacy
have not been established in
children.

CONTRAINDICATIONS
Hypersensitivity to arformoterol, or
its components.

DRUG INTERACTIONS
Drug
β-blockers: May interfere with each
other's effects.

**Methylxanthines (e.g.,
aminophylline, theophylline),
steroids, diuretics:** May potentiate
hypokalemic effects.
**Tricyclic antidepressants,
drugs that prolong QT interval:**
May potentiate cardiovascular
effects.

DIAGNOSTIC TEST EFFECTS
None known.

SIDE EFFECTS/ADVERSE REACTIONS
Occasional (2%-10%)
Pain, chest pain, back pain, sinusitis,
rash, leg cramps, dyspnea, peripheral
edema.
Rare (< 2%)
Oral candidiasis, pulmonary
congestion.

SERIOUS REACTIONS
• May increase the risk of asthma-
related death.
• May exacerbate cardiovascular
conditions including arrhythmias
and hypertension.
• Hypersensitivity reactions including
urticaria, angioedema, rash, bronchospasm, and anaphylaxis may occur.

PRECAUTIONS & CONSIDERATIONS
Use with caution in patients with
acutely deteriorating COPD,
cardiovascular disorders, convulsive
disorders, diabetes mellitus,
hypokalemia, thyrotoxicosis. Do not
coadminister with other long-acting
β_2 agonists.
Storage
Before dispensing, store in protective
foil pouch in the refrigerator. After
dispensing, unopened foil pouches
may be stored at room temperature
up to 6 wks. Remove from foil pouch
immediately before use. Solution
should be colorless; discard any vial
that is not.

Administration

Administered with a standard jet nebulizer connected to an air compressor. May be administered with mouthpiece or face mask. Administer undiluted; do not mix with other medications in nebulizer.

Argatroban

ar-gat′tro-ban
(Acova)
Do not confuse with Aggrestat or Organan.

CATEGORY AND SCHEDULE

Pregnancy Risk Category: B

Classification: Anticoagulants, thrombin inhibitors

MECHANISM OF ACTION

A direct thrombin inhibitor that reversibly binds to thrombin-active sites. Inhibits thrombin-catalyzed or thrombin-induced reactions, including fibrin formation, activation of coagulant factors V, VIII, and XIII; also inhibits protein C formation and platelet aggregation. *Therapeutic Effect:* Produces anticoagulation.

PHARMACOKINETICS

Following IV administration, distributed primarily in extracellular fluid. Protein binding: 54%. Metabolized in the liver. Primarily excreted in the feces, presumably through biliary secretion. *Half-life:* 39-51 min.

AVAILABILITY

Injection: 100 mg/mL.

INDICATIONS AND DOSAGES
▸ **To prevent and treat heparin-induced thrombocytopenia**

IV INFUSION
Adults, Elderly. Initially, 2 mcg/kg/min administered as a continuous infusion. After initial infusion, dose may be adjusted until steady state aPTT is 1.5-3 times initial baseline value, not to exceed 100 s. Maximum dose 10 mcg/kg/min.
▸ **During percutaneous coronary intervention**
IV INFUSION
Adults, Elderly. Initially, give a loading dose of 350 mcg/kg by slow IV injection over 3-5 min, *follow* with IV infusion of 25 mg/kg/min. ACT checked in 5-10 min following bolus. If ACT is < 300 s, give additional bolus 150 mcg/kg, increase infusion to 30 mcg/kg/min. If ACT is > 450 s, decrease infusion to 15 mcg/kg/min. Once ACT of 300-450 s achieved, proceed with procedure.
▸ **Dosage in hepatic impairment**
Adults, Elderly. Initially, 0.5 mcg/kg/min.

CONTRAINDICATIONS

Overt major bleeding.

INTERACTIONS

Drug
Antiplatelet agents, thrombolytics, other anticoagulants: May increase the risk of bleeding.

DIAGNOSTIC TEST EFFECTS

Increases aPTT, International Normalized Ratio, and PT.

Ⓦ IV INCOMPATIBILITIES

Do not mix with other medications or solutions.

SIDE EFFECTS

Frequent (3%-8%)
Dyspnea, hypotension, chest pain, fever, diarrhea, nausea, pain, vomiting, infection, cough, minor bleeding.

SERIOUS REACTIONS
• Ventricular tachycardia and atrial fibrillation occur occasionally.
• Major bleeding and sepsis occur rarely.

PRECAUTIONS & CONSIDERATIONS
Caution is warranted with congenital or acquired bleeding disorders, hepatic impairment, severe hypertension, and ulcerations. Also, use argatroban cautiously immediately following administration of spinal anesthesia, lumbar puncture, and major surgery. It is unknown whether argatroban is excreted in breast milk; use in breastfeeding is not recommended. Safety and efficacy of argatroban have not been established in children younger than 18 yr of age. No age-related precautions have been noted in elderly patients. An electric razor and soft toothbrush should be used to prevent bleeding.

Notify the physician of abdominal pain, bleeding at surgical site, black or red stool, coffee-ground vomitus, red or dark urine, or blood-tinged mucus from cough. Activated coagulation time, aPTT, PT, platelet count, BP, pulse rate, and menstrual flow should be monitored.

Storage
Before reconstitution, store at room temperature. Following reconstitution, the solution is stable for 24 h at room temperature and for 48 h if refrigerated. Avoid exposing the solution to direct sunlight. Discard the solution if it appears cloudy or has an insoluble precipitate.

Administration
Before infusion, dilute the solution 100-fold in 0.9% NaCl, D5W, or lactated Ringer's solution to provide a final concentration of 1 mg/mL. Mix the solution by repeatedly inverting the diluent bag for 1 min. Following reconstitution, the solution may briefly appear hazy because of formation of microprecipitates. These rapidly dissolve when the solution is mixed. Administer as an IV infusion.

Aripiprazole
ara-pip′rah-zole
(Abilify)

CATEGORY AND SCHEDULE
Pregnancy Risk Category: C

Classification: Antipsychotics

MECHANISM OF ACTION
An antipsychotic agent that provides partial agonist activity at dopamine and serotonin (5-HT_{1A}) receptors and antagonist activity at serotonin (5-HT_{2A}) receptors. *Therapeutic Effect:* Diminishes schizophrenic behavior.

PHARMACOKINETICS
Well absorbed through the GI tract. Protein binding: 99% (primarily albumin). Reaches steady levels in 2 wks. Metabolized in the liver. Eliminated primarily in feces and, to a lesser extent, in urine. Not removed by hemodialysis. *Half-life:* 75 h (increased in CYP2D6 poor metabolizers).

AVAILABILITY
Injection Solution: 7.5 mg/mL.
Oral Solution: 1 mg/mL.
Tablets, Orally Disintegrating: 10 mg, 15 mg.
Tablets: 2 mg, 5 mg, 10 mg, 15 mg, 20 mg, 30 mg.

INDICATIONS AND DOSAGES
▶ **Acute agitation associated with schizophrenia or bipolar disorder**
IM
Adults. 9.75 mg as a single dose (range 5.25-15 mg); repeated doses

may be given at intervals of at least 2 h to a maximum of 30 mg/day.

▸ **Bipolar disorder**

PO

Adult. Elderly. 15 mg once daily. May increase to 30 mg once daily.

Children 10 yr of age and older: 2 mg daily for 2 days, followed by 5 mg daily for 2 days with a further increase to a target dose of 10 mg daily; subsequent dose increases may be made in 5 mg increments up to a maximum dose of 30 mg/day.

▸ **Depression, adjunctive therapy**

PO

Adult, Elderly. Initial dose of 2-5 mg/day, with adjustments of 5 mg/day at intervals of at least 1 wk. Usual dose range 2-15 mg/day.

▸ **Schizophrenia**

PO

Adults, Elderly. Initially, 10-15 mg once a day. May increase up to 30 mg/day. At least 2 wks should elapse between dosage adjustments.

Adolescents 13 yr of age and older: 2 mg daily for 2 days, followed by 5 mg daily for 2 days with a further increase to a target dose of 10 mg daily; subsequent dose increases may be made in 5 mg increments up to a maximum dose of 30 mg/day.

OFF-LABEL USES

Schizoaffective disorder.

CONTRAINDICATIONS

Hypersensitivity.

INTERACTIONS

Drug

Carbamazepine: May decrease the aripiprazole blood concentration.

Strong CYP3A4, CY2D6 inhibitors, such as fluoxetine, ketoconazole, quinidine, paroxetine: May increase the aripiprazole blood concentration.

Herbal

St. John's wort: May decrease aripiprazole levels.

Kava kava, gotu kola, valerian: May incease CNS depression.

DIAGNOSTIC TEST EFFECTS

None known.

SIDE EFFECTS

Frequent (5%-11%)

Weight gain, headache, insomnia, vomiting.

Occasional (3%-4%)

Light-headedness, nausea, akathisia, somnolence.

Rare (2% or less)

Blurred vision, constipation, asthenia or loss of energy and strength, anxiety, fever, rash, cough, rhinitis, orthostatic hypotension, hyperglycemia.

SERIOUS REACTIONS

• Extrapyramidal symptoms and neuroleptic malignant syndrome occur rarely.

PRECAUTIONS & CONSIDERATIONS

Caution is warranted with cardiovascular or cerebrovascular diseases (because it may induce hypotension), dementia-related psychosis (increased risk of death with use of atypical antipsychotics), history of seizures or conditions that may lower the seizure threshold (such as Alzheimer's disease), hepatic or renal impairment, and Parkinson disease (because of potential for exacerbation). Use with caution in patients with diabetes or with risk factors for diabetes. CNS depressants and alcohol should be avoided during therapy. It is unknown whether aripiprazole crosses the placenta. Because this drug may be distributed in breast milk, female patients should avoid breastfeeding during therapy. The safety and efficacy of aripiprazole have not been established in children < 10 yr of age. Antidepressants have been observed to increase the risk of suicidal thinking and behavior in children, adolescents, and young adults with major depressive disorder and other psychiatric disorders. No age-related precautions have been noted in elderly patients. Extrapyramidal symptoms and tardive dyskinesia, manifested as chewing or puckering of the mouth, puffing of the cheeks, or tongue protrusion, should be monitored. BP, pulse rate, weight, and therapeutic response should also be monitored. Hydration and hypovolemia should be corrected before beginning therapy.

Storage
Store at room temperature.
Administration
Take aripiprazole without regard to food. Injectable for IM administration only; inject slowly into deep muscle mass.

Arsenic Trioxide
ar′sen-ik try-ox′ide
(Trisenox)
Do not confuse with Trimox.

CATEGORY AND SCHEDULE
Pregnancy Risk Category: D

Classification: Antineoplastics, miscellaneous

MECHANISM OF ACTION
An antineoplastic that produces morphologic changes and DNA fragmentation in promyelocytic leukemia cells. *Therapeutic Effect:* Produces cell death.

AVAILABILITY
Injection: 1 mg/mL in glass ampules.

INDICATIONS AND DOSAGES
▶ **Acute promyelocytic leukemia**
IV INFUSION
Adults, Elderly, Children 5 yr of age and older. Induction: 0.15 mg/kg/day until bone marrow remission. Begin consolidation treatment. Do not exceed 60 induction doses. 3-6 wks after completion of induction therapy, 0.15 mg/kg/day for 25 doses over a period of up to 5 wks.

CONTRAINDICATIONS
Hypersensitivity to arsenic.

INTERACTIONS
Drug
Amphotericin B, diuretics: May produce electrolyte imbalances.
Antiarrhythmics, thioridazine: May prolong QT interval.

DIAGNOSTIC TEST EFFECTS
May decrease hemoglobin levels, serum calcium and magnesium levels, and platelet and WBC counts. May increase AST (SGOT) and ALT (SGPT) levels.

Ⓘ IV INCOMPATIBILITIES
Do not mix arsenic trioxide with any other medications.

SIDE EFFECTS
Expected (50%-75%)
Nausea, cough, fatigue, fever, headache, vomiting, abdominal pain, tachycardia, diarrhea, dyspnea.
Frequent (30%-43%)
Dermatitis, insomnia, edema, rigors, prolonged QT interval, sore throat, pruritus, arthralgia, paresthesia, anxiety.
Occasional (20%-28%)
Constipation, myalgia, hypotension, epistaxis, anorexia, dizziness, sinusitis.

Occasional (8%-15%)
Ecchymosis, nonspecific pain, weight gain, herpes simplex, wheezing, flushing, diaphoresis, tremor, hypertension, palpitations, dyspepsia, eye irritation, blurred vision, asthenia, diminished breath sounds, crackles.
Rare
Confusion, petechiae, dry mouth, oral candidiasis, incontinence, rhonchi.

SERIOUS REACTIONS

• Seizures, GI hemorrhage, renal impairment or failure, pleural or pericardial effusion, hemoptysis, and sepsis occur rarely.
• Prolonged QT interval, complete AV block, unexplained fever, dyspnea, weight gain, and effusion are evidence of arsenic toxicity. If arsenic toxicity is apparent, stop arsenic trioxide treatment and begin steroid treatment as ordered.

PRECAUTIONS & CONSIDERATIONS
Caution is warranted with cardiac abnormalities and renal impairment. Arsenic trioxide is distributed in breast milk and may cause fetal harm. It should not be used by pregnant or breastfeeding women.
Notify the physician if confusion, muscle weakness, fever, vomiting, difficulty breathing, or rapid pulse rate occurs. CBC, creatinine, 12-lead ECG, hepatic function test results, blood chemistry values, serum electrolyte levels (hypokalemia is more common than hyperkalemia), and blood glucose levels (hyperglycemia is more common than hypoglycemia) should be assessed before and during therapy.
Storage
Store the drug at room temperature. The diluted solution is stable for 24 h at room temperature and 48 h if refrigerated.

Administration
! A central venous line is not required for administration of arsenic; the drug may be infused through a peripheral line.
After withdrawing the drug from ampule, dilute it with 100-250 mL D5W or 0.9% NaCl. Infuse the solution over 1-2 h. The duration of the infusion may be extended up to 4 h.

Ascorbic Acid (Vitamin C)
a-skor′bic
(Apo-C [CAN], Cecon, Cenolate, Pro-C [AUS], Redoxon [CAN])

CATEGORY AND SCHEDULE
Pregnancy Risk Category: A (C if used in doses above recommended daily allowance)
OTC

Classification: Vitamins/minerals

MECHANISM OF ACTION
Assists in collagen formation and tissue repair and is involved in oxidation-reduction reactions and other metabolic reactions. *Therapeutic Effect:* Involved in carbohydrate use and metabolism, as well as synthesis of carnitine, lipids, and proteins. Preserves blood vessel integrity.

PHARMACOKINETICS
Readily absorbed from the GI tract. Protein binding: 25%. Metabolized in the liver. Excreted in urine. Removed by hemodialysis.

AVAILABILITY
Capsules: 500 mg, 1 g.
Capsules (Controlled-Release): 500 mg, 1 g.

Crystals for Oral Solution: 3.6 g/tsp, 4 g/tsp.
Liquid: 500 mg/5 mL.
Lozenge: 25 mg.
Oral Solution: 90 mg/mL, 500 mg/5 mL.
Powder for Oral Solution: 4 g/tsp, 4 g/5 mL, 4.3 g/5 mL, 5 g/5 mL.
Tablets: 100 mg, 250 mg, 500 mg, 1 g.
Tablets (Chewable): 100 mg, 250 mg, 500 mg.
Tablets (Controlled-Release): 500 mg, 1 g, 1500 mg.
Injection: 250 mg/mL, 500 mg/mL.

INDICATIONS AND DOSAGES
▸ **Dietary supplement**
PO
Adults, Elderly. 50-200 mg/day.
Children. 35-100 mg/day.
▸ **Acidification of urine**
PO
Adults, Elderly. 4-12 g/day in 3-4 divided doses.
Children. 500 mg q6-8h.
▸ **Scurvy**
PO
Adults, Elderly. 100-250 mg 1-2 times a day.
Children. 100-300 mg/day in divided doses.
▸ **Prevention and reduction of severity of colds**
PO
Adults, Elderly. 1-3 g/day in divided doses.

OFF-LABEL USES
Prevention of common cold, control of idiopathic methemoglobinemia, urine acidifier.

CONTRAINDICATIONS
None known.

INTERACTIONS
Drug
Deferoxamine: May increase iron toxicity.

Herbal
None known.
Food
None known.

DIAGNOSTIC TEST EFFECTS
May decrease serum bilirubin level and urinary pH. May increase urine, uric acid, and urine oxalate levels.

⊘ IV INCOMPATIBILITIES
No information available for Y-site administration.

⊘ IV COMPATIBILITIES
Calcium gluconate, heparin.

SIDE EFFECTS
Rare
Abdominal cramps, nausea, vomiting, diarrhea, increased urination with doses exceeding 1 g. Parenteral: Flushing, headache, dizziness, sleepiness or insomnia, soreness at injection site.

SERIOUS REACTIONS
• Ascorbic acid may acidify urine, leading to crystalluria.
• Large doses of IV ascorbic acid may lead to deep vein thrombosis.
• Abrupt discontinuation after prolonged use of large doses may produce rebound ascorbic acid deficiency.

PRECAUTIONS & CONSIDERATIONS
Caution is warranted in patients with diabetes mellitus, patients with a history of renal calculi, persons on sodium-restricted diet, and those receiving warfarin or daily doses of salicylate. Ascorbic acid crosses the placenta and is excreted in breast milk. Large doses of ascorbic acid taken during pregnancy may produce scurvy in neonates. No age-related precautions have been noted in children or in elderly patients. Eating foods rich in vitamin C, including citrus

fruits, green peppers, brussel sprouts, rose hips, spinach, strawberries, and watercress, is encouraged.

Clinical improvement, such as improved wound healing, should be assessed. Signs and symptoms of recurring vitamin C deficiency, including bleeding gums, digestive difficulties, gingivitis, poor wound healing, and arthralgia, should also be monitored.

Storage
Oral dosage forms: Store at room temperature. Protect from moisture.

Refrigerate vials and protect them from freezing and sunlight.

Administration
Take oral ascorbic acid without regard to food. Reduce the dosage gradually because abrupt discontinuation may produce rebound deficiency.

Injection may be given undiluted or may be diluted in D5W, 0.9% NaCl, or lactated Ringer's solution. For IV push, dilute with an equal volume of D5W or 0.9% NaCl and infuse over 10 min. For IV solution, infuse over 4-12 h.

May also be given IM or SC.

Asparaginase
a-spare′a-gi-nase
(Elspar, Kidrolase [CAN], Leunase [AUS])
Do not confuse with pegaspargase.

CATEGORY AND SCHEDULE
Pregnancy Risk Category: C

Classification: Antineoplastics, enzymes

MECHANISM OF ACTION
An enzyme that inhibits DNA, RNA, and protein synthesis by breaking down asparagine, thus depriving tumor cells of this essential amino acid. Cell cycle-specific for G_1 phase of cell division. *Therapeutic Effect:* Kills leukemic cells.

PHARMACOKINETICS
Metabolized by the reticuloendothelial system through slow sequestration. *Half-life:* 39-49 h IM; 8-30 h IV.

AVAILABILITY
Powder for Injection: 10,000 International Units.

INDICATIONS AND DOSAGES
▸ **Acute lymphocytic leukemia**
IV
Adults, Elderly, Children. 1000 units/ kg/day for 10 days as combination therapy or 200 units/kg/day for 28 days as monotherapy.
IM
Adults, Elderly, Children. 6000 units/m^2/dose 3 times/wk for 3 wks as combination therapy.

OFF-LABEL USES
Treatment of acute myelocytic leukemia, acute myelomonocytic leukemia, chronic lymphocytic leukemia, Hodgkin's disease, lymphosarcoma, melanosarcoma, and reticulum cell sarcoma.

CONTRAINDICATIONS
History of hypersensitivity to asparaginase, history of pancreatitis, serious thrombosis, or serious hemorrhagic events with prior aparaginase treatment.

INTERACTIONS
Drug
Antigout medications: May decrease the effects of these drugs.

Live-virus vaccines: May potentiate virus replication, increase vaccine side effects, and decrease the patient's antibody response to the vaccine.

Methotrexate: May block effects of methotrexate.

Steroids, vincristine: May increase the risk of neuropathy and disturbances of erythropoiesis; may enhance hyperglycemic effect of asparaginase.

Herbal and Food
None known.

DIAGNOSTIC TEST EFFECTS

May increase BUN, blood ammonia, and blood glucose levels; serum alkaline phosphatase, bilirubin, uric acid, AST (SGOT), and ALT (SGPT) levels; platelet count; PT; activated partial thromboplastin time; and thrombin time. May decrease blood-clotting factors (including antithrombin, plasma fibrinogen, and plasminogen) as well as serum albumin, calcium, and cholesterol levels.

⚕ IV INCOMPATIBILITIES

None known.

SIDE EFFECTS

Frequent
Allergic reaction (rash, urticaria, arthralgia, facial edema, hypotension, respiratory distress) pancreatitis (severe stomach pain, nausea, and vomiting).

Occasional
CNS effects (confusion, drowsiness, depression, anxiety, and fatigue), stomatitis, hypoalbuminemia or uric acid nephropathy (manifested as edema of feet or lower legs), hyperglycemia.

Rare
Hyperthermia (including fever or chills), thrombosis, seizures.

SERIOUS REACTIONS

• Hepatotoxicity usually occurs within 2 wks of initial treatment.
• The risk of an allergic reaction, including anaphylaxis, increases after repeated therapy.
• Myelosuppression may be severe.

PRECAUTIONS & CONSIDERATIONS

Caution is warranted with diabetes mellitus, current or recent chickenpox, gout, herpes zoster, infection, hepatic or renal impairment, and in those who have recently had cytotoxic or radiation therapy. Asparaginase use should be avoided during pregnancy, especially during the first trimester and during breastfeeding. No age-related precautions have been noted in children or the elderly. Immunizations and coming in contact with those who have recently received a live-virus vaccine should be avoided.
! Expect to discontinue asparaginase at the first sign or symptom of renal failure (oliguria, anuria) or pancreatitis (abdominal pain, nausea and vomiting, elevated serum amylase and lipase levels). Adequate hydration should be maintained to help prevent kidney problems.

Signs and symptoms of hematologic toxicity, such as excessive fatigue and weakness, ecchymosis, fever, signs of local infection, sore throat, and unusual bleeding from any site, should be assessed. Baseline CNS function should be assessed and a comprehensive blood chemistry should be obtained before therapy begins and whenever more than 1 wk has elapsed between doses.

Storage
Refrigerate the powder for the injected form. Reconstituted solutions are stable for 8 h if refrigerated.

Administration

! Asparaginase dosage is individualized based on clinical response and the tolerance of the drug's adverse effects. When administering this drug in combination therapy, consult specific protocols for optimum dosage and sequence of drug administration. Asparaginase may be carcinogenic, mutagenic, or teratogenic. Handle with extreme care during preparation and administration. Treat urine as infectious waste. Asparaginase powder or solution may irritate the skin on contact. Wash the affected area for 15 min if contact occurs.

! Administer an intradermal test dose (2 International Units) before beginning asparaginase therapy and when more than 1 wk has elapsed between doses. To prepare the test solution, reconstitute 10,000-unit vial with 5 mL sterile water for injection or 0.9% NaCl and shake to dissolve. Withdraw 0.1 mL and inject it into another vial containing 9.9 mL of the same diluent to produce a concentration of 20 International Units/mL. After injecting the test dose, observe the site for 1 h for the appearance of erythema or a wheal. Keep antihistamines, epinephrine, IV corticosteroid, and oxygen equipment readily available before administering asparaginase.

If gelatinous, fiber-like particles develop in the solution, remove them by using a 5-μm filter during administration. For IV use, reconstitute the 10,000-unit vial with 5 mL sterile water for injection or 0.9% NaCl to provide a concentration of 2000 International Units/mL. Shake gently to ensure complete dissolution. Vigorous shaking will produce foam and cause some loss of potency. For IV

injection, administer asparaginase solution into the tubing of free-flowing IV solution of D5W or 0.9% NaCl over at least 30 min. For IV infusion, further dilute with up to 1000 mL D5W or 0.9% NaCl.

For IM use, add 2 mL 0.9% NaCl to 10,000-unit vial to provide a concentration of 5000 International Units/mL. Administer no more than 2 mL at any one site.

Aspirin/ Acetylsalicylic Acid

as′pir-in/ah-seet-il-sill-ic as′id
(Ascriptin, Aspro [AUS], Bayer, Bex [AUS], Bufferin, Disprin [AUS], Ecotrin, Entrophen [CAN], Half-prin, Novasen [CAN], Solprin [AUS], Spren [AUS])
Do not confuse with aspirin or Ascriptin with Aricept, Afrin, or Asendin, or Ecotrin with Edecrin.

CATEGORY AND SCHEDULE

Pregnancy Risk Category: C (D if full dose used in third trimester of pregnancy)
OTC

Classification: Analgesics, non-narcotic, antipyretics, salicylates

MECHANISM OF ACTION

A nonsteroidal salicylate that inhibits prostaglandin synthesis, acts on the hypothalamus heat-regulating center, and interferes with the production of thromboxane A, a substance that stimulates platelet aggregation. *Therapeutic Effect:* Reduces inflammatory response and intensity of pain; decreases fever; inhibits platelet aggregation.

PHARMACOKINETICS

Route	Onset	Peak	Duration
PO	1 h	2-4 h	24 h

Rapidly and completely absorbed from GI tract; enteric-coated absorption delayed; rectal absorption delayed and incomplete. Protein binding: High. Widely distributed. Rapidly hydrolyzed to salicylate. *Half-life:* 15-20 min (aspirin); 2-3 h (salicylate at low dose); more than 20 h (salicylate at high dose).

AVAILABILITY

Tablets (Bayer): 325 mg, 500 mg.
Tablets (Chewable [Bayer and St. Joseph]): 81 mg.
Tablets (Controlled Release [Bayer, ZORprin]): 81 mg, 650 mg, 800 mg.
Tablets (Enteric-Coated [Bayer, Ecotrin, St. Joseph]): 81 mg, 325 mg, 500 mg, 650 mg.
Tablets (Gum [Aspergum]): 227.5 mg.
Tablets (Hafprin): 162 mg.
Caplet (Bayer): 81 mg, 325 mg, 500 mg.
Gelcap (Bayer): 325 mg, 500 mg.
Suppository: 60 mg, 120 mg, 125 mg, 200 mg, 325 mg, 600 mg, 650 mg.

INDICATIONS AND DOSAGES
▶ **Analgesia, fever**
PO, RECTAL
Adults, Elderly. 325-1000 mg q4-6h.
Children. 10-15 mg/kg/dose q4-6h.
Maximum: 4 g/day.
▶ **Anti-inflammatory**
PO
Adults, Elderly. Initially, 2.4-3.6 g/day in divided doses; then 3.6-5.4 g/day.
▶ **Juvenile rheumatoid arthritis**
Children. Initially, 60-90 mg/kg/day in divided doses; then 80-100 mg/kg/day. Adjust to target salicylate concentration of 15-30 mg/dL.

▶ **Suspected myocardial infarction (MI)**
PO
Adults, Elderly. 160-325 mg as soon as the MI is suspected, then daily for 30 days after the MI.
▶ **Prevention of MI**
PO
Adults, Elderly. 75-325 mg/day.
▶ **Prevention of stroke after transient ischemic attack**
PO
Adults, Elderly. 50-325 mg/day.
▶ **Kawasaki disease**
PO
Children. 80-100 mg/kg/day in divided doses during acute phase, then decrease to 3-5 mg/kg/day for maintenance. Discontinue after 6 wks if no cardiac abnormalities; otherwise continue.
▶ **Coronary artery bypass graft**
PO
Adults, Elderly. 75-325 mg/day starting 6 h following procedure.
▶ **Percutaneous transluminal coronary angioplasty**
PO
Adults, Elderly. 80-325 mg/day starting 2 h before procedure.
▶ **Stent implantation**
PO
Adults, Elderly. 325 mg 2 h before implantation and 160-325 mg daily thereafter.
▶ **Carotid endarterectomy**
Adults, Elderly. 81-325 mg/day preoperatively and daily thereafter.
▶ **Acute ischemic stroke**
PO
Adults, Elderly. 160-325 mg/day, initiated within 48 h in patients who are not candidates for thrombolytics and are not receiving systemic anticoagulation.

OFF-LABEL USES
Prevention of thromboembolism, treatment of Kawasaki disease.

CONTRAINDICATIONS

Allergy to tartrazine dye, bleeding disorders, chickenpox, or flu in children and teenagers, GI bleeding or ulceration, hepatic impairment, history of hypersensitivity to aspirin or NSAIDs.

INTERACTIONS

Drug

Alcohol, NSAIDs: May increase the risk of adverse GI effects, including ulceration.

Antacids, urinary alkalinizers: Increase the excretion of aspirin.

Anticoagulants, heparin, thrombolytics: Increase the risk of bleeding.

Insulin, oral antidiabetics: May increase the effects of these drugs (with large doses of aspirin).

Methotrexate, zidovudine: May increase the risk of toxicity of these drugs.

Ototoxic medications, vancomycin: May increase the risk of ototoxicity.

Platelet aggregation inhibitors, valproic acid: May increase the risk of bleeding.

Probenecid, sulfinpyrazone: May decrease the effects of these drugs.

Herbal

None known.

Food

None known.

DIAGNOSTIC TEST EFFECTS

May alter serum alkaline phosphatase, uric acid, AST (SGOT), and ALT (SGPT) levels. May prolong PT and bleeding time. May decrease serum cholesterol, serum potassium, and T3 and T4 levels.

SIDE EFFECTS

Occasional

GI distress (including abdominal distention, cramping, heartburn, and mild nausea); allergic reaction (including bronchospasm, pruritus, and urticaria).

SERIOUS REACTIONS

• High doses of aspirin may produce GI bleeding and gastric mucosal lesions.

• Dehydrated, febrile children may experience aspirin toxicity quickly. Reye syndrome may occur in children with chickenpox or the flu.

• Low-grade toxicity characterized by tinnitus, generalized pruritus (possibly severe), headache, dizziness, flushing, tachycardia, hyperventilation, diaphoresis, and thirst.

• Marked toxicity is characterized by hyperthermia, restlessness, seizures, abnormal breathing patterns, respiratory failure, and coma.

PRECAUTIONS & CONSIDERATIONS

Caution is warranted with chronic renal insufficiency, vitamin K deficiency, and the "aspirin triad" of asthma, nasal polyps, and rhinitis. Aspirin readily crosses the placenta and is distributed in breast milk. Pregnant women should not take aspirin during the last trimester of pregnancy because the drug may prolong gestation and labor and cause adverse effects in the fetus, such as premature closure of the ductus arteriosus, low birth weight, hemorrhage, stillbirth, and death. Caution should be used giving aspirin to children with acute febrile illness. Do not give aspirin to children with chickenpox or the flu because this increases their risk of developing Reye syndrome. Know that behavioral changes and vomiting may be early signs of Reye syndrome. Lower aspirin dosages are recommended for elderly patients because they are more susceptible to aspirin toxicity. Withhold the drug and contact the physician if respirations are 12/min or lower (20/min or lower in children). Alcohol and NSAIDs should be avoided because of increased risk of GI bleeding.

Notify the physician if ringing in the ears (tinnitus) or persistent abdominal or GI pain occurs. Temperature should be taken just before and 1 h after giving the drug. Urine pH should be monitored for signs of sudden acidification, indicated by a pH of 6.5-5.5: sudden acidification may cause the serum salicylate level to greatly increase, leading to toxicity. Be aware the therapeutic serum aspirin level for antiarthritic effect is 20-30 mg/dL; the toxic serum level is over 30 mg/dL. Be aware the anti-inflammatory effect should occur within 1-3 wks.
Storage
Tablets: Store at room temperature, tightly closed. Protect from moisture.

Refrigerate suppositories.
Administration
Do not give aspirin to children or teenagers with chickenpox or the flu because this increases their risk of developing Reye syndrome. Do not use aspirin that smells of vinegar because this odor indicates chemical breakdown of the drug. Do not crush or break enteric-coated or extended-release tablets. Take aspirin with water, milk, or meals if GI distress occurs.

For rectal use, if the suppository is too soft, refrigerate it for 30 min or run cold water over the foil wrapper. Remove foil wrapper before use. Moisten the suppository with cold water before inserting it well into the rectum.

Atazanavir Sulfate
ah-tah-zan´-ah-veer sul´-fate
(Reyataz)
Do not confuse Reyataz with Retavase.

CATEGORY AND SCHEDULE
Pregnancy Risk Category: B

Classification: Antiretroviral, HIV-1 protease inhibitor

MECHANISM OF ACTION
An antiviral that acts as an HIV-1 protease inhibitor, selectively preventing the processing of viral precursors found in cells infected with HIV-1. *Therapeutic Effect:* Prevents the formation of mature HIV virions.

PHARMACOKINETICS
Rapidly absorbed after PO administration. Protein binding: 86%. Extensively metabolized in the liver. Excreted primarily in urine and, to a lesser extent, in feces. *Half-life:* 5-8 h.

AVAILABILITY
Capsules: 100 mg, 150 mg, 200 mg, 300 mg.

INDICATIONS AND DOSAGES
▶ **HIV-1 infection (therapy-naïve)**
PO
Adults, Elderly. 400 mg once a day with food. If given with ritonavir, dosage is 300 mg once daily.
Children 6-17 yr of age (15 kg to < 25 kg). 150 mg with ritonavir; 80 mg once a day with food.
Children 6-17 yr of age (25 to < 32 kg). 200 mg with ritonavir; 100 mg once a day with food.
Children 6-17 yr of age (32 to < 39 kg). 250 mg with ritonavir; 100 mg once a day with food.

Children 6-17 yr of age (at least 39 kg). 300 mg with ritonavir; 100 mg once a day with food.
▶ **HIV-1 infection (therapy-naïve; concurrent therapy with efavirenz, tenofovir, H$_2$ receptor antagonist, or proton pump inhibitor)**
PO
Adults, Elderly. 300 mg atazanavir with 100 mg ritonavir as a single daily dose with food.
▶ **HIV-1 infection (treatment-experienced)**
PO
Adults, Elderly. 300 mg with ritonavir (Norvir) 100 mg once a day. *Children 6-17 yr of age (25 to < 32 kg).* 200 mg with ritonavir; 100 mg once a day with food. *Children 6-17 yr of age (32 to < 39 kg).* 250 mg with ritonavir; 100 mg once a day with food. *Children 6-17 yr of age (at least 39 kg).* 300 mg with ritonavir; 100 mg once a day with food.
▶ **HIV-1 infection (treatment-experienced; concurrent therapy with H$_2$ receptor antagonist)**
PO
Adults, Elderly. 300 mg with ritonavir; 100 mg as a single daily dose with food.
▶ **HIV-1 infection (treatment-experienced; concurrent therapy with H$_2$ receptor antagonist and tenofovir)**
PO
Adults, Elderly. 400 mg with ritonavir; 100 mg as a single daily dose with food.
▶ **HIV-1 infection in patients with moderate hepatic impairment**
PO
Adults, Elderly. 300 mg once a day with food.
▶ **HIV-1 infection in treatment-naïve patients with end-stage renal disease managed with hemodialysis**
PO
Adults, Elderly. 300 mg with ritonavir; 100 mg once a day with food.

CONTRAINDICATIONS
Hypersensitivity, concurrent use with cisapride, ergot derivatives, indinavir, irinotecan, lovastatin, midazolam, pimozide, rifampin, simvastatin, triazolam, and St. John's wort.

INTERACTIONS
Drugs
Antacids, didanosine, buffered medications: Take atazanavir 2 h before or 1 h after.
Amiodarone, clarithromycin, cyclosporine, ergot derivatives, fentanyl, fluticasone, irinotecan, lapatinib, lovastatin, midazolam, rifabutin, sildenafil, simvastatin, sirolimus, tacrolimus, tadalafil, trazodone, triazolam, tenofovir, vardenafil: May increase concentrations of these drugs and increase risk of toxicity.
H$_2$ receptor antagonists: Take atazanavir with or 10 h after the H$_2$ antagonist.
Nevirapine, tenofovir: May reduce atazanavir concentrations.
Proton pump inhibitor: Take 12 h prior to atazanavir in therapy naïve; avoid use with atazanavir in treatment-experienced patients.
β-blockers, calcium channel blockers, cisapride, clarithromycin, pimozide, ranolazine: Increased risk of arrhythmias.
Warfarin: Increased risk of bleeding; monitor INR.
Herbal
St. John's wort: May reduce atazanavir concentrations. Contraindicated.
Food
All foods: Atazanavir bioavailability increased when taken with food.

DIAGNOSTIC TEST EFFECTS
Increased amylase, bilirubin, cholesterol, CPK, glucose, hepatic transaminases, lipase, triglycerides; decreased hemoglobin, neutrophils.

SIDE EFFECTS
Frequent (> 10%)
Nausea, rash, cough, headache.
Occasional (2%-10%)
Dizziness, jaundice, vomiting,
depression, diarrhea, abdominal
pain, fever, lipodystrophy, peripheral
neuropathy, hyperbilirubinemia.
Rare
Insomnia, fatigue, back pain.

SERIOUS REACTIONS
• A severe hypersensitivity reaction
(marked by angioedema and chest
pain) and jaundice may occur.
• Nephrolithiasis.
• Lactic acidosis.

PRECAUTIONS & CONSIDERATIONS
Prolongs PR interval. Use with
caution in preexisting conduction
disorders, diabetes mellitus,
hyperglycemia, hepatic impairment,
and renal impairment; monitor
liver function, HBV infection, and
redistribution of body fat; do not
breastfeed infants.
Storage
Store at room temperature.
Administration
Administer with food.
Swallow capsules whole.

Atenolol
a-ten'oh-lol
(Apo-Atenol [CAN], AteHexal
[AUS], Noten [AUS], Tenolin [CAN],
Tenormin, Tensig [AUS])
**Do not confuse atenolol with
albuterol or timolol.**

CATEGORY AND SCHEDULE
Pregnancy Risk Category: D

Classification: Antiadrenergics,
β-blocking

MECHANISM OF ACTION
A β_1-adrenergic blocker that acts
as an antianginal, antiarrhythmic,
and antihypertensive agent by
blocking β_1-adrenergic receptors
in cardiac tissue. *Therapeutic
Effect:* Slows sinus node heart
rate, decreasing cardiac output and
BP. Decreases myocardial oxygen
demand.

PHARMACOKINETICS

Route	Onset	Peak	Duration
PO	1 h	2-4 h	24 h

Incompletely absorbed from the
GI tract. Protein binding: 6%-16%.
Minimal liver metabolism. Primarily
excreted unchanged in urine.
Removed by hemodialysis. *Half-life:*
6-7 h (increased in impaired renal
function).

AVAILABILITY
Tablets: 25 mg, 50 mg, 100 mg.

INDICATIONS AND DOSAGES
▶ **Hypertension**
PO
Adults. Initially, 25-50 mg once a
day. May increase dose up to 100 mg
once a day.
Elderly. Usual initial dose, 25 mg
a day.
Children. Initially, 0.5-1 mg/kg/dose
given once a day. Range:
0.5-1.5 mg/kg/day. Maximum:
2 mg/kg/day or 100 mg/day.
▶ **Angina pectoris**
PO
Adults. Initially, 50 mg once a day.
May increase dose up to 200 mg
once a day.
Elderly. Usual initial dose, 25 mg a
day. Range same as for adults.
▶ **Dosage in renal impairment**
Dosage interval is modified based on
creatinine clearance.

Creatinine Clearance (mL/min)	Maximum Dosage and Interval
15-35	50 mg a day
< 15	25 mg/day

OFF-LABEL USES

Improved survival in diabetics with heart disease; treatment of hypertrophic cardiomyopathy, pheochromocytoma, and syndrome of mitral valve prolapse; prevention of migraine, thyrotoxicosis, and tremors.

CONTRAINDICATIONS

Cardiogenic shock, overt heart failure, second- or third-degree heart block, severe bradycardia.

INTERACTIONS

Drug

Cimetidine: May increase atenolol blood concentration.

Diuretics, other antihypertensives: May increase hypotensive effect of atenolol.

Insulin, oral hypoglycemics: May mask symptoms of hypoglycemia and prolong hypoglycemic effect of insulin and oral hypoglycemics.

NSAIDs: May decrease antihypertensive effect of atenolol.

Sympathomimetics, xanthines: May mutually inhibit effects.

Herbal

None known.

Food

None known.

DIAGNOSTIC TEST EFFECTS

May increase serum antinuclear antibody titer and BUN, glucose, serum creatinine, potassium, lipoprotein, triglyceride, and uric acid levels.

SIDE EFFECTS

Atenolol is generally well tolerated, with mild and transient side effects.

Frequent

Hypotension manifested as cold extremities, constipation or diarrhea, diaphoresis, dizziness, fatigue, headache, and nausea.

Occasional

Insomnia, flatulence, urinary frequency, impotence or decreased libido, mental depression.

Rare

Rash, arthralgia, myalgia, confusion (especially in the elderly), altered taste.

SERIOUS REACTIONS

• Overdose may produce profound bradycardia and hypotension.

• Abrupt atenolol withdrawal may result in diaphoresis, palpitations, headache, and tremors.

• Atenolol administration may precipitate CHF or MI in patients with cardiac disease; thyroid storm in those with thyrotoxicosis; and peripheral ischemia in those with existing peripheral vascular disease.

• Hypoglycemia may occur in patients with previously controlled diabetes.

• Thrombocytopenia, manifested as unusual bruising or bleeding, occurs rarely.

PRECAUTIONS & CONSIDERATIONS

Caution is warranted with bronchospastic disease, diabetes, hyperthyroidism, impaired renal or hepatic function, inadequate cardiac function, and peripheral vascular disease. Atenolol readily crosses the placenta and is distributed in breast milk. Atenolol use should be avoided in pregnant women after the first trimester because it may result in low-birth-weight infants. The drug may also produce apnea, bradycardia, hypoglycemia, and hypothermia during childbirth. No age-related precautions have been noted in children. Use cautiously in elderly patients, who may have age-related peripheral vascular disease and impaired renal function. Be aware that salt and alcohol intake should be restricted. Nasal decongestants or OTC cold preparations (stimulants) should not be used without physician approval.

Orthostatic hypotension may occur, so rise slowly from a lying to sitting position and dangle the legs from the bed momentarily before standing. Notify the physician of confusion, depression, dizziness, rash, or unusual bruising or bleeding. BP for hypotension, respiratory status for shortness of breath, and pulse for quality, rate, and rhythm should be monitored during treatment. If pulse rate is 60 beats/min or lower or systolic BP is < 90 mm Hg, withhold the medication and contact the physician. Signs and symptoms of CHF, such as decreased urine output, distended neck veins, dyspnea (particularly on exertion or lying down), night cough, peripheral edema, and weight gain should also be assessed.

Storage
Store at room temperature.

Administration
Take oral atenolol without regard to meals. Crush tablets if necessary. Do not abruptly discontinue the drug. Compliance is essential to control angina and hypertension.

Atomoxetine
at-o-mox-e-teen
(Strattera)

CATEGORY AND SCHEDULE
Pregnancy Risk Category: C

Classification: Selective norepinephrine reuptake inhibitor

MECHANISM OF ACTION
A norepinephrine reuptake inhibitor that enhances noradrenergic function by selective inhibition of the presynaptic norepinephrine transporter. *Therapeutic Effect:* Improves symptoms of attention-deficit hyperactivity disorder (ADHD).

PHARMACOKINETICS
Rapidly absorbed after PO administration. Protein binding: 98% (primarily to albumin). Eliminated primarily in urine and, to a lesser extent, in feces. Not removed by hemodialysis. *Half-life:* 4-5 h in general population, 22 h in 7% of white patients and 2% of African Americans (increased in moderate to severe hepatic insufficiency).

AVAILABILITY
Capsules: 10 mg, 18 mg, 25 mg, 40 mg, 60 mg, 80 mg, 100 mg.

INDICATIONS AND DOSAGES
▸ ADHD
PO
Adults, Children weighing 70 kg and more. 40 mg once a day. May increase after at least 3 days to 80 mg as a single daily dose or in divided doses. Maximum: 100 mg.
Children weighing < 70 kg. Initially, 0.5 mg/kg/day. May increase after at least 3 days to 1.2 mg/kg/day.

Maximum: 1.4 mg/kg/day or
100 mg.
▶ **ADHD with concomitant therapy
with CYP2D6 strong inhibitors
(fluoxetine, paroxetine, quinidine) or
in known poor CYP2D6 metabolizers**
PO
*Adults, Children weighing 70 kg and
more.* 40 mg once a day. Only increase
to usual target dose of 80 mg/day if
symptoms fail to improve after 4 wks
and initial dose is well tolerated.
Children weighing < 70 kg. Initially,
0.5 mg/kg/day. Only increase to
usual target dose of 1.2 mg/kg/day if
symptoms fail to improve after 4 wks
and initial dose is well tolerated.
▶ **Dosage in hepatic impairment**
Expect to administer 50% of normal
atomoxetine dosage to patients with
moderate hepatic impairment and
25% of normal dosage to those with
severe hepatic impairment.

OFF-LABEL USES
Treatment of depression.

CONTRAINDICATIONS
Angle-closure glaucoma,
hypersensitivity, use within 14 days
of MAOIs.

INTERACTIONS
Drug
Albuterol: Cardiovascular effects of
albuterol may be potentiated.
**CYPD26 inhibitors, such as
fluoxetine, paroxetine, quinidine:**
May increase atomoxetine blood
concentration. Adjust dose.
MAOIs: May increase the risk of
toxic effects. Contraindicated.
Herbal
None known.
Food
None known.

DIAGNOSTIC TEST EFFECTS
None known.

SIDE EFFECTS
Frequent
Headache, dyspepsia, nausea,
vomiting, fatigue, decreased appetite,
dizziness, altered mood.
Occasional
Tachycardia, hypertension, weight
loss, delayed growth in children,
irritability.
Rare
Insomnia, sexual dysfunction
in adults, fever, aggressiveness,
hostility.

SERIOUS REACTIONS
• Hepatotoxicity.
• Priapism.
• Urine retention or urinary hesitance
may occur.

PRECAUTIONS & CONSIDERATIONS
Caution is warranted with
cardiovascular disease, tachycardia,
hypertension, moderate or severe
hepatic impairment, and a risk
of urine retention. Be aware that
concurrent use of medications
that can increase heart rate or BP
should be avoided. It is unknown
whether atomoxetine is excreted
in breast milk. The safety and
efficacy of atomoxetine have
not been established in children
younger than 6 yr. A thorough
cardiovascular assessment is
recommended before initiation
of therapy in pediatric patients;
assessment should include medical
history, family history, and physical
examination with consideration
of ECG testing. Atomoxetine
increased the risk of suicidal
ideation in short-term studies
in children or adolescents with
ADHD. Age-related cardiovascular
or cerebrovascular disease and
hepatic or renal impairment may
increase the risk of side effects in
elderly patients.

Dizziness may occur, so avoid tasks that require mental alertness and motor skills. Notify the physician if fever, irritability, palpitations, or vomiting occurs. BP, pulse rate, mood changes, urine output, and fluid and electrolyte status should be monitored.

Storage

Store at room temperature.

Administration

Take atomoxetine without regard to food. Take the last daily dose of atomoxetine early in the evening to avoid insomnia. Swallow capsules whole. Do not chew, crush, or open.

Atorvastatin

a-tor'va-sta-tin
(Lipitor)
Do not confuse Lipitor with Levatol.

CATEGORY AND SCHEDULE

Pregnancy Risk Category: X

Classification: Antihyperlip-idemics, HMG CoA reductase inhibitors.

MECHANISM OF ACTION

An antihyperlipidemic that inhibits HMG-CoA reductase, the enzyme that catalyzes the early step in cholesterol synthesis. *Therapeutic Effect:* Decreases LDL and VLDL cholesterol and plasma triglyceride levels; increases HDL cholesterol concentration.

PHARMACOKINETICS

Poorly absorbed from the GI tract. Protein binding is > 98%. Metabolized in the liver. Minimally eliminated in urine. Plasma levels are markedly increased in chronic alcoholic hepatic disease but are unaffected by renal disease. *Half-life:* 14 h.

AVAILABILITY

Tablets: 10 mg, 20 mg, 40 mg, 80 mg.

INDICATIONS AND DOSAGES

▶ **Hyperlipidemia, reduction of risk of myocardial infarction (MI), angina revascularization procedures**
PO
Adults, Elderly. Initially, 10-40 mg a day given as a single dose. Dose range: 10-80 mg/day. Increase at 2- to 4-wks intervals to maximum of 80 mg/day.
Children 10-17 yr. Initially, 10 mg/day, may increase to 20 mg/day.
▶ **Familial hypercholesterolemia**
PO
Children 10-17 yr. Initially, 10 mg/day. May increase to 20 mg/day.

CONTRAINDICATIONS

Active hepatic disease, lactation, pregnancy, unexplained elevated hepatic function test results, rhabdomyolysis.

INTERACTIONS

Drug
Antacids, colestipol: Decrease atorvastatin absorption.
Gemfibrozil, nicotinic acid: Increase the risk of myopathy or rhabdomyolysis.
Cyclosporine, erythromycin, itraconazole: CYP3A4 inhibitors increase atorvastatin blood concentration and increase the risk of myopathy or rhabdomyolysis.
Digoxin: Increased digoxin levels.
Herbal
St. John's wort: May reduce atorvastatin concentrations.

Food
Fiber, oat bran, pectin: May reduce atorvastatin absorption; separate time of administration.
Grapefruit juice: May increase the bioavailability of atorvastatin resulting in an increased risk of myopathy or rhabdomyolysis.

DIAGNOSTIC TEST EFFECTS

May increase serum CK and transaminase concentrations.

SIDE EFFECTS

Atorvastatin is generally well tolerated. Side effects are usually mild and transient.
Frequent (16%)
Headache.
Occasional (2%-5%)
Myalgia, rash or pruritus, allergy.
Rare (1%-2%)
Flatulence, dyspepsia.

SERIOUS REACTIONS

• Cataracts may develop, and photosensitivity may occur.
• Hepatotoxicity or rhabdomyolysis occur rarely.

PRECAUTIONS & CONSIDERATIONS

Caution is warranted with a history of hepatic disease, hypotension, major surgery, severe acute infection, substantial alcohol consumption, trauma, those receiving anticoagulant therapy, and those with severe acute infection, uncontrolled seizures, or severe endocrine, electrolyte, or metabolic disorders. Atorvastatin is distributed in breast milk. It is contraindicated during pregnancy because it may produce skeletal malformation. Pregnancy should be determined before beginning therapy. Safety and efficacy of atorvastatin have not been established in children younger than 10 yr of age. No age-related precautions have been noted in elderly patients.

Notify the physician of headache, malaise, pruritus, or rash. Laboratory results and serum cholesterol and triglyceride levels and hepatic function test results should be documented before therapy. Serum cholesterol and triglyceride levels should be monitored periodically during therapy. Be aware that diet is an important part of treatment.
Storage
Store at room temperature.
Administration
May be taken without regard to food. Do not break film-coated tablets.

Atovaquone
a-toe′va-kwone
(Mepron, Wellvone [AUS])

CATEGORY AND SCHEDULE
Pregnancy Risk Category: C

Classification: Antiprotozoals

MECHANISM OF ACTION

A systemic anti-infective that inhibits the mitochondrial electron-transport system at the cytochrome bc1 complex (complex III), which interrupts nucleic acid and adenosine triphosphate synthesis. *Therapeutic Effect:* Antiprotozoal and antipneumocystic activity.

PHARMACOKINETICS

Absorption increased with a high-fat meal. Protein binding: > 99%. Metabolized in liver. Primarily excreted in feces. *Half-life:* 2-3 days.

AVAILABILITY

Oral Suspension: 750 mg/5 mL.

INDICATIONS AND DOSAGES

▸ *Pneumocystis carinii* **pneumonia (PCP)**
PO
Adults, adolescents 13 yr of age and older. 750 mg twice a day with food for 21 days.
▸ **Prevention of PCP**
PO
Adults, adolescents 13 yr of age and older. 1500 mg once a day with food.

OFF-LABEL USES

Malaria, babesiosis, foxoplasmosis.

CONTRAINDICATIONS

Development or history of potentially life-threatening allergic reaction to the drug.

INTERACTIONS

Drug
Rifampin or rifabutin: May decrease atovaquone blood concentration and increase rifampin blood concentration.
Herbal
None known.
Food
Ingestion with a fatty meal increases absorption.

DIAGNOSTIC TEST EFFECTS

May increase serum alkaline phosphatase, amylase, AST (SGOT), and ALT (SGPT) levels. May decrease serum sodium levels.

SIDE EFFECTS

Frequent (> 10%)
Rash, nausea, diarrhea, headache, vomiting, fever, insomnia, cough.
Occasional (< 10%)
Abdominal discomfort, thrush, asthenia, anemia, neutropenia.

SERIOUS REACTIONS

• Anemia occurs rarely.

PRECAUTIONS & CONSIDERATIONS

Caution is warranted with chronic diarrhea, malabsorption syndromes, and severe PCP and in elderly patients, who require close monitoring because of age-related cardiac, hepatic, and renal impairment. Safety and effectiveness have not been established in pediatric patients < 13 yr of age.

Notify the physician if diarrhea, rash, or other new symptoms occur. Pattern of daily bowel activity and stool consistency and skin for rash should be monitored. Hemoglobin levels, intake and output, and renal function should be assessed. Medical history for problems that may interfere with the drug's absorption, such as GI disorders, should be determined before beginning therapy.
Storage
Store at room temperature. Do not freeze.
Administration
Shake suspension well before using. Administer with meals. Take atovaquone for the full course of treatment.

Atropine

a′troe-peen
(Atropine Sulfate, Atropt [AUS])
Do not confuse with Akarpine or Aplisol.

CATEGORY AND SCHEDULE

Pregnancy Risk Category: C

Classification: Antiarrhythmics, anticholinergics, antidotes, cycloplegics, mydriatics, ophthalmics, preanesthetics

MECHANISM OF ACTION

An acetylcholine antagonist that inhibits the action of acetylcholine by competing with acetylcholine for common binding sites on muscarinic receptors, which are located on exocrine glands, cardiac and smooth-muscle ganglia, and intramural neurons. This action blocks all muscarinic effects. *Therapeutic Effect:* Decreases GI motility and secretory activity and genitourinary muscle tone (ureter, bladder); produces ophthalmic cycloplegia and mydriasis.

PHARMACOKINETICS

Rapidly absorbed after oral administration. Crosses blood-brain barrier. Renally eliminated. *Half-life:* 2.5 h.

AVAILABILITY

Injection: 0.05 mg/mL, 0.1 mg/mL, 0.3 mg/mL, 0.4 mg/mL, 0.5 mg/mL, 0.8 mg/mL, 1 mg/mL.
Injection (Autoinjectors): 0.5 mg, 1 mg, 2 mg.
Ophthalmic Ointment: 1%.
Ophthalmic Solution: 0.5%, 1%, 2%.
Tablets: 0.4 mg.

INDICATIONS AND DOSAGES
▸ **Asystole, slow pulseless electrical activity**
IV
Adults, Elderly. 1 mg; may repeat q3-5min up to total dose of 0.04 mg/kg. Normal maximum: 3 mg total.
▸ **Preanesthetic**
IV/IM/SC
Adults, Elderly. 0.4-0.6 mg 30-60 min preoperatively.
Children weighing 5 kg or more. 0.01-0.02 mg/kg/dose to maximum of 0.4 mg/dose.
Children weighing < 5 kg. 0.02 mg/kg/dose 30-60 min preoperatively.
▸ **Bradycardia**

IV
Adults, Elderly. 0.5-1 mg q5min not to exceed 2 mg or 0.04 mg/kg.
Children. 0.02 mg/kg with a minimum of 0.1 mg to a maximum of 0.5 mg in children and 1 mg in adolescents. May repeat in 5 min. Maximum total dose: 1 mg in children, 2 mg in adolescents.
▸ **Reduction salivation and bronchial secretions**
PO
Adults. 0.4 mg.
Children. Weight-based doses: 7-16 lb, 0.1 mg; 17-24 lb, 0.15 mg; 24-40 lb, 0.2 mg; 40-65 lb, 0.3 mg; 65-90 lb, 0.4 mg; over 90 lb, 0.4 mg.
▸ **Cycloplegia/mydriasis**
OPHTHALMIC
Adults. 1 drop of solution in the eye 3 times a day or small amount of ointment in the eye once or twice daily.

CONTRAINDICATIONS

Cardiospasm, intestinal atony, narrow-angle glaucoma, obstructive disease of the GI tract, paralytic ileus, severe ulcerative colitis, tachycardia secondary to cardiac insufficiency or thyrotoxicosis, toxic megacolon, unstable cardiovascular status in acute hemorrhage,s myasthenia gravis in those not treated with neostigmine, bladder neck obstruction due to prostatic hypertrophy.

INTERACTIONS
Drug
Antacids, antidiarrheals: May decrease absorption of atropine.
Anticholinergics: May increase effects of atropine.
Ketoconazole: May decrease absorption of ketoconazole.
Potassium chloride: May increase severity of GI lesions (wax matrix).
Herbal and Food
None known.

DIAGNOSTIC TEST EFFECTS
None known.

⚠️ IV INCOMPATIBILITIES
Diazepam, pentothal (Thiopental), phenytoin.

🔋 IV COMPATIBILITIES
Diphenhydramine (Benadryl), droperidol (Inapsine), fentanyl (Sublimaze), glycopyrrolate (Robinul), heparin, hydromorphone (Dilaudid), midazolam (Versed), morphine, potassium chloride.

SIDE EFFECTS
Frequent
Dry mouth, nose, and throat that may be severe; decreased sweating, constipation, irritation at subcutaneous or IM injection site.
Occasional
Swallowing difficulty, blurred vision, bloated feeling, impotence, urinary hesitancy.
Rare
Allergic reaction, including rash and urticaria; mental confusion or excitement, particularly in children, fatigue.

SERIOUS REACTIONS
• Overdosage may produce tachycardia; palpitations; hot, dry, or flushed skin; absence of bowel sounds; increased respiratory rate; nausea; vomiting; confusion; somnolence; slurred speech; dizziness; and CNS stimulation.
• Overdosage may also produce psychosis as evidenced by agitation, restlessness, rambling speech, visual hallucinations, paranoid behavior, and delusions, followed by depression.

PRECAUTIONS & CONSIDERATIONS
Extreme caution should be used with autonomic neuropathy,
diarrhea, known and suspected GI infections, and mild to moderate ulcerative colitis. Caution is also warranted with CHF, COPD, coronary artery disease, esophageal reflux or hiatal hernia associated with reflux esophagitis, gastric ulcer, hepatic or renal disease, hypertension, hyperthyroidism, and tachyarrhythmias. Use atropine cautiously in the elderly and in infants.

Warm, dry, flushing feeling may occur upon administration. The patient should urinate before taking this drug to reduce the risk of urine retention. BP, pulse rate, temperature, pattern of daily bowel activity and stool consistency, intake and output, and skin turgor and mucous membranes should be assessed.
Storage
Store at room temperature.
Administration
❗ Notify physician and expect to discontinue atropine immediately if blurred vision, dizziness, or increased pulse rate occurs.
For IV use, give the drug rapidly, to prevent paradoxical slowing of the heart rate. Atropine may also be given by IM or subcutaneous injection.

Auranofin
ah-ran'oh-fin
(Ridaura)
Do not confuse Ridaura with Cardura.

CATEGORY AND SCHEDULE
Pregnancy Risk Category: C

Classification: Disease-modifying antirheumatic drugs, gold compounds.

MECHANISM OF ACTION
Gold compounds that alter cellular mechanisms, collagen biosynthesis, enzyme systems, and immune responses. *Therapeutic Effect:* Suppress synovitis in the active stage of rheumatoid arthritis.

PHARMACOKINETICS
Auranofin (29% gold): Moderately absorbed from the GI tract. Protein binding: 60%. Rapidly metabolized. Primarily excreted in urine. *Half-life:* 21-31 days.

AVAILABILITY
Capsules (Ridaura): 3 mg.

INDICATIONS AND DOSAGES
▸ **Rheumatoid arthritis**
PO
Adults, Elderly. 6 mg/day as a single or 2 divided doses. If there is no response in 6 mo, may increase to 9 mg/day in 3 divided doses. If response is still inadequate, discontinue.

CONTRAINDICATIONS
Bone marrow aplasia, history of gold-induced pathologies (including blood dyscrasias, exfoliative dermatitis, necrotizing enterocolitis, and pulmonary fibrosis), severe blood dyscrasias.

INTERACTIONS
Drug
Bone marrow depressants; hepatotoxic and nephrotoxic medications: May increase the risk of aurothioglucose toxicity.
Penicillamine: May increase the risk of hematologic or renal adverse effects.
Herbal
None known.
Food
None known.

DIAGNOSTIC TEST EFFECTS
May decrease hemoglobin level, hematocrit, and WBC and platelet counts. May increase urine protein level. May alter hepatic function test results.

SIDE EFFECTS
Frequent
Diarrhea (50%), pruritic rash (26%), abdominal pain (14%), stomatitis (13%), nausea (10%).

SERIOUS REACTIONS
• Signs and symptoms of gold toxicity, the primary serious reaction, include decreased hemoglobin level, decreased granulocyte count ($< 150,000/mm^3$), proteinuria, hematuria, stomatitis, blood dyscrasias (anemia, leukopenia [WBC count $< 4000/mm^3$], thrombocytopenia, and eosinophilia), glomerulonephritis, nephrotic syndrome, and cholestatic jaundice.

PRECAUTIONS & CONSIDERATIONS
Caution is warranted with blood dyscrasias, compromised cerebral or cardiovascular circulation, eczema, a history of sensitivity to gold compounds, marked hypertension, renal or liver impairment, severe debilitation, Sjögren syndrome in rheumatoid arthritis, and systemic lupus erythematosus. Auranofin crosses the placenta and is distributed in breast milk. These drugs should be used only when their benefits outweigh the possible risks to the fetus. Safety and effectiveness have not been established in children. Use these drugs cautiously in patients who may have age-related renal impairment. Avoid exposure to sunlight, which may turn skin gray or blue. Oral hygiene should be diligently maintained to help prevent stomatitis.

Notify the physician if GI symptoms (nausea, vomiting, or abdominal cramps), metallic taste, sore mouth, pruritus, or rash occurs. Pattern of daily bowel activity and stool consistency, urine for hematuria and proteinuria, CBC (particularly hemoglobin level, hematocrit, and WBC and platelet counts), renal and liver function tests (especially BUN level and serum alkaline phosphatase, creatinine, AST [SGOT], and ALT [SGPT] levels), skin for rash, and oral mucous membranes for stomatitis should be monitored. Therapeutic response, including improved grip strength, increased joint mobility, reduced joint tenderness, and relief of pain, stiffness, and swelling, should also be assessed.

Administration
Take without regard to food. Taking with food may help GI tolerance. Therapeutic response to the drug may occur in 3-6 mo.

Aurothioglucose/ Gold Sodium Thiomalate

ah-row-thigh-oh-glue′cose
(Gold-50 [AUS], Solganal);
(Myochrysine, Myocrisin [AUS])

CATEGORY AND SCHEDULE
Pregnancy Risk Category: C

Classification: Antirheumatic agents, gold compounds

MECHANISM OF ACTION
Aurothioglucose
A gold compound that alters cellular mechanisms, collagen biosynthesis, enzyme systems, and immune responses. *Therapeutic Effect:* Suppresses synovitis of the active stage of rheumatoid arthritis.
Gold Sodium Thiomalate
A gold compound whose mechanism of action is unknown. May decrease prostaglandin synthesis or alter cellular mechanisms by inhibiting sulfhydryl systems. *Therapeutic Effect:* Decreases synovial inflammation, retards cartilage and bone destruction, suppresses or prevents, but does not cure, arthritis, synovitis.

PHARMACOKINETICS
Aurothioglucose (50% gold)
Slow, erratic absorption after IM administration. Protein binding: 95%-99%. Primarily excreted in urine. *Half-life:* 3-27 days (half-life increased with increased number of doses).
Gold Sodium Thiomalate
Well absorbed. Protein binding: 95%. Widely distributed. Metabolized in liver. Excreted in urine and feces. Not removed by hemodialysis. *Half-life:* 5 days.

AVAILABILITY
Aurothioglucose
Injection: 50 mg/mL suspension (Solganal).
Gold Sodium Thiomalate
Injection: 50 mg/mL (Myochrysine).

INDICATIONS AND DOSAGES
▸ **Rheumatoid arthritis**
Aurothioglucose
IM
Adults, Elderly. Initially, 10 mg, then 25 mg for 2 doses, then 50 mg weekly thereafter until total dose of

0.8-1 g given. If patient improves and there are no signs of toxicity, may give 50 mg at 3- to 4-wks intervals for many months.

Children. 0.25 mg/kg, may increase by 0.25 mg/kg/week. Maintenance: 0.75-1 mg/kg/dose. Maximum: 25-mg dose for total of 20 doses, then q2-4wk.

Gold Sodium Thiomalate
IM
Adults, Elderly. Initially, 10 mg, then 25 mg for second dose. Follow with 25-50 mg/wk until improvement noted or total of 1 g administered. Maintenance: 25-50 mg q2wk for 2-20 wks; if stable, may increase to q3-4wk intervals.
Children. Initially, 10 mg, then 1 mg/kg/wk. Maximum single dose: 50 mg. Maintenance: 1 mg/kg/dose at 2- to 4-wks intervals.

▸ **Dosage in renal impairment**

Creatinine Clearance (mL/min)	Dosage
50-80	50% of usual dosage
< 50	Not recommended

CONTRAINDICATIONS
Aurothioglucose
Bone marrow aplasia, history of gold-induced pathologies, including blood dyscrasias, exfoliative dermatitis, necrotizing enterocolitis, and pulmonary fibrosis, serious adverse effects with previous gold therapy, severe blood dyscrasias.
Gold Sodium Thiomalate
Colitis; concurrent use of antimalarials, immunosuppressive agents, penicillamine, or phenylbutazone; congestive heart failure (CHF); exfoliative dermatitis; history of blood dyscrasias; severe liver or renal impairment; systemic lupus erythematosus.

INTERACTIONS
Drug
Bone marrow depressants; hepatotoxic, nephrotoxic medications: May increase risk of aurothioglucose toxicity.
Penicillamine: May increase risk of hematologic or renal adverse effects of aurothioglucose.
Herbal
None known.
Food
None known.

DIAGNOSTIC TEST EFFECTS
May decrease hemoglobin, hematocrit, platelets, WBC count. May alter liver function tests. May increase urine protein.

SIDE EFFECTS
Frequent
Aurothioglucose: Rash, stomatitis, diarrhea.
Gold sodium thiomalate: Pruritic dermatitis; stomatitis, marked by erythema, redness, shallow ulcers of oral mucous membranes, sore throat; and difficulty swallowing; diarrhea or loose stools; abdominal pain; nausea.
Occasional
Aurothioglucose: Nausea, vomiting, anorexia, abdominal cramps.
Gold sodium thiomalate: Vomiting, anorexia, flatulence, dyspepsia, conjunctivitis, photosensitivity.
Rare
Gold sodium thiomalate: Constipation, urticaria, rash.

SERIOUS REACTIONS
• Gold toxicity is the primary serious reaction. Signs and symptoms of gold toxicity include decreased hemoglobin, leukopenia (WBC count < 4000/mm^3), reduced granulocyte counts (< 150,000/mm^3), proteinuria, hematuria, stomatitis (sores, ulcers, and white spots in the mouth and

throat), blood dyscrasias (anemia, leukopenia, thrombocytopenia, and eosinophilia), glomerulonephritis, nephritic syndrome, and cholestatic jaundice.

PRECAUTIONS & CONSIDERATIONS

Caution is warranted with blood dyscrasias, compromised cerebral or cardiovascular circulation, eczema, a history of sensitivity to gold compounds, marked hypertension, renal or liver impairment, severe debilitation, Sjögren's syndrome in rheumatoid arthritis, and systemic lupus erythematosus. Gold salts have been considered to cross the placenta and be distributed in the breast milk. There are no age-related precautions noted in children. Use cautiously in elderly patients, who may have decreased renal function. Maintain diligent oral hygiene to prevent stomatitis. Avoid exposure to sunlight because it may cause a gray to blue pigment to appear on the skin.

Determine if the patient is pregnant before beginning treatment. Check the results of complete blood count (CBC), particularly BUN, hematocrit, hemoglobin, platelet count, serum alkaline phosphatase, creatinine, SGOT (AST), and SGPT (ALT) levels to assess renal and liver function and urinalysis, before and during therapy. If indigestion, metallic taste, pruritus, rash, or sore mouth occurs, notify the physician.

Storage
Store at room temperature and protect from light.

Administration
Be aware to give as weekly injections. Give in upper outer quadrant of gluteus maximus. Therapeutic response of the drug may be expected in 3-6 mo.

Azacitidine
ay-zah-sigh'tih-deen
(Vidaza)

CATEGORY AND SCHEDULE
Pregnancy Risk Category: D

Classification: Antineoplastics, antimetabolites

MECHANISM OF ACTION
An antineoplastic agent that exerts a cytotoxic effect on rapidly dividing cells by causing demethylation of DNA in abnormal hematopoietic cells in the bone marrow.
Therapeutic Effect: Restores normal function to tumor-suppressor genes regulating cellular differentiation and proliferation.

PHARMACOKINETICS
Rapidly absorbed after subcutaneous administration. Metabolized by the liver. Eliminated in urine. *Half-life:* 4 h.

AVAILABILITY
Powder for Injection: 100 mg.

INDICATIONS AND DOSAGES
▸ **Myelodysplastic syndrome**
IV, SC
Adults, Elderly. 75 mg/m^2/day for 7 days every 4 wks. Dosage may be increased after 2 cycles to 100 mg/m^2 if initial dose is insufficient and toxicity is manageable.

OFF-LABEL USES
Acute myelogenous leukemia, chronic myelogenous leukemia.

CONTRAINDICATIONS
Advanced malignant hepatic tumors, hypersensitivity to mannitol.

INTERACTIONS
Drug
Bone marrow suppressants: May increase myelosuppression.

DIAGNOSTIC TEST EFFECTS
May decrease hemoglobin level, hematocrit, and WBC, RBC, and platelet counts. May increase serum creatinine and potassium levels.

SIDE EFFECTS
Frequent (29%-71%)
Nausea, vomiting, fever, diarrhea, fatigue, injection site erythema, constipation, ecchymosis, cough, dyspnea, weakness.
Occasional (16%-26%)
Rigors, petechiae, injection site pain, pharyngitis, arthralgia, headache, limb pain, dizziness, peripheral edema, back pain, erythema, epistaxis, weight loss, myalgia.
Rare (8%-13%)
Anxiety, abdominal pain, rash, depression, tachycardia, insomnia, night sweats, stomatitis.

SERIOUS REACTIONS
• Hematologic toxicity, manifested most commonly as anemia, leukopenia, neutropenia, and thrombocytopenia, is a common adverse effect.

PRECAUTIONS & CONSIDERATIONS
Caution is warranted with hepatic or renal impairment. Azacitidine may be embryotoxic, causing developmental abnormalities in the fetus. Barrier contraception should be used while receiving azacitidine. Women of childbearing age should avoid becoming pregnant while taking azacitidine. Breastfeeding while taking azacitidine should be avoided. The safety and efficacy of azacitidine have not been established in children. Age-related renal impairment may increase the risk of renal toxicity in elderly patients.

Notify the physician of nausea and vomiting, bleeding, and any signs of infection, including fever and flulike symptoms. Blood counts should be obtained before each dosing cycle to monitor the response and assess for drug toxicity.

Storage
Store vials at room temperature. The reconstituted solution may be stored for up to 1 h at room temperature or up to 8 h if refrigerated. After removing from refrigeration, allow the drug suspension to return to room temperature and use it within 30 min.

Administration
For subcutaneous administration, use strict aseptic technique when preparing the drug. Reconstitute azacitidine with 4 mL sterile water for injection. The reconstituted suspension will appear cloudy. Divide doses > 4 mL equally into two syringes. To resuspend the contents, invert the syringe 2 or 3 times and roll it between your palms for 30 s immediately before administration. For SC injection, rotate injection sites among the abdomen, upper arm, and thigh for each injection. Administer each new injection at least 1 inch from a previous injection site. If azacitidine comes into contact with skin, immediately wash with soap and water.

For IV infusion: Dilute the appropriate dose in 50-100 mL of 0.9% NACL or lactated Ringer's injection. Administer IV infusion over 10-40 min; infusion must be completed within 1 h of reconstitution.

Azathioprine
ay-za-thye′oh-preen
(Alti-Azathioprine [CAN],
Azasan, Imuran, Thioprine [AUS])
**Do not confuse azathioprine
with Azulfidine, or Imuran with
Elmiron or Imferon.**

CATEGORY AND SCHEDULE
Pregnancy Risk Category: D

Classification: Disease-
modifying antirheumatic drugs,
immunosuppressives

MECHANISM OF ACTION
An immunologic agent that
antagonizes purine metabolism
and inhibits DNA, protein, and
RNA synthesis. *Therapeutic
Effect:* Suppresses cell-mediated
hypersensitivities; alters antibody
production and immune response
in transplant recipients; reduces the
severity of arthritis symptoms.

AVAILABILITY
Tablets (Azasan): 75 mg, 100 mg.
Tablets (Imuran): 50 mg.
Injection: 100-mg vial.

INDICATIONS AND DOSAGES
▸ **Adjunct in prevention of renal
allograft rejection**
PO, IV
Adults, Elderly, Children.
3-5 mg/kg/day on day of
transplant, then 1-3 mg/kg/day as
maintenance dose.
▸ **Rheumatoid arthritis**
PO
Adults. Initially, 1 mg/kg/day as a
single dose or in 2 divided doses.
May increase by 0.5 mg/kg/day after
6-8 wks at 4-wks intervals up
to maximum of 2.5 mg/kg/day.
Maintenance: Lowest effective

dosage. May decrease dose by
0.5 mg/kg or 25 mg/day q4wk
(while other therapies, such as rest,
physiotherapy, and salicylates, are
maintained).
Elderly. Initially, 1 mg/kg/day
(50-100 mg); may increase by
25 mg/day until response or toxicity.
▸ **Dosage in renal impairment**
Dosage is modified based on
creatinine clearance.

Creatinine Clearance (mL/min)	Dose
10-50	75% of usual dose
< 10	50% of usual dose

OFF-LABEL USES
Treatment of biliary cirrhosis,
chronic active hepatitis,
glomerulonephritis, inflammatory
bowel disease, inflammatory
myopathy, multiple sclerosis,
myasthenia gravis, nephrotic
syndrome, pemphigoid, pemphigus,
polymyositis, systemic lupus
erythematosus.

CONTRAINDICATIONS
Pregnant patients with rheumatoid
arthritis.

INTERACTIONS
Drug
ACE inhibitors: May increase risk
of anemia and severe leukopenia.
Allopurinol: May increase
activity and risk of toxicity of
azathioprine.
Anticoagulants: May
decrease anticoagulant activity.
Bone marrow depressants: May
increase myelosuppression.
Live-virus vaccines: May potentiate
virus replication, increase the
vaccine's side effects, and decrease
the patient's antibody response to the
vaccine.

Other immunosuppressants: May increase the risk of infection.
Herbal
None known.
Food
None known.

DIAGNOSTIC TEST EFFECTS

May decrease serum albumin, Hgb, and serum uric acid levels. May increase serum alkaline phosphatase, amylase, bilirubin, AST (SGOT), and ALT (SGPT) levels.

ⓘ IV INCOMPATIBILITIES

Methylparabens and propylparabens, phenol.

SIDE EFFECTS

Frequent
Nausea, vomiting, anorexia (particularly during early treatment and with large doses).
Occasional
Rash.
Rare
Severe nausea and vomiting with diarrhea, abdominal pain, hypersensitivity reaction.

SERIOUS REACTIONS

• Azathioprine use increases the risk of developing neoplasia (new abnormal-growth tumors).
• Significant leukopenia and thrombocytopenia may occur, particularly in those undergoing kidney transplant rejection.
• Hepatotoxicity occurs rarely.

PRECAUTIONS & CONSIDERATIONS

Azathioprine should be used cautiously in immunosuppressed patients, those who have undergone previous treatment for rheumatoid arthritis with alkylating agents (such as chlorambucil, cyclophosphamide, and melphalan), and patients with current or recent chickenpox. Avoid pregnancy during treatment.

Notify the physician if abdominal pain, fever, mouth sores, sore throat, or unusual bleeding occurs. CBC (especially platelet count) and serum hepatic enzyme levels should be monitored weekly during the first month of therapy, twice monthly during the second and third months of treatment, and monthly thereafter. The dosage should be reduced or discontinued if the WBC count falls rapidly. Therapeutic response, including improved grip strength, increased joint mobility, reduced joint tenderness, and relief of pain, stiffness, and swelling, should be assessed in rheumatoid arthritis patients.
Storage
Store the tablets at room temperature. Store the parenteral form at room temperature. After reconstitution, the IV solution is stable for 24 h at room temperature.
Administration
Take oral azathioprine during or after meals to reduce the risk of GI disturbances. The drug's therapeutic response may take up to 12 wks to appear.

For IV use, reconstitute the 100-mg vial with 10 mL sterile water for injection to provide a concentration of 10 mg/mL. Swirl the vial gently to dissolve the solution. The solution may be further diluted in 50 mL D5W or 0.9% NaCl. Infuse the solution over 30-60 min (range is 5 min to 8 h).

Azelaic Acid
aye-zeh-lay´-ick as´-id
(Azelex, Finacea, Finevin)

CATEGORY AND SCHEDULE
Pregnancy Risk Category: B

Classification: Topical
antimicrobial, antiacne

MECHANISM OF ACTION
The exact mechanism of action
of azelaic acid is not known.
Possesses antimicrobial activity
against *Propionibacterium acnes*
and *Staphylococcus epidermidis.*
Therapeutic Effect: Inhibits
microbial cellular protein
synthesis.

PHARMACOKINETICS
Minimal absorption after topical
administration. Metabolized in liver.
Excreted in urine as unchanged drug.
Half-life: 12 h.

AVAILABILITY
Cream: 20%.
Gel: 15%.

INDICATIONS AND DOSAGES
▸ **Mild-to-moderate acne**
TOPICAL
Adults, Adolescents. Apply cream to
affected area twice daily (morning
and evening).
▸ **Mild to moderate rosacea**
TOPICAL
Adults. Apply gel to affected
area twice daily (morning and
evening).

CONTRAINDICATIONS
Hypersensitivity to azelaic acid
or any component of the
formulation.

DRUG INTERACTIONS
Drug
None known.
Herbal
None known.
Food
None known.

DIAGNOSTIC TEST EFFECTS
None known.

SIDE EFFECTS
Occasional
Pruritus, stinging, burning, tingling,
erythema, dryness, rash, peeling,
irritation, contact dermatitis.
Rare
Worsening of asthma, vitiligo
depigmentation, small depigmented
spots, hypertrichosis, reddening
(signs of keratosis pilaris),
exacerbation of recurrent cold sore,
fever blister, or oral herpes simplex.

SERIOUS REACTIONS
• None reported.

PRECAUTIONS & CONSIDERATIONS
Monitor for early signs of
hypopigmentation, particularly in
patients with dark complexions.
Storage
Store at room temperature.
Administration
Massage a thin layer into the affected
area. Avoid contact with the eyes,
mouth, and mucous membranes.
Cosmetics may be applied after the
gel has dried.

Azelastine
a´zel-ah-steen
(Astelin, Optivar)
Do not confuse Optivar with Optiray.

CATEGORY AND SCHEDULE
Pregnancy Risk Category: C

Classification: Antihistamines, H1, inhalation, ophthalmics

MECHANISM OF ACTION
An antihistamine that competes with histamine for histamine receptor sites on cells in the blood vessels, GI tract, and respiratory tract. *Therapeutic Effect:* Relieves symptoms associated with seasonal allergic rhinitis such as increased mucus production and sneezing and symptoms associated with allergic conjunctivitis, such as redness, itching, and excessive tearing.

PHARMACOKINETICS

Route	Onset	Peak	Duration
Nasal spray	0.5-1 h	2-3 h	12 h
Ophthalmic	N/A	3 min	8 h

Well absorbed through nasal mucosa. Primarily excreted in feces. *Half-life:* 22 h.

AVAILABILITY
Nasal Spray (Astelin): 137 mcg.
Ophthalmic Solution (Optivar): 0.05%.

INDICATIONS AND DOSAGES
▸ **Allergic rhinitis**
NASAL
Adults, Elderly, Children 12 yr and older. 2 sprays in each nostril twice a day.
Children 5-11 yr. 1 spray in each nostril twice a day.

▸ **Allergic conjunctivitis**
Ophthalmic
Adults, Elderly, Children 3 yr or older. 1 drop into affected eye twice a day.

CONTRAINDICATIONS
History of hypersensitivity to antihistamines.

INTERACTIONS
Drug
Alcohol, other CNS depressants: May increase CNS depression.
Cimetidine: May increase azelastine blood concentration.
Herbal
None known.
Food
None known.

DIAGNOSTIC TEST EFFECTS
May increase ALT (SGPT) levels. May suppress flare and wheal reactions to antigen skin testing unless drug is discontinued 4 days before testing.

SIDE EFFECTS
Frequent (15%-20%)
Headache, bitter taste.
Rare
Nasal burning, paroxysmal sneezing. Ophthalmic: Transient eye burning or stinging, bitter taste, headache.

SERIOUS REACTIONS
• Epistaxis occurs rarely with nasal administration.

PRECAUTIONS & CONSIDERATIONS
Caution is warranted with renal impairment. It is unknown whether azelastine crosses the placenta or is distributed in breast milk. Do not use azelastine during the third trimester of pregnancy. The safety and efficacy of azelastine have not been established in children younger

than 3 yr. No age-related precautions have been noted in elderly patients. Avoid drinking alcoholic beverages during therapy.

Storage

Store at room temperature.

Administration

For intranasal use, prime the pump with 4 sprays or until a fine mist appears before using the nasal spray the first time. After the first use and if the pump has not been used for 3 or more days, prime the pump with 2 sprays or until a fine mist appears. To administer the spray, clear nasal passages as much as possible before use. Tilt head slightly forward. Insert the applicator tip into one nostril, pointing the tip toward the nasal passage and away from the nasal septum. While holding the other nostril closed, spray into the nostril and inhale at the same time to deliver the drug as high into the nasal passages as possible. Repeat in the other nostril. Wipe the applicator tip with a clean, damp tissue and replace cap immediately after use. Avoid spraying nasal drug into the eyes.

For ophthalmic use, tilt head back and instill the solution in the conjunctival sac of the affected eye. Close the eye; then press gently on the lacrimal sac for 1 min.

Azithromycin
ay-zi-thro-mye´sin
(Zithromax, Zithromax TRI-PAK, Zithromax Z-PAK)
Do not confuse azithromycin with erythromycin.

CATEGORY AND SCHEDULE
Pregnancy Risk Category: B

Classification: Antibiotics, macrolides

MECHANISM OF ACTION
A macrolide antibiotic that binds to ribosomal receptor sites of susceptible organisms, inhibiting RNA-dependent protein synthesis. *Therapeutic Effect:* Bacteriostatic or bactericidal, depending on the drug dosage.

PHARMACOKINETICS
Rapidly absorbed from the GI tract. Protein binding: 7%-50%. Widely distributed. Eliminated primarily unchanged by biliary excretion. *Half-life:* 68 h.

AVAILABILITY
Ophthalmic Solutions: 1%.
Oral Suspension: 100 mg/5 mL, 200 mg/5 mL.
Oral Suspension, Extended-Release: 2 g.
Tablets: 250 mg, 500 mg, 600 mg.
Tri-Pak: 500 mg (3 tablets). Z-Pak: 250 mg (6 tablets).
Injection: 500 mg.

INDICATIONS AND DOSAGES
▸ **Respiratory tract, skin, and skin-structure infections**
PO
Adults, Elderly. 500 mg once, then 250 mg/day for 4 days.
Children 6 mo and older. 10 mg/kg once (maximum 500 mg), then 5 mg/kg/day for 4 days (maximum 250 mg).
▸ **Acute bacterial exacerbations of COPD**
PO
Adults. 500 mg/day for 3 days.
▸ **Otitis media**
PO
Children 6 mo and older. 10 mg/kg once (maximum 500 mg), then 5 mg/kg/day for 4 days (maximum 250 mg). Single dose: 30 mg/kg. Maximum: 1500 mg. Three-day regimen: 10 mg/kg/day as

single daily dose. Maximum:
500 mg/day.

▶ **Pharyngitis, tonsillitis**
PO
Children older than 2 yr. 12 mg/kg/
day (maximum 500 mg) for 5 days.

▶ **Chancroid**
PO
Adults, Elderly. 1 g as single dose.
Children. 20 mg/kg as single dose.
Maximum: 1 g.

▶ **Treatment of *Mycobacterium avium* complex (MAC)**
PO
Adults, Elderly. 500 mg/day in
combination.
Children. 5 mg/kg/day (maximum
250 mg) in combination.

▶ **Prevention of MAC**
PO
Adults, Elderly. 1200 mg/wk alone or
with rifabutin.
Children. 5 mg/kg/day (maximum
250 mg) or 20 mg/kg/wk (maximum
1200 mg) alone or with rifabutin.

▶ **Nongonococcal urethritis and cervicitis due to *Chlamydia trachomatis***
PO
Adults. 1 g as a single dose.

▶ **Bacterial conjunctivitis**
OPHTHALMIC
Adults, Elderly, Children 1 yr and older. 1 drop in the affected eye twice
daily, 8-12 h apart for the first 2 days,
then instill 1 drop in the affected eye
once daily for the next 5 days.

▶ **Usual pediatric dosage**
PO
Children older than 6 mo. 10 mg/kg
once (maximum 500 mg)
then 5 mg/kg/day for 4 days
(maximum 250 mg).

▶ **Usual parenteral dosage (community-acquired pneumonia, PID)**
IV
Adults. 500 mg/day, followed by oral
therapy.

OFF-LABEL USES
Chlamydial infections, gonococcal
pharyngitis, uncomplicated
gonococcal infections of the cervix,
urethra, and rectum.

CONTRAINDICATIONS
Hypersensitivity to azithromycin or
other macrolide antibiotics.

INTERACTIONS
Drug
**Aluminum- or magnesium-
containing antacids:** May decrease
azithromycin blood concentration.
**Carbamazepine, cyclosporine,
theophylline, warfarin:** May
increase the serum concentrations of
these drugs.
Herbal
None known.
Food
None known.

DIAGNOSTIC TEST EFFECTS
May increase serum CK, AST
(SGOT), and ALT (SGPT) levels.

ⓓ IV INCOMPATIBILITIES
Information is not available.

⬛ IV COMPATIBILITIES
None known; don't mix with other
medications.

SIDE EFFECTS
Occasional
PO, IV: Nausea, vomiting, diarrhea,
abdominal pain.
Ophthalmic: eye irritation, burning,
staining.
Rare
PO, IV: Headache, dizziness, allergic
reaction.

SERIOUS REACTIONS
• Antibiotic-associated colitis and
other superinfections may result from
altered bacterial balance.

• Acute interstitial nephritis and hepatotoxicity occur rarely.

PRECAUTIONS & CONSIDERATIONS

Caution is warranted with hepatic or renal dysfunction. Determine whether there is a history of hepatitis or allergies to azithromycin or other macrolides before beginning therapy. It is unknown whether azithromycin is distributed in breast milk. The safety and efficacy of azithromycin have not been established in children younger than 16 yr for IV use and younger than 6 mo for oral use. No age-related precautions have been noted in elderly patients with normal renal function.

GI discomfort, nausea, or vomiting should be assessed. Evaluate for signs and symptoms of superinfection, including genital or anal pruritus, sore mouth or tongue, and moderate to severe diarrhea. Assess for signs and symptoms of hepatotoxicity, such as abdominal pain, fever, GI disturbances, and malaise. Liver function tests should be monitored.

Storage

Store the oral suspension at room temperature. The immediate release suspension is stable for 10 days after reconstitution. The extended-release suspension should be consumed within 12 h of reconstitution. Store injection vials at room temperature. After reconstitution, the injectable solution is stable for 24 h at room temperature or 7 days if refrigerated. Store unopened ophthalmic solution in refrigerator. Once opened, store in refrigerator or at room temperature for up to 14 days.

Administration

Give immediate release tablets without regard to food; tolerability may be improved by administration with food. Do not administer the oral suspension with food. Give it at least 1 h before or 2 h after a meal. Take the oral suspension with 8 oz of water at least 1 h before or 2 h after consuming any food or beverages. Azithromycin should be taken 1 h before or 2 h after antacids. Space doses evenly around the clock and continue taking for the full course of treatment.

For IV use, reconstitute each 500-mg vial with 4.8 mL sterile water for injection to provide a concentration of 100 mg/mL. Shake well to ensure dissolution. Further dilute the solution with 250 or 500 mL 0.9% NaCl or D5W to provide a final concentration of 2 mg/mL or 1 mg/mL, respectively. Infuse the drug over 60 min.

Shake ophthalmic solution before each use.

Aztreonam
az-tree´oo-nam
(Azactam)

CATEGORY AND SCHEDULE

Pregnancy Risk Category: B

Classification: Antibacterial, monobactams

MECHANISM OF ACTION

A monobactam antibiotic that inhibits bacterial cell wall synthesis. *Therapeutic Effect:* Bactericidal.

PHARMACOKINETICS

Completely absorbed after IM administration. Protein binding: 56%-60%. Partially metabolized by hydrolysis. Primarily excreted unchanged in urine. Removed by hemodialysis.

Half-life: 1.4-2.2 h (increased in impaired renal or hepatic function).

AVAILABILITY
Injection Powder for Reconstitution: 500 mg, 1 g, 2 g.

INDICATIONS AND DOSAGES
▸ **Urinary tract infections**
IV, IM
Adults, Elderly. 500 mg to 1 g q8-12h.
▸ **Moderate to severe systemic infections**
IV, IM
Adults, Elderly. 1-2 g q8-12h.
▸ **Severe or life-threatening infections**
IV
Adults, Elderly. 2 g q6-8h.
▸ **Cystic fibrosis**
IV
Children. 50 mg/kg/dose q6-8hr up to 200 mg/kg/day. Maximum: 8g/day.
▸ **Mild to severe infections in children**
IV
Children. 30 mg/kg q6-8hr. Maximum: 120 mg/kg/day.
Neonates. 60-120 mg/kg/day q6-12h.
▸ **Dosage in renal impairment**
Dosage and frequency are modified based on creatinine clearance and the severity of the infection.

Creatinine Clearance (mL/min)	Adult Dosage
10-30	1-2 g initially, then ½ usual dose at usual intervals
< 10	1-2 g initially; then ¼ usual dose at usual intervals

OFF-LABEL USES
Treatment of bone and joint infections.

CONTRAINDICATIONS
Hypersensitivity.

INTERACTIONS
Drug
None known.
Herbal
None known.
Food
None known.

DIAGNOSTIC TEST EFFECTS
May increase serum alkaline phosphatase, creatinine, LDH, AST (SGOT), and ALT (SGPT) levels. Produces a positive Coombs' test.

Ⓓ IV INCOMPATIBILITIES
Acyclovir (Zovirax), amphotericin (Fungizone), daunorubicin (Cerubidine), ganciclovir (Cytovene), lorazepam (Ativan), metronidazole (Flagyl), nafcillin, vancomycin (Vancocin).

Ⓓ IV COMPATIBILITIES
Aminophylline, ampicillin, bumetanide (Bumex), calcium gluconate, cefazolin, cimetidine (Tagamet), clindamycin, diltiazem (Cardizem), dobutamine (Dobutrex), dopamine (Intropin), famotidine (Pepcid), furosemide (Lasix), gentamicin, heparin, hydromorphone (Dilaudid), insulin (regular), magnesium sulfate, morphine, potassium chloride, propofol (Diprivan), tobramycin.

SIDE EFFECTS
Occasional (< 3%)
Discomfort and swelling at IM injection site, nausea, vomiting, diarrhea, rash.
Rare (< 1%)
Phlebitis or thrombophlebitis at IV injection site, abdominal cramps, headache, hypotension.

SERIOUS REACTIONS

• Antibiotic-associated colitis and other superinfections may result from altered bacterial balance.
• Severe hypersensitivity reactions, including anaphylaxis, occur rarely.

PRECAUTIONS & CONSIDERATIONS

Caution is warranted with hepatic or renal impairment or a history of allergies, especially to antibiotics. Aztreonam crosses the placenta and is distributed in amniotic fluid and in low concentrations in breast milk. The safety and efficacy of aztreonam have not been established in children < 9 months old. Age-related renal impairment may require a dosage adjustment in the elderly. History of allergies, especially to antibiotics, should be determined before giving aztreonam.

GI discomfort, nausea, and vomiting may occur. Pattern of daily bowel activity and stool consistency and skin for rash should be assessed. Signs and symptoms of phlebitis, such as heat, pain, red streaking over the vein, and pain at the IM injection site, should also be assessed. Be alert for signs and symptoms of superinfection, including anal or genital pruritus, black hairy tongue, vomiting, diarrhea, fever, sore throat, and ulceration or changes of oral mucosa.

Storage

Store vials at room temperature. The solution normally appears colorless to light yellow. After reconstitution, the solution is stable for 48 h at room temperature and 7 days if refrigerated. Discard the solution if a precipitate forms. Discard unused portions of solution. After reconstitution for IM injection, the solution is stable for 48 h at room temperature and 7 days if refrigerated.

Administration

For IV push, dilute each gram with 6-10 mL of sterile water for injection. Administer IV push, over 3-5 min. For intermittent IV infusion, further dilute with 50-100 mL of D5W or 0.9% NaCl. Administer IV infusion over 20-60 min.

For IM use, shake the vial immediately and vigorously after adding the diluent. Inject the drug deep into a large muscle mass.

Bacitracin
Bacitracin
bass-i-tray′sin
(Baciguent, Baci-IM, Bacitracin)
**Do not confuse bacitracin with
Bactrim or Bactroban.**

CATEGORY AND SCHEDULE
Pregnancy Risk Category: C
Rx/OTC

Classification: Anti-infective,
antibiotic

MECHANISM OF ACTION
An antibiotic that interferes with
plasma membrane permeability and
inhibits bacterial cell wall synthesis
in susceptible bacteria. *Therapeutic
Effect:* Bacteriostatic.

PHARMACOKINETICS
Poorly absorbed from mucous
membranes or intact or denuded skin.
Rapidly and completely absorbed
following IM administration. Not
absorbed with bladder irrigation but
can be absorbed with mediastinal or
peritoneal lavage. Excreted slowly by
glomerular filtration.

AVAILABILITY
Powder for Injection: 50,000 units.
Ophthalmic Ointment: 500 units/g.
Topical Ointment: 500 units/g.

INDICATIONS AND DOSAGES
▸ **Superficial ocular infections**
OPHTHALMIC
Adults: ½-inch ribbon in conjunctival
sac q3-4h.
▸ **Skin abrasions, superficial skin
infections**
TOPICAL
Adults, Children. Apply to affected
area 1-5×/day.

▸ **Surgical treatment and
prophylaxis**
IRRIGATION
Adults, Elderly. 50,000-150,000
units, as needed.
▸ **Pneumonia and empyema caused
by susceptible staphylococci**
IM
Infants weighing < 2500 g. 900 units/
kg/24 h in 2-3 divided doses.
Infants weighing more than 2500 g.
1000 units/kg/24 h in 2-3 divided
doses.

CONTRAINDICATIONS
None known.

INTERACTIONS
Drug
**Aminoglycosides, polymyxin B,
colistin, neomycin:** Avoid
concurrent use of other nephrotoxic
medications.
Herbal
None known.
Food
None known.

DIAGNOSTIC TEST EFFECTS
None known.

SIDE EFFECTS
Rare
IM: Rash, nausea, vomiting, pain at
injection site.
Ophthalmic: Burning, itching,
redness, swelling, pain.
Topical: Hypersensitivity
reaction (allergic contact
dermatitis, burning, inflammation,
pruritus).

SERIOUS REACTIONS
• Severe hypersensitivity reactions,
including apnea and hypotension,
occur rarely.
• Renal failure due to glomerular and
tubular necrosis.

B

! When administering a fixed-combination product containing bacitracin, be familiar with the side effects of each of the product's drug components. History of allergies, especially to bacitracin, should be determined before giving the drug.

Burning, itching, increased irritation, and rash should be reported immediately. Be alert for signs and symptoms of hypersensitivity, such as burning, inflammation, and pruritus. When using preparations containing corticosteroids, closely monitor the patient for any unusual signs or symptoms because corticosteroids may mask clinical signs.

Monitor renal function closely with use of the injectable. Maintain adequate hydration. Discontinue therapy if renal toxicity occurs.
Storage
Store unreconstituted powder for injection in refrigerator. Reconstituted solutions are stable for 1 wk when stored in the refrigerator.
Administration
For ophthalmic use, place a gloved finger on the lower eyelid and pull it out until a pocket is formed between the eye and lower lid. Place ¼ to ½ inch of the ointment in the pocket. Close the eye gently for 1-2 min and roll the eyeball to increase the drug's contact with the eye. Remove excess ointment around the eye with a tissue.

For IM use, dilute powder for injection with NS containing 2% procaine HCl to a concentration between 5000 and 10,000 units/mL. IM injections should be given in the upper outer quadrant of the buttocks, alternating right and left and avoiding multiple injections in the same region.

Baclofen
bak'loe-fen
(Apo-Baclofen [CAN], Baclo [AUS], Clofen [AUS], Lioresal, Liotec [CAN], Stelax [AUS])
Do not confuse baclofen with Bactroban or Beclovent.

CATEGORY AND SCHEDULE
Pregnancy Risk Category: C

Classification: Skeletal muscle relaxant, central acting

MECHANISM OF ACTION
A direct-acting skeletal muscle relaxant that inhibits transmission of reflexes at the spinal cord level. *Therapeutic Effect:* Relieves muscle spasticity.

PHARMACOKINETICS
Well absorbed from the GI tract. Protein binding: 30%. Partially metabolized in the liver. Primarily excreted in urine. *Half-life:* 2.5-4 h; intrathecal: 1.5 h.

AVAILABILITY
Tablets: 10 mg, 20 mg.
Tablets, Orally Disintegrating: 10 mg, 20 mg.
Intrathecal Injection: 50 mcg/mL, 500 mcg/mL, 2000 mcg/mL.

INDICATIONS AND DOSAGES
▸ **Spasticity**
PO
Adults. Initially, 5 mg 3×/day. May increase by 15 mg/day at 3-day intervals. Range: 40-80 mg/day. Maximum: 80 mg/day.
Elderly. Initially, 5 mg 2-3×/day. May gradually increase dosage.

B

USUAL MAINTENANCE
INTRATHECAL DOSAGE
*Adults, Elderly, Children older than
12 yr.* 300-800 mcg/day.
Children 12 yr and younger.
100-300 mcg/day.

OFF-LABEL USES
Treatment of trigeminal neuralgia,
hiccups.

CONTRAINDICATIONS
Hypersensitivity.

INTERACTIONS
Drug
Alcohol, other CNS depressants:
May increase CNS depression.
**Morphine epidural (when
intrathecal baclofen used):** Increased
risk for hypotension or dyspnea.
Herbal
None known.
Food
None known.

DIAGNOSTIC TEST EFFECTS
May increase blood glucose level and
serum alkaline phosphatase, AST
(SGOT), and ALT (SGPT) levels.

SIDE EFFECTS
Frequent (> 10%)
Transient somnolence, asthenia,
dizziness, light-headedness, nausea,
vomiting.
Occasional (2%-10%)
Headache, paresthesia, constipation,
anorexia, hypotension, confusion,
nasal congestion.
Rare (< 1%)
Paradoxical CNS excitement or restlessness, slurred speech, tremor, dry
mouth, diarrhea, nocturia, impotence.

SERIOUS REACTIONS
• Abrupt discontinuation of baclofen
may produce hallucinations and
seizures.

• Overdose results in blurred vision,
seizures, myosis, mydriasis, severe
muscle weakness, strabismus,
respiratory depression, and vomiting.

PRECAUTIONS & CONSIDERATIONS
Caution is warranted with diabetes
mellitus, epilepsy, impaired renal
function, preexisting psychiatric
disorders, and a history of CVA. It is
unknown whether baclofen crosses the
placenta or is distributed in breast milk.
The safety and efficacy of baclofen
have not been established in children
younger than 12 yr for the oral, and 4 yr
for intrathecal, forms. Elderly patients
may require decreased dosage because
of age-related renal impairment. They
are also at increased risk for CNS
toxicity, manifested by confusion,
hallucinations, depression, and sedation.
   Drowsiness may occur but is
usually diminished with continued
therapy. Avoid alcohol, CNS
depressants, and tasks that require
mental alertness or motor skills.
Blood counts and liver and renal
function tests should be obtained
periodically for those on long-term
therapy. Therapeutic response, such
as decreased intensity of skeletal
muscle pain, should be assessed.
Storage
Oral: Room temperature. Keep
tightly closed.
Intrathecal: Do not freeze. Do not
heat sterilize.
Administration
Take baclofen without regard to
food. Crush tablets as needed. Do not
abruptly discontinue the drug after
long-term therapy.
   Prepare intrathecal baclofen by
dilution with preservative-free NS.
Administer intrathecal baclofen in a
screening trial before implantation
of an intrathecal pump. Specifically
approved for intrathecal Lioresal
administration.

Balsalazide
ball-sal'a-zide
(Colazal)

CATEGORY AND SCHEDULE
Pregnancy Risk Category: B

Classification: Anti-inflammatory,
GI antiinflammatory,
5-aminosalicylates

MECHANISM OF ACTION
A 5-aminosalicylic acid derivative
that changes intestinal microflora,
altering prostaglandin production
and inhibiting function of natural
killer cells, mast cells, neutrophils,
and macrophages. *Therapeutic
Effect:* Diminishes inflammatory
effect in colon.

PHARMACOKINETICS
PO
Drug reaches colon intact;
bacterial azoreductases release
5-aminobenzyl-*B*-analine and
mesalamine (active metabolite); low,
variable systemic absorption; peak
concentration 1-2 h, protein binding
≈99%; < 1% renal excretion; most
excreted in feces (65%).

AVAILABILITY
Capsules: 750 mg.

INDICATIONS AND DOSAGES
▶ **Ulcerative colitis**
PO
Adults, Elderly. Three 750-mg
capsules 3 times/day for 8-12 wks.
Children 5-17 yr of age. Three
750-mg capsules 3 times/day or one
750 mg capsule 3 times/day for 8 wks.

CONTRAINDICATIONS
Hypersensitivity to 5-aminosalicylates,
and salicylates.

SIDE EFFECTS
Frequent (6%-8%)
Headache, abdominal pain, nausea,
diarrhea.
Occasional (2%-4%)
Vomiting, arthralgia, rhinitis,
insomnia, fatigue, flatulence,
coughing, dyspepsia.

SERIOUS REACTIONS
• Liver toxicity occurs rarely.

PRECAUTIONS & CONSIDERATIONS
Caution is warranted with hepatic
or renal impairment. Notify the
physician if abdominal pain, severe
headache or chest pain, or unresolved
diarrhea occurs. Serum chemistry
laboratory values, including BUN,
alkaline phosphatase, bilirubin,
creatinine, AST (SGOT), and ALT
(SGPT) levels, should be obtained
before treatment.
Storage
Store at room temperature.
Administration
For patients with difficulty
swallowing, the capsules may be
opened and the contents sprinkled
on applesauce and immediately
consumed. The contents may be
chewed if necessary. Teeth and
tongue staining may occur in some
patients taking balsalazide sprinkled
on applesauce.

Basiliximab
bay-zul-ix'ah-mab
(Simulect)
Do not confuse with daclizumab.

CATEGORY AND SCHEDULE
Pregnancy Risk Category: B

Classification: Immunosuppressives, monoclonal antibodies

MECHANISM OF ACTION
A monoclonal antibody that binds to and blocks the receptor of interleukin-2, a protein that stimulates the proliferation of T lymphocytes, which play a major role in organ transplant rejection. *Therapeutic Effect:* Prevents lymphocytic activity and impairs response of the immune system to antigens, which prevents acute renal transplant rejection.

PHARMACOKINETICS
Half-life: Adults, 4-10 days; children, 5-17 days.

AVAILABILITY
Powder for Injection: 10 mg, 20 mg.

INDICATIONS AND DOSAGES
▸ **Prevention of acute organ rejection in patients receiving a kidney transplant**
IV
Adults, Elderly, Children weighing 35 kg or more. 20 mg within 2 hr before transplant surgery and 20 mg 4 days after transplant.
Children weighing < 35 kg. 10 mg within 2 hr before transplant surgery and 10 mg 4 days after transplant.

CONTRAINDICATIONS
Hypersensitivity to basiliximab, murine proteins, or any component of the formulation.

INTERACTIONS
Drug
Live virus vaccines: Defer until immune function improves.

DIAGNOSTIC TEST EFFECTS
May increase BUN and serum cholesterol, creatinine, and uric acid levels. May decrease platelet count and serum magnesium and phosphate levels. May increase or decrease blood glucose, hematocrit, hemoglobin level, and serum calcium and potassium levels.

ⓘ IV INCOMPATIBILITIES
Specific information is not available. Do not infuse other drugs through the same IV line.

SIDE EFFECTS
Frequent (> 10%)
GI disturbances (constipation, diarrhea, dyspepsia), CNS effects (dizziness, headache, insomnia, tremor), respiratory tract infection, dysuria, acne, leg or back pain, peripheral edema, hypertension.
Occasional (3%-10%)
Angina, neuropathy, abdominal distention, tachycardia, rash, hypotension, urinary disturbances (urinary frequency, genital edema, hematuria), arthralgia, hirsutism, myalgia.

SERIOUS REACTIONS
• Serious hypersensitivity, including anaphylactic shock; risk increases with repeat cycles.

PRECAUTIONS & CONSIDERATIONS
Caution is warranted in patients with infection and a history of malignancy. It is unknown whether basiliximab crosses the placenta or is distributed in breast milk. Basiliximab is not recommended for breastfeeding or pregnant women; avoid pregnancy. No age-related precautions have been noted in children or in elderly patients.
   Notify the physician of fever, sore throat, unusual bleeding or bruising, difficulty breathing or swallowing, itching, rapid heartbeat, rash, swelling of lower extremities, or weakness. BUN, blood glucose, serum calcium,

creatinine, alkaline phosphatase, potassium, uric acid levels, vital signs, particularly BP and pulse rate, should be assessed before and during therapy. Patients previously administered basiliximab should only be re-exposed with extreme caution.

Storage
Refrigerate unopened vials. Do not freeze. Use drug within 4 h after reconstitution (within 24 h if refrigerated).

Administration
Discard the solution if a precipitate forms. Reconstitute with 5 mL sterile water for injection. Shake gently to dissolve. If administered as injection, further dilution is not needed. Further dilute with 50 mL 0.9% NaCl or D5W if going to give as IV infusion. Gently invert to avoid foaming. Infuse over 20-30 min.

BCG, Intravesical
(TheraCys, Tice BCG)

CATEGORY AND SCHEDULE
Pregnancy Risk Category: D

Classification: Antineoplastics, biological response modifiers

---

MECHANISM OF ACTION
An antineoplastic that produces a local inflammatory reaction with histiocytic and leukocytic infiltration in the urinary bladder. *Therapeutic Effect:* Decreases superficial cancerous lesions in the urinary bladder.

AVAILABILITY
Parenteral Vials: 50 mg, 81 mg.

INDICATIONS AND DOSAGES
▸ **Treatment and prevention of bladder carcinoma in situ; prophylaxis of primary or recurrent stage Ta and/or T1 papillary tumors following transurethral resection**
INTRAVESICAL (THERACYS)
Adults, Elderly. One dose in 50 mL 0.9% NaCl once weekly for 6 wks, then repeated 3, 6, 12, 18, and 24 mo after initial treatment. Begin 7-14 days after biopsy or transurethral resection.
INTRAVESICAL (TICE BCG)
Adults, Elderly. One dose in 50 mL 0.9% NaCl once weekly for 6 wks; may repeat once. Thereafter, continue monthly for 6-12 mo.

CONTRAINDICATIONS
Compromised immune system, concurrent corticosteroid or immunosuppressive therapy, fever from infection or undetermined cause, HIV infection, active tuberculosis, or urinary tract infection.

INTERACTIONS
Drug
Bone marrow depressants, immunosuppressants: May decrease the immune response and increase the risk of osteomyelitis and disseminated BCG infection.
Live-virus vaccines: May potentiate virus replication, increase vaccine side effects, and decrease the patient's antibody response to the vaccine.

DIAGNOSTIC TEST EFFECTS
Falsely positive tuberculin reaction.

B

SIDE EFFECTS
Frequent
Dysuria, urinary frequency, hematuria, hypersensitivity reaction (manifested as malaise, fever, chills).
Occasional
Cystitis, urinary urgency, nausea, vomiting, anorexia, diarrhea, myalgia, arthralgia.

SERIOUS REACTIONS
• Disseminated BCG infection is usually characterized by a fever higher than 103° F (or persistently higher than 101° F for more than 2 days), chills, and severe malaise.

PRECAUTIONS & CONSIDERATIONS
Before beginning treatment, establish renal status; obtain a urine specimen for culture and sensitivity tests to rule out a urinary tract infection; determine medications the person is taking concurrently, especially corticosteroids and immunosuppressants; and determine whether the person has a compromised immune system, has a fever, or is HIV positive. Immunizations and coming in contact with those who have recently received a live-virus vaccine should be avoided during BCG treatment.

Notify the physician if blood in urine, chills, fever, frequent or painful urination, joint pain, or nausea or vomiting occurs. Adequate hydration should be maintained within 4 h of administration. The patient should void immediately before the drug is given. During the first hour of drug administration, the patient should lie in different positions (supine, prone, and both sides) for 15 min each to allow the drug to come in contact with all parts of the bladder. The patient should try to retain the solution for 2 h. The patient should sit while voiding after instillation to avoid spraying or splashing the infected urine. All urine should be disinfected when expelled within 6 h of drug instillation with an equal volume of 5% hypochlorite solution (undiluted household bleach) and allowed to stand 15 min. before flushing. Renal status should be diligently monitored. Dysuria, hematuria, urinary frequency, and urinalysis should be assessed to check for urinary tract infection.

Storage
Store vials in refrigerator. Store reconstituted solution in refrigerator and use within 2 h.

Administration
! Be aware that BCG contains live, attenuated mycobacteria. Treat the drug as infectious material, and use protective gear when reconstituting it. Avoid contact with the drug if immunocompromised.

For intravesical use, reconstitute the powder immediately before administration. Discard any unused portion within 2 h of reconstitution. After adding diluent to the powder, gently swirl the solution, or repeatedly inject and withdraw the solution from the vial until the solution is mixed. Avoid vigorous shaking, which could cause foaming. Do not give BCG intravenously or subcutaneously; plan to deliver the drug by urethral catheter.

Becaplermin
beh-cap-lear-min
(Regranex)

CATEGORY AND SCHEDULE
Pregnancy Risk Category: C

Classification: Topical wound repair, growth factor

MECHANISM OF ACTION
A platelet-derived growth factor that heals open wounds. *Therapeutic Effect:* Stimulates body to grow new tissue.

PHARMACOKINETICS
None reported.

AVAILABILITY
Gel: 0.01% (Regranex).

INDICATIONS AND DOSAGES
▶ **Diabetic foot ulcer and decubitus ulcers**
TOPICAL
Adults, Elderly. Apply once daily (spread evenly; cover with saline-moistened gauze dressing). After 12 h, rinse ulcer, re-cover with saline gauze.

CONTRAINDICATIONS
Neoplasms at site of application, hypersensitivity to becaplermin or any component of the formulation.

INTERACTIONS
Drug
None known.
Herbal
None known.
Food
None known.

DIAGNOSTIC TEST EFFECTS
None known.

SIDE EFFECTS
Occasional
Local rash near ulcer.

SERIOUS REACTIONS
• Increased mortality from cancer.

PRECAUTIONS & CONSIDERATIONS
Caution should be used on wounds showing exposed joints, tendons, ligaments, or bones. It is unknown whether becaplermin crosses the placenta or is distributed in breast milk. Safety and efficacy have not been established in children < 16 yr of age. There are no age-related precautions noted in elderly patients.
Storage
Refrigerate gel. Do not freeze.
Administration
Measure gel on a clean, nonabsorbable surface. Transfer to ulcer and spread as a thin, continuous layer onto the ulcer. Cover site with saline-moistened dressing for approx. 12 h. Remove and wash any residual gel from ulcer and replace with new gauze pad moistened with 0.9% NaCl until next application. Dose requires recalculation weekly or biweekly, depending on the rate of change in the width and length of ulcer.

Beclomethasone Dipropionate
be-kloe-meth′a-sone di-pro′pi-o-nate
(Aldecin [AUS], Aldecin Hayfever Aqueous Nasal Spray [AUS], Beclodisk [CAN], Becloforte Inhaler [CAN], Beconase AQ, Becotide [AUS], Qvar)
Do not confuse Becloforte or Beconase AQ with baclofen.

CATEGORY AND SCHEDULE
Pregnancy Risk Category: C

Classification: Corticosteroids, halogenated

MECHANISM OF ACTION
An adrenocorticosteroid that prevents or controls inflammation by controlling the rate of protein synthesis, decreasing migration of polymorphonuclear leukocytes and fibroblasts, and reversing

capillary permeability. *Therapeutic Effect:* Inhalation: Inhibits bronchoconstriction, produces smooth muscle relaxation, decreases mucus secretion. Intranasal: Decreases response to seasonal and perennial rhinitis.

PHARMACOKINETICS

Rapidly absorbed from pulmonary, nasal, and GI tissue. Undergoes extensive first-pass metabolism in the liver. Protein binding: 87%. Primarily eliminated in feces. *Half-life:* 15 h.

AVAILABILITY

Oral Inhalation (QVAR): 40 mcg per inhalation, 80 mcg/inhalation.
Nasal spray (Beconase AQ): 42 mcg/inhalation.

INDICATIONS AND DOSAGES
▸ **Long-term control of bronchial asthma, reduces need for oral corticosteroid therapy for asthma**
ORAL INHALATION
Adults, Elderly, Children 12 yr and older. 40-160 mcg twice a day. Maximum: 320 mcg twice a day.
Children 5-11 yr. 40 mcg twice a day. Maximum: 80 mcg twice a day.
▸ **Relief of seasonal or perennial rhinitis, prevention of nasal polyp recurrence after surgical removal, treatment of nonallergic rhinitis**
NASAL INHALATION
Adults, Children older than 12 yr. 1-2 sprays in each nostril twice a day.
Children 6-12 yr. 1 spray in each nostril twice a day. May increase up to 2 sprays in each nostril twice a day.

OFF-LABEL USES

Prevention of seasonal rhinitis (nasal form).

CONTRAINDICATIONS

Hypersensitivity to beclomethasone, status asthmaticus.

INTERACTIONS
Drug
None known.
Herbal
None known.
Food
None known.

DIAGNOSTIC TEST EFFECTS
None known.

SIDE EFFECTS
Frequent
Inhalation (4%-14%): Throat irritation, dry mouth, hoarseness, cough.
Intranasal: Nasal burning, mucosal dryness.
Occasional
Inhalation (2%-3%): Localized fungal infection (thrush).
Intranasal: Nasal-crusting epistaxis, sore throat, ulceration of nasal mucosa.
Rare
Inhalation: Transient bronchospasm, esophageal candidiasis.
Intranasal: Nasal and pharyngeal candidiasis, eye pain.

SERIOUS REACTIONS
• An acute hypersensitivity reaction, as evidenced by urticaria, angioedema, and severe bronchospasm, occurs rarely.
• A transfer from systemic to local steroid therapy may unmask previously suppressed bronchial asthma condition.
• Potential adrenal insufficiency if used to replace systemic corticosteriod use.
• Signs and symptoms of hypercorticism.
• Nasal septum perforation with chronic use and improper technique.

PRECAUTIONS & CONSIDERATIONS

Caution is warranted with cirrhosis, glaucoma, hypothyroidism, osteoporosis, tuberculosis, and untreated systemic infections. Avoid nasal corticosteroid use in patients with recent nasal septal ulcers, nasal surgery, or nasal trauma until healing has occurred. It is unknown whether beclomethasone crosses the placenta or is distributed in breast milk. In children, prolonged treatment and high doses may decrease cortisol secretion and the short-term growth rate. No age-related precautions have been noted in elderly patients.

Those receiving beclomethasone by inhalation should maintain fastidious oral hygiene; notify the physician or nurse if sore throat or mouth develops. If using a bronchodilator inhaler concomitantly with a steroid inhaler, use the bronchodilator several minutes before using the corticosteroid to help the steroid penetrate into the bronchial tree. Those using beclomethasone intranasally should notify the physician if nasal irritation occurs or if symptoms, such as sneezing, fail to improve. Persons who are using drugs that suppress the immune system are more susceptible to infections than healthy individuals are.

Administration

For inhalation, first shake the container well. Exhale completely and place the mouthpiece between the lips. Inhale and hold the breath for as long as possible before exhaling. Allow at least 1 min between inhalations. Rinse mouth after each use to decrease dry mouth and hoarseness and prevent fungal infection of the mouth. Do not change the beclomethasone dosage schedule or stop taking the drug

abruptly; taper dosage gradually under medical supervision.

For intranasal use, clear nasal passages as much as possible. Insert the spray tip into the nostril, pointing toward the nasal passages, away from the nasal septum. Spray beclomethasone into the nostril while holding the other nostril closed, and at the same time, inhale through the nose to deliver the medication as high into the nasal passages as possible. Do not change the beclomethasone dosage schedule or stop taking the drug abruptly; taper dosage gradually under medical supervision.

Belladonna Alkaloids; Phenobarbital

bell-a-don-a al-kuh-loydz
(Antispas, Antispasmodic, Barbidonna, Barophen, Bellalphen, Bellatal, Chardonna-2, Donnapine, Donnatal, Donnatal Extentabs, D-Tal, Haponal, Spacol, Spasmolin, Spasquid)

CATEGORY AND SCHEDULE

Pregnancy Risk Category: C

Classification: Anticholinergic, antispasmodic, gastrointestinal

MECHANISM OF ACTION

Competitive inhibitors of the muscarinic actions of acetylcholine act at receptors located in exocrine glands, smooth and cardiac muscle, and intramural neurons. Composed of 3 main constituents: atropine, scopolamine, and hyoscyamine. Scopolamine exerts greater effects on the CNS, eye, and secretory glands than the constituents

B

atropine and hyoscyamine. Atropine exerts more activity on the heart, intestine, and bronchial muscle and exhibits a more prolonged duration of action compared with scopolamine. Hyoscyamine exerts similar actions to atropine but has more potent central and peripheral nervous system effects. *Therapeutic Effect:* Peripheral anticholinergic and antispasmodic action, mild sedation.

PHARMACOKINETICS
None known.

AVAILABILITY
Combination products:
Tablets: 40 mg phenobarbital, 0.6 mg ergotamine tartrate, 0.2 mg levorotatory alkaloids of belladonna (Bellergal, Bellergal-S, Bellergal-R, Spasmolin, Bellalphen, Antispas, Spacol, Chardonna-2, Barbidonna).
Tablets: Hyoscyamine sulfate 0.1037 mg, atropine sulfate 0.0194 mg, scopolamine hydrobromide 0.0065 mg, and phenobarbital 16.2 mg (Donnatal, Spasmolin).
Tablets, Extended Release: Hyoscyamine sulfate 0.3111 mg, atropine sulfate 0.0582 mg, scopolamine hydrobromide 0.0195 mg, and phenobarbital 48.6 mg (Donnatal Extendtabs).
Elixir: Hyoscyamine sulfate 0.1037 mg, atropine sulfate 0.0194 mg, scopolamine hydrobromide 0.0065 mg, and phenobarbital 16.2 mg per 5 mL (Barophen, Donnapine, Antispasmodic, Spacol, Donnatal, D-Tal, Spasquid).
Tablets: Belladonna alkaloids 15 mg and butarbital sodium 15 mg.
Elixir: Belladonna alkaloids 15 mg and butalbital sodium 15 mg per 5 mL.

INDICATIONS AND DOSAGES
▶ **Irritable bowel syndrome, acute enterocolitis**
PO
Adults. 1-2 tablets or capsules 3-4 times daily or 1-2 tsp of elixir 3-4 times daily according to conditions and severity of symptoms.

CONTRAINDICATIONS
Narrow-angle glaucoma, obstructive uropathy, obstructive disease of tract, paralytic ileus, intestinal atony of the elderly or debilitated patient, tachycardia, acute myocardial ischemia, unstable cardiovascular status in acute hemorrhage, severe ulcerative colitis, especially if complicated by toxic megacolon, myasthenia gravis, hiatal hernia associated with reflux esophagitis, hypersensitivity to any component of the formulation, acute intermittent porphyria.

INTERACTIONS
Drug
Oral medications: Belladonna decreases gastric emptying time therefore affecting absorption of orally administered agents.
Anticholinergic drugs: May enhance anticholinergic effect.
Ambenonium, arbutamine, belladonna, cisapride, cromolyn, halothane, methacholine, procainamide: May enhance effects of atropine constituent of belladonna alkaloids.
Tricyclic antidepressants: May enhance anticholinergic effect.
Cisapride: Atropine may decrease effects of cisapride.
Antiarrhythmics: May result in additive antivagal effects on atrioventricular nodal conduction.
Alcohol: May result in additive CNS depression.

Herbal
Anticholinergic herbs: May
enhance anticholinergic effect.
Food
None known.

DIAGNOSTIC TEST EFFECTS
None known.

SIDE EFFECTS
Frequent
Dry mouth, urinary retention, flushing,
pupillary dilation, constipation,
confusion, redness of the skin,
flushing, dry skin, allergic contact
dermatitis, headache, excitement,
agitation, dizziness, light-headedness,
drowsiness, unsteadiness,
confusion, slurred speech, sedation,
hyperreflexia, convulsions, vertigo,
coma, mydriasis, photophobia, blurred
vision, dilation of pupils.
Rare
Hallucinations, acute psychosis,
Stevens-Johnson syndrome,
photosensitivity.

SERIOUS REACTIONS
• Signs and symptoms of overdose
include headache, nausea, vomiting,
blurred vision, dilated pupils, hot and
dry skin, dizziness, dryness of the
mouth, difficulty in swallowing, and
CNS stimulation, coma.

PRECAUTIONS & CONSIDERATIONS
Caution is warranted with ulcerative
colitis or intestinal disease, coronary
artery disease, dehydration,
diarrhea caused by poisoning,
Down syndrome, acute dysentery,
glaucoma, hepatic and renal function
impairment, hiatal hernia, prostatic
hyperplasia, urinary retention,
asthma, COPD, and brain damage.
Belladonna alkaloids cross the
placenta and are distributed into
breast milk. Safety and efficacy have
not been established in children

younger than 6 yr. Infants and young
children may be more susceptible
to adverse effects of belladonna
alkaloids. Elderly patients may
be more susceptible to the
anticholinergic effects; avoid use
in this population.
Constipation, difficulty urinating,
decreased sweating, drowsiness,
dry mouth, increased heart rate,
headache, orthostatic hypotension
may occur. Change positions slowly
to avoid light-headedness. Avoid
alcohol, CNS depressants, and tasks
that require mental alertness.
Administration
Dose should be adjusted to the
needs of the individual to assume
symptomatic control with minimum
adverse effects. Do not crush
extended-release tablets.

Belladonna and Opium
bell-a-don′a
(B&O Supprettes 15-A, B&O
Supprettes 16-A, PMS-Opium &
Belladonna [CAN])

CATEGORY AND SCHEDULE
Pregnancy Risk Category: C
Controlled Substance: Schedule II

Classification: Analgesics,
narcotic, anticholinergics

MECHANISM OF ACTION
Anticholinergic alkaloids that
inhibit the action of acetylcholine
at postganglionic (muscarinic)
receptor sites. Morphine (10% of
opium) depresses cerebral cortex,

hypothalamus, and medullary centers. *Therapeutic Effect:* Decreases digestive secretions, increases GI muscle tone, reduces GI force, and alters pain perception and emotional response to pain.

PHARMACOKINETICS
Onset of action occurs within 30 min. Absorption is dependent on body hydration. Metabolized in liver to form glucuronide metabolites.

AVAILABILITY
Suppository: 16.2 mg belladonna extract/30 mg opium (B&O Supprettes 15-A), 16.2 mg belladonna extract/60 mg opium (B&O Supprettes 16-A).

INDICATIONS AND DOSAGES
▸ **Analgesic, antispasmodic**
RECTAL
Adults, Elderly. 1 suppository 1-2 times/day. Maximum: 4 doses/day.

OFF-LABEL USES
None known.

CONTRAINDICATIONS
Glaucoma, severe renal or hepatic disease, bronchial asthma, respiratory depression, convulsive disorders, acute alcoholism, premature labor, hypersensitivity to belladonna or opium or its components.

INTERACTIONS
Drug
Alcohol, CNS depressants: May increase CNS or respiratory depression, hypotension.
Anticholinergics: May increase the effects of belladonna and opium.
Phenothiazines: May decrease the antipsychotic effects of these drugs.
Herbal
None known.

Food
None known.

DIAGNOSTIC TEST EFFECTS
May increase serum SGOT (AST) and SGPT (ALT) levels.

SIDE EFFECTS
Frequent
Dry mouth, nose, skin, and throat; decreased sweating; constipation; irritation at site of administration; drowsiness; urinary retention; dizziness.
Occasional
Blurred vision, decreased flow of breast milk, bloated feeling, drowsiness, headache, intolerance to light, nervousness, and flushing.
Rare
Dizziness, faintness, pruritus, urticaria.

SERIOUS REACTIONS
• Respiratory depression, increased intraocular pain, loss of memory, orthostatic hypotension, tachycardia, and ventricular fibrillation rarely occur.
• Tolerance to the drug's analgesic effect and physical dependence may occur with repeated use.

PRECAUTIONS & CONSIDERATIONS
Extreme caution should be used with acute alcoholism, anoxia, CNS depression, hypercapnia, respiratory depression or dysfunction, seizures, shock, and untreated myxedema. Caution is also warranted with acute abdominal conditions, Addison disease, chronic obstructive pulmonary disease (COPD), hypothyroidism, impaired liver function, increased intracranial pressure, prostatic hypertrophy, and urethral stricture. It is unknown whether belladonna and opium cross the placenta or are distributed in

breast milk. Children may be more susceptible to respiratory depression; not recommended for use in children < 12 yr of age. Elderly patients may also be more susceptible to respiratory depression, and the drug may cause paradoxical excitement. Age-related prostatic hypertrophy or obstruction and renal impairment may increase the risk of urinary retention, and dosage adjustment is recommended for elderly patients. Alcohol, tasks that require mental alertness and motor skills, hot baths, and saunas should be avoided.

Storage
Store at room temperature.
Administration
Moisten finger and suppository before rectal insertion.

Benazepril

be-naze′a-pril
(Lotensin)
Do not confuse benazepril with Benadryl, or Lotensin with Loniten or lovastatin.

CATEGORY AND SCHEDULE
Pregnancy Risk Category: C (D if used in second or third trimester)

Classification: Angiotensin-converting enzyme inhibitors

MECHANISM OF ACTION
An ACE inhibitor that decreases the rate of conversion of angiotensin I to angiotensin II, a potent vasoconstrictor. Reduces peripheral arterial resistance. *Therapeutic Effect:* Lowers BP.

PHARMACOKINETICS

Route	Onset	Peak	Duration
PO	1 h	2-4 h	24 h

Partially absorbed from the GI tract. Protein binding: 97%. Metabolized in the liver to active metabolite. Primarily excreted in urine. Minimal removal by hemodialysis. *Half-life:* 35 min; metabolite 10-11 h.

AVAILABILITY
Tablets: 5 mg, 10 mg, 20 mg, 40 mg.

INDICATIONS AND DOSAGES
▸ **Hypertension (monotherapy)**
PO
Adults. Initially, 10 mg/day. Maintenance: 20-40 mg/day as single dose or in 2 divided doses. Maximum: 80 mg/day.
Elderly. Initially, 5-10 mg/day. Range: 20-40 mg/day.
Children 6 yr of age and older. Initially 0.2 mg/kg once daily (maximum: initially: 5 mg/day). Maintenance 0.1-0.6 mg/kg once daily. Maximum 0.6 mg/kg (40 mg)/day.
▸ **Hypertension (combination therapy)**
PO
Adults. May discontinue diuretic 2-3 days before initiating benazepril, then dose as noted above. If unable to discontinue diuretic, begin benazepril at reduced dose of 5 mg/day.
▸ **Dosage in renal impairment**
For adult patients with creatinine clearance < 30 mL/min, initially, 5 mg/day titrated up to maximum of 40 mg/day. Not recommended in children with creatinine clearances < 30 mL/min.

OFF-LABEL USES
Treatment of congestive heart failure, diabetic neuropathy.

B

CONTRAINDICATIONS
History of angioedema from previous treatment with ACE inhibitors.

INTERACTIONS
Drug
Alcohol, antihypertensives, diuretics: May increase the effects of benazepril.
Lithium: May increase the lithium blood concentration and risk of lithium toxicity.
NSAIDs: May decrease the effects of benazepril.
Potassium-sparing diuretics, potassium supplements: May cause hyperkalemia. Avoid when possible.
Herbal
None known.
Food
None known.

DIAGNOSTIC TEST EFFECTS
May increase BUN, serum alkaline phosphatase, serum bilirubin, serum potassium, AST (SGOT), and ALT (SGPT) levels. May decrease serum sodium levels. May cause positive antinuclear antibody titer.

SIDE EFFECTS
Frequent (3%-6%)
Cough, headache, dizziness.
Occasional (2%)
Fatigue, somnolence or drowsiness, nausea.
Rare (< 1%)
Rash, fever, myalgia, diarrhea, loss of taste.

SERIOUS REACTIONS
• Excessive hypotension ("first-dose syncope") may occur in patients with CHF and in those who are severely salt or volume depleted.
• Angioedema (swelling of the face and lips) and hyperkalemia occur rarely.

• Agranulocytosis and neutropenia may be noted in those with collagen vascular disease, including scleroderma and systemic lupus erythematosus, and impaired renal function.
• Nephrotic syndrome may be noted in patients with history of renal disease.
• Hyperkalemia.

PRECAUTIONS & CONSIDERATIONS
Caution is warranted with cerebrovascular and coronary insufficiency, diabetes mellitus, hypovolemia, renal impairment, and sodium depletion as well as persons on dialysis and in those receiving diuretics. Benazepril crosses the placenta, and it is unknown whether it is distributed in breast milk. Benazepril may cause fetal or neonatal morbidity or mortality with exposure during the second or third trimesters. Safety and efficacy of benazepril have not been established in children < 6 yr of age. Elderly patients may be more sensitive to the hypotensive effects of benazepril.

Dizziness and orthostatic hypotension may occur. Rise slowly from lying to sitting position, and permit legs to dangle from the bed momentarily before standing to reduce the hypotensive effect of benazepril. Full therapeutic effect of benazepril may take 2-4 wks. BP should be obtained immediately before giving each benazepril dose, in addition to regular monitoring. Be alert to fluctuations in BP. If an excessive reduction in BP occurs, place the person in the supine position with legs elevated. CBC and blood chemistry should be obtained before beginning benazepril therapy, then every 2 wks for the next 3 mo, and periodically thereafter in patients with autoimmune disease or renal impairment and in those who are taking drugs that affect immune response or leukocyte count.

Administration
May take without regard to food. Do not skip doses.

Bentoquatam
ben'toe-kwa-tam
(IvyBlock)

CATEGORY AND SCHEDULE
Pregnancy Risk Category: NR

Classification: Rhus dermatitis protectant

MECHANISM OF ACTION
An organoclay substance that absorbs and binds to urushiol, the active principle in poison oak, ivy, and sumac. *Therapeutic Effect:* Blocks urushiol skin contact and absorption.

PHARMACOKINETICS
None reported.

AVAILABILITY
Lotion: 5% (IvyBlock).

INDICATIONS AND DOSAGES
▸ **Contact dermatitis prophylaxis caused by poison oak, ivy, or sumac**
TOPICAL
Adults, Elderly, Children 6 yr and older. Apply thin film over skin at least 15 min before potential exposure. Re-apply q4hr or sooner if needed.

CONTRAINDICATIONS
Hypersensitivity to bentoquatam or any of its components such as methylparabens.

INTERACTIONS
Drug
None known.
Herbal
None known.
Food
None known.

DIAGNOSTIC TEST EFFECTS
None known.

SIDE EFFECTS
Occasional
Erythema.

SERIOUS REACTIONS
• None reported.

PRECAUTIONS & CONSIDERATIONS
Caution is necessary in patients with a history of allergic-type responses to medications, especially topical formulations, open wounds, psoriatic lesions, or other cutaneous conditions. The use of bentoquatam has not been studied in pregnancy. There are no age-related precautions noted in children or in elderly patients.
Storage
Store at room temperature.
Administration
Bentoquatam is for external use only. Bentoquatam is a protectant, not a treatment, for poison oak, ivy, or sumac. Shake well before use. Apply 15 min before exposure. Do not apply after exposure. Reapply every 4 h or sooner if needed to maintain protection.

B

Benzocaine
ben'zoe-kane
(Americaine Anesthetic Lubricant,
Americaine Otic, Anbesol,
Anbesol Baby Gel, Anbesol
Maximum Strength, Babee
Teething, Benzodent, Cepacol,
Cetacaine, Chiggerex, Chiggertox,
Cylex, Dermoplast, Detaine,
Foille, Foille Medicated First
Aid, Foille Plus, HDA Toothache,
Hurricane, Lanacane, Mycinettes,
Omedia, Orabase-B, Orajel, Orajel
Baby, Orajel Baby Nighttime,
Orajel Maximum Strength, Orasol,
Otricaine, Otocain, Retre-Gel,
Solarcaine, Topicaine [AUS],
Trocaine, Zilactin, Zilactin Baby).

CATEGORY AND SCHEDULE
Pregnancy Risk Category: C

Classification: Topical ester
local anesthetic

MECHANISM OF ACTION
A local anesthetic that blocks nerve
conduction in the autonomic, sensory,
and motor nerve fibers. Competes
with calcium ions for membrane
binding. Reduces permeability of
resting nerves to potassium and
sodium ions. *Therapeutic Effect:*
Produces local analgesic effect.

PHARMACOKINETICS
Poorly absorbed by topical
administration. Well absorbed from
mucous membranes and traumatized
skin. Metabolized in liver and by
hydrolysis with cholinesterase.
Minimal excretion in urine.

AVAILABILITY
Cream: 5%, 20% (Lanacane).
Lozenge: 10 mg (Cepacol, Trocaine),
15 mg (Cyclex, Mycinettes).

Oral Aerosol: 14% (Cetacaine), 20%
(Hurricane).
Oral Gel: 6.3% (Anbesol), 6.5%
(HDA Toothache), 7.5% (Anbesol
Baby, Detaine, Orajel Baby), 10%
(Orajel, Orajel Baby Nighttime,
Zilactin-B, Zilactin Baby), 20%
(Anbesol Maximum Strength,
Hurricane).
Oral Liquid: 6.3% (Anbesol), 7.5%
(Orajel Baby), 10% (Orajel), 20%
(Anbesol Maximum Strength,
Hurricane).
Oral Lotion: 2.5% (Babee Teething).
Oral Ointment: 20% (Benzadent).
Otic Solution: 20% (Americane Otic,
Omedia, Oticaine, Otocain).
Paste: 20% (Orabase-B).
Topical Aerosol: 5% (Foille,
Foille Plus), 20% (Dermoplast,
Solarcaine).
Topical Gel: 5% (Retre-Gel), 20%
(Americaine Anesthetic Lubricant).
Topical Liquid: 2% (Chiggertox).
Topical Ointment: 2%
(Chiggerex), 5% (Foille Medicated
First Aid).

INDICATIONS AND DOSAGES
▶ **Canker sores**
TOPICAL
*Adults, Elderly, Children older
than 2 yr.* Apply gel, liquid, or
ointment to affected area. Maximum:
4 times/day.
▶ **Denture irritation**
TOPICAL
Adults, Elderly. Apply a thin layer of
gel to affected area up to 4 times/day
or until pain is relieved.
▶ **General lubrication**
TOPICAL
*Adults, Elderly, Children older
than 2 yr.* Apply gel to exterior of
tube or instrument before use.
▶ **Otitis externa, otitis media**
OTIC
*Adults, Elderly, Children older
than 1 yr.* Instill 4-5 drops into

external ear canal of affected ears. Repeat q1-2h as needed.
▸ **Pain and itching associated with sunburn, insect bites, minor cuts, scrapes, minor burns, minor skin irritations**
TOPICAL
Adults, Elderly, Children older than 2 yr. Apply to affected area 3-4 times/day.
▸ **Pharyngitis**
PO
Adults, Elderly. 1 lozenge q2hr. Maximum 8 lozenges/day.
▸ **Toothache/teething pain**
TOPICAL
Adults, Elderly, Children older than 2 yr. Apply gel, liquid, or ointment to affected areas. Maximum: 4 times/day. Do not use for more than 7 days.
▸ **Anesthesia**
TOPICAL
Adults, Elderly. Apply aerosol, gel, ointment, liquid q4-12h as needed.

CONTRAINDICATIONS

Hypersensitivity to benzocaine or ester-type local anesthetics, perforated tympanic membrane or ear discharge (otic preparations).

INTERACTIONS

Drug
Hyaluronidase: May increase the incidence of systemic reaction to benzocaine, when used at same sites.
Herbal
None known.
Food
None known.

DIAGNOSTIC TEST EFFECTS

None known.

SIDE EFFECTS

Occasional
Burning, stinging, angioedema, contact dermatitis, taste disorders.

SERIOUS REACTIONS

• Methemoglobinemia occurs rarely in infants and young children.

PRECAUTIONS & CONSIDERATIONS
Caution should be used with children younger than 2 yr and infants and with inflamed skin or open wounds. It is unknown whether benzocaine crosses the placenta or is distributed in breast milk. Safety and efficacy of this drug have not been established in children younger than 2 yr for topical preparations and younger than 1 yr for otic solutions. There are no age-related precautions for elderly patients. Avoid contact with eyes.

An allergic reaction with blue color around mouth, fingers, or toes; fast breathing; redness; pain or swelling; or unusual tiredness or weakness should be reported immediately (may signal methemoglobinemia).
Administration
Oral, topical, or dental use: Do not eat 1 h before topical oral administration. Rinse mouth well before reinserting dentures. Do not use for more than 1 wk.

Clean area before applying topical aerosol benzocaine. For external use only. Hold can 6-12 in. away from affected area. If applying to face, spray in palm of hand and then apply to affected area. Do not spray for longer than 2 seconds.

Benzonatate
ben-zoe′na-tate
(Tessalon Perles)

CATEGORY AND SCHEDULE
Pregnancy Risk Category: C

Classification: Antitussive, nonnarcotic, ester, local anesthetic

MECHANISM OF ACTION
A nonnarcotic antitussive that anesthetizes stretch receptors in respiratory passages, lungs, and pleura. *Therapeutic Effect:* Reduces cough.

PHARMACOKINETICS
PO onset 15-20 min; duration 3-8 h; metabolized by liver, excreted in urine.

AVAILABILITY
Capsules: 100 mg, 200 mg.

INDICATIONS AND DOSAGES
▸ **Antitussive**
PO
Adults, Elderly, Children older than 10 yr. 100 mg 3 times/day only if needed, may give up to q4h (maximum: 600 mg/day).

OFF-LABEL USES
Intractable hiccups.

CONTRAINDICATIONS
Hypersensitivity.

INTERACTIONS
Drug
CNS depressants: May increase the effects of benzonatate.
Herbal
None known.
Food
None known.

DIAGNOSTIC TEST EFFECTS
None known.

SIDE EFFECTS
Occasional
Mild somnolence, mild dizziness, constipation, GI upset, skin eruptions, nasal congestion.

SERIOUS REACTIONS
• A paradoxical reaction, including restlessness, insomnia, euphoria, nervousness, and tremor, has been noted, especially in overdose.
• Severe hypersensitivity (rare).

PRECAUTIONS & CONSIDERATIONS
Caution is warranted with a productive cough. Dizziness and drowsiness are common side effects. Avoid tasks that require mental alertness or motor skills until response to the drug has been established. Fluid intake and environmental humidity should be increased to lower the viscosity of secretions.
Administration
Take benzonatate without regard to food. Swallow the capsules whole; chewing them or dissolving them in the mouth may produce temporary local anesthesia or choking, which may compromise the airway.

Benzoyl Peroxide

ben′zoe-ill per-ox′ide
(Acetoxyl [CAN], Benoxyl [CAN],
Benzac, Benzac AC, Benzac
AC Wash, Benzac W, Benzac
W Wash, Benzagel, Benzagel
Wash, Benzashave, Brevoxyl,
Brevoxyl Cleansing, Brevoxyl
Wash, Clearplex, Clinac BPO, Del
Aqua, Desquam-E, Desquam-X,
Exact Acne Medication, Fostex
10% BPO, Loroxide, Neutrogena
Acne Mask, Neutrogena On The
Spot Acne Treatment, Oxy [AUS],
Oxy 10 Balanced Medicated
Face Wash, Oxy 10 Balance Spot
Treatment, Palmer's Skin Success
Acne, Oxyderm [CAN], PanOxyl,
PanOxyl-AQ, PanOxyl Aqua Gel,
PanOxylBar, Seba-Gel, Solugel
[CAN], Triaz, Triaz Cleanser,
Zapzyt).

CATEGORY AND SCHEDULE

Pregnancy Risk Category: C
OTC

Classification: Antiacne agent,
topical; keratolytic, topical

MECHANISM OF ACTION

A keratolytic agent that releases
free-radical oxygen, which oxidizes
bacterial proteins in the sebaceous
follicles, decreasing the number of
anaerobic bacteria and decreasing
irritating-type free fatty acids.
Therapeutic Effect: Bactericidal
action against *Propionibacterium
acnes* and *Staphylococcus
epidermidis.*

PHARMACOKINETICS

Minimal absorption through skin.
Gel is more penetrating than cream.
Metabolized to benzoic acid in skin.
Excreted in urine as benzoate.

AVAILABILITY

Cream, Topical: 2.5% (Neutrogena
On The Spot Acne Treatment), 3.5%
(NeoBenz Micro), 5% (Benzashave,
Exact Acne Medication, Neutrogena
Acne Mask), 5.5% (NeoBenz
Micro), 8.5% (NeoBenz Micro),
10% (Benzashave, Clearasil).
Gel, Topical: 2.5% (Benzac, Benzac
AC, Benzac W, Desquam-E), 4%
(Brevoxyl), 4.5% (Zoderm), 5%
(Benzac, Benzac AC, Benzac W,
Benzagel, Clearplex, Desquam-E,
Desquam-X, Oxy 10 Balance Spot
Treatment, PanOxyl, PanOxyl AQ,
Seba-Gel), 6% (Triaz, Triaz Cleanser),
6.5% (Zoderm), 7% (Clinac BPO),
8% (Brevoxyl), 8.5% (Zoderm), 9%
(Triaz), 10% (Benzac, Benzac AC,
Benzac W, Benzagel, Benzagel Wash,
Clearplex, Desquam-E, Desquam-X,
Fostex, Oxy 10 Balance Spot
Treatment, PanOxyl, PanOxyl AQ,
PanOxyl Aqua Gel, Seba-Gel, Triaz,
Triaz Cleanser, Zapzyt).
Liquid, Topical: 2.5% (Benzac AC
Wash), 3% (Triaz), 4% (Brevoxyl),
5% (Benzac AC Wash, Benzac W
Wash, Del-Aqua, Desquam-X), 6%
(Triaz), 8% (Brevoxyl), 9% (Triaz),
10% (Benzac AC Wash, Benzac W
Wash, Del-Aqua, Oxy-10 Balance
Medicated Face Wash).
Lotion, Topical: 3% (Triaz Cleanser),
4% (Brevoxyl Cleansing, Brevoxyl
Wash), 5%, 5.5% (Loroxide), 6% (Triaz
Cleanser), 8% (Brevoxyl Cleansing,
Brevoxyl Wash), 10% (Fostex, Palmerís
Skin Success Acne, Triaz Cleanser).
Soap Bar, Topical: 5% (PanOxyl
Bar), 10% (Desquam-X, Fostex,
PanOxyl Bar).

INDICATIONS AND DOSAGES
▸ **Acne**
TOPICAL
Adults. Apply 2.5%-10%
concentration 1-2 times/day;
cleansers used 1-2 times/day.

OFF-LABEL USES
Dermal ulcers, seborrheic dermatitis, surgical wounds, tinea pedis, tinea versicolor.

CONTRAINDICATIONS
Hypersensitivity to benzoyl peroxide or any component of the formulation.

INTERACTIONS
Drug
Sunscreens containing PABA: May cause skin to change color when both agents are used concomitantly.
Tretinoin: May increase skin irritation.
Herbal
None known.
Food
None known.

DIAGNOSTIC TEST EFFECTS
None known.

SIDE EFFECTS
Occasional
Irritation, dryness, burning, peeling, stinging, contact dermatitis, bleaching of hair.

SERIOUS REACTIONS
• Hypersensitivity reactions have been reported with benzoyl peroxide use.

PRECAUTIONS & CONSIDERATIONS
Caution should be used on skin because benzoyl peroxide may cause contact dermatitis, hair bleaching, and seborrhea. Caution should also be used around the eyes, lips, mucous membranes, and highly inflamed skin. Sun exposure may increase skin irritation. Be aware that cross-sensitization may occur with benzoic acid derivatives such as cinnamon and other topical anesthetics. It is unknown whether benzoyl peroxide crosses the placenta or is distributed in breast milk. Safety and efficacy of benzoyl peroxide have not been established in children younger than 12 yr. There are no age-related precautions noted for elderly patients.

Mild stinging and redness may occur. Be aware that benzoyl peroxide may bleach hair and fabric.
Storage
Store at room temperature.
Administration
Control frequency or concentration of benzoyl peroxide by the amount of drying or peeling. If excessive dryness or peeling occurs, decrease dose. Avoid eyes and mucous membranes. Follow directions for specific product type.

Benztropine
benz'troe-peen
(Apo-Benztropine [CAN], Bentrop [AUS], Cogentin)
Do not confuse benztropine with bromocriptine.

CATEGORY AND SCHEDULE
Pregnancy Risk Category: C

Classification: Anticholinergic, antidyskinetic

MECHANISM OF ACTION
An antiparkinson agent that selectively blocks central cholinergic receptors, helping to balance cholinergic and dopaminergic activity. *Therapeutic Effect:* Reduces the incidence and severity of akinesia, rigidity, and tremor.

PHARMACOKINETICS
IM/IV: Onset 15 min, duration 6-10 h.
PO: onset 1 h, duration 6-10 h.

AVAILABILITY
Tablets: 0.5 mg, 1 mg, 2 mg.
Injection: 1 mg/mL.

INDICATIONS AND DOSAGES
▸ **Parkinsonism**
PO
Adults. 0.5-6 mg/day as a
single dose or in 2 divided doses.
Titrate by 0.5 mg at 5- to 6-day
intervals.
Elderly. Initially, 0.5 mg once or
twice a day. Titrate by 0.5 mg
at 5- to 6-day intervals. Maximum:
4 mg/day.
▸ **Drug-induced extrapyramidal
symptoms**
PO, IM
Adults. 1-4 mg once or twice a day.
Children older than 3 yr.
0.02-0.05 mg/kg/dose once or twice
a day.
▸ **Acute dystonic reactions**
IM, IV (IM PREFERRED)
Adults. Initially, 1-2 mg; then 1-2 mg
PO twice a day to prevent recurrence.

⚈ IV INCOMPATIBILITIES
Diazepam, Furosemide, Phenytoin.

CONTRAINDICATIONS
Angle-closure glaucoma,
benign prostatic hyperplasia,
children younger than 3 yr, GI
obstruction, intestinal atony,
megacolon, myasthenia gravis,
paralytic ileus, severe ulcerative
colitis.

INTERACTIONS
Drug
Alcohol, other CNS depressants:
May increase sedation.
**Amantadine, anticholinergics,
MAOIs:** May increase the effects of
benztropine.
Antacids, antidiarrheals: May
decrease the absorption and effects
of benztropine.

**Phenothiazines, tricyclic
antidepressants:** May increase
the risk of heat intolerance,
hyperthermia, and heat stroke.

DIAGNOSTIC TEST EFFECTS
None known.

SIDE EFFECTS
Frequent
Somnolence, dry mouth, blurred
vision, constipation, decreased
sweating or urination, GI upset,
photosensitivity.
Occasional
Headache, memory loss, muscle
cramps, anxiety, peripheral
paresthesia, orthostatic hypotension,
abdominal cramps.
Rare
Rash, confusion, eye pain.

SERIOUS REACTIONS
• Overdose may produce severe
anticholinergic effects, such as
unsteadiness, somnolence, tachycardia,
dyspnea, skin flushing, and severe
dryness of the mouth, nose, or throat.
• Severe paradoxical reactions, marked
by hallucinations, tremor, seizures, and
toxic psychosis, may occur.

PRECAUTIONS & CONSIDERATIONS
Caution is warranted with
arrhythmias, heart disease,
hypertension, hepatic or renal
impairment, obstructive diseases
of the GI or genitourinary tracts,
urine retention, benign prostatic
hyperplasia, tachycardia, and treated
open-angle glaucoma. Caution is
advised in hot weather; benztropine
may increase risk of hyperthermia
and heat stroke. Elderly (older than 60
yr) patients are more likely to develop
agitation, disorientation, confusion,
and psychotic-like symptoms.
Dizziness, drowsiness, and dry
mouth are expected responses to

the drug. Alcohol and tasks that require mental alertness or motor skills should be avoided. Notify the physician of agitation, headache, somnolence, or confusion.

Administration
Oral: May give without regard to meals. Initial doses usually given at bedtime or dose may be divided throughout the day to treat tremors. Improvement usually occurs in 1-2 days.

Beractant
ber-akt′ant
(Survanta)
Do not confuse Survanta with Sufenta.

CATEGORY AND SCHEDULE
Pregnancy Risk Category: This drug is not indicated for use in pregnant women.

Classification: Surfactants, lung

MECHANISM OF ACTION
A natural bovine lung extract that reduces alveolar surface tension, stabilizing alveoli. *Therapeutic Effect:* Improves lung compliance and respiratory gas exchange.

PHARMACOKINETICS
Not absorbed systemically.

AVAILABILITY
Intratracheal Suspension for Inhalation: 25 mg/mL vials.

INDICATIONS AND DOSAGES
▶ **Prevention and rescue treatment of respiratory distress syndrome (RDS) or hyaline membrane disease in premature infants**
ENDOTRACHEAL
Infants. 100 mg of phospholipids/kg birth weight (4 mL/kg).

Give within 15 min of birth if infant weighs < 1250 g and has evidence of surfactant deficiency; give within 8 h when RDS is confirmed by x-ray and requires mechanical ventilation. May repeat 6 h or longer after preceding dose. Maximum: 4 doses in the first 48 h of life.

CONTRAINDICATIONS
None known.

INTERACTIONS
Drug
None known.
Herbal
None known.
Food
None known.

DIAGNOSTIC TEST EFFECTS
None known.

SIDE EFFECTS
Frequent
Transient bradycardia, oxygen (O_2) desaturation, increased carbon dioxide (CO_2) retention.
Occasional
Endotracheal tube reflux.
Rare
Apnea, endotracheal tube blockage, hypotension or hypertension, pallor, vasoconstriction.

SERIOUS REACTIONS
• Life-threatening nosocomial sepsis may occur but is a risk factor for the population in general.

PRECAUTIONS & CONSIDERATIONS
Caution should be used in persons at risk for circulatory overload. This drug is for use only in neonates. No age-related precautions have been noted.

The infant should be monitored with arterial or transcutaneous measurement of systemic O_2 and CO_2. Visitors should be limited during treatment. Handwashing and other infection control measures should be monitored to minimize the risk of nosocomial infections.

Storage

Refrigerate vials. Unopened, unused vials may be returned to the refrigerator only once and within 8 h after having been warmed to room temperature.

Administration

Administer beractant in a highly supervised setting. Clinicians caring for the neonate must be experienced with intubation and ventilator management.

Warm the vial by letting it stand at room temperature for 20 min or warming in your hand for 8 min. Gently swirl the vial, if needed, to redisperse contents. Do not shake it. The solution normally appears off-white to light brown. Enter each single-use vial only once; discard unused suspension. Use a 20-gauge or larger needle to withdraw the proper dose from the vial. Do not filter.

Instill the drug through a catheter inserted into the infant's endotracheal tube in 4 quarter doses, with the infant in a different position for each quarter dose. Do not instill it into the mainstem bronchus. Monitor the infant for bradycardia and decreased arterial O_2 saturation during administration. Stop the procedure, as prescribed, if the infant experiences these effects, and take appropriate measures before reinstituting therapy.

Betamethasone

bay-ta-meth′a-sone
(glucocorticoid, synthetic, corticosteroid, systemic, corticosteroid, topical)
(Alphatrex, Betaderm [CAN], Betatrex, Beta-Val, Betnesol [CAN], Celestone, Diprolene, Luxiq, Maxivate)

CATEGORY AND SCHEDULE

Pregnancy Risk Category: C (D if used in first trimester)

Classification: Corticosteroid

MECHANISM OF ACTION

An adrenocortical steroid that controls the rate of protein synthesis, depresses the migration of polymorphonuclear leukocytes and fibroblasts, reduces capillary permeability, and prevents or controls inflammation. *Therapeutic Effect:* Decreases tissue response to inflammatory process.

PHARMACOKINETICS

PO: Onset 1-2 h, peak 1 h, duration 3 days. IM/IV: onset 10 min, peak 4-8 h, duration 1-1.5 days. Metabolized in liver, excreted in urine as steroids, crosses the placenta.

AVAILABILITY

Tablet (Celestone): 0.6 mg.
Cream (Alphatrex, Diprolene, Maxivate): 0.05%.
Cream (Betatrex, Beta-Val): 0.1%.
Foam (Luxiq): 0.12%.
Gel (Diprolene): 0.05%.
Lotion: (Alphatrex, Diprolene, Maxivate): 0.05%.
Lotion (Betatrex; Beta-Val): 0.1%.
Ointment (Alphatrex, Diprolene, Maxivate): 0.05%.

Ointment (Betatrex): 0.1%.
Syrup (Celestone): 0.6 mg/5 mL.
Injection (Celestone, Soluspan):
6 mg/mL.

INDICATIONS AND DOSAGES

▸ **Anti-inflammation,
immunosuppression, corticosteroid
replacement therapy**
PO
Adults, Elderly. 0.6-7.2 mg/day.
Children. 0.063-0.25 mg/kg/day in
3-4 divided doses.
IM
Adults. 0.6-9 mg/day (generally, ⅓
to ½ of oral dose) divided every
12-24 h.
Children. 0.0175-0.125 mg/kg/day
divided every 6-12 h or 0.5-7.5 mg
base/m²/day divided every 6-12 h.
▸ **Relief of inflamed and pruritic
dermatoses**
TOPICAL
Adults, Elderly. 1-2 times a day.
Foam: Apply twice a day.
INTRADERMAL
Adults. 0.2 mL/cm²/dose. Maximum
dose 1 mL/wk.
▸ **Rheumatoid arthritis/osteoarthritis**
INTRA-ARTICULAR
Adults. 0.5-2 mL; 1-2 mL in very
large joints (hip), 1 mL in large joints
(knee, ankle, or shoulder), 0.5-1 mL
in medium joints (wrist, elbow), and
0.25-0.5 mL in small joints (hand,
chest).
▸ **Bursitis**
INTRABURSAL
Adult. 0.5-1 mL depending on
affected area.

OFF-LABEL USES

Fetal lung maturation to prophylax;
anticipate neonatal respiratory
immaturity (IM dosage).

CONTRAINDICATIONS

Hypersensitivity to betamethasone,
systemic fungal infections.

INTERACTIONS

Drug
Amphotericin; Diuretics: May
increase hypokalemia.
Digoxin: May increase digoxin
toxicity secondary to hypokalemia.
Insulin, oral hypoglycemics: May
decrease the effects of these drugs.
(example: Rifampin)
Hepatic enzyme inducers: May
decrease the systemic effect of
betamethasone.
Live virus vaccines: May decrease
the patient's antibody response
to vaccine, and potentiate virus
replication.

DIAGNOSTIC TEST EFFECTS

May increase blood glucose levels
and serum lipids, amylase, and
sodium levels. May decrease serum
calcium, potassium, and thyroxine
levels.

SIDE EFFECTS

Frequent
Systemic: Increased appetite,
abdominal distention, nervousness,
insomnia, false sense of well-being.
Topical: Burning, stinging, pruritus.
Occasional
Systemic: Dizziness, facial flushing,
diaphoresis, decreased or blurred
vision, mood swings.
Topical: Allergic contact dermatitis,
purpura or blood-containing blisters,
thinning of skin with easy bruising,
telangiectases or raised dark red
spots on skin.

SERIOUS REACTIONS

• Systemic hypercorticism and
adrenal suppression.

PRECAUTIONS & CONSIDERATIONS

Caution is warranted with persons at
increased risk for peptic ulcer disease
and in those with cirrhosis, diabetes,
heart failure, hypothyroidism,

Smyasthenia gravis, osteoporosis, renal impairment, or nonspecific ulcerative colitis. Monitor the growth and development of children receiving long-term steroid therapy.

Mood swings, ranging from euphoria to depression, may occur. Initially, tuberculosis skin test, x-rays, and ECG should be evaluated. Blood glucose level, BP, serum electrolyte levels, height, and weight should be monitored before and during therapy. Injectable form should not be given intravenously.

Storage
Store all forms at room temperature.

Administration
Give oral betamethasone with milk or food to decrease GI upset. Give single doses in the morning before 9 AM; give multiple doses at evenly spaced intervals. Do not abruptly discontinue the drug.

For topical use, gently cleanse area before applying drug. Apply sparingly and rub into area thoroughly. Use occlusive dressings only as ordered. When using aerosol, spray area for 3 s from a 15-cm distance; avoid inhalation. Do not use topical form on broken skin or in areas of infection, and do not apply to the face or inguinal areas or to wet skin.

For injection, shake well before using. If coadministration of a local anesthetic is desired, betamethasone sodium phosphate/ betamethasone acetate injectable suspension may be mixed with 1% or 2% lidocaine hydrochloride or similar local anesthetics, using the formulations which do not contain parabens.

Betaxolol
bay-tax′oh-lol
(Betoptic-S, Betoquin [AUS], Kerlone)
Do not confuse betaxolol with bethanechol.

CATEGORY AND SCHEDULE
Pregnancy Risk Category: C (D if used in second or third trimester)

Classification: Antihypertensive, selective β_1-blocker

MECHANISM OF ACTION
An antihypertensive and antiglaucoma agent that blocks β_1-adrenergic receptors in cardiac tissue. Reduces aqueous humor production. *Therapeutic Effect:* Slows sinus heart rate, decreases BP, and reduces intraocular pressure (IOP).

PHARMACOKINETICS
PO: peak 3-4 h. *Half-life:* 14-22 hr; protein binding 50%; some hepatic metabolism; excreted in urine mostly unchanged.

AVAILABILITY
Tablets (Kerlone): 10 mg, 20 mg.
Ophthalmic Solution (Betoptic): 0.5%.
Ophthalmic Suspension (Betoptic-S): 0.25%.

INDICATIONS AND DOSAGES
▸ **Hypertension**
PO
Adults. Initially, 5-10 mg/day. May increase to 20 mg/day after 7-14 days. Maximum: 40 mg/day.
Elderly. Initially, 5 mg/day, then titrate as per adult dose.
▸ **Chronic open-angle glaucoma and ocular hypertension**

B

SOLUTION-EYEDROPS
Adults, Elderly: 1-2 drop(s) twice a day in affected eye(s).
SUSPENSION EYEDROPS (BETOPTIC-S)
1 drop twice a day in affected eyes.
▸ **Oral dosage in renal impairment**
Adult and elderly patients on dialysis. Initially give 5 mg/day; increase by 5 mg/day q2wk. Maximum: 20 mg/day.

OFF-LABEL USES

Treatment of angle-closure glaucoma during or after iridectomy, malignant glaucoma, secondary glaucoma; with miotics, to decrease IOP in acute and chronic angle-closure glaucoma.

CONTRAINDICATIONS

Cardiogenic shock, overt cardiac failure, second- or third-degree heart block, sinus bradycardia, hypersensitivity.

INTERACTIONS

Drug
Cimetidine: May increase betaxolol blood concentration.
Diuretics, other antihypertensives: May increase hypotensive effect of betaxolol.
Insulin, oral hypoglycemics: May mask signs & symptoms of hypoglycemia from these drugs.
NSAIDs: May decrease antihypertensive effect.
Sympathomimetics, xanthines: May mutually inhibit hypotensive effects and may mask symptoms of hypoglycemia.

DIAGNOSTIC TEST EFFECTS

May increase serum antinuclear antibody titer and BUN, serum lipoprotein, creatinine, potassium, uric acid, and triglyceride levels.

SIDE EFFECTS

Betaxolol is generally well tolerated, with mild and transient side effects.

Frequent
Systemic: Hypotension manifested as dizziness, nausea, diaphoresis, headache, fatigue, constipation or diarrhea, dyspnea.
Ophthalmic: Eye irritation, visual disturbances.
Occasional
Systemic: Insomnia, flatulence, urinary frequency, impotence or decreased libido, bradycardia, bronchospasm
Ophthalmic: Increased light sensitivity, watering of eye.
Rare
Systemic: Rash, arrhythmias, arthralgia, myalgia, confusion, altered taste, increased urination.
Ophthalmic: Dry eye, conjunctivitis, eye pain.

SERIOUS REACTIONS

• Overdose may produce profound bradycardia, hypotension, and bronchospasm.
• Abrupt withdrawal may result in diaphoresis, palpitations, headache, and tremors.
• Betaxolol administration may precipitate CHF or MI in patients with cardiac disease; thyroid storm in those with thyrotoxicosis; and peripheral ischemia in those with existing peripheral vascular disease.
• Hypoglycemia may occur in patients with previously controlled diabetes.
• Ophthalmic overdose may produce bradycardia, hypotension, bronchospasm, and acute cardiac failure.

PRECAUTIONS & CONSIDERATIONS

Caution is warranted with diabetes, hyperthyroidism, impaired hepatic or renal function, inadequate cardiac function, and peripheral vascular disease. Betaxolol is excreted in breast milk; use with caution in nursing mothers.

Orthostatic hypotension may occur, so rise slowly from a lying to sitting position and dangle the legs from the bed momentarily before standing. Notify the physician of fatigue, headache, prolonged dizziness, and shortness of breath. BP for hypotension, respiratory status for shortness of breath, pattern of daily bowel activity and stool consistency, and pulse for quality, rate, and rhythm should be monitored during treatment. If pulse rate is 60 beats/min or lower or systolic BP is < 90 mm Hg, withhold the medication and contact the physician. Signs and symptoms of CHF, such as decreased urine output, distended neck veins, dyspnea (particularly on exertion or lying down), night cough, peripheral edema, and weight gain should also be assessed.

Storage
Store at room temperature (all forms).
Administration
To assess tolerance for betaxolol, obtain a standing systolic BP 1 h after giving the drug. Do not abruptly discontinue betaxolol. Compliance is essential to control glaucoma and hypertension.

Shake ophthalmic suspension well before using. After administration, perform nasolacrimal occlusion to reduce systemic absorption. Remove contact lens before administration and wait 15 min before reinserting. If other ophthalmic solutions are being used concurrently, administer at least 10 min before instilling the suspension.
Oral: May give without regard to food.

Bethanechol
be-than′e-kole
(Duvoid [CAN], Myotonachol [CAN], Urecholine, Urocarb [AUS])
Do not confuse bethanechol with betaxolol.

CATEGORY AND SCHEDULE
Pregnancy Risk Category: C

Classification: Cholinergic stimulant

MECHANISM OF ACTION
A cholinergic that acts directly at cholinergic receptors in the smooth muscle of the urinary bladder and GI tract. Increases detrusor muscle tone. *Therapeutic Effect:* May initiate micturition and bladder emptying. Improves gastric and intestinal motility.

PHARMACOKINETICS
PO onset 30-90 min, duration 6 h. SC onset 5-15 min, duration 2 h; excreted by kidneys.

AVAILABILITY
Tablets: 5 mg, 10 mg, 25 mg, 50 mg.

INDICATIONS AND DOSAGES
▶ **Postoperative and postpartum urine retention, neurogenic atony of bladder with retention**
PO
Adults, Elderly. 10-50 mg 3-4 times a day. Minimum effective dose determined by giving 5-10 mg initially, then repeating same amount at 1-h intervals until desired response is achieved, or maximum of 50 mg is reached.

B

OFF-LABEL USES
Treatment of congenital megacolon, gastroesophageal reflux, postoperative gastric atony.

CONTRAINDICATIONS
Active or latent bronchial asthma, acute inflammatory GI tract conditions, anastomosis, bladder wall instability, cardiac or coronary artery disease, epilepsy, hypertension, hyperthyroidism, hypotension, GI or urinary tract obstruction, parkinsonism, peptic ulcer, pronounced bradycardia, recent GI resection, vasomotor instability.

INTERACTIONS
Drug
Cholinesterase inhibitors: May increase the effects and risk of toxicity of bethanechol.
Procainamide, quinidine: May decrease the effects of bethanechol.
Herbal
None known.
Food
None known.

DIAGNOSTIC TEST EFFECTS
May increase serum amylase, lipase, and AST (SGOT) levels.

SIDE EFFECTS
Occasional
Belching, blurred or changed vision, diarrhea, urinary urgency.

SERIOUS REACTIONS
• Overdosage produces CNS stimulation (including insomnia, anxiety, and orthostatic hypotension) and cholinergic stimulation (such as headache, increased salivation, diaphoresis, nausea, vomiting, flushed skin, abdominal pain, and seizures).

PRECAUTIONS & CONSIDERATIONS
Notify the physician of difficulty breathing, irregular heartbeat, muscle weakness, nausea and vomiting, diarrhea, severe abdominal pain, and increased salivation or sweating. Intake and output and vital signs should be monitored. Not recommended in nursing mothers. Use with caution in patients with hypertension, urinary retention. Safety and effectiveness not established in children.
Administration
Take 1 h before meals or 2 h after meals to reduce nausea.

Bevacizumab
beh-vah-sif′zoo-mab
(Avastin)

CATEGORY AND SCHEDULE
Pregnancy Risk Category: C

Classification: Antineoplastics, monoclonal antibody; vascular endothelial growth factor (VEGF) inhibitor.

MECHANISM OF ACTION
An antineoplastic that binds to and inhibits vascular endothelial growth factor, a protein that plays a major role in the formation of new blood vessels to tumors. *Therapeutic Effect:* Inhibits metastatic disease progression.

PHARMACOKINETICS
Clearance varies by body weight, gender, and tumor burden. *Half-life:* 20 days (range, 11-50 days).

AVAILABILITY
Injection: 25 mg/mL vial.

INDICATIONS AND DOSAGES

▶ **First-line treatment of metastatic carcinoma of the colon or rectum in combination with 5-fluorouracil (5-FU)**

IV INFUSION

Adults, Elderly. 5 mg/kg once every 14 days when used with bolus irinotecan/5-FU/leucovorin; 10 mg/kg once every 14 days when used with 5-FU/leucovorin/oxaliplatin.

▶ **Nonsquamous non–small cell lung cancer**

IV INFUSION

Adults, Elderly. 15 mg/kg once every 3 wks.

▶ **Metastatic HER2-negative breast cancer**

IV INFUSION

Adults, Elderly. 10 mg/kg once every 14 days. Used in a regimen with paclitaxel.

OFF-LABEL USES

Age-related macular degeneration, renal cell carcinoma.

CONTRAINDICATIONS

Bevacizumab therapy should be permanently discontinued in patients developing GI perforation, hypertensive crisis, nephrotic syndrome, fistula, serious bleeding, wound dehiscence requiring medical intervention.

INTERACTIONS

Drug
Sunitinib: May cause hemolytic anemia; avoid combination.
Herbal
None known.
Food
None known.

DIAGNOSTIC TEST EFFECTS

May decrease serum potassium, sodium, and hemoglobin levels; hematocrit; and WBC and platelet counts.

⊘ IV INCOMPATIBILITIES

Do not mix bevacizumab with dextrose solutions.

SIDE EFFECTS

Frequent (25%-73%)
Asthenia, vomiting, anorexia, hypertension, epistaxis, stomatitis, constipation, headache, dyspnea.
Occasional (15%-21%)
Altered taste, dry skin, exfoliative dermatitis, dizziness, flatulence, excessive lacrimation, skin discoloration, weight loss, myalgia.
Rare (6%-8%)
Nail disorder, skin ulcer, alopecia, confusion, abnormal gait, dry mouth.

SERIOUS REACTIONS

• Urinary tract infections, manifested as urinary frequency or urgency and proteinuria, occur frequently.
• Congestive heart failure, deep vein thrombosis, GI perforation, hypertensive crisis, nephrotic syndrome, and severe hemorrhage are the most serious reactions that occur.
• Anemia, neutropenia, and thrombocytopenia occur occasionally.
• Hypersensitivity reactions occur rarely.

PRECAUTIONS & CONSIDERATIONS

Caution is warranted with congestive heart failure, epistaxis, hypertension, proteinuria, and renal insufficiency. Bevacizumab should be permanently discontinued in patients developing GI perforation, fistula formation, wound dehiscence, serious bleeding, a severe arterial thromboembolic event, nephrotic syndrome, hypertensive crisis, or hypertensive encephalopathy. Therapy should be temporarily suspended in patients with moderate to severe proteinuria, with severe hypertension, or undergoing surgery. Bevacizumab is teratogenic and has the potential to impair fertility. Its use by pregnant women may decrease maternal and fetal body weight and increase the risk of fetal skeletal abnormalities. Breastfeeding women should not take bevacizumab. The safety and efficacy of bevacizumab have not been established in children. Patients older than 65 yr have a higher incidence of serious adverse reactions. Avoid receiving immunizations without the physician's approval and avoid contact with crowds, people with known infections, and anyone who has recently received a live-virus vaccine because bevacizumab lowers the body's resistance to infection.

Notify the physician if asthenia (loss of energy), abdominal pain, chills, fever, or nausea and vomiting occur. BP, CBC, serum potassium, and sodium levels should be monitored before and regularly during bevacizumab treatment. Urine should be assessed for proteinuria. Persons with a urine dipstick reading of 2+ or more should have a 24-h urine collection. Pattern of daily bowel activity and stool consistency should be monitored.

Storage
Refrigerate vials. Do not freeze. The diluted solution may be refrigerated for up to 8 h.

Administration
! Do not give bevacizumab by IV push or IV bolus. Withdraw the amount of bevacizumab needed for a dose and dilute it in 100 mL 0.9% NaCl. Do not administer or mix with dextrose solutions. Discard any unused portion. Infuse the initial dose of bevacizumab over 90 min after chemotherapy. If the person tolerates the first infusion well, the second infusion may be administered over 60 min.

Bexarotene
beks-air′oh-teen
(Targretin)

CATEGORY AND SCHEDULE
Pregnancy Risk Category: X

Classification: Antineoplastic, retinoids

MECHANISM OF ACTION
This retinoid antineoplastic agent binds to and activates retinoid X receptor subtypes, which regulate the genes that control cellular differentiation and proliferation. *Therapeutic Effect:* Inhibits growth of tumor cell lines of hematopoietic and squamous cell origin and induces tumor regression.

PHARMACOKINETICS
Moderately absorbed from the GI tract. Protein binding: > 99%. Metabolized in the liver. Primarily eliminated through the hepatobiliary system. *Half-life:* 7 h.

AVAILABILITY
Capsules, Soft Gelatin: 75 mg.
Gel, Topical: 1%.

INDICATIONS AND DOSAGES
▸ **Cutaneous T-cell lymphoma refractory to at least one prior systemic therapy**
PO
Adults. 300 mg/m^2/day. If no response and initial dose is well tolerated, may be increased to 400 mg/m^2/day. If not tolerated, may decrease to 200 mg/m^2/day, then to 100 mg/m^2/day. Round doses to nearest 75 mg.
TOPICAL
Adults. Initially apply once every other day. May increase at weekly

intervals up to 4 times/day. Most patients tolerate and maintain 2-4 times/day application.

OFF-LABEL USES
Treatment of diabetes mellitus; head, neck, lung, and renal cell carcinomas; Kaposi sarcoma.

CONTRAINDICATIONS
Hypersensitivity, pregnancy.

INTERACTIONS
Drug
Antidiabetics: May enhance the effects of these drugs.
Erythromycin, itraconazole, ketoconazole: May increase bexarotene blood concentrations.
Phenytoin, rifampin: May decrease bexarotene blood concentrations.
Oral contraceptives: May reduce efficacy of hormonal contraceptive contraceptives.
Vitamin A supplements and other retinoids: Increased toxicity; avoid concurrent use.
Food
Grapefruit juice: May increase bexarotene blood concentration and risk of toxicity.

DIAGNOSTIC TEST EFFECTS
May increase serum cholesterol, triglyceride, and total and LDL cholesterol levels. May increase CA-125 assay value in patients with ovarian cancer. May decrease serum HDL cholesterol levels, total thyroxine, and thyroid-stimulating hormone levels. May produce abnormal liver function test results.

SIDE EFFECTS
Frequent
Hyperlipidemia (79%), headache (30%), hypothyroidism (29%), asthenia (20%).

Occasional
Rash (17%); nausea (15%); peripheral edema (13%); dry skin, abdominal pain (11%); chills, exfoliative dermatitis (10%); diarrhea (7%).

SERIOUS REACTIONS
• Pancreatitis, hepatic failure, and pneumonia occur rarely.

PRECAUTIONS & CONSIDERATIONS
Caution is warranted with diabetes mellitus, lipid abnormalities, and hepatic impairment. Bexarotene use should be avoided during pregnancy because the drug may cause fetal harm. Pregnancy should be determined before beginning oral or topical treatment. Two reliable contraceptive methods (one nonhormonal) should be used during therapy and for 1 mo afterward. Notify the physician if she plans to become or becomes pregnant. It is unknown if bexarotene is distributed in breast milk; however, breastfeeding is not recommended. The safety and efficacy of bexarotene have not been established in children. No age-related precautions have been noted in the elderly. Abrasive, drying, or medicated soaps should be avoided during therapy. DEET-containing insect repellants should not be used concurrently due to an increased risk of DEET toxicity.

Baseline lipid profile, liver function, thyroid function, and WBC count should be determined. Serum cholesterol and triglyceride levels, CBC, and liver and thyroid function test results should be monitored during therapy.
Storage (all forms)
Store at room temperatures. Protect from light and moisture. Avoid high temperatures.

Administration
Take oral bexarotene with a fat-containing meal. Avoid application of topical bexarotene to normal skin. Cover lesion with generous coating; avoid occlusive dressings. Allow to dry before applying clothing.

Bicalutamide
bye-ka-loo′ta-mide
(Casodex, Cosudex [AUS])

CATEGORY AND SCHEDULE
Pregnancy Risk Category: X

Classification: Nonsteroidal antiandrogen, antineoplastic

MECHANISM OF ACTION
An antiandrogen antineoplastic agent that competitively inhibits androgen action by binding to androgen receptors in target tissue. *Therapeutic Effect:* Decreases growth of prostatic carcinoma.

PHARMACOKINETICS
Well absorbed from the GI tract. Protein binding: 96%. Metabolized in the liver to inactive metabolite. Excreted in urine and feces. Not removed by hemodialysis. *Half-life:* 5.8 days (prolonged in severe liver disease).

AVAILABILITY
Tablets: 50 mg.

INDICATIONS AND DOSAGES
▸ **Prostatic carcinoma**
PO
Adults, Elderly. 50 mg once a day in morning or evening, given concurrently with a luteinizing hormone-releasing hormone (LHRH) analogue or after surgical castration.

CONTRAINDICATIONS
Pregnancy, use in women, hypersensitivity to any component of the formulation.

INTERACTIONS
Drug
Potent CYP3A4 inhibitors: May increase bicalutamide exposure.
Warfarin: May increase warfarin's effects.
Herbal
St. John's wort: May decrease bicalutamide concentrations.

DIAGNOSTIC TEST EFFECTS
May increase BUN level and serum alkaline phosphatase, bilirubin, AST (SGOT), and ALT (SGPT) levels. May decrease blood hemoglobin level and WBC count.

SIDE EFFECTS
Frequent
Hot flashes (49%), breast pain (38%), muscle pain (27%), constipation (17%), diarrhea (10%), asthenia (15%), nausea (11%).
Occasional (8%-9%)
Nocturia, abdominal pain, peripheral edema.
Rare (3%-7%)
Vomiting, weight loss, dizziness, insomnia, rash, impotence, gynecomastia.

SERIOUS REACTIONS
• Sepsis, CHF, hypertension, hepatotoxicity, and iron deficiency anemia may occur.

PRECAUTIONS & CONSIDERATIONS
Caution is warranted with moderate to severe hepatic impairment. Liver function test results should be obtained before beginning therapy. Bicalutamide may inhibit spermatogenesis; this drug is not used in women. The safety and

efficacy of bicalutamide have not been established in children. No age-related precautions have been noted in elderly patients.

Potential side effects, such as diarrhea, nausea, and vomiting, may occur. Notify the physician if nausea and vomiting persist.

Administration
Give oral bicalutamide at the same time each day and without regard to food. Avoid abruptly discontinuing the drug. Both bicalutamide and the LHRH analogue must be continued to achieve the desired therapeutic effect.

Bimatoprost
bye-mat'-oh-prost
(Lumigan, Latisse)

CATEGORY AND SCHEDULE
Drug Class: A prostamide (synthetic structural analog of prostaglandin), antiglaucoma agents

MECHANISM OF ACTION
A synthetic analogue of prostaglandin with ocular hypotensive activity. *Therapeutic Effect:* Reduces intraocular pressure (IOP) by increasing the outflow of aqueous humor, increases eyelash growth.

PHARMACOKINETICS
Absorbed through the cornea and hydrolyzed to the active free acid form. Protein binding: 88%. Moderately distributed into body tissues. Metabolized in liver. Primarily excreted in urine; some elimination in feces. *Half-life:* 45 min.

AVAILABILITY
Ophthalmic solution: 0.03%

INDICATIONS AND DOSAGES
▸ **Glaucoma, Ocular Hypertension**
OPHTHALMIC
Adults, Elderly. 1 drop in affected eye(s) once daily, in the evening.
▸ **Hypotrichosis of eyelashes**
Adults. 1 drop to each eye at night, applied to the upper eyelid margin.

CONTRAINDICATIONS
Hypersensitivity to bimatoprost or any other component of the formulation.

DIAGNOSTIC TEST EFFECTS
None known.

SIDE EFFECTS
Frequent
Conjunctival hyperemia, growth of eyelashes, increased iris pigmentation, and ocular pruritus.
Occasional
Ocular dryness, visual disturbance, ocular burning, foreign body sensation, eye pain, pigmentation of the periocular skin, blepharitis, cataract, superficial punctate keratitis, eyelid erythema, ocular irritation, and eyelash darkening.
Rare
Intraocular inflammation (iritis).

SERIOUS REACTIONS
• Systemic adverse events, including infections (colds and upper respiratory tract infections), headaches, asthenia, and hirsutism, have been reported.

PRECAUTIONS & CONSIDERATIONS
May permanently increase pigmentation in iris and eyelid and produce changes in eye color and changes in eyelashes (color, length, shape). Use with caution in patients with uveitis or risk factors for macular edema. Effects in pregnancy and lactation not known; use with caution

and only if clearly needed in women who are pregnant or breastfeeding. Safety and effectiveness have not been established in children. Remove contact lenses to apply; wait 15 min after administration to reinsert.

Storage
Store at room temperature.

Administration
If more than 1 topical ophthalmic agent is being used, wait at least 5 min between administration of each.

Latisse administration is different from that of lumigan.

Follow product directions carefully for best use.

Bisacodyl
bis-ah-koe′dill
(Alophen, Apo-Bisacodyl [CAN], Bisalax [AUS], Dulcolax, Femilax, Gentlax, Modane, Veracolate)
Do not confuse Doxidan with doxepin, Veracolate with Accolate, or Modane with Mudrane.

CATEGORY AND SCHEDULE
Pregnancy Risk Category: C
OTC

Classification: laxative, stimulant

MECHANISM OF ACTION
A GI stimulant that has a direct effect on colonic smooth musculature by stimulating the intramural nerve plexi. *Therapeutic Effect:* Promotes fluid and ion accumulation in the colon, increasing peristalsis and producing a laxative effect.

PHARMACOKINETICS

Route	Onset	Peak	Duration
PO	6-12 h	N/A	N/A
Rectal	15-60 min	N/A	N/A

Minimal absorption following oral and rectal administration. Absorbed drug is excreted in urine; remainder is eliminated in feces.

AVAILABILITY
Tablets, Enteric-Coated: 5 mg.
Tablets, Delayed-Release: 10 mg.
Suppositories, Rectal: 10 mg.

INDICATIONS AND DOSAGES
▸ **Treatment of constipation**
PO
Adults, Children older than 12 yr.
5-15 mg as needed. Maximum: 30 mg.
Children 6-12 yr. 5-10 mg or 0.3 mg/kg at bedtime or after breakfast.
RECTAL
Adults, Children 12 yr and older.
10 mg to induce bowel movement.
Children 3-11 yr. 5-10 mg as a single dose.
Children younger than 3 yr. 5 mg.

CONTRAINDICATIONS
Abdominal pain, appendicitis, intestinal obstruction, nausea, undiagnosed rectal bleeding, vomiting.

INTERACTIONS
Drug
Antacids, H_2-blockers, proton-pump inhibitors: May cause rapid dissolution of bisacodyl, producing gastric irritation or dyspepsia, possible vomiting.
Oral medications: May decrease transit time of concurrently administered oral medications.
Food
Milk: May cause rapid dissolution of bisacodyl, increasing stomach irritation.

DIAGNOSTIC TEST EFFECTS
None known.

SIDE EFFECTS
Frequent
Some degree of abdominal discomfort, nausea, mild cramps, and faintness.
Occasional
Rectal administration: burning of rectal mucosa, mild proctitis.

SERIOUS REACTIONS
• Long-term use may result in laxative dependence, chronic constipation, and loss of normal bowel function.
• Prolonged use or overdose may result in electrolyte or metabolic disturbances (such as hypokalemia, hypocalcemia, and metabolic acidosis or alkalosis) as well as persistent diarrhea, vomiting, muscle weakness, malabsorption, and weight loss.

PRECAUTIONS & CONSIDERATIONS
Excessive use of bisacodyl may lead to fluid and electrolyte imbalance. It is unknown whether bisacodyl crosses the placenta or is distributed in breast milk. Avoid oral bisacodyl use in children younger than 6 yr of age because this population is usually unable to describe symptoms or more severe side effects. Rectal use ok in younger children with medical supervision. Repeated use of bisacodyl in elderly patients may cause orthostatic hypotension and weakness because of electrolyte loss.

Increasing fluid intake, exercising, and eating a high-fiber diet should be instituted to promote defecation. Notify the physician if unrelieved constipation, dizziness, muscle cramps or pain, rectal bleeding, or weakness occurs. Electrolyte levels, hydration status, daily bowel activity, stool consistency, and record time of evacuation should be assessed.
Administration
Take oral bisacodyl on an empty stomach for faster action. Offer 6-8 glasses of water a day to aid in stool softening. Administer tablets whole; do not chew or crush them. Avoid taking within 1 h of antacids, milk, or other oral medications.

For rectal use, if suppository is too soft, chill for 30 min in refrigerator or run cold water over wrapper. Unwrap and moisten suppository with cold water before inserting deep into rectum.

Bismuth Subsalicylate
bis′muth sub-sal-ih′sah-late
(Bismed [CAN], Colo-Fresh, Devrom, Kaopectate, Pepto-Bismol)

CATEGORY AND SCHEDULE
Pregnancy Risk Category: C
OTC

Classification: Antidiarrheal, salicylates

MECHANISM OF ACTION
An antinauseant and antiulcer agent that absorbs water and toxins in the large intestine and forms a protective coating in the intestinal mucosa. Also possesses antisecretory and antimicrobial effects. *Therapeutic Effect:* Prevents diarrhea. Helps treat *Helicobacter pylori*–associated peptic ulcer disease.

AVAILABILITY
Caplet (Devrom): 200 mg.
Liquid (Kaopectate, Pepto-Bismol): 87 mg/5 mL, 130 mg/15 mL, 262 mg/15 mL, 524 mg/15 mL, 525 mg/15 mL.

Suspension (Kapectolin, Maalox Total Stomach Relief):
525 mg/15 mL.
Tablet (Kaopectate, Pepto-Bismol): 262 mg.
Tablet (Chewable [Devrom]): (Devrom): 200 mg.
Tablet (Chewable [Pepto-Bismol, Diotame]): 262 mg.

INDICATIONS AND DOSAGES
▶ **Diarrhea, gastric distress**
PO
(Doses based on 262 mg/15 mL liquid or 262 mg tablets)
Adults, Children over 12 yrs of age. 2 tablets (30 mL) q30-60 min. Maximum: 8 doses in 24 h.
▶ **H. pylori–associated duodenal ulcer, gastritis**
PO
Adults, Elderly. 525 mg 4 times a day, for 14 days. Combined with metronidazole, tetracycline, and acid-suppressive therapy.

OFF-LABEL USES
Prevention of traveler's diarrhea.

CONTRAINDICATIONS
Bleeding ulcers, gout, hemophilia, hemorrhagic states, renal impairment, pregnancy (third trimester); children and teenagers who have or are recovering from chickenpox, influenza symptoms, or influenza because of the risk of Reye syndrome. Not a suitable treatment for dysentery.

INTERACTIONS
Drug
Anticoagulants, heparin, thrombolytics: May increase the risk of bleeding.
Aspirin, other salicylates: May increase the risk of salicylate toxicity.
Insulin, oral antidiabetics: Large dose may increase the effects of insulin and oral antidiabetics.

Tetracyclines: May decrease the absorption of tetracyclines.
Herbal
None known.
Food
None known.

DIAGNOSTIC TEST EFFECTS
May alter serum alkaline phosphatase, AST (SGOT), ALT (SGPT), and uric acid levels. May decrease serum potassium level. May prolong PT.

SIDE EFFECTS
Frequent
Grayish black stools.
Rare
Constipation.

SERIOUS REACTIONS
• Debilitated patients may develop impaction.
• Tinnitus, confusion, dizziness, high tone deafness, delirium, psychosis.

PRECAUTIONS & CONSIDERATIONS
Caution is warranted with diabetes and in elderly patients. Avoid bismuth if taking aspirin or other salicylates because of increased risk of toxicity. Also, inform the physician if taking anticoagulants because this drug combination can dangerously prolong bleeding time. Be aware that stool may appear black or gray; may cause darkening of the tongue. Pattern of daily bowel activity and stool consistency should be monitored. Due to risk of Reye syndrome and lack of clinical data to support use, do not use in infants and children < 12 yrs of age.
Administration
Shake liquid/suspension well before administration.

Chew the chewable tablet before swallowing. Alternatively, allow the chewable tablet to dissolve before swallowing.

Bisoprolol
bis-ope'pro-lal
(Zebeta)
Do not confuse Zebeta with DiaBeta.

CATEGORY AND SCHEDULE
Pregnancy Risk Category: C (D if used in second or third trimester)

Classification: Antihypertensive, selective β_1-blocker

MECHANISM OF ACTION
An antihypertensive that blocks β_1-adrenergic receptors in cardiac tissue. *Therapeutic Effect:* Slows sinus heart rate and decreases BP.

PHARMACOKINETICS
Well absorbed from the GI tract. Protein binding: 26%-33%. Metabolized in the liver. Primarily excreted in urine. Not removed by hemodialysis. *Half-life:* 9-12 h (increased in impaired renal function).

AVAILABILITY
Tablets: 5 mg, 10 mg.

INDICATIONS AND DOSAGES
▸ **Hypertension**
PO
Adults. Initially, 5 mg/day. May increase up to 20 mg/day.
Elderly. Initially, 2.5-5 mg/day. May increase by 2.5-5 mg/day. Maximum: 20 mg/day.

▸ **Dosage in renal or hepatic impairment**
For adults and elderly patients with cirrhosis or hepatitis or whose creatinine clearance is < 40 mL/min; initially give 2.5 mg/day, then titrate.

OFF-LABEL USES
Angina pectoris, heart failure, premature ventricular contractions, supraventricular arrhythmias.

CONTRAINDICATIONS
Cardiogenic shock, overt cardiac failure, second- or third-degree heart block (except in patients with functioning artificial pacemaker), marked sinus bradycardia, acute pulmonary edema.

INTERACTIONS
Drug
Cimetidine: May increase bisoprolol blood concentration.
Diuretics, other antihypertensives: May increase the hypotensive effect of bisoprolol.
Insulin, oral hypoglycemics: May mask symptoms of hypoglycemia and prolong the hypoglycemic effect of these drugs.
NSAIDs: May decrease antihypertensive effect.
Sympathomimetics, xanthines: May mutually inhibit effects.
Herbal
None known.
Food
None known.

DIAGNOSTIC TEST EFFECTS
May increase antinuclear antibody titer and BUN, serum lipoprotein, creatinine, potassium, uric acid, and triglyceride levels.

B

SIDE EFFECTS
Frequent
Hypotension manifested as dizziness, nausea, diaphoresis, headache, cold extremities, fatigue, constipation, or diarrhea.
Occasional
Insomnia, flatulence, urinary frequency, impotence, or decreased libido.
Rare
Rash, arthralgia, myalgia, confusion (especially in the elderly), altered taste.

SERIOUS REACTIONS
• Overdose may produce profound bradycardia and hypotension.
• Abrupt withdrawal may result in diaphoresis, palpitations, headache, and tremulousness.
• Bisoprolol administration may precipitate congestive heart failure and myocardial infarction in patients with heart disease; thyroid storm in those with thyrotoxicosis; and peripheral ischemia in those with existing peripheral vascular disease.
• Hypoglycemia may occur in patients with previously controlled diabetes.
• Thrombocytopenia, including unusual bruising and bleeding, occurs rarely.

PRECAUTIONS & CONSIDERATIONS
Caution is warranted with bronchospastic disease, diabetes, hyperthyroidism, impaired hepatic or renal function, inadequate cardiac function, and peripheral vascular disease. Bisoprolol readily crosses the placenta and is distributed in breast milk. Bisoprolol use should be avoided in pregnant women after the first trimester because it may result in low-birth-weight infants. The drug may also produce apnea, bradycardia, hypoglycemia, or hypothermia at birth. The safety and efficacy of bisoprolol have not been established in children. In elderly patients, age-related peripheral vascular disease may increase the risk of decreased peripheral circulation. Be aware that salt and alcohol intake should be restricted. Nasal decongestants or OTC cold preparations (stimulants) should not be used without physician approval.

Orthostatic hypotension may occur, so rise slowly from a lying to sitting position and dangle the legs from the bed momentarily before standing. Tasks that require mental alertness or motor skills should be avoided. BP for hypotension, respiratory status for shortness of breath, pattern of daily bowel activity and stool consistency, and pulse for quality, rate, and rhythm should be monitored. If pulse rate is 60 beats/min or lower or systolic BP is < 90 mm Hg, withhold the medication and contact the physician. Signs and symptoms of CHF, such as decreased urine output, distended neck veins, dyspnea (particularly on exertion or lying down), night cough, peripheral edema, and weight gain, should also be assessed.
Administration
Bisoprolol may be taken without regard to food. Tablets are not scored. Do not abruptly discontinue bisoprolol. Compliance is essential to control hypertension.

Bivalirudin
bye-val'i-roo-din
(Angiomax)

CATEGORY AND SCHEDULE
Pregnancy Risk Category: B

Classification: Anticoagulants,
thrombin inhibitors

MECHANISM OF ACTION
An anticoagulant that specifically
and reversibly inhibits thrombin
by binding to its receptor sites.
Therapeutic Effect: Decreases acute
ischemic complications in patients
with unstable angina pectoris.

PHARMACOKINETICS

Route	Onset	Peak	Duration
IV	Immediate	N/A	1 h

Primarily eliminated by kidneys.
A total of 25% removed by
hemodialysis. *Half-life:* 25 min
(increased in moderate to severe
renal impairment).

AVAILABILITY
Injection, Lyophilized Powder:
250 mg.

INDICATIONS AND DOSAGES
▸ **Anticoagulant in patients with
unstable angina who are undergoing
percutaneous transluminal coronary
angioplasty (PTCA) or percutaneous
coronary intervention (PCI); patients
undergoing PCI with (or at risk of)
heparin-induced thrombocytopenia/
thrombosis syndrome**
IV
Adults, Elderly. 0.75 mg/kg
as IV bolus, followed by
continuous infusion of 1.75 mg/kg/h
for the duration of the procedure

and up to 4 h postprocedure. Infusion
may be continued beyond the initial
4 h at 0.2 mg/kg/h for up to 20 h.
▸ **Dosage in renal impairment**

GFR	Infusion Dose Reduced to
10-29 mL/min	1 mg/kg/h
Dialysis	0.25 mg/kg/h

CONTRAINDICATIONS
Active major bleeding,
hypersensitivity.

INTERACTIONS
Drug
**Platelet aggregation inhibitors
thrombolytics, warfarin:** May
increase the risk of bleeding
complications.
Herbal
Ginkgo biloba: May increase the
risk of bleeding.
Food
None known.

DIAGNOSTIC TEST EFFECTS
Prolongs aPTT and PT.

Ⓓ IV INCOMPATIBILITIES
Do not mix with other medications.

SIDE EFFECTS
Frequent (42%)
Back pain.
Occasional (12%-15%)
Nausea, headache, hypotension,
generalized pain.
Rare (4%-8%)
Injection site pain, insomnia,
hypertension, anxiety, vomiting,
pelvic or abdominal pain,
bradycardia, nervousness, dyspepsia,
fever, urine retention.

SERIOUS REACTIONS
• A hemorrhagic event occurs rarely
and is characterized by a fall in BP
or hematocrit.

PRECAUTIONS & CONSIDERATIONS

Caution is warranted with conditions associated with increased risk of bleeding, including bacterial endocarditis, cerebrovascular accident, hemorrhagic diathesis, intracerebral surgery, recent major bleeding, recent major surgery, stroke, severe hypertension, and severe hepatic or renal impairment. It is unknown whether bivalirudin is distributed in breast milk or crosses the placenta. Safety and efficacy of bivalirudin have not been established in children. In elderly patients, age-related renal impairment may require dosage adjustment. Elderly patients experience more bleeding events than younger patients. Women should be aware that menstrual flow may be heavier than usual.

Notify the physician of bleeding from femoral vein site, blood in urine or stool, or discomfort or pain (especially chest pain) after treatment. Pulse rate, BP, aPTT, hematocrit, BUN and serum creatinine levels, and stool or urine cultures for occult blood should be monitored.

Storage

Store unreconstituted vials at room temperature. Reconstituted solution may be refrigerated for no more than 24 h. Diluted drug with a concentration of 0.5-5 mg/mL is stable at room temperature for 24 h or less.

Administration

! Bivalirudin is intended for use with aspirin, 300-325 mg daily. Treatment should be initiated immediately before angioplasty.

To each 250-mg vial, add 5 mL sterile water for injection. Gently swirl until all material is dissolved. Further dilute each vial in 50 mL D5W or 0.9% NaCl to yield final concentration of 5 mg/mL: 1 vial in 50 mL, 2 vials in 100 mL, 5 vials in 250 mL. If low-rate infusion is used after the initial infusion, reconstitute the 250-mg vial as directed and further dilute in 500 mL D5W or 0.9% NaCl to yield final concentration of 0.5 mg/mL. Diluting produces a clear, colorless solution; do not use solution if it is cloudy or contains a precipitate. Expect to adjust IV infusion based on aPTT or person's body weight.

Bleomycin Sulfate
blee-oh-my'-sin sull'-fate
(Blenamax [AUS], Blenoxane)

CATEGORY AND SCHEDULE
Pregnancy Risk Category: D

Drug Class: Antineoplastic, Natural antineoplastics

MECHANISM OF ACTION
A glycopeptide antibiotic whose mechanism of action is unknown. Is most effective in the G2 phase of cell division. *Therapeutic Effect:* Appears to inhibit DNA synthesis and, to a lesser extent, RNA and protein synthesis.

PHARMACOKINETICS
Half-life: 2 h; when creatinine clearance is > 35 mL/min, half-life is increased in lower clearance; metabolized in liver, 50% excreted in urine (unchanged).

AVAILABILITY
Powder for Injection: 15 units, 30 units.

INDICATIONS AND DOSAGES
▸ **For monotherapy or in combination therapy for testicular carcinoma; lymphomas (including Hodgkin's disease, choriocarcinoma, reticulum**

cell sarcoma, and lymphosarcoma); and squamous cell carcinomas of the head and neck (including mouth, tongue, tonsil, nasopharynx, oropharynx, sinus, palate, lip, buccal mucosa, gingiva, epiglottis, and larynx)

IV, IM, SC

Adults, Elderly. 10-20 units/m^2 (0.25-0.5 unit/kg) 1-2 times/wk. For Hodgkin's disease, after a 50% response is obtained, the maintenance dose is usually 1 unit/day or 5 units/week. NOTE: Other dosing regimens have been used for selected cancers, and bleomycin dosing in such regimens varies with the concurrent usage of other chemotherapy along with bleomycin.

▸ **As a sclerosing agent to treat malignant pleural effusions and prevent recurrent pleural effusions**

INTRAPLEURAL

Adults, Elderly. 60 units as a single injection.

▸ **General dose in renal impairment (adults)**

IV/IM/SC

CrCl 40-50 mL/min. 70% of normal dose.
CrCl 30-40 mL/min. 60% of normal dose.
CrCl 20-30 mL/min. 55% of normal dose.
CrCl 10-20 mL/min. 45% of normal dose.
CrCl 5-10 mL/min. 40% of normal dose.

CONTRAINDICATIONS

Hypersensitivity.

INTERACTIONS

Drug
Digoxin: May reduce digoxin serum concentrations.
Phenytoin: May reduce phenytoin serum concentrations.

Tobacco: Smoking increases pulmonary toxicity risk.
Herbal
None known.
Food
None known.

DIAGNOSTIC TEST EFFECTS

None known.

SIDE EFFECTS

Frequent

Anorexia, weight loss, erythematous skin swelling, urticaria, rash, striae, vesiculation, hyperpigmentation (particularly at areas of pressure, skinfolds, cuticles, IM injection sites, and scars), stomatitis (usually evident 1-3 wks after initial therapy); may also be accompanied by decreased skin sensitivity followed by skin hypersensitivity, nausea, vomiting, alopecia, and (with parenteral form) fever or chills (typically occurring a few hours after large single dose and lasting 4-12 h).

SERIOUS REACTIONS

• Interstitial pneumonitis occurs in 10% of patients and occasionally progresses to pulmonary fibrosis. This condition appears to be dose or age related, occurring more often in patients receiving a total dose > 400 units and those older than 70 yr.
• Nephrotoxicity and hepatotoxicity occur infrequently.
• Idiosyncratic reaction consisting of hypertension, mental confusion, fever, chills, and wheezing has been reported in 1% of lymphoma patients treated with bleomycin.

PRECAUTIONS & CONSIDERATIONS

Use with caution in patients with renal impairment, compromised pulmonary function. Avoid use in pregnant or lactating women.

Storage
Store unreconstituted powder for injection in the refrigerator. Diluted solution stable for 24 h at room temperature.

Administration
For IM, IV, or subcutaneous administration. Reconstituted with sterile water for injection or NS; do not reconstitute or dilute with dextrose-containing solutions. Test dose should be administered to patients with lymphoma.

Bortezomib
bor-teh′zoe-mib
(Velcade)

CATEGORY AND SCHEDULE
Pregnancy Risk Category: D

Classification: Antineoplastics, proteasome inhibitors

MECHANISM OF ACTION
A proteasome inhibitor and antineoplastic agent that degrades conjugated proteins required for cell-cycle progression and mitosis, disrupting cell proliferation. *Therapeutic Effect:* Produces antitumor and chemosensitizing activity and cell death.

PHARMACOKINETICS
Distributed to tissues and organs, with highest level in the GI tract and liver. Protein binding: 83%. Primarily metabolized by enzymatic action. Rapidly cleared from the circulation. Significant biliary excretion, with lesser amount excreted in the urine. *Half-life:* 9-15 h.

AVAILABILITY
Powder for Injection: 3.5 mg.

INDICATIONS AND DOSAGES
▸ **Relapsed multiple myeloma, mantle cell lymphoma**
IV
Adults, Elderly. Treatment cycle consists of 1.3 mg/m² twice weekly on days 1, 4, 8, and 11 for 2 wks followed by a 10-day rest period on days 12-21. Consecutive doses separated by at least 72 h. Therapy beyond 8 cycles may be given once weekly for 4 wks (days 1, 8, 15, and 22) followed by a 13-day rest (days 23-35).
▸ **Dosage adjustment guidelines**
Therapy is withheld at onset of grade 3 nonhematologic or grade 4 hematologic toxicities, excluding neuropathy. When symptoms resolve, therapy is restarted at a 25% reduced dosage.
 For grade 1 with pain or grade 2 (interfering with function but not activities of daily living [ADLs]), 1 mg/m². For grade 2 with pain or grade 3 (interfering with ADLs), withhold drug until toxicity is resolved, then reinitiate with 0.7 mg/m². For grade 4 (permanent sensory loss that interferes with function), discontinue bortezomib.

CONTRAINDICATIONS
Hypersensitivity to bortezomib, boron, or mannitol.

INTERACTIONS
Drug
Oral antidiabetics: May alter the response of these drugs.
Potent CYP3A4 inhibitors (e.g., ketoconazole, ritonavir): May increase bortezomib exposure. Closely monitor.
Herbal
St. John's wort: may decrease bortezomib levels, may

significantly decrease blood hemoglobin and hematocrit levels and neutrophil, platelet, and WBC counts.

SIDE EFFECTS

Expected (36%-65%)
Fatigue, malaise, asthenia, nausea, diarrhea, anorexia, constipation, fever, vomiting.
Frequent (21%-28%)
Headache, insomnia, arthralgia, limb pain, edema, paresthesia, dizziness, rash.
Occasional (11%-18%)
Dehydration, cough, anxiety, bone pain, muscle cramps, myalgia, back pain, abdominal pain, taste alteration, dyspepsia, pruritus, hypotension (including orthostatic hypotension), rigors, blurred vision.

SERIOUS REACTIONS

• Thrombocytopenia occurs in 40% of patients. Platelet count peaks at day 11 and returns to baseline by day 21. GI and intracerebral hemorrhage are associated with drug-induced thrombocytopenia.
• Anemia occurs in 32% of patients.
• New-onset or worsening neuropathy occurs in 37% of patients. Symptoms may improve in some patients when bortezomib is discontinued.
• Reversible posterior leukoencephalopathy syndrome.
• Pneumonia occurs occasionally; rare reports of pneumonitis, interstitial pneumonia, lung infiltration, and acute respiratory distress syndrome.
• New-onset or exacerbation of heart failure, new onset of decreased left ventricular ejection fraction.
• Tumor Lysis Syndrome, acute hepatic failure (rare).

PRECAUTIONS & CONSIDERATIONS

Caution is warranted with history of syncope, risk factors for heart disease, diabetes, hepatic impairment. Caution should also be used with any medication that increases the risk of dehydration, hypotension, and hepatic or renal function impairment. Bortezomib may induce degenerative effects in the ovaries and testes and may affect male and female fertility. Breastfeeding is not recommended. The safety and efficacy of bortezomib have not been established in children. Elderly patients are at increased risk for grade 3 and 4 thrombocytopenia.

Notify the physician of orthostatic hypotension, fever, pregnancy, nausea, vomiting, or diarrhea. Tasks that require mental alertness or motor skills should be avoided until response to the drug is established. Signs and symptoms of peripheral neuropathy, including a burning sensation, hyperesthesia, neuropathic pain, and paresthesia of the extremities, should be assessed. CBC, especially platelet count, should be monitored before and throughout bortezomib treatment. Intake and output and BP should also be monitored. Adequate hydration should be maintained to prevent dehydration. IM injections or rectal medications and performing other procedures that may induce trauma and bleeding should be avoided.
Storage
Store unopened vials at room temperature. The reconstituted solution is stable at room temperature for up to 8 h.
Administration
Reconstitute the vial with 3.5 mL 0.9% NaCl. Give bortezomib as a 3- to 5-s bolus IV injection.

Bosentan
bo′sen-tan
(Tracleer)
Do not confuse with Tricor.

CATEGORY AND SCHEDULE
Pregnancy Risk Category: X

Classification: Antihypertensive;
endothelin receptor antagonist

MECHANISM OF ACTION
An endothelin receptor antagonist
that blocks endothelin-1, the
neurohormone that constricts
pulmonary arteries. *Therapeutic
Effect:* Improves exercise ability
and slows clinical worsening of
pulmonary arterial hypertension
(PAH).

PHARMACOKINETICS
Highly bound to plasma
proteins, mainly albumin.
Metabolized in the liver. Eliminated
by biliary excretion. *Half-life:*
Approximately 5 h.

AVAILABILITY
Tablets: 62.5 mg, 125 mg.

INDICATIONS AND DOSAGES
▸ **PAH in those with World Health
Organization Class III or IV
symptoms**
PO
*Adults, Elderly weighing more than
40 kg.* 62.5 mg twice a day for 4 wks;
then increase to maintenance dosage
of 125 mg twice a day.
Adults, Elderly, weighing < 40 kg.
62.5 mg twice a day.

CONTRAINDICATIONS
Administration with cyclosporine or
glyburide, pregnancy, hypersensitivity,
moderate or severe liver impairment.

INTERACTIONS
Drug
**Atorvastatin, hormonal
contraceptives (including oral,
injectable, and implantable),
lovastatin, simvastatin, warfarin:**
May decrease the plasma
concentrations of these drugs.
**Cyclosporine, ketoconazole,
tacrolimus:** Increases plasma
concentration of bosentan.
Cyclosporine is contraindicated.
Glyburide: Increased risk of liver
injury. Bosentan also decreases
glyburide concentrations. Glyburide
is contraindicated.
Herbal
St. John's wort: May decrease
bosentan serum concentrations.
Food
Grapefruit juice: May increase
bosentan serum concentrations.

DIAGNOSTIC TEST EFFECTS
May increase serum bilirubin, AST
(SGOT), and ALT (SGPT) levels.
May decrease blood hemoglobin and
hematocrit levels.

SIDE EFFECTS
Occasional
Headache, nasopharyngitis, flushing.
Rare
Dyspepsia (heartburn, epigastric
distress), fatigue, pruritus,
hypotension, lower extremity edema,
low sperm counts.

SERIOUS REACTIONS
• Abnormal hepatic function, and
palpitations occur rarely.
• Major birth defects.

PRECAUTIONS & CONSIDERATIONS
Bosentan administration may induce
atrophy of seminiferous tubules of
the testes, cause male infertility,
or reduced sperm count. Bosentan
causes fetal harm and has teratogenic

effects on the fetus, including malformations of the face, head, large vessels, and mouth. Breastfeeding is not recommended. The safety and efficacy of bosentan use in children have not been established. Use cautiously in elderly patients because the higher frequency of decreased cardiac, hepatic, and renal function is more common in this age group.

Because pregnancy must be avoided during bosentan therapy, it should be ruled out before the start of therapy. A negative result from a urine or serum pregnancy test should be performed during the first 5 days of a normal menstrual period and at least 11 days after the last act of sexual intercourse before drug therapy begins. Monthly pregnancy tests should be performed during bosentan therapy. Female patients should not rely on hormonal contraceptives as sole birth control method.

Hepatic enzyme levels (serum aminotransferase, serum alkaline phosphatase, bilirubin, AST [SGOT], and ALT [SGPT]) should be monitored before bosentan therapy begins and monthly thereafter. Changes in monitoring and treatment should be initiated if an elevation in hepatic enzyme levels occurs. Treatment should be stopped if clinical symptoms of hepatic injury, including abdominal pain, fatigue, jaundice, nausea, and vomiting, occur or if bilirubin level increases. Blood hemoglobin level at 1 and 3 mo should also be obtained after treatment begins and every 3 mo thereafter; a decrease in blood hematocrit and hemoglobin levels signifies anemia.

Administration

Take bosentan in the morning and evening, with or without food. Do not break or crush film-coated tablets. Swallow the film-coated tablets whole, and avoid chewing them.

Botulinum Toxin Type A

bot′yoo-lin-num toks′in type a
(Botox, Dysport [AUS])

CATEGORY AND SCHEDULE
Pregnancy Risk Category: C

Classification: Miscellaneous CNS agents.

MECHANISM OF ACTION
A neurotoxin that blocks neuromuscular conduction by binding to receptor sites on motor nerve endings and inhibiting the release of acetylcholine, resulting in muscle denervation. *Therapeutic Effect:* Reduces muscle activity.

AVAILABILITY
Injection: 100 units/vial.

INDICATIONS AND DOSAGES
▶ **Cervical dystonia in patients who have previously tolerated botulinum toxin type A**
IM
Adults, Elderly. Mean dose of 236 units (range: 198-300 units) divided among the affected muscles, based on patient's head and neck position, localization of pain, muscle hypertrophy, patient response, and adverse reaction history.
▶ **Cervical dystonia in patients who have not previously been treated with botulinum toxin type A**
IM
Adults, Elderly. Administer at lower dosage than for patients who have previously tolerated the drug. Limit total dose injected into the sternocleidomastoid muscles to 100 units or less to decrease incidence of dysphagia.

> **Strabismus**

IM

Adults, Children older than 12 yr. 1.25-2.5 units into any one muscle.
Children 2 mo to 12 yr. 1-2.5 units into any one muscle.

> **Blepharospasm**

IM

Adults. Initially, 1.25-2.5 units. May increase up to 2.5-5.0 units at repeat treatments. Maximum: 5 units per injection or cumulative dose of 200 units over a 30-day period.

> **Improvement of brow furrow/ glabellar lines**

IM

Adults 65 yr and younger. 20 units total dose injected over 5 sites.

> **Axillary hyperhidrosis**

INTRADERMAL

Adults. 50 units per axilla.

OFF-LABEL USES

Treatment of dynamic muscle contracture in children with cerebral palsy, focal task-specific dystonia, head and neck tremor unresponsive to drug therapy, hemifacial spasms, laryngeal dystonia, oromandibular dystonia, spasmodic torticollis, writer's cramp.

CONTRAINDICATIONS

Infection at proposed injection sites, hypersensitivity to albumin, botulinum toxin, or any component of the formulation.

INTERACTIONS

Drug

Aminoglycoside antibiotics, other drugs that interfere with neuromuscular transmission (such as curare-like compounds): May potentiate the effects of botulinum toxin type A.

Herbal

None known.

Food

None known.

DIAGNOSTIC TEST EFFECTS

None known.

SIDE EFFECTS

Frequent (11%-15%)

Localized pain, tenderness, or bruising at injection site; localized weakness in injected muscle; upper respiratory tract infection; neck pain; headache.

Occasional (2%-10%)

Increased cough, flulike symptoms, back pain, rhinitis, dizziness, hypertonia, soreness at injection site, asthenia, dry mouth, nausea, somnolence.

Rare

Stiffness, numbness, diplopia, ptosis.

SERIOUS REACTIONS

• Mild to moderate dysphagia occurs in approximately 20% of patients.

• Arrhythmias and severe dysphagia (manifested as aspiration, pneumonia, and dyspnea) occur rarely.

• Overdose produces systemic weakness and muscle paralysis, respiratory failure, death.

PRECAUTIONS & CONSIDERATIONS

Caution is warranted with neuromuscular junctional disorders, such as amyotrophic lateral sclerosis, Lambert-Eaton syndrome, motor neuropathy, and myasthenia gravis, because they may experience significant systemic effects, including respiratory compromise, and severe dysphagia. Be aware of signs of dysphagia and aspiration pneumonia, including fever, sputum production, and adventitious breath sounds after treatment.

Safety and effectiveness are not established in children < 12 yr for blepharospasm or strabismus, < 16 yr for cervical dystonia, and < 18 yr for hyperhidrosis.

Clinical improvement should begin within 2 wks of the injection, but the drug's maximum benefit will appear approximately 6 wks after the injection. Resume normal activity slowly and carefully. Seek medical attention immediately if respiratory, speech, or swallowing difficulties occur.

Storage

Store drug vials in the refrigerator. The reconstituted solution may be refrigerated for up to 4 h. Administer the drug within 4 h after reconstitution. The solution normally appears as clear and colorless; discard the solution if particulate matter is present.

Administration

! Plan to have a physician inject the drug into the affected muscle.

Expect to administer the drug at the lowest effective dosage and at the longest effective dosing interval to avoid formation of neutralizing antibodies. Dilute drug with 0.9% NaCl. For a resulting dose of units/0.1 mL, draw up 1 mL of diluent to provide 10 units per 0.1 mL, 2 mL to provide 5 units per 0.1 mL, 2.5 mL to provide 4 units per 0.1 mL, 4 mL to provide 2.5 units per 0.1 mL, or 8 mL to provide 1.25 units per 0.1 mL. Slowly and gently inject the diluent into the vial to avoid producing bubbles. Then rotate the vial gently to mix the drug. If a vacuum does not pull the diluent into the vial, discard it. For IM use, assist the physician, as necessary, while he or she injects the drug into the affected muscles using a 25-, 27-, or 30-gauge needle for superficial muscles and a 22-gauge needle for deeper muscles. For intradermal injection, inject each dose at a 45-degree angle to a depth of approximately 2 mm.

Botulinum Toxin Type B
bot′yoo-lin-num toks′in type b
(Myobloc)

CATEGORY AND SCHEDULE
Pregnancy Risk Category: C

Classification: Miscellaneous CNS agents

MECHANISM OF ACTION
A neurotoxin that inhibits acetylcholine release at the neuromuscular junction.
Therapeutic Effect: Produces flaccid paralysis.

AVAILABILITY
Injection: 2500 units, 5000 units, 10,000 units.

INDICATIONS AND DOSAGES
▸ **To reduce the severity of symptoms in patients with cervical dystonia who have previously tolerated botulinum toxin type B**
IM
Adults, Elderly. 2500-5000 units divided among the affected muscles.
▸ **To reduce the severity of symptoms in patients with cervical dystonia who have not previously been treated with botulinum toxin type B**
IM
Adults, Elderly. Administer at lower dosage than for patients who have previously tolerated the drug.

CONTRAINDICATIONS

Infection at proposed injection site, hypersensitivity to albumin, botulinum toxin, or any component of the formulation.

INTERACTIONS

Drug

Aminoglycoside antibiotics, other drugs that interfere with neuromuscular transmission (such as curare-like compounds): May potentiate the effects of botulinum toxin type B.

Herbal

None known.

Food

None known.

DIAGNOSTIC TEST EFFECTS

None known.

SIDE EFFECTS

Frequent (12%-19%)

Infection, neck pain, headache, injection site pain, dry mouth.

Occasional (4%-10%)

Flu-like symptoms, generalized pain, increased cough, back pain, myasthenia.

Rare

Dizziness, nausea, rhinitis, headache, vomiting, edema, allergic reaction.

SERIOUS REACTIONS

• Mild to moderate dysphagia occurs in approximately 10% of patients.
• Arrhythmias and severe dysphagia (manifested as aspiration, pneumonia, and dyspnea) occur rarely.
• Overdose produces systemic weakness and muscle paralysis, respiratory failure, death.

PRECAUTIONS & CONSIDERATIONS

Caution is warranted with neuromuscular junctional disorders, such as amyotrophic lateral sclerosis, Lambert-Eaton syndrome, motor neuropathy, and myasthenia gravis, because they may experience significant systemic effects, including respiratory compromise and severe dysphagia. Be aware of signs of dysphagia and aspiration pneumonia, including fever, sputum production, and adventitious breath sounds after treatment. Safety and effectiveness have not been established for use in children.

Resume normal activity slowly and carefully. Seek medical attention immediately if respiratory, speech, or swallowing difficulties occur.

Storage

Unreconstituted vials may be refrigerated for up to 21 mo. Do not freeze. The reconstituted solution may be stored in the refrigerator for up to 4 h. Administer the drug within 4 h after reconstitution. The solution normally appears clear and colorless; discard it if particulate matter is present.

Administration

! Plan to have a physician inject the drug into the affected muscle.

Dilute drug with 0.9% NaCl. Slowly and gently inject the diluent into the vial to avoid producing bubbles. Then rotate the vial gently to mix the drug. If a vacuum does not pull the diluent into the vial, discard it. For IM use, assist the physician as necessary while he or she injects the drug into the affected muscles using a 25-, 27-, or 30-gauge needle for superficial muscles and a 22-gauge needle for deeper muscles. Know that drug's effect lasts for 12-16 wks at doses of 5000 or 10,000 units.

Bretylium
bre-tilee-um
(Bretylium Tosylate-Dextrose,
Bretylate [CAN])
Discontinued in the United States

CATEGORY AND SCHEDULE
Pregnancy Risk Category: C

Classification: Antiarrhythmics,
class III

MECHANISM OF ACTION
An antiarrhythmic that directly
affects myocardial cell membranes.
Therapeutic Effect: Contributes to
suppression of ventricular tachycardia.

PHARMACOKINETICS
Absorption is not expected to
be present in peripheral blood at
recommended doses. Protein binding:
1%-6%. Not metabolized. Excreted
unchanged in urine. Removed by
hemodialysis. *Half-life:* 6-13.5 h.

AVAILABILITY
Injection: 50 mg/mL (Bretylium
Tosylate).
Premix Solutions: 500 mg/250 mL,
1000 mg/250 mL (Bretylium
Tosylate-Dextrose).

INDICATIONS AND DOSAGES
▸ **Ventricular arrhythmias,
immediate, life threatening**
IV
Adults, Elderly. 5 mg/kg undiluted
by rapid IV injection. May increase
to 10 mg/kg, repeat as needed.
Maintenance: 5-10 mg/kg diluted
over 8 min or longer, q6h or IV
infusion at 1-2 mg/min.
Children. 5 mg/kg, then 10 mg/kg at
15- to 30-min intervals. Maximum:
30 mg/kg total dose. Maintenance:
5-10 mg/kg q6h.

▸ **Ventricular arrhythmias, other**
IM
Adults, Elderly. 5-10 mg/kg
undiluted, may repeat at 1- to
2-h intervals. Maintenance:
5-10 mg/kg q6-8h.
IV
Adults, Elderly. 5-10 mg/kg diluted
over 8 min or longer, may repeat at
1- to 2-h intervals. Maintenance:
5-10 mg/kg q6h or IV infusion at
1-2 mg/min.
Children. 5-10 mg/kg/dose diluted
q6h.

OFF-LABEL USES
Treatment of cervical dystonia
in patients who have developed
resistance to botulinum toxin type A.

CONTRAINDICATIONS
None known.

INTERACTIONS
Drug
**Arsenic trioxide, antipsychotics,
Class I, IA, and III
antiarrhythmics, dolasetron,
fluoroquinolones, halofantrine,
tricyclic antidepressants:** May
increase risk of cardiotoxicity (QT
prolongation, torsades de pointes,
cardiac arrest).
Digoxin: May increase digoxin
toxicity (due to initial norepinephrine
release).
Herbal
None known.
Food
None known.

DIAGNOSTIC TEST EFFECTS
None known.

SIDE EFFECTS
Frequent
Transitory hypertension followed
by postural and supine hypotension
in 50% of patients, observed

as dizziness, light-headedness, faintness, vertigo.
Occasional
Diarrhea, loose stools, nausea, vomiting.
Rare
Angina, bradycardia.

SERIOUS REACTIONS
• Respiratory depression from possible neuromuscular blockade.

PRECAUTIONS & CONSIDERATIONS
Extreme cautions should be used with digitalis-induced arrhythmias and fixed cardiac output such as severe pulmonary hypertension and aortic stenosis. Caution is also warranted with impaired renal function, hyperthermia, hypotension, and sinus bradycardia. It is unknown whether bretylium crosses the placenta or is distributed in breast milk. There are no age-related precautions noted in children, although experience in this population is limited. Elderly patients are more susceptible to the drug's hypotensive effect. Tolerance to hypotensive effects usually occurs within several days of initial therapy. Rise slowly from lying to sitting position and permit legs to dangle from bed for at least 5 min before standing 1 h after dose administration.
Storage
Store vials at room temperature.
Administration
Maintain supine position during infusion.
 Do not dilute solution for IM injection. Do not give more than 5 mL into one site (over 3 mL may cause pain at injection site). Same-site injection may cause muscular atrophy and necrosis; rotate injection sites.

 Reconstitute solution for injection by diluting vials with at least 50 mL D5W or 0.9% NaCl. Give injection undiluted over 1 min.
 For intermittent IV infusion (piggyback), infuse over at least 8 min (too rapid IV produces nausea and vomiting).
 For IV infusion, give 1-2 mg/min of diluted solution.

Brimonidine
bry-mo′-nih-deen
(Alphagan P)
Do not confuse with bromocriptine.

CATEGORY AND SCHEDULE
Pregnancy Risk Category: B

Classification: β-adrenergic receptor agonist

MECHANISM OF ACTION
An ophthalmic agent that is a selective β_2-adrenergic agonist.
Therapeutic Effect: Reduces intraocular pressure (IOP).

PHARMACOKINETICS
Plasma concentrations peak within 0.5–2.5 h after ocular administration. Distributed into aqueous humor. Metabolized in liver. Primarily excreted in urine. *Half-life:* 3 h.

AVAILABILITY
Ophthalmic Solution (Alphagan P): 0.1%, 0.15%.
Ophthalmic Solution: 0.2%.

INDICATIONS AND DOSAGES
▸ **Glaucoma, Ocular Hypertension**
Ophthalmic
Adults, Eldery, Children 2 yr and older. 1 drop in affected eye(s) 3 times a day.

CONTRAINDICATIONS
Concurrent use of MAOI therapy, hypersensitivity to brimonidine tartrate or any other component of the formulation.

INTERACTIONS
Drug
CN5 depressants: Potential additive effects.
Antihypertensives, β-blockers, cardiac glycosides: Caution because brimonidine may also reduce heart rate and blood pressure.
MAOIs: Contraindicated.

SIDE EFFECTS
Occasional
Allergic conjunctivitis, conjunctival hyperemia, eye pruritus, burning sensation, conjunctival folliculosis, oral dryness, visual disturbances.

SERIOUS REACTIONS
• Bradycardia; hypotension; iritis; miosis; skin reactions, including erythema, eyelid, pruritus, rash; vasodilation; and tachycardia have been reported.

PRECAUTIONS & CONSIDERATIONS
Brimonidine should be used with caution in patients with severe cardiovascular disease, depression, cerebral or coronary insufficiency, Raynaud phenomenon, orthostatic hypotension, or thromboangiitis obliterans. Use not recommended in children younger than 2 yr. Somnolence occurs more frequently in children 2-6 yr of age than in older children.
Storage
Store at room temperature.
Administration
Nasolacrimal occlusion is advised to reduce systemic exposure. If more than 1 topical ophthalmic product is to be used, administration should be separated by at least 5 min. Wait 15 min after using before inserting contact lenses.

Brinzolamide
brin-zol'-ah-mide
(Azopt)

CATEGORY AND SCHEDULE
Pregnancy Risk Category: C

Classification: Carbonic anhydrase inhibitor

MECHANISM OF ACTION
An ophthalmic agent that inhibits carbonic anhydrase. Decreases aqueous humor secretion. *Therapeutic Effect:* Reduces intraocular pressure (IOP).

PHARMACOKINETICS
Systemically absorbed to some degree. Protein binding: 60%. Distributed extensively in red blood cells. Site of metabolism has not been established. Metabolized to active and inactive metabolites. Primarily excreted unchanged in urine.

AVAILABILITY
Ophthalmic Suspension: 1%.

INDICATIONS AND DOSAGES
▶ **Glaucoma, Ocular Hypertension**
OPHTHALMIC
Adults, Elderly. Instill 1 drop in affected eye(s) 3 times a day.

CONTRAINDICATIONS
Hypersensitivity to brinzolamide, sulfonamides, or any of the product ingredients.

INTERACTIONS
Drug
Carbonic anhydrase inhibitors:
Concurrent use with oral carbonic anhydrase inhibitors may lead to additive toxicity.
Herbal
None known.
Food
None known.

DIAGNOSTIC TEST EFFECTS
None known.

SIDE EFFECTS
Frequent (5%-10%)
Blurred vision; bitter, sour, or unusual taste.
Occasional (1%-5%)
Blepharitis, dermatitis, dry eye, ocular discharge, ocular discomfort and pain, ocular pruritus, headache, rhinitis, hyperemia.
Rare (< 1%)
Allergic reactions, alopecia, chest pain, conjunctivitis, diarrhea, diplopia, dizziness, dry mouth, dyspnea, dyspepsia, eye fatigue, hypertonia, keratoconjunctivitis, keratopathy, kidney pain, lid margin crusting or sticky sensation, nausea, pharyngitis, tearing, urticaria.

SERIOUS REACTIONS
• Electrolyte imbalance, development of an acidotic state, and possible CNS effects may occur.

• Systemic effects including blood dyscrasias, Stevens-Johnson syndrome, toxic epidermal necrolysis, and fulminant hepatic necrosis possible.

PRECAUTIONS & CONSIDERATIONS
Use with caution in patients with renal impairment, hepatic impairment. Safety and effectiveness have not been established in children or during pregnancy or lactation.
Storage
Store at room temperature.
Administration
Shake well before using. If more than one ophthalmic agent is being used, separate administration by at least 10 min. Administer solutions before suspensions. Remove contact lenses before instillation; may reinsert 15 min after instillation.

Bromocriptine
broe-moe-krip′teen
(Apo-Bromocriptine [CAN], Bromohexal [AUS], Kripton [AUS], Parlodel)
Do not confuse bromocriptine with benztropine, or Parlodel with pindolol.

CATEGORY AND SCHEDULE
Pregnancy Risk Category: C

Classification: Dopamine receptor agonist

MECHANISM OF ACTION
A dopamine agonist that directly stimulates dopamine receptors in the corpus striatum and inhibits prolactin secretion. Also suppresses secretion of growth hormone. *Therapeutic Effect:* Improves symptoms of parkinsonism, suppresses galactorrhea, and reduces serum growth hormone concentrations in acromegaly.

PHARMACOKINETICS

Indication	Onset	Peak	Duration
Prolactin lowering	2 h	8 h	24 h
Antiparkinson	0.5-1.5 h	2 h	N/A
Growth hormone suppressant	1-2 h	4-8 wks	4-8 h

Minimally absorbed from the GI tract. Protein binding: 90%-96%. Metabolized in the liver. Excreted in feces by biliary secretion.
Half-life: 15 h.

AVAILABILITY
Capsules: 5 mg.
Tablets: 2.5 mg.

INDICATIONS AND DOSAGES
▸ **Hyperprolactinemia**
PO
Adults, Elderly. Initially, 1.25-2.5 mg/day. May increase by 2.5 mg/day at 3- to 7-day intervals. Range: 2.5 mg 2-3 times a day.
▸ **Parkinson disease**
PO
Adults, Elderly. Initially, 1.25 mg twice a day. May increase by 2.5 mg/day every 14-28 days. Range: 30-90 mg/day.
▸ **Acromegaly**
PO
Adults, Elderly. Initially, 1.25-2.5 mg. May increase at 3-7 day intervals. Usual dose 20-30 mg/day. Maximum: 100 mg/day.

OFF-LABEL USES
Treatment of cocaine addiction, hyperprolactinemia associated with pituitary adenomas, neuroleptic malignant syndrome.

CONTRAINDICATIONS
Hypersensitivity to ergot alkaloids, peripheral vascular disease, pregnancy, severe ischemic heart disease, uncontrolled hypertension.

INTERACTIONS
Drug
Alcohol: May produce a disulfiram-like reaction (chest pain, confusion, flushed face, nausea, vomiting).
Erythromycin, clarithromycin, ritonavir, protease inhibitors, itraconazole, ketoconazole: May increase bromocriptine blood concentration and risk of toxicity.
Emot alkaloids: Concurrent use is not recommended.
Estrogens, progestins: May decrease the effects of bromocriptine.
Haloperidol, MAOIs, phenothiazines, risperidone: May decrease bromocriptine's prolactin-lowering effect.
Hypotension-producing medications: May increase hypotension.
Levodopa: May increase the effects of bromocriptine.
Sibutramine: May increase the risk of serotonin syndrome.
Herbal
St. John's wort: May reduce bromocriptine levels.
Food
None known.

DIAGNOSTIC TEST EFFECTS
May increase plasma growth hormone concentration.

SIDE EFFECTS
Frequent
Nausea (49%), headache (19%), dizziness (17%).
Occasional (3%-7%)
Fatigue, light-headedness, vomiting, abdominal cramps, diarrhea, constipation, nasal congestion, somnolence, dry mouth.

B

Rare
Muscle cramps, urinary hesitancy.

SERIOUS REACTIONS
• Visual or auditory hallucinations have been noted in patients with Parkinson disease.
• Somnolence and sudden sleep onset.
• Long-term, high-dose therapy may produce continuing rhinorrhea, syncope, GI hemorrhage, peptic ulcer, and severe abdominal pain.

PRECAUTIONS & CONSIDERATIONS
Caution is warranted with cardiac, renal, or hepatic function impairment, hypertension, and psychiatric disorders. Be aware the incidence of side effects is high, especially at the beginning of therapy and with high dosages. Bromocriptine use is not recommended during pregnancy or breastfeeding. Nonhormonal contraceptives are recommended to women during treatment. When used in the treatment of hyperprolactinemia, bromocriptine should be withdrawn when pregnancy is diagnosed. The safety and efficacy of bromocriptine have not been established in children. Elderly patients are more prone to CNS adverse effects.

Dizziness, drowsiness, and dry mouth are expected responses to the drug. Alcohol and tasks that require mental alertness or motor skills should be avoided. Also, change positions slowly and dangle the legs momentarily before standing to avoid light-headedness. Notify the physician if watery nasal discharge occurs. Constipation should be assessed during treatment.

Storage
Store at room temperature. Protect from light.

Administration
Lie down before taking the first dose to avoid light-headedness.

Take with food to decrease the incidence of nausea.

Brompheniramine
brome-fen-ir′a-meen
(BroveX, BroveX CT, Codimal A, Colhist, Dimetane, Dimetane Extentabs, Dimetapp, Lodrane 12 Hour, Nasahist B, ND Stat)

CATEGORY AND SCHEDULE
Pregnancy Risk Category: B
Rx

Classification: Antihistamines, H_1-receptor antagonist

MECHANISM OF ACTION
An alkylamine that competes with histamine at histaminic receptor sites. Inhibits central acetylcholine. *Therapeutic Effect:* Results in anticholinergic, antipruritic, antitussive, antiemetic effects. Produces antidyskinetic, sedative effect.

PHARMACOKINETICS
Rapidly absorbed after PO administration. Widely distributed. Metabolized in liver. Primarily excreted in urine. *Half-life:* 25 h.

AVAILABILITY
Capsule, Extended-Release: 12 mg (Lodrane 24).
Tablets: 4 mg (Dimetane).
Tablets, Chewable: 12 mg (BroveX CT).
Tablets, Extended-Release: 6 mg (Bidhist, LoHist, Lodrane 12 Hour).
Tablets, Timed-Release: 8 mg, 12 mg (Dimetane Extentabs).
Elixir: 2 mg/5 mL (VaZol).
Oral Suspension: 4 mg/5 mL (J-Tan), 8 mg/5 mL (Lodrane XR, TanaCof-XR), 10 mg/5 mL (P-tex), 12 mg/5 mL (BroveX).

INDICATIONS AND DOSAGES
▸ **Allergic rhinitis, anaphylaxis, urticarial transfusion reactions, urticaria**
PO
Adults, Elderly, Children 12 yr and older. Extended-release tablets: 6-12 mg every 12 h; chewable tablets: 12-24 mg every 12 h (up to 48 mg/24 h); extended-release capsules: 12-24 mg once daily; oral suspension: 12-24 mg every 12 h (up to 48 mg/24 h); oral liquid: 4 mg 4 times daily; Lodane XR suspension: 8 mg every 12 h.
Children 6 yr to younger than 12 yr. Extended-release tablets: 6 mg every 12 h; chewable tablets: 6-12 mg every 12 h (up to 24 mg/24 h); extended-release capsules: 12 mg once daily; oral suspension: 12 mg every 12 h (up to 24 mg/24 h); oral liquid: 2 mg 4 times daily; Lodrane XR suspension: 4 mg every 12 h.
Children 2-6 yr. Chewable tablets: 6 mg every 12 h (up to 12 mg/24 h); oral suspension: 6 mg every 12 h (up to 12 mg/24 h); oral liquid: 1 mg 4 times daily; Lodrane XR suspension: 2 mg every 12 h.
Children 12 mo to 2 yr. Oral suspension 3 mg every 12 h (up to 6 mg/24 h); oral liquid 0.5 mg/kg/ day in divided doses 4 times daily.

CONTRAINDICATIONS
Concurrent MAOI therapy, focal CNS lesions, newborn or premature infants, nursing mothers, hypersensitivity to brompheniramine or related drugs.

INTERACTIONS
Drug
Anticholinergics: May increase anticholinergic effects.
MAOIs: May increase anticholinergic and CNS depressant effects.

Procarbazine: May increase CNS depressant effects.
Herbal
None known.
Food
None known.

DIAGNOSTIC TEST EFFECTS
May suppress wheal and flare reactions to antigen skin testing unless antihistamines are discontinued 4 days before testing.

SIDE EFFECTS
Frequent
Drowsiness; dizziness; dry mouth, nose, or throat; urinary retention; thickening of bronchial secretions.
Elderly: Sedation, dizziness, hypotension.
Occasional
Epigastric distress, flushing, blurred vision, tinnitus, paresthesia, sweating, chills.

SERIOUS REACTIONS
• Children may experience dominant paradoxical reactions, including restlessness, insomnia, euphoria, nervousness, and tremors.
• Overdosage in children may result in hallucinations, seizures, and death.
• Hypersensitivity reactions, such as eczema, pruritus, rash, cardiac disturbances, and photosensitivity, may occur.

PRECAUTIONS & CONSIDERATIONS
Caution is warranted with asthma, narrow-angle glaucoma, increased intraocular pressure, hyperthyroidism, cardiovascular disease, hypertension, pyloroduodenal or bladder neck obstruction, glucose-6-phosphate dehydrogenase (G6PD) deficiency, or prostatic hypertrophy. It is unknown whether brompheniramine crosses the placenta or is detected in breast milk. There is an increased

risk of seizures in neonates and premature infants if the drug is used during the third trimester of pregnancy. Brompheniramine use is not recommended in newborns or premature infants because these groups are at an increased risk of experiencing paradoxical reaction. Elderly patients are at an increased risk of developing confusion, dizziness, hyperexcitability, hypotension, and sedation.

Dizziness, drowsiness, and dry mouth are expected side effects of brompheniramine. Avoid alcohol during therapy.

Storage

Store at room temperature. Protect from light to prevent discoloration.

Administration

Give oral brompheniramine with meals to minimize GI upset.

Budesonide
bu-dess'ah-nide
(Entocort EC, Pulmicort Flexhaler, Pulmicort Respules, Pulmicort Turbuhaler, Rhinocort Aqua, Rhinocort Aqueous [AUS], Rhinocort Hayfever [AUS])

CATEGORY AND SCHEDULE
Pregnancy Risk Category: B

Classification: Corticosteroids, inhalation

MECHANISM OF ACTION
A glucocorticoid that inhibits the accumulation of inflammatory cells and decreases and prevents tissues from responding to the inflammatory process. *Therapeutic Effect:* Relieves symptoms of allergic rhinitis or Crohn disease.

PHARMACOKINETICS
Minimally absorbed from nasal tissue; moderately absorbed from inhalation. Protein binding: 88%. Primarily metabolized in the liver. *Half-life:* 2-3 h.

AVAILABILITY
Capsules (Entocort EC): 3 mg.
Powder for Oral Inhalation (Pulmicort Flexhaler): 90 mcg per inhalation, 180 mcg per inhalation.
Powder for Oral Inhalation (Pulmicort Turbuhaler): 200 mcg per inhalation.
Suspension for Oral Inhalation (Pulmicort Respules): 0.25 mg/ 2 mL, 0.5 mg/2 mL, 1 mg/2 mL.
Nasal Spray (Rhinocort Aqua): 32 mcg/spray.

INDICATIONS AND DOSAGES
▸ **Allergic or vasomotor rhinitis**
INTRANASAL (RHINOCORT AQUA)
Adults, Elderly, Children 6 yr and older. 1 spray in each nostril once a day. Maximum: 4 sprays/nostril for adults and children 12 yr and older; 2 sprays/nostril for children younger than 12 yr.
▸ **Bronchial asthma**
NEBULIZATION
Children 12 mo to 8 yr.
0.25-1 mg/day titrated to lowest effective dosage.
INHALATION
Adults, Elderly, Children 6 yr and older. Turbuhaler: Initially, 200-400 mcg twice a day. Maximum: Adults: 800 mcg twice a day. Children: 400 mcg twice a day.
Adults, Elderly, Children 6 yr and older. Flexhaler: Initially 180-360 mcg twice daily. Maximum: Adults: 720 mcg twice a day. Children: 360 mcg twice a day.

▸ **Crohn disease**
PO
Adults, Elderly. 9 mg once a day for
up to 8 wks.

CONTRAINDICATIONS

Hypersensitivity to any
corticosteroid or its components,
persistently positive sputum cultures
for *Candida albicans,* primary
treatment of status asthmaticus,
systemic fungal infections, untreated
localized infection involving nasal
mucosa.

INTERACTIONS

Drug
Cimetidine: May increase the serum
concentrations of budesonide.
CYP3A4 inhibitors: May increase
the serum level and toxicity of
budesonide.
Herbal
St. John's wort: May decrease
levels of budesonide.
Food
Grapefruit juice: May double
systemic exposure to oral budesonide.

DIAGNOSTIC TEST EFFECTS

None known.

SIDE EFFECTS

Frequent (≥3%)
Nasal: Mild nasopharyngeal
irritation, burning, stinging, or
dryness; headache; cough.
Inhalation: Flulike symptoms,
headache, pharyngitis.
Occasional (1%-3%)
Nasal: Dry mouth, dyspepsia, rebound
congestion, rhinorrhea, loss of taste.
Inhalation: Back pain, vomiting,
altered taste, voice changes,
abdominal pain, nausea, dyspepsia.

SERIOUS REACTIONS

• An acute hypersensitivity reaction
marked by urticaria, angioedema,
and severe bronchospasm; occurs
rarely.
• Nasal septum perforation with
chronic use or improper technique.

PRECAUTIONS & CONSIDERATIONS

Caution is warranted with adrenal
insufficiency, cirrhosis, glaucoma,
hypothyroidism, osteoporosis,
tuberculosis, and untreated infection.
It is unknown whether budesonide
crosses the placenta or is distributed
in breast milk. In children, prolonged
treatment and high doses may
decrease cortisol secretion and
short-term growth rate. No
age-related precautions have been
noted in elderly patients.
    Symptoms should improve in
24 h, but the drug's full effect may
take 3-7 days to appear. Those using
budesonide intranasally should
notify the physician if nasal irritation
occurs or if symptoms, such as
sneezing, fail to improve.
Storage
Store all budesonide dosage forms
at room temperature. Once foil
envelope for inhalation suspension
has been opened, all ampules must be
used within 2 wks. Discard Flexhaler
when dose indicator displays zero.
Discard nasal spray after 120 sprays.
Administration
Oral capsule should be swallowed
whole. Do not crush or chew.
For inhalation, prime inahler before
first use. Exhale completely and
place the mouthpiece between the
lips. Inhale and hold breath for as
long as possible before exhaling.
Allow at least 1 min between
inhalations. Rinse mouth after
each use to decrease dry mouth
and hoarseness and prevent fungal
infection of the mouth.
Inhalation suspension for
nebulization should be shaken
well before using. Administer with

B

jet nebulizer connected to an air compressor; do not use ultrasonic nebulizer. Do not mix with other medications in nebulizer. Rinse mouth after each use; wash face if using face mask.

For intranasal use, clear nasal passages as much as possible. Shake gently before use. Prime before first use by actuating 8 times. If not used for 2 consecutive days, reprime with 1 spray or until a fine spray appears. If not used for 14 days, rinse applicator and reprime with 2 sprays or until a fine spray appears. Tilt the head slightly forward. Insert the spray tip into the nostril, pointing toward the nasal passages, away from the nasal septum. Spray budesonide into the nostril while holding the other nostril closed, and at the same time inhale through the nose to deliver the medication as high into the nasal passages as possible.

Bumetanide
byoo-met′a-nide
(Bumex, Burinex [CAN])

CATEGORY AND SCHEDULE
Pregnancy Risk Category:
C (D if used in pregnancy-induced hypertension)

Classification: Diuretics, loop

MECHANISM OF ACTION
A loop diuretic that enhances excretion of sodium, chloride, and, to lesser degree, potassium, by direct action at the ascending limb of the loop of Henle and in the proximal tubule. *Therapeutic Effect:* Produces diuresis.

PHARMACOKINETICS

Route	Onset	Peak	Duration
PO	30-60	60-120 min	4-6 h
IV	Rapid	15-30 min	2-3 h
IM	40	60-120 min	4-6 h

Completely absorbed from the GI tract (absorption decreased in CHF and nephrotic syndrome). Protein binding: 94%-96%. Partially metabolized in the liver. Primarily excreted in urine. Not removed by hemodialysis. *Half-life:* 1-1.5 h in adults; prolonged in neonates and infants.

AVAILABILITY
Tablets: 0.5 mg, 1 mg, 2 mg.
Injection: 0.25 mg/mL.

INDICATIONS AND DOSAGES
▶ **Edema**
PO
Adults. 0.5-2 mg as a single dose in the morning. May repeat q4-5h.
Elderly. 0.5 mg/day, increased as needed.
IV, IM
Adults, Elderly. 0.5-2 mg/dose; may repeat in 2-3 hr. Or 0.5-1 mg/h by continuous IV infusion. Maximum: 10 mg/day.
▶ **Hypertension**
PO
Adults, Elderly. Initially, 0.5 mg/day. Range: 1-4 mg/day. Maximum: 5 mg/day. Larger doses may be given 2-3 doses/day.
▶ **Usual pediatric dosage**
PO, IV, IM
Children. 0.015-0.1 mg/kg/dose q6-24h. Maximum: 10 mg/day.

OFF-LABEL USES
Treatment of hypercalcemia.

CONTRAINDICATIONS

Anuria, hepatic coma, severe electrolyte depletion, hypersensitivity to bumetanide.

INTERACTIONS

Drug

Amphotericin B, nephrotoxic and ototoxic medications: May increase the risk of nephrotoxicity and ototoxicity.

Anticoagulants, heparin: May decrease the effects of these drugs.

Lithium: May increase the risk of lithium toxicity.

Other hypokalemia-causing medications: May increase the risk of hypokalemia.

Herbal

None known.

Food

None known.

DIAGNOSTIC TEST EFFECTS

May increase blood glucose, BUN, serum uric acid, and urinary phosphate levels. May decrease serum calcium, chloride, magnesium, potassium, and sodium levels.

ⓓ IV INCOMPATIBILITIES

Diazepam, Midazolam (Versed).

ⓓ IV COMPATIBILITIES

Aztreonam (Azactam), cefepime (Maxipime), diltiazem (Cardizem), dobutamine (Dobutrex), furosemide (Lasix), lorazepam (Ativan), milrinone (Primacor), morphine, piperacillin and tazobactam (Zosyn), propofol (Diprivan).

SIDE EFFECTS

Expected

Increased urinary frequency and urine volume.

Frequent

Orthostatic hypotension, dizziness.

Occasional

Blurred vision, diarrhea, headache, anorexia, premature ejaculation, impotence, dyspepsia.

Rare

Rash, urticaria, pruritus, asthenia, muscle cramps, nipple tenderness.

SERIOUS REACTIONS

• Vigorous diuresis may lead to profound water and electrolyte depletion, resulting in hypokalemia, hyponatremia, dehydration, coma, and circulatory collapse.

• Ototoxicity, manifested as deafness, vertigo, or tinnitus, may occur, especially in patients with severe renal impairment and those taking other ototoxic drugs.

• Blood dyscrasias and acute hypotensive episodes have been reported.

PRECAUTIONS & CONSIDERATIONS

Caution is warranted with diabetes mellitus, hypersensitivity to sulfonamides, hepatic or renal impairment, and in elderly and debilitated patients. It is unknown wehther bumetanide is distributed in breast milk. The safety and efficacy of bumetanide have not been established in children. Bumetanide is a potent displacer of bilirubin; avoid use in neonates at risk for kernicterus. Elderly patients are at increased risk for circulatory collapse or thromboembolic episodes and may be more sensitive to the drug's hypotensive and electrolyte effects. Age-related renal impairment may require reduced dosage or an extended dosage interval in older patients. Consuming foods high in potassium such as apricots, bananas, legumes, meat, orange juice, raisins, whole grains, including cereals, and white and sweet potatoes, is encouraged.

An increase in the frequency and volume of urination and hearing abnormalities, such as a sense of fullness or ringing in the ears, may occur. BP, vital signs, electrolytes, intake and output, and weight should be monitored before and during treatment. Be aware of signs of electrolyte disturbances such as hypokalemia or hyponatremia. Hypokalemia may cause arrhythmias, altered mental status, muscle cramps, asthenia, and tremor. Hyponatremia may result in cold and clammy skin, confusion, and thirst.

Storage
Store vials at room temperature. Protect from light.

Administration
Take bumetanide with food to avoid GI upset, preferably with breakfast to help prevent nocturia.
Bumetanide is compatible with D5W, 0.9% NaCl, and lactated Ringer's solution, but it may also be given undiluted. The solution remains stable for 24 h if diluted. Administer the drug by IV push over 1-2 min. Bumetanide may also be given as a continuous infusion.

Bupivacaine
byoo-piv'a-caine
(Marcaine, Marcaine Spinal, Sensorcaine, Sensorcaine-MPF)

CATEGORY AND SCHEDULE
Pregnancy Risk Category: C

Classification: Anesthetics, local

MECHANISM OF ACTION
An amide-type anesthetic that stabilizes neuronal membranes and prevents initiation and transmission of nerve impulses, thereby effecting local anesthetic actions. *Therapeutic Effect:* Produces local analgesia.

PHARMACOKINETICS
Onset of action occurs within 4-10 min, depending on route of administration. Duration is 1.5-8.5 h. Well absorbed. Protein binding: 95%. Metabolized in liver. Excreted in urine. *Half-life:* 1.5-5.5 h (Adults), 8.1 h (Neonates).

AVAILABILITY
Injection: 0.25% (Marcaine, Sensorcaine-MPF), 0.5% (Marcaine, Sensorcaine-MPF), 0.75% (Marcaine, Marcaine Spinal, Sensorcaine-MPF).

INDICATIONS AND DOSAGES
Dose varies with procedure, depth of anesthesia, vascularity of tissues, duration of anesthesia, and condition of patient.
▸ **Analgesic, epidural (partial to moderate motor blockade)**
IV
Adults, Elderly. 10-20 mL (25-50 mg) of a 0.25% solution. Repeat once q3hr as needed.
Children > 10 kg. 1-2.5 mg/kg single dose as a 0.125% or 0.25% solution or 0.2-0.4 mg/kg/h continuous infusion as a 0.1%, 0.125%, or 0.25% solution. Maximum: 0.4 mg/kg/h.
Children < 10 kg. 1-1.25 mg/kg single dose as a 0.125% or 0.25% solution or 0.1-0.2 mg/kg/h continuous infusion as a 0.1%, 0.125%, or 0.25% solution. Maximum: 0.2 mg/kg/h.

▸ **Analgesic, epidural (moderate to complete motor blockade)**

IV

Adults, Elderly. 10-20 mL (50-100 mg) as a 0.5% solution. Repeat once q3h as needed.

Children > 10 kg. 1-2.5 mg/kg single dose as a 0.125% or 0.25% solution or 0.2-0.4 mg/kg/h continuous infusion as a 0.1%, 0.125%, or 0.25% solution. Maximum: 0.4 mg/kg/h.

Children < 10 kg. 1-1.25 mg/kg single dose as a 0.125% or 0.25% solution or 0.1-0.2 mg/kg/h continuous infusion as a 0.1%, 0.125%, or 0.25% solution. Maximum: 0.2 mg/kg/h.

▸ **Analgesic, epidural (complete motor blockade)**

IV

Adults. 10-20 mL (75-150 mg) as a 0.75% solution. Repeat once q3h as needed.

Children weighing >10 kg. 1-2.5 mg/kg single dose as a 0.125% or 0.25% solution or 0.2-0.4 mg/kg/h continuous infusion as a 0.1%, 0.125%, or 0.25% solution. Maximum: 0.4 mg/kg/h.

Children weighing < 10 kg. 1-1.25 mg/kg single dose as a 0.125% or 0.25% solution or 0.1-0.2 mg/kg/h continuous infusion as a 0.1%, 0.125%, or 0.25% solution. Maximum: 0.2 mg/kg/h.

▸ **Analgesic, intrapleural**

IV

Adults, Elderly. 10-30 mL bolus of 0.25%, 0.375%, or 0.5% q4-8h or 0.375% solution with epinephrine continuous infusion at 6 mL/h after 20 mL loading dose.

▸ **Analgesic, caudal (moderate to complete blockade)**

IV

Adults, Elderly. 15-30 mL of 0.5% solution (75-150 mg) or 0.25% solution (37.5-75 mg), repeated once every 3 h as needed.

Children weighing > 10 kg. 1-2.5 mg/kg single dose as a 0.125% or 0.25% solution or 0.2-0.4 mg/kg/h continuous infusion as a 0.1%, 0.125%, or 0.25% solution. Maximum: 0.4 mg/kg/h.

Children weighing < 10 kg. 1-1.25 mg/kg single dose as a 0.125% or 0.25% solution or 0.1-0.2 mg/kg/h continuous infusion as a 0.1%, 0.125%, or 0.25% solution. Maximum: 0.2 mg/kg/h.

▸ **Analgesic, dental**

IV

Adults, Elderly. 1.8-3.6 mL of 0.5% solution (9-18 mg) with epinephrine. A second dose of 9 mg may be administered. Maximum: 90 mg total dose.

▸ **Analgesic, peripheral nerve block (moderate to complete motor blockade)**

IV

Adults, Elderly. 5-37.5 mL (25-175 mg) of 0.5% solution or 5-70 mL (12.5-175 mg) of 0.25% solution. Repeat q3h as needed. Maximum: up to 400 mg/day.

Children 12 yr and older. 0.3-2.5 mg/kg as a 0.25% or 0.5% solution. Maximum: 1 mL/kg of 0.25% solution or 0.5 mL/kg of 0.5% solution.

▸ **Analgesic, retrobulbar (complete motor blockade)**

IV

Adults, Elderly. 2-4 mL (15-30 mg) of 0.75% solution.

▸ **Analgesic, sympathetic blockade**

IV

Adults, Elderly. 20-50 mL (50-125 mg) of 0.25% (no epinephrine) solution. Repeat once q3h as needed.

▸ **Analgesic, hyperbaric spinal (obstetric, normal vaginal delivery)**

IV

Adults, Elderly. 0.8 mL (6 mg) bupivacaine in dextrose as 0.75% solution.

▶ **Analgesic, hyperbaric spinal (obstetrical, cesarean section)**
IV
Adults, Elderly. 1-1.4 mL
(7.5-10.5 mg) bupivacaine in
dextrose as 0.75% solution.

▶ **Anesthesia, hyperbaric spinal (surgical, lower extremity, and perineal procedures)**
IV
Adults, Elderly. 1 mL (7.5 mg)
bupivacaine in dextrose as 0.75%
solution.
Children 12 yr and older.
0.3-0.6 mg/kg bupivacaine in
dextrose as a 0.75% solution.

▶ **Anesthesia, spinal (surgical, lower abdominal procedures)**
IV
Adults, Elderly. 1.6 mL (12 mg)
bupivacaine in dextrose as 0.75%
solution.
Children 12 yr and older.
0.3-0.6 mg/kg bupivacaine in
dextrose as a 0.75% solution.

▶ **Anesthesia, spinal (surgical, hyperbaric, upper abdominal procedures)**
IV
Adults, Elderly. 2 mL (15 mg)
bupivacaine in dextrose administered
in horizontal position.
Children 12 yr and older.
0.3-0.6 mg/kg bupivacaine in
dextrose as a 0.75% solution.

▶ **Analgesic, local infiltration**
IV
Adults, Elderly. 0.25% solution.
Maximum: 225 mg with epinephrine
or 175 mg without epinephrine.
Children 12 yr and older. 0.5-2.5 mg/kg
as a 0.25% or 0.5% solution. Maximum:
1 mL/kg of 0.25% solution or
0.5 mL/kg of 0.5% solution.

CONTRAINDICATIONS
Local infection at the site of
proposed lumbar puncture (spinal
anesthesia), obstetric paracervical
block anesthesia, septicemia (spinal
anesthesia), severe hemorrhage,
severe hypotension or shock,
arrhythmias such as complete
heart block, which severely restrict
cardiac output (spinal anesthesia),
sulfite allergy (epinephrine-
containing solutions only),
hypersensitivity to bupivacaine
products or to other amide-type
anesthetics.

INTERACTIONS
Drug
Angiotensin-converting enzyme inhibitors: May
increase risk of bradycardia and
hypotension as well as loss of
consciousness.
β-Blockers, ergot-type oxytocics, MAO inhibitors, TCAs, phenothiazines, vasopressors:
May increase the risk of bupivacaine
toxicity.
Cisatracurium, rapacuronium: May
increase neuromuscular blocking
action.
Hyaluronidase: May increase
incidence of systemic reaction to
bupivacaine.
Propofol: May increase hypnotic
effect of propofol.
Ropivacaine: May prolong effect of
intrathecal bupivacaine.
Verapamil: May increase risk of
heart block.
Herbal
St. John's wort: May increase
risk of cardiovascular collapse
and/or delay emergence from
anesthesia.
Food
None known.

DIAGNOSTIC TEST EFFECTS
None known.

Ⓥ IV INCOMPATIBILITIES
None known.

🔌 IV COMPATIBILITIES

Fentanyl, hydromorphone (Dilaudid), morphine.

SIDE EFFECTS

Occasional

Hypotension, bradycardia, palpitations, respiratory depression, dizziness, headache, vomiting, nausea, restlessness, weakness, blurred vision, tinnitus, apnea.

SERIOUS REACTIONS

• Arterial hypotension, bradycardia, ventricular arrhythmias, CNS depression and excitation, convulsions, respiratory arrest, tinnitus have been reported.

• Solutions with epinephrine contain metabisulfite, a sulfite that may cause allergic-type reactions, including anaphylaxis.

PRECAUTIONS & CONSIDERATIONS

Caution is warranted with pregnancy as well as obstetrical epidural anesthesia. Only concentrations lower than 0.75% should be used for obstetrical anesthesia. Caution should be used with regional IV anesthesia (Bier block), hyperthyroidism, hepatic disease, impaired cardiovascular function, hypertension, and heart block because there is a higher risk for developing bupivacaine toxicity. Solutions containing vasoconstrictors should be used cautiously in areas with limited blood supply, in the presence of disease that may adversely affect the cardiovascular system, or with peripheral vascular disease. Caution should also be used with retrobulbar blocks because bupivacaine has caused respiratory arrest.

Solutions containing epinephrine or other vasopressors should not be used concomitantly with ergot-type oxytocic drugs. Use in extreme caution in persons receiving MAOIs or tricyclic antidepressants because severe hypertension can occur. Spinal anesthetics should not be injected during uterine contractions. Local anesthetic solutions containing antimicrobial preservatives should not be used for caudal or epidural anesthesia. Reduced doses should be given to debilitated, elderly, acutely ill, and young people. It is unknown if bupivacaine is a triggering agent for malignant hyperthermia. Bupivacaine may cause severe disturbances of cardiac rhythm, shock, or heart block after spinal anesthesia. Severe dose-related cardiac arrhythmias may occur if preparations containing a vasoconstrictor such as epinephrine are used during or following the administration of chloroform, cyclopropane, halothane, trichloroethylene, or other related agents.

Bupivicaine is distributed in breast milk. Fetal bradycardia frequently follows obstetrical paracervical block with some amide-type local anesthetics and may be associated with fetal acidosis. Bupivacaine spinal with dextrose is not recommended in children younger than 18 yr. Some elderly may require dosage adjustment.

Storage

Store at room temperature. Protect from light. Bupivacaine 1.25 mg/mL in 0.9% NaCl injection is stable for up to 32 days when refrigerated.

Administration

Solutions containing preservatives should be used for epidural or caudal blocks. Dosage varies with anesthetic procedure, area to be anesthetized, vascularity of the tissues, number of neuronal segments to be blocked, depth of anesthesia and degree and muscle relaxation required, duration of anesthesia desired, individual tolerance, and physical condition of the person. The 0.75% solutions should not used for obstetric epidural anesthesia due to reports of cardiac arrest and death occurring with this concentration. Repeated doses of bupivacaine may cause significant increases in blood levels with each repeated dose due to accumulation of the drug or its metabolites or to slow metabolic degradation. Concentrated solutions (0.5%-0.75%) should be given in incremental doses of 3-5 mL with sufficient time between doses to detect toxic manifestations of unintentional intravascular or intrathecal injection during epidural administration. Bupivacaine should be used in dextrose only for spinal analgesia. The lowest bupivacaine dosage that gives effective anesthesia should be used to avoid high plasma levels and serious systemic side effects.

Buprenorphine
byoo-pre-nor'feen
(Buprenex, Subutex, Temgesic
[CAN])

CATEGORY AND SCHEDULE
Pregnancy Risk Category: C
Controlled Substance: Schedule III

Classification: Opioid
agonist-antagonist

MECHANISM OF ACTION
An opioid agonist-antagonist that binds with opioid receptors in the CNS. *Therapeutic Effect:* Alters the perception of and emotional response to pain; blocks the effects of heroin and produces minimal opioid withdrawal symptoms.

PHARMACOKINETICS
IM onset 15-30 min, duration 4-6 h; absorption 90%-100%; hepatic metabolism; excreted in feces (68%-71%); also renal excretion.

AVAILABILITY
Tablets, Sublingual: 2 mg, 8 mg.
Injection: 0.3 mg/mL.

INDICATIONS AND DOSAGES
▸ **Analgesia**
IV, IM
Adults, Children older than 12 yr.
0.3 mg q6-8h as needed. May repeat once in 30-60 min. Range: 0.15-0.6 mg q4-8h as needed.
Children 2-12 yr. 2-6 mcg/kg q4-6h as needed.
Elderly. 0.15 mg q6h as needed.
▸ **Opioid dependence**
SUBLINGUAL
Adults, Elderly, Children older than 16 yr. Initially, 12-16 mg/day, beginning at least 4 h after last use of heroin or short-acting opioid. Maintenance: 16 mg/day. Range: 4-24 mg/day. Patients should be switched to buprenorphine and naloxone combination, which is preferred for maintenance treatment to defer abuse.

CONTRAINDICATIONS
Hypersensitivity to buprenorphine; hypersensitivity to naloxone for those receiving the fixed combination product containing naloxone (Suboxone).

INTERACTIONS
Drug
CNS depressants, MAOIs: May increase CNS or respiratory depression and hypotension.
Other opioid analgesics: May decrease the effects of other opioid analgesics.
Herbal
Kava kava, St. John's wort, valerian: May increase CNS depression.
Food
None known.

DIAGNOSTIC TEST EFFECTS
May increase serum amylase and lipase levels.

SIDE EFFECTS
Frequent
Tablet: Headache, pain, insomnia, anxiety, depression, nausea, abdominal pain, constipation, back pain, weakness, rhinitis, withdrawal syndrome, infection, diaphoresis.
Injection (more than 10%): Sedation.
Occasional
Injection: Hypotension, respiratory depression, dizziness, headache, vomiting, nausea, vertigo.

SERIOUS REACTIONS
• Overdose results in cold and clammy skin, weakness, confusion, severe respiratory depression, cyanosis, pinpoint pupils, and extreme somnolence progressing to seizures, stupor, and coma.

PRECAUTIONS & CONSIDERATIONS
Caution is warranted with hepatic impairment and possible neurologic injury. Dizziness may occur, so change positions slowly and avoid tasks that require mental alertness or motor skills. BP, pulse rate, respiratory status, and clinical improvement should be monitored.
Administration
Place the tablet under the tongue until dissolved. If two or more tablets are needed, all may be placed under the tongue at the same time.
For IV use, administer buprenorphine slowly, over at least 2 min.

Bupropion
byoo-proe′-pee-on
(Wellbutrin, Wellbutrin SR, Wellbutrin XL, Zyban, Zyban sustained release [AUS])
Do not confuse bupropion with buspirone, Wellbutrin with Wellcovorin or Wellferon, or Zyban with Zagam.

CATEGORY AND SCHEDULE
Pregnancy Risk Category: B

Classification: Antidepressant

MECHANISM OF ACTION
An aminoketone that blocks the reuptake of neurotransmitters, including serotonin and norepinephrine at CNS presynaptic membranes, increasing their availability at postsynaptic receptor sites. Also reduces the firing rate of noradrenergic neurons. *Therapeutic Effect:* Relieves depression and nicotine withdrawal symptoms.

PHARMACOKINETICS
Rapidly absorbed from the GI tract. Protein binding: 84%. Crosses the blood-brain barrier. Undergoes extensive first-pass metabolism in the liver to active metabolite. Primarily excreted in urine. *Half-life:* 14 h.

AVAILABILITY
Tablets (Wellbutrin): 75 mg, 100 mg.
*Tablets, Sustained-Release
(Wellbutrin SR, Zyban):* 100 mg,
150 mg.
*Tablets, Extended-Release
(Wellbutrin XL):* 150 mg, 300 mg.

INDICATIONS AND DOSAGES
▸ **Depression**
PO (IMMEDIATE-RELEASE)
Adults. Initially, 100 mg twice
a day. May increase to 100 mg
3 times a day no sooner than
3 days after beginning therapy.
Maximum: 450 mg/day.
Elderly. 37.5 mg twice a day. May
increase by 37.5 mg q3-4 days.
Maintenance: Lowest effective
dosage.
PO (SUSTAINED-RELEASE)
Adults, Elderly. Initially, 150
mg/day as a single dose in the
morning. May increase to 150 mg
twice a day as early as day 4 after
beginning therapy. Maximum:
400 mg/day.
PO (EXTENDED-RELEASE)
Adults. 150 mg once a day.
May increase to 300 mg once a day.
Maximum: 450 mg once a day.
▸ **Smoking Cessation**
PO (ZYBAN)
Adults. Initially, 150 mg a day for 3
days; then 150 mg twice a day for 7-12
wks. Longer duration of maintenance
therapy may be considered. Do not
exceed 300 mg/day.

CONTRAINDICATIONS
Current or prior diagnosis of
anorexia nervosa or bulimia,
seizure disorder, use within
14 days of MAOIs.

INTERACTIONS
Drug
**Carbamazepine, nevirapine,
phenobarbital, phenytoin,**
rifampin: Decreased bupropion
levels.
Desipramine, paroxetine, sertraline:
May increase bupropion levels.
**Tricyclic antidepressants,
phenothiazines, benzodiazepines,
alcohol, haloperidol, and
trazodone:** Increased seizure risk.
Herbal
None known.
Food
None known.

DIAGNOSTIC TEST EFFECTS
None known.

SIDE EFFECTS
Frequent
Constipation, weight gain or loss,
nausea, vomiting, anorexia, dry
mouth, headache, diaphoresis,
tremors, sedation, insomnia,
dizziness, agitation.
Occasional
Diarrhea, akinesia, blurred vision,
tachycardia, confusion, hostility,
fatigue.

SERIOUS REACTIONS
• The risk of seizures increases
in patients taking more than
150 mg/dose of bupropion, in
patients with a history of bulimia
or seizure disorders, and in patients
discontinuing drugs that may lower
the seizure threshold.

PRECAUTIONS & CONSIDERATIONS
Bupropion should be used with
caution in patients with renal and
hepatic disease, bipolar disorder,
recent myocardial infarction,
cranial trauma, undergoing
electroconvulsive therapy, and in
elderly patients. Initial and maximum
doses are reduced in patients with
severe hepatic cirrhosis. Use in
pregnancy only if the potential
benefit outweighs the possible risks.

Is excreted in breast milk; use is not recommended in nursing mothers. Bupropion is not FDA approved for use in children. A thorough cardiovascular assessment is recommended before initiation of therapy in pediatric patients; assessment should include medical history, family history, and physical examination with consideration of ECG testing. In addition, antidepressants have been associated with an increased risk of suicidal thinking and behavior in children, adolescents, and young adults with major depressive disorder and other psychiatric disorders. Elderly patients may be at greater risk of accumulation with chronic dosing.
Administration
May take without regard to food. Swallow sustained release and extended-release tablets whole; do not crush or chew.

Buspirone
byoo-spir'own
(BuSpar, Buspirex [CAN], Bustab [CAN])
Do not confuse buspirone with bupropion.

CATEGORY AND SCHEDULE
Pregnancy Risk Category: B

Classification: Anxiolytics

MECHANISM OF ACTION
Although its exact mechanism of action is unknown, this nonbarbiturate is thought to bind to serotonin and dopamine receptors in the CNS. The drug may also increase norepinephrine metabolism in the locus ceruleus. *Therapeutic Effect:* Produces anxiolytic effect.

PHARMACOKINETICS
Rapidly and completely absorbed from the GI tract. Protein binding: 95%. Undergoes extensive first-pass metabolism. Metabolized in the liver to active metabolite. Primarily excreted in urine. Not removed by hemodialysis. *Half-life:* 2-3 h.

AVAILABILITY
Tablets: 5 mg, 7.5 mg, 10 mg, 15 mg, 30 mg.

INDICATIONS AND DOSAGES
▸ **Generalized anxiety disorders**
PO
Adults. 5 mg 2-3 times a day or 7.5 mg twice a day. May increase by 5 mg/day every 2-4 days. Maintenance: 15-30 mg/day in 2-3 divided doses. Maximum: 60 mg/day.
Elderly. Initially, 5 mg twice a day. May increase by 5 mg/day every 2-3 days. Maximum: 60 mg/day.
Children 6 yr and older. Initially, 2.5-5 mg/day. May increase by 5 mg/day at weekly intervals. Usual maintenance dose: 15-30 mg/day in divided doses.

OFF-LABEL USES
Management of panic attack.

CONTRAINDICATIONS
Concurrent use of MAOIs, severe hepatic or renal impairment.

INTERACTIONS
Drug
Erythromycin, itraconazole: May increase buspirone blood concentration and risk of toxicity.
MAOIs: May increase BP. Contraindicated.
Other CNS depressants: Potentiates effects of buspirone and may increase sedation.

Herbal
Kava kava: May increase sedation.
St. John's wort: May decrease buspirone levels.
Food
Alcohol: Potentiates effects of buspirone and may increase sedation.
Grapefruit, grapefruit juice: May increase buspirone blood concentration and risk of toxicity. Avoid concurrent use.

DIAGNOSTIC TEST EFFECTS
None known.

SIDE EFFECTS
Frequent (6%-12%)
Dizziness, somnolence, nausea, headache.
Occasional (2%-5%)
Nervousness, fatigue, insomnia, dry mouth, light-headedness, mood swings, blurred vision, poor concentration, diarrhea, paresthesia.
Rare
Muscle pain and stiffness, nightmares, chest pain, involuntary movements.

SERIOUS REACTIONS
• Overdose may produce severe nausea, vomiting, dizziness, drowsiness, abdominal distention, and excessive pupil contraction.

PRECAUTIONS & CONSIDERATIONS
Caution is warranted with impaired renal or hepatic function. It is unknown whether buspirone crosses the placenta or is distributed in breast milk. The safety and efficacy of buspirone have not been established in children under 6 yr of age. No age-related precautions have been noted in children. No age-related precautions have been noted in elderly patients.

Drowsiness may occur but usually disappears with continued therapy. Change positions slowly from recumbent, to sitting, before standing to prevent dizziness. Alcohol and tasks that require mental alertness or motor skills should also be avoided. Autonomic responses, such as cold, clammy hands and diaphoresis, and motor responses, such as agitation, trembling, and tension, should be assessed. Hepatic and renal function should be monitored in long-term therapy.
Administration
Take buspirone consistently either with or without food. Crush tablets if needed. Improvement may be noticed within 7-10 days of starting therapy, but optimum therapeutic effect generally takes 3-4 wks to appear.

Busulfan
byoo-sull'-fan
(Busulfex, Myleran)
Do not confuse Myleran with Alkeran, Leukeran, or Mylicon.

CATEGORY AND SCHEDULE
Pregnancy Risk Category: D

Classification: Antineoplastic

MECHANISM OF ACTION
An alkylating agent that interferes with DNA replication and RNA synthesis. Cell cycle-phase nonspecific. *Therapeutic Effect:* Disrupts nucleic acid function and causes myelosuppression.

PHARMACOKINETICS
Completely absorbed from the GI tract. Protein binding: 33%.

Metabolized in the liver. Primarily excreted in urine. Minimally removed by hemodialysis.
Half-life: 2.5 h.

AVAILABILITY
Tablets: 2 mg.
Injection solution: 6 mg/mL.

INDICATIONS AND DOSAGES
▸ **Remission induction in chronic myelogenous leukemia (CML)**
PO
Adults, Elderly. 4-8 mg/day; up to 12 mg/day. Maintenance: 1-4 mg/day to 2 mg/wks. Continue until WBC count is 10,000-20,000/mm^3, and resume when WBC count reaches 50,000/mm^3.
Children. 0.06-0.12 mg/kg/day. Maintenance: Titrate to maintain leukocyte count above 40,000/mm^3, reduce dose by 50% if count is 30,000-40,000/mm^3, and discontinue if the count is 20,000/mm^3 or less.
▸ **Marrow ablative conditioning for bone marrow transplantation**
IV
Adults, Elderly, Children weighing more than 12 kg. 0.8 mg/kg/dose q6h for total of 16 doses. (Use IBW or ABW, whichever is lower.)
Children weighing 12 kg or less. 1.1 mg/kg/dose (IBW) q6h for 16 doses.
PO
Adults, Elderly, Children. 1 mg/kg/dose (IBW) q6h for 16 doses.

ⓘ IV INCOMPATIBILITIES
Do *not* dilute in dextrose 5% because it is incompatible.

CONTRAINDICATIONS
Disease resistance to previous therapy with this drug; hypersensitivity to any component of the formulation.

INTERACTIONS
Drug
Acetaminophen: Reduced busulfan clearance if used within 72 h before or concurrently with busulfan.
Itraconazole, ketoconazole: Increased busulfan levels.
Metronidazole: Increased busulfan trough concentrations and increased toxicity.
Herbal
St. John's wort: May decrease busulfan levels.
Food
Alcohol: May increase GI irritation.

DIAGNOSTIC TEST EFFECTS
Therapy associated with severe myelosuppression; AST elevation; increased creatinine, bilirubin, glucose; reduced calcium, potassium, magnesium.

SIDE EFFECTS
Expected
Nausea, stomatitis, vomiting, anorexia, insomnia, diarrhea, fever, abdominal pain, anxiety.
Frequent
Headache, rash, asthenia, infection, chills, tachycardia, dyspepsia.
Occasional
Constipation, dizziness, edema, pruritus, cough, dry mouth, depression, abdominal enlargement, pharyngitis, hiccups, back pain, alopecia, myalgia.
Rare
Injection site pain, arthralgia, confusion, hypotension, lethargy.

SERIOUS REACTIONS
• Busulfan's major adverse effect is myelosuppression, resulting in hematologic toxicity, as evidenced by anemia, severe leukopenia, and severe thrombocytopenia.
• Very high busulfan dosages may produce blurred vision, muscle twitching, and tonic-clonic seizures.

High concentrations are also associated with increased risk of hepatic veno-occlusive disease.
• Long-term therapy (more than 4 yr) may produce pulmonary syndrome ("busulfan lung"), characterized by persistent cough, congestion, crackles, and dyspnea.
• Hyperuricemia may produce uric acid nephropathy, renal calculi, and acute renal failure.

PRECAUTIONS & CONSIDERATIONS
Severe bone marrow suppression is common; may result in prolonged pancytopenia and severe neutropenia, thrombocytopenia, and/or anemia. Secondary malignancies have been observed following busulfan therapy. Seizures have been associated with use; initiate prophylactic anticonvulsant therapy before high-dose treatment. Solvent in the IV formulation has been associated with impaired fertility, hepatotoxicity, hallucinations, somnolence, lethargy, and confusion. Busulfan may cause fetal harm if administered during pregnancy. Women of childbearing potential should avoid pregnancy while receiving busulfan. Breastfeeding is not recommended during busulfan therapy.

Storage
Store unopened injectable in refrigerator. Final solution stable 8 h at room temperature; complete infusion within the 8 h. Dilution in NS is stable for 12 h in refrigerator; infusion must be completed within the 12 h. Store tablet at room temperature.

Administration
Dilute injectable with NS or D5W. Final concentration usually 0.5 mg/mL. IV dose should be administered as a 2-h infusion via a central line.

Administer oral tablets 1 h before or 2 h after meals.

Butabarbital Sodium
byoo-tah-bar′-bi-tal
(Butisol)

CATEGORY AND SCHEDULE
Pregnancy Risk Category: D
Controlled Substance: Schedule III

Classification: Anticonvulsant; antihyperbilirubinemic; sedative-hypnotic

MECHANISM OF ACTION
A barbiturate and nonselective CNS depressant that binds at GABA receptor complex, enhancing GABA activity. *Therapeutic Effect:* Produces hypnotic effect due to CNS depression.

PHARMACOKINETICS
Widely distributed. Metabolized in liver. Minimally excreted unchanged in urine. *Half-life:* 34-100 h.

AVAILABILITY
Tablets: 15 mg, 30 mg, 50 mg.
Elixir: 30 mg/5 mL.

INDICATIONS AND DOSAGES
▸ **Insomnia, short-term**
PO
Adults. 50-100 mg at bedtime.
▸ **Preoperative sedation**
PO
Adults. 50-100 mg, 60-90 min before surgery.
Children. 2-6 mg/kg. Maximum: 100 mg.
▸ **Sedation, daytime**
PO
Adults. 15-30 mg 3-4 times a day.

CONTRAINDICATIONS
Porphyria, barbiturate sensitivity.

INTERACTIONS
Drug
Alcohol, CNS depressants: May be increased sedative and respiratory depressant effects.
Corticosteroids, cyclosporine, doxycyline, lamotrigine, methadone, oral contraceptives, quinidine, theophylline, tricyclic antidepressants, warfarin: Increased metabolism of these agents may reduce their therapeutic effects.
Herbal
None known.
Food
None known.

DIAGNOSTIC TEST EFFECTS
None known.

SIDE EFFECTS
Occasional (1%-3%)
Somnolence.
Rare (< 1%)
Confusion, dizziness, agitation, nausea, vomiting, constipation, headache, hypotension, acne.

SERIOUS REACTIONS
• Skin eruptions appear as hypersensitivity reaction.
• Blood dyscrasias, liver disease, and hypocalcemia occur rarely.

PRECAUTIONS & CONSIDERATIONS
Use with caution in patients with depression, a history of drug abuse, hepatic or renal impairment, respiratory disease, and in elderly patients and children. Acute withdrawal symptoms may occur in neonates following in utero exposure near term. Excreted in breast milk; use with caution in nursing mothers. Paradoxical reactions, including agitation and hyperactivity, have been observed in patients with pain and pediatric patients.

B

Butenafine
byoo-ten′a-feen
(Lotrimin Ultra, Mentax)

CATEGORY AND SCHEDULE
OTC/Rx
Pregnancy Risk Category: B

Classification: Antifungals, topical, dermatologics

MECHANISM OF ACTION
An antifungal agent that locks biosynthesis of ergosterol, essential for fungal cell membrane. Fungicidal. *Therapeutic Effect:* Relieves athlete's foot.

PHARMACOKINETICS
Total amount absorbed into systemic circulation has not been determined. Metabolized in liver. Excreted in urine. *Half-life:* 35 h.

AVAILABILITY
Cream: 1% (Lotrimin Ultra, Mentax).

INDICATIONS AND DOSAGES
▸ **Tinea corporis, tinea cruris, tinea versicolor**
TOPICAL
Adults, Elderly, Children 12 yr and older. Apply to affected area and immediate surrounding skin once daily for 2 wks.
▸ **Tinea pedis**
TOPICAL
Adults, Elderly, Children 12 yr and older. Apply to affected area and immediate surrounding skin twice daily for 7 days or once daily for 4 wks.

B

CONTRAINDICATIONS
Hypersensitivity to butenafine or any component of the formulation.

INTERACTIONS
Drug
None known.
Herbal
None known.
Food
None known.

DIAGNOSTIC TEST EFFECTS
None known.

SIDE EFFECTS
Occasional (2%)
Contact dermatitis, burning/stinging, worsening of the condition.
Rare (≤2%)
Erythema, irritation, pruritus.

SERIOUS REACTIONS
• None known.

PRECAUTIONS & CONSIDERATIONS
Caution should be used with sensitivity to naftifine or other allylamine antifungals. It is unknown whether butenafine is excreted in breast milk. Safety and efficacy of butenafine have not been established in children younger than 12 yr. There are no age-related precautions noted for elderly patients. Avoid contact with eyes, nose, mouth, or other mucous membranes.
Administration
Gently cleanse area prior to application. Use occlusive dressings only as ordered. Apply sparingly and rub into area thoroughly. Use for full course of treatment or until symptoms improve.

Butoconazole
byoo-toe-ko'na-zole
(Gynazole-1, Femstat One [CAN], Mycelex-3 2%)

CATEGORY AND SCHEDULE
Pregnancy Risk Category: C

Classification: Antifungals, topical, dermatologics

MECHANISM OF ACTION
An antifungal similar to imidazole derivatives that inhibits the steroid synthesis, a vital component of fungal cell formation, thereby damaging the fungal cell membrane. *Therapeutic Effect:* Fungistatic.

PHARMACOKINETICS
Not known.

AVAILABILITY
Cream: 2% (Mycelex-3, OTC).
Cream: 2% (Gynazole-1, Rx).

INDICATIONS AND DOSAGES
▶ **Treatment of vaginal candidiasis**
TOPICAL
Adults, Elderly. Insert one applicatorful intravaginally as a single dose or at bedtime for up to 3 or 6 days.

CONTRAINDICATIONS
Hypersensitivity to butoconazole or any of its components.

INTERACTIONS
Drug
Not known.
Herbal
Not known.
Food
Not known.

SIDE EFFECTS

Occasional

Vaginal itching, burning, irritation.

SERIOUS REACTIONS

• Soreness, swelling, pelvic pain, or cramping rarely occurs.

PRECAUTIONS & CONSIDERATIONS

Be aware that butoconazole contains mineral oil, which may weaken latex or rubber products such as condoms. Tampons should not be used while using butoconazole because tampons can absorb and decrease the efficacy of the medication. The OTC preparation should not be used if abdominal pain, fever, or foul-smelling discharge is present. It is unknown whether butoconazole crosses the placenta or is distributed in breast milk. Limit use during pregnancy to the second and third trimesters.

Administration

Insert one applicatorful intravaginally as a single dose or at bedtime for 3 consecutive days.

Butorphanol

byoo-tor′fa-nole
(Stadol, Stadol NS)
Do not confuse butorphanol with butabarbital or Stadol with Haldol.

CATEGORY AND SCHEDULE

Pregnancy Risk Category: C, D if used for prolonged time, high dose at term
Controlled Substance: Schedule IV

Classification: Analgesics, narcotic agonist-antagonist

MECHANISM OF ACTION

An opioid that binds to opiate receptor sites in the central nervous system (CNS). Reduces the intensity of pain stimuli incoming from sensory nerve endings. *Therapeutic Effect:* Alters pain perception and emotional response to pain.

PHARMACOKINETICS

Route	Onset (min)	Peak	Duration (h)
IM	10-30	30-60 min	3-4
IV	< 1	30 min	2-4
Nasal	15	1-2 h	4-5

Rapidly absorbed after IM injection. Protein binding: 80%. Extensively metabolized in the liver. Primarily excreted in urine. *Half-life:* 2.5-4 h.

AVAILABILITY

Injection: 1 mg/mL, 2 mg/mL.
Nasal Spray: 10 mg/mL.

INDICATIONS AND DOSAGES

▶ **Analgesia**

IM

Adults. 1-4 mg q3-4h as needed.
Elderly. 1 mg q4-6h as needed.

IV

Adults. 0.5-2 mg q3-4h as needed.
Elderly. 1 mg q4-6h as needed.

▶ **Migraine**

NASAL

Adults. 1 mg or 1 spray in one nostril. May repeat in 60-90 min. May repeat 2-dose sequence q3-4h as needed. Alternatively, 2 mg or one spray each nostril if patient remains recumbent; may repeat in 3-4 h.

CONTRAINDICATIONS

CNS disease that affects respirations, physical dependence on other opioid analgesics, preexisting respiratory depression, pulmonary disease.

INTERACTIONS
Drug
Alcohol, CNS depressants: May increase CNS or respiratory depression and hypotension.
Buprenorphine: Effects may be decreased with buprenorphine.
MAOIs: May produce severe, fatal reaction unless dose is reduced by one fourth.
Sumatriptan nasal spray: May reduce butorphanol levels; may increase risk of transient high BP.
Herbal
None known.
Food
None known.

DIAGNOSTIC TEST EFFECTS
None known.

ⓥ IV INCOMPATIBILITIES
Amphotericin B complex (Abelcet, AmBisome, Amphotec).

ⓥ IV COMPATIBILITIES
Atropine, diphenhydramine (Benadryl), droperidol (Inapsine), hydroxyzine (Vistaril), morphine, promethazine (Phenergan), propofol (Diprivan).

SIDE EFFECTS
Frequent
Parenteral: Somnolence (43%), dizziness (19%).
Nasal: Nasal congestion (13%), insomnia (11%).
Occasional
Parenteral (3%-9%): Confusion, diaphoresis, clammy skin, lethargy, headache, nausea, vomiting, dry mouth.

Nasal (3%-9%): Vasodilation, constipation, unpleasant taste, dyspnea, epistaxis, nasal irritation, upper respiratory tract infection, tinnitus.
Rare
Parenteral: Hypotension, pruritus, blurred vision, sensation of heat, CNS stimulation, insomnia.
Nasal: Hypertension, tremor, ear pain, paresthesia, depression, sinusitis.

SERIOUS REACTIONS
• Abrupt withdrawal after prolonged use may produce symptoms of narcotic withdrawal, such as abdominal cramping, rhinorrhea, lacrimation, anxiety, increased temperature, and piloerection or goose bumps.
• Overdose results in severe respiratory depression, skeletal muscle flaccidity, cyanosis, and extreme somnolence progressing to seizures, stupor, and coma.
• Tolerance to analgesic effect and physical dependence may occur with chronic use.

PRECAUTIONS & CONSIDERATIONS
Caution is warranted with head injury, hypertension, impaired liver or renal function, or myocardial infarction, before biliary tract surgery (because the drug produces spasm of sphincter of Oddi), and in elderly or debilitated patients. During labor, assess fetal heart tones and uterine contractions. Be aware that the safety and efficacy of butorphanol have not been established in children younger than 18 yr of age. Be aware that elderly patients may be more sensitive to effects. Adjust drug dose and interval for elderly patients.

Dizziness and drowsiness may occur, so change positions slowly and

avoid alcohol, CNS depressants, and
tasks that require mental alertness
or motor skills until response to the
drug is established. BP, pulse rate
and quality, respirations, and clinical
improvement of pain should be
monitored.

Storage

Store at room temperature.

Administration

! May be given by IM or IV push.
For intranasal use, blow nose to
clear nasal passages as much as
possible. Before first use, prime
pump 7-8 times. If unit not used
for > 48 h, then reprime by pumping
1-2 times. Spray into nostril while
holding other nostril closed and
concurrently inspire through nose to
permit medication as high into nasal
passages as possible.

For IV use, butorphanol may be
given undiluted. Administer over
3-5 min.

Cabergoline
cab-err-go-leen
(Dostinex)

CATEGORY AND SCHEDULE
Pregnancy Risk Category: B

Classification: Dopamine
agonist; antihyperprolactinemic

MECHANISM OF ACTION
Agonist at dopamine D_2 receptors
suppressing prolactin secretion.
Therapeutic Effects: Shrinks
prolactinomas, restores gonadal
function.

PHARMACOKINETICS
Cabergoline is administered orally
and undergoes significant first-pass
metabolism following systemic
absorption. Extensively metabolized
in the liver. Elimination is primarily
in the feces. *Half-life:* 80 h.

AVAILABILITY
Tablet: 0.5 mg.

INDICATIONS AND DOSAGES
▸ **Hyperprolactemia (idiopathic or
primary pituitary adenomas)**
PO

Adults, Elderly. 0.25 mg 2 times per
week, titrate by 0.25 mg/dose no
more than every 4 wks up to 1 mg
2 times per week. Serum prolactin
level guides dose adjustment.

OFF-LABEL USES
Parkinson's disease, restless leg
syndrome (RLS).

CONTRAINDICATIONS
Hypersensitivity to cabergoline,
ergot alkaloids or any one of its
components.
Uncontrolled hypertension.

INTERACTIONS
Drug
Antihypertensives: May increase
hypotensive effect.
**Cimetidine, haloperidol,
loxapine, MAOIs, methyldopa,
metoclopramide, molindone,
olanzapine, phenothiazines,
pimozide, reserpine,
risperidone, thiothixene,
tricyclic antidepressants:**
Antagonizes the prolactin-
lowering effect of cabergoline.
**Antipsychotics,
phenothiazine-type
antiemetics:** Cabergoline may
diminish the effects of these
dopamine agonists.
Levodopa: Additive neurologic
effects are possible.
Ergot alkaloids: May lead to ergot
toxicity.
Antiretroviral drugs: May lead to
ergot toxicity.
Imatinib: May increase
the risk of ergot-related side
effects.
Herbal
None known.
Food
None known.

DIAGNOSTIC TEST EFFECTS
None known.

SIDE EFFECTS
Frequent
Nausea, orthostatic hypotension,
confusion, dyskinesia,
hallucinations, peripheral
edema.
Occasional
Headache, vertigo, dizziness,
dyspepsia, postural hypotension,
constipation, asthenia, fatigue,
abdominal pain, drowsiness.
Rare
Vomiting, dry mouth, diarrhea,
flatulence, anxiety, depression,

dysmenorrhea, dyspepsia, mastalgia, paresthesias, vertigo, visual impairment, pleuropulmonary changes, pleural effusion, pulmonary fibrosis, heart failure, peptic ulcer.

SERIOUS REACTIONS
• Overdosage may produce nasal congestion, syncope, or hallucinations.

PRECAUTIONS & CONSIDERATIONS
Dopamine agonist use is not recommended for postpartum lactation inhibition or suppression. Caution is advised in patients with hepatic impairment. Orthostatic hypotension frequently reported; risk increased with initial doses > 1 mg and concurrent use of other blood pressure–lowering medications. It is unknown whether cabergoline crosses the placenta or is distributed into breast milk. In general, dopamine agonists like cabergoline are not used in pregnant women. Safety and efficacy have not been established in children or in elderly patients.

Nausea, headache, constipation, and dizziness may occur during therapy.

Administration
Take without regard to meals.

Caffeine Citrate
kaf′een
(Cafcit)

CATEGORY AND SCHEDULE
Pregnancy Risk Category: C

Classification: Analeptics, stimulants, central nervous system, xanthine derivatives.

MECHANISM OF ACTION
A methylxanthine and competitive inhibitor of phosphodiesterase that blocks antagonism of adenosine receptors. *Therapeutic Effect:* Stimulates respiratory center, increases minute ventilation, decreases threshold of or increases response to hypercapnia, increases skeletal muscle tone, decreases diaphragmatic fatigue, increases metabolic rate, and increases oxygen consumption.

PHARMACOKINETICS
Protein binding: 36%. Widely distributed through the tissues and CSF. Metabolized in liver; limited metabolism in preterm neonates. Excreted in urine. *Half-life:* 4-5 h in adults, children, and older infants; 3-4 days in neonates.

AVAILABILITY
Intravenous Solution: 20 mg/mL (Cafcit).
Oral Solution: 20 mg/mL (Cafcit).

INDICATIONS AND DOSAGES
▸ **Neonatal apnea**
IV/PO
Dosage given as caffeine citrate. *Infants between 28 and 33 wks gestational age.* Loading dose: 20 mg/kg over 30 min. Maintenance: 5 mg/kg/day over 10 min or orally beginning 24 h after loading dose.

CONTRAINDICATIONS

Hypersensitivity to caffeine, xanthines, or any other component of the formulation.

INTERACTIONS

Drug
Cimetidine: May increase effects of caffeine citrate.
Ketoconazole: May increase effects of caffeine citrate.
Phenobarbital: May decrease effects of caffeine citrate.
Phenytoin: May decrease effects of caffeine citrate.
Theophylline: May increase theophylline concentrations and toxicity.
Herbal
None known.
Food
None known.

DIAGNOSTIC TEST EFFECTS

May report false decreases in phenobarbital levels.

⊘ IV INCOMPATIBILITIES

Furosemide, Lorazepam, Nitroglycerin, Pantoprazole.

⊌ IV COMPATIBILITIES

Amino acid solutions, D5W, IV fat emulsion, antipyrine, calcium, dopamine, fentanyl, heparin, D50W.

SIDE EFFECTS

Occasional
Feeding intolerance, irritability, restlessness.
Rare
Necrotizing enterocolitis, rash, tachycardia, increased ventricular output, increased stroke volume, GI intolerance, hypo/hyperglycemia, increased creatinine clearance, increased sodium and calcium excretion.

SERIOUS REACTIONS

• Accidental injury, sepsis, hemorrhage, gastritis, GI hemorrhage, disseminated intravascular coagulation, acidosis, abnormal healing, cerebral hemorrhage, dyspnea, lung edema, dry skin, retinopathy, and kidney failure have been reported.
• Overdosage includes symptoms of fever, tachypnea, jitteriness, insomnia, fine tremor of the extremities, hypertonia, opisthotonos, tonic-clonic movements, nonpurposeful jaw and lip movements, vomiting, hyperglycemia, elevated blood urea nitrogen, and elevated total leukocyte concentration.

PRECAUTIONS & CONSIDERATIONS

Caution should be used in infants with cardiovascular disorders, hepatic or renal impairment, and seizure disorders. Caffeine readily crosses the placenta and is excreted in breast milk. Safety and efficacy in long-term treatment of infants have not been established. Be aware that necrotizing enterocolitis may occur in infants. There are no age-related precautions noted in elderly patients.
Storage
Store at room temperature.
Administration
! Be aware that 20 mg of caffeine citrate = 10 mg caffeine base. Take care in calculating dosage. Do not administer if visible particulate matter or discoloration is visible; discard vial. Available as preservative-free solution in single-dose vial; discard unused portion. Administer IV using a syringe pump over 10 min. Oral administration: May give with formula feedings.

Calcipotriene
kal-sip′oh-tri-een
(Dovonex)

C

CATEGORY AND SCHEDULE
Pregnancy Risk Category: C

Classification: Dermatologics,
topical vitamin D analogs

MECHANISM OF ACTION
A synthetic vitamin D_3 analogue
that regulates skin cell (keratinocyte)
production and development.
Therapeutic Effect: Preventing
abnormal growth and production
of psoriasis (abnormal keratinocyte
growth).

PHARMACOKINETICS
Minimal absorption through intact
skin. Metabolized in liver.

AVAILABILITY
Cream: 0.005% (Dovonex).
Ointment: 0.005% (Dovonex).
Topical Solution: 0.005%
(Dovonex).

INDICATIONS AND DOSAGES
▶ **Psoriasis**
TOPICAL
*Adults, Elderly, Children 12 yr
and older.* Apply thin layer to
affected skin twice daily (morning
and evening); rub in gently and
completely.
▶ **Scalp psoriasis**
TOPICAL SOLUTION
*Adults, Elderly, Children 12 yr and
older.* Apply to lesions twice daily
after combing hair.

CONTRAINDICATIONS
Hypercalcemia or evidence of
vitamin D toxicity, use on face,
hypersensitivity to calcipotriene or
any component of the formulation.
Scalp solution also contraindicated
in patients with acute psoriatic
eruptions.

INTERACTIONS
Drug
None known.
Herbal
None known.
Food
None known.

DIAGNOSTIC TEST EFFECTS
Excessive use may increase serum
calcium level.

SIDE EFFECTS
Frequent
Burning, itching, skin irritation.
Occasional
Erythema, dry skin, peeling, rash,
worsening of psoriasis, dermatititis.
Rare
Skin atrophy, hyperpigmentation,
folliculitis.

SERIOUS REACTIONS
• Potential for hypercalcemia may
occur.

PRECAUTIONS & CONSIDERATIONS
Caution should be used with
history of nephrolithiasis. It is
unknown whether calcipotriene
crosses the placenta or is
distributed in breast milk. Be
aware that children and elderly
patients are at greater risk for skin
reactions. Improvement is usually
noted after 2 wks of therapy and
marked improvement after 8 wks
of therapy.
Storage
Store at room temperature.
Administration
Apply cream or ointment by
rubbing gently into the affected and
surrounding area twice daily (in

C

morning and in the evening). Wash hands after application.

Apply scalp solution after combing hair to remove scaly debris and part the hair. Apply solution only to lesions and rub in gently and completely. Avoid spread of solution to the forehead.

Calcitonin

kal-si-toe′nin
(Calcimar, Caltine [CAN], Miacalcin)
Do not confuse calcitonin with calcitriol.

CATEGORY AND SCHEDULE

Pregnancy Risk Category: C

Classification: Hormones/hormone modifiers

MECHANISM OF ACTION

A synthetic hormone that decreases osteoclast activity in bones, decreases tubular reabsorption of sodium and calcium in the kidneys, and increases absorption of calcium in the GI tract. *Therapeutic Effect:* Regulates serum calcium concentrations.

PHARMACOKINETICS

Injection form rapidly metabolized (primarily in kidneys); primarily excreted in urine. Nasal form rapidly absorbed. *Half-life:* 70-90 min (injection); 43 min (nasal).

AVAILABILITY

Injection: 200 international units/mL (calcitonin-salmon).
Nasal Spray: 200 international units/activation (calcitonin-salmon).

INDICATIONS AND DOSAGES

▸ **Skin testing before treatment in patients with suspected sensitivity to calcitonin-salmon**

Adults, Elderly. Prepare a 10-international units/mL dilution; withdraw 0.05 mL from a 200-international units/mL vial in a tuberculin syringe; fill up to 1 mL with 0.9% NaCl. Take 0.1 mL and inject intracutaneously on inner aspect of forearm. Observe after 15 min; a positive response is the appearance of more than mild erythema or wheal.

▸ **Paget's disease**

IM, SUBCUTANEOUS
Adults, Elderly. Initially, 100 international units/day. Maintenance: 50 international units/day or 50-100 international units every 1-3 days.
INTRANASAL
Adults, Elderly. 200-400 international units/day.

▸ **Postmenopausal osteoporosis**

IM, SUBCUTANEOUS
Adults, Elderly. 100 international units every other day with adequate calcium and vitamin D intake.
INTRANASAL
Adults, Elderly. 200 international units/day as a single spray, alternating nostrils daily.

▸ **Hypercalcemia**

IM, SUBCUTANEOUS
Adults, Elderly. Initially, 4 international units/kg q12h; may increase to 8 international units/kg q12h if no response in 2 days; may further increase to 8 international units/kg q6h if no response in another 2 days.

OFF-LABEL USES

Treatment of secondary osteoporosis due to drug therapy or hormone disturbance, osteogenesis imperfection.

CONTRAINDICATIONS

Hypersensitivity to calcitomin-salmon or salmon protein.

INTERACTIONS
Drug
Lithium: May decrease lithium levels by increasing renal clearance.
Herbal
None known.
Food
None known.

DIAGNOSTIC TEST EFFECTS
None known.

SIDE EFFECTS
Frequent
IM, subcutaneous (10%):
Nausea (may occur 30 min after injection, usually diminishes with continued therapy), inflammation at injection site.
NASAL (10%-12%):
Rhinitis, nasal irritation, redness, sores.
Occasional
IM, subcutaneous (2%-5%):
Flushing of face or hands.
NASAL (3%-5%):
Back pain, arthralgia, epistaxis, headache.
Rare
IM, subcutaneous:
Epigastric discomfort, dry mouth, diarrhea, flatulence.
Nasal: Itching of earlobes, edema of feet, rash, diaphoresis.

SERIOUS REACTIONS
• Patients with a protein allergy may develop a hypersensitivity reaction.
• Severe nasal ulcertion.

PRECAUTIONS & CONSIDERATIONS
Caution is warranted with history of allergy. Calcitonin does not cross the placenta, and it is unknown whether the drug is distributed in breast milk; its safety in breastfeeding women has not been established. The safety and efficacy of this drug have not been established in children. Elderly patients may experience a higher incidence of nasal adverse events with the nasal spray.

Nausea may occur but usually decreases with continued therapy. Notify the physician if itching, rash, shortness of breath, or significant nasal irritation occurs. Electrolyte levels should be checked. Improvement in biochemical abnormalities and bone pain usually occurs in the first few months of treatment; with neurologic lesions, improvement may take more than a year.

Storage
Refrigerate the unopened nasal spray and injection; do not freeze. Nasal spray may be stored at room temperature 30-35 days once the pump has been activated.

Administration
Calcitonin may be administered as IM or subcutaneous injection. No more than 2 mL should be given IM at any one site. Bedtime administration may reduce flushing and nausea.

For intranasal use, clear nasal passages as much as possible. Tilt head slightly forward and insert the spray tip into the nostril, pointing toward the nasal passages and away from the septum. Spray into the nostril while holding the other nostril closed, and at the same time inhale through the nose to deliver the drug as high into the nasal passage as possible. Bring to room temperature and prime pump before first use.

C

Calcitriol
kal-si-trye'ole
(Calcijex, Rocaltrol Vectical)

CATEGORY AND SCHEDULE
Pregnancy Risk Category: A (D if used in doses above RDA)

Classification: Vitamins/minerals, vitamin D analogs

MECHANISM OF ACTION
A fat-soluble vitamin that is essential for absorption, utilization of calcium phosphate, and normal calcification of bone. *Therapeutic Effect:* Stimulates calcium and phosphate absorption from small intestine, promotes secretion of calcium from bone to blood, promotes renal tubule phosphate resorption, and acts on bone cells to stimulate skeletal growth and on parathyroid gland to suppress hormone synthesis and secretion.

PHARMACOKINETICS
Rapidly absorbed from small intestine. Extensive metabolism in kidneys. Primarily excreted in feces; minimal excretion in urine. *Half-life:* 5-8 h (prolonged in children and patients on hemodialysis).

AVAILABILITY
Capsule: 0.25 mcg, 0.5 mcg (Rocaltrol).
Injection: 1 mcg/mL, 2 mcg/mL (Calcijex).
Oral Solution: 1 mcg/mL (Rocaltrol).
Ointment (Vectical): 3 mcg/g.

INDICATIONS AND DOSAGES
▸ **Renal failure on dialysis**
PO
Adults, Elderly. 0.25 mcg/day or every other day; increase dose at 4- to 8-wks intervals. Usual range 0.5-1 mcg/day.
Children. 0.25-2 mcg/day with hemodialysis.
IV
Adults, Elderly. 0.5 mcg/day (0.01 mcg/kg) 3 times/wk. Dose range: 0.5-3 mcg (0.01-0.05 mcg/kg) 3 times/wk. Adjust dose at 2- to 4-wks intervals.
Children. 0.01-0.05 mcg/kg 3 times/wk with hemodialysis.
▸ **Renal Failure Predialysis**
PO
Adults, Children 3 yr and older. Initially 0.25 mcg daily, may increase to 0.5 mcg daily.
Children < 3 yr of age. Initially 0.01-0.015 mcg/kg once daily.
▸ **Hypoparathyroidism/ pseudohypoparathyroidism**
PO
Adults, Elderly, Children 6 yr and older. Initial dose 0.25 mcg/day, range 0.5-2 mcg once daily.
Children 1-5 yr. 0.25-0.75 mcg once daily.
Children < 1 yr. 0.04-0.08 mcg/kg once daily.
▸ **Vitamin D–dependent rickets**
PO
Adults, Elderly, Children. 1 mcg once daily.
▸ **Vitamin D–resistant rickets**
PO
Adults, Elderly, Children. 0.015-0.02 mcg/kg once daily. Maintenance: 0.03-0.06 mcg/kg once daily. Maximum: 2 mcg once daily.
▸ **Psoriasis**
TOPICAL
Adults: Apply ointment twice daily to affected areas. Maximum: 200 g/wk.

CONTRAINDICATIONS
Hypercalcemia, vitamin D toxicity, hypersensitivity to other vitamin D products or analogues.

INTERACTIONS
Drug
Aluminum-containing antacid (long-term use): May increase aluminum concentration and aluminum bone toxicity.
Calcium-containing preparations, thiazide diuretics: May increase the risk of hypercalcemia.
Magnesium-containing antacids: May increase magnesium concentration.
Herbal
None known.
Food
None known.

DIAGNOSTIC TEST EFFECTS
May increase serum cholesterol, calcium, magnesium, and phosphate levels. May decrease serum alkaline phosphatase.

SIDE EFFECTS
Occasional
Hypercalcemia, headache, irritability, constipation, metallic taste, nausea, polyuria.

SERIOUS REACTIONS
• Early signs of overdosage are manifested as weakness, headache, somnolence, nausea, vomiting, dry mouth, constipation, muscle and bone pain, and metallic taste sensation.
• Later signs of overdosage are evidenced by polyuria, polydipsia, anorexia, weight loss, nocturia, photophobia, rhinorrhea, pruritus, disorientation, hallucinations, hyperthermia, hypertension, and cardiac arrhythmias.

PRECAUTIONS & CONSIDERATIONS
Caution is warranted with coronary artery disease, kidney stones, malabsorption syndrome, and renal impairment.

It is unknown whether calcitriol crosses the placenta. It is distributed in breast milk; breastfeeding is not recommended. Children may be more sensitive to the effects of calcitriol. Unique age-related precautions have not been observed in elderly patients. Serum alkaline phosphatase, BUN, serum calcium, serum creatinine, serum magnesium, serum phosphate, and urinary calcium levels should be monitored. Therapeutic serum calcium level is 9-10 mg/dL. Daily dietary calcium intake should be estimated; minimum intake should be 600 mg daily. Maintain adequate fluid intake.
Storage
Store at room temperature. Protect from light.
Administration
IV May be administered undiluted as bolus through catheter at the end of hemodialysis.
Give oral calcitriol without regard to food. Swallow the drug whole and avoid crushing, chewing, or opening the capsules.

Calcium Salts
(PhosLo)(Apo-Cal [CAN], Calsan [CAN], Calsup [AUS], Caltrate, Dicarbosil, OsCal, Titralac, Tums) (Calciject) (Calcitrate, Citracal) (Calcione, Calciquid)
Do not confuse OsCal with Asacol, Citracal with Citrucel, or PhosLo with PhosChol.

CATEGORY AND SCHEDULE
Pregnancy Risk Category: C
OTC (acetate, carbonate, citrate, glubionate, gluconate [tablets only])

Classification: Minerals and electrolytes

C

MECHANISM OF ACTION

An electrolyte that is essential for the function and integrity of the nervous, muscular, and skeletal systems. Calcium plays an important role in normal cardiac and renal function, respiration, blood coagulation, and cell membrane and capillary permeability. It helps to regulate the release and storage of neurotransmitters and hormones, and it neutralizes or reduces gastric acid (increased pH). Calcium acetate combines with dietary phosphate to form insoluble calcium phosphate. *Therapeutic Effect:* Replaces calcium in deficiency states; controls hyperphosphatemia in end-stage renal disease.

PHARMACOKINETICS

Moderately absorbed from the small intestine (absorption depends on presence of vitamin D metabolites and patient's pH). Primarily eliminated in feces.

AVAILABILITY

Calcium Acetate
Gelcap (PhosLo): 667 mg (equivalent to 169 mg elemental calcium).
Tablet (PhosLo): 667 mg (equivalent to 169 mg elemental calcium).
Calcium Carbonate
Tablets: (Caltrate 600): Equivalent to 600 mg elemental calcium.
Tablets (OsCal 500): Equivalent to 500 mg elemental calcium.
Tablets (Chewable [OsCal 500]): Equivalent to 500 mg elemental calcium.
Tablets (Chewable [Tums]): Equivalent to 200 mg elemental calcium.
Calcium Chloride
Injection: 10% (100 mg/mL) equivalent to 27.2 mg [1.36 mEq] elemental calcium per milliliter.
Calcium Citrate
Tablets: (Calcitrate): 250 mg

(equivalent to 53 mg elemental calcium).
Tablets: (Citracal): 950 mg (equivalent to 200 mg elemental calcium).
Calcium Glubionate
Syrup: 1.8 g/5 mL (equivalent to 115 mg of elemental calcium per 5 mL).
Calcium Gluconate
Injection: 10% (equivalent to 9 mg [0.45-0.48 mEq] elemental calcium per mL).

INDICATIONS AND DOSAGES

▸ **Hyperphosphatemia**
PO (CALCIUM ACETATE)
Adults, Elderly. 2 tablets 3 times a day with meals.
▸ **Hypocalcemia**
PO (CALCIUM CARBONATE)
Adults, Elderly. 1-2 g/day in 3-4 divided doses.
Children. 45-65 mg/kg/day in 3-4 divided doses.
PO (CALCIUM GLUBIONATE)
Adults, Elderly. 16-18 g/day in 4-6 divided doses.
Children, Infants. 0.6-2 g/kg/day in 4 divided doses.
Neonates. 1.2 g/kg/day in 4-6 divided doses.
IV (CALCIUM CHLORIDE)
Adults, Elderly. 0.5-1 g repeated q4-6h as needed.
Children, 2.5-5 mg/kg/dose q4-6h.
IV (CALCIUM GLUCONATE)
Adults, Elderly. 2-15 g/24 h.
Children. 200-500 mg/kg/day.
▸ **Antacid**
PO (CALCIUM CARBONATE)
Adults, Elderly. 1-2 tablets (5-10 mL) q2h as needed.
▸ **Osteoporosis**
PO (CALCIUM CARBONATE)
Adults, Elderly. 1200 mg/day.
▸ **Cardiac arrest**
IV (CALCIUM CHLORIDE)
Adults, Elderly. 2-4 mg/kg. May repeat q10min.

Children. 20 mg/kg. May repeat in 10 min.

▸ **Hypocalcemia tetany**
IV (CALCIUM CHLORIDE)
Adults, Elderly. 1 g may repeat in 6 h.
Children. 10 mg/kg over 5-10 min. May repeat in 6-8 h.
IV (CALCIUM GLUCONATE)
Adults, Elderly. 1-3 g until therapeutic response achieved.
Children. 100-200 mg/kg/dose q6-8h.

OFF-LABEL USES
Treatment of hyperphosphatemia (calcium carbonate).

CONTRAINDICATIONS
Calcium renal calculi, digoxin toxicity, hypercalcemia, hypercalciuria, sarcoidosis, ventricular fibrillation.
Calcium acetate: Decreased renal function, hypoparathyroidism.

INTERACTIONS
Drug
Digoxin: May increase the risk of arrhythmias.
Etidronate, gallium: May antagonize the effects of these drugs.
Fuoroguinolone antibiotics, ketoconazole, phenytoin, tetracyclines: May decrease the absorption of these drugs.
Magnesium (parenteral), methenamine: May decrease the effects of these drugs.
Herbal
None known.
Food
None known.

DIAGNOSTIC TEST EFFECTS
May increase blood pH and serum gastrin and calcium levels. May decrease serum phosphate and potassium levels.

💊 IV INCOMPATIBILITIES
Calcium chloride: amphotericin B complex (Abelcet, AmBisome, Amphotec), propofol (Diprivan), sodium bicarbonate, sodium or potassium phosphate (concentration dependent).
Calcium gluconate: amphotericin B complex (Abelcet, AmBisome, Amphotec), fluconazole (Diflucan), sodium or potassium phosphate (concentration dependent).

💉 IV COMPATIBILITIES
Calcium chloride: Amikacin (Amikin), dobutamine (Dobutrex), lidocaine, milrinone (Primacor), morphine, norepinephrine (Levophed).
Calcium gluconate: Ampicillin, aztreonam (Azactam), cefazolin (Ancef), cefepime (Maxipime), ciprofloxacin (Cipro), dobutamine (Dobutrex), enalapril (Vasotec), famotidine (Pepcid), furosemide (Lasix), heparin, lidocaine, magnesium sulfate, meropenem (Merrem IV), midazolam (Versed), milrinone (Primacor), norepinephrine (Levophed), piperacillin and tazobactam (Zosyn), potassium chloride, propofol (Diprivan).

SIDE EFFECTS
Frequent
PO: Chalky taste.
Parenteral: Hypotension; flushing; feeling of warmth; nausea; vomiting; pain, rash, redness, or burning at injection site; diaphoresis.
Occasional
PO: Mild constipation, fecal impaction, peripheral edema, metabolic alkalosis (muscle pain, restlessness, slow breathing, altered taste).
Calcium carbonate: Milk-alkali syndrome (headache, decreased appetite, nausea, vomiting, unusual tiredness).

Rare
Difficult or painful urination.

SERIOUS REACTIONS
• Hypercalcemia is a serious adverse
effect of calcium acetate use.
Early signs include constipation,
headache, dry mouth, increased
thirst, irritability, decreased appetite,
metallic taste, fatigue, weakness,
and depression. Later signs
include confusion, somnolence,
hypertension, photosensitivity,
arrhythmias, nausea, vomiting, and
increased painful urination.

PRECAUTIONS & CONSIDERATIONS
Caution is warranted with chronic
renal impairment, decreased
cardiac function, dehydration,
history of renal calculi, and
ventricular fibrillation during cardiac
resuscitation. Calcium acetate is
distributed in breast milk; it is
unknown whether calcium chloride
and gluconate are distributed
in breast milk. Restrict IV use
in children because their small
vasculature increases the risk of
developing extreme irritation and
possible tissue necrosis or sloughing.
Oral absorption may be decreased
in the elderly. Avoid consuming
excessive amounts of alcohol,
caffeine, and tobacco.

Adequate hydration should
be maintained. BP, ECG, serum
magnesium, phosphate and
potassium levels, urine calcium
concentrations, and renal function
test results should be monitored.
Storage
Store vials and oral products at room
temperature.
Administration
Take tablets with a full glass of water
30 min to 1 h after meals. Dilute the
syrup in juice or water and administer
it before meals to increase absorption.

Chew the chewable tablets well before
swallowing them. Do not take calcium
within 2 h of consuming other oral
drugs or fiber-containing foods.

Calcium chloride may be given
undiluted or may be diluted with an
equal amount 0.9% NaCl or sterile
water for injection.

Calcium gluconate may be given
undiluted or may be diluted in up to
1000 mL 0.9% NaCl. Give calcium
chloride by slow IV push (0.5-1 mL/
min). Rapid administration may
produce bradycardia, hypotension,
peripheral vasodilation, a chalky
or metallic taste, and a feeling of
warmth. Give calcium gluconate by
IV push at a rate of 0.5-1 mL/min.
Rapid administration may produce
arrhythmias, hypotension,
myocardial infarction, and
vasodilation. When administering
calcium gluconate by intermittent IV
infusion, the maximum rate is
200 mg/min.

Calfactant
cal-fac′tant
(Infasurf)

CATEGORY AND SCHEDULE
Pregnancy Risk Category: This
drug is not indicated for use in
pregnant women.

Classification: Surfactants, lung

MECHANISM OF ACTION
A natural lung extract that reduces
alveolar surface tension, stabilizing
the alveoli. *Therapeutic Effect:*
Restores surface activity to infant
lungs, improves lung compliance and
respiratory gas exchange.

PHARMACOKINETICS
No studies have been performed.

AVAILABILITY
Intratracheal Suspension:
35-mg/mL vials.

INDICATIONS AND DOSAGES
▸ **Respiratory distress syndrome (RDS)**
INTRATRACHEAL
Neonates. 3 mL/kg of birth weight administered as soon as possible after birth in 2 doses of 1.5 mL/kg. Repeat 3-mL/kg doses, up to a total of 4 doses each given 12 h apart.

CONTRAINDICATIONS
None known.

INTERACTIONS
Drug
None known.
Herbal
None known.
Food
None known.

DIAGNOSTIC TEST EFFECTS
None known.

SIDE EFFECTS
Frequent
Cyanosis (65%), airway obstruction (39%), bradycardia (34%), reflux of surfactant into endotracheal tube (21%), need for manual ventilation (16%).
Occasional
Need for reintubation (3%).

SERIOUS REACTIONS
• Cyanosis, airway obstruction, bradycardia, and reflux of surfactant into endotracheal tube may occur.

PRECAUTIONS & CONSIDERATIONS
Caution is warranted with a hypersensitivity to calfactant. This drug is for use only in neonates. No age-related precautions have been noted.

The neonate's oxygenation and ventilation should be monitored

using arterial or transcutaneous measurement of systemic oxygen (O_2) and carbon dioxide (CO_2). Visitors should be limited during treatment. Handwashing and other infection control measures should be monitored to minimize the risk of nosocomial infections.
Storage
Refrigerate vials. Unopened, unused vials may be returned to refrigerator within 24 h after having been warmed to room temperature. Repeated warming to room temperature should be avoided. Warming before administration is not necessary.
Administration
Gently swirl the vial, if needed, to redisperse contents. Do not shake it. Enter each single use vial only once; discard unused suspension. Instill the drug intratracheally through a side port adapter into the infant's endotracheal tube. Give each aliquot over 20-30 ventilatory breaths. Administer only during the inspiratory cycle. Between aliquot dosages, turn the infant so that the opposite lung is in the dependent position.

Candesartan
kan-de-sar′tan
(Atacand)

CATEGORY AND SCHEDULE
Pregnancy Risk Category: C (D if used in second or third trimester)

Classification: Angiotensin II receptor antagonists

MECHANISM OF ACTION
An angiotensin II receptor, type AT1, antagonist that blocks the vasoconstrictor and aldosterone-secreting

effects of angiotensin II, inhibiting the binding of angiotensin II to the AT1 receptors. *Therapeutic Effect:* Causes vasodilation, decreases peripheral resistance, and decreases BP.

PHARMACOKINETICS

Route	Onset	Peak	Duration
PO	2-3 h	6-8 h	24 h

Rapidly, completely absorbed. Protein binding: > 99%. Undergoes minor hepatic metabolism to inactive metabolite. Excreted unchanged in urine and in the feces through the biliary system. Not removed by hemodialysis. *Half-life:* 9 h.

AVAILABILITY

Tablets: 4 mg, 8 mg, 16 mg, 32 mg.

INDICATIONS AND DOSAGES
▸ **Hypertension alone or in combination with other antihypertensives**
PO
Adults, Elderly. Initially, 16 mg once a day in those who are not volume depleted. Can be given once or twice a day with total daily doses of 8-32 mg. Give lower initial dosage in those treated with diuretics or with impaired renal function or moderate hepatic disease.
▸ **Heart Failure**
PO
Adults, Elderly. Initially 4 mg once daily. Target dose of 32 mg once daily can be reached by doubling dose approximately every 2 wks as tolerated.

CONTRAINDICATIONS

Hypersensitivity to candesartan.

INTERACTIONS
Drug
None known.
Herbal
None known.
Food
None known.

DIAGNOSTIC TEST EFFECTS

May increase BUN, serum alkaline phosphatase, serum bilirubin, serum creatinine, potassium, AST (SGOT), and ALT (SGPT) levels. May decrease blood hemoglobin and hematocrit levels.

SIDE EFFECTS
Occasional (3%-6%)
Upper respiratory tract infection, dizziness, back and leg pain.
Rare (1%-2%)
Pharyngitis, rhinitis, headache, fatigue, diarrhea, nausea, dry cough, peripheral edema.

SERIOUS REACTIONS

• Overdosage may manifest as hypotension and tachycardia. Bradycardia occurs less often. Institute supportive measures.

PRECAUTIONS & CONSIDERATIONS

Caution is warranted with hepatic and renal impairment, renal artery stenosis, severe congestive heart failure, and dehydration. It is unknown whether candesartan is distributed in breast milk. Candesartan may cause fetal or neonatal morbidity or mortality. Safety and efficacy of candesartan have not been established in children. No age-related precautions have been noted in elderly patients.

Apical pulse and BP should be assessed immediately before each candesartan dose and regularly throughout therapy. Be alert to fluctuations in apical pulse and BP. If

an excessive reduction in BP occurs, place the patient in the supine position with feet slightly elevated and notify the physician. Tasks that require mental alertness or motor skills should be avoided. Blood hemoglobin and hematocrit and BUN, serum alkaline phosphatase, serum bilirubin, serum creatinine, AST (SGOT), and ALT (SGPT) levels should be obtained before and during therapy. Also monitor potassium in heart failure patients. Maintain adequate hydration; exercising outside during hot weather should be avoided in order to decrease the risk of dehydration and hypotension.
Storage
Store at room temperature.
Administration
Take candesartan without regard to food.

Capecitabine
ka-pe-site′-a-been
(Xeloda)
Do not confuse Xeloda with Xenical.

CATEGORY AND SCHEDULE
Pregnancy Risk Category: D

Classification: Antineoplastics, antimetabolites

MECHANISM OF ACTION
An antimetabolite that is enzymatically converted to 5-fluorouracil. Inhibits enzymes necessary for synthesis of essential cellular components. *Therapeutic Effect:* Interferes with DNA synthesis, RNA processing, and protein synthesis.

PHARMACOKINETICS
Readily absorbed from the GI tract. Protein binding: < 60%. Metabolized in the liver. Primarily excreted in urine. *Half-life:* 45 min.

AVAILABILITY
Tablets: 150 mg, 500 mg.

INDICATIONS AND DOSAGES
▸ **Metastatic breast cancer, colon cancer**
PO
Adults, Elderly. Initially, 2500 mg/m^2/day in 2 equally divided doses approximately q12h for 2 wks. Follow with a 1-wk rest period; given in 3-wk cycles.
▸ **Dosage in moderate renal impairment (CrCl 30-50 mL/min)**
PO
Adults, Elderly. Initally 950 mg/m^2 twice daily. If creatinine clearance is less than 30 mL/min, contraindicated.

CONTRAINDICATIONS
Severe renal impairment, hypersensitivity to capecitabine, fluorouracil, or any component of the formulation; known deficiency of dihydropyrimidine dehydrogenase.

INTERACTIONS
Drug
Phenytoin: May increase phenytoin levels.
Warfarin: May increase the effects of warfarin.
Herbal
None known.
Food
None known.

DIAGNOSTIC TEST EFFECTS
May increase serum alkaline phosphatase, bilirubin, AST (SGOT), and ALT (SGPT) levels. May decrease blood hematocrit, hemoglobin level, and WBC count.

SIDE EFFECTS

Frequent (> 5%)
Diarrhea (sometimes severe), nausea, vomiting, stomatitis, hand and foot syndrome (painful palmar-plantar swelling with paresthesia, erythema, and blistering), fatigue, anorexia, dermatitis.

Occasional (< 5%)
Constipation, dyspepsia, nail disorder, headache, dizziness, insomnia, edema, myalgia.

SERIOUS REACTIONS

• Serious reactions may include myelosuppression (evidenced by neutropenia, thrombocytopenia, and anemia), cardiovascular toxicity (marked by angina, cardiomyopathy, and deep vein thrombosis), respiratory toxicity (marked by dyspnea, epistaxis, and pneumonia), and lymphedema.

PRECAUTIONS & CONSIDERATIONS

Use cautiously in patients with a history of coronary artery disease, concomitant coumarin-derived anticoagulant therapy, concomitant phenytoin therapy, renal impairment, or liver dysfunction due to liver metastases. Caution is also warranted in elderly patients. Avoid use in pregnant women. It is unknown whether capecitabine is distributed in breast milk. Safety and efficacy of capecitabine have not been established in children. Monitor for signs of infection. Monitor for symptoms of hand-and-foot syndrome.

Storage
Store at room temperature; keep tightly closed.

Administration
Take capecitabine within 30 min after a meal.

Capreomycin
kap-ree-oh-mye′sin
(Capastat [aus], Capastat Sulfate)
Do not confuse with Captopril, Capsaicin, or Kanamycin.

CATEGORY AND SCHEDULE
Pregnancy Risk Category: C

Classification:
Antimycobacterials

MECHANISM OF ACTION
A cyclic polypeptide antimicrobial but the mechanism of action is not well understood. *Therapeutic Effect:* Suppresses mycobacterial multiplication.

PHARMACOKINETICS
Not well absorbed from the gastrointestinal (GI) tract. Undergoes little metabolism. Primarily excreted unchanged in urine. *Half-life:* 4-6 h (half-life is increased with impaired renal function).

AVAILABILITY
Injection: 100 mg/mL (Capastat Sulfate).

INDICATIONS AND DOSAGES
▸ **Tuberculosis**
IM/IV
Adults, Elderly. 1 g daily (not to exceed 20 mg/kg/day) for 60-120 days, followed by 1 g 2-3 times/wk.
▸ **Dosage in renal impairment**
CrCl > 100 mL/min: 13-15 mg/kg every 24 h.
CrCl 80-100 mL/min: 10-13 mg/kg every 24 h.
CrCl 60-80 mL/min: 7-10 mg/kg every 24 h.
CrCl 40-60 mL/min: 11-14 mg/kg every 48 h.

CrCl 20-40 mL/min: 10-14 mg/kg every 72 h.
CrCl < 20 mL/min: 4-7 mg/kg every 72 h.

OFF-LABEL USES
Treatment of atypical mycobacterial infections.

CONTRAINDICATIONS
Hypersensitivity to capreomycin.

INTERACTIONS
Drug
Aminoglycosides: May increase the risk of aminoglycoside toxicity.
Nondepolarizing neuromuscular blocking agents: May increase neuromuscular blockade.
Herbal
None known.
Food
None known.

DIAGNOSTIC TEST EFFECTS
None known.

SIDE EFFECTS
Frequent
Ototoxicity, nephrotoxicity.
Occasional
Eosinophilia.
Rare
Rash, fever, urticaria, hypokalemia, thrombocytopenia, vertigo.

SERIOUS REACTIONS
• Renal failure, ototoxicity, and thrombocytopenia can occur.

PRECAUTIONS & CONSIDERATIONS
Cautiously use with preexisting hearing impairment, renal dysfunction, or concurrent use of other ototoxic or nephrotoxic drugs. It is unknown whether capreomycin crosses the placenta and is excreted in breast milk. Age-related renal impairment may require dosage

adjustment in elderly patients. Complete blood count (CBC) and renal and liver function test results should be obtained before the initiation of therapy. Hearing changes must be reported immediately. Renal function, electrolytes, and acid-base balance should be monitored during therapy.
Administration
Reconstitute by dissolving the vial contents (1 g) in 2 mL of 0.9% NaCl injection or sterile water for injection. Allow 2-3 min for complete dissolution. Further dilute in NS 100 mL for IV administration. Administer IV over 60 min. Administer deep IM into large muscle mass.

The solution for injection may acquire a pale straw color and darken with time. This is not associated with a loss of potency or development of toxicity.

Capsaicin
cap-say'sin
(Zostrix)
Do not confuse with Zovirax.

CATEGORY AND SCHEDULE
Pregnancy Risk Category: C
OTC

Classification: Analgesics, topical, dermatologics

MECHANISM OF ACTION
A topical analgesic that depletes and prevents reaccumulation of the chemomediator of pain impulses (substance P) from peripheral sensory neurons to CNS. *Therapeutic Effect:* Relieves pain.

C

PHARMACOKINETICS
None reported.

AVAILABILITY
Cream: 0.025%, 0.035%, 0.075%, 0.1%, 0.25%.
Gel: 0.025%, 0.05%.
Lotion: 0.025%, 0.075%.
Roll-on: 0.075%.

INDICATIONS AND DOSAGES
▸ **Treatment of neuralgia, osteoarthritis, rheumatoid arthritis**
TOPICAL
Adults, Elderly, Children older than 2 yr. Apply directly to affected area 3-4 times/day. Continue for optimal clinical response.

CONTRAINDICATIONS
Hypersensitivity to capsaicin or any component of the formulation.

INTERACTIONS
Drug
Anticoagulants, antiplatelet agents, low-molecular-weight heparins, thrombolytic agents: May increase risk of bleeding.
Herbal
None known.
Food
None known.

DIAGNOSTIC TEST EFFECTS
None known.

SIDE EFFECTS
Frequent
Burning, stinging, erythema at site of application.

SERIOUS REACTIONS
• None known.

PRECAUTIONS & CONSIDERATIONS
Caution is warranted with concurrent use of nephrotoxic agents, dehydration, fluid and electrolyte imbalance, neurologic abnormalities, and renal or hepatic impairment. It is unknown whether capsaicin crosses the placenta or is distributed in breast milk. Safety and efficacy have not been established in children < 2 yr of age. There are no age-related precautions noted for elderly patients.

Transient burning may occur on application and usually disappears after 72 h with continued use.
Storage
Store at room temperature.
Administration
Capsaicin is for external use only. Avoid eye or mucous membrane contact. Wash hands immediately after application, unless used on arthritic hands, then wait 30 min, then wash. If there is no improvement or condition deteriorates after 28 days, discontinue use and consult physician.

Captopril
cap-toe-pril
(Acenorm [AUS], Capoten, Captohexal [AUS], Novo-Captoril [CAN], Topace [AUS])
Do not confuse captopril with Capitrol.

CATEGORY AND SCHEDULE
Pregnancy Risk Category: C (D if used in second or third trimester)

Classification: Angiotensin-converting enzyme (ACE) inhibitors

MECHANISM OF ACTION

An ACE inhibitor that suppresses the renin-angiotensin-aldosterone system and prevents conversion of angiotensin I to angiotensin II, a potent vasoconstrictor; may also inhibit angiotensin II at local vascular and renal sites. Decreases plasma angiotensin II, increases plasma renin activity, and decreases aldosterone secretion. *Therapeutic Effect:* Reduces peripheral arterial resistance, pulmonary capillary wedge pressure; improves cardiac output and exercise tolerance.

PHARMACOKINETICS

Route	Onset	Peak	Duration
PO	0.25 h	0.5-1.5 h	Dose related

Rapidly, well absorbed from the GI tract (absorption is decreased in the presence of food). Protein binding: 25%-30%. Metabolized in the liver. Primarily excreted in urine. Removed by hemodialysis. *Half-life:* < 3 h (increased in those with impaired renal function).

AVAILABILITY

Tablets: 12.5 mg, 25 mg, 50 mg, 100 mg.

INDICATIONS AND DOSAGES
▶ **Hypertension**
PO
Adults, Elderly. Initially, 12.5-25 mg 2-3 times a day. After 1-2 wks, may increase to 50 mg 2-3 times a day. Diuretic may be added if no response in additional 1-2 wks. If taken in combination with diuretic, may increase to 100-150 mg 2-3 times a day after 1-2 wks. Maintenance: 25-150 mg 2-3 times a day. Maximum: 450 mg/day.

▶ **Congestive heart failure**
PO
Adults, Elderly. Initially, 6.25-25 mg 3 times a day. Increase to 50 mg 3 times a day. After at least 2 wks, may increase to 50-100 mg 3 times a day. Maximum: 450 mg/day.
▶ **Post-myocardial infarction, left ventricular dysfunction**
PO
Adults, Elderly. 6.25 mg a day, then 12.5 mg 3 times a day. Increase to 25 mg 3 times a day over several days up to 50 mg 3 times a day over several weeks.
▶ **Diabetic nephropathy**
PO
Adults, Elderly. 25 mg 3 times a day.
▶ **Usual pediatric dose**
Children. Initially 0.3-0.5 mg/kg/dose titrated up to a maximum of 6 mg/kg/day in 2-4 divided doses. *Neonates.* Initially, 0.05-0.1 mg/kg/dose q8-24h titrated up to 0.5 mg/kg/dose given q6-24h. Maximum: 2 mg/kg/day.
▶ **Dosage in renal impairment (Adults)**
Creatinine clearance 10-50 mL/min. 75% of normal dosage.
Creatinine clearance < 10 mL/min. 50% of normal dosage.

OFF-LABEL USES

Diagnosis of anatomic renal artery stenosis, hypertensive urgency.

CONTRAINDICATIONS

History of angioedema from previous treatment with ACE inhibitors.

INTERACTIONS
Drug
Alcohol, antihypertensives, diuretics: May increase the effects of captopril.
Lithium: May increase lithium blood concentration and risk of lithium toxicity.

NSAIDs: May decrease the effects of captopril.
Potassium-sparing diuretics, potassium supplements: May cause hyperkalemia.
Herbal
None known.
Food
All food: Food significantly reduces drug absorption by 30%-40%.

DIAGNOSTIC TEST EFFECTS

May increase BUN, serum alkaline phosphatase, serum bilirubin, serum creatinine, serum potassium, AST (SGOT), and ALT (SGPT) levels. May decrease serum sodium levels. May cause positive antinuclear antibody titer.

SIDE EFFECTS

Frequent (4%-7%)
Rash.
Occasional (2%-4%)
Pruritus, dysgeusia (change in sense of taste).
Rare (0.5%-< 2%)
Headache, cough, insomnia, dizziness, fatigue, paresthesia, malaise, nausea, diarrhea or constipation, dry mouth, tachycardia.

SERIOUS REACTIONS

• Excessive hypotension (first-dose syncope) may occur in patients with CHF and in those who are severely salt and volume depleted.
• Angioedema (swelling of face and lips) and hyperkalemia occur rarely.
• Agranulocytosis and neutropenia may be noted in those with collagen vascular disease, including scleroderma and systemic lupus erythematosus, and impaired renal function.
• Nephrotic syndrome may be noted in those with history of renal disease.

PRECAUTIONS & CONSIDERATIONS

Caution is warranted with cerebrovascular or coronary insufficiency, hypovolemia, renal impairment, sodium depletion, those on dialysis and/or receiving diuretics, and in elderly patients. Captopril crosses the placenta, is distributed in breast milk, and may cause fetal or neonatal morbidity or mortality. Safety and efficacy of captopril have not been established in children. Elderly patients may be more sensitive to the hypotensive effects of captopril.

Dizziness may occur. BP should be obtained immediately before giving each captopril dose, in addition to regular monitoring. Be alert to fluctuations in BP. If an excessive reduction in BP occurs, place the person in the supine position with legs elevated. CBC and blood chemistry should be obtained before beginning captopril therapy, then every 2 wks for the next 3 mo, and periodically thereafter in patients with autoimmune disease or renal impairment and in those who are taking drugs that affect immune response or leukocyte count. Skin for rash and urinalysis for proteinuria should also be assessed. CBC, BUN, serum creatinine, and serum potassium should be monitored in those who are receiving a diuretic. Full therapeutic effect of captopril may take several weeks.
Administration
! Give captopril 1 h before meals for maximum absorption because food significantly decreases drug absorption.

Crush tablets if necessary. Do not skip doses.

Carbachol
kar´-ba-kole
(Caroptic, Isopto Carbachol, Miostat)

CATEGORY AND SCHEDULE
Pregnancy Risk Category: C

Classification: Antiglaucoma agent, ophthalmic; Antihypertensive agent, ocular, postsurgical; Miotic

MECHANISM OF ACTION
A direct-acting parasympathomimetic agent that stimulates cholinergic receptors resulting in muscarinic and nicotinic effects. Indirectly promotes release of acetylcholine. *Therapeutic Effect:* Produces contraction of the iris sphincter muscle, resulting in miosis and reduction in intraocular pressure associated with decreased resistance to aqueous humor outflow.

PHARMACOKINETICS
None reported.

AVAILABILITY
Ophthalmic Solution: 0.75%, 1.5%, 2.25%, 3%.
Solution for Intraocular Administration: 0.01%.

INDICATIONS AND DOSAGES
▶ Glaucoma
OPHTHALMIC
Adults, Elderly. Instill 1–2 drops of 0.75%–3% solution in affected eye(s) up to 3 times a day.
▶ Miosis, Ophthalmic Surgery
OPHTHALMIC
Adults, Elderly. Instill 0.5 mL of 0.01% solution into anterior chamber before or after securing sutures.

CONTRAINDICATIONS
Acute iritis, hypersensitivity to carbachol or any component of the formulation.

INTERACTIONS
Drugs
None known.
Herbal
None known.
Food
None known.

DIAGNOSTIC TEST EFFECTS
None known.

SIDE EFFECTS
Occasional
Blurred vision, burning/irritation of eye, decreased night vision, headache.
Rare
Diaphoresis, abdominal cramps, diaphoresis.

SERIOUS REACTIONS
Retinal detachment.

PRECAUTIONS & CONSIDERATIONS
Intraocular carbachol 0.01% should be used with caution in patients with acute cardiac failure, bronchial asthma, peptic ulcer, hyperthyroidism, GI spasm, urinary tract obstruction, and Parkinson disease. Safety and effectiveness have not been established in children.
Storage
Store at room temperature.
Administration
Use nasolacrimal occlusion following topical instillation to reduce systemic side effects.

Sterile technique must be used for intraocular administration. Instill no more than 0.5 mL into the anterior chamber. Discard unused portion.

Carbamazepine

kar-ba-maz′e-peen

(Apo-Carbamazepine [CAN], Carbatrol, Epitol, Tegretol, Tegretol CR [AUS], Tegretol XR, Teril [AUS])

Do not confuse Tegretol with Cartrol, Toradol, or Trental.

CATEGORY AND SCHEDULE

Pregnancy Risk Category: D

Classification:
Anticonvulsants, antipsychotics

MECHANISM OF ACTION

An iminostilbene derivative that decreases sodium and calcium ion influx into neuronal membranes, reducing posttetanic potentiation at synapses. *Therapeutic Effect:* Reduces seizure activity.

PHARMACOKINETICS

Slowly and completely absorbed from the GI tract. Protein binding: 75%. Metabolized in the liver to active metabolite. Primarily excreted in urine. Not removed by hemodialysis. *Half-life:* 25-65 h (decreased with chronic use).

AVAILABILITY

Capsules (Extended-Release [Carbatrol, Equetro]): 100 mg, 200 mg, 300 mg.
Suspension (Tegretol): 100 mg/5 mL.
Tablets (Epitol, Tegretol): 200 mg.
Tablets (Chewable [Tegretol]): 100 mg.
Tablets (Extended-Release [Tegretol XR]): 100 mg, 200 mg, 400 mg.

INDICATIONS AND DOSAGES
▸ **Seizure control**
PO
Adults, Children older than 12 yr. Initially, 200 mg twice a day. May increase dosage by 200 mg/day at weekly intervals. Range: 400-1200 mg/day in 2-4 divided doses. Maximum: 1.6-2.4 g/day.
Children 6-12 yr. Initially, 100 mg twice a day. May increase by 100 mg/day at weekly intervals. Range: 20-30 mg/kg/day. Maxiumum: 1000 mg/day.
Children younger than 6 yr. Initially 5 mg/kg/day. May increase at weekly intervals to 10 mg/kg/day up to 20 mg/kg/day. Do not use extended-release forms.
Elderly. Initially 100 mg 1-2 times a day. May increase by 100 mg/day at weekly intervals. Usual dose 400-1000 mg/day.
▸ **Trigeminal neuralgia, diabetic neuropathy**
PO
Adults. Initially, 100 mg twice a day. May increase by 100 mg twice a day up to 400-800 mg/day. Maxiumum: 1200 mg/day.
Elderly. Initially 100 mg 1-2 times a day. May increase by 100 mg/day at weekly intervals. Usual dose 400-1000 mg/day.
▸ **Bipolar disorder**
PO
Adults. Initially 200 mg twice a day. May increase by 200 mg/day. Maximum: 1600 mg/day.

OFF-LABEL USES

Diabetes insipidus, psychotic disorders.

CONTRAINDICATIONS

Concomitant use of MAOIs or nefazodone, history of myelosuppression, hypersensitivity to carbamazepine or tricyclic antidepressants.

INTERACTIONS

Drug
Anticoagulants, clarithromycin, diltiazem, erythromycin, estrogens,

propoxyphene, quinidine, steroids: May decrease the effects of these drugs.

Antipsychotics, haloperidol, tricyclic antidepressants: May increase CNS depressant effects.

Cimetidine: May increase carbamazepine blood concentration and risk of toxicity.

Isoniazid: May increase metabolism of isoniazid; may increase carbamazepine blood concentration and risk of toxicity.

MAOIs: May cause seizures and hypertensive crisis. Contraindicated.

Nefazodone, Delavirdine, Carbamazepine: Decreased concentrations to negligible; do not give.

Other anticonvulsants, barbiturates, benzodiazepines, valproic acid: May increase the metabolism of these drugs.

Verapamil: May increase the toxicity of carbamazepine.

Herbal
None known.

Food
Grapefruit: May increase the absorption and blood concentration of carbamazepine.

DIAGNOSTIC TEST EFFECTS

May increase BUN and blood glucose levels and serum alkaline phosphatase, bilirubin, AST (SGOT), ALT (SGPT), protein, cholesterol, HDL, and triglyceride levels. May decrease serum calcium and thyroid hormone (T3, T4, T4 index) levels. Therapeutic serum level is 4-12 mcg/mL; toxic serum level is > 12 mcg/mL.

SIDE EFFECTS

Frequent
Drowsiness, dizziness, nausea, vomiting.

Occasional
Visual abnormalities (spots before eyes, difficulty focusing, blurred vision), dry mouth or pharynx, tongue irritation, headache, fluid retention, diaphoresis, constipation or diarrhea, behavioral changes in children.

SERIOUS REACTIONS

• Toxic reactions may include blood dyscrasias (such as aplastic anemia, agranulocytosis, thrombocytopenia, leukopenia, leukocytosis, and eosinophilia), cardiovascular disturbances (such as CHF, hypotension or hypertension, thrombophlebitis and arrhythmias), and dermatologic effects (such as rash, urticaria, pruritus, photosensitivity, Stevens-Johnson syndrome, and toxic epidermal necrolysis).
• Abrupt withdrawal may precipitate status epilepticus.

PRECAUTIONS & CONSIDERATIONS

Caution is warranted with impaired cardiac, hepatic, and renal function. Be aware that carbamazepine crosses the placenta and accumulates in fetal tissue. It is also distributed in breast milk. Children are more likely than adults to develop behavioral changes. Elderly patients are more susceptible to agitation, AV block, bradycardia, confusion, and syndrome of inappropriate antidiuretic hormone secretion. Individuals who possess a genetic susceptibility marker known as the HLA-B*1502 allele have an increased risk of developing Stevens-Johnson syndrome and/or toxic epidermal necrolysis compared with persons without this genotype. The presence of this genetic variant exists in up to 15% of people of Asian descent, varying from < 1% in Japanese and Koreans, to 2%-4% of South Asians and Indians, to 10%-15%

of populations from China, Taiwan, Malaysia, and the Philippines. This variant is virtually absent in those of white, African-American, Hispanic, or European ancestry. Genetic testing is recommended before initiation of therapy in most patients of Asian ancestry for the presence of this genetic marker. A positive result should preclude use of carbamazepine unless the benefit exceeds risk. An increased risk of suicidal behavior and suicidal ideation has been observed in patients receiving antiepileptic therapies. Monitor for anxiety, depression, or changes in behavior. Grapefruit juice should be avoided because it may increase the drug's blood concentration.

Drowsiness may occur but disappears with continued therapy, so tasks that require mental alertness or motor skills should be avoided. Notify the physician if visual disturbances, fever, joint pain, mouth ulcerations, sore throat, or unusual bleeding occur. Seizure disorder, including the duration, frequency, and intensity of seizures, should be assessed before and during therapy. BUN level, CBC, serum iron determination, and urinalysis should be obtained before and periodically during carbamazepine therapy.
Storage
Store the tablets, capsules, and oral suspension at room temperature.
Administration
! If the patient must change to another anticonvulsant, plan to decrease the carbamazepine dose gradually as therapy begins with a low dose of the replacement drug. When transferring from tablets to suspension, expect to divide the total daily tablet dose into smaller, more frequent doses of suspension. Also plan to administer

extended-release tablets in 2 divided doses. Therapeutic serum level of carbamazepine is 4-12 mcg/mL.

Take carbamazepine with meals to reduce the risk of GI distress. Shake the oral suspension well. Do not administer it simultaneously with any other liquid medicine. Do not crush extended-release tablets. May open extended-release capsules and administer beads sprinkled on applesauce; however, do not crush or chew.

Carbamide Peroxide
(Auro Ear Drops, Debrox, ERO Ear, GlyOxide, Mollifene Ear Wax Removing, Murine Ear Drops, Orajel Perioseptic, Proxigel) (gel, solution)

CATEGORY AND SCHEDULE
Pregnancy Risk Category: C

Classification: Cerumenolytic; topical oral anti-inflammatory

MECHANISM OF ACTION
A cerumenolytic that releases oxygen on contact with moist mouth tissues to provide cleansing effects, reduce inflammation, relieve pain, and inhibit odor-forming bacteria. In the ear, oxygen is released and hydrogen peroxide is reduced to water, which enables the chemical reaction.
Therapeutic Effect: Relieves inflammation of gums and lips. Emulsifies and disperses ear wax.

PHARMACOKINETICS
Not known.

AVAILABILITY
Gel, Oral: 10% (Proxigel).
Solution, Oral: 10% (Gly-Oxide), 15% (Orajel Perioseptic).

Solution, Otic: 6.5% (Auro Ear Drops, Debrox, ERO Ear, Mollifene Ear Wax Removing, Murine Ear Drops).

INDICATIONS AND DOSAGES
▶ **Earwax removal**
OTIC SOLUTION
Adults, Elderly, Children 12 yr or older. Tilt head and administer 5-10 drops twice a day for up to 4 days.
Children 12 yr or younger. Tilt head and administer 1-5 drops twice a day for up to 4 days.
▶ **Oral lesions**
TOPICAL, GEL
Adults, Elderly, Children. Apply to affected area 4 times a day.
TOPICAL, SOLUTION
Adults, Elderly, Children. Apply several drops undiluted on affected area 4 times a day after meals and at bedtime.

CONTRAINDICATIONS
Dizziness, ear discharge or drainage, ear injury, ear pain, irritation, or rash, hypersensitivity to carbamide peroxide or any one of its components.

INTERACTIONS
Drug
None known.
Herbal
None known.
Food
None known.

DIAGNOSTIC TEST EFFECTS
Not known.

SIDE EFFECTS
Occasional
Oral: Gingival sensitivity.

SERIOUS REACTIONS
• Opportunistic infections caused by organisms like *Candida albicans* are possible with prolonged use.

PRECAUTIONS & CONSIDERATIONS
With prolonged use of oral carbamide peroxide, there is a potential for overgrowth of opportunistic organisms, damage to periodontal tissues, and delayed wound healing; should not be used for longer than 7 days. Otic solution should not be used for longer than 4 days. It is unknown whether carbamide peroxide crosses the placenta or is distributed in breast milk. There are no age-related precautions noted in elderly patients.
Administration
Use several drops after a meal or at bedtime. Mix with saliva, swish for several minutes, and expectorate. Do not drink or rinse mouth after use.

Tilt the patient's head sideways to instill in ear. Keep drops in ear for several minutes by keeping head tilted and placing cotton in ear. Tip of the applicator should not enter the ear canal.

Carbidopa and Levodopa
kar-bee-doe′pa; lee-voe-doe′pa
(Apo-Levocarb [CAN], Kinson [AUS], Sinemet, Sinemet CR)

CATEGORY AND SCHEDULE
Pregnancy Risk Category: C

Classification: Antiparkinson agents, dopaminergics

MECHANISM OF ACTION

Levodopa is converted to dopamine in the basal ganglia, thus increasing dopamine concentration in the brain and inhibiting hyperactive cholinergic activity. Carbidopa prevents peripheral breakdown of levodopa, allowing more levodopa to be available for transport into the brain. *Therapeutic Effect:* Reduces tremor.

PHARMACOKINETICS

Carbidopa is rapidly and completely absorbed from the GI tract. Widely distributed. Excreted primarily in urine. Levodopa is converted to dopamine. Excreted primarily in urine. *Half-life:* 1-2 h (carbidopa); 1-3 h (levodopa).

AVAILABILITY

Tablets: 10 mg carbidopa/100 mg levodopa, 25 mg carbidopa/100 mg levodopa, 25 mg carbidopa/250 mg levodopa.
Tablets (Extended-Release): 25 mg carbidopa/100 mg levodopa, 50 mg carbidopa/200 mg levodopa.
Tablets (Orally Disintegrating): 10 mg carbidopa/100 mg levodopa, 25 mg carbidopa/100 mg levodopa, 25 mg carbidopa/250 mg levodopa.

INDICATIONS AND DOSAGES

▸ **Parkinsonism**
PO
Adults. Initially, 25/100 mg 2-4 times a day. May increase up to 200/2000 mg daily.
Elderly. Initially, 25/100 mg twice a day. May increase as necessary.
When converting a patient from Sinemet to Sinemet CR (50 mg/200 mg), dosage is based on the total daily dose of levodopa:

Sinemet (mg)	Sinemet CR
300-400	1 tablet twice a day
500-600	1.5 tablets twice a day or 1 tablet 3 times a day
700-800	4 tablets in 3 or more divided doses
900-1000	5 tablets in 3 or more divided doses

Intervals between doses of Sinemet CR should be 4-8 h while awake.

CONTRAINDICATIONS

Angle-closure glaucoma, use within 14 days of MAOIs.

INTERACTIONS

Drug
Anticonvulsants, benzodiazepines, haloperidol, phenothiazines: May decrease the effects of carbidopa and levodopa.
MAOIs: May increase the risk of hypertensive crisis. Contraindicated.
Selegiline: May increase levodopa-induced dyskinesias, nausea, orthostatic hypotension, confusion, and hallucinations.
Iron salts: May reduce levodopa absorption.
Herbal
None known.
Food
Protein: Avoid high-protein diet. Distribute dietary protein throughout the day to avoid fluctuations in levodopa absorption.
Pyridoxine/Vitamin B_6: may reduce levodopa's effect at high doses.

DIAGNOSTIC TEST EFFECTS

May increase BUN level and serum LDH, alkaline phosphatase, bilirubin, AST (SGOT), and ALT (SGPT) levels.

C

SIDE EFFECTS
Frequent (10%-90%)
Uncontrolled movements of the face, tongue, arms, or upper body; nausea and vomiting (80%); anorexia (50%).
Occasional
Depression, anxiety, confusion, nervousness, urine retention, palpitations, dizziness, light-headedness, decreased appetite, blurred vision, constipation, dry mouth, flushed skin, headache, insomnia, diarrhea, unusual fatigue, darkening of urine and sweat.
Rare
Hypertension, ulcer, hemolytic anemia (marked by fatigue).

SERIOUS REACTIONS
• Patients on long-term therapy have a high incidence of involuntary choreiform, dystonic, and dyskinetic movements.
• Numerous mild to severe CNS and psychiatric disturbances may occur, including reduced attention span, anxiety, nightmares, daytime somnolence, euphoria, fatigue, paranoia, psychotic episodes, depression, and hallucinations.

PRECAUTIONS & CONSIDERATIONS
Caution is warranted with active peptic ulcer, severe cardiac, endocrine, hepatic, pulmonary, or renal impairment, treated open-angle glaucoma, a history of myocardial infarction, bronchial asthma (because of tartrazine sensitivity), and emphysema. It is unknown whether carbidopa and levodopa cross the placenta or are distributed in breast milk. However, this drug may inhibit lactation. Women should not breastfeed while taking this drug. The safety and efficacy of carbidopa and levodopa have not been established in children younger than 18 yr. Elderly patients are more sensitive to levodopa's effects. Elderly patients receiving anticholinergics are at increased risk for adverse CNS effects, such as anxiety, confusion, and nervousness. Dizziness, drowsiness, dry mouth, and darkened urine may occur. Alcohol and tasks that require mental alertness or motor skills should be avoided. Notify the physician if agitation, headache, lethargy, or confusion occurs. Relief of symptoms, such as improvement of masklike facial expression, muscular rigidity, shuffling gait, and resting tremors of the hands and head, should be assessed.
Administration
! Plan to discontinue levodopa at least 12 h before giving carbidopa and levodopa. Expect the initial dose to provide at least 25% of the previous levodopa dose. Void before giving carbidopa and levodopa to reduce the risk of urine retention.

Take carbidopa and levodopa without regard to food. If GI upset occurs, take with food. Scored tablets may be crushed as needed. Extended-release tablets may be cut in half but not crushed. Orally disintegrating tablets should be allowed to dissolve on the tongue and then swallowed with saliva. Therapeutic effects may be delayed from several weeks to months.

Carboplatin
car-bow´play-tin
(Paraplatin)
Do not confuse carboplatin with Cisplatin or Platinol.

CATEGORY AND SCHEDULE
Pregnancy Risk Category: D

Classification: Antineoplastics, platinum agents

C

MECHANISM OF ACTION

A platinum coordination complex that inhibits DNA synthesis by cross-linking with DNA strands, preventing cell division. Cell cycle-phase nonspecific. *Therapeutic Effect:* Interferes with DNA function.

PHARMACOKINETICS

Protein binding: Low. Hydrolyzed in solution to active form. Primarily excreted in urine. *Half-life:* 2.6-5.9 h.

AVAILABILITY

Powder for Injection: 50 mg, 150 mg, 450 mg.
Injection Solution: 10 mg/mL.

INDICATIONS AND DOSAGES

▸ **Ovarian carcinoma (monotherapy)**
IV INFUSION
Adults. 360 mg/m² on day 1, every 4 wks. Do not repeat dose until neutrophil and platelet counts are within acceptable levels. Adjust drug dosage in previously treated patients based on lowest posttreatment platelet or neutrophil count. Increase dosage only once to no more than 125% of starting dose.
▸ **Ovarian carcinoma (combination therapy)**
IV INFUSION
Adults. 300 mg/m² (with cyclophosphamide) on day 1, every 4 wks. Do not repeat dose until neutrophil and platelet counts are within acceptable levels.
Children. 300-600 mg/m² every 4 wks for solid tumor, or 175 mg/m² every 4 wks for brain tumor.
▸ **Calvert formula for AUC-based dosing as an alternative method of dosing for ovarian cancer:**
Total dose (mg) = Target AUC × (GFR + 25)

▸ **Dosage in renal impairment**
Initial dosage is based on creatinine clearance; subsequent dosages are based on the patient's tolerance and degree of myelosuppression.

Creatinine Clearance (mL/min)	Dosage Day 1 (mg/m²)
≥ 60	360
41-59	250
16-40	200

OFF-LABEL USES

Treatment of bony and soft tissue sarcoma; germ cell tumor; neuroblastoma pediatric brain tumor; small cell lung cancer; solid tumors of the bladder, cervix, and testes; squamous cell carcinoma of the esophagus.

CONTRAINDICATIONS

History of severe allergic reaction to cisplatin, platinum compounds, or mannitol; severe bleeding; severe myelosuppression.

INTERACTIONS

Drug
Bone marrow depressants: May increase myelosuppression.
Live-virus vaccines: May potentiate virus replication and decrease the patient's antibody response to the vaccine.
Nephrotoxic, ototoxic medications: May increase the risk of nephrotoxicity/ototoxicity.
Phenytoin: Phenytoin levels may be reduced
Warfarin: The effects of warfarin may be increased.
Herbal and Food
None known.

DIAGNOSTIC TEST EFFECTS

May decrease serum electrolyte levels, including calcium, magnesium, potassium, and sodium.

High dosages (more than 4 times the recommended dosage) may elevate BUN and serum alkaline phosphatase, bilirubin, creatinine, and AST SGOT levels.

IV INCOMPATIBILITIES
Amphotericin B complex (Abelcet, AmBisome, Amphotec), diazepam Lansoprazole, Phenytoin.

IV COMPATIBILITIES
Etoposide (VePesid), granisetron (Kytril), ondansetron (Zofran), paclitaxel (Taxol).

SIDE EFFECTS
Frequent
Nausea (75%-80%), vomiting (65%).
Occasional
Generalized pain (17%), diarrhea or constipation (6%), peripheral neuropathy (4%).
Rare (2%-3%)
Alopecia, asthenia, hypersensitivity reaction (erythema, pruritus, rash, urticaria, and rarely bronchospasm and hypotension).

SERIOUS REACTIONS
• Myelosuppression may be severe, resulting in anemia, infection (sepsis, pneumonia), and bleeding.
• Prolonged treatment may result in peripheral neurotoxicity.
• High doses may be associated with reversible vision loss.

PRECAUTIONS & CONSIDERATIONS
Caution is warranted in renal impairment. Be aware that prior aminoglycoside therapy may potentiate carboplatin-induced renal toxicity. Use cautiously in elderly patients who were previously treated with cisplatin; they are at an increased risk of developing carboplatin-induced peripheral neuropathy. Avoid using carboplatin in pregnant women. The use of a contraceptive is recommended during therapy. It is unknown whether carboplatin is distributed in breast milk. Safety and efficacy have not been established in children. Tell the patient of the possibility of hair loss and that normal hair growth should resume after treatment has ended.
Storage
Store at room temperature. Diluted solutions are stable for 8 h at room temperature.
Administration
Be aware that aluminum reacts with carboplatin to form an inactive precipitate; intravenous sets and needles containing aluminum that may come in contact with carboplatin should not be used. Given as an IV infusion.

Carboprost
kar'boe-prost
(Hemabate)

CATEGORY AND SCHEDULE
Pregnancy Risk Category: X

Classification: Abortifacients, oxytocics, prostaglandins, stimulants, uterine

MECHANISM OF ACTION
A prostaglandin similar to prostaglandin F2α (dinoprost) that directly acts on myometrium and stimulates contraction in gravid uterus. *Therapeutic Effect:* Produces cervical dilation and softening.

PHARMACOKINETICS
None reported.

AVAILABILITY
Injection: 250 mcg carboprost and 83 mcg tromethamine/mL (Hemabate).

C

INDICATIONS AND DOSAGES
▸ **Abortion**
IM
Adults. Initially, 100-250 mcg, may repeat at 1.5- to 3.5-h intervals. May increase up to 500 mcg if uterine contractility inadequate. Maximum: 12 mg total dose or continuous administration for more than 2 days.
▸ **Postpartum uterine hemorrhage**
IM
Adults. Initially, 250 mcg, may repeat at 15- to 90-min intervals. Maximum: 2 mg total dose.

OFF-LABEL USES
Treatment of incomplete abortion.

CONTRAINDICATIONS
Acute pelvic inflammatory disease, active cardiac disease, pulmonary disease, renal disease, hepatic disease, hypersensitivity to carboprost or other prostaglandins.

INTERACTIONS
Drug
Oxytocin, oxytocics: May cause uterine hypertonus leading to uterine rupture or cervical lacerations.
Herbal
None known.
Food
None known.

DIAGNOSTIC TEST EFFECTS
None known.

SIDE EFFECTS
Frequent
Nausea, transient pyrexia, vomiting, diarrhea.
Occasional
Facial flushing.
Rare
Endometritis.

SERIOUS REACTIONS
• Excessive dosing may cause uterine hypertonicity with spasm and tetanic contraction, leading to cervical laceration/perforation and uterine rupture and hemorrhage.

PRECAUTIONS & CONSIDERATIONS
Caution is warranted in patients with a history of hypotension or hypertension, anemia, jaundice, diabetes mellitus, epilepsy, compromised (scarred) uterus, cardiovascular disease, adrenal disease, or hepatic disease. Be aware that carboprost tromethamine use is contraindicated during pregnancy and that small amounts of the drug are found in breast milk. There is no information available on carboprost tromethamine use in children or in elderly patients. Avoid smoking because of added effects of vasoconstriction.

Strength, duration, and frequency of contractions as well as vital signs should be monitored every 15 min until stable, then hourly until abortion is complete. Fever, chills, foul-smelling/increased vaginal discharge, and uterine cramps/pain should be reported immediately.
Storage
Refrigerate ampules. Do not freeze.
Administration
Be aware that carboprost tromethamine should not be injected IV because it may result

in bronchospasm, hypertension, vomiting, and anaphylaxis.

Carisoprodol
kar'i-so-pro'dol
(Soma)

CATEGORY AND SCHEDULE
Pregnancy Risk Category: C

Classification: Skeletal muscle relaxant, central acting

MECHANISM OF ACTION
A centrally acting skeletal muscle relaxant whose exact mechanism is unknown. Effects may be due to its CNS depressant actions. *Therapeutic Effect:* Relieves muscle spasms and pain.

PHARMACOKINETICS
Onset 2 h; duration 4-6 h. *Half-life:* 2.5 h. Meprobamate *Half-life:* 10 h. Metabolized in liver to meprobamate by the CYP2C19 isoenzyme; excreted by kidneys.

AVAILABILITY
Tablets: 250 mg, 350 mg.

INDICATIONS AND DOSAGES
▶ **Adjunct to rest, physical therapy, analgesics, and other measures for relief of discomfort from acute, painful musculoskeletal conditions**
PO
Adults, Elderly, Adolescents over 16 yr of age. 250-350 mg 4 times a day. Duration of therapy should be limited to 2-3 wks.

CONTRAINDICATIONS
Acute intermittent porphyria, sensitivity to meprobamate or other carbanates.

INTERACTIONS
Drug
Alcohol, other CNS depressants: May increase CNS depression.
Herbal
None known.
Food
None known.

DIAGNOSTIC TEST EFFECTS
None known.

SIDE EFFECTS
Frequent (> 10%)
Somnolence.
Occasional (1%-10%)
Tachycardia, facial flushing, dizziness, headache, light-headedness, dermatitis, nausea, vomiting, abdominal cramps, dyspnea.

SERIOUS REACTIONS
• Overdose may cause CNS and respiratory depression, shock, and coma.
• Rarely idiosyncratic reaction appears within minutes or hours of the first dose. Symptoms reported include extreme weakness, transient quadriplegia, dizziness, ataxia, temporary loss of vision, diplopia, mydriasis, dysarthria, agitation, euphoria, confusion, and disorientation.

PRECAUTIONS & CONSIDERATIONS
Caution is warranted in patients with hepatic and renal impairment and addictive personalities and in elderly patients. Drowsiness or dizziness may occur. Avoid alcohol, CNS depressants, and tasks that require mental alertness or motor skills. Liver and renal function tests should be obtained at baseline and periodically for those on long-term therapy. Therapeutic response, such as relief of muscle spasm and pain, should be assessed.

C

Storage
Store at room temperaure.
Administration
Take carisoprodol without regard to food. Take the last dose at bedtime.

Carmustine
kar-muss´-teen
(BiCNU, Gliadel)

CATEGORY AND SCHEDULE
Pregnancy Risk Category: D

Classification: Antineoplastic, nitrosureas, alkylating agent

MECHANISM OF ACTION
An alkylating agent and nitrosourea that inhibits DNA and RNA synthesis by cross-linking with DNA and RNA strands, preventing cell division. Cell cycle–phase nonspecific. *Therapeutic Effect:* Interferes with DNA and RNA function.

PHARMACOKINETICS
Degraded within 15 min; crosses blood-brain barrier; 70% excreted in urine within 96 h; 10% excreted as CO_2; fate of 20% is unknown. *Half-life:* 20 min (active metabolites half-life 67 h).

AVAILABILITY
Powder for Injection: 100 mg.
Wafer: 7.7 mg.

INDICATIONS AND DOSAGES
▸ **Disseminated Hodgkin disease, non-Hodgkin lymphoma, multiple myeloma, and primary and metastatic brain tumors in previously untreated patients (monotherapy)**
IV (BiCNU) INFUSION

NOTE: Dosages and regimens depend on type of cancer and use in combination with other agents. See prescribing information.
Adults, Elderly. 150–200 mg/m² as a single dose or 75–100 mg/m² on 2 successive days.
Children with brain tumors. 200–250 mg/m² every 4-6 wks as a single dose.
IMPLANTATION (GLIADEL) FOR BRAIN TUMOR INDICATIIONS
Adults, Elderly, Children. Up to 8 wafers may be placed in resection cavity.

CONTRAINDICATIONS
Hypersenstivity to carmustine.

INTERACTIONS
Drug
Cimetidine: May increase concentrations and toxic effects of carmustine.
Digoxin: May reduce digoxin concentrations.
Phenytoin: May reduce phenytoin concentrations.

DIAGNOSTIC TEST EFFECTS
Increases in bilirubin, alkaline phosphatase, AST; decreases in leukocytes, platelets.

SIDE EFFECTS
Frequent
Nausea and vomiting within min to 2 h after administration (may last up to 6 h); myelosuppression.
Occasional
Diarrhea, esophagitis, anorexia, dysphagia.
Rare
Thrombophlebitis.

SERIOUS REACTIONS
• Hematologic toxicity due to myelosuppression occurs frequently. Thrombocytopenia occurs about 4 wks after carmustine treatment begins and lasts 1-2 wks.

• Leukopenia is evident 5-6 wks after treatment begins and lasts 1-2 wks. Anemia occurs less frequently and is less severe.
• Mild, reversible hepatotoxicity also occurs frequently.
• Prolonged high-dose carmustine therapy may produce impaired renal function and pulmonary toxicity (pulmonary infiltrate or fibrosis).

PRECAUTIONS & CONSIDERATIONS
Administer with caution to patients with depressed platelet, leukocyte, or erythrocyte counts or with renal or hepatic impairment. Pretreatment pulmonary function testing is advised. Nausea and vomiting occur frequently with carmustine therapy; prophylactic antiemetics are advised. Women of childbearing potential should be advised to avoid pregnancy. Not recommended for use in breastfeeding.
Storage
Store powder for injection in refrigerator. Reconstituted and diluted solutions may be stored at room temperature for up to 8 h. Store wafers in freezer. Unopened foil pouches may be held at room temperature for up to 6 h.
Administration
To prepare injectable, dilute powder with 3 mL of absolute alcohol. Further dilute with 27 mL of sterile water for injection to a concentration of 3.3 mg/mL. May further dilute with D5W. Displays significant absorption to PVC containers; administer in glass or polyolefin containers. Infuse over 1-2 h. Protect from light.
    For wafers: Wear surgical gloves to handle. See specialized instructions to avoid loss of sterility or unitented exposure, which may cause burns and depigmentation of skin.

Carteolol
kar-tee′oh-lole
(Ocupress)
Do not confuse with carvedilol.

CATEGORY AND SCHEDULE
Pregnancy Risk Category: C/D if after first trimester

Classification: β-adrenergic blocker

MECHANISM OF ACTION
An antihypertensive that blocks β_1-adrenergic receptor at normal doses and β_2-adrenergic receptors at large doses. Predominantly blocks β_1-adrenergic receptors in cardiac tissue. Reduces aqueous humor production. *Therapeutic Effect:* Slows sinus heart rate, decreases cardiac output, decreases BP, increases airway resistance, decreases intraocular pressure (IOP).

PHARMACOKINETICS
Well absorbed from the GI tract. Protein binding: unknown. Minimally metabolized in liver. Primarily excreted unchanged in urine. Not removed by hemodialysis. *Half-life:* 6 h (increased in decreased renal function).

AVAILABILITY
Ophthalmic Solution: 1% (Ocupress).
▸ **Open-angle glaucoma, ocular hypertension**
OPHTHALMIC
Adults, Elderly. 1 drop 2 times a day to affected eye(s).

OFF-LABEL USES
Combination with miotics decreases IOP in acute/chronic angle-closure

glaucoma, treatment of secondary glaucoma, malignant glaucoma, angle-closure glaucoma during or after iridectomy.

CONTRAINDICATIONS
Bronchial asthma, COPD, bronchospasm, overt cardiac failure, cardiogenic shock, heart block greater than first degree, persistently severe bradycardia.

INTERACTIONS
Diuretics, other hypotensives: May increase hypotensive effect.
Insulin, oral hypoglycemics: May mask symptoms of hypoglycemia and prolong hypoglycemic effect of these drugs.

DIAGNOSTIC TEST EFFECTS
May increase serum ANA titer, BUN, serum LDH, lipoprotein, alkaline phosphatase, bilirubin, creatinine, potassium, triglyceride, uric acid, SGOT (AST), and SGPT (ALT) levels.

SIDE EFFECTS
Frequent
Oral: Hypotension manifested as dizziness, nausea, diaphoresis, headache, cold extremities, fatigue, constipation, or diarrhea.
Ophthalmic: Redness of eye or inside of eyelids, decreased night vision.
Occasional
Oral: Insomnia, flatulence, urinary frequency, impotence, or decreased libido.
Ophthalmic: Blepharoconjunctivitis, edema, droopy eyelid, staining of cornea, blurred vision, brow ache, increased light sensitivity, burning, stinging.
Rare
Rash, arthralgia, myalgia, confusion (especially elderly), taste disturbances.

SERIOUS REACTIONS
• Abrupt withdrawal (particularly in those with coronary artery disease) may produce angina or precipitate myocardial infarction. (systemic)
• May precipitate thyroid crisis in those with thyrotoxicosis. (systemic)
• β-blockers may mask signs and symptoms of acute hypoglycemia (tachycardia, BP changes) in diabetic patients.

PRECAUTIONS & CONSIDERATIONS
Caution is warranted with impaired renal, cardiac, or liver function; hypothyroidism; hypothermia during delivery; and small-birth-weight infants. Be aware that carteolol crosses the placenta and is distributed in small amounts in breast milk. Safety and efficacy of carteolol have not been established in children. Age-related peripheral vascular disease may increase susceptibility to decreased peripheral circulation in the elderly.

Do not abruptly discontinue carteolol. If carteolol is stopped suddenly, it may cause chest pain or heart attack.

Restrict salt and avoid alcohol and tasks that require mental alertness or motor skills. In addition, avoid nasal decongestants and over-the-counter (OTC) cold preparations, especially those containing stimulants, without physician approval.

Stinging or discomfort is common with ophthalmic use.
Storage
Store ophthalmic solution at room temperature.
Administration
To use ophthalmic preparation, wash hands before instilling. Sit or lie down to instill. Open eye, look at ceiling, and instill prescribed

amount. Close eye and apply gentle pressure to inner corner of eye. Do not let tip of applicator touch eye.

Carvedilol
kar-vea′die-lole
(Coreg, Coreg CR Dilatrend [AUS])
Do not confuse carvedilol with carteolol.

CATEGORY AND SCHEDULE
Pregnancy Risk Category: C (D if used in the second or third trimester)

Classification: Antiadrenergics, β-blocking

MECHANISM OF ACTION
An antihypertensive that possesses nonselective β-blocking and α-adrenergic blocking activity. Causes vasodilation. *Therapeutic Effect:* Reduces cardiac output, exercise-induced tachycardia, and reflex orthostatic tachycardia; reduces peripheral vascular resistance.

PHARMACOKINETICS

Route	Onset	Peak	Duration
PO	30 min	1-2 h	24 h

Rapidly and extensively absorbed from the GI tract. Protein binding: 98%. Metabolized in the liver. Excreted primarily via bile into feces. Minimally removed by hemodialysis. *Half-life:* 7-10 h. Food delays rate of absorption.

AVAILABILITY
Capsules (Extended-Release):
10 mg, 20 mg, 40 mg, 80 mg.
Tablets: 3.125 mg, 6.25 mg, 12.5 mg, 25 mg.

INDICATIONS AND DOSAGES
▸ **Hypertension**
PO (IMMEDIATE-RELEASE)
Adults, Elderly. Initially, 6.25 mg twice a day. May double at 7- to 14-day intervals to highest tolerated dosage. Maximum: 50 mg/day.
PO (EXTENDED-RELEASE)
Adults, Elderly. Initially 20 mg once daily. May double at 7- to 14-day intervals to highest tolerated dosage. Maximum 80 mg/day.
▸ **Congestive heart failure**
PO (IMMEDIATE RELEASE)
Adults, Elderly. Initially, 3.125 mg twice a day. May double at 2-wks intervals to highest tolerated dosage. Maximum: For patients weighing more than 85 kg, give 50 mg twice a day for those weighing 85 kg or less, give 25 mg twice a day.
PO (EXTENDED RELEASE)
Adults, Elderly. Initially 10 mg once daily for 2 wks. May double at 2-wks intervals to highest tolerated dosage. Maximum 80 mg/day.
▸ **Left ventricular dysfunction**
PO (IMMEDIATE-RELEASE)
Adults, Elderly. Initially, 3.125-6.25 mg twice a day. May increase at intervals of 3-10 days up to 25 mg twice a day.
PO (EXTENDED RELEASE)
Adults, Elderly. Initially 10-20 mg once daily. May increase at intervals of 3-10 days up to 80 mg once daily.

OFF-LABEL USES
Treatment of angina pectoris, idiopathic cardiomyopathy.

CONTRAINDICATIONS

Bronchial asthma or related bronchospastic conditions, cardiogenic shock, pulmonary edema, second- or third-degree AV block, severe bradycardia, clinical hepatic impairment.

INTERACTIONS

Drug

Alcohol: Alcohol may affect the extended-release properties resulting in fasting absorption and a higher peak. Avoid alcohol, including alcohol in prescription and nonprescription medications, for at least 2 h after carvedilol extended-release administration.

Calcium blockers: Increase risk of conduction disturbances.

Clonidine: May potentiate BP effects.

Cimetidine: May increase carvedilol blood concentration.

Digoxin: Increases concentrations of this drug.

Diuretics, other antihypertensives: May increase hypotensive effect.

Insulin, oral hypoglycemics: May mask symptoms of hypoglycemia and prolong hypoglycemic effect of these drugs.

Rifampin: Decreases carvedilol blood concentration.

Herbal

None known.

Food

None known.

DIAGNOSTIC TEST EFFECTS

Increases in AST and ALT.

SIDE EFFECTS

Carvedilol is generally well tolerated, with mild and transient side effects.

Frequent (4%-6%)

Fatigue, dizziness.

Occasional (2%)

Diarrhea, bradycardia, rhinitis, back pain.

Rare (< 2%)

Orthostatic hypotension, somnolence, urinary tract infection, viral infection.

SERIOUS REACTIONS

• Overdose may produce profound bradycardia, hypotension, bronchospasm, cardiac insufficiency, cardiogenic shock, and cardiac arrest.

• Abrupt withdrawal may result in diaphoresis, palpitations, headache, and tremors.

• Carvedilol administration may precipitate congestive heart failure (CHF) and myocardial infarction (MI) in patients with heart disease, thyroid storm in those with thyrotoxicosis, and peripheral ischemia in those with existing peripheral vascular disease.

• Hypoglycemia may occur in patients with previously controlled diabetes.

PRECAUTIONS & CONSIDERATIONS

Caution should be used in those undergoing anesthesia and in those with CHF controlled with ACE inhibitor, digoxin, or diuretics; diabetes mellitus; hypoglycemia; impaired hepatic function; peripheral vascular disease; and thyrotoxicosis. It is unknown whether carvedilol crosses the placenta or is distributed in breast milk. Carvedilol use should be avoided in pregnant women after the first trimester because it may result in low-birth-weight infants. The drug may also produce apnea, bradycardia, hypoglycemia, or hypothermia during childbirth. The safety and efficacy of carvedilol have not been established in children. In elderly patients, the incidence of dizziness may be increased. Be aware that salt and alcohol intake should be restricted. Nasal decongestants or OTC cold preparations (stimulants) should not be used without physician approval.

Orthostatic hypotension may occur, so rise slowly from a lying to sitting position and dangle the legs from the bed momentarily before standing. Tasks that require mental alertness or motor skills should be avoided. Apical pulse and BP should be assessed immediately before giving carvedilol. BP for hypotension; respiratory status for shortness of breath, pattern of daily bowel activity and stool consistency; ECG for arrhythmias; and pulse for quality, rate, and rhythm should be monitored during treatment. If pulse rate is 60 beats/min or lower or systolic BP is < 90 mm Hg, withhold the medication and contact the physician. Signs and symptoms of CHF, such as decreased urine output, distended neck veins, dyspnea (particularly on exertion or lying down), night cough, peripheral edema, and weight gain, should also be assessed.

Administration

Take carvedilol tablets with food to slow the rate of absorption and reduce the risk of orthostatic hypotension. Swallow carvedilol extended-release capsules whole, without crushing or chewing, or capsules may be opened and the contents sprinkled on applesauce. Carvedilol extended-release capsules should be taken once daily in the morning with food. To assess tolerance for carvedilol, assess a standing systolic BP 1 h after giving the drug.

Patients can be converted from immediate release to extended-release carvedilol at the following doses:

Twice-daily dose (mg)	Once-daily dose (mg) (coreg-CR)
3.125	10
6.25	20
12.5	40
25	80

Caspofungin Acetate
kas-poe-fun′jin
(Cancidas)

CATEGORY AND SCHEDULE
Pregnancy Risk Category: C

Classification: Antifungal, systemic, echinocandins

MECHANISM OF ACTION
An antifungal that inhibits the synthesis of glucan, a vital component of fungal cell formation, thereby damaging the fungal cell membrane. *Therapeutic Effect:* Fungicidal.

PHARMACOKINETICS
Distributed in tissue. Extensively bound to albumin. Protein binding: 97%. Slowly metabolized in liver to active metabolite. Excreted primarily in urine and to a lesser extent in feces. Not removed by hemodialysis. *Half-life:* 40-50 h.

AVAILABILITY
Powder for Injection: 50-mg, 70-mg vials.

INDICATIONS AND DOSAGES
▶ **Aspergillosis**
IV INFUSION
Adults, Elderly, Children older than 12 yr. Give single 70-mg loading

C

dose on day 1, followed by 50 mg/day thereafter.

▸ **Invasive candidiasis**
IV INFUSION
Adults, Elderly. Initially, 70 mg followed by 50 mg daily.

▸ **Esophageal candidiasis**
IV INFUSION
Adult, Elderly. 50 mg a day.

▸ **Empirical therapy, neutropenic patients**
IV INFUSION
Adults, Elderly. Give single 70-mg loading dose on day 1, followed by 50 mg/day thereafter. If 50-mg dose is tolerated, but does not provide adequate clinical response, it can increase dose to 70 mg/day.

▸ **Dosage in hepatic impairment**
IV INFUSION
Adults, Elderly with moderate hepatic impairment. Reduce daily dose to 35 mg. Loading dose, when indicated, remains 70 mg.

CONTRAINDICATIONS
Hypersensitivity to any of the product ingredients.

INTERACTIONS
Drug
Carbamazepine, dexamethasone, efavirenz, nelfinavir, nevirapine, phenytoin, rifampin: May decrease blood concentration of caspofungin.
Cyclosporine: May increase caspofungin concentrations and increase incidence of hepatic transaminase elevations.
Tacrolimus: May decrease the effect of tacrolimus.
Herbal
None known.
Food
None known.

DIAGNOSTIC TEST EFFECTS
May increase PT as well as serum alkaline phosphatase, serum bilirubin, serum creatinine, LDH, SGOT (AST), SGPT (ALT), serum uric acid, urine pH, urine protein, urine RBC, and urine WBC levels. May decrease hemoglobin, hematocrit, platelet count, and serum albumin, serum bicarbonate, serum protein, and serum potassium levels.

Ⓦ IV INCOMPATIBILITIES
Do not mix caspofungin with any other medication or use dextrose as a diluent.

SIDE EFFECTS
Frequent (26%)
Fever.
Occasional (4%-11%)
Headache, nausea, phlebitis.
Rare (3% or less)
Paresthesia, vomiting, diarrhea, abdominal pain, myalgia, chills, tremor, insomnia.

SERIOUS REACTIONS
• Hypersensitivity reactions (characterized by rash, facial swelling, pruritus, and a sensation of warmth) may occur.

PRECAUTIONS & CONSIDERATIONS
Caution is warranted for patients with liver function impairment. Be aware that caspofungin crosses the placental barrier, may be embryotoxic, and is distributed in breast milk. Be aware that the safety and efficacy of caspofungin have not been established in children. In elderly patients, age-related moderate renal impairment may require dosage adjustment.

Baseline temperature, liver function test results, and history of allergies should be obtained before giving the drug. Signs and symptoms of liver function should be assessed. If increased shortness of breath, itching, facial swelling, or a rash occurs, notify the physician. Report pain, burning, or swelling at the IV infusion site.

Storage
Refrigerate but warm it to room temperature before preparing it with the diluent. The reconstituted solution, before it is prepared as the patient infusion solution, may be stored at room temperature for 1 h before infusion. The final infusion solution can be stored at room temperature for 24 h. Discard the solution if it contains particulate or is discolored.

Administration
For a 50- to 70-mg loading dose, add 10.5 mL 0.9% NaCl to the 50- or 70-mg vial. Transfer 10 mL of the reconstituted solution to 250 mL 0.9% NaCl. For 35-mg dose in persons with moderate liver insufficiency, add 10.5 mL 0.9% NaCl to the 50-mg vial. Transfer 7 mL to 100 or 250 mL 0.9% NaCl. Infuse over 60 min.

Castor Oil
(Emulsoil, Purge)

CATEGORY AND SCHEDULE
Pregnancy Risk Category: X
OTC

Classification: Laxative, stimulant

MECHANISM OF ACTION
A laxative prepared from the bean of the castor plant; the exact mechanism of action is unknown. Acts primarily in the small intestine. May be hydrolyzed to ricinoleic acid, which reduces net absorption of fluid and electrolytes and stimulates peristalsis.
Therapeutic Effect: Increases peristalsis, promotes laxative effect.

PHARMACOKINETICS
Minimal absorption by the GI tract. May be metabolized like other fatty acids.

AVAILABILITY
Emulsion: 36.4%.
Oral liquid: 95% (Emulsoil, Purge).

INDICATIONS AND DOSAGES
▸ **Constipation**
PO
Adults, Elderly, Children 12 yr and older. 15-60 mL as a single dose.
Children 2-12 yr. 5-15 mL as a single dose.
Children < 2 yr. 1-2 mL as a single dose. Maximum: 5 mL as a single dose.

CONTRAINDICATIONS
Abdominal pain, appendicitis, intestinal obstruction, nausea, vomiting, pregnancy.

INTERACTIONS
Drug
None known
Herbal
Licorice: May increase risk of hypokalemia.
Food
None known.

DIAGNOSTIC TEST EFFECTS
None known.

SIDE EFFECTS
Occasional
Some degree of abdominal discomfort, nausea, mild cramps, griping, faintness.

C

SERIOUS REACTIONS

• Long-term use may result in laxative dependence, chronic constipation, and loss of normal bowel function.

• Chronic use or overdosage may result in electrolyte disturbances, such as hypokalemia, hypocalcemia, metabolic acidosis or alkalosis, persistent diarrhea, malabsorption, and weight loss. Electrolyte disturbance may produce vomiting and muscle weakness.

PRECAUTIONS & CONSIDERATIONS

Caution should be used for extended periods (> 1 wk) of castor oil use. Be aware that castor oil is contraindicated in pregnancy. It is unknown whether castor oil is distributed in breast milk. Safety and efficacy of castor oil have not been established in children younger than 2 yr of age. No age-related precautions have been noted in elderly patients, but monitor for signs of dehydration and electrolyte loss. Avoid taking within 1 h of other oral medication because it decreases drug absorption.

Storage

Store at room temperature.

Administration

Take castor oil on an empty stomach for faster results. Drink at least 6-8 glasses of water a day to aid in stool softening.

Cefaclor

sef′a-klor

(Apo-Cefaclor [CAN], Ceclor, Ceclor CD, Cefkor [AUS], Cefkor CD [AUS], Keflor [AUS])

CATEGORY AND SCHEDULE

Pregnancy Risk Category: B

Classification: Antibiotics, cephalosporin (second generation)

MECHANISM OF ACTION

A second-generation cephalosporin that binds to bacterial cell membranes and inhibits cell wall synthesis. *Therapeutic Effect:* Bactericidal.

PHARMACOKINETICS

Well absorbed from the GI tract. Protein binding: 25%. Widely distributed. Primarily excreted unchanged in urine. Moderately removed by hemodialysis. *Half-life:* 0.6-0.9 h (increased in impaired renal function).

AVAILABILITY

Capsules (Ceclor): 250 mg, 500 mg.
Oral Suspension (Ceclor): 125 mg/ 5 mL, 187 mg/5 mL, 250 mg/5 mL, 375 mg/5 mL.
Tablets, Extended Release (Ceclor CD): 375 mg, 500 mg.
Tablets, Chewable (Raniclor): 125 mg, 187 mg, 250 mg, 375 mg.

INDICATIONS AND DOSAGES

▸ **Bronchitis**

PO

Adults, Elderly (extended release). 500 mg q12h for 7 days.

▸ **Lower respiratory tract infections**

PO

Adults, Elderly. 250-500 mg q8h.

▸ **Otitis media**
PO
Children. 20-40 mg/kg/day in 2-3 divided doses. Maximum: 1 g/day.
▸ **Pharyngitis, skin/skin structure infections, tonsillitis**
PO
Adults, Elderly (extended release). 375 mg q12h.
Adults, Elderly (regular release). 250-500 mg q8h.
Children. 20-40 mg/kg/day in 2-3 divided doses. Maximum: 1 g/day.
▸ **Urinary tract infections**
PO
Adults, Elderly. 250-500 mg q8h.
Children. 20-40 mg/kg/day in 2-3 divided doses q8h. Maximum: 1 g/day.
PO (EXTENDED-RELEASE TABLETS)
Adults, Children older than 16 yr. 375-500 mg q12h.
▸ **Otitis media**
PO
Children older than 1 mo. 40 mg/kg/day in divided doses q8h. Maximum: 1 g/day.
▸ **Dosage in renal impairment**
Decreased dosage may be necessary in patients with creatinine clearance < 40 mL/min.

CONTRAINDICATIONS
History of anaphylactic reaction to penicillins or hypersensitivity to cephalosporins.

INTERACTIONS
Drug
Probenecid: May increase cefaclor blood concentration.
Herbal
None known.
Food
None known.

DIAGNOSTIC TEST EFFECTS
May increase BUN level and serum alkaline phosphatase, bilirubin, creatinine, LDH, AST (SGOT), and ALT (SGPT) levels. May cause a positive direct or indirect Coombs' test.

SIDE EFFECTS
Frequent
Oral candidiasis, mild diarrhea, mild abdominal cramping, vaginal candidiasis.
Occasional
Nausea, serum sickness-like reaction (marked by fever and joint pain; usually occurs after the second course of therapy and resolves after the drug is discontinued)
Rare
Allergic reaction (pruritus, rash, and urticaria).

SERIOUS REACTIONS
• Antibiotic-associated colitis and other superinfections may result from altered bacterial balance.
• Nephrotoxicity may occur, especially in patients with preexisting renal disease.
• Patients with a history of allergies, especially to penicillin, are at increased risk for developing a severe hypersensitivity reaction, marked by severe pruritus, angioedema, bronchospasm, and anaphylaxis.

PRECAUTIONS & CONSIDERATIONS
Caution is warranted with a history of GI disease (especially antibiotic-associated colitis or ulcerative colitis), renal impairment, and concurrent use of nephrotoxic medications. Be aware that cefaclor readily crosses the placenta and is distributed in breast milk. No age-related precautions have been noted in children older than 1 mo. In elderly patients, age-related renal impairment may require dosage adjustment.

Although mild GI effects may be tolerable, an increase in their

C

severity may indicate the onset of antibiotic-associated colitis. Assess the mouth for white patches on the mucous membranes and tongue, the pattern of daily bowel activity and stool consistency, signs and symptoms of superinfection including abdominal pain, moderate to severe diarrhea, severe anal or genital pruritus, and severe mouth soreness. Renal function should be assessed.

Storage
After reconstitution, oral solution is stable for 14 days if refrigerated.
Administration
Take without regard to meals; if GI upset occurs, give with food or milk. Do not cut, crush, or chew extended-release tablets.

Shake oral suspension well before using.

Cefadroxil
sef-a-drox'ill
(Duricef)

CATEGORY AND SCHEDULE
Pregnancy Risk Category: B

Classification: Antibiotics, cephalosporin (first generation)

MECHANISM OF ACTION
A first-generation cephalosporin that binds to bacterial cell membranes and inhibits cell wall synthesis. *Therapeutic Effect:* Bactericidal.

PHARMACOKINETICS
Well absorbed from the GI tract. Protein binding: 15%-20%. Widely distributed. Primarily excreted unchanged in urine.

Removed by hemodialysis. *Half-life:* 1.2-1.5 h (increased in impaired renal function).

AVAILABILITY
Capsules: 500 mg.
Oral Suspension: 125 mg/5 mL, 250 mg/5 mL, 500 mg/5 mL.
Tablets: 1000 mg.

INDICATIONS AND DOSAGES
▸ **Urinary tract infection**
PO
Adults, Elderly. 1-2 g/day as a single dose or in 2 divided doses.
Children. 30 mg/kg/day in 2 divided doses. Maximum: 2 g/day.
▸ **Skin and skin-structure infections, group A β-hemolytic streptococcal pharyngitis, tonsillitis**
PO
Adults, Elderly. 1-2 g in 2 divided doses.
Children. 30 mg/kg/day in 2 divided doses. Maximum: 2 g/day.
▸ **Impetigo**
PO
Children. 30 mg/kg/day as a single or in 2 divided doses. Maximum: 2 g/day.
▸ **Dosage in renal impairment (adults)**
After an initial 1-g dose, dosage and frequency are modified based on creatinine clearance and the severity of the infection.

Creatinine Clearance (mL/min)	Dosage Interval
25-50	500 mg q12h
10-25	500 mg q24h
0-10	500 mg q36h

CONTRAINDICATIONS
History of anaphylactic reaction to penicillins or hypersensitivity to cephalosporins.

INTERACTIONS
Drug
Probenecid: Increases cefadroxil blood concentration.
Herbal
None known.
Food
None known.

DIAGNOSTIC TEST EFFECTS
May increase BUN level and serum alkaline phosphatase, bilirubin, creatinine, LDH, AST (SGOT), and ALT (SGPT) levels. May cause a positive direct or indirect Coombs' test.

SIDE EFFECTS
Frequent
Oral candidiasis, mild diarrhea, mild abdominal cramping, vaginal candidiasis.
Occasional
Nausea, unusual bruising or bleeding, serum sickness-like reaction (marked by fever and joint pain; usually occurs after the second course of therapy and resolves after the drug is discontinued).
Rare
Allergic reaction (rash, pruritus, urticaria), thrombophlebitis (pain, redness, swelling at injection site).

SERIOUS REACTIONS
• Antibiotic-associated colitis and other superinfections may result from altered bacterial balance.
• Nephrotoxicity may occur, especially in patients with preexisting renal disease.
• Patients with a history of allergies, especially to penicillin, are at increased risk for developing a severe hypersensitivity reaction, marked by severe pruritus, angioedema, bronchospasm, and anaphylaxis.

PRECAUTIONS & CONSIDERATIONS
Caution is warranted for patients with a history of GI disease (especially antibiotic-associated colitis or ulcerative colitis), renal impairment, and concurrent use of nephrotoxic medications. Be aware that cefadroxil readily crosses the placenta and is distributed in breast milk. No age-related precautions have been noted for children. In elderly patients, age-related renal impairment may require dosage adjustment.

Although mild GI effects may be tolerable, an increase in their severity may indicate the onset of antibiotic-associated colitis. Assess the mouth for white patches on the mucous membranes and tongue, pattern of daily bowel activity and stool consistency, signs and symptoms of superinfection including abdominal pain, moderate to severe diarrhea, severe anal or genital pruritus, and severe mouth soreness. Renal function should be assessed.
Storage
After reconstitution, oral solution is stable for 14 days if refrigerated.
Administration
Take without regard to meals; if GI upset occurs, give with food or milk.
Shake oral suspension well before using.

C

Cefazolin
sef-a′zoe-lin
(Ancef, Kefzol)
Do not confuse cefazolin with cefprozil or Cefzil.

CATEGORY AND SCHEDULE
Pregnancy Risk Category: B

Classification: Antibiotics, cephalosporin (first generation)

MECHANISM OF ACTION
A first-generation cephalosporin that binds to bacterial cell membranes and inhibits cell wall synthesis. *Therapeutic Effect:* Bactericidal.

PHARMACOKINETICS
Widely distributed. Protein binding: 85%. Primarily excreted unchanged in urine. Moderately removed by hemodialysis. *Half-life:* 1.4-1.8 h (increased in impaired renal function).

AVAILABILITY
Powder for Injection: 500 mg, 1 g, 5 g, 10 g, 20 g.

INDICATIONS AND DOSAGES
▸ **Uncomplicated UTIs**
IV, IM
Adults, Elderly. 1 g q12h.
▸ **Mild to moderate infections**
IV, IM
Adults, Elderly. 250-500 mg q8-12h.
▸ **Severe infections**
IV, IM
Adults, Elderly. 0.5-1 g q6-8h.
▸ **Life-threatening infections**
IV, IM
Adults, Elderly. 1-1.5 g q6h.
Maximum: 12 g/day.

▸ **Perioperative prophylaxis**
IV, IM
Adults, Elderly. 1 g 30-60 min before surgery, 0.5-1 g during surgery, and q6-8h for up to 24 h postoperatively.
▸ **Usual pediatric dosage**
Children. 50-100 mg/kg/day in divided doses q8h. Maximum: 6 g/day.
Neonates older than 7 days. 40-60 mg/kg/day in divided doses q8-12h.
Neonates 7 days and younger. 40 mg/kg/day in divided doses q12h.
▸ **Dosage in renal impairment (adults)**
Dosing frequency is modified based on creatinine clearance.

Creatinine Clearance (mL/min)	Dosage Interval
10-30	Usual dose q12h
< 10	Usual dose q24h

CONTRAINDICATIONS
History of anaphylactic reaction to penicillins or hypersensitivity to cephalosporins.

INTERACTIONS
Drug
Probenecid: Increases cefazolin blood concentration.
Warfarin: May increase response to warfarin.
Herbal
None known.
Food
None known.

DIAGNOSTIC TEST EFFECTS
May increase INR, BUN level, and serum alkaline phosphatase, bilirubin, creatinine, LDH, AST (SGOT), and ALT (SGPT) levels. May cause a positive direct or indirect Coombs' test.

🞇 IV INCOMPATIBILITIES
Amikacin (Amikin), amiodarone (Cordarone), hydromorphone (Dilaudid).

🞇 IV COMPATIBILITIES
Calcium gluconate, diltiazem (Cardizem), famotidine (Pepcid), heparin, insulin (regular), lidocaine, magnesium sulfate, midazolam (Versed), morphine, multivitamins, potassium chloride, propofol (Diprivan), vecuronium (Norcuron).

SIDE EFFECTS
Frequent
Discomfort with IM administration, oral candidiasis, mild diarrhea, mild abdominal cramping, vaginal candidiasis.
Occasional
Nausea, serum sickness-like reaction (marked by fever and joint pain; usually occurs after the second course of therapy and resolves after the drug is discontinued).
Rare
Allergic reaction (rash, pruritus, urticaria), thrombophlebitis (pain, redness, swelling at injection site).

SERIOUS REACTIONS
• Antibiotic-associated colitis and other superinfections may result from altered bacterial balance.
• Nephrotoxicity may occur, especially in patients with pre-existing renal disease.
• Patients with a history of allergies, especially to penicillin, are at increased risk for developing a severe hypersensitivity reaction, marked by severe pruritus, angioedema, bronchospasm, and anaphylaxis.

PRECAUTIONS & CONSIDERATIONS
Caution is warranted with a history of GI disease (especially antibiotic-associated colitis or ulcerative colitis), seizure disorder, renal impairment, and concurrent use of nephrotoxic medications. May be associated with increased INR, especially in nutritionally deficient patients, prolonged treatment, hepatic or renal disease. Be aware that cefazolin readily crosses the placenta and is distributed in breast milk. No age-related precautions have been noted in children. In elderly patients, age-related renal impairment may require dosage adjustment.

Although mild GI effects may be tolerable, an increase in their severity may indicate the onset of antibiotic-associated colitis. Assess the mouth for white patches on the mucous membranes and tongue, pattern of daily bowel activity and stool consistency, signs and symptoms of superinfection including abdominal pain, moderate to severe diarrhea, severe anal or genital pruritus, and severe mouth soreness. Renal function should be assessed.
Storage
Solution normally appears light yellow to yellow. IV infusion (piggyback) is stable for 24 h at room temperature and 10 days if refrigerated. Discard solution if precipitate forms.
Administration
To minimize discomfort, give IM injection deep and slowly. To minimize injection site discomfort, give the IM injection in the gluteus maximus rather than lateral aspect of thigh. Administer cefazolin for the full length of treatment and evenly space doses around the clock. For IV use, reconstitute each 1 g with at least 10 mL sterile water for injection. May further dilute in 50-100 mL D5W or 0.9% NaCl to decrease the incidence of thrombophlebitis. For IV push,

C

administer over 3-5 min. For intermittent IV infusion (piggyback), infuse over 20-30 min.

Cefdinir
sef'di-neer
(Omnicef)

CATEGORY AND SCHEDULE
Pregnancy Risk Category: B

Classification: Antibiotics, cephalosporin (third generation)

MECHANISM OF ACTION
A third-generation cephalosporin that binds to bacterial cell membranes and inhibits cell wall synthesis. *Therapeutic Effect:* Bactericidal.

PHARMACOKINETICS
Moderately absorbed from the GI tract. Protein binding: 60%-70%. Widely distributed. Not appreciably metabolized. Primarily excreted unchanged in urine. Minimally removed by hemodialysis. *Half-life:* 1-2 h (increased in impaired renal function).

AVAILABILITY
Capsules: 300 mg.
Oral Suspension: 125 mg/5 mL, 250 mg/5 mL.

INDICATIONS AND DOSAGES
▸ **Community-acquired pneumonia**
PO
Adults, Elderly, Children 13 yr and older. 300 mg q12h for 10 days.
▸ **Acute exacerbation of chronic bronchitis**
PO
Adults, Elderly. 300 mg q12h for 5-10 days.

▸ **Acute maxillary sinusitis**
PO
Adults, Elderly, Children 13 yr and older. 300 mg q12h or 600 mg q24h for 10 days.
Children 6 mo to 12 yr. 7 mg/kg q12h or 14 mg/kg q24h for 10 days.
▸ **Pharyngitis or tonsillitis**
PO
Adults, Elderly, Children 13 yr and older. 300 mg q12h for 5-10 days or 600 mg q24h for 10 days.
Children 6 mo to 12 yr. 7 mg/kg q12h for 5-10 days or 14 mg/kg q24h for 10 days.
▸ **Uncomplicated skin or skin-structure infections**
PO
Adults, Elderly, Children 13 yr and older. 300 mg q12h for 10 days.
Children 6 mo to 12 yr. 7 mg/kg q12h for 10 days.
▸ **Acute bacterial otitis media**
PO (CAPSULES)
Children 6 mo to 12 yr. 7 mg/kg q12h or 14 mg/kg q24h for 10 days.
▸ **Usual pediatric dosage for oral suspension**
Children weighing 81-95 lb (37-43 kg). 12.5 mL (2.5 tsp) q12h or 25 mL (5 tsp) q24h.
Children weighing 61-80 lb (28-36 kg). 10 mL (1.5 tsp) q12h or 20 mL (4 tsp) q24h.
Children weighing 41-60 lb (19-27 kg). 7.5 mL (1 tsp) q12h or 15 mL (3 tsp) q24h.
Children weighing 20-40 lb (9-18 kg). 5 mL (1 tsp) q12h or 10 mL (2 tsp) q24h.
Infants weighing < 20 lb (9 kg). 2.5 mL (½ tsp) q12h or 5 mL (1 tsp) q24h.
▸ **Dosage in renal impairment (adults)**
For patients with creatinine clearance < 30 mL/min, dosage is 300 mg/day as single daily dose.

For hemodialysis patients, dosage is 300 mg every other day.

CONTRAINDICATIONS
History of anaphylactic reaction to penicillins or hypersensitivity to cephalosporins.

INTERACTIONS
Drug
Antacids: Decrease cefdinir blood concentration.
Magnesium or iron supplements: Decrease cefinir blood concentration.
Probenecid: Increases cefdinir blood concentration.
Herbal
None known.
Food
None known.

DIAGNOSTIC TEST EFFECTS
May increase serum alkaline phosphatase, bilirubin, LDH, AST (SGPT), and ALT (SGOT) levels. May produce a false-positive reaction for ketones in urine.

SIDE EFFECTS
Frequent
Oral candidiasis, mild diarrhea, mild abdominal cramping, vaginal candidiasis.
Occasional
Nausea, serum sickness-like reaction (marked by fever and joint pain; usually occurs after the second course of therapy and resolves after the drug is discontinued).
Rare
Allergic reaction (rash, pruritus, urticaria).

SERIOUS REACTIONS
• Antibiotic-associated colitis and other superinfections may result from altered bacterial balance.

• Nephrotoxicity may occur, especially in patients with preexisting renal disease.
• Patients with a history of allergies, especially to penicillin, are at increased risk for developing a severe hypersensitivity reaction, marked by severe pruritus, angioedema, bronchospasm, and anaphylaxis.

PRECAUTIONS & CONSIDERATIONS
Caution is warranted for patients with hypersensitivity to penicillins or other drugs, a history of GI disease (especially antibiotic-associated colitis or ulcerative colitis), and liver or renal impairment. Be aware that cefdinir readily crosses the placenta and is not detected in breast milk. Be aware that infants and newborns may have lower renal clearance of cefdinir. In elderly patients, age-related decreases in renal function may require decreased cefdinir dosage or increased dosing interval.

Although mild GI effects may be tolerable, an increase in their severity may indicate the onset of antibiotic-associated colitis. Assess the mouth for white patches on the mucous membranes and tongue, pattern of daily bowel activity and stool consistency, signs and symptoms of superinfection including abdominal pain, moderate to severe diarrhea, severe anal or genital pruritus, and severe mouth soreness. Renal function should be assessed.
Storage
Store mixed suspension at room temperature. Discard unused portion after 10 days.
Administration
Take without regard to meals; if GI upset occurs, give with food or milk. Reconstitute oral suspension according to package label.

Shake oral suspension well before administering. Continue therapy for the full length of treatment and evenly space doses around the clock.

Cefditoren
seff-di-tore'en
(Spectracef)

CATEGORY AND SCHEDULE
Pregnancy Risk Category: B

Classification: Antibiotics, cephalosporin (third generation)

MECHANISM OF ACTION
A third-generation cephalosporin that binds to bacterial cell membranes and inhibits cell wall synthesis. *Therapeutic Effect:* Bactericidal.

PHARMACOKINETICS
Moderately absorbed from the GI tract. Protein binding: 88%. Not metabolized. Excreted in the urine. Minimally removed by hemodialysis. *Half-life:* 1.6 h (half-life increased with impaired renal function).

AVAILABILITY
Tablets: 200 mg, 400 mg.

INDICATIONS AND DOSAGES
▶ **Pharyngitis, tonsillitis, skin infections**
PO
Adults, Elderly, Children older than 12 yr. 200 mg twice a day for 10 days.
▶ **Acute exacerbation of chronic bronchitis**
PO
Adults, Elderly, Children older than 12 yr. 400 mg twice a day for 10 days.

▶ **Community-acquired pneumonia**
PO
Adults, Elderly, Children older than 12 yr. 400 mg twice a day for 14 days.
▶ **Dosage in renal impairment**
Dosage and frequency are modified based on creatinine clearance.

Creatinine Clearance (mL/min)	Dosage
50-80	No adjustment necessary
30-49	200 mg twice a day
< 30	200 mg once a day

CONTRAINDICATIONS
Carnitine deficiency or inborn errors of metabolism that may result in carnitine deficiency, known allergy to cephalosporins, or anaphylactic reactions to penicillins, hypersensitivity to milk protein.

INTERACTIONS
Drug
Antacids containing magnesium or aluminum, H$_2$ receptor antagonists: May decrease the absorption of cefditoren.
Probenecid: May increase the absorption of cefditoren.
Warfarin: May increase response to warfarin.
Herbal
None known.
Food
High-fat meals: Increase the cefditoren plasma concentration.

DIAGNOSTIC TEST EFFECTS
May cause a positive direct or indirect Coombs' test and a false-positive reaction to glycosuria. May increase INR, alkaline phosphatase, bilirubin, LDH, creatinine. May cause pancytopenia, neutropenia, and agranulocytosis.

SIDE EFFECTS
Occasional (11%)
Diarrhea.
Rare (1%-4%)
Nausea, headache, abdominal pain, vaginal candidiasis, dyspepsia, vomiting.

SERIOUS REACTIONS
• Antibiotic-associated colitis and other superinfections may occur.
• Patients with a history of allergies, especially to penicillin, are at increased risk for developing a severe hypersensitivity reaction, marked by severe pruritus, angioedema, bronchospasm, and anaphylaxis.

PRECAUTIONS & CONSIDERATIONS
Caution is warranted with allergies, renal impairment, seizure disorder, a history of GI disease, and hypersensitivity to penicillins or other drugs. May be associated with increased INR, especially in nutritionally deficient patients, prolonged treatment, hepatic or renal disease. It is unknown whether cefditoren is distributed in breast milk. The safety and efficacy of cefditoren have not been established in children younger than 12 yr. Age-related renal impairment may require a dosage adjustment in elderly patients.

Although mild GI effects may be tolerable, an increase in their severity may indicate the onset of antibiotic-associated colitis. Assess the mouth for white patches on the mucous membranes and tongue; also check the pattern of daily bowel activity and stool consistency, signs and symptoms of superinfection including abdominal pain, moderate to severe diarrhea, severe anal or genital pruritus, and severe mouth soreness. Renal function should be assessed.

Storage
Store at room temperature. Protect from light and moisture.
Administration
Take with meals to enhance drug absorption. Take for the full length of treatment. Do not skip doses.

Cefepime
sef′e-peem
(Maxipime)
Do not confuse with ceftidine.

CATEGORY AND SCHEDULE
Pregnancy Risk Category: B

Classification: Antibiotics, cephalosporin (fourth generation)

MECHANISM OF ACTION
A fourth-generation cephalosporin that binds to bacterial cell membranes and inhibits cell wall synthesis.
Therapeutic Effect: Bactericidal.

PHARMACOKINETICS
Well absorbed after IM administration. Protein binding: 20%. Widely distributed. Primarily excreted unchanged in urine. Removed by hemodialysis. *Half-life:* 2-2.3 h (increased in impaired renal function and in elderly patients).

AVAILABILITY
Powder for Injection: 500 mg, 1 g, 2 g.

INDICATIONS AND DOSAGES
▶ **Pneumonia**
IV
Adults, Elderly. 1-2 g q12h for 7-10 days.
Children 2 mo and older. 50 mg/kg q12h. Maximum: 2 g/dose.

▸ **Intra-abdominal infections**
IV
Adults, Elderly. 2 g q12h for 10 days.
▸ **Skin and skin-structure infections**
IV
Adults, Elderly. 2 g q12h for 10 days.
Children 2 mo and older. 50 mg/kg
q12h. Maximum: 2 g/dose.
▸ **Urinary tract infections**
IV/IM
Adults, Elderly. 0.5-2 g q12h for
7-10 days.
Children 2 mo and older. 50 mg/kg
q12h. Maximum: 2 g/dose.
▸ **Febrile neutropenia**
IV
Adults, Elderly. 2 g q8h.
Children 2 mo and older. 50 mg/kg
q8h. Maximum: 2 g/dose.
▸ **Dosage in renal impairment**
Dosage and frequency are modified
based on creatinine clearance and
the severity of the infection, and the
initial dosage given.

CONTRAINDICATIONS
History of anaphylactic reaction to
penicillins or hypersensitivity to
cephalosporins.

INTERACTIONS
Drug
Aminoglycosides, loop diuretics:
Increased risk of nephrotoxicity.
Probenecid: May increase cefepime
blood concentration.
Warfarin: May increase response to
warfarin.
Herbal
None known.
Food
None known.

DIAGNOSTIC TEST EFFECTS
May increase serum alkaline
phosphatase, bilirubin, INR, LDH,
AST (SGOT), and ALT (SGPT)
levels. May cause a positive direct or
indirect Coombs' test.

ⓘ IV INCOMPATIBILITIES
Acyclovir (Zovirax), amphotericin
(Fungizone), cimetidine (Tagamet),
ciprofloxacin (Cipro), cisplatin
(Platinol), dacarbazine (DTIC),
daunorubicin (Cerubidine), diazepam
(Valium), diphenhydramine
(Benadryl), dobutamine (Dobutrex),
dopamine (Intropin), doxorubicin
(Adriamycin), droperidol (Inapsine),
famotidine (Pepcid), ganciclovir
(Cytovene), haloperidol (Haldol),
magnesium, magnesium sulfate,
mannitol, meperidine (Demerol),
metoclopramide (Reglan), morphine,
ofloxacin (Floxin), ondansetron
(Zofran), vancomycin (Vancocin).

ⓘ IV COMPATIBILITIES
Bumetanide (Bumex), calcium
gluconate, furosemide (Lasix),
hydromorphone (Dilaudid), lorazepam
(Ativan), propofol (Diprivan).

SIDE EFFECTS
Frequent
Discomfort with IM administration,
oral candidiasis, mild diarrhea,
mild abdominal cramping, vaginal
candidiasis.
Occasional
Nausea, serum sickness-like reaction
(marked by fever and joint pain;
usually occurs after the second
course of therapy and resolves after
the drug is discontinued).
Rare
Allergic reaction (rash, pruritus,
urticaria), thrombophlebitis (pain,
redness, swelling at injection site).

SERIOUS REACTIONS
• Antibiotic-associated colitis
manifested and other superinfections
may result from altered bacterial
balance.
• Nephrotoxicity may occur,
especially in patients with
preexisting renal disease.

• Patients with a history of allergies, especially to penicillin, are at increased risk for developing a severe hypersensitivity reaction, marked by severe pruritus, angioedema, bronchospasm, and anaphylaxis.

PRECAUTIONS & CONSIDERATIONS

Caution is warranted with renal impairment, seizure disorder. May be associated with increased INR, especially in nutritionally efficient patients, prolonged treatment, hepatic or renal disease. It is unknown whether cefepime is distributed in breast milk. No age-related precautions have been noted in children older than 2 mo. Age-related renal impairment may require dosage adjustment in elderly patients.

Although mild GI effects may be tolerable, an increase in their severity may indicate the onset of antibiotic-associated colitis. Assess the pattern of daily bowel activity and stool consistency, the mouth for white patches on the mucous membranes and tongue, signs and symptoms of superinfection including abdominal pain, moderate to severe diarrhea, severe anal or genital pruritus, and severe mouth soreness. Renal function should also be assessed.

Storage

Solution is stable for 24 h at room temperature or 7 days if refrigerated.

Administration

For IM use, add 1.3 mL sterile water for injection, 0.9% NaCl, or D5W to 500-mg vial (2.4 mL for 1-g and 2-g vials). To minimize the pain experienced by the patient, give IM injection slowly and deeply into a large muscle mass (e.g., upper gluteus maximus) instead of the lateral aspect of the thigh.

For IV use, add 5 mL to 500-mg vial (10 mL for 1-g and 2-g vials). Further dilute with 50-100 mL 0.9% NaCl, or D5W. For IV push, administer over 3-5 min. For intermittent IV infusion (piggyback), infuse over 30 min.

Cefixime

sef-ix′ime
(Suprax)
Do not confuse Suprax with Sporanox, Surbex, or Surfak.

CATEGORY AND SCHEDULE

Pregnancy Risk Category: B

Classification: Antibiotics, cephalosporin (third generation)

MECHANISM OF ACTION

A third-generation cephalosporin that binds to bacterial cell membranes and inhibits cell wall synthesis. *Therapeutic Effect:* Bactericidal.

PHARMACOKINETICS

Moderately absorbed from the GI tract. Protein binding: 65%-70%. Widely distributed. Primarily excreted unchanged in urine. Minimally removed by hemodialysis. *Half-life:* 3-4 h (increased in renal impairment).

AVAILABILITY

Oral Suspension: 100 mg/5 mL, 200 mg/5 mL.
Tablets: 400 mg.

INDICATIONS AND DOSAGES

▸ **Otitis media, acute bronchitis, acute exacerbations of chronic bronchitis, pharyngitis, tonsillitis, and uncomplicated urinary tract infections**
PO
Adults, Elderly, Children weighing more than 50 kg. 400 mg/day as a single dose or in 2 divided doses.
Children 6 mo to 12 yr weighing < 50 kg. 8 mg/kg/day as a single dose or in 2 divided doses.
Maximum: 400 mg/day.
▸ **Uncomplicated gonorrhea**
PO
Adults. 400 mg as a single dose.
▸ **Dosage in renal impairment**
Dosage is modified based on creatinine clearance.

Creatinine Clearance (mL/min)	% of Usual Dose
20-60	75
< 20	50

CONTRAINDICATIONS

History of anaphylactic reaction to penicillins, hypersensitivity to cephalosporins.

INTERACTIONS

Drug
Aminoglycosides, loop diuretics: May increase risk of nephrotoxicity.
Carbamazepine: May increase carbamazepine concentrations.
Probenecid: Increases serum concentration of cefixime.
Warfarin: Increases prothrombin time.
Herbal
None known.
Food
None known.

DIAGNOSTIC TEST EFFECTS

May increase BUN and serum alkaline phosphatase, bilirubin, creatinine, AST (SGOT), and ALT (SGPT) levels. May increase LDH level. May cause a positive direct or indirect Coombs' test.

SIDE EFFECTS

Frequent
Oral candidiasis, mild diarrhea, mild abdominal cramping, vaginal candidiasis.
Occasional
Nausea, serum sickness-like reaction (marked by arthralgia and fever; usually occurs after second course of therapy and resolves after drug is discontinued).
Rare
Allergic reaction (rash, pruritus, urticaria).

SERIOUS REACTIONS

• Antibiotic-associated colitis and other superinfections may result from altered bacterial balance.
• Nephrotoxicity may occur, especially in patients with preexisting renal disease.
• Patients with a history of allergies, especially to penicillin, are at increased risk for developing a severe hypersensitivity reaction, marked by severe pruritus, angioedema, bronchospasm, and anaphylaxis.

PRECAUTIONS & CONSIDERATIONS

Caution is warranted with hypersensitivity to penicillin, history of gastrointestinal disease (particularly colitis), and renal impairment. Cefixime crosses the placenta. It is not known whether it is distributed in breast milk. No age-related precautions have been noted in children. Age-related renal impairment in elderly may require dose adjustment.

Stool changes, abdominal cramps, diarrhea, nausea, vomiting, headache, sore mouth or tongue may occur. If fever, skin itching, rash, or swelling occurs, notify the physician immediately.

Storage

Suspension is stable at room temperature or under refrigeration for 14 days. Flavor improves with refrigeration.

Store tablets at room temperature.

Administration

For otitis media, give suspension only. Shake well before using. Take tablets or suspension with food if GI irritation occurs. Continue for the full length of treatment.

Cefotaxime

sef-oh-taks'eem

(Claforan)

Do not confuse cefotaxime with cefoxitin, ceftizoxime, cefuroxime, or Claritin.

CATEGORY AND SCHEDULE

Pregnancy Risk Category: B

Classification: Antibiotics, cephalosporin (third generation)

MECHANISM OF ACTION

A third-generation cephalosporin that binds to bacterial cell membranes and inhibits cell wall synthesis. *Therapeutic Effect:* Bactericidal.

PHARMACOKINETICS

Widely distributed, including to CSF. Protein binding: 30%-50%. Partially metabolized in the liver to active metabolite. Primarily excreted in urine. Moderately removed by hemodialysis.

Half-life: 1 h (increased in impaired renal function).

AVAILABILITY

Powder for Injection: 500 mg, 1 g, 2 g, 10 g.

Injection: 1 g, 2 g.

INDICATIONS AND DOSAGES

▸ **Uncomplicated infections**

IV, IM

Adults, Elderly. 1 g q12h.

▸ **Mild to moderate infections**

IV, IM

Adults, Elderly. 1-2 g q8h.

▸ **Severe infections**

IV, IM

Adults, Elderly. 2 g q6-8h.

▸ **Life-threatening infections**

IV

Adults, Elderly. 2 g q4h.

▸ **Gonorrhea**

IM

Adults. (Male).1 g as a single dose. (Female): 0.5 g as a single dose.

▸ **Perioperative prophylaxis**

IV, IM

Adults, Elderly. 1 g 30-90 min before surgery.

▸ **Cesarean section**

IV

Adults. 1 g as soon as umbilical cord is clamped, then 1 g 6 and 12 h after first dose.

▸ **Usual pediatric dosage**

Children weighing 50 kg or more. 1-2 g q6-8h; 29 mg 4 h for life-threatening infection.

Children 1 mo to 12 yr weighing < 50 kg. 100-200 mg/kg/day in divided doses q6-8h.

▸ **Dosage in renal impairment**

For patients with creatinine clearance < 20 mL/min, give half of dose at usual dosing intervals.

OFF-LABEL USES

Treatment of Lyme disease.

C

CONTRAINDICATIONS

History of anaphylactic reaction to penicillins or hypersensitivity to cephalosporins.

INTERACTIONS

Drug
Aminoglycosides, loop diuretics: May increase risk of nephrotoxicity.
Probenecid: May increase cefotaxime blood concentration.
Herbal
None known.
Food
None known.

DIAGNOSTIC TEST EFFECTS

May increase liver function test results and produce a positive direct or indirect Coombs' test.

ⓘ IV INCOMPATIBILITIES

Allopurinol (Aloprim), filgrastim (Neupogen), fluconazole (Diflucan), hetastarch (Hespan), pentamidine (Pentam IV), vancomycin (Vancocin).

ⓘ IV COMPATIBILITIES

Diltiazem (Cardizem), famotidine (Pepcid), hydromorphone (Dilaudid), lorazepam (Ativan), magnesium sulfate, midazolam (Versed), morphine, propofol (Diprivan).

SIDE EFFECTS

Frequent
Discomfort with IM administration, oral candidiasis, mild diarrhea, mild abdominal cramping, vaginal candidiasis.
Occasional
Nausea, serum sickness-like reaction (marked by fever and joint pain; usually occurs after the second course of therapy and resolves after the drug is discontinued).

Rare
Allergic reaction (rash, pruritus, urticaria), thrombophlebitis (pain, redness, swelling at injection site).

SERIOUS REACTIONS

• Antibiotic-associated colitis and other superinfections may result from altered bacterial balance.
• Nephrotoxicity may occur, especially in patients with preexisting renal disease.
• Patients with a history of allergies, especially to penicillin, are at increased risk for developing a severe hypersensitivity reaction, marked by severe pruritus, angioedema, bronchospasm, and anaphylaxis.
• Granulocytopenia and rarely granulocytosis have occurred with prolonged therapy (i.e., longer than 10 days).

PRECAUTIONS & CONSIDERATIONS

Caution is warranted with history of GI disease (especially antibiotic-associated or ulcerative colitis) and renal impairment. Cefotaxime readily crosses the placenta and is distributed in breast milk. No age-related precautions have been noted for use in children. Age-related renal impairment may require dosage adjustment in elderly patients.

Although mild GI effects may be tolerable, an increase in their severity may indicate the onset of antibiotic-associated colitis. The pattern of daily bowel activity and stool consistency, the mouth for white patches on the mucous membranes and tongue, signs and symptoms of superinfection including abdominal pain, moderate to severe diarrhea, severe anal or genital pruritus, and severe mouth soreness should be assessed. Renal function should be assessed.

Storage

Store powder for injection at room temperature and premixed solutions in the freezer. The solution for IV use normally appears light yellow to amber. The IV infusion (piggyback) may become darker, but this does not affect potency. The IV infusion (piggyback) prepared from the powder for injection is stable for 24 h at room temperature, 5 day if refrigerated, and 13 wks if frozen. Thawed previously frozen premixed bags are stable for 24 h at room temperature or 10 days if refrigerated. Discard the solution if a precipitate forms.

Administration

For IV use, add 10 mL of sterile water for injection to each 500-mg, 1-g, or 2-g vial to provide a concentration of 50, 95, or 180 mg/mL, respectively. The resulting solution may be further diluted with 50-100 mL of 0.9% NaCl or D5W. Administer the IV push over 3-5 min. More rapid IV administration through a central line has been associated with a high incidence of cardiac arrhythmias. Administer the intermittent IV infusion (piggyback) over 20-30 min.

For IM use, reconstitute the drug with sterile water for injection or bacteriostatic water for injection. Add 2, 3, or 5 mL to each 500-mg, 1-g, or 2-g vial, respectively, to yield a concentration of 230, 300, or 330 mg/mL, respectively. To minimize patient discomfort, slowly inject the drug deep into the gluteus maximus rather than the lateral aspect of the thigh. Administer a 2-g IM dose at two separate sites.

Cefotetan

sef'oh-tee-tan
(Cefotan)
Do not confuse cefotetan with cefoxitin or Ceftin.

CATEGORY AND SCHEDULE

Pregnancy Risk Category: B

Classification: Antibiotics, cephalosporin (second generation)

MECHANISM OF ACTION

A second-generation cephalosporin that binds to bacterial cell membranes and inhibits cell wall synthesis. *Therapeutic Effect:* Bactericidal.

PHARMACOKINETICS

Protein binding: 78%-91%. Primarily excreted unchanged in urine. Minimally removed by hemodialysis. *Half-life:* 3-4.6 h (increased in impaired renal function).

AVAILABILITY

Powder for Injection: 1 g, 2 g, 10 g.

INDICATIONS AND DOSAGES
▶ **Urinary tract infections**
IV, IM
Adults, Elderly. 1-2 g in divided doses q12-24h.
▶ **Mild to moderate infections**
IV, IM
Adults, Elderly. 1-2 g q12h.
▶ **Severe infections**
IV
Adults, Elderly. 2 g q12h.
▶ **Life-threatening infections**
IV
Adults, Elderly. 3 g q12h.
▶ **Perioperative prophylaxis**
IV
Adults, Elderly. 1-2 g 30-60 min before surgery.

▸ **Cesarean section**
IV
Adults. 1-2 g as soon as umbilical cord is clamped.
▸ **Usual pediatric dosage**
Children. 40-80 mg/kg/day in divided doses q12h. Maximum: 6 g/day.
▸ **Dosage in renal impairment**
Dosing frequency is modified based on creatinine clearance and the severity of the infection.

Creatinine Clearance (mL/min)	Dosage Interval
10-30	Usual dose q24h
< 10	Usual dose q48h

CONTRAINDICATIONS

History of anaphylactic reaction to penicillins or hypersensitivity to cephalosporins.

INTERACTIONS

Drug
Alcohol: May produce a disulfiram-like reaction (facial flushing, headache, nausea, pruritus, tachycardia).
Heparin, warfarin, other anticoagulants: May increase the risk of bleeding.
Herbal
None known.
Food
None known.

DIAGNOSTIC TEST EFFECTS

May increase BUN level and serum alkaline phosphatase, creatinine, AST (SGOT), and ALT (SGPT) levels. May prolong PT and produce a positive direct or indirect Coombs' test. Interferes with crossmatching procedures and hematologic tests.

ⓘ IV INCOMPATIBILITIES

Vancomycin (Vancocin).

ⓘ IV COMPATIBILITIES

Diltiazem (Cardizem), famotidine (Pepcid), heparin, insulin (regular), morphine, propofol (Diprivan).

SIDE EFFECTS

Frequent
Discomfort with IM administration, oral candidiasis, mild diarrhea, mild abdominal cramping, vaginal candidiasis.
Occasional
Nausea, unusual bleeding or bruising, serum sickness-like reaction (marked by fever and joint pain; usually occurs after the second course of therapy and resolves after the drug is discontinued).
Rare
Allergic reaction (rash, pruritus, urticaria), thrombophlebitis (pain, redness, swelling at injection site).

SERIOUS REACTIONS

• Antibiotic-associated colitis and other superinfections may result from altered bacterial balance.
• Nephrotoxicity may occur, especially in patients with preexisting renal disease.
• Patients with a history of allergies, especially to penicillin, are at increased risk for developing a severe hypersensitivity reaction, marked by severe pruritus, angioedema, bronchospasm, and anaphylaxis.
• Hemolytic anemia.

PRECAUTIONS & CONSIDERATIONS

Caution is warranted with history of GI disease (especially antibiotic-associated or ulcerative colitis), renal impairment, and concurrent use of nephrotoxic drugs. May be associated with increased INR, especially in nutritionally deficient patients, prolonged treatment, hepatic or renal disease. Cefotetan readily crosses the placenta and is distributed in breast milk. The safety and efficacy have not been established in children. Age-related renal impairment may require dosage adjustment in elderly patients.

Although mild GI effects may be tolerable, an increase in their severity may indicate the onset of antibiotic-associated colitis. Assess the pattern of daily bowel activity and stool consistency, the mouth for white patches on the mucous membranes and tongue, signs and symptoms of superinfection including abdominal pain, moderate to severe diarrhea, severe anal or genital pruritus, and severe mouth soreness. Renal function should also be assessed.

Storage

The solution normally appears colorless to light yellow. A deeper yellow does not indicate loss of potency. The IV infusion (piggyback) is stable for 24 h at room temperature, 96 h if refrigerated, and 12 wks if frozen. Discard the solution if a precipitate forms.

Administration

! Give by IM injection, IV push, or intermittent IV infusion (piggyback) only.

For IV use, reconstitute each 1-g vial with 10 mL of sterile water for injection to provide a concentration of 95 mg/mL. The resulting solution may be further diluted with 50-100 mL of 0.9% NaCl or D5W. Administer IV push over 3-5 min. Administer intermittent IV infusion (piggyback) over 20-30 min.

For IM use, add 2 mL of sterile water for injection or other appropriate diluent to each 1-g vial, or 3 mL to each 2-g vial, to provide a concentration of 400 mg/mL or 500 mg/mL, respectively. To minimize discomfort, slowly inject the drug deep into the gluteus maximus rather than the lateral aspect of the thigh.

Cefoxitin
se-fox′i-tin
(Mefoxin)
Do not confuse cefoxitin with cefotaxime, cefotetan, or Cytoxan.

CATEGORY AND SCHEDULE
Pregnancy Risk Category: B

Classification: Antibiotics, cephalosporins

MECHANISM OF ACTION
A second-generation cephalosporin that binds to bacterial cell membranes and inhibits cell wall synthesis. *Therapeutic Effect:* Bactericidal.

AVAILABILITY
Powder for Injection: 1 g, 2 g, 10 g.
Premixed Injection, Frozen: 1 g, 2 g.

INDICATIONS AND DOSAGES
▸ **Mild to moderate infections**
IV
Adults, Elderly. 1-2 g q6-8h.
▸ **Severe infections**
IV
Adults, Elderly. 1 g q4h or 2 g q6-8h up to 2 g q4h.
▸ **Perioperative prophylaxis**
IV
Adults, Elderly. 2 g 30-60 min before surgery, then q6h for up to 24 h after surgery.
Children older than 3 mo.
30-40 mg/kg 30-60 min before surgery, then q6h for up to 24 h after surgery.
▸ **Cesarean section**
IV
Adults. 2 g as soon as umbilical cord is clamped, then 2 g 4 and 8 h after first dose, then q6h for up to 24 h.

▸ **Usual pediatric dosage**

Children older than 3 mo. 80-160 mg/kg/day in 4-6 divided doses. Maximum: 12 g/day.

Neonates. 90-100 mg/kg/day in divided doses q8h.

▸ **Dosage in renal impairment (adults)**

After a loading dose of 1-2 g, dosage and frequency are modified based on creatinine clearance and the severity of the infection.

Creatinine Clearance (mL/min)	Dosage
30-50	1-2 g q8-12h
10-29	1-2 g q12-24h
5-9	500 mg-1 g q12-24h
< 5	500 mg-1 g q24-48h

CONTRAINDICATIONS

History of anaphylactic reaction to penicillins or hypersensitivity to cephalosporins.

INTERACTIONS

Drug

Aminoglycosides, loop diuretics: May increase risk of nephrotoxicity.

Probenecid: Increases serum concentration of cefoxitin.

Herbal

None known.

Food

None known.

DIAGNOSTIC TEST EFFECTS

May increase BUN level and serum alkaline phosphatase, creatinine, AST (SGOT), and ALT (SGPT) levels. May produce a positive direct or indirect Coombs' test. Interferes with crossmatching procedures and hematologic tests.

ⓘ IV INCOMPATIBILITIES

Filgrastim (Neupogen), pentamidine (Pentam IV), vancomycin (Vancocin).

ⓘ IV COMPATIBILITIES

Diltiazem (Cardizem), famotidine (Pepcid), heparin, hydromorphone (Dilaudid), magnesium sulfate, morphine, multivitamins, propofol (Diprivan).

SIDE EFFECTS

Frequent

Oral candidiasis, mild diarrhea, mild abdominal cramping, vaginal candidiasis.

Occasional

Nausea, serum sickness-like reaction (marked by fever and joint pain; usually occurs after the second course of therapy and resolves after the drug is discontinued).

Rare

Allergic reaction (pruritus, rash, urticaria), thrombophlebitis (pain, redness, swelling at injection site).

SERIOUS REACTIONS

• Antibiotic-associated colitis and other superinfections may result from altered bacterial balance.

• Nephrotoxicity may occur, especially in patients with preexisting renal disease.

• Patients with a history of allergies, especially to penicillin, are at increased risk for developing a severe hypersensitivity reaction, marked by severe pruritus, angioedema, bronchospasm, and anaphylaxis.

PRECAUTIONS & CONSIDERATIONS

Caution is warranted with history of GI disease (especially antibiotic-associated or ulcerative colitis), renal impairment, and concurrent use of nephrotoxic drugs.

Although mild GI effects may be tolerable, an increase in their severity may indicate the onset of antibiotic-associated colitis. Assess the pattern of daily bowel activity and stool consistency, the mouth for white

patches on the mucous membranes
and tongue, signs and symptoms of
superinfection including abdominal
pain, moderate to severe diarrhea,
severe anal or genital pruritus,
and severe mouth soreness. Renal
function should also be assessed.

Storage
The solution normally appears
colorless to light amber; a darker
color does not indicate loss of
potency. Reconstituted solution is
stable for 6 h at room temperature
and 7 days if refrigerated. The IV
infusion (piggyback) is stable for
24 h at room temperature and 48 h
if refrigerated. Thawed, previously
frozen premixed solution is stable for
24 h at room temperature or 21 days
if refrigerated. Discard the solution if
a precipitate forms.

Administration
! Give by intermittent IV infusion
(piggyback) or IV push. Space doses
evenly around the clock.

For IV use, reconstitute each 1-g
vial with 10 mL of sterile water for
injection to provide a concentration of
95 mg/mL. The resulting solution may
be further diluted with 50-100 mL of
sterile water for injection, 0.9% NaCl,
or D5W. Administer IV push over
3-5 min. Administer intermittent IV
infusion (piggyback) over 10-60 min.

Cefpodoxime
sef-pod′ox-ime
(Vantin)
**Do not confuse Vantin with
Ventolin.**

CATEGORY AND SCHEDULE
Pregnancy Risk Category: B

Classification: Antibiotics,
cephalosporin (third generation)

MECHANISM OF ACTION
A third-generation cephalosporin
that binds to bacterial cell
membranes and inhibits cell wall
synthesis. *Therapeutic Effect:*
Bactericidal.

PHARMACOKINETICS
Well absorbed from the GI tract
(food increases absorption).
Protein binding: 21%-40%. Widely
distributed. Primarily excreted
unchanged in urine. Partially
removed by hemodialysis. *Half-life:*
2.3 h (increased in impaired renal
function and elderly patients).

AVAILABILITY
Oral Suspension: 50 mg/5 mL,
100 mg/5 mL.
Tablets: 100 mg, 200 mg.

INDICATIONS AND DOSAGES
▶ **Chronic bronchitis, pneumonia**
PO
*Adults, Elderly, Children older than
13 yr.* 200 mg q12h for 10-14 days.
▶ **Gonorrhea (men and women),
rectal gonococcal infection (female
patients only)**
PO
Adults, Children older than 13 yr.
200 mg as a single dose.
▶ **Skin and skin-structure infections**
PO
*Adults, Elderly, Children older than
13 yr.* 400 mg q12h for 7-14 days.
▶ **Pharyngitis, tonsillitis**
PO
*Adults, Elderly, Children older than
13 yr.* 100 mg q12h for 5-10 days.
Children 6 mo to 13 yr.
5 mg/kg q12h for 5-10 days.
Maximum: 100 mg/dose.
▶ **Acute maxillary sinusitis**
PO
*Adults, Children older than
13 yr.* 200 mg twice a day for
10 days.

Children 2 mo to 13 yr. 5 mg/kg q12h for 10 days. Maximum: 400 mg/day.

▶ **Urinary tract infection**
PO
Adults, Elderly, Children older than 13 yr. 100 mg q12h for 7 days.

▶ **Acute otitis media**
PO
Children 6 mo to 13 yr. 5 mg/kg q12h for 5 days. Maximum: 400 mg/dose.

▶ **Dosage in renal impairment**
For patients with creatinine clearance < 30 mL/min, usual dose is given q24h. For patients on hemodialysis, usual dose is given 3 times/wk after dialysis.

CONTRAINDICATIONS

History of anaphylactic reaction to penicillins or hypersensitivity to cephalosporins.

INTERACTIONS

Drug
Antacids, H_2 antagonists: May decrease cefpodoxime absorption.
Probenecid: May increase cefpodoxime blood concentration.
Herbal
None known.
Food
None known.

DIAGNOSTIC TEST EFFECTS

May increase BUN level and serum alkaline phosphatase, bilirubin, creatinine, LDH, AST (SGOT), and ALT (SGPT) levels. May produce a positive direct or indirect Coombs' test.

SIDE EFFECTS

Frequent
Oral candidiasis, mild diarrhea, mild abdominal cramping, vaginal candidiasis.

Occasional
Nausea, serum sickness-like reaction (marked by fever and joint pain; usually occurs after the second course of therapy and resolves after the drug is discontinued).
Rare
Allergic reaction (pruritus, rash, urticaria).

SERIOUS REACTIONS

• Antibiotic-associated colitis and other superinfections may result from altered bacterial balance.
• Nephrotoxicity may occur, especially in patients with preexisting renal disease.
• Patients with a history of allergies, especially to penicillin, are at increased risk for developing a severe hypersensitivity reaction, marked by severe pruritus, angioedema, bronchospasm, and anaphylaxis.

PRECAUTIONS & CONSIDERATIONS

Caution is warranted with history of GI disease (especially antibiotic-associated or ulcerative colitis), renal impairment, and concurrent use of nephrotoxic drugs. Cefpodoxime readily crosses the placenta and is distributed in breast milk. The safety and efficacy of cefpodoxime have not been established in children younger than 6 mo. Age-related renal impairment may require a dosage adjustment in elderly patients.

Although mild GI effects may be tolerable, an increase in their severity may indicate the onset of antibiotic-associated colitis. Assess the pattern of daily bowel activity and stool consistency, the mouth for white patches on the mucous membranes and tongue, signs and symptoms of superinfection including abdominal pain, moderate to severe diarrhea, severe anal or genital pruritus, and severe mouth soreness. Renal function should also be assessed.

Storage
After reconstitution, the oral suspension is stable for 14 days if refrigerated.

Administration
Administer cefpodoxime tablets with food to enhance drug absorption; suspension may be taken without regard to food. Shake suspension well.

Cefprozil
sef-pro′zil
(Cefzil)
Do not confuse cefprozil with Cefazolin, Cefol, Ceftin, or Kefzol.

CATEGORY AND SCHEDULE
Pregnancy Risk Category: B

Classification: Antibiotics, cephalosporin (second generation)

MECHANISM OF ACTION
A second-generation cephalosporin that binds to bacterial cell membranes and inhibits cell wall synthesis. *Therapeutic Effect:* Bactericidal.

PHARMACOKINETICS
Well absorbed from the GI tract. Protein binding: 36%-45%. Widely distributed. Primarily excreted unchanged in urine. Moderately removed by hemodialysis. *Half-life:* 1.3 h (increased in impaired renal function).

AVAILABILITY
Oral Suspension: 125 mg/5 mL, 250 mg/5 mL.
Tablets: 250 mg, 500 mg.

INDICATIONS AND DOSAGES
▸ **Pharyngitis, tonsillitis**
PO
Adults, Elderly. 500 mg q24h for 10 days.
Children 2-12 yr. 7.5 mg/kg q12h for 10 days.
▸ **Acute bacterial exacerbation of chronic bronchitis, secondary bacterial infection of acute bronchitis**
PO
Adults, Elderly. 500 mg q12h for 10 days.
▸ **Skin and skin-structure infections**
PO
Adults, Elderly. 250-500 mg q12h for 10 days.
Children. 20 mg/kg q24h for 10 days.
▸ **Acute sinusitis**
PO
Adults, Elderly. 250-500 mg q12h for 10 days.
Children 6 mo to 12 yr. 7.5-15 mg/kg q12h for 10 days.
▸ **Otitis media**
PO
Children 6 mo to 12 yr. 15 mg/kg q12h for 10 days. Maximum: 1 g/day.
▸ **Dosage in renal impairment**
Patients with creatinine clearance < 30 mL/min receive 50% of usual dose at usual interval.

CONTRAINDICATIONS
History of anaphylactic reaction to penicillins or hypersensitivity to cephalosporins.

INTERACTIONS
Drug
Probenecid: Increases serum concentration of cefprozil.
Herbal
None known.
Food
None known.

DIAGNOSTIC TEST EFFECTS

May increase liver function test results. May produce a positive direct or indirect Coombs' test. Interferes with crossmatching procedures and hematologic tests.

SIDE EFFECTS

Frequent
Oral candidiasis, mild diarrhea, mild abdominal cramping, vaginal candidiasis.
Occasional
Nausea, serum sickness reaction (marked by fever and joint pain; usually occurs after the second course of therapy and resolves after the drug is discontinued).
Rare
Allergic reaction (pruritus, rash, urticaria).

SERIOUS REACTIONS

• Antibiotic-associated colitis and other superinfections may result from altered bacterial balance.
• Nephrotoxicity may occur, especially in patients with preexisting renal disease.
• Patients with a history of allergies, especially to penicillin, are at increased risk for developing a severe hypersensitivity reaction, marked by severe pruritus, angioedema, bronchospasm, and anaphylaxis.

PRECAUTIONS & CONSIDERATIONS

Caution is warranted with history of GI disease (especially antibiotic-associated or ulcerative colitis), renal impairment, and concurrent use of nephrotoxic drugs. Cefprozil readily crosses the placenta and is distributed in breast milk. The safety and efficacy of cefprozil have not been established in children younger than 6 mo. Age-related renal impairment may require a dosage adjustment in elderly patients.

Although mild GI effects may be tolerable, an increase in their severity may indicate the onset of antibiotic-associated colitis. Assess the pattern of daily bowel activity and stool consistency, the mouth for white patches on the mucous membranes and tongue, signs and symptoms of superinfection including abdominal pain, moderate to severe diarrhea, severe anal or genital pruritus, and severe mouth soreness. Renal function should be assessed.
Storage
After reconstitution, the oral suspension is stable for 14 days if refrigerated.
Administration
Shake the oral suspension well before using. Take cefprozil without regard to meals; however, if GI upset occurs, give it with food or milk.

Ceftazidime

sef-taz′i-deem
(Ceptaz, Fortaz, Fortum [AUS], Tazicef, Tazidime)
Do not confuse ceftazidime with ceftizoxime.

CATEGORY AND SCHEDULE

Pregnancy Risk Category: B

Classification: Antibiotic, cephalosporin (third generation)

MECHANISM OF ACTION

A third-generation cephalosporin that binds to bacterial cell membranes and inhibits cell wall synthesis. *Therapeutic Effect:* Bactericidal.

PHARMACOKINETICS

Widely distributed (including to CSF). Protein binding: 5%-17%. Primarily excreted unchanged in urine. Removed by hemodialysis. *Half-life:* 2 h (increased in impaired renal function).

AVAILABILITY

Powder for Injection (Fortaz, Tazicef, Tazidime): 500 mg, 1 g, 2 g, 6 g.
Premixed Injection, Frozen: 1 g, 2 g.

INDICATIONS AND DOSAGES

▸ **Urinary tract infection**
IV, IM
Adults. 250-500 mg q8-12h.
▸ **Mild to moderate infections**
IV, IM
Adults. 1 g q8-12h.
▸ **Uncomplicated pneumonia, skin and skin-structure infections**
IV, IM
Adults. 0.5-1 g q8h.
▸ **Bone and joint infections**
IV
Adults. 2 g q12h.
▸ **Meningitis, serious gynecologic and intra-abdominal infections**
IV
Adults. 2 g q8h.
▸ **Pseudomonal pulmonary infections in patients with cystic fibrosis**
IV
Adults. 30-50 mg/kg q8h. Maximum: 6 g/day.
▸ **Usual elderly dosage**
Elderly (with normal renal function). 500 mg-1 g q12h.
▸ **Usual pediatric dosage**
Children 1 mo to 12 yr.
100-150 mg/kg/day in divided doses q8h. Maximum: 6 g/day.
Neonates 0-4 wks. 100-150 mg/kg/day in divided doses q8-12h.
▸ **Dosage in renal impairment**
After an initial 1-g dose, dosage and frequency are modified based on creatinine clearance and the severity of the infection.

Creatinine Clearance (mL/min)	Adult Dosage
30-50	1 g q12h
16-30	1 g q24h
6-15	500 mg q24h
< 5	500 mg q48h

CONTRAINDICATIONS

History of anaphylactic reaction to penicillins or hypersensitivity to cephalosporins.

INTERACTIONS

Drug
Warfarin: May increase warfarin effect.
Herbal
None known.
Food
None known.

DIAGNOSTIC TEST EFFECTS

May increase BUN level and serum alkaline phosphatase, creatinine, INR, LDH, AST (SGOT), and ALT (SGPT) levels. May produce a positive direct or indirect Coombs' test. Interferes with crossmatching procedures and hematologic tests.

ⓓ IV INCOMPATIBILITIES

Amphotericin B complex (Abelcet, AmBisome, Amphotec), doxorubicin liposomal (Doxil), fluconazole (Diflucan), idarubicin (Idamycin), midazolam (Versed), pentamidine (Pentam IV), vancomycin (Vancocin).

ⓓ IV COMPATIBILITIES

Diltiazem (Cardizem), famotidine (Pepcid), heparin, hydromorphone (Dilaudid), morphine, propofol (Diprivan).

C

SIDE EFFECTS

Frequent

Discomfort with IM administration, oral candidiasis, mild diarrhea, mild abdominal cramping, vaginal candidiasis.

Occasional

Nausea, serum sickness-like reaction (marked by fever and joint pain; usually occurs after the second course of therapy and resolves after the drug is discontinued).

Rare

Allergic reaction (pruritus, rash, urticaria), thrombophlebitis (pain, redness, swelling at injection site).

SERIOUS REACTIONS

• Antibiotic-associated colitis and other superinfections may result from altered bacterial balance.

• Nephrotoxicity may occur, especially in patients with preexisting renal disease.

• Patients with a history of allergies, especially to penicillin, are at increased risk for developing a severe hypersensitivity reaction, marked by severe pruritus, angioedema, bronchospasm, and anaphylaxis.

PRECAUTIONS & CONSIDERATIONS

Caution is warranted with history of GI disease (especially antibiotic-associated or ulcerative colitis), seizure disorder, renal impairment, and concurrent use of nephrotoxic drugs. May be associated with increased INR, especially in nutritionally deficient patients, prolonged treatment, and hepatic or renal disease. Ceftazidime readily crosses the placenta and is distributed in breast milk. No age-related precautions have been noted in children. Age-related renal impairment may require a dosage adjustment in elderly patients.

Although mild GI effects may be tolerable, an increase in their severity may indicate the onset of antibiotic-associated colitis. Assess the pattern of daily bowel activity and stool consistency, the mouth for white patches on the mucous membranes and tongue, signs and symptoms of superinfection including abdominal pain, moderate to severe diarrhea, severe anal or genital pruritus, and severe mouth soreness. Renal function should also be assessed.

Storage

The solution normally appears light yellow to amber, but it tends to darken; color change does not indicate loss of potency. Reconstituted solution is stable for 24 h at room temperature, 7 days if refrigerated, or 12 wks if frozen. The IV infusion (piggyback) is stable for 24 h at room temperature and 7 days if refrigerated. Thawed premixed frozen solutions are stable for 24 h at room temperature and 7 days if refrigerated. Discard the solution if a precipitate forms.

Administration

! Give ceftazidime by IM injection, direct IV injection, or intermittent IV infusion (piggyback).

For IV use, add 10 mL of sterile water for injection to each 1-g vial to provide a concentration of 90 mg/mL. The resulting solution may be further diluted with 50-100 mL of 0.9% NaCl, D5W, or another compatible diluent. Administer IV push over 3-5 min. Administer intermittent IV infusion (piggyback) over 15-30 min.

For IM use, to reconstitute, add 1.5 mL of sterile water for injection or lidocaine 1% to 500-mg vial, if prescribed, or 3 mL to 1-g vial to provide a concentration of 280 mg/mL. To minimize patient discomfort, slowly inject the drug deep into the gluteus maximus rather than into the lateral aspect of the thigh.

Ceftibuten
cef'te-bute-in
(Cedax)

CATEGORY AND SCHEDULE
Pregnancy Risk Category: B

Classification: Antibiotic,
cephalosporin (third generation)

MECHANISM OF ACTION
A third-generation cephalosporin
that binds to bacterial cell
membranes and inhibits cell wall
synthesis. *Therapeutic Effect:*
Bactericidal.

PHARMACOKINETICS
Rapidly absorbed from the
gastrointestinal tract. Excreted
primarily in urine. *Half-life:*
2-3 h.

AVAILABILITY
Capsules: 400 mg.
Oral Suspension: 90 mg/5 mL.

INDICATIONS AND DOSAGES
▶ **Chronic bronchitis**
PO
Adults, Elderly. 400 mg/day once a
day for 10 days.
▶ **Pharyngitis, tonsillitis**
PO
Adults, Elderly. 400 mg once a day
for 10 days.
Children 6 mo of age and older.
9 mg/kg once a day for 10 days.
Maximum: 400 mg/day.
▶ **Otitis media**
PO
Children 6 mo of age and older.
9 mg/kg once a day for 10 days.
Maximum: 400 mg/day.
▶ **Dosage in renal impairment**
Dosage is modified based on
creatinine clearance.

Creatinine Clearance (mL/min)	Dosage
50 (and higher)	400 mg or 9 mg/kg q24h
30-49	200 mg or 4.5 mg/kg q24h
< 30	100 mg or 2.25 mg/kg q24h

CONTRAINDICATIONS
History of anaphylactic reaction to
penicillins or hypersensitivity to
cephalosporins.

INTERACTIONS
Drug
Aminoglycosides: Increased risk of
nephrotoxicity.
Probenecid: Increases serum
ceftibuten level.
Herbal
None known.
Food
None known.

DIAGNOSTIC TEST EFFECTS
May increase BUN level and serum
alkaline phosphatase, bilirubin,
creatinine, LDH, AST (SGOT), and
ALT (SGPT), levels. May produce a
positive direct or indirect Coombs'
test.

SIDE EFFECTS
Frequent
Oral candidiasis, mild diarrhea
(discharge, itching).
Occasional
Nausea, serum sickness-like
reaction (marked by fever and
joint pain; usually occurs after
the second course of therapy
and resolves after the drug is
discontinued).
Rare
Allergic reaction (rash, pruritus,
urticaria).

C

SERIOUS REACTIONS
• Antibiotic-associated colitis and other superinfections may result from altered bacterial balance.
• Nephrotoxicity may occur, especially in patients with preexisting renal disease.
• Patients with a history of allergies, especially to penicillin, are at increased risk for developing a severe hypersensitivity reaction, marked by severe pruritus, angioedema, bronchospasm, and anaphylaxis.

PRECAUTIONS & CONSIDERATIONS
Caution is warranted with history of GI disease (especially antibiotic-associated or ulcerative colitis), renal impairment, and allergies to penicillins or other drugs.

Although mild GI effects may be tolerable, an increase in their severity may indicate the onset of antibiotic-associated colitis. Assess the pattern of daily bowel activity and stool consistency, the mouth for white patches on the mucous membranes and tongue, signs and symptoms of superinfection including abdominal pain, moderate to severe diarrhea, severe anal or genital pruritus, and severe mouth soreness. Renal function should also be assessed.

Storage
Reconstituted suspension is stable for 14 days if refrigerated.

Administration
! Use oral suspension when treating otitis media to achieve higher peak blood levels.

Take capsule without regard to food; may take with food or milk if GI upset occurs. Take suspension 1 h before or 2 h after a meal. Take a full course of treatment, and space drug doses evenly around the clock. Shake suspension well.

Ceftizoxime
sef-ti-zox′eem
(Cefizox)
Do not confuse ceftizoxime with cefotaxime or ceftazidime.

CATEGORY AND SCHEDULE
Pregnancy Risk Category: B

Classification: Antibiotics, cephalosporin (third generation)

MECHANISM OF ACTION
A third-generation cephalosporin that binds to bacterial cell membranes and inhibits cell wall synthesis. *Therapeutic Effect:* Bactericidal.

PHARMACOKINETICS
Widely distributed (including to CSF). Protein binding: 30%. Primarily excreted unchanged in urine. Moderately removed by hemodialysis. *Half-life:* 1.7 h (increased in impaired renal function).

AVAILABILITY
Powder for Injection: 500 mg, 1 g, 2 g, 10 g.
Premixed Injection, Frozen: 1 g, 2 g.

INDICATIONS AND DOSAGES
▸ **Uncomplicated urinary tract infection**
IV, IM
Adults, Elderly. 500 mg q12h.
▸ **Mild, moderate, or severe infections of the biliary, respiratory, and genitourinary tracts; skin, bone, and intra-abdominal infections; meningitis; and septicemia**
IV, IM
Adults, Elderly. 1-2 g q8-12h.
▸ **Life-threatening infections of the biliary, respiratory, and genitourinary tracts; skin, bone,**

and intra-abdominal infections;
meningitis; and septicemia
IV
Adults, Elderly. 3-4 g q8h, up to
2 g q4h.
▸ **Pelvic inflammatory disease (PID)**
IV
Adults. 2 g q4-8h.
▸ **Uncomplicated gonorrhea**
IM
Adults. 1 g one time.
▸ **Usual pediatric dosage**
Children older than 6 mo. 50 mg/kg
q6-8h. Maximum: 12 g/day.
▸ **Dosage in renal impairment**
After a loading dose of 0.5-1 g,
dosage and frequency are modified
based on creatinine clearance and the
severity of the infection.

Creatinine Clearance (mL/min)	Adult Dosage
50-79	0.5 g-1.5 g q8h
5-49	0.25 g-1 g q12h
< 5	0.25-0.5 g q24h or 0.5 g-1 g q48h

CONTRAINDICATIONS
History of anaphylactic reaction to
penicillins or hypersensitivity to
cephalosporins.

INTERACTIONS
Drug
Aminoglycosides: May increase risk
of nephrotoxicity.
Probenecid: Increases serum
concentration of ceftizoxime.
Herbal
None known.
Food
None known.

DIAGNOSTIC TEST EFFECTS
May increase BUN level and
serum alkaline serum phosphatase,
creatinine, AST (SGOT), and ALT
(SGPT) levels. May produce a positive
direct or indirect Coombs' test.

IV INCOMPATIBILITIES
Filgrastim (Neupogen).

IV COMPATIBILITIES
Hydromorphone (Dilaudid),
morphine, propofol (Diprivan).

SIDE EFFECTS
Frequent
Discomfort with IM administration,
oral candidiasis, mild diarrhea,
mild abdominal cramping, vaginal
candidiasis.
Occasional
Nausea, serum sickness-like reaction
(fever, joint pain; usually occurs
after the second course of therapy
and resolves after the drug is
discontinued).
Rare
Allergic reaction (rash, pruritus,
urticaria), thrombophlebitis (pain,
redness, swelling at injection site).

SERIOUS REACTIONS
• Antibiotic-associated colitis
manifested and other superinfections
may result from altered bacterial
balance.
• Nephrotoxicity may occur,
especially in patients with
preexisting renal disease.
• Patients with a history of allergies,
especially to penicillin, are at
increased risk for developing a
severe hypersensitivity reaction,
marked by severe pruritus,
angioedema, bronchospasm, and
anaphylaxis.

PRECAUTIONS & CONSIDERATIONS
Caution is warranted with history
of GI disease (especially antibiotic-
associated or ulcerative colitis)
and hepatic or renal impairment.
Ceftizoxime readily crosses the
placenta and is distributed in breast
milk. Ceftizoxime use in children is
associated with transient elevations

of blood eosinophil count and serum CK, AST (SGOT), and ALT (SGPT) levels. Age-related renal impairment may require a dosage adjustment in elderly patients.

Although mild GI effects may be tolerable, an increase in their severity may indicate the onset of antibiotic-associated colitis. Assess the pattern of daily bowel activity and stool consistency, the mouth for white patches on the mucous membranes and tongue, signs and symptoms of superinfection including abdominal pain, moderate to severe diarrhea, severe anal or genital pruritus, and severe mouth soreness. Renal function should also be assessed.

Storage

The solution normally appears clear to pale yellow. A change from yellow to amber does not indicate loss of potency. The IV infusion (piggyback) is stable for 24 h at room temperature and 96 h if refrigerated. Thawed premixed frozen solution is stable for 24 h at room temperature and 10 days if refrigerated. Discard the solution if a precipitate forms.

Administration

For IV use, to reconstitute, add 5 mL of sterile water for injection to each 0.5-g vial to provide a concentration of 95 mg/mL. The resulting solution may be further diluted with 50-100 mL of 0.9% NaCl, D5W, or another compatible fluid. Administer IV push over 3-5 min. Infuse intermittent IV infusion (piggyback) over 15-30 min.

For IM use, add 1.5 mL of sterile water for injection to each 0.5-g vial to provide a concentration of 270 mg/mL. Give deep IM injections slowly to minimize patient discomfort. When giving a 2-g dose, divide the dose and give in different large muscle masses.

Ceftriaxone
sef-try-ax′one
(Rocephin)

CATEGORY AND SCHEDULE
Pregnancy Risk Category: B

Classification: Antibiotics, cephalosporin (third generation)

MECHANISM OF ACTION
A third-generation cephalosporin that binds to bacterial cell membranes and inhibits cell wall synthesis. *Therapeutic Effect:* Bactericidal.

PHARMACOKINETICS
Widely distributed (including to CSF). Protein binding: 83%-96%. Primarily excreted unchanged in urine. Not removed by hemodialysis. *Half-life:* 4.3-4.6 h IV; 5.8-8.7 h IM (increased in impaired renal function).

AVAILABILITY
Powder for Injection: 250 mg, 500 mg, 1 g, 2 g, 10 g.
Premixed Injection: 1 g, 2 g.

INDICATIONS AND DOSAGES
▸ **Mild to moderate infections**
IV, IM
Adults, Elderly. 1-2 g as a single dose or in 2 divided doses.
▸ **Serious infections**
IV, IM
Adults, Elderly. Up to 4 g/day in 2 divided doses.
Children. 50-75 mg/kg/day in divided doses q12h. Maximum: 2 g/day.
▸ **Skin and skin-structure infections**
IV, IM
Children. 50-75 mg/kg/day as a single dose or in 2 divided doses. Maximum: 2 g/day.

▸ **Meningitis**

IV

Children. Initially 100 mg/kg, then 100 mg/kg/day as a single dose or in divided doses q12h. Maximum: 4 g/day.

▸ **Lyme disease**

IV

Adults, Elderly. 2-4 g a day for 10-14 days.

▸ **Acute bacterial otitis media**

IM

Children. 50 mg/kg as a single dose.

▸ **Perioperative prophylaxis**

IV, IM

Adults, Elderly. 1 g 0.5-2 h before surgery.

▸ **Uncomplicated gonorrhea**

IM

Adults. 250 mg plus azithromycin or doxycycline one time.

▸ **Dosage in renal impairment**

Dosage modification is usually unnecessary, but liver and renal function test results should be monitored in persons with both renal and liver impairment or severe renal impairment.

CONTRAINDICATIONS

History of anaphylactic reaction to penicillins or hypersensitivity to cephalosporins; hyperbilirubinemic neonates; concomitant use with calcium-containing solutions or products.

INTERACTIONS

Drug

Calcium-containing solutions: Ceftriaxone may precipitate with calcium when mixed. Avoid coadministration, even via separate infusion lines or at different times. Do not administer calcium-containing solutions or products within 48 h after the last dose of ceftriaxone.

Warfarin: May increase the effects of warfarin.

Herbal

None known.

Food

None known.

DIAGNOSTIC TEST EFFECTS

May increase BUN level, INR, and serum alkaline phosphatase, bilirubin, creatinine, AST (SGOT), and ALT (SGPT) levels. May produce a positive direct or indirect Coombs' test. Interferes with crossmatching procedures and hematologic tests.

Ⓦ IV INCOMPATIBILITIES

Aminophylline, amphotericin B complex (Abelcet, AmBisome, Amphotec), calcium, filgrastim (Neupogen), fluconazole (Diflucan), labetalol (Normodyne), pentamidine (Pentam IV), vancomycin (Vancocin).

Ⓦ IV COMPATIBILITIES

Diltiazem (Cardizem), heparin, lidocaine, morphine, propofol (Diprivan).

SIDE EFFECTS

Frequent

Discomfort with IM administration, oral candidiasis, mild diarrhea, mild abdominal cramping, vaginal candidiasis.

Occasional

Nausea, serum sickness-like reaction (marked by fever and joint pain; usually occurs after the second course of therapy and resolves after the drug is discontinued).

Rare

Allergic reaction (rash, pruritus, urticaria), thombophlebitis (pain, redness, swelling at injection site).

SERIOUS REACTIONS

• Antibiotic-associated colitis and other superinfections may result from altered bacterial balance.

• Nephrotoxicity may occur, especially in patients with preexisting renal disease.

• Patients with a history of allergies, especially to penicillin, are at increased risk for developing a severe hypersensitivity reaction, marked by severe pruritus, angioedema, bronchospasm, and anaphylaxis.

• Renal and pulmonary ceftriaxone-calcium precipitations, including some fatalities in neonates.

PRECAUTIONS & CONSIDERATIONS

Caution is warranted in patients with a history of GI disease (especially antibiotic-associated or ulcerative colitis), hepatic or renal impairment, and concurrent use of nephrotoxic drugs. May be associated with increased INR, especially in nutritionally deficient patients or those who have undergone prolonged treatment or have hepatic or renal disease. Ceftriaxone readily crosses the placenta and is distributed in breast milk. Ceftriaxone use in children may displace serum bilirubin from serum albumin. Use ceftriaxone cautiously in neonates, who may become hyperbilirubinemic; use is contraindicated in neonates with hyperbilirubinemia. Age-related renal impairment may require a dosage adjustment in elderly patients.

Although mild GI effects may be tolerable, an increase in their severity may indicate the onset of antibiotic-associated colitis. Assess the pattern of daily bowel activity and stool consistency, the mouth for white patches on the mucous membranes and tongue, signs and symptoms of superinfection including abdominal pain, moderate to severe diarrhea, severe anal or genital pruritus, and severe mouth soreness. Renal function should also be assessed.

Storage

The solution normally appears light yellow to amber. The IV infusion (piggyback) is stable for 3 days at room temperature and 10 days if refrigerated. Thawed premixed frozen solutions are stable for 3 days at room temperature or 21 days if refrigerated. Discard the solution if a precipitate forms.

Administration

For IV use, add 2.4 mL of sterile water for injection to each 250-mg vial, 4.8 mL to each 500-mg vial, 9.6 mL to each 1-g vial, and 19.2 mL to each 2-g vial to provide a concentration of 100 mg/mL. The resulting solution may be further diluted with 50-100 mL of 0.9% NaCl or D5W. Infuse the intermittent IV infusion (piggyback) over 15-30 min for adults and over 10-30 min for children or neonates. Alternate IV sites and use large veins to reduce the risk of phlebitis.

For IM use, add 0.9 mL of sterile water for injection, 0.9% NaCl, D5W, bacteriostatic water and 0.9% benzyl alcohol, or lidocaine to each 250-mg vial; 1.8 mL to each 500-mg vial; 3.6 mL to each 1-g vial; and 7.2 mL to each 2-g vial to provide a concentration of 250 mg/mL. To minimize patient discomfort, slowly inject the drug deep into the gluteus maximus rather than the lateral aspect of the thigh.

Cefuroxime

sef-yoor-ox'eem
(Ceftin, Zinnat [AUS]) (Kefurox, Zinacef)

Do not confuse cefuroxime with cefotaxime, Cefzil, or deferoxamine.

CATEGORY AND SCHEDULE
Pregnancy Risk Category: B

Classification: Antibiotics, cephalosporin (second generation)

MECHANISM OF ACTION
A second-generation cephalosporin that binds to bacterial cell membranes and inhibits cell wall synthesis. *Therapeutic Effect:* Bactericidal.

PHARMACOKINETICS
Rapidly absorbed from the GI tract. Protein binding: 33%-50%. Widely distributed (including to CSF). Primarily excreted unchanged in urine. Moderately removed by hemodialysis. *Half-life:* 1.3 h (increased in impaired renal function).

AVAILABILITY
Oral Suspension: 125 mg/5 mL, 250 mg/5 mL.
Tablets: 125 mg, 250 mg, 500 mg.
Powder for Injection: 750 mg, 1.5 g, 7.5 g.
Premixed Injection: 750 mg, 1.5 g.

INDICATIONS AND DOSAGES
▸ **Ampicillin-resistant influenza; bacterial meningitis; early Lyme disease; genitourinary tract, gynecologic, skin, and bone infections; septicemia; gonorrhea; and other gonococcal infections**
IV, IM
Adults, Elderly. 750 mg-1.5 g q8h.

Children. 75-100 mg/kg/day divided q8h. Maximum: 8 g/day.
Neonates. 50-100 mg/kg/day divided q12h.
PO
Adults, Elderly. 125-500 mg twice a day, depending on the infection. For uncomplicated gonorrhea, give a 1-g single dose.
▸ **Pharyngitis, tonsillitis**
PO
Children 3 mo to 12 yr. 125 mg (tablets) q12h or 20 mg/kg/day (suspension) in 2 divided doses.
▸ **Acute otitis media, acute bacterial maxillary sinusitis, impetigo**
PO
Children 3 mo to 12 yr. 250 mg (tablets) q12h or 30 mg/kg/day (suspension) in 2 divided doses.
▸ **Bacterial meningitis**
IV
Children 3 mo to 12 yr. 200-240 mg/kg/day in divided doses q6-8h.
▸ **Perioperative prophylaxis**
IV
Adults, Elderly. 1.5 g 30-60 min before surgery and 750 mg q8h after surgery.
▸ **Dosage in renal impairment**
Adult dosage and frequency are modified based on creatinine clearance and the severity of the infection. The usual initial (loading dose) is given, followed by maintenance as follows:

Creatinine Clearance (mL/min)	Adult Dosage
> 20	Use usual dose
10-20	750 mg q12h
< 10	750 mg q24h

CONTRAINDICATIONS
History of anaphylactic reaction to penicillins or hypersensitivity to cephalosporins.

C

INTERACTIONS

Drug
Antacids, H$_2$ antagonists: May reduce cefuroxime absorption.
Probenecid: Increases serum concentration of cefuroxime.
Herbal
None known.
Food
None known.

DIAGNOSTIC TEST EFFECTS

May increase serum alkaline phosphatase, bilirubin, LDH, AST (SGOT), and ALT (SGPT) levels. May produce a positive direct or indirect Coombs' test. Interferes with crossmatching procedures, hematologic tests.

IV INCOMPATIBILITIES

Filgrastim (Neupogen), fluconazole (Diflucan), midazolam (Versed), vancomycin (Vancocin).

IV COMPATIBILITIES

Diltiazem (Cardizem), hydromorphone (Dilaudid), morphine, propofol (Diprivan).

SIDE EFFECTS

Frequent
Discomfort with IM administration, oral candidiasis, mild diarrhea, mild abdominal cramping, vaginal candidiasis.
Occasional
Nausea, serum sickness–like reaction (marked by fever and joint pain; usually occurs after the second course of therapy and resolves after the drug is discontinued).
Rare
Allergic reaction (rash, pruritus, urticaria), thrombophlebitis (pain, redness, swelling at injection site).

SERIOUS REACTIONS

• Antibiotic-associated colitis and other superinfections may result from altered bacterial balance.
• Nephrotoxicity may occur, especially in patients with preexisting renal disease.
• Patients with a history of allergies, especially to penicillin, are at increased risk for developing a severe hypersensitivity reaction, marked by severe pruritus, angioedema, bronchospasm, and anaphylaxis.

PRECAUTIONS & CONSIDERATIONS

Caution is warranted for patients with a history of GI disease (especially antibiotic-associated or ulcerative colitis), renal impairment, and concurrent use of nephrotoxic drugs. May be associated with increased INR, especially in nutritionally deficient patients, prolonged treatment, hepatic or renal disease. Cefuroxime readily crosses the placenta and is distributed in breast milk. No age-related precautions have been noted in children. Age-related renal impairment may require a dosage adjustment in elderly patients.

Although mild GI effects may be tolerable, an increase in their severity may indicate the onset of antibiotic-associated colitis. Assess the pattern of daily bowel activity and stool consistency, the mouth for white patches on the mucous membranes and tongue, signs and symptoms of superinfection including abdominal pain, moderate to severe diarrhea, severe anal or genital pruritus, and severe mouth soreness. Renal function should also be assessed.
Storage
Reconstituted oral suspension is stable for 10 days at room

temperature or refrigerated. The injection solution normally appears light yellow to amber; a darker color does not indicate loss of potency. Reconstituted solution is stable for 24 h at room temperature and 48 h if refrigerated. The IV infusion (piggyback) is stable for 24 h at room temperature, 7 days if refrigerated, and 26 wks if frozen. Thawed previously frozen premixed solution is stable for 24 h at room temperature and 21 days if refrigerated. Discard the solution if a precipitate forms.

Administration

Cefuroxime axetil tablets and powder for oral suspension are not bioequivalent and are therefore not substitutable on a mg/mg basis; bioavailability is greater with the tablets. Take cefuroxime tablets without regard to food. However, if GI upset occurs, give with food or milk. Avoid crushing tablets because they have a bitter taste. Give the oral suspension with food.

For IV use, to reconstitute, add 8 mL of sterile water for injection to each 750-mg vial, or 14 mL to each 1.5-g vial to provide a concentration of 100 mg/mL. For intermittent IV infusion (piggyback), further dilute with 50-100 mL of 0.9% NaCl or D5W. Administer the IV push over 3-5 min. Infuse the intermittent IV infusion (piggyback) over 15-60 min.

For IM use, to minimize patient discomfort, slowly inject the drug deep into the gluteus maximus rather than the lateral aspect of the thigh.

Celecoxib

sel-eh-cox′ib
(Celebrex, DisperDose, Panixine)
Do not confuse Celebrex, with Cerebyx, or Celexa.

CATEGORY AND SCHEDULE

Pregnancy Risk Category: C (D if used in third trimester or near delivery)

Classification: Nonsteroidal anti-inflammatory, analgesic, COX-2 inhibitor

MECHANISM OF ACTION

An NSAID that inhibits cyclo-oxygenase-2, the enzyme responsible for prostaglandin synthesis. Mechanism of action in treating familial adenomatous polyposis is unknown. *Therapeutic Effect:* Reduces inflammation and relieves pain.

PHARMACOKINETICS

Widely distributed. Protein binding: 97%. Metabolized in the liver. Primarily eliminated in feces. *Half-life:* 11.2 h.

AVAILABILITY

Capsules: 50 mg, 100 mg, 200 mg, 400 mg.

INDICATIONS AND DOSAGES
▶ **Osteoarthritis**
PO
Adults, Elderly. 200 mg/day as a single dose or 100 mg twice a day.
▶ **Rheumatoid arthritis**
PO
Adults, Elderly. 100-200 mg twice a day.
▶ **Acute pain, primary dysmenorrhea**
PO
Adults, Elderly. Initially, 400 mg with additional 200 mg on day 1, if

needed. Maintenance: 200 mg twice a day as needed.

▸ **Familial adenomatous polyposis**
PO
Adults, Elderly. 400 mg twice daily (with food).

▸ **Juvenile rheumatoid arthritis**
PO
Children 2 yr and older and weighing 10-25 kg. 50 mg twice daily.
Children 2 yr and older and weighing more than 25 kg. 100 mg twice daily.

▸ **Ankylosing spondylitis**
PO
Adults. 200 mg once daily or 100 mg twice daily. May increase to 400 mg/day.

▸ **Dose in moderate hepatic impairment**
Reduce dose 50%.

CONTRAINDICATIONS

Hypersensitivity to aspirin, NSAIDs, or sulfonamides; perioperative pain in the setting of coronary artery bypass graft surgery.

INTERACTIONS

Drug
Fluconazole: May increase celecoxib blood level.
Lithium: May increase lithium blood levels.
Warfarin: May increase the risk of bleeding.
Herbal
None known.
Food
None known.

DIAGNOSTIC TEST EFFECTS

May increase AST (SGOT) and ALT (SGPT) levels.

SIDE EFFECTS

Frequent (> 5%)
Diarrhea, dyspepsia, headache, hypertension, upper respiratory tract infection.

Occasional (1%-5%)
Abdominal pain, flatulence, nausea, back pain, peripheral edema, dizziness, rash.

SERIOUS REACTIONS

• None known.

PRECAUTIONS & CONSIDERATIONS

Be aware of the potential for increased risk of cardiovascular events and GI bleeding associated with celecoxib use. Caution is warranted with smokers and patients with active alcoholism, who have a history of peptic ulcer disease, who are receiving anticoagulant or steroid therapy, and who are elderly. It is unknown whether celecoxib crosses the placenta or is distributed in breast milk. Celecoxib should not be used during the third trimester of pregnancy because it may cause adverse effects in the fetus, such as premature closure of the ductus arteriosus. The safety and efficacy of celecoxib have not been established in children younger than 18 yr. No age-related precautions have been noted in elderly patients. Alcohol and aspirin should be avoided during celecoxib therapy because these substances increase the risk of GI bleeding.

Therapeutic response, such as decreased pain, stiffness, swelling, and tenderness, improved grip strength, and increased joint mobility, should be evaluated.

Administration
Celecoxib at dosages up to 200 mg twice daily can be administered without regard to timing of meals. Administer higher dosages (400 mg twice daily). with food to improve absorption. For patients with difficulty swallowing, the capsules may be opened and the contents sprinkled on applesauce.

Cellulose Sodium Phosphate
(Calcibind)
Do not confuse with cellulite.

CATEGORY AND SCHEDULE
Pregnancy Risk Category: C

Classification: Metabolics

MECHANISM OF ACTION
A nonabsorbable compound that alters urinary composition of calcium, magnesium, phosphate, and oxalate. Calcium binds to cellulose sodium phosphate, therefore preventing intestinal absorption of it. *Therapeutic Effect:* Prevents the formation of kidney stones.

PHARMACOKINETICS
Not absorbed from the GI tract. Eliminated in the feces.

AVAILABILITY
Powder for Reconstitution: 300 g (Calcibind).

INDICATIONS AND DOSAGES
▶ **Absorptive hypercalciuria type I**
PO
Adults, Elderly. Initially, 15 g/day (5 g with each meal). Decrease dosage to 10 g/day when urinary calcium is < 150 mg/day.

OFF-LABEL USES
Absorptive hypercalciuria type II.

CONTRAINDICATIONS
Primary or secondary hyperparathyroidism, including renal hypercalciuria (renal calcium leak), hypomagnesemic states (serum magnesium < 1.5 mg/dL), bone disease (osteoporosis, osteomalacia, osteitis), hypocalcemic states (e.g., hypoparathyroidism, intestinal malabsorption), normal or low intestinal absorption and renal excretion of calcium, enteric hyperoxaluria, and patients with high fasting urinary calcium or hypophosphatemia.

INTERACTIONS
Drug
Calcium-containing medications: May decrease effectiveness of cellulose sodium phosphate.
Magnesium: May decrease effectiveness of magnesium. Separate administration by 1 hour.
Herbal
None known.
Food
Milk, dairy products: May decrease effectiveness of cellulose sodium phosphate.
Foods high in oxalate (spinach, rhubarb, chocolate, brewed tea): May increase risk of hyperoxaluria, which decreases the effect of cellulose sodium phosphate.

DIAGNOSTIC TEST EFFECTS
None known.

SIDE EFFECTS
Occasional
GI disturbance, manifested by poor taste of the drug, loose bowel movements, diarrhea, dyspepsia.

SERIOUS REACTIONS
• Hyperoxaluria and hypomagnesiuria, which negate the beneficial effect of hypocalciuria on new stone formation, magnesium depletion, and depletion of trace metals (copper, zinc, iron) may occur.

PRECAUTIONS & CONSIDERATIONS
Caution should be used in patients with congestive heart failure or ascites.

Cellulose sodium phosphate is not recommended in pregnant women. It is unknown whether cellulose sodium phosphate is distributed in breast milk. Safety and efficacy of cellulose sodium phosphate have not been established in children < 16 yr of age.

Reduction in urinary calcium (< 200 mg/day) should be assessed every 3-6 mo. Magnesium, copper, zinc, iron, parathyroid hormone, and complete blood count (CBC) should be checked every 3-6 mo. Serum PTH should also be monitored at least once between the first 2 wks to 3 mo of treatment and adjusted or stopped if there is a rise in serum PTH above normal. Reduction in renal stone formation during therapy should be assessed.

Administration

Take with meals or within 30 min of meals. Cellulose sodium phosphate is usually taken with magnesium to replace dietary magnesium; however, the magnesium supplement should be taken 1 h before or after the cellulose sodium phosphate dose. Mix cellulose sodium phosphate with a large glass of water, fruit juice, or soft drink. Do not mix with milk or products that have electrolytes, such as Gatorade or Powerade.

Cephalexin

sef-a-lex'in
(Apo-Cephalex [CAN], Biocef, Ceporex [AUS], Ibilex [AUS], Keflex, Keftab, Novolexin [CAN])

CATEGORY AND SCHEDULE

Pregnancy Risk Category: B

Classification: Antibiotics, cephalosporin (first generation)

MECHANISM OF ACTION

A first-generation cephalosporin that binds to bacterial cell membranes and inhibits cell wall synthesis. *Therapeutic Effect:* Bactericidal.

PHARMACOKINETICS

Rapidly absorbed from the GI tract. Protein binding: 10%-15%. Widely distributed. Primarily excreted unchanged in urine. Moderately removed by hemodialysis. *Half-life:* 0.9-1.2 h (increased in impaired renal function).

AVAILABILITY

Powder for Oral Suspension: 125 mg/5 mL, 250 mg/5 mL.
Capsules or Tablets: 250 mg, 500 mg.

INDICATIONS AND DOSAGES

▸ **Bone infections, prophylaxis of rheumatic fever, follow-up to parenteral therapy**
PO
Adults, Elderly. 250-500 mg q6h up to 4 g/day.
▸ **Streptococcal pharyngitis, skin and skin-structure infections, uncomplicated cystitis**
PO
Adults, Elderly. 500 mg q12h.
▸ **Usual pediatric dosage**
Children. 25-100 mg/kg/day in 2-4 divided doses.
▸ **Otitis media**
PO
Children. 75-100 mg/kg/day in 4 divided doses.
▸ **Dosage in renal impairment**
After usual initial dose, dosing frequency is modified based on creatinine clearance and the severity of the infection.

Creatinine Clearance (mL/min)	Dosage Interval
10-40	Usual dose q8-12h
< 10	Usual dose q12-24h

CONTRAINDICATIONS
History of anaphylactic reaction to penicillins or hypersensitivity to cephalosporins.

INTERACTIONS
Drug
Probenecid: Increases serum concentration of cephalexin.
Herbal
None known.
Food
None known.

DIAGNOSTIC TEST EFFECTS
May increase INR, serum alkaline phosphatase, AST (SGOT), and ALT (SGPT) levels. May produce a positive direct or indirect Coombs' test. Interferes with crossmatching procedures and hematologic tests.

SIDE EFFECTS
Frequent
Oral candidiasis, mild diarrhea, mild abdominal cramping, vaginal candidiasis.
Occasional
Nausea, serum sickness-like reaction (marked by fever and joint pain; usually occurs after the second course of therapy and resolves after the drug is discontinued).
Rare
Allergic reaction (rash, pruritus, urticaria).

SERIOUS REACTIONS
• Antibiotic-associated colitis and other superinfections may result from altered bacterial balance.

• Nephrotoxicity may occur, especially in patients with preexisting renal disease.
• Patients with a history of allergies, especially to penicillin, are at increased risk for developing a severe hypersensitivity reaction, marked by severe pruritus, angioedema, bronchospasm, and anaphylaxis.

PRECAUTIONS & CONSIDERATIONS
Caution is warranted with history of GI disease (especially antibiotic-associated or ulcerative colitis), renal impairment, and concurrent use of nephrotoxic drugs. May be associated with increased INR, especially in nutritionally deficient patients, those undergoing prolonged treatment, and patients with hepatic or renal disease. Cephalexin readily crosses the placenta and is distributed in breast milk. No age-related precautions have been noted in children. Age-related renal impairment may require a dosage adjustment in elderly patients.

Although mild GI effects may be tolerable, an increase in their severity may indicate the onset of antibiotic-associated colitis. Assess the pattern of daily bowel activity and stool consistency, the mouth for white patches on the mucous membranes and tongue, signs and symptoms of superinfection including abdominal pain, moderate to severe diarrhea, severe anal or genital pruritus, and severe mouth soreness. Renal function should be assessed.
Storage
After reconstitution, the oral suspension is stable for 14 days if refrigerated.
Administration
! Space drug doses evenly around the clock.

Shake the oral suspension well before using. Take oral cephalexin without regard to meals. However, if GI upset occurs, give with food or milk.

Cetirizine
si-tear'a-zeen
(Reactine [CAN], Zyrtec)
Do not confuse Zyrtec with Zantac or Zyprexa.

CATEGORY AND SCHEDULE
Pregnancy Risk Category: B
OTC

Classification: Antihistamines, H_1, low sedating

MECHANISM OF ACTION
A second-generation piperazine that competes with histamine for H_1-receptor sites on effector cells in the GI tract, blood vessels, and respiratory tract. *Therapeutic Effect:* Prevents allergic response, produces mild bronchodilation, and blocks histamine-induced bronchitis.

PHARMACOKINETICS

Route	Onset	Peak	Duration
PO	< 4-8 h	< 1 h	24 h

Rapidly and almost completely absorbed from the GI tract (absorption not affected by food). Protein binding: 93%. Undergoes low first-pass metabolism; not extensively metabolized. Primarily excreted in urine (more than 80% as unchanged drug). *Half-life:* 6.5-10 h.

AVAILABILITY
Oral Solution: 5 mg/5 mL.
Tablets: 5 mg, 10 mg.
Tablets (Chewable): 5 mg, 10 mg.

INDICATIONS AND DOSAGES
▸ **Allergic rhinitis, urticaria**
PO
Adults, Elderly, Children older than 5 yr. Initially, 5-10 mg/day as a single or in 2 divided doses.
Children 2-5 yr. 2.5 mg/day. May increase up to 5 mg/day as a single or in 2 divided doses.
Children 12-23 mo. Initially, 2.5 mg/day. May increase up to 5 mg/day in 2 divided doses.
Children 6-11 mo. 2.5 mg once a day.
▸ **Dosage in renal or hepatic impairment**
For adult and elderly patients with renal impairment (creatinine clearance of 11-31 mL/min), receiving hemodialysis (creatinine clearance of < 7 mL/min), and those with hepatic impairment, dosage is decreased to 5 mg once a day.

CONTRAINDICATIONS
Hypersensitivity to cetirizine or hydroxyzine.

INTERACTIONS
Drug
Alcohol, other CNS depressants: May increase CNS depression.
Herbal
None known.
Food
None known.

DIAGNOSTIC TEST EFFECTS
May suppress wheal and flare reactions to antigen skin testing, unless drug is discontinued 4 days before testing.

SIDE EFFECTS
Occasional (2%-10%)
Pharyngitis; dry mucous membranes, nose, or throat; nausea and vomiting; abdominal pain;

headache; dizziness; fatigue; thickening of mucus; somnolence; photosensitivity; urine retention.

SERIOUS REACTIONS

• Children may experience paradoxical reactions, including restlessness, insomnia, euphoria, nervousness, and tremor.
• Dizziness, sedation, and confusion are more likely to occur in elderly patients.

PRECAUTIONS & CONSIDERATIONS

Caution is warranted with renal or hepatic impairment. Cetirizine use is not recommended during the early months of pregnancy. It is unknown whether cetirizine is excreted in breast milk. Breastfeeding is not recommended. Cetirizine is less likely to cause anticholinergic effects in children. Elderly patients are more likely to experience anticholinergic effects, such as dry mouth and urine retention, as well as dizziness, sedation, and confusion. Avoid drinking alcoholic beverages, prolonged exposure to sunlight, and tasks that require alertness or motor skills until response to the drug is established.

Drowsiness may occur at dosages > 10 mg/day. Therapeutic response should be monitored.

Storage

All dosage forms can be stored at room temperature.

Administration

Take cetirizine without regard to food. Chewable tablets should be throughly chewed.

Cetuximab
ceh-tux'ih-mab
(Erbitux)

C

CATEGORY AND SCHEDULE
Pregnancy Risk Category: C

Classification: Antineoplastics, monoclonal antibodies

MECHANISM OF ACTION
A monoclonal antibody that binds to the epidermal growth factor receptor (EGFR), a glycoprotein on normal and tumor cells, thus inhibiting cell growth and inducing apoptosis. *Therapeutic Effect:* Inhibits the growth and survival of tumor cells that overexpress EGFR.

PHARMACOKINETICS
Reaches steady-state levels by the third weekly infusion. Clearance decreases as dose increases. *Half-life:* 114 h (range, 75-188 h).

AVAILABILITY
Injection: 2 mg/mL.

INDICATIONS AND DOSAGES
▶ **Metastatic colorectal carcinoma, squamous cell carcinoma of the head and neck**
IV INFUSION
Adults, Elderly. Initially, 400 mg/m² over 2 h as a loading dose. Maintenance: 250 mg/m² infused over 60 min weekly.

CONTRAINDICATIONS
None known.

INTERACTIONS
Drug
None known.
Herbal
None known.

Food
None known.

DIAGNOSTIC TEST EFFECTS
May decrease WBC count, magnesium, calcium, potassium, hematocrit, and hemoglobin level.

Ⓓ IV INCOMPATIBILITIES
Do not mix cetuximab with any other medications.

SIDE EFFECTS
Frequent (25%-90%)
Acneiform rash, malaise, fever, nausea, diarrhea, constipation, headache, abdominal pain, anorexia, vomiting.
Occasional (10%-16%)
Nail disorder, back pain, stomatitis, peripheral edema, pruritus, cough, insomnia.
Rare (5%-9%)
Weight loss, depression, dyspepsia, conjunctivitis, alopecia.

SERIOUS REACTIONS
• Anemia occurs in 10% of patients.
• A severe infusion reaction, characterized by rapid onset of airway obstruction, a precipitous drop in blood pressure, and severe urticaria, occurs rarely.
• Dermatologic toxicity, pulmonary embolus, interstitial lung disease, leukopenia, and renal failure occur rarely.
• Cardiopulmonary arrest has been reported in patients receiving cetuximab in conjunction with radiation therapy.

PRECAUTIONS & CONSIDERATIONS
Caution is warranted with hypersensitivity to murine proteins and in patients with a history of coronary artery disease, heart failure, arrhythmias, or lung disease. Cetuximab crosses the placental barrier and may cause fetal harm or spontaneous abortion. Women should not breastfeed while taking cetuximab. The safety and efficacy of cetuximab have not been established in children. No age-related precautions have been noted in elderly patients. Vaccinations and contact with crowds, persons with a known infection, and anyone who has recently received a live-virus vaccine should be avoided. Sun exposure should be limited and sunscreen should be worn outdoors during cetuximab therapy because sunlight can exacerbate skin reactions.

Signs and symptoms of an infusion reaction, such as rapid onset of bronchospasm, hoarseness, hypotension, stridor, and urticaria, should be monitored. The first severe infusion reaction may occur during subsequent infusions. Skin should be assessed for evidence of dermatologic toxicity, such as dry skin, exfoliative dermatitis or rash, and inflammatory sequelae. Electrolytes, hemoglobin levels, and hematocrit levels should be monitored.
Storage
Refrigerate vials. Preparations in infusion containers are stable for up to 8 h at room temperature or 12 h if refrigerated. Discard any unused portion. The solution should appear clear and colorless; it may contain a small amount of visible white particulates.
Administration
! Premedicate the patient with 50 mg diphenhydramine IV. Cetuximab may be used as monotherapy or in combination with irinotecan. Do not give cetuximab by IV push or bolus.

Do not shake or dilute the vials. Infuse the drug using a low-protein-binding 0.22-μm in-line filter.

Give the first dose as a 120-min IV infusion. Administer maintenance infusions over 60 min. The maximum infusion rate is 5 mL/min. When administered in conjunction with radiation therapy in head and neck carcinoma, first dose is given 1 wk before initiation of radiation therapy and maintenance therapy is administered for the duration of radiation therapy with each infusion completed 1 h before radiation. Patient should be monitored closely for 1 h after each infusion.

Cevimeline

sev-im'el-ine
(Evoxac)
Do not confuse Evoxac with Eurax.

CATEGORY AND SCHEDULE

Pregnancy Risk Category: C

Classification: Cholinergic (muscarinic) agonist

MECHANISM OF ACTION

A cholinergic agonist that binds to muscarinic receptors of effector cells, thereby increasing secretion of exocrine glands, such as salivary glands. *Therapeutic Effect:* Relieves dry mouth.

PHARMACOKINETICS

Rapid absorption after oral administration, peak levels 1.5-2 h. Protein binding: 20%. Metabolized in liver by CYP2D6 and CYP3A4 isoenzymes. *Half-life:* 5 h. 84% excreted in urine within 24 h.

AVAILABILITY

Capsules: 30 mg.

INDICATIONS AND DOSAGES
▶ **Dry mouth associated with sjögren's syndrome**
PO
Adults. 30 mg 3 times a day.

CONTRAINDICATIONS

Acute iritis, angle-closure glaucoma, uncontrolled asthma.

INTERACTIONS

Drug
Amiodarone, diltiazem, erythromycin, fluoxetine, itraconazole, ketoconazole, paroxetine, quinidine, ritonavir, verapamil: May increase the effects of cevimeline.
Atropine, phenothiazines, tricyclic antidepressants: May decrease the effects of cevimeline.
β-Blockers: May increase the risk of conduction disturbances.
Herbal
None known.
Food
All foods: Decreases the absorption rate of cevimeline.

DIAGNOSTIC TEST EFFECTS

None known.

SIDE EFFECTS

Frequent (11%-19%)
Diaphoresis, headache, nausea, sinusitis, rhinitis, upper respiratory tract infection, diarrhea.
Occasional (3%-10%)
Dyspepsia, abdominal pain, cough, urinary track infection, vomiting, back pain, rash, dizziness, fatigue.
Rare (1%-2%)
Skeletal pain, insomnia, hot flashes, excessive salivation, rigors, anxiety.

SERIOUS REACTIONS

• Cevimeline use may result in decreased visual acuity, especially at night, and impaired depth perception.

PRECAUTIONS & CONSIDERATIONS

Caution is warranted in patients with cardiovascular disease, congestive heart failure, asthma, chronic bronchitis, COPD, cholecystitis, biliary obstruction, cholelithiasis, GI ulcers, seizure disorders, Parkinson disease, urinary tract or bladder obstruction, and a history of nephrolithiasis. Avoid driving at night or performing hazardous duties in reduced lighting because cevimeline use may decrease visual acuity or impair depth perception. Adequate hydration should be maintained to prevent dehydration. Vital signs should be monitored.

Storage
Store at room temperature.

Administration
Take cevimeline without regard to food. Administration with food may decrease GI upset.

Charcoal, Activated
(Actidose-Aqua, Actidose with Sorbitol, Aqueous Charcodote [CAN], CharcoAid-G, Charcoal Plus DS, Charcocaps, EZ-Char, Kerr Insta-Char, Liqui-Char)

CATEGORY AND SCHEDULE
Pregnancy Risk Category: C

Classification: Antidiarrheal, antidote, antiflatulent

MECHANISM OF ACTION
An antidote that adsorbs (detoxifies) ingested toxic substances, irritants, intestinal gas. *Therapeutic Effect:* Inhibits GI absorption and absorbs intestinal gas.

PHARMACOKINETICS
Not orally absorbed from the GI tract. Not metabolized. Excreted in feces as charcoal. *Half-life:* Unknown.

AVAILABILITY
Capsules, Activated: 260 mg (Charcocaps).
Granules, Activated: 15 g (CharcoAid-G).
Liquid, Activated: 15 g (Actidose-Aqua, Liqui-Char), 25 g (Actidose-Aqua, Kerr Insta-Char, Liqui-Char), 50 g (Actidose-Aqua, Kerr Insta-Char).
Liquid, Activated: 25 g (Actidose with Sorbitol, Liqui-Char, Kerr Insta-Char), 50 g (Actidose with Sorbitol, Liqui-Char, Kerr Insta-Char).
Pellets, Activated: 25 g (EZ-Char).
Powder for Suspension, Activated: 30 g, 240 g.
Tablets, Activated: 250 mg (Charcoa Plus DS).

INDICATIONS AND DOSAGES
▸ **Acute poisoning**
PO
Adults, Elderly, Children 12 yr and older. Give 30-100 g as slurry (30 g in at least 8 oz H_2O) or 12.5-50 g in aqueous or sorbitol suspension. Usually given as single dose.
Children more than 1 yr and < 12 yr. 25-50 g as a single dose. Smaller doses (10-25 g) may be used in children aged 1-5 yr because of smaller gut lumen capacity.

CONTRAINDICATIONS
Intestinal obstruction, GI tract that is not anatomically intact, patients at risk of hemorrhage or GI perforation. If use would increase risk and severity of aspiration; not effective for cyanide, mineral acids, caustic alkalis, organic solvents, iron, ethanol, methanol poisoning, lithium. Do not use charcoal with sorbitol in patients with fructose intolerance; charcoal with sorbitol not recommended in children

younger than 1 yr of age or in persons with access hypersensitivity to charcoal or any component of the formation.

INTERACTIONS
Drug
Orally administered medications: May decrease absorption of orally administered medications.
Ipecac: May decrease the effect of ipecac.
Herbal
None known.
Food
Ice cream, sherbet, marmalade, milk: May reduce the effects of charcoal.

DIAGNOSTIC TEST EFFECTS
None known.

SIDE EFFECTS
Occasional
Diarrhea, GI discomfort, intestinal gas.

SERIOUS REACTIONS
• Hypernatremia, hypokalemia, and hypermagnesemia may occur with coadministration of cathartics.

PRECAUTIONS & CONSIDERATIONS
Caution should be used with decreased peristalsis. It is unknown whether charcoal crosses the placenta or is distributed in breast milk. Safety and efficacy of charcoal have not been established in children < 1 yr old. There are no age-related precautions noted for elderly patients. Be aware that charcoal causes the stools to turn black.

Be aware that charcoal may cause vomiting, which is hazardous in petroleum distillate and caustic ingestions. Be aware that vomiting should be induced with ipecac before administering activated charcoal because charcoal absorbs ipecac

syrup. Be aware that if charcoal and sorbitol are administered, doses should be limited to prevent excessive fluid and electrolyte loss.
Storage
Store in closed container because it absorbs gases from air.
Administration
Charcoal is most effective when administered within 1 h of ingestion for most ingestions. Flavoring agents, such as chocolate, can enhance charcoal's palatability.

Be aware that about 10 g of activated charcoal for each 1 g of toxin is considered adequate but may require multiple doses. If sorbitol is also used, sorbitol dose should not exceed 1.5 g/kg. When using multiple doses of charcoal, sorbitol should be given with every other dose (not to exceed 2 doses/day).

Be aware that if treatment includes ipecac syrup, vomiting should be induced before administration of charcoal.

Chloral Hydrate
klor-al hye'drate
(Aquachloral Supprettes, PMS-Chloral Hydrate [CAN], Somnote)

CATEGORY AND SCHEDULE
Pregnancy Risk Category: C
DEA Schedule IV

Classification: Sedatives/hypnotics

MECHANISM OF ACTION
A nonbarbiturate chloral derivative that produces CNS depression. *Therapeutic Effect:* Induces quiet, deep sleep, with only a slight decrease in respiratory rate and BP.

C

PHARMACOKINETICS
Rapid absorption after oral administration, peak levels 30-45 min. Duration: 2-5 h. Metabolized to trichloroethanol in liver and other tissues and, to a lesser extent, trichloroacetic acid, in liver. *Half-life:* 7-9.5 h. Glucuronide conjugate excreted in urine.

AVAILABILITY
Capsules (Somnote): 500 mg.
Syrup: 250 mg/5 mL, 500 mg/5 mL.
Suppositories (Aquachloral Supprettes): 3254 mg, 500 mg, 650 mg.

INDICATIONS AND DOSAGES
▶ **Premedication for dental or medical procedures**
PO, RECTAL
Adults. 0.5-1 g. Maximum: 2g.
Children. 75 mg/kg up to 1 g total.
▶ **Premedication for EEG, CT scan, etc**
PO, RECTAL
Adults. 0.5-1.5 g. Maximum: 2g.
Children. 25-50 mg/kg/dose 30-60 min prior to EEG. May repeat in 30 min. Maximum: 1.5 g for children.

CONTRAINDICATIONS
Gastritis, marked hepatic or renal impairment, severe cardiac disease.

INTERACTIONS
Drug
Alcohol, other CNS depressants: May increase the effects of chloral hydrate.
Furosemide (IV): May alter BP and cause diaphoresis if given within 24 h after chloral hydrate.
Warfarin: May increase the effect of warfarin.
Herbal
None known.
Food
None known.

DIAGNOSTIC TEST EFFECTS
None known.

SIDE EFFECTS
Occasional
Gastric irritation (nausea, vomiting, flatulence, diarrhea), rash, sleepwalking.
Rare
Headache, paradoxical CNS hyperactivity or nervousness in children, excitement or restlessness in elderly patients, particularly in patients with pain.

SERIOUS REACTIONS
• Overdose may produce somnolence, confusion, slurred speech, severe incoordination, respiratory depression, and coma.

PRECAUTIONS & CONSIDERATIONS
Caution is warranted in patients with clinical depression, patients with a history of drug abuse, patients with porphyria, and neonates. Do not drive if taking chloral hydrate before a procedure. BP, pulse rate, and respiratory rate, rhythm, and depth should be assessed immediately before and during chloral hydrate use. Elderly patients should be monitored for paradoxical reactions, such as excitability.
Storage
Store suppositories at room temperature; do not refrigerate them. Store capsules and syrup at room temperature.
Administration
! Always verify a child's mg/kg dosage to avoid serious overdose. Take chloral hydrate capsules with a full glass of water or fruit juice. Swallow the capsules whole and do not chew them. Dilute the dose of syrup in water to minimize gastric irritation. May dilute in juice to mask unpleasant taste.

For rectal use, if the suppository is too soft to insert, chill in the refrigerator for 30 min or run cold water over it before removing the foil wrapper. First remove the foil wrapper and moisten the suppository with cold water. Lie down on side and use finger to push the suppository well up into the rectum.

Chloramphenicol
klor-am-fen'i-kole
(Chloromycetin, Chlorsig [AUS])
Do not confuse chloramphenicol with chlorambucil.

CATEGORY AND SCHEDULE
Pregnancy Risk Category: C

Classification: Anti-infectives, ophthalmics, otics, antibiotics, chloramphenicol and derivatives

MECHANISM OF ACTION
A dichloroacetic acid derivative that inhibits bacterial protein synthesis by binding to bacterial ribosomal receptor sites. *Therapeutic Effect:* Bacteriostatic (may be bactericidal in high concentrations).

PHARMACOKINETICS
Widely distributed, crosses blood-brain barrier. Extensively metabolized to inactive metabolites, primarily via glucuronidation. *Half-life:* 1.6-3.3 h (prolonged in renal and hepatic impairment).

AVAILABILITY
Powder for Injection: 100 mg/mL.

INDICATIONS AND DOSAGES
▸ **Mild to moderate infections caused by organisms resistant to other less toxic antibiotics**

IV
Adults, Elderly. 50-100 mg/kg/day in divided doses q6h. Maximum: 4 g/day.
Children older than 1 mo. 50-75 mg/kg/day in divided doses q6h. Maximum: 4 g/day.
▸ **Meningitis**
IV
Adults, Children older than 1 mo. 75-100 mg/kg/day in divided doses q6h.

CONTRAINDICATIONS
Hypersensitivity to chloramphenicol.

INTERACTIONS
Drug
Anticonvulsants, bone marrow depressants: May increase myelosuppression.
Clindamycin, erythromycin: May antagonize the effects of these drugs.
Oral antidiabetics: May increase the effects of these drugs.
Phenobarbital, phenytoin, Warfarin: May increase blood concentrations of these drugs.
Vitamin B_{12}: May decrease the effects of vitamin B_{12} in patients with pernicious anemia.
Herbal
None known.
Food
None known.

DIAGNOSTIC TEST EFFECTS
Therapeutic blood level: 10-20 mcg/mL; toxic blood level: > 25 mcg/mL. When administered with iron salts, may increase serum iron levels.

🚫 IV INCOMPATIBILITIES
In general, do not mix chloramphenicol with other medications.

SIDE EFFECTS

Occasional
Systemic: Nausea, vomiting, diarrhea.

Rare
"Gray baby" syndrome in neonates (abdominal distention, blue-gray skin color, cardiovascular collapse, unresponsiveness), rash, shortness of breath, confusion, headache, optic neuritis (blurred vision, eye pain), peripheral neuritis (numbness and weakness in feet and hands).

SERIOUS REACTIONS

• Superinfection from bacterial or fungal overgrowth may occur.
• There is a narrow margin between effective therapy and toxic levels producing blood dyscrasias.
• Myelosuppression, with resulting aplastic anemia, hypoplastic anemia, and pancytopenia, may occur weeks or months later.
• Opticneuritis may cause blindness.

PRECAUTIONS & CONSIDERATIONS

Caution is warranted with myelosuppression, glucose-6-phosphate dehydrogenase deficiency, or renal or hepatic impairment, and in those who have previously undergone cytotoxic drug therapy or radiation therapy. Caution should be used in children younger than 2 yr.

Concurrent use of other drugs that cause myelosuppression should be determined before therapy because chloramphenicol should not be given concurrently with these drugs, if possible. Baseline blood studies should also be determined before beginning chloramphenicol therapy.

Nausea, vomiting, and visual disturbances should be reported. Pattern of daily bowel activity and stool consistency, mental status, and skin for rash should be assessed. Be alert for signs and symptoms of superinfection, such as anal or genital pruritus, a change in the oral mucosa, diarrhea, and increased fever. Know and monitor the drug's therapeutic blood level, which is 10-20 mcg/mL; toxic blood level is > 25 mcg/mL.

Storage
Store vials at room temperature.

Administration
Space drug doses evenly around the clock and continue for the full course of treatment.

Expect to change therapy to an antibiotic of less risk as soon as possible. Prepare IV injection by adding 10 mL of sterile water for injection on dextrose 5 % into the 1-g vial (concentration: 100 mg/mL). Withdraw correct dose. Inject dose over at least a 1-min interval.

Chlordiazepoxide

klor-dye-az-e-pox′ide
(Apo-Chlordiazepoxide [CAN], Librium, Novopoxide [CAN])
Do not confuse Librium with Librax.

CATEGORY AND SCHEDULE

Pregnancy Risk Category: D
Controlled substance schedule IV

Classification: Anxiolytics, benzodiazepines

MECHANISM OF ACTION

A benzodiazepine that enhances the action of the inhibitory neurotransmitter γ-aminobutyric acid in the CNS. *Therapeutic Effect:* Produces anxiolytic effect.

PHARMACOKINETICS
Slow onset after oral
administration, peak levels 2 h.
Metabolized in liver (active
metabolites). *Half-life:* 24-48 h.
Metabolites excreted in urine.

AVAILABILITY
Capsules: 5 mg, 10 mg, 25 mg.

INDICATIONS AND DOSAGES
▸ **Alcohol withdrawal symptoms**
PO
Adults, Elderly. 50-100 mg. May
repeat q2-4h. Maximum:
300 mg/24 h.
▸ **Anxiety**
PO
Adults. 15-100 mg/day in
3-4 divided doses.
Elderly. 5 mg 2-4 times a day.
▸ **Preoperative apprehension
and anxiety**
PO
Adults. 5-10 mg 3-4 times/day on
days preceding surgery.
▸ **Usual pediatric dose (anxiety)**
Children 6 yr of age and older.
5 mg 2-4 times/daily, may increase to
10 mg 2-3 times/daily.
Adjustment for renal impairment:
If creatinine clearance is less than
10 mL/min, reduce usual dose
by 50%.

CONTRAINDICATIONS
Acute alcohol intoxication, acute
angle-closure glaucoma.

INTERACTIONS
Drug
Other CNS depressants: May
increase CNS depression.
Herbal
Kava kava, valerian: May increase
CNS depression.
Food
Alcohol: May increase CNS
depression.

DIAGNOSTIC TEST EFFECTS
None known. Therapeutic serum
drug level is 1-3 mcg/mL; toxic
serum drug level is > 5 mcg/mL.

SIDE EFFECTS
Frequent
Somnolence, ataxia, dizziness,
confusion (particularly in elderly or
debilitated patients).
Occasional
Rash, peripheral edema, GI
disturbances.
Rare
Paradoxical CNS reactions, such
as hyperactivity or nervousness
in children and excitement or
restlessness in elderly patients
(generally noted during first 2 wks of
therapy, particularly in presence of
uncontrolled pain).

SERIOUS REACTIONS
• Abrupt or too rapid withdrawal may
result in pronounced restlessness,
irritability, insomnia, hand tremors,
abdominal or muscle cramps,
diaphoresis, vomiting, and seizures.
• Overdosage results in somnolence,
confusion, diminished reflexes, and
coma.

PRECAUTIONS & CONSIDERATIONS
Caution is warranted with impaired
renal or hepatic function. Drowsiness
may occur. Change positions slowly
from recumbent to sitting before
standing to prevent dizziness.
Alcohol and tasks that require mental
alertness or motor skills should also
be avoided. Autonomic responses,
such as cold, clammy hands and
diaphoresis, and motor responses,
such as agitation, trembling, and
tension, should be assessed. BP,
pulse rate, and respiratory rate,
rhythm, and depth should be
monitored immediately before giving
the drug.

C

Administration
! Expect to use the smallest effective chlordiazepoxide dose in elderly or debilitated patients and those with hepatic disease.

Take orally without regard to meals.

Do not abruptly discontinue after long-term therapy.

Chlorhexidine Gluconate
klor-hex´-ih-deen gloo´-ko-nate
(Chlorhexidine Mouthwash [AUS], Chlorhexidine Obstetric Lotion[AUS], Chlorohex Gel [AUS], Chlorohex Gel Forte [AUS], Chlorohex Mouth Rinse [AUS], Peridex, PerioChip, PerioGard, Perisol)

CATEGORY AND SCHEDULE
Pregnancy Risk Category: C

Classification: Anti-infective

MECHANISM OF ACTION
An antiseptic and antimicrobial agent that is active against a broad spectrum of microbes. The chlorhexidine molecule, due to its positive charge, reacts with the microbial cell surface, destroys the integrity of the cell membrane, penetrates the cell, and precipitates the cytoplasm, and the cell dies. *Therapeutic Effect:* Causes cell death.

PHARMACOKINETICS
Initially, the chlorhexidine gluconate dental chip releases approximately 40% of the drug within the first 24 h, then releases the remainder in an almost linear fashion for 7–10 days.

Approximately 30% of the active ingredient, chlorhexidine gluconate, is retained in the oral cavity following oral rinsing. This retained drug is slowly released into the oral fluids. Poorly absorbed from the GI tract. Primarily excreted in feces. *Half-life:* Unknown.

AVAILABILITY
Chip: 2.5 mg.
Oral Rinse: 0.12%.
Topical Solution: 2%, 4%.
Topical Rinse: 0.5%.
Topical Wipes: 0.5%.
Topical Sponge: 4%.

INDICATIONS AND DOSAGES
▸ **Gingivitis**
ORAL RINSE
Adults, Elderly. Swish and spit for 30 s twice daily.
▸ **Periodontitis**
DENTAL IMPLANT (PERIOCHIP)
Adults, Elderly. One chip is inserted into a periodontal pocket; insert a new chip q3mo; maximum of 8 chips per dental visit.
▸ **Topical cleansing of skin**
CLEANSER
Rinse with water, apply chlorhexidine and wash, rinse with water.
PREOPERATIVE SKIN PREPARATION
Apply to site and swab for 2 min. Dry with sterile towel. Repeat.

OFF-LABEL USES
Acute aphthous ulcers and denture stomatitis. (dental rinse).

CONTRAINDICATIONS
Hypersensitivity to chlorhexidine gluconate or any component of the formulation.

INTERACTIONS
Drug
None known.
Herbal and Food
None known.

DIAGNOSTIC TEST EFFECTS
None known.

SIDE EFFECTS
Occasional
Oral rinse: Altered taste, staining of tooth, toothache, increased tartar on teeth.
Topical: Skin erythema and roughness, dryness, sensitization, allergic reactions.

SERIOUS REACTIONS
• Anaphylaxis has been reported.

PRECAUTIONS & CONSIDERATIONS
Oral rinse not intended for periodontitis. Topical solution should not be used for preoperative preparation of the face, head, or lumbar puncture sites. Avoid use of topical solution in children < 2 yr of age.
Storage
Store oral rinse, dental implant, and topical solutions at room temperature. Protect from light and freezing.
Administration
Avoid flossing for 10 days after chip insertion.

Chloroquine/ Chloroquine Phosphate
klor'oh-kwin
(Aralen [CAN], Aralen hydrochloride) (Aralen phosphate)

CATEGORY AND SCHEDULE
Pregnancy Risk Category: C

Classification: Antimalarial, antiprotazoal.

MECHANISM OF ACTION
An amebecide that concentrates in parasite acid vesicles and may interfere with parasite protein synthesis. *Therapeutic Effect:* Increases pH and inhibits parasite growth.

PHARMACOKINETICS
Rate of absorption is variable. Chloroquine is almost completely absorbed from the GI tract. Protein binding: 50%-65%. Widely distributed into body tissues such as eyes, heart, kidneys, liver, and lungs. Partially metabolized to active de-ethylated metabolites (principal metabolite is desethylchloroquine). Excreted in urine. Removed by hemodialysis. *Half-life:* 1-2 mo.

AVAILABILITY
Tablets: 250 mg, 500 mg (Aralen).

INDICATIONS AND DOSAGES
▸ **Chloroquine phosphate**
Treatment of malaria (acute attack): Dose (mg base)
PO

Dose	Time	Adults (mg)	Children (mg/kg)
Initial	Day 1	600	10
Second	6 h later	300	5
Third	Day 2	300	5
Fourth	Day 3	300	5

▸ **Malaria prophylaxis**
PO
Adults. 300 mg (base)/wk on same day each week beginning 2 wks before exposure; continue for 6-8 wks after leaving endemic area.
Children. 5 mg (base)/kg/wk with start duration as for adults.
▸ **Amebiasis**
PO
Adults. 1 g (600 mg base) daily for 2 days; then 500 mg (300 mg base)/day for at least 2-3 wks.

OFF-LABEL USES

Treatment of rheumatoid arthritis, discoid lupus erythematosus, solar urticaria.

CONTRAINDICATIONS

Hypersensitivity to 4-aminoquinoline compounds, retinal or visual field changes.

INTERACTIONS

Drug
Alcohol: May increase GI irritation.
Ampicillin: May reduce the absorption of ampicillin. Separate administration by 2 h.
Antacids and kaolin: May be decreased due to GI binding with kaolin or magnesium trisilicate.
Cimetidine: May increase levels of chloroquine.
Cyclosporine: May increase cyclosporine concentrations.
CYP2D6 inhibitors (chlorpromazine, delavirdine, fluoxetine, miconazole, paroxetine, pergolide, quinidine, quinine, ritonavir, ropinirole): May increase the levels and effects of chloroquine.
CYP2D6 substrates (amphetamines, selected β-blockers, dextromethorphan, fluoxetine, lidocaine, mirtazapine, nefazodone, paroxetine, risperidone, ritonavir, thioridazine, tricyclic antidepressants, venlafaxine): May increase the levels and effects of CYP2D6 substrates.
CYP2D6 prodrug substrates: Chloroquine may decrease the levels and effects of CYP2D6 prodrug substrates.
CYP3A4 inducers (aminoglutethimide, carbamazepine, nafcillin, nevirapine, phenobarbital, phenytoin, and rifamycins): CYP3A4 inducers may decrease the levels and effects of chloroquine.

CYP3A4 inhibitors (azole antifungals, ciprofloxacin, clarithromycin, diclofenac, doxycycline, erythromycin, imatinib, isoniazid, nefazodone, nicardipine, propofol, protease inhibitors, quinidine, and verapamil): May increase the levels and effects of chloroquine.
Mefloguine: May increase risk of convulsions.
Penicillamine: May increase concentration of penicillamine and increase risk of hematologic, renal, or severe skin reaction.
Praziquantel: May decrease praziquantel concentrations.
Herbal and Food
None known.

DIAGNOSTIC TEST EFFECTS

Acute decrease in hematocrit, hemoglobin, and RBC count may occur.

SIDE EFFECTS

Frequent
Mild transient headache, anorexia, nausea, vomiting.
Occasional
Visual disturbances (blurring, difficulty focusing); nervousness; fatigue; pruritus, especially of palms, soles, scalp; bleaching of hair; irritability; personality changes; diarrhea; skin eruptions.
Rare
Abdominal cramps, headache, hypotension.

SERIOUS REACTIONS

• Ocular toxicity and ototoxicity have been reported.
• Prolonged therapy: Peripheral neuritis and neuromyopathy, hypotension, ECG changes, agranulocytosis, aplastic anemia, thrombocytopenia, convulsions, psychosis.

• Overdosage includes symptoms of headache, vomiting, visual disturbance, drowsiness, convulsions, hypokalemia followed by cardiovascular collapse, and death.

PRECAUTIONS & CONSIDERATIONS
Caution is warranted with alcoholism, severe blood disorders, liver disease, neurologic disorders, auditory damage, porphyria, psoriasis, and G6PD deficiency. It is unknown whether chloroquine crosses the placenta or is distributed in breast milk. Be aware that children are especially susceptible to chloroquine fatalities. There are no age-related precautions noted in elderly patients.

History of allergies, especially to antibiotics, should be determined before giving chloroquine.

Visual disturbances should be reported immediately.
Storage
Store tablets at room temperature.
Administration
Chloroquine PO_4 500 mg = 300 mg base.

Give oral chloroquine with food or milk to minimize GI irritation. May mix with chocolate syrup or enclose in gelatin capsules to mask the bitter taste.

Chlorothiazide
klor-oh-thye'a-zide
(Diuril)

CATEGORY AND SCHEDULE
Pregnancy Risk Category: C

Classification: Diuretics, thiazide

MECHANISM OF ACTION
A sulfonamide derivative that acts as a thiazide diuretic and antihypertensive. As a diuretic, it blocks the reabsorption of water and the electrolytes sodium and potassium at the cortical diluting segment of the distal tubule. As an antihypertensive, it reduces plasma; extracellular fluid volume decreases peripheral vascular resistance (PVR) by direct effect on blood vessels.
Therapeutic Effect: Promotes diuresis, reduces BP.

PHARMACOKINETICS
Poorly absorbed from the GI tract. Not metabolized. Primarily excreted unchanged in urine. Not removed by hemodialysis.
Half-life: 45-120 min.

AVAILABILITY
Powder for Injection, Lyophilized: 0.5 g.
Oral Suspension: 250 mg/5 mL (Diuril).
Tablets: 250 mg, 500 mg (Diuril).

INDICATIONS AND DOSAGES
▸ **Edema, hypertension**
PO
Adults. 0.5-1 g 1-2 times/day for hypertension. For edema, may give every other day or 3-5 days/wk.
Children 12 yr and older.
10-20 mg/kg/dose in divided doses q8-12h. Maximum: 2 g/day.
Children 2-12 yr. 10-20 mg/kg/day in divided doses q12-24 h; not to exceed 1 g/day.
Children 6 mo to 2 yr.
10-20 mg/kg/day in divided doses q12-24h. Maximum: 375 mg/day.
Children younger than 6 mo.
20-30 mg/kg/day in divided doses q12h. Maximum: 375 mg/day.
▸ **Hypertension/Edema**
IV
Adults. 0.5-1 g in divided doses q12-24h. For edema, may give every other day on 3-5 days/wk.

OFF-LABEL USES

Treatment of diabetes insipidus, prevention of calcium-containing renal stones.

CONTRAINDICATIONS

Anuria, history of hypersensitivity to sulfonamides or thiazide diuretics, renal decompensation.

INTERACTIONS

Drug

Cholestyramine, colestipol: May decrease the absorption and effects of chlorothiazide.

Digoxin: May increase the risk of toxicity of digoxin caused by hypokalemia.

Lithium: May increase the risk of toxicity of lithium.

NSAIDs: May decrease the absorption and effects of chlorothiazide.

Probenecid: May increase concentrations of chlorothiazide.

Herbal

Ginkgo biloba: May increase BP.

Licorice: May increase risk of hypokalemia and decrease effectiveness of chlorothiazide.

Ma huang: May decrease hypotensive effect of chlorothiazide.

Yohimbe: May decrease effects of chlorothiazide.

Food

None known.

DIAGNOSTIC TEST EFFECTS

None known.

SIDE EFFECTS

Expected. Increase in urine frequency and volume.

Frequent

Potassium depletion.

Occasional

Postural hypotension, headache, GI disturbances, photosensitivity reaction, muscle spasms, alopecia, rash, urticaria.

SERIOUS REACTIONS

• Vigorous diuresis may lead to profound water loss and electrolyte depletion, resulting in hypokalemia, hyponatremia, and dehydration.

• Acute hypotensive episodes may occur.

• Hyperglycemia may be noted during prolonged therapy.

• GI upset, pancreatitis, dizziness, paresthesias, headache, blood dyscrasias, pulmonary edema, allergic pneumonitis, and dermatologic reactions occur rarely.

• Overdosage can lead to lethargy and coma without changes in electrolytes or hydration.

PRECAUTIONS & CONSIDERATIONS

Caution should be used with diabetes mellitus, electrolyte imbalance, hyperuricemia or gout, hypotension, systemic lupus erythematosus, hypercholesterolemia, impaired liver function, and severe renal disease. Chlorothiazide crosses the placenta, and a small amount is distributed in breast milk. Breastfeeding is not recommended in this patient population. Safety and efficacy of IV chlorothiazide have not been established in children and infants. Be aware that elderly patients may be more sensitive to the drug's electrolyte and hypotensive effects. Age-related renal impairment may require caution in elderly patients.

Frequency and volume of urination are expected to increase. Be aware that chlorothiazide may aggravate digitalis toxicity. Be aware that sensitivity reactions may occur with or without history of allergy or asthma. Skin should be protected from sunlight.

Hypokalemia may result in change in mental status, muscle

cramps, nausea, tachycardia, tremor, vomiting, and weakness.

Hyponatremia may result in clammy and cold skin, confusion, and thirst. Be especially alert for potassium depletion in persons taking digoxin, such as cardiac arrhythmias. Foods high in potassium, such as apricots, bananas, legumes, meat, orange juice, white and sweet potatoes, and raisins, and whole grains, such as cereals, should be eaten during treatment.

Storage

Store at room temperature.

Administration

May take with food or milk if GI upset occurs, preferably with breakfast to help prevent nocturia. Shake oral suspension well before use.

A fresh solution for injection should be prepared before each administration because chlorothiazide does not contain preservatives. Discard unused portion. Do not administer subcutaneously or intramuscularly. May be given slowly by direct IV injection or infusion. Reconstitute with 18 mL sterile water for injection for a final concentration of 28 mg/mL. For IV infusion, may add to dextrose 5% or 0.9% Nacl injection solutions.

Chlorpheniramine
klor-fen-ir´a-meen
(Aller-Chlor, Chlor-Trimeton, Chlor-Trimeton Allergy, Chlor-Trimeton Allergy 12 Hour, Chlorphen, Chlorate, Chlor-Trimeton Allergy 8 Hour, Chlor-Tripolon [CAN], Diabetic Tussin Allergy Relief)
Do not confuse with chlorpromazine or chlorpropamide.

CATEGORY AND SCHEDULE
Pregnancy Risk Category: C
OTC (tablets, syrup)

Classification: Antihistamines, H₁

MECHANISM OF ACTION
A propylamine derivative antihistamine that competes with histamine for histamine receptor sites on cells in the blood vessels, GI tract, and respiratory tract. *Therapeutic Effect:* Inhibits symptoms associated with seasonal allergic rhinitis such as increased mucus production and sneezing.

PHARMACOKINETICS
Well absorbed after PO administration. Food delays absorption. Widely distributed. Metabolized in liver. Primarily excreted in urine. Not removed by dialysis. *Half-life:* 20 h.

AVAILABILITY
Syrup: 2 mg/5 mL (Aller-Chlor, Diabetic Tussin Allergy Relief [sugar free]).
Tablets: 4 mg (Aller-Chlor, Chlorate, Chlorphen) Chlor-Trimeton.
Tablets (Sustained-Release): 8 mg (Chlor-Trimeton Allergy 8 Hour), 12 mg (Chlor-Trimeton Allergy 12 Hour), 16 mg (Efidac 24).

Tablets (Chewable): 2 mg.
Capsules (Extended Release):
8 mg, 12 mg.
Suspension: 4 mg/5 mL, 8 mg/5 mL.
also *Oral Drops Suspension:* 2 mg/mL.

INDICATIONS AND DOSAGES
▸ **Allergic rhinitis, common cold**
PO
Adults, Elderly. 4 mg q6-8h or
8-12 mg (sustained-release) q8-12h
or 16 mg (sustained release) q24h.
Maximum: 24 mg/day.
Children 12 yr and older. 4 mg
q6-8h or 8 mg (sustained-release)
q12h. Maximum: 24 mg/day.
Children 6-11 yr. 2 mg q4-6h.
Maximum: 12 mg/day.

CONTRAINDICATIONS
Hypersensitivity to chlorpheniramine
or its components; MAOI therapy;
breastfeeding; newborn or premature
infants.

INTERACTIONS
Drug
**Alcohol, central nervous system
(CNS) depressants:** May increase
CNS depressant effects.
Anticholinergics: May increase
anticholinergic effects.
MAOIs: May increase anticholinergic
and CNS depressant effects.
Phenytoin, fosphenytoin: May
increase the risk of phenytoin toxicity.
Procarbazine: May increase CNS
depressant effects.
Herbal and Food
None known.

DIAGNOSTIC TEST EFFECTS
None known.

SIDE EFFECTS
Frequent
Drowsiness; dizziness; muscular
weakness; hypotension; dry mouth,
nose, throat, and lips; urinary

retention; thickening of bronchial
secretions.
Elderly: Sedation, dizziness,
hypotension.
Occasional
Epigastric distress, flushing, visual
or hearing disturbances, paresthesia,
diaphoresis, chills.

SERIOUS REACTIONS
• Children may experience dominant
paradoxical reactions, including
restlessness, insomnia, euphoria,
nervousness, and tremors.
• Overdosage in children may result
in hallucinations, seizures, and death.
• Hypersensitivity reactions, such
as eczema, pruritus, rash, cardiac
disturbances, and photosensitivity,
may occur.
• Overdosage may vary from CNS
depression, including sedation,
apnea, hypotension, cardiovascular
collapse, and death, to severe
paradoxical reaction, such as
hallucinations, tremor, and seizures.

PRECAUTIONS & CONSIDERATIONS
Caution is warranted with
asthma, cardiovascular disease,
chronic obstructive pulmonary
disease (COPD), hypertension,
hyperthyroidism, narrow-angle
glaucoma, increased intraocular
pressure (IOP), peptic ulcer
disease, prostatic hypertrophy,
pyloroduodenal or bladder
neck obstruction, and seizure
disorders. It is unknown whether
chlorpheniramine crosses the
placenta or is detected in breast milk.
Be aware that chlorpheniramine use
is not recommended in newborns
or premature infants since these
groups are at an increased risk
of experiencing paradoxical
reaction. Be aware that elderly
patients are at an increased risk of
developing confusion, dizziness,

hyperexcitability, hypotension, and sedation.

Dizziness, drowsiness, and dry mouth are expected side effects. Mental alertness or motor skills should be avoided. Tolerance to the drug's sedative effects can occur.

Storage
Store at room temperature.

Administration
Give oral chlorpheniramine without regard to meals. Do not crush, break, or chew sustained-release tablets. Shake suspensions drops well before use.

Chlorpromazine
klor-proe′ma-zeen
(Chlorpromanyl [CAN], Largactil [CAN], Thorazine)
Do not confuse chlorpromazine with chlorpropamide, clomipramine, or prochlorperazine, or Thorazine with thiamide or thioridazine.

CATEGORY AND SCHEDULE
Pregnancy Risk Category: C

Classification: Phenothiazine, antiemetic, antipsychotic

MECHANISM OF ACTION
A phenothiazine that blocks dopamine neurotransmission at postsynaptic dopamine receptor sites. Possesses strong anticholinergic, sedative, and antiemetic effects; moderate extrapyramidal effects; and slight antihistamine action. *Therapeutic Effect:* Relieves nausea and vomiting; improves psychotic conditions; controls intractable hiccups and porphyria.

PHARMACOKINETICS
Rapidly absorbed after oral or IM administration. Protein binding: 92%-97%. Metabolized in the liver. Excreted in urine. *Half-life:* 6 h.

AVAILABILITY
Tablets: 10 mg, 25 mg, 50 mg, 100 mg, 200 mg.
Injection (Thorazine): 25 mg/mL.

INDICATIONS AND DOSAGES
▸ **Severe nausea or vomiting**
PO
Adults, Elderly. 10-25 mg q4-6h.
Children. 0.55 mg/kg q4-6h.
IM
Adults, Elderly. 25 mg; may repeat 25-50 mg q3-4h as needed until vomiting stops. Then switch to oral dosage.
Children. 0.55 mg/kg q6-8h.
▸ **Psychotic disorders**
PO
Adults, Elderly. 75-800 mg/day 3-4 divided doses.
Children older than 6 mo. 0.55 mg/kg q4-6h.
IM, IV
Adults, Elderly. Initially, 25 mg; may repeat in 1-4 h. May gradually increase to 400 mg q4-6h. Maximum: 300-800 mg/day.
Children older than 6 mo. 0.5-1 mg/kg q6-8h. Maximum: 75 mg/day for children 5-12 yr; 40 mg/day for children younger than 5 yr.
▸ **Intractable hiccups**
PO, IM
Adults. 25-50 mg PO 3 times a day. If symptoms persist after 2-3 days, try a single 25-50 mg IM dose.
▸ **Acute intermittent porphyria**
PO
Adults. 25-50 mg 3-4 times a day.
IM
Adults, Elderly. 25 mg 3-4 times a day.

▸ **Preoperative apprehension and anxiety**
PO
Adults. 25-50 mg, single dose 2-3 h before surgery.
Children. 0.5 mg/kg, single dose 2-3 h before surgery.

INDICATIONS AND DOSAGES
▸ **Tetanus**
IM
Adults: 25-50 mg 3-4 times/day; in conjunction with barbiturates.
Children: 0.55 mg q6-8h.
If<23 kg, do not exceed 40 mg. day. If 23-45 kg, do not exceed 75 mg/day.

OFF-LABEL USES
Treatment of choreiform movement of Huntington disease,

CONTRAINDICATIONS
Comatose states, myelosuppression, severe cardiovascular disease, severe CNS depression, subcortical brain damage hypersensitivity to phenothiazine.

INTERACTIONS
Drug
Alcohol, other CNS depressants: May increase respiratory depression and the hypotensive effects of chlorpromazine.
Antithyroid agents: May increase the risk of agranulocytosis.
Extrapyramidal symptom-producing medications: Increased risk of extrapyramidal symptoms.
Hypotensives: May increase hypotension.
Levodopa: May decrease the effects of levodopa.
Lithium: May decrease the absorption of chlorpromazine and produce adverse neurologic effects.

MAOIs, tricyclic antidepressants: May increase the anticholinergic and sedative effects of chlorpromazine.
Herbal
None known.
Food
None known.

DIAGNOSTIC TEST EFFECTS
May produce false-positive pregnancy and phenylketonuria (PKU) test results. May cause ECG changes, including Q- and T-wave disturbances. Therapeutic serum drug level is 50-300 mcg/mL; toxic serum drug level is > 750 mcg/mL.

SIDE EFFECTS
Frequent
Somnolence, blurred vision, hypotension, color vision or night vision disturbances, dizziness, decreased sweating, constipation, dry mouth, nasal congestion.
Occasional
Urinary retention, photosensitivity, rash, decreased sexual function, swelling or pain in breasts, weight gain, nausea, vomiting, abdominal pain, tremors.

SERIOUS REACTIONS
• Extrapyramidal symptoms appear to be dose related and are divided into three categories: akathisia (including inability to sit still, tapping of feet), parkinsonian symptoms (such as masklike face, tremors, shuffling gait, hypersalivation), and acute dystonias (including torticollis, opisthotonos, and oculogyric crisis). A dystonic reaction may also produce diaphoresis and pallor.
• Tardive dyskinesia, including tongue protrusion, puffing of the cheeks, and puckering of the mouth,

is a rare reaction that may be irreversible.

• Abrupt discontinuation after long-term therapy may precipitate nausea, vomiting, gastritis, dizziness, and tremors.

• Blood dyscrasias, particularly agranulocytosis and mild leukopenia, may occur.

• Chlorpromazine may lower the seizure threshold.

PRECAUTIONS & CONSIDERATIONS

Caution is warranted with alcoholism; glaucoma; history of seizures; hypocalcemia (increases susceptibility to dystonias); impaired cardiac, hepatic, renal, or respiratory function; benign prostatic hyperplasia; and urine retention. Increased mortality has been observed in elderly patients with dementia-related psychosis treated with antipsychotics. Alcohol, tasks that require mental alertness or motor skills, and excessive exposure to sunlight should be avoided. Skin should not come in contact with the injection solution because it can cause contact dermatitis.

Drowsiness may occur, and urine may darken. Notify the physician of visual disturbances. CBC, calcium, hydration status, and skin should be assessed.

Storage

All products should be stored at room temperature. Do not freeze. A slight yellow color to injection is acceptable.

Administration

! Do not give chlorpromazine by the subcutaneous route because severe tissue necrosis may occur. Be aware that the therapeutic serum level for chlorpromazine is 50-300 mcg/mL and the toxic serum level is > 750 mcg/mL.

For IM use, to prevent irritation at the injection site, dilute the injection solution with sodium chloride for injection or add 2% procaine, as prescribed. Inject IM slowly deep into upper outer quadrant of buttock keep point recumbent for at least 30 min after injection.

! The IV route is reserved for severe hiccups, tetanus, and surgery and requires specialized instructions for patients care.

Chlorpropamide
klor-pro′pa-mide
(Apo-Chlorpropamide [CAN], Diabinese)
Do not confuse with chlorpromazine.

CATEGORY AND SCHEDULE
Pregnancy Risk Category: C

Classification: Antidiabetic agents, sulfonylureas, first generation.

MECHANISM OF ACTION
A first-generation sulfonylurea that promotes release of insulin from β cells of pancreas. *Therapeutic Effect:* Lowers blood glucose concentration.

PHARMACOKINETICS
Rapidly absorbed from the gastrointestinal (GI) tract. Protein binding: 60%-90%. Extensively metabolized in liver. Excreted primarily in urine. Removed by hemodialysis. *Half-life:* 30-42 h.

AVAILABILITY
Tablets: 100 mg, 250 mg (Diabinese).

C

INDICATIONS AND DOSAGES

▸ **Diabetes mellitus, type 2**

PO

Adults. Initially, 250 mg once a day. Maintenance: 250-500 mg once a day. Maximum: 750 mg/day.

Elderly. Initially, 100-125 mg once a day. Maintenance: 100-250 mg once a day. Increase or decrease by 50-125 mg/day for 3- to 5-day intervals.

▸ **Renal function impairment**

Creatinine clearance 50-80 mL/min: Reduce dosage by 50%. If Creatinine clearance is less than 50 mL/min, do not use.

OFF-LABEL USES

Neurogenic diabetes insipidus.

CONTRAINDICATIONS

Diabetic complications, such as ketosis, acidosis, and diabetic coma, severe liver or renal impairment, sole therapy for type 1 diabetes mellitus, or hypersensitivity to sulfonylureas.

INTERACTIONS

Drug

Alcohol: Disulfiram-like reactions may occur. Symptoms of low blood sugar, including sweating, shaking, weakness, drowsiness, and trouble concentrating, will occur.

β-Blockers, MAOIs, NSAIDs, salicylates: May increase hypoglycemic effect.

Fluoroquinolone antibiotics: May increase the risk of hypoglycemia.

Glucocorticoids, thiazide diuretics: May increase blood glucose.

Oral contraceptives: May increase blood glucose.

Herbal

Bitter melon: May increase the risk of hypoglycemia.

St. John's wort: May increase the risk of hypoglycemia.

Food

None known.

DIAGNOSTIC TEST EFFECTS

None known.

SIDE EFFECTS

Frequent

Headache, upper respiratory tract infection.

Occasional

Sinusitis, myalgia (muscle aches), pharyngitis, aggravated diabetes mellitus.

SERIOUS REACTIONS

• Possible increased risk of cardiovascular mortality with this class of drugs.

• Overdosage can cause severe hypoglycemia prolonged by extended half-life.

PRECAUTIONS & CONSIDERATIONS

Caution is necessary with elderly patients and those with liver function impairment. Chlorpropamide should be avoided in elderly patients because of the high risk of hypoglycemia. Blood glucose should be checked before giving chlorpropamide. Chlorpropamide crosses the placenta and is distributed in breast milk and is not recommended in pregnant or breastfeeding women. Abdominal or chest pain, dark urine or light stool, hypoglycemic reactions, fever, nausea, palpitations, rash, vomiting, or yellowing of the eyes or skin should be reported immediately.

Be alert to conditions that alter blood glucose requirements, such as fever, increased activity, stress, or a surgical procedure. Hypoglycemia, such as anxiety, cool, wet skin, diplopia, dizziness, headache, hunger, numbness in mouth, tachycardia, and tremors, and hyperglycemia, including deep, rapid breathing, dim vision, fatigue, nausea, polydipsia, polyphagia, polyuria, and vomiting, can occur. Blood glucose levels, hemoglobin levels, and liver function tests should be monitored during therapy. Candy, sugar packets, or other sugar supplements for immediate response to hypoglycemia should be carried.

Administration

Give chlorpropamide with or without regard to meals. Usually given in the morning with breakfast.

Chlorthalidone

klor-thal'i-doan
(Apo-Chlorthalidone [CAN], Hygroton [AUS], Thalitone)

CATEGORY AND SCHEDULE

Pregnancy Risk Category: B (D if used in pregnancy-induced hypertension)

Classification: Diuretics, thiazide, and derivatives, antihypertensive

MECHANISM OF ACTION

A thiazide diuretic that blocks reabsorption of sodium, potassium, and water at the distal convoluted tubule; also decreases plasma and extracellular fluid volume and peripheral vascular resistance. *Therapeutic Effect:* Produces diuresis; lowers BP.

PHARMACOKINETICS

Route	Onset	Peak	Duration
PO (diuretic)	2 h	2-6 h	Up to 36 h

Rapidly absorbed from the GI tract. Excreted unchanged in urine. *Half-life:* 35-50 h. Onset of antihypertensive effect: 3-4 days; optimal *Therapeutic Effect:* 3-4 wks.

AVAILABILITY

Tablets: 15 mg, 25 mg, 50 mg, 100 mg.

INDICATIONS AND DOSAGES

▸ **Hypertension**

PO

Adults. Initially 15 mg once daily; may increase to 30 mg and then 45-50 mg once daily.
Elderly. 12.5-25 mg/day or every other day.

▸ **Edema**

PO

Adults. Initially 30-60 mg once daily or 60 mg on alternate days. Some patients may require increase to 90 mg or 120 mg.

CONTRAINDICATIONS

Anuria, history of hypersensitivity to sulfonamides or thiazide diuretics, renal decompensation.

INTERACTIONS

Drug

Cholestyramine, colestipol: May decrease the absorption and effects of chlorthalidone.
Digoxin: May increase the risk of digoxin toxicity associated with chlorthalidone-induced hyperkalemia.
Lithium: May increase the risk of lithium toxicity.
Herbal
None known.
Food
None known.

DIAGNOSTIC TEST EFFECTS

May increase blood glucose and serum cholesterol, LDL, bilirubin, calcium, creatinine, uric acid, and triglyceride levels. May decrease urinary calcium and serum magnesium, potassium, and sodium levels.

SIDE EFFECTS

Expected
Increase in urinary frequency and
urine volume.
Frequent
Potassium depletion (rarely produces
symptoms).
Occasional
Anorexia, impotence, diarrhea,
orthostatic hypotension, GI
disturbances, photosensitivity.
Rare
Rash.

SERIOUS REACTIONS

• Vigorous diuresis may lead to
profound water and electrolyte
depletion, resulting in hypokalemia,
hyponatremia, and dehydration.
• Acute hypotensive episodes may
occur.
• Hyperglycemia may occur during
prolonged therapy.
• Overdose can lead to lethargy and
coma without changes in electrolytes
or hydration.

PRECAUTIONS & CONSIDERATIONS

Caution is warranted with
diabetes mellitus, gout,
hypercholesterolemia, hepatic
impairment, and severe renal disease
and in elderly and debilitated
patients. It is unknown whether
chlorthalidone is distributed in
breast milk. Chlorthalidone crosses
the placenta, and a small amount
is distributed in breast milk.
Breastfeeding is not recommended
for patients taking this drug. No
age-related precautions have been
noted in children. Elderly patients
may be more sensitive to the drug's
hypotensive and electrolyte effects.
Consuming foods high in potassium,
such as apricots, bananas, legumes,
white and sweet potatoes, meat,
orange juice, and raisins, and whole
grains, including cereals, and
is encouraged. Avoid prolonged
exposure to sunlight.

Dizziness or light-headedness may
occur, so change positions slowly
to reduce the drug's hypotensive
effect. An increase in the frequency
and volume of urination may also
occur. BP, vital signs, electrolytes,
intake and output, and weight should
be monitored before and during
treatment. Blood glucose levels
should be checked after prolonged
therapy, because hyperglycemia
may occur. Be aware of the signs
of electrolyte disturbances, such as
hypokalemia. Hypokalemia may
cause arrhythmias, altered mental
status, muscle cramps, asthenia, and
tremor.
Administration
Take chlorthalidone with food or
milk if GI upset occurs, preferably
with breakfast to help prevent
nocturia. Crush scored tablets if
needed.

Chlorzoxazone
klor-zox′a-zone
(Parafon Forte DSC, Remular,
Remular-S)
**Do not confuse with
chlorthalidone.**

CATEGORY AND SCHEDULE
Pregnancy Risk Category: C

Classification: Skeletal muscle
relaxant, centrally acting

MECHANISM OF ACTION
A skeletal muscle relaxant that
inhibits transmission of reflexes at
the spinal cord level. *Therapeutic
Effect:* Relieves muscle spasticity.

PHARMACOKINETICS
Readily absorbed from the GI tract. Metabolized in liver. Primarily excreted in urine. *Half-life:* 1.1 h.

AVAILABILITY
Caplets: 500 mg (Parafon Forte DSC).
Tablets: 250 mg.

INDICATIONS AND DOSAGES
▸ **Musculoskeletal pain**
PO
Adults, Elderly. 250-500 mg 3-4 times/day. Maximum: 750 mg 3-4 day.

CONTRAINDICATIONS
Hypersensitivity to chlorzoxazone or any one of its components.

INTERACTIONS
Drug
Alcohol, central nervous system (CNS) depressants: May increase CNS depression.
Herbal
Garlic: May decrease the effectiveness of chlorzoxazone.
Kava: May increase CNS depression.
St. John's wort: May decrease the effectiveness of chlorzoxazone.
Food
None known.

DIAGNOSTIC TEST EFFECTS
False-positive for serum aprobarbital when using Toxi-Lab Screen.

SIDE EFFECTS
Frequent
Drowsiness, fever, headache.
Occasional
Nausea, vomiting, stomach cramps, rash.

SERIOUS REACTIONS
• Overdosage results in nausea, vomiting, diarrhea, and hypotension.

PRECAUTIONS & CONSIDERATIONS
Caution is necessary with liver impairment. Blood counts and liver and renal function tests should be performed periodically for those on long-term therapy. There is an increased risk of central nervous system (CNS) toxicity, manifested as confusion, hallucinations, mental depression, and sedation in elderly patients. Age-related renal impairment may require a decreased dosage.

Drowsiness may occur during treatment but usually diminishes with continued therapy. Tasks that require mental alertness or motor skills should be avoided until response to drug is established. Alcohol and CNS depressants should be avoided.
Administration
Take without regard to meals.
Storage
Store at room temperature.

Cholestyramine Resin
koe-less-tir′a-meen
(Novo-Cholamine [CAN], Prevalite, Questran [CAN], Questran Lite [AUS])
Do not confuse Questran with Quarzan.

CATEGORY AND SCHEDULE
Pregnancy Risk Category: B

Classification: Antihyperlipidemics, bile acid sequestrants

MECHANISM OF ACTION

An antihyperlipoproteinemic that binds with bile acids in the intestine, forming an insoluble complex. Binding results in partial removal of bile acid from enterohepatic circulation. *Therapeutic Effect:* Removes LDL cholesterol from plasma.

PHARMACOKINETICS

Not absorbed from the GI tract. Decreases in serum LDL apparent in 5-7 days and in serum cholesterol in 1 mo. Serum cholesterol returns to baseline levels about 1 mo after drug is discontinued.

AVAILABILITY

Powder for Oral Suspension: 4 g.

INDICATIONS AND DOSAGES

▸ **Primary hypercholesterolemia**
PO
Adults, Elderly. 3-4 g 3-4 times a day. Maximum: 24 g/day in 2-4 divided doses.
Children older than 10 yr. 2 g/day. Maximum: 8 g/day in 2 or more divided doses.
▸ **Pruritius associated with biliary stasis**
PO
Adults, Elderly. 4 g 1-2 times a day. Maintenance: Up to 16 g/day in divided doses.

OFF-LABEL USES

Treatment of diarrhea (due to bile acids), hyperoxaluria.

CONTRAINDICATIONS

Complete biliary obstruction, bowel obstruction hypersensitivity to cholestyramine or tartrazine (frequently seen in aspirin hypersensitivity).

INTERACTIONS

Drug
Anticoagulants: May increase effects of these drugs by decreasing level of vitamin K.
Digoxin, folic acid, penicillins, propranolol, tetracyclines, thiazides, thyroid hormones, other medications: May bind and decrease absorption of these drugs.
Oral vancomycin: Binds and decreases the effects of oral vancomycin.
Warfarin: May decrease warfarin absorption.
Herbal
None known.
Food
Vitamins A, D, E, K: cholestyramine may interfere with absorption.

DIAGNOSTIC TEST EFFECTS

May increase serum alkaline phosphatase, serum magnesium, AST (SGOT), and ALT (SGPT) levels. May decrease serum calcium, potassium, and sodium levels. May prolong prothrombin time.

SIDE EFFECTS

Frequent
Constipation (may lead to fecal impaction), nausea, vomiting, abdominal pain, indigestion.
Occasional
Diarrhea, belching, bloating, headache, dizziness.
Rare
Gallstones, peptic ulcer disease, malabsorption syndrome.

SERIOUS REACTIONS

• GI tract obstruction, hyperchloremic acidosis, and osteoporosis secondary to calcium excretion may occur.
• High dosage may interfere with fat absorption, resulting in steatorrhea.

PRECAUTIONS & CONSIDERATIONS

Caution is warranted with bleeding disorders, GI dysfunction (especially constipation), hemorrhoids, and osteoporosis. Cholestyramine is not systemically absorbed and may interfere with maternal absorption of fat-soluble vitamins. No age-related precautions have been noted in children. Cholestyramine use is limited in children younger than 10 yr of age. Elderly patients are at increased risk for experiencing adverse nutritional effects and GI side effects.

Notify the physician of abdominal discomfort, flatulence, and food intolerance. Pattern of daily bowel activity and stool consistency should be assessed. High-fiber foods, such as fruits, whole grain cereals, and vegetables, will reduce the risk of constipation. History of hypersensitivity to aspirin, cholestyramine, and tartrazine should be determined before beginning cholestyramine therapy. Serum cholesterol and triglyceride levels should be checked at baseline and periodically thereafter.

Administration

Take other drugs at least 1 h before or 4-6 h after cholestyramine, because this drug is capable of binding drugs in the GI tract. Do not take cholestyramine in its dry form because it is highly irritating and may cause choking. Mix with 3-6 oz fruit juice, milk, soup, or water. Allow the powder to sit on the surface of the liquid for 1-2 min to prevent lumping, then mix thoroughly. Mixing with carbonated beverages is NOT recommended. Take before meals.

Choline Magnesium Trisalicylate

koe′leen mag-nees′ee-um
tri-sal′eh-cye′late
(Tricosal, Trilisate)

C

CATEGORY AND SCHEDULE

Pregnancy Risk Category: C (D if full dose used in third trimester of pregnancy)

Classification: Analgesics, nonnarcotic, salicylates

MECHANISM OF ACTION

A nonsteroidal salicylate that inhibits prostaglandin synthesis and acts on the hypothalamus heat-regulating center. *Therapeutic Effect:* Reduces inflammatory response and intensity of pain stimulus reaching sensory nerve endings.

PHARMACOKINETICS

Rapidly absorbed from the GI tract. Oral route onset 1 h, peak 2 h, and duration 9-17 h. Protein binding: High. Widely distributed. Excreted in the urine. *Half-life:* 2-3 h.

AVAILABILITY

Tablets: 500 mg, 750 mg, 1000 mg (Tricosal, Trilisate).
Liquid: 500 mg/5 mL (Trilisate).

INDICATIONS AND DOSAGES
▸ **Analgesic, acute painful shoulder, anti-inflammatory, antipyretic**
PO
Adults, Elderly. Initially, 500-1500 mg q8-12h or 3g at bedtime, then 1-4.5 g/day.
Children weighing < 37 kg. 50 mg/kg/day in divided doses.

C

CONTRAINDICATIONS

Allergy to tartrazine dye, bleeding disorders, GI bleeding or ulceration, history of hypersensitivity to choline magnesium trisalicylate, aspirin, or other salicylates.

INTERACTIONS

Drug

Alcohol, NSAIDs: May increase the risk of adverse GI effects, including ulceration.

Antacids, urinary alkalinizers: Increase the excretion of choline magnesium trisalicylate.

Anticoagulants, heparin, thrombolytics: Increase the risk of bleeding.

Platelet aggregation inhibitors, valproic acid: May increase the risk of bleeding.

Probenecid: May decrease the effect of these drugs.

Herbal

Cat's claw, dong quai, evening primrose, feverfew, garlic, ginger, ginkgo, red clover, horse chestnut, green tea, ginseng: May increase the risk of bleeding.

Food

Curry powder, paprika, licorice, Benedictine liqueur, prunes, raisins, tea, gherkins: May increase the risk of salicylate accumulation.

DIAGNOSTIC TEST EFFECTS

May yield false-negative results for glucose oxidase urinary glucose tests (Clinitest); false-positive results using the cupric sulfate method (Clinitest). May interfere with Gerhardt test (urinary ketone analysis). May decrease T3 and T4 levels.

SIDE EFFECTS

Side effects appear less frequently with short-term treatment.

Occasional

Nausea, dyspepsia (heartburn, indigestion, epigastric pain), tinnitus.

Rare

Anorexia, headache, vomiting, flatulence, dizziness, somnolence, insomnia, fatigue, hearing impairment.

SERIOUS REACTIONS

• High doses may produce GI bleeding.

• Overdosage may be characterized by ringing in ears, generalized pruritus (may be severe), headache, dizziness, flushing, tachycardia, hyperventilation, sweating, and thirst.

PRECAUTIONS & CONSIDERATIONS

Caution should be used with dehydration, erosive gastritis, peptic ulcer disease, and chronic renal insufficiency. Caution is also warranted in children with acute febrile illness because choline magnesium trisalicylate increases the risk of developing Reye syndrome. Choline magnesium trisalicylate crosses the placenta and is distributed in breast milk. It should be avoided during the last trimester of pregnancy because the drug may adversely affect the fetal cardiovascular system, causing premature closure of ductus arteriosus. Lower choline magnesium trisalicylate dosages are recommended in elderly patients because this age group may be more susceptible to toxicity.

Administration

Take choline magnesium trisalicylate with meals to avoid GI upset. Liquid may be mixed with fruit juice or water just before drinking.

Ciclesonide
Sye-kles′-oh-nide
(Alvesco, Omnaris)

CATEGORY AND SCHEDULE
Pregnancy Risk Category: C

Classification: Corticosteroid

MECHANISM OF ACTION
Corticosteroid prodrug, activated by esterases in the respiratory tract, to active des-ciclesonide. Des-ciclesonide is a glucocorticoid that inhibits the accumulation of inflammatory cells and decreases and prevents tissues from responding to the inflammatory process. *Therapeutic Effect:* Inhalation: Inhibits bronchoconstriction, produces smooth muscle relaxation, decreases mucus secretion. Intranasal: Decreases response to seasonal and perennial rhinitis.

PHARMACOKINETICS
Oral bioavailability < 1%; extensive first-pass metabolism. Primarily excreted in the feces. *Half-life:* 0.71 h ciclesonide; 6-7 h des-ciclesonide.

AVAILABILITY
Nasal Spray: 50 mcg (120 metered sprays).
Inhalation Aerosol: 80 mcg per actuation (60 actuations), 160 mcg per actuation (60 or 120 actuations).

INDICATIONS AND DOSAGES
▸ **Maintenance treatment of asthma**
ORAL INHALATION
Adults, Elderly, Children 12 yr and older. Starting dose 80 mcg twice daily in patients previously treated with bronchodilators alone or previously treated with another inhaled corticosteroid, with titration as needed. Lowest effective dose should be used. Maximum recommended dose is 160 mcg twice daily in patients previously treated with bronchodilators alone and 320 mcg twice daily in patients previouly treated with inhaled corticosteroids. In patients receiving oral corticosteroids, ciclesonide dose is 320 mcg twice daily.
▸ **Perennial allergic rhinitis**
INTRANASAL
Adults, Elderly, Children 12 yr and older. 200 mcg per day administered as two 50-mcg sprays per nostril once daily.
▸ **Seasonal allergic rhinitis**
INTRANASAL
Adults, Elderly, Children 6 yr and older. 200 mcg per day administered as two 50-mcg sprays per nostril once daily.

CONTRAINDICATIONS
Hypersensitivity to ciclesonide or any of the product ingredients, status asthmaticus (inhaled).

INTERACTIONS
Drug
Ketoconazole: May increase concentrations of des-ciclesonide.
Herbal
None known.
Food
None known.

DIAGNOSTIC TEST EFFECTS
None known.

SIDE EFFECTS
Frequent (> 3%)
Oral inhalation: Headache, nasopharyngitis, sinusitis, pharyngolaryngeal pain, upper respiratory infection, arthralgia,

nasal congestion, pain in extremity, back pain.
Nasal: Headache, epistaxis, nasopharyngitis, pharyngolaryngeal pain.
Occasional
Oral inhalation: Nasal: ear pain.

SERIOUS REACTIONS

• An acute hypersensitivity reaction, as evidenced by urticaria, angioedema, and severe bronchospasm, occurs rarely.
• A transfer from systemic to local steroid therapy may unmask previously suppressed bronchial asthma condition.
• Potential adrenal insufficiency if used to replace systemic corticosteroid.
• Signs and symptoms of hypercorticism.

PRECAUTIONS & CONSIDERATIONS

Caution is warranted for patients with glaucoma, hypothyroidism, osteoporosis, tuberculosis, and untreated systemic infections. Avoid nasal corticosteroid use in patients with recent nasal septal ulcers, nasal surgery, or nasal trauma until healing has occurred. It is unknown whether ciclesonide or des-ciclesonide crosses the placenta or is distributed in breast milk. In children, prolonged treatment and high doses may decrease cortisol secretion and the short-term growth rate. Safety and effectiveness have not been established in children under the age of 12 yr for the inhalation or under the age of 6 yr for the nasal spray. No age-related precautions have been noted in elderly patients.

Those receiving beclomethasone by inhalation should maintain fastidious oral hygiene; notify the physician or nurse if sore throat or mouth develops. If using a bronchodilator inhaler concomitantly with a steroid inhaler, use the bronchodilator several minutes before using the corticosteroid to help the steroid penetrate into the bronchial tree. Those using beclomethasone intranasally should notify the physician if nasal irritation occurs or if symptoms, such as sneezing, fail to improve. Persons who are using drugs that suppress the immune system are more susceptible to infections than healthy individuals.

Storage
Store at room temperature. Discard inhaler when dose indicator displays zero. Discard nasal spray after 120 sprays after initial priming or 4 mo after removal from the foil pouch.

Administration
For inhalation, prime before first use and when not used for more than 10 days by actuating 3 times. Exhale completely and place the mouthpiece between the lips. Inhale and hold breath for as long as possible before exhaling. If more than one inhalation is necessary, allow at least 1 min between inhalations. Rinse mouth after each use to decrease dry mouth and hoarseness and prevent fungal infection of the mouth.

For intranasal use, clear nasal passages as much as possible. Prime before first use by actuating 8 times. Prime if not used for more than 4 consecutive days by actuating once or until a fine spray appears. Shake gently before use. Insert the spray tip into the nostril, pointing toward the nasal passages, away from the nasal septum. Spray into the nostril while holding the other nostril closed, and at the same time, inhale through the nose to deliver the medication as high into the nasal passages as possible.

Ciclopirox
sye-kloe-peer′ox
(Loprox, Penlac)
Do not confuse ciclopirox with ciprofloxacin.

CATEGORY AND SCHEDULE
Pregnancy Risk Category: B

Classification: Antifungals, topical

MECHANISM OF ACTION
An antifungal that inhibits the transport of essential elements in the fungal cell, thereby interfering with biosynthesis in fungi. *Therapeutic Effect:* Results in fungal cell death.

PHARMACOKINETICS
Absorbed through intact skin. Distributed to epidermis and dermis, including hair, hair follicles, and sebaceous glands. Protein binding: 98%. Primarily excreted in urine and to a lesser extent in feces. *Half-life:* 1.7 h.

AVAILABILITY
Cream: 0.77% (Loprox).
Gel: 0.77% (Loprox).
Lotion: 0.77% (Loprox TS).
Shampoo: 1% (Loprox).
Topical Solution, Nail Lacquer: 8% (Penlac).

INDICATIONS AND DOSAGES
▶ **Tinea pedis**
TOPICAL
Adults, Elderly, Children 10 yr and older. Apply 2 times a day until signs and symptoms significantly improve. Usually for 4 wks.
▶ **Tinea cruris, tinea corporis**
TOPICAL
Adults, Elderly, Children 10 yr and older. Apply 2 times a day until signs and symptoms significantly improve. Usually 2-4 wks.

▶ **Onychomycosis**
TOPICAL (SOLUTION)
Adults, Elderly, Children 10 yr and older. Apply to the affected area (nails) daily. Remove with alcohol every 7 days. May require months of treatment.
▶ **Seborrheic dermatitis**
GEL
Adults, Elderly, Children 10 yr and older. Apply to affected scalp areas 2 times a day, in the morning and evening for 4 wks.
SHAMPOO
Adults, Elderly, Children 10 yr and older. Apply 5 mL (1 teaspoonful) to wet hair; lather, and leave in place about 3 min; rinse. May use up to 10 mL for longer hair. Repeat twice weekly for 4 wks; allow a minimum of 3 days between applications.

CONTRAINDICATIONS
Hypersensitivity to ciclopirox or any one of its components.

INTERACTIONS
Drug
Not known.
Herbal
Not known.
Food
Not known.

DIAGNOSTIC TEST EFFECTS
None known.

SIDE EFFECTS
Rare
Topical: Irritation, burning, redness, pain at the site of application.

SERIOUS REACTIONS
• None known.

PRECAUTIONS & CONSIDERATIONS
Avoid use of occlusive wrappings or dressings. Avoid contact with eyes. If local irritation occurs, ciclopirox should be discontinued.

It is unknown whether ciclopirox crosses the placenta or is distributed in breast milk. Safety and efficacy have not been established in children younger than 10 yr old. No age-related precautions have been noted for elderly patients.

Administration

Apply topical formulation by rubbing gently into the affected and surrounding area twice daily until signs and symptoms improve.

Apply nail lacquer once daily, preferably at bedtime or 8 h before washing, to the affected nails with the applicator brush provided. Cover evenly over the entire nail plate. Ciclopirox should not be removed on a daily basis. Daily applications should be made over the previous coat. Remove with alcohol every 7 days. Repeat cycle throughout the duration of therapy. File away with emery board loose nail material, and trim nails every 7 days after ciclopirox is removed with alcohol.

Apply gel to affected scalp areas twice daily, in the morning and evening for 4 wks, or use the shampoo twice weekly for 4 wks. Clinical improvement usually occurs within the first week, with continuing resolution of signs and symptoms through the fourth week of treatment.

Cidofovir
ci-dah′fo-veer
(Vistide)

CATEGORY AND SCHEDULE
Pregnancy Risk Category: C

Classification: Antivirals

MECHANISM OF ACTION
An anti-infective that inhibits viral DNA synthesis by incorporating itself into the growing viral DNA chain. *Therapeutic Effect:* Suppresses replication of cytomegalovirus (CMV).

PHARMACOKINETICS
Protein binding: < 6%. Excreted primarily unchanged in urine. Effect of hemodialysis unknown. *Elimination Half-Life:* 1.4-3.8 h.

AVAILABILITY
Injection: 75 mg/mL (5-mL ampule).

INDICATIONS AND DOSAGES
▸ **CMV retinitis in patients with AIDS (in combination with probenecid)**
IV INFUSION
Adults. Induction: 5 mg/kg at constant rate over 1 h once weekly for 2 consecutive weeks. Give 2 g of PO probenecid 3 h before cidofovir dose, and then give 1 g 2 h and 8 h after completion of the 1-h cidofovir infusion (total of 4 g). In addition, give 1 L of 0.9% NaCl over 1-2 h immediately before the cidofovir infusion. If tolerated, a second liter may be infused over 1-3 h at the start of the infusion or *immediately* afterward. *Maintenance:* 5 mg/kg cidofovir at constant rate over 1 h once every 2 wks.
▸ **Dosage in renal impairment**
Patients with CrCl ≤ or = 55 mL/min before treatment must not receive cidofovin. Once treatment starts in other patients, decrease dose to 3 mg/kg if Scr increases 0.3-0.4 mg/dL above baseline. Discontinue if a rise in Scr is 0.5 mg/dL or more.

OFF-LABEL USES
Treatment of ganciclovir-resistant cytomegalovirus (CMV),

foscarnet-resistant CMV, adenovirus, and acyclovir-resistant herpes simplex virus or varicella-zoster virus.

CONTRAINDICATIONS

Direct intraocular injection, history of clinically severe hypersensitivity to probenecid or other sulfa-containing drugs, hypersensitivity to cidofovir, renal function impairment (serum creatinine level > 1.5 mg/dL, creatinine clearance of 55 mL/min or less, or urine protein level > 100 mg/dL), use with or within 7 days of other nephrotoxic medications.

INTERACTIONS

Drug
Nephrotoxic medications (such as aminoglycosides, amphotericin B, foscarnet, Tacrolimus IV pentamidine): Increase the risk of nephrotoxicity. Discontinue these at least 7 days before cidofovir treatmet.
Tenofovir: Cidofovir may increase tenofovir serum concentrations.
Zidovudine: For persons also taking zidovudine (AZT), expect to discontinue zidovudine administration temporarily or to decrease AZT dose by 50% on days of cidofovir infusion. Be aware that concurrent probenecid use reduces the metabolic clearance of zidovudine.
Herbal
None known.
Food
None known.

DIAGNOSTIC TEST EFFECTS

May decrease neutrophil count and serum bicarbonate, phosphate, and uric acid levels. May elevate serum creatinine levels.

⚙ IV INCOMPATIBILITIES

No information available for Y-site administration.

SIDE EFFECTS

Frequent
Nausea, vomiting (65%), fever (57%), asthenia (46%), rash (30%), diarrhea (27%), headache (27%), alopecia (25%), chills (24%), anorexia (22%), dyspnea (22%), abdominal pain (17%).

SERIOUS REACTIONS

• Serious adverse reactions may include proteinuria (80%), nephrotoxicity (53%), neutropenia (31%), elevated serum creatinine levels (29%), infection (24%), anemia (20%), ocular hypotony (a decrease in intraocular pressure, 12%), and pneumonia (9%).
• Concurrent use of probenecid may produce a hypersensitivity reaction characterized by a rash, fever, chills, and anaphylaxis.
• Acute renal failure occurs rarely.

PRECAUTIONS & CONSIDERATIONS

Caution is warranted with preexisting diabetes. Be aware that cidofovir is embryotoxic and results in reduced fetal body weight in animals. Females of childbearing age should use effective contraception during and for 1 mo after cidofovir treatment; male patients should practice barrier contraceptive methods during and for 3 mo after treatment. Be aware that it is unknown whether cidofovir is excreted in breast milk. Do not administer to breastfeeding women. Breastfeeding is not recommended in this population because of the possibility of HIV transmission. Be aware that the safety and efficacy of cidofovir have not been established in children. In elderly patients, age-related renal impairment may require dosage adjustment.

Renal function should be closely monitored through serum creatinine levels and urinalysis during therapy. Urine protein and white blood cell (WBC) count should also be monitored. Visual acuity and ocular symptoms should be evaluated.

Storage
Store cidofovir at room temperature. Refrigerate admixtures for no longer than 24 h. Allow refrigerated admixtures to warm to room temperature before use.

Administration
! Do not exceed the recommended dosage, frequency, or infusion rate. Dilute in 100 mL 0.9% NaCl and infuse over 1 h. Prepare to administer IV hydration with 0.9% NaCl and give oral probenecid with each cidofovir infusion to minimize the risk of nephrotoxicity. Eat food before each dose of probenecid to help reduce nausea and vomiting. As prescribed, administer an antiemetic to reduce the risk of nausea. Give cidofovir IV infusion over 60 min.

Cilostazol
sil-os′tah-zol
(Pletal)
Do not confuse Pletal with Plendil.

CATEGORY AND SCHEDULE
Pregnancy Risk Category: C

Classification: Platelet inhibitors

MECHANISM OF ACTION
A phosphodiesterase III inhibitor that inhibits platelet aggregation. Dilates vascular beds with greatest dilation in femoral beds. *Therapeutic Effect:*
Improves walking distance in patients with intermittent claudication.

PHARMACOKINETICS
Moderately absorbed from the GI tract. Protein binding: 95%-98%. Extensively metabolized in the liver. Excreted primarily in the urine and, to a lesser extent, in the feces. Not removed by hemodialysis. *Half-life:* 11-13 h. Therapeutic effect is usually noted in 2-4 wks but may take as long as 12 wks.

AVAILABILITY
Tablets: 50 mg, 100 mg.

INDICATIONS AND DOSAGES
▶ **Intermittent claudication**
PO
Adults, Elderly. 100 mg twice a day at least 30 min before or 2 h after meals. Reduce dose to 50 mg twice a day with concurrent CYP3A4 or CYP2C19 inhibitors.

CONTRAINDICATIONS
Congestive heart failure of any severity, hemostatic disorders or active bleeding, hypersensitivity to cilostazol or any of the product ingredients.

INTERACTIONS
Drug
CYP3A4 inhibitors (azole antifungals, clarithromycin, diltiazem, erythromycin, fluoxetine, nefazodone, protease inhibitors, quinidine, sertraline, telithromycin, and verapamil): May increase cilostazol concentration.
CYP2C19 inhibitors (delavirdine, fluconazole, fluvoxamine, omeprazole, and ticlopidine): May increase cilostazol concentration.
Aspirin: May potentiate inhibition of platelet aggregation.

Herbal
None known.
Food
Grapefruit juice: May increase blood concentration and risk of toxicity of cilostazol.
High-fat meal: May increase cilostazol peak concentration up to 90%.

DIAGNOSTIC TEST EFFECTS
May increase BUN and serum creatinine levels. May decrease hemoglobin and hematocrit.

SIDE EFFECTS
Frequent (10%-34%)
Headache, diarrhea, palpitations, dizziness, pharyngitis.
Occasional (3%-7%)
Nausea, rhinitis, back pain, peripheral edema, dyspepsia, abdominal pain, tachycardia, cough, flatulence, myalgia.
Rare (1%-2%)
Leg cramps, paresthesia, rash, vomiting.

SERIOUS REACTIONS
• Signs and symptoms of overdose are noted by severe headache, diarrhea, hypotension, and cardiac arrhythmias.
• Leukopenia and thrombocytopenia, with progression to agranulocytosis when cilostazol was not immediately discontinued.

PRECAUTIONS & CONSIDERATIONS
Use with caution in patients with heart disease and renal or hepatic impairment. It is unknown whether cilostazol crosses the placenta or is distributed in breast milk. Safety and efficacy of cilostazol have not been established in children. No age-related precautions have been noted in elderly patients. Hemoglobin, hematocrit, and platelet counts should be obtained before and periodically during treatment.
Administration
Take cilostazol at least 30 min before or 2 h after meals. Do not give with grapefruit juice, because grapefruit juice may increase the drug's blood concentration and risk of toxicity.

Cimetidine
sye-met′i-deen
(Apo-Cimetidine [CAN], Cimehexal [AUS], Magicul [AUS], Novocimetine [CAN], Peptol [CAN], Sigmetadine [AUS], Tagamet, Tagamet HB)
Do not confuse cimetidine with simethicone.

CATEGORY AND SCHEDULE
Pregnancy Risk Category: B
OTC Tablets: 100 mg

Classification: H_2 histamine receptor antagonist

MECHANISM OF ACTION
An antiulcer agent and gastric acid secretion inhibitor that inhibits histamine action at H_2 receptor sites of parietal cells. *Therapeutic Effect:* Inhibits gastric acid secretion during fasting, at night, or when stimulated by food, caffeine, or insulin.

PHARMACOKINETICS
Well absorbed from the GI tract. Protein binding: 15%-20%. Widely distributed. Metabolized in the liver. Primarily excreted in urine. Not removed by hemodialysis. *Half-life:* 2 h; increased with impaired renal function.

AVAILABILITY
Tablets (Tagamet HB): 200 mg.
Tablets (Tagamet): 300 mg, 400 mg, 800 mg.
Liquid: 300 mg/5 mL.
Injection: 150 mg/mL.
Injection Solution Premixed: 300 mg, 900 mg, 1200 mg.

INDICATIONS AND DOSAGES
▸ **Active ulcer**
PO
Adults, Elderly. 300 mg 4 times a day or 400 mg twice a day or 800 mg at bedtime.
IM, IV
Adults, Elderly. 300 mg q6h or 150 mg as single dose followed by 37.5 mg/h continuous infusion.
▸ **Prevention of duodenal ulcer**
PO
Adults, Elderly. 400-800 mg at bedtime.
▸ **Gastric hypersecretory secretions**
PO, IV, IM
Adults, Elderly. 300-600 mg q6h. Maximum: 2400 mg/day.
Children. 20-40 mg/kg/day in divided doses q6h.
Infants. 10-20 mg/kg/day in divided doses q6-12h.
Neonates. 5-10 mg/kg/day in divided doses q8-12h.
▸ **Gastrointestinal reflux disease**
PO
Adults, Elderly. 800 mg twice a day or 400 mg 4 times a day for 12 wks.
▸ **OTC use**
PO
Adults, Elderly. 100 mg up to 30 min before meals. Maximum: 2 doses/day.
▸ **Prevention of upper GI bleeding**
IV INFUSION
Adults, Elderly. 50 mg/h.
▸ **Dosage in renal impairment**
Dosage is based on a 300-mg dose in adults. Dosage interval is modified based on creatinine clearance.

Creatinine Clearance (mL/min)	Dosage Interval
> 40	q6h
20-40	q8h or decrease dose by 25%
< 20	q12h or decrease dose by 50%

Give after hemodialysis and q12h between dialysis sessions.

OFF-LABEL USES
Prevention of aspiration pneumonia; treatment of acute urticaria, chronic warts, upper GI bleeding.

CONTRAINDICATIONS
Hypersensitivity to cimetidine or other H_2-antagonists.

INTERACTIONS
Drug
Antacids: May decrease the absorption of cimetidine.
Calcium channel blockers, cyclosporine, lidocaine, metoprolol, metronidazole, oral anticoagulants, oral antidiabetics, phenytoin, propranolol, theophylline, tricyclic antidepressants: May decrease the metabolism and increase the blood concentrations of these drugs.
CYP 1A2, 2C19, 2D6, 3A4, 2C9, and 2E1 substrates: Cimetidine inhibits these isoenzymes and may decrease the metabolism and increase the blood concentrations of substrates of these isoenzymes.
Ketoconazole: May decrease the absorption of ketoconazole.
Herbal
St. John's wort: May decrease cimetidine levels.
Food
None known.

DIAGNOSTIC TEST EFFECTS

Interferes with skin tests using allergen extracts. May increase prolactin, serum creatinine, and transaminase levels. May decrease parathyroid hormone concentration.

⊘ IV INCOMPATIBILITIES

Allopurinol (Aloprim), amphotericin B complex (Abelcet, AmBisome, Amphotec), cefepime (Maxipime).

⚕ IV COMPATIBILITIES

Aminophylline, diltiazem (Cardizem), furosemide (Lasix), heparin, hydromorphone (Dilaudid), insulin (regular), lidocaine, lorazepam (Ativan), midazolam (Versed), morphine, potassium chloride, propofol (Diprivan).

SIDE EFFECTS

Occasional (2%-4%)
HEADACHE
Elderly and severely ill patients, patients with impaired renal function: Confusion, agitation, psychosis, depression, anxiety, disorientation, hallucinations. Effects reverse 3-4 days after discontinuance.
Rare (< 2%)
Diarrhea, dizziness, somnolence, nausea, vomiting, gynecomastia, rash, impotence.

SERIOUS REACTIONS

• Rapid IV administration may produce cardiac arrhythmias and hypotension.

PRECAUTIONS & CONSIDERATIONS

Caution is warranted for patients with impaired hepatic or renal function and in elderly patients. Cimetidine crosses the placenta and is distributed in breast milk. Cimetidine use in infants may suppress gastric acidity, inhibit drug metabolism, and produce CNS stimulation. Long-term use in children may induce cerebral toxicity and affect the hormonal system. Elderly patients are more likely to experience confusion, especially those with impaired renal function. Do not take antacids within 1 h of oral cimetidine administration. Avoid smoking. Tasks that require mental alertness or motor skills should also be avoided until response to the drug has been established. Alcohol and aspirin, both of which may cause GI distress, should also be avoided during cimetidine therapy.

Notify the physician if blood in emesis or stool or dark, tarry stool occurs. Pattern of daily bowel activity and stool consistency, electrolytes, and hydration status should be monitored.

Storage
Store parenteral form at room temperature. Reconstituted IV solution is stable for 48 h at room temperature.

Administration
Dilute each 300 mg (2 mL) injection with 18 mL 0.9% NaCl, 0.45% NaCl, 0.2% NaCl, D5W, D10W, Ringer's solution, or lactated Ringer's solution to a total volume of 20 mL. For IV push, administer over not < 2 min to prevent arrhythmias and hypotension. For intermittent IV (piggyback) administration, infuse over 15-20 min. For IV infusion, dilute with 100-1000 mL 0.9% NaCl, D5W, or other compatible solution and infuse over 24 h.

For IM use, administer undiluted. Inject deep into large muscle mass, such as the gluteus maximus muscle. IM administration may produce transient discomfort at the injection site.

Take oral cimetidine with meals.

Cinacalcet
sin-a-cal′set
(Sensipar)

CATEGORY AND SCHEDULE
Pregnancy Risk Category: C

Classification: Calcimimetic agent

MECHANISM OF ACTION
A calcium receptor agonist that increases the sensitivity of the calcium-sensing receptor on the parathyroid gland to extracellular calcium, thus lowering the parathyroid hormone (PTH) level. *Therapeutic Effect:* Decreases serum calcium and PTH levels.

PHARMACOKINETICS
Extensively distributed after PO administration. Protein binding: 93%-97%. Rapidly and extensively metabolized by multiple enzymes. Primarily eliminated in urine with a lesser amount excreted in feces. *Half-life:* 30-40 h.

AVAILABILITY
Tablets: 30 mg, 60 mg, 90 mg.

INDICATIONS AND DOSAGES
▸ **Hypercalcemia in parathyroid carcinoma**
PO
Adults, Elderly. Initially, 30 mg twice a day. Titrate dosage sequentially (60 mg twice a day, 90 mg twice a day, and 90 mg 3-4 times a day) every 2-4 wks as needed to normalize serum calcium levels.
▸ **Secondary hyperparathyroidism in patients on dialysis**
PO
Adults, Elderly. Initially, 30 mg once a day. Titrate dosage sequentially (60, 90, 120, and 180 mg once a day) every 2-4 wks.

CONTRAINDICATIONS
Hypersensitivity.

INTERACTIONS
Drug
Amitriptyline: Increases amitriptyline plasma concentration.
Flecainide, thioridazine, tricyclic antidepressants, vinblastine: May require dosage adjustment of these drugs.
CYP2D6 substrates (e.g., dextromethorphan, fluoxetine, lidocaine, mirtazapine, nefazodone, paroxetine, risperidone, ritonavir, thioridazine, tricyclic antidepressants, venlafaxine): Increased concentrations of CYP2D6 substrates.
CYP2D6 inhibitors (e.g., azole antifungals, clarithromycin, erythromycin, nefazodone, protease inhibitors, quinidine, telithromycin, and verapamil): Increase cinacalcet plasma concentration.
Herbal
None known.
Food
High-fat meals: Increase cinacalcet plasma concentration.

DIAGNOSTIC TEST EFFECTS
Reduces serum calcium level.

SIDE EFFECTS
Frequent (21%-31%)
Nausea, vomiting, diarrhea.
Occasional (10%-15%)
Myalgia, dizziness.
Rare (5%-7%)
Asthenia, hypertension, anorexia, noncardiac chest pain.

SERIOUS REACTIONS
• Overdose may lead to hypocalcemia.
• Hypotension and heart failure have been reported in patients with cardiovascular disease.

PRECAUTIONS & CONSIDERATIONS

Caution is warranted in patients with cardiovascular disease, seizure disorder, chronic kidney disease not on hemodialysis, or hepatic impairment. Cinacalcet may cross the placental barrier. Cinacalcet's safe use during breastfeeding has not been established; the drug may cause adverse reactions in breastfed infants. The safety and efficacy of cinacalcet have not been established in children. No age-related precautions have been noted in elderly patients.

Notify the physician if diarrhea or vomiting occurs. Serum electrolyte levels and pattern of daily bowel activity and stool consistency should be monitored.

Storage
Store tablets at room temperature.
Administration
Do not break or crush film-coated tablets. Take the drug with food or shortly after a meal.

Ciprofloxacin

sip-ro-floks'a-sin
(C-Flox [AUS], Ciloquin [AUS], Ciloxan, Cipro, Ciproxin [AUS])
Do not confuse ciprofloxacin or Ciproxin with Ciloxan, cinoxacin, or Cytoxan.

CATEGORY AND SCHEDULE

Pregnancy Risk Category: C

Classification: Anti-infectives, ophthalmics, antibiotics, quinolones

MECHANISM OF ACTION

A fluoroquinolone that inhibits the enzyme DNA gyrase in susceptible bacteria, interfering with bacterial cell replication. *Therapeutic Effect:* Bactericidal.

PHARMACOKINETICS

Well absorbed from the GI tract (food delays absorption). Protein binding: 20%-40%. Widely distributed (including to CSF). Metabolized in the liver to active metabolite. Primarily excreted in urine. Minimal removal by hemodialysis. *Half-life:* 4-6 h (increased in patients with impaired renal function and in elderly patients).

AVAILABILITY

Tablets (Cipro): 100 mg, 250 mg, 500 mg, 750 mg.
Tablets, Extended-Release (Cipro XR): 500 mg, 1000 mg.
Infusion: 200 mg/100 mL, 400 mg/200 mL.
Injection Solution: 10 mg/mL.
Ophthalmic Ointment (Ciloxan): 0.3%.
Ophthalmic Suspension (Ciloxan): 0.3%.
Oral Suspension: 250 mg/5 mL, 500 mg/5 mL.

INDICATIONS AND DOSAGES
▸ **Mild to moderate urinary tract infection (UTI)**
PO
Adults, Elderly. 250 mg q12h.
IV
Adults, Elderly. 200 mg q12h.
▸ **Complicated UTIs, mild to moderate respiratory tract, bone, joint, skin, and skin-structure infections; infectious diarrhea**
PO
Adults, Elderly. 500 mg q12h.
IV
Adults, Elderly. 400 mg q12h.
▸ **Severe, complicated infections**
PO
Adults, Elderly. 750 mg q12h.
IV
Adults, Elderly. 400 mg q12h.

C

▸ **Prostatitis**
PO
Adults, Elderly. 500 mg q12h for 28 days.
▸ **Uncomplicated bladder infection**
PO
Adults. 100 mg twice a day for 3 days.
▸ **Acute sinusitis**
PO
Adults. 500 mg q12h.
▸ **Uncomplicated gonorrhea**
PO
Adults. 250 mg as a single dose.
▸ **Cystic fibrosis**
IV
Children. 30 mg/kg/day in 2-3 divided doses. Maximum: 1.2 g/day.
PO
▸ **Corneal ulcer**
OPHTHALMIC
Adults, Elderly. 2 drops q15min for 6 h, then 2 drops q30min for the remainder of first day, 2 drops q1h on second day, and 2 drops q4h on days 3-14.
▸ **Conjunctivitis**
OPHTHALMIC
Adults, Elderly. 1-2 drops q2h for 2 days, then 2 drops q4h for next 5 days.
▸ **Dosage in renal impairment**
Dosage and frequency are modified based on creatinine clearance and the severity of the infection.

Creatinine Clearance	Dosage Interval
< 30 mL/min	Usual dose q18-24h

▸ **Hemodialysis**
250-500 mg q24h (after dialysis).
▸ **Peritoneal dialysis**
250-500 mg q24h (after dialysis).

OFF-LABEL USES
Treatment of chancroid.

CONTRAINDICATIONS
Hypersensitivity to ciprofloxacin or other quinolones, concurrent tizanidine; for ophthalmic administration: vaccinia, varicella, epithelial herpes simplex, keratitis, mycobacterial infection, fungal disease of ocular structure, use after uncomplicated removal of a foreign body.

INTERACTIONS
Drug
Antacids, iron preparations, calcium or magnesium supplement, sucralfate: May decrease ciprofloxacin absorption. Separate times of administration.
Caffeine, oral anticoagulants: May increase the effects of these drugs.
Theophylline: Decreases clearance and may increase blood concentration and risk of toxicity of theophylline.
Herbal
None known.
Food
Enteral feedings: Reduce ciprofloxacin absorption.

DIAGNOSTIC TEST EFFECTS
May increase BUN and serum alkaline phosphatase, bilirubin, creatinine, LDH, AST (SGOT), and ALT (SGPT) levels.

ⓦ IV INCOMPATIBILITIES
Aminophylline, ampicillin and sulbactam (Unasyn), cefepime (Maxipime), dexamethasone (Decadron), furosemide (Lasix), heparin, hydrocortisone (Solu-Cortef), methylprednisolone (Solu-Medrol), phenytoin (Dilantin), sodium bicarbonate.

ⓦ IV COMPATIBILITIES
Calcium gluconate, diltiazem (Cardizem), dobutamine (Dobutrex),

dopamine (Intropin), lidocaine, lorazepam (Ativan), magnesium, midazolam (Versed), potassium chloride.

SIDE EFFECTS
Frequent (2%-5%)
Nausea, diarrhea, dyspepsia, vomiting, constipation, flatulence, confusion, crystalluria.
Ophthalmic: Burning, crusting in corner of eye.
Occasional (< 2%)
Abdominal pain or discomfort, headache, rash.
Ophthalmic: Bad taste, sensation of something in eye, eyelid redness or itching.
Rare (< 1%)
Dizziness, confusion, tremors, hallucinations, hypersensitivity reaction, insomnia, dry mouth, paresthesia.

SERIOUS REACTIONS
• Superinfection (especially enterococcal or fungal), nephropathy, cardiopulmonary arrest, chest pain, tendon inflammation/rupture, and cerebral thrombosis may occur.
• Hypersensitivity reactions, including photosensitivity (as evidenced by rash, pruritus, blisters, edema, and burning skin), have occurred in patients receiving fluoroquinolones.
• Arthropathy may occur if the drug is given to children younger than 18 yr.
• Sensitization to the ophthalmic form of the drug may contraindicate later systemic use of ciprofloxacin.

PRECAUTIONS & CONSIDERATIONS
Caution is warranted in patients with CNS disorders, renal impairment, seizures, risk factors for QT prolongation, and those

taking caffeine or theophylline. Be aware that the oral suspension should not be administered by nasogastric tube. It is unknown whether ciprofloxacin is distributed in breast milk. If possible, pregnant or breastfeeding women should avoid taking the drug because of the risk of arthropathy in the fetus or infant. The safety and efficacy of ciprofloxacin have not been established in children younger than 18 yr. Age-related renal impairment may require a dosage adjustment in elderly patients.

Dizziness, headache, tremors, visual problems, and chest and joint pain should be reported. Food tolerance and pattern of daily bowel activity and stool consistency should be assessed. A crystal precipitate may form when using the ophthalmic preparation but resolves in 1-7 days. History of hypersensitivity to ciprofloxacin and other quinolones should be determined before therapy.

Storage
The oral suspension may be stored for 14 days at room temperature. Store the injection form at room temperature. The solution normally appears clear and colorless or slightly yellow.

Administration
Oral ciprofloxacin may be taken without regard to food, but the preferred administration time is 2 h after a meal. Shake the oral suspension well before taking it, and do not chew the microcapsules in the suspension. Do not administer antacids containing aluminum or magnesium within 2 h of ciprofloxacin. Take full course of therapy, and do not skip doses.

For IV use, after withdrawing the drug from a 200- or 400-mg vial, further dilute it with D5W or 0.9% NaCl for injection to a final concentration of 1-2 mg/mL. Infuse the drug over 60 min. IV ciprofloxacin is also available prediluted in ready-to-use infusion containers.

For ophthalmic use, tilt the head back and place the solution in the conjunctival sac of the affected eye. Close the eye and then press gently on the lacrimal sac for 1 min. Unless the infection is very superficial, systemic administration generally accompanies ophthalmic use.

Cisplatin
sis-plah´-tin
(Platinol-AQ)
Do not confuse cisplatin with carboplatin, or Platinol-AQ with Paraplatin or Patanol.

CATEGORY AND SCHEDULE
Pregnancy Risk Category: D

Classification: Platinum coordination complex; antineoplastic

MECHANISM OF ACTION
A platinum coordination complex that inhibits DNA and, to a lesser extent, RNA, protein synthesis by cross-linking with DNA strands, preventing cell division. Cell cycle–phase nonspecific. *Therapeutic Effect:* Interferes with DNA function.

PHARMACOKINETICS
Widely distributed. Protein binding: > 90%. Undergoes rapid nonenzymatic conversion to inactive metabolite. Excreted in urine. Removed by hemodialysis. *Half-life:* 58-73 h (increased with impaired renal function).

AVAILABILITY
Injection Solution: 1 mg/mL.

INDICATIONS AND DOSAGES
▸ **Advanced bladder carcinoma, metastatic ovarian tumors, metastatic testicular tumors**
IV INFUSION
Adults, Elderly, Children. For intermittent dosage schedule, 37-75 mg/m^2 once every 2-3 wks or 50-100 mg/m^2 over 4-8 h once every 21-28 days. For daily dosage schedule, 15-20 mg/m^2/day for 5 days every 3-4 wks.

CONTRAINDICATIONS
Hearing impairment; myelosuppression; pregnancy; hypersensitivity to cisplatin or other platinum compounds, creatinine clearance less than 50 mL/min, preexisting renal impairment.

INTERACTIONS
Drug
Nephrotoxic, ototoxic medications: May increase the risk of nephrotoxicity/ototoxicity.
Herbal and Food
None known.

DIAGNOSTIC TEST EFFECTS
Increased hepatic transaminases, BUN, serum creatinine; decreased serum sodium, calcium, magnesium, uric acid.

Ⓘ IV INCOMPATIBILITIES
Amphotericin B, Cefepime, Dentrolene, Diazepam, Gallium, Insulin, Lansoprazole, Mesna, Pantoprazole, Poperacillin-Tazobactam, Thiotepa, TPN. Refer to specialized references to check compatibility with other medications and solutions.

SIDE EFFECTS
Frequent
Nausea, vomiting (generally beginning 1-4 h after administration and lasting up to 24 h); myelosuppression (affecting 25%-30% of patients, with

recovery generally occurring in
18-23 days); mild alopecia;
ototoxicity; nephrotoxicity.
Occasional
Peripheral neuropathy (with
prolonged therapy [4-7 mo]).
Pain or redness at injection site, loss
of taste or appetite.
Rare
Hemolytic anemia, blurred vision,
stomatitis.

SERIOUS REACTIONS

• An anaphylactic reaction
manifested as angioedema, wheezing,
tachycardia, and hypotension may
occur in the first few min of IV
administration in patients previously
exposed to cisplatin.
• Nephrotoxicity occurs in 28%-36%
of patients treated with a single
dose of cisplatin, usually during the
second week of therapy.
• Ototoxicity, including tinnitus and
hearing loss, occurs in 31% of patients
treated with a single dose of cisplatin.
It may be more severe in children and
may become more frequent or severe
with repeated doses.

PRECAUTIONS & CONSIDERATIONS

Cisplatin therapy is highly
emetogenic; all patients must receive
prophylactic antiemetic therapy. Use
with caution in patients with renal
impairment and in elderly patients,
who may be more susceptible
to peripheral neuropathy and
nephrotoxicity. Avoid use in pregnant
women.
Storage
Cisplatin injection solution should
be stored at room temperature.
Diluted solutions for infusion
are stable for up to 24 h at room
temperature.
Administration
Verify any cisplatin doses
> 100 mg/m² per course; such

high doses are rarely used.
Aluminum needles or IV sets
containing aluminum should
not be used for cisplatin
preparation or administration,
because aluminum reacts with
cisplatin to form a precipitate,
causing loss of potency. Infuse
over no more than 1 mg/min.
Hydration with 0.9% NaCl is
usually begun before the infusion
and continued after. Cioplatin
is quite emetogenic, so expect
pretreatment with a 5HT-3
astagonist and corticosteroids.

Citalopram
sye-tal'oh-pram
(Celexa, Cipramil [AUS])
**Do not confuse Celexa with
Celebrex, Zyprexa, or Cerebyx.**

CATEGORY AND SCHEDULE
Pregnancy Risk Category: C

Classification: Antidepressants, serotonin-specific reuptake
inhibitors

MECHANISM OF ACTION
A selective serotonin reuptake
inhibitor that blocks the uptake of the
neurotransmitter serotonin at CNS
presynaptic neuronal membranes,
increasing its availability at
postsynaptic receptor sites. *Therapeutic
Effect:* Relieves depression.

PHARMACOKINETICS
Well absorbed after PO
administration. Protein binding:
80%. Primarily metabolized in the
liver. Primarily excreted in feces with
a lesser amount eliminated in urine.
Half-life: 35 h.

C

AVAILABILITY
Oral Solution: 10 mg/5 mL.
Tablets: 10 mg, 20 mg, 40 mg.

INDICATIONS AND DOSAGES
▸ **Depression**
PO
Adults. Initially, 20 mg once a day in the morning or evening. May increase in 20-mg increments at intervals of no < 1 wk. Maximum: 60 mg/day.
Elderly, Patients with hepatic impairment. 20 mg/day. May titrate to 40 mg/day only for nonresponding patients.

OFF-LABEL USES
Treatment of anxiety, obsessive-compulsive disorder hot flashes, premenstrual dysphoric disorder, Panic disorder, Post-traumatic stress.

CONTRAINDICATIONS
Sensitivity to citalopram, use within 14 days of MAOIs.

INTERACTIONS
Drug
Antifungals, cimetidine, macrolide antibiotics: May increase the citalopram plasma level.
Carbamazepine: May decrease the citalopram plasma level.
MAOIs: May cause serotonin syndrome, marked by autonomic hyperactivity, coma, diaphoresis, excitement, hyperthermia, and rigidity, and neuroleptic malignant syndrome.
Metoprolol: Increases the metoprolol plasma level.
Anticoagulants, antiplatelet agents, NSAIDs, aspirin: May increase bleeding risk.
Nefazodone, triptans, sibutramine, trazodone, venlafaxine: May increase risk of serotonin syndrome.

Herbal
Valerian, St. John's wort, SAM-e, kava kava, and gotu kola: May increase CNS depression.
Food
None known.

DIAGNOSTIC TEST EFFECTS
May reduce serum sodium level.

SIDE EFFECTS
Frequent (11%-21%)
Nausea, dry mouth, somnolence, insomnia, diaphoresis.
Occasional (4%-8%)
Tremor, diarrhea, abnormal ejaculation, dyspepsia, fatigue, anxiety, vomiting, anorexia.
Rare (2%-3%)
Sinusitis, sexual dysfunction, menstrual disorder, abdominal pain, agitation, decreased libido.

SERIOUS REACTIONS
• Overdose is manifested as dizziness, drowsiness, tachycardia, somnolence, confusion, and seizures.
• SIADH and hyponatremia have been reported rarely, most commonly in elderly patients.

PRECAUTIONS & CONSIDERATIONS
Caution is warranted in patients with hepatic and renal impairment and in those with a history of hypomania, mania, and seizures. Citalopram is distributed in breast milk. Citalopram use in children may increase anticholinergic effects and hyperexcitability. Antidepressants have been reported to increase the risk of suicidal thinking and behavior in children, adolescents, and young adults (18-24 yr of age) with major depressive disorder (MDD) and other psychiatric disorders. Patients should be closely monitored for clinical worsening, suicidality, or unusual

changes in behavior, particularly during the initial 1-2 mo of therapy or following dosage adjustments. Elderly patients are more sensitive to the drug's anticholinergic effects, such as dry mouth, and are more likely to experience confusion, dizziness, hyperexcitability, and sedation.

Alcohol and tasks that require mental alertness or motor skills should be avoided. CBC and blood chemistry tests should be performed before and periodically during therapy, especially with long-term use. Citalopram may impair platelet aggregation.

Administration

! Make sure that at least 14 days elapse between the use of MAOIs and citalopram.

Take citalopram without regard to food. Crush scored tablets, if necessary. Do not abruptly discontinue citalopram or increase the dosage.

Clarithromycin
clare-i-thro-mye′sin
(Biaxin, Biaxin XL, Klacid [AUS])

CATEGORY AND SCHEDULE
Pregnancy Risk Category: C

Classification: Antibiotics, macrolides

MECHANISM OF ACTION
A macrolide that binds to ribosomal receptor sites of susceptible organisms, inhibiting protein synthesis of the bacterial cell wall. *Therapeutic Effect:* Bacteriostatic; may be bactericidal with high

dosages or very susceptible microorganisms.

PHARMACOKINETICS
Well absorbed from the GI tract. Protein binding: 65%-75%. Widely distributed. Metabolized in the liver to active metabolite. Primarily excreted in urine. Not removed by hemodialysis. *Half-life:* 3-7 h; metabolite 5-7 h (increased in impaired renal function).

AVAILABILITY
Oral Suspension: 125 mg/5 mL, 250 mg/5 mL.
Tablets: 250 mg, 500 mg.
Tablets (Extended-Release): 500 mg.

INDICATIONS AND DOSAGES
▸ **Bronchitis**
PO
Adults, Elderly. 500 mg q12h for 7-14 days or extended-release tablets 1g q24h for 7 days.
▸ **Skin, soft-tissue infections**
PO
Adults, Elderly. 250 mg q12h for 7-14 days.
Children.
7.5 mg/kg q12h for 10 days.
▸ **MAC prophylaxis**
PO
Adults, Elderly. 500 mg 2 times/day.
Children.
7.5 mg/kg q12h. Maximum: 500 mg 2 times/day.
▸ **MAC treatment**
PO
Adults, Elderly. 500 mg 2 times/day in combination.
Children. 7.5 mg/kg q12h in combination. Maximum: 500 mg 2 times/day.
▸ **Pharyngitis, tonsillitis**
PO
Adults, Elderly. 250 mg q12h for 10 days.
Children. 7.5 mg/kg q12h for 10 days.

▶ **Pneumonia**
PO
Adults, Elderly. 250 mg q12h for
7-14 days or extended-release tablets
1g q24h for 7 days.
Children. 7.5 mg/kg q12h.

▶ **Maxillary sinusitis**
PO
Adults, Elderly. 500 mg q12h for
14 days or extended-release tablets
1g q24h for 14 days.
Children. 7.5 mg/kg q12h.
Maximum: 500 mg 2 times/day.

▶ **Helicobacter pylori**
PO
Adults, Elderly. 500 mg q12h for
10-14 days in combination.

▶ **Acute otitis media**
PO
Children. 7.5 mg/kg q12h for
10 days.

▶ **Dosage in renal impairment**
For patients with creatinine
clearance < 30 mL/min, reduce
dose by 50% and administer once or
twice a day. Further adjustment is
needed in patients taking ritonavir
concurrently.

CONTRAINDICATIONS

Hypersensitivity to clarithromycin
or other macrolide antibiotics;
concurrent ergot use.

INTERACTIONS

Drug
**Carbamazepine, digoxin,
theophylline:** May increase blood
concentration and toxicity of these
drugs.
Rifampin: May decrease
clarithromycin blood concentration.
Ritonavir: Increases clarithromycin
concentrations; reduce
clarithromycin dose.
Warfarin: May increase warfarin
effects.
Zidovudine: May decrease blood
concentration of zidovudine.

Herbal
St. John's wort: May decrease
clarithromycin blood concentration.
Food
None known.

DIAGNOSTIC TEST EFFECTS

May (rarely) increase BUN, AST
(SGOT), and ALT (SGPT) levels.

SIDE EFFECTS

Occasional (3%-6%)
Diarrhea, nausea, altered taste,
abdominal pain.
Rare (1%-2%)
Headache, dyspepsia.

SERIOUS REACTIONS

• Antibiotic-associated colitis and
other superinfections may result from
altered bacterial balance.
• Hepatotoxicity and
thrombocytopenia occur rarely.

PRECAUTIONS & CONSIDERATIONS

Caution is warranted in patients
with hepatic or renal dysfunction
and in elderly patients with
severe renal impairment.
Determine whether there is a
history of hepatitis or allergies to
clarithromycin or other macrolides
before beginning therapy.
Macrolides have been associated
with QTc prolongation; use with
caution in patients with risk
factors for QT prolongation. It is
unknown whether clarithromycin is
distributed in breast milk. The safety
and efficacy of clarithromycin have
not been established in children
younger than 6 mo. Age-related
renal impairment may require a
dosage adjustment in older patients.
    Daily bowel activity and stool
consistency should be assessed.
Mild GI effects may be tolerable, but
severe symptoms may indicate the
onset of antibiotic-associated colitis.

Be alert for signs and symptoms of superinfection, including abdominal pain, anal or genital pruritus, moderate to severe diarrhea, and mouth soreness.

Storage

Store at room temperature. Reconstitued oral suspension is stable for 14 days at room temperature. Do not refrigerate; suspension may gel.

Administration

Shake suspension well before use, Take tablets and oral suspension with or without food; take extended release tablets with food. Take clarithromycin tablets with 8 oz of water. Do not crush or break extended-release tablets. Space doses evenly around the clock, and continue taking clarithromycin for the full course of therapy.

Clemastine

klem'as-teen
(Dayhist Allergy, Tavist Allergy)

CATEGORY AND SCHEDULE

Pregnancy Risk Category: B
OTC (1.34 mg tablet)

Classification: Antihistamines, H_1-receptor antagonist

MECHANISM OF ACTION

An ethanolamine that competes with histamine on effector cells in the GI tract, blood vessels, and respiratory tract. *Therapeutic Effect:* Relieves allergy symptoms, including urticaria, rhinitis, and pruritus.

PHARMACOKINETICS

Route	Onset	Peak	Duration
PO	15-60 min	5-7 h	10-12 h

Well absorbed from the GI tract. Metabolized in the liver. Excreted primarily in urine.

AVAILABILITY

Syrup (Daytist, Allergy, Tavist):
0.67 mg/5 mL.
Tablets (Dayhist, Tavist, Allergy):
1.34 mg (OTC), 2.68 mg.

INDICATIONS AND DOSAGES
▶ **Allergic rhinitis, urticaria**
PO
Adults, Children 12 years and older:
1.34 mg twice a day up to 2.68 mg 3 times a day. Maximum:
8.04 mg/day.
Children 6-11 yr. 0.67-1.34 mg twice a day. Maximum: 4.02 mg/day.
Children younger than 6 yr.
0.05 mg/kg/day divided into 2-3 doses per day. Maximum: 1.34 mg/day.
Elderly. 1.34 mg 1-2 times a day.

CONTRAINDICATIONS

Angle-closure glaucoma, hypersensitivity to clemastine, use within 14 days of MAOIs.

INTERACTIONS

Drug
Alcohol, other CNS depressants:
May increase CNS depression.
MAOIs: May increase the anticholinergic and CNS depressant effects of clemastine.
Herbal and Food
None known.

DIAGNOSTIC TEST EFFECTS

May suppress wheal and flare reactions to antigen skin testing unless drug is discontinued 4 days before testing.

SIDE EFFECTS

Frequent
Somnolence, dizziness, urine retention, thickening of bronchial

secretions, dry mouth, nose, or throat; in elderly, sedation, dizziness, hypotension.

Occasional

Epigastric distress, flushing, blurred vision, tinnitus, paresthesia, diaphoresis, chills.

SERIOUS REACTIONS

• A hypersensitivity reaction, marked by eczema, pruritus, rash, cardiac disturbances, angioedema, and photosensitivity, may occur.

• Overdose symptoms may vary from CNS depression, including sedation, apnea, cardiovascular collapse, and death, to severe paradoxical reaction, such as hallucinations, tremor, and seizures.

• Children may experience paradoxical reactions, such as restlessness, insomnia, euphoria, nervousness, and tremors.

• Overdose in children may result in hallucinations, seizures, and death.

PRECAUTIONS & CONSIDERATIONS

Caution is warranted with increased intraocular pressure, renal disease, cardiac disease, hypertension, seizure disorder, hyperthyroidism, asthma, GI or genitourinary obstruction, peptic ulcer disease, and benign prostatic hyperplasia. Clemastine is excreted in breast milk and should not be used in breastfeeding women. The safety and efficacy of clemastine have not been established in children younger than 6 yr. Age-related renal impairment may require a dosage adjustment in elderly patients. Avoid drinking alcoholic beverages and tasks that require alertness or motor skills until response to the drug is established.

Drowsiness, dizziness, and dry mouth may occur; tolerance may develop to the sedative effects. BP and therapeutic response should be monitored.

Administration

❗ Take clemastine without regard to food. Crush scored tablets as needed.

Clindamycin

klin-da-mye′sin
(Cleocin, Dalacin [CAN]), Clindesse, Cleocin-T, Clindamax

CATEGORY AND SCHEDULE

Pregnancy Risk Category: B

Classification: Lincomycin derivative anti-infective

MECHANISM OF ACTION

A lincosamide antibiotic that inhibits protein synthesis of the bacterial cell wall by binding to bacterial ribosomal receptor sites. Topically, it decreases fatty acid concentration on the skin. *Therapeutic Effect:* Bacteriostatic. Prevents outbreaks of acne vulgaris.

PHARMACOKINETICS

Rapidly absorbed from the GI tract. Protein binding: 92%-94%. Widely distributed. Metabolized in the liver to some active metabolites. Primarily excreted in urine. Not removed by hemodialysis. *Half-life:* 2.4-3 h (increased in impaired renal function and premature infants).

AVAILABILITY

Capsules: 75 mg, 150 mg, 300 mg.
Oral Solution: 75 mg/5 mL.
Injection: 150 mg/mL.
Injection solution premixed: 300 mg, 600 mg, 900 mg.
Topical Gel: 1%.
Topical Foam: 1%.
Topical Lotion: 1%.

Topical Solution: 1%.
Vaginal Cream: 2%.
Vaginal Suppository: 100 mg.

INDICATIONS AND DOSAGES
▸ **Chronic bone and joint, respiratory tract, skin and soft-tissue, intra-abdominal, and female genitourinary infections; endocarditis; septicemia**
PO
Adults, Elderly. 150-450 mg/dose q6-8h.
Children. 10-30 mg/kg/day in 3-4 divided doses. Maximum: 1.8 g/day.
IV, IM
Adults, Elderly. 1.2-1.8 g/day in 2-4 divided doses. Maximum: 4.8 g/day.
Children. 25-40 mg/kg/day in 3-4 divided doses.
▸ **Bacterial vaginosis**
PO
Adults, Elderly. 300 mg twice a day for 7 days.
INTRAVAGINAL
Adults. One applicatorful at bedtime for 3-7 days or 1 suppository at bedtime for 3 days. A one-dose reqimen is also available (Clindesse).
▸ **Acne vulgaris**
TOPICAL
Adults. Apply thin layer to affected area twice a day; foam once daily.

OFF-LABEL USES
Treatment of malaria, otitis media, *Pneumocystis carinii* pneumonia, toxoplasmosis, dental abscess.

CONTRAINDICATIONS
History of antibiotic-associated colitis, regional enteritis, or ulcerative colitis; hypersensitivity to clindamycin or lincomycin; known allergy to tartrazine dye.

INTERACTIONS
Drug
Adsorbent antidiarrheals: May delay absorption of clindamycin.

Chloramphenicol, erythromycin: May antagonize the effects of clindamycin.
Neuromuscular blockers: May increase the effects of these drugs.
Herbal and Food
None known.

DIAGNOSTIC TEST EFFECTS
May increase serum alkaline phosphatase, AST (SGOT), and ALT (SGPT) levels.

Ⓙ IV INCOMPATIBILITIES
Allopurinol (Aloprim), filgrastim (Neupogen), fluconazole (Diflucan), idarubicin (Idamycin).

Ⓙ IV COMPATIBILITIES
Amiodarone (Cordarone), diltiazem (Cardizem), heparin, hydromorphone (Dilaudid), magnesium sulfate, midazolam (Versed), morphine, multivitamins, propofol (Diprivan).

SIDE EFFECTS
Frequent
Systemic: Abdominal pain, nausea, vomiting, diarrhea.
Topical: Dry scaly skin.
Vaginal: Vaginitis, pruritus.
Occasional
Systemic: Phlebitis or thrombophlebitis with IV administration, pain and induration at IM injection site, allergic reaction, urticaria, pruritus.
Topical: Contact dermatitis, abdominal pain, mild diarrhea, burning or stinging.
Vaginal: Headache, dizziness, nausea, vomiting, abdominal pain.
Rare
Vaginal: Hypersensitivity reaction.

SERIOUS REACTIONS

• Antibiotic-associated colitis and other superinfections may occur during and several weeks after clindamycin therapy (including the topical form).
• Blood dyscrasias (leukopenia, thrombocytopenia) and nephrotoxicity (proteinuria, azotemia, oliguria) occur rarely.

PRECAUTIONS & CONSIDERATIONS

Caution is warranted with severe renal or hepatic dysfunction and in patients using neuromuscular blockers concurrently. Do not apply topical preparations to abraded areas or near the eyes. Systemic clindamycin readily crosses the placenta and is distributed in breast milk. It is unknown whether the topical and vaginal forms of clindamycin are distributed in breast milk. Use clindamycin cautiously in children < 1 mo-old. No age-related precautions have been noted in elderly patients. Use caution when applying topical clindamycin concurrently with abrasive, peeling acne agents, soaps, or alcohol-containing cosmetics to avoid a cumulative effect. Sexual intercourse during treatment with the vaginal form of clindamycin should be avoided.

Diarrhea should be reported promptly to the physician because of the potential for developing serious colitis (even with topical or vaginal clindamycin). Pattern of daily bowel activity and stool consistency should be assessed. Skin should be assessed for dryness, irritation, and rash. Be alert for signs and symptoms of superinfection, such as anal or genital pruritus, a change in oral mucosa, increased fever, and severe diarrhea. History of allergies, particularly to aspirin, clindamycin, or lincomycin, should be determined before beginning drug therapy. Use of neuromuscular blockers should also be determined because their concurrent use should be avoided, if possible.

Storage
Store capsules and topical formulations at room temperature. After reconstitution, the oral solution is stable for 2 wks at room temperature. Do not refrigerate the oral solution to avoid thickening it. The IV infusion (piggyback) is stable at room temperature for up to 16 days.

Administration
Take capsules and solution with water and without regard to food.

The IV infusion (piggyback) is stable at room temperature for up to 16 days. Dilute 300-600 mg with 50 mL D5W or 0.9% NaCl (900-1200 mg with 100 mL). Never exceed a concentration of 18 mg/mL. Infuse 50-mL (300- to 600-mg) piggyback solution over 10-20 min; infuse 100-mL (900-mg to 1.2-g) piggyback solution over 30-40 min. Be aware that severe hypotension or cardiac arrest can occur with too-rapid administration. Do not administer more than 1.2 g in a single infusion.

For IM use, do not exceed 600 mg/dose. Give by deep IM injection.

Do not apply topical or intravaginal preparations near the eyes or on abraded areas. Rinse eyes with copious amounts of cool tap water if these forms of clindamycin accidentally come in contact with eyes. For intravaginal use, use provided applicators to insert dosage.

Clioquinol, Hydrocortisone

klee-oh-kwee′nole
(Ala-Quin, Dek-Quin, Vioform-Hydrocortisone Cream, Vioform-Hydrocortisone Mild Cream, Vioform-Hydrocortisone Mild Ointment, Vioform-Hydrocortisone Ointment)

CATEGORY AND SCHEDULE
Pregnancy Risk Category: C

Classification: Anti-infectives, topical, antifungals, topical, corticosteroids, topical, dermatologics

MECHANISM OF ACTION
Clioquinol is a broad-spectrum antibacterial agent, but the mechanism of action is unknown. Hydrocortisone is a corticosteroid that diffuses across cell membranes, forms complexes with specific receptors, and further binds to DNA and stimulates transcription of mRNA (messenger RNA) and subsequent protein synthesis of various enzymes thought to be ultimately responsible for the anti-inflammatory effects of corticosteroids applied topically to the skin. *Therapeutic Effect:* Alters membrane function and produces antibacterial activity.

PHARMACOKINETICS
Clioquinol is absorbed through the skin; absorption may be increased with use of an occlusive dressing.

AVAILABILITY
Cream: 3% clioquinol and 0.5% hydrocortisone (Ala-Quin, Vioform-Hydrocortisone Mild Cream), 3% clioquinol and 1% hydrocortisone (Dek-Quin, Vioform-Hydrocortisone Cream).

Ointment: 3% clioquinol and 1% hydrocortisone (Vioform-Hydrocortisone Mild Ointment).

INDICATIONS AND DOSAGES
▸ **Antibacterial, antifungal skin conditions**
TOPICAL
Adults, Elderly, Children 12 yr and older. Apply to skin 3-4 times/day. Typical duration is 2-4 wks.

CONTRAINDICATIONS
Lesions of the eye, tuberculosis of skin, diaper rash, children < 2 yr of age; hypersensitivity to clioquinol or hydrocortisone or any other component of the formulation.

INTERACTIONS
Drug
None known.
Herbal
None known.
Food
None known.

DIAGNOSTIC TEST EFFECTS
May alter thyroid function tests. Clioquinol may produce false-positive ferric chloride test results for phenylketonuria (PKU).

SIDE EFFECTS
Occasional
Blistering, burning, itching, peeling, skin rash, redness, swelling.

SERIOUS REACTIONS
• Thinning of skin with easy bruising may occur with prolonged use.

PRECAUTIONS & CONSIDERATIONS
Caution is warranted with herpes simplex, eczema vaccinatum, varicella, or other viral infections of the skin as well as intolerance to chloroxine, iodine, or iodine-containing preparations. It is

unknown whether clioquinol and hydrocortisone cross placenta or are distributed in breast milk. No age-related precautions have been noted in children or elderly patients.
This medication may stain fabrics, skin, hair, and nails yellow. The affected area should be kept clean and dry. Light clothing should be worn to promote ventilation.

Storage
Store at room temperature.

Administration
Before applying, wash affected area with soap and water and dry thoroughly. Apply a thin layer to affected area. Wash hands after application.

Clobetasol
klo-bet′a-sol
(Alti-Clobetasol [CAN], Cormax, Dermovate [CAN], Gen-Clobetasol [CAN], Olux, Novo-Clobetasol [CAN], Temovate)

CATEGORY AND SCHEDULE
Pregnancy Risk Category: C

Classification: Topical corticosteroid, very high potency

MECHANISM OF ACTION
A corticosteroid that inhibits accumulation of inflammatory cells at inflammation sites, phagocytosis, lysosomal enzyme release, and synthesis or release of mediators of inflammation. *Therapeutic Effect:* Decreases or prevents tissue response to inflammatory process.

PHARMACOKINETICS
May be absorbed from intact skin. Metabolized in liver. Excreted in the urine.

AVAILABILITY
Cream: 0.05% (Cormax, Temovate).
Cream, in emollient base: 0.05% (Temovate).
Foam: 0.05% (Olux).
Gel: 0.05% (Temovate).
Lotion: 0.05% (Clobex).
Ointment: 0.05% (Cormax, Temovate).
Shampoo: 0.05% (Clobex).
Topical Solution: 0.05% (Clobex, Cormax, Temovate).

INDICATIONS AND DOSAGES
▶ **Anti-inflammatory, corticosteroid replacement therapy**
TOPICAL
Adults, Elderly, Children 12 yr and older. Apply 2 times/day for 2 wks.
FOAM
Adults, Elderly, Children 12 yr and older. Apply 2 times/day for 2 wks.
SHAMPOO
Adults, Elderly. Apply thin film to dry scalp once daily; leave in place for 15 min, and then add water, lather; rinse thoroughly.

CONTRAINDICATIONS
Hypersensitivity to clobetasol or other corticosteroids.

INTERACTIONS
Drug
None known.
Herbal
None known.
Food
None known.

DIAGNOSTIC TEST EFFECTS
None known.

SIDE EFFECTS
Frequent
Local irritation, dry skin, itching, redness.

Occasional
Allergic contact dermatitis.
Rare
Cushing syndrome, numbness of fingers, skin atrophy.

SERIOUS REACTIONS
• Overdosage can occur from topically applied clobetasol propionate absorbed in sufficient amounts to produce systemic effects producing reversible adrenal suppression, manifestations of Cushing syndrome, hyperglycemia, and glucosuria in some patients.

PRECAUTIONS & CONSIDERATIONS
Avoid use of occlusive dressings on affected area. Skin irritation should be reported. HPA axis suppression should be evaluated by ACTH stimulation test, AM plasma cortisol test, or urinary free cortisol test. It is unknown whether clobetasol propionate crosses the placenta or is distributed in breast milk. Safety and efficacy of clobetasol propionate have not been established in children. No age-related precautions have been noted in elderly patients.
Administration
Apply sparingly to skin or scalp and rub into area thoroughly. Use for 2 wks. If using for the scalp, part the hair and apply to the area.

Clocortolone
klo-kort′o-lone
(Cloderm, Cloderm [CAN])

CATEGORY AND SCHEDULE
Pregnancy Risk Category: C

Classification: Corticosteroids, topical group III medium potency

MECHANISM OF ACTION
A topical corticosteroid that inhibits accumulation of inflammatory cells at inflammation sites, suppresses mitotic activity, and causes vasoconstriction. *Therapeutic Effect:* Decreases or prevents tissue response to inflammatory process.

PHARMACOKINETICS
Absorption is variable and dependent upon many factors, including the integrity of skin, dose, vehicle used, and use of occlusive dressings. Small amounts may be absorbed from the skin. Metabolized in liver. Excreted in the urine and feces.

AVAILABILITY
Cream: 0.1%.

INDICATIONS AND DOSAGES
▶ **Dermatoses**
TOPICAL
Adults, Elderly, Children 12 yr and older. Apply 1-4 times/day.

CONTRAINDICATIONS
Hypersensitivity to clocortolone pivalate or other corticosteroids; viral, fungal, or tubercular skin lesions.

INTERACTIONS
Drug, Herbal, and Food
None known.

DIAGNOSTIC TEST EFFECTS
None known.

SIDE EFFECTS
Occasional
Local irritation, burning, itching, redness, allergic contact dermatitis.
Rare
Hypertrichosis, hypopigmentation, maceration of skin, miliaria, perioral dermatitis, skin atrophy, striae.

C

SERIOUS REACTIONS

• Overdosage can occur from topically applied clocortolone pivalate absorbed in sufficient amounts to produce systemic effects in some patients.

PRECAUTIONS & CONSIDERATIONS

Avoid use of occlusive dressings on affected area. Skin irritation should be reported. HPA axis suppression should be evaluated by ACTH stimulation test, AM plasma cortisol test, or urinary free cortisol test. It is unknown whether clocortolone crosses the placenta or is distributed in breast milk. Safety and efficacy of clocortolone have not been established in children. No age-related precautions have been noted in elderly patients.

Administration

Apply topical preparation sparingly. Do not use on broken skin. Avoid use of occlusive dressings.

Clofarabine

kloe-far′-ah-been
(Clolar)

CATEGORY AND SCHEDULE

Pregnancy Risk Category: D

Classification: Antineoplastic, purine analogs

MECHANISM OF ACTION

An antineoplastic agent that inhibits DNA synthesis by decreasing deoxynucleotide triphosphate pools. It inhibits ribonucleoside reductase, terminates elongation of the DNA chain, and inhibits repair through incorporation into the DNA chain by competitive inhibition of DNA polymerases. *Therapeutic Effect:* Inhibits synthesis of DNA.

PHARMACOKINETICS

Protein binding: 47%. Negligible liver metabolism. Primarily excreted in urine. *Half-life:* 5.2 h.

AVAILABILITY

Injection Solution: 1 mg/mL.

INDICATIONS AND DOSAGES
▸ **ALL**
IV

Young Adults and Children 1-21 yr.
52 mg/m^2 over 2 h daily for 5 consecutive days. Repeat every 2–6 wks following recovery or return to baseline organ function.

CONTRAINDICATIONS

Hypersensitivity to clofarabine or its components.

INTERACTIONS

Drug, Herbal, and Food
None known.

DIAGNOSTIC TEST EFFECTS

Increased AST, ALT, potassium, uric acid, creatinine.

⊘ IV INCOMPATIBILITIES

Do not administer with any other medications through the same IV line.

⬗ IV COMPATIBILITIES

Dextrose 5%, 0.9% Sodium Chloride. No other information available.

SIDE EFFECTS

Frequent
Infection, vomiting, nausea, febrile neutropenia, diarrhea, pruritus, headache, ALT increased, dermatitis, pyrexia, AST increased, rigors, abdominal pain, fatigue, pericardial effusion, tachycardia, epistaxis, anorexia, petechiae, hypotension, pain in limb, left ventricular systolic dysfunction, anxiety, constipation, edema, pain, cough, erythema, flushing,

mucosal inflammation, hematuria, dizziness, bilirubin increased, jaundice, gingival bleeding, hepatomegaly, injection site pain, myalgia, respiratory distress, palmar-plantar sore throat, back pain, dyspnea, erythrodysesthesia syndrome, staphylococcal infection, oral candidiasis, appetite decreased, cellulitis, depression, irritability, arthralgia, herpes simplex, hypertension, lethargy.

Occasional

Somnolence, weight gain, tremor, pleural effusion, pneumonia, systemic inflammatory response syndrome (SIRS)/capillary leak syndrome, transfusion reaction, bacteremia, creatinine increased.

SERIOUS REACTIONS

• Tumor lysis syndrome may occur.
• Severe bone marrow suppression, including neutropenia, anemia, and thrombocytopenia, has been observed.

PRECAUTIONS & CONSIDERATIONS

Use with caution in renal or hepatic impairment. Safety and effectiveness have not been established in patients over 21 yr of age. High emetic potential; all patients should receive prophylactic antiemetics. Prophylactic corticosteroids should be considered to SIRS/capillary leak syndrome; prophylactic allopurinol may be considered if tumor lysis is anticipated. Avoid clofarabine use in pregnancy and breastfeeding. Women of childbearing potential should be advised to use an effective contraceptive.

Storage

Store vials at room temperature. Reconstituted solution stable 24 h at room temperature.

Administration

Administer as IV infusion over 2 h.

Injection should be filtered through a 0.2 μm syringe filter and then diluted with D5%W or 0.9% NaCl (Final concentration: 0.15-0.4 mg/mL.)

Clomiphene

kloe′mi-feen
(Clomhexal [AUS], Clomid, Clomid [CAN], Milophene, Milophene [CAN], Serophene, Serophene [CAN])
Do not confuse clomiphene with chlomipramine.

CATEGORY AND SCHEDULE

Pregnancy Risk Category: X

Classification: Nonsteroidal ovulatory stimulant, antiestrogen

MECHANISM OF ACTION

An ovulation stimulator that promotes release of pituitary gonadotropins. *Therapeutic Effect:* Stimulates ovulation.

PHARMACOKINETICS

Readily absorbed. Time to peak occurs within 6.5 h. Undergoes enterohepatic recirculation. Primarily excreted in feces. *Half-life:* 5-7 days.

AVAILABILITY

Tablets: 50 mg (Clomid, Milophene, Serophene).

INDICATIONS AND DOSAGES

▶ **Ovulatory failure, females**
PO
Adults. 50 mg/day for 5 days (first course); start the regimen on the fifth day of cycle. Increase dose only if unresponsive to cyclic 50 mg. Maximum: 100 mg/day for 5 days. Do not exceed 6 courses of treatment.

OFF-LABEL USES

Infertility in men.

CONTRAINDICATIONS

Liver dysfunction, abnormal uterine bleeding, enlargement or development of ovarian cyst,

C

uncontrolled thyroid or adrenal dysfunction in the presence of an organic intracranial lesion such as pituitary tumor, pregnancy, hypersensitivity to clomiphene.

INTERACTIONS
Drug
Danazol: May decrease the response of clomiphene.
Estradiol: May decrease estradiol.
Herbal
None known.
Food
None known.

DIAGNOSTIC TEST EFFECTS
Altered levels of thyroid function tests.

SIDE EFFECTS
Frequent (10%-13%)
Hot flashes, ovarian enlargement.
Occasional (2%-5%)
Abdominal/pelvic discomfort, bloating, nausea, vomiting, breast discomfort (females).
Rare (< 1%)
Vision disturbances, abnormal menstrual flow, breast enlargement (males), headache, mental depression, ovarian cyst formation, thromboembolism, uterine fibroid enlargement.

SERIOUS REACTIONS
• Thrombophlebitis, alopecia, and polyuria occur rarely.

PRECAUTIONS & CONSIDERATIONS
Caution should be used with liver dysfunction, polycystic ovary disease, and multiple pregnancies. Clomiphene use should be avoided during pregnancy, and it is distributed in breast milk. Safety and efficacy have not been established in children or in elderly patients. Pregnancy should be immediately reported.

Visual disturbances, dizziness, light-headedness may occur.
Administration
Take clomiphene without meals. Encourage coitus to coincide with ovulation.

Clomipramine
klom-ip′ra-meen
(Anafranil, Apo-Clomipramine [CAN], Clopram [AUS], Novo-Clopamine [CAN], Placil [AUS])
Do not confuse clomipramine with chlorpromazine or clomiphene, or Anafranil with alfentanil, enalapril, or nafarelin.

CATEGORY AND SCHEDULE
Pregnancy Risk Category: C

Classification: Antidepressants, tricyclic

MECHANISM OF ACTION
A tricyclic antidepressant that blocks the reuptake of neurotransmitters, such as norepinephrine and serotonin, at CNS presynaptic membranes, increasing their availability at postsynaptic receptor sites. *Therapeutic Effect:* Reduces obsessive-compulsive behavior.

PHARMACOKINETICS
Well absorbed from GI tract. Protein binding: 97%. Principally bound to albumin. Distributed into cerebrospinal fluid. Metabolized in the liver. Undergoes extensive first-pass effect. Excreted in urine and feces. *Half-life:* 19-37 h.

AVAILABILITY
Capsules: 25 mg, 50 mg, 75 mg.

INDICATIONS AND DOSAGES
▶ **Obsessive-compulsive disorder**
PO
Adults, Elderly. Initially, 25 mg/day.
May gradually increase to 100 mg/
day in the first 2 wks. Maximum:
250 mg/day.
Children 10 yr and older.
Initially, 25 mg/day. May gradually
increase up to maximum of 200 mg/day.
OFF-LABEL USES
Treatment of bulimia nervosa,
cataplexy associated with narcolepsy,
mental depression, neurogenic pain,
panic disorder.

CONTRAINDICATIONS
Acute recovery period after MI,
use within 14 days of MAOIs,
hypersensitivity to TCAs.

INTERACTIONS
Drug
Antithyroid agents: May increase
the risk of agranulocytosis.
Cimetidine: May increase
clomipramine blood concentration
and risk of toxicity.
Clonidine, guanadrel: May
decrease the effects of these drugs.
MAOIs: May increase the risk of
neuroleptic malignant syndrome,
seizures, hyperpyresis, and
hypertensive crisis. Contraindicated.
Other CNS depressants: May
increase CNS and respiratory
depression and the hypotensive
effects of clomipramine.
Phenothiazines: May increase the
anticholinergic and sedative effects
of clomipramine.
Sympathomimetics: May increase
the risk of cardiac effects.
Herbal
None known.
Food
Alcohol: May increase CNS and
respiratory depression and the
hypotensive effects of clomipramine.

Grapefruit juice: May increase
clomipramine concentrations.

DIAGNOSTIC TEST EFFECTS
May alter the blood glucose level and
ECG readings.

SIDE EFFECTS
Frequent
Somnolence, fatigue, dry mouth,
blurred vision, constipation, sexual
dysfunction (42%), ejaculatory
failure (20%), impotence, weight
gain (18%), delayed micturition,
orthostatic hypotension, diaphoresis,
impaired concentration, increased
appetite, urine retention.
Occasional
GI disturbances (such as nausea, GI
distress, and metallic taste), asthenia,
aggressiveness, muscle weakness.
Rare
Paradoxical reactions (agitation,
restlessness, nightmares, insomnia),
extrapyramidal symptoms,
(particularly fine hand tremor),
laryngitis, seizures.

SERIOUS REACTIONS
• Overdose may produce seizures;
cardiovascular effects, such as severe
orthostatic hypotension, dizziness,
tachycardia, palpitations, and
arrhythmias; and altered temperature
regulation, including hyperpyrexia or
hypothermia.
• Abrupt discontinuation after
prolonged therapy may produce
headache, malaise, nausea, vomiting,
and vivid dreams.
• Anemia and agranulocytosis have
been noted.

PRECAUTIONS & CONSIDERATIONS
Caution is warranted in patients with
cardiac disease, diabetes mellitus,
glaucoma, hiatal hernia, history
of seizures, history of urinary
obstruction or urine retention,

hyperthyroidism, increased intraocular pressure, benign prostatic hyperplasia, renal or hepatic disease, and schizophrenia. Clomipramine is minimally distributed in breast milk. Clomipramine use is not recommended for children younger than 10 yr. Antidepressants have been reported to increase the risk of suicidal thinking and behavior in children, adolescents, and young adults (18-24 yr of age) with major depressive disorder (MDD) and other psychiatric disorders. Patients should be closely monitored for clinical worsening, suicidality, or unusual changes in behavior, particularly during the initial 1-2 mo of therapy or following dosage adjustments. A lower dosage should be given to elderly patients, who are at increased risk for drug toxicity.

Dizziness may occur, so change positions slowly and avoid alcohol and tasks that require mental alertness or motor skills. CBC to detect signs of anemia and agranulocytosis and ECG to detect arrhythmias should be performed before and periodically during therapy.

Administration
! Make sure at least 14 days elapse between the use of MAOIs and clomipramine.

Take clomipramine with food or milk if GI distress occurs. Administer in divided doses with food during dose titration; final dose may be administered once daily at bedtime to minimize daytime sedation. Full therapeutic effect may be noted in 2-4 wks. Do not abruptly discontinue clomipramine.

Clonazepam
kloe-na′zi-pam
(Apo-Clonazepam [CAN], Clonapam [CAN], Klonopin, Paxam [AUS], Rivotril [CAN])
Do not confuse clonazepam with clonidine or lorazepam.

CATEGORY AND SCHEDULE
Pregnancy Risk Category: D
Controlled Substane Schedule IV

Classification: Anxiolytic, anticonvulsant, benzodiazepines

MECHANISM OF ACTION
A benzodiazepine that depresses all levels of the CNS, inhibits nerve impulse transmission in the motor cortex, and suppresses abnormal discharge in petit mal seizures. *Therapeutic Effect:* Produces anxiolytic and anticonvulsant effects.

PHARMACOKINETICS
Well absorbed from the GI tract. Protein binding: 85%. Metabolized in the liver. Excreted in urine. Not removed by hemodialysis. *Half-life:* 18-50 h.

AVAILABILITY
Tablets: 0.5 mg, 1 mg, 2 mg.
Tablets (Disintegrating): 0.125 mg, 0.25 mg, 0.5 mg, 1 mg, 2 mg.

INDICATIONS AND DOSAGES
▸ **Adjunctive treatment of Lennox-Gastaut syndrome (petit mal variant) and akinetic, myoclonic, and absence (petit mal) seizures**
PO
Adults, Elderly, Children 10 yr and older. 1.5 mg/day; may be increased in 0.5- to 1-mg increments every 3 days until seizures are controlled.

Do not exceed maintenance dosage of 20 mg/day.

Infants, Children younger than 10 yr or weighing < 30 kg. 0.01-0.03 mg/kg/day in 2-3 divided doses; may be increased by up to 0.5 mg every 3 days until seizures are controlled. Do not exceed maintenance dosage of 0.2 mg/kg/day.

▶ **Panic disorder**

PO

Adults, Elderly. Initially, 0.25 mg twice a day; increased in increments of 0.125-0.25 mg twice a day every 3 days. Maximum: 4 mg/day.

OFF-LABEL USES

Adjunctive treatment of seizures; treatment of simple, complex partial, and tonic-clonic seizures.

CONTRAINDICATIONS

Narrow-angle glaucoma, significant hepatic disease.

INTERACTIONS

Drug

Alcohol, other CNS depressants: May increase CNS depressant effect.
Ketoconazole, itraconazole, fluconazole, protease inhibitors, nefazodone: May increase clonazepam serum levels.

Herbal

Kava kava: May increase sedation.
St. John's wort: May decrease clonazepam concentrations.

Food

None known.

DIAGNOSTIC TEST EFFECTS

None known.

SIDE EFFECTS

Frequent

Mild, transient drowsiness; ataxia; behavioral disturbances (aggression, irritability, agitation), especially in children.

Occasional

Rash, ankle, or facial edema, nocturia, dysuria, change in appetite or weight, dry mouth, sore gums, nausea, blurred vision.

Rare

Paradoxical CNS reactions, including hyperactivity or nervousness in children and excitement or restlessness in elderly patients (particularly in the presence of uncontrolled pain).

SERIOUS REACTIONS

• Abrupt withdrawal may result in pronounced restlessness, irritability, insomnia, hand tremors, abdominal or muscle cramps, diaphoresis, vomiting, and status epilepticus.
• Overdose results in somnolence, confusion, diminished reflexes, and coma.

PRECAUTIONS & CONSIDERATIONS

Caution is warranted with chronic respiratory disease and impaired renal and hepatic function. Clonazepam crosses the placenta and may be distributed in breast milk. Chronic clonazepam use during pregnancy may produce withdrawal symptoms and CNS depression in neonates. Long-term clonazepam use may adversely affect the mental and physical development of children. Elderly patients are usually more sensitive to clonazepam's CNS effects, such as ataxia, dizziness, and oversedation. Expect to give them a lower dosage and increase it gradually. Alcohol, smoking, and tasks that require mental alertness or motor skills should be avoided.

Drowsiness and dizziness may occur. History of the seizure disorder, including the duration, frequency, and intensity of seizures, should be assessed. Autonomic responses, such as cold or clammy hands and diaphoresis, and motor responses, such as agitation, trembling, and tension, in those with panic disorder should also be assessed. CBC and blood chemistry tests and hepatic and renal function should be periodically monitored.

Administration

! If the patient must switch to another anticonvulsant, expect to decrease the clonazepam dose gradually as therapy begins with a low dose of the replacement drug.

Take clonazepam without regard to meals. Crush tablets as needed. Do not abruptly discontinue the drug after long-term therapy. Strict maintenance of drug therapy is essential for seizure control.

For disintegrating tablets: place in mouth, allow to dissolve. Swallow with or without water.

Clonidine

klon'ih-deen
(Catapres, Catapres TTS, Dixarit [CAN], Duraclon)
Do not confuse clonidine with clomiphene, Klonopin, or quinidine, or Catapres with Cetapred.

CATEGORY AND SCHEDULE

Pregnancy Risk Category: C

Classification: Antihypertensive, central α-adrenergic agonist

MECHANISM OF ACTION

An antiadrenergic, sympatholytic agent that prevents pain signal transmission to the brain and produces analgesia at pre- and post-α-adrenergic receptors in the spinal cord. *Therapeutic Effect:* Reduces peripheral resistance; decreases BP and heart rate.

PHARMACOKINETICS

Route	Onset	Peak	Duration
PO	0.5-1 h	2-4 h	Up to 8 h

Well absorbed from the GI tract. Transdermal best absorbed from the chest and upper arm; least absorbed from the thigh. Protein binding: 20%-40%. Metabolized in the liver. Primarily excreted in urine. Minimally removed by hemodialysis. *Half-life:* 12-16 h (increased with impaired renal function).

AVAILABILITY

Tablets (Catapres): 0.1 mg, 0.2 mg, 0.3 mg.
Transdermal Patch (Catapres TTS): 2.5 mg (release at 0.1 mg/24 h), 5 mg (release at 0.2 mg/24 h), 7.5 mg (release at 0.3 mg/24 h).
Injection (Duraclon): 100 mcg/mL, 500 mcg/mL.

INDICATIONS AND DOSAGES
▸ **Hypertension**
PO
Adults. Initially, 0.1 mg twice a day. Increase by 0.1-0.2 mg q2-4 days. Maintenance: 0.2-1.2 mg/day in 2-4 divided doses up to maximum of 2.4 mg/day.
Elderly. Initially, 0.1 mg at bedtime. May increase gradually.
Children. 5-25 mcg/kg/day in divided doses q6h. Increase at 5- to 7-day intervals. Maximum: 0.9 mg/day.
TRANSDERMAL
Adults, Elderly. System delivering 0.1 mg/24 h up to 0.6 mg/24 h q7 days.
▸ **Attention deficit hyperactivity disorder (ADHD)**
PO
Children. Initially 0.05 mg/day. May increase by 0.05 mg/day q3-7 days. Maximum: 0.3-0.4 mg/day.

▶ **Severe pain**
EPIDURAL
Adults, Elderly. 30-40 mcg/h.
Children. Initially, 0.5 mcg/kg/h, not
to exceed adult dose.

OFF-LABEL USES
ADHD, diagnosis of
pheochromocytoma, opioid
withdrawal, prevention of
migraine headaches, treatment
of dysmenorrhea or menopausal
flushing.

CONTRAINDICATIONS
Epidural contraindicated in those
patients with bleeding diathesis or
infection at the injection site, and
in those receiving anticoagulation
therapy.

INTERACTIONS
Drug
β-Blockers: Discontinuing these
drugs may increase risk of clonidine-
withdrawal hypertensive crisis.
Tricyclic antidepressants: May
decrease effect of clonidine.
Herbal
None known.
Food
None known.

DIAGNOSTIC TEST EFFECTS
None known.

SIDE EFFECTS
Frequent
Dry mouth (40%), somnolence
(33%), dizziness (16%), sedation,
constipation (10%).
Occasional (1%-5%)
Tablets, injection: Depression,
swelling of feet, loss of appetite,
decreased sexual ability, itching
eyes, dizziness, nausea, vomiting,
nervousness.
Transdermal: Itching, reddening or
darkening of skin.

Rare (< 1%)
Nightmares, vivid dreams, cold
feeling in fingers and toes.

SERIOUS REACTIONS
• Overdose produces profound
hypotension, irritability, bradycardia,
respiratory depression, hypothermia,
miosis (pupillary constriction),
arrhythmias, and apnea.
• Abrupt withdrawal may result in
rebound hypertension associated
with nervousness, agitation, anxiety,
insomnia, hand tingling, tremor,
flushing, and diaphoresis.

PRECAUTIONS & CONSIDERATIONS
Caution is warranted with
cerebrovascular disease, chronic
renal failure, Raynaud disease,
recent myocardial infarction,
severe coronary insufficiency,
and thromboangiitis obliterans.
Clonidine crosses the placenta
and is distributed in breast milk.
Children are more sensitive to
clonidine's effects. Use clonidine
with caution in children. A thorough
cardiovascular assessment is
recommended before initiation
of therapy in pediatric patients;
assessment should include medical
history, family history, and physical
examination with consideration of
ECG testing. Elderly patients may
be more sensitive to the hypotensive
effect of clonidine. Age-related renal
impairment may require dosage
adjustment in elderly patients.
Dizziness and light-headedness
may occur. Rise slowly from a
lying to a sitting position and
permit legs to dangle momentarily
before standing to avoid clonidine's
hypotensive effect. BP should
be obtained immediately before
giving each dose, in addition to
regular monitoring. Be alert for BP
fluctuations. Daily bowel activity

and stool consistency should also be assessed. Expect concurrent β-blocker therapy to be discontinued several days before discontinuing clonidine therapy to prevent clonidine withdrawal hypertensive crisis; and clonidine dosage should be reduced over 2-4 days.

Administration

Take oral clonidine without regard to food. Tablets may be crushed. Take last oral dose just before bedtime. Avoid skipping doses or voluntarily discontinuing clonidine because it can produce severe, rebound hypertension.

For transdermal use, apply the system to dry, hairless area of intact skin on upper arm or chest. Rotate sites to prevent skin irritation. Do not trim patch to adjust dose.

Epidural injection must be diluted in 0.9% NaCL injection to a concentration of 100 mcg/mL before use.

Clopidogrel

clo-pid′o-grill
(Iscover [AUS], Plavix)
Do not confuse Plavix with Paxil.

CATEGORY AND SCHEDULE

Pregnancy Risk Category: B

Classification: Platelet aggregation inhibitor

MECHANISM OF ACTION

A thienopyridine derivative that inhibits binding of the enzyme adenosine phosphate (ADP) to its platelet receptor and subsequent ADP-mediated activation of a glycoprotein complex. *Therapeutic Effect:* Inhibits platelet aggregation.

PHARMACOKINETICS

Route	Onset	Peak	Duration
PO	1 h	2 h	N/A

Rapidly absorbed. Protein binding: 98%. Extensively metabolized by the liver. Eliminated equally in the urine and feces. *Half-life:* 8 h.

AVAILABILITY

Tablets: 75 mg, 300 mg.

INDICATIONS AND DOSAGES

▸ **Myocardial infarction (MI), stroke reduction**
PO
Adults, Elderly. 75 mg once a day.
▸ **Acute coronary syndrome**
PO
Adults, Elderly. Initially, 300 mg loading dose, then 75 mg once a day (in combination with aspirin).

CONTRAINDICATIONS

Active bleeding, coagulation disorders, severe hepatic disease.

INTERACTIONS

Drug
Anticoagulants: May increase the risk of bleeding.
Clarithromycin, erythromycin: May reduce the effects of clopidogrel.
Fluvastatin, NSAIDs, phenytoin, tamoxifen, tolbutamide, torsemide, warfarin: May interfere with metabolism of these drugs.
Herbal
Ginger, ginkgo biloba, white willow: May increase the risk of bleeding.
Food
None known.

DIAGNOSTIC TEST EFFECTS

Prolongs bleeding time.

SIDE EFFECTS

Frequent (15%)
Skin disorders.
Occasional (6%-8%)
Upper respiratory tract infection,
chest pain, flu-like symptoms,
headache, dizziness, arthralgia.
Rare (3%-5%)
Fatigue, edema, hypertension,
abdominal pain, dyspepsia, diarrhea,
nausea, epistaxis, dyspnea, rhinitis.

SERIOUS REACTIONS

• Thrombotic thrombocytopenic
purpura.
• GI hemorrhage.

PRECAUTIONS & CONSIDERATIONS

Caution is warranted with
hematologic disorders, history of
bleeding, hypertension, hepatic
or renal impairment, and in
preoperative persons. Be aware that
it may take longer to stop bleeding
during drug therapy.
  Notify the physician of unusual
bleeding. Also, notify dentists and
other physicians before surgery
is scheduled or when new drugs
are prescribed. Platelet count for
thrombocytopenia, hemoglobin
level, WBC count, and BUN,
serum bilirubin, creatinine, AST
(SGOT) and ALT (SGPT) levels
should be monitored. Platelet
count should be obtained before
clopidogrel therapy, every 2
days during the first week of
treatment, and weekly thereafter
until therapeutic maintenance dose
is reached. Be aware that abrupt
discontinuation of clopidogrel
produces an elevated platelet count
within 5 days.
Administration
Take clopidogrel without regard to
food. Do not crush coated tablets.

Clorazepate

klor-az'e-pate
(Novoclopate [CAN], Tranxene,
Tranxene SD, Tranxene SD Half-
Strength, T-Tab)
**Do not confuse clorazepate with
clofibrate.**

CATEGORY AND SCHEDULE
Pregnancy Risk Category: D
Controlled Substance Schedule IV

Classification: Benzodiazepine

MECHANISM OF ACTION
A benzodiazepine that depresses
all levels of the CNS, including
limbic and reticular formation,
by binding to benzodiazepine
receptor sites on the γ-aminobutyric
acid (GABA) receptor complex.
Modulates GABA, a major
inhibitory neurotransmitter in the
brain. *Therapeutic Effect:* Produces
anxiolytic effect, suppresses seizure
activity.

PHARMACOKINETICS
Well absorbed after oral
administration. Rapidly metabolized
by liver to nordiazepam, which
is slowly eliminated. *Half-life:*
40-50 h. Protein binding of
nordiazepam: 97%-98%. Metabolites
(nordiazepam, oxazepam, and
glucuronide conjugates) excreted in
urine.

AVAILABILITY
Tablets (Tranxene, T-Tab): 3.75 mg,
7.5 mg, 15 mg.
*Tablets (Extended Release [Tranxene
SD]):* 22.5 mg.
*Tablets (Extended-Release [Tranxene
SD Half-Strength]):* 11.25 mg.

C

INDICATIONS AND DOSAGES
▸ **Anxiety**
PO
Adults, Elderly. (Regular release): 7.5-15 mg 2-4 times a day. (Sustained release): 11.25 mg or 22.5 mg once a day at bedtime.
▸ **Anticonvulsant (adjunct)**
PO
Adults, Elderly, Children older than 12 yr. Initially, 7.5 mg 2-3 times a day. May increase by 7.5 mg at weekly intervals. Maximum: 90 mg/day.
Children 9-12 yr. Initially, 3.75-7.5 mg twice a day. May increase by 2.75 mg at weekly intervals. Maximum: 60 mg/day.
▸ **Alcohol withdrawal**
PO
Adults, Elderly. Initially, 30 mg, then 15 mg 2-4 times a day on first day. Gradually decrease dosage over subsequent days. Maximum: 90 mg/day.

CONTRAINDICATIONS
Acute narrow-angle glaucoma.

INTERACTIONS
Drug
Other CNS depressants: May increase CNS depressant effects.
Herbal
Kava kava, St. John's wort, valerian: May increase CNS depression.
Food
Alcohol: May increase CNS depressant effects.
Grapefruit juice: Clorazepate concentrations may be increased.

DIAGNOSTIC TEST EFFECTS
Decreased hematocrit; abnormal liver and renal function tests. Therapeutic serum drug level is 0.12-1.5 mcg/mL; toxic serum drug level is > 5 mcg/mL.

SIDE EFFECTS
Frequent
Somnolence.
Occasional
Dizziness, GI disturbances, nervousness, blurred vision, dry mouth, headache, confusion, ataxia, rash, irritability, slurred speech.
Rare
Paradoxical CNS reactions, such as hyperactivity or nervousness in children and excitement or restlessness in elderly or debilitated patients (generally noted during first 2 wks of therapy, particularly in the presence of uncontrolled pain).

SERIOUS REACTIONS
• Abrupt or too-rapid withdrawal may result in pronounced restlessness, irritability, insomnia, hand tremors, abdominal or muscle cramps, diaphoresis, vomiting, and seizures.
• Overdose results in somnolence, confusion, diminished reflexes, and coma.

PRECAUTIONS & CONSIDERATIONS
Caution is warranted in patients with acute alcohol intoxication and renal and hepatic impairment. Women should use effective contraception during therapy and notify their physician immediately if they become or may be pregnant.

Drowsiness and dizziness may occur. Change positions slowly from recumbent to sitting, before standing, to prevent dizziness. Alcohol, smoking, and tasks that require mental alertness or motor skills should also be avoided. Autonomic responses, such as cold, clammy hands and diaphoresis, and motor responses, such as agitation, trembling, and tension, should be assessed. Seizure frequency and intensity should be assessed.

Administration
! If the person must change to another anticonvulsant, plan to decrease clorazepate dosage gradually as low-dose therapy begins with the replacement drug. Be aware the therapeutic peak serum level is 0.12-1.5 mcg/mL; the toxic serum level is > 5 mcg/mL.

Do not abruptly discontinue the medication after long-term use, because this may precipitate seizures. Strict compliance with the drug regimen is essential for seizure control.

Clotrimazole
kloe-try-mah-zole
(Canesten [CAN], Clotrimaderm [CAN], Gyne-Lotrimin, Lotrimin, Mycelex, Mycelex OTC, Trivagizole 3)

CATEGORY AND SCHEDULE
Pregnancy Risk Category: B (topical), C (troches)
OTC/Rx

Classification: Imidazole, antifungal

MECHANISM OF ACTION
An antifungal that binds with phospholipids in fungal cell membrane. The altered cell membrane permeability. *Therapeutic Effect:* Inhibits yeast growth.

PHARMACOKINETICS
Poorly, erratically absorbed from GI tract. Bound to oral mucosa. Absorbed portion metabolized in liver. Eliminated in feces. Topical: Minimal systemic absorption (highest concentration in stratum corneum). Intravaginal: Small amount systemically absorbed. *Half-life:* 3.5-5 h.

AVAILABILITY
Combination Pack: Vaginal tablet 100 mg and vaginal cream 1% (Mycelex-7).
Lotion: 1% (Lotrimin).
Topical Cream: 1% (Lotrimin, Lotrimin AF, Mycelex, Mycelex OTC).
Topical Solution: 1% (Lotrimin, Lotrimin AF, Mycelex, Mycelex OTC).
Troches: 10 mg (Mycelex).
Vaginal Cream: 1% (Gyne-Lotrimin, Mycelex-7), 2% (Gyne-Lotrimin 3, Mycelex-3, Trivagizole 3).
Vaginal Tablets: 100 mg, 500 mg (Gyne-Lotrimin, Mycelex-7).

INDICATIONS AND DOSAGES
▸ **Oropharyngeal candidiasis treatment**
PO
Adults, Elderly. 10 mg 5 times/day for 14 days.
▸ **Oropharyngeal candidiasis prophylaxis**
PO
Adults, Elderly. 10 mg 3 times/day.
▸ **Dermatophytosis, cutaneous candidiasis**
TOPICAL
Adults, Elderly. 2 times/day. Therapeutic effect may take up to 8 wks.
▸ **Vulvovaginal candidiasis**
VAGINAL (TABLETS)
Adults, Elderly. 1 tablet (100 mg) at bedtime for 7 days; 2 tablets (200 mg) at bedtime for 3 days; or 500-mg tablet one time.
VAGINAL (CREAM)
Adults, Elderly. 1 applicatorful at bedtime for 7-14 days.

OFF-LABEL USES
Topical: Treatment of paronychia, tinea barbae, tinea capitis.

CONTRAINDICATIONS
Hypersensitivity to clotrimazole or any component of the formulation, children < 3 yr.

INTERACTIONS
Drug
Benzodiazepines: May increase benzodiazepine serum concentrations and increase risk of toxicity.
Ergot derivatives: May increase risk of ergotism (nausea, vomiting, vasospastic ischemia).
Fentanyl: May increase or prolong opioid effects (CNS depression).
Tacrolimus: May increase risk of tacrolimus toxicity.
Trimetrexate: May increase risk of trimetrexate toxicity.
Herbal
None known.
Food
None known.

DIAGNOSTIC TEST EFFECTS
May increase SGOT (AST).

SIDE EFFECTS
Frequent
Oral: Nausea, vomiting, diarrhea, abdominal pain.
Occasional
Topical: Itching, burning, stinging, erythema, urticaria.
Vaginal: Mild burning (tablets/cream); irritation, cystitis (cream).
Rare
Vaginal: Itching, rash, lower abdominal cramping, headache.

SERIOUS REACTIONS
• None reported.

PRECAUTIONS & CONSIDERATIONS
Caution is warranted in patients with hepatic disorder with oral therapy. It is unknown whether clotrimazole crosses the placenta or is distributed in breast milk. Be aware that clotrimazole use is contraindicated in children < 3 y of age. No age-related precautions have been noted in children more than 5 yr old or in elderly patients. Refrain from sexual intercourse or advise partner to use condom during clotrimazole therapy. Separate personal items and linens.

Itching, burning, and stinging may occur with topical preparations. Vulvovaginal irritation, abdominal cramping, urinary frequency, and discomfort may occur with vaginal therapy.
Administration
Lozenges must be dissolved in mouth more than 15-30 min for oropharyngeal therapy. Swallow saliva.

When using topical preparation, rub well into affected, surrounding areas. Do not apply occlusive covering or other preparations. Keep area clean and dry. Wear light clothing to promote ventilation.

To use vaginally, use vaginal applicator and insert high in vagina. Continue to use during menses.

Clozapine
klo′za-peen
(Clopine [AUS], Clozaril, FazaClo)
Do not confuse clozapine with Cloxapen or clofazimine, or Clozaril with Clinoril, or Colazal.

CATEGORY AND SCHEDULE
Pregnancy Risk Category: B

Classification. Antipsychotic, atypical

MECHANISM OF ACTION
A dibenzodiazepine derivative that interferes with the binding of dopamine at dopamine receptor sites;

binds primarily at nondopamine receptor sites. *Therapeutic Effect:* Diminishes schizophrenic behavior.

PHARMACOKINETICS

Absorbed rapidly and almost completely. Distributed rapidly and extensively. Crosses the blood-brain barrier. Protein binding: 95%. Metabolized in the liver. Excreted in urine and feces. *Half-life:* 8 h.

AVAILABILITY

Tablets (Clozaril): 25 mg, 50 mg, 100 mg, 200 mg.
Oral disintegrating tablets (FazaClo): 12.5 mg, 25 mg, 100 mg.

INDICATIONS AND DOSAGES

▸ **Schizophrenic disorders, reduce suicidal behavior**
PO
Adults. Initially, 25 mg once or twice a day. May increase by 25-50 mg/day over 2 wks until dosage of 300-450 mg/day is achieved. May further increase by 50-100 mg/day no more than once or twice a week.
Range: 200-600 mg/day. Maximum: 900 mg/day.
Elderly. Initially, 25 mg/day. May increase by 25 mg/day. Maximum: 450 mg/day.

CONTRAINDICATIONS

Coma, concurrent use of other drugs that may suppress bone marrow function, history of clozapine-induced agranulocytosis or severe granulocytopenia, myeloproliferative disorders, severe CNS depression.

INTERACTIONS

Drug
Alcohol, other CNS depressants: May increase CNS depressant effects.
Bone marrow depressants: May increase myelosuppression.
Lithium: May increase the risk of confusion, dyskinesia, and seizures.
Phenobarbital: Decreases clozapine blood concentration.
Herbal
St. John's wort: May decrease clozapine levels.
Kava kava, gotu kola, valerian, St. John's wort: May increase CNS depression.
Food
None known.

DIAGNOSTIC TEST EFFECTS

May increase serum glucose levels.

SIDE EFFECTS

Frequent
Somnolence (39%), salivation (31%), tachycardia (25%), dizziness (19%), constipation (14%).
Occasional
Hypotension (9%); headache (7%); tremor, syncope, diaphoresis, dry mouth (6%); nausea, visual disturbances (5%); nightmares, restlessness, akinesia, agitation, hypertension, abdominal discomfort or heartburn, weight gain (4%).
Rare
Rigidity, confusion, fatigue, insomnia, diarrhea, rash.

SERIOUS REACTIONS

• Seizures occur in about 3% of patients.
• Overdose produces CNS depression (including sedation, coma, and delirium), respiratory depression, and hypersalivation.
• Blood dyscrasias, particularly agranulocytosis and mild leukopenia, may occur.
• Myocarditis.

C

PRECAUTIONS & CONSIDERATIONS

Caution is warranted in patients with alcohol withdrawal and in those with cardiovascular disease, glaucoma, diabetes, history of seizures, benign prostatic hyperplasia, myocarditis, myasthenia gravis, urine retention, and impaired hepatic, renal, or respiratory function.

Drowsiness may occur but generally subsides with continued therapy. Increased mortality has been observed in elderly patients with dementia-related psychosis treated with antipsychotics. Alcohol and tasks that require mental alertness or motor skills should be avoided. BP for hypertension or hypotension, heart rate for tachycardia, and CBC for blood dyscrasias (particularly agranulocytosis and mild leukopenia) should be assessed. WBC count should be monitored every week for the first 6 mo of continuous therapy, then biweekly when WBC counts are acceptable.

Administration

Take clozapine without regard to food. Do not abruptly discontinue clozapine. It is required to monitor blood work before prescription can be filled. Orally disintegrating tablets should be allowed to dissolve on tongue; swallow saliva. If dosing requires splitting orally disintegrating tablet, discard unused portion.

Co-Trimoxazole (Sulfamethoxazole and Trimethoprim)

koe-trye-mox′a-zole
(Apo-Sulfatrim [CAN], Bactrim, Bactrim DS, Cosig Forte [AUS], Novotrimel [CAN], Resprim [AUS], Resprim Forte [AUS], Sulfatrim Pediatric, Septra, Septra DS, Septrin [AUS], Septrin Forte [AUS])
Do not confuse Bactrim with bacitracin, co-trimoxazole with clotrimazole, or Septra with Sectral or Septa.

CATEGORY AND SCHEDULE

Pregnancy Risk Category: C

Classification: Antibiotics, folate antagonists, sulfonamides

MECHANISM OF ACTION

A sulfonamide and folate antagonist that blocks bacterial synthesis of essential nucleic acids. *Therapeutic Effect:* Bactericidal in susceptible microorganisms.

PHARMACOKINETICS

Rapidly and well absorbed from the GI tract. Protein binding: 45%-60%. Widely distributed. Metabolized in the liver. Excreted in urine. Minimally removed by hemodialysis. *Half-life:* Sulfamethoxazole 6-12 h, trimethoprim 8-10 h (increased in impaired renal function).

AVAILABILITY

! All dosage forms have same 5:1 ratio of sulfamethoxazole (SMX) to trimethoprim (TMP).
Oral Suspension (Septra, Sulfatrim Pediatric): SMX 200 mg/5 mL and TMP 40 mg/5 mL.
Tablets (Bactrim, Septra): SMX 400 mg and TMP 80 mg.

Tablets, double strength (Bactrim DS, Septra DS): SMX 800 mg and TMP 160 mg.
Injection (Septra): SMX 80 mg/mL and TMP 16 mg/mL.

INDICATIONS AND DOSAGES
▸ **Mild to moderate infections**
PO
Adults, Elderly. 160 mg TMP/800 mg SMX q12hr.
Children older than 2 mo. 8-12 mg/kg/day based on the TMP component in divided doses q12hr.
IV
Adults, Elderly, Children older than 2 mo. 8-12 mg/kg/day based on the TMP component in divided doses q6-12h.
▸ **Serious infections, *Pneumocystis carinii* pneumonia (PCP)**
PO, IV
Adults, Elderly, Children older than 2 mo. 15-20 mg/kg/day based on the TMP component in divided doses q6-8h.
▸ **Prevention of PCP**
PO
Adults. 160 mg TMP/800 mg SMX each day.
Children. 150 mg/m^2/day based on the TMP component in two divided doses on 3 consecutive days/wk.
▸ **Traveler's diarrhea**
PO
Adults, Elderly. 160 mg TMP/800 mg SMX q12h for 5 days.
▸ **Acute exacerbation of chronic bronchitis**
PO
Adults, Elderly. 160 mg TMP/800 mg SMX q12h for 14 days.
▸ **Prevention of urinary tract infection**
PO
Adults, Elderly, Children older than 2 mo. 2 mg/kg/dose once a day.
▸ **Dosage in renal impairment**
Dosage and frequency are modified based on creatinine clearance, the severity of the infection, and the serum concentration of the drug. For those with creatinine clearance of 15-30 mL/min, a 50% dosage reduction is recommended.

OFF-LABEL USES
Treatment of bacterial endocarditis; gonorrhea; meningitis; septicemia; sinusitis; and biliary tract, bone, joint, chancroid, chlamydial, intra-abdominal, skin, and soft-tissue infections.

CONTRAINDICATIONS
Hypersensitivity to trimethoprim or any sulfonamides, infants younger than 2 mo, megaloblastic anemia due to folate deficiency.

INTERACTIONS
Drug
Cyclosporine: May decrease cyclosporine levels and increase risk of nephrotoxicity.
Hemolytics: May increase the risk of toxicity.
Hepatotoxic medications: May increase the risk of hepatotoxicity.
Hydantoin anticonvulsants, oral antidiabetics, warfarin: May increase or prolong the effects of these drugs and increase their risk of toxicity.
Methenamine: May form a precipitate.
Methotrexate: May increase the effects of methotrexate.
Warfarin: Potentiates anticoagulant effect of warfarin.
Herbal and Food
None known.

DIAGNOSTIC TEST EFFECTS
May increase BUN and serum alkaline phosphatase, creatinine, potassium, AST (SGOT), and ALT (SGPT) levels; decreases glucose.

ⓘ IV INCOMPATIBILITIES

Fluconazole (Diflucan), foscarnet (Foscavir), midazolam (Versed), vinorelbine (Navelbine).

SIDE EFFECTS

Frequent
Anorexia, nausea, vomiting, rash (generally 7-14 days after therapy begins), urticaria.
Occasional
Diarrhea, abdominal pain, pain or irritation at the IV infusion site.
Rare
Headache, vertigo, insomnia, seizures, hallucinations, depression.

SERIOUS REACTIONS

• Rash, fever, sore throat, pallor, purpura, cough, and shortness of breath may be early signs of serious adverse reactions.
• Fatalities have occasionally occurred after Stevens-Johnson syndrome, toxic epidermal necrolysis, fulminant hepatic necrosis, agranulocytosis, aplastic anemia, and other blood dyscrasias in patients taking sulfonamides.
• Myelosuppression, decreased platelet count, and severe dermatologic reactions may occur, especially in elderly patients.

PRECAUTIONS & CONSIDERATIONS

Caution is warranted with impaired renal or hepatic function or glucose-6-phosphate dehydrogenase deficiency. Co-trimoxazole use is contraindicated during pregnancy at term and during breastfeeding. Co-trimoxazole readily crosses the placenta and is distributed in breast milk. Co-trimoxazole use is contraindicated in children younger than 2 mo old; if given to newborns, it may produce kernicterus. Elderly patients have an increased risk of developing myelosuppression, decreased platelet count, and severe skin reactions.

History of bronchial asthma, hypersensitivity to trimethoprim or any sulfonamide, or sulfite sensitivity should be determined before beginning drug therapy. Report any new symptoms, especially bleeding, bruising, fever, sore throat, and a rash or other skin changes. Intake and output, pattern of daily bowel activity and stool consistency, skin for rash, renal and liver function, CNS symptoms such as hallucinations, headache, insomnia, and vertigo should be assessed. Vital signs should be monitored at least twice a day.

Storage
Store tablets and oral suspension at room temperature. Be aware that the piggyback IV infusion solution is stable for 2-6 h. Discard the solution if it is cloudy or contains a precipitate.

Administration
! Be aware that drug potency is expressed in terms of trimethoprim content.

Take the oral form with 8 oz water on an empty stomach. Have the patient drink several additional glasses of water each day.

For piggyback IV infusion, dilute each 5-mL vial with 75-125 mL D5W. Do not mix co-trimoxazole with other drugs or solutions. Infuse the solution over 60-90 min. Avoid bolus or rapid infusion and IM injection. Ensure that the patient is adequately hydrated.

Codeine

koe'deen

(Actacode [AUS], Codeine
Phosphate Injection, Codeine
Linctus [AUS])(Contin [CAN])

**Do not confuse codeine with
Cardene or Lodine.**

CATEGORY AND SCHEDULE

Pregnancy Risk Category: C (D if
used for prolonged periods or at
high dosages at term)
Controlled Substance: Schedule II
(analgesic), III (fixed-combination
form)

Classification: Analgesics,
narcotic, antitussives

MECHANISM OF ACTION

An opioid agonist that binds to
opioid receptors at many sites in the
CNS, particularly in the medulla.
This action inhibits the ascending
pain pathways. *Therapeutic
Effect:* Alters the perception of
and emotional response to pain,
suppresses cough reflex.

PHARMACOKINETICS

Well absorbed after oral
administration; rapidly metabolized
by liver/10% methylated to the
active analgesic morphine. *Half-life:*
2.5-3 h. Metabolites excreted in
urine.

AVAILABILITY

Tablets: 15 mg, 30 mg, 60 mg.
Oral Solution: 15 mg/5 mL.
Injection: 15 mg/mL, 30 mg/mL.

INDICATIONS AND DOSAGES
▶ **Analgesia**
PO, IM, SUBCUTANEOUS
Adults, Elderly. 30 mg q4-6h.
Range: 15-60 mg.

Children. 0.5-1 mg/kg q4-6h.
Maximum: 60 mg/dose.
▶ **Cough**
PO
*Adults, Elderly, Children 12 yr and
older.* 10-20 mg q4-6h.
Children 6-11 yr. 5-10 mg q4-6h.
Children 2-5 yr. 2.5-5 mg q4-6h.
▶ **Dosage in renal impairment**
Dosage is modified based on
creatinine clearance.

| Creatinine
Clearance (mL/min)	Dosage
10-50	75% of usual dose
< 10	50% of usual dose

OFF-LABEL USES

Treatment of diarrhea.

CONTRAINDICATIONS

None known.

INTERACTIONS
Drug
Alcohol, other CNS depressants:
May increase hypotension an CNS or
respiratory depression.
MAOIs: May produce a severe,
sometimes fatal reaction; plan to
administer a test dose, which is one-
quarter of usual codeine dose.
**CYP2D6 inhibitors
(chlorpromazine, delavirdine,
fluoxetine, miconazole,
paroxetine, pergolide, quinidine,
quinine, ritonavir, and
ropinirole):** May decrease the
effects of codeine.
Herbal
**St. John's wort, valerian, kava
kava, gotu kola:** Increase CNS
depression.
St. John's wort: may reduce codeine
concentrations; speed conversion to
the metabolite.
Food
None known.

C

DIAGNOSTIC TEST EFFECTS

May increase serum amylase and lipase levels.

SIDE EFFECTS

Frequent

Constipation, somnolence, nausea, vomiting.

Occasional

Paradoxical excitement, confusion, palpitations, facial flushing, decreased urination, blurred vision, dizziness, dry mouth, headache, hypotension (including orthostatic hypotension), decreased appetite, injection site redness, burning, or pain.

Rare

Hallucinations, depression, abdominal pain, insomnia.

SERIOUS REACTIONS

• Too-frequent use may result in paralytic ileus.

• Overdose may produce cold and clammy skin, confusion, seizures, decreased BP, restlessness, pinpoint pupils, bradycardia, respiratory depression, decreased LOC, and severe weakness.

• The patient who uses codeine repeatedly may develop a tolerance to the drug's analgesic effect as well as physical dependence.

PRECAUTIONS & CONSIDERATIONS

Extreme caution should be used in patients with acute alcoholism, anoxia, CNS depression, hypercapnia, respiratory depression or dysfunction, seizures, shock, and untreated myxedema. Caution is also warranted in patients with acute abdominal conditions, Addison disease, COPD, hypothyroidism, hepatic impairment, increased intracranial pressure, benign prostatic hyperplasia, and urethral stricture. Codeine crosses the placenta and is distributed in breast milk. Regular use of opioids during pregnancy may produce withdrawal symptoms in the neonate, such as diarrhea, excessive crying, fever, hyperactive reflexes, irritability, seizures, sneezing, tremors, vomiting, and yawning. Codeine may prolong labor if it is administered in the latent phase of the first stage of labor or before the cervix is dilated 4-5 cm. The neonate may develop respiratory depression if the mother receives codeine during labor. Nursing infants may be exposed to high levels of the codeine metabolite morphine in breast milk. Caution is advised with use in breastfeeding. Infant should be closely monitored for signs of toxicity. Children and elderly patients are more prone to experience paradoxical excitement. Children younger than 2 yr and elderly patients are more susceptible to the drug's respiratory depressant effects. In elderly patients, age-related renal impairment may increase the risk of codeine-induced urine retention.

Dizziness and drowsiness may occur, so change positions slowly and avoid alcohol, CNS depressants, and tasks that require mental alertness or motor skills until response to the drug is established. Vital signs, pattern of daily bowel activity and stool consistency, and clinical improvement of pain should be monitored.

Administration

! Be aware that ambulatory patients and patients not in severe pain may be more prone to dizziness, hypotension, nausea, and vomiting than patients in the supine position and those in severe pain. Expect to reduce the initial dosage in elderly and debilitated patients; those with hypothyroidism, Addison disease, or renal insufficiency; and those using other CNS depressants concurrently.

For oral use, take codeine with food or milk to minimize adverse GI effects.

For IM and subcutaneous use, inspect drug for cloudiness or precipitate. If present, discard the drug.

Colchicine
kol'chi-seen
(Colchicine, Colgout [AUS])

CATEGORY AND SCHEDULE
Pregnancy Risk Category: D

Classification: Antigout agents

MECHANISM OF ACTION
An alkaloid that decreases leukocyte motility, phagocytosis, and lactic acid production. *Therapeutic Effect:* Decreases urate crystal deposits and reduces inflammatory process.

PHARMACOKINETICS
Rapidly absorbed from the GI tract. Highest concentration is in the liver, spleen, and kidney. Protein binding: 30%-50%. Reenters the intestinal tract by biliary secretion and is reabsorbed from the intestines. Partially metabolized in the liver. Eliminated primarily in feces.

AVAILABILITY
Tablets: 0.6 mg.
Injection: 0.5 mg/mL, 1 mg.

INDICATIONS AND DOSAGES
▶ **Acute gouty arthritis**
PO
Adults, Elderly. 0.6-1.2 mg; then 0.6 mg q1-2h or 1-1.2 mg q2h, until pain is relieved or nausea, vomiting, or diarrhea occurs. Total dose: 4-8 mg.

IV
Adults, Elderly. Initially, 2 mg; then 0.5 mg q6h until satisfactory response. Maximum: 4 mg/wk or 4 mg/one course of treatment. If pain recurs, may give 1-2 mg/day for several days but no sooner than 7 days after a full course of IV therapy (total of 4 mg).
▶ **Chronic gouty arthritis**
PO
Adults, Elderly. 0.5-0.6 mg daily, weekly up to once daily, depending on number of attacks per year.

OFF-LABEL USES
To reduce the frequency of recurrence of familial Mediterranean fever; treatment of acute calcium pyrophosphate deposition, amyloidosis, biliary cirrhosis, recurrent pericarditis, sarcoid arthritis.

CONTRAINDICATIONS
Blood dyscrasias; severe cardiac, GI, hepatic, or renal disorders.

INTERACTIONS
Drug
Bone marrow depressants: May increase the risk of blood dyscrasias.
Clarithromycin, erythromcyin, telithromycin: May decrease colchicine metabolism, resulting in increased colchicine toxicity.
NSAIDs: May increase the risk of bone marrow depression, neutropenia, and thrombocytopenia.
Herbal
None known.
Food
Vitamin B_{12}: Vitamin B_{12} absorption may be reduced.

DIAGNOSTIC TEST EFFECTS
May increase serum alkaline phosphatase and AST (SGOT) levels. May decrease platelet count.

Ⓓ IV INCOMPATIBILITIES
Dextrose 5%.

SIDE EFFECTS
Frequent
PO: Nausea, vomiting, abdominal discomfort.
Occasional
PO: Anorexia.
Rare
Hypersensitivity reaction, including angioedema.
Parenteral: Nausea, vomiting, diarrhea, abdominal discomfort, pain or redness at injection site, neuritis in the injected arm.

SERIOUS REACTIONS
• Bone marrow depression, including aplastic anemia, agranulocytosis, and thrombocytopenia, may occur with long-term therapy.
• Overdose initially causes a burning feeling in the skin or throat, severe diarrhea, and abdominal pain. The patient then experiences fever, seizures, delirium, and renal impairment, marked by hematuria and oliguria. The third stage of overdose causes hair loss, leukocytosis, and stomatitis.

PRECAUTIONS & CONSIDERATIONS
Caution is warranted with impaired hepatic function and in elderly or debilitated patients. It is unknown whether colchicine crosses the placenta or is distributed in breast milk. Safety and efficacy of colchicine have not been established in children. Elderly patients may be more susceptible to cumulative toxicity, and age-related renal impairment may increase the risk of myopathy. The drug should be discontinued immediately if GI symptoms occur. Limit intake of high-purine foods, such as fish and organ meats, and drink 8-10 eight-oz glasses of fluid daily while taking colchicine.

Notify the physician if fever, numbness, skin rash, sore throat, fatigue, unusual bleeding or bruising, or weakness occurs. The drug should be discontinued as soon as gout pain is relieved or at the first appearance of diarrhea, nausea, or vomiting. High fluid intake (3000 mL/day) should be encouraged; intake and output should be monitored; output should be at least 2000 mL/day. Signs and symptoms of a therapeutic response, including improved joint range of motion and reduced joint tenderness, redness, and swelling, should be evaluated.

Storage
Store at room temperature.
Administration
Take colchicine without regard to meals.
For IV use, may dilute with 0.9% NaCl or sterile water for injection; do not dilute with D5W. Administer over 2-5 min. Irritating. Do not administer by IM or subcutaneous injection.

Colesevelam
koh-le-sev′e-lam
(Welchol)

CATEGORY AND SCHEDULE
Pregnancy Risk Category: B

Classification: Antihyperlipidemics, bile acid sequestrants

MECHANISM OF ACTION
A bile acid sequestrant and nonsystemic polymer that binds with bile acids in the intestines, preventing their reabsorption and removing them from the body. *Therapeutic Effect:* Decreases LDL cholesterol.

PHARMACOKINETICS

Insignificant absorption. 0.05% of dose excreted in urine after 1 mo of chronic use.

AVAILABILITY

Tablets: 625 mg.

INDICATIONS AND DOSAGES

▸ **To decrease LDL cholesterol level in primary hypercholesterolemia (Fredrickson type IIa); adjunctive therapy for type 2 diabetes mellitus**
PO
Adults, Elderly. 3 tablets with meals twice a day or 6 tablets once a day with a meal.

CONTRAINDICATIONS

Complete biliary obstruction, hypersensitivity to colesevelam.

INTERACTIONS

Drug
Aspirin, clindamycin, digoxin, furosemide, glipizide, hydrocortisone, imipramine, NSAIDs, phenytoin, propranolol, tetracyclines, thiazide diuretics, vitamin A, vitamin D, vitamin E, vitamin K: May decrease the absorption of these drugs.
Herbal
None known.
Food
None known.

DIAGNOSTIC TEST EFFECTS

None known.

SIDE EFFECTS

Frequent (8%-12%)
Flatulence, constipation, infection, dyspepsia (heartburn, epigastric distress).

SERIOUS REACTIONS

• GI tract obstruction may occur.

PRECAUTIONS & CONSIDERATIONS

Caution is warranted in patients with dysphagia, patients with severe GI motility disorders, patients who have had major GI tract surgery, and those susceptible to fat-soluble vitamin deficiency. Colesevelam is not absorbed systemically. It may decrease proper maternal vitamin absorption and may affect breastfeeding infants. Safety and efficacy of colesevelam have not been established in children. No age-related precautions have been noted in elderly patients.

Pattern of daily bowel activity and stool consistency should be assessed. Serum cholesterol and triglyceride levels should be checked at baseline and periodically thereafter.
Administration
Take with meals and with a full glass of liquid.

Colestipol

koe-les'ti-pole
(Colestid, Colestid [CAN])

CATEGORY AND SCHEDULE

Pregnancy Risk Category: C

Classification: Antihyperlipi-demics, bile acid sequestrants

MECHANISM OF ACTION

An antihyperlipoproteinemic that binds with bile acids in the intestine, forming an insoluble complex. Binding results in partial removal of bile acid from enterohepatic circulation. *Therapeutic Effect:* Removes low-density lipoproteins (LDLs) and cholesterol from plasma.

PHARMACOKINETICS

Not absorbed from the GI tract. Excreted in the feces.

C

AVAILABILITY
Granules: 5 g packet (Colestid).
Tablet: 1 g (Colestid).

INDICATIONS AND DOSAGES
▸ **Primary hypercholesterolemia**
PO, GRANULES
Adults, Elderly. Initially, 5 g
1-2 times/day. Range: 5-30 g/day
once or in divided doses.
PO, TABLETS
Adults, Elderly. Initially, 2 g
1-2 times/day. Range: 2-16 g/day.

OFF-LABEL USES
Treatment of diarrhea (due to bile
acids); hyperoxaluria.

CONTRAINDICATIONS
Complete biliary obstruction,
hypersensitivity to bile acid
sequestering resins.

INTERACTIONS
Drug
Anticoagulants: May increase
effects of these drugs by decreasing
vitamin K.
**Digoxin, folic acid, penicillins,
propranolol, tetracyclines,
thiazides, thyroid hormones, and
other medications:** May bind and
decrease absorption of these drugs.
Oral vancomycin: Binds and
decreases the effects of oral
vancomycin.
Warfarin: May decrease warfarin
absorption.
Herbal
Vitamin A, vitamin E: May
decrease vitamin A and vitamin E
absorption.
Food
None known.

DIAGNOSTIC TEST EFFECTS
May decrease serum calcium,
potassium, and sodium levels.
May prolong prothrombin time.

SIDE EFFECTS
Frequent
Constipation (may lead to fecal
impaction), nausea, vomiting,
stomach pain, indigestion.
Occasional
Diarrhea, belching, bloating,
headache, dizziness.
Rare
Gallstones, peptic ulcer,
malabsorption syndrome.

SERIOUS REACTIONS
• GI tract obstruction,
hyperchloremic acidosis, and
osteoporosis secondary to calcium
excretion may occur.
• High dosage may interfere with fat
absorption, resulting in steatorrhea.

PRECAUTIONS & CONSIDERATIONS
Caution is warranted in patients with
bleeding disorders, GI dysfunction
(especially constipation),
hemorrhoids, and osteoporosis.
Abdominal discomfort, flatulence,
and food tolerance may occur during
therapy. Colestipol may interfere
with maternal absorption of fat-
soluble vitamins. No age-related
precautions have been noted in
children. Elderly patients are at
an increased risk of experiencing
adverse nutritional effects and GI
side effects. Electrolytes and serum
cholesterol and triglyceride levels
should be monitored during therapy.
Administration
Take other drugs at least 1 h before
or 4-6 h after colestipol because this
drug is capable of binding drugs in
the GI tract. Do not take colestipol
in its dry form because it is highly
irritating. Mix with 3-6 oz fruit juice,
milk, soup, or water. Place powder on
the surface of the liquid for 1-2 min
to prevent lumping, and then mix
thoroughly. When mixing the powder
with carbonated beverages, use an

extra large glass and stir the liquid slowly to avoid excessive foaming. Take before meals. Drink water between meals. High-fiber foods such as fruits, whole-grain cereals, and vegetables are encouraged to reduce the risk of constipation.

Conivaptan
con-ih-vap´-tan
(Vaprisol)

CATEGORY AND SCHEDULE
Pregnancy Risk Category: C

Classification: Vasopressin antagonist

MECHANISM OF ACTION
An arginine vasopressin (AVP) V1A and V2 selective antagonist that inhibits vasopressin binding V1A in the liver and V1 and V2 sites in renal collecting ducts. Results in excretion of free water. *Therapeutic Effect:* Restores normal fluid and electrolyte status.

PHARMACOKINETICS
Protein binding: 99%. Metabolized in liver; CYP450 3A4 is responsible for primary metabolism. Primarily eliminated in feces (approximately 83%); minimal excretion in urine (about 12%). *Half-life:* 3.6–8.6 h.

AVAILABILITY
Injection Solution: 5 mg/mL.

INDICATIONS AND DOSAGES
▸ **Hyponatremia**
IV
Adults. Initially, a loading dose of 20 mg given over 30 min. Maintenance: 20 mg/day as

continuous infusion over 24 h for an additional 1-3 days. May titrate to maximum dose of 40 mg/day; total duration should not exceed 4 days after loading dose.
Children. Safety and efficacy have not been established in children.

CONTRAINDICATIONS
Hypersensitivity to conivaptan or its components.
Use with ketoconazole, itraconazole, clarithromycin, ritonavir, and indinavir is contraindicated.

INTERACTIONS
Drug
CYP3A4 inducers: May decrease the levels and effects of conivaptan.
CYP3A4 inhibitors (e.g., erythromycin): May increase the levels and effects of conivaptan.
CYP3A4 substrates: Conivaptan may increase the levels and effects of CYP3A4 substrates.
Digoxin: May increase the levels of digoxin.
Herbal
St. John's wort: May reduce conivaptan levels.

Ⓘ IV INCOMPATIBILITIES
Lactated Ringer's and 0.9% sodium chloride. Do not mix or infuse with other medications, since no other information available.

🔋 IV COMPATIBILITIES
Dextrose 5%.

DIAGNOSTIC TEST EFFECTS
Increased sodium.

SIDE EFFECTS
Frequent
Injection site reaction, headache.
Occasional
Hypokalemia, thirst, vomiting, diarrhea, hypertension, orthostatic

hypotension, polyuria, phlebitis, constipation, dry mouth, anemia, fever, nausea, confusion, erythema, insomnia, atrial fibrillation, hyperglycemia or hypoglycemia, hyponatremia, pneumonia, urinary tract infection, hypomagnesemia, pain, dehydration, oral candidiasis, hematuria.

SERIOUS REACTIONS
• Atrial fibrillation has been reported.

PRECAUTIONS & CONSIDERATIONS
Use with caution in patients with hyponatremia with underlying congestive heart failure or renal or hepatic impairment.
Storage
Store ampules at room temperature. Prepared solution for IV infusion is stable for up to 24 h at room temperature.
Administration
Administer loading dose over 30 min, followed by continous IV drip. Do not administer undiluted. For IV use only; infuse into large veins and change infusion site every 24 h to minimize vascular irritation. Dilute *only* with Dextrose 5%.

Cortisone
kor′ti-sone
(Cortate [AUS], Cortone [CAN])
Do not confuse cortisone with Cort-Dome.

CATEGORY AND SCHEDULE
Pregnancy Risk Category: C
(D if used in the first trimester)

Classification: Glucocorticoid, short-acting

MECHANISM OF ACTION
An adrenocortical steroid that inhibits the accumulation of inflammatory cells at inflammation sites, phagocytosis, lysosomal enzyme release and synthesis, and release of mediators of inflammation. *Therapeutic Effect:* Prevents or suppresses cell-mediated immune reactions. Decreases or prevents tissue response to inflammatory process.

PHARMACOKINETICS
Slowly absorbed. Hepatic metabolism to inactive metabolites. *Half-life:* 0.5-2 h.

AVAILABILITY
Tablets: 25 mg.

INDICATIONS AND DOSAGES
Dosage is dependent on the condition being treated and patient response.
▸ **Anti-inflammation, immunosuppression**
PO
Adults, Elderly. 25-300 mg/day in divided doses q12-24h.
Children. 2.5-10 mg/kg/day in divided doses q6-8h.
▸ **Physiologic replacement**
PO
Adults, Elderly. 25-35 mg/day.
Children. 0.5-0.75 mg/kg/day in divided doses q8h.

CONTRAINDICATIONS
Hypersensitivity to corticosteroids, administration of live virus vaccine, peptic ulcers (except in life-threatening situations), systemic fungal infection.

INTERACTIONS
Drug
Amphotericin: May increase hypokalemia.

Digoxin: May increase digoxin toxicity caused by hypokalemia.
Diuretics, insulin, oral hypoglycemics, potassium supplements: May decrease the effects of these drugs.
Hepatic enzyme inducers: May decrease the effects of cortisone.
Live virus vaccines: May decrease the patient's antibody response to vaccine, increase vaccine side effects, and potentiate virus replication.
Herbal
None known.
Food
None known.

DIAGNOSTIC TEST EFFECTS

May increase blood glucose and serum lipid, amylase, and sodium levels. May decrease serum calcium, potassium, and thyroxine levels.

SIDE EFFECTS

Frequent
Insomnia, heartburn, anxiety, abdominal distention, increased diaphoresis, acne, mood swings, increased appetite, facial flushing, delayed wound healing, increased susceptibility to infection, diarrhea or constipation.
Occasional
Headache, edema, change in skin color, frequent urination.
Rare
Tachycardia, allergic reaction (such as rash and hives), psychologic changes, hallucinations, depression.

SERIOUS REACTIONS

• Long-term therapy may cause hypocalcemia, hypokalemia, muscle wasting in arms and legs, osteoporosis, spontaneous fractures, amenorrhea, cataracts, glaucoma, peptic ulcer disease, and congestive heart failure.

Abrupt withdrawal following long-term therapy may cause anorexia, nausea, fever, headache, joint pain, rebound inflammation, fatigue, weakness, lethargy, dizziness, and orthostatic hypotension.

PRECAUTIONS & CONSIDERATIONS

Caution is warranted with diabetes, cirrhosis, congestive heart failure, glaucoma, history of tuberculosis (cortisone may reactivate tuberculosis disease), hypertension, hypothyroidism, nonspecific ulcerative colitis, osteoporosis, psychosis, seizure disorders, and thromboembolic disorders. Monitor growth and development of children receiving long-term corticosteroid therapy. Dentist or other physicians should be informed of cortisone therapy if taken within the past 12 mo.

Mood swings, ranging from euphoria to depression, may occur. Notify the physician of fever, muscle aches, sore throat, and sudden weight gain or swelling. Blood glucose level, BP, serum electrolyte levels, height, and weight should be monitored before and during therapy. Be alert to signs and symptoms of infection caused by reduced immune response, including fever, sore throat, and vague symptoms. In long-term therapy, signs and symptoms of hypocalcemia (such as muscle twitching, cramps, and positive Chvostek's or Trousseau's signs) or hypokalemia (such as ECG changes, nausea and vomiting, irritability, weakness and muscle cramps, and numbness or tingling, especially in the lower extremities) should be assessed.
Administration
Do not change the dosage of or schedule for cortisone. Do not abruptly discontinue the drug; the drug must be withdrawn gradually under medical supervision. May be taken with food to reduce GI irritation.

Cosyntropin
kos-syn-troe′pin
(Cortrosyn)

CATEGORY AND SCHEDULE
Pregnancy Risk Category: C

Classification: Hormones/
hormone modifiers

MECHANISM OF ACTION
A glucocorticoid that stimulates
initial reaction in synthesis of
adrenal steroids from cholesterol.
Therapeutic Effect: Increases
endogenous corticoid synthesis.

PHARMACOKINETICS
Time to peak for IM and IV push
dose about 1 h. Plasma cortisol
levels rise within 5 min; peak plasma
cortisol levels are reached within
45-60 min.

AVAILABILITY
Powder for Reconstitution: 0.25 mg
(Cortrosyn).

INDICATIONS AND DOSAGES
▸ **Screening test for adrenal function**
IM
*Adults, Elderly, Children 2 yr and
older.* 0.25-0.75 mg one time.
Children < 2 yr. 0.125 mg one time.
Neonates. 0.015 mg/kg/dose.
IV, INFUSION
Adults. 0.25 mg in D5W or 0.9%
NaCl infused at rate of 0.04 mg/h.

CONTRAINDICATIONS
Hypersensitivity to cosyntropin or
corticotrophin.

INTERACTIONS
Drug
Bupropion: May lower seizure
threshold.

Fluoroquinolones: May increase
risk for tendon rupture.
Itraconazole: May increase
cosyntropin plasma concentrations
and side effects.
Rotavirus vaccine: May increase
risk of infection by live vaccine.
Herbal
Echinacea, ma huang: May
decrease effectiveness of cosyntropin.
Licorice: May increase risk of
corticosteroid side effects.
Saiboku-to: May increase and
prolong effect of cosyntropin.
Food
None known.

DIAGNOSTIC TEST EFFECTS
None known.

SIDE EFFECTS
Occasional
Nausea, vomiting.
Rare
Hypersensitivity reaction (fever,
pruritus).

SERIOUS REACTIONS
• None reported.

PRECAUTIONS & CONSIDERATIONS
Be aware that short duration for
diagnostic use does not produce
effects of long-term cosyntropin
therapy. It is unknown whether
cosyntropin crosses the placenta or
is distributed in breast milk. No age-
related precautions have been noted
in children or in elderly patients.

If an allergic reaction with
itching, hives, swelling in face or
hands, swelling or tingling in mouth
or throat, tightness in chest, and
trouble breathing occurs, notify the
physician.

The following criteria may be used
as guidelines to determine whether
there has been a normal response to
cosyntropin:

- Morning control plasma cortisol concentration exceeds 5 mcg (0.005 mg) per 100 mL.
- 30-min cortisol concentration shows an increase of at least 7 mcg (0.007 mg) per 100 mL above the control level.
- 30-min cortisol concentration exceeds 18 mcg (0.018 mg) per 100 mL.
- If a 60-min test interval is used, a normal response to cosyntropin is shown by a plasma cortisol concentration that is approximately 2 times the baseline concentration.

Storage

When constituted with 0.9% NaCl, cosyntropin is stable for 24 h at room temperature. It is stable for up to 21 days when refrigerated under a nitrogen atmosphere.

Administration

Each 0.25 mg of cosyntropin is equivalent to 25 units of corticotrophin. Peak plasma cortisol concentrations usually occur 45-60 min after cosyntropin administration.

For IM injection, 1 mL of diluent provided (0.9% NaCl injection) should be added to the vial containing 250 mcg (0.025 mg) of cosyntropin. The resultant solution contains 250 mcg (0.025 mg) of cosyntropin per mL.

For IV infusion, cosyntropin may be further diluted with D5W or 0.9% NaCl injection. Administer 0.25 mg in D5W or 0.9% NaCl infused at rate of 0.04 mg/h.

Cromolyn

kroe'moe-lin
(Apo-Cromolyn [CAN], Crolom, Gastrocrom, Intal, Nasalcrom, Opticrom, Rynacrom [AUS])

CATEGORY AND SCHEDULE
Pregnancy Risk Category: B

Classification: Antiasthmatic, mast cell stabilizer

MECHANISM OF ACTION
An antiasthmatic and antiallergic agent that prevents mast cell release of histamine, leukotrienes, and slow-reacting substances of anaphylaxis by inhibiting degranulation after contact with antigens. *Therapeutic Effect:* Helps prevent symptoms of asthma, allergic rhinitis, mastocytosis, and exercise-induced bronchospasm.

PHARMACOKINETICS
Minimal absorption after PO, inhalation, or nasal administration. Absorbed portion excreted in urine or by biliary system. *Half-life:* 80-90 min.

AVAILABILITY
Oral Concentrate (Gastrocrom): 100 mg/5 mL.
Nasal Spray (Nasalcrom): 40 mg/mL.
Solution for Nebulization: 10 mg/mL.
Solution for Oral Inhalation (Intal): 800 mcg/inhalation.
Ophthalmic Solution (Crolom, Opticrom): 4%.

INDICATIONS AND DOSAGES
▸ **Asthma**
INHALATION (NEBULIZATION)
Adults, Elderly, Children older than 2 yr. 20 mg 3-4 times a day.

C

AEROSOL SPRAY

Adults, Elderly, Children 12 yr and older. Initially, 2 sprays 4 times a day. Maintenance: 2-4 sprays 3-4 times a day.

Children 5-11 yr. Initially, 2 sprays 4 times a day, then 1-2 sprays 3-4 times a day.

▸ **Prevention of bronchospasm**

INHALATION (NEBULIZATION)

Adults, Elderly, Children older than 2 yr. 20 mg within 1 h before exercise or exposure to allergens.

AEROSOL SPRAY

Adults, Elderly, Children older than 5 yr. 2 sprays within 1 h before exercise or exposure to allergens.

▸ **Food allergy, inflammatory bowel disease**

PO

Adults, Elderly, Children older than 12 yr. 200-400 mg 4 times a day.

Children 2-12 yr. 100-200 mg 4 times a day. Maximum: 40 mg/kg/day.

▸ **Allergic rhinitis**

INTRANASAL

Adults, Elderly, Children older than 6 yr. 1 spray each nostril 3-4 times a day. May increase up to 6 times a day.

▸ **Systemic mastocytosis**

PO

Adults, Elderly, Children older than 12 yr. 200 mg 4 times a day.

Children 2-12 yr. 100 mg 4 times a day. Maximum: 40 mg/kg/day.

Children younger than 2 yr. 20 mg/kg/day in 4 divided doses. Maximum: 30 mg/kg/day (children 6 mo to 2 yr).

▸ **Conjunctivitis**

OPHTHALMIC

Adults, Elderly, Children older than 4 yr. 1-2 drops in both eyes 4-6 times a day.

CONTRAINDICATIONS

Status asthmaticus.

INTERACTIONS

Drug
None known.
Herbal
None known.
Food
None known.

DIAGNOSTIC TEST EFFECTS

None known.

SIDE EFFECTS

Frequent
PO: Headache, diarrhea.
Inhalation: Cough, dry mouth and throat, stuffy nose, throat irritation, unpleasant taste.
Nasal: Nasal burning, stinging, or irritation; increased sneezing.
Ophthalmic: Eye burning or stinging.
Occasional
PO: Rash, abdominal pain, arthralgia, nausea, insomnia.
Inhalation: Bronchospasm, hoarseness, lacrimation.
Nasal: Cough, headache, unpleasant taste, postnasal drip.
Ophthalmic: Lacrimation and itching of eye.
Rare
Inhalation: Dizziness, painful urination, arthralgia, myalgia, rash.
Nasal: Epistaxis, rash.
Ophthalmic: Chemosis or edema of conjunctiva, eye irritation.

SERIOUS REACTIONS

• Anaphylaxis occurs rarely when cromolyn is given by the inhalation, nasal, or oral route.

PRECAUTIONS & CONSIDERATIONS

Caution is warranted with arrhythmias and coronary artery disease. When discontinuing the drug, taper the dosage cautiously because symptoms may recur. It is unknown whether cromolyn crosses the placenta or is distributed in breast milk. No age-related precautions have been noted in children. Age-related hepatic and renal impairment may require a dosage adjustment in elderly patients. Drink plenty of fluids to decrease the thickness of lung secretions.

Baseline exercise and activity tolerance should be established. Pulse rate and quality and respiratory rate, depth, rhythm, and type should be monitored. Observe for cyanosis manifested as lips and fingernails with a blue or dusky color in light-skinned patients, a gray color in dark-skinned patients.

Administration
Take oral cromolyn at least 30 min before meals. Pour contents of capsule into hot water and stir until completely dissolved; add an equal amount of cold water while stirring. Do not mix the drug with food, fruit juice, or milk.

For inhalation, first shake the container well. Exhale completely and place the mouthpiece between the lips. Inhale and hold breath for as long as possible before exhaling. Allow 1-10 s before inhaling a second dose to promote deeper bronchial penetration. Rinse mouth after each use to decrease dry mouth and hoarseness and prevent fungal infection of the mouth.

For intranasal use, clear nasal passages as much as possible; a nasal decongestant may be required. Tilt the head slightly forward. Insert the spray tip into the nostril, pointing toward the nasal passages, away from the nasal septum. Spray into the nostril while holding the other nostril closed, and at the same time, inhale through the nose to deliver the medication as high into the nasal passages as possible.

For ophthalmic use, place a finger on the lower eyelid and pull it down until a pocket is formed between the eye and lower lid. Hold the dropper above the pocket and instill the prescribed number of drops into the pocket. Close the eyes gently so that the drug is not squeezed out of the lacrimal sac. Apply gentle finger pressure to the lacrimal sac at the inner canthus for 1 min after installation to lessen the risk of systemic absorption.

Crotamiton
kroe-tam′i-ton
(Eurax)
Do not confuse Eurax with Euflex, Eulexin, or Evoxac.

CATEGORY AND SCHEDULE
Pregnancy Risk Category: C

Classification: Anti-infectives, topical, dermatologics, scabicides/pediculicides

MECHANISM OF ACTION
A scabicidal agent whose exact mechanism is unknown. *Therapeutic Effect:* Scabicidal activity against *Sarcoptes scabiei.*

PHARMACOKINETICS
Not known.

AVAILABILITY
Cream: 10% (Eurax).
Lotion: 10% (Eurax).

INDICATIONS AND DOSAGES
▸ **Treatment of scabies**
TOPICAL
Adults, Elderly, Children. Wash and scrub away loose scales and towel

dry. Apply a thin layer and massage into the skin over the entire body with special attention to skinfolds, creases, and interdigital spaces. Repeat application in 24 h. Take a cleansing bath 48 h after the final application. Treatment may be repeated after 7-10 days if live mites are still present.

▸ **Pruritus**
TOPICAL
Adults, Elderly, Children. Massage into affected areas until medication is completely absorbed. Repeat as needed.

OFF-LABEL USES
Folliculitis, pediculosis.

CONTRAINDICATIONS
Hypersensitivity to crotamiton or any one of its components.

INTERACTIONS
Drug
None known.
Herbal
None known.
Food
None known.

DIAGNOSTIC TEST EFFECTS
None known.

SIDE EFFECTS
Occasional
Itching, burning, irritation, warm sensation, contact dermatitis.

SERIOUS REACTIONS
• None known.

PRECAUTIONS & CONSIDERATIONS
All contaminated clothing and bed linens should be cleaned to avoid reinfestation. It is unknown whether crotamiton crosses the placenta or is distributed in breast milk. Safety and efficacy of crotamiton have not

been established in children. No age-related precautions have been noted in elderly patients.

Administration
Avoid contact with eyes. Shake lotion well before using. Apply a thin layer and massage onto the entire body from the neck to the toes, especially to skinfolds, digits, and creases.

Cyanocobalamin (Vitamin B$_{12}$)
sye-an-oh-koe-bal'a-min
(Bedoz [CAN], Cytamen [AUS])

CATEGORY AND SCHEDULE
Pregnancy Risk Category: A (C if used in doses above recommended daily allowance)

Classification: Vitamin B$_{12}$, water-soluble vitamin

MECHANISM OF ACTION
Acts as a coenzyme for various metabolic functions, including fat and carbohydrate metabolism and protein synthesis. *Therapeutic Effect:* Necessary for cell growth and replication, hematopoiesis, and myelin synthesis.

PHARMACOKINETICS
In the presence of calcium, absorbed systemically in lower half of ileum. Initially, bound to intrinsic factor; this complex passes down intestine, binding to receptor sites on ileal mucosa. Protein binding: High. Metabolized in the liver. Primarily eliminated unchanged in urine. *Half-life:* 6 days.

AVAILABILITY

Lozenge: 50 mcg, 100 mcg, 250 mcg, 500 mcg.
Tablets: 50 mcg, 100 mcg, 250 mcg, 500 mcg, 1000 mcg, 5000 mcg.
Tablet (Extended-Release): 1000 mcg, 1500 mcg.
Tablet (Sublingual): 1000 mcg, 2500 mcg, 5000 mcg.
Injection: 1000 mcg/mL.
Nasal solution: 25 mcg/0.1 mL actuation, 500 mcg/0.1 mL actuation.

INDICATIONS AND DOSAGES

▶ **Pernicious anemia**
IM, SUBCUTANEOUS
Adults, Elderly. 100 mcg/day for 7 days, then every other day for 7 days, then every 3-4 days for 2-3 wks. Maintenance: 100 mcg/mo (oral 1000-2000 mcg/day).
Children. 30-50 mcg/day for 2 or more weeks. Maintenance: 100 mcg/mo.
Neonates. 1000 mcg/day for 2 or more weeks. Maintenance: 50 mcg/mo.
▶ **Uncomplicated vitamin B$_{12}$ deficiency**
PO
Adults, Elderly. 1000-2000 mcg/day.
IM, SUBCUTANEOUS
Adults, Elderly. 100 mcg/day for 5-10 days, followed by 100-200 mcg/mo.
NASAL (NASCOBAL)
Adults. 500 mcg in one nostril once weekly.
NASAL (CALOMIST)
Adults. Maintenance therapy following correction with IM cyanocobalamin: 25 mcg in each nostril daily (50 mcg/day). If inadequate response, 25 mcg in each nostril twice daily (100 mcg/day).
▶ **Complicated vitamin B$_{12}$ deficiency**
IM, SUBCUTANEOUS
Adults, Elderly. 1000 mcg (with IM or IV folic acid 15 mg) as a single dose, then 1000 mcg/day plus oral folic acid 5 mg/day for 7 days.

CONTRAINDICATIONS

Folic acid deficiency anemia, hereditary optic nerve atrophy, history of allergy to cobalamins.

INTERACTIONS

Drug
Alcohol, colchicines: May decrease the absorption of cyanocobalamin.
Ascorbic acid: May destroy cyanocobalamin.
Folic acid (large doses): May decrease cyanocobalamin blood concentration.
Herbal
None known.
Food
None known.

DIAGNOSTIC TEST EFFECTS

None known.

SIDE EFFECTS

Occasional
Diarrhea, pruritus.

SERIOUS REACTIONS

• Impurities in preparation may cause a rare allergic reaction.
• Peripheral vascular thrombosis, pulmonary edema, hypokalemia, and congestive heart failure may occur.

PRECAUTIONS & CONSIDERATIONS

Cyanocobalamin crosses the placenta and is excreted in breast milk. No age-related precautions have been noted in children or in elderly patients. Eating foods rich in vitamin B$_{12}$, including clams, dairy products, egg yolks, fermented cheese, herring, muscle and organ meats, oysters, and red snapper, is encouraged.

Notify the physician of symptoms of infection. Serum potassium level,

C

which normally ranges from 3.5 to 5 mEq/L, and serum cyanocobalamin level, which normally ranges from 200 to 800 mcg/mL, should be monitored. Also, watch for a rise in the blood reticulocyte count, which peaks in 5-8 days. Reversal of deficiency symptoms (anorexia, ataxia, fatigue, hyporeflexia, insomnia, irritability, loss of positional sense, pallor, and palpitations on exertion) should also be assessed. A therapeutic response to treatment usually occurs within 48 h.

Administration

Take cyanocobalamin with meals to increase absorption.

Before the initial dose, activate Nascobal spray nozzle by pumping until first appearance of spray, and then prime twice more. The unit must be reprimed once immediately before each subsequent use. Administer 1 h before or after ingestion of hot foods or liquids.

Prime Calomist unit by spraying 7 times. If 5 or more days since use, reprime with 2 sprays. Separate from other intranasal medications by several hours.

Cyclobenzaprine

sye-kloe-ben′za-preen
(Flexeril, Flexitec [CAN], Novo-Cycloprine [CAN])
Do not confuse cyclobenzaprine with cycloserine or cyproheptadine, or Flexeril with Floxin.

CATEGORY AND SCHEDULE
Pregnancy Risk Category: B

Classification: Skeletal muscle relaxant, centrally acting tricyclic

MECHANISM OF ACTION
A centrally acting skeletal muscle relaxant that reduces tonic somatic muscle activity at the level of the brainstem. *Therapeutic Effect:* Relieves local skeletal muscle spasm.

PHARMACOKINETICS

Route	Onset	Peak	Duration
PO	1 h	3-4 h	12-24 h

Well but slowly absorbed from the GI tract. Protein binding: 93%. Metabolized in the GI tract and the liver. Primarily excreted in urine. *Half-life:* 1-3 days.

AVAILABILITY
Capsule (Extended-Release): 15 mg, 30 mg.
Tablets: 5 mg, 7.5 mg, 10 mg.

INDICATIONS AND DOSAGES
▸ **Acute, painful musculoskeletal conditions**
PO
Adults. Initially, 5 mg 3 times a day. May increase to 10 mg 3 times a day OR 15 mg extended-release capsule once daily. May increase to 30 mg once daily.
Elderly. 5 mg 3 times a day; extended-release capsules not recommended in elderly patients.
▸ **Dosage in hepatic impairment**
Mild: 5 mg 3 times a day; extended-release capsules not recommended in hepatic impairment. Moderate and severe: Not recommended.

OFF-LABEL USES
Treatment of fibromyalgia.

CONTRAINDICATIONS
Acute recovery phase of MI, arrhythmias, congestive heart failure, heart block, conduction disturbances,

hyperthyroidism, use within 14 days of MAOIs.

INTERACTIONS
Drug
Alcohol, other CNS depression–producing medications (such as tricyclic antidepressants): May increase CNS depression.
MAOIs: May increase the risk of hypertensive crisis and severe seizures. Contraindicated.
Herbal
Valerian, kava kava, gotu kola: May increase CNS depression.

DIAGNOSTIC TEST EFFECTS
None known.

SIDE EFFECTS
Frequent
Somnolence (39%), dry mouth (27%), dizziness (11%).
Rare (1%-3%)
Fatigue, asthenia, blurred vision, headache, nervousness, confusion, nausea, constipation, dyspepsia, unpleasant taste.

SERIOUS REACTIONS
• Overdose may result in visual hallucinations, hyperactive reflexes, muscle rigidity, vomiting, and hyperpyrexia.

PRECAUTIONS & CONSIDERATIONS
Caution is warranted with angle-closure glaucoma, impaired hepatic or renal function, increased intraocular pressure, and history of urine retention. It is unknown whether cyclobenzaprine crosses the placenta or is distributed in breast milk. The safety and efficacy of cyclobenzaprine have not been established in children. Elderly patients have an increased sensitivity to the drug's anticholinergic effects, such as confusion and urine retention.

Drowsiness may occur but usually diminishes with continued therapy. Avoid alcohol, CNS depressants, and tasks that require mental alertness or motor skills. Change positions slowly to help avoid the drug's hypotensive effects. Therapeutic response, such as decreased skeletal muscle pain, stiffness, and tenderness and improved mobility, should be assessed.
Administration
! Do not administer cyclobenzaprine for longer than 2-3 wks. Take cyclobenzaprine without regard to food.

Cyclophosphamide
sye-kloe-foss´-fa-mide
(Cycloblastin [AUS], Cytoxan, Endoxan Asta [AUS], Endoxon Asta [AUS], Neosar, Procytox [CAN])
Do not confuse Cytoxan with cefoxitin, Ciloxan, cyclosporine, or Cytotec.

CATEGORY AND SCHEDULE
Pregnancy Risk Category: D

Classification: Antineoplastic alkylating agent

MECHANISM OF ACTION
An alkylating agent that inhibits DNA and RNA protein synthesis by cross-linking with DNA and RNA strands, preventing cell growth. Cell cycle-phase nonspecific.
Therapeutic Effect: Potent immunosuppressant.

PHARMACOKINETICS
Well absorbed from the GI tract. Protein binding: Low. Crosses the

blood-brain barrier. Metabolized in the liver to active metabolites. Primarily excreted in urine. Removed by hemodialysis. *Half-life:* 3-12 h.

AVAILABILITY

Injection, Powder for Solution: 500 mg, 1 g, 2 g.
Tablets: 25 mg, 50 mg.

INDICATIONS AND DOSAGES

Ovarian adenocarcinoma, breast carcinoma, Hodgkin disease, non-Hodgkin's lymphoma, multiple myeloma, leukemia (acute lymphoblastic, acute myelogenous, acute monocytic, chronic granulocytic, chronic lymphocytic), mycosis fungoides, disseminated neuroblastoma, retinoblastoma.
PO
Adults. 1-5 mg/kg/day.
Children. Initially, 2-8 mg/kg/day. Maintenance: 2-5 mg/kg twice a week.
IV
Adults. 40-50 mg/kg in divided doses over 2-5 days, 10-15 mg/kg every 7-10 days, or 3-5 mg/kg twice a week.
Children. 2-8 mg/kg/day for 6 days or total dose for 7 days once a week.
▸ **Biopsy-proven minimal-change nephrotic syndrome**
PO
Adults, Children. 2.5-3 mg/kg/day for 60-90 days.

CONTRAINDICATIONS

Severely depressed bone marrow function; hypersensitivity to cyclophosphamide.

INTERACTIONS

Drug
Allopurinol: increased cyclophosphamide levels.
Cyclosporine: decreased cyclosporine levels.
Succinylcholine: prolonged succinylcholine effects.

Vaccines, Live: increased risk of infection by live vaccine.
Warfarin: increased risk elevated INR and bleeding.
Herbal
St. John's wort: reduced cyclophosphamide effectiveness.

DIAGNOSTIC TEST EFFECTS

Myelosuppression risk, monitor CBC with differential and platelets; nephrotoxicity risk, monitor BUN, urinalysis, and serum creatinine.

Ⓓ IV INCOMPATIBILITIES

Amphotericin B cholesteryl sulfate complex.

SIDE EFFECTS

Expected
Marked leukopenia 8-15 days after initial therapy.
Frequent
Nausea, vomiting (beginning about 6 h after administration and lasting about 4 h), alopecia.
Occasional
Diarrhea, darkening of skin and fingernails, stomatitis, headache, diaphoresis.
Rare
Pain or redness at injection site.

SERIOUS REACTIONS

• Cyclophosphamide's major toxic effect is myelosuppression resulting in blood dyscrasias, such as leukopenia, anemia, thrombocytopenia, and hypoprothrombinemia.
• Expect leukopenia to resolve in 17-28 days. Anemia generally occurs after large doses or prolonged therapy. Thrombocytopenia may occur 10-15 days after drug initiation.
• Hemorrhagic cystitis occurs commonly in long-term therapy, especially in pediatric patients.

• Pulmonary fibrosis and cardiotoxicity have been noted with high doses.
• Amenorrhea, azoospermia, and hyperkalemia may also occur.

PRECAUTIONS & CONSIDERATIONS
Ensure adequate fluid intake and frequent voiding to reduce occurrence of hemorrhagic cystitis. Use with caution in patients with leukopenia, thrombocytopenia, tumor cell infiltration of bone marrow, previous radiation therapy, previous therapy with other cytotoxic agents, impaired hepatic function, or impaired renal function. Emetic potential ranges from very high with high doses to moderate with oral therapy. Women of childbearing potential should be advised to avoid becoming pregnant. Avoid use in nursing mothers. No unique precautions in pediatric patients or in elderly patients.

Storage
Store vials at room temperature. Product reconstituted with Bacteriostatic Water for injection should be used within 24 h if stored at room temperature or within 6 days if stored under refrigeration. Product reconstituted with Sterile Water for Injection should be used within 6 h.

Administration
Reconstitute lyophilized cyclophosphamide with bacteriostatic water for Injection, USP (paraben preserved only) or sterile water for injection, USP. Do not crush or cut tablets. Administer during or after meals. To reduce risk of bladder irritation, do not administer tablets at bedtime.

Cycloserine
sye-kloe-ser'een
(Closina [AUS], Seromycin)

CATEGORY AND SCHEDULE
Pregnancy Risk Category: C

Classification:
Antimycobacterials

MECHANISM OF ACTION
An antitubercular that inhibits cell wall synthesis by competing with the amino acid, D-alanine, for incorporation into the bacterial cell wall. *Therapeutic Effect:* Causes disruption of bacterial cell wall. Bactericidal or bacteriostatic.

PHARMACOKINETICS
Readily absorbed from the GI tract. No protein binding. Widely distributed (including cerebrospinal fluid [CSF]). Metabolized in liver. Primarily excreted in urine. Removed by hemodialysis. *Half-life:* 10 h.

AVAILABILITY
Capsules: 250 mg (Seromycin).

INDICATIONS AND DOSAGES
▶ **Tuberculosis**
Adults, Elderly. 250 mg q12h for 14 days, then 500 mg to 1g/day in 2 divided doses for 18-24 mo. Maximum: 1 g as a single daily dose.
Children. 10-20 mg/kg/day in 2 divided doses. Maximum: 1000 mg/day for 18-24 mo.
▶ **Dosage in renal impairment**

Creatinine Clearance (mL/min)	Dosage Interval
10-50	q24h
< 10	q36-48h

OFF-LABEL USES

Gaucher's disease, acute urinary tract infections.

CONTRAINDICATIONS

Epilepsy, depression, severe anxiety, psychosis, severe renal insufficiency, excessive concurrent use of alcohol, history of hypersensitivity reactions with previous cycloserine therapy.

INTERACTIONS

Drug
Alcohol: May increase CNS effects.
Isoniazid, ethionamide: May increase cycloserine toxicity.
Phenytoin: May increase the risk of epileptic seizures.
Herbal
Vitamin B$_{12}$: May decrease vitamin B$_{12}$.
Folic acid: May decrease folic acid.

DIAGNOSTIC TEST EFFECTS

None known.

SIDE EFFECTS

Occasional
Drowsiness, headache, dizziness, vertigo, seizures, confusion, psychosis, paresis, tremor, vitamin B$_{12}$ deficiency, folate deficiency, cardiac arrhythmias, increased liver enzymes.

SERIOUS REACTIONS

• Neurotoxicity, as evidenced by confusion, agitation, CNS depression, psychosis, coma, and seizures, occurs rarely.
• Neurotoxic effects of cycloserine may be treated and prevented with the administration of 200-300 mg of pyridoxine daily.

PRECAUTIONS & CONSIDERATIONS

Caution is warranted with epilepsy, depression, severe anxiety, psychosis, severe renal disease, and chronic alcoholism. Hypersensitivity

reactions to cycloserine should be determined before starting treatment. Cycloserine crosses the placenta and is excreted in breast milk. No age-related precautions have been noted in children or in elderly patients. Cycloserine concentrations should be monitored. Toxicity is greatly increased at levels more than 30 mcg/mL.

Drowsiness, mental confusion, dizziness, or tremors may occur during treatment. Excessive amounts of alcoholic beverages should be avoided.

Administration
May be taken with food. Vitamin B$_{12}$ and folic acid dietary requirements may need to be increased during therapy.

Cyclosporine

sye-kloe-spor'in
(Cysporin [AUS], Gengraf, Neoral, Restasis, Sandimmune, Sandimmune Neoral [AUS])
Do not confuse cyclosporine with cycloserine, cyclophosphamide, or Cyklokapron.

CATEGORY AND SCHEDULE

Pregnancy Risk Category: C

Classification: Immunologic agents

MECHANISM OF ACTION

A cyclic polypeptide that inhibits both cellular and humoral immune responses by inhibiting interleukin-2, a proliferative factor needed for T-cell activity. *Therapeutic Effect:* Prevents organ rejection and relieves symptoms of psoriasis and arthritis.

PHARMACOKINETICS

Variably absorbed from the GI tract. Protein binding: 90%. Widely distributed. Metabolized in the liver. Eliminated primarily by biliary or fecal excretion. Not removed by hemodialysis. *Half-life:* Adults, 10-27 h; children, 7-19 h.

AVAILABILITY

Capsules, Softgel (Sandimmune): 25 mg, 100 mg.
Capsules, Softgel [modified] (Gengraf, Neoral): 25 mg, 100 mg.
Oral Solution (Sandimmune): 100 mg/mL in 50-mL bottle with calibrated liquid measuring device.
Oral Solution [modified] (Gengraf, Neoral): 100 mg/mL.
Injection (Sandimmune): 50 mg/mL.
Ophthalmic Emulsion (Restasis): 0.05%.

INDICATIONS AND DOSAGES

Sandimmune capsules and oral solution have decreased bioavailability compared with the Gengraf and Neoral modified capsules and oral solution. Gengraf, Neoral, and generic modified cyclosporine formulations are not bioequivalent to Sandimmune. Blood concentration monitoring should be used to guide dosing changes and conversion between formulations.

▶ **Transplantation, prevention of organ rejection**
PO
Adults, Elderly, Children. 10-18 mg/kg/dose given 4-12h before organ transplantation. Maintenance: 5-15 mg/kg/day in divided doses, then tapered to 3-10 mg/kg/day.
IV
Adults, Elderly, Children. Initially, 5-6 mg/kg/dose given 4-12h before organ transplantation. Maintenance: 2-10 mg/kg/day in divided doses.

▶ **Rheumatoid arthritis**
PO
Adults, Elderly. Initially, 2.5 mg/kg/day in 2 divided doses. May increase by 0.5-0.75 mg/kg/day. Maximum: 4 mg/kg/day.

▶ **Psoriasis**
PO
Adults, Elderly. Initially, 2.5 mg/kg/day in 2 divided doses. May increase by 0.5 mg/kg/day. Maximum: 4 mg/kg/day.

▶ **Dry eye**
OPHTHALMIC
Adults, Elderly. Instill 1 drop in each affected eye q12h.

OFF-LABEL USES

Treatment of alopecia areata, aplastic anemia, atopic dermatitis, Behçet's disease, biliary cirrhosis, prevention of corneal transplant rejection.

CONTRAINDICATIONS

History of hypersensitivity to cyclosporine or polyoxyethylated castor oil; contraindicated in psoriasis and rheumatoid arthritis patients with abnormal renal function, uncontrolled hypertension, or malignancies; contraindicated with concurrent PUVA or UVB therapy, methotrexate or other immunosuppressives, coal tar, or radiation therapy in psoriasis patients; ophthalmic contraindicated in patients with active ocular infection.

INTERACTIONS

Drug
ACE inhibitors, potassium-sparing diuretics, potassium supplements: May cause hyperkalemia.
Cimetidine, danazol, diltiazem, erythromycin, ketoconazole, itraconazole, methotrexate, protease inhibitors, voriconazole: May increase cyclosporine concentration and risk of hepatotoxicity and nephrotoxicity.

Immunosuppressants: May increase risk of infection and lymphoproliferative disorders.

Live-virus vaccines: May increase vaccine side effects, potentiate virus replication, and decrease the patient's antibody response to the vaccine.

HMG-CoA reductase inhibitors: Cyclosporine may increase statin levels and increase the risk of acute renal failure and rhabdomyolysis.

Carbamazepine, oxcarbazepine, phenobarbital, phenytoin, rifampin, sulfasalazine, ticlopidine: May decrease cyclosporine levels.

Herbal

St. John's wort: May decrease cyclosporine plasma levels. Contraindicated.

Food

Grapefruit, grapefruit juice: May increase the absorption and risk of toxicity of cyclosporine.

DIAGNOSTIC TEST EFFECTS

May increase BUN and serum alkaline phosphatase, amylase, bilirubin, creatinine, potassium, uric acid, AST (SGOT), and ALT (SGPT) levels. May decrease serum magnesium level. Therapeutic peak serum level is 50-300 ng/mL; toxic serum level is > 400 ng/mL.

ⓓ IV INCOMPATIBILITIES

Amphotericin B complex (Abelcet, AmBisome, Amphotec), magnesium.

ⓤ IV COMPATIBILITIES

Propofol (Diprivan).

SIDE EFFECTS

Frequent

Mild to moderate hypertension (26%), hirsutism (21%), tremor (12%).

Occasional (2%-4%)

Acne, leg cramps, gingival hyperplasia (marked by red, bleeding, and tender gums), paresthesia, diarrhea, nausea, vomiting, headache.

Rare (< 1%)

Hypersensitivity reaction, abdominal discomfort, gynecomastia, sinusitis.

SERIOUS REACTIONS

• Mild nephrotoxicity occurs in 25% of renal transplant patients, 38% of cardiac transplant patients, and 37% of liver transplant patients, generally 2-3 mo after transplantation (more severe toxicity generally occurs soon after transplantation). Hepatotoxicity occurs in 4% of renal transplant patients, 7% of cardiac transplant patients, and 4% of liver transplant patients, generally within the first month after transplantation. Both toxicities usually respond to dosage reduction.

• Severe hyperkalemia and hyperuricemia occur occasionally.

PRECAUTIONS & CONSIDERATIONS

Caution is warranted in patients with cardiac impairment, chickenpox, herpes zoster infection, hypokalemia, malabsorption syndrome, renal or hepatic impairment, and pregnant women. Cyclosporine readily crosses the placenta and is distributed in breast milk. Women taking this drug should not breastfeed. No age-related precautions have been noted in transplant children. Elderly patients are at increased risk for hypertension and an increased serum creatinine level. Avoid consuming grapefruit and grapefruit juice because they increase the drug's blood concentration and risk of side effects.

Headache, excessive hair growth, gum disease, and tremor may occur. Good oral hygiene should be maintained to prevent gingivitis. Blood test results, including renal function studies, liver function tests, and drug blood levels, should be monitored before beginning cyclosporine therapy and regularly during treatment. Mild toxicity is characterized by a slow rise in serum levels; more overt toxicity, by a rapid rise in serum levels. Hematuria is also noted in nephrotoxicity. Know that the therapeutic peak serum level of cyclosporine is 50-300 ng/mL and the toxic serum level is over 400 ng/mL; the dose should be taken after a trough serum level has been drawn. Serum potassium level for hyperkalemia and BP for hypertension should also be assessed.

Storage

The capsules should be kept in original foil wrapping and stored in a dry, cool environment, away from direct light. Do not refrigerate the oral solution because it may separate. The liquid form should be kept in the amber-colored glass container. Discard the oral solution 2 mo after the bottle has been opened. Store the parenteral form at room temperature and protect it from light. After diluted, solution is stable for 24 h. Store ophthalmic emulsion at room temperature.

Administration

! The oral solution is available in 50-mL bottles and comes with a calibrated liquid measuring device. Expect to begin therapy with the oral form as soon as possible. Expect to give cyclosporine with adrenal corticosteroids. Know that administering other immuno-suppressive agents with cyclosporine increases the patient's susceptibility to infection and lymphoma.

In a glass container, mix Sandimmune oral solution with room-temperature milk, chocolate milk, or orange juice or mix Neoral or Gengraf oral solution with room temperature orange or apple juice. Stir the mixture well, and have the patient drink it immediately. Avoid using Styrofoam containers because the liquid form of the drug may adhere to the wall of the container. Add more diluent to the glass container and mix it with the remaining solution to ensure that the total amount of cyclosporine is swallowed. Dry the outside of the measuring device before replacing it in its cover. Do not rinse it with water. Take the drug at the same time each day. All oral cyclosporine dosage forms should be taken consistently with regard to time of day and relation to meals.

For IV use, dilute each milliliter of concentrate with 20-100 mL 0.9% NaCl or D5W. Infuse the solution over 2-6 h. Monitor continuously for the first 30 min of the infusion and frequently thereafter for a hypersensitivity reaction, marked by facial flushing and dyspnea.

For ophthalmic use, invert vial several times to obtain a uniform suspension. Remove any contact lenses before administration. May reinsert lenses 15 min after drug administration. May use with artificial tears. Single-use vial; discard after use.

Cyproheptadine
si-proe-hep′ta-deen
(Periactin)

CATEGORY AND SCHEDULE
Pregnancy Risk Category: B

Classification: Antihistamines, H_1 receptor antagonist

MECHANISM OF ACTION
An antihistamine that competes with histamine at histaminic receptor sites. Anticholinergic effects cause

drying of nasal mucosa. *Therapeutic Effect:* Relieves allergic conditions (urticaria, pruritus).

PHARMACOKINETICS

Well absorbed from GI tract. Metabolized in liver. Primarily eliminated in feces. *Half-life:* 16 h.

AVAILABILITY

Syrup: 2 mg/5 mL (Periactin).
Tablets: 4 mg (Periactin).

INDICATIONS AND DOSAGES
▸ **Allergic condition**
PO
Adults, Children older than 15 yr.
4 mg 3 times/day. May increase dose but do not exceed 0.5 mg/kg/day.
Children 7-14 yr. 4 mg 2-3 times/day, or 0.25 mg/kg daily in divided doses.
Children 2-6 yr. 2 mg 2-3 times/day, or 0.25 mg/kg daily in divided doses.
Elderly. Usual elderly dosage.
PO
Initially, 4 mg 2 times/day.

CONTRAINDICATIONS

Acute asthmatic attack, patients receiving MAOIs, history of hypersensitivity to antihistamines.

INTERACTIONS

Drug
Alcohol, central nervous system (CNS) depressants: May increase CNS depression.
Fluoxetine, paroxetine: May decrease fluoxetine efficacy.
MAOIs: May increase anticholinergic and CNS depressant effects.
Protirelin: May decrease TSH response.
Herbal
None known.
Food
None known.

DIAGNOSTIC TEST EFFECTS

May suppress flare and wheal reaction to antigen skin testing unless drug is discontinued 4 days before testing. May increase SGPT (AST) levels.

SIDE EFFECTS

Frequent
Drowsiness, dizziness, muscular weakness, dry mouth/nose/throat/lips, urinary retention, thickening of bronchial secretions.
▸ **Elderly**
Frequent
Sedation, dizziness, hypotension.
Occasional
Epigastric distress, flushing, visual disturbances, hearing disturbances, paresthesia, sweating, chills.

SERIOUS REACTIONS

• Children may experience dominant paradoxical reaction (restlessness, insomnia, euphoria, nervousness, tremors).
• Overdosage in children may result in hallucinations, convulsions, death.
• Hypersensitivity reaction (eczema, pruritus, rash, cardiac disturbances, angioedema, photosensitivity) may occur.
• Overdosage may vary from CNS depression (sedation, apnea, cardiovascular collapse, death) to severe paradoxical reaction (hallucinations, tremor, seizures).

PRECAUTIONS & CONSIDERATIONS

Caution is warranted with narrow-angle glaucoma, peptic ulcer, prostatic hypertrophy, pyloroduodenal or bladder neck obstruction, asthma, COPD, increased intraocular pressure, cardiovascular disease, hyperthyroidism, hypertension, and seizure disorders. It is unknown whether cyproheptadine crosses the placenta or is distributed in breast milk. Safety and efficacy of cyproheptadine have not been established in newborns. Be aware that elderly patients are more likely to experience dizziness, sedation, confusion, and hypotension.

Dry mouth, drowsiness, and dizziness are expected side effects. Tolerance to sedative effects may occur. Avoid alcohol and tasks that require alertness and motor skills.

Administration

Give without regard to meals. Scored tablets may be crushed.

Cytarabine
sye-tare´a-been
(Ara-C, Cytosar [CAN], Cytosar-U)
Do not confuse cytarabine with Cytadren, Cytovene, or vidarabine.

CATEGORY AND SCHEDULE
Pregnancy Risk Category: D

Classification: Antineoplastics, antimetabolites

MECHANISM OF ACTION
An antimetabolite that is converted intracellularly to a nucleotide. Cell cycle-specific for S phase of cell division. *Therapeutic Effect:* May inhibit DNA synthesis. Potent immunosuppressive activity.

PHARMACOKINETICS
Widely distributed; moderate amount crosses the blood-brain barrier. Protein binding: 15%. Primarily excreted in urine. *Half-life:* 1-3 h.

AVAILABILITY
Injection Powder: 100 mg, 500 mg, 1 g, 2 g.
Injection Solution: 20 mg/mL, 100 mg/mL.

INDICATIONS AND DOSAGES
▸ **To induce remission in acute lymphocytic leukemia, acute and chronic myelocytic leukemia, meningeal leukemia, or non-Hodgkin lymphoma in children**
IV
Adults, Elderly, Children.
200 mg/m^2/day for 5 days q2wk as monotherapy or 100-200 mg/m^2/day for 5- to 10-day course of therapy every q2-4wk in combination therapy.
INTRATHECAL
Adults, Elderly, Children.
5-7.5 mg/m^2 every 2-7 days.
▸ **To maintain remission in acute lymphocytic leukemia, acute and chronic myelocytic leukemia, meningeal leukemia, or non-Hodgkin lymphoma in children**
IV
Adults, Elderly, Children. 70-200 mg/m^2/day for 2-5 days every month.
IM, SUBCUTANEOUS
Adults, Elderly, Children. 1-1.5 mg/m^2 as single dose q1-4wk.
INTRATHECAL
Adults, Elderly, Children. 5-7.5 mg/m^2 every 2-7 days.

OFF-LABEL USES
Treatment of Hodgkin disease, myelodysplastic syndrome.

CONTRAINDICATIONS
None known.

INTERACTIONS
Drug
Antigout medications: May decrease the effects of these drugs.
Bone marrow depressants: May increase myelosuppression.
Cyclophosphamide: May increase the risk of cardiomyopathy.
Digoxin: May decrease levels of digoxin.

C

Flucytosine: May decrease therapeutic effect of flucytosine.
Live-virus vaccines: May potentiate virus replication, increase vaccine side effects, and decrease the patient's antibody response to the vaccine.
Herbal
None known.
Food
None known.

DIAGNOSTIC TEST EFFECTS

May increase serum alkaline phosphatase, bilirubin, uric acid, and AST (SGOT) levels.

ⓦ IV INCOMPATIBILITIES

Amphotericin B complex (Abelcet, AmBisome, Amphotec), ganciclovir (Cytovene), insulin (regular).

ⓦ IV COMPATIBILITIES

Dexamethasone (Decadron), diphenhydramine (Benadryl), filgrastim (Neupogen), granisetron (Kytril), hydromorphone (Dilaudid), lorazepam (Ativan), morphine, ondansetron (Zofran), potassium chloride, propofol (Diprivan).

SIDE EFFECTS

Frequent
IV, Subcutaneous (16%-33%): Asthenia, fever, pain, altered taste and smell, nausea, vomiting (risk greater with IV push than with continuous IV infusion).
   Intrathecal (11%-28%): Headache, asthenia, altered taste and smell, confusion, somnolence, nausea, vomiting.
Occasional
IV, subcutaneous (7%-11%): Abnormal gait, somnolence, constipation, back pain, urinary incontinence, peripheral edema, headache, confusion.
   Intrathecal (3%-7%): Peripheral edema, back pain, constipation, abnormal gait, urinary incontinence.

SERIOUS REACTIONS

• Myelosuppression may result in blood dyscrasias, such as leukopenia, anemia, thrombocytopenia, megaloblastosis, and reticulocytopenia, after a single IV dose.
• Leukopenia, anemia, and thrombocytopenia should be expected with daily or continuous IV therapy.
• Cytarabine syndrome (as evidenced by fever, myalgia, rash, conjunctivitis, malaise, and chest pain) and hyperuricemia/tumor lysis syndrome may occur.
• Acute pancreatitis has been reported in patients receiving continuous infusions.
• High-dose cytarabine therapy may produce severe CNS, GI, and pulmonary toxicity.

PRECAUTIONS & CONSIDERATIONS

Caution is warranted in cardiomyopathy, hepatic impairment, and preexisting drug-induced bone marrow suppression. Caution should also be used in women of childbearing age. The use of contraception should be advised. It is unknown whether cytarabine is distributed in breast milk. Monitor leukocyte and platelet counts daily during the induction phase. Perform bone marrow examinations and liver and kidney function tests periodically. Monitor uric acid serum concentrations.
Storage
Unopened vials may be stored at room temperature. Reconstituted solutions are stable at room temperature for 48 h.
Administration
Avoid using diluents containing benzyl alcohol; preservative-free 0.9% NaCL is usually used. Administer as IV infusion over 1-3 h or as continuous infusion: continuous infusion may be associated with fewer GI effects.

Dacarbazine
da-kar′ba-zeen
(DTIC [CAN], DTIC-Dome)
**Do not confuse dacarbazine with
Dicarbosil or procarbazine.**

CATEGORY AND SCHEDULE
Pregnancy Risk Category: C

Classification: Antineoplastics,
alkylating agents

MECHANISM OF ACTION
An alkylating antineoplastic agent
that forms methyldiazonium
ions, which attack nucleophilic
groups in DNA. Cross-links
DNA strands. *Therapeutic Effect:*
Inhibits DNA, RNA, and protein
synthesis.

PHARMACOKINETICS
Minimally crosses the blood-brain
barrier. Protein binding: 5%.
Metabolized in the liver.
Excreted in urine. *Half-life:* 5 h
(increased in impaired renal
function).

AVAILABILITY
Powder for Injection: 100-mg vials,
200-mg vials.

INDICATIONS AND DOSAGES
▶ **Malignant melanoma**
IV
Adults, Elderly. 2-4.5 mg/kg/day for
10 days, repeated q4wk; or
250 mg/m^2/day for 5 days,
repeated q3wk.
▶ **Hodgkin's disease**
IV
Adults, Elderly. 150 mg/m^2/day for
5 days, repeated q4wk; or
375 mg/m^2 once, repeated every
15 days (as combination
therapy).

OFF-LABEL USES
Treatment of islet cell carcinoma,
neuroblastoma, soft tissue
sarcoma.

CONTRAINDICATIONS
Demonstrated hypersensitivity to
dacarbazine.

INTERACTIONS
Drug
Bone marrow depressants: May
enhance myelosuppression.
Live-virus vaccines: May potentiate
virus replication, and decrease the
patient's antibody response to the
vaccine.
Herbal
None known.
Food
None known.

DIAGNOSTIC TEST EFFECTS
May increase BUN, serum alkaline
phosphatase, AST (SGOT), and ALT
(SGPT) levels.

⚠ IV INCOMPATIBILITIES
Allopurinol (Aloprim), cefepime
(Maxipime), heparin, piperacillin,
and tazobactam (Zosyn).

⚠ IV COMPATIBILITIES
Etoposide (VePesid), granisetron
(Kytril), ondansetron (Zofran),
paclitaxel (Taxol).

SIDE EFFECTS
Frequent (90%)
Nausea, vomiting, anorexia (occurs
within 1 h of initial dose, may last up
to 12 h).
Occasional
Facial flushing, paresthesia,
alopecia, flulike symptoms
(fever, myalgia, malaise),
dermatologic reactions, confusion,
blurred vision, headache,
lethargy.

Rare
Diarrhea, stomatitis,
photosensitivity.

SERIOUS REACTIONS

• Myelosuppression may result in
blood dyscrasias, such as leukopenia
and thrombocytopenia, generally
2-4 wks after the last dacarbazine
dose.
• Hepatotoxicity occurs rarely.

PRECAUTIONS & CONSIDERATIONS

Caution is warranted with hepatic
or renal impairment. Because
dacarbazine is highly emetogenic,
antiemetic therapy for the prevention
of acute and delayed emesis is
recommended. Because of the risk
of fetal harm, pregnant women
should not take dacarbazine,
especially during the first trimester.
Breastfeeding women also should
not take this drug. The safety and
efficacy of dacarbazine have not
been established in children. In
elderly patients, age-related renal
impairment may require a dosage
adjustment. Immunizations and
coming in contact with those who
have recently received a live-virus
vaccine should be avoided during
treatment.

Notify the physician if easy
nausea and vomiting, bruising, fever,
signs of local infection, sore throat,
or unusual bleeding from any site
occurs. Adequate hydration should
be maintained to avoid dehydration
from vomiting. Erythrocyte,
leukocyte, and platelet counts for
evidence of myelosuppression should
be monitored.

Storage
Refrigerate unopened vials and
protect them from light. The
reconstituted solution containing
10 mg/mL is stable for up to 8 h at
room temperature or up to 72 h if
refrigerated. Solutions further diluted
with D5W or 0.9% NaCl are stable
for up to 8 h at room temperature or
up to 24 h if refrigerated.

Administration
! Dacarbazine dosage is
individualized based on clinical
response and tolerance of the drug's
adverse effects. When administering
this drug in combination therapy,
consult specific protocols for
optimum dosage and sequence of
drug administration.
! Give dacarbazine by IV push or
IV infusion, as prescribed. Because
dacarbazine may be carcinogenic,
mutagenic, or teratogenic, handle
the drug with extreme care during
preparation and administration.

For IV use, reconstitute the 100-
mg vial with 9.9 mL (or the 200-mg
vial with 19.7 mL) sterile water for
injection to provide a concentration
of 10 mg/mL. Give by IV push
over 2-3 min. Because IV push
administration may cause severe pain
along the injected vein, IV infusion
may be preferred. For IV infusion,
further dilute in 250 mL D5W or
0.9% NaCl. Infuse the drug over
15-30 min. Discard it if the color
changes from ivory to pink, because
this indicates decomposition. Apply
hot packs if the patient develops a
burning sensation, irritation, or local
pain at the injection site. Monitor the
injection site for signs and symptoms
of extravasation, including coolness,
stinging, swelling, and slight or no
blood return.

Daclizumab
da-kliz′yoo-mab
(Zenapax)

CATEGORY AND SCHEDULE
Pregnancy Risk Category: C

Classification: Immunosuppressives, monoclonal antibodies

MECHANISM OF ACTION
A humanized monoclonal antibody that binds to the interleukin-2 (IL-2) receptor complex, inhibiting the IL-2-mediated activation of T lymphocytes, a critical pathway in the cellular immune response involved in allograft rejection. *Therapeutic Effect:* Prevents organ rejection.

PHARMACOKINETICS
Half-life: Adults, 20 days. Children, 13 days.

AVAILABILITY
Injection: 25 mg/5 mL.

INDICATIONS AND DOSAGES
▶ **Prevention of acute renal transplant rejection (in combination with immunosuppressives that include cyclosporine and corticosteroids)**
IV
Adults, Children. 1 mg/kg over 15 min q14 days for 5 doses, beginning first dose no more than 24 h before transplantation.

OFF-LABEL USES
Treatment of graft vs. host disease. Prevention of heart, kidney-pancreas, liver transplant rejection.

CONTRAINDICATIONS
Hypersensitivity to the durg or to murine proteins.

INTERACTIONS
Drug
None known.
Herbal
None known.
Food
None known.

DIAGNOSTIC TEST EFFECTS
Elevated blood glucose.

Ⓓ IV INCOMPATIBILITIES
Do not mix daclizumab with any other drugs.

SIDE EFFECTS
Frequent (> 5%)
Constipation, nausea, diarrhea, vomiting, abdominal pain, dyspepsia, edema, headache, dizziness, tremor, fever, chest pain, pain, fatigue, insomnia, hypertension, hypotension, impaired wound healing, acne, cough, dysuria, tachycardia, thrombosis, bleeding.
Occasional (> 2%)
Flatulence, dehydration, renal impairment, diaphoresis, arthralgia, myalgia, shivering, weakness.

SERIOUS REACTIONS
• Hypersensitivity reaction, which occurs rarely, may include bronchospasm, hypotension, dyspnea, tachycardia, peripheral edema, cardiac arrest, respiratory arrest, loss of consciousness, rash, and pruritus.

PRECAUTIONS & CONSIDERATIONS
Comment: Only physicans with experience with daclizumab should prescribe. Should only be administered by trained personnel with adequate laboratory and supportive medical resources.
　Use as part of immunosuppressive regimen may increase risk of mortality.

D

Risk of lymphoproliferative disease and opportunistic infections.

Severe, acute hypersensitivity reactions, including anaphylaxis, have occurred within first 24 h of administration and reexposure.

Long-term effects on immune system unknown.

Caution is warranted with an infection and history of malignancy. Pregnancy should be avoided before, during, and for 4 mo after completion of therapy. It is unknown whether daclizumab crosses the placenta or is distributed in breast milk. No age-related precautions have been noted in children or elderly patients. Avoid crowded areas and other circumstances that increase risk for infection.

Notify the physician of GI disturbances, urinary changes, difficulty breathing or swallowing, itching or swelling of the lower extremities, rash, rapid heartbeat, or weakness. Laboratory values, including a CBC, and vital signs, particularly BP and pulse rate, should be monitored.

Storage

Refrigerate vials and protect them from light. Once reconstituted, the solution is stable for 4 h at room temperature, 24 h if refrigerated.

Administration

! Daclizumab is given in combination with an immunosuppresive regimen (cyclosporine, corticosteriods) for prevention of organ rejection.

For IV use, dilute the drug in 50 mL 0.9% NaCl. Invert the bag gently. Avoid shaking it. Infuse the drug over 15 min.

Dalteparin
doll'teh-pare-in
(Fragmin)

CATEGORY AND SCHEDULE
Pregnancy Risk Category: B

Classification: Anticoagulants, low-molecular-weight heparins

MECHANISM OF ACTION
A low-molecular-weight heparin that enhances inhibition of factor Xa and thrombin by antithrombin. Only slightly influences platelet aggregation, PT, and aPTT. *Therapeutic Effect:* Produces anticoagulation.

PHARMACOKINETICS

Route	Onset	Peak	Duration
Subcuta-neous	1-2 h	4 h	12 h

Protein binding: < 10%. *Half-life:* 3-5 h.

AVAILABILITY
Single-Dose Syringe:
2500 international units/0.2 mL,
5000 international units/0.2 mL,
7500 international units/0.3 mL,
10,000 international units/0.4 mL,
10,000 international units/mL,
12,500 international units/0.5 mL,
15,000 international units/0.6 mL,
18,000 international units/0.72 mL
Multiple-Dose Vial:
10,000 international units/mL,

25,000
international units/mL

INDICATIONS AND DOSAGES
▸ **Prophylaxis of deep vein thrombosis (DVT), low- to moderate-risk abdominal surgery**
SUBCUTANEOUS
Adults, Elderly. 2500 international units 1-2 h before surgery, then daily for 5-10 days.
▸ **Prophylaxis of DVT, high-risk abdominal surgery**
SUBCUTANEOUS
Adults, Elderly. 5000 international units the evening before surgery, then 5000 international units/day for 5-10 days. In patients with malignancy, 2500 international units 1-2 h before surgery, then 2500 international units 12 h later, then 5000 international units daily for 5-10 days.
▸ **Prophylaxis of DVT, total hip surgery**
SUBCUTANEOUS
Adults, Elderly. 2500 international units 1-2 h before surgery, then 2500 units 4-8 h after surgery, then 5000 units/day for 5-10 days; or 2500 international units 4-8 h after surgery, then 5000 international units/day for 5-10 days; or 5000 international units 10-12 h before surgery, then 5000 international units 4-8 h after surgery, then 5000 units/day for 5-10 days.
▸ **Unstable angina, non–Q-wave MI**
SUBCUTANEOUS
Adults, Elderly. 120 international units/kg q12h (maximum: 10,000 international units/dose) given with aspirin until clinically stable; usual duration 5-8 days.
▸ **Prophylaxis of DVT or pulmonary embolism in the acutely ill patient**
SUBCUTANEOUS
Adults, Elderly. 5000 international units once a day. Usual duration 12-14 days.

▸ **Extended treatment of symptomatic venous thromboembolism (VTE) in patients with cancer**
SUBCUTANEOUS
Adults, Elderly. 200 international units/kg once daily (maximum 18,000 international units/day for first 30 days). 150 international units/kg once daily (maximum 18,000 international units/day for months 2-6).
Doses for patients with cancer and symptomatic VTE with platelet counts 50,000-100,000/mm³: Reduce dose by 2500 international units daily until platelet count recovers to 100,000/mm³. Discontinue if platelet count <50,000/mm³.
Dose for renal insufficiency in patients with cancer and symptomatic VTE: Target anti-xa range 0.5-1.5 international units/mL (sample 4-6 h after dose after patient has received 3-4 doses).

CONTRAINDICATIONS
Active major bleeding; concurrent heparin therapy; hypersensitivity to dalteparin, heparin, or pork products; thrombocytopenia associated with positive in vitro test for antiplatelet antibody; treatment for cancer, unstable angina, or non–Q-wave myocardial infarction indications if receiving regional anesthesia.

INTERACTIONS
Drug
Anticoagulants, platelet inhibitors, thrombolytics: May increase risk of bleeding.
Herbal
Supplements with antiplatelet or anticoagulant effects (e.g., feverfew, garlic, ginger, ginkgo biloba, ginseng, red clover, sweet clover, white willow, etc.).
Food
None known.

D

DIAGNOSTIC TEST EFFECTS

Increases (reversible) LDH, serum alkaline phosphatase, AST (SGOT), and ALT (SGPT) levels.

SIDE EFFECTS

Occasional (3%-7%)
Hematoma at injection site.
Pain at injection site.
Rare (< 1%)
Hypersensitivity reaction (chills, fever, pruritus, urticaria, asthma, rhinitis, lacrimation, headache); mild, local skin irritation.

SERIOUS REACTIONS

- Major bleeding occurs rarely.
- Overdose may lead to bleeding complications ranging from local ecchymoses to major hemorrhage.
- Thrombocytopenia occurs rarely.

PRECAUTIONS & CONSIDERATIONS

Caution is warranted with neuraxial (spinal/epidural) anesthesia or spinal puncture, bacterial endocarditis, conditions with increased risk of hemorrhage, history of heparin-induced thrombocytopenia, recent GI ulceration and hemorrhage, hypertensive or diabetic retinopathy, impaired hepatic or renal function, and uncontrolled arterial hypertension. Dalteparin should be used with caution in pregnant women, particularly during the last trimester and immediately postpartum because it increases the risk of maternal hemorrhage. Even with additional doses of protamine, the APTT may remain more prolonged than would usually be found following administration of conventional heparin. In all cases, the anti-Factor Xa activity is never completely neutralized (maximum about 60%-75%). It is unknown whether dalteparin is distributed in breast milk. Safety and efficacy of dalteparin have not been established in children. No age-related precautions have been noted in elderly patients. Other medications, including OTC drugs, should be avoided.

Notify the physician of signs of bleeding, breathing difficulty, bruising, dizziness, fever, itching, light-headedness, rash, or swelling. Baseline CBC and BP should be established. CBC and stool for occult blood should be monitored throughout therapy.
Storage
Store drug at room temperature.
Administration
Administer subcutaneously. Do not inject intramuscularly. The patient should sit or lie down before administering by deep subcutaneous injection. Inject into U-shaped area around the navel, upper outer side of thigh, or upper outer quadrangle of buttock. Use a fine needle (25- to 26-gauge) to minimize tissue trauma. Introduce the entire length of the needle (½-inch) into skinfold held between the thumb and forefinger, holding the needle during injection at a 45- to 90-degree angle. Do not rub the injection site after administration to avoid bruising. Alternate administration site with each injection. The usual length of dalteparin therapy is 5-10 days. Perform an ice massage at the injection site shortly before injection to prevent excessive bruising.

Danazol

da′na-zole
(Cyclomen [CAN])

CATEGORY AND SCHEDULE

Pregnancy Risk Category: X

Classification: Hormones/hormone modifiers, and androgenic anti-estrogenic

MECHANISM OF ACTION

A testosterone derivative that suppresses the pituitary-ovarian axis by inhibiting the output of pituitary gonadotropins. Causes atrophy of both normal and ectopic endometrial tissue in endometriosis. Follicle-stimulating hormone (FSH) and luteinizing hormone (LH) are depressed in fibrocystic breast disease. Inhibits steroid synthesis and binding of steroids to their receptors in breast tissues. Increases serum levels of esterase inhibitor. *Therapeutic Effect:* Produces anovulation and amenorrhea, reduces the production of estrogen, corrects biochemical deficiency as seen in hereditary angioedema.

PHARMACOKINETICS

Well absorbed from the GI tract. Metabolized in liver, primarily to 2-hydroxymethylethisterone. Excreted in urine. *Half-life:* 4.5 h.

AVAILABILITY

Capsules: 50 mg, 100 mg, 200 mg.

INDICATIONS AND DOSAGES

▸ **Endometriosis**
PO
Adults. Initially, 200-400 mg/day in 2 divided doses; usual maintenance 800 mg/day in 2 divided doses for 3-9 mo.

▸ **Fibrocystic breast disease**
PO
Adults. 100-400 mg/day in 2 divided doses.

▸ **Hereditary angioedema**
PO
Adults. Initially, 200 mg 2-3 times/day. Decrease dose by 50% or less at 1- to 3-mo intervals. If attack occurs, increase dose by up to 200 mg/day.

OFF-LABEL USES

Treatment of gynecomastia, menorrhagia, precocious puberty, premenstrual syndrome.

CONTRAINDICATIONS

Cardiac impairment, pregnancy, breastfeeding, severe liver or renal disease, undiagnosed genital bleeding, porphyria.

INTERACTIONS

Drug
Carbamazepine, cyclosporine, tacrolimus, and warfarin: May increase serum levels and increase risk of toxicity of these drugs.
HMG-CoA reductase inhibitors: May increase chance of developing myopathy or rhabdomyolysis.
Hormonal contraceptives: May decrease effectiveness of contraceptives.
Hypoglycemic agents: May increase the risk of hypoglycemia.
Herbal
None known.
Food
Food: May delay time to peak.
High-fat meal: Increases plasma concentration.

DIAGNOSTIC TEST EFFECTS

May increase blood hemoglobin and hematocrit levels, LDL concentrations, serum alkaline phosphatase, bilirubin, calcium, potassium, SGOT (AST) levels, and sodium levels. May decrease HDL concentrations. May alter levels of testosterone, androstenedione, and dehydroepiandrosterone.

SIDE EFFECTS

Frequent
Females: Amenorrhea, breakthrough bleeding/spotting, decreased breast size, increased weight, irregular menstrual periods.

Males: Semen abnormalities, spermatogenesis reduction.
Occasional
Males/females: Edema, rhabdomyolysis (muscle cramps, unusual fatigue), virilism (acne, oily skin), flushed skin, altered moods.
Rare
Males/females: Hematuria, gingivitis, carpal tunnel syndrome, cataracts, severe headache, vomiting, rash, photosensitivity, anxiety, depression, sleep disorders.
Females: Enlarged clitoris, hoarseness, deepening voice, hair growth, monilial vaginitis.
Males: Decreased testicle size.

SERIOUS REACTIONS
• Jaundice may occur in those receiving 400 mg/day or more. Liver dysfunction, eosinophilia, thrombocytopenia, pancreatitis occur rarely.
• Peliosis and benign hepatic adenoma have occurred with long-term use.
• Benign intracranial hypertension (pseudotumor cerebri) occurs rarely. Monitor for papilledema, headache, nausea and vomiting, and visual disturbances.
• Thromboembolism, thrombotic, and thrombophlebitic events have occurred.

PRECAUTIONS & CONSIDERATIONS
Caution should be used with seizure disorder, migraine, or conditions influenced by edema. Be aware that danazol use is contraindicated during lactation. If pregnancy is suspected, notify the physician. Safety and efficacy of danazol have not been established in children. Be aware that danazol should be used with caution in elderly patients. Breast cancer should be ruled out before starting therapy for fibrocystic breast disease. Monitor liver function.

If masculinizing effects, weight gain, muscle cramps, or fatigue occurs, notify the physician. Spotting or bleeding may occur in the first months of therapy. Nonhormonal contraceptives should be used during therapy.
Storage
Store at room temperature.
Administration
Take full course of treatment as prescribed by the physician. In females, be aware that therapy should be initiated during menstruation or when patient is not pregnant. Administration with meals may lessen GI upset.

Dantrolene
dan′troe-leen
(Dantrium)
Do not confuse Dantrium with Daraprim.

CATEGORY AND SCHEDULE
Pregnancy Risk Category: C

Classification: Musculoskeletal agents, relaxants, skeletal muscle

MECHANISM OF ACTION
A skeletal muscle relaxant that reduces muscle contraction by interfering with release of calcium ion. Reduces calcium ion concentration. *Therapeutic Effect:* Dissociates excitation-contraction coupling. Interferes with catabolic process associated with malignant hyperthermic crisis.

PHARMACOKINETICS
Poorly absorbed from the GI tract. Protein binding: High. Metabolized in the liver. Primarily excreted in

urine. *Half-life:* IV 4-8 h;
PO 8.7 h.

AVAILABILITY
Capsules: 25 mg, 50 mg, 100 mg.
Powder for Injection: 20-mg vial.

INDICATIONS AND DOSAGES
▶ **Spasticity**
PO
Adults, Elderly. Initially, 25 mg/day.
Increase to 25 mg 2-4 times a day,
then by 25-mg increments every
4-7 days up to 100 mg 2-4 times a
day.
Children. Initially, 0.5 mg/kg twice a
day. Increase to 0.5 mg/kg 3-4 times
a day, then in increments of
0.5 mg/kg/day up to 3 mg/kg 2-4 times
a day. Maximum: 400 mg/day.
▶ **Prevention of malignant**
hyperthermic crisis
PO
Adults, Elderly, Children.
4-8 mg/kg/day in 3-4 divided doses
1-2 days before surgery; give last
dose 3-4 h before surgery.
IV
Adults, Elderly, Children. 2.5 mg/kg
about 1.25 h before surgery.
▶ **Management of malignant**
hyperthermic crisis
IV
Adults, Elderly, Children. Initially a
minimum of 1 mg/kg rapid IV; may
repeat up to total cumulative dose
of 10 mg/kg. May follow with 4-8
mg/kg/day PO in 4 divided doses up
to 3 days after crisis.

OFF-LABEL USES
Relief of exercise-induced pain in
patients with muscular dystrophy,
treatment of flexor spasms and
neuroleptic malignant syndrome,
heat stroke.

CONTRAINDICATIONS
Active hepatic disease.

INTERACTIONS
Drug
CNS depressants: May increase
CNS depression with short-term use.
Liver toxic medications, estrogens:
May increase the risk of liver toxicity
with chronic use.
CYP3A4 inducers/inhibitors: May
alter dantrolene plasma levels.
Herbal
St. John's wort: May decrease
plasma level of dantrolene.
Food
None known.

DIAGNOSTIC TEST EFFECTS
May alter liver function test results.

Ⓓ IV INCOMPATIBILITIES
Alfentanil (Alfenta), amikacin
(Amikar), aminophylline,
amphotericin B cholesteryl sulfate
complex (Amphotec), ampicillin,
ampicillin/sulbactam (Unasyn),
ascorbic acid, atracurium (Tracrium),
atropine, azathioprine, aztreonam
(Azactam), benztropine (Cogentin),
bivalirudin (Angiomax), bretylium,
bumetanide (Bumex), buprenorphine
(Buprenex), butorphanol (Stadol),
calcium chloride, calcium
gluconate, caspofungin (Cancidas),
cefazolin, cefotaxime (Claforan),
cefotetan (Cefotan), cefoxitin
(Mefoxin), ceftazidime (Ceptaz,
Fortaz, Tazicef, Tazidime),
ceftizoxime (Cefizox), ceftriaxone
(Rocephin), cefuroxime (Zinacef),
chloramphenicol, chlorpromazine,
cimetidine (Tagamet), cisplatin,
clindamycin (Cleocin),
cyanocobalamin, cyclosporine
(Sandimmune), dactinomycin
(Cosmegen), daptomycin (Cubicin),
dexamethasone sodium phosphate,
digoxin (Lanoxin), diltiazem
(Cardizem), diphenhydramine
(Benadryl), dobutamine,
docetaxel (Taxotere), dopamine

(Intropin), enalaprilat, ephedrine, epinephrine, epoetin alfa (Procrit), ertapenem (Invanz), erythromycin lactobionate, esmolol (Brevibloc), etoposide phosphate (Etopophos), famotidine (Pepcid), fenoldopam (Corlopam), fentanyl (Sublimaze), fluconazole (Diflucan), fludarabine (Fludara), folic acid, furosemide (Lasix), ganciclovir (Cytovene), gemcitabine (Gemzar), gentamicin, granisetron (Kytril), haloperidol (Haldol), heparin, hydrocortisone sodium succinate (Solu-Cortef), hydromorphone (Dilaudid), hydroxyzine, imipenem/cilastatin (Primaxin), insulin (Humulin R, Novolin R, regular), ketorolac, labetalol, lidocaine, linezolid (Zyvox), lorazepam (Ativan), magnesium sulfate, mannitol, meperidine (Demerol), methicillin, methylprednisolone sodium succinate, metoclopramide (Reglan), metoprolol (Lopressor), metronidazole (Flagyl), midazolam (Versed), milrinone (Primacor), minocycline (Minocin), mitoxantrone (Novantrone), morphine, multiple vitamin injection, nafcillin, nalbuphine (Nubain), naloxone (Narcan), nitroglycerin, nitroprusside sodium (Nitropress), norepinephrine (Levophed), ondansetron (Zofran), oxacillin, oxaliplatin (Eloxatin), oxytocin (Pitocin), pemetrexed (Alimta), penicillin G potassium, penicillin G sodium, phenytoin, phytonadione, piperacillin, piperacillin/tazobactam, potassium chloride, procainamide, prochloperazine, promethazine, propranolol, ranitidine (Zantac), sodium acetate, sodium bicarbonate, streptokinase, succinylcholine, sufentanil (Sufenta), tacrolimus (Prograf), teniposide (Vumon), ticarcillin (Ticar), ticarcillin/clavulanate (Timentin), tigecycline (Tygacil), tirofibran (Aggrastat), tobramycin, vancomycin, vasopressin, vecuronium (Norcuron), verapamil, vinorelbine (Navelbine), voriconazole (Vfend).

▯ IV COMPATIBILITIES
Acyclovir (Zovirax), paclitaxel (Taxol), palonosetron (Aloxi).

SIDE EFFECTS
Frequent (> 10%)
Drowsiness, dizziness, weakness, general malaise, diarrhea (mild), rash, nausea.
Occasional
Confusion, diarrhea (may be severe), headache, insomnia, constipation, urinary frequency.
Rare
Paradoxical CNS excitement or restlessness, paresthesia, tinnitus, slurred speech, tremor, blurred vision, dry mouth, nocturia, impotence, rash, pruritus.

SERIOUS REACTIONS
• There is a risk of liver toxicity, most notably in women, those 35 yr of age and older, and those taking other medications concurrently.
• Overt hepatitis noted most frequently between 3rd and 12th mo of therapy.
• Overdosage results in vomiting, muscular hypotonia, muscle twitching, respiratory depression, and seizures.

PRECAUTIONS & CONSIDERATIONS
Caution is warranted for patients with a history of previous liver disease and impaired cardiac or pulmonary function. Be aware that dantrolene readily crosses the placenta and should not be used in breastfeeding mothers. No age-related precautions have been noted in children 5 yr and older. There is no

information available on dantrolene use in elderly patients.

Drowsiness may occur but usually diminishes with continued therapy. Avoid alcohol, CNS depressants, and tasks that require mental alertness or motor skills. Notify the physician if bloody or tarry stools, continued weakness, diarrhea, fatigue, itching, nausea, or skin rash occurs. Blood tests, such as liver and renal function tests, should be performed before and during therapy. Therapeutic response, such as decreased intensity of skeletal muscle pain or spasm, should be assessed.

Storage
Store at room temperature. Use within 6 h after reconstitution. Solution normally appears clear, colorless; discard if cloudy or precipitate is present.

Administration
! Begin with low-dose therapy, as prescribed, then increase gradually at 4- to 7-day intervals to reduce incidence of side effects.

Take oral dantrolene without regard to meals.

For IV use, reconstitute 20-mg vial with 60 mL sterile water for injection to provide a concentration of 0.33 mg/mL. For IV infusion, administer over 1 h. Diligently monitor for extravasation because of high pH of IV preparation. May produce severe complications.

Dapsone
dap´sone
(Aczone, Dapsone)
Do not confuse with Diprosone

CATEGORY AND SCHEDULE
Pregnancy Risk Category: C

Classification: Antiprotazoal

MECHANISM OF ACTION
An antibiotic that is a competitive antagonist of para-aminobenzoic acid (PABA); it prevents normal bacterial utilization of PABA for synthesis of folic acid. *Therapeutic Effect:* Inhibits bacterial growth.

AVAILABILITY
Tablets: 25 mg, 100 mg.
Topical Gel: 5%

INDICATIONS AND DOSAGES
▸ **Leprosy**
PO
Adults, Elderly. 50-100 mg/day for 3-10 yr.
Children. 1-2 mg/kg/24 h.
Maximum: 100 mg/day.
▸ **Dermatitis herpetiformis**
PO
Adults, Elderly. Initially, 50 mg/day. May increase up to 300 mg/day.
▸ *Pneumocystis carinii* **pneumonia (PCP)**
PO
Adults, Elderly. 100 mg/day in combination with trimethoprim for 21 days.
▸ **Prevention of PCP**
PO
Adults, Elderly. 100 mg/day.
Children older than 1 mo. 2 mg/kg/day. Maximum: 100 mg/day.
Alternate dosing: 4 mg/kg/dose once weekly. Maximum 200 mg.
▸ **ACNE**
TOPICAL GEL
Adults and children 12 yr and older: Apply thin layer twice daily to affected areas.

OFF-LABEL USES
Malaria prophylaxis, PCP prophylaxis and treatment, toxoplasmosis prophylaxis.

CONTRAINDICATIONS
None significant.

D

INTERACTIONS
Drug
CYP2C9 and CYP3A4 inhibitors:
May increase levels and effects of
dapsone.
CYP2C9 and CYP3A4 inducers:
May decrease levels and effects of
dapsone.
Methotrexate: May increase
hematologic reactions.
Probenecid: May decrease the
excretion of dapsone.
**Protease inhibitors (including
ritonavir):** May increase dapsone
blood concentration.
Rifampin: May decrease rifampin
blood concentration.
Trimethoprim: May increase the
risk of toxic effects of both drugs.
Herbal
St. John's wort: May decrease
dapsone blood concentration.
Food
None significant.

DIAGNOSTIC TEST EFFECTS
Hemoglobin decrease.

SIDE EFFECTS
Frequent (> 10%)
Hemolytic anemia,
methemoglobinemia, rash.
Occasional (1%-10%)
Hemolysis, photosensitivity reaction,
tachycardia, headache, insomnia,
dermatitis, abdominal pain, nausea.

SERIOUS REACTIONS
• Agranulocytosis, aplastic anemia,
and blood dyscrasias may occur.
• Stevens-Johnson syndrome has
occurred rarely.
• Drug-induced hepatitis.

PRECAUTIONS & CONSIDERATIONS
Caution is warranted with
agranulocytosis, severe anemia,
aplastic anemia, glucose-6-phosphate
dehydrogenase deficiency,
hemoglobin M deficiency, or a
hypersensitivity to dapsone or
its derivatives (such as sulfoxone
sodium). Overexposure to sun or
ultraviolet light should be avoided.

Baseline CBC should be obtained.
Hypersensitivity to dapsone or its
derivatives should be determined
before therapy. Skin should be
assessed for a dermatologic reaction.
Signs and symptoms of hemolysis,
such as jaundice, should be
monitored. Persistent fatigue, fever,
or sore throat should be reported.
Storage
Store at room temperature; do not
freeze.
Administration
Take dapsone without regard to food.
Topical gel: apply thin layer to
affected areas: rub in gently and
completely. Gel is gritty. Wash hands
after applying.

Daptomycin
dap'toe-my-sin
(Cubicin)

CATEGORY AND SCHEDULE
Pregnancy Risk Category: B

Classification: Anti-infectives
lipopeptides

MECHANISM OF ACTION
A lipopeptide antibacterial agent
that binds to bacterial membranes
and causes a rapid depolarization of
the membrane potential. The loss of
membrane potential leads to inhibition
of protein, DNA, and RNA synthesis.
Therapeutic Effect: Bactericidal.

PHARMACOKINETICS
Widely distributed. Protein binding:
90%. Primarily excreted unchanged
in urine. Moderately removed

by hemodialysis. *Half-life:* 7-8 h (increased in impaired renal function).

AVAILABILITY
Powder for Injection: 500 mg/vial.

INDICATIONS AND DOSAGES
▶ **Complicated skin and skin-structure infections (SSSI)**
IV INFUSION
Adults, Elderly. 4 mg/kg every 24 h for 7-14 days.
▶ **Bacteremia from *Staphylococcus aureus* (MSSA or MRSA), including right-sided endocarditis**
IV INFUSION
Adults, Elderly. 6 mg/kg every 24 h for 2-6 wks.
▶ **Dosage in renal impairment**
For patients with creatinine clearance of < 30 mL/min, dosage is 4 mg/kg q48h for 7-14 days for skin infections. For patients with creatinine clearance of < 30 mL/min, dosage is 6 mg/kg q48h for 2-6 wks for bacteremia.

OFF-LABEL USES
Nonpulmonary infections caused by vancomycin-resistant entero cocci (VRE).

CONTRAINDICATIONS
Hypersensitivity.

INTERACTIONS
Drug
HMG-CoA reductase inhibitors: May cause myopathy.
Tobramycin: Increases the serum concentration of daptomycin.
Herbal
None known.
Food
None known.

DIAGNOSTIC TEST EFFECTS
May increase serum CPK levels.
May alter liver function test results.
May alter serum potassium levels.

ⓘ IV INCOMPATIBILITIES
Diluents containing dextrose. If the same IV line is used to administer different drugs, the line should be flushed with 0.9% NaCl.
Acyclovir (Zovirax), allopurinol (Aloprim), amphotericin B cholesteryl sulfate complex (Amphotec), amphotericin B lipid complex (Abelcet), gemcitabine (Gemzar), impipenem/cilastatin (Primaxin), methotrexate, metronidazole (Flagyl), minocycline (Minocin), mitomycin (Mutamycin), nesiritide (Natrecor), nitroglycerin, pantoprazole (Protonix), pentobarbital, phenytoin, remifentanil (Ultiva), streptozocin, sufentanil (Sufenta), thiopental (Thioplex).

ⓘ IV COMPATIBILITIES
Alfentanil (Alfenta), amifostine (Ethyol), amikacin (Amikar), aminophylline, amiodarone, amphotericin B liposomal (AmBisome), ampicillin, ampicillin/sulbactam (Unasyn), argatroban, arsenic trioxide (Trisenox), atenolol, atracurium (Tracrium), azithromycin (Zithromax), aztreonam (Azactam), bivalirudin (Angiomax), bleomycin (Blenoxane), bretylium, bumetanide (Bumex), buprenorphine (Buprenex), busulfan (Busulfex), butorphanol (Stadol), calcium chloride, calcium gluconate, carboplatin, carmustine (BiCNU), caspofungin (Cancidas), cefazolin, cefepime (Maxipime), cefotaxime (Claforan), cefotetan (Cefotan), cefoxitin (Mefoxin), ceftazidime (Ceptaz, Fortaz, Tazicef, Tazidime), ceftizoxime (Cefizox), ceftriaxone (Rocephin), cefuroxime (Zinacef), chloramphenicol, chlorpromazine, cimetidine (Tagamet), ciprofloxacin (Cipro), cisatracurium (Nimbex), cisplatin, clindamycin (Cleocin), cyclophosphamide (Cytoxan),

cyclosporine (Sandimmune), dacarbazine (DTIC-Dome), dactinomycin (Cosmegen), daunorubicin (Cerubidine), dexamethasone sodium phosphate, dexmedetomidine (Precedex), dexrazoxane (Zinecard), diazepam (Valium), digoxin (Lanoxin), diltiazem (Cardizem), diphenhydramine (Benadryl), dobutamine (Dobutrex), docetaxel (Taxotere), dolasetron (Anzemet), dopamine (Intropin), doripenem (Doribax), doxorubicin (Adriamycin), doxorubicin liposomal (Doxil), droperidol, enalaprilat, ephedrine, epinephrine, epirubicin (Ellence), eptifibitide (Integrilin), ertapenem (Invanz), erythromycin lactobionate, esmolol (Brevibloc), etoposide (Vepesid), etoposide phosphate (Etopophos), famotidine (Pepcid), fenoldopam (Corlopam), fentanyl (Sublimaze), fluconazole (Diflucan), fludarabine (Fludara), foscarnet (Foscavir), fosphenytoin (Cerebyx), furosemide (Lasix), gentamicin, granisetron (Kytril), haloperidol (Haldol), heparin, hydralazine, hydrocortisone sodium succinate (Solu-Cortef), hydromorphone (Dilaudid), hydroxyzine, idarubicin (Idamycin PFS), ifosfamide (Ifex), insulin (Humulin R, Novolin R, Regular), irinotecan (Camptosar), isoproterenol (Isuprel), ketorolac, labetalol, leucovorin, levofloxacin (Levaquin), lidocaine, linezolid (Zyvox), lorazepam (Ativan), magnesium sulfate, mannitol, melphalan (Alkeran), meperidine (Demerol), meropenem (Merrem), mesna (Mesnex), methylprednisolone sodium succinate, metoclopramide (Reglan), metoprolol (Lopressor), midazolam (Versed), milrinone (Primacor), mitoxantrone (Novantrone), mivacurium (Mivacron), morphine, moxifloxacin (Avelox), nafcillin, nalbuphine (Nubain), naloxone (Narcan), nicardipine (Cardene), nitroprusside sodium (Nitropress), norepinephrine (Levophed), ondansetron (Zofran), oxaliplatin (Eloxatin), oxytocin (Pitocin), paclitaxel (Taxol), palonosetron (Aloxi), pancuronium, pemetrexed (Alimta), phenobarbital, phytonadione, piperacillin/tazobactam (Zosyn), potassium acetate, potassium chloride, potassium phosphates, procainamide, prochloperazine, promethazine, propranolol, quinupristin/dalfopristin (Synercid), ranitidine (Zantac), succinylcholine, tacrolimus (Prograf), teniposide (Vumon), theophylline, thiotepa (Thioplex), ticarcillin (Ticar), ticarcillin/clavulanate (Timentin), tigecycline (Tygacil), tirofibran (Aggrastat), tobramycin, topotecan (Hycamtim), vasopressin, vecuronium (Norcuron), verapamil, vinblastine (Velban), vincristine (Vincasar), vinorelbine (Navelbine), voriconazole (Vfend), zidovudine (Retrovir), zoledronic acid (Zometa).

SIDE EFFECTS

Frequent (5%-13%)
Constipation, nausea, peripheral injection site reactions, headache, diarrhea, vomiting, anemia, peripheral edema, chest pain, hypertension, hypotension, insomnia.
Occasional (3%-4%)
Insomnia, rash, vomiting, abdominal pain, injection site reaction.
Rare (< 3%)
Pruritus, dizziness.

SERIOUS REACTIONS

• Skeletal muscle myopathy, characterized by muscle pain and weakness, particularly of the distal extremities, occurs rarely.

D

- Antibiotic-associated colitis and other superinfections may result from altered bacterial balance.
- Renal failure has occurred.
- Hypersensitivity.

PRECAUTIONS & CONSIDERATIONS

Daptomycin should not be used to treat pneumonia as the drug is inactivated by pulmonary surfactant. Caution is warranted with pregnancy, musculoskeletal disorders, and renal impairment. Avoid concurrent use of HMG-CoA reductase inhibitors because they may cause myopathy. It is unknown whether daptomycin is distributed in breast milk. The safety and efficacy of this drug have not been established in children younger than 18 yr of age. No age-related precautions have been noted in elderly patients.

Report headache, dizziness, nausea, rash, severe diarrhea, new muscle weakness, or any other new symptoms. Mild GI effects may be tolerable, but severe symptoms may indicate the onset of antibiotic-associated colitis. Pattern of daily bowel activity and stool consistency should be monitored. Culture and sensitivity tests should be obtained before giving the first dose of daptomycin; therapy may begin before the test results are known. Check for white patches on the mucous membranes and tongue. Be alert for signs and symptoms of superinfection, including abdominal pain, moderate to severe diarrhea, severe anal or genital pruritus, and severe mouth soreness.

Storage

Store the drug in the refrigerator. The reconstituted and diluted solutions are stable for 12 h at room temperature and up to 48 h if refrigerated.

Administration

The drug normally appears as a pale yellow to light brown lyophilized cake. Discard the solution if it contains particulate matter. Reconstitute the 250-mg vial with 5 mL 0.9% NaCl and the 500-mg vial with 10 mL 0.9% NaCl. Further dilute in 50 mL 0.9% NaCl. Infuse the intermittent IV (piggyback) infusion over 30 min.

Darbepoetin Alfa

dar-beh-poe′ee-tin
(Aranesp)
Do not confuse Aranesp with Aricept.

CATEGORY AND SCHEDULE

Pregnancy Risk Category: C

Classification: Hematopoietic agents

MECHANISM OF ACTION

A glycoprotein that stimulates formation of red blood cells in bone marrow; increases the serum half-life of epoetin. *Therapeutic Effect:* Induces erythropoiesis and release of reticulocytes from bone marrow.

PHARMACOKINETICS

Well absorbed after subcutaneous (SC) administration. *Half-life (CRF):* IV 21 h, SC 48.5 h. *Half-life (cancer):* SC Adults 74 h, Children 49 h.

AVAILABILITY

Injection, Single-Dose Vials: 25 mcg/mL, 40 mcg/mL, 60 mcg/mL, 100 mcg/mL, 150 mcg/mL, 200 mcg/mL, 300 mcg/mL.
Injection, Pre-Filled Syringes: 25 mcg/0.42 mL, 40 mcg/0.4 mL, 60 mcg/0.3 mL, 100 mcg/0.5 mL,

D

150 mcg/0.3 mL, 200 mcg/0.4 mL, 300 mcg/0.6 mL, 500 mcg/1 mL

INDICATIONS AND DOSAGES
▸ **Anemia in chronic renal failure**
IV BOLUS, SUBCUTANEOUS
Adults, Elderly. Initially,
0.45 mcg/kg once weekly. Adjust dosage to achieve and maintain a target hemoglobin level not to exceed 12 g/dL (target 10-12 g/dL). Do not increase dosage more frequently than once monthly. Limit increases in hemoglobin level by < 1 g/dL over any 2-wk period. IV route preferred in hemodialysis patients.
Children >1 yr. Convert from epoetin alfa based on manufacturer dosing table.
Dosage adjustment: If hemoglobin level approaches 12 g/dL or increases >1 g/dL in any 2-wk period, decrease dose by 25%. If it continues to rise, discontinue therapy temporarily, then resume with 25% reduction. If hemoglobin level does not increase by 1 g/dL after 4 wks, increase dose by 25%.
▸ **Anemia associated with chemotherapy**
IV, SUBCUTANEOUS
Adults, Elderly. 2.25 mcg/kg/dose once a week or 500 mcg every 3 wks. Adjust dosage to achieve and maintain a target hemoglobin level not to exceed 12 g/dL.
Dosage adjustment: If hemoglobin exceeds 12 g/dL, withhold dose and then restart at 40% dose reduction. If hemoglobin increases 1 g/dL in any 2-wk period, decrease dose by 40%. If hemoglobin does not increase by 1 g/dL after 6 wks, increase dose up to 4.5 mcg/kg once a week.

CONTRAINDICATIONS
History of sensitivity to hamster cell-derived products or human albumin, uncontrolled hypertension.

INTERACTIONS
Drug, Herbal, Food
None known.

DIAGNOSTIC TEST EFFECTS
May increase BUN, serum phosphorus, serum potassium, serum creatinine, serum uric acid, and serum sodium levels. May decrease bleeding time, serum iron concentration, and serum ferritin.

ⓘ IV INCOMPATIBILITIES
Do not mix with other medications.

SIDE EFFECTS
Frequent (11%-33%)
Myalgia, fatigue, edema, fever, dizziness, constipation, vomiting, nausea, abdominal pain, arthralgia, infection, hypertension or hypotension, headache, diarrhea.
Occasional (3%-10%)
Angina, rash, injection site pain, vascular access infection, flulike syndrome, reaction at administration site, asthenia, dizziness.

SERIOUS REACTIONS
• Vascular access thrombosis, congestive heart failure (CHF), sepsis, arrhythmias, thrombosis, myocardial infarction (MI), stroke, transient ischemic attack (TIA), and anaphylactic reaction occur rarely.
• Pure red blood cell aplasia and severe anemia, with or without other cytopenias, associated with neutralizing antibodies to erythropoietin have occurred, predominantly in patients with CRF receiving darbepoetin by subcutaneous administration.
• Erythropoiesis-stimulating agents (ESAs) increase the risk for death and serious cardiovascular events in controlled clinical trials when administered to target a hemoglobin of more than 12 g/dL and in cancer

patients receiving chemotherapy. There is an increased risk of serious arterial and venous thromboembolic reactions, including MI, stroke, CHF, and hemodialysis graft occlusion. To reduce cardiovascular risks, use the lowest dose of ESAs that will gradually increase the hemoglobin concentration to a level sufficient to avoid the need for red blood cell (RBC) transfusion. The hemoglobin concentration should not exceed 12 g/dL; the rate of hemoglobin increase should not exceed 1 g/dL in any 2-wks period.

• ESAs have shortened time to tumor progression and reduced survival time in solid tumor patients with target hemoglobin >12 g/dL.

PRECAUTIONS & CONSIDERATIONS

Caution is warranted with hemolytic anemia, a history of seizures, known porphyria (impairment of erythrocyte formation in bone marrow), sickle cell anemia, and thalassemia. It is unknown whether darbepoetin alfa crosses the placenta or is distributed in breast milk. Safety and efficacy of darbepoetin alfa have not been established in children. In elderly patients, age-related renal impairment may require dosage adjustment. Avoid tasks that require mental alertness or motor skills until response to the drug is established.

Notify the physician of severe headache. Hematocrit level should be monitored diligently. The dosage should be reduced if hematocrit level increases more than 4 points in 2 wks. CBC with differential, hemoglobin, reticulocyte count, BUN, phosphorus, potassium, serum creatinine, and serum ferritin levels should also be monitored before and during therapy. In addition, BP must be monitored aggressively for an increase because 25% of persons taking darbepoetin alfa require antihypertensive therapy and dietary restrictions. Keep in mind that most patients will eventually need supplemental iron therapy.

Storage

Refrigerate vials. Do not shake vials vigorously because doing so may denature medication, rendering it inactive. Do not freeze. Protect from light.

Administration

! Avoid excessive agitation of vial; do not shake because it will cause foaming.

For IV use, reconstitution is not necessary. May be given as an IV bolus. IV administration is preferred route for patients with renal failure.

For subcutaneous administration, use one dose per vial; do not reenter vial. Discard unused portion. Also available in prefilled syringes or auto-injectors.

Do not inject into an area that is red, bruised, hard, or tender. Rotate sites of SC administration with each injection.

Darifenacin Hydrobromide
dare-ih-fen′ah-sin
(Enablex)

CATEGORY AND SCHEDULE
Pregnancy Risk Category: C

Classification: Anti muscarinics

MECHANISM OF ACTION
A urinary antispasmodic agent that acts as a direct antagonist at muscarinic receptor sites in cholinergically

innervated organs. Blockade of the receptors limits bladder contractions. *Therapeutic Effect:* Reduces symptoms of bladder irritability and overactivity; improves bladder capacity.

AVAILABILITY
Tablets (Extended-Release): 7.5 mg, 15 mg.

INDICATIONS AND DOSAGES
▸ **Overactive bladder**
PO
Adults, Elderly. Initially, 7.5 mg once daily. If response is not adequate after at least 2 wks, dosage may be increased to 15 mg once daily. Dose should not exceed 7.5 mg once daily with concomitant CYP3A4 inhibitors.
▸ **Dosage in hepatic impairment**
For patients with moderate hepatic impairment, maximum dosage is 7.5 mg once daily.

CONTRAINDICATIONS
GI or gastrourinary obstruction, paralytic ileus, severe hepatic impairment, uncontrolled angle-closure glaucoma, urine retention.

INTERACTIONS
Drug
Aminoglutethimide, carbamazepine, nafcillin, nevirapine, phenobarbital, phenytoin, rifamycins, CYP3A4 inducers: May decrease the effects and blood level of darifenacin.
Amphetamines, β-blockers (selected), dextromethorphan, fluoxetine, lidocaine, mirtazapine, nefazodone, paroxetine, risperidone, ritonavir, thioridazine, tricyclic antidepressants, venlafaxine, CYP2D6 substrates: May increase the effects and blood levels of these drugs.
Anticholinergic agents: Anticholinergic side effects may be increased.

Azole antifungals, ciprofloxacin, clarithromycin, diclofenac, doxycycline, erythromycin, imatinib, isoniazid, nefazodone, nicardipine, propofol, protease inhibitors, quinidine, verapamil, CYP3A4 inhibitors: May increase the effects and blood level of darifenacin. Maximum dose 7.5 mg daily with potent CYP3A4 inhibitors.
Codeine, hydrocodone, oxycodone, tramadol, CYP2D6 prodrug substrates: May decrease the effects and blood levels of these drugs.
Digoxin: Increased digoxin levels.
Herbal
St. John's wort: May decrease effects and blood level of darifenacin.
Food
None known.

DIAGNOSTIC TEST EFFECTS
None known.

SIDE EFFECTS
Frequent (21%-35%)
Dry mouth, constipation.
Occasional (4%-8%)
Dyspepsia, headache, hypertension, peripheral edema, nausea, abdominal pain.
Rare (2%-3%)
Asthenia, diarrhea, dizziness, dry eyes.

SERIOUS REACTIONS
• Urinary tract infection occurs occasionally.
• Heat prostration may occur.

PRECAUTIONS & CONSIDERATIONS
Caution is warranted with bladder outflow obstruction, constipation, controlled angle-closure glaucoma, decreased GI motility, GI obstructive disorders, hiatal hernia, myasthenia gravis, nonobstructive prostatic hyperplasia, reflux esophagitis, ulcerative colitis, moderate hepatic dysfunction, and urine

retention. Safety and efficacy have not been established in pediatric patients. Effects in pregnancy and breastfeeding are unknown.

Administration

Take darifenacin without regard to food. Swallow extended-release tablets whole; do not cut or crush them.

Dasatinib

da-sa′ti-nib
(Sprycel)

CATEGORY AND SCHEDULE

Pregnancy Risk Category: D

Classification: Antineoplastic

MECHANISM OF ACTION

Inhibits BCR-ABL tyrosine kinase, an enzyme created by the Philadelphia chromosome abnormality found in patients with chronic myeloid leukemia (CML). Also inhibits SRC family kinases. *Therapeutic Effect:* Suppresses tumor growth during the three stages of CML: blast crisis, accelerated phase, and chronic phase.

PHARMACOKINETICS

Protein binding: 96%. Metabolized in liver, primarily by CYP450 3A4. Primarily eliminated in feces (85%, 19% as unchanged); minimal excretion in urine (4%, 0.1% unchanged). *Half-life:* 3-5 h.

AVAILABILITY

Tablets: 20 mg, 50 mg, 70 mg, 100 mg.

INDICATIONS AND DOSAGES

▸ **ALL, Philadelphia chromosome–positive, resistant or intolerant to prior therapy**
PO
Adults. 70 mg twice a day (morning and evening).

▸ **CML, accelerated, or myeloid, or lymphoid blast phase**
Adults. 70 mg twice a day (morning and evening).
▸ **CML, chronic phase**
Adults. 100 mg PO once daily.

CONTRAINDICATIONS

Hypersensitivity to dasatinib or its components, hypokalemia, hypomagnesemia, use with antiarrhythmic medication, patients at risk for fluid retention.

INTERACTIONS

Drug
H2 antagonists, proton pump inhibitors: Decreased dasatinib absorption.
Anticoagulants, NSAIDs: Increased risk of bleeding.
CYP3A4 inhibitors (e.g., clarithromycin, erythromycin, azole antifungals): May increase the levels and adverse effects of dasatinib. Consider dasatinib dose reduction.
CYP3A4 substrates (midazolam, triazolam): Increased plasma concentrations of these drugs with increased CNS depression.
QTc-prolonging medications: Additive effects.
Herbal
St. John's wort: decrease dasatinib levels.
Food
Grapefruit juice: May increase dasatinib levels and adverse effects. Do not drink grapefruit juice while taking dasatinib.

DIAGNOSTIC TEST EFFECTS

Myelosuppression, QTc prolongation.

SIDE EFFECTS

Frequent
Neutropenia, thrombocytopenia, diarrhea, headache, musculoskeletal

pain, fatigue, fever, superficial
edema, rash, nausea, dyspnea, upper
respiratory infection, abdominal
pain, pleural effusion, vomiting,
arthralgia, asthenia, loss of appetite,
inflammatory disease of mucous
membrane, GI hemorrhage,
constipation, weight loss, dizziness,
chest pain, neuropathy, myalgia,
weight increased, cardiac dysrhythmia,
pruritus, pneumonia, swollen
abdomen, pneumonia, shivering.

Occasional
Febrile neutropenia, CHF, pericardial
effusion, pulmonary edema,
prolonged QT interval, anemia.

Rare
Pulmonary hypertension, CNS
hemorrhage, ascites.

SERIOUS REACTIONS
• Severe CNS hemorrhage, including
fatalities, have been reported.
• Dasatinib may cause severe bone
marrow suppression (thrombocytopenia, neutropenia, anemia).
• Fluid retention, including pleural
and pericardial effusion, severe
ascites, and generalized edema, has
been reported.

PRECAUTIONS & CONSIDERATIONS
Use with caution in patients
with impaired hepatic function,
cardiovascular disease, pulmonary
disease, and patients with QTc
prolongation or at risk for QT
prolongation including those with
hypokalemia, hypomagnesemia,
congenital long QT syndrome,
taking other medications known
to prolong QTc, or receiving
cumulative high-dose anthracycline
therapy. Safety and effectiveness
have not been established in
children. Fluid retention may occur
more often in the elderly. Men and
women of childbearing potential
should be advised to use adequate

contraception. Breast milk excretion
unknown; do not breast feed.

Storage
Store at room temperature.

Administration
Tablets should be swallowed whole,
not crushed or cut. May be taken
without regard to food. Dosage
adjustments are recommended based
on tolerability and potential drug
interactions.

Daunorubicin
daw-noe-roo′bi-sin
(Cerubidine, DaunoXome)
**Do not confuse daunorubicin
with dactinomycin or
doxorubicin.**

CATEGORY AND SCHEDULE
Pregnancy Risk Category: D

Classification: Antineoplastics,
anthracyclines

MECHANISM OF ACTION
An anthracycline antibiotic that
inhibits DNA and DNA-dependent
RNA synthesis by binding with DNA
strands. Liposomal encapsulation
increases uptake by tumors, prolongs
drug action, and may decrease
toxicity. *Therapeutic Effect:* Prevents
cell division.

PHARMACOKINETICS
Widely distributed. Protein binding:
High. Does not cross the blood-brain
barrier. Metabolized in the liver to
active metabolite. Excreted in urine;
eliminated by biliary excretion. *Half-
life:* 18.5 h; metabolite: 26.7 h.

AVAILABILITY
Cerubidine (daunorubicin
hydrochloride)

Powder for Injection: 20 mg.
Solution for Injection: 5 mg/mL.
DaunoXome (liposomal daunorubicin)
Injection: 2 mg/mL.

INDICATIONS AND DOSAGES
▸ **Acute lymphocytic leukemia (ALL)**
IV
Adults. 45 mg/m^2 on days 1-3 of induction course.
Children <2 or BSA <0.5. 2.1 mg/kg/ dose per protocol.
Children >2 and BSA >0.5. 25 mg/m^2 on day 1 each week for 4-6 cycles.
▸ **Acute myeloid leukemia (AML)**
IV
Adults <60 yr. 45 mg/m^2 on days 1-3 of first cycle and on days 1 and 2 of subsequent courses.
Adults >60 yr. 30 mg/m^2 on days 1-3 of induction course and on days 1 and 2 of subsequent cycles.
Children <2 or BSA <0.5. 2.1 mg/kg/ dose per protocol.
Children >2 and BSA >0.5. 30-60 mg/m^2 on days 1-3 of cycle.
▸ **Acute nonlymphocytic leukemia (ANLL)**
IV
Adults <60 yr. 45 mg/m^2 on days 1-3 of first cycle and on days 1 and 2 of subsequent courses.
Adults >60 yr. 30 mg/m^2 on days 1-3 of induction course and on days 1 and 2 of subsequent cycles.
▸ **Kaposi sarcoma**
IV
Adults. 40 mg/m^2 (DaunoXome) over 1 h repeated q2wk.
▸ **Dosage in renal impairment**
ALL, AML, ANLL
Adults, Children. Serum creatinine > 3 mg/dL. 50% of normal dose.
Kaposi sarcoma (DaunoXome)

Serum creatinine > 3 mg/dL. 50% of normal dose.
▸ **Dosage in hepatic impairment**
ALL, AML, ANLL
Bilirubin 1.2-3 mg/dL. 75% of normal dose.
Bilirubin 3.1-5 mg/dL. 50% of normal dose.
Bilirubin > 5 mg/dL. Daunorubicin is not recommended for use in this patient population.
Kaposi sarcoma (DaunoXome).
Bilirubin 1.2-3 mg/dL. 75% of normal dose.
Bilirubin > 3 mg/dL. 50% of normal dose.

OFF-LABEL USES
Treatment of chronic myelocytic leukemia, Ewing sarcoma, neuroblastoma, non-Hodgkin lymphoma, Wilms tumor.

CONTRAINDICATIONS
Hypersensitivity to daunorubicin.

INTERACTIONS
Drug
Antigout medications: May decrease the effects of these drugs.
Bevacizumab, trastuzumab, cyclophosphamide: May increase cardiotoxic effects.
Bone marrow depressants: May enhance myelosuppression.
Live-virus vaccines: May potentiate virus replication, increase vaccine side effects, and decrease the patient's antibody response to the vaccine.
Killed vaccines: May decrease the patient's antibody response to the vaccine.
Herbal and Food
None known.

DIAGNOSTIC TEST EFFECTS
May increase serum alkaline phosphatase, bilirubin, uric acid, and AST (SGOT) levels.

IV INCOMPATIBILITIES

Daunorubicin hydrochloride:
Allopurinol (Aloprim), amphotericin B liposomal (AmBisome), aztreonam (Azactam), cefepime (Maxipime), dexamethasone sodium phosphate, heparin, ertapenem (Invanz), fludarabine (Fludara), lanosprazole (Prevacid), levofloxacin (Levaquin), pantoprazole (Protonix), pemetrexed (Alimta), piperacillin/tazobactam (Zosyn).

DaunoXome: Do not mix with any other solution, especially NaCl or bacteriostatic agents (such as benzyl alcohol).

Rituximab (Rituxan), tigecycline (Tygacil).

IV COMPATIBILITIES

Daunorubicin hydrochloride:
Amifostine (Ethyol), anidulafungin (Eraxis), bivalirudin (Angiomax), carboplatin, caspofungin (Cancidas), cisplatin, cyclophosphamide (Cytoxan), cytarabine (Cytosar), dactinomycin (Cosmegen), daptomycin (Cubicin), dexmedetomidine (Precedex), etoposide (VePesid), etoposide phosphate (EtopoPhos), fenoldopam (Corlopam), filgrastim (Neupogen), gemcitabine (Gemzar), granisetron (Kytril), hydrocortisone sodium succinate, melphalan (Alkeran), meperidine (Demerol), methotrexate, ondansetron (Zofran), oxaliplatin (Eloxatin), paclitaxel (Taxol), palonosetron (Aloxi), quinupristin/dalfopristin (Synercid), rituximab (Rituxan), sodium acetate, sodium bicarbonate, teniposide (Vumon), thiotepa (Thioplex), tigecycline (Tygacil), trastuzumab (Herceptin), vincristine (Vincasar), vinorelbine (Navelbine), voriconazole (Vfend).

DaunoXome: Bivalirudin (Angiostat), meperidine (Demerol), sodium acetate, tirofibran (Aggrastat), trastuzumab (Herceptin).

SIDE EFFECTS

Frequent (> 15%)
Complete alopecia (scalp, axillary, pubic), nausea, vomiting (beginning a few hours after administration and lasting 24-48 h), discoloration of bodily fluids.
DaunoXome: Mild to moderate nausea, fatigue, diarrhea, fever, abdominal pain, anorexia, headache, rigors, back pain, cough, dyspnea.
Occasional (5%-14%)
Diarrhea, abdominal pain, esophagitis, stomatitis, transverse pigmentation of fingernails and toenails
Rare (< 5%)
Transient fever, chills, hypertension, palpitation, tachycardia, anxiety, confusion.

SERIOUS REACTIONS

• Myelosuppression may cause hematologic toxicity, manifested as severe leukopenia, anemia, and thrombocytopenia. Platelet and WBC counts typically nadir in 10-14 days and return to normal levels by the third week of daunorubicin treatment. Neutropenic fever commonly occurs.
• Allergic reactions (DanuoXome) in 25% of patients.
• The risk of cardiotoxicity (either acute, manifested as transient ECG abnormalities, or chronic, manifested as congestive heart failure [CHF]) increases when the total cumulative dose exceeds 550 mg/m^2 in adults, 400 mg/m^2 in adults receiving chest radiation, 300 mg/m^2 in children older than 2 yr, or 10 mg/kg in children younger than 2 yr. Monitor LV function at baseline and periodically.
• Severe, local tissue damage leading to ulceration and necrosis can occur with extravasation.

D

- Secondary malignancy may occur when used in combination with chemotherapy or radiation.

PRECAUTIONS & CONSIDERATIONS

Caution is warranted in elderly patients, preexisting cardiac disease, CHF, hepatic or renal function impairment, myelosuppression, hyperuricemia, and concomitant radiation. Avoid using daunorubicin in pregnant women. It is unknown whether daunorubicin is distributed in breast milk. Cardiac, hepatic, and renal function should be monitored prior to each cycle.

Storage

Daunorubicin hydrochloride: Store vials of powder at room temperature, vials of solution in refrigerator. Reconstituted solutions are stable for 4 days at room temperature. Protect from light. Daunorubicin liposomal (DaunoXome): Store vials in refrigerator. Protect from light. Diluted solution stable in refrigerator for 6 h.

Administration

Do not administer IM or SC. Avoid extravasation, potent vesicant. Daunorubicin hydrochloride: Reconstitute by adding 4 mL of sterile water for injection to the vial and shaking gently to dissolve to produce 5 mg of daunorubicin per mL. Daunorubicin liposomal (DaunoXome): Only dilute with D5W to 1 mg/mL. Do not filter.

Decitabine

de-sye´ta-been
(Dacogen)

CATEGORY AND SCHEDULE

Pregnancy Risk Category: D

Classification: Antineoplastic

MECHANISM OF ACTION

A pyrimidine antimetabolite that is incorporated into DNA and inhibits DNA methyltransferase causing hypomethylation and subsequent cell death. *Therapeutic Effect:* Restores normal function to tumor-suppressor genes regulating cellular differentiation and proliferation.

PHARMACOKINETICS

No information is available regarding the pharmacokinetics of decitabine.

AVAILABILITY

Powder for injection: 50 mg.

INDICATIONS AND DOSAGES
▸ **Myelodysplastic Syndrome (MDS)**
IV
Adults. 15 mg/m^2 over 3 h; repeat every 8 h for 3 days; repeat cycle every 6 wks for a minimum of 4 cycles.

CONTRAINDICATIONS

Hypersensitivity to decitabine or its components.

INTERACTIONS

Drug
None reported.
Herbal
None known.
Food
None known.

DIAGNOSTIC TEST EFFECTS

Myelosuppression, hyperglycemia, increased liver enzymes.

🜚 IV COMPATIBILITIES

Stable in NS, D5W, and lactated Ringer's.

SIDE EFFECTS

Frequent
Neutropenia, thrombocytopenia, anemia, fever, nausea, cough,

petechiae, constipation, diarrhea, hyperglycemia, headache, febrile neutropenia, leukopenia, insomnia, peripheral edema, hypomagnesemia, hypoalbuminemia, vomiting, pallor, bruising, hypokalemia, rigors, pneumonia, arthralgia, rash, limb pain, edema, dizziness, back pain, cardiac murmur, anorexia, pharyngitis, appetite decreased, abdominal pain, lung crackles, hyperbilirubinemia, erythema, pain, hyperkalemia, hyponatremia, oral mucosal lymphadenopathy, confusion, lethargy, cellulitis, stomatitis, dyspepsia, anxiety, hypoesthesia, lesions, pruritus, alkaline phosphatase increased, tenderness.

Occasional

Candidal infection, ascites, increased AST, breath sounds diminished, hyperuricemia, hypoxia, rales, LDH increased, hemorrhoids, alopecia, catheter infection, gingival bleeding, chest discomfort, urinary tract infection, chest wall pain, loose stools, staphylococcal infection, transfusion reaction, tongue ulceration, dysphagia, oral candidiasis, dysuria, facial swelling, hypotension, musculoskeletal discomfort, blurred vision, bicarbonate increased, dehydration, hypochloremia, pulmonary edema, urticaria, malaise, hematoma, thrombocythemia, bacteremia, polyuria, hypobilirubinemia, site erythema, catheter site pain, injection site swelling, lip ulceration, abdominal distention, bicarbonate decreased, hypoproteinemia, crepitation, myalgia, gastroesophageal reflux, glossodynia, postnasal drip, sinusitis.

Rare

Anaphylactic reaction, atrial fibrillation, cardiomyopathy, congestive heart failure, cholecystitis, dyspnea, fungal infection, hemorrhage, gingival pain, mental status change, mucosal inflammation, mycobacterium avium complex infection, peridiverticular abscess, pseudomonal lung infection, pulmonary embolism, renal failure, respiratory arrest, respiratory tract infection, sepsis, splenomegaly, supraventricular tachycardia, weakness.

SERIOUS REACTIONS

• Neutropenia and thrombocytopenia are expected to occur.

PRECAUTIONS & CONSIDERATIONS

Use with caution in patients with bone marrow depression, or renal or hepatic impairment. Safety and effectiveness have not been established in children. No unique precautions were observed in the elderly. Advise women of childbearing potential to avoid becoming pregnant while receiving treatment. Advise men not to father a child while receiving decitabine or for 2 months after discontinuation of therapy. Not known if excreted in breast milk; do not breast feed.

Storage

Store vials at room temperature. Use within 15 min of reconstitution. Solution prepared with cold infusion fluids may be stored in the refrigerator for up to 7 h.

Administration

Reconstitute with sterile water for injection and further dilute with NS, D5W, or Ringer's lactate injection. Administer by continuous IV infusion over 3 h.

Moderately emetogenic; consider antiemetic pretreatment. Dosing may be delayed or reduced based on tolerability.

Deferoxamine
de-fer-ox′a-meen
(Desferal [CAN], Desferal
Mesylate)

CATEGORY AND SCHEDULE
Pregnancy Risk Category: C

Classification: Antidotes,
chelators

MECHANISM OF ACTION
An antidote that binds with iron to
form complex. *Therapeutic Effect:*
Promotes urine excretion of acute
iron poisoning or chronic iron
overload.

PHARMACOKINETICS
Well absorbed after IM or SC
administration. Widely distributed.
Rapidly metabolized in tissues,
plasma. Excreted in urine,
eliminated in feces via biliary
excretion. Removed by hemodialysis.
Half-life: 6 h.

AVAILABILITY
Injection: 500 mg, 2 g.

INDICATIONS AND DOSAGES
▸ Acute iron intoxication
IM (PREFERRED)
Children > 3yr. 90 mg/kg/dose
every 8 h. Maximum: 6 g/day.
Adults. 1000 mg initially, then
500 mg q4h for up to 2 doses.
Subsequent doses have been given
every 4-12 h. Maximum: 6 g/day.
IV (FOR PATIENTS IN SHOCK)
Adults. 1000 mg initially, then
500 mg q4h for up to 2 doses.
Subsequent doses have been
given. Every 4-12 h. Maximum:
6 g/day.
Children. 15 mg/kg/h. Maximum:
6 g/day.

▸ Chronic iron overload
SUBCUTANEOUS (VIA SC
INFUSION PUMP)
Adults. 1-2 g/day (20-40 mg/kg) over
8-24 h.
Children. 20-40 mg/kg/day over
8-24 h. Maximum 1000-2000 mg/
24 h.
IM/IV
Adults. 0.5-1 g/day IM. In addition to
IM, 2 g infused at rate not to exceed
15 mg/kg/h for each unit of blood
transfused. Maximum: 1 g/day if not
transfused; 6 g/day on transfusion
days.
Children (IV). 15 mg/kg/h.

OFF-LABEL USES
Diagnosis and treatment of aluminum
toxicity in chronic kidney disease.

CONTRAINDICATIONS
Severe renal disease, anuria,
primary hemochromatosis,
hypersensitivity to deferoxamine
mesylate or any component of the
formulation.

INTERACTIONS
Drug
Vitamin C: May increase effect of
deferoxamine.
Prochlorperazine: May cause loss
of consciousness.
Herbal and Food
None known.

DIAGNOSTIC TEST EFFECTS
May cause a falsely high total iron-
binding capacity (TIBC).

Ⓓ IV INCOMPATIBILITIES
Do not mix with any other
intravenous medications.

SIDE EFFECTS
Frequent
Pain, induration at injection site,
urine color change (to orange-rose).

Occasional

Abdominal discomfort, diarrhea, leg cramps, impaired vision.

SERIOUS REACTIONS

• Neurotoxicity, including high-frequency hearing loss, and seizures have been reported.

• Adult respiratory distress syndrome with high doses.

• Infusion reactions (flushing, hypotension, urticaria, shock) with rapid infusion.

• Ocular disturbances with prolonged or high doses.

PRECAUTIONS & CONSIDERATIONS

Caution should be used with aluminum overload or aluminum-related encephalopathy.

It is unknown whether drug crosses the placenta or is distributed in breast milk. Use only when absolutely necessary. Be aware that skeletal anomalies may present in neonate. Safety and efficacy have not been evaluated in children < 3 yr of age. Monitor children for growth retardation. Be aware that age-related renal impairment may require caution. Reddish urine may occur.

Administration

In general, IM route is preferred unless in shock. Reconstitute each 500-mg vial with 2 mL sterile water for injection to provide a concentration of 250 mg/mL or dilute each 2-g vial with 8 mL of sterile water for injection.

For IM administration, inject deeply into upper outer quadrant of buttock. May give undiluted.

For subcutaneous injection, administer very slowly. May give undiluted. An SC infusion pump is utilized.

For IV administration, further dilute with 0.9% NaCl, D5W, or lactated Ringer's and administer at maximum rate of 15 mg/kg/h. A too-rapid IV administration may produce skin flushing, urticaria, hypotension, or shock.

Delavirdine
deh-la′ver-deen
(Rescriptor)

CATEGORY AND SCHEDULE
Pregnancy Risk Category: C

Do not confuse Rescriptor with Retrovin or Ritonavir.

Classification: Antiretrovirals, non-nucleoside reverse transcriptase inhibitors

MECHANISM OF ACTION

A nonnucleoside reverse transcriptase inhibitor that binds directly to HIV-1 reverse transcriptase and blocks RNA- and DNA-dependent DNA polymerase activities. *Therapeutic Effect:* Interrupts HIV replication, slowing the progression of HIV infection.

PHARMACOKINETICS

Rapidly absorbed after PO administration. Protein binding: 98%. Primarily distributed in plasma. Metabolized in the liver. Eliminated in feces and urine. *Half-life:* 2-11 h.

AVAILABILITY

Tablets: 100 mg, 200 mg.

INDICATIONS AND DOSAGES

▸ **HIV infection (in combination with other antiretrovirals)**

PO

Adults. 400 mg 3 times a day.

CONTRAINDICATIONS

Concomitant use with alprazolam, cisapride, ergot alkaloids, midazolam, pimozide, rifampin, or triazolam.

INTERACTIONS
Drug
Antacids, H₂ blockers, proton pump inhibitors: May reduce absorption of lansoprazole. Separate antacids by at least 1 h. Concurrent use with H₂ blockers and proton pump inhibitors is not recommended.
Benzodiazepines, calcium channel blockers: May cause life-threatening adverse reactions. See contraindications.
Carbamazepine, phenobarbital, phenytoin, CYP3A4: May decrease delavirdine blood concentration.
Corticosteroids, inhaled: May increase systemic effects of corticosteroids.
CYP2C9, CYP2C19, CYP2D6, CYP3A4 substrates: Levels and effects of substrates may be increased by delavirdine.
Didanosine: Decreased concentrations of both drugs. Separate administration by 1 h.
Protease inhibitors: Delavirdine has been reported to increase the serum concentrations of amprenavir, indinavir, nelfinavir, ritonavir, and saquinavir. Decreased delavirdine concentrations may occur when used with amprenavir and nelfinavir. Dose reduction of indinavir and saquinavir should be considered.
Rifampin: May decrease delavirdine blood concentrations. Contraindicated.
Sildenafil, lovastatin, simvastatin: Increased levels and side effects of these medications may occur. Avoid use.
Herbal
St. John's wort: May decrease delavirdine levels and efficacy. Avoid.
Food
None known.

DIAGNOSTIC TEST EFFECTS
May increase AST (SGOT) and ALT (SGPT), bilirubin, and amylase levels. Prothrombin time may increase. May decrease neutrophil count or hemoglobin.

SIDE EFFECTS
Frequent (> 18%)
Rash, pruritus, headache, nausea.
Occasional (> 2%)
Vomiting, fever, depression, diarrhea, fatigue, anorexia, anxiety.

SERIOUS REACTIONS
• Severe skin rashes, including Stevens-Johnson syndrome, have been reported.

PRECAUTIONS & CONSIDERATIONS
Caution should be used with impaired liver function. It is unknown whether delavirdine crosses the placenta or is distributed in breast milk. Be aware that the safety and efficacy of delavirdine have not been established in children younger than 16 yr and elderly patients. Delavirdine is not a cure for HIV infection, nor does it reduce the risk of transmission to others.

Expect to obtain baseline laboratory testing, especially liver function tests, before beginning therapy and at periodic intervals during therapy. Assess for any nausea or vomiting and for skin rash. Determine the pattern of bowel activity and stool consistency. Monitor eating pattern and weight loss. Consume small, frequent meals to help offset anorexia and nausea. Medications, including OTC drugs, should not be taken without consulting the physician.
Administration
May take without regard to food. May disperse 100-mg tablets in water before consumption. Add four tablets to at least 3 oz of water and allow

D

to stand for a few minutes, then stir well. Drink promptly. Refill glass with water, and swallow to ensure full dose. Do not dissolve 200-mg tablets. Persons with achlorhydria should take delavirdine with orange juice or cranberry juice. Do not administer within 1 h of antacids or didanosine.

Demeclocycline
dem-e-kloe-sye'kleen
(Declomycin, Ledermycin [AUS])

CATEGORY AND SCHEDULE
Pregnancy Risk Category: D

Classification: Antibiotics, tetracyclines

MECHANISM OF ACTION
A broad-spectrum tetracycline antibiotic that inhibits bacterial protein synthesis by binding to ribosomal receptor sites; also inhibits ADH-induced water reabsorption. *Therapeutic Effect:* Bacteriostatic; also produces water diuresis.

AVAILABILITY
Tablets: 150 mg, 300 mg.

INDICATIONS AND DOSAGES
▸ **Mild to moderate infections, including acne, pertussis, chronic bronchitis, and urinary tract infection**
PO
Adults, Elderly. 150 mg 4 times a day or 300 mg 2 times a day.
Children older than 8 yr.
8-12 mg/kg/day in 2-4 divided doses.
▸ **Uncomplicated gonorrhea**
PO
Adults. Initially, 600 mg, then 300 mg q12hr for 4 days for total of 3 g.

▸ **Syndrome of inappropriate ADH secretion (SIADH)**
PO
Adults, Elderly. Initially, 900-1200 mg/day in 3-4 divided doses, then decrease dose to 600-900 mg/day in divided doses.

CONTRAINDICATIONS
Children 8 yr and younger, pregnancy, hypersensitivity to tetracyclines.

INTERACTIONS
Drug
Antacids or supplements containing aluminum, calcium, or magnesium; laxatives containing magnesium; oral iron preparations; zinc: Impair the absorption of demeclocycline. Take demeclocycline 1 h before or 2 h after meals.
Cholestyramine, colestipol: May decrease demeclocycline absorption.
Methotrexate: May decrease clearance of methotrexate.
Oral contraceptives: May decrease the effects of oral contraceptives.
Penicillins: Concomitant therapy may decrease efficacy. Avoid.
Herbal
None known.
Food
Dairy products: May decrease demeclocycline absorption. Take demeclocycline 1 h before or 2 h after meals.

DIAGNOSTIC TEST EFFECTS
May increase BUN and serum alkaline phosphatase, amylase, bilirubin, AST (SGOT), and ALT (SGPT) levels.

SIDE EFFECTS
Frequent
Anorexia, nausea, vomiting, diarrhea, dysphagia, possibly severe

photosensitivity (with moderate to high demeclocycline dosage).
Occasional
Urticaria; rash; diabetes insipidus syndrome, marked by polydipsia, polyuria, and weakness (with long-term therapy).

SERIOUS REACTIONS
• Superinfection (especially fungal), anaphylaxis, and benign intracranial hypertension occur rarely.
• Bulging fontanelles occur rarely in infants.
• Nephropathy can occur if expired.
• Pseudotumor cerebri has been reported rarely.

PRECAUTIONS & CONSIDERATIONS
Caution is warranted with renal and hepatic impairment, and in those who can't avoid sun or ultraviolet exposure, because such exposure may produce a severe photosensitivity reaction. Should be avoided in children < 8 yr because can cause permanent tooth discoloration, damage to tooth enamel. Do not use during pregnancy because of effects on bone and tooth development.

History of allergies, especially to tetracyclines, should be determined before drug therapy. Pattern of daily bowel activity, stool consistency, food intake and tolerance, renal function, and skin for rash should be assessed. Be alert for signs and symptoms of superinfection, such as anal or genital pruritus, diarrhea, and ulceration or changes of the oral mucosa or tongue. BP and LOC should be monitored because of the potential for increased intracranial pressure.
Administration
Take demeclocycline doses on an empty stomach with a full glass of water. Space drug doses evenly around the clock and continue taking demeclocycline for the full course of treatment. Take antacids containing aluminum, calcium, or magnesium; laxatives containing magnesium; or oral iron preparations 1-2 h before or after demeclocycline because they may impair the drug's absorption.

Desipramine
dess-ip'ra-meen
(Apo-Desipramine [CAN], Norpramin, Novo-Desipramine [CAN], Pertofran [AUS])
Do not confuse desipramine with disopyramide or imipramine.

CATEGORY AND SCHEDULE
Pregnancy Risk Category: C

Classification: Antidepressants, tricyclic

MECHANISM OF ACTION
A tricyclic antidepressant that blocks the reuptake of neurotransmitters, such as norepinephrine and serotonin, at presynaptic membranes, increasing their availability at postsynaptic receptor sites. Also has strong anticholinergic activity. *Therapeutic Effect:* Relieves depression.

PHARMACOKINETICS
Rapidly and well absorbed from the GI tract. Protein binding: 90%. Metabolized in the liver. Primarily excreted in urine. Minimally removed by hemodialysis. *Half-life:* 12-27 h.

AVAILABILITY
Tablets: 10 mg, 25 mg, 50 mg, 75 mg, 100 mg, 150 mg.

INDICATIONS AND DOSAGES
▸ **Depression**
PO
Adults. 75 mg/day. May gradually increase to 150-200 mg/day. Maximum: 300 mg/day.
Elderly. Initially, 10-25 mg/day. May gradually increase to 75-100 mg/day. Maximum: 300 mg/day.
Children older than 12 yr. Initially, 25-50 mg/day. May gradually increase to 100 mg/day. Maximum: 150 mg/day.
Children 6-12 yr. 1-3 mg/kg/day. Maximum: 5 mg/kg/day.

OFF-LABEL USES
Treatment of bulimia nervosa, cataplexy associated with narcolepsy, neurogenic pain, panic disorder, social phobia.

CONTRAINDICATIONS
Angle-closure glaucoma, use within 14 days of MAOIs, use in postmyocardial infarction period, hypersensitivity to TCAs.

INTERACTIONS
Drug
Alcohol, other CNS depressants: May increase CNS and respiratory depression and the hypotensive effects of desipramine.
Anticholinergic agents: May increase toxicity.
Antithyroid agents: May increase the risk of agranulocytosis.
Carbamazepine: May decrease desipramine levels. Desipramine may increase carbamazepine levels.
Cimetidine, ritonavir: May increase desipramine blood concentration and risk of toxicity.
Clonidine, guanadrel: May decrease the effects of these drugs.

CYP2D6 inhibitors: May increase effects of desipramine.
Fluoxetine: May increase desipramine levels and toxicity. Reduce desipramine dose by 75%.
MAOIs: May increase the risk of neuroleptic malignant syndrome, hyperpyrexia, hypertensive crisis, and seizures. Contraindicated.
Phenothiazines: May increase the anticholinergic and sedative effects of desipramine.
Phenytoin: May decrease the desipramine blood concentration.
Sympathomimetics: May increase the risk of cardiac effects.
Serotonergic agents, SSRIs, sibutramine: Concomitant use may increase serotonergic effects and risk for serotonin syndrome.
Herbal
St. John's wort: May increase desipramine's pharmacologic effects and risk of toxicity, specifically serotonin syndrome.
Food
None known.

DIAGNOSTIC TEST EFFECTS
May alter blood glucose level and ECG readings. Therapeutic serum drug level is 50-300 ng/mL; toxic serum drug level is > 400 ng/mL.

SIDE EFFECTS
Frequent
Somnolence, fatigue, dry mouth, blurred vision, constipation, delayed micturition, orthostatic hypotension, diaphoresis, impaired concentration, increased appetite, urine retention.
Occasional
GI disturbances (such as nausea, GI distress, metallic taste).
Rare
Paradoxical reactions (agitation, restlessness, nightmares, insomnia), extrapyramidal symptoms (particularly fine hand tremor).

SERIOUS REACTIONS

• Overdose may produce confusion, seizures, somnolence, arrhythmias, fever, hallucinations, dyspnea, vomiting, and unusual fatigue or weakness.

• Abrupt discontinuation after prolonged therapy may produce severe headache, malaise, nausea, vomiting, and vivid dreams.

• Tricyclics may cause bone marrow suppression (rare).

• Orthostatic hypotension may occur.

PRECAUTIONS & CONSIDERATIONS

Antidepressants increase the risk of suicidal thinking and behavior in children, adolescents, and young adults (18-24 yr of age) with major depressive disorder (MDD) and other psychiatric disorders. Caution is warranted with cardiac conduction disturbances, cardiovascular disease, hyperthyroidism, diabetes, hepatic and renal dysfunction, seizure disorders, urine retention, and in those taking thyroid replacement therapy. Desipramine crosses the placenta and is minimally distributed in breast milk. Desipramine use is not recommended for children younger than 6 yr. Expect to administer lower dosages to elderly patients because they are at increased risk for drug toxicity.

Anticholinergic, sedative, and hypotensive effects may occur during early therapy, but tolerance to these effects usually develops. Because dizziness may occur, change positions slowly and avoid alcohol and avoid tasks that require mental alertness or motor skills. CBC and blood chemistry tests to assess hepatic and renal function and ECG to detect arrhythmias should be performed before and periodically during therapy.

Administration

! Make sure at least 14 days elapse between the use of MAOIs and desipramine. Be aware that the therapeutic serum level for desipramine is 50-300 ng/mL, and the toxic serum level is > 400 ng/mL.

Take desipramine with food or milk if GI distress occurs. Full therapeutic effect may be noted in 2-4 wks. Do not abruptly discontinue desipramine. May administer at bedtime.

Desloratadine

des-loer-at′ah-deen
(Aerius, Clarinex, Clarinex Reditabs)
Do not confuse with Claritin.

CATEGORY AND SCHEDULE

Pregnancy Risk Category: C

Classification: Antihistamines, nonsedating

MECHANISM OF ACTION

A nonsedating antihistamine that exhibits selective peripheral histamine H_1 receptor blocking action. Competes with histamine at receptor sites. *Therapeutic Effect:* Prevents allergic responses mediated by histamine, such as rhinitis and urticaria.

PHARMACOKINETICS

Rapidly and almost completely absorbed from the GI tract. Distributed mainly in liver, lungs, GI tract, and bile. Metabolized in the liver to active metabolite and undergoes extensive first-pass metabolism. Eliminated in urine and feces. *Half-life:* 27 h (increased in elderly patients and in those with renal or hepatic impairment).

AVAILABILITY

Syrup: 0.5 mg/mL.
Tablets: 5 mg.
Tablets (Orally Disintegrating [Reditabs]): 2.5 mg, 5 mg.

INDICATIONS AND DOSAGES
▶ **Urticaria**
PO
Adults, Elderly, Children 12 yr and older. 5 mg once a day.
Children 6-11 mo. 1 mg once a day.
Children 12 mo to 5 yr. 1.25 mg once a day.
Children 6-11 yr. 2.5 mg once a day.
▶ **Seasonal or perennial allergic rhinitis**
PO
Adults, Elderly, Children 12 yr and older. 5 mg once a day.
Children 2-5 years. 1.25 mg once a day.
Children 6-11 yr. 2.5 mg once a day.
▶ **Dosage in hepatic or renal impairment**
Adult dosage is decreased to 5 mg every other day.

CONTRAINDICATIONS
None known.

INTERACTIONS
Drug
Erythromycin, ketoconazole:
May increase desloratadine blood concentration.
Herbal
None known.
Food
None known.

DIAGNOSTIC TEST EFFECTS
May suppress wheal and flare reactions to antigen skin testing unless the drug is discontinued 4 days before testing.

SIDE EFFECTS
Frequent (> 10%)
Headache.
Occasional (9%-39%)
Dry mouth, fatigue, dizziness, nausea.
Rare (< 3%)
Dysmenorrhea, myalgia, diarrhea, somnolence.

SERIOUS REACTIONS
• None known.

PRECAUTIONS & CONSIDERATIONS
Caution is warranted in patients with hepatic and renal impairment. Desloratadine is excreted in breast milk and should not be used by breastfeeding women. The safety and efficacy of desloratadine have not been established in children younger than 6 mo. Children and elderly patients are more sensitive to the drug's anticholinergic effects, such as dry mouth, nose, and throat. Avoid drinking alcoholic beverages and performing tasks that require alertness or motor skills until response to the drug is established. Desloratadine orally disintegrating tablets contain phenylalanine 1.75 mg per tablet.

Drowsiness may occur. Increase fluid intake with upper respiratory allergies to decrease the viscosity of secretions, offset thirst, and replace fluids lost from diaphoresis. Therapeutic response should be monitored.
Storage
Store at room temperature. Keep disentegrating tablets in blister packaging until ready to use.
Administration
Do not crush or break film-coated tablets. Place rapidly disintegrating tablets on the tongue immediately after opening the blister; tablet disintegration occurs rapidly. Administer with or without water. Oral solution often used for children's doses.

! Desloratadine is 2.5-4 times more potent than its parent compound, loratadine.

Desmopressin
des-moe-press′in
(DDAVP, Minirin [AUS], Octostim [CAN], Stimate)

CATEGORY AND SCHEDULE
Pregnancy Risk Category: B

Classification: Antidiuretics, hormones/hormone modifiers

MECHANISM OF ACTION
A synthetic pituitary hormone that increases reabsorption of water by increasing permeability of collecting ducts of the kidneys. Also serves as a plasminogen activator. *Therapeutic Effect:* Increases plasma factor VIII (antihemophilic factor). Decreases urinary output.

PHARMACOKINETICS

Route	Onset	Peak	Duration
PO	1 h	2-7 h	6-8 h
IV	15-30 min	1.5-3 h	N/A
Intra-nasal	15 min to 1 h	1-5 h	5-21 h

Poorly absorbed after oral or nasal administration. Metabolism: Unknown. *Half-life:* Oral: 1.5-2.5 h. Intranasal: 3.3-3.5 h. IV: 0.4-4 h.

AVAILABILITY
Tablets (DDAVP): 0.1 mg, 0.2 mg.
Injection (DDAVP): 4 mcg/mL.
Nasal Solution (DDAVP): 100 mcg/mL.
Nasal Spray (Stimate): 1.5 mg/mL (150 mcg/spray).
Nasal Spray (DDAVP): 100 mcg/mL (10 mcg/spray).

INDICATIONS AND DOSAGES
▶ **Primary nocturnal enuresis**
PO
Children 6 yr and older. 0.2-0.6 mg once before bedtime.
INTRANASAL
Children 6 yr and older. Initially, 20 mcg (0.2 mL) at bedtime; use one-half dose in each nostril. Adjust to maximum of 40 mcg/day.
▶ **Central cranial diabetes insipidus**
PO
Adults, Elderly, Children 12 yr and older. Initially, 0.05 mg twice a day. Range: 0.1-1.2 mg/day in 2-3 divided doses.
Children at least 4 yr. Initially, 0.05 mg; then twice a day. Range: 0.1-1.2 mg daily in 2-3 divided doses.
INTRANASAL
Adults, Elderly, Children older than 12 yr. 5-40 mcg (0.05-0.4 mL) in 1-3 doses/day.
Children 3 mo to 12 yr. Initially, 5 mcg (0.05 mL)/day in 1-2 divided doses. Range: 5-30 mcg (0.05-0.3 mL)/day.
IV, SUBCUTANEOUS
Adults, Elderly, Children older than 12 yr. 2-4 mcg/day in 2 divided doses or 1/10 of maintenance intranasal dose.
▶ **Hemophilia A, von Willebrand disease (type I)**
IV INFUSION
Adults, Elderly, Children 3 mo and older weighing 10 kg or more. 0.3 mcg/kg diluted in 50 mL 0.9% NaCl.
Children weighing < 10 kg. 0.3 mcg/kg diluted in 10 mL 0.9% NaCl.
INTRANASAL (STIMATE)
Adults, Elderly, Children 11 mo and older weighing 50 kg or more. 300 mcg; use 1 spray in each nostril.

D

Adults, Elderly, Children 11 mo and older weighing < 50 kg. 150 mcg as a single spray.

CONTRAINDICATIONS

Hyponatremia, moderate to severe renal dysfunction. (Creatinine clearance less than 50 mL/min).

INTERACTIONS

Drug
Carbamazepine, chlorpropamide, clofibrate: May increase the effects of desmopressin.
Demeclocycline, lithium, norepinephrine: May decrease effects of desmopressin.
Herbal
None known.
Food
None known.

DIAGNOSTIC TEST EFFECTS

May increase AST and ALT.

SIDE EFFECTS

Occasional
IV: Pain, redness, or swelling at injection site; headache; abdominal cramps; vulval pain; flushed skin; mild BP elevation or decrease; nausea with high dosages.
Nasal: Rhinorrhea, nasal congestion, slight BP elevation, dizziness, rhinitis.

SERIOUS REACTIONS

• Water intoxication or hyponatremia, marked by headache, somnolence, confusion, decreased urination, rapid weight gain, seizures, and coma, may occur in overhydration. Children, elderly patients, and infants are especially at risk. As a result of FDA review, intranasal desmopressin is no longer indicated for treatment of primary nocturnal enuresis. Tablets may be used, but treatment should be stopped during acute illness or conditions with increased water consumption.

Caution is warranted with fluid or electrolyte imbalances, coronary artery disease, hypertensive cardiovascular disease, and predisposition to thrombus formation. Use cautiously in neonates younger than 3 mo because this age-group is at increased risk for fluid balance problems. Hemophilia A with factor VIII levels < 5%; hemophilia B; severe type I, type IIB, or platelet-type von Willebrand disease are precautions for use. Careful fluid restrictions are recommended in infants. Fluid intake should be restricted for 1 h prior to dose and for 8 h after administration. Caution should be used in patients with polydipsia or SIADH. Elderly patients are at increased risk for hyponatremia and water intoxication. Avoid overhydration.

Notify the physician of abdominal cramps, headache, heartburn, nausea, or shortness of breath. Signs and symptoms of diabetes insipidus should be monitored. Also, serum electrolyte levels, fluid intake, serum osmolality, urine volume, urine specific gravity, and weight should be assessed. Factor VIII antigen level, aPTT, and factor VIII activity level should be assessed for hemophilia.
Storage
Store oral desmopressin away from light and excessive heat. Refrigerate desmopressin for injection; it is stable for 2 wks at room temperature. Refrigerate DDAVP nasal solution and Stimate nasal spray. DDAVP nasal solution and Stimate nasal spray are stable for 3 wks at room temperature if unopened; DDAVP nasal spray is stable at room temperature.

Administration
For IV infusion, dilute in 10-50 mL 0.9% NaCl and prepare to infuse over 15-30 min. For preoperative use, administer 30 min before procedure, as prescribed. Monitor BP and pulse during infusion. Remember that the IV dose is one tenth the intranasal dose.

To administer nasal solution, draw up a measured quantity of desmopressin with a calibrated catheter (Rhinyle). Insert one end in nose and blow on the other end to deposit the solution deep in the nasal cavity. For infants, young children, and obtunded patients, an air-filled syringe may be attached to the catheter to deposit the solution.

For subcutaneous use, estimate therapeutic response by adequacy of sleep duration. Expect to adjust morning and evening dosages separately.

! Stimate Nasal spray and DDAVP nasal spray are not exchangeable because of significant differences in concentration. Follow patient package insert for correct administration techniques.

Desonide
dess'oh-nide
(Desocrot [CAN], Desonate, DesOwen, LoKara, Scheinpharm Desonide [CAN], Verdeso)

CATEGORY AND SCHEDULE
Pregnancy Risk Category: C

Classification: Corticosteroids, topical, dermatologics

MECHANISM OF ACTION
A topical corticosteroid that has anti-inflammatory, antipruritic, and vasoconstrictive properties. The exact mechanism of the anti-inflammatory process is unclear.

Therapeutic Effect: Reduces or prevents tissue response to the inflammatory process.

PHARMACOKINETICS
Large variation in absorption determined by many factors. Metabolized in the liver. Primarily excreted by the kidneys and small amounts in the bile.

AVAILABILITY
Lotion: 0.05% (DesOwen, LoKara).
Cream: 0.05% (DesOwen).
Ointment: 0.05% (DesOwen).
Foam: 0.05% (Verdeso).
Gel: 0.05% (Desonate).

INDICATIONS AND DOSAGES
▸ **Corticosteroid-responsive dermatoses**
TOPICAL (LOTION)
Adults, Elderly. Apply sparingly 2-3 times/day. *Cream/Ointment:* Apply sparingly 2-4 times/day.
▸ **Atopic dermatitis**
TOPICAL (AEROSOL/GEL)
Adults, Elderly, Children >3 mo. Apply sparingly 2-4 times/day.

CONTRAINDICATIONS
History of hypersensitivity to desonide.

INTERACTIONS
Drug
None known.
Herbal
None known.
Food
None known.

DIAGNOSTIC TEST EFFECTS
None known.

SIDE EFFECTS
Occasional
Burning and stinging at site of application, dryness, skin peeling, contact dermatitis.

SERIOUS REACTIONS

• The serious reactions of long-term therapy and the addition of occlusive dressings are reversible hypothalamic-pituitary-adrenal (HPA) axis suppression, manifestations of Cushing syndrome, hyperglycemia, and glucosuria.

PRECAUTIONS & CONSIDERATIONS

Caution should be used over large surface areas, with prolonged use, and in addition to occlusive dressings as well as uncontrolled or untreated infections. Avoid use of occlusive dressings on affected area. Skin irritation should be reported. It is unknown whether desonide crosses the placenta or is distributed in the breast milk. Children may absorb larger amounts of the topical form and may be more susceptible to toxicity. No age-related precautions have been noted in elderly patients. Treatment should not exceed 4 consecutive weeks.

Administration

Gently cleanse area before topical application. Use occlusive dressings only as directed. Apply sparingly and rub into area gently and thoroughly. Do not apply foam directly to face; dispense into hands and apply. Shake lotion well before use.

Desoximetasone

des-ox-i-met′a-sone
(Taro-Desoximetason [CAN], Topicort, Topicort-LP)
Do not confuse desoximetasone with dexamethasone.

CATEGORY AND SCHEDULE

Pregnancy Risk Category: C

Classification: Corticosteroids, topical, dermatologics

MECHANISM OF ACTION

A high potency, fluorinated topical corticosteroid that has anti-inflammatory, antipruritic, and vasoconstrictive properties. The exact mechanism of the anti-inflammatory process is unclear. *Therapeutic Effect:* Reduces tissue response to the inflammatory process.

PHARMACOKINETICS

Large variation in absorption among sites. Protein binding in varying degrees. Metabolized in liver. Primarily excreted in urine.

AVAILABILITY

Cream: 0.25% (Topicort), 0.05% (Topicort-LP).
Gel: 0.05% (Topicort).
Ointment: 0.25% (Topicort).

INDICATIONS AND DOSAGES

▸ **Corticosteroid-responsive dermatoses**
TOPICAL
Adults, Elderly. Apply sparingly 2 times/day.
Children >10 yr. Apply sparingly 1-2 times/day.

CONTRAINDICATIONS
History of hypersensitivity to desoximetasone, topical fungal infections.

INTERACTIONS
Drug
None known.
Herbal
None known.
Food
None known.

DIAGNOSTIC TEST EFFECTS
None known.

SIDE EFFECTS
Frequent
Itching, redness, irritation, burning at site of application.
Occasional
Dryness, folliculitis, hypertrichosis, acneiform eruptions, hypopigmentation, perioral dermatitis.
Rare
Allergic contact dermatitis, adrenal suppression, atrophy, striae, miliaria, photosensitivity.

SERIOUS REACTIONS
• Serious reactions of long-term therapy and addition of occlusive dressings are reversible hypothalamic-pituitary-adrenal (HPA) axis suppression, manifestations of Cushing syndrome, hyperglycemia, and glucosuria.
• Abruptly withdrawing the drug after long-term therapy may require supplemental systemic corticosteroids.

PRECAUTIONS & CONSIDERATIONS
Urinary free cortisol test and ACTH stimulation test should be evaluated before therapy. It is unknown whether desoximetasone is excreted in breast milk. No age-related precautions have been established for elderly patients. Pediatric patients may absorb larger amounts and may be more susceptible to toxicity. Safety and efficacy have not been evaluated in children younger than 10 yr.

Caution should be used over large surface areas, with prolonged use, and addition of occlusive dressings.
Administration
Gently cleanse area before application. Use occlusive dressings only as directed. Apply sparingly. Rub into area gently and thoroughly.

Dexamethasone
dex-a-meth′a-sone
(Decadron, Dexasone [can], Dexmethsone [AUS], Diodex [CAN], Hexadrol [CAN], Maxidex)
Do not confuse dexamethasone with desoximetasone or dextromethorphan, or Maxidex with Maxzide.

CATEGORY AND SCHEDULE
Pregnancy Risk Category: C (D if used in the first trimester)

Classification: Corticosteroids, ophthalmic, dermatologics

MECHANISM OF ACTION
A long-acting glucocorticoid that inhibits accumulation of inflammatory cells at inflammation sites, phagocytosis, lysosomal enzyme release and synthesis, and release of mediators of inflammation. *Therapeutic Effect:* Prevents and suppresses cell and tissue immune reactions and inflammatory process.

D

PHARMACOKINETICS

Rapidly, completely absorbed from the GI tract after oral administration. Widely distributed. Protein binding: High. Metabolized in the liver. Primarily excreted in urine. Minimally removed by hemodialysis. *Half-life:* 3-4.5 h.

AVAILABILITY

Elixir: 0.5 mg/5 mL.
Ophthalmic Suspension, Solution: 0.1% drops.
Oral Solution: 0.5 mg/5 mL, 0.5 mg/0.5 mL, 1 mg/mL.
Tablets: 0.5 mg, 0.75 mg, 1 mg, 1.5 mg, 2 mg, 4 mg, 6 mg.
Topical: Aerosol, cream.
Injection: 4 mg/mL, 10 mg/mL.

INDICATIONS AND DOSAGES
▸ **Anti-inflammatory**
PO/IV/IM
Adults, Elderly. 0.75-9 mg/day in divided doses q6-12h.
Children. 0.08-0.3 mg/kg/day in divided doses q6-12h.
▸ **Cerebral edema**
IV
Adults, Elderly. Initially, 10 mg, then 4 mg (IM/IV) q6h.
IV/IM
Children. Loading dose of 1-2 mg/kg, then 1-1.5 mg/kg/day in divided doses q4-6h.
▸ **Nausea and vomiting in chemotherapy patients**
IV
Adults, Elderly. 8-20 mg once, then 4 mg (PO) q4-6hr or 8 mg q8h. Many dosage regimens available.
Children. 10 mg/m^2/dose (Maximum: 20 mg), then 5 mg/m^2/dose q6h.
▸ **Physiologic replacement**
PO/IV/IM
Children, Adults. 0.03-0.15 mg/kg/day in divided doses q6-12h.

▸ **Usual ophthalmic dosage, ocular inflammatory conditions**
SUSPENSION/SOLUTION
Adults, Elderly, Children. Initially, 2 drops q1h while awake and q2h at night for 1 day, then reduce to 1 drop q4h, then 3-4 times/day.

CONTRAINDICATIONS

Active untreated systemic infections; fungal, tuberculosis, or viral diseases of the eye.

INTERACTIONS
Drug
Amphotericin: May increase hypokalemia.
Aprepitant: May increase levels and effects of dexamethasone.
CYP3A4 inhibitors/inducers: May increase/decrease effects of dexamethasone.
CYP3A4 substrates, cyclosporine: Dexamethasone may decrease levels and effects of substrates.
Digoxin: May increase digoxin toxicity caused by hypokalemia.
Diuretics, insulin, oral hypoglycemics, potassium supplements: May decrease the effects of these drugs.
Hepatic enzyme inducers: May decrease the effects of dexamethasone.
Live virus vaccines: May decrease the patient's antibody response to vaccine, increase vaccine side effects, and potentiate virus replication.
Killed vaccines: May decrease patient's antibody response to vaccine.
Salicylates: Salicylates may increase the GI adverse effects of corticosteroids.
Thalidomide: May increase risk of DVT.

Warfarin: May alter effects of warfarin.
Herbal
None known.
Food
None known.

DIAGNOSTIC TEST EFFECTS

May increase blood glucose and serum lipid, amylase, and sodium levels. May decrease serum calcium, potassium, and thyroxine levels.

ⓘ IV INCOMPATIBILITIES

Calcium chloride, calcium gluconate, caspofungin (Cancidas), cefuroxime (Zinacef), chlorpromazine, ciprofloxacin (Cipro), dantrolene, diazepam (Valium), diphenhydramine (Benadryl), daunorubicin (Cerubidine), dobutamine, epirubicin (Ellence), erythromycin lactobionate, esmolol (Brevibloc), fenoldopam (Corlopam), gentamicin, haloperidol (Haldol), hydroxyzine, idarubicin (Idamycin), labetalol, magnesium sulfate, midazolam (Versed), minocycline (Minocin), mitoxantrone (Novantrone), pantoprazole (Protonix), phenytoin, prochlorperazine, promethazine, protamine, quinupristin/dalfopristin (Synercid), rocuronium (Zemuron), sulfamethoxazole-trimethoprim, tobramycin, topotecan (Hycamtin).

ⓘ IV COMPATIBILITIES

Acyclovir (Zovirax), alfentanil (Alfenta), allopurinol (Aloprim), amifostine (Ethyol), amikacin (Amikar), aminophylline, amphotericin B cholesteryl complex (Amphotec), amphotericin B liposomal (AmBisome), anidulafungin (Eraxis), ascorbic acid, atracurium (Tracrium), atropine, aztreonam (Azactam), benztropine

(Cogentin), bleomycin (Blenoxane), bivalirudin (Angiomax), bretylium, bumetanide (Bumex), buprenorphine (Buprenex), butorphanol (Stadol), carboplatin, cefazolin, cefepime (Maxipime), cefotaxime (Claforan), cefotetan (Cefotan), cefoxitin (Mefoxin), ceftazidime (Ceptaz, Fortaz, Tazicef, Tazidime), ceftizoxime (Cefizox), ceftriaxone (Rocephin), chloramphenicol, cimetidine (Tagamet), cisplatin, cyclophosphamide (Cytoxan), cytarabine (Cytosar), dactinomycin (Cosmegen), daptomycin (Cubicin), dexmedetomidine (Precedex), digoxin (Lanoxin), diltiazem (Cardizem), docetaxel (Taxotere), dopamine (Intropin), doripenem (Doribax), doxorubicin (Adriamycin), doxorubicin liposomal (Doxil), enalaprilat, ephedrine, epinephrine, epoetin alfa (Procrit), ertapenem (Invanz), etoposide (VePesid), etoposide phosphate (Etopophos), famotidine (Pepcid), fentanyl (Sublimaze), filgrastim (Neupogen), fluconazole (Diflucan), fludarabine (Fludara), fluorouracil, folic acid, foscarnet (Foscavir), furosemide (Lasix), ganciclovir (Cytovene), gemcitabine (Gemzar), granisetron (Kytril), heparin, hydromorphone (Dilaudid), imipenem/cilastatin (Primaxin), insulin (Regular, Humulin R, Novolin R), ketorolac, lanosprazole (Prevacid), levofloxacin (Levaquin), lidocaine, linezolid (Zyvox), mannitol, melphalan (Alkeran), meropenem (Merrem), methylprednisolone sodium succinate, metoclopramide (Reglan), metoprolol (Lopressor), metronidazole (Flagyl), milrinone (Primacor), mitomycin (Mutamycin), morphine, multiple vitamins injection, nafcillin, nalbuphine (Nubain), naloxone

(Narcan), nitroglycerin, nitroprusside sodium (Nitropress), norepinephrine (Levophed), ondansetron (Zofran), oxacillin, oxycodone, oxytocin (Pitocin), paclitaxel (Taxol), palonosetron (Aloxi), pemetrexed (Alimta), penicillin G potassium, penicillin G sodium, pentobarbital, phytonadione, piperacillin, piperacillin/tazobactam (Zosyn), potassium chloride, procainamide, propofol (Diprivan), propranolol, ranitidine (Zantac), remifentanil (Ultiva), rituximab (Rituxan), sargramostim, sodium acetate, sodium bicarbonate, streptokinase, sufentanil (Sufenta), tacrolimus (Prograf), teniposide (Vumon), theophylline, thiotepa (Thioplex), ticarcillin (Ticar), ticarcillin/clavulanate (Timentin), tigecycline (Tygacil), tirofibran (Aggrastat), trastuzumab (Herceptin), vasopressin, vecuronium (Norcuron), verapamil, vincristine (Vincasar), vinorelbine (Navelbine), vitamin B complex with C, voriconazole (Vfend), zidovudine (Retrovir).

SIDE EFFECTS
Frequent
Inhalation: Cough, dry mouth, hoarseness, throat irritation.
Intranasal: Burning, mucosal dryness.
Ophthalmic: Blurred vision.
Systemic: Insomnia, facial swelling or cushingoid appearance, moderate abdominal distention, indigestion, increased appetite, nervousness, facial flushing, diaphoresis.
Occasional
Inhalation: Localized fungal infection, such as thrush.
Intranasal: Crusting inside nose, nosebleed, sore throat, ulceration of nasal mucosa.

Ophthalmic: Decreased vision, watering of eyes, eye pain, burning, stinging, redness of eyes, nausea, vomiting.
Systemic: Dizziness, decreased or blurred vision.
Topical: Allergic contact dermatitis, purpura or blood-containing blisters, thinning of skin with easy bruising, telangiectasis or raised dark red spots on skin.
Rare
Inhalation: Increased bronchospasm, esophageal candidiasis.
Intranasal: Nasal and pharyngeal candidiasis, eye pain.
Systemic: General allergic reaction (such as rash and hives); pain, redness, or swelling at injection site; psychologic changes; false sense of well-being; hallucinations; depression.

SERIOUS REACTIONS
• Long-term therapy may cause immunosuppression, Kaposi sarcoma, muscle wasting (especially in the arms and legs), osteoporosis, spontaneous fractures, amenorrhea, cataracts, glaucoma, peptic ulcer disease, and congestive heart failure (CHF).
• The ophthalmic form may cause glaucoma, ocular hypertension, and cataracts.
• May cause adrenal suppression with high doses or extended treatment periods. Taper therapy slowly to avoid adrenal crisis.
• Abrupt withdrawal following long-term therapy may cause severe joint pain, severe headache, anorexia, nausea, fever, rebound inflammation, fatigue, weakness, lethargy, dizziness, and orthostatic hypotension.
• May cause psychiatric disturbances, depression, euphoria, insomnia.

PRECAUTIONS & CONSIDERATIONS

Caution is warranted with
cirrhosis, hepatic impairment,
renal impairment, CHF, diabetes
mellitus, high thromboembolic risk,
hypertension, hyperthyroidism,
adrenal insufficiency, myasthenia
gravis, ocular herpes simplex,
osteoporosis, peptic ulcer disease,
respiratory tuberculosis, seizure
disorders, ulcerative colitis, and
untreated systemic infections. The
ophthalmic form should be used
cautiously in long-term therapy
because prolonged use may
result in cataracts or glaucoma.
Dexamethasone crosses the placenta
and is distributed in breast milk.
Prolonged treatment with high
dosages may decrease the short-term
growth rate and cortisol secretion
in children. Elderly patients are
at higher risk for developing
hypertension or osteoporosis. Severe
stress, including serious infection,
surgery, or trauma, may require an
increase in dexamethasone dosage.
Dentists or other physicians should
be informed of dexamethasone
therapy if taken within the past
12 mo.

Mood swings, ranging from
euphoria to depression, may occur.
Notify the physician of fever, muscle
aches, sore throat, and sudden weight
gain or swelling. Blood glucose
level, intake and output, BP, serum
electrolyte levels, height, and weight
should be monitored before and
during therapy. Be alert to signs and
symptoms of infection caused by
reduced immune response, including
fever, sore throat, and vague
symptoms. In long-term therapy,
signs and symptoms of hypocalcemia
(such as muscle twitching, cramps,
and positive Chvostek's or
Trousseau's sign) or hypokalemia
(such as ECG changes, nausea and

vomiting, irritability, weakness and
muscle cramps, and numbness or
tingling, especially in the lower
extremities) should be assessed.

Administration

Take oral dexamethasone with milk
or food. Do not abruptly discontinue
the drug or change the dosage or
schedule.

! Dexamethasone sodium phosphate
may be given by IV push or IV
infusion.

For IV push, give over 1-4 min.
For IV infusion, mix with 0.9%
NaCl or D5W and infuse over
15-30 min. If administering
to a neonate, solution must be
preservative free. IV solution must
be used within 24 h.

May give deep IM, preferably in
the gluteus maximus.

Shake ophthalmic suspension
well before use. For ophthalmic
use, to administer the solution or
suspension, place a gloved finger
on the lower eyelid and pull it out
until a pocket is formed between
the eye and lower lid. Hold the
dropper above the pocket and place
the correct number of drops into the
pocket. Close the eye gently. For the
ophthalmic solution, apply digital
pressure to the lacrimal sac for
1-2 min to minimize drainage to the
nose and throat, thereby reducing
the risk of systemic effects. Remove
excess solution around the eye with
a tissue. Expect to taper the dosage
slowly when discontinuing the drug.

For topical use, gently cleanse
the area before applying the drug.
Apply sparingly and rub into area
thoroughly after bath or shower
for best absorption. Use occlusive
dressings only as ordered.

Dexchlorpheniramine
dex′klor-fen-eer′a-meen

CATEGORY AND SCHEDULE
Pregnancy Risk Category: B

Classification: Antihistamines, H₁ receptor antagonist

MECHANISM OF ACTION
A propylamine derivative that competes with histamine for H_1-receptor sites on effector cells in the GI tract, blood vessels, and respiratory tract. Dexchlorpheniramine is the dextro-isomer of chlorpheniramine and is approximately two times more active. *Therapeutic Effect:* Prevents allergic response, produces mild bronchodilation, blocks histamine-induced bronchitis.

PHARMACOKINETICS

Route	Onset	Peak	Duration
PO	0.5 h	1-2 h	3-6 h

Well absorbed from the GI tract. Protein binding: 70%. Widely distributed. Metabolized in liver to active metabolite; undergoes extensive first-pass metabolism. Excreted primarily in urine. Not removed by hemodialysis. *Half-life:* 20 h.

AVAILABILITY
Extended-Release Tablets: 4 mg.
Syrup: 2 mg/5 mL.

INDICATIONS AND DOSAGES
▸ **Allergic rhinitis, common cold, angioedema, urticaria, vasomotor rhinitis**
PO
Adults, Elderly, Children 12 yr or older. 2 mg q4-6h or 4-6 mg (timed release) at bedtime or q8-10h.
Children 6-11 yr. 4 mg (timed release) at bedtime or 1 mg q4-6h. (oral syrup)
Children 2-5 yr. 0.5 mg q4-6h. Do not use timed release.

CONTRAINDICATIONS
History of hypersensitivity to antihistamines, newborn or premature infants, third trimester of pregnancy, MAOIs.

INTERACTIONS
Drug
Alcohol, central nervous system (CNS) depressants: May increase CNS depression.
MAOIs: May cause severe hypotension.
Methacholine: May interfere with interpretation of pulmonary function tests after a methacholine bronchial challenge.
Procarbazine: May increase CNS depression.
Herbal
None known.
Food
None known.

DIAGNOSTIC TEST EFFECTS
May interfere with the interpretation of the pulmonary function tests after a methacholine bronchial challenge test.

SIDE EFFECTS
Frequent
Drowsiness; dizziness; headache; dry mouth, nose, or throat; urinary retention; thickening of bronchial secretions; sedation; hypotension.
Occasional
Epigastric distress, flushing, blurred vision, tinnitus, paresthesia, sweating, chills.

SERIOUS REACTIONS
• Children may experience dominant paradoxical reactions, including restlessness, insomnia, euphoria, nervousness, and tremors.
• Hypersensitivity reaction, such as eczema, pruritus, rash, cardiac disturbances, and photosensitivity, may occur.
• Overdosage may vary from CNS depression, including sedation, apnea, hypotension, cardiovascular collapse, or death, to severe paradoxical reaction, such as hallucinations, tremor, and seizures.

PRECAUTIONS & CONSIDERATIONS
Caution is warranted with asthma, cardiovascular disease, chronic obstructive pulmonary disease (COPD), narrow-angle glaucoma, peptic ulcer disease, prostatic hypertrophy, pyloroduodenal or bladder neck obstruction, thyroid disease, and severe CNS depression or coma. Be aware that timed-release tablets should be avoided in children 5 yr and younger. It is unknown whether dexchlorpheniramine crosses the placenta or is distributed in breast milk. Dexchlorpheniramine should not be used in patients during the third trimester of pregnancy or while breastfeeding. No age-related precautions have been noted in elderly patients, although they may be more sensitive to adverse effects.

Dizziness, drowsiness, and dry mouth are expected side effects of dexchlorpheniramine. Tasks that require mental alertness or motor skills should be avoided until the effects are established. Alcohol should be avoided during therapy.
Administration
Take without regard to meals.

Do not crush, chew, or break timed-release tablets.

Dexmedetomidine Hydrochloride
decks-meh-deh-tome′ih-deen (Precedex)
Do not confuse Precedex with Peridex or Percocet.

CATEGORY AND SCHEDULE
Pregnancy Risk Category: C

Classification: Adrenergic agonists, sedatives/hypnotics

MECHANISM OF ACTION
A selective α_2-adrenergic agonist. *Therapeutic Effect:* Produces analgesic, hypnotic, and sedative effects.

PHARMACOKINETICS
Protein binding 94%. Metabolized in liver. Excreted primarily in urine. Half-life 6 min, terminal 2 h. Onset of action is rapid.

AVAILABILITY
Injection: 100 mcg/mL.

INDICATIONS AND DOSAGES
▸ **Sedation before, during, and after intubation and mechanical ventilation while in the intensive care unit (ICU)**
IV
Adults. Loading dose of 1 mcg/kg over 10 min followed by maintenance infusion of 0.2-0.7 mcg/kg/h.
Elderly. May require decreased dosage. No guidelines available.

CONTRAINDICATIONS
None known.

INTERACTIONS
Drug
Anesthetics, opioids, other

sedative-hypnotics: May enhance the effects of dexmedetomidine.

CYP2D6 substrates:
Dexmedetomidine may increase levels/effects of substrates.

Herbal
None known.

Food
None known.

DIAGNOSTIC TEST EFFECTS
May increase serum potassium, alkaline phosphatase, AST (SGOT), and ALT (SGPT) levels.

ⓘ IV INCOMPATIBILITIES
Do not mix dexmedetomidine with Amphotericin, blood, serum, or plasma.
Diazepam (Valium), pantoprazole (Protonix), phenytoin.

ⓘ IV COMPATIBILITIES
Acyclovir (Zovirax), alfentanil (Alfenta), allopurinol (Aloprim), amifostine (Ethyol), amikacin (Amikar), aminophylline, amiodarone, amphotericin B liposomal (AmBisome), ampicillin, ampicillin/sulbactam (Unasyn), atracurium (Tracrium), atropine, azithromycin (Zithromax), aztreonam (Azactam), bivalirudin (Angiomax), bleomycin (Blenoxane), bretylium, bumetanide (Bumex), buprenorphine (Buprenex), busulfan (Busulfex), butorphanol (Stadol), calcium chloride, calcium gluconate, carboplatin, carmustine (BiCNU), caspofungin (Cancidas), cefazolin, cefepime (Maxipime), cefotaxime (Claforan), cefotetan (Cefotan), cefoxitin (Mefoxin), ceftazidime (Ceptaz, Fortaz, Tazicef, Tazidime), ceftizoxime (Cefizox), ceftriaxone (Rocephin), cefuroxime (Zinacef), chlorpromazine, cimetidine (Tagamet), ciprofloxacin (Cipro), cisatracurium (Nimbex), cisplatin, clindamycin (Cleocin), cyclophosphamide (Cytoxan), cyclosporine (Sandimmune), dactinomycin (Cosmegen), daptomycin (Cubicin), dexamethasone sodium phosphate, dexrazoxane (Zinecard), digoxin (Lanoxin), diltiazem (Cardizem), diphenhydramine (Benadryl), dobutamine (Dobutrex), docetaxel (Taxotere), dolasetron (Anzemet), dopamine (Intropin), doxorubicin (Adriamycin), droperidol, enalaprilat, ephedrine, epinephrine, ertapenem (Invanz), erythromycin lactobionate, esmolol (Brevibloc), etomidate, etoposide (VePesid), etoposide phosphate (Etopophos), famotidine (Pepcid), fenoldopam (Corlopam), fentanyl (Sublimaze), fluconazole (Diflucan), fludarabine (Fludara), foscarnet (Foscavir), fosphenytoin (Cerbyx), furosemide (Lasix), ganciclovir, gemcitabine (Gemzar), gentamicin, granisetron (Kytril), haloperidol (Haldol), heparin, hydrocortisone sodium phosphate, hydrocortisone sodium succinate (Solu-Cortef), hydromorphone (Dilaudid), hydroxyzine, idarubicin (Idamycin), ifosfamide (Ifex), imipenem/cilastatin (Primaxin), insulin (Regular, Humulin R, Novolin R), isoproterenol (Isuprel), ketorolac, labetalol, leucovorin, levofloxacin (Levaquin), lidocaine, linezolid (Zyvox), lorazepam (Ativan), magnesium sulfate, mannitol, meperidine (Demerol), meropenem (Merrem), mesna (Mesnex), methotrexate, methylprednisolone sodium succinate, metoclopramide (Reglan), metoprolol (Lopressor), metronidazole (Flagyl), midazolam (Versed), milrinone (Primacor), minocycline (Minocin), mitoxantrone (Novantrone), morphine, nalbuphine (Nubain), naloxone

(Narcan), nicardipine (Cardene), nitroglycerin, nitroprusside sodium (Nitropress), norepinephrine (Levophed), ondansetron (Zofran), oxaliplatin (Eloxatin), oxytocin (Pitocin), paclitaxel (Taxol), palonosetron (Aloxi), pancuronium, pemetrexed (Alimta), pentobarbital, phenobarbital, piperacillin, piperacillin/tazobactam (Zosyn), potassium chloride, potassium phosphates, procainamide, prochloperazine, promethazine, propofol (Diprivan), propranolol, quinupristin/dalfopristin (Synercid), ranitidine (Zantac), remifentanil (Ultiva), rocuronium (Zemuron), sodium acetate, sodium bicarbonate, sodium phosphates, succinylcholine, sufentanil (Sufenta), sulfamethoxazole/trimethoprim, tacrolimus (Prograf), teniposide (Vumon), theophylline, ticarcillin (Ticar), ticarcillin/clavulanate (Timentin), tigecycline (Tygacil), tirofibran (Aggrastat), tobramycin, topotecan (Hycamtin), vancomycin, vasopressin, vecuronium (Norcuron), verapamil, vinblastine (Velban), vincristine (Vincasar), vinorelbine (Navelbine), voriconazole (Vfend), zidovudine (Retrovir).

SIDE EFFECTS

Frequent
Hypotension (30%), hypertension (16%), nausea (11%).
Occasional (2%-5%)
Pain, fever, vomiting, dry mouth, oliguria, thirst.

SERIOUS REACTIONS

• Bradycardia, hypotension, and sinus arrest may occur with too-rapid IV infusion.
• Atrial fibrillation, tachycardia, arrhythmia, hypoxia, anemia, hemorrhage, and pleural effusion have occurred.

PRECAUTIONS & CONSIDERATIONS

! Use only in intensive care setting. Caution is warranted with CHF, advanced heart block, hypovolemia, chronic hypertension, ventricular dysfunction, diabetes hepatic or renal impairment, and those on a continuous cardiac monitor and pulse oximeter. Be aware that dexmedetomidine will provide relaxation and sedation before, during, and after insertion of the endotracheal tube, and during mechanical ventilation. Comfort measures, such as mouth care and repositioning, should be provided. Transient hypertension may occur initially and may require reduction in infusion rate.

Before dexmedetomidine use, baseline vital signs, ECG, and liver function tests should be obtained. ECG for atrial fibrillation, BP for hypotension and level of sedation, pulse rate for bradycardia, and respiratory rate and rhythm should be monitored during therapy.
Storage
Store vials at room temperature.
Administration
! Do not infuse the drug for longer than 24 h.

For IV use, dilute 2 mL of dexmedetomidine with 48 mL of 0.9% NaCl. (Final concentration: 4 mcg/mL.) Administer the drug as a maintenance infusion using a controlled infusion device, as prescribed. Titrate dose to desired clinical effect for individual patient. The rate of maintenance infusion should be adjusted to achieve desired level of sedation. Dexmedetomidine has been continuously infused in mechanically ventilated patients before, during, and after extubation. It is not necessary to discontinue dexmedetomidine before extubation provided the infusion does not exceed 24 h.

Dexmethylphenidate
dex-meth-ill-fen'i-date
(Focalin, Focalin XR)

CATEGORY AND SCHEDULE
Pregnancy Risk Category: C
Controlled Substance Schedule: II

Classification: Stimulants,
central nervous system (CNS)

MECHANISM OF ACTION
A CNS stimulant that blocks the
reuptake of norepinephrine and
dopamine into presynaptic neurons,
increasing the release of these
neurotransmitters into the synaptic
cleft. *Therapeutic Effect:* Decreases
motor restlessness and fatigue;
increases motor activity, mental
alertness, and attention span;
elevates mood.

PHARMACOKINETICS
Readily absorbed from the GI tract.
Plasma concentrations increase rapidly.
Time to peak: 1-1.5 h (tablet); 1.5 h
and 6.5 h (extended-release capsule).
Metabolized in the liver. Excreted as
metabolites in urine. *Half-life:* 2.2 h.
Duration of action: 4-5 h (tablet), 12 h
(extended-release capsule).

AVAILABILITY
Tablets: 2.5 mg, 5 mg, 10 mg.
Capsules (Extended Release): 5 mg,
10 mg, 15 mg, 20 mg.

INDICATIONS AND DOSAGES
▸ **Attention-deficit-hyperactivity
disorder (ADHD)**
PO
Adults. Patients new to
dexmethylphenidate or
methylphenidate. *Tablets:* 2.5 mg
twice a day (5 mg/day). May adjust
dosage in 2.5- to 5-mg increments.

Maximum: 20 mg/day. *Capsule:*
10 mg daily. May adjust dose in
10-mg increments at weekly intervals.
Maximum dose: 20 mg/day.
Children 6 yr and older. Patients
new to dexmethylphenidate or
methylphenidate. *Tablets:* 2.5 mg
twice a day (5 mg/day). May
adjust dosage in 2.5- to 5-mg
increments. Maximum dose:
20 mg/day. *Capsule:* 5 mg daily. May
adjust dose in 5-mg increments at
weekly intervals. Maximum dose:
20 mg/day.
*Patients currently taking
methylphenidate.* Half the
methylphenidate dosage. Maximum
dose: 20 mg/day.
*Patients changing from
dexmethylphenidate immediate-
release tablets to dexmethylphenidate
extended release.* Convert at same
daily dose. Capsules are given once
daily.

CONTRAINDICATIONS
Diagnosis or family history of
Tourette syndrome; glaucoma;
history of marked agitation, anxiety,
or tension; motor tics; use within
14 days of MAOIs.

INTERACTIONS
Drug
**Amitriptyline, phenobarbital,
phenytoin, primidone,
anticonvulsants:** Dosage of these
drugs may need to be decreased.
Antihypertensives: Decreased
effect of antihypertensives may
occur.
Clonidine: Severe toxic reactions
occur with methylphenidate.
MAOIs, linezolid: May increase the
effects of dexmethylphenidate such
as severe hypertensive episodes.
MAOIs are contraindicated.
Other CNS stimulants: May have
an additive effect.

Warfarin: May inhibit the metabolism of warfarin.
Herbal
None known.
Food
None known.

DIAGNOSTIC TEST EFFECTS
None known.

SIDE EFFECTS
Frequent
Headache, abdominal pain, nausea, anorexia, fever, restlessness.
Occasional
Tachycardia, arrhythmias, palpitations, insomnia, twitching.
Rare
Blurred vision, rash, arthralgia, insomnia.

SERIOUS REACTIONS
• Withdrawal after prolonged therapy may unmask symptoms of the underlying disorder.
• CNS stimulant use associated with serious cardiovascular events and sudden death in patients with cardiac abnormalities or serious heart problems.
• Dexmethylphenidate may lower the seizure threshold in those with a history of seizures.
• Overdose produces excessive sympathomimetic effects, including vomiting, tremor, hyperreflexia, seizures, confusion, hallucinations, and diaphoresis.
• Prolonged administration to children may delay growth.

PRECAUTIONS & CONSIDERATIONS
Caution is warranted with cardiovascular disease, structural cardiac abnormalities, or other cardiac problems, psychosis, seizure disorders, hypertension, and history of substance abuse. It is unknown whether dexmethylphenidate is excreted in breast milk; avoid breastfeeding. Children are more prone to develop abdominal pain, insomnia, anorexia, and weight loss. Long-term dexmethylphenidate use may inhibit growth in children. In psychotic children, dexmethylphenidate use may exacerbate behavior disturbances and abnormal thoughts. No age-related precautions have been noted in elderly patients.

Tasks that require mental alertness and motor skills should be avoided until response to the drug is established. CBC, WBC count with differential, and platelets should be monitored. Baseline height and weight should be obtained at the beginning and periodically throughout therapy.
Administration
Take dexmethylphenidate without regard to food. Capsules may be opened and sprinkled over cool applesauce. Take the last dose of the day several hours before bedtime to prevent insomnia. Do not crush or chew capsule contents.

Dextran
dex'tran
(Gentran, Rheomacrodex [CAN])
Do not confuse with Genprine.

CATEGORY AND SCHEDULE
Pregnancy Risk Category: C

Classification: Plasma expanders

MECHANISM OF ACTION
A branched polysaccharide that produces plasma volume expansion as a result of high colloidal

osmotic effect. Draws interstitial fluid into the intravascular space. May also increase blood flow in microcirculation. *Therapeutic Effect:* Increases central venous pressure, cardiac output, stroke volume, BP, urine output, capillary perfusion, and pulse pressure. Decreases heart rate, peripheral resistance, and blood viscosity. Corrects hypovolemia.

AVAILABILITY

Injection (High Molecular Weight [Gentran]): 6% dextran 70 in 500 mL 0.9% NaCl.
Injection (Low Molecular Weight [Gentran LMD]): 10% dextran 40 in 500 mL D5W, 10% dextran 40 in 500 mL 0.9% NaCl.

INDICATIONS AND DOSAGES
▸ **Volume expansion, shock**
IV
Adults, Elderly (Dextran 40 or 70). 500-1000 mL at a rate of 20-40 mL/min. Maximum dose: 20 mL/kg for first 24 h and 10 mL/kg thereafter.
Children (Dextran 40 or 70). Total dose not to exceed 20 mL/kg on day 1 and 10 mL/kg/day thereafter.
▸ **Prevention of venous thrombosis/ pulmonary embolism**
IV (DEXTRAN 40)
Adults. 50-100 g on day of surgery, then 50 g every 2-3 days as needed based on risk, up to 2 wks.

CONTRAINDICATIONS

Hypervolemia, renal failure with severe oliguria or anuria, severe bleeding disorders, severe cardiac decompensation, severe thrombocytopenia.

INTERACTIONS
Drug
None known.

Herbal
None known.
Food
None known.

DIAGNOSTIC TEST EFFECTS

Prolongs bleeding time and depresses platelet count. Decreases clotting factors V, VIII, and IX. May falsely elevate glucose assays.

ⓘ IV INCOMPATIBILITIES

Do not add medications to dextran solution.

SIDE EFFECTS
Occasional
Mild hypersensitivity reaction, including urticaria, nasal congestion, wheezing.

SERIOUS REACTIONS

• Severe or fatal anaphylaxis, manifested by marked hypotension and cardiac or respiratory arrest, may occur early during IV infusion, generally in those not previously exposed to IV dextran.
• Renal failure has occurred.

PRECAUTIONS & CONSIDERATIONS

Caution is warranted with chronic hepatic disease and extreme dehydration and in patients with active hemorrhage. Observe for bleeding, and monitor hematocrit to keep above 30%. Fluid overload can occur; use with caution in patients with hypovolemia. Be aware of signs and symptoms of fluid overload, such as peripheral or pulmonary edema, and impending congestive heart failure. Women may experience a heavier menstrual flow than usual. An electric razor and soft toothbrush should be used to prevent bleeding during dextran therapy. Do not take any medications, including OTC drugs (especially aspirin), without physician approval.

Notify the physician of bleeding from the surgical site, chest pain, dyspnea, black or red stool, coffee-ground emesis, dark or red urine, or red-speckled mucus from cough. Urine output, vital signs, and laboratory values, such as bleeding time, platelet count, and clotting factors, should be monitored. Central venous pressure (CVP) should also be assessed to detect blood volume overexpansion.

Storage

Store at room temperature. Use only clear solutions, and discard partially used containers.

Administration

! Therapy should not continue longer than 5 days.

Give by IV infusion only. Monitor closely during first 15 min of infusion for anaphylactic reaction. Monitor vital signs every 5 min. Monitor urine flow rate during administration. Discontinue dextran 40 and give an osmotic diuretic, as prescribed, if oliguria or anuria occurs to minimize vascular overloading. If dextran is given by rapid injection, monitor CVP. Immediately discontinue the drug and notify the physician if CVP rises precipitously. Monitor BP diligently during infusion. Stop the infusion immediately if marked hypotension occurs, a sign of imminent anaphylactic reaction. If evidence of blood volume overexpansion occurs, discontinue the drug until blood volume is adjusted by diuresis.

Dextroamphetamine

dex-troe-am-fet′a-meen
(Dexamphetamine [AUS],
Dexedrine, Dexedrine Spansule,
Dextrostat)
Do not confuse dextroamphetamine with dextromethorphan, or Dexedrine with Dextran or Excedrin.

D

CATEGORY AND SCHEDULE

Pregnancy Risk Category: C
Controlled Substance Schedule: II

Classification: Adrenergic agonists, amphetamines, stimulants

MECHANISM OF ACTION

An amphetamine that enhances the action of dopamine and norepinephrine by blocking their reuptake from synapses; also inhibits monoamine oxidase and facilitates the release of catecholamines. *Therapeutic Effect:* Increases motor activity and mental alertness; decreases motor restlessness, drowsiness, and fatigue; suppresses appetite.

AVAILABILITY

Capsules, Sustained-Release (Dexedrine, Spansule): 5 mg, 10 mg, 15 mg.
Tablets (Dextrostat, Dextroamphetamine): 5 mg, 10 mg.

INDICATIONS AND DOSAGES
▸ **Narcolepsy**
PO
Adults, Children older than 12 yr.
Initially, 10 mg/day. Increase by 10 mg/day at weekly intervals until therapeutic response is achieved. Maximum 60 mg/day.
Children 6-12 yr. Initially, 5 mg/day. Increase by 5 mg/day at weekly

intervals until therapeutic response is achieved. Maximum dose: 60 mg/day.

▸ **Attention-deficit-hyperactivity disorder (ADHD)**

PO

Adults: Initially, 5 mg once or twice daily. Titrate at weekly intervals. Usual Maximum: 60 mg/day.

Children 6 yr and older. Initially, 5 mg once or twice a day. Increase by 5 mg/day at weekly intervals until therapeutic response is achieved. Maximum 40 mg/day. Usual dose: 5-20 mg/day.

Children 3-5 yr. Initially, 2.5 mg/day. Increase by 2.5 mg/day at weekly intervals until therapeutic response is achieved. Maximum dose: 40 mg/day. Usual range 0.1-0.5 mg/kg/day.

▸ **Appetite suppressant**

PO

Adults, Children older than 12 yr. 5-30 mg daily in divided doses of 5-10 mg each, given 30-60 min before meals; or 1 extended-release capsule in the morning. Usually no longer than 3-6 wks.

CONTRAINDICATIONS

Advanced arteriosclerosis, agitated states, glaucoma, history of drug abuse, hypersensitivity to sympathomimetic amines, hyperthyroidism, moderate to severe hypertension, symptomatic cardiovascular disease, use within 14 days of MAOIs.

INTERACTIONS

Drug

Antihypertensives: May decrease efficacy of antihypertensives.
Antipsychotics: Efficacy of antipsychotics may be decreased.
β-Blockers: May increase the risk of bradycardia, heart block, and hypertension.
Digoxin: May increase the risk of arrhythmias.

MAOIs, linezolid: May prolong and intensify the effects of dextroamphetamine, including severe hypertensive episodes.
Meperidine: May increase the risk of hypotension, respiratory depression, seizures, and vascular collapse.
Other CNS stimulants: May increase the effects of dextroamphetamine.
SSRIs: May increase risk of serotonin syndrome.
Thyroid hormones: May increase the effects of either drug.
Tricyclic antidepressants: May increase cardiovascular effects.
Herbal
None known.
Food
None known.

DIAGNOSTIC TEST EFFECTS

May increase plasma corticosteroid concentrations.

SIDE EFFECTS

Frequent
Irregular pulse, increased motor activity, talkativeness, nervousness, mild euphoria, insomnia.
Occasional
Headache, chills, dry mouth, GI distress, worsening depression in patients who are clinically depressed, tachycardia, palpitations, chest pain, dizziness, decreased appetite.

SERIOUS REACTIONS

• CNS stimulant use associated with serious cardiovascular events and sudden death in patients with cardiac abnormalities or serious heart problems.
• Overdose may produce skin pallor or flushing, arrhythmias, and psychosis.
• Abrupt withdrawal after prolonged use of high doses may produce lethargy lasting for weeks.

• Prolonged administration to children with ADHD may inhibit growth.

PRECAUTIONS & CONSIDERATIONS
Caution is warranted in debilitated and elderly patients; in those with hypertension, psychiatric disorders, seizure disorder, and Tourette syndrome; and in those who are tartrazine sensitive. Safety and efficacy have not been established in children. Distributed in breast milk; breastfeeding should be avoided. Mental status, BP, and weight should be assessed. Tasks that require mental alertness or motor skills should be avoided until response to the drug has been established. Notify the physician if decreased appetite, dizziness, dry mouth, or pronounced nervousness occurs.

Administration
Take the last dose of the day several hours before bedtime to prevent insomnia. Tolerance to the drug's appetite-suppressant and mood-elevating effects usually occurs within a few weeks. Dexedrine Spansule is not for initial therapy; patients should be established on regular-release formulations first. Spansule is administered once daily. Safety and efficacy have not been established for children < 6 yr. Maximum spansule dose in children > 6 yr is 45 mg/day for ADHD, 60 mg/day for narcolepsy.

Dextromethorphan
dex-troe-meth-or´fan
(Babee Cof Syrup, Buckley's DM Cough, Buckley's Mixture, Creomulsion Cough, Creomulsion for Children, Creo-Terpin, Delsym 12-Hour, ElixSure Cough, PediaCare Long-Acting Cough, Robitussion [AUS], Robitussin CoughGels, Robafen, Robitussin Honey Cough, Robitussin Maximum Strength Cough, Robitussin Pediatric Cough, Scot-Tussin Diabetes CF, Silphen DM, Vicks 44 Cough Relief, Triaminic Long-Acting Cough, Tylenol Children's Simply Cough, Zicam Cool Mist Spray)

CATEGORY AND SCHEDULE
Pregnancy Risk Category: C
OTC

Classification: Antitussive, nonnarcotic

MECHANISM OF ACTION
A chemical relative of morphine without the narcotic properties that acts on the cough center in the medulla oblongata by elevating the threshold for coughing. *Therapeutic Effect:* Suppresses cough.

PHARMACOKINETICS
Rapidly absorbed from the GI tract. Distributed into cerebrospinal fluid (CSF). Extensively and poorly metabolized in liver to dextrorphan (active metabolite). Excreted unchanged in urine. *Half-life:* 1.4-3.9 h (parent compound), 3.4-5.6 h (dextrorphan). Onset of action: 15-30 min.

AVAILABILITY

Gelcap: 15 mg (Robafen, Robitussin CoughGels).
Liquid: 5 mg/5 mL (Tylenol Children's Simply Cough), 10 mg/5 mL (Vicks 44 Cough Relief), 10 mg/15 mL (Creo-Terpin), 10 mg/5 mL (Scot-Tussin Diabetes CF).
Solution: 2.2 mg, 3.3 mg (Zicam Concentrated Cough Kids Cool Mist Spray), 6 mg/spray (Zicam Cool Mist Spray).
Suspension (Extended Release): 30 mg/5 mL (Delsym).
Syrup: 5 mg/5 mL (Creomulsion for Children), 7.5 mg/5 mL (Babee Cof Syrup, ElixSure cough, PediAcare Long-Acting, Robitussin Pediatric Cough, Triaminic Long-Acting Cough), 10 mg/5 mL (Robitussin Honey Cough, Silphen DM), 12.5 mg/5 mL (Buckley's DM), 15 mg/5 mL (Robitussin Maximum Strength Cough), 20 mg/15 mL (Creomulsion Cough), 30 mg/15 mL (Vicks Formula 44).

INDICATIONS AND DOSAGES
▸ **Cough**
PO
Adults, Elderly, Children 12 yr and older. 10-20 mg q4h or 30 mg q6-8h or extended release 60 mg twice a day. Maximum: 120 mg/day.
Children 6-12 yr. 5-10 mg q4h or 15 mg q6-8h or extended release 30 mg twice a day. Maximum: 60 mg/day.
Children 2-5 yr. 2.5-7.5 mg q4-8h or extended release 15 mg twice a day. Maximum: 30 mg/day.

OFF-LABEL USES
N-Methyl-D-aspartate (NMDA) antagonist in cerebral injury.

CONTRAINDICATIONS

Coadministration with monoamine oxidase inhibitors (MAOIs), hypersensitivity to dextromethorphan or its components.

INTERACTIONS
Drug
MAOIs, phenelzine, SSRIs, sibutramine: May increase the risk of serotonin syndrome. MAOIs are contraindicated.
Haloperidol, quinidine, CYP2D6 inhibitors: May increase adverse effects associated with dextromethorphan.
Herbal
None known.
Food
None known.

DIAGNOSTIC TEST EFFECTS
None known.

SIDE EFFECTS
Rare
Abdominal discomfort, constipation, dizziness, drowsiness, GI upset, nausea.

SERIOUS REACTIONS
• Overdosage may result in muscle spasticity, increase or decrease in BP, blurred vision, blue fingernails and lips, nausea, vomiting, hallucinations, and respiratory depression.

PRECAUTIONS & CONSIDERATIONS
Dextromethorphan has become a drug of abuse. Be aware that dextromethorphan should not be used for chronic and persistent cough accompanying a disease state or cough associated with excessive secretions. It is unknown whether dextromethorphan crosses the placenta or is distributed in breast milk. Be aware that

dextromethorphan is not recommended for use in children younger than 2 yr of age. No age-related precautions have been noted in elderly patients. If fever, rash, headache, or sore throat persists, notify the physician.

Storage

Store syrup, suspension, liquid, lozenges, or gelcaps at room temperature.

Administration

Give dextromethorphan without regard to meals.

Shake oral suspension well before use.

Diazepam

dye-az′e-pam

(Antenex [AUS], Apo-Diazepam [CAN], Diastat, Diazemuls [CAN], Diazepam Intensol, Ducene [AUS],Valium, Valpam [AUS], Vivol [CAN])

Do not confuse diazepam with diazoxide or Ditropan, or Valium with Valcyte.

CATEGORY AND SCHEDULE

Pregnancy Risk Category: D
Controlled Substance: Schedule IV

Classification: Anxiolytics, benzodiazepines, relaxants, skeletal muscle

MECHANISM OF ACTION

A benzodiazepine that depresses all levels of the central nervous system (CNS) by enhancing the action of γ-aminobutyric acid, a major inhibitory neurotransmitter in the brain. *Therapeutic Effect:* Produces anxiolytic effect, elevates the seizure threshold, produces skeletal muscle relaxation.

PHARMACOKINETICS

Route	Onset	Peak	Duration
PO	30 min	1-2 h	2-3 h
IV	1-5 min	15 min	15-60 min
IM	15 min	30-90 min	30-90 min

Well absorbed from the GI tract. Widely distributed. Protein binding: 98%. Metabolized in the liver to active metabolite. Excreted in urine. Minimally removed by hemodialysis. *Half-life:* 20-70 h (increased in patients with hepatic dysfunction and in elderly patients).

AVAILABILITY

Oral Concentrate (Diazepam Intensol): 5 mg/mL.
Oral Solution: 5 mg/5 mL.
Tablets (Valium): 2 mg, 5 mg, 10 mg.
Injection: 5 mg/mL.
Rectal Gel (Diastat): 5 mg/mL (10 mg, 20 mg). 2.5 mg/mL (2.5 mg).

INDICATIONS AND DOSAGES

▸ **Anxiety, skeletal muscle relaxation**
PO
Adults. 2-10 mg 2-4 times a day.
Elderly. 2.5 mg twice a day.
Children. 0.12-0.8 mg/kg/day in divided doses q6-8h.
IV, IM
Adults. 2-10 mg repeated in 3-4 h.
Children. 0.04-0.3 mg/kg/dose q2-4h. *Maximum:* 0.6 mg/kg in an 8-h period.
▸ **Preanesthesia**
IV
Adults, Elderly. 5-15 mg 5-10 min before procedure.

Children. 0.2-0.3 mg/kg. Maximum: 10 mg.

▸ **Alcohol withdrawal**
PO
Adults, Elderly. 10 mg 3-4 times during first 24 h, then reduced to 5-10 mg 3-4 times a day as needed.
IV, IM
Adults, Elderly. Initially, 10 mg, followed by 5-10 mg q3-4h as needed.

▸ **Status epilepticus**
IV
Adults, Elderly. 5-10 mg q10-15 min up to 30 mg/8 h.
Children 5 yr and older. 0.05-0.3 mg/kg/dose q15-30 min. Maximum: 10 mg/dose.
Children 1 mo to 5 yr. 0.05-0.3 mg/kg/dose q15-30 min. Maximum: 5 mg/dose.

▸ **Control of increased seizure activity in patients with refractory epilepsy who are on stable regimens of anticonvulsants**
RECTAL GEL
Adults, Elderly, Children 12 yr and older. 0.2 mg/kg; may be repeated in 4-12 h. Round dose up to nearest dosage form for adults and down for elderly.
Children 6-11 yr. 0.3 mg/kg; may be repeated in 4-12 h.
Children 2-5 yr. 0.5 mg/kg; may be repeated in 4-12 h.

▸ **Dose in hepatic dysfunction (cirrhosis)**
Consider reduced dosage, but no specific recommendations are available.

OFF-LABEL USES
Treatment of panic disorder, tremors, benzodiazepine withdrawal, insomnia.

CONTRAINDICATIONS
Angle-closure glaucoma, coma, children younger than 6 mo, pregnancy.

INTERACTIONS
Drug
Alcohol, other CNS depressants: May increase CNS depression.
CYP2C19, CYP3A4 inhibitors: May increase levels/effects of diazepam.
CYP2C19, CYP3A4 inducers: May decrease levels/effects of diazepam.
Herbal
Kava kava, valerian: May increase CNS depression.
Food
Grapefruit juice: May increase sedative effect by increasing diazepam levels.

DIAGNOSTIC TEST EFFECTS
May elevate serum LDH, alkaline phosphatase, bilirubin, AST (SGOT), and ALT (SGPT) levels. May produce abnormal renal function test results. Therapeutic serum drug level is 0.5-2 mcg/mL; toxic serum drug level is > 3 mcg/mL.

⊘ IV INCOMPATIBILITIES
Acyclovir (Zovirax), alfentanil (Alfenta), amikacin (Amikar), aminophylline, amphotericin B cholesteryl (Amphotec), amphotericin B liposomal (AmBisome), ampicillin, ampicillin/sulbactam (Unasyn), ascorbic acid, atracurium (Tracrium), atropine, azathioprine, aztreonam (Azactam), benztropine (Cogentin), bivalirudin (Angiomax), bretylium, bumetanide (Bumex), buprenorphine (Buprenex), butorphanol (Stadol), calcium chloride, calcium gluconate, carboplatin, caspofungin (Cancidas), cefazolin, cefepime (Maxipime), cefotaxime (Claforan), cefotetan (Cefotan), cefoxitin (Mefoxin), ceftazidime (Ceptaz, Fortaz, Tazicef, Tazidime), ceftizoxime (Cefizox),

ceftriaxone (Rocephin), cefuroxime (Zinacef), chloramphenicol, chlorpromazine, cimetidine (Tagamet), cisplatin, clindamycin (Cleocin), cyanocobalamin, cyclophosphamide (Cytoxan), cyclosporine (Sandimmune), dactinomycin (Cosmegen), dantrolene, dexamethasone sodium phosphate, dexmedetomidine (Precedex), digoxin (Lanoxin), diltiazem (Cardizem), diphenhydramine (Benadryl), dopamine (Intropin), doripenem (Doribax), doxorubicin (Adriamycin), enalaprilat, ephedrine, epinephrine, epirubicin (Ellence), epoetin alfa (Procrit), ertapenem (Invanz), erythromycin lactobionate, esmolol (Brevibloc), etoposide phosphate (Etopophos), famotidine (Pepcid), fenoldopam (Corlopam), fluconazole (Diflucan), fludarabine (Fludara), fluorouracil, folic acid, foscarnet (Foscavir), furosemide (Lasix), ganciclovir, gemcitabine (Gemzar), gentamicin, granisetron (Kytril), haloperidol (Haldol), heparin, hydralazine, hydrocortisone sodium succinate (Solu-Cortef), hydroxyzine, imipenem/cilastatin (Primaxin), insulin (regular, Humulin R, Novolin R), isoproterenol (Isuprel), ketorolac, labetalol, lansoprazole (Prevacid), levofloxacin (Levaquin), lidocaine, linezolid (Zyvox), magnesium sulfate, mannitol, meperidine (Demerol), meropenem (Merrem IV), methicillin, methotrexate, methylprednisolone sodium succinate, metoclopramide (Reglan), metoprolol (Lopressor), metronidazole (Flagyl), midazolam (Versed), milrinone (Primacor), minocycline (Minocin), mitoxantrone (Novantrone), multiple vitamins injection, nalbuphine (Nubain), naloxone (Narcan), nitroglycerin, nitroprusside sodium (Nitropress), norepinephrine (Levophed), oxacillin, oxaliplatin (Eloxatin), oxytocin (Pitocin), paclitaxel (Taxol), palonosetron (Aloxi), pancuronium, pemetrexed (Alimta), pencillin G potassium, penicillin G sodium, pentobarbital, phenobarbital, phenytoin, piperacillin, potassium chloride, procainamide, prochloperazine, promethazine propofol (Diprivan), propranolol, quinupristin/dalfopristin (Synercid), ranitidine (Zantac), rocuronium (Zemuron), sodium acetate, sodium bicarbonate, streptokinase, succinylcholine, sulfamethoxazole/trimethoprim, tacrolimus (Prograf), theophylline, ticarcillin (Ticar), ticarcillin/clavulanate (Timentin), tigecycline (Tygacil), tirofibran (Aggrastat), tobramycin, vancomycin, vasopressin, vecuronium (Norcuron), verapamil, vincristine (Vincasar), vinorelbine (Navelbine), vitamin B complex with C, voriconazole (Vfend), hetastarch, lactated Ringer's.

IV COMPATIBILITIES

Daptomycin (Cubicin), docetaxel (Taxotere), fentanyl, methadone, morphine, piperacillin/tazobactam (Zosyn), teniposide (Vumon).

SIDE EFFECTS

Frequent
Pain with IM injection, somnolence, fatigue, ataxia.
Occasional
Slurred speech, confusion, depression, orthostatic hypotension, headache, hypoactivity, constipation, nausea, blurred vision.
Rare
Paradoxical CNS reactions, such as hyperactivity or nervousness

in children and excitement or restlessness in elderly or debilitated patients (generally noted during first 2 wks of therapy, particularly in presence of uncontrolled pain).

SERIOUS REACTIONS
• IV administration may produce pain, swelling, thrombophlebitis, and carpal tunnel syndrome.
• Abrupt or too-rapid withdrawal may result in pronounced restlessness, irritability, insomnia, hand tremor, abdominal or muscle cramps, diaphoresis, vomiting, and seizures.
• Anterograde amnesia may occur.
• Abrupt withdrawal in patients with epilepsy may produce an increase in the frequency or severity of seizures.
• Overdose results in somnolence, confusion, diminished reflexes, and coma.

PRECAUTIONS & CONSIDERATIONS
Caution is warranted in patients with hypoalbuminemia, hepatic and renal impairment, impaired gag reflex, respiratory depression, uncontrolled pain, history of drug abuse, depression, and in those who are taking other CNS depressants. Diazepam crosses the placenta and is distributed in breast milk. Diazepam may increase the risk of fetal abnormalities if administered during the first trimester of pregnancy. Chronic diazepam use during pregnancy may produce withdrawal symptoms in the patient and CNS depression in the neonate. For children and elderly patients, expect to administer a reduced dose initially and to increase dosage gradually to prevent ataxia and excessive sedation.

Females should use effective contraception during therapy and notify the physician immediately if they become or suspect they are pregnant.

Drowsiness and dizziness may occur. Change positions slowly from recumbent to sitting before standing to prevent dizziness. Alcohol, caffeine, and tasks that require mental alertness or motor skills should also be avoided. Autonomic responses, such as cold, clammy hands and diaphoresis, and motor responses, such as agitation, trembling, and tension, should be assessed. Seizure frequency and intensity should be assessed. BP, pulse rate, and respiratory rate, rhythm, and depth should be obtained immediately before giving diazepam. The duration, location, onset, and type of pain should be recorded, and immobility, stiffness, and swelling should be assessed in those being treated for musculoskeletal spasm.

Storage
Store unopened vials at room temperature.

Administration
Take oral diazepam without regard to food. Crush tablets as needed, but do not crush or break capsules. Dilute the oral concentrate with juice, water, or a carbonated beverage or mix it with a semisolid food, such as applesauce or pudding.

For IV use, administer IV push into the tubing of a free-flowing IV solution as close to the vein insertion point as possible. Be aware of solution incompatibilities, which are many. Administer directly into a large vein to reduce the risk of phlebitis and thrombosis. Do not use small veins, such as those of the wrist or dorsum of the hand. Administer IV at a rate not exceeding

5 mg/min (adults). For children, give over a 3-min period because a too-rapid IV may result in hypotension and respiratory depression. Monitor respirations every 5-15 min for 2 h. Stay recumbent for up to 3 h after parenteral administration to reduce the drug's hypotensive effect.

For IM use, inject the IM dose deep into the deltoid muscle. IM injection may be painful.

! For rectal use, do not administer the rectal gel more often than once every 5 days or 5 times a month. See specialized instructions for use.

Diclofenac
dye-kloe′fen-ak
(Cataflam, Diclohexal [AUS], Diclotek [CAN], Fenac [AUS], Flector, Novo-Difenac [CAN], Solaraze, Voltaren Emulgel [AUS], Voltaren Ophthalmic, Voltaren Rapid [AUS], Voltaren XR)
Do not confuse diclofenac with Diflucan or Duphalac, or Voltaren with Verelan.

CATEGORY AND SCHEDULE
Pregnancy Risk Category: B (topical), C (oral, transdermal; D if used in third trimester or near delivery), C (ophthalmic solution)

Classification: Analgesics, nonnarcotic, nonsteroidal anti-inflammatory drugs, ophthalmics

MECHANISM OF ACTION
An NSAID that inhibits prostaglandin synthesis, reducing the intensity of pain. Also constricts the iris sphincter. May inhibit angiogenesis (the formation of blood vessels) by inhibiting substance P or blocking the angiogenic effects of prostaglandin E. *Therapeutic Effect:* Produces analgesic and anti-inflammatory effects. Prevents miosis during cataract surgery. May reduce angiogenesis in inflamed tissue.

PHARMACOKINETICS

Route	Onset	Peak	Duration
PO	30 min	2-3 h	Up to 8 h

Completely absorbed from the GI tract; penetrates cornea after ophthalmic administration (may be systemically absorbed). Topical gel absorption 6%-10%. Protein binding: > 99%. Widely distributed. Metabolized in the liver. Primarily excreted in urine. Minimally removed by hemodialysis. *Half-life:* 1.2-2 h, transdermal patch 12 h. Diclofenac potassium more rapid onset than diclofenac sodium.

AVAILABILITY
Topical Gel (Solaraze): 3%.
Topical Gel (Voltaren): 1%.
Topical Patch (Flector): 1.3%.
Tablets (Cataflam): 50 mg.
Tablets (Enteric-Coated, Delayed-Release Diclofenac Sodium): 25 mg, 50 mg, 75 mg.
Tablets (Extended Release [Voltaren XR]): 100 mg.
Ophthalmic Solution (Voltaren Ophthalmic): 0.1%.

INDICATIONS AND DOSAGES
▸ **Osteoarthritis**
PO (CATAFLAM, DICLOFENAC DELAYED RELEASE)
Adults, Elderly. 50 mg 2-3 times a day or delayed release 75 mg twice a day.
PO (VOLTAREN XR)
Adults, Elderly. 100 mg/day as a single dose.

D

TOPICAL GEL(VOLTAREN GEL)
Adults. Apply 4 g to knee, ankle, foot 4 times a day (maximum 16 g/joint daily). Apply 2 g to elbow, hand, wrist 4 times a day (maximum 8 g/joint a day). Maximum 32 g/day total for all joints.

▸ **Rheumatoid arthritis**
PO (CATAFLAM, DICLOFENAC DELAYED RELEASE)
Adults, Elderly. 50 mg 2-4 times a day or delayed release 75 mg twice a day. Maximum: 225 mg/day.
PO (VOLTAREN XR)
Adults, Elderly. 100 mg once a day. Maximum: 100 mg twice a day.

▸ **Ankylosing spondylitis**
PO (DICLOFENAC DELAYED RELEASE)
Adults, Elderly. 100-125 mg/day in 4-5 divided doses.

▸ **Analgesia, primary dysmenorrhea**
PO (CATAFLAM)
Adults, Elderly. 50 mg 3 times a day.

▸ **Usual pediatric dosage**
PO
Children. 2-3 mg/kg/day in 2-4 divided doses.

▸ **Actinic keratoses**
TOPICAL GEL (SOLARAZE)
Adults, Adolescents. Apply twice a day to lesion for 60-90 days.

▸ **Cataract surgery**
OPHTHALMIC
Adults, Elderly. Apply 1 drop to eye 4 times a day commencing 24 h after cataract surgery. Continue for 2 wks afterward.

▸ **Pain, relief of photophobia in patients undergoing corneal refractive surgery**
OPHTHALMIC
Adults, Elderly. Apply 1 drop to affected eye 1 h before surgery, within 15 min after surgery, then 4 times a day for 3 days.

▸ **Acute pain from sprains, contusions**

TRANSDERMAL PATCH
Adults. Apply patch twice a day to the affected area.

OFF-LABEL USES
Treatment of vascular headaches (oral); to reduce the occurrence and severity of cystoid macular edema after cataract surgery (ophthalmic form).

CONTRAINDICATIONS
Hypersensitivity to aspirin, diclofenac, and other NSAIDs; perioperative use with CABG.

INTERACTIONS
Drug
Acetylcholine, carbachol: May decrease the effects of these drugs (with ophthalmic diclofenac).
Antihypertensives, diuretics: May decrease the effects of these drugs.
Aspirin, other salicylates: May increase the risk of GI side effects such as bleeding.
Bone marrow depressants: May increase the risk of hematologic reactions.
Cyclosporine: Diclofenac may increase risk for nephrotoxicity.
Epinephrine, other antiglaucoma medications: May decrease the antiglaucoma effect of these drugs.
Heparin, oral anticoagulants, thrombolytics: May increase the effects of these drugs.
Lithium: May increase the blood concentration and risk of toxicity of lithium.
Methotrexate: May increase the risk of methotrexate toxicity.
Probenecid: May increase diclofenac blood concentration.
Herbal
Supplements with antiplatelet or anticoagulant effects. (e.g., feverfew,

garlic, ginger, ginkgo biloba, ginseng, red clover, sweet clover, white willow): May increase effects on platelets or risk of bleeding.
Food
None known.

DIAGNOSTIC TEST EFFECTS

May increase BUN level; urine protein level; and serum LDH, potassium, alkaline phosphatase, creatinine, AST (SGOT), and ALT (SGPT) levels. May decrease serum uric acid level.

SIDE EFFECTS

Frequent (4%-9%)
PO: Headache, abdominal cramps, constipation, diarrhea, nausea, dyspepsia.
Ophthalmic (6%-30%): Lacrimation, keratitis, increased intraocular pressure, burning or stinging on instillation, ocular discomfort.
Topical: Pruritus, rash, dry skin, pain, numbness.
Occasional (1%-3%)
PO: Flatulence, dizziness, epigastric pain.
Ophthalmic (5%-10%): Ocular itching or tearing, corneal changes, blurred/abnormal vision, eyelid swelling.
Rare (< 1%)
PO: Rash, peripheral edema or fluid retention, visual disturbances, vomiting, drowsiness.

SERIOUS REACTIONS

• Overdose may result in acute renal failure.
• Rare reactions with long-term use include peptic ulcer disease, GI bleeding, gastritis, a severe hepatic reaction (jaundice), nephrotoxicity (hematuria, dysuria, proteinuria), and a severe hypersensitivity

reaction (bronchospasm or angioedema).

PRECAUTIONS & CONSIDERATIONS

Caution is warranted with hepatic or renal impairment, a predisposition to fluid retention, and history of GI tract disease such as active peptic ulcer disease, chronic inflammation of GI tract, GI bleeding or ulceration. Use the lowest effective dose for the shortest time. Anaphylactoid reactions have occurred in patients with aspirin triad hypersensitivity. Do not use in patients with aspirin-sensitive asthma. Cardiovascular event risk may be increased with duration of use or preexisting cardiovascular risk factors or disease. Use caution with fluid retention, heart failure, or hypertension. Concurrent administration of ibuprofen, and potentially other nonselective NSAIDs, may interfere with aspirin's cardioprotective effect. Use the lowest effective dose for the shortest time. Discontinue at first sign of rash since NSAIDs have been associated with Stevens-Johnson syndrome. Risk of myocardial infarction and stroke may be increased following coronary artery bypass graft surgery. Do not administer within 4-6 half-lives before surgical procedures. Do not use diclofenac topical gel on children, infants, or neonates. Avoid applying the gel around eyes or on open skin wounds, infected areas, or areas affected by exfoliative dermatitis. Diclofenac crosses the placenta; it is unknown whether the drug is distributed in breast milk. Notify the physician of pregnancy. Diclofenac should not be used during the last trimester of pregnancy because it may cause adverse effects in the fetus, such as premature closure of the ductus arteriosus. The safety and efficacy of diclofenac have not been established in children. In elderly patients, GI bleeding or ulceration is more likely to cause serious complications, and age-related renal impairment may increase the risk of hepatotoxicity or renal toxicity; a decreased drug dosage is therefore recommended. Avoid alcohol and aspirin during therapy because these substances increase the risk of GI bleeding.

Notify the physician of persistent headache, black stools, changes in vision, pruritus, rash, or weight gain. Pattern of daily bowel activity and stool consistency should be assessed. Therapeutic response, such as decreased pain, stiffness, swelling, tenderness, improved grip strength, and increased joint mobility, should be evaluated.

Administration
Do not crush or break enteric-coated tablets. Take diclofenac with food, milk, or antacids if GI distress occurs.

For ophthalmic use, place a finger on the lower eyelid and pull it out until a pocket is formed between the eye and lower lid. Hold the dropper above the pocket, and place the prescribed number of drops in the pocket. Gently close the eye, and apply digital pressure to the lacrimal sac for 1-2 min to minimize drainage into the nose and throat, reducing the risk of systemic effects. Remove excess solution with a tissue. Do not use Hydrogel soft contact lenses during ophthalmic therapy.

Topical gels: Follow prescribed use. Voltaren gel has dose card to measure dosage. Wash hands after application.

Topical patch: Remove liner before adhering to normal intact skin. Patct should be applied to affected area. Apply only 1 patch at a time.

Dicloxacillin
dye-klox′a-sill-in
Do not confuse dicloxacillin with dicyclomine.

CATEGORY AND SCHEDULE
Pregnancy Risk Category: B

Classification: Antibiotics, antistaphylococcal penicillins

MECHANISM OF ACTION
A penicillin that acts as a bactericidal in susceptible microorganisms. *Therapeutic Effect:* Inhibits bacterial cell wall synthesis.

PHARMACOKINETICS
Absorption 35%-76% from the GI tract. Rate and extent reduced by food. Distributed throughout body, including CSF (low). Protein binding: 96%. Partially metabolized in liver. Primarily excreted in feces and urine. Not removed by hemodialysis. *Half-life:* 0.7 h.

AVAILABILITY
Capsules: 250 mg, 500 mg.

INDICATIONS AND DOSAGES
▸ **Respiratory tract infection, staphylococcal and streptococcal infections**
PO
Adults, Elderly, Children weighing more than 40 kg. 125-250 mg q6h.
Children weighing < 40 kg. 25-50 mg/kg/day divided q6h.

CONTRAINDICATIONS
Hypersensitivity to any penicillin.

INTERACTIONS
Drug
Oral contraceptives: May decrease the effects of oral contraceptives.

Probenecid: May increase blood concentration and risk for dicloxacillin toxicity.
Warfarin: May decrease effects of warfarin.

DIAGNOSTIC TEST EFFECTS
May cause positive Coombs' test.

SIDE EFFECTS
Frequent
GI disturbances (mild diarrhea, nausea, or vomiting), headache.
Occasional
Generalized rash, urticaria.

SERIOUS REACTIONS
• Altered bacterial balance may result in potentially fatal superinfections and antibiotic-associated colitis as evidenced by abdominal cramps, watery or severe diarrhea, and fever.
• Severe hypersensitivity reactions, including anaphylaxis and acute interstitial nephritis, occur rarely. Immediate reactions occur within 20 min to 48 h and include anaphylaxis, pruritus, urticaria, hypotension, laryngospasm. Delayed allergic reactions occur after 48 h and include serum sickness-like symptoms.
• Neurotoxic reactions may occur with large intravenous doses, especially in patients with renal dysfunction.

PRECAUTIONS & CONSIDERATIONS
Be aware that dicloxacillin crosses the placenta and is distributed in breast milk in low concentrations. Be aware that dicloxacillin use should be avoided in neonates. No age-related precautions have been noted for elderly patients. History of allergies, especially to cephalosporins or penicillins, should be determined before

giving the drug. If diarrhea, rash, or symptoms occur during treatment, notify the physician.
Storage
Store at room temperature.
Administration
Best to take on empty stomach, 1 h before or 2 h after meals. Continue dicloxacillin for the full length of treatment.

D

Dicyclomine
dye-sye'kloe-meen
(Bentyl, Bentylol [CAN], Formulex [CAN], Lomine [CAN], Merbentyl [AUS])
Do not confuse dicyclomine with doxycycline or dyclomine, or Bentyl with Aventyl or Benadryl.

CATEGORY AND SCHEDULE
Pregnancy Risk Category: B

Classification: Anticholinergics, gastrointestinals

MECHANISM OF ACTION
A GI antispasmodic and anticholinergic agent that directly acts as a relaxant on smooth muscle. *Therapeutic Effect:* Reduces tone and motility of GI tract.

PHARMACOKINETICS

Route	Onset	Peak	Duration
PO	1-2 h	N/A	4 h

Readily absorbed from the GI tract. Widely distributed. Metabolized in the liver. *Half-life:* 9-10 h.

D

AVAILABILITY
Capsules: 10 mg.
Tablets: 20 mg.
Syrup, Solution: 10 mg/5 mL.
Injection: 10 mg/mL.

INDICATIONS AND DOSAGES
▸ **Functional disturbances of GI motility**
PO
Adults. 20 mg 4 times a day, then increase up to 40 mg 4 times/day.
Children older than 2 yr. 10 mg 3-4 times a day.
Children 6 mo to 2 yr. 5 mg 3-4 times a day.
Elderly. 10-20 mg 4 times a day. May increase up to 160 mg/day.
IM
Adults. 20 mg 4 times a day for 1-2 days, switch to PO as soon as possible.

CONTRAINDICATIONS
Bladder neck obstruction, myasthenia gravis in patients not treated with neostigmine, narrow-angle glaucoma, obstructive disease of the GI tract, paralytic ileus, severe ulcerative colitis, tachycardia, unstable cardiovascular status in acute hemorrhage, reflux esophagitis, breastfeeding, infants <6 mo.

INTERACTIONS
Drug
Antacids, antidiarrheals: May decrease the absorption of dicyclomine.
Digoxin: May increase absorption of digoxin.
Ketoconazole: May decrease the absorption of ketoconazole.
Other anticholinergics: May increase the effects of dicyclomine.
Potassium chloride: May increase the severity of GI lesions with the wax matrix formulation of potassium chloride.

Herbal
None known.
Food
None known.

DIAGNOSTIC TEST EFFECTS
None known.

SIDE EFFECTS
Frequent
Dry mouth (sometimes severe), dizziness, constipation, blurred vision, nausea, diminished sweating ability.
Occasional
Photophobia; urinary hesitancy; somnolence (with high dosage); agitation, excitement, confusion, or somnolence noted in elderly patients (even with low dosages); transient light-headedness (with IM route), irritation at injection site (with IM route).
Rare
Confusion, hypersensitivity reaction, increased intraocular pressure, vomiting, unusual fatigue.

SERIOUS REACTIONS
• Overdose may produce temporary paralysis of ciliary muscle; pupillary dilation; tachycardia; palpitations; hot, dry, or flushed skin; absence of bowel sounds; hyperthermia; increased respiratory rate; ECG abnormalities; nausea; vomiting; rash over face or upper trunk; central nervous system (CNS) stimulation
• Psychosis (marked by agitation, restlessness, rambling speech, visual hallucinations, paranoid behavior, and delusions, followed by depression).

PRECAUTIONS & CONSIDERATIONS
Extreme caution should be used with autonomic neuropathy,

diarrhea, known or suspected GI infections, and mild to moderate ulcerative colitis. Caution is also warranted with congestive heart failure, chronic obstructive pulmonary disease, coronary artery disease, or hiatal hernia associated with reflux esophagitis, gastric ulcer, hyperthyroidism, hypertension, hepatic or renal disease, tachyarrhythmias, prostatic hypertrophy, and in elderly patients. It is unknown whether dicyclomine crosses the placenta or is distributed in breast milk. Infants and young children are more susceptible to the drug's toxic effects. Dicyclomine use in elderly patients may cause agitation, confusion, somnolence, or excitement. Avoid hot baths, saunas, and becoming overheated while exercising in hot weather because this may cause heat stroke. Tasks that require mental alertness or motor skills should also be avoided until response to the drug has been established. Antacids or antidiarrheals should not be taken within 1 h of taking dicyclomine because they will decrease dicyclomine's effectiveness.

BP, body temperature, pattern of daily bowel activity and stool consistency, and hydration status should be monitored. The patient should void before taking the drug to reduce the risk of urine retention.

Storage
Store capsules, tablets, syrup, and parenteral form at room temperature. Do not freeze.

Administration
For oral use, dilute syrup with an equal volume of water just before administration. Dicyclomine may be given without regard to meals.

The injection normally appears colorless. Do not administer IV or subcutaneously. Inject IM deep into large muscle mass. Do not give for longer than 2 days, as prescribed.

Didanosine (ddI)
dye-dan'o-seen
(Videx, Videx-EC)

CATEGORY AND SCHEDULE
Pregnancy Risk Category: B

Classification: Antivirals, nucleoside reverse transcriptase inhibitors

MECHANISM OF ACTION
A purine nucleoside analogue that is intracellularly converted into a triphosphate, which interferes with RNA-directed DNA polymerase (reverse transcriptase). *Therapeutic Effect:* Inhibits replication of retroviruses, including HIV.

PHARMACOKINETICS
Variably absorbed from the GI tract. Protein binding: < 5%. Rapidly metabolized intracellularly to active form. Primarily excreted in urine. Partially (20%) removed by hemodialysis. *Half-life:* 1.5 h; metabolite: 8-24 h.

AVAILABILITY
Capsules (Delayed Release): 125 mg, 200 mg, 250 mg, 400 mg.
Pediatric Powder for Oral Solution: 10 mg/mL.

INDICATIONS AND DOSAGES
▸ **HIV infection (in combination with other antiretrovirals)**
DELAYED-RELEASE CAPSULES
Adults, Children 13 yr and older, weighing 60 kg or more. 400 mg once a day.

Adults, Children 13 yr and older, weighing < 60 kg. 250 mg once a day.
PEDIATRIC POWDER FOR ORAL SOLUTION
Adults, Children 13 yr and older weighing 60 kg or more. 250 mg q12h.
Adults, Children 13 yr and older weighing < 60 kg.
167 mg q12h.
PEDIATRIC POWDER FOR ORAL SOLUTION
Children 2 wks to 8 mo. 100 mg/m² twice daily.
Children > 8 mo. 120 mg/m² twice daily.

▶ **Dosage in renal impairment**
For adults or adolescents weighing 60 kg or more.

CrCl (mL/min)	Powder for Oral Solution	Delayed-Release Capsule
30-59	100 mg twice daily	200 mg daily
10-29	167 mg daily	125 mg daily
< 10	100 mg daily	125 mg daily

For adults or adolescents weighing < 60 kg:

CrCl (mL/min)	Powder for Oral Solution	Delayed-Release Capsule
30-59	100 mg twice daily	125 mg daily
10-29	100 mg daily	125 mg daily
< 10	100 mg daily	Do not use capsule

CONTRAINDICATIONS
Hypersensitivity to didanosine or any of its components.

INTERACTIONS
Drug
Allopurinol: May increase didanosine concentration.
Atazanavir: Levels of both drugs may be decreased.
Dapsone, fluoroquinolones, itraconazole, ketoconazole, tetracyclines: May decrease absorption of these drugs.
Delavirdine, indinavir: Levels of these agents may be decreased. Administer 1 h before didanosine.
Medications producing pancreatitis or peripheral neuropathy: May increase the risk of pancreatitis or peripheral neuropathy.
Methadone: Decreased didanosine levels may occur.
Stavudine: May increase the risk of fatal lactic acidosis in pregnancy.
Tenofovir, ribavirin: Increased levels of didanosine and toxicity including pancreatitis, hyperglycemia, lactic acidosis, and peripheral neuropathy.
Herbal
None known.
Food
All foods: Decreases absorption of didanosine.

DIAGNOSTIC TEST EFFECTS
May increase serum alkaline phosphatase, amylase, bilirubin, lipase, triglyceride, AST (SGOT), ALT (SGPT), and uric acid levels. May decrease serum potassium levels.

SIDE EFFECTS
Frequent
Adults (> 10%): Diarrhea, neuropathy, chills, and fever.
Children (> 25%): Chills, fever, decreased appetite, pain, malaise, nausea, vomiting, diarrhea, abdominal pain, headache, nervousness, cough, rhinitis, dyspnea, asthenia, rash, pruritus.

Occasional
Adults (2%-9%)
Rash, pruritus, headache, abdominal
pain, nausea, vomiting, pneumonia,
myopathy, decreased appetite, dry
mouth, dyspnea.
Children (10%-25%)
Failure to thrive, weight loss,
stomatitis, oral thrush, ecchymosis,
arthritis, myalgia, insomnia,
epistaxis, pharyngitis.

SERIOUS REACTIONS

• Pneumonia and opportunistic
infections occur occasionally.
• Peripheral neuropathy, potentially
fatal pancreatitis, lactic acidosis,
severe hepatomegaly with steatosis,
retinal changes, and optic neuritis are
the major toxic effects.
• Myocardial infarction.

PRECAUTIONS & CONSIDERATIONS

Extreme caution should be used in
patients with history of pancreatitis.
Caution is warranted with
alcoholism, elevated triglycerides,
and renal or liver dysfunction,
T-cell counts < 100 cells/mm^3,
and phenylketonuria and sodium-
restricted diets because didanosine
contains phenylalanine and sodium.
Myocardial infarction risk may be
greatest in patients with recent use
and those with existing risk factors
for heart. Be aware that didanosine
should be used during pregnancy
only if clearly needed and that
breastfeeding should be discontinued
during didanosine therapy. Be aware
that didanosine is well tolerated in
children older than 3 mo. Elderly
patients are at higher risk for
pancreatitis. In elderly patients,
age-related renal impairment
may require dosage adjustment.
Didanosine is not a cure for HIV
infection, nor does it reduce risk of
transmission to others. Avoid alcohol.

! Contact the physician if abdominal
pain, elevated serum amylase or
triglycerides, nausea, and vomiting
before administering the medication
occur, because these symptoms may
indicate pancreatitis. Assess for
signs and symptoms of peripheral
neuropathy, including burning
feet, "restless legs syndrome"
(unable to find comfortable
position for legs and feet), and
lack of coordination, and for signs
and symptoms of opportunistic
infections, including cough or other
respiratory symptoms, fever, or
oral mucosa changes. Assess for
nausea, abdominal pain, vomiting,
and weight loss as well as visual
or hearing difficulty. Expect to
obtain baseline values for complete
blood count (CBC), renal and liver
function tests, vital signs, and
weight.
Storage
Store at room temperature. Pediatric
powder for oral solution following
reconstitution, as directed, is stable
for 30 days refrigerated.
Administration
Take oral didanosine 1 h before
or 2 h after meals because food
decreases the rate and extent of
didanosine absorption.
  Add 100-200 mL water to 2 or
4 g of the unbuffered pediatric
powder, respectively, to provide
a concentration of 20 mg/mL.
Immediately mix with an equal
amount of an antacid to provide a
concentration of 10 mg/mL. Shake
thoroughly before removing each
dose. Recommended antacid:
Maximum strength mylanta. Keep in
mind antacids decrease absorption of
some medications and may need to
separate administration times.
  Swallow enteric-coated capsules
whole; take them on an empty
stomach.

Diethylpropion
die-ethyl-prop′ion

CATEGORY AND SCHEDULE
Pregnancy Risk Category: B
Controlled Substance: Schedule IV

Classification: Anorexiants, stimulants, central nervous system

MECHANISM OF ACTION
A sympathomimetic amine that stimulates the release of norepinephrine and dopamine. *Therapeutic Effect:* Decreases appetite.

PHARMACOKINETICS
Rapidly absorbed from the GI tract. Widely distributed. Metabolized in liver to active metabolite and undergoes extensive first-pass metabolism. Excreted in urine. Unknown whether removed by hemodialysis. *Half-life:* 4-6 h.

AVAILABILITY
Tablets: 25 mg.
Tablets (Extended Release): 75 mg.

INDICATIONS AND DOSAGES
▸ **Obesity**
PO
Adults. 25 mg 3 times/day before meals *or* Extended Release: 75 mg at midmorning.

CONTRAINDICATIONS
Agitated states, use of MAOIs within 14 days, glaucoma, history of drug abuse, hyperthyroidism, advanced arteriosclerosis or severe cardiovascular disease, severe hypertension, pulmonary hypertension, glaucoma, history of drug abuse, other anorectic agents, and hypersensitivity to sympathomimetic amines.

INTERACTIONS
Drug
Anorectic agents, sympathomimetics: May increase the risk of cardiac effects of diethylpropion.
Anesthetics: May increase the risk of arrhythmias.
Antidiabetic agents, insulin: May alter blood glucose concentrations.
Guanethidine: May decrease the effects of guanethidine.
MAOIs, linezolid: May increase the risk of hypertensive crisis. MAOI use is contraindicated.
Phenothiazines: May decrease the effects of diethylpropion.
Tricyclic antidepressants: May increase the cardiac and CNS effects of diethylpropion.
Herbal
None known.
Food
None known.

DIAGNOSTIC TEST EFFECTS
Urine screen for amphetamines.

SIDE EFFECTS
Frequent
Elevated blood pressure, nervousness, insomnia.
Occasional
Dizziness, drowsiness, tremor, headache, nausea, stomach pain, fever, rash.
Rare
Blurred vision.

SERIOUS REACTIONS
• Overdose may produce agitation, tachycardia, palpitations, cardiac irregularities, chest pain, psychotic episode, seizures, and coma.
• Hypersensitivity reactions, psychosis, cerebrovascular accident, seizures, and blood dyscrasias occur rarely.

• Primary pulmonary hypertension and valvular heart disease have been associated with anorexients.

PRECAUTIONS & CONSIDERATIONS

Caution is required in patients with diabetes, epilepsy, Tourette syndrome, hypertension, and cardiovascular disease. Diethylpropion crosses the placenta and is distributed in breast milk. No age-related precautions have been noted in elderly patients. Safety and efficacy have not been evaluated in pediatric patients. Alcohol should be avoided during therapy. Should not be used if other anorexients used within the past year.

Administration

Generally, do not take in the afternoon or evening because the drug can cause insomnia. Do not crush or break sustained-release capsules. Take immediate-release tablets 1 h before meals. Expect to reassess weight loss after 4 wks to determine risk: benefit of continued use.

Diflorasone
die-floor'a-sone
(Florone [CAN], Apexicon, Psorcon-e)

CATEGORY AND SCHEDULE
Pregnancy Risk Category: C

Classification: Corticosteroids, topical; dermatologics, high-potency

MECHANISM OF ACTION
A high-potency, fluorinated corticosteroid that decreases inflammation by suppression of migration of polymorphonuclear leukocytes and reversal of increased capillary permeability. The exact mechanism of the anti-inflammatory process is unclear. *Therapeutic Effect:* Decreases or prevents tissue response to the inflammatory process.

PHARMACOKINETICS
Poor absorption; occlusive dressings increase absorption. Metabolized in liver. Primarily excreted in urine.

AVAILABILITY
Cream: 0.05%.
Ointment: 0.05%.

INDICATIONS AND DOSAGES
▸ **Corticosteroid-responsive dermatoses**
TOPICAL
Adults, Elderly. Cream: Apply sparingly 2-4 times/day. Ointment: Apply sparingly 1-3 times/day. Maximum: 50q/wk topically.

CONTRAINDICATIONS
History of hypersensitivity to diflorasone or other corticosteroids.

INTERACTIONS
Drug
None known.
Herbal
None known.
Food
None known.

DIAGNOSTIC TEST EFFECTS
None known.

SIDE EFFECTS
Rare
Itching, redness, dryness, irritation, burning at site of application, arthralgia, folliculitis, maceration, muscle atrophy, secondary infection.

SERIOUS REACTIONS
• Overdosage symptoms include moon face, central obesity, hypertension, diabetes, hyperlipidemia, peptic ulcer, increased susceptibility to infection, electrolyte and fluid imbalance, psychosis, and hallucinations.
• The serious reactions of long-term therapy and the addition of occlusive dressings are reversible hypothalamic-pituitary-adrenal (HPA) axis suppression, manifestations of Cushing syndrome, hyperglycemia, and glucosuria.
• Kaposi sarcoma has been reported with prolonged treatment with corticosteroids.

PRECAUTIONS & CONSIDERATIONS
Caution should be used over large surface areas, with prolonged use, addition of occlusive dressings, and uncontrolled infections. Skin irritation should be reported. HPA axis suppression should be evaluated by ACTH stimulation test, AM plasma cortisol test, or urinary free cortisol test. It is unknown whether diflorasone diacetate crosses the placenta or is distributed in breast milk. Children may absorb larger amounts and may be more susceptible to toxicity. Safety and efficacy of diflorasone diacetate have not been established in children or in elderly patients.

Administration
Diflorasone diacetate ointments are recommended for dry, scaly lesions; creams are recommended for moist lesions. Gently cleanse area before application. Use occlusive dressings only as directed. Apply a thin film over affected area and rub into area gently and thoroughly. Wash hands after application. In general, avoid face, groin, and axillae.

Diflunisal
dye-floo'ni-sal
(Apo-Diflunisal [CAN], Dolobid, Novo-Diflunisal [CAN])
Do not confuse diflunisal with Dicarbosil, or Dolobid with Slo-bid.

CATEGORY AND SCHEDULE
Pregnancy Risk Category: C (D if used in third trimester or near delivery)

Classification: Analgesics, nonnarcotic, salicylates

MECHANISM OF ACTION
A nonsteroidal anti-inflammatory that inhibits prostaglandin synthesis, reducing inflammatory response and intensity of pain stimulus reaching sensory nerve endings. *Therapeutic Effect:* Produces analgesic and anti-inflammatory effect.

PHARMACOKINETICS

Route	Onset	Peak	Duration
PO	1 h	2-3 h	8-12 h

Completely absorbed from the GI tract. Widely distributed. Protein binding: > 99%. Metabolized in liver. Primarily excreted in urine as metabolites. Not removed by hemodialysis. *Half-life:* 8-12 h.

AVAILABILITY
Tablets: 500 mg.

INDICATIONS AND DOSAGES
▸ **Mild to moderate pain**
PO
Adults, Elderly. Initially, 0.5-1 g, then 250-500 mg q8-12h. Maximum: 1.5 g/day.
▸ **Rheumatoid arthritis, osteoarthritis**

PO
Adults, Elderly. 0.5-1 g/day in 2
divided doses. Maximum:
1.5 g/day.

OFF-LABEL USES
Treatment of psoriatic arthritis,
migraine, vascular headache.

CONTRAINDICATIONS
Active GI bleeding, hypersensitivity
to aspirin or NSAIDs, perioperative
use with coronary artery bypass graft.

INTERACTIONS
Drug
Antihypertensives, diuretics: May
decrease the effects of these drugs.
Aspirin, antiplatelets, salicylates:
May increase the risk of GI bleeding
and side effects.
Bisphosphonates, corticosteroids:
Increased risk of GI ulceration.
Bone marrow depressants: May
increase the risk of hematologic
reactions.
Cyclosporine, pemetrexed: May
increase levels and effects of
cyclosporine, pemetrexed.
**Heparin, oral anticoagulants,
thrombolytics:** May increase the
effects of these drugs.
Lithium: May increase the blood
concentration and risk of toxicity of
lithium.
Methotrexate: May increase the risk
of toxicity of methotrexate.
Probenecid: May increase diflunisal
blood concentration.
Herbal
Supplements with antiplatelet
or anticoagulant effects. (e.g.,
feverfew, garlic, ginger, ginkgo
biloba, ginseng, red clover, sweet
clover, white willow, etc.,) May
increase effects on platelets or risk of
bleeding.
Food
None known.

DIAGNOSTIC TEST EFFECTS
May increase serum AST (SGOT)
and ALT (SGPT) levels. May
decrease serum uric acid levels.

SIDE EFFECTS
Side effects are less common with
short-term treatment.
Occasional (0%-3%)
Nausea, dyspepsia (heartburn,
indigestion, epigastric pain),
diarrhea, headache, rash.
Rare (1%-3%)
Vomiting, constipation, flatulence,
dizziness, somnolence, insomnia,
fatigue, tinnitus.

SERIOUS REACTIONS
• Overdosage may produce
drowsiness, vomiting, nausea,
diarrhea, hyperventilation, tachycardia,
diaphoresis, stupor, and coma.
• Peptic ulcer, GI bleeding, gastritis,
and severe hepatic reaction, including
cholestasis, jaundice occur rarely.
• Nephrotoxicity, including
dysuria, hematuria, proteinuria, and
nephrotic syndrome, and severe
hypersensitivity reaction, marked
by bronchospasm and angioedema,
occur rarely.

PRECAUTIONS & CONSIDERATIONS
Caution is warranted with hepatic or
renal impairment, a predisposition
to fluid retention, and a history of
GI tract disease such as active peptic
ulcer disease, chronic inflammation
of GI tract, GI bleeding or ulceration.
Use the lowest effective dose for the
shortest duration. Anaphylactoid
reactions have occurred in patients
with aspirin triad hypersensitivity.
Do not use in patients with aspirin-
sensitive asthma. Cardiovascular
event risk may be increased with
duration of use or preexisting
cardiovascular risk factors or disease.
Use caution with fluid retention,

heart failure, or hypertension. Concurrent administration of ibuprofen, and potentially other nonselective NSAIDs, may interfere with aspirin's cardioprotective effect. Use the lowest effective dose for the shortest duration. Discontinue at first sign of rash, since NSAIDs have been associated with Stevens-Johnson syndrome. Risk of myocardial infarction and stroke may be increased following coronary artery bypass graft surgery. Do not administer within 4-6 half-lives before surgical procedures.

Caution is also warranted in patients with factor VII or factor IX deficiencies, platelet and bleeding disorders, and vitamin K deficiency. Be aware that diflunisal crosses the placenta and is distributed in breast milk. Avoid diflunisal use during the last trimester of pregnancy, since the drug may adversely affect the fetal cardiovascular system, causing premature closure of the ductus arteriosus. Be aware that the safety and efficacy of this drug have not been established in children. Reye syndrome is possible with diflunisal. In elderly patients, GI bleeding or ulceration is more likely to cause serious adverse effects. In elderly patients, age-related renal impairment may increase risk of liver or renal toxicity; a decreased drug dosage is recommended.

Notify the physician if GI distress, headache, or rash occurs. Baseline laboratory tests, including PT, aPTT, renal and liver function studies, and CBC, should be obtained. Skin for rash, pattern of daily bowel activity and stool consistency, and therapeutic response should be assessed.

Administration

Take diflunisal with meals, milk, or water. Do not crush or break film-coated tablets.

Digoxin
di-jox′in
(Digitek, Lanoxin, Sigmaxin [AUS])
Do not confuse digoxin with Desoxyn or doxepin, or Lanoxin with Levsinex or Lonox.

CATEGORY AND SCHEDULE
Pregnancy Risk Category: C

Classification: Antiarrhythmics, cardiac glycosides, inotropes

MECHANISM OF ACTION
A cardiac glycoside that increases the influx of calcium from extracellular to intracellular cytoplasm. *Therapeutic Effect:* Potentiates the activity of the contractile cardiac muscle fibers and increases the force of myocardial contraction. Slows the heart rate by decreasing conduction through the SA and AV nodes.

PHARMACOKINETICS

Route	Onset	Peak	Duration
PO	0.5-2 h	2-8 h	3-4 days
IV	5-30 min	1-4 h	3-4 days

Readily absorbed from the GI tract. Widely distributed. Protein binding: 30%. Partially metabolized in the liver. Primarily excreted in urine. Minimally removed by hemodialysis. *Half-life (adults):* 36-48 h (increased with impaired renal function and in elderly patients).

AVAILABILITY
Elixir: 50 mcg/mL.
Tablets (Digitek, Lanoxin): 125 mcg, 250 mcg.
Injection (Lanoxin): 250 mcg/mL, 100 mcg/mL.

D

INDICATIONS AND DOSAGES
▶ **Rapid loading dose for the management and treatment of CHF; control of ventricular rate in patients with atrial fibrillation; treatment and prevention of recurrent paroxysmal atrial tachycardia**
PO
Adults, Elderly. Initially, 0.5-0.75 mg, additional doses of 0.125-0.375 mg at 6- to 8-h intervals. Range: 0.75-1.25 mg.
Children older than 10 yr. 10-15 mcg/kg.
Children 5-10 yr. 20-35 mcg/kg.
Children 2-5 yr. 30-40 mcg/kg.
Children 1-24 mo. 35-60 mcg/kg.
Neonate, full-term. 25-35 mcg/kg.
Neonate, premature. 20-30 mcg/kg.
One-half of loading dose given initially, followed by equal portions of the remaining dose at 4- to 8-h intervals.
IV
Adults, Elderly. 0.6-1 mg. See titration as with PO dosing.
Children older than 10 yr. 8-12 mcg/kg.
Children 5-10 yr. 15-30 mcg/kg.
Children 2-5 yr. 25-35 mcg/kg.
Children 1-24 mo. 30-50 mcg/kg.
Neonates, full-term. 20-30 mcg/kg.
Neonates, premature. 15-25 mcg/kg.
One-half of loading dose given initially, followed by equal portions of the remaining dose at 4- to 8-h intervals.
▶ **Maintenance dosage for CHF; control of ventricular rate in patients with atrial fibrillation; treatment and prevention of recurrent paroxysmal atrial tachycardia**
PO, IV
Adults, Elderly. 0.125-0.375 mg/day.
Children. 25%-35% loading dose (20%-30% for premature neonates) divided every 12 h in children <10 yr.
▶ **Dosage in renal impairment**
Dosage adjustment is based on creatinine clearance. Total digitalizing dose: decrease by 50% in end-stage renal disease.

Creatinine Clearance	Adult Dosage
10-50 mL/min	25%-75% usual or every 36 h
Less than 10 mL/min	10%-25% usual or every 48 h

CONTRAINDICATIONS
Ventricular fibrillation, ventricular tachycardia unrelated to congestive heart failure.

INTERACTIONS
Drug
Amiodarone: May increase digoxin blood concentration and risk of toxicity; may have an additive effect on the SA and AV nodes. Reduce digoxin dose by 50% when initiating amiodarone.
Amphotericin, glucocorticoids, potassium-depleting diuretics: May increase risk of toxicity due to hypokalemia.
Antiarrhythmics, parenteral calcium, sympathomimetics: May increase risk of arrhythmias.
Antidiarrheals, cholestyramine, colestipol, sucralfate: May decrease absorption of digoxin.
β-Blockers: May have additive effect on heart rate.
Carvedilol, diltiazem, fluoxetine, quinidine, verapamil: May increase digoxin blood concentration. Reduce dose 25%-50% when initiating quinidine. Reduce digoxin dose with others.
Cyclosporine, itraconazole: May increase digoxin levels.
Parenteral magnesium: May cause cardiac conduction changes and heart block.

Herbal
Siberian ginseng: May increase serum digoxin levels.
Licorice: Hypokalemic effects may increase digoxin toxicity.
Food
None known.

DIAGNOSTIC TEST EFFECTS
None known.

ⓘ IV INCOMPATIBILITIES
Amiodarone, amphotericin B cholesteryl (Amphotec), amphotericin B liposomal (AmBisome), caspofungin (Cancidas), dantrolene, diazepam (Valium), doxorubicin (Adriamycin), fluconazole (Diflucan), foscarnet (Foscavir), lansoprazole (Prevacid), minocycline (Minocin), mitoxantrone (Novantrone), paclitaxel (Taxol), phenytoin, propofol (Diprivan), quinupristin/dalfopristin (Synercid), sulfamethoxazole/trimethoprim.

ⓘ IV COMPATIBILITIES
Acyclovir (Zovirax), alfentanil (Alfenta), amikacin (Amikar), aminophylline, anidulafungin (Eraxis), ascorbic acid, atracurium (Tracrium), atropine, aztreonam (Azactam), benztropine (Cogentin), bivalirudin (Angiomax), bretylium, bumetanide (Bumex), buprenorphine (Buprenex), butorphanol (Stadol), calcium chloride, calcium gluconate, carboplatin, cefazolin, cefotaxime (Claforan), cefotetan (Cefotan), cefoxitin (Mefoxin), ceftazidime (Ceptaz, Fortaz, Tazicef, Tazidime), ceftizoxime (Cefizox), ceftriaxone (Rocephin), cefuroxime (Zinacef), chloramphenicol, chlorpromazine, cimetidine (Tagamet), ciprofloxacin (Cipro), cisatracurium (Nimbex), cisplatin, clindamycin (Cleocin), cyanocobalamin, cyclophosphamide (Cytoxan), cyclosporine (Sandimmune), dactinomycin (Cosmegen), daptomycin (Cubicin), dexamethasone sodium phosphate, diltiazem (Cardizem), diphenhydramine (Benadryl), dobutamine (Dobutrex), docetaxel (Taxotere), dopamine (Intropin), doripenem (Doribax), enalaprilat, ephedrine, epinephrine, epirubicin (Ellence), epoetin alfa (Procrit), ertapenem (Invanz), erythromycin lactobionate, esmolol (Brevibloc), etoposide phosphate (Etopophos), famotidine (Pepcid), fenoldopam (Corlopam), fentanyl (Sublimaze), fludarabine (Fludara), fluorouracil, furosemide (Lasix), ganciclovir, gemcitabine (Gemzar), gentamicin, granisetron (Kytril), heparin, hydrocortisone sodium succinate (Solu-Cortef), hydromorphone (Dilaudid), hydroxyzine, imipenem/cilastatin (Primaxin), isoproterenol (Isuprel), ketorolac, labetalol, levofloxacin (Levaquin), lidocaine, linezolid (Zyvox), lorazepam (Ativan), magnesium sulfate, mannitol, meperidine (Demerol), meropenem (Merrem), methicillin, methotrexate, methylprednisolone sodium succinate, metoclopramide (Reglan), metoprolol (Lopressor), metronidazole (Flagyl), midazolam (Versed), milrinone (Primacor), morphine, multiple vitamins injection, nafcillin, nalbuphine (Nubain), naloxone (Narcan), nesiritide (Natrecor), nitroglycerin, nitroprusside sodium (Nitropress), norepinephrine (Levophed), ondansetron (Zofran), oxacillin, oxaliplatin (Eloxatin), oxytocin (Pitocin), palonosetron (Aloxi), pantoprazole (Protonix), pemetrexed (Alimta), penicillin G potassium, penicillin G sodium, pentobarbital, phenobarbital, piperacillin, piperacillin/tazobactam (Zosyn),

potassium chloride, procainamide, prochloperazine, promethazine, propranolol, ranitidine (Zantac), remifentanil (Ultiva), rituximab (Rituxan), sodium acetate, sodium bicarbonate, streptokinase, succinylcholine, sufentanil (Sufenta), tacrolimus (Prograf), teniposide (Vumon), theophylline, thiotepa (Thioplex), ticarcillin (Ticar), ticarcillin/clavulanate (Timentin), tigecycline (Tygacil), tirofibran (Aggrastat), tobramycin, trastuzumab (Herceptin), vancomycin, vasopressin, vecuronium (Norcuron), verapamil, vincristine (Vincasar), vinorelbine (Navelbine), vitamin B complex with C, voriconazole (Vfend).

SIDE EFFECTS

Most side effects occur at doses greater than needed for therapeutic effect. However, there is a very narrow margin of safety between a therapeutic and a toxic result. Long-term therapy may produce mammary gland enlargement in women, but this is reversible when the drug is withdrawn.
Occasional (< 10%)
Dizziness, headache, mental disturbances, diarrhea, nausea, rash.

SERIOUS REACTIONS

• The most common early manifestations of digoxin toxicity are GI disturbances (anorexia, nausea, vomiting) and neurologic abnormalities (fatigue, headache, depression, weakness, drowsiness, confusion, nightmares). In children, the early signs are cardiac arrhythmias, including sinus bradycardia.
• Facial pain, personality change, and ocular disturbances (photophobia, light flashes, halos around

bright objects, yellow or green color perception) may be noted.
• Proarrhythmic effects occur with digoxin.

D

PRECAUTIONS & CONSIDERATIONS

Caution is warranted in patients who have had an acute myocardial infarction (i.e., within 6 mo), advanced cardiac disease, heart failure, cor pulmonale, hypokalemia, hypomagnesemia, hypothyroidism, impaired hepatic or renal function, incomplete AV block, sinus nodal disease, or pulmonary disease. Digoxin crosses the placenta and is distributed in breast milk. Premature infants are more susceptible to toxicity. Keep in mind that infants and children experience signs of overdose differently than adults do. The first sign of overdose in children is usually an arrhythmia, such as bradycardia, followed by nausea, vomiting, diarrhea, anorexia, and CNS disturbances. In elderly patients, age-related hepatic or renal function impairment may require dosage adjustment. Also, there is an increased risk of loss of appetite in this age group. Withhold or reduce dose 1-2 days before elective electrical cardioversion.

Notify the physician if decreased appetite, diarrhea, nausea, visual changes, or vomiting occurs. Apical pulse should be assessed for 60 s or 30 s if the person is receiving maintenance therapy. If the pulse rate is 60 beats/min or lower in adults or 70 beats/min or lower in children, withhold the drug and contact the physician. Blood samples for digoxin level should be obtained 6-8 h after digoxin administration or just before administration of the next digoxin dose. Be aware that signs and symptoms of digoxin toxicity are GI disturbances and neurologic abnormalities.

Storage
Store at room temperature.
Administration
! Avoid giving digoxin by the IM route, because the drug may cause severe local irritation and is erratically absorbed (IV preferred). Only if no other route is possible, give deep into the muscle followed by massage. Give no more than 2 mL at any one site. Expect to adjust the digoxin dosage in elderly patients and in those with renal dysfunction. Know that larger digoxin doses are often required for adequate control of ventricular rate with atrial fibrillation or flutter. Administer digoxin loading dosage in several doses at 4- to 8-h intervals, as prescribed.

May take oral digoxin without regard to meals. Crush tablets if necessary. Do not increase or skip digoxin doses. Carefully measure oral solution to ensure accurate dosage.

For IV use, give undiluted or dilute with at least a fourfold volume of sterile water for injection, NS, or D5W, because using less than this amount may cause a precipitate to form. Use immediately. Give IV slowly over at least 5 min.

Digoxin Immune Fab
di-jox′in
(Digibind, DigiFab)
Do not confuse digoxin with Desoxyn or doxepin.

CATEGORY AND SCHEDULE
Pregnancy Risk Category: C

Classification: Antidotes

MECHANISM OF ACTION
An antidote that binds molecularly to digoxin in the extracellular space and the complex is excreted by kidneys. *Therapeutic Effect:* Makes digoxin unavailable for binding at its site of action on cells in the body.

PHARMACOKINETICS

Route	Onset	Peak	Duration
IV	30 min	N/A	3-4 days

Widely distributed into extracellular space. Excreted in urine. *Half-life:* 15-20 h.

AVAILABILITY
Powder for Injection (Digibind): 38-mg vial.
Powder for Injection (DigiFab): 40-mg vial.

INDICATIONS AND DOSAGES
▶ **Potentially life-threatening digoxin overdose**
IV
Adults, Elderly, Children. Dosage varies according to amount of digoxin to be neutralized. Refer to manufacturer's dosing calculation guidelines.

CONTRAINDICATIONS
None known.

INTERACTIONS
Drug
None known.
Herbal
None known.
Food
None known.

DIAGNOSTIC TEST EFFECTS
May alter serum potassium level. Serum digoxin concentration may increase precipitously and persist for up to 1 wk until FAB/digoxin complex is eliminated from the body.

Ⓓ IV INCOMPATIBILITIES
None known.

SIDE EFFECTS
Allergic reaction, phlebitis.

SERIOUS REACTIONS
• Hyperkalemia may occur as a result of digitalis toxicity. Signs and symptoms of hyperkalemia include diarrhea, paresthesia of extremities, heaviness of legs, decreased BP, cold skin, grayish pallor, hypotension, mental confusion, irritability, flaccid paralysis, tented T waves, widening QRS interval, and ST depression.
• Hypokalemia may develop rapidly when the effect of digitalis is reversed. Signs and symptoms of hypokalemia include muscle cramping, nausea, vomiting, hypoactive bowel sounds, abdominal distention, difficulty breathing, and orthostatic hypotension.
• Low cardiac output and congestive heart failure exacerbations may occur rarely when digoxin level is reduced.

PRECAUTIONS & CONSIDERATIONS
Caution is warranted with impaired cardiac and renal function. Be aware of signs and symptoms of digoxin toxicity, including anorexia, nausea,

and vomiting, as well as visual changes. It is unknown whether digoxin immune Fab crosses the placenta or is distributed in breast milk. No age-related precautions have been noted in children. In elderly patients, age-related renal impairment may require cautious use.

BP, ECG, serum potassium level, and temperature should be monitored during and after drug administration. Changes from the initial assessment should be assessed. Hypokalemia may result in cardiac arrhythmias, changes in mental status, muscle cramps, muscle strength changes, or tremor. Hyperkalemia may result in cold and clammy skin, confusion, and diarrhea. Signs and symptoms of an arrhythmia (such as palpitations) or heart failure (such as dyspnea and edema) should also be assessed if the digoxin level falls below the therapeutic level.

Storage
Refrigerate vials. After reconstitution, use the solution immediately. If it is not used immediately, store the solution in the refrigerator for up to 4 h.

Administration
Serum digoxin level should be obtained before administering the drug. If the serum digoxin level was drawn < 6 h before the last digoxin dose, the serum digoxin level may be unreliable. Impaired renal function may require more than 1 wk before serum digoxin assay is reliable; however, this fact does not alter recommendations for acute treatment. Monitor for prolonged toxicity.

Reconstitute each 38-mg vial with 4 mL sterile water for injection to provide a concentration of 9.5 mg/mL. Reconstitute each 40-mg vial with 4 mL of sterile water for injection to provide a concentration of 10 mg/mL. Further dilute with 50 mL 0.9% NaCl.

Infuse over 30 min. It is recommended that the solution be infused through a 0.22-μm filter. If cardiac arrest is imminent, may give drug by IV push. In children, may need to watch for fluid overload, depending on the number of vials to be given.

Dihydroergotamine
dye-hye-droe-er-got′a-meen
(D.H.E. 45, Dihydergot [AUS], Ergomar [CAN], Migranal)

CATEGORY AND SCHEDULE
Pregnancy Risk Category: X

Classification: Ergot alkaloids and derivatives

MECHANISM OF ACTION
An ergotamine derivative, α-adrenergic blocker that directly stimulates vascular smooth muscle. May also have antagonist effects on serotonin. *Therapeutic Effect:* Peripheral and cerebral vasoconstriction.

PHARMACOKINETICS
Slow, incomplete absorption from the GI tract; rate of absorption of intranasal varies. Protein binding: > 90%. Undergoes extensive first-pass metabolism in liver. Metabolized to active metabolite. Eliminated in feces via biliary system. *Half-life:* 7-9 h.

AVAILABILITY
Injection: 1 mg/mL (D.H.E. 45).
Nasal Spray: 4 mg/mL (0.5 mg/spray) (Migranal).

INDICATIONS AND DOSAGES
▸ **Migraine headaches, cluster headaches**

IM/SUBCUTANEOUS
Adults, Elderly. 1 mg at onset of headache; repeat hourly. Maximum: 3 mg/day; 6 mg/wk.
IV
Adults, Elderly. 1 mg at onset of headache; repeat hourly. Maximum: 2 mg/day; 6 mg/wk.
INTRANASAL
Adults, Elderly. 1 spray (0.5 mg) into each nostril; repeat in 15 min, up to 4 sprays. Maximum: 6 sprays/day; 8 sprays/wk.

OFF-LABEL USES
Orthostatic hypotension.

CONTRAINDICATIONS
Coronary artery disease, angina, hypertension, impaired liver or renal function, malnutrition, peripheral vascular diseases, such as thromboangiitis obliterans, syphilitic arteritis, severe arteriosclerosis, thrombophlebitis, coronary artery vasospasm/Prinzmetal's angina, hemiplegic or basilar migraine, Raynaud disease, sepsis, severe pruritus (biliary disease), high-dose aspirin therapy, potent CYP3A4 inhibitors, within 24 h of serotonin agonists, within 2 wks of MAOIs, pregnancy, breastfeeding.

INTERACTIONS
Drug
β-Blockers, erythromycin: May increase the risk of vasospasm.
CYP3A4 inhibitors: May increase toxicity of dihydroergotamine. Contraindicated.
Ergot alkaloids, systemic vasoconstrictors: May increase pressor effect.
Fluoxetine: May increase risk of ergotism.
MAOIs, serotonin agonists, sibutramine: May increase

risk of serotonin syndrome. Contraindicated.

Nitroglycerin: May decrease the effect of nitroglycerin.

Protease inhibitors: May increase the risk of toxicity of dihydroergotamine.

Herbal
None known.

Food
None known.

DIAGNOSTIC TEST EFFECTS
None known.

SIDE EFFECTS
Frequent (> 25%)
Nasal spray: Rhinitis.
Occasional
Nasal spray: Nausea, cough, dizziness, altered taste, throat and nose irritation.
Rare
Muscle pain, fatigue, diarrhea, upper respiratory infection, dyspepsia.

SERIOUS REACTIONS
• Prolonged administration or excessive dosage may produce ergotamine poisoning manifested as nausea, vomiting, weakness of legs, pain in limb muscles, numbness and tingling of fingers or toes, precordial pain, tachycardia or bradycardia, and hypertension or hypotension.
• Coronary artery vasospasm, myocardial ischemia, myocardial infarction, ventricular tachycardia, ventricular fibrillation, cerebrovascular hemorrhage, stroke.
• Localized edema and itching due to vasoconstriction of peripheral arteries and arterioles may occur.
• Feet or hands will become cold, pale, and numb.
• Muscle pain will occur when walking and later, even at rest.

• Gangrene may occur.
• Pleural and retroperitoneal fibrosis have occurred with prolonged daily use.
• Occasionally confusion, depression, drowsiness, and seizures appear.

PRECAUTIONS & CONSIDERATIONS
Dihydroergotamine use is contraindicated in pregnancy because it produces uterine stimulant action, resulting in possible fetal death or retarded fetal growth, and it increases vasoconstriction of placental vascular bed. It is distributed in breast milk and may prohibit lactation.

Dihydroergotamine use may produce diarrhea or vomiting in the neonate. It may be used safely in children older than 6 yr, but use only when the patient is unresponsive to other medication. In elderly patients, age-related occlusive peripheral vascular disease increases the risk of peripheral vasoconstriction. In elderly patients, age-related renal impairment may require caution.

Irregular heartbeat, nausea, numbness or tingling of the fingers and toes, pain or weakness of the extremities, and vomiting should be reported.

Storage
Do not refrigerate or freeze injection formulation or nasal spray.

Administration
Take injection at the first signs of acute migraine or cluster headache.

Before intranasal administration, nasal spray must be primed (pumped 4 times). Use no more than 4 inhalations (2 mg) for a single administration; do not use > 6 sprays in a 24-h period or 8 sprays in a week. Inhale deeply through the nose while spraying or immediately after spraying to allow the drug to be absorbed through the skin in the nose. Do not tilt the head back or inhale through the nose. Initiate treatment at the first sign of symptom of an attack. Nasal spray may be administered at any time during a migraine attack. Once spray is prepared, use within 8 h. Discard unused solution.

Diltiazem
dil-tye′a-zem
(Apo-Diltiaz [CAN], Auscard [AUS], Cardcal [AUS], Cardizem, Cardizem CD, Cardizem LA, Cartia XT, Coras [AUS], Dilacor XR, Diltahexal [AUS], Diltia XT, Diltiamax [AUS], Dilzem [AUS], Novo-Diltiazem [CAN], Taztia XT, Tiazac, Vasocardal CD [AUS])
Do not confuse Cardizem with Cardene or Cardene SR, or Tiazac with Ziac.

CATEGORY AND SCHEDULE
Pregnancy Risk Category: C

Classification: Antiarrhythmics, class IV, calcium channel blockers

MECHANISM OF ACTION
An antianginal, antihypertensive, and antiarrhythmic agent that inhibits calcium movement across cardiac and vascular smooth-muscle cell membranes. This action causes the dilation of coronary arteries, peripheral arteries, and arterioles. *Therapeutic Effect:* Decreases BP, heart rate, and myocardial contractility; slows SA and AV conduction; and decreases total peripheral vascular resistance by vasodilation.

PHARMACOKINETICS

Route	Onset	Peak	Dura-tion
PO	0.5-1 h	2-3 h	N/A
PO	2-3 h	10-18 h N/A (extended-release)	
IV	3 min	15 min N/A	

Well absorbed from the GI tract. Protein binding: 70%-80%. Undergoes first-pass metabolism in the liver to active metabolite. Primarily excreted in urine. Not removed by hemodialysis. *Half-life* (immediate-release tablet): 3-4.5 h. *Half-life* (extended-release tablet): 6-9 h. *Half-life* (extended-release capsules): 5-10 h.

AVAILABILITY
Capsules (Sustained Release [Diltiazem Sustained Release]): 60 mg, 90 mg, 120 mg.
Capsules (Extended Release [Cardizem CD]): 120 mg, 180 mg, 240 mg, 300 mg, 360 mg.
Capsules (Extended Release [Cartia XT]): 120 mg, 180 mg, 240 mg, 300 mg.
Capsules (Extended Release [Dilacor XR]): 120 mg, 180 mg, 240 mg.
Capsules (Extended Release [Diltia XT]): 120 mg, 180 mg, 240 mg.
Capsules (Extended Release [Taztia XT]): 120 mg, 180 mg, 240 mg, 300 mg, 360 mg.
Capsules (Extended Release [Tiazac]): 120 mg, 180 mg, 240 mg, 300 mg, 360 mg, 420 mg.
Tablets (Cardizem): 30 mg, 60 mg, 90 mg, 120 mg.
Tablets (Extended Release [Cardizem LA]): 120 mg, 180 mg, 240 mg, 300 mg, 360 mg, 420 mg.

Injection (Solution): 5 mg/mL.
Injection (Powder): 100 mg.

INDICATIONS AND DOSAGES
▸ **Angina related to coronary artery spasm (Prinzmetal's variant), chronic stable angina (effort-associated)**
PO
Adults, Elderly. Initially, 30 mg 4 times a day. Increase up to 180-360 mg/day in 3-4 divided doses at 1- to 2-day intervals.
Adults, Elderly (Cardizem LA). Initially, 180 mg/day. May increase at intervals of 7-14 days up to 360 mg/day.
Adults, Elderly (Cardizem CD, Cartia XT, Dilacor XR, Diltia XT, Tiazac). Initially, 120-180 mg/day; titrate over 7-14 days. Range: Up to 480 mg/day.
▸ **Essential hypertension**
PO
Adults, Elderly. (Cardizem CD, Cartia XT, Dilacor XR, Diltia XT): Initially, 180-240 mg once a day. May increase at 2-wk intervals. Maintenance 240-360 mg/day. Maximum: 480 mg once a day (Cardizem CD, Cartia XT, Dilacor XR). Maximum: 540 mg once a day (Diltia XT). (Cardizem LA): Initially, 180-240 mg once a day. May increase at 2-wk intervals. Maintenance: 120-540 mg/day. (Taztia XT, Tiazac): Initially, 120-240 mg once a day. May increase at 2-wk intervals. Maximum: 540 mg once a day.
▸ **Temporary control of rapid ventricular rate in atrial fibrillation or flutter, rapid conversion of paroxysmal supraventricular tachycardia to normal sinus rhythm**
IV PUSH
Adults, Elderly. Initially, 0.25 mg/kg actual body weight over 2 min. May repeat in 15 min at dose of 0.35 mg/kg actual body weight. Subsequent doses individualized.
IV INFUSION
Adults, Elderly. After initial bolus injection, may begin infusion at 5-10 mg/h; may increase by 5 mg/h up to a maximum of 15 mg/h. Infusion duration should not exceed 24 h.

OFF-LABEL USES
Migraine prophylaxis.

CONTRAINDICATIONS
Acute myocardial infarction, pulmonary congestion, severe hypotension (< 90 mm Hg, systolic), sick sinus syndrome, second- or third-degree AV block (except in the presence of a pacemaker), IV administration within hour of IV β-blockers, ventricular tachycardia, hypersinsitivity

INTERACTIONS
Drug
α-Blockers: Increased hypotensive effect.
Aprepitant/fosaprepitant: May increase levels of each drug.
β-Blockers: May have additive effect.
Carbamazepine: May decrease levels of diltiazem. May increase levels of carbamazepine.
Cyclosporine: Levels of each drug may be increased.
CYP3A4 inhibitors/inducers: May increase or decrease levels and effects of diltiazem, respectively.
CYP3A4 substrates, HMG-CoA reductase inhibitors: Diltiazem may increase levels of substrates.
Digoxin: May increase serum digoxin concentration.
Procainamide, quinidine: May increase risk of QT-interval prolongation.

D

Herbal
St. John's wort: May decrease levels of diltiazem.
Food
None known.

DIAGNOSTIC TEST EFFECTS
PR interval may be increased.

Ⓓ IV INCOMPATIBILITIES
Acetazolamide (Diamox), acyclovir (Zovirax), allopurinol (Aloprim), aminophylline, amphotericin B liposomal (AmBisome), ampicillin, ampicillin/sulbactam (Unasyn), cefepime (Maxipime), chloramphenicol, dantrolene, diazepam (Valium), fluorouracil, furosemide (Lasix), ganciclovir (Cytovene), heparin, insulin, ketorolac, lansoprazole (Prevacid), methotrexate, nafcillin, pantoprazole (Protonix), pentobarbital, phenobarbital, phenytoin (Dilantin), piperacillin/tazobactam (Zosyn), rifampin (Rifadin), sodium bicarbonate, thiopental.

Ⓓ IV COMPATIBILITIES
Albumin, alfentanil (Alfenta), amifostine (Ethyol), amikacin (Amikar), amiodarone, argatroban, atenolol, atracurium (Tracrium), aztreonam (Azactam), bivalirudin (Angiomax), bretylium, bumetanide (Bumex), buprenorphine (Buprenex), busulfan (Busulfex), butorphanol (Stadol), calcium chloride, calcium gluconate, carboplatin, caspofungin (Cancidas), cefazolin (Ancef), cefotaxime (Claforan), cefotetan (Cefotan), cefoxitin (Mefoxin), ceftazidime (Ceptaz, Fortaz, Tazicef, Tazidime), ceftizoxime (Cefizox), ceftriaxone (Rocephin), cefuroxime (Zinacef), chlorpromazine, cimetidine (Tagamet), ciprofloxacin (Cipro), cisatracurium (Nimbex), cisplatin, clindamycin (Cleocin),

cyclophosphamide (Cytoxan), cyclosporine (Sandimmune), dactinomycin (Cosmegen), daptomycin (Cubicin), dexamethasone sodium phosphate, dexmedetomidine (Precedex), digoxin (Lanoxin), diphenhydramine (Benadryl), dobutamine (Dobutrex), docetaxel (Taxotere), dopamine (Intropin), doripenem (Doribax), doxorubicin (Adriamycin), doxycycline, droperidol, enalaprilat, ephedrine, epinephrine, epirubicin (Ellence), ertapenem (Invanz), erythromycin lactobionate, esmolol (Brevibloc), etoposide phosphate (Etopophos), famotidine (Pepcid), fenoldopam (Corlopam), fentanyl (Sublimaze), fluconazole (Diflucan), fludarabine (Fludara), foscarnet (Foscavir), fosphenytoin (Cerbyx), gemcitabine (Gemzar), granisetron (Kytril), haloperidol (Haldol), hydrocortisone sodium succinate (Solu-Cortef), gentamicin (Garamycin), hydromorphone (Dilaudid), hydroxyzine, imipenem/cilastatin (Primaxin), isoproterenol (Isuprel), labetalol, levofloxacin (Levaquin), lidocaine, linezolid (Zyvox), lorazepam (Ativan), magnesium sulfate, mannitol, melphalan (Alkeran), meperidine (Demerol), meropenem (Merrem), metoclopramide (Reglan), metoprolol (Lopressor), metronidazole (Flagyl), midazolam (Versed), milrinone (Primacor), minocycline (Minocin), mitoxantrone (Novantrone), morphine, multivitamins, nalbuphine (Nubain), naloxone (Narcan), nesiritide (Natrecor), nicardipine (Cardene), nitroglycerin, nitroprusside sodium (Nitropress), norepinephrine (Levophed), ondansetron (Zofran), oxacillin, oxaliplatin (Eloxatin), oxytocin (Pitocin), paclitaxel (Taxol), palonosetron (Aloxi), pancuronium, pemetrexed (Alimta), penicillin G potassium, piperacillin, potassium chloride, potassium phosphate, prochlorperazine, promethazine, propranolol, quinupristin/dalfopristin (Synercid), ranitidine (Zantac), remifentanil (Ultiva), sodium acetate, succinylcholine, sufentanil (Sufenta), sulfamethoxazole/trimethoprim, tacrolimus (Prograf), teniposide (Vumon), theophylline, thiotepa (Thioplex), ticarcillin (Ticar), ticarcillin/clavulanate (Timentin), tigecycline (Tygacil), tirofibran (Aggrastat), tobramycin, vancomycin, vasopressin, vecuronium (Norcuron), verapamil, vincristine (Vincasar), vinorelbine (Navelbine), voriconazole (Vfend), zidovudine (Retrovir).

SIDE EFFECTS

Frequent (1%-5%)
Peripheral edema, dizziness, light-headedness, headache, pain, bradycardia, asthenia (loss of strength, weakness), dyspepsia.
Occasional (2%-5%)
Nausea, constipation, flushing, ECG changes, injection site reactions (burning, itching).
Rare (< 2%)
Rash, micturition disorder (polyuria, nocturia, dysuria, frequency of urination), abdominal discomfort, somnolence.

SERIOUS REACTIONS

• Abrupt withdrawal may increase frequency or duration of angina.
• Congestive heart failure (CHF) and second- and third-degree AV block and sinus bradycardia occur rarely.
• Overdose produces nausea, somnolence, confusion, slurred speech, and profound bradycardia.

PRECAUTIONS & CONSIDERATIONS

Caution is warranted in patients with CHF, hypertrophic obstructive cardiomyopathy, and impaired hepatic or renal function. It is unclear whether diltiazem crosses the placenta. It should be used during pregnancy only if the benefit to the mother outweighs the risk to the fetus. Diltiazem is distributed in breast milk. No age-related precautions have been noted in children. In elderly patients, age-related renal impairment may require cautious use. Tasks that require alertness and motor skills should also be avoided.

Dizziness or light-headedness may occur. Rise slowly from a lying to a sitting position and wait momentarily before standing to avoid diltiazem's hypotensive effect. Notify the physician of constipation, irregular heartbeat, nausea, pronounced dizziness, or shortness of breath. The onset, type (sharp, dull, or squeezing), radiation, location, intensity, and duration of anginal pain and its precipitating factors, such as exertion and emotional stress, should be documented before therapy. Pulse, BP, and renal and hepatic function test results should be monitored before and during therapy. Skin should be assessed for flushing and peripheral edema, especially behind the medial malleolus.

Storage
Refrigerate single-use solution for injection (may store at room temperature 1 mo). Store single-use syringe at room temperature. Store powder for reconstitution at room temperature. After dilution, solution is stable for 24 h.

Administration
Take oral immediate-release diltiazem before meals and at bedtime. Taztia

XT and Tiazac capsules may be opened and sprinkled on applesauce. Do not crush or open other sustained-release capsules. In general administer at the same time each day for extended-release dosage forms. Dilacor XR or Diltior XT should be given on an empty stomach. Other extended-release capsules are taken without regard to food.

! Refer to manufacturer's information for dose concentration and infusion rates.

IV bolus given over 2 min. Add 125 mg to 100 mL D5W or 0.9% NaCl to provide a concentration of 1 mg/mL. Add 250 mg to 250 or 500 mL diluent to provide a concentration of 0.83 mg/mL or 0.45 mg/mL, respectively. The maximum concentration is 1.25 g/250 mL or 5 mg/mL. Infuse per dilution or rate chart provided by manufacturer.

Dimenhydrinate
dye-men-hye′dri-nate
(Dramamine)

CATEGORY AND SCHEDULE
Pregnancy Risk Category: B

Classification: Anticholinergics, antiemetics/antivertigo
OTC, RX

MECHANISM OF ACTION
An antihistamine and anticholinergic that competes for H_1 receptor sites on effector cells of the GI tract, blood vessels, and respiratory tract. The anticholinergic action diminishes vestibular stimulation and depresses labyrinthine function. *Therapeutic Effect:* Prevents symptoms of motion sickness.

AVAILABILITY
Tablets Chewable: 50 mg.
Tablets: 50 mg.
Injection: 50 mg/mL.

INDICATIONS AND DOSAGES
▸ **Motion sickness**
PO
Adults, Elderly, Children older than 12 yr. 50-100 mg q4-6h. Maximum: 400 mg/day.
Children 6-12 yr. 25-50 mg q6-8h. Maximum: 150 mg/day.
Children 2-5 yr. 12.5-25 mg q6-8h. Maximum: 75 mg/day.
IM/IV
Adults. 50 mg as needed every 4 h. Maximum: 300 mg/day.
Children. 1.25 mg/kg or 37.5 mg/m^2 4 times daily. Maximum 300 mg a day. Do not use in neonates.

CONTRAINDICATIONS
Hypersensitivity to dimenhydrinate. Do not use in neonates because injectable product contains benzyl alcohol.

INTERACTIONS
Drug
Alcohol, other central nervous system (CNS) depressants: May increase CNS depression.
Aminoglycosides: Masks signs and symptoms of ototoxicity associated with aminoglycosides.
Other anticholinergics: Increases anticholinergic effect.

DIAGNOSTIC TEST EFFECTS
None known.

SIDE EFFECTS
Frequent
Dry mouth, drowsiness.
Occasional
Hypotension, palpitations, tachycardia, headache, somnolence, dizziness, paradoxical stimulation

(especially in children), anorexia, constipation, dysuria, blurred vision, tinnitus, wheezing, chest tightness.
Rare
Photosensitivity, rash, urticaria.

SERIOUS REACTIONS
• None significant.

PRECAUTIONS & CONSIDERATIONS
Caution is warranted in patients with asthma, bladder neck obstruction, cardiovascular disease, history of seizures, angle-closure glaucoma, thyroid dysfunction, and benign prostatic hyperplasia. Alcohol, tasks that require mental alertness or motor skills, and excessive exposure to sunlight should be avoided. Skin should not come in contact with the oral concentrate and syrup, because it can cause contact dermatitis. Should not be used in children younger than 2 yr. Elderly patients are more susceptible to side effects.

Drowsiness, dizziness, and dry mouth may occur. BP should be monitored. Be alert for paradoxical reactions, especially in children, and signs and symptoms of motion sickness.
Administration
Tablets may be swallowed whole, chewed, or allowed to dissolve. For motion sickness, take dimenhydrinate 1-2 h before the activity that may cause motion sickness.
IM: Inject into large muscle mass.
IV: Dilute dose in 10 mL of 0.9% Nacl; give by slow IV push over 2 min.

Dimercaprol
dye-mer-kap′role
(BAL in Oil)

CATEGORY AND SCHEDULE
Pregnancy Risk Category: C

Classification: Antidotes, chelators

MECHANISM OF ACTION
A chelating agent that contains two sulfhydryl groups that form a stable, nontoxic chelate 5-membered heterocyclic ring with heavy metals. *Therapeutic Effect:* Prevents the metal from combining with sulfhydryl groups on physiologic proteins and keeps them inactive until they can be excreted.

PHARMACOKINETICS
Time to peak after IM administration occurs in 30-60 min. Widely distributed to all tissues, including the brain and, mainly, intracellular space. Rapidly metabolized by the liver to inactive metabolites. Excreted in the urine and bile. Removed by hemodialysis. *Half-life:* 4 h.

AVAILABILITY
Injection, Oil: 100 mg/mL (BAL in Oil).

INDICATIONS AND DOSAGES
▸ **Poisoning, arsenic (mild)**
IM
Adults, Elderly, Children. 2.5 mg/kg 4 times/day for 2 days, 2 times on day 3, then once daily for 10 days or recovery.
▸ **Poisoning, arsenic (severe)**
IM
Adults, Elderly, Children. 3 mg/kg q4h for 2 days, 4 times on day 3, then

twice daily for 10 days or until recovery.

▸ **Poisoning, gold (mild)**
IM
Adults, Elderly, Children. 2.5 mg/kg 4 times/day for 2 days, 2 times on day 3, then once daily for 10 days or until recovery.

▸ **Poisoning, gold (severe)**
IM
Adults, Elderly, Children. 3 mg/kg q4h for 2 days, 4 times on day 3, then twice daily for 10 days or until recovery.

▸ **Poisoning, lead (mild)**
IM
Adults, Elderly, Children. Initially, 4 mg/kg, then 3 mg/kg q4h for 2-7 days in combination with edetate calcium disodium injection beginning with second dose at different injection sites.

▸ **Poisoning, lead (severe)**
IM
Adults, Elderly, Children. 4 mg/kg q4h usually for 5 days. In combination with edetate calcium disodium injection beginning with second dose at different injection sites. A second 5-day course may be used in severe poisoning. Wait at least 5-7 days before administering a third course, if needed.

▸ **Poisoning, mercury**
IM
Adults, Elderly, Children. 5 mg/kg for 1 day, followed by 2.5 mg/kg 1 or 2 times/day for 10 days.

▸ **Dosage in renal impairment**
Quantitative dosage recommendations are not available. The manufacturer states the drug should be discontinued or used with extreme caution if acute renal insufficiency occurs during treatment.

OFF-LABEL USES
Antimony poisoning, bismuth poisoning, selenium poisoning, silver poisoning, vanadium poisoning.

CONTRAINDICATIONS
Hepatic insufficiency (unless due to arsenic poisoning; use in iron, cadmium, or selenium poisoning; hypersensitivity to dimercaprol or any component of the formulations, such as peanut oil.

INTERACTIONS
Drug
Gold compounds: Compromise anti-inflammators effect by chelatins gold.
Iron, cadmium, selenium, uranium: May increase risk of toxicity, especially to the kidneys.

DIAGNOSTIC TEST EFFECTS
Iodine (^{131}I) thyroidal uptake values may be decreased. May result in false-positive reaction with nitroprusside test. May increase ALT and AST values.

Ⓘ IV INCOMPATIBILITIES
Edetate calcium disodium.

SIDE EFFECTS
Frequent
Hypertension, dose-related tachycardia, headache.
Occasional
Nausea, vomiting.
Rare
Burning eyes, lips, mouth, throat, and penis; nervousness; pain at injection site; salivation; fever; dysuria.

SERIOUS REACTIONS
• Abscess formation at injection site, blepharospasm, convulsions, thrombocytopenia, and transient neutropenia occur rarely.
• Fever may occur and persist in children.

PRECAUTIONS & CONSIDERATIONS
Caution is warranted with hypotension because of dose-related increase in blood pressure

and heart rate; renal impairment including oliguria; and glucose 6-phosphate dehydrogenase (G6PD) deficiency. Contains peanut oil. Ensure alkalinization of urine to protect the kidney. Caution is also necessary with people receiving iron supplementation. Avoid use until 24 h after last dose of dimercaprol.

Be aware that dimercaprol is effective for acute poisoning by mercury salts if therapy is initiated within 1-2 h after ingestion. Dimercaprol is not effective for chronic mercury poisoning. Serum alkaline phosphatase concentration, blood urea nitrogen (BUN) concentration, serum calcium, creatinine, electrolyte concentrations, hemoglobin (especially in mercury toxicity), and phosphorus concentrations should be monitored.

Storage
Store ampules at room temperature.

Administration
Be careful not to mix in the same syringe with edetate calcium disodium. Administer at different sites.

Administer deep IM injection only. Adjust dose if receiving dialysis.

The injection is painful and causes a sterile abscess in some patients.

Dinoprostone (PGE₂)
dye-noe-prost′one
(Cervidil, Prepidil Gel, Prostin E2)
Do not confuse Cervidil or Prepidil with bepridil, or Prostin with Prostigmin.

CATEGORY AND SCHEDULE
Pregnancy Risk Category: C

Classification: Oxytocics, prostaglandins, stimulants, uterine

MECHANISM OF ACTION
A prostaglandin that directly acts on the myometrium, causing softening and dilation effect of the cervix. *Therapeutic Effect:* Stimulates myometrial contractions in gravid uterus, promotes cervical ripening.

PHARMACOKINETICS
Undergoes rapid enzymatic deactivation, primarily in maternal lungs. Protein binding: 73%. Primarily excreted in urine. *Half-life:* < 5 min. Onset of action (vaginal suppository): within 10 min. Duration (vaginal insert): 12 h. Duration (vaginal suppository): 2-3 h.

AVAILABILITY
Vaginal Gel (Prepidil): 0.5 mg.
Vaginal Inserts (Cervidil): 10 mg.
Vaginal Suppositories (Prostin E2): 20 mg.

INDICATIONS AND DOSAGES
▶ **Abortifacient**
INTRAVAGINAL
Adults. 20 mg (one suppository) high into vagina. May repeat at 3- to 5-h intervals until abortion occurs. Do not administer for > 2 days.
▶ **Ripening of unfavorable cervix**
INTRACERVICAL
Adults. Initially, 0.5 mg (2.5 mL) (Prepidil); if no cervical or uterine response, may repeat 0.5-mg dose in 6 h. Maximum: 1.5 mg (7.5 mL) for a 24-h period. Or 10 mg (Cervidil) over 12-h period; remove upon onset of active labor or 12 h after insertion.

CONTRAINDICATIONS
Suppository: Active cardiac, hepatic, pulmonary, or renal disease; acute pelvic inflammatory disease; hypersensitivity to dinoprostone or other prostaglandins.

Gel, insert: Fetal malpresentation/ distress; hypersensitivity to dinoprostone or other prostaglandins; significant cephalopelvic disproportion; more than 6 previous term pregnancies; unexplained vaginal bleeding; obstetrical emergencies.

INTERACTIONS
Drug
Oxytocics: May cause uterine hypertonus, possibly resulting in uterine rupture or cervical laceration. Wait 6-12 h after dinoprostone gel administration or at least 30 min after removal of vaginal insert before initiating oxytocin.

DIAGNOSTIC TEST EFFECTS
None known.

SIDE EFFECTS
Frequent
Vomiting (66%), temperature elevations (50%), diarrhea (40%), nausea (33%).
Occasional
Headache (10%), chills or shivering (10%), transient diastolic BP decrease (10%), hives, bradycardia, increased uterine pain accompanying abortion, peripheral vasoconstriction.
Rare
Flushing, vulvar edema.

SERIOUS REACTIONS
• Overdose may cause uterine hypertonicity with spasm and tetanic contraction, leading to cervical laceration or perforation, and uterine rupture or hemorrhage.
• Uterine hyperstimulation with or without fetal distress.

PRECAUTIONS & CONSIDERATIONS
Suppository: Caution is warranted in patients with anemia, cardiovascular disease, cervicitis, compromised or scarred uterus, diabetes mellitus, epilepsy, hepatic disease, history of asthma, hypertension or hypotension, infected endocervical lesions or acute vaginitis, jaundice, renal disease, and uterine fibroids. Notify the physician if chills, fever, foul-smelling or increased vaginal discharge, or uterine cramps or pain occurs.

Gel, vaginal insert: Caution is warranted with ruptured membranes, nonsingle pregnancy, glaucoma, asthma, nonvertex pregnancy, renal and hepatic impairment.

The character of the cervix, including dilation and effacement, fetal status, including heart rate as well as uterine activity, including the onset of uterine contractions, should be monitored in those receiving the vaginal gel. Bishop score should be monitored before and after therapy.

Uterine tone and duration, frequency, and strength of contractions should be checked if receiving the suppository form. Vital signs should be monitored every 15 min until stable and then hourly until abortion is complete. Expect to give medications to relieve GI adverse effects, if indicated, or abdominal cramps in those receiving the suppository form.
Storage
Refrigerate gel; bring to room temperature just before use to avoid forcing warming process. Keep suppository frozen (< 4° F [15.6° C]); bring to room temperature just before use. Remove foil wrapper after suppository reaches room temperature. Vaginal insert should be stored in freezer.
Administration
Use gel with caution when handling to prevent skin contact. Wash hands thoroughly with soap and water following administration. Assemble

dosing apparatus as described in manufacturer's insert. Place the person in the dorsal position, and use a speculum to visualize the cervix. Introduce gel into cervical canal just below level of internal os. After administration, remain in the supine position for at least 15-30 min to minimize leakage of the drug from the cervical canal.

Administer suppository only in a hospital setting, with emergency equipment available. Avoid skin contact because of risk of absorption. Insert high in the vagina. Remain supine for 10 min after administration.

Diphenhydramine
dye-fen-hye′dra-meen
(Allerdryl [CAN], Altaryl, Banophen, Benadryl, Ben-Tann, Diphedryl, Diphenhist, Dytan, ElixSure, Genahist, Hydramine Nytol [CAN], Nytol, Pediacare Nighttime, Q-Dryl, Quenalin, Siladryl, Silphen, Sominex, Unisom Sleepgels [AUS])
Do not confuse diphenhydramine with dimenhydrinate, or Benadryl with benazepril, Bentyl, or Benylin, or Banophen with Baclophen.

CATEGORY AND SCHEDULE
Pregnancy Risk Category: B
OTC (capsules, tablets, chewable tablets, orally disintegrating tablets, syrup, elixir, strips, cream, spray)

Classification: Antihistamines, anti-Parkinson agent, antiana-phylactic (adjunct), antipruritic, antivertigo agent, hypnotic

MECHANISM OF ACTION
An ethanolamine that competitively blocks the effects of histamine at peripheral H_1 receptor sites. *Therapeutic Effect:* Produces anticholinergic, antipruritic, antitussive, antiemetic, antidyskinetic, and sedative effects.

PHARMACOKINETICS

Route	Onset	Peak	Duration
PO	15-30 min	1-4 h	4-6 h
IV, IM	< 15 min	1-4 h	4-6 h

Well absorbed after PO or parenteral administration. Protein binding: 98%-99%. Widely distributed. Metabolized in the liver. Primarily excreted in urine. *Half-life:* 2-10 h.

AVAILABILITY
Capsules (Banophen, Benadryl, Diphedryl, Diphenhist, Genahist, Q-Dryl): 25 mg, 50 mg (generic).
Capsules (Nytol, Unisom): 50 mg.
Elixir (Banophen): 12.5 mg/5 mL.
Oral solution (Altaryl, Banophen, Benadryl, Diphenhist, ElixSure, Genahist, Hydramine, Pediacare Nighttime, Q-Dryl, Siladryl): 12.5 mg/5 mL.
Oral Suspension (Ben-Tann, Dytan): 25 mg/5 mL.
Syrup (Quenalin, Silphen): 12.5 mg/5 mL.
Tablets (Banophen, Benadryl, Diphedryl, Diphenhist, Genahist): 25 mg.
Tablets (Nytol, Sominex): 25 mg, 50 mg.
Chewable Tablets: 12.5 mg (Benadryl Allergy), 25 mg (DiphenMax, Dytan)
Orally Disintegrating Tablets (Benadryl Fastmelt): 19 mg.

*Strips, Oral Dissolving Film
(Benadryl Quick Dissolve):* 12.5 mg,
25 mg.
Injection: 50 mg/mL.
Cream (Benadryl): 2%.
Topical Gel (Benadryl): 2%.
*Topical Solution (Benadryl
Stick):* 2%.
Spray: 2%.

INDICATIONS AND DOSAGES
▸ **Moderate to severe allergic
reaction**
PO, IV, IM
Adults, Elderly. 10-50 mg q4-6h.
Maximum: 400 mg/day.
Children. 5 mg/kg/day in divided
doses q6-8h. Maximum:
300 mg/day.
▸ **Dystonic reaction**
IV, IM
Adults, Elderly. 10-50 mg/single dose.
May repeat in 20-30 min if needed.
Children. 0.5-1 mg/kg/dose.
▸ **Motion sickness, minor allergic
rhinitis**
PO
*Adults, Elderly, Children 12 yr and
older.* 25-50 mg q4-6h. Maximum:
300 mg/day.
Children 6-11 yr. 12.5-25 mg
q4-6h. Maximum: 150 mg/day.
Children 2-5 yr. 6.25 mg q4-6h.
Maximum: 37.5 mg/day.
▸ **Antitussive**
PO
*Adults, Elderly, Children 12 yr and
older.* 25 mg q4h. Maximum:
150 mg/day.
Children 6-11 yr. 12.5 mg q4h.
Maximum: 75 mg/day.
Children 2-5 yr. 6.25 mg q4h.
Maximum: 37.5 mg/day. NOTE: The
FDA recommends against use in
children < 6 years of age (2008).
▸ **Nighttime sleep aid**
PO
*Adults, Elderly, Children 12 yr and
older.* 50 mg at bedtime.

Children 2-11 yr. 1 mg/kg/dose.
Do not exceed: 50 mg. (FDA
recommends OTC cough and cold
products not be used as sleep aid for
children.).
▸ **Pruritus**
TOPICAL
*Adults, Elderly, Children 2 yr and
older.* Apply 2% cream or spray 3-4
times a day.

CONTRAINDICATIONS
Acute exacerbation of asthma,
use within 14 days of MAOIs,
newborn or premature infants,
breastfeeding, narrow-angle
glaucoma, prostatic hypertrophy,
bladder neck obstruction,
pyloroduodenal obstruction,
stenosing peptic ulcer.

INTERACTIONS
Drug
**Alcohol, other central nervous
system (CNS) depressants:**
May increase CNS-depressant
effects.
Anticholinergics: May increase
anticholinergic effects.
CYP2D6 substates: Levels of
substrates may be increased.
MAOIs: May increase the
anticholinergic and CNS-depressant
effects of diphenhydramine.
Herbal and Food
None known.

DIAGNOSTIC TEST EFFECTS
May suppress wheal and flare
reactions to antigen skin testing
unless the drug is discontinued
4 days before testing.

ⓦ IV INCOMPATIBILITIES
Allopurinol (Aloprim),
aminophylline, amphotericin
B cholesteryl (Amphotec),
ampicillin, azathioprine,
cefazolin, cefepime (Maxipime),

cefotaxime (Claforan), cefotetan (Cefotan), cefoxitin (Mefoxin), ceftazidime (Ceptaz, Fortaz, Tazicef, Tazidime), ceftriaxone (Rocephin), cefuroxime (Zinacef), chloramphenicol, dantrolene, dexamethasone (Decadron), diazepam (Valium), fluorouracil, foscarnet (Foscavir), furosemide (Lasix), ganciclovir (Cytovene), insulin (regular, Humulin R, Novolin R), ketorolac, lansoprazole (Prevacid), methylprednisolone sodium succinate (Solu-Medrol), metronidazole (Flagyl), milrinone (Primacor), nitroprusside sodium (Nitropress), pantoprazole (Protonix), pentobarbital, phenobarbital, phenytoin, sodium bicarbonate, sulfamethoxazole/trimethoprim.

🗲 IV COMPATIBILITIES

Abciximab (ReoPro), acyclovir (Zovirax), aldesleukin (Proleukin), alfentanil (Alfenta), allopurinol (Aloprim), amifostine (Ethyol), amikacin (Amikar), amphotericin B liposomal (AmBisome), argatroban, ascorbic acid, atracurium (Tracrium), atropine, azithromycin (Zithromax), bivalirudin (Angiomax), bretylium, bumetanide (Bumex), buprenorphine (Buprenex), butorphanol (Stadol), calcium chloride, calcium gluconate, carboplatin, ceftizoxime (Cefizox), chlorpromazine, cimetidine (Tagamet), ciprofloxacin (Cipro), cisatracurium (Nimbex), cisplatin, cladribine (Leustatin), clindamycin (Cleocin), cyclophosphamide (Cytoxan), cyclosporine (Sandimmune), cytarabine (Ara-C), dactinomycin (Cosmegen), daptomycin (Cubicin), dexmedetomidine (Precedex), digoxin (Lanoxin), diltiazem (Cardizem), dobutamine (Dobutrex), docetaxel (Taxotere), dopamine,

doripenem (Doribax), doxorubicin (Adriamycin), doxorubicin liposomal (Doxil), doxycycline, droperidol (Inapsine), enalaprilat, ephedrine, epinephrine, epirubicin (Ellence), epoetin alfa (Procrit), ertapenem (Invanz), erythromycin lactobionate, esmolol (Brevibloc), etoposide phosphate (Etopophos), famotidine (Pepcid), fenoldopam (Corlopam), fentanyl (Sublimaze), glycopyrrolate (Robinul), filgrastim (Neupogen), fluconazole (Diflucan), fludarabine (Fludara), folic acid, gemcitabine (Gemzar), gentamicin, granisetron (Kytril), hydromorphone (Dilaudid), hydroxyzine, idarubicin (Idamycin), imipenem/cilastatin (Primaxin), isoproterenol (Isuprel), labetalol, levofloxacin (Levaquin), lidocaine, linezolid (Zyvox), magnesium sulfate, mannitol, melphalan (Alkeran), meperidine (Demerol), meropenem (Merrem), methadone, methicillin, methotrexate, metoprolol (Lopressor), midazolam (Versed), minocycline (Minocin), mitoxantrone (Novantrone), morphine, nalbuphine (Nubain), naloxone (Narcan), nitroglycerin, norepinephrine (Levophed), ondansetron (Zofran), oxaliplatin (Eloxatin), oxytocin (Pitocin), paclitaxel (Taxol), palonosetron (Aloxi), pemetrexed (Alimta), penicillin G potassium, penicillin G sodium, piperacillin, piperacillin/tazobactam (Zosyn), potassium chloride, procainamide, prochlorperazine, promethazine, propofol (Diprivan), propranolol, quinupristin/dalfopristin (Synercid), ranitidine (Zantac), remifentanil (Ultiva), rituximab (Rituxan), sargramostim (Leukine), sodium acetate, streptokinase, succinylcholine, sufentanil (Sufenta), tacrolimus (Prograf), teniposide (Vumon), theophylline, thiotepa

(Thioplex), ticarcillin (Ticar), ticarcillin/clavulanate (Timentin), tigecycline (Tygacil), tirofiban (Aggrastat), tobramycin, trastuzumab (Herceptin), vancomycin, vasopressin, vecuronium (Norcuron), verapamil, vincristine (Vincasar), vinorelbine (Navelbine), vitamin B complex with C, voriconazole (Vfend).

SIDE EFFECTS

Frequent

Somnolence, dizziness, muscle weakness, hypotension, urine retention, thickening of bronchial secretions, dry mouth, nose, throat, or lips; in elderly, sedation, dizziness, hypotension.

Occasional

Epigastric distress, flushing, visual or hearing disturbances, paresthesia, diaphoresis, chills.

SERIOUS REACTIONS

• Hypersensitivity reactions, eczema, pruritus, rash, cardiac disturbances, and photosensitivity may occur.

• Overdose symptoms may vary from CNS depression, including sedation, apnea, hypotension, cardiovascular collapse, and death, to severe paradoxical reactions, such as hallucinations, tremor, and seizures.

• Children and neonates may experience paradoxical reactions, including restlessness, insomnia, euphoria, nervousness, and tremors.

• Overdosage in children may result in hallucinations, seizures, and death.

PRECAUTIONS & CONSIDERATIONS

Caution is warranted in patients with asthma, cardiovascular disease, chronic obstructive pulmonary disease (COPD), hypertension, hyperthyroidism, angle-closure glaucoma, increased intraocular pressure, peptic ulcer disease, benign prostatic hyperplasia, pyloroduodenal or bladder neck obstruction, and seizure disorders. Diphenhydramine crosses the placenta and appears in breast milk. Its use by breastfeeding women may inhibit lactation and produce irritability in breastfeeding infants. Use of the drug during the third trimester of pregnancy increases the risk of seizures in neonates and premature infants. Diphenhydramine is not recommended for children, neonates, or premature infants because they are at an increased risk for paradoxical reactions. The FDA recommends that OTC cough and cold medications should not be used in children < 2 yr old. Elderly patients are at increased risk for developing confusion, dizziness, hyperexcitability, hypotension, and sedation. Avoid drinking alcoholic beverages and performing tasks that require alertness or motor skills until response to the drug is established.

Drowsiness, dizziness, and dry mouth may occur; tolerance usually develops to sedative effects. Respiratory rate, depth, and rhythm; pulse rate and quality; BP; and therapeutic response should be monitored.

Administration

Take diphenhydramine without regard to food. Crush scored tablets as needed. Do not crush, break, or open capsules or film-coated tablets.

For IM use, inject diphenhydramine deep into a large muscle mass.

For IV use, diphenhydramine may be given undiluted.

Administer IV injection no faster than 25 mg/min.

Diphenoxylate and Atropine

dye-fen-ox′i-late
(Lofenoxal [AUS], Lomotil, Lonox)
Do not confuse Lomotil with Lamictal, or Lofenoxal or Lonox with Lanoxin, Loprox, or Lovenox.

CATEGORY AND SCHEDULE

Pregnancy Risk Category: C

Classification: Anticholinergics, antidiarrheals

MECHANISM OF ACTION

A meperidine derivative that acts locally and centrally on gastric mucosa. *Therapeutic Effect:* Reduces intestinal motility.

PHARMACOKINETICS

Well absorbed from the GI tract. Metabolized in the liver to active metabolite. Primarily eliminated in feces. *Half-life:* 2.5 h; metabolite, 12-24 h. Onset: 45-60 min. Duration 3-4 h.

AVAILABILITY

Tablets (Lomotil, Lonox):
2.5 mg/0.025 mg.
Liquid (Lomotil): 2.5 mg/0.025 mg per 5 mL.

INDICATIONS AND DOSAGES

▶ **Diarrhea**
PO
Adults, Elderly. Initially, 5 mg 4 times a day, then reduce dose to 2.5 mg 2-3 times per day. Maximum: 20 mg/day.
Children 2-12 yr. 0.3-0.4 mg/kg/day in 4 divided doses, then reduce dose. Maximum: 10 mg/day. Use liquid form only.

CONTRAINDICATIONS

Children younger than 2 yr, obstructive jaundice, narrow-angle glaucoma, diarrhea from pseudomembranous colitis, or enterotoxin-producing bacteria.

INTERACTIONS

Drug
Alcohol, other CNS depressants: May increase CNS-depressant effects.
Anticholinergics: May increase the effects of atropine.
MAOIs: May precipitate hypertensive crisis.
Herbal
None known.
Food
None known.

DIAGNOSTIC TEST EFFECTS

May increase serum amylase level.

SIDE EFFECTS

Frequent
Somnolence, light-headedness, dizziness, nausea.
Occasional
Headache, dry mouth.
Rare
Flushing, tachycardia, urine retention, constipation, paradoxical reaction (marked by restlessness and agitation), blurred vision.

SERIOUS REACTIONS

• Hypersensitivity reactions, including pruritus, gum swelling, urticaria, anaphylaxis.
• Dehydration may aggravate dehydration or electrolyte imbalance.

D

Correct fluid balance before administering.
• Paralytic ileus and toxic megacolon (marked by constipation, decreased appetite, and stomach pain with nausea or vomiting) occur rarely.
• Severe anticholinergic reaction, manifested by severe lethargy, hypotonic reflexes, and hyperthermia, may result in severe respiratory depression and coma.

PRECAUTIONS & CONSIDERATIONS

Caution is warranted in patients with acute ulcerative colitis, cirrhosis, hepatic or renal disease, and renal impairment. It is unknown whether diphenoxylate crosses the placenta or is distributed in breast milk. Diphenoxylate is not recommended for use in children because of the increased risk of toxicity, which can lead to respiratory depression. Use extreme caution in young children. Elderly patients are more susceptible to the anticholinergic effects of diphenoxylate, and they may experience confusion and respiratory depression. Tasks that require mental alertness or motor skills should be avoided until response to the drug has been established. Alcohol and barbiturates should also be avoided during drug therapy.

Notify the physician if abdominal distention, fever, palpitations, or persistent diarrhea occurs. Pattern of daily bowel activity and stool consistency and hydration status should be monitored.

Administration

Take without regard to meals. If GI irritation occurs, give with food. Administer only the liquid form to children 2-12 yr of age using a graduated dropper for accurate measurement.

Dipyridamole

dye-peer-id′a-mole
(Apo-Dipyridamole [CAN], Novodipiradol [CAN], Persantin [AUS], Persantin 100 [AUS], Persantin SR [AUS], Persantine)
Do not confuse dipyridamole with disopyramide or Persantin with Periactin.

CATEGORY AND SCHEDULE
Pregnancy Risk Category: B

Classification: Platelet inhibitors

MECHANISM OF ACTION
A blood modifier and platelet aggregation inhibitor that inhibits the activity of adenosine deaminase and phosphodiesterase, enzymes causing accumulation of adenosine and cyclic adenosine monophosphate. *Therapeutic Effect:* Inhibits platelet aggregation; may cause coronary vasodilation.

PHARMACOKINETICS
Slowly, variably absorbed from the GI tract. Widely distributed. Protein binding: 91%-99%. Metabolized in the liver. Primarily eliminated via biliary excretion. *Half-life:* 10-15 h.

AVAILABILITY
Tablets: 25 mg, 50 mg, 75 mg.
Injection: 5 mg/mL.

INDICATIONS AND DOSAGES
▶ **Prevention of thromboembolic disorders after cardiac valve replacement**
PO
Adults, Elderly, Children 12 yr and older. 75-100 mg four times/day. In combination with other medications.

▸ **Diagnostic aid, coronary artery disease**

IV

Adults, Elderly (based on weight).
0.142 mg/kg/min infused over 4 min; although a maximum has not been determined, doses > 60 mg have been determined to be unnecessary for any patient.

OFF-LABEL USES

Prevention of myocardial reinfarction, treatment of transient ischemic attacks.

CONTRAINDICATIONS

None known.

INTERACTIONS

Drug
Anticoagulants, aspirin, heparin, salicylates, thrombolytics: May increase the risk of bleeding with these drugs.
Adenosine: Effects may be increased.
Herbal
None known.
Food
None known.

DIAGNOSTIC TEST EFFECTS

None known.

Ⓓ IV INCOMPATIBILITIES

No information available via Y-site administration. Do not mix with other medications.

SIDE EFFECTS

Oral:
FREQUENT (14%)
Dizziness.
OCCASIONAL (2%-6%)
Abdominal distress, headache, rash.
RARE (< 2%)
Diarrhea, vomiting, flushing, pruritus.
Injection:
FREQUENT (12%-20%)

Angina pectoris exacerbation, dizziness, headache.
OCCASIONAL (2%-10%)
Hypotension, ECG changes, nausea, pain, flushing, hypertension.
RARE (< 2%).
Fatigue, paresthesia.

SERIOUS REACTIONS

• Overdose produces peripheral vasodilation, resulting in hypotension.
• Hepatic failure and enzyme elevations have occurred.

PRECAUTIONS & CONSIDERATIONS

Caution is warranted in patients with hypotension, unstable angina, recent myocardial infarction, or hepatic impairment. Dipyridamole is distributed in breast milk. Safety and efficacy of dipyridamole have not been established in children. No age-related precautions have been noted in elderly patients. Avoid alcohol because it increases the risk of stomach bleeding and dizziness, possibly resulting in a fall.

Dizziness may occur. Do not rise suddenly from a lying or sitting position. Notify the physician of unusual bleeding or chest pain. BP for hypotension and skin for erythema and rash should be monitored.
Storage
Store inection and tablets at room temperature.
Administration
Take oral dipyridamole on an empty stomach with full glass of water. Therapeutic response may not be achieved before 2-3 mo of continuous therapy.

For IV use, dilute to at least 1:2 ratio with 0.9% NaCl or D5W for total volume of 20-50 mL because undiluted solution may cause irritation. Infuse over 4 min.

D

Inject thallium within 5 min after dipyridamole infusion has ended, as prescribed.

Disopyramide

dye-soe-peer′a-mide
(Norpace, Norpace CR, Rythmodan [CAN])
Do not confuse disopyramide with desipramine or dipyridamole, or Rythmodan with Rythmol.

CATEGORY AND SCHEDULE
Pregnancy Risk Category: C

Classification: Antiarrhythmics, class IA

MECHANISM OF ACTION
An antiarrhythmic that prolongs the refractory period of the cardiac cell by direct effect, decreasing myocardial excitability and conduction velocity. *Therapeutic Effect:* Depresses myocardial contractility. Has anticholinergic and negative inotropic effects.

AVAILABILITY
Capsules (Norpace): 100 mg, 150 mg.
Capsules (Extended Release [Norpace CR]): 100 mg, 150 mg.

INDICATIONS AND DOSAGES
▶ **Suppression and prevention of ventricular ectopy, unifocal or multifocal premature ventricular contractions, paired ventricular contractions (couplets), and episodes of ventricular tachycardia**
PO
! Do not use extended-release capsules for rapid control.

Adults, Elderly weighing 50 kg and more. 150 mg q6h (300 mg q12h with extended-release capsules).
Adults, Elderly weighing < 50 kg. 100 mg q6h (200 mg q12h with extended-release capsules).
▶ **Rapid control of arrhythmias**
PO
Adults, Elderly weighing 50 kg and more. Initially, 300 mg (immediate release), then 150 mg q6h or 300 mg (controlled release) q12h.
Adults, Elderly weighing < 50 kg. Initially, 200 mg (immediate release), then 100 mg q6h or 200 mg (controlled release) q12h.
▶ **Severe refractory arrhythmias**
NOTE: Patient should be hospitalized during the initial treatment period.
PO
Adults, Elderly. Up to 400 mg q6h.
Children 12-18 yr. 6-15 mg/kg/day in divided doses q6h.
Children 5-12 yr. 10-15 mg/kg/day in divided doses q6h.
Children 1-4 yr. 10-20 mg/kg/day in divided doses q6h.
Children younger than 1 yr. 10-30 mg/kg/day in divided doses q6h.
▶ **Dosage in renal impairment**
With or without loading dose of 150 mg:

Creatinine Clearance (mL/min)	Dosage
≥ 40	100 mg q6h (extended-release, 200 mg q12h)
30-39	100 mg q8h
15-29	100 mg q12h
< 15	100 mg q24h

▶ **Dosage in liver impairment**
Adults, Elderly weighing 50 kg and more. 100 mg q6h (200 mg q12h with extended-release capsules).

▸ **Dosage in cardiomyopathy, cardiac decompensation**

Adults, Elderly weighing 50 kg and more. No loading dose; 100 mg q6-8h with gradual dosage adjustments.

OFF-LABEL USES

Prophylaxis and treatment of supraventricular tachycardia (atrial fibrillation, atrial flutter).

CONTRAINDICATIONS

Cardiogenic shock, narrow-angle glaucoma (unless patient is undergoing cholinergic therapy), preexisting second- or third-degree atrioventricular (AV) block, congenital QT syndrome.

INTERACTIONS

Drug

CYP3A4 inducers/inhibitors: May decrease/increase levels and effects of disopyramide.

Other antiarrhythmics, including diltiazem, propranolol, verapamil: May prolong cardiac conduction, decrease cardiac output.

Pimozide: May increase cardiac arrhythmias.

QT-prolonging agents: May increase risk for QT prolongation.

Herbal and Food

None known.

DIAGNOSTIC TEST EFFECTS

May decrease blood glucose levels. May cause ECG changes. May increase serum cholesterol and triglyceride levels. Therapeutic serum level is 2-8 mcg/mL, and the toxic serum level is > 8 mcg/mL.

SIDE EFFECTS

Frequent (> 9%)

Dry mouth (32%), urinary hesitancy, constipation.

Occasional (3%-9%)

Blurred vision; dry eyes, nose, or throat; urinary retention; headache; dizziness; fatigue; nausea.

Rare (< 1%)

Impotence, hypotension, edema, weight gain, shortness of breath, syncope, chest pain, nervousness, diarrhea, vomiting, decreased appetite, rash, itching.

SERIOUS REACTIONS

• May produce or aggravate congestive heart failure (CHF).
• May produce severe hypotension, shortness of breath, chest pain, syncope (especially in patients with primary cardiomyopathy or CHF).
• May cause arrhythmias, monitor for QT prolongation.
• Hepatotoxicity occurs rarely.

PRECAUTIONS & CONSIDERATIONS

Caution is warranted in patients with atrial fibrillation or flutter, bundle-branch block, CHF, impaired liver or renal function, myasthenia gravis, prostatic hypertrophy (avoid use), glaucoma (avoid use), sick sinus syndrome (sinus bradycardia alternating with tachycardia), and Wolff-Parkinson-White syndrome. Nasal decongestants or OTC cold preparations, especially those containing stimulants, should be avoided without the physician's approval. Alcohol and salt consumption should also be avoided. Dizziness and light-headedness may occur. Notify the physician if cough or shortness of breath occurs. The patient should urinate before taking this drug to reduce the risk of urine retention. BP; ECG for cardiac changes; blood glucose; liver enzyme; and serum alkaline phosphatase, bilirubin, potassium, AST (SGOT), and ALT (SGPT) levels should be assessed.

Disopyramide's therapeutic serum level is 2-8 mcg/mL and toxic serum level is > 8 mcg/mL.

Administration
Dosage must be individualized. Do not chew or break extended-release capsules.

Disulfiram
die-sul′fi-ram
(Antabuse)

CATEGORY AND SCHEDULE
Pregnancy Risk Category: C

Classification: Aldehyde dehydrogenase inhibitor

MECHANISM OF ACTION
A thiuram derivative and an irreversible aldehyde dehydrogenase inhibitor. When taken with alcohol, there is an increase in serum acetaldehyde levels. *Therapeutic Effect:* Produces an acute sensitivity to alcohol.

PHARMACOKINETICS
Slowly absorbed from the GI tract. Metabolized in liver. Primarily excreted in urine. Up to 20% of dose remains in body for at least 1 wk. *Half-life:* Unknown.

AVAILABILITY
Tablets: 250 mg, 500 mg

INDICATIONS AND DOSAGES
▸**Adjunct in management of selected chronic alcoholic patients who want to remain in state of enforced sobriety**
PO
Adults, Elderly. Initially, administer maximum of 500 mg daily given as a single dose for 1-2 wks.

Maintenance: 250 mg daily (normal range: 125-500 mg). Do not exceed maximum daily dose of 500 mg.

CONTRAINDICATIONS
Severe heart disease, psychosis, hypersensitivity to disulfiram or any component of the formulation; patients receiving or using ethanol, metronidazole, paraldehyde, or ethanol-containing products.

DRUG INTERACTIONS
Alcohol, alcohol-containing syrups, elixers, solutions: Increased disulfiram reaction.
Long-acting benzodiazepines: Increased central nervous system (CNS) depression.
Metronidazole (do not use), tricyclic antidepressants: Risk of psychosis.
Phenytoin: Increased phenytoin levels.
Food
Alcohol-containing extracts, vinegars, ciders, foods: Increased disulfiram reaction.

DIAGNOSTIC TEST EFFECTS
Increased liver enzymes.

SIDE EFFECTS/ADVERSE REACTIONS
Frequent
Drowsiness.
Occasional
Headache, restlessness, optic neuritis (impaired color perception, altered vision), peripheral neuropathy, metallic or garlic taste, rash.

SERIOUS REACTIONS
• Disulfiram-alcohol reactions to ingestion of alcohol in any form include flushing/throbbing in head and neck, throbbing headache, nausea, copious vomiting, diaphoresis, dyspnea, hyperventilation, tachycardia, hypotension, marked

uneasiness, vertigo, blurred vision, confusion, and death.

PRECAUTIONS & CONSIDERATIONS

Never administer to patient in state of alcohol intoxication or without patient's full knowledge. Do not administer until patient has abstained from alcohol for at least 12 hours. Fully inform patient of the disulfiram-alcohol reaction. Advise patients to avoid all alcohol containing products including mouthwashes, OTC products, and skin products. Use with caution in patients with diabetes mellitus, hypothyroidism, seizure disorders, cerebral damage, chronic or acute nephritis, or hepatic disease. Safety and effectiveness have not been established in children. Unique precautions have not been observed in the elderly. Not known if excreted in breast milk; do not breast feed.
Storage
Store at room temperature.
Administration
May be taken in the evening if causes sedation. Tablets may be crushed and mixed with water or juice.

Dobutamine
doe-byoo'ta-meen
Do not confuse dobutamine with Dopamine.

CATEGORY AND SCHEDULE
Pregnancy Risk Category: B

Classification: Adrenergic agonists, inotropes

MECHANISM OF ACTION
A direct-acting inotropic agent acting primarily on β_2-adrenergic receptors. *Therapeutic Effect:* Decreases preload and afterload, and enhances myocardial contractility, stroke volume, and cardiac output. Improves renal blood flow and urine output indirectly.

PHARMACOKINETICS

Route	Onset	Peak	Duration
IV	1-2 min	10 min	Length of infusion

Metabolized in the liver and tissues. Primarily excreted in urine. Not removed by hemodialysis. *Half-life:* 2 min.

AVAILABILITY
Injection (Premix with Dextrose):
1000 mg/250 mL, 250 mg/250 mL, 250 mg/500 mL, 500 mg/250 mL, 500 mg/500 mL.
Injection: 12.5-mg/mL vial.

INDICATIONS AND DOSAGES
▶ **Short-term management of cardiac decompensation**
IV INFUSION
Adults, Elderly, Children.
2.5-15 mcg/kg/min. Rarely, drug can be infused at a rate of up to 40 mcg/kg/min to increase cardiac output.

CONTRAINDICATIONS
Idiopathic hypertrophic subaortic stenosis, sulfite sensitivity.

INTERACTIONS
Drug
β-Blockers: May antagonize the effects of dobutamine.
Digoxin: May increase the risk of arrhythmias and enhance the inotropic effect of both drugs.
MAOIs, oxytocics, tricyclic antidepressants: May increase the adverse effects of dobutamine, such as arrhythmias and hypertension. MAOIs are contraindicated.
Herbal and Food
None known.

D

DIAGNOSTIC TEST EFFECTS
Decreases serum potassium level.

⚠️ IV INCOMPATIBILITIES
Acyclovir (Zovirax), alteplase (Activase), aminophylline, amphotericin B cholesteryl (Amphotec), amphotericin B liposomal (AmBisome), ampicillin, ampicillin/sulbactam (Unasyn), azathioprine, cefazolin, cefotetan (Cefotan), cefoxitin (Mefoxin), ceftriaxone (Rocephin), cefuroxime (Zinacef), chloramphenicol, dantrolene, dexamethasone sodium phosphate, ertapenem (Invanz), fluorouracil, folic acid, foscarnet (Foscavir), ganciclovir, hydrocortisone sodium succinate (Solu-Cortef), indomethacin, ketorolac, lansoprazole (Prevacid), methicillin, methotrexate, micafungin (Mycamine), oxacillin, pantoprazole (Protonix), pemetrexed (Alimta), penicillin G potassium, penicillin G sodium, pentobarbital, phenobarbital, phenytoin, piperacillin, piperacillin/tazobactam (Zosyn), sodium bicarbonate, sulfamethoxazole/trimethoprim, ticarcillin (Ticar), ticarcillin/clavulanate (Timentin), warfarin.

💉 IV COMPATIBILITIES
Alfentanil (Alfenta), alprostadil (Prostin VR), amifostine (Ethyol), amikacin (Amikar), amiodarone (Cordarone), anidulafungin (Eraxis), argatroban, ascorbic acid, atracurium (Tracrium), atropine, aztreonam (Azactam), benztropine (Cogentin), bretylium, buprenorphine (Buprenex), butorphanol (Stadol), calcium chloride, carboplatin, caspofungin (Cancidas), chlorpromazine, cimetidine (Tagamet), ciprofloxacin (Cipro), cisatracurium (Nimbex), cisplatin, cladribine (Leustatin), clonidine, cyanocobalamin, cyclophosphamide (Cytoxan), cyclosporine (Sandimmune), dactinomycin (Cosmegen), daptomycin (Cubicin), dexmedetomidine (Precedex), digoxin (Lanoxin), diltiazem (Cardizem), diphenhydramine (Benadryl), docetaxel (Taxotere), doxorubicin (Adriamycin), doxorubicin liposomal (Doxil), enalaprilat, ephedrine, epinephrine, epirubicin (Ellence), erythromycin lactobionate, etoposide phosphate (Etopophos), famotidine (Pepcid), fenoldopam (Corlopam), fentanyl (Sublimaze), fluconazole (Diflucan), fludarabine (Fludara), gemcitabine (Gemzar), gentamicin, granisetron (Kytril), hydromorphone (Dilaudid), hydroxyzine, isoproterenol (Isuprel), labetalol, levofloxacin (Levaquin), lidocaine, linezolid (Zyvox), lorazepam (Ativan), mannitol, meperidine (Demerol), methylprednisolone sodium succinate, metoclopramide (Reglan), metoprolol (Lopressor), milrinone (Primacor), minocycline (Minocin), mitoxantrone (Novantrone), morphine, nafcillin, nalbuphine (Nubain), naloxone (Narcan), nicardipine (Cardene), nitroglycerin, norepinephrine (Levophed), ondansetron (Zofran), oxaliplatin (Eloxatin), oxytocin (Pitocin), paclitaxel (Taxol), palonosetron (Aloxi), pancuronium, potassium chloride, procainamide, prochlorperazine, promethazine, propofol (Diprivan), propranolol, ranitidine (Zantac), remifentanil (Ultiva), rituximab (Rituxan), sodium acetate, streptokinase, succinylcholine, sufentanil (Sufenta), tacrolimus (Prograf), teniposide (Vumon), theophylline, thiotepa (Thioplex),

tigecycline (Tygacil), tirofibran (Aggrastat), tobramycin, trastuzumab (Herceptin), vancomycin, vasopressin, vecuronium (Norcuron), verapamil, vincristine (Vincasar), vinorelbine (Navelbine), voriconazole (Vfend), zidovudine (Retrovir).

SIDE EFFECTS

Frequent (> 5%)
Increased heart rate, increased BP.
Occasional (3%-5%)
Pain at injection site, phlebitis.
Rare (1%-3%)
Nausea, headache, anginal pain, shortness of breath, fever.

SERIOUS REACTIONS

• Overdose may produce a marked increase in heart rate (by 30 beats/min or higher), marked increase in BP (by 50 mm Hg or higher), anginal pain, and premature ventricular contractions (PVCs).
• May cause hypotension in some patients. Tachycardia, marked increases in BP, or ventricular ectopy may occur.

PRECAUTIONS & CONSIDERATIONS

Caution is warranted in patients with atrial fibrillation, aortic stenosis, hypovolemia, post myocardial infarction, and hypertension. It is unknown whether dobutamine crosses the placenta or is distributed in breast milk; therefore, it is not administered to pregnant women. No age-related precautions have been noted in children or in elderly patients. Start at lower end of dosage range for elderly patients.

Notify the physician of chest pain or palpitations during infusion or pain or burning at the IV site. Cardiac monitoring should be performed continuously to check for arrhythmias. BP, heart rate, urine

output, and respiration should be checked before and during treatment. Serum potassium and dobutamine plasma levels should be monitored; keep in mind that dobutamine's therapeutic range is 40-190 ng/mL.
Storage
Store at room temperature because freezing produces crystallization. Pink discoloration of the solution, caused by oxidation, does not indicate loss of potency if the solution is used within the recommended period. Further diluted solution for infusion must be used within 24 h.
Administration
! Dobutamine dosage is determined by the patient's response to the drug. Plan to correct hypovolemia with volume expanders before dobutamine infusion. Expect to administer digoxin to patients with atrial fibrillation before infusion. Administer by IV infusion only.

For IV use, further dilute the injection concentrate with either D5%W or 0.9% NaCl. Usual final concentrations are 2000 mcg/mL or 4000 mcg/mL. Maximum should not exceed 5000 mcg/mL. Infuse into a large vein. Also available in pre-mixed solutions for infusion.

During CPR, may be infused via the intraosseous route if IV is not available. Use infusion pump to control flow rate. Titrate dosage to individual response, as prescribed.

Docosanol
do-cos′ah-nole
(Abreva)

CATEGORY AND SCHEDULE
Pregnancy Risk Category: B

Classification: Synthetic lipophilic alcohol

MECHANISM OF ACTION
A highly lipophilic, fatty alcohol that prevents fusion of lipid-enveloped viruses with cell membranes, thereby blocking viral replication.

PHARMACOKINETICS
Topical: Negligible absorption.

AVAILABILITY
Cream: 10%.

INDICATIONS AND DOSAGES
▸**Recurrent herpes labialis**
TOPICAL
Adult, Children older than 12 yr.
Apply a small amount to the affected area on the face or lips or at the first sign of lesion 5 times a day until healed.

CONTRAINDICATIONS
Hypersensitivity.

INTERACTIONS
Drug
None reported.

SIDE EFFECTS
CNS: Headache.
Integument: Site reaction, rash, pruritus, dry skin, acne.

PRECAUTIONS & CONSIDERATIONS
Avoid application into eyes or mouth; for external use only. Not for use in children less than 12 years of age.
Storage
Store at room temperature. Do not freeze.
Administration
Wash hands before and after use.

Docusate
dok′yoo-sate
(Coloxyl [AUS], Apo-Docusate [CAN], Colace, Colax-C [CAN], Correctol, Diocto, Docusoft-S, DOK, D.O.S., Dulcolax, Novo-Ducosate [CAN], Phillips', PMS-Docusate [CAN], Regulex [CAN], Selax [CAN], Soflax [CAN], Silace, Sulfolax)

CATEGORY AND SCHEDULE
Pregnancy Risk Category: C
OTC

Classification: Laxatives, Stool softeners

MECHANISM OF ACTION
A bulk-producing laxative that decreases surface film tension by mixing liquid and bowel contents. *Therapeutic Effect:* Increases infiltration of liquid to form a softer stool.

PHARMACOKINETICS
Minimal absorption from the GI tract. Acts in small and large intestines. Results usually occur 1-2 days after first dose but may take 3-5 days.

AVAILABILITY
Capsules (Docusate Sodium; Colace, D.O.S., DOK): 50 mg, 100 mg, 250 mg.
Capsules (Docusoft-S): 100 mg.
Capsules, Liquid Filled (Correctol, Doc-Q-Lace, Dulcolax, Phillips'): 100 mg.
Capsules (Docusate Calcium; Sulfolax, Sur-Q-Lax): 240 mg.
Capsules, Liquid Filled (Docusate Calcium; DC Softgel, Kao-Tin, Kaopectate): 240 mg.
Liquid, Docusate Sodium: 10 mg/1 mL (Colace), 50 mg/5 mL, 150 mg/ 15 mL (Doc-Q-Lace).

Syrup (Colace, Diocto): 50 mg/5 mL, 60 mg/15 mL, 20 mg/5 mL (Silace).

INDICATIONS AND DOSAGES
▶ **Stool softener**
PO
Adults, Elderly, Children 12 yr and older. 50-300 mg/day in 1-4 divided doses.
Children 6-11 yr. 40-150 mg/day in 1-4 divided doses.
Children 3-5 yr. 20-60 mg/day in 1-4 divided doses.
Children younger than 3 yr. 10-40 mg/day in 1-4 divided doses.

CONTRAINDICATIONS
Acute abdominal pain, concomitant use of mineral oil, intestinal obstruction, nausea, vomiting, hypersensitivity.

INTERACTIONS
Drug
Mineral oil: May increase the absorption of mineral oil.
Herbal and Food
None known.

DIAGNOSTIC TEST EFFECTS
None known.

SIDE EFFECTS
Occasional
Mild GI cramping, throat irritation (with liquid preparation), diarrhea.
Rare
Rash.

SERIOUS REACTIONS
• None known.

PRECAUTIONS & CONSIDERATIONS
It is unknown whether docusate is distributed in breast milk, considered compatible with breastfeeding. No age-related precautions have been noted in elderly patients.

Notify the physician if unrelieved constipation, dizziness, muscle cramps or pain, rectal bleeding, or weakness occurs. Maintain adequate fluid intake. Monitor pattern of daily bowel activity and stool consistency.
Administration
Drink 6-8 glasses of water a day to aid in stool softening. Take each dose with full glass of water or fruit juice. Administer docusate liquid with infant formula, fruit juice, or milk to mask the bitter taste. To promote defecation, increase fluid intake, exercise, and eat a high-fiber diet.

Dofetilide
doe-fet′ill-ide
(Tikosyn)

CATEGORY AND SCHEDULE
Pregnancy Risk Category: C

Classification: Antiarrhythmics, class III

MECHANISM OF ACTION
A selective potassium channel blocker that prolongs repolarization without affecting conduction velocity by blocking one or more time-dependent potassium currents. Dofetilide has no effect on sodium channels or adrenergic α or β receptors. *Therapeutic Effect:* Terminates reentrant tachyarrhythmias, preventing reinduction.

AVAILABILITY
Capsules: 125 mcg, 250 mcg, 500 mcg.

INDICATIONS AND DOSAGES
▸ **Maintain normal sinus rhythm after conversion from atrial fibrillation or flutter**
PO
Adults, Elderly. Individualized using a seven-step dosing algorithm dependent on calculated creatinine clearance and QT-interval measurements. See prescribing information. Usual range: 125-500 mcg twice daily. Maximum: 500 mcg twice daily.
▸ **Starting dosage in renal impairment**
CrCl > 60 mL/min: 500 mcg twice a day.
CrCl 40-60 mL/min: 250 mcg twice a day.
CrCl 20-39 mL/min: 125 mcg twice a day.
CrCl < 20 mL/min: Do not use.

CONTRAINDICATIONS
Concurrent use of drugs that prolong the QT interval; concurrent use of amiodarone, cimetidine, hydrochlorothiazide, megestrol, metformin, prochlorperazine, trimethoprim, or verapamil; congenital or acquired prolonged QT syndrome; paroxysmal atrial fibrillation; severe renal impairment.

INTERACTIONS
Drug
Amiloride, megestrol, metformin, prochlorperazine, triamterene: May increase plasma levels of dofetilide. Contraindicated.
Bepridil, phenothiazines, tricyclic antidepressants, other QT-interval prolonging agents: May prolong the QT interval.
Cimetidine, verapamil: Increases levels of dofetilide. Contraindicated.
Diuretics, drugs that deplete potassium or magnesium: May increase dofetilide toxicity. Hydrochlorothiazide contraindicated.
Ketoconazole, itraconazole, trimethoprim: Increase plasma concentration of dofetilide. Contraindicated.
Food
Grapefruit juice: Can increase dofetilide plasma levels.

DIAGNOSTIC TEST EFFECTS
None known.

SIDE EFFECTS
Occasional (< 15%)
Headache, chest pain, dizziness, dyspnea, nausea, insomnia, back and abdominal pain, diarrhea, rash.

SERIOUS REACTIONS
• Angioedema, bradycardia, cerebral ischemia, facial paralysis, and serious ventricular arrhythmias or various forms of heart block may be noted.

PRECAUTIONS & CONSIDERATIONS
Continuous cardiac and BP monitoring should be instituted. ECG for ventricular arrhythmias and for prolongation of the QT interval and serum creatinine level for changes should be monitored. Patients must have continuous ECG monitoring for 3 days, and drug should be initiated in hospital setting. Should reserve dofetilide for symptomatic atrial fibrillation/flutter. Avoid in patients with 2nd- or 3rd-degree heart block or sinus sick syndrome. Correct electrolyte imbalances before and during dofetilide therapy. Caution is warranted in hepatic and renal impairment. Safety and efficacy have not been evaluated in children. Notify the physician if dizziness, severe diarrhea, or other adverse effects occur.
Administration
! Expect patient to be hospitalized for a minimum of 3 days when treatment is instituted. Administer dofetilide at the same times each

day without regard to food. Follow dosing instructions diligently.

If dofetilide needs to be discontinued to allow for dosing of potentially interacting drugs, a 2-day washout period should be followed before starting the other drug.

Dolasetron
doe-lass'eh-tron
(Anzemet)
Do not confuse Anzemet with Aldomet.

CATEGORY AND SCHEDULE
Pregnancy Risk Category: B

Classification: Antiemetics, serotonin receptor antagonists.

MECHANISM OF ACTION
A 5-HT3 receptor antagonist that acts centrally in the chemoreceptor trigger zone and peripherally at the vagal nerve terminals. *Therapeutic Effect:* Prevents nausea and vomiting.

PHARMACOKINETICS
Readily absorbed from the GI tract after PO administration. Protein binding: 69%-77%. Metabolized in the liver. Primarily excreted in urine. Unknown if removed by hemodialysis. *Half-life:* 5-10 h.

AVAILABILITY
Tablets: 50 mg, 100 mg.
Injection: 20 mg/mL in single-use 0.625-mL amps, 0.625-mL fill-in 2-mL Carpuject and 5-mL vials.

INDICATIONS AND DOSAGES
▸ **Prevention of chemotherapy-induced nausea and vomiting**
PO
Adults. 100 mg within 1 h of chemotherapy.
Children 2-16 yr. 1.8 mg/kg within 1 h of chemotherapy. Maximum: 100 mg.
IV
Adults, Children 2-16 yr. 1.8 mg/kg as a single dose 30 min before chemotherapy. Maximum: 100 mg.
▸ **Treatment (IV) or prevention of postoperative nausea or vomiting (IV/PO)**
PO
Adults. 100 mg within 2 h of surgery.
Children. 2-16 yr. 1.2 mg/kg within 2 h of surgery. Maximum: 100 mg.
IV
Adults. 12.5 mg 15 min before cessation of anesthesia or as soon as nausea occurs.
Children. 2-16 yr. 0.35 mg/kg 15 min before cessation of anesthesia or as soon as nausea occurs. Maximum: 12.5 mg.

OFF-LABEL USES
Radiation therapy-induced nausea and vomiting.

CONTRAINDICATIONS
Hypersensitivity.

INTERACTIONS
Drug
Agents that cause QTc prolongation: Caution should be used with these agents.

DIAGNOSTIC TEST EFFECTS
May transiently increase AST (SGOT) and ALT (SGPT) levels.

⚕ IV INCOMPATIBILITIES
Amphotericin B liposomal
(AmBisome), pantoprazole
(Protonix).

⚕ IV COMPATIBILITIES
Azithromycin (Zithromax),
bivalirudin (Angiomax),
caspofungin (Cancidas), cefazolin,
cefepime (Maxipime), cefotaxime
(Claforan), cyclophosphamide
(Cytoxan), daptomycin (Cubicin),
dexmedetomidine (Precedex),
doxorubicin (Adriamycin),
epirubicin (Ellence), ertapenem
(Invanz), fenoldopam (Corlopam),
levofloxacin (Levaquin), linezolid
(Zyvox), mannitol, meperidine
(Demerol), oxaliplatin (Eloxatin),
oxytocin (Pitocin), pemetrexed
(Alimta), quinupristin/dalfopristin
(Synercid), sodium acetate,
tacrolimus (Prograf), tigecycline
(Tygacil), tirofiban (Aggrastat),
vecuronium (Norcuron), vincristine
(Vincasar), voriconazole (Vfend).

SIDE EFFECTS
Frequent (4%-24%)
Headache, diarrhea, fatigue,
hypotension.
Occasional (1%-5%)
Fever, dizziness, pruritus,
bradycardia, tachycardia,
hypertension, dyspepsia.

SERIOUS REACTIONS
• Overdose may produce a
combination of central nervous
system (CNS) stimulant and
depressant effects.
• Changes in ECG intervals, including
QT, have occurred within hours after
IV administration and rarely lead to
heart block or arrhythmia.

PRECAUTIONS & CONSIDERATIONS
Caution is warranted in patients
with congenital prolonged QT
interval syndrome, hypokalemia,
hypomagnesemia, and prolonged
cardiac conduction intervals.
Caution should also be used
with concurrent use of diuretics,
because this can cause electrolyte
disturbances, antiarrhythmics that
may lead to prolonged QT interval,
and high doses of anthracyclines.
It is unknown whether dolasetron
is distributed in breast milk. The
safety and efficacy of this drug have
not been established in children
younger than 2 yr. No age-related
precautions have been noted in
elderly patients.
Storage
Store vials at room temperature.
After dilution, store solution for up
to 24 h at room temperature or up to
48 h if refrigerated.
Administration
Do not cut, break, or chew film-
coated tablets. For children aged
2-16 yr, the injection form may be
mixed in apple or apple-grape juice
and given orally, if needed; see
children's oral dosage. May be at
room temperature for 2 h.
    For IV use, dilute the injection in
0.9% NaCl, D5W, dextrose 5% in
0.45% NaCl, lactated Ringer's (LR)
solution, D5LR, or 10% mannitol
injection to 50 mL. Administer by IV
push as rapidly as 100 mg/30 s or by
intermittent or piggyback IV infusion
over 15 min.

Donepezil
dah-nep'eh-zil
(Aricept)
**Do not confuse Aricept with
Aciphex or Ascriptin.**

CATEGORY AND SCHEDULE
Pregnancy Risk Category: C

Classification: Cholinesterase
inhibitors

MECHANISM OF ACTION
A cholinesterase inhibitor
that inhibits the enzyme
acetylcholinesterase, thus increasing
the concentration of acetylcholine at
cholinergic synapses and enhancing
cholinergic function in the central
nervous system (CNS). *Therapeutic
Effect:* Slows the progression of
Alzheimer disease.

PHARMACOKINETICS
Well absorbed after PO
administration. Protein binding: 96%.
Extensively metabolized. Eliminated
in urine and feces. *Half-life:* 70 h.

AVAILABILITY
Tablets: 5 mg, 10 mg.
Orally Disintegrating Tablets: 5 mg,
10 mg.

INDICATIONS AND DOSAGES
▸ **Alzheimer disease**
PO
Adults, Elderly. 5-10 mg/day as a
single dose. If initial dose is 5 mg, do
not increase to 10 mg for 4-6 wks.

CONTRAINDICATIONS
History of hypersensitivity to
donepezil or piperidine derivatives,
acute jaundice, active GI bleeding.

INTERACTIONS
Drug
Anticholinergics: May decrease the
effect of donepezil.
**Cholinergic agonists,
neuromuscular blockers,
succinylcholine:** May increase
cholinergic effects.
**Ketoconazole, quinidine, CYP3A4
inhibitors:** May inhibit the
metabolism of donepezil.
NSAIDs: Increase GI irritation.
Monitor for GI bleeding.
Paroxetine, CYP2D6 inhibitors:
May decrease the metabolism and
increase the blood concentration of
donepezil.
Herbal
None known.
Food
None known.

DIAGNOSTIC TEST EFFECTS
May increase blood glucose, alkaline
phosphatase, and serum creatinine
kinase and LDH concentrations.
May decrease the serum potassium
level.

SIDE EFFECTS
Frequent (8%-19%)
Nausea, diarrhea, headache,
insomnia, nonspecific pain,
dizziness, infection, anorexia.
Occasional (3%-6%)
Mild muscle cramps, fatigue,
vomiting, ecchymosis.
Rare (2%-3%)
Depression, abnormal dreams,
weight loss, hypertension, arthritis,
somnolence, syncope, frequent
urination.

SERIOUS REACTIONS
• Vagotonic effects may include
bradycardia, heart block, and
syncopal episodes.
• Overdose may result in
cholinergic crisis, characterized

D

by severe nausea, increased salivation, diaphoresis, bradycardia, hypotension, flushed skin, abdominal pain, respiratory depression, seizures, and cardiorespiratory collapse. Increasing muscle weakness may result in death if respiratory muscles are involved. The antidote is 1-2 mg IV atropine sulfate with subsequent doses based on therapeutic response.

PRECAUTIONS & CONSIDERATIONS

Caution is warranted with asthma; bladder outflow obstruction; prostatic hypertrophy; chronic obstructive pulmonary disease (COPD); peptic ulcer disease; history of seizures, sick sinus syndrome, or other supraventricular conduction disturbances (bradycardia); and concurrent use of NSAIDs. It is unknown whether donepezil is distributed in breast milk. Donepezil is not prescribed for children. No age-related precautions have been noted in elderly patients. Be aware that donepezil is not a cure for Alzheimer disease but may slow the progression of its symptoms. Safety and efficacy have not been evaluated in children.

Notify the physician if abdominal pain, diarrhea, excessive sweating or salivation, dizziness, or nausea and vomiting occur. Baseline vital signs should be assessed. Cholinergic reactions, such as diaphoresis, dizziness, excessive salivation, facial warmth, abdominal cramps or discomfort, lacrimation, pallor, and urinary urgency, should be monitored.

Administration
Take donepezil without regard to food. The drug may be given in the morning or evening; however, best results (limited side effects) may be achieved if it is given at bedtime.

Allow orally disintegrating tablet to dissolve on tongue. They can be given with or without liquid.

Dopamine
doe′pa-meen
(Dopamine Injection [AUS])
Do not confuse dopamine with dobutamine or Dopram

CATEGORY AND SCHEDULE
Pregnancy Risk Category: C

Classification: Adrenergic agonists, inotropes

MECHANISM OF ACTION
A sympathomimetic (adrenergic agonist) that stimulates adrenergic receptors. Effects are dose dependent. Low dosages (0.5-2 mcg/kg/min) stimulate dopaminergic receptors, causing renal vasodilation. Low to moderate dosages (2-10 mcg/kg/min) have a positive inotropic effect by direct action and release of norepinephrine. High dosages (> 10 mcg/kg/min) stimulate α-receptors. *Therapeutic Effect:* With low dosages, increases renal blood flow, urine flow, and sodium excretion. With low to moderate dosages, increases myocardial contractility, stroke volume, and cardiac output. With high dosages, increases peripheral resistance, renal vasoconstriction, and systolic and diastolic BP.

PHARMACOKINETICS

Route	Onset	Peak	Duration
IV	1-2 min	N/A	< 10 min

Widely distributed. Does not cross blood-brain barrier. Metabolized in the liver, kidney, and plasma. Primarily excreted in urine. Not removed by hemodialysis. *Half-life:* 2 min.

AVAILABILITY

Injection: 40 mg/mL, 80 mg/mL, 160 mg/mL.
Injection (Premix With Dextrose): 80 mg/100 mL, 160 mg/100 mL, 200 mg/250 mL, 320 mg/100 mL, 400 mg/250 mL, 400 mg/500 mL, 800 mg/250 mL, 800 mg/500 mL.

INDICATIONS AND DOSAGES

▶ **Treatment and prevention of acute hypotension; shock (associated with cardiac decompensation, myocardial infarction, open heart surgery, renal failure, or trauma); treatment of low cardiac output; treatment of congestive heart failure**
IV

Adults, Elderly. 1-5 mcg/kg/min up to 50 mcg/kg/min titrated to desired response. Increase rate by 1-4 mcg/kg/min at 10- to 30-min intervals.
Children. 1-20 mcg/kg/min. Maximum: 20 mcg/kg/min. Rates > 20 mcg/kg/min in children and infants may result in excessive vasoconstriction.
Neonates. 1-20 mcg/kg/min. Effects are dose-dependent (see Mechanism of Action).

CONTRAINDICATIONS

Pheochromocytoma, sulfite sensitivity, uncorrected tachyarrhythmias, ventricular fibrillation.

INTERACTIONS

Drug
β-Blockers: May decrease the effects of dopamine.

Digoxin: May increase the risk of arrhythmias.
Ergot alkaloids: May increase vasoconstriction.
MAOIs: May increase cardiac stimulation and vasopressor effects.
Tricyclic antidepressants, oxytocics: May increase cardiovascular effects.
Herbal and Food
None known.

DIAGNOSTIC TEST EFFECTS
None known.

🚫 IV INCOMPATIBILITIES

Acyclovir (Zovirax), amphotericin B cholesteryl (Amphotec), amphotericin B liposomal (AmBisome), ampicillin, azathioprine, cefazolin, cefepime (Maxipime), chloramphenicol, dantrolene, diazepam (Valium), ganciclovir (Cytovene), furosemide (Lasix), indomethacin, lansoprazole (Prevacid), methotrexate, phenytoin, sodium bicarbonate, sulfamethoxazole/trimethoprim.

💉 IV COMPATIBILITIES

Alfentanil (Alfenta), alprostadil (Prostin VR), amifostine (Ethyol), amikacin (Amikar), aminophylline, amiodarone (Cordarone), anidulafungin (Eraxis), argatroban, ascorbic acid, atracurium (Tracrium), atropine, aztreonam (Azactam), benztropine (Cogentin), bivalirudin (Angiomax), bretylium, bumetanide (Bumex), buprenorphine (Buprenex), butorphanol (Stadol), calcium chloride, calcium gluconate, carboplatin, caspofungin (Cancidas), cefotaxime (Claforan), cefotetan (Cefotan), cefoxitin (Mefoxin), ceftazidime (Ceptaz, Fortaz, Tazicef, Tazidime), ceftizoxime (Cefizox), ceftriaxone (Rocephin), cefuroxime

D

(Zinacef), chlorpromazine, cimetidine (Tagamet), ciprofloxacin (Cipro), cisatracurium (Nimbex), cisplatin, clindamycin (Cleocin), clonidine, cyclophosphamide (Cytoxan), cyclosporine (Sandimmune), dactinomycin (Cosmegen), daptomycin (Cubicin), dexamethasone sodium phosphate, dexmedetomidine (Precedex), digoxin (Lanoxin), diltiazem (Cardizem), diphenhydramine (Benadryl), dobutamine (Dobutrex), docetaxel (Taxotere), doripenem (Doribax), doxorubicin (Adriamycin), doxorubicin liposomal (Doxil), droperidol, enalaprilat, ephedrine, epinephrine, epirubicin (Ellence), epoetin alfa (Procrit), ertapenem (Invanz), erythromycin lactobionate, esmolol (Brevibloc), etoposide phosphate (Etopophos), famotidine (Pepcid), fenoldopam (Corlopam), fentanyl (Sublimaze), fluconazole (Diflucan), fludarabine (Fludara), fluorouracil, folic acid, foscarnet (Foscavir), gemcitabine (Gemzar), gentamicin, granisetron (Kytril), heparin, hydrocortisone sodium phosphate, hydrocortisone sodium succinate (Solu-Cortef), hydromorphone (Dilaudid), hydroxyzine, imipenem/cilastatin (Primaxin), isoproterenol (Isuprel), ketorolac, labetalol, levofloxacin (Levaquin), lidocaine, linezolid (Zyvox), lorazepam (Ativan), magnesium sulfate, mannitol, meperidine (Demerol), methicillin, methylprednisolone (Solu-Medrol), metoclopramide (Reglan), metoprolol (Lopressor), micafungin (Mycamine), midazolam (Versed), milrinone (Primacor), minocycline (Minocin), mitoxantrone (Novantrone), morphine, nafcillin, nalbuphine (Nubain), naloxone (Narcan), nicardipine (Cardene), nitroglycerin, nitroprusside sodium (Nitropress), norepinephrine (Levophed), ondansetron (Zofran), oxacillin, oxaliplatin (Eloxatin), oxytocin (Pitocin), paclitaxel (Taxol), palonosetron (Aloxi), pancuronium, pemetrexed (Alimta), penicillin G sodium, pentobarbital, phenobarbital, piperacillin, piperacillin tazobactam (Zosyn), potassium chloride, procainamide, prochloperazine, promethazine, propofol (Diprivan), propranolol, ranitidine (Zantac), remifentanil (Ultiva), rituximab (Rituxan), sargramostim (Leukine), sodium acetate, streptokinase, succinylcholine, sufentanil (Sufenta), tacrolimus (Prograf), teniposide (Vumon), theophylline, thiotepa (Thioplex), ticarcillin (Ticar), ticarcillin/clavulanate (Timentin), tigecycline (Tygacil), tirofibran (Aggrastat), tobramycin, trastuzumab (Herceptin), vancomycin, vasopressin, vecuronium (Norcuron), verapamil, vincristine (Vincasar), vinorelbine (Navelbine), vitamin B complex with C, voriconazole (Vfend), warfarin, zidovudine (Retrovir).

SIDE EFFECTS

Frequent
Headache, ectopic beats, tachycardia, anginal pain, palpitations, vasoconstriction, hypotension, nausea, vomiting, dyspnea.
Occasional
Piloerection or goose bumps, bradycardia, widening of QRS complex.

SERIOUS REACTIONS

• High doses may produce ventricular arrhythmias, tachycardia.
• Patients with occlusive vascular disease are at high risk for further compromise of circulation to the extremities, which may result in gangrene.

• Tissue necrosis with sloughing may occur with extravasation of IV solution.

PRECAUTIONS & CONSIDERATIONS

Caution is warranted in patients with ischemic heart disease, cardiac arrhythmias, post myocardial infarction, and occlusive vascular disease. Be aware that dopamine dosage may have to be reduced if MAOIs were taken within the last 2-3 wks. It is unknown whether dopamine crosses the placenta or is distributed in breast milk. Closely monitor children, because gangrene attributable to extravasation has been reported. No age-related precautions have been noted in elderly patients.

Cardiac monitoring should be performed continuously to check for arrhythmias. BP, heart rate, urine output, and respiration should be checked before and during treatment. Notify the physician of chest pain, palpitations, arrhythmias, decreased peripheral circulation (marked by cold, pale, or mottled extremities), decreased urine output, or significant changes in BP or heart rate, or burning at the IV site.

Storage

Unopened vials are stored at room temperature.

Dopamine is stable for 24 h after dilution. Do not use solutions darker than slightly yellow or solutions that have discolored to brown or pink to purple, because these discolorations indicate decomposition of drug.

Administration

! Expect to correct blood volume depletion before administering dopamine. Blood volume replacement may occur simultaneously with dopamine infusion.

For IV use, dilute 200-400 mg vial in 250-500 mL 0.9% NaCl, D5W/0.45% NaCl, D5W/lactated Ringer's, or lactated Ringer's. Keep in mind that the concentration is dependent on the dosage and the patient's fluid requirements. Remember that a 200 mg/250 mL solution yields 800 mcg/mL and that a 200 mg/500 mL solution yields 400 mcg/mL. The maximum infusion concentration is 3200 mcg/mL. The drug is available prediluted in 250 or 500 mL of D5W. Administer into large vein, such as the antecubital or subclavian vein, to prevent drug extravasation. Use an infusion pump to control rate of flow. Titrate dosage to the desired hemodynamic values or optimum urine flow, as prescribed. If extravasation occurs, immediately infiltrate the affected tissue with 10-15 mL 0.9% NaCl solution containing 5-10 mg phentolamine mesylate, as ordered.

During CPR, if IV is not available, may be administered by intraosseous infusion.

Dornase Alfa
door'nace al'fa
(Pulmozyme)

CATEGORY AND SCHEDULE
Pregnancy Risk Category: B

Classification: Enzymes, respiratory, mucolytics, recombinant DNA origin

MECHANISM OF ACTION
An enzyme that selectively splits and hydrolyzes DNA in sputum. *Therapeutic Effect:* Reduces sputum viscosity and elasticity.

AVAILABILITY
Inhalation: 2.5-mg ampules for nebulization.

INDICATIONS AND DOSAGES
▸ **To improve management of pulmonary function in patients with cystic fibrosis**
NEBULIZATION
Adults, Children 3 mo and older.
2.5 mg (1 ampule) once daily by recommended nebulizer. May increase to 2.5 mg twice daily.

CONTRAINDICATIONS
Sensitivity to dornase alfa.

INTERACTIONS
Drug, Herbal, and Food
None known.

DIAGNOSTIC TEST EFFECTS
None known.

SIDE EFFECTS
Frequent (> 10%)
Pharyngitis, fever, rhinitis, dyspnea, chest pain or discomfort, voice changes.
Occasional (3%-10%)
Conjunctivitis, hoarseness, rash.

SERIOUS REACTIONS
• None significant.

PRECAUTIONS & CONSIDERATIONS
Hoarseness, chest pain, and sore throat may occur during dornase alfa therapy. Viscosity of pulmonary secretions should be checked. Drink plenty of fluids. Use in children < 5 yr is limited.
Storage
Refrigerate unopened ampules and protect them from light. Keep in foil pouch until ready to use.
Administration
For nebulization, do not mix any other medications in the nebulizer with dornase alfa.

Doxapram
dox′a-pram
(Dopram)
Do not confuse doxapram with doxepin or ultram.

CATEGORY AND SCHEDULE
Pregnancy Risk Category: B

Classification: Analeptics, stimulants, central nervous system (CNS)

MECHANISM OF ACTION
A CNS stimulant that directly stimulates the respiratory center in the medulla or indirectly by effects on the carotid. *Therapeutic Effect:* Increases pulmonary ventilation by increasing resting minute ventilation, tidal volume, respiratory frequency, and inspiratory neuromuscular drive and enhances the ventilatory response to carbon dioxide.

PHARMACOKINETICS
IV onset 20-40, peak 1-2 min, duration 5-12 min. Metabolized in the liver to metabolites, ketodoxapram (active), and desethyldoxapram (inactive). Partially excreted in the urine. Not removed by hemodialysis. *Half-life:* 2.4-9.9 h.

AVAILABILITY
Injection: 20 mg/mL (Dopram).

INDICATIONS AND DOSAGES
▸ **Chronic obstructive pulmonary disease (COPD)**
IV INFUSION
Adults, Elderly, Children older than 12 yr. Initially, 1-2 mg/min. Maximum: 3 g/day for no more than 2 h.

▶ Drug-induced CNS depression
IV INJECTION
Adults, Elderly, Children older than 12 yr. Initially, 1-2 mg/kg, repeat after 5 min. May repeat at 1- to 2-h intervals, until sustained consciousness.
Maximum: 3 g/day.
IV INFUSION
Adults, Elderly, Children older than 12 yr. Initially, bolus dose of 1-2 mg/kg, repeat after 5 min. If no response, wait 1-2 h and repeat. If stimulation is noted, initiate infusion at 1-3 mg/min. Infusion should not be continued for more than 2 h.
Maximum: 3 g/day.

▶ Respiratory depression following anesthesia
IV INJECTION
Adults, Elderly, Children older than 12 yr. Initially, 0.5-1 mg/kg. May repeat at 5-min intervals in patients who demonstrate initial response.
Maximum: 2 mg/kg.
IV INFUSION
Adults, Elderly, Children older than 12 yr. Initially, 5 mg/min until adequate response or adverse effects are seen. Decrease to 1-3 mg/min.
Maximum: 4 mg/kg.

OFF-LABEL USES

Apnea of prematurity, sleep apnea, congenital central hypoventilation syndrome, obesity-hypoventilation syndrome, post-anesthetic respiratory depression, shivering.

CONTRAINDICATIONS

Convulsive disorders, cardiovascular impairment, cerebral edema, head injury or cerebrovascular accident, severe hypertension, pulmonary embolism, mechanical ventilation disorders, hypersensitivity to doxapram.

INTERACTIONS
Drug
Cyclopropane, enflurane, halothane: May increase catecholamine release. Delay the initiation of doxapram therapy for at least 10 min following discontinuation of these anesthetics known to sensitize the myocardium.
CNS-stimulant medications: May increase risk of stimulation to excessive levels, causing nervousness, insomnia, irritability, or possibly cardiac arrhythmias or seizures.
Monoamine oxidase (MAO) inhibitors, sympathomimetic agents: May increase the pressor effects of these medications or doxapram.
Herbal
None known.
Food
None known.

DIAGNOSTIC TEST EFFECTS

May decrease hemoglobin, hematocrit, or red blood cell counts. May further decrease WBC in the presence of pre-existing leukopenia. May increase BUN and albuminuria.

🚫 IV INCOMPATIBILITIES

Alkaline solutions, aminophylline (Theophylline), ascorbic acid, cefotaxime (Claforan), cefotetan (Cefotan), cefuroxime (Zinacef), clindamycin (Cleocin), dexamethasone sodium phosphate, diazepam (Valium), digoxin, dobutamine, folic acid, furosemide (Lasix), hydrocortisone sodium succinate (Solu-Cortef), ketamine (Ketalar), methylprednisolone, minocycline (Minocin), sodium bicarbonate, thiopental (Pentothal), ticarcillin (Ticar).

📋 IV COMPATIBILITIES

Amikacin (Amikin), ampicillin, bumetanide (Bumex), caffeine citrate (Cafcit), calcium chloride, calcium gluconate, cefazolin, ceftazidime (Ceptaz, Fortaz, Tazicef, Tazidime), chlorpromazine, cimetidine (Tagamet), cisplatin, cyclophosphamide (Cytosar), deslanoside, dopamine, doxycycline (Doxy-100), epinephrine, erythromycin lactobionate, fentanyl (Sublimaze), gentamicin, heparin, insulin (regular, Humulin R, Novolin R), hydroxyzine, isoniazid (Nydrazid), lincomycin (Lincocin), methotrexate, metoclopramide (Reglan), metronidazole (Flagyl), oxacillin, phenobarbital, phytonadione, pyridoxine, ranitidine (Zantac), terbutaline (Brethine), thiamine, tobramycin (Nebcin), vancomycin, vincristine.

SIDE EFFECTS

Occasional

Flushing, sweating, pruritus, disorientation, headache, dizziness, hyperactivity, convulsions, dyspnea, cough, tachypnea, hiccough, rebound hypoventilation, phlebitis, variations in heart rate, arrhythmias, chest pain, nausea, vomiting, diarrhea, stimulation of urinary bladder with spontaneous voiding.

SERIOUS REACTIONS

• Overdosage may produce extensions of the pharmacologic effects of the drug. Excessive pressor effect, skeletal muscle hyperactivity, tachycardia, and enhanced deep tendon reflexes may be early signs of overdosage.
• May cause severe CNS toxicity, including seizures.

PRECAUTIONS & CONSIDERATIONS

Caution is warranted with hypermetabolic states, such as hyperthyroidism and pheochromocytoma as well as arrhythmias, diabetes mellitus, glaucoma, hypertension, impaired renal or liver function, peptic ulcer disease. It is unknown whether doxapram crosses the placenta or is excreted in breast milk, so it is not administered to pregnant women. Be aware that doxapram is contraindicated in neonates. No age-related precautions have been noted for the elderly. Safety and efficacy have not been evaluated in children younger than 12 yr. Benzyl alcohol may cause gasping syndrome in neonates.

Administration

Doxapram dosage is determined by response to the drug. Discontinue if sudden hypotension or dyspnea develops. The rate of infusion should not be increased in severely ill patients with chronic obstructive pulmonary disease (COPD). Monitor closely during administration and for some time afterward until the patient is fully alert for 30-60 min to ensure that reflexes have been restored and to prevent rebound hypoventilation. Before doxapram administration, ensure adequate airway and oxygenation in postanesthetic or drug-induced respiratory depression. Avoid extravasation or use a single injection site over an extended period. Local irritation or thrombophlebitis may result. Doxapram is stable and compatible with D5W, D10W, or 0.9% NaCl.

Doxepin
dox´eh-pin
(Deptran [AUS], Novo-Doxepin [CAN], Prudoxin, Zonalon)
Do not confuse doxepin with doxapram, doxazosin, or Doxidan, or Sinequan with saquinavir.

CATEGORY AND SCHEDULE
Pregnancy Risk Category: C (B for topical form)

Classification: Antidepressants, tricyclic; dermatologics

MECHANISM OF ACTION
A tricyclic antidepressant, antianxiety agent, antineuralgic agent, antipruritic agents, and antiulcer agent that increases synaptic concentrations of norepinephrine and serotonin. *Therapeutic Effect:* Produces antidepressant and anxiolytic effects.

PHARMACOKINETICS
Rapidly and well absorbed from the GI tract. Protein binding: 80%-85%. Metabolized in the liver to active metabolite. Primarily excreted in urine. Not removed by hemodialysis. *Half-life:* 6-8 h. *Topical:* Absorbed through the skin to levels similar to those of oral administration. Distributed to body tissues. Metabolized to active metabolite. Excreted in urine.

AVAILABILITY
Capsules: 10 mg, 25 mg, 50 mg, 75 mg, 100 mg, 150 mg.
Oral Concentrate: 10 mg/mL.
Cream (Prudoxin, Zonalon): 5%.

INDICATIONS AND DOSAGES
▸ **Depression, anxiety**
PO
Adults. 25-150 mg/day at bedtime or in 2-3 divided doses. May increase to 300 mg/day.
Elderly. Initially, 10-25 mg at bedtime. May increase by 10-25 mg/day every 3-7 days. Maximum: 75 mg/day.
Adolescents. Initially, 25-50 mg/day as a single dose or in divided doses. May increase to 100 mg/day.
▸ **Pruritus associated with eczema**
TOPICAL
Adults, Elderly. Apply thin film 4 times a day with at least 3-4 h between applications.

OFF-LABEL USES
Treatment of neurogenic pain, panic disorder; prevention of vascular headache, pruritus in idiopathic urticaria.

CONTRAINDICATIONS
Angle-closure glaucoma, hypersensitivity to other tricyclic antidepressants, urine retention, acute post myocardial infarction period.

INTERACTIONS
Drug
Alcohol, other central nervous system (CNS) depressants: May increase CNS and respiratory depression and the hypotensive effects of doxepin.
Anticholinergics: Additive anticholinergic effects may occur.
Antithyroid agents: May increase the risk of agranulocytosis.
Bupropion: May increase doxepin levels.
Cimetidine: May increase doxepin blood concentration and risk of toxicity.
Clonidine, guanadrel: May decrease the effects of these drugs.
CYP1A2 inducers/inhibitors: May decrease/increase levels and effects of doxepin.

D

CYP2D6 inhibitors: May increase levels and effects of doxepin.

CYP3A4 inducers/inhibitors: May decrease/increase levels and effects of doxepin.

Lithium: Increased risk of neurotoxicity.

MAOIs, linezolid: May increase the risk of seizures, hyperpyrexia, and hypertensive crisis. MAOIs are contraindicated.

Phenothiazines: May increase the anticholinergic and sedative effects of doxepin.

Sympathomimetics: May increase cardiac effects.

QT-prolonging agents: May increase risk of QT prolongation of tricyclics.

Herbal and Food
None known.

DIAGNOSTIC TEST EFFECTS

May alter blood glucose levels and ECG readings. Therapeutic serum drug level is 110-250 ng/mL; toxic serum drug level is > 300 ng/mL.

SIDE EFFECTS

Frequent
Oral: Orthostatic hypotension, somnolence, dry mouth, headache, increased appetite, weight gain, nausea, unusual fatigue, unpleasant taste.
Topical: Drowsiness; edema; increased itching, eczema, burning, or stinging at application site; altered taste; dizziness; somnolence; dry skin; dry mouth; fatigue; headache; thirst.

Occasional
Oral: Blurred vision, confusion, constipation, hallucinations, difficult urination, eye pain, irregular heartbeat, fine muscle tremors, nervousness, impaired sexual function, diarrhea, diaphoresis, heartburn, insomnia.

Topical: Anxiety, skin irritation or cracking, nausea.

Rare
Oral: Allergic reaction, alopecia, tinnitus, breast enlargement.
Topical: Fever, photosensitivity.

SERIOUS REACTIONS

• Overdose may produce confusion; seizures; severe somnolence; fast, slow, or irregular heartbeat; fever; hallucinations; agitation; dyspnea; vomiting; and unusual fatigue or weakness.

• Abrupt withdrawal after prolonged therapy may produce headache, malaise, nausea, vomiting, and vivid dreams.

PRECAUTIONS & CONSIDERATIONS

Antidepressants increase the risk of suicidal ideation in children, adolescents, and young adults with depression and psychiatric disorders. Closely monitor when initiating therapy, especially the first 2 mo.

Caution is warranted with cardiac disease, diabetes mellitus, glaucoma, hiatal hernia, history of seizures, history of urinary obstruction or urine retention, hyperthyroidism, increased intraocular pressure, renal or hepatic disease, benign prostatic hyperplasia, mania, bipolar disorder, and schizophrenia. Doxepin crosses the placenta and is distributed in breast milk. The safety and efficacy of this drug have not been established in children. Lower doxepin dosages are recommended for elderly patients because they are at increased risk for toxicity. Exposure to sunlight or artificial light sources should be avoided.

Drowsiness and dizziness may occur. Change positions slowly from recumbent to sitting, before standing, to prevent dizziness. Alcohol, caffeine, and tasks that require mental alertness or motor skills should also be avoided. BP, pulse rate, weight, and ECG should also be monitored. Appearance, behavior, level of interest, mood, and speech pattern should be assessed.

Administration

Take doxepin with food or milk if GI distress occurs. Dilute the oral concentrate in 8 oz fruit juice (such as grapefruit, orange, pineapple, or prune), milk, or water. Avoid diluting in carbonated drinks because they are incompatible with doxepin. An improvement should occur within 2-5 days of starting therapy, but the maximum therapeutic effect usually takes 2-3 wks to appear. The therapeutic serum level for doxepin is 110-250 ng/mL; the toxic serum level is > 300 ng/mL.

Doxercalciferol
dox-er-cal-sif'er-ol
(Hectorol)

CATEGORY AND SCHEDULE
Pregnancy Risk Category: B

Classification: Vitamins/minerals, vitamin D analogs

MECHANISM OF ACTION
A fat-soluble vitamin that is essential for absorption, utilization of calcium phosphate, and normal calcification of bone. *Therapeutic Effect:* Stimulates calcium and phosphate absorption from small intestine, promotes secretion of calcium from bone to blood, promotes renal tubule phosphate resorption, acts on bone cells to stimulate skeletal growth

and on parathyroid gland to suppress hormone synthesis and secretion.

PHARMACOKINETICS
Readily absorbed from small intestine. Metabolized in liver. Partially eliminated in urine. Not removed by hemodialysis. *Half-life:* up to 96 h.

AVAILABILITY
Capsule: 0.5 mcg, 2.5 mcg.
Injection: 2 mcg/mL.

INDICATIONS AND DOSAGES
▶ **Secondary hyperparathyroidism, dialysis patients**
IV

Adults, Elderly. Titrate dose to lower immunoreactive parathyroid hormone (iPTH) to 150-300 pg/mL. Adjust dose at 8-wks intervals to a maximum dose of 18 mcg/wk. Initially, if iPTH level is more than 400 pg/mL, give 4 mcg 3 times/wk after dialysis, administered as a bolus dose.

Dose titration

The iPTH level decreased by 50% and more than 300 pg/mL: Dose may be increased by 1-2 mcg at 8-wks intervals as needed.
iPTH level 150-300 pg/mL: Maintain the current dose.
iPTH level < 100 pg/mL: Suspend drug for 1 wk and resume at a reduced dose of at least 1 mcg lower.
PO

Adults, Elderly. Dialysis patients: Titrate dose to lower iPTH to 150-300 pg/mL. Adjust dose at 8-wks intervals to a maximum dose of 20 mcg 3 times/wk. Initially, if iPTH is more than 400 pg/mL, give 10 mcg 3 times/wk at dialysis.

Dose titration:

Level decreased by 50% and more than 300 pg/mL: Increase dose to 12.5 mcg 3 times/wk for 8 wks or longer. This titration process may

D

continue at 8-wks intervals. Each increase should be by 2.5 mcg/dose. iPTH level 150-300 pg/mL: Maintain current dose.
iPTH level < 100 pg/mL: Suspend drug for 1 wk and resume at a reduced dose. Decrease each dose by at least 2.5 mcg.

▸ **Secondary hyperparathyroidism, predialysis patients**
PO
Adults, Elderly. Titrate dose to lower iPTH to 35-70 pg/mL with stage 3 disease or to 70-110 pg/mL with stage 4 disease. Dose may be adjusted at 2-wk intervals with a maximum dose of 3.5 mcg/day. Begin with 1 mcg/day.
Dose titration:
iPTH level more than 70 pg/mL with stage 3 disease or more than 110 pg/mL with stage 4 disease: Increase dose by 0.5 mcg every 2 wks as needed.
iPTH level 35-70 pg/mL with stage 3 disease or 70-110 pg/mL with stage 4 disease: Maintain current dose.
iPTH level is < 35 pg/mL with stage 3 disease or < 70 pg/mL with stage 4 disease: Suspend drug for 1 wk, then resume at a reduced dose of at least 0.5 mcg lower.

CONTRAINDICATIONS
Hypercalcemia, vitamin D toxicity, hypersensitivity to doxercalciferol or other vitamin D analogues.

INTERACTIONS
Drug
Aluminum-containing antacid (long-term use): May increase aluminum concentration and aluminum bone toxicity.
Calcium-containing preparations, thiazide diuretics: May increase the risk of hypercalcemia.
Magnesium-containing antacids: May increase magnesium concentration.

Vitamin D, other supplements: May increase risk of toxicity.
Herbal
None known.
Food
None known.

DIAGNOSTIC TEST EFFECTS
May increase serum cholesterol, calcium, magnesium, and phosphate levels. May decrease serum alkaline phosphatase.

SIDE EFFECTS
Occasional
Edema (34%), headache (28%), malaise (28%), dizziness (12%), nausea (24%), vomiting (24%), dyspnea (12%).
Rare (< 10%)
Bradycardia, sleep disorder, pruritus, anorexia, constipation.

SERIOUS REACTIONS
• Excessive vitamin D may cause progressive hypercalcemia, hypercalciuria, hyperphosphatemia, and adynamic bone disease.
• Early signs of overdosage are manifested as weakness, headache, somnolence, nausea, vomiting, dry mouth, constipation, muscle and bone pain, and metallic taste sensation.
• Later signs of overdosage are evidenced by polyuria, polydipsia, anorexia, weight loss, nocturia, photophobia, rhinorrhea, pruritus, disorientation, hallucinations, hyperthermia, hypertension, and cardiac arrhythmias.

PRECAUTIONS & CONSIDERATIONS
Caution is necessary with coronary artery disease, kidney stones, and hepatic impairment. Correct hyperphosphatemia before starting therapy. Mineral oil should be avoided during doxercalciferol use. It is unknown whether doxercalciferol

crosses the placenta or is distributed in breast milk. Safety and efficacy have not been established in children. No age-related precautions have been noted in elderly patients. Consume foods rich in vitamin D, including eggs, leafy vegetables, margarine, meats, milk, vegetable oils, and vegetable shortening.

Storage
Store at room temperature. Protect from light.

Administration
Individualize dosing based on serum iPTH levels. Injection for IV use only. Give oral doxercalciferol without regard to food. Swallow whole and avoid crushing, chewing, or opening the capsules. During titration, iPTH, serum calcium, and serum phosphorus levels should be obtained weekly. If hypercalcemia, hyperphosphatemia, or a serum calcium × phosphorus product > 70 is noted, the drug should be immediately suspended until these parameters are appropriately lowered, then, the drug should be restarted at a dose which is 1.0 mcg lower.

Doxorubicin
dox-oh-roo′bi-sin
(Adriamycin, Doxil)
Do not confuse with Daunorubicin, Idamycin, or Idarubicin.

CATEGORY AND SCHEDULE
Pregnancy Risk Category: D

Classification: Anthracycline antibiotic; antineoplastic

MECHANISM OF ACTION
An anthracycline antibiotic that inhibits DNA and DNA-dependent RNA synthesis by binding with DNA strands. Liposomal encapsulation increases uptake by tumors, prolongs action, and may decrease toxicity. *Therapeutic Effect:* Prevents cellular division.

PHARMACOKINETICS
Widely distributed. Protein binding: Unknown. Metabolized in liver. Minimal excretion in urine. *Half-life:* 45-55 h.

AVAILABILITY
Injection, Powder for Solution: 10 mg, 20 mg, 50 mg, 150 mg.
Injection, Solution: 2 mg/mL.
Liposomal Injection: 2 mg/mL.

INDICATIONS AND DOSAGES
▸ **AIDS-related Kaposi sarcoma**
IV INFUSION
Adults. Liposomal doxorubicin 20 mg/m² over 30 min q3wk.
Neoplastic conditions (ovarian, breast, prostate, thyroid, gastric, lung cancers; lymphomas)
IV INFUSION
Adults. Conventional doxorubicin. As a single agent, 60-75 mg/m² q3wk. In combination with other chemotherapy, 40-60 mg/m² q3-4 wk.
▸ **Ovarian cancer**
IV INFUSION
Adults. Liposomal doxorubicin. 50 mg/m² q 4 wk
▸ **Dosage in Hepatic Impairment**
If serum bilirubin 1.2-3 mg/dL, give 50% of usual dose. If serum bilirubin > 3 mg/dL, give 25% of usual dose.

CONTRAINDICATIONS
Myelosuppression; previous receipt of complete cumulative doses of doxorubicin, daunorubicin, idarubicin or other anthracyclines; Nursing mothers, hypersensitivity

to doxorubicin compounds or daunorubicin.

DRUG INTERACTIONS

Cyclosporine: Increased doxorubicin concentrations and toxicity.
Live vaccines: Increased risk infection by vaccine.

IV INCOMPATIBILITIES

Conventional doxorubicin: allopurinol, aminophylline, cephalothin, dexamethasone, diazepam, etoposide, fluorouracil, furosemide, gallium nitrate, heparin, hydrocortisone, piperacillin sodium/ tazobactam, vincristine.
Liposomal doxorubicin: benzyl alcohol. Doxorubicin liposomal should not be mixed with any other medications.

SIDE EFFECTS

Frequent
Nausea, vomiting, alopecia, mucositis, myelosuppression.
Occasional
Anorexia, diarrhea, hyperpigmentation of nailbeds, phalangeal and dermal creases.
Rare
Fever, chills, urticaria, conjunctivitis, lacrimation.
Liposomal doxorubicin.
Frequent (>20%)
Asthenia, fatigue, fever, anorexia, nausea, vomiting, stomatitis, diarrhea, constipation, hand and foot syndrome, rash, neutropenia, thrombocytopenia, anemia.

SERIOUS REACTIONS

• Bone marrow depression manifested as hematologic toxicity (principally leukopenia and, to a lesser extent, anemia, thrombocytopenia) may occur.
• Cardiotoxicity noted as either acute, transient abnormal ECG findings or cardiomyopathy manifested as congestive heart failure may occur.
• Acute infusion-related reactions with liposomal doxorubicin.

PRECAUTIONS & CONSIDERATIONS

Probability of cardiac toxicity increases with higher total cumulative dose. Risk of cardiotoxicity increased in patients with prior mediastinal irradiation, concurrent cyclophosphamide therapy, concurrent calcium channel blocker therapy, preexisting heart disease, or early or advanced age. Monitor cardiac function. Use with caution in patients with impaired hepatic function. Women of childbearing potential should be advised to avoid becoming pregnant. Excreted in breast milk; do not breast-feed.
Storage
Store lyophilized powder at room temperature. Protect from light. Reconstituted solution stable 7 days at room temperature and 15 days in the refrigerator.
    Store conventional solution in the refrigerator. Protect from light.
    Store liposomal solution in the refrigerator.
Administration
Reconstitute lyophilized powder with NS. Do not administer IM or SubQ. Severe local tissue damage will occur with IV extravasation. Slowly administer into tubing of a freely running IV infusion of NS or D5W into a large vein. Administer over at least 3 to 5 min.
    Do not substitute liposomal doxorubicin for conventional doxorubicin on a mg per mg basis. Do not use in-line filter with liposomal formulation. Dilute liposomal doxorubicin with D5W. Administer over at least 1 hr.

Doxycycline
dox-i-sye′kleen
(Adoxa, Alodox, Apo-Doxy [CAN],
Doryx, Doxsig [AUS], Doxy-100,
Doxycin [CAN], Doxyhexal [AUS],
Doxylin [AUS], Monodox, Oraxyl,
Periostat, Vibramycin, Vibra-Tabs)
**Do not confuse doxycycline with
dicyclomine or doxylamine, or
Monodox with Monopril.**

CATEGORY AND SCHEDULE
Pregnancy Risk Category: D

Classification: Antibiotics,
tetracyclines

MECHANISM OF ACTION
A tetracycline antibiotic that inhibits
bacterial protein synthesis by binding
to ribosomes. *Therapeutic Effect:*
Bacteriostatic.

PHARMACOKINETICS
Well absorbed after oral
administration. Protein binding:
90%. Widely distributed except in
the central nervous system (CNS;
poor). Excreted in urine and feces.
Half-life: 12-15 h.

AVAILABILITY
Capsules (Doxycycline, Monodox):
50 mg, 75 mg, 100 mg.
Capsules (Vibramycin): 100 mg.
Capsules (Adoxa): 150 mg.
Capsules (Oraxyl): 20 mg.
Capsules, Delayed Release: 75 mg,
100 mg.
Oral Suspension (Vibramycin):
50 mg/5 mL, 25 mg/5 mL.
Syrup (Vibramycin): 50 mg/5 mL.
Tablets (Adoxa): 50 mg, 75 mg,
100 mg, 150 mg.
Tablets (Alodox, Periostat):
20 mg.
Tablets (Vibra-Tabs): 100 mg.

Tablet, Delayed Release (Doryx):
75 mg, 100 mg.
*Injection, Powder for Reconstitution
(Doxy-100):* 100 mg.

INDICATIONS AND DOSAGES
▸ **Respiratory, skin, and soft-tissue
infections; urinary tract infection;
pelvic inflammatory disease (PID);
brucellosis; trachoma; Rocky
Mountain spotted fever; typhus;
Q fever; rickettsia; severe acne
(Adoxa); smallpox; psittacosis;
ornithosis; granuloma inguinale;
lymphogranuloma venereum;
intestinal amebiasis (adjunctive
treatment); prevention of rheumatic
fever**
PO
*Adults, Elderly, Children older than
8 yr and weighing > 100 lb.* Initially,
100 mg q12h, then 100 mg/day as
single dose or 50 mg q12h or 100 mg
q12h for severe infections.
*Children older than 8 yr and
weighing < 45 kg.* Initially, 4 mg/
kg/day, then 2-4 mg/kg/day divided
q12-24h. Maximum: 200 mg/day.
IV
*Adults, Elderly, Children older than
8 yr and weighing > 100 lb.* Initially,
200 mg as 1-2 infusions; then 100-
200 mg/day in 1-2 divided doses.
Children older than 8 yr and <45 kg.
2-4 mg/kg/day divided q12-24h.
Maximum: 200 mg/day.
▸ **Acute gonococcal infections**
PO
Adults. 100 mg twice daily for
7 days.
▸ **Syphilis**
PO, IV
Adults. 200 mg/day in divided doses
for 14-28 days.
▸ **Traveler's diarrhea, prophylaxis**
PO
Adults, Elderly. 100 mg/day during
a period of risk (up to 14 days) and
for 2 days after returning home.

D

> **Periodontitis**

PO

Adults (Periostat, Alodox, Oraxyl).
20 mg twice a day.

> **Malaria, prophylaxis**

PO

Adults. 100 mg once a day
beginning 1-2 days before travel,
during travel, and 4 wks after
returning home.

Children over 8 yr. 2 mg/kg once
a day beginning 1-2 days before
travel, during travel, and 4 wks after
returning home.

OFF-LABEL USES

Treatment of atypical
mycobacterial infections, rheumatoid
arthritis, gonorrhea, and malaria;
prevention of Lyme disease; prevention
or treatment of traveler's diarrhea.

CONTRAINDICATIONS

Children 8 yr and younger,
hypersensitivity to tetracyclines or
sulfites, pregnancy, severe hepatic
dysfunction.

INTERACTIONS

Drug

**Antacids and supplements
containing aluminum, calcium,
or magnesium and Oral iron
preparations; laxatives containing
magnesium:** Decrease doxycycline
absorption; separate administration.

**Barbiturates, carbamazepine,
phenytoin:** May decrease
doxycycline blood concentrations.

Cholestyramine, colestipol: May
decrease doxycycline absorption;
separate administration.

Methotrexate: May increase levels
of methotrexate.

Oral contraceptives: May
decrease the effects of oral
contraceptives.

Warfarin: May increase
anticoagulation of warfarin.

Herbal
None known.
Food
None known.

DIAGNOSTIC TEST EFFECTS

May increase serum alkaline
phosphatase, amylase, bilirubin, AST
(SGOT), and ALT (SGPT) levels.
May alter CBC.

Ⓘ IV INCOMPATIBILITIES

Allopurinol (Aloprim),
amphotericin B cholesteryl
(Amphotec), amphotericin B
liposomal (AmBisome), ampicillin,
ampicillin/sulbactam (Unasyn),
cefazolin, cefotetan (Cefotan),
cefoxitin (Mefoxin), ceftazidime
(Ceptaz, Fortaz, Tazicef, Tazidime),
ceftizoxime (Cefizox), cefuroxime
(Zinacef), chloramphenicol,
dantrolene, diazepam, erythromycin
lactobionate, fluorouracil, folic acid,
furosemide (Lasix), ganciclovir
(Cytovene), heparin, hydrocortisone
sodium succinate (Solu-Cortef),
indomethacin, ketorolac, methicillin,
methotrexate, methylprednisolone
sodium succinate, nafcillin, oxacillin,
palonosetron (Aloxi), pemetrexed
(Alimta), penicillin G potassium,
penicillin G sodium, pentobarbital,
phenytoin, piperacillin, piperacillin/
tazobactam (Zosyn), sodium
bicarbonate, sulfamethoxazole/
trimethoprim.

Ⓘ IV COMPATIBILITIES

Acyclovir (Zovirax), alfentanil
(Alfenta), amifostine (Ethyol),
amikacin (Amikar), aminophylline,
amiodarone, ascorbic acid,
atracurium (Tracrium), atropine,
aztreonam (Azactam), benztropine
(Cogentin), bivalirudin (Angiomax),
bretylium, bumetanide (Bumex),
buprenorphine (Buprenex),
butorphanol (Stadol), calcium

chloride, calcium gluconate, carboplatin, caspofungin (Cancidas), cefotaxime (Claforan), ceftriaxone (Rocephin), chlorpromazine, cimetidine (Tagamet), cisatracurium (Nimbex), cisplatin, clindamycin (Cleocin), cyclophosphamide (Cytoxan), cyclosporine (Sandimmune), dactinomycin (Cosmegen), daptomycin (Cubicin), dexmedetomidine (Precedex), digoxin (Lanoxin), diltiazem (Cardizem), diphenhydramine (Benadryl), dobutamine (Dobutrex), docetaxel (Taxotere), dopamine (Intropin), doxorubicin (Adriamycin), enalaprilat, ephedrine, epinephrine, epirubicin (Ellence), ertapenem (Invanz), esmolol (Brevibloc), etoposide phosphate (Etopophos), famotidine (Pepcid), fenoldopam (Corlopam), fentanyl (Sublimaze), filgrastim (Neupogen), fluconazole (Diflucan), fludarabine (Fludara), gemcitabine (Gemzar), gentamicin, granisetron (Kytril), hydromorphone (Dilaudid), hydroxyzine, imipenem/cilastatin (Primaxin), insulin (regular, Humulin R, Novolin R), isoproterenol (Isuprel), labetalol, levofloxacin (Levaquin), lidocaine, linezolid (Zyvox), lorazepam (Ativan), magnesium sulfate, mannitol, melphalan (Alkeran), metoclopramide (Reglan), metoprolol (Lopressor), metronidazole (Flagyl), midazolam (Versed), milrinone (Primacor), minocycline (Minocin), mitoxantrone (Novantrone), morphine, nalbuphine (Nubain), naloxone (Narcan), nitroglycerin, nitroprusside sodium (Nitropress), norepinephrine (Levophed), ondansetron (Zofran), oxaliplatin (Eloxatin), oxytocin (Pitocin), paclitaxel (Taxol), pantoprazole (Protonix), potassium chloride, procainamide, prochloperazine, promethazine, propofol (Diprivan), propranolol, quinupristin/dalfopristin (Synercid), ranitidine (Zantac), remifentanil (Ultiva), rituximab (Rituxan), sargramostim (Leukin), sodium acetate, streptokinase, succinylcholine, sufentanil (Sufenta), tacrolimus (Prograf), teniposide (Vumon), theophylline, thiotepa (Thioplex), ticarcillin (Ticar), ticarcillin/clavulanate (Timentin), tigecycline (Tygacil), tirofibran (Aggrastat), tobramycin, trastuzumab (Herceptin), vancomycin, vasopressin, vecuronium (Norcuron), verapamil, vincristine (Vincasar), vinorelbine (Navelbine), voriconazole (Vfend).

SIDE EFFECTS

Frequent

Anorexia, nausea, vomiting, diarrhea, dysphagia, possibly severe photosensitivity.

Occasional

Rash, urticaria.

SERIOUS REACTIONS

• Superinfection (especially fungal) and benign intracranial hypertension (headache, visual changes) may occur.

• Hepatoxicity, fatty degeneration of the liver, and pancreatitis occur rarely. Autoimmune syndromes have been reported.

PRECAUTIONS & CONSIDERATIONS

Caution should be used in those who cannot avoid sun or ultraviolet exposure, because such exposure, may produce a severe photosensitivity reaction.

History of allergies, especially to tetracyclines or sulfites, should be determined before drug therapy. Caution is warranted in renal impairment. Avoid use in children, because it may cause permanent tooth discoloration, enamel hypoplasia. Pattern of daily bowel activity, stool consistency, food intake and tolerance, renal function, and skin for rash should be assessed. Be alert for signs and symptoms of superinfection, such as anal or genital pruritus, diarrhea, and ulceration or changes of the oral mucosa or tongue. Loss of consciousness should be monitored because of the potential for increased intracranial pressure.

Storage

Store capsules and tablets at room temperature. Store oral suspension for up to 2 wks at room temperature. After reconstitution, the IV piggyback infusion may be stored for up to 12 h at room temperature or up to 72 h if refrigerated. Protect the drug from direct sunlight. Discard it if a precipitate forms.

Administration

Take oral doxycycline with a full glass of fluid. It may also be given with food or milk. Take oral doxycycline 1-2 h before or after antacids that contain aluminum, calcium, or magnesium; laxatives that contain magnesium; or oral iron preparations, because these drugs may impair doxycycline absorption. Shake suspension well before use.

! Do not administer doxycycline IM or subcutaneously. Space doses evenly around the clock. Reconstitute each 100-mg vial with 10 mL of sterile water for injection to yield a concentration of 10 mg/mL. Further dilute each 100 mg with at least 100 mL to concentration of 0.1 mg/mL to 1 mg/mL with D5W, 0.9% NaCl, or lactated Ringer's

solution. Give the intermittent IV (piggyback) infusion over 1-4 h. Avoid extravasation.

Dronabinol
droe-nab′i-nol
(Marinol)
Do not confuse dronabinol with droperidol.

CATEGORY AND SCHEDULE
Pregnancy Risk Category: C
Controlled Substance Schedule: III

Classification: Antiemetics/antivertigo, appetite stimulant

MECHANISM OF ACTION
An antiemetic and appetite stimulant that may act by inhibiting vomiting control mechanisms in the medulla oblongata. *Therapeutic Effect:* Inhibits vomiting and stimulates appetite.

PHARMACOKINETICS
Well absorbed after oral administration. Distributes to adipose tissue. Protein binding > 97%. Metabolized in liver, extensive first-pass effect. *Half-life:* 25-36 h. Primarily excreted in feces. Onset of action: 1 h. Duration of appetite stimulation: 24 h.

AVAILABILITY
Capsules (Gelatin): 2.5 mg, 5 mg, 10 mg.

INDICATIONS AND DOSAGES
▸ **Prevention of chemotherapy-induced nausea and vomiting**
PO
Adults, Children. Initially, 5 mg/m^2 1-3 h before chemotherapy, then q2-4h after chemotherapy for total of

4-6 doses a day. May increase by 2.5 mg/m^2 up to 15 mg/m^2 per dose.
▸ **Appetite stimulant**
PO
Adults. Initially, 2.5 mg twice a day (before lunch and dinner). Range: 2.5-20 mg/day.

CONTRAINDICATIONS

Hypersensitivity to marijauna or any cannabinoid or sesame oil.

INTERACTIONS

Drug
Alcohol, other CNS depressants:
May increase CNS depression.
Amphetamines, cocaine, sympathomimetics: Hypertension, tachycardia, cardiotoxicity may occur.
Anticholinergics, antihistamines:
Additive tachycardia drowsiness may occur.
Tricyclic antidepressants:
Tachycardia, hypertension, or drowsiness may occur.
Herbal
None known.
Food
None known.

DIAGNOSTIC TEST EFFECTS

None known.

SIDE EFFECTS

Frequent (3%-24%)
Euphoria, dizziness, paranoid reaction, somnolence, abnormal thinking
Occasional (1%-3%)
Asthenia, ataxia, confusion, abdominal pain, depersonalization
Rare (< 1%)
Diarrhea, depression, nightmares, speech difficulties, headache, anxiety, tinnitus, flushed skin.

SERIOUS REACTIONS

• Withdrawal symptoms may occur upon abrupt discontinuation.

• Mild intoxication may produce increased sensory awareness (including taste, smell, and sound), altered time perception, reddened conjunctiva, dry mouth, and tachycardia.
• Moderate intoxication may produce memory impairment and urine retention.
• Severe intoxication may produce lethargy, decreased motor coordination, slurred speech, and orthostatic hypotension.

PRECAUTIONS & CONSIDERATIONS

Caution is warranted in patients with heart disease, hypertension, a history of drug or alcohol abuse, hepatic impairment, seizure disorder, depression, mania, and schizophrenia. Use with caution in elderly patients because postural hypotension can occur.

Dronabinol use is not recommended for children with AIDS-related anorexia. Alcohol, barbiturates, other CNS depressants, and tasks that require mental alertness or motor skills should be avoided. BP, heart rate, and behavioral and mood reactions should be monitored.
Storage
Keep tightly closed. Store in refrigerator (46°-59° F). Protect from freezing.
Administration
Take dronabinol before lunch and dinner to stimulate appetite. Relief from nausea and vomiting generally occurs within 15 min of drug administration.

D

Droperidol
droe-pear'ih-dall
(Inapsine)

CATEGORY AND SCHEDULE
Pregnancy Risk Category: C

Classification: Antiemetics/
antivertigo; anxiolytics; sedatives/
hypnotics

MECHANISM OF ACTION
A general anesthetic and
antiemetic agent that antagonizes
dopamine neurotransmission at
synapses by blocking postsynaptic
dopamine receptor sites; partially
blocks adrenergic receptor
binding sites. *Therapeutic Effect:*
Produces tranquilization, antiemetic
effect.

PHARMACOKINETICS
Onset of action occurs within 3-10
min, peak 30 min. Well absorbed.
Metabolized in liver. Excreted in
urine and feces. Duration of action:
2-4 h. *Half-life:* 2.3 h.

AVAILABILITY
Injection: 2.5 mg/mL.

INDICATIONS AND DOSAGES
▸ **Prevention of nausea and vomiting
with surgery**
IM/IV
*Adults, Elderly, Children 12 yr
and older.* Initially, up to 2.5 mg.
Additional doses of 1.25 mg may be
given.
Children 2-12 yr. Initially, up to
0.1 mg/kg.

CONTRAINDICATIONS
Known or suspected QT
prolongation, hypersensitivity to
droperidol or any component of

the formulation. Droperidol is not
recommended for any use other than
for the treatment of perioperative
nausea and vomiting in patients
for whom other treatments are
ineffective or inappropriate.

INTERACTIONS
Drug
**Central nervous system (CNS)
depressants:** May increase CNS-
depressant effect.
**Class I, IA, or III antiarrhythmics,
cisapride, cyclobenzaprine,
phenothiazines, pimozide,
quinolone antibiotics, tricylic
antidepressants:** May increase risk
of QT prolongation.
Hypotensive agents: May increase
hypotension.
Metoclopramide: Increased risk for
extrapyramidal symptoms.
Propofol: Increased nausea and
vomiting.
Herbal
None known.
Food
None known.

ⓘ IV INCOMPATIBILITIES
Allopurinol (Aloprim),
amphotericin B cholesteryl
(Amphotec), amphotericin B
liposomal (AmBisome), cefepime
(Maxipime), ertapenem (Invanz),
fluorouracil, foscarnet (Foscavir),
furosemide (Lasix), lansoprazole
(Prevacid), leucovorin, nafcillin,
pantoprazole (Protonix), pemetrexed
(Alimta), piperacillin/tazobactam
(Zosyn).

ⓘ IV COMPATIBILITES
Amifostine (Ethyol), azithromycin
(Zithromax), aztreonam (Azactam),
bivalirudin (Angiomax), bleomycin
(Blenoxane), carboplatin,
caspofungin (Cancidas),
cisatracurium (Nimbex),

cisplatin, cladribine (Leustatin), cyclophosphamide (Cytoxan), cytarabine, dactinomycin (Cosmegen), daptomycin (Cubicin), dexmedetomidine (Precedex), diltiazem (Cardizem), docetaxel (Taxotere), dopamine (Intropin), doxorubicin (Adriamycin), doxorubicin liposomal (Doxil), epirubicin (Ellence), famotidine (Pepcid), fenoldopam (Corlopam), fentanyl (Sublimaze), filgrastim (Neupogen), fluconazole (Diflucan), fludarabine (Fludara), gemcitabine (Gemzar), granisetron (Kytril), hydrocortisone sodium succinate (Solu-Cortef), hydromorphone (Dilaudid), idarubicin (Idamycin), ketamine (Ketalar), levofloxacin (Levaquin), linezolid (Zyvox), lorazepam (Ativan), melphalan (Alkeran), meperidine (Demerol), metoclopramide (Reglan), milrinone (Primacor), mitoxantrone (Novantrone), oxaliplatin (Eloxatin), oxytocin (Pitocin), paclitaxel (Taxol), palonosetron (Aloxi), potassium chloride, quinupristin/dalfopristin (Synercid), rituximab (Rituxan), sargramostim (Leukine), tacrolimus (Prograf), teniposide (Vumon), thiotepa (Thioplex), tigecycline (Tygacil), tirofiban (Aggrastat), trastuzumab (Herceptin), vasopressin, vecuronium (Norcuron), vinblastine (Velban), vincristine (Vincasar), vinorelbine (Navelbine), vitamin B complex with C, voriconazole (Vfend).

SIDE EFFECTS

Frequent
Mild to moderate hypotension.
Occasional
Tachycardia, postoperative drowsiness, dizziness, chills, shivering.
Rare
Postoperative nightmares, facial sweating, bronchospasm.

SERIOUS REACTIONS

• Extrapyramidal symptoms may appear as akathisia (motor restlessness) and dystonias: torticollis (neck muscle spasm), opisthotonos (rigidity of back muscles), and oculogyric crisis (rolling back of eyes).
• Overdosage includes symptoms of hypotension, tachycardia, hallucinations, and extrapyramidal symptoms.
• Prolonged QT interval (> 10%), torsade de pointes, seizures, neuroleptic malignant syndrome, orthostatic hypotension, and arrhythmias have been reported.

PRECAUTIONS & CONSIDERATIONS

Caution is warranted in patients with impaired hepatic, renal, or cardiac function, bradycardia, seizure disorder, pheochromocytoma, myasthenia gravis, or glaucoma. Droperidol readily crosses the placenta, and it is unknown whether droperidol is distributed in breast milk. Be aware that dystonias are more likely in children. Be aware that elderly patients may be more susceptible to sedative and hypotensive effects. Safety and efficacy have not been established in children < 2 yr of age. Monitor ECG.

Change positions slowly to avoid orthostatic hypotension and avoid tasks that require mental alertness or motor skills.
Storage
Store parenteral form at room temperature. Diluted solutions may be stored for 7 days at room temperature.
Administration
Be aware that the person must remain recumbent for 30-60 min in

head-low position with legs raised, to minimize hypotensive effect.

For IM administration, inject slow and deep into upper outer quadrant of gluteus maximus.

For IV administration, may give undiluted as IV push at a rate of 10 mg or less over 1 min. Dose for high-risk persons should be added to D5W or lactated Ringer's injection to a concentration of 1 mg/50 mL and given as an IV infusion.

Drotrecogin Alfa
droh-tree-koh′gen
(Xigris)

CATEGORY AND SCHEDULE
Pregnancy Risk Category: C

Classification: Thrombolytics

MECHANISM OF ACTION
A recombinant form of human-activated protein C that exerts an antithrombotic effect by inhibiting factors Va and VIIIa and may exert an indirect profibrinolytic effect by inhibiting plasminogen activator inhibitor-1 and limiting the generation of activated thrombin-activatable fibrinolysis-inhibitor. The drug may also exert an anti-inflammatory effect by inhibiting tumor necrosis factor (TNF) production by monocytes, by blocking leukocyte adhesion to selectins, and by limiting thrombin-induced inflammatory responses. *Therapeutic Effect:* Produces anti-inflammatory, antithrombotic, and profibrinolytic effects.

PHARMACOKINETICS
Inactivated by endogenous plasma protease inhibitors. Clearance occurs within 2 h of initiating infusion. *Half-life:* 1.6 h.

AVAILABILITY
Powder for Infusion: 5 mg, 20 mg.

INDICATIONS AND DOSAGES
▸ **Severe sepsis (Apache II score > or = 25)**
IV INFUSION
Adults, Elderly. 24 mcg/kg/h for 96 h. Dose is based on actual body weight.

CONTRAINDICATIONS
Active internal bleeding, evidence of cerebral herniation, intracranial neoplasm or mass lesion, presence, of an epidural catheter, recent (within the past 3 mo) hemorrhagic stroke, recent (within the past 2 mo) intracranial or intraspinal surgery or severe head trauma, trauma with an increased risk of life-threatening bleeding.

INTERACTIONS
Drug
Antiplatelets, anticoagulants, thrombolytics: May increase risk for bleeding.
Herbal
None known.
Food
None known.

DIAGNOSTIC TEST EFFECTS
May prolong aPTT.

ⓓ IV INCOMPATIBILITIES
Do not mix drotrecogin alfa with other medications.

🔋 IV COMPATIBILITIES
Lactated Ringer's solution, 0.9% NaCl and dextrose are the only solutions that can be administered through the same line.

SIDE EFFECTS
Occasional
Bleeding, bruising.

SERIOUS REACTIONS
• Bleeding (intrathoracic, retroperitoneal, GI, genitourinary, intra-abdominal, intracranial) occurs in about 2% of patients.

PRECAUTIONS & CONSIDERATIONS
Caution is warranted in patients with chronic, severe hepatic disease, intracranial aneurysm, platelet count < 30,000/mm^3, INR > 3, or prolonged PT, and in those who have had GI bleeding within the past 6 wks. Caution should be used in those who are using heparin concurrently and in those who have had thrombolytic therapy within the past 3 days or anticoagulant or aspirin therapy within the past 7 days. Caution should also be used when administering other drugs that affect hemostasis. It is unknown whether drotrecogin alfa causes fetal harm or is excreted in breast milk. The safety and efficacy of drotrecogin alfa have not been established in children or in elderly patients.

The following criteria must be met before initiating drotrecogin alfa therapy: age of at least 18 yr; weight < 135 kg; no pregnancy or breastfeeding; 3 or more systemic inflammatory response criteria (fever, heart rate > 90 beats/min, respiratory rate > 20 breaths/min, increased WBC count); and at least 1 sepsis-induced organ or system failure (cardiovascular, hepatic, renal, respiratory, or unexplained metabolic acidosis). Monitor for hemorrhagic complications. Bleeding may occur for up to 28 days after treatment. Notify the physician if signs and symptoms of unusual bleeding occur. Study in pediatric patients was terminated early due to lack of efficacy and increased side effects.

Storage
Store unreconstituted vials at room temperature. Reconstituted vials should be used within 3 hr to prepare infusion.

Administration
! If clinically important bleeding occurs, immediately stop the infusion.
Reconstitute the 5- and 20-mg vials by slowly adding 2.5 mL or 10 mL of sterile water for injection, respectively, to yield a concentration of 2 mg/mL. Swirl the vial gently to mix; do not shake or invert it. Add the reconstituted drug to an infusion bag containing 0.9% NaCl, and dilute to a final concentration of 100-200 mcg/mL. Direct the stream to the side of the bag to minimize agitation. Invert the infusion bag to mix the solution. Start the infusion within 3 h after reconstitution. Administer the drug through a dedicated IV line or a dedicated lumen of a multilumen central venous catheter at a rate of 24 mcg/kg/h for 96 h. If the infusion is interrupted, restart it at 24 mcg/kg/h, as prescribed. Stop infusion 2 h before invasive procedures. Resume immediately after minimally invasive procedures; delay for 12 h after major invasive procedures or surgery.

Duloxetine
du-lox′uh-teen
(Cymbalta)

CATEGORY AND SCHEDULE
Pregnancy Risk Category: C

Classification: Antidepressants, Selective serotonin/norepinephrine (SNRI) reuptake inhibitor

MECHANISM OF ACTION
An antidepressant that appears to inhibit serotonin and norepinephrine reuptake at neuronal presynaptic membranes; is a less potent inhibitor of dopamine reuptake. *Therapeutic Effect:* Relieves depression.

PHARMACOKINETICS
Well absorbed from the GI tract. Protein binding: > 90%. Extensively metabolized to active metabolites. Excreted primarily in urine and, to a lesser extent, in feces. *Half-life:* 8-17 h.

AVAILABILITY
Capsules, Delayed Release: 20 mg, 30 mg, 60 mg.

INDICATIONS AND DOSAGES
▶ **Major depressive disorder**
PO
Adults. 20 mg twice a day, increased up to 60 mg/day as a single dose or in 2 divided doses. Maximum: 120 mg/day.
▶ **Diabetic neuropathy**
PO
Adults. 60 mg once daily. Maximum: 120 mg/day.
▶ **Fibromyalgia**
PO
Adults. 30 mg/day, titrated to 60 mg/day after 1 wk. Maximum 120 mg/day.

▶ **Generalized anxiety**
Adults. 60 mg once daily (may start at 30 mg once daily for 1 wk, then titrate). Maximum: 120 mg/day.
▶ **Dosage in renal impairment**
Consider lower starting dosage. If creatinine clearance < 30 mL/min, use is not recommended.

OFF-LABEL USES
Chronic pain syndromes, stress incontinence.

CONTRAINDICATIONS
Uncontrolled angle-closure glaucoma; use within 14 days of MAOIs.

INTERACTIONS
 Drug
Alcohol: Increases the risk of hepatic injury.
Buspirone, meperidine, serotonin agonists, SSRIs/SNRIs, sibutramine, tramadol, trazodone: May increase risk of serotonin syndrome.
CYP1A2 inhibitors/inducers: May increase/decrease duloxetine levels and effects.
Fluoxetine, fluvoxamine, paroxetine, quinidine, quinolone antimicrobials, CYP2D6 inhibitors: May increase duloxetine plasma concentration.
MAOIs, linezolid: May cause serotonin syndrome, characterized by autonomic hyperactivity, coma, diaphoresis, excitement, hyperthermia, and rigidity. MAOIs are contraindicated.
Thioridazine: May produce ventricular arrhythmias.
Warfarin: May increase the warfarin plasma concentration.
 Herbal
St John's wort: May increase adverse effects.

DIAGNOSTIC TEST EFFECTS

May increase serum bilirubin, AST (SGOT), and ALT (SGPT) levels.

SIDE EFFECTS

Frequent (11%-20%)
Nausea, dry mouth, diarrhea, constipation, insomnia, somnolence, headache.
Occasional (9%-59%)
Dizziness, fatigue, anorexia, diaphoresis/hyperhidrosis, vomiting.
Rare (2%-4%)
Blurred vision, erectile dysfunction, delayed or failed ejaculation, anorgasmia, anxiety, decreased libido, hot flashes.

SERIOUS REACTIONS

• Duloxetine use may slightly increase the patient's heart rate or cause orthostatic hypotension.
• Colitis, dysphagia, gastritis, hepatotoxicity, and irritable bowel syndrome occur rarely.
• Activation of mania or hypomania in bipolar patients can occur. Monotherapy is not recommended in these patients.
• SIADH and hyponatremia occur with SSRIs and SNRIs.
• Withdrawal syndrome may occur with abrupt discontinuation. Gradually taper dose.

PRECAUTIONS & CONSIDERATIONS

Antidepressants increase the risk of suicidal ideation in children, adolescents, and young adults with depression and psychiatric disorders. Closely monitor when initiating therapy, especially the first 2 mo.

Caution is warranted with conditions that may slow gastric emptying, hepatic impairment, history of anemia, history of seizures, renal impairment, mania, hypomania, bipolar, and suicidal tendencies. Be aware that duloxetine use in pregnant women may produce neonatal adverse reactions, including constant crying, feeding difficulty, hyperreflexia, and irritability. Be aware that duloxetine is distributed in breast milk. Breastfeeding is not recommended. Be aware that the safety and efficacy of duloxetine have not been established in children. Exercise caution when increasing duloxetine doses in elderly patients.

Drowsiness and dizziness may occur, so avoid alcohol and tasks that require mental alertness or motor skills. Blood chemistry tests to assess hepatic and renal function should be performed before and periodically during therapy.
Administration
Take without regard to meals. Take with food or milk if GI distress occurs. Do not crush or chew enteric-coated capsules. Do not sprinkle capsule contents on food or mix with liquids. The therapeutic effects will be noted within 1-4 wk. Do not abruptly discontinue duloxetine.

Dutasteride
du-tas′tur-ide
(Avodart)

CATEGORY AND SCHEDULE
Pregnancy Risk Category: X

Classification: 5-α-Reductase inhibitors, antiandrogens, hormones/hormone modifiers

MECHANISM OF ACTION
An androgen hormone inhibitor that inhibits 5-α reductase, an intracellular enzyme that converts testosterone into dihydrotestosterone (DHT) in the prostate gland,

reducing the serum DHT level.
Therapeutic Effect: Reduces size
of the prostate gland and BPH
symptoms.

PHARMACOKINETICS

Route	Onset	Peak	Duration
PO	24 h	N/A	3-8 wks

Moderately absorbed after PO
administration; can be absorbed
through skin. Widely distributed.
Protein binding: 99%. Metabolized
in the liver. Primarily excreted in
feces. *Half-life:* Up to 5 wks.

AVAILABILITY

Capsule: 0.5 mg.

INDICATIONS AND DOSAGES
▸ **Benign prostatic hyperplasia (BPH)**
PO
Adults, Elderly. 0.5 mg once a day.

OFF-LABEL USES

Treatment of hair loss.

CONTRAINDICATIONS

Females, physical handling of capsules
by those who are or may be pregnant,
hypersensitivity to dutasteride or other
5-α reductase inhibitors, children.

INTERACTIONS
Drug
**Calcium channel antagonists,
cimetidine, CYP3A4 inhibitors:**
May increase dutasteride
concentrations.
Herbal
None known.
Food
None known.

DIAGNOSTIC TEST EFFECTS

Decreases the serum prostate-specific
antigen (PSA) level, testosterone
increased, TSH increased.

SIDE EFFECTS
Occasional
Gynecomastia, sexual dysfunction
(decreased libido, impotence,
and decreased volume of
ejaculate).

SERIOUS REACTIONS
• Toxicity may be manifested as
rash, diarrhea, and abdominal pain.
• Allergic reaction, angioedema,
pruritus, rash, urticaria may occur.

PRECAUTIONS & CONSIDERATIONS
Caution is warranted with hepatic
impairment, preexisting sexual
dysfunction (such as impotence
and decreased libido), and
obstructive uropathy. The drug
has a pregnancy risk category of
X and carries the risk of causing
anomalies in the male fetus. Pregnant
women or women trying to conceive
should not consume or handle
dutasteride.
  Dutasteride may cause impotence
and decrease ejaculate volume.
Serum PSA determinations should
be obtained before and periodically
during therapy. A new baseline must
be established after 3-6 mo of use.
Intake and output and improvement
in BPH signs and symptoms should
also be monitored. Avoid blood
donation during therapy and for 6 mo
after last dose. Safety and efficacy
have not been established in children;
contraindicated.
Storage
Store at room temperature of 77° F
or lower. Higher temps may cause
capsules to become soft, leak, or
stick together.
Administration
Do not break, crush, or open
capsules. Take dutasteride without
regard to food. Urinary flow may
not improve for up to 6 mo after
beginning treatment.

Dyphylline
dye′fi-lin
(Dylix, Lufyllin)
Do not confuse dyphylline with Dilacor.

D

CATEGORY AND SCHEDULE
Pregnancy Risk Category: C

Classification: Bronchodilators, xanthine derivatives

MECHANISM OF ACTION
A xanthine derivative that acts as a bronchodilator by directly relaxing smooth muscle of the bronchial airway and pulmonary blood vessels similar to theophylline. *Therapeutic Effect:* Relieves bronchospasm, increases vital capacity, produces cardiac and skeletal muscle stimulation.

PHARMACOKINETICS
Rapid absorption after PO administration. Protein binding: Unknown. Not metabolized to theophylline in vivo. Excreted in urine. *Half-life:* 2 h.

AVAILABILITY
Elixir: 100 mg/15 mL (Dylix).
Tablet: 200 mg, 400 mg (Lufyllin).

INDICATIONS AND DOSAGES
▶ **Chronic bronchospasm, asthma**
PO
Adults, Elderly. 15 mg/kg 4 times/day.
▶ **Dosage in renal impairment:**

Creatinine Clearance (mL/min)	Dosage Percent
50-80	Administer 75% of dose
10-50	Administer 50% of dose
<10	Administer 25% of dose

CONTRAINDICATIONS
History of hypersensitivity to dyphylline, related xanthine derivatives, or any component of the formulation.

INTERACTIONS
Drug
Adenosine, benzodiazepines: Effects may be decreased by dyphylline.
β-Blockers, non-selective: May decrease bronchodilator effects of dyphylline.
Cimetidine, ciprofloxacin, erythromycin, norfloxacin, probenecid: May increase dyphylline blood concentrations and risk of toxicity.
Glucocorticoids: May produce hypernatremia.
Phenytoin, primidone, rifampin: May increase dyphylline metabolism.
Smoking: May decrease dyphylline blood concentrations.
Herbal
Ma huang, ephedra: Increased CNS stimulation.
Food
Caffeine: Increased CNS stimulation.

SIDE EFFECTS
Frequent
Tachycardia, nervousness, restlessness.
Occasional
Heartburn, vomiting, headache, mild diuresis, insomnia, nausea.

SERIOUS REACTIONS
• Ventricular arrhythmias, hypotension, circulatory failure, seizures, hyperglycemia, and syndrome of inappropriate antidiuretic hormone (SIADH) have been reported.

PRECAUTIONS & CONSIDERATIONS
Uncontrolled arrhythmias, hyperthyroidism.

D

Caution is necessary with congestive heart failure (CHF), hypertension, impaired cardiac or renal function, hyperthyroidism, peptic ulcer disease, and seizure disorder. Be aware that dyphylline is equivalent to 70% theophylline. Dyphylline should not be used to treat status asthmaticus. Serious dosing errors can occur if dyphylline serum levels are monitored by theophylline serum assay. Smoking, charcoal-broiled food, and a high-protein, low-carbohydrate diet may decrease dyphylline level. Caffeine derivatives such as chocolate, coffee, cola, cocoa, and tea should be avoided.

Oxygen depletion may occur and is evident by blue or gray lips, blue or dusky-colored fingernails in light-skinned patients, and gray fingernails in dark-skinned persons.

Storage

Store at room temperature.

Administration

Give oral dyphylline with food to avoid GI distress. Give with plenty of water.

Econazole
e-kone′a-zole
(Ecostatin [CAN], Spectazole)

CATEGORY AND SCHEDULE
Pregnancy Risk Category: C

Classification: Antifungals, topical, dermatologics

MECHANISM OF ACTION
An imidazole derivative that changes the permeability of the fungal cell wall. *Therapeutic Effect:* Inhibits fungal biosynthesis of triglycerides, phospholipids. Fungistatic.

PHARMACOKINETICS
Low systemic absorption. Protein binding: 98%. Metabolized in liver to more than 20 metabolites. Primarily excreted in urine; minimal excretion in feces (< 1% of applied dose recovered in urine or feces). Not removed by hemodialysis.

AVAILABILITY
Cream: 1%.

INDICATIONS AND DOSAGES
▶ **Treatment of tinea pedis, tinea cruris, tinea corporis, tinea versicolor**
TOPICAL
Adults, Elderly, Children. Apply once daily to affected area for 2-4 wks. Tinea pedis for 1 mo.
▶ **Treatment of cutaneous candidiasis**
TOPICAL
Adults, Elderly, Children. Apply twice daily to affected area for 2 wks.

CONTRAINDICATIONS
Hypersensitivity to econazole.

INTERACTIONS
Drug
None known.
Herbal
None known.
Food
None known.

DIAGNOSTIC TEST EFFECTS
None known.

SIDE EFFECTS
Occasional (1%-10%)
Burning, itching, stinging, redness at application site.
Vulvar/vaginal burning.
Rare (< 1%)
Itching and burning of sexual partner, polyuria, vulvar itching, soreness, edema, discharge.

SERIOUS REACTIONS
• None known.

PRECAUTIONS & CONSIDERATIONS
Caution should be used during pregnancy. Econazole should be avoided during the first trimester of pregnancy. Use only if clearly needed in the second and third trimesters. Other agents are preferred. It is unknown whether econazole is distributed in breast milk.
Storage
Store at room temperature. Protect from heat and light.
Administration
Apply and rub gently into affected areas. Prolonged therapy over weeks or months may be necessary. Avoid occlusive dressings and wear light clothing for ventilation. Avoid getting in the eyes.

Edetate Calcium Disodium (Calcium EDTA)

ed-eh-tate kal-see-um dye-sow-dee-um

(Calcium Disodium Versenate)

Do not confuse with edetate disodium.

Do not use EDTA as abbreviation to avoid potential confusion.

CATEGORY AND SCHEDULE

Pregnancy Risk Category: B

Classification: Antidotes, heavy metal

MECHANISM OF ACTION

A chelating agent that reduces the blood concentration of heavy metals, especially lead, forming stable complexes. *Therapeutic Effect:* Allows heavy metal excretion in urine.

PHARMACOKINETICS

Well absorbed after parenteral administration; poorly absorbed from the GI tract. Penetrates to extracellular fluid and slowly diffuses into cerebrospinal fluid (CSF). No metabolism occurs. Excreted in the urine either unchanged or as the metal chelates. *Half-life:* 20-60 min (IV), 1.5 h (IM). Onset for chelation of lead: 1 h.

AVAILABILITY

Injection: 200 mg/mL.

INDICATIONS AND DOSAGES
▸ **Diagnosis of lead poisoning**
IM/IV

Adults, Elderly for 8-h or 24-h mobilization test. 500 mg/m^2 IV over 1 h or IM. (Maximum: 1 g).
Adults, Eldery for 8-h mobilization test. 50 mg/kg (Maximum: 1g) IM as one dose is alternate.
IM/IV

Children for 24-h mobilization test. 500 mg/m^2 as single dose IV over 1hr, or 500 mg/m^2 IMdivided into two doses at 12-h intervals (maximum: 1 g).
Note: Mobilization tests should not be performed in symptomatic patients or those with blood levels > 55 mcg/dL as therapy is indicated.

▸ **Symptomatic (without encephalopathy), or asymptomatic lead poisoning with blood lead levels > 70 mcg/dL**
IM/IV

Adults, Elderly, Children. 1-1.5 g/m^2 daily as 8-24 h IV infusion or divided every 12 h or 167 mg/m^2 IM every 4 h for 3-5 days (if blood lead concentration > 70 mcg/dL, calcium edetate usually given with dimercaprol until levels < 50 mcg/dL). Allow at least 2-4 days, up to 2-3 wks, between courses of therapy. Adults should not be given more than 2 courses of therapy.

▸ **Lead poisoning (with encephalopathy) with or without blood lead levels > 70 mcg/dL**
IM

Adults, Elderly, Children. Initially, dimercaprol 4 mg/kg; then give dimercaprol 4 mg/kg and calcium EDTA 250 mg/m^2 IM 4 h later and q4h for 5 days. Can also be given IV 50 mg/kg/day as 24-h continuous infusion or 1-1.5 g/m^2 as 8- to 24-h infusion or divided into 2 doses every 12 h. Allow at least 2 days before considering repeating course. Give dimercaprol for at least first 3 days.

▸ **Asymptomatic lead poisoning in children with blood lead level 45-69 mcg/dL**
IV

1 g/m^2/day IV infusion over 8-24 h is preferred regimen. 25 mg/kg/day

for 5 days as an 8- to 24-h infusion or divided into 2 doses every 12 h. May also give dose IM at 8- to 12-h intervals.

CONTRAINDICATIONS

Anuria, severe renal disease, hepatitis, hypersensitivity to EDTA or any component of the formulation.

INTERACTIONS

Drug
Insulin preparations: May bind to zinc components of some insulin preparations increasing active amount of insulin while decreasing duraction of action.
Zinc: May decrease the effects of zinc.
Herbal and Food
None known.

✪ IV INCOMPATIBILITIES

Amphotericin B cholesteryl (Amphotec), hydralazine, dextrose 10%, lactated Ringer's, Ringer's.

✪ IV COMPATIBILITIES

Epinephrine.

SIDE EFFECTS

Frequent
Chills, fever, anorexia, headache, histamine-like reaction (sneezing, stuffy nose, watery eyes), decreased BP, nausea, vomiting, thrombophlebitis, pain at IM injection site.
Rare
Frequent urination, secondary gout (severe pain in feet, knees, elbows).

SERIOUS REACTIONS

• Drug may produce same signs of renal damage as severe acute lead poisoning (proteinuria, microscopic hematuria). Transient anemia/bone marrow depression, hypercalcemia (constipation, drowsiness, dry mouth, metallic taste) occur occasionally.

Edetate calcium disodium is capable of producing toxic effects that can be fatal. Dosage schedules should be followed, and at no time should the recommended daily dose be increased. It is unknown whether EDTA is distributed in breast milk. Lead encephalopathy is usually rare in adults but occurs more often in children. No age-related precautions have been noted in children or elderly patients. Edetate calcium disodium can produce the same renal damage as lead poisoning, such as proteinuria and microscopic hematuria. Discontinue if severe oliguria or anuria occurs. Monitor for cardiac arrhythmias.

Do not confuse with edetate disodium. The FDA recommends that edetate disodium never be given for chelation therapy as fatal hypocalcemia can occur if edetate disodium is used instead of edetate calcium disodium for chelation. Do not use abbreviation EDTA. Only edetate calcium disodium should be used for lead intoxication.
Administration
Be aware that when administering IV, calcium EDTA may be given in 2 divided doses at 12 h intervals or 8- to 24-h infusions; when administered IM and used alone, it may be given in divided doses at 8- to 12-h intervals; when given IM with dimercaprol in divided doses, administer at 4-h intervals.

Be aware that total dose is dependent on severity of lead poisoning, patient response, and tolerance to medication. Consult specific protocols.

For IV administration, Add total daily dose to 250-500 mL of 0.9% NaCl or D5W. Preferably infused over 8-12 hr.

E

Patients with lead encephalopathy and cerebral edema may experience a lethal increase in intracranial pressure following IV infusion; the IM route is preferred for these patients. In cases where the IV route is necessary, avoid rapid infusion. The dosage schedule should be followed, and at no time should the recommended daily dose be exceeded. Rapid IV infusion may be lethal due to increased intracranial pressure.

For IM injection, should add lidocaine or prilocaine to injection: 1 mL of 1% procaine hydrochloride or lidocaine 1% to each milliliter of edetate calcium disodium to minimize pain at injection site. The total daily dose is usually divided into equal doses given 8-12 h apart.

Edetate Disodium
ed′eh-tate dye-sow-dee-um
Do not confuse with edetate calcium disodium.
Do not use EDTA as abbreviation to avoid potential confusion.

CATEGORY AND SCHEDULE
Pregnancy Risk Category: C

Classification: Antidotes, chelators

MECHANISM OF ACTION
A chelating agent that forms a soluble chelate with calcium, resulting in rapid decrease in plasma calcium concentrations. *Therapeutic Effect:* Allows calcium to be excreted in urine.

PHARMACOKINETICS
Distributed in extracellular fluid and does not appear in red blood cells. No metabolism occurs. Rapidly excreted in the urine. *Half-life:* 1.4-3 h. Prolonged in renal impairment. Chelation occurs in 24-48 h.

AVAILABILITY
Injection: 150 mg/mL.

INDICATIONS AND DOSAGES
▶ **Digitalis toxicity (ventricular arrhythmia), hypercalcemia**
IV
Adults, Elderly. 50 mg/kg/day over 3 h or more, daily for 5 days, skip 2 days, repeat as needed up to 15 doses. Maximum: 3 g/day.
Children. 40 mg/kg/day over 3 h or more, daily for 5 days, skip 5 days, repeat as needed. Maximum: 70 mg/kg/day.

CONTRAINDICATIONS
Anuria, renal impairment, hypersensitivity to edetate disodium or any component of the formulation.

INTERACTIONS
Drug
Insulin: May increase the effects of some forms of insulin containing zinc.
Herbal
None known.
Food
None known.

SIDE EFFECTS
Frequent
Abdominal cramps or pain, diarrhea, nausea, vomiting, circumoral paresthesia, headache, numbness, postural hypotension.
Rare
Exfoliative dermatitis, toxic skin and mucous membrane reactions, thrombophlebitis (at injection site).

SERIOUS REACTIONS
• Nephrotoxicity may occur with excessive dosages.
• Hypomagnesemia may occur with prolonged use.
• Hypokalemia can occur as potassium excretion may increase.

PRECAUTIONS & CONSIDERATIONS
Caution is warranted in patients with diabetes mellitus, clinical or subclinical hypokalemia, intracranial lesions, seizures, renal impairment, and limited cardiac reserve or incipient congestive heart failure. Be aware that edetate sodium is recommended only when the severity of the clinical condition justifies the aggressive measures associated with this type of therapy. It is unknown whether edetate disodium is distributed in breast milk. No age-related precautions have been noted in children or elderly patients.

Stop edetate sodium immediately and notify physician if frequent or sudden urges to urinate occur.

Do not confuse with edetate calcium disodium. The FDA recommends that edetate disodium never be given for chelation therapy as fatal hypocalcemia can occur if edetate disodium is used instead of edetate calcium disodium for chelation. Do not use abbreviation EDTA. Only edetate calcium disodium should be used for lead intoxication.

Administration
Be aware that edetate disodium is rarely used to treat digitalis-induced ventricular arrhythmias because other, more effective agents are available. It should only be used in emergency situations. It is not for IM use.

Dilute solution for injection with 500 mL of D5W or 0.9% NaCl before IV administration; in pediatric patients, concentration should not exceed 3% (30 mg/mL). Administer by IV infusion only after dilution. Be careful not to exceed recommended dose or rate of administration (over at least 3 h). A precipitous drop in serum calcium concentrations may occur. Calcium replacement suitable for IV administration should be instantly available.

Efalizumab
(Raptiva)

CATEGORY AND SCHEDULE
Pregnancy Risk Category: C

Classification: Immunosuppressives, monoclonal antibodies

MECHANISM OF ACTION
A monoclonal antibody that interferes with lymphocyte activation by binding to the lymphocyte antigen, inhibiting the adhesion of leukocytes to other cell types. *Therapeutic Effect:* Prevents the release of cytokines and the growth and migration of circulating total lymphocytes, predominant in psoriatic lesions.

PHARMACOKINETICS
Clearance is affected by body weight, not by gender or race, after subcutaneous injection. Serum concentration reaches steady state at 4 wks. Estimated 50% bioavailability after subcutaneous injection. Mean time to elimination: 25 days.

AVAILABILITY
Powder for Injection: One single-use vial designed to deliver 125 mg of efalizumab with one single-use prefilled diluent syringe containing 1.3 mL sterile water for injection.

E

INDICATIONS AND DOSAGES
▶ **Psoriasis**
Subcutaneous
Adults, Elderly. Initially, 0.7 mg/kg
followed by weekly doses of
1 mg/kg. Maximum: 200 mg
(single dose).

OFF-LABEL USES
Atopic dermatitis (severe,
recalcitrant).

CONTRAINDICATIONS
Hypersensitivity to efalizumab.

INTERACTIONS
Drug
Immunosuppressive agents:
Increase the risk of infection.
Live-virus vaccines: Decrease the
immune response to vaccination.
Avoid acellular, live, and live-
attenuated vaccines.
Herbal and Food
None known.

DIAGNOSTIC TEST EFFECTS
May increase the lymphocyte
count. Alkaline phosphatase
increased.

SIDE EFFECTS
Frequent (10%-32%)
Headache, first-dose reaction (fever,
chills, headache, myalgia, nausea
within 2 days), infections, chills,
nausea, injection site pain.
Occasional (5%-9%)
Myalgia, flulike symptoms,
hypersensitivity reaction, flulike
syndrome, fever.
Rare (4%)
Back pain, acne.

SERIOUS REACTIONS
• Hypersensitivity reaction,
malignancies, serious infections
(abscess, cellulitis, postoperative
wound infection, pneumonia),
thrombocytopenia, hemolytic
anemia, and worsening of psoriasis
occur rarely.

PRECAUTIONS & CONSIDERATIONS
Concurrent use of immuno-
suppressive agents or live vaccines
should be avoided. Safety and
efficacy have not been established
in patients with hepatic or renal
dysfunction. Caution is warranted
in patients with asthma, chronic
infections, a history of allergic
reactions, and a history of
malignancy. It is unknown whether
efalizumab is distributed in breast
milk. Efalizumab is not indicated
for use in children. Age-related
increased incidence of infection
requires cautious use in elderly
patients. Phototherapy treatments
should be avoided.

Notify the physician of bleeding
from gums, bruising or petechiae of
the skin, or signs of infection. Skin
should be examined throughout
therapy, and improvement or
worsening of psoriasis lesions should
be documented. CBC, lymphocyte,
and platelet counts should be
obtained before beginning therapy
and periodically thereafter.
Storage
Refrigerate unopened vials. Protect
from light. Reconstituted solution
may be stored at room temperature
for up to 8 h.
Administration
For subcutaneous use, slowly inject
1.3 mL of sterile water for injection
into the efalizumab vial using the
provided prefilled diluent syringe.
Swirl the vial gently to dissolve; do
not shake it because foaming will
occur. Dissolution takes < 5 min.
Administer the injection into the
abdomen, buttocks, thigh, or upper
arm. Discard unused reconstituted
solution. Rotate injection sites.

Efavirenz
e-fahv′er-ins
(Stocrin [AUS], Sustiva)
Do not confuse with Survanta.

CATEGORY AND SCHEDULE
Pregnancy Risk Category: D

Classification: Antiretroviral, non-nucleoside reverse transcriptase inhibitor

MECHANISM OF ACTION
A nonnucleoside reverse transcriptase inhibitor that inhibits the activity of HIV reverse transcriptase of HIV-1 and the transcription of HIV-1 RNA to DNA. *Therapeutic Effect:* Interrupts HIV replication, slowing the progression of HIV infection.

PHARMACOKINETICS
Rapidly absorbed after PO administration, increased by fatty meals. Protein binding: 99% (primarily albumin). Metabolized to inactive metabolites in the liver via CYP3A4 and CYP2B6. Eliminated in urine and feces. *Half-life:* 40-55 h.

AVAILABILITY
Capsules: 50 mg, 200 mg.
Tablets: 600 mg.

INDICATIONS AND DOSAGES
▸ **HIV infection (in combination with other antiretrovirals)**
PO
Adults, Elderly, Children 3 yrs and older weighing 40 kg or more. 600 mg once a day at bedtime.
Children 3 yrs and older weighing 32.5 kg to < 40 kg. 400 mg once a day.
Children 3 yrs and older weighing 25 kg to < 32.5 kg. 350 mg once a day.
Children 3 yrs and older weighing 20 kg to < 25 kg. 300 mg once a day.
Children 3 yrs and older weighing 15 kg to < 20 kg. 250 mg once a day.
Children 3 yrs and older weighing 10 kg to < 15 kg. 200 mg once a day.
Dosage adjustment with voriconazole: The voriconazole maintenance dose should be increased to 400 mg every 12 h, and the efavirenz dose should be decreased to 300 mg once daily using the capsule formulation (one 200-mg and two 50-mg capsules or six 50-mg capsules).

CONTRAINDICATIONS
Concurrent use with ergot derivatives, midazolam, triazolam, or standard doses of voriconazole; efavirenz as monotherapy; hypersensitivity to efavirenz.

INTERACTIONS
Drug
Alcohol, benzodiazepines, psychoactive drugs: May produce additive central nervous system (CNS) effects.
Amprenavir, atazanavir, diltiazem, HMG-CoA reductase inhibitors, indinavir, itraconazole, lopinavir, methadone, saquinavir, sertraline, voriconazole: Decreases the plasma concentrations of these drugs. Some of these medications significantly increase efavirenz concentrations.
Carbamazepine: Levels of carbamazepine and/or efavirenz may decrease.
Clarithromycin: Decreases clarithromycin plasma levels.
CYP2B6, CYP3A4 inducers: May decrease concentration of efavirenz.
CYP2C9, CYP2C19 substrates: May increase concentration of substrates.
CYP3A4 substrates: Concentration of substrates may be altered.

E

E

Ergot derivatives, midazolam, triazolam: May cause serious or life-threatening reactions, such as arrhythmias, prolonged sedation, or respiratory depression. Contraindicated.
Nelfinavir, ritonavir, ethinyl estradiol: Increases the plasma concentrations of these drugs.
Phenobarbital, rifabutin, rifampin: Lowers efavirenz plasma concentration.
Warfarin: Alters warfarin plasma concentration.
Herbal
St. John's wort: May decrease efavirenz concentration.
Food
High-fat meals: May increase drug absorption.

DIAGNOSTIC TEST EFFECTS

May produce false-positive urine test results for cannabinoid and increased total cholesterol, AST (SGOT), ALT (SGPT), and serum triglyceride levels.

SIDE EFFECTS

Frequent (52%)
Mild to severe: Dizziness, vivid dreams, insomnia, confusion, impaired concentration, amnesia, agitation, depersonalization, hallucinations, euphoria, somnolence (mild symptoms do not interfere with daily activities; severe symptoms interrupt daily activities).
Occasional
Mild to moderate: Maculopapular rash (27%); nausea, fatigue, headache, diarrhea, fever, cough (< 26%) (moderate symptoms may interfere with daily activities).

SERIOUS REACTIONS

• Convulsions and immune reconstitution syndrome rarely occur. Psychiatric symptoms, including aggressive behavior, paranoid reactions, severe depression, suicidal ideations, and manic reactions, may occur.

PRECAUTIONS & CONSIDERATIONS

Caution is warranted in patients with a history of liver impairment, mental illness, or substance abuse. Be aware of breastfeeding while taking efavirenz; breastfeeding is not recommended for mothers with HIV-1 infection. Reports of neural tube defects in infants born to women with first trimester exposure, including three cases of meningomyelocele and one Dandy-Walker syndrome, indicate that efavirenz may cause fetal harm when administered during the first trimester. Pregnancy should be avoided in women receiving efavirenz. The safety and efficacy of efavirenz have not been established in children younger than 3 yr. In children, there may be an increased incidence of rash. No age-related precautions have been noted in elderly patients. Efavirenz is not a cure for HIV infection, nor does it reduce risk of transmission to others.

Expect to obtain history of all prescription and nonprescription medications before giving the drug because efavirenz interacts with several drugs. Monitor for signs and symptoms of adverse CNS psychological side effects, such as abnormal dreams, dizziness, impaired concentration, insomnia, severe acute depression including suicidal ideation or attempts, and somnolence. Avoid tasks that require mental alertness or motor skills until response to the drug is established. Insomnia may begin during the first or second day of therapy and generally resolves in 2-4 wks. Fat redistribution or severe rash can occur.
Storage
Store at room temperature.

Administration
Take on empty stomach at bedtime. Do not take with high-fat meals because it may increase drug absorption and side effects. For adults and elderly patients, take efavirenz at bedtime during the first 2-4 wks because of the increased risk of temporary CNS side effects. Take the medication every day as prescribed. Do not alter the dose or discontinue the medication without first notifying the physician.

Eflornithine
eh-floor-nigh-theen
(Vaniqa)

CATEGORY AND SCHEDULE
Pregnancy Risk Category: C

Classification: Antiprotozoals, depilatory agents, dermatologics

MECHANISM OF ACTION
A topical antiprotozoal that inhibits ornithine decarboxylase cell division and synthetic function in the skin. *Therapeutic Effect:* Reduces rate of hair growth.

PHARMACOKINETICS
Absorption is < 1% from intact skin. Not metabolized. Primarily excreted as unchanged drug in urine. *Half-life:* 8 h.

AVAILABILITY
Cream: 13.9%.

INDICATIONS AND DOSAGES
▸ **For reduction of unwanted facial hair in women**
TOPICAL
Adults, Elderly. Apply a thin layer to affected area of the face and adjacent involved areas under chin; rub in thoroughly. Use twice daily at least 8 h apart. Do not wash area for at least 4 h.

OFF-LABEL USES
None.

CONTRAINDICATIONS
Hypersensitivity to eflornithine or any component of the formulation.

INTERACTIONS
Drug, Herbal, and Food
None known.

DIAGNOSTIC TEST EFFECTS
May elevate serum transaminases.

SIDE EFFECTS
Frequent (> 10%)
Acne, pseudofolliculitis barbae.
Occasional (2%-10%)
Headache, stinging/burning skin, tingling skin, dry skin, pruritus, erythema, dyspepsia.
Rare (< 1%)
Bleeding skin, rash, herpes simplex, folliculitis, rosacea.

SERIOUS REACTIONS
• Bleeding skin, cheilitis, contact dermatitis, herpes simplex, lip swelling, nausea, and weakness have been reported.

PRECAUTIONS & CONSIDERATIONS
It is unknown whether eflornithine is distributed in breast milk. Safety and efficacy of eflornithine have not been established in children. No age-related precautions have been noted in elderly patients.
 Transient stinging or burning may occur when applied to broken or abraded skin.
Administration
Continue to use other hair-removal techniques in conjunction with eflornithine. Apply eflornithine more

E

than 5 min after hair removal. Avoid application on abraded or broken skin. Cosmetics or sunscreen may be applied over treated areas after cream has dried. Therapeutic improvement noted in 4-8 wks. Condition may return to pretreatment levels 8 wks after discontinuing treatment.

Eletriptan
(Relpax)

CATEGORY AND SCHEDULE
Pregnancy Risk Category: C

Classification: Serotonin receptor agonists

MECHANISM OF ACTION
A serotonin receptor agonist that binds selectively to vascular serotonin 5-HT1B, 5-HT1D, and 5-HT1F receptors, producing a vasoconstrictive effect on cranial blood vessels. *Therapeutic Effect:* Relieves migraine headache.

PHARMACOKINETICS
Well absorbed after PO administration (50% bioavailability), peaks with 1.5 h. Metabolized by the liver to inactive metabolite by CYP3A4. Eliminated in urine (90%). *Half-life:* 4.4 h increased in patients with hepatic impairment and in elderly patients (older than 65 yrs).

AVAILABILITY
Tablets: 20 mg, 40 mg.

INDICATIONS AND DOSAGES
▸ **Acute migraine headache with or without aura**
PO
Adults, Elderly. 20-40 mg. If headache improves but then returns, dose may be repeated after 2 h. Maximum: 80 mg/day.

OFF-LABEL USES
None known.

CONTRAINDICATIONS
Arrhythmias associated with angina, conduction disorders, coronary artery disease, ischemic heart disease, history of myocardial infarction, cerebrovascular disease, peripheral vascular disease, ischemic bowel disease, hemiplegic or basilar migraine, severe hepatic impairment, uncontrolled hypertension. eletriptan should not be used within 24 h of another serotonin agonist (triptan) or an ergot-type medication, use within 72 hr of a potent CYP3A4 inhibitor.

INTERACTIONS
Drug
Clarithromycin, itraconazole, ketoconazole, nefazodone, nelfinavir, ritonavir, CYP3A4 inhibitors: May decrease eletriptan metabolism. Contraindicated within 72 hr of eletriptan use.
Ergotamine-containing medications: May produce a vasospastic reaction.
Sibutramine: May produce serotonin syndrome (marked by altered level of consciousness, CNS irritability, motor weakness, myoclonus, and shivering).
Serotonin reuptake inhibitors/ serotonin agonists (triptans): May increase risk of serotonin syndrome.
Herbal and Food
None known.

DIAGNOSTIC TEST EFFECTS
None known.

SIDE EFFECTS
Occasional (5%-6%)
Dizziness, somnolence, asthenia, nausea.
Rare (2%-4%)
Paresthesia, headache, dry mouth, warm or hot sensation, dyspepsia, dysphagia.

SERIOUS REACTIONS
• Cardiac reactions (including ischemia, coronary artery vasospasm, and myocardial infarction) and noncardiac vasospasm-related reactions (such as hemorrhage and cerebrovascular accident [CVA]) occur rarely, particularly in patients with hypertension, diabetes, or a strong family history of coronary artery disease; obese patients; smokers; males older than 40 yrs; and postmenopausal women. Serotonin syndrome has occurred; avoid concomitant use of serotonergic drugs. Increased BP and hypertensive crisis have occurred in patients with and without a history of hypertension.

PRECAUTIONS & CONSIDERATIONS
Caution is warranted in patients with controlled hypertension, mild to moderate hepatic or renal impairment, and a history of CVA. Eletriptan should not be given to patients with risk factors predictive of coronary artery disease unless clinical evaluation demonstrates that the patient is free of cardiovascular disease. Eletriptan is distributed in breast milk, and caution should be exercised in lactating women. Eletriptan effects in pregnancy are unknown and may suppress ovulation. The safety and efficacy of eletriptan have not been established in children younger than 18 yrs. Elderly patients

are at increased risk for hypertension. Tasks that require mental alertness or motor skills should be avoided.

Notify the physician immediately if palpitations, pain or tightness in the chest or throat, pain or weakness in the extremities, or sudden or severe abdominal pain occurs. BP for evidence of uncontrolled hypertension should be assessed before treatment. Migraines and associated symptoms, including nausea and vomiting, photophobia, and phonophobia (sound sensitivity), should be assessed before and during treatment.
Storage
Store at room temperature. Protect from light and moisture.
Administration
! Don't administer eletriptan within 72 h of clarithromycin, erythromycin, itraconazole, ketoconazole, nefazodone, nelfinavir, or ritonavir.

Take film-coated tablets whole with fluids; don't crush or break them.

Emedastine
eh-med´-ah-steen
(Emadine)

CATEGORY AND SCHEDULE
Pregnancy Risk Category: B

Classification: Ophthalmic antihistamine

MECHANISM OF ACTION
An ophthalmic H_1-receptor antagonist that inhibits histamine-stimulated vascular permeability in the conjunctiva. *Therapeutic Effect:* Relieves ocular itching associated with allergic conjunctivitis.

PHARMACOKINETICS
Negligible absorption after ophthalmic administration.

Metabolized into inactive metabolites. Excreted in urine.
Half-life: 6.6 h.

AVAILABILITY
Ophthalmic Solution: 0.05%.

INDICATIONS AND DOSAGES
▶ **Allergic conjunctivitis**
OPHTHALMIC
Adults, Elderly, Children 3 yr and older. 1 drop in affected eye(s) up to 4 times daily.

CONTRAINDICATIONS
Hypersensitivity to emedastine or any other component of the formulation.

DRUG INTERACTIONS
Drug
None reported.
Herbal and Food
None known.

SIDE EFFECTS
Frequent
Headache.
Occasional
Abnormal dreams, asthenia (loss of strength, energy), bad taste, blurred vision, burning or stinging, dry eyes, foreign body sensation, tearing.

SERIOUS REACTIONS
• Somnolence and malaise occur rarely.

PRECAUTIONS & CONSIDERATIONS
For topical ophthalmic use only. Safety and effectiveness have not been established in children < 3 years of age. Not known to what extent it is distributed in breast milk; use with caution.
Storage
Store at room temperature. Do not use if solution becomes discolored.

Administration
Wait at least 10 min after use before inserting contact lenses.

Emtricitabine
(Emtriva)

CATEGORY AND SCHEDULE
Pregnancy Risk Category: B

Classification: Antiretroviral, nucleoside reverse transcriptase inhibitors

MECHANISM OF ACTION
An antiretroviral that inhibits HIV-1 reverse transcriptase by incorporating itself into viral DNA, resulting in chain termination.
Therapeutic Effect: Interrupts HIV replication, slowing the progression of HIV infection.

PHARMACOKINETICS
Rapidly and extensively absorbed from the GI tract. Bioavailability of capsules 93%, oral solution 75%. Relative bioavailability of oral solution approximately 80% of capsules. Excreted primarily in urine (86%) and, to a lesser extent, in feces (14%); 30% removed by hemodialysis. Unknown whether removed by peritoneal dialysis.
Half-life: 10 h, children 5-18 h.

AVAILABILITY
Capsules: 200 mg.
Oral Solution: 10 mg/mL.

INDICATIONS AND DOSAGES
▶ **HIV infection (in combination with other antiretrovirals)**
PO
Adults, Elderly. 200 mg capsule or 240 mg (24 mL) oral solution once a day.

Children 3 months to 17 yr.
6 mg/kg (maximum: 240 mg) of oral
solution once daily.
Infants 0-3 months. 3mg/kg once
daily (oral solution).
▸ **Adult dosage in renal impairment**
Dosage and frequency are modified
based on creatinine clearance.

Creatinine Clearance (mL/min)	Capsule Dosage	Oral Solution Dosage
30-49	200-mg capsule q24h	120 mg (12 mL) q24h
15-29	200-mg capsule q72h	80 mg (8 mL) q24h
<15	200-mg capsule q72h	60 mg (6 mL) q24h

▸ **Hemodialysis patients
(give after hemodialysis)**
Adults. 200 mg q96h capsule or
60 mg q24h oral solution.

OFF-LABEL USES
Hepatitis B infection, part of non-
occupational and occupational
postexposure prophylaxis regimen for
HIV infection (Adults and children),
reduction of perinatal transmission
from HIV infected mother to newborn.

CONTRAINDICATIONS
Hypersensitivity.

INTERACTIONS
Drug
Ribavirin, interferons: Risk of
hepatic decompensation may be
increased.
Herbal and Food
None known.

DIAGNOSTIC TEST EFFECTS
May elevate serum amylase,
lipase, ALT (SGPT), AST (SGOT),
creatinine kinase, and triglyceride
levels. May alter blood glucose levels.

SIDE EFFECTS
Frequent (13%-23%)
Headache, rhinitis, rash,
diarrhea, nausea, fever, skin
hyperpigmentation (especially
children).
Occasional (4%-14%)
Cough, vomiting, abdominal
pain, insomnia, abnormal dreams,
depression, paresthesia, fatigue,
dizziness, peripheral neuropathy,
dyspepsia, myalgia.
Rare (2%-3%)
Arthralgia.

SERIOUS REACTIONS
• Lactic acidosis and hepatomegaly
with steatosis occur rarely and may
be severe. Severe acute exacerbations
of hepatitis B may occur. Anemia
has been reported more commonly in
children.

PRECAUTIONS & CONSIDERATIONS
Caution is warranted in patients
with impaired liver and dosage
adjustments recommended for
renal dysfunction. Be aware that
breastfeeding is not recommended. In
elderly patients, age-related decreased
renal function may require dosage
adjustment. Emtricitabine use may
cause the redistribution of body fat.
Emtricitabine is not a cure for HIV
infection, nor does it reduce risk of
transmission to others. Emtricitabine is
not indicated for hepatitis B. Patients
with hepatitis B have experienced
flare-ups on discontinuation of
emtricitabine, and liver function
should be monitored closely.
Treatment with medications for
hepatitis B if co-infection is present
may be necessary.
    Expect to obtain baseline laboratory
testing, especially liver function tests

E

and triglycerides, before beginning emtricitabine therapy and at periodic intervals during therapy. Assess for any nausea or vomiting and skin for rash and urticaria. Determine pattern of bowel activity and stool consistency.
Administration
Take without regard to food, at approximately the same time daily. Continue emtricitabine therapy for the full length of treatment.

Enalapril
en-al'a-pril
(Alphapril [AUS], Amprace [AUS], Apo-Enalapril [CAN], Auspril [AUS], Renitec [AUS], Vasotec)
Do not confuse with Anafranil, Eldepryl, or ramipril.

CATEGORY AND SCHEDULE
Pregnancy Risk Category: D (C if used in first trimester)

Classification: Angiotensin-converting enzyme inhibitors

MECHANISM OF ACTION
This angiotensin-converting enzyme (ACE) inhibitor suppresses the renin-angiotensin-aldosterone system and prevents conversion of angiotensin I to angiotensin II, a potent vasoconstrictor; it may inhibit angiotensin II at local vascular, renal sites. Decreases plasma angiotensin II, increases plasma renin activity, and decreases aldosterone secretion. *Therapeutic Effect:* In hypertension, reduces peripheral arterial resistance. In congestive heart failure (CHF), increases cardiac output; decreases peripheral vascular resistance, BP, pulmonary capillary wedge pressure, heart size.

PHARMACOKINETICS

Route	Onset	Peak	Duration
PO	1 h	4-6 h	24 h
IV	15 min	1-4 h	6 h

Readily absorbed from the GI tract (not affected by food). Protein binding: 50%-60%. Enalaprilat, the IV form rapidly converted to active metabolite. Primarily excreted in urine. Removed by hemodialysis. *Half-life:* 11 h (half-life is increased in those with impaired renal function).

AVAILABILITY
Tablets: 2.5 mg, 5 mg, 10 mg, 20 mg.
Injection: 1.25 mg/mL.

INDICATIONS AND DOSAGES
▶ **Hypertension alone or in combination with other antihypertensives**
PO
Adults, Elderly. Initially, 2.5-5 mg/day. Range: 10-40 mg/day in 1-2 divided doses.
Children > 1 mo. 0.08 mg/kg/day (up to 5 mg) in 1-2 divided doses. *Maximum:* 0.58 mg/kg/day (not to exceed 40 mg).
IV
Adults, Elderly. 0.625-1.25 mg q6h up to 5 mg q6h.
Children, Infant >1mo.
5-10 mcg/kg/dose q8-24h.
▶ **Adjunctive therapy for congestive heart failure**
PO
Adults, Elderly. Initially, 2.5-5 mg/day. Range: 5-20 mg/day in 2 divided doses. Maximum dose: 40 mg/day in 2 divided doses.
▶ **Adult oral dosage in renal impairment**
Dosage is modified based on creatinine clearance.

Creatinine Clearance (mL/min)	% Usual PO Dose
10-50	75-100
< 10	50

Enalapril should not be used in children with CrCl ≤ 30 mL/min.

OFF-LABEL USES

Treatment of diabetic nephropathy, nondiabetic kidney disease, or renal crisis in scleroderma, left ventricular dysfunction after myocardial infarction, Raynaud phenomenon.

CONTRAINDICATIONS

Hypersensitivity or history of angioedema from previous treatment with ACE inhibitors, idiopathic or hereditary angioedema, bilateral renal artery stenosis.

INTERACTIONS

Drug

Alcohol, antihypertensives, diuretics: May increase the effects of enalapril.

Aspirin: May decrease effectivenss of enalapril.

Lithium: Increased risk of lithium toxicity.

NSAIDs: Renal adverse effects may be increased.

Potassium-sparing diuretics, potassium supplements: Increased risk of hyperkalemia.

Herbal ane Food

None known.

DIAGNOSTIC TEST EFFECTS

May increase BUN and serum alkaline phosphatase, serum bilirubin, serum creatinine, serum potassium, SGOT (AST), and SGPT (ALT) levels. May decrease serum sodium levels. May cause positive ANA titer.

IV INCOMPATIBILITIES

Amphotericin B (Fungizone), caspofungin (Cancidas), cefepime (Maxipime), dantrolene, diazepam (Valium), lansoprazole (Prevacid), nesiritide (Natrecor), phenytoin.

IV COMPATIBILITIES

Acyclovir (Zovirax), alfentanil (Alfenta), allopurinol (Aloprim), amifostine (Ethyol), amikacin (Amikar), aminophylline, amphotericin B liposome (AmBisome), ascorbic acid, atracurium (Tracrium), atropine, azathioprine, aztreonam (Azactam), benztropine (Cogentin), bivalirudin (Angiomax), bretylium, bumetanide (Bumex), buprenorphine (Buprenex), butorphanol (Stadol), calcium chloride, calcium gluconate, carboplatin, cefazolin, ceftazidime (Ceptaz, Fortaz, Tazicef, Tazidime), ceftizoxime (Cefizox), ceftriaxone (Rocephin), cefuroxime (Zinacef), chloramphenicol, cimetidine, cisatracurium (Nimbex), cisplatin, cladribine (Leustatin), clindamycin (Cleocin), cyclophosphamide (Cytoxan), cyclosporine (Prograf), dactinomycin (Cosmegen), daptomycin (Cubicin), dextran 40, digoxin (Lanoxin), diltiazem, diphenhydramine (Benadryl), dobutamine (Dobutrex), docetaxel (Taxotere), dopamine (Intropin), doripenem (Doribax), doxorubicin liposomal (Doxil), ephedrine, epinephrine, erythromycin lactobionate, esmolol (Brevibloc), etoposide phosphate (Etopophos), famotidine (Pepcid), fentanyl (Sublimaze), filgrastim (Neupogen), fluconazole (Diflucan), fludarabine (Fludara), fluorouracil, folic acid, furosemide, ganciclovir (Cytovene), gemcitabine (Gemzar), gentamicin, granisetron (Kytril), heparin, hetastarch, hydrocortisone sodium succinate (Solu-Cortef), hydromorphone (Dilaudid), hydroxyzine, imipenem/cilastatin (Primaxin), insulin (regular; Humulin R, Novolin R), isoproterenol (Isuprel), ketorolac, labetalol, levofloxacin (Levaquin), lidocaine, linezolid (Zyvox), lorazepam (Ativan), magnesium sulfate, melphalan (Alkeran), meropenem (Merrem), methicillin, methotrexate, methylprednisolone sodium succinate, metoclopramide (Reglan), metoprolol (Lopressor), metronidazole (Flagyl), minocycline (Minocin), mitoxantrone (Novantrone), morphine, nafcillin, nalbuphine (Nubain), naloxone (Narcan), nicardipine (Cardene), nitroglycerin, nitroprusside sodium (Nitropress), norepinephrine (Levophed), ondansetron (Zofran), oxacillin, oxaliplatin (Eloxatin), oxytocin (Pitocin), paclitaxel (Taxol), penicillin G potassium, phenobarbital, piperacillin, piperacillin/tazobactam (Zosyn), potassium chloride, potassium phosphate, promethazine, propofol (Diprivan), propranolol, protamine, quinupristin/dalfopristin (Synercid), ranitidine (Zantac), remifentanil (Ultiva), rituximab (Rituxan), sodium acetate, sodium bicarbonate, streptokinase, succinylcholine (Anectine, Quelicin), tacrolimus (Prograf), teniposide (Vumon), theophylline, thiotepa (Thioplex), tigecycline (Tygacil), tirofiban (Aggrastat), tobramycin, trastuzumab (Herceptin), vancomycin, vecuronium (Norcuron), verapamil, vincristine (Vincasar), vinorelbine (Navelbine), voriconazole (Vfend).

SIDE EFFECTS

Frequent (5%-7%)
Headache, dizziness, hypotension, increased serum creatinine.

Occasional (2%-3%)
Orthostatic hypotension, fatigue, diarrhea, cough, syncope.
Rare (< 2%)
Angina, abdominal pain, vomiting, nausea, rash, asthenia (loss of strength, energy), syncope.

SERIOUS REACTIONS

• Excessive hypotension (first-dose syncope) may occur in patients with CHF and in those who are severely salt or volume depleted.
• Angioedema (swelling of face, lips; especially after first dose).
• Hyperkalemia may occur, especially with concomitant potassium-altering agents.
• Agranulocytosis and neutropenia may be noted in collagen vascular diseases, including scleroderma and systemic lupus erythematosus, and impaired renal function.
• Nephrotic syndrome may be noted in those with history of renal disease.
• Cholestatic jaundice, which may progress to hepatic necrosis. Discontinue if abnormal liver function tests.
• Renal dysfunction may occur. Increases in serum creatinine may occur after initiation of therapy. Monitor serum creatinine and discontinue if progressive or severe decline in function.

PRECAUTIONS & CONSIDERATIONS

Caution is warranted with cerebrovascular and coronary insufficiency, hypovolemia, renal impairment, unilateral renal artery stenosis, valvular stenosis, sodium depletion, and those on dialysis or receiving diuretics or anesthesia. Be aware that enalapril crosses the placenta and is distributed in breast milk. Enalapril may cause fetal or neonatal morbidity or mortality and should not be used during pregnancy.

Discontinue as soon as pregnancy is detected. Be aware that the safety and efficacy of enalapril have not been established in children. Elderly patients may be more susceptible to the hypotensive effects of enalapril.

Dizziness may occur. BP should be obtained immediately before giving each enalapril dose in addition to regular monitoring. Be alert to fluctuations in BP. If an excessive reduction in BP occurs, place the person in the supine position with legs elevated. CBC and blood chemistry should be obtained before beginning enalapril therapy, then every 2 wks for the next 3 mo, and periodically thereafter in patients with autoimmune disease or renal impairment and in those who are taking drugs that affect immune response or leukocyte count. BUN, serum creatinine, and serum potassium should also be monitored in those who are receiving a diuretic.
Administration
Tablets: May administer without regard to meals.

W: May be administered undiluted, or in up to 50 mL of a compatible IV solution (e.g., D5%W, 0.9% NaCl). Expect diuretics to be withheld a few days while enalapril initiated. If needed for BP control, they may be reinitiated a few days later.

Enfuvirtide
en-few′vir-tide
(Fuzeon)
Do not confuse with Furoxone.

CATEGORY AND SCHEDULE
Pregnancy Risk Category: B

Classification: Antivirals, fusion inhibitors

MECHANISM OF ACTION
A fusion inhibitor that interferes with the entry of HIV-1 into CD4+ cells by inhibiting the fusion of viral and cellular membranes. *Therapeutic Effect:* Impairs HIV replication, slowing the progression of HIV infection.

PHARMACOKINETICS
Comparable absorption when injected into subcutaneous tissue of abdomen, arm, or thigh. Protein binding: 92% (mainly albumin). Undergoes catabolism to amino acids. *Half-life:* 3.8 h.

AVAILABILITY
Powder for Injection: 108 mg (approximately 90 mg/mL when reconstituted) single-use vials.

INDICATIONS AND DOSAGES
▶ **HIV infection (in combination with other antiretrovirals)**
SUBCUTANEOUS
Adults, Elderly. 90 mg (1 mL) twice a day.
Children 6-16 yrs. 2 mg/kg twice a day. Maximum: 90 mg twice a day.
▶ **Pediatric dosing guidelines**
90 mg/mL when reconstituted.

Weight: kg (lb)	Dosage (mg/mL)
11-15.5 (24-34)	27 (0.3) (give BID)
15.6-20 (35-44)	36 (0.4) (give BID)
20.1-24.5 (45-54)	45 (0.5) (give BID)
24.6-29 (55-64)	54 (0.6) (give BID)
29.1-33.5 (65-74)	63 (0.7) (give BID)
33.6-38 (75-84)	72 (0.8) (give BID)
38.1-42.5 (85-94)	81 (0.9) (give BID)
> 42.5 (> 94)	90 (1) (give BID)

CONTRAINDICATIONS
Hypersensitivity to enfuvirtide or any of its components.

E

INTERACTIONS
None known.

DIAGNOSTIC TEST EFFECTS
May elevate blood glucose and serum amylase, CK, lipase, triglyceride, AST (SGOT), and ALT (SGPT) levels. May decrease blood hemoglobin levels and WBC count.

SIDE EFFECTS
Expected (98%)
Local injection site reactions (pain, discomfort, induration, erythema, nodules, cysts, pruritus, ecchymosis).
Frequent (16%-26%)
Diarrhea, nausea, fatigue.
Occasional (4%-11%)
Insomnia, peripheral neuropathy, depression, cough, decreased appetite or weight loss, sinusitis, anxiety, asthenia, myalgia, cold sores, infections.
Rare (2%-3%)
Constipation, influenza, upper abdominal pain, anorexia, conjunctivitis, infection at injection site, flulike syndrome.

SERIOUS REACTIONS
• Enfuvirtide use may potentiate bacterial pneumonia.
• Hypersensitivity (rash, fever, chills, rigors, hypotension), thrombocytopenia, neutropenia, and renal insufficiency or failure may occur rarely.

PRECAUTIONS & CONSIDERATIONS
Caution is warranted in patients with liver function impairment. Breastfeeding is not recommended in this patient population because of the possibility of HIV transmission. Be aware that the safety and efficacy of enfuvirtide have not been established in children younger than 6 yrs of age. No age-related precautions have been noted in elderly patients. Increased rate of bacterial pneumonia has occurred with enfuvirtide use. Seek medical attention if cough with fever, rapid breathing, or shortness of breath occurs. Enfuvirtide is not a cure for HIV infection, nor does it reduce risk of transmission to others.

Expect to obtain baseline laboratory testing, especially liver function tests and serum triglyceride levels, before beginning enfuvirtide therapy and at periodic intervals during therapy. Assess for hypersensitivity reaction and local injection site reaction, fatigue or nausea, depression, and insomnia.
Storage
Store at room temperature or in a refrigerator. Do not freeze. Refrigerate reconstituted solution; use within 24 h.

Bring reconstituted solution to room temperature before injection.
Administration
Reconstitute with 1.1 mL sterile water for injection. Gently tap vial for 10 s and then gently roll between the hands to avoid foaming and to ensure that all particles of drug are in contact with the liquid and no drug remains on the vial wall. The vial should then be allowed to stand until the powder goes completely into solution, which could take up to 45 min. Reconstitution time can be reduced by gently rolling the vial between the hands until the product is completely dissolved. Visually inspect vial for particulate matter; if present, do not use. Ensure solution is clear, colorless, and without bubbles. Discard unused portion. Administer subcutaneously into the upper abdomen, anterior thigh, or upper arm. Administer each injection at a different site

than the preceding injection site and only where there is no injection site reaction. Continue taking enfuvirtide for the full length of treatment.

Enoxaparin
e-nox-ah-pair'in
(Klexane [CAN], Lovenox)
Do not confuse Lovenox with Lotronex.

CATEGORY AND SCHEDULE
Pregnancy Risk Category: B

Classification: Anticoagulants low-molecular-weight heparins

MECHANISM OF ACTION
A low-molecular-weight heparin that potentiates the action of antithrombin III and inactivates coagulation factor Xa. *Therapeutic Effect:* Produces anticoagulation. Does not significantly influence bleeding time, PT, or aPTT.

PHARMACOKINETICS

Route	Onset	Peak	Duration
Subcuta-neous	N/A	3-5 h	12 h

Well absorbed after subcutaneous (SC) administration. Eliminated primarily in urine. Not removed by hemodialysis. *Half-life:* 4.5 h.

AVAILABILITY
Injection: 30 mg/0.3 mL, 40 mg/0.4 mL, 60 mg/0.6 mL, 80 mg/0.8 mL, 100 mg/mL, 120 mg/0.8 mL, 150 mg/mL in prefilled syringes. Mulitdose vial 100 mg/mL (3 mL).

INDICATIONS AND DOSAGES
▸ **Prevention of deep vein thrombosis (DVT) after hip and knee surgery**
SC
Adults, Elderly. 30 mg twice a day, generally for 7-10 days. Initial dose 12-24 h after surgery (if hemostasis established). For hip replacement, initial dose may be given 12 h before surgery. After initial thromboprophylaxis in hip replacement, 40 mg once daily for 3 wks is recommended.
▸ **Prevention of DVT after abdominal surgery**
SC
Adults, Elderly. 40 mg once a day for 7-10 days. Initial dose given 2 h before surgery.
▸ **Prevention of long-term DVT in nonsurgical acute illness**
SC
Adults, Elderly. 40 mg once a day for 6-11 days, up to 14 days in clinical trials.
▸ **Prevention of ischemic complications of unstable angina and non-Q-wave MI (with oral aspirin therapy)**
SC
Adults, Elderly. 1 mg/kg q12h. Should be given for minimum of 2 days and until clinical stabilization, usual duration 2-8 days.
▸ **Treatment of acute ST-segment elevation myocardial infarction**
IV/SUBCUTANEOUS
Adults. Bolus 30 mg IV once followed by 1 mg/kg SC, then 1 mg/kg SC q12h (maximum 100 mg for first two doses, followed by 1 mg/kg dosing for remaining doses).
Elderly > 75 yrs. Do not give IV bolus. Start with 0.75 mg/kg SC q12h (maximum 75 mg for the first two doses, followed by 0.75 mg/kg dosing for remaining doses).
When administered in conjunction with a thrombolytic (fibrin-specific

E

or nonfibrin specific), give between 15 min before and 30 min after the start of fibrinolytic therapy. All patients should receive acetylsalicylic acid (ASA) as soon as they are identified as having STEMI and maintained with 75-325 mg once daily unless contraindicated. Treatment duration 8 days or until hospital discharge. For patients managed with percutaneous coronary intervention (PCI): If the last SC administration was given < 8 h before balloon inflation, no additional dosing is needed. If the SC administration was given more than 8 h before balloon inflation, an IV bolus of 0.3 mg/kg should be administered.

▶ **Acute DVT**

SC

Adults, Elderly. 1 mg/kg q12h or 1.5 mg/kg once daily. Initiate warfarin within 72 h. Continue enoxaparin for minimun of 5 days and until therapeutic INR achieved (INR 2-3).

▶ **Usual pediatric dosage**

SC

Children > 2 mo to 18 yrs. 0.5 mg/kg q12h (prophylaxis); 1 mg/kg q12h (treatment).

▶ **Dosage in renal impairment**

Clearance of enoxaparin is decreased when creatinine clearance is < 30 mL/min. Monitor patient and adjust dosage as necessary. When enoxaparin is used in abdominal, hip, or knee surgery or acute illness, the adult dosage in renal impairment is 30 mg once a day. When enoxaparin is used to treat DVT, angina, or non-Q-wave MI, the dosage in renal impairment is 1 mg/kg once a day. Treatment of acute ST-segment elevation myocardial infarction (MI; in patients < 75 yrs of age) dose is 30 mg IV bolus plus 1 mg/kg SC dose followed by 1 mg/kg SC once daily. Treatment of acute ST-segment elevation MI (> 75 yrs) is 1 mg/kg SC once daily.

ⓘ IV INCOMPATIBILITIES

Do not mix with other medications.

OFF-LABEL USES

Prevention of DVT following general surgical procedures, acute arterial thrombosis, prevention of thrombosis with hemodialysis, lichen planus, thrombophilia in pregnancy.

CONTRAINDICATIONS

Active major bleeding, concurrent heparin therapy, hypersensitivity to heparin or pork products, hypersensitivity to benzyl alcohol (multidose vial), thrombocytopenia associated with positive in vitro test for antiplatelet antibodies.

INTERACTIONS

Drug

Anticoagulants, platelet inhibitors: May increase bleeding.

Herbal

Supplements with antiplatelet or anticoagulant effects (e.g., feverfew, garlic, ginger, ginkgo biloba, ginseng, red clover, sweet clover, white willow, etc.): May increase effects on platelets or risk of bleeding.

Food

None known.

DIAGNOSTIC TEST EFFECTS

Increases (reversible) LDH, serum alkaline phosphatase, AST (SGOT), ALT (SGPT) and anti-factor Xa levels. May decrease platelet counts.

SIDE EFFECTS

Occasional (1%-4%)

Injection site hematoma, fever, nausea, hemorrhage, peripheral edema.

SERIOUS REACTIONS

• Overdose may lead to bleeding complications ranging from local ecchymoses to major hemorrhage.

Antidote: Protamine sulfate (1% solution) equal to the dose of enoxaparin injected. 1 mg protamine sulfate neutralizes 1 mg enoxaparin. A second dose of 0.5 mg protamine sulfate per 1 mg enoxaparin may be given if aPTT tested 2-4 h after first injection remains prolonged.

• Spinal or epidural hematomas resulting in paralysis have occurred. Risk is increased in patients with postoperative indwelling epidural catheters.

• Heparin-induced thrombocytopenia.

PRECAUTIONS & CONSIDERATIONS

Caution is warranted in patients with conditions associated with increased risk of hemorrhage (e.g., bacterial endocarditis, congenital or acquired bleeding disorders, active ulcerative and angiodysplastic GI disease, hemorrhagic stroke, or shortly after brain, spinal, or ophthalmologic surgery, or in patients treated concomitantly with platelet inhibitors), history of recent GI ulceration and hemorrhage, history of heparin-induced thrombocytopenia, impaired renal function, uncontrolled arterial hypertension, thrombocytopenia, indwelling epidural catheters, and in elderly patients. Enoxaparin should be used with caution in pregnant women, particularly during the last trimester and immediately postpartum, because it increases the risk of maternal hemorrhage. It is unknown whether enoxaparin is excreted in breast milk. Safety and efficacy of enoxaparin have not been established in children. Elderly patients may be more susceptible to bleeding. Women may experience heavier menstrual flow. Other medications, including OTC drugs, should be avoided. An electric razor and soft toothbrush should be used to prevent bleeding during therapy.

Notify the physician of abdominal or back pain, severe headache, black or red stool, coffee-ground vomitus, dark or red urine, or red-speckled mucus from cough. CBC and stool for occult blood should be periodically monitored. Be aware of signs of bleeding, including bleeding at injection or surgical sites or from gums, blood in stool, bruising, hematuria, and petechiae.

Storage

Store at room temperature.

Administration

! Do not mix with other injections or infusions. Do not give IM. Give initial dose as soon as possible after surgery but not more than 24 h after surgery.

Parenteral form normally appears clear and colorless to pale yellow. The patient should lie down before administering by deep subcutaneous injection. Inject between the left and right anterolateral and left and right posterolateral abdominal wall. Introduce entire length of needle (one-half inch) into skinfold held between thumb and forefinger, holding skinfold during injection. Duration of therapy varies by indication.

Entacapone
en-tak'a-pone
(Comtan)

CATEGORY AND SCHEDULE

Pregnancy Risk Category: C

Classification: Antiparkinson agents, COMT inhibitors

E

MECHANISM OF ACTION
An antiparkinson agent that inhibits the enzyme, catechol *O*-methyltransferase (COMT), potentiating dopamine activity and increasing the duration of action of levodopa. *Therapeutic Effect:* Decreases signs and symptoms of Parkinson's disease.

PHARMACOKINETICS
Rapidly absorbed after PO administration (peak effect 1 h). Protein binding: 98% (primarily albumin). Metabolized in the liver. Primarily eliminated by biliary excretion. Not removed by hemodialysis. *Half-life:* 2.4 h.

AVAILABILITY
Tablets: 200 mg.

INDICATIONS AND DOSAGES
▸ **Adjunctive treatment of Parkinson's disease**
PO
Adults, Elderly. 200 mg concomitantly with each dose of carbidopa and levodopa up to a maximum of 8 times a day (1600 mg).

CONTRAINDICATIONS
Hypersensitivity, use within 14 days of non-selective MAOIs.

INTERACTIONS
Drug
Ampicillin, cholestyramine, erythromycin, probenecid: May decrease the excretion of entacapone.
Bitolterol, dobutamine, dopamine, epinephrine, isoetharine, isoproterenol, epinephrine, methyldopa, norepinephrine: May increase the risk of arrhythmias and changes in BP.
Nonselective MAOIs (including phenelzine): May inhibit catecholamine metabolism and increase risk of cardiovascular side effects such as hypertensive crisis. Contraindicated.
Other central nervous system (CNS) depressants: May increase CNS depression.
Herbal
None known.
Food
None known.

DIAGNOSTIC TEST EFFECTS
None known.

SIDE EFFECTS
Frequent (> 10%)
Dyskinesia, hyperkinesia, nausea, dark yellow or orange urine and sweat, diarrhea.
Occasional (3%-9%)
Abdominal pain, vomiting, constipation, hallucinations, dry mouth, fatigue, back pain.
Rare (< 2%)
Anxiety, somnolence, agitation, dyspepsia, flatulence, diaphoresis, asthenia, dyspnea.

SERIOUS REACTIONS
• Rhabdomyolysis and neuroleptic malignant syndrome have occurred rarely.

PRECAUTIONS & CONSIDERATIONS
Caution is warranted with hepatic or renal impairment, dyskinesia, orthostatic hypotension, and syncope. It is unknown whether entacapone is distributed in breast milk. This drug is not indicated for children. No age-related precautions have been noted in elderly patients.

Dizziness, drowsiness, dry mouth, and darkened sweat and urine may occur. Tasks that require mental alertness or motor skills should be avoided. Notify the physician if uncontrolled movement of the hands, arms, legs, eyelids, face, mouth, or tongue occurs. Baseline vital signs should be obtained. Relief of symptoms, such as improvement of masklike facial expression, muscular rigidity, shuffling gait, and resting tremors of the hands and head, should be assessed during treatment. Dyskinesia, diarrhea, and orthostatic hypotension should also be monitored. Do not withdraw abruptly as rapid withdrawal may lead to hyperpyrexia and confusion resembling neuroleptic malignant syndrome.

Administration

! Always administer entacapone with carbidopa and levodopa.

Take entacapone without regard to food.

Ephedrine
eh-fed′rin
(Pretz-D)
Do not confuse with epinephrine.

CATEGORY AND SCHEDULE
Pregnancy Risk Category: C

Classification: Adrenergic agonists; bronchodilators; decongestants, nasal

MECHANISM OF ACTION
An adrenergic agonist that stimulates α-adrenergic receptors causing vasoconstriction and pressor effects, β_1-adrenergic receptors, resulting in cardiac stimulation, and β_2-adrenergic receptors, resulting in bronchial dilation and vasodilation. *Therapeutic Effect:* Increases BP and pulse rate.

PHARMACOKINETICS
Well absorbed after oral, nasal, and parenteral absorption. Metabolized in liver to small extent. Excreted in urine. *Half-life:* 3-6 h. Onset of bronchodilation: 15 min to 1h. Duration (oral): 3-6 h.

E

AVAILABILITY
Injection: 50 mg/mL.
Intranasal Spray: 0.25% (Pretz-D).

INDICATIONS AND DOSAGES
▸ **Asthma**
IM/IV/SQ
Adults. 12.5-25 mg. Maximum dose 150 mg/day.
Children > 2 yrs. 2-3 mg/kg/day or 100 mg/m^2/day divided into 4-6 doses/day.
▸ **Hypotension**
IM
Adults. 25-50 mg as a single dose. Maximum 150 mg/day.
IV
Adults. 5 mg/dose slow IVP as prevention. 10-25 mg/dose slow IVP repeated q5-10min as treatment. Maximum: 150 mg/day.
Children. 0.2-0.3 mg/kg/dose slow IVP q4-6h.
SUBCUTANEOUS
Adults. 25-50 q4-6h. Maximum 150 mg/day.
Children. 3 mg/kg/day in divided doses q4-6 h.
▸ **Nasal congestion**
NASAL
Adults, Children 12 yrs and older. 2-3 sprays into each nostril q4h.
Children 6-12 yrs. 1-2 sprays into each nostril q4h.

OFF-LABEL USES
Obesity, orthostatic hypotension, propofol-induced pain, radiocontrast media reactions.

E

CONTRAINDICATIONS

Anesthesia with cyclopropane or halothane, diabetes (ephedrine injection), hypersensitivity to ephedrine or other sympathomimetic amines, hypertension or other cardiovascular disorders, myocardial infarction, angina, arrhythmias, pregnancy with maternal blood pressure above 130/80, thyrotoxicosis, angle-closure glaucoma.

INTERACTIONS

Drug
Atropine, MAOIs, oxytocics, tricyclic antidepressants: May increase cardiovascular effects.
α-adrenergic, β-adrenergic blockers: May blunt ephedrine vasopressor effects.
Caffeine: May increase cardiac stimulation.
Cardiac glycosides, sympathomimetics, theophylline, general anesthetics: May increase toxic cardiac stimulation.
Herbal
Ephedra (ma huang), bitter orange, yohimbe: May increase central nervous system (CNS) and cardiovascular stimulation and effects.
Food
None known.

DIAGNOSTIC TEST EFFECTS

May result in false-positive amphetamine EMIT assay.
Lactic acid serum values may be increased.

ⓘ IV INCOMPATIBILITIES

Hydrocortisone sodium succinate (Solu-Cortef), phenobarbital (Luminal), secobarbital (Seconal), thiopental (Thioplex).

ⓘ IV COMPATIBILITIES

Chloramphenicol, etomidate (Amidate), fenoldopam (Corlopam), lidocaine, methotrexate, milrinone (Primacor), tigecycline (Tygacil), vecuronium (Norcuron), nafcillin (Unipen), penicillin G, propofol (Diprivan), tetracycline.

SIDE EFFECTS

Frequent
Hypertension, anxiety, agitation.
Occasional
Nausea, vomiting, palpitations, tremor, chest pain, BP changes, tachycardia, hallucinations, restlessness, diaphoresis, xerostomia.
Nasal: Burning, stinging, runny nose.
Rare
Psychosis, decreased/painful urination, necrosis at injection site from repeated injections.

SERIOUS REACTIONS

• Excessive doses may cause hypertension, intracranial hemorrhage, anginal pain, and fatal arrhythmias (including ventricular tachycardia), myocardial infarction, cardiac arrest.
• Stroke, transient ischemic attack, seizures.
• Prolonged or excessive use may result in metabolic acidosis as a result of increased serum lactic acid concentrations.
• Observe for disorientation, weakness, hyperventilation, headache, nausea, vomiting, and diarrhea.

PRECAUTIONS & CONSIDERATIONS

Caution is warranted with angina, coronary artery disease, diabetes, hypoxia (lack of oxygen), heart attack, psychiatric disorders, tachycardia, severe liver or kidney impairment, seizure disorder, thyroid disorders, prostatic hypertrophy, and in elderly patients. Epinephrine crosses the placenta and is distributed in breast milk and breastfeeding should be avoided. Excessive amounts of caffeine such as in chocolate, cocoa, coffee, cola, or tea should be avoided. Changes in vital signs and proper lung function should be monitored. Slight burning or stinging may be experienced when ophthalmic solution is administered to the eye. New symptoms such as dizziness, shortness of breath, or tachycardia (decreased heart rate) experienced with the ophthalmic solution should be reported immediately because they may indicate absorption by the body.

Storage
Injectable and intranasal forms should be stored at room temperature and protected from light.

Administration
Ampule should be shaken thoroughly. Solution should not be used if it appears discolored or contains a precipitate (separation of particles from liquid). A tuberculin syringe for subcutaneous injection into lateral deltoid muscle region should be used and injection site massaged. For injection, each 1 mg of 1:1000 solution is diluted with 10 mL 0.9% NaCl to provide 1:10,000 solution, and injected as each 1 mg or fraction thereof over more than 1 min. For infusion, preparation should be further diluted with 250-500 D5W. Maximum concentration is 64 mg/250 mL, the recommended rate of IV infusion is 1-10 mcg/min, adjusted to desired response.

For intranasal administration, before using spray, blow nose gently.

Keep head in the upright position and spray into each nostril. Blow nose well 3-5 min after using ephedrine. Do not administer more frequently than every 4 h. Do not use for more than 3 days to avoid rebound nasal congestion.

Epinastine
(Elestat)

CATEGORY AND SCHEDULE
Pregnancy Risk Category: C

Classification: Antihistamines, H_1, ophthalmics

MECHANISM OF ACTION
An ophthalmic H_1 receptor antagonist that inhibits the release of histamine from the mast cell. *Therapeutic Effect:* Prevents pruritus associated with allergic conjunctivitis.

PHARMACOKINETICS
Low systemic exposure. Protein binding: 64%. Less than 10% is metabolized. Excreted primarily in urine and, to a lesser extent, in feces. *Half-life:* 12 h.

AVAILABILITY
Ophthalmic Solution: 0.05% (5 mL).

INDICATIONS AND DOSAGES
▸ **Allergic conjunctivitis**
OPHTHALMIC
Adults, Elderly, Children 3 yrs and older. 1 drop in each eye twice a day. Continue treatment until period of exposure (pollen

season, exposure to offending allergen) is over.

CONTRAINDICATIONS
Hypersensitivity to epinastine or any of its components.

INTERACTIONS
Drug
None known.
Herbal
None known.
Food
None known.

DIAGNOSTIC TEST EFFECTS
None known.

SIDE EFFECTS
Occasional
Ocular (1%-10%): Burning sensation in the eye, hyperemia, pruritus. Nonocular (10%): Cold symptoms, upper respiratory tract infection.
Rare (1%-3%)
Headache, rhinitis, sinusitis, increased cough, pharyngitis.

SERIOUS REACTIONS
• None known.

PRECAUTIONS & CONSIDERATIONS
It is not known whether epinastine is distributed in breast milk. The safety and efficacy of epinastine have not been established in children younger than 3 yrs. No age-related precautions have been noted in elderly patients.
Drowsiness, dizziness, and dry mouth may occur; tolerance usually develops to sedative effects. Therapeutic response should be monitored.
Administration
For ophthalmic use, place a finger on the lower eyelid, and pull it out until a pocket is formed between the eye and lower lid. Don't let the applicator tip touch any surface. Hold the dropper above the pocket, and place the prescribed number of drops in the pocket. Close the affected eye gently so the medication won't squeeze out of the lacrimal sac. Apply gentle pressure to the lacrimal sac at the inner canthus for 1 min after installation to lessen the risk of systemic absorption. Remove contact lenses before instilling epinastine because the lenses may absorb the drug's preservatives. The lenses may be reinserted 10 min after administration unless the treated eye is red.

Epinephrine
ep-i-nef´rin
(Adrenalin, Adrenaline Injection [AUS], AsthmaNephrin, EpiPen, microNephrin, Primatene Mist, Raphon, S2, Twinject).
Do not confuse epinephrine with ephedrine.

CATEGORY AND SCHEDULE
Pregnancy Risk Category: C
Rx: Injection, Topical solution
OTC: Inhalation solution, Oral aerosol

Classification: Adrenergic agonists, bronchodilators, inotropes

MECHANISM OF ACTION
A sympathomimetic, adrenergic agonist that stimulates β-adrenergic receptors, causing vasoconstriction and pressor effects, β_1-adrenergic receptors, resulting in cardiac

stimulation, and β_2-adrenergic receptors, resulting in bronchial dilation and vasodilation.
Therapeutic Effect: Relaxes smooth muscle of the bronchial tree, produces cardiac stimulation, and dilates skeletal muscle vasculature.

PHARMACOKINETICS

Route	Onset (min)	Peak (min)	Dura-tion (h)
IM	5-10	20	1-4
Subcutane-ous	5-10	20	1-4
Inhalation	1-5	20	1-3

Well absorbed after parenteral administration; minimally absorbed after inhalation. Metabolized in the liver, other tissues, and sympathetic nerve endings. Excreted in urine. Vasoconstriction occurs within 5 min and lasts < 1 h.

AVAILABILITY

Injection: 0.1 mg/mL, 1 mg/mL.
Injection (EpiPen): 0.3 mg/0.3 mL, 0.15 mg/0.3 mL.
Injection (Twinject): 0.15 mg/0.15 mL.
Inhalation, Aerosol (Primatene Mist): 0.22 mg/inhalation.
Inhalation, Solution: 1%, 2.25% (racepinephrine).

INDICATIONS AND DOSAGES
▸ **Asystole**
IV
Adults, Elderly. 1 mg q3-5min up to 0.1 mg/kg q3-5min.
Infants, Children. 0.01 mg/kg (0.1 mL/kg of 1:10,000 solution). May repeat q3-5min. Subsequent doses of 0.1 mg/kg (0.1 mL/kg) of a 1:1000 solution q3-5min. Maximum 1 mg (10 mL).
ENDOTRACHEAL
Adults. 2-2.5 mg via ET, may repeat every 3-5 min.

Children, Infants. 0.1 mg/kg (0.1 mL/kg of 1:1000 solution). May repeat q3-5min. (maximum 10 mg).
▸ **Bradycardia**
IV INFUSION
Adults, Elderly. 1-10 mcg/min titrated to desired effect.
IV
Infants, Children. 0.01 mg/kg (0.1 mL/kg of 1:10,000 solution) q3-5min. Maximum: 1 mg (10 mL).
▸ **Bronchodilation**
IM, SUBCUTANEOUS
Adults, Elderly. 0.3-0.5 mg (1:1000) q20min to 4 h for 3 doses.
SUBCUTANEOUS
Children. 10 mcg/kg (0.01 mL/kg of 1:1000). Maximum: 0.5 mg every 5 min up to 3 doses.
INHALATION
Adults, Elderly, Children 4 yrs and older. 1 inhalation, may repeat in at least 1 min. Give subsequent doses no sooner than 3-4 h.
NEBULIZER
Adults, Elderly, Children 4 yrs and older. 1-3 deep inhalations. Give subsequent doses no sooner than 3 h.
▸ **Hypersensitivity reaction**
IM, SUBCUTANEOUS
Adults, Elderly. 0.3-0.5 mg q15-20min.
SUBCUTANEOUS
Children. 0.01 mg/kg q15min for 2 doses, then q4h. Maximum single dose: 0.5 mg.
AUTOINJECTORS
Adults. Twinject (Subcutaneous/IM) 0.3 mg. EpiPen (IM) 0.3 mg. May repeat once after 10-20 min.
Children 15-30 kg. Twinject (Subcutaneous/IM) 0.15 mg. EpiPen (IM) 0.15 mg.
Children > 30 kg. Twinject (Subcutaneous/IM) 0.3 mg. EpiPen (IM) 0.3 mg.

OFF-LABEL USES
Systemic: Treatment of gingival or pulpal hemorrhage, priapism.

E

CONTRAINDICATIONS
Cardiac arrhythmias, cerebrovascular insufficiency, hypertension, hyperthyroidism, ischemic heart disease, labor, narrow-angle glaucoma, shock (except anaphylactic).

INTERACTIONS
Drug
β-Blockers: May decrease the effects of β-blockers.
Digoxin, sympathomimetics, halogenated inhalational anesthetics: May increase the risk of arrhythmias and toxicity.
Ergonovine, methergine, oxytocin: May increase vasoconstriction.
MAOIs, tricyclic antidepressants: May increase cardiovascular effects. Contraindicated within 2 wks of MAOI.
Herbal
Ephedra (ma huang), bitter orange, yohimbe: May increase central nervous system (CNS) and cardiovascular stimulation and effects.
Food
None known.

DIAGNOSTIC TEST EFFECTS
May decrease serum potassium level.

⑩ IV INCOMPATIBILITIES
Acyclovir (Zovirax), aminophylline, azathioprine, ampicillin (Omnipen, Polycillin), dantrolene, diazepam (Valium), fluorouracil, ganciclovir (Cytovene), indomethacin, micafungin (Mycamine), pantoprazole (Protonix), pentobarbital, phenobarbital, phenytoin, thiopental, sodium bicarbonate, sulfamethoxazole/ trimethoprim.

⑩ IV COMPATIBILITIES
Alfentanil (Alfenta), amikacin (Amikar), amiodarone, amphotericin B liposomal (AmBisome), anidulafungin (Eraxis), ascorbic acid, atracurium (Tracrium), atropine, aztreonam (Azactam), benztropine (Cogentin), bivalirudin (Angiomax), bretylium, bumetanide (Bumex), bupivacaine, calcium chloride, calcium gluconate, carboplatin, caspofungin (Cancidas), cefazolin, cefotaxime (Claforan), cefotetan (Cefotan), cefoxitin (Mefoxin), ceftazidime (Ceptaz, Fortaz, Tazicef, Tazidime), ceftizoxime (Cefizox), ceftriaxone (Rocephin), cefuroxime (Zinacef), chloramphenicol, chlorpromazine, cimetidine (Tagamet), cisatracurium (Nimbex), cisplatin, clindamycin (Cleocin), clonidine, cyanocobalamin, cyclophosphamide (Cytoxan), cyclosporine (Sandimmune), dactinomycin (Cosmegen), daptomycin (Cubicin), dexamethasone sodium phosphate, dexmedetomidine (Precedex), digoxin (Lanoxin), diltiazem (Cardizem), diphenhydramine (Benadryl), dobutamine (Dobutrex), docetaxel (Taxotere), dopamine (Intropin), doxorubicin (Adriamycin), edetate calcium disodium, enalaprilat, ephedrine, epirubicin (Ellence), epoetin alfa (Procrit), ertapenem (Invanz), erythromycin lactobionate, esmolol (Brevibloc), etoposide phosphate (Etopophos), famotidine (Pepcid), fenoldopam (Corlopam), fentanyl (Sublimaze), fluconazole (Diflucan), fludarabine (Fludara), folic acid, furosemide (Lasix), gemcitabine (Gemzar), gentamicin, granisetron (Kytril), heparin, hydrocortisone sodium succinate (Solu-Cortef), hydromorphone (Dilaudid), hydroxyzine, imipenem/cilastatin (Primaxin), isoproterenol (Isuprel), ketorolac, labetalol, levofloxacin (Levaquin), lidocaine, linezolid (Zyvox), lorazepam (Ativan),

magnesium sulfate, mannitol, meperidine (Demerol), methicillin, methotrexate, methylprednisolone sodium succinate, metoclopramide (Reglan), metoprolol (Lopressor), metronidazole (Flagyl), midazolam (Versed), milrinone (Primacor), minocycline (Minocin), mitoxantrone (Novantrone), morphine, multiple vitamins injection, nafcillin, nalbuphine (Nubain), naloxone (Narcan), nicardipine (Cardene), nitroglycerin, nitroprusside sodium (Nitropress), norepinephrine (Levophed), ondansetron (Zofran), oxacillin, oxaliplatin (Eloxatin), oxytocin (Pitocin), paclitaxel (Taxol), pancuronium, pemetrexed (Alimta), penicillin G potassium, penicillin G sodium, phytonadione, potassium chloride, procainamide, prochlorperazine, promethazine, propofol (Diprivan), propranolol, quinupristin/dalfopristin (Synercid), ranitidin (Zantac), remifentanil (Ultiva), streptokinase, succinylcholine, sufentanil (Sufenta), tacrolimus (Prograf), teniposide (Vumon), ticarcillin (Ticar), ticarcillin/clavulanate (Timentin), tigecycline (Tygacil), tirofiban (Aggrastat), tobramycin, vancomycin, vasopressin, vecuronium (Norcuron), verapamil, vincristine (Vincasar), vinorelbine (Navelbine), vitamin B complex with C, voriconazole (Vfend), warfarin.

SIDE EFFECTS

Frequent
Systemic: Tachycardia, palpitations, nervousness, dizziness.
Ophthalmic: Headache, eye irritation, watering of eyes.
Occasional
Systemic: Dizziness, lightheadedness, facial flushing, headache, diaphoresis, increased BP, nausea, trembling, insomnia, vomiting, fatigue, urinary retention.
Ophthalmic: Blurred or decreased vision, eye pain.
Rare
Systemic: Chest discomfort or pain, arrhythmias, bronchospasm, dry mouth or throat.

SERIOUS REACTIONS

• Excessive doses may cause acute hypertension or arrhythmias or cerebrovascular hemorrhage.
• Prolonged or excessive use may result in metabolic acidosis as a result of increased serum lactic acid concentrations. Metabolic acidosis may cause disorientation, fatigue, hyperventilation, headache, nausea, vomiting, and diarrhea.

PRECAUTIONS & CONSIDERATIONS

Caution is warranted with angina, diabetes, coronary artery disease, cerebrovascular disease, thyroid disease, seizure disorders, prostatic hypertrophy, hypoxia (lack of oxygen), heart attack, psychiatric disorders, tachycardia, severe liver or kidney impairment, and in elderly patients. Avoid extravasation as tissue necrosis can occur. Epinephrine crosses the placenta and is distributed in breast milk. Excessive amounts of caffeine, such as in chocolate, cocoa, coffee, cola, or tea, should be avoided. Changes in vital signs and proper lung function should be monitored.
Storage
Injectable solutions should be stored at room temperature.
Administration
Ampule should be shaken thoroughly. Solution should not be used if it appears discolored or

E

contains a precipitate (separation of particles from liquid). A tuberculin syringe for subcutaneous injection into lateral deltoid muscle region should be used and injection site massaged.

For injection, each 1 mg of 1:1000 solution is diluted with 10 mL 0.9% NaCl to provide 1:10,000 solution, and injected as each 1 mg or fraction thereof over more than 1 min. For infusion, preparation should be further diluted with 250-500 D5W. Maximum concentration is 64 mg/250 mL; the recommended rate of IV infusion is 1-10 mcg/min, adjusted to desired response.

Eplerenone
e-plear′a-nown
(Inspra)

CATEGORY AND SCHEDULE
Pregnancy Risk Category: B

Classification: Selective aldosterone receptor antagonist

MECHANISM OF ACTION
An aldosterone receptor antagonist that binds to the mineralocorticoid receptors in the kidney, heart, blood vessels, and brain, blocking the binding of aldosterone. *Therapeutic Effect:* Reduces BP.

PHARMACOKINETICS
Absorption is unaffected by food. Protein binding: 50%. Metabolized by CYP3A4. No active metabolites. Excreted in the urine with a lesser amount eliminated in the feces. Not removed by hemodialysis. *Half-life:* 4-6 h. Onset of full hypertensive effect may take 4 wks.

AVAILABILITY
Tablets: 25 mg, 50 mg.

INDICATIONS AND DOSAGES
▸ **Hypertension**
PO
Adults, Elderly. 50 mg once a day. If 50 mg once a day produces an inadequate BP response, may increase dosage to 50 mg twice a day (max dose). If patient is concurrently receiving erythromycin, saquinavir, verapamil, or fluconazole, reduce initial dose to 25 mg once a day.
▸ **Congestive heart failure following myocardial infarction**
PO
Adults, Elderly. Initially, 25 mg once a day. If tolerated, titrate up to 50 mg once a day within 4 wks. If potassium < 5 mEq/L, increase the dose from 25 mg every other day to 25 mg daily or increase dose from 25 to 50 mg daily. No dose adjustment if potassium 5-5.4 mEq/L. If potassium 5.5-5.9 mEq/L, decrease the dose from 50 to 25 mg daily or from 25 mg daily to 25 mg every other day or 25 mg every other day to withhold. If potassium > 6 mEq/L, withhold dose until potassium < 5.5 mEq/L, then give 25 mg every other day.

CONTRAINDICATIONS
Concurrent use of potassium supplements or potassium-sparing diuretics (such as amiloride, spironolactone, and triamterene), or strong inhibitors of the cytochrome P450 3A4 enzyme system (including ketoconazole and

itraconazole), creatinine clearance < 50 mL/min, serum creatinine level > 2 mg/dL in men or 1.8 mg/dL in women, serum potassium level > 5.5 mEq/L, type 2 diabetes mellitus with microalbuminuria.

INTERACTIONS
Drug
ACE inhibitors, angiotensin II antagonists, potassium-sparing diuretics, potassium supplements: Increases the risk of hyperkalemia.
CYP3A4 inhibitors such as calcium channel blockers, erythromycin, fluconazole, saquinavir, verapamil: May increase levels and toxicity such as hyperkalemia. Strong inhibitors such as clarithromycin, itraconazole, and ketoconazole should not be used concomitantly.
CYP3A4 inducers: May decrease levels of eplerenone.
NSAIDs: May decrease antihypertensive effect.
Herbal
St. John's wort: Decreases eplerenone effectiveness.
Food
Grapefruit juice: Produces small increase in exposure to eplerenone (25%).

DIAGNOSTIC TEST EFFECTS
May increase serum potassium level, serum creatinine, triglycerides, cholesterol, ALT, and GGT levels. May decrease serum sodium level.

SIDE EFFECTS
Rare (1%-3%)
Dizziness, diarrhea, cough, fatigue, flulike symptoms, abdominal pain, abnormal vaginal bleeding, mastodynia.

SERIOUS REACTIONS
• Hyperkalemia may occur, particularly in patients with type 2 diabetes mellitus and microalbuminuria. Monitor closely.

PRECAUTIONS & CONSIDERATIONS
Caution is warranted with hyperkalemia and hepatic or renal impairment. It is unknown whether eplerenone crosses the placenta or is distributed in breast milk. The safety and efficacy of eplerenone have not been established in children. No age-related precautions have been noted in elderly patients. Exercising outside during hot weather should be avoided because of the risks of dehydration and hypotension.

Dizziness and lightheadedness may occur. Tasks that require mental alertness or motor skills should be avoided. Apical heart rate and BP should be obtained immediately before each dose, in addition to regular monitoring. Be alert to BP fluctuations. If an excessive reduction in BP occurs, place in the supine position with feet slightly elevated, and notify the physician. Pattern of daily bowel activity and stool consistency and potassium and sodium levels should also be monitored.
Administration
Film-coated tablets should not be broken, crushed, or chewed. May give without regard to food.

E

Epoetin Alfa (Erythropoietin)

eh-poh'ee-tin al'fa
(Epogen, Eprex [CAN], Procrit)
Do not confuse Epogen with Neupogen.

CATEGORY AND SCHEDULE

Pregnancy Risk Category: C

Classification: Hematopoietic agents

MECHANISM OF ACTION

A glycoprotein that stimulates division and differentiation of erythroid progenitor cells in bone marrow. *Therapeutic Effect:* Induces erythropoiesis and releases reticulocytes from bone marrow to raise hemoglobin and hematocrit.

PHARMACOKINETICS

Well absorbed after subcutaneous (SC) administration. Following administration, an increase in reticulocyte count occurs within 10 days, and increases in hemoglobin, hematocrit, and RBC count are seen within 2-6 wks. *Half-life:* 4-13 h.

AVAILABILITY

Injection, Single-Dose Vials:
2000 units/mL, 3000 units/mL, 4000 units/mL, 10,000 units/mL, 40,000 units/mL.
Injection, Multiple Dose Vials:
10,000 units/mL, 20,000 units/mL.

INDICATIONS AND DOSAGES

▸ **Treatment of anemia in chemotherapy patients**
IV, SC
Adults, Elderly. 150 units/kg/dose SC 3 times/wk. Maximum: 1200 units/kg/wk. Weekly dosing: 40,000 units SC weekly. Reduce dose by 25% when hemoglobin approaches 12 g/dL or increases by more than 1 g/dL in any 2-wks period. If hemoglobin exceeds 12 g/dL, hold dose until hemoglobin is < 11 g/dL and restart at 25% reduction in previous dose. If hemoglobin does not increase 1 g/dL or more after 4 wks for weekly dosing, increase dose to 60,000 units/wk. If hemoglobin does not increase with 3 times/wk dosing, after 8 wks increase dose to 300 units/kg 3 times/wk.
Children: 600 units/kg IV once per week. Maximum: 40,000 units/kg/dose. If hemoglobin does not increase 1 g/dL or more after 4 wks, increase dose to 900 units/kg IV weekly.
▸ **Reduction of allogenic blood transfusions in elective surgery**
SC
Adults, Elderly. 300 units/kg/day 10 days before, the day of, and 4 days after surgery. Alternate dose: 600 units/kg once weekly (21, 14, and 7 days before surgery) and the day of surgery.
▸ **Chronic renal failure**
IV bolus, SC
Adults, Elderly. Initially, 50-100 units/kg 3 times a week. Target hemoglobin for patients not on dialysis 10-12 g/dL. Hematocrit range: 30%-36%. Adjust dosage no earlier than 1-mo intervals unless prescribed. Decrease dosage if hemoglobin is approaching 12 g/dL, reduce dose by 25%. If level continues to increase, withhold dose until hemoglobin decreases and restart at 25% reduction. If increase in hemoglobin is < 1 g/dL in 4 wks (with adequate iron stores), increase dose by 25% of previous dose. Maintenance: For patients on dialysis: 75 units/kg 3 times/wk. Range: 12.5-525 units/kg. For patients not on dialysis: 75-150 units/kg/wk.

Children on Dialysis. Initially, 50 units/kg 3 times/wk. Maintenance: For children on hemodialysis, median dose of 167 units/kg/wk administered in divided doses 2-3 times weekly. For children on peritoneal dialysis, median dose of 76 units/kg/wk in divided doses 2-3 times weekly.

▸ **HIV infection in patients treated with Zidovudine (AZT)**

IV, SC

Adults. Initially, 100 units/kg 3 times a week for 8 wks; may increase by 50-100 units/kg 3 times a week. Evaluate response q4-8wk thereafter. Adjust dosage by 50-100 units/kg 3 times/wk. If dosages larger than 300 units/kg 3 times/wk are not eliciting response, it is unlikely patient will respond. Maintenance: Titrate to maintain desired hematocrit; hemoglobin not to exceed 12 g/dL.

OFF-LABEL USES

Prevention of anemia in patients donating blood before elective surgery or autologous transfusion, treatment of anemia associated with neoplastic diseases, treatment of anemia in critical illness, uremic pruritus.

CONTRAINDICATIONS

History of sensitivity to hamster cell–derived products or human albumin, uncontrolled hypertension.

INTERACTIONS

Drug

Heparin: An increase in RBC volume may enhance blood clotting. Heparin dosage may need to be increased.

Herbal

None known.

Food

None known.

DIAGNOSTIC TEST EFFECTS

May increase BUN, serum phosphorus, serum potassium, serum creatinine, serum uric acid, and sodium levels. May decrease bleeding time, iron concentration, and serum ferritin levels.

E

🚫 IV INCOMPATIBILITIES

Do not mix with other medications. Amphotericin B cholesteryl sulfate complex (Amphotec), chlorpromazine, dantrolene, diazepam (Valium), haloperidol (Haldol), midazolam, minocycline (Minocin), phenytoin, prochlorperazine, sulfamethoxazole/trimethoprim, vancomycin.

💧 IV COMPATIBILITIES

Alfentanil (Alfenta), amikacin (Amikar), aminophylline, ascorbic acid, atracurium (Tracrium), atropine, azathioprine, aztreonam (Azactam), benztropine (Cogentin), bretylium, bumetanide (Bumex), buprenorphine (Buprenex), butorphanol (Stadol), calcium chloride, calcium gluconate, cefazolin, cefotaxime (Claforan), cefotetan (Cefotan), cefoxitin (Mefoxin), ceftazidime (Ceptaz, Fortaz, Tazicef, Tazidime), ceftizoxime (Cefizox), ceftriaxone (Rocephin), cefuroxime (Zinacef), chloramphenicol, cimetidine (Tagamet), clindamycin (Cleocin), cyanocobalamin, cyclosporine (Sandimmune), dexamethasone sodium phosphate, digoxin (Lanoxin), diltiazem (Cardizem), diphenhydramine (Benadryl), dobutamine (Dobutrex), dopamine (Intropin), enalaprilat, ephedrine, epinephrine, erythromycin lactobionate, esmolol (Brevibloc), famotidine (Pepcid), fentanyl (Sublimaze), fluconazole (Diflucan), folic acid, furosemide (Lasix), ganciclovir (Cytovene), heparin, hydrocortisone sodium succinate (Solu-Cortef), hydroxyzine, imipenem/cilastatin (Primaxin), insulin (regular, Humulin R, Novolin R), isoproterenol (Isuprel), ketorolac, labetalol, lidocaine, magnesium sulfate, mannitol, meperidine (Demerol), methicillin, methylprednisolone sodium succinate, metoclopramide (Reglan), metoprolol (Lopressor), metronidazole (Flagyl), morphine, multiple vitamins injection, nafcillin, nalbuphine (Nubain), naloxone (Narcan), nitroglycerin, nitroprusside sodium (Nitropress), norepinephrine (Levophed), ondansetron (Zofran), oxacillin, oxytocin (Pitocin), penicillin G potassium, penicillin G sodium, pentobarbital, phenobarbital, phytonadione, potassium chloride, procainamide, promethazine, propranolol, ranitidin (Zantac), sodium bicarbonate, streptokinase, succinylcholine, sufentanil (Sufenta), theophylline, ticarcillin (Ticar), ticarcillin/clavulanate (Timentin), tobramycin, vasopressin, verapamil.

SIDE EFFECTS

▸ **Patients receiving chemotherapy**

Frequent (17%-20%)
Fever, diarrhea, nausea, vomiting, edema.
Occasional (11%-13%)
Asthenia, shortness of breath, paresthesia.
Rare (3%-5%)
Dizziness, trunk pain.

▸ **Patients with chronic renal failure**

Frequent (11%-24%)
Hypertension, headache, nausea, arthralgia.
Occasional (7%-9%)
Fatigue, edema, diarrhea, vomiting, chest pain, skin reactions at administration site, asthenia, dizziness, clotted access.

▸ **Patients with HIV infection treated with AZT**

Frequent (15%-38%)
Fever, fatigue, headache, cough, diarrhea, rash, nausea.
Occasional (9%-14%)
Shortness of breath, asthenia, skin reaction at injection site, dizziness.

SERIOUS REACTIONS

• Hypertensive encephalopathy, thrombosis, cerebrovascular accident, myocardial infarction (MI), and seizures have occurred rarely.
• Epoetin alfa increased the risk for death and serious cerebrovascular events in controlled clinical trials when administered to target a hemoglobin of more than 12 g/dL and in cancer patients receiving chemotherapy. There is increased risk of serious arterial and venous thromboembolic reactions, including MI, stroke, congestive heart failure (CHF), and hemodialysis graft occlusion. To reduce cerebrovascular risks, use the lowest dose of epoetin alfa that will gradually increase the hemoglobin concentration to a level sufficient to avoid the need for RBC transfusion. The hemoglobin concentration should not exceed 12 g/dL; the rate of hemoglobin increase should not exceed 1 g/dL in any 2-wks period.
• Epoetin alfa has shortened time to tumor progression and reduced survival time in solid tumor patients with target hemoglobin >12 g/dL.
• Hyperkalemia occurs occasionally in patients with chronic renal failure, usually in those who do not conform to medication regimen, dietary guidelines, and frequency of dialysis regimen.
• Cases of pure red cell aplasia and severe anemia, with or without other cytopenias, associated with neutralizing antibodies to

erythropoietin, have been reported in patients treated with epoetin alfa. This has been reported predominantly in patients with chronic renal failure (CRF) receiving epoetin alfa by SC administration.

PRECAUTIONS & CONSIDERATIONS

Caution is warranted with a history of seizures and known porphyria (an impairment of erythrocyte formation in bone marrow). It is unknown whether epoetin alfa crosses the placenta or is distributed in breast milk. Safety and efficacy of epoetin alfa have not been established in children 1 mo of age and younger. No age-related precautions have been noted in elderly patients. Avoid potentially hazardous activities during the first 90 days of therapy. There is an increased risk of seizure development in those with chronic renal failure during the first 90 days of therapy.

Notify the physician of severe headache. Hematocrit level should be monitored diligently. The dosage should be reduced if hematocrit level increases more than 4 points in 2 wks. Hemoglobin should not exceed 12 g/dL or increase by 1 g/dL in any 2-wks period. CBC should also be monitored before and during therapy. In addition BP must be monitored aggressively for an increase because 25% of persons taking epoetin alfa require antihypertensive therapy and dietary restrictions. Keep in mind that most patients will eventually need supplemental iron therapy. Body temperature, especially in persons receiving chemotherapy and in those with HIV infection treated with zidovudine, and serum BUN, serum phosphorus, serum potassium, serum creatinine, and serum uric acid levels, especially in persons with chronic renal failure.

Storage
Refrigerate vials. Do not shake vials.
Administration
! Avoid excessive agitation of vial; do not shake because it can cause foaming. Also, vigorous shaking may denature medication, rendering it inactive. Patients receiving AZT who have serum erythropoietin levels > 500 milliunits are not likely to respond to therapy. IV route is preferred for patients on hemodialysis.

For IV use, reconstitution is not necessary. May be given as an IV bolus.

For SC administration, use one dose per vial; do not reenter vial. Discard unused portion. May be mixed in a syringe with bacteriostatic 0.9% NaCl with benzyl alcohol 0.9% or bacteriostatic saline at a 1:1 ratio. Benzyl alcohol acts as a local anesthetic and may reduce injection site discomfort.

Epoprostenol (Prostacyclin)
e-poe-pros'ten-ol
(Flolan)

CATEGORY AND SCHEDULE
Pregnancy Risk Category: B

Classification: Platelet inhibitors, vasodilators

MECHANISM OF ACTION
An antihypertensive that directly dilates pulmonary and systemic arterial vascular beds and inhibits platelet aggregation.

Therapeutic Effect: Reduces right and left ventricular afterload; increases cardiac output and stroke volume.

AVAILABILITY

Injection, Powder for Reconstitution: 0.5 mg, 1.5 mg.

INDICATIONS AND DOSAGES

▸ **Long-term treatment of New York Heart Association Class III and IV primary pulmonary hypertension and pulmonary hypertension associated with scleroderma spectrum of disease in New York Heart Association Class II and IV who do not respond adequately to conventional therapy**

IV INFUSION

Adults, Elderly. Procedure to determine dose range: Initially, 2 ng/kg/min, increased in increments of 2 ng/kg/min q15min until dose-limiting adverse effects occur.

Increments in dose should be considered if symptoms of pulmonary hypertension persist or recur after improving. The infusion should be increased by 1- to 2-ng/kg/min increments at intervals sufficient to allow assessment of clinical response; these intervals should be at least 15 min. In clinical trials, incremental increases in dose occurred at intervals of 24-48 h or longer. Avoid abrupt withdrawal or sudden large dose reductions.

OFF-LABEL USES

Primary pulmonary arterial hypertension in children.

CONTRAINDICATIONS

Long-term use in patients with CHF (severe ventricular systolic dysfunction) or chronically in patients who develop pulmonary edema during initiation.

INTERACTIONS

Drug

Acetate in dialysis fluids, other vasodilators, antihypertensives, diuretics: May increase hypotensive effect.

Anticoagulants, antiplatelets: May increase the risk of bleeding.

Vasoconstrictors: May decrease effects of epoprostenol.

Herbal

Supplements with antiplatelet or anticoagulant effects (e.g., feverfew, garlic, ginger, ginkgo biloba, ginseng, red clover, sweet clover, white willow, etc.): May increase effects on platelets or risk of bleeding.

Food

None known.

DIAGNOSTIC TEST EFFECTS

None known.

Ⓓ IV INCOMPATIBILITIES

Do not mix epoprostenol with other medications.

🖫 IV COMPATIBILITIES

Bivalirudin (Angiomax).

SIDE EFFECTS

Frequent

Acute phase: Flushing (58%), headache (49%), nausea (32%), vomiting (32%), hypotension (16%), anxiety (11%), chest pain (11%), dizziness (8%).

Chronic phase (> 20%): Dyspnea, asthenia, dizziness, headache, chest pain, nausea, vomiting, palpitations, edema, jaw pain, tachycardia, flushing, myalgia, nonspecific muscle pain, diarrhea, anxiety, chills, fever, or flulike symptoms.

Occasional

Acute phase (2%-5%): Bradycardia, abdominal pain, muscle pain, dyspnea, back pain.

Chronic phase (10%-20%): Rash, depression, hypotension, paresthesia, pallor, syncope, bradycardia, ascites, tachycardia.

Rare

Acute phase: Paresthesia, diaphoresis, dyspepsia, tachycardia.

SERIOUS REACTIONS

• Angina, myocardial infarction, and thrombocytopenia occur rarely.
• Abrupt withdrawal, including a large reduction in dosage or interruption in drug delivery, may produce rebound pulmonary hypertension as evidenced by dyspnea, dizziness, and asthenia.
• Sepsis during long-term follow-up.

PRECAUTIONS & CONSIDERATIONS

Interruptions in the IV infusion should be avoided because even a short break in the infusion can result in rebounding pulmonary hypertension. The patient should be closely monitored during initiation of therapy. Use epoprostenol cautiously in elderly patients.

Before beginning therapy, a backup infusion pump and IV infusion sets should be obtained to avoid interruptions in therapy. A central venous catheter must be in place. Vital signs should be monitored before and during therapy. Standing and supine BP should be monitored for several hr after a dosage adjustment. Therapeutic evidence is evidenced by decreased chest pain, dyspnea on exertion, fatigue, pulmonary arterial pressure, pulmonary vascular resistance, and syncope, and improved pulmonary function.

Storage

Store unopened vial at room temperature. Do not freeze.

Reconstituted solutions are stable for up to 48 h if refrigerated. Discard if frozen or if reconstituted > 48 h.

Administration

! Infuse epoprostenol continuously through an indwelling central venous catheter. If necessary and on a temporary basis, infuse through a peripheral vein. Use only the diluent provided by the manufacturer.

Follow instructions of manufacturer for dilution to specific concentrations. Give as pump infusion only. Adjustments to dose should only be done by physician.

E

Eprosartan
eh-pro-sar'tan
(Teveten)

CATEGORY AND SCHEDULE
Pregnancy Risk Category: C (D if used in second or third trimester)

Classification: Angiotensin II receptor antagonists

MECHANISM OF ACTION
An angiotensin II receptor antagonist that blocks the vasoconstrictor and aldosterone-secreting effects of angiotensin II, inhibiting the binding of angiotensin II to the AT1 receptors. *Therapeutic Effect:* Causes vasodilation, decreases peripheral resistance, and decreases BP.

PHARMACOKINETICS
Rapidly absorbed after PO administration. Protein binding: 98%. Minimally metabolized in liver. Excreted in urine (90%) and biliary system. Minimally removed by hemodialysis. *Half-life:* 5-9 h.

E

AVAILABILITY
Tablets: 400 mg, 600 mg.

INDICATIONS AND DOSAGES
▸ **Hypertension**
PO
Adults, Elderly. Initially, 600 mg/day (given in one or two doses). Range: 400-800 mg/day.

CONTRAINDICATIONS
Hypersensitivity to eprosartan.

INTERACTIONS
Drug
Potassium-sparing diuretics, potassium supplements: May increase risk of hyperkalemia.
Herbal
Licorice, ma huang, yohimbine: May increase the effectiveness of eprosartan.
Food
None known.

DIAGNOSTIC TEST EFFECTS
May increase BUN, serum alkaline phosphatase, serum bilirubin, serum creatinine, potassium, AST (SGOT), and ALT (SGPT) levels. May decrease blood hemoglobin levels.

SIDE EFFECTS
Occasional (2%-8%)
Upper respiratory infection, rhinitis, cough, abdominal pain.
Rare (< 2%)
Muscle pain, fatigue, diarrhea, urinary tract infection, depression, hypertriglyceridemia.

SERIOUS REACTIONS
• Overdosage may manifest as hypotension and tachycardia. Bradycardia occurs less often.

PRECAUTIONS & CONSIDERATIONS
Caution is warranted with preexisting renal insufficiency, significant aortic and mitral stenosis, hyperaldosteronism, and bilateral or unilateral renal artery stenosis. Salt and volume-depletion should be corrected before starting therapy. Eprosartan has caused fetal or neonatal morbidity or mortality. Also, because of the potential for adverse effects on the infant, patients taking eprosartan should not breastfeed. Safety and efficacy of eprosartan have not been established in children. No age-related precautions have been noted in elderly patients. Sodium consumption and alcohol should be avoided.

Apical pulse and BP should be assessed immediately before each eprosartan dose and regularly throughout therapy. Be alert to fluctuations in apical pulse and BP. If an excessive reduction in BP occurs, place the person in the supine position with feet slightly elevated and notify the physician. Tasks that require mental alertness or motor skills should be avoided. BUN, serum electrolytes, serum creatinine levels, heart rate for tachycardia, and urinalysis results should be obtained before and during therapy.
Administration
Take eprosartan without regard to food. Do not crush or break tablets.

Eptifibatide
ep-tih-fib′ah-tide
(Integrilin)

CATEGORY AND SCHEDULE
Pregnancy Risk Category: B

Classification: Platelet inhibitors

MECHANISM OF ACTION
A glycoprotein IIb/IIIa inhibitor that rapidly inhibits platelet aggregation by preventing binding of fibrinogen to receptor sites on platelets. *Therapeutic Effect:* Prevents closure of treated coronary arteries. Also prevents acute cardiac ischemic complications.

AVAILABILITY
Injection Solution: 0.75 mg/mL, 2 mg/mL.

INDICATIONS AND DOSAGES
▸ **Adjunct to percutaneous coronary intervention (PCI)**
IV BOLUS, IV INFUSION
Adults, Elderly. 180 mcg/kg bolus (maximum 22.6 mg) before PCI initiation; then continuous drip of 2 mcg/kg/min and a second 180 mcg/kg bolus (maximum 22.6 mg) 10 min after the first. Maximum: 15 mg/h. Continue until hospital discharge or for up to 18-24 h. Minimum 12 h is recommended. Concurrent aspirin and heparin therapy is recommended.
▸ **Acute coronary syndrome**
IV BOLUS, IV INFUSION
Adults, Elderly. 180 mcg/kg bolus (max 22.6 mg) then 2 mcg/kg/min until discharge or coronary artery bypass graft, up to 72 h. Maximum: 15 mg/h. Concurrent aspirin and heparin therapy is recommended.
▸ **Dosage in renal impairment**
Serum creatinine 2-4 mg/dL or CrCl < 50 mL/min. Use 180 mcg/kg bolus (maximum 22.6 mg) and 1 mcg/kg/min infusion (maximum: 7.5 mg/h). For PCI, a second bolus dose should be administered (180 mcg/kg, maximum 22.6 mg) 10 min after the first bolus.

CONTRAINDICATIONS
Active internal bleeding within previous 30 days, history of stroke within 30 days, or any history of hemorrhagic stroke, recent (6 wks or less) surgery or trauma, severe uncontrolled hypertension, thrombocytopenia (< 100,000 cells/μL), renal dialysis, administration of another parenteral GP IIb/IIIa inhibitor, hypersensitivity.

INTERACTIONS
Drug
Anticoagulants, heparin: May increase the risk of hemorrhage.
Dextran, drotrecogin alfa, other platelet aggregation inhibitors (such as aspirin), thrombolytic agents: May increase the risk of bleeding.
Herbal
None known.
Food
None known.

DIAGNOSTIC TEST EFFECTS
Increases aPTT, PT, and clotting time. Decreases platelet count.

Ⓜ IV INCOMPATIBILITIES
Administer in separate line; do not add other medications to infusion solution.
Furosemide (Lasix).

🖊 IV COMPATIBILITIES
Alteplase (Activase), amiodarone, argatroban, atropine, bivalirudin (Angiomax), daptomycin (Cubicin), dobutamine, ertapenem (Invanz), heparin, lidocaine, meperidine (Demerol), metoprolol (Lopressor), micafungin (Mycamine), midazolam, morphine, nitroglycerin, oxytocin (Pitocin), palonosetron (Aloxi), potassium chloride, teniposide (Vumon), tigecycline (Tygacil), tirofiban (Aggrastat), verapamil, 0.9% NaCl, 0.9% NaCl-D5%W.

SIDE EFFECTS
Occasional (7%)
Hypotension.

E

SERIOUS REACTIONS

• Minor to major bleeding complications may occur, most commonly at arterial access site for cardiac catheterization.
• Thrombocytopenia, intracranial hemorrhage and stroke, anaphylaxis have occurred rarely

PRECAUTIONS & CONSIDERATIONS

Caution is warranted in patients with PTCA < 12 h from the onset of symptoms of acute myocardial infarction, prolonged PTCA that is > 70 min, and failed PTCA. Caution should also be used in persons who weigh < 75 kg or are older than 65 yrs; have a history of GI disease or GI or genitourinary bleeding; have an AV malformation or aneurysm, intracranial tumors, platelet count < 100,000, renal dysfunction, hemorrhagic retinopathy; or are receiving aspirin, heparin, or thrombolytics. It is unknown whether eptifibatide causes fetal harm or can affect reproduction capacity. It is unknown whether eptifibatide is distributed in breast milk. Safety and efficacy of eptifibatide have not been established in children. In elderly patients, the risk of major bleeding is increased.

Hemoglobin, hematocrit, and platelet count should be obtained before treatment. If platelet count is < 90,000/mm^3, additional platelet counts should be obtained routinely to avoid development of thrombocytopenia. Nasogastric tube and urinary catheter use should be avoided, if possible.

Storage
Store vials in refrigerator. Vials may be stored at room temperature for up to 2 mo.

Administration
Solution normally appears clear and is colorless. Do not shake. Discard unused portions. Also discard if preparation contains any opaque particles. Withdraw bolus dose from 10-mL vial (2 mg/mL); for IV infusion, withdraw from 100-mL vial (0.75 mg/mL). May give IV push and infusion undiluted. Give bolus dose IV push over 1-2 min. Infusion should be given via a controlled infusion pump.

Ergoloid Mesylates
ur-go-loyd mess-ah-lates
(Hydergine [CAN])

CATEGORY AND SCHEDULE
Pregnancy Risk Category: C

Classification: Ergot alkaloids and derivatives

MECHANISM OF ACTION
There is no specific evidence that clearly establishes the mechanism by which ergoloid mesylates preparations produce mental effects, nor is there conclusive evidence that the drug particularly affects cerebral arteriosclerosis or cerebrovascular insufficiency.

PHARMACOKINETICS
Rapidly, incompletely absorbed from GI tract. Metabolized in liver. Eliminated primarily in feces. *Half-life:* 2-5 h.

AVAILABILITY
Tablets: 1 mg.

INDICATIONS AND DOSAGES
▸ **Age-related decline in mental capacity**
PO
Adults, Elderly. Initially, 1 mg 3 times/day. Range: 1.5-12 mg/day. Usual dose: 1-2 mg 3 times/day.

CONTRAINDICATIONS
Acute or chronic psychosis (regardless of etiology), hypersensitivity to ergoloid mesylates, or any component of the formulation; pregnancy.

INTERACTIONS
Drug
Potent CYP450 3A4 inhibitors: May increase risk of ergotism (nausea, vomiting, vasospastic ischemia).
Frovatriptan, naratriptan, rizatriptan, sumatriptan, zolmitriptan, other serotonergic agents: May prolong vasospastic reactions (ergot derivatives).
Herbal
None known.
Food
Grapefruit juice: May increase risk of ergotism (nausea, vomiting, vasospastic ischemia).

SIDE EFFECTS
Occasional
GI distress, transient nausea, sublingual irritation.

SERIOUS REACTIONS
• Overdose may produce blurred vision, dizziness, syncope, headache, flushed face, nausea, vomiting, decreased appetite, stomach cramps, and stuffy nose.

PRECAUTIONS & CONSIDERATIONS
It is unknown whether ergoloid mesylates cross the placenta or are distributed in breast milk. Most ergot alkaloids are excreted into breast milk and are considered contraindicated during pregnancy because of their oxytocic and uterine stimulant properties. Be aware that the safety and efficacy of ergoloid mesylates have not been established in children. There are no age-related

precautions noted in elderly patients.

Clinical improvement is gradual, and results may not be noted for 3-4 wks.
Storage
Store at room temperature.
Administration
Give with food to avoid GI upset.

E

Ergonovine
er-goe-noe-veen
(Ergotrate)

CATEGORY AND SCHEDULE
Pregnancy Risk Category: X

Classification: Ergot alkaloids and derivatives; oxytocics, stimulants, uterine

MECHANISM OF ACTION
An oxytoxic agent that directly stimulates uterine muscle. Stimulates α-adrenergic, serotonin receptors producing arterial vasoconstriction. Causes vasospasm of coronary arteries. *Therapeutic Effect:* Increases force and frequency of contractions. Induces cervical contractions.

PHARMACOKINETICS
Onset of action 2-5 min (IM), 6-15 min (PO). Duration 3 h (IM, PO), 45 min (IV). Metabolized in liver. Excreted primarily in feces. *Half-life* 0.5-3.5 h.

AVAILABILITY
Injection: 0.2 mg/mL.
Tablet: 0.2 mg.

E

INDICATIONS AND DOSAGES
▸ **Prevention and treatment of postabortal or postpartum bleeding due to uterine atony**
IM/IV
Adults. Initially, 0.2 mg. May repeat no more than q2-4h for no more than 5 doses total.
PO/SUBLINGUAL
Adults. 0.2-0.4 mg every 6-12 h until danger of uterine atony has passed (usually max 48 h).

OFF-LABEL USES
Treatment of incomplete abortion, diagnosis of Prinzmetal angina.

CONTRAINDICATIONS
Induction of labor, threatened spontaneous abortions, hypersensitivity to ergonovine maleate or any component of the formulation.

INTERACTIONS
Drug
Vasoconstrictors, vasopressors, β-blockers: May increase effects of ergonovine maleate.
CYP3A4 inhibitors: May increase level of ergonovine.
CYP3A4 inducers: May decrease level of ergnovine.
Serotonergic agents such as SSRIs, SNRIs, triptans, MAOIs: May increase risk of serotonin syndrome.
Herbal
St. John's wort: May decrease the level of ergonovine or increase the risk of serotonin syndrome.
Food
None known.

DIAGNOSTIC TEST EFFECTS
May decrease prolactin.

⊘ IV INCOMPATIBILITIES
Procaine.

🖥 IV COMPATIBILITIES
Epinephrine.

SIDE EFFECTS
Frequency not defined.
Uterine cramping.
Diarrhea, dizziness, abdominal pain, hallucinations, pruritus, nasal congestion, sweating, ringing in ears. Headache, nausea, vomiting, allergic reaction, thrombophlebitis.

SERIOUS REACTIONS
• Severe hypertensive episodes may result in cerebrovascular accident, serious arrhythmias, seizures; hypertensive effects more frequent with rapid IV administration, concurrent regional anesthesia or vasoconstrictors.
• Peripheral ischemia may lead to gangrene. Ergotism (intense vasoconstriction) usually with overdose or prolonged use.
• Overdose includes symptoms of angina, bradycardia, confusion, drowsiness, fast, weak pulse; miosis, severe peripheral vasoconstriction (numbness in arms or legs, blue skin color), seizures, tachycardia, thirst, and severe uterine cramping.

PRECAUTIONS & CONSIDERATIONS
Caution is warranted in patients with heart disease, hepatic dysfunction, calcium deficiency, hypertension, mitral valve stenosis, obliterative vascular disease, renal impairment, sepsis, and venoarterial shunts. Ergonovine maleate use is contraindicated during pregnancy, and small amounts of the drug are found in breast milk. No information is available on ergonovine maleate use in children or in elderly patients.
Uterine contractions (frequency, strength, duration), bleeding, BP, and pulse should be monitored every 15 min until stable (about 1-2 h).

If uterine cramps occur, notify the physician because dosage reduction may be required.

Storage

Store injection in refrigerator. Stable for up to 60 days at room temperature. Do not use if discoloration occurs. Protect from light. Tablets are stored at room temperature.

Administration

Give IM injection deep in muscle.

Be aware that for IV administration, it should only be used with severe uterine bleeding or other life-threatening emergency situations. Administer slowly, over a period of at least 1 min. May administer undiluted or dilute in 0.9% NaCl to 5 mL.

Ergotamine

er-got′a-meen

(Cafergot [CAN], Ergodryl Mono [AUS], Ergomar, Ergostat)

CATEGORY AND SCHEDULE

Pregnancy Risk Category: X

Classification: Ergot alkaloids and derivatives

MECHANISM OF ACTION

An ergotamine derivative and α-adrenergic blocker that directly stimulates vascular smooth muscle, resulting in peripheral and cerebral vasoconstriction. May also have antagonist effects on serotonin. *Therapeutic Effect:* Suppresses vascular headaches.

PHARMACOKINETICS

Slowly and incompletely absorbed from the GI tract; rapidly and extensively absorbed after rectal administration. Protein binding: > 90%. Undergoes extensive first-pass metabolism in the liver to active metabolite. Eliminated in feces by the biliary system. *Half-life:* 2 h.

AVAILABILITY

Tablets (Sublingual [Ergomar]): 2 mg.

Tablets (Ergotamine and Caffeine [Cafergot]): 1 mg, with 100 mg caffeine.

Suppositories (Ergotamine and Caffeine [Migergot]): 2 mg, with 100 mg caffeine.

INDICATIONS AND DOSAGES

▸ **Vascular headaches**

PO (CAFERGOT [FIXED-COMBINATION OF ERGOTAMINE AND CAFFEINE])

Adults, Elderly. 1-2 tablets at onset of headache, then 1-2 tablets q30min. Maximum: 6 tablets/episode; 10 tablets/wk.

Children. 1 tablet at onset of headache, then 1 tab q30 min as needed. Maximum 3 mg/episode.

SUBLINGUAL (ERGOMAR)

Adults, Elderly. 1 tablet at onset of headache, then 1 tablet q30min as needed. Maximum: 3 tablets/24 h; 5 tablets/wk.

SUBLINGUAL (ERGOMAR)

Children > 10 yrs. 1 mg at onset of headache, then 1 mg q30min. Maximum: 3 mg/episode.

RECTAL (MIGERTOL)

Adults, Elderly. 1 suppository at onset of headache; may repeat dose in 1 h. Maximum: 2 suppositories/episode; 5 suppositories/wk.

Children > 10 yrs. One fourth to one half of suppository; may repeat dose in 1 h. Maximum: 2 mg ergotamine/attack.

CONTRAINDICATIONS

Coronary artery disease, hypertension, impaired hepatic or renal function, malnutrition, peripheral vascular

E

diseases (such as thromboangiitis obliterans, syphilitic arteritis, severe arteriosclerosis, thrombophlebitis, and Raynaud disease), sepsis, severe pruritus, sepsis, pregnancy.

INTERACTIONS
Drug
β-blockers, erythromycin: May increase the risk of vasospasm.
CYP3A4 inhibitors: May increase levels and effects of ergotamine.
Ergot alkaloids, systemic vasoconstrictors: May increase pressor effect.
MAOIs, serotonergic agonists, SSRIs: May increase risk of serotonin syndrome.
Nitroglycerin: May decrease the effects of nitroglycerin.
Herbal
None known.
Food
Caffeine and grapefruit: May increase levels.

DIAGNOSTIC TEST EFFECTS
None known.

SIDE EFFECTS
Frequent (6%-10%)
Nausea, vomiting.
Occasional (2%-5%)
Cough, dizziness.
Rare (< 2%)
Myalgia, fatigue, diarrhea, dry mouth, upper respiratory tract infection, dyspepsia, confusion, drowsiness.

SERIOUS REACTIONS
• Prolonged administration or excessive dosage may produce ergotamine poisoning, manifested as nausea and vomiting; paresthesia, muscle pain, or weakness; precordial pain; angina; tachycardia or bradycardia; and hypertension or hypotension. Vasoconstriction of peripheral arteries and arterioles may result in localized edema and pruritus. Muscle pain will occur when walking and later, even at rest. Other rare effects include confusion, depression, drowsiness, seizures, pancreatitis, ischemic colitis, myocardial infarction, and gangrene. Ergotismy can occur at does < 5 mg but are most likely to occur with > 15 mg/24 h or 40 mg in a few days.

PRECAUTIONS & CONSIDERATIONS
Ergotamine use is contraindicated in pregnancy because it may result in fetal harm and even death. Ergotamine is distributed in breast milk and may inhibit lactation. Ergotamine use may produce diarrhea or vomiting in neonates; it may be used safely in children 10 yr and older but should be used only when patient is unresponsive to other drugs. In elderly patients, age-related occlusive peripheral vascular disease increases the risk of peripheral vasoconstriction; in addition, age-related renal impairment may require cautious use.

Notify the physician immediately if the drug does not relieve the headache or if irregular heartbeat, nausea or vomiting, numbness or tingling of the fingers and toes, or pain or weakness of the extremities occurs. Peripheral circulation, including the temperature, color, and strength of pulses in the extremities, should be assessed.
Administration
! Do not exceed daily, per attack, or weekly dosage limits. Patients should not use serotonin agonist (triptans) within 24 h of ergot use.
For sublingual use, place the sublingual tablet under the tongue, let it dissolve, and swallow the saliva. Do not administer it with water.

Tablets may be taken with fluids. For rectal suppository, if too soft, run wrapper under cool water. Remove wrapper; moisten with water before insertion.

Erlotinib
er-low'tih-nib
(Tarceva)

CATEGORY AND SCHEDULE
Pregnancy Risk Category: D

Classification: Antineoplastics, miscellaneous

MECHANISM OF ACTION
A human epidermal growth factor that inhibits tyrosine kinases (TK) associated with transmembrane cell surface receptors found on both normal and cancer cells. One such receptor is epidermal growth factor receptor (EGFR). *Therapeutic Effect:* TK activity appears to be vitally important to cell proliferation and survival.

AVAILABILITY
Tablets: 25 mg, 100 mg, 150 mg.

INDICATIONS AND DOSAGES
▶ **Locally advanced or metastatic non–small cell lung cancer after failure of first-line therapy**
PO
Adults, Elderly. 150 mg/day.
▶ **Locally advanced, unresectable, or metastatic pancreatic cancer, first-line therapy**
Adults, Elderly. 100 mg/day with gemcitabine.
▶ **Concomitant therapy with strong CYP3A4 inhibitor**
Consider erlotinib dose reduction if adverse reactions occur.

▶ **Concomitant therapy with strong CYP3A4 inducer**
Consider treatments lacking CYP3A4-inducing activity or consider dose > 150 mg.
▶ **Dosage-hepatic impairment**
Expect to interrupt or reduce dose treatment if severe changes in total bilirubin or liver transaminase levels occur.

OFF-LABEL USES
Metastatic renal cell carcinoma.

CONTRAINDICATIONS
Pregnancy.

INTERACTIONS
Drug
CYP3A4 inducers, aminoglutethimide, carbamazepine, nafcillin, nevirapine, phenobarbital, phenytoin, rifampin: May decrease the levels and effects of erlotinib.
CYP3A4 inhibitors, azole antifungals, ciprofloxacin, clarithromycin, diclofenac, doxycycline, erythromycin, imatinib, isoniazid, ketoconazole, nefazodone, nicardipine, propofol, protease inhibitors, quinidine, verapamil: May increase the levels and effects of erlotinib.
Herbal
St. John's wort: May increase metabolism and decrease serum erlotinib concentration. Avoid.
Food
All foods: Give erlotinib at least 1 h before or 2 h after ingestion of food. Bioavailability without food 60%, with food 100%.
Other
Cigarette smoking: Decreases erlotinib exposure. Advise patients to quit smoking.

DIAGNOSTIC TEST EFFECTS
May increase hepatic enzyme levels.

SIDE EFFECTS
Frequent (10%-88%)
Acneiform rash, pruritus, diarrhea, fatigue, pyrexia, anorexia, nausea, edema, constipation, bone pain, anxiety, headache, dry skin, vomiting, mucositis, dry mouth, depression, dizziness, insomnia, erythema, alopecia, dyspepsia, weight loss, abdominal pain, myalgia, arthralgia, rigors, paresthesia, dyspnea, cough, infection.
Occasional (4%-9%)
Keratitis, pneumonitis, deep vein thrombosis.

SERIOUS REACTIONS
• Interstitial lung disease has been reported.
• Myocardial infarction, cerebrovascular accident, and microangiopathic hemolytic anemia with thrombocytopenia.

PRECAUTIONS & CONSIDERATIONS
Caution is warranted with hepatic or severe renal impairment. Safety and efficacy have not been established in children. No age-related precautions have been noted in elderly patients.
Administration
Take erlotinib at least 1 h before or 2 h after ingestion of food.

Ertapenem
er-ta-pen'em
(Invanz)

CATEGORY AND SCHEDULE
Pregnancy Risk Category: B

Classification: Antibiotics, carbapenems

MECHANISM OF ACTION
A carbapenem that penetrates the bacterial cell wall of microorganisms and binds to penicillin-binding proteins, inhibiting cell wall synthesis. *Therapeutic Effect:* Produces bacterial cell death.

PHARMACOKINETICS
Almost completely absorbed after IM administration. Protein binding: 85%-95%. Widely distributed. Primarily excreted in urine with smaller amount eliminated in feces. Removed by hemodialysis. *Half-life:* 4 h.

AVAILABILITY
Injection Powder for Reconstitution: 1 g.

INDICATIONS AND DOSAGES
▸ **Intra-abdominal infection**
IM, IV
Adults, Elderly, Children 13 yr and older. 1 g/day for 5-14 days.
Children 3 mo to 12 yrs.
15 mg/kg twice daily (maximum 1 g/day) for 5-14 days.
▸ **Skin and skin structure infection**
IM, IV
Adults, Elderly, Children 13 yr and older. 1 g/day for 7-14 days.
Children 3 mo to 12 yrs. 15 mg/kg twice daily (maximum 1 g/day) for 7-14 days.
▸ **Community acquired pneumonia, urinary tract infection (UTI)**
IM, IV
Adults, Elderly, Children 13 yr and older. 1 g/day for 10-14 days.
Children 3 mo to 12 yrs. 15 mg/kg twice daily (maximum 1 g/day) for 10-14 days.
▸ **Pelvic/gynecologic infection**
IM, IV
Adults, Elderly, Children 13 yr and older. 1 g/day for 3-10 days.
Children 3 mo to 12 yrs. 15 mg/kg twice daily (maximum 1 g/day) for 3-10 days.

> **Prophylaxis of surgical site infection following colorectal surgery**
IV
Adults, Elderly. 1 g given 1 h before surgical incision.

> **Dosage in renal impairment**
For adults and elderly patients with creatinine clearance ≤ 30 mL/min or on hemodialysis, dosage is 500 mg once a day.

CONTRAINDICATIONS
History of hypersensitivity to other carbapenems (imipenem, meropenem) or anaphylaxis to beta-lactams, hypersensitivity to lidocaine or amide-type local anesthetics (IM).

INTERACTIONS
Drug
Probenecid: Reduces renal excretion of ertapenem, increases concentation.
Valproic acid: Reduces serum levels of valproic acid. Monitor levels and adjust dose.
Herbal and Food
None known.

DIAGNOSTIC TEST EFFECTS
May increase serum alkaline phosphatase, AST (SGOT) and ALT (SGPT) levels. May decrease platelet count, blood hematocrit and hemoglobin levels, and serum potassium level.

🚫 IV INCOMPATIBILITIES
Do not use diluents or IV solutions containing dextrose.
Allopurinol (Aloprim), amiodarone, amphotericin B cholesteryl sulfate complex (Amphotec), anidulafungin (Eraxis), caspofungin (Cancidas), chlorpromazine, dantrolene, daunorubicin (Cerubidine), diazepam (Valium), dobutamine, doxorubicin (Adriamycin), droperidol, epirubicin (Ellence), hydralazine, hydroxyzine, idarubicin (Idamycin PFS), midazolam, minocycline (Minocin), mitoxantrone (Novantrone), nicardipine (Cardene), ondansetron (Zofran), phenytoin, prochlorperazine, promethazine, quinupristin/dalfopristin (Synercid), topotecan (Hycamtin), verapamil.

💧 IV COMPATIBILITIES
Acyclovir (Zovirax), alfentanil (Alfenta), amifostine (Ethyol), amikacin (Amikar), aminocaproic acid, aminophylline, amphotericin B lipid complex (Abelcet), amphotericin B liposome (AmBisome), argatroban, aresenic trioxide (Trisenox), atenolol, atracurium (Tracrium), azithromycin (Zithromax), aztreonam (Azactam), bivalirudin (Angiomax), bleomycin (Blenoxane), bretylium, bumetanide (Bumex), buprenorphine (Buprenex), busulfan (Bulsulfex), butorphanol (Stadol), calcium chloride, calcium gluconate, carboplatin, carmustine (BiCNU), cimetidine (Tagamet), ciprofloxacin (Cipro), cisatracurium (Nimbex), cisplatin, cyclophosphamide (Cytoxan), cyclosporine (Sandimmune), cytarabine (Tarabine), dacarbazine (DTIC-Dome), dactinomycin (Cosmegen), daptomycin (Cubicin), dexamethasone sodium phosphate, dexrazoxane (Zinecard), digoxin (Lanoxin), diltiazem (Cardizem), diphenhydramine (Benadryl), docetaxel (Taxotere), dopamine, enalaprilat, ephedrine, epinephrine, eptifibatide (Integrilin), erythromycin lactobionate, esmolol (Brevibloc), etoposide (VePesid), etoposide phosphate (Etopophos), famotidine (Pepcid), fenoldopam (Corlopam), fluconazole (Diflucan), fludarabine (Fludara), fluorouracil, foscarnet (Foscavir), fosphenytoin (Cerebyx), furosemide (Lasix), ganciclovir

(Cytovene), gemcitabine (Gemzar), gentamicin, granisetron (Kytril), haloperidol lactate (Haldol), heparin, hetastarch in NS, hydrocortisone sodium succinate (Solu-Cortef), hydromorphone (Dilaudid), ifosfamide (Ifex), insulin (regular, Humulin R, Novolin R), irinotecan (Camptosar), isoproterenol (Isuprel), ketorolac, labetalol, leucovorin, levofloxacin (Levaquin), lidocaine, linezolid (Zyvox), lorazepam (Ativan), magnesium sulfate, melphalan (Alkeran), meperidine (Demerol), mesna (Mesnex), methotrexate, methylprednisolone sodium succinate, metoclopramide (Reglan), metronidazole (Flagyl), milrinone (Primacor), mitomycin (Mutamycin), morphine, moxifloxacin (Avelox), nalbuphine (Nubain), naloxone (Narcan), nesiritide (Natrecor), nitroglycerin, nitroprusside sodium (Nitropress), norepinephrine (Levophed), oxaliplatin (Eloxatin), oxytocin (Pitocin), paclitaxel (Taxol), pamidronate (Aredia), pantoprazole (Protonix), pemetrexed (Alimta), pentobarbital, phenobarbital, phenylephrine, potassium acetate, potassium chloride, potassium phosphates, procainamide, propranolol, ranitidine (Zantac), remifentanil (Ultiva), rocuronium (Zemuron), sodium acetate, sodium phosphates, succinylcholine (Anectine, Quelicin), sufentanil (Sufenta), tacrolimus (Prograf), teniposide (Vumon), theophylline, thiotepa (Thioplex), tigecycline (Tygacil), tirofibran (Aggrastat), tobramycin, vancomycin, vasopressin, vecuronium (Norcuron), vinblastine (Velban), vincristine (Vincasar), vinorelbine (Navelbine), voriconazole (Vfend), water for injection, 0.9% NaCl, zidovudine (Retrovir), zolendronic acid (Zometa)

SIDE EFFECTS

Frequent (6%-10%)
Diarrhea, nausea, headache, infused vein complications.
Occasional (2%-5%)
Altered mental status, insomnia, rash, abdominal pain, constipation, vomiting, edema, fever.
Rare (< 2%)
Dizziness, cough, oral candidiasis, anxiety, tachycardia, hypertension, hypotension, phlebitis at IV site, extravasation.

SERIOUS REACTIONS

• Antibiotic-associated colitis and other superinfections may occur.
• Anaphylactic reactions have been reported.
• Seizures may occur in those with central nervous system (CNS) disorders (including patients with brain lesions or a history of seizures), bacterial meningitis, or severe renal impairment.

PRECAUTIONS & CONSIDERATIONS

Caution is warranted with CNS disorders (particularly with brain lesions or history of seizures), a hypersensitivity to cephalosporins, penicillins, or other allergens, and impaired renal function. Be aware that ertapenem is distributed in breast milk. Be aware that the safety and efficacy of ertapenem have not been established in children younger than 3 mo. In elderly patients, advanced renal insufficiency and end-stage renal insufficiency may require dosage adjustment. Methicillin-resistant *Staphylococcus, Enterococcus* spp., penicillin-resistant strains of *Streptococcus pneumoniae,* β-lactamase-positive strains of *Haemophilus influenzae* are resistant to ertapenem, as are most *Pseudomonas aeruginosa.*

History of allergies, particularly to β-lactams, cephalosporins, and penicillins should be obtained before beginning drug therapy. Hydration status, nausea, vomiting, skin for rash, sleep pattern, and mental status should be evaluated. Report any diarrhea, rash, seizures, tremors, or other new symptoms.

Storage

Store vials at room temperature. Solution normally appears colorless to yellow (variation in color does not affect potency). Discard if solution contains precipitate. Reconstituted solution is stable for 6 h at room temperature, 24 h if refrigerated and used within 4 h after removing.

Administration

For IM use, reconstitute with 3.2 mL 1% lidocaine HCl injection (without epinephrine). Shake vial thoroughly. Give deep IM injections slowly to minimize patient discomfort. To further minimize discomfort, administer IM injections into the gluteus maximus instead of the lateral aspect of the thigh. Administer suspension within 1 h after preparation.

For IV use, dilute 1-g vial with 10 mL, 0.9% NaCl or bacteriostatic water for injection. Shake well to dissolve. Further dilute with 50 mL 0.9% NaCl to concentration 20 mg/mL or less. Give by intermittent IV infusion (piggyback). Do not give IV push. Infuse over 20-30 min. Dextrose solutions are not compatible with ertapenem.

Erythromycin
er-ith-roe-mye′sin
(Akne-Mycin, Apo-Erythro Base [CAN], EES, Emcin, Emgel, Ery, Eryacne [AUS], Erybid [CAN], Eryc LD [AUS], EryDerm, Erygel, EryPed, Ery-Tab, Erythrocin, Erythromid [CAN], My-E, PCE)
Do not confuse with Emcet, azithromycin, Ethmozine, or Pedialyte.

CATEGORY AND SCHEDULE
Pregnancy Risk Category: B

Classification: Anti-infectives, ophthalmics, topical, antibiotics, macrolides

MECHANISM OF ACTION
A macrolide that reversibly binds to bacterial ribosomes, inhibiting bacterial protein synthesis.
Therapeutic Effect: Bacteriostatic.

PHARMACOKINETICS
Variably absorbed from the GI tract (depending on dosage form used; better with salt forms than base form). Protein binding: 70%-90%. Widely distributed. Metabolized in the liver by CYP3A4. Primarily eliminated in feces by bile. Not removed by hemodialysis. *Half-life:* 1.4-2 h (increased in impaired renal function).

AVAILABILITY
Topical Gel (Emgel, Erygel): 2%.
Injection Powder for Reconstitution (Erythrocin): 500 mg, 1 g.
Ophthalmic Ointment: 5 mg/g (0.5%).
Topical Ointment (Akne-Mycin): 2%.
Oral Suspension (EryPed, EES): 200 mg/5 mL, 400 mg/5 mL.
Topical Solution (EryDerm): 2%.
Capsule (Delayed Release): 250 mg.

E

Tablets (Ery-Tab): 250 mg,
333 mg, 500 mg.
Tablets (EES): 400 mg.
Tablets (Erythrocin): 250 mg, 500 mg.
Tablets (PCE): 333 mg, 500 mg.
*Topical Medicated Pledget (Emcin
Clear, Ery):* 2%.

INDICATIONS AND DOSAGES
> **Mild to moderate infections of the
upper and lower respiratory tract,
pharyngitis, skin infections**
PO
Adults, Elderly (base). 250 mg
q6h, 500 mg q12h, or 333 mg q8h.
Maximum: 4 g/day.
Adults, Elderly (ethylsuccinate).
400-800 mg q6-12h. Maximum 4 g/day.
Children. 30-50 mg/kg/day in 2-4
divided doses up to 60-100 mg/kg/day
for severe infections.
IV
Adults, Elderly, Children.
15-20 mg/kg/day in divided doses
q6h or 500-1000 mg q6h. Maximum:
4 g/day.
> **Preoperative intestinal antisepsis**
PO
Adults, Elderly. 1 g at 1 PM, 2 PM,
and 11 PM on the day before surgery
(with neomycin).
Children. 20 mg/kg at 1 PM, 2 PM,
and 11 PM on day before surgery
(with neomycin).
> **Acne vulgaris**
TOPICAL
Adults, Children. Apply thin layer to
affected area twice a day.
PO
Adults. 250 mg four times daily.
> **Gonococcal ophthalmia
neonatorum prevention**
OPHTHALMIC
Neonates. 0.5-2 cm to each eye no later
than 1 h after delivery.

OFF-LABEL USES
Systemic: Chancroid, *Campylobacter
enteritis,* gastroparesis, Lyme disease.

Topical: Treatment of minor bacterial
skin infections.
Ophthalmic: Treatment of
blepharitis, conjunctivitis, keratitis,
chlamydial trachoma.

CONTRAINDICATIONS
Administration of fixed-combination
product; history of hepatitis due
to macrolides; hypersensitivity to
macrolides; pre-existing hepatic
disease (estolate only).

INTERACTIONS
Drug
**Buspirone, cyclosporine,
felodipine, lovastatin,
simvastatin:** May increase the blood
concentration and toxicity of these
drugs.
Carbamazepine: May inhibit the
metabolism of carbamazepine.
Chloramphenicol, clindamycin:
May decrease the effects of these
drugs.
Hepatotoxic medications: May
increase the risk of hepatotoxicity.
Theophylline: May increase the risk
of theophylline toxicity.
Warfarin: May increase warfarin's
effects.
Herbal and Food
None known.

DIAGNOSTIC TEST EFFECTS
May increase serum alkaline
phosphatase, bilirubin, AST (SGOT),
and ALT (SGPT) levels.

Ⓓ IV INCOMPATIBILITIES
Amphotericin B cholesteryl
sulfate complex (Amphotec),
amphotericin B liposome
(AmBisome), ascorbic acid,
aztreonam (Azactam), cefazolin,
cefepime (Maxipime), cefoxitin
(Mefoxin), chloramphenicol,
dantrolene, dexamethasone
sodium phosphate, diazepam

(Valium), fluconazole (Diflucan), furosemide (Lasix), ganciclovir (Cytovene), indomethacin, ketorolac, linezolid (Zyvox), minocycline (Minocin), nitroprusside sodium (Nitropress), pemetrexed (Alimta), pentobarbital, phenobarbital, phenytoin, rocuronium (Zemuron), sulfamethoxazole/trimethoprim, ticarcillin (Ticar), ticarcillin/ clavulanate (Timentin).

IV COMPATIBILITIES

Acyclovir (Zovirax), alfentanil (Alfenta), amikacin (Amikar), aminophylline, amiodarone (Cordarone), anidulafungin (Eraxis), atracurium (Tracrium), atropine, azathioprine, benztropine (Cogentin), bivalirudin (Angiomax), bretylium, bumetanide (Bumex), buprenorphine (Buprenex), butorphanol (Stadol), calcium chloride, calcium gluconate, carboplatin caspofungin (Cancidas), cefotaxime (Claforan), ceftriaxone (Rocephin), cefuroxime (Zinacef), chlorpromazine, cimetidine (Tagamet), cisplatin, cyclophosphamide (Cytoxan), cyclosporine (Sandimmune), dactinomycin (Cosmegen), daptomycin (Cubicin), digoxin (Lanoxin), diltiazem (Cardizem), diphenhydramine (Benadryl), dobutamine (Dobutrex), docetaxel (Taxotere), dopamine (Intropin), doxorubicin (Adriamycin), enalaprilat, ephedrine, epinephrine, epirubicin (Ellence), epoetin alfa (Procrit), ertapenem (Invanz), esmolol (Brevibloc), etoposide phosphate (Etopophos), famotidine (Pepcid), fenoldopam (Corlopam), fentanyl (Sublimaze), fludarabine (Fludara), fluorouracil, folic acid, foscarnet (Foscavir), gemcitabine (Gemzar), gentamicin, granisetron (Kytril), hydrocortisone sodium succinate, hydromorphone (Dilaudid), hydroxyzine, idarubicin (Idamycin), imipenem/cilastatin (Primaxin), insulin (regular, Humulin R, Novolin R), isoproterenol (Isuprel), labetalol, levofloxacin (Levaquin), lidocaine, lorazepam (Ativan), meperidine (Demerol), methicillin, methotrexate, methylprednisolone sodium succinate, metoclopramide (Reglan), metronidazole (Flagyl), midazolam (Versed), milrinone, mitoxantrone (Novantrone), morphine, multivitamins, nafcillin, nalbuphine (Nubain), naloxone (Narcan), nicardipine (Cardene), nitroglycerin, norepinephrine (Levophed), ondansetron (Zofran), oxacillin, oxaliplatin (Eloxatin), oxytocin (Pitocin), paclitaxel (Taxol), palonosetron (Aloxi), perphenazine, piperacillin, piperacillin/tazobactam (Zosyn), procainamide, prochlorperazine, promethazine, propranolol, protamine, pyridoxine, ranitidine, sodium acetate, sodium bicarbonate, streptokinase, succinylcholine, sufentanil (Sufenta), tacrolimus (Prograf), teniposide (Vumon), theophylline, thiotepa (Thioplex), tigecycline (Tygacil), tirofiban (Aggrastat), tobramycin, vancomycin, vasopressin, vecuronium (Norcuron), verapamil, vincristine (Vincasar), vinorelbine (Navelbine), voriconazole (Vfend), zidovudine (Retrovir).

SIDE EFFECTS
Frequent
IV: Abdominal cramping or discomfort, phlebitis or thrombophlebitis.
Topical: Dry skin (50%).
Occasional
Nausea, vomiting, diarrhea, rash, urticaria.

Rare

Ophthalmic: Sensitivity reaction with increased irritation, burning, itching, and inflammation.

Topical: Urticaria.

SERIOUS REACTIONS

• Antibiotic-associated colitis and other superinfections may occur.

• High dosages in patients with renal or hepatic impairment may lead to reversible hearing loss.

• Anaphylaxis and hepatotoxicity occur rarely.

• Ventricular arrhythmias and prolonged QT interval occur rarely with the IV drug form.

PRECAUTIONS & CONSIDERATIONS

Caution is warranted with hepatic dysfunction. Caution should also be used with the combination drug Pediazole (erythromycin and sulfisoxazole) cautiously in patients with impaired renal or hepatic function, severe allergies, bronchial asthma, or glucose-6-phosphate dehydrogenase deficiency. Major inhibitor of CYP3A4, which may lead to serious drug interactions. Use with caution in patients with myasthenia gravis (aggravation of disease). Infantile hypertrophic pyloric stenosis has occurred in infants. Determine whether there is a history of hepatitis or allergies to erythromycin or other macrolides before beginning therapy. Erythromycin crosses the placenta and is distributed in breast milk. Erythromycin estolate may increase liver function test results in pregnant women. Elderly patients may be at increased risk for hearing loss or torsade de pointes at doses > 4 g/day.

WBC should be monitored to determine whether the infection is improving. Diarrhea, GI discomfort, headache, nausea, pattern of daily bowel activity and stool consistency, as well as signs and symptoms of superinfection, including anal or genital pruritus, moderate to severe diarrhea, abdominal cramps, fever, and sore mouth or tongue, should be assessed. Signs of hearing loss should be monitored because high dosages can cause hearing loss with hepatic and renal dysfunction.

Storage

Store capsules and tablets at room temperature. The oral suspension is stable for 14 days at room temperature. Store the parenteral form at room temperature. The initial reconstituted solution in vial is stable for 8 h at room temperature and 2 wks if refrigerated. Diluted IV solutions are stable for 8 h at room temperature and 24 h if refrigerated. Discard the solution if a precipitate forms.

Administration

Administer erythromycin base or stearate 1 h before or 2 h after a meal. Erythromycin estolate and ethylsuccinate may be given without regard to food but are absorbed better when given on an empty stomach. Give tablets or capsules with 8 oz of water. If the patient has difficulty swallowing, sprinkle the capsule contents in a teaspoonful of applesauce and follow with water. Chew or crush chewable tablets.

For IV use, reconstitute each 500-mg vial with 10 mL or each 1-g vial with 20 mL sterile water for injection without a preservative to provide a concentration of 50 mg/mL. Further dilute with 100-250 mL D5W or 0.9% NaCl. Administer intermittent IV infusion (piggyback) over 20-60 min. Administer continuous infusion over 6-24 h. Assess for pain along vein frequently. For topical use, gently cleanse and dry area before application. Apply thin film. Avoid eyes and mucous membranes.

For ophthalmic use, place a gloved finger on the lower eyelid and pull it out until a pocket is formed between the eye and the lower lid. Place ¼ to ½ inch of ointment into the pocket. Close the eye for 1-2 min and roll the eyeball gently to increase the drug's distribution. Remove excess ointment around the eye with tissue.

Escitalopram
es-sy-tal′oh-pram
(Lexapro)

CATEGORY AND SCHEDULE
Pregnancy Risk Category: C

Classification: Antidepressants, serotonin specific reuptake inhibitors

MECHANISM OF ACTION
A selective serotonin reuptake inhibitor that blocks the uptake of the neurotransmitter serotonin at neuronal presynaptic membranes, increasing its availability at postsynaptic receptor sites. *Therapeutic Effect:* Relieves depression.

PHARMACOKINETICS
Well absorbed after PO administration. Primarily metabolized in the liver. Primarily excreted in feces, with a lesser amount eliminated in urine. *Half-life:* 35 h, extended with hepatic impairment. Oral solution and tablet bioequivalent.

AVAILABILITY
Oral Solution: 1 mg/mL (240 mL).
Tablets: 5 mg, 10 mg, 20 mg.

INDICATIONS AND DOSAGES
▶ **Depression, general anxiety disorder (GAD)**
PO
Adults. Initially, 10 mg once a day in the morning or evening. May increase to 20 mg after a minimum of 1 wk.
Elderly. Patients with hepatic impairment. 10 mg/day.

OFF-LABEL USES
Trichotillomania, panic disorder.

CONTRAINDICATIONS
Use within 14 days of MAOIs, hypersensitivity to eitalopram or escitalopram.

INTERACTIONS
Drug
Alcohol, other CNS depressants: May increase CNS depression.
Anticoagulants, antiplatelets, NSAIDs: May increase risk of bleeding.
Antifungals, cimetidine, macrolide antibiotics, CYP3A4 inhibitors: May increase plasma level of escitalopram.
Carbamazepine, CYP2C19 inducers, CYP3A4 inducers: May decrease plasma level of escitalopram.
CYP2C19 inhibitors, delavirdine, fluconazole, gemfibrozil, omeprazole: May increase plasma level of escitalopram.
MAOIs, linezolid, meperidine, selegiline: May cause serotonin syndrome, marked by autonomic hyperactivity, coma, diaphoresis, excitement, hyperthermia, and rigidity, and neuroleptic malignant syndrome. Avoid combination with MAOIs and allow 14-day washout.
Metoprolol: Increases plasma level of metoprolol.

E

SSRIs, SNRIs, buspirone, sibutramine, tramadol, triptans: May increase risk for serotonin syndrome.
Herbal
St. John's wort: May increase risk for serotonin syndrome and/or decrease escitalopram plasma level.
Food
None known.

DIAGNOSTIC TEST EFFECTS
May reduce serum sodium level.

SIDE EFFECTS
Frequent (9%-21%)
Nausea, dry mouth, somnolence, insomnia, abnormal ejaculation.
Occasional (4%-8%)
Tremor, diarrhea, diaphoresis, dyspepsia, fatigue, anxiety, decreased libido.
Rare (2%-3%)
Sinusitis, vomiting, constipation, anorexia, sexual dysfunction, menstrual disorder, abdominal pain, agitation.

SERIOUS REACTIONS
• Overdose is manifested as dizziness, drowsiness, tachycardia, somnolence, confusion, and seizures.
• Serotonin syndrome, activation of hypomania/mania, abnormal bleeding, hyponatremia/SIADH.

PRECAUTIONS & CONSIDERATIONS
Antidepressants increased the risk of suicidal thinking and behavior (suicidality) in short-term studies in children and adolescents with depression and other psychiatric disorders. Caution is warranted with hepatic or severe renal impairment; those with a history of hypomania, mania, or seizures; and patients concurrently using CNS depressants. Neonates exposed to escitalopram late in the third trimester have developed complications requiring prolonged hospitalization, respiratory support, and tube feeding. Consider tapering escitalopram in the third trimester of pregnancy. Escitalopram is distributed in breast milk. Escitalopram use may increase anticholinergic effects and hyperexcitability in children. Elderly patients are more sensitive to the drug's anticholinergic effects, such as dry mouth, and are more likely to experience confusion, dizziness, hyperexcitability, and sedation.

Alcohol and tasks that require mental alertness or motor skills should be avoided. CBC and liver and renal function tests should be performed before and periodically during therapy, especially with long-term use. Gradual discontinuation is advised to avoid withdrawal symptoms.
Administration
! Make sure at least 14 days elapse between the use of MAOIs and escitalopram.

Take escitalopram without regard to food. Do not crush film-coated tablets. Do not abruptly discontinue escitalopram or increase the dosage.

Esmolol
ess'moe-lol
(Brevibloc)

CATEGORY AND SCHEDULE
Pregnancy Risk Category: C

Classification: Antiadrenergics, β-blocking; antiarrhythmics, class II

MECHANISM OF ACTION
An antiarrhythmic that selectively blocks β₁-adrenergic receptors.
Therapeutic Effect: Slows sinus heart rate, decreases cardiac output, reducing BP.

AVAILABILITY
Injection: 10 mg/mL (250 mL, 10 mL), 20 mg/mL (5 mL, 100 mL).

INDICATIONS AND DOSAGES
▶ **Arrhythmias**
IV

Adults, Elderly. Initially, a loading dose of 500 mcg/kg over 1 min, followed by 50 mcg/kg/min for 4 min. If optimum response is not attained in 5 min, give a second loading dose of 500 mcg/kg/min for 1 min, followed by infusion of 100 mcg/kg/min for 4 min. An additional loading dose can be given and infusion increased by 50 mcg/kg/min, up to 200 mcg/kg/min, for 4 min. Once the desired response is attained, cease loading dose and decrease infusion by no more than 25 mcg/kg/min at 10-min intervals. Infusion is usually administered over 24-48 h in most patients. Range: 50-200 mcg/kg/min, with average dose of 100 mcg/kg/min.

▶ **Intraoperative tachycardia or hypertension (immediate control)**
IV

Adults, Elderly. Initially, 80 mg over 30 s, then 150 mcg/kg/min infusion up to 300 mcg/kg/min. Titrate to desired heart rate and/or BP.

OFF-LABEL USES
Postoperative hypertension and SVT in children.

CONTRAINDICATIONS
Cardiogenic shock, overt cardiac failure, second- and third-degree heart block, sinus bradycardia, pregnancy (2nd and 3rd trimesters)

INTERACTIONS
Drug
Calcium channel blockers: Effects of verapamil, nifedipine may be potentiated. Diltiazem, felodipine, nicardipine may increase esmolol effects.
Digoxin: Increase in digoxin levels.
Insulin, oral hypoglycemics: May mask symptoms of hypoglycemia and prolong hypoglycemic effect of these drugs.
MAOIs: May cause significant hypertension or bradycardia.
Morphine: Increase in esmolol levels.
Succinylcholine: Prolonged duration of neuromuscular blockade.
Sympathomimetics, xanthines: May mutually inhibit effects.
Herbal
None known.
Food
None known.

DIAGNOSTIC TEST EFFECTS
None known.

🚫 IV INCOMPATIBILITIES
Acyclovir (Zovirax), amphotericin B cholesteryl sulfate complex (Amphotec), azathioprine, cefotetan (Cefotan), dantrolene, dexamethasone sodium phosphate, diazepam (Valium), furosemide (Lasix), ganciclovir (Cytovene), indomethacin, ketorolac, lansoprazole (Prevacid), minocycline (Minocin), oxacillin, pantoprazole (Protonix), pentobarbital, phenobarbital.

💉 IV COMPATIBILITIES
Alfentanil (Alfenta), amikacin (Amikar), aminophylline, amiodarone (Cordarone), amphotericin B liposomal (AmBisome), ascorbic acid, atracurium (Tracrium), atropine, aztreonam (Azactam), benztropine (Cogentin), bivalirudin (Angiomax), bretylium, bumetanide (Bumex), buprenorphine (Buprenex),

E

butorphanol (Stadol), calcium chloride, calcium gluconate, carboplatin, caspofungin (Cancidas), cefazolin, cefotaxime (Claforan), cefoxitin (Mefoxin), ceftazidime (Ceptaz, Fortaz, Tazicef, Tazidime), ceftizoxime (Cefizox), ceftriaxone (Rocephin), cefuroxime (Zinacef), chlorpromazine, cimetidine (Tagamet), cisatracurium (Nimbex), cisplatin, clindamycin (Cleocin), cyanocobalamin, cyclophosphamide (Cytoxan), cyclosporine (Sandimmune), dactinomycin (Cosmegen), daptomycin (Cubicin), dexmedetomidine (Precedex), digoxin (Lanoxin), diltiazem (Cardizem), diphenhydramine (Benadryl), dobutamine (Dobutrex), docetaxel (Taxotere), dopamine (Intropin), doxorubicin (Adriamycin), enalaprilat, ephedrine, epinephrine, epoetin alfa (Procrit), ertapenem (Invanz), erythromycin lactobionate, etoposide phosphate (Etopophos), famotidine (Pepcid), fenoldopam (Corlopam), fentanyl (Sublimaze), fluconazole (Diflucan), fludarabine (Fludara), fluorouracil, folic acid, gemcitabine (Gemzar), gentamicin, granisetron (Kytril), heparin, hydromorphone (Dilaudid), hydroxyzine, imipenem/cilastatin (Primaxin), insulin (regular, Humulin R, Novolin R), isoproterenol (Isuprel), labetalol, levofloxacin (Levaquin), lidocaine, linezolid (Zyvox), lorazepam (Ativan), magnesium sulfate, mannitol, meperidine (Demerol), methicillin, methotrexate, metoclopramide (Reglan), metoprolol (Lopressor), metronidazole (Flagyl), micafungin (Mycamine), midazolam (Versed), mitoxantrone (Novantrone), morphine, multiple vitamins injection, nalbuphine (Nubain), naloxone (Narcan), nicardipine (Cardene), nitroglycerin, nitroprusside sodium (Nitropress), norepinephrine (Levophed), ondansetron (Zofran), oxaliplatin (Eloxatin), oxytocin (Pitocin), paclitaxel (Taxol), palonosetron (Aloxi), pancuronium, pemetrexed (Alimta), penicillin G potassium, penicillin G sodium, phytonadione, potassium chloride, prochloperazine, promethazine, propofol (Diprivan), propranolol, quinupristin/dalfopristin (Synercid), ranitidin (Zantac), remifentanil (Ultiva), sodium bicarbonate, streptokinase, succinylcholine, sufentanil (Sufenta), tacrolimus (Prograf), teniposide (Vumon), theophylline, thiotepa (Thioplex), ticarcillin (Ticar), ticarcillin/clavulanate (Timentin), tigecycline (Tygacil), tirofibran (Aggrastat), tobramycin, vancomycin, vasopressin, vecuronium (Norcuron), verapamil, vincristine (Vincasar), voriconazole (Vfend), warfarin.

SIDE EFFECTS

Esmolol is generally well tolerated, with transient and mild side effects.
Frequent (> 10%)
Hypotension (systolic BP < 90 mm Hg) asymptomatic or symptomatic manifested as dizziness, nausea, diaphoresis, headache, cold extremities, fatigue.
Occasional
Nausea, dizziness, anxiety, drowsiness, flushed skin, vomiting, confusion, pain or inflammation at injection site, fever.

SERIOUS REACTIONS

• Overdose may produce profound hypotension, bradycardia, dizziness, syncope, drowsiness, breathing difficulty, bluish fingernails or palms of hands, and seizures.
• Esmolol administration may potentiate insulin-induced hypoglycemia in diabetic patients.

PRECAUTIONS & CONSIDERATIONS

Caution is warranted in patients with bronchial asthma, conduction disorder (e.g., sinus sick syndrome), bronchitis, congestive heart failure, diabetes, emphysema, history of allergy, myasthenia gravis, depression, peripheral vascular disease, and impaired renal function. Extravasation may cause tissue necrosis. Safety and efficacy have not been evaluated in children.

Notify the physician of cold extremities, dizziness, faintness, or nausea. BP for hypotension, respiratory status for shortness of breath, pattern of daily bowel activity and stool consistency, ECG for arrhythmias, and pulse for quality, rate and rhythm should be monitored during treatment. If pulse rate is 60 beats/min or lower or systolic BP is < 90 mm Hg, withhold the medication and contact the physician. Signs and symptoms of congestive heart failure, such as decreased urine output, distended neck veins, dyspnea (particularly on exertion or lying down), night cough, peripheral edema, and weight gain should also be assessed.

Storage

After dilution, solution is stable for 24 h. Store at room temperature.

Administration

! Give esmolol by IV infusion. Avoid using butterfly needles and very small veins.

For IV administration, use only clear and colorless to light yellow solution. Discard solution if it is discolored or if precipitate forms. For IV infusion, make sure the prescribed amount of esmolol is diluted to provide a concentration of 10 mg/mL or 20 mg/mL. Premixed bags are available. Administer by controlled infusion device, and titrate according to the patient's tolerance and response. Infuse IV loading dose over 1-2 min. Monitor the patient for hypotension (a systolic BP of < 90 mm Hg), especially during the first 30 min of infusion.

E

Esomeprazole
es-om-eh-pray'zole
(Nexium)

CATEGORY AND SCHEDULE
Pregnancy Risk Category: B

Classification: Gastrointestinals, proton pump inhibitors

MECHANISM OF ACTION

A proton pump inhibitor that is converted to active metabolites that irreversibly bind to and inhibit hydrogen-potassium adenosine triphosphates, an enzyme on the surface of gastric parietal cells. Inhibits hydrogen ion transport into gastric lumen. *Therapeutic Effect:* Increases gastric pH, reducing gastric acid production.

PHARMACOKINETICS

Well absorbed after oral administration. Protein binding: 97%. Extensively metabolized by the liver by CYP219 and CYP3A4. Primarily excreted in urine. *Half-life:* 1-1.5 h.

AVAILABILITY

Capsules (Delayed-Release): 20 mg, 40 mg.
Suspension (Delayed-Release): 10 mg/packet, 20 mg/packet, 40 mg/packet.
Injection, Powder for Reconstitution: 20 mg, 40 mg.

E

INDICATIONS AND DOSAGES
▶ **Erosive esophagitis healing**
PO
Adults, Elderly, Adolescents.
20-40 mg once daily for 4-8 wks.
Children 1-11 yr of age weighing
< 20 kg. 10 mg once daily for up to
8 wks.
Children 1-11 yr of age weighing
> 20 kg. 10-20 mg once daily for up
to 8 wks.
▶ **To maintain healing of erosive**
esophagitis
PO
Adults, Elderly. 20 mg/day.
▶ **Gastroesophageal reflux**
disease
PO
Adults, Elderly. 20 mg once a day for
4-8 wks.
Adolescents aged 12-17 yrs.
20-40 mg once daily for up to 8 wks.
Children aged 1-11 yrs. 10 mg once
daily for up to 8 wks.
IV
Adults, Elderly. 20-40 mg once
daily.
▶ **Duodenal ulcer caused by**
Helicobacter pylori
PO
Adults, Elderly. 40 mg
(esomeprazole) once a day,
with amoxicillin 1000 mg and
clarithromycin 500 mg twice a day
for 10-14 days.
▶ **Prevention of NSAID-induced**
gastric ulcer
PO
Adults, Elderly. 20-40 mg once daily
for up to 6 mo.
▶ **Hypersecretory conditions (e.g.,**
Zollinger-Ellison syndrome)
PO
Adults, Elderly. 40 mg twice daily.
▶ **Dose in hepatic impairment**
(Child-Pugh Class C)
PO
Adults, Elderly. Dose should not
exceed 20 mg/day.

CONTRAINDICATIONS
Hypersensitivity to other PPIs or
esomeprazole.

INTERACTIONS
Drug
Digoxin, iron, ketoconazole,
atazanavir, indinavir: May decrease
the concentration of digoxin, iron,
atazanavir, indinavir, and ketoconazole.
Benzodiazepines
(diazepam, midazolam, triazolam):
May increase levels of benzodiazepines
metabolized by oxidation.
CYP2C19 inducers: May decrease
esomeprazole level.
CYP2C19 inhibitors: May increase
esomeprazole level.
Methotrexate: May decrease
excretion of methotrexate, monitor
for side effects.
Herbal
None known.
Food
None known.

DIAGNOSTIC TEST EFFECTS
None known.

💧 IV COMPATIBILITIES
Doripenem (Doribax).

SIDE EFFECTS
Frequent (> 10%)
Headache.
Occasional (2%-9%)
Diarrhea, abdominal pain,
flatulence, nausea, hypertension,
pain, anxiety, insomnia, local
injection site reaction (IV).
Rare (< 2%)
Dizziness, dyspepsia, asthenia or loss
of strength, vomiting, constipation,
rash, cough, anemia.

SERIOUS REACTIONS
• Pancreatitis, Stevens-Johnson
syndrome, toxic epidermal necrolysis,
erythema multiforme occur rarely.

PRECAUTIONS & CONSIDERATIONS

It is unknown whether esomeprazole crosses the placenta or is distributed in breast milk. However, omeprazole is distributed in breast milk. Safety and efficacy of esomeprazole have not been established in children < 1 yr-old. No age-related precautions have been noted in elderly patients. Notify the physician if headache, diarrhea, discomfort, or nausea occurs during esomeprazole therapy.

Storage

Controlled room temperature; protect IV from light.

Administration

Take 1 h or more before eating. Do not crush or open capsule; swallow the capsule whole. May open the capsule and mix pellets with 1 tbsp of applesauce; swallow the spoonful without chewing. Mix contents of oral suspension packet with 1 tbsp (15 mL) of water, then leave 2-3 min to thicken. Stir and drink within 30 min. If any material remains after drinking, add more water, stir, and drink immediately.

Estazolam
es-tay-zoe-lam

CATEGORY AND SCHEDULE
Pregnancy Risk Category: X
Controlled Substance: Schedule IV

Classification: Sedatives/ hypnotics

MECHANISM OF ACTION
A benzodiazepine that enhances action of gamma aminobutyric acid (GABA) neurotransmission in the central nervous system (CNS). *Therapeutic Effect:* Produces depressant effect at all levels of central nervous system (CNS).

PHARMACOKINETICS
Rapidly absorbed from the GI tract. Onset of action 1 h. Protein binding: 93%. Metabolized in liver extensively. Primarily excreted in urine, minimal in feces. *Half-life:* 10-24 h.

AVAILABILITY
Tablets: 1 mg, 2 mg.

INDICATIONS AND DOSAGES
▶ **Insomnia**
PO
Adults (older than 18 yrs). 1-2 mg at bedtime.
Elderly, debilitated, liver disease, low serum albumin. 0.5-1 mg at bedtime.

CONTRAINDICATIONS
Pregnancy, hypersensitivity to other benzodiazepines.

INTERACTIONS
Drug
Alcohol, CNS depressants: May increase CNS and respiratory depression and have hypotensive effects.
Herbal
Kava kava, valerian: May increase CNS depressant effect.
Food
None known.

SIDE EFFECTS
Frequent
Drowsiness, sedation, hypokinesia, rebound insomnia (may occur for 1-2 nights after drug is discontinued), dizziness, confusion, euphoria, abnormal coordination.
Occasional
Weakness, anorexia, diarrhea.

E

Rare
Paradoxical CNS excitement, restlessness (particularly noted in elderly or debilitated patients).

SERIOUS REACTIONS

• Overdosage results in somnolence, confusion, diminished reflexes, and coma.
• Hypersensitivity reactions, including anaphylaxis and angioedema, have been reported.

PRECAUTIONS & CONSIDERATIONS

Caution should be used with impaired renal or liver function, respiratory disease, decreased gag reflex, or depression. Be aware that estazolam is contraindicated in pregnancy. Estazolam crosses the placenta and is distributed in breast milk. Safety and efficacy of estazolam have not been established in children. Use small initial doses and gradually increase them to avoid excessive sedation or ataxia as evidenced by muscular incoordination in elderly patients. Patients taking benzodiazepines are at risk for falls. Rebound insomnia may occur when drug is discontinued after short-term therapy. Avoid alcohol.
Storage
Store at room temperature.
Administration
Take at bedtime. May be taken without regard to meals.

Estradiol
ess-tra-dye′ole
(Aerodil [AUS], Alora, Climara, Delestrogen, Depo-Estradiol, Divigel, Elestrin, Estrace, Estraderm, Estraderm MX [AUS], Estradot [CAN], Estrasorb, EstroGel, Estring, Evamist, Femring, Femtrace, Gynodiol, Kliovance [AUS], Menostar, Oesclim [CAN], Sandrena Gel [AUS], Vagifem, Vivelle-Dot, Zumenon [AUS]).
Do not confuse Estraderm with Testoderm.

CATEGORY AND SCHEDULE
Pregnancy Risk Category: X

Classification: Estrogens, hormones/hormone modifiers

MECHANISM OF ACTION
An estrogen that increases the synthesis of DNA, RNA, and proteins in target tissues; reduces release of gonadotropin-releasing hormone from the hypothalamus; and reduces follicle-stimulating hormone and luteinizing hormone (LH) release from the pituitary. *Therapeutic Effect:* Promotes normal growth, promotes development of female sex organs, and maintains genitourinary function and vasomotor stability. Prevents accelerated bone loss by inhibiting bone resorption, restoring balance of bone resorption and formation. Inhibits LH and decreases serum testosterone concentration.

PHARMACOKINETICS
Well absorbed from the GI tract. Widely distributed. Protein binding: 50%-80%. Metabolized in the liver. Primarily excreted in urine.
Half-life: 1-2 h.

AVAILABILITY

Tablets (micronized, Estrace, Femtrace, Gynodiol): 0.5 mg, 1 mg, 1.5 mg, 2 mg.
Tablets (acetate, Femtrace): 0.45 mg, 0.9 mg, 1.8 mg.
Emulsion (Topical [Estrasorb]): 2.5 mg/g (0.25%).
Injection (Cypionate [Depo-Estradiol]): 5 mg/mL.
Injection (Valerate [Delestrogen]): 10 mg/mL, 20 mg/mL, 40 mg/mL.
Topical Gel (Divigel, Elestrin, EstroGel): 0.06%, 0.1%.
Topical Spray (Evamist): 1.53 mg/actuation.
Transdermal System (Alora): twice weekly: 0.025 mg, 0.05 mg, 0.075 mg, 0.1 mg.
Transdermal System (Climara): once weekly: 0.025 mg, 0.0375 mg, 0.05 mg, 0.06 mg, 0.075 mg, 0.1 mg.
Transdermal System (Estraderm): twice weekly: 0.05 mg, 0.1 mg.
Transdermal System (Menostar): once a week: 1 mg estradiol (14 mcg/24 h).
Transdermal System (Vivelle Dot): twice weekly: 0.025 mg, 0.0375 mg, 0.05 mg, 0.075 mg, 0.1 mg.
Vaginal Cream (Estrace): 0.1 mg/g (0.01%).
Vaginal Ring (Estring): 2 mg.
Vaginal Ring (Femring): 0.05 mg, 0.1 mg.
Vaginal Tablet (Vagifem): 25 mcg.

INDICATIONS AND DOSAGES

▸ **Prostate cancer (palliative)**
IM (VALERATE)
Adults, Elderly. 30 mg or more q1-2-wk.
PO
Adults, Elderly. 10 mg 3 times a day for at least 3 mo.

▸ **Breast cancer (palliative)**
PO
Adults, Elderly. 10 mg 3 times a day for at least 3 mo.

▸ **Osteoporosis prophylaxis in postmenopausal females**
PO If intact uterus, give 14 days progestin every 6-12 mo.
Adults, Elderly. 0.5 mg/day cyclically (3 wks on, 1 wk off).
TRANSDERMAL (CLIMARA)
Adults, Elderly. Initially, 0.025 mg weekly, adjust dose as needed.
TRANSDERMAL (ALORA, VIVELLE-DOT)
Adults, Elderly. Initially, 0.025 mg patch twice weekly, adjust dose as needed.
TRANSDERMAL (ESTRADERM)
Adults, Elderly. 0.05 mg twice weekly.
TRANSDERMAL (MENOSTAR)
Adults, Elderly. 1 mg weekly.

▸ **Female hypoestrogenism**
PO
Adults, Elderly. 1-2 mg/day, adjust dose as needed.
IM (CYPIONATE)
Adults, Elderly. 1.5-2 mg monthly.
IM (VALERATE)
Adults, Elderly. 10-20 mg q4wk.
TRANSDERMAL (CLIMARA)
Adults, Elderly. 0.025 mg once weekly.

▸ **Vasomotor symptoms associated with menopause**
PO
Adults, Elderly. 1-2 mg/day cyclically (3 wks on, 1 wk off), adjust dose as needed.
IM (CYPIONATE)
Adults, Elderly. 1-5 mg q3-4wk.
IM (VALERATE)
Adults, Elderly. 10-20 mg q4wk.
TOPICAL EMULSION (ESTRASORB)
Adults, Elderly. 3.84 g once a day in the morning.
TOPICAL GEL (ESTROGEL)
Adults, Elderly. 1.25 g/day.
TOPICAL GEL (DIVIGEL)
Adults, Elderly. 0.25 g/day. Range 0.25-1 g/day.

E

E

TOPICAL GEL (ELESTRIN)
Adults, Elderly. 0.87 g/day.
TOPICAL SPRAY (EVAMIST)
Adults, Elderly. One spray/day.
Range 1-3 sprays/day based on
response.
TRANSDERMAL (CLIMARA)
Adults, Elderly. 0.025 mg weekly.
Adjust dose as needed.
TRANSDERMAL (ALORA,
ESCLIM, ESTRADERM,
VIVELLE-DOT)
Adults, Elderly. 0.05 mg twice a week.
VAGINAL RING (FEMRING)
Adults, Elderly. 0.05 mg once
q90 days. May increase to 0.1 mg if
needed.
▸ **Vaginal atrophy**
VAGINAL RING (ESTRING)
Adults, Elderly. 2 mg once q90 days.
VAGINAL CREAM (ESTRACE)
Adults, Elderly. 2-4 g/day for 2 wks,
then reduce to ½ initial dose for
2 wks, then 1 g 1-3 times a week.
TOPICAL GEL (ESTROGEL)
Adults, Elderly. 1.25 g/day.
TOPICAL GEL (ELESTRIN)
Adults, Elderly. 0.87 g/day.
TRANSDERMAL (CLIMARA)
Adults, Elderly. 0.025 mg/ once a
week.
▸ **Atrophic vaginitis**
VAGINAL TABLET (VAGIFEM)
Adults, Elderly. Initially, 1 tablet/day
for 2 wks. Maintenance: 1 tablet
twice a week.

OFF-LABEL USES
Treatment of Turner syndrome.

CONTRAINDICATIONS
Abnormal vaginal bleeding,
active arterial thrombosis, blood
dyscrasias, estrogen-dependent
cancer, known or suspected breast
cancer, pregnancy, thrombophlebitis
or thromboembolic disorders,
thyroid dysfunction, severe hepatic
dysfunction.

INTERACTIONS
Drug
Aromatase inhibitors: May
interfere with effects of aromatase
inhibitors.
Bromocriptine: May interfere with
the effects of bromocriptine.
Corticosteroids: May increase
effects of hydrocortisone and
prednisone.
Cyclosporine: May increase
blood cyclosporine concentration
and the risk of hepatotoxicity and
nephrotoxicity.
CYP3A4 inducers/inhibitors: May
alter levels of estradiol.
**Hepatotoxic medications,
cyclosporine:** May increase the risk
of hepatotoxicity. May increase the
level of cyclosporine.
Thyroid medications: May decrease
effects of thyroid medications.
Herbal
Saw palmetto: Increases the effects
of saw palmetto.
St. John's wort: May decrease
effects of estradiol.
Food
None known.

DIAGNOSTIC TEST EFFECTS
May increase blood glucose,
HDL, serum calcium, and
triglyceride levels. May decrease
serum cholesterol levels and
LDH concentrations. May affect
metapyrone testing and thyroid
function tests.

SIDE EFFECTS
Frequent
Anorexia, nausea, swelling of
breasts, peripheral edema marked by
swollen ankles and feet.
Transdermal: Skin irritation, redness.
Occasional
Vomiting, especially with high
doses; headache that may be severe;
intolerance to contact lenses;

E

hypertension; glucose intolerance; brown spots on exposed skin.
Vaginal: Local irritation, vaginal discharge, changes in vaginal bleeding, including spotting, and breakthrough or prolonged bleeding.

Rare

Chorea or involuntary movements, hirsutism or abnormal hairiness, loss of scalp hair, depression.

SERIOUS REACTIONS

• Prolonged administration increases the risk of gallbladder disease, thromboembolic disease, and breast, cervical, vaginal, endometrial, and hepatic carcinoma.
• Myocardial infarction, stroke, venous thromboembolism.
• Cholestatic jaundice occurs rarely.
• Retinal vascular thrombosis.

PRECAUTIONS & CONSIDERATIONS

Estrogen therapy should not be used to prevent cardiovascular disease, and other options for osteoporosis should be considered if being used solely for prevention of osteoporosis because it increases the risk of cardiovascular events. Use with caution in patients with cardiovascular disease. Use with caution in patients with history of cholestatic jaunice with past estrogen use or pregnancy. Estrogen therapy should be used for the shortest duration and lowest dose possible. Caution is warranted in patients with diseases exacerbated by fluid retention and with hepatic or renal insufficiency and with gallbladder disease, hypocalcemia, porphyria, or lupus. Should be discontinued at least 4 wks before and for 2 wks following surgical procedures or prolonged immobilizations (risk of thromboembolism). Estradiol is distributed in breast milk and may be harmful to the infant. Estradiol should not be used during breastfeeding. Estradiol should be used cautiously in children whose bone growth is not complete because the drug may accelerate epiphyseal closure. The risk of dementia is increased in postmenopausal women aged > 65 yrs.

Avoid smoking because of the increased risk of blood clot formation and myocardial infarction. Limit alcohol and caffeine intake.

Notify the physician of calf or chest pain, depression, numbness or weakness of an extremity, severe abdominal pain, shortness of breath, speech or vision disturbance, sudden headache, unusual bleeding, or vomiting. BP, weight, blood glucose, hepatic enzyme, and serum calcium levels should be monitored.

Administration

Take oral estradiol at the same time each day. Apply gel and spray at the same time each day topically as directed.

For IM use, rotate the vial to disperse drug in solution. Give deep IM injection into the gluteus maximus.

For vaginal use, apply estradiol cream at bedtime for best absorption. To administer, insert the end of the filled applicator into the vagina, directing the applicator slightly toward the sacrum; push the plunger down completely. To prevent topical absorption of the drug, do not allow the cream to contact the skin.

! Transdermal Climara is administered once weekly; other transdermal forms of estradiol are applied twice weekly.

To apply the transdermal system, remove the old patch and select a new site. Consider using the

E

buttocks as an alternative application site. Peel off the protective strip on the patch to expose the adhesive surface. Apply to clean, dry, intact skin on the trunk of the body in an area with as little hair as possible. Press in place for at least 10 s. Do not apply the patch to breasts or waistline.

Estrogens, Conjugated

ess'troe-jenz

(Cenestin, C.E.S. [CAN], Congest [CAN], Enjuvia, Premarin, Premarin Créme [AUS])

Do not confuse with Primaxin or Remeron.

CATEGORY AND SCHEDULE
Pregnancy Risk Category: X

Classification: Estrogens, hormones/hormone modifiers

MECHANISM OF ACTION
An estrogen that increases the synthesis of DNA, RNA, and various proteins in target tissues; reduces release of gonadotropin-releasing hormone from the hypothalamus; and reduces follicle-stimulating hormone (FSH) and luteinizing hormone (LH) release from the pituitary gland. *Therapeutic Effect:* Promotes normal growth, promotes development of female sex organs, and maintains genitourinary function and vasomotor stability. Prevents accelerated bone loss by inhibiting bone resorption, restoring balance of bone resorption and formation. Inhibits LH and

decreases serum concentration of testosterone.

PHARMACOKINETICS
Well absorbed from the GI tract. Widely distributed. Protein binding: 50%-80%. Metabolized in the liver. Primarily excreted in urine. *Half-life (metabolite):* 27 h.

AVAILABILITY
Tablets (Cenestin, Premarin): 0.3 mg, 0.45 mg, 0.625 mg, 0.9 mg, 1.25 mg.
Tablets (Enjuvia): 0.3 mg, 0.45 mg, 0.625 mg, 0.9 mg, 1.25 mg.
Injection: 25 mg.
Vaginal Cream: 0.625 mg/g.

INDICATIONS AND DOSAGES
▸ **Vasomotor symptoms associated with menopause, atrophic vaginitis, kraurosis vulvae**
PO
Adults, Elderly. 0.3-0.625 mg/day cyclically (21 days on, 7 days off) or continuously.
INTRAVAGINAL
Adults, Elderly. 0.5-2 g/day cyclically, such as 21 days on and 7 days off.
▸ **Female hypogonadism**
PO
Adults. 0.3-0.625 mg/day in divided doses for 20 days; then a rest period of 10 days.
▸ **Female castration, primary ovarian failure**
PO
Adults. Initially, 1.25 mg/day cyclically. Adjust dosage, upward or downward, according to severity of symptoms and patient response. For maintenance, adjust dosage to lowest level that will provide effective control.
▸ **Osteoporosis**
PO
Adults, Elderly. 0.3-0.625 mg/day, cyclically, such as 25 days on and 5 days off.

▸ **Breast cancer palliation**
PO
Adults, Elderly. 10 mg 3 times a day
for at least 3 mo.
▸ **Prostate cancer (palliative)**
PO
Adults, Elderly. 1.25-2.5 mg 3 times
a day.
▸ **Abnormal uterine bleeding**
PO
Adults. 1.25 mg q4h for 24 h, then
1.25 mg/day for 7-10 days.
IV, IM
Adults. 25 mg; may repeat once in
6-12 h.

OFF-LABEL USES
Prevention of estrogen deficiency–
induced premenopausal osteoporosis.
Cream: Prevention of nosebleeds.

CONTRAINDICATIONS
Breast cancer (with some
exceptions), severe hepatic disease,
thrombophlebitis or thromboembolic
disorders, undiagnosed vaginal
bleeding, active arterial thrombosis,
blood dyscrasias, estrogen-dependent
cancer, pregnancy, thrombophlebitis
or thromboembolic disorders, thyroid
dysfunction.

INTERACTIONS
Drug
Aromatase inhibitors: May interfere
with effects of aromatase inhibitors.
Bromocriptine: May interfere with
the effects of bromocriptine.
Corticosteroids: May increase
effects of hydrocortisone and
prednisone.
Cyclosporine: May increase
blood cyclosporine concentration
and the risk of hepatotoxicity and
nephrotoxicity.
CYP3A4 inducers/inhibitors: May
alter levels of estrogens.
Hepatotoxic medications: May
increase the risk of hepatotoxicity.

Thyroid medications: May decrease
effects of thyroid medications.
Herbal
St. John's wort: May decrease the
effects of estrogens.
Food
None known.

DIAGNOSTIC TEST EFFECTS
May increase blood glucose, HDL,
serum calcium, and triglyceride
levels. May decrease serum
cholesterol levels and LDH
concentrations. May affect serum
metapyrone testing and thyroid
function tests.

ⓘ IV INCOMPATIBILITIES
Pantoprazole.

ⓘ IV COMPATIBILITIES
Heparin, hydrocortisone sodium
succinate, potassium chloride,
vitamin B complex with C.

SIDE EFFECTS
Frequent
Vaginal bleeding, such as spotting or
breakthrough bleeding; breast pain or
tenderness; gynecomastia.
Occasional
Headache, hypertension, intolerance
to contact lenses.
High doses: Anorexia, nausea.
Rare
Loss of scalp hair, depression.

SERIOUS REACTIONS
• Prolonged administration may
increase the risk of gallbladder
disease, thromboembolic disease,
and breast, cervical, vaginal,
endometrial, and hepatic
carcinoma.
• Myocardial infarction, stroke,
venous thromboembolism.
• Cholestatic jaundice occurs
rarely.
• Retinal vascular thrombosis.

E

PRECAUTIONS & CONSIDERATIONS

Estrogen therapy should not be used to prevent cardiovascular disease; because of the increased risk of cardiovascular disease, other options for osteoporosis should be considered if it is being used solely for prevention of osteoporosis. Use with caution in patients with cardiovascular disease. Use with caution in patients with a history of cholestatic jaunice with past estrogen use or pregnancy. Estrogen therapy should be used for the shortest duration and lowest dose possible. Caution is warranted in patients with diseases exacerbated by fluid retention, such as asthma, cardiac dysfunction, diabetes mellitus, epilepsy, migraine headaches, heart failure, and renal impairment. Caution is warranted in patients with hepatic and with gallbladder disease, hypocalcemia, porphyria, lupus. Should be discontinued at least 4 wks before and for 2 wks following surgical procedures or prolonged immobilizations (risk of thromboembolism). Conjugated estrogens are distributed in breast milk and may be harmful to the infant. The drug should be discontinued in a pregnant woman. Estrogens should not be used during breastfeeding. Safety and efficacy of conjugated estrogens have not been established in children. Estradiol should be used cautiously in children whose bone growth is not complete because the drug may accelerate epiphyseal closure. The risk of dementia is increased in postmenopausal women aged > 65 yrs. Avoid smoking because of the increased risk of blood clot formation and MI. Limit alcohol and caffeine intake.

Notify the physician of weight gain of more than 5 lb in a week, abnormal vaginal bleeding, depression, or signs and symptoms of blood clots. Also, signs and symptoms of thromboembolic or thrombotic disorders, including loss of coordination, numbness or weakness of an extremity, shortness of breath, speech or vision disturbance, sudden severe headache, and pain in the chest, leg, or groin, should be reported immediately. Breast self-examinations should be made monthly. Weight and BP should be monitored.

Storage
Refrigerate vials. The reconstituted solution is stable for 60 days refrigerated. Do not use if solution darkens or precipitate forms.

Administration
Take at the same time each day with food or milk if nausea occurs. Administer vaginal cream at bedtime to reduce side effects.

For IV and IM use, reconstitute with 5 mL sterile water for injection containing benzyl alcohol (provided). Slowly add diluent, shaking gently. Avoid vigorous shaking. For the IV form, give slowly to prevent flushing.

Estrogens, Esterified
ess'troe-jenz
(Menest, Neo-Estrone [CAN])

CATEGORY AND SCHEDULE
Pregnancy Risk Category: X

Classification: Estrogens, hormones/hormone modifiers

MECHANISM OF ACTION
A combination of sodium salts of sulfate esters of estrogenic substances (principal component is estrone) that increases synthesis of DNA, RNA, and various proteins in

responsive tissues. Reduces release of gonadotropin-releasing hormone, reducing follicle-stimulating hormone (FSH) and luteinizing hormone (LH). *Therapeutic Effect:* Promotes vasomotor stability, maintains genitourinary function, normal growth, development of female sex organs. Prevents accelerated bone loss by inhibiting bone resorption, restoring balance of bone resorption and formation.

PHARMACOKINETICS

Readily absorbed from the GI tract. Widely distributed. Protein binding: 50%-80%. Rapidly metabolized in liver and GI tract to estrone sulfate and conjugated and unconjugated metabolites. Excreted in urine and bile. *Half-life:* Unknown.

AVAILABILITY

Tablets: 0.3 mg, 0.625 mg, 1.25 mg.

INDICATIONS AND DOSAGES

▸ **Vasomotor symptoms associated with menopause, atrophic vaginitis, kraurosis vulvae**
PO
Adults, Elderly. 0.3-1.25 mg/day cyclically.
▸ **Female hypogonadism**
PO
Adults. 2.5-7.5 mg/day in divided doses for 20 days; rest 10 days.
▸ **Female castration, primary ovarian failure**
PO
Adults. Initially, 1.25 mg/day cyclically.
▸ **Breast cancer palliation**
PO
Adults, Elderly. 10 mg 3 times/day for at least 3 mo.
▸ **Prostate cancer**
PO
Adults, Elderly. 1.25-2.5 mg 3 times/day.

▸ **Osteoporosis in postmenopausal women**
PO
Adults, Elderly. 0.3-1.25 mg/day cyclically.

CONTRAINDICATIONS

Breast cancer (with some exceptions), liver disease, thrombophlebitis or thromboembolic disorders, undiagnosed vaginal bleeding, active arterial thrombosis, blood dyscrasias, estrogen-dependent cancer, pregnancy, thyroid dysfunction, severe hepatic dysfunction.

INTERACTIONS

Drug
Aromatase inhibitors: May interfere with effects of aromatase inhibitors.
Bromocriptine: May interfere with effects of bromocriptine.
Corticosteroids: May increase effects of hydrocortisone and prednisone.
Cyclosporine: May increase blood concentration and liver and nephrotoxicity of cyclosporine.
Liver toxic medications: May increase the risk of liver toxicity.
CYP3A4 inducers/inhibitors: May alter levels of estradiol.
Thyroid medications: May decrease effects of thyroid medications.
Herbal
St. John's wort: May decrease levels of esterified estrogens.
Black cohosh, dong quai: May increase estrogenic activity.
Red clover, saw palmetto, ginseng: May increase hormonal effects.

DIAGNOSTIC TEST EFFECTS

May affect metapyrone testing, thyroid function tests. May decrease serum cholesterol levels and LDH concentrations. May increase blood glucose levels, HDL concentrations, serum calcium and triglyceride levels.

E

SIDE EFFECTS
Frequent
Change in vaginal bleeding, such as spotting or breakthrough bleeding, breast pain or tenderness, gynecomastia.
Occasional
Headache, increased BP, intolerance to contact lenses, nausea.
Rare
Loss of scalp hair, clinical depression.

SERIOUS REACTIONS
• Prolonged administration may increase risk of gallbladder, thromboembolic disease, breast, cervical, vaginal, endometrial, and liver carcinoma.
• Myocardial infarction, stroke, venous thromboembolism.
• Cholestatic jaundice occurs rarely.
• Retinal vascular thrombosis.

PRECAUTIONS & CONSIDERATIONS
Estrogen therapy should not be used to prevent cardiovascular disease. Other options for osteoporosis should be considered if estrogen therapy is being used solely for prevention of osteoporosis because of the increased risk of cardiovascular events. Use with caution in patients with cardiovascular disease. Use with caution in patients with history of cholestatic jaundice with past estrogen use or pregnancy. Estrogen therapy should be used for the shortest duration and lowest dose possible. Caution is warranted in patients with diseases exacerbated by fluid retention, such as asthma, cardiac dysfunction, diabetes mellitus, epilepsy, migraine headaches, and renal impairment. Caution is warranted with hepatic insufficiency and with gallbladder disease, hypocalcemia, porphyria, or lupus. Should be discontinued at least 4 wks before and for 2 wks following surgical procedures or prolonged immobilizations (risk of thromboembolism). Be aware that esterified estrogen is distributed in breast milk and may be harmful to infant. Esterified estrogen should not be used during breastfeeding or pregnancy. Be aware that the safety and efficacy of this drug have not been established in children. Esterified estrogen should be used cautiously in children whose bone growth is not complete because the drug may accelerate epiphyseal closure. The risk of dementia is increased in postmenopausal women aged > 65 yrs. Smoking should be strongly discouraged because of increased risk of blood clot formation and myocardial infarction. Limit alcohol and caffeine intake.

Signs and symptoms of thromboembolic or thrombotic disorders are evident by loss of coordination; numbness or weakness of an extremity; pain in the chest, leg, or groin; shortness of breath; speech or vision disturbance; or sudden severe headache. Abnormal vaginal bleeding, tenderness, and swelling may be signs and symptoms of blood clots.
Administration
Administer at the same time each day. Give esterified estrogen with food or milk if the patient experiences nausea.

Estropipate
es-tro-pip'ate
(Genoral [AUS], Ogen, Ortho-Est)

CATEGORY AND SCHEDULE
Pregnancy Risk Category: X

Classification: Estrogens,
hormones/hormone modifiers

MECHANISM OF ACTION
An estrogen that increases synthesis
of DNA, RNA, and proteins in
target tissues; reduces release of
gonadotropin-releasing hormone
from the hypothalamus; and reduces
follicle-stimulating hormone (FSH)
and luteinizing hormone (LH) from
the pituitary. *Therapeutic Effect:*
Promotes normal growth, promotes
development of female sex organs
and maintains genitourinary function
and vasomotor stability. Prevents
accelerated bone loss by inhibiting
bone resorption, restoring balance
of bone resorption and formation.
Inhibits LH and decreases serum
testosterone concentration.

AVAILABILITY
Tablets (Ogen, Ortho-Est): 0.625 mg
(0.75 mg estropipate), 1.25 mg
(1.5 mg estropipate), 2.5 mg (3 mg
estropipate).

INDICATIONS AND DOSAGES
▸ **Vasomotor symptoms, atrophic
vaginitis, kraurosis vulvae**
PO
Adults, Elderly. 0.625-5 mg/day
(0.75-6 mg estropipate) cyclically.
▸ **Female hypogonadism, castration,
primary ovarian failure**
PO
Adults, Elderly. 1.25-7.5 mg/day
(1.5-9 mg estropipate) for 21 days;
then off for 8-10 days. Repeat if
bleeding does not occur by end of
off cycle.
▸ **Prevention of osteoporosis**
PO
Adults, Elderly. 0.625 mg/day
(0.75 mg estropipate) (25 days of
31-day cycle).

CONTRAINDICATIONS
Abnormal vaginal bleeding, active
arterial thrombosis, blood dyscrasias,
estrogen-dependent cancer, known or
suspected breast cancer, pregnancy,
thrombophlebitis or thromboembolic
disorders, thyroid dysfunction, severe
liver disease.

INTERACTIONS
Drug
Aromatase inhibitors: May
interfere with effects of aromatase
inhibitors.
Bromocriptine: May interfere with
the effects of bromocriptine.
Corticosteroids: May increase
effects of hydrocortisone and
prednisone.
Cyclosporine: May increase blood
cyclosporine concentration and the risk
of hepatotoxicity and nephrotoxicity.
CYP3A4 inducers/inhibitors: May
alter levels of estropipate.
Hepatotoxic medications: May
increase the risk of hepatotoxicity.
Thyroid medications: May decrease
effects of thyroid medications.
Herbal
Saw palmetto: Increases the effects
of saw palmetto.
St. John's wort: May decrease
levels of estropipate.
Food
None known.

DIAGNOSTIC TEST EFFECTS
May increase blood glucose, HDL,
serum calcium, and triglyceride
levels. May decrease serum

E

cholesterol and LDH concentrations. May affect metapyrone testing and thyroid function tests.

SIDE EFFECTS

Frequent
Anorexia, nausea, swelling of breasts, peripheral edema marked by swollen ankles and feet.

Occasional
Vomiting, especially with high doses; headache that may be severe; intolerance to contact lenses; hypertension; glucose intolerance; brown spots on exposed skin.
Vaginal: Local irritation, vaginal discharge, changes in vaginal bleeding, including spotting, and breakthrough or prolonged bleeding.

Rare
Chorea or involuntary movements, hirsutism or abnormal hairiness, loss of scalp hair, depression.

SERIOUS REACTIONS

• Prolonged administration increases the risk of gallbladder disease; thromboembolic disease; and breast, cervical, vaginal, endometrial, and hepatic carcinoma.
• Myocardial infarction, stroke, venous thromboembolism.
• Retinal vascular thrombosis.
• Cholestatic jaundice occurs rarely.

PRECAUTIONS & CONSIDERATIONS

Estrogen therapy should not be used to prevent cardiovascular disease. Because of the increased risk for cardiovascular events, other options for osteoporosis should be considered if estrogen therapy is being used solely for the prevention of osteoporosis. Use with caution in patients with cardiovascular disease. Use with caution in patients with a history of cholestatic jaundice with past estrogen use or pregnancy. Estrogen therapy should be used for the shortest duration and lowest dose possible. Caution is warranted with diseases exacerbated by fluid retention such as asthma, cardiac dysfunction, diabetes, epilepsy, migraine headaches, and renal insufficiency. Caution is warranted in patients with hepatic insufficiency and with gallbladder disease, hypocalcemia, porphyria, or lupus. Should be discontinued at least 4 wks before and for 2 wks following surgical procedures or prolonged immobilizations (risk of thromboembolism). Estropipate is distributed in breast milk and may be harmful to the infant. Estropipate should not be used during breastfeeding. Estropipate should be used cautiously in children whose bone growth is not complete because the drug may accelerate epiphyseal closure. The risk of dementia is increased in postmenopausal women aged > 65 yrs. Limit alcohol and caffeine intake. Avoid smoking because of the increased risk of blood clot formation and myocardial infarction.

Notify the physician of depression or abnormal vaginal bleeding. Signs and symptoms of thromboembolic or thrombotic disorders, including peripheral paresthesia, shortness of breath, speech or vision disturbance, and sudden headache, should be immediately reported. BP, weight, and blood glucose, hepatic enzyme, and serum calcium levels should be monitored.

Storage
Store in a tightly-closed container at room temperature.

Administration
Take estropipate at the same time each day. Administration with food may decrease GI upset.

Eszopiclone
es-zoe-pick'lone
(Lunesta)

CATEGORY AND SCHEDULE
Pregnancy Risk Category: C

Classification: Sedatives/
hypnotics

MECHANISM OF ACTION
A nonbenzodiazepine that may
interact with GABA-receptor
complexes at binding domains
located close to or allosterically
coupled to benzodiazepine
receptors. *Therapeutic Effect:*
Induces sleep and helps maintain
sleep at night.

AVAILABILITY
Tablets (Film-Coated): 1 mg, 2 mg,
3 mg.

INDICATIONS AND DOSAGES
▶ **Insomnia**
PO
Adults. 2 mg immediately before
bedtime. Maximum: 3 mg.
*Adults using CYP3A4 inhibitors
concurrently.* 1 mg before bedtime;
may be increased to 2 mg if needed.
Elderly (difficulty falling asleep).
1 mg before bedtime. Maximum:
2 mg.
*Adults, Elderly (difficulty
maintaining sleep).* 2 mg before
bedtime. Maximum: 3 mg.
▶ **Severe hepatic impairment**
PO
Adults. Initially, 1 mg at bedtime.
Maximum 2 mg.

CONTRAINDICATIONS
None known.

INTERACTIONS
Drug
Alcohol, olanzapine: May lead to
decreased psychomotor function.
**Aminoglutethimide, carbamazepine,
nafcillin, nevirapine, phenobarbital,
phenytoin, rifampicin, CYP3A4
inducers:** May decrease the blood
level and effects of eszopiclone.
**Clarithromycin, ketoconazole,
nefazodone, nelfinavir, ritonavir,
traconazole, troleandomycin,
CYP3A4 inhibitors:** May increase
the blood level and effects of
eszopiclone.
CNS depressants: May increase
adverse effects.
Herbal
**Gotu kola, kava kava, St. John's
wort, valerian:** May increase CNS
depression.
Food
Heavy meals: May reduce onset of
eszopiclone action if taken with or
immediately after a heavy meal.

DIAGNOSTIC TEST EFFECTS
None known.

SIDE EFFECTS
Frequent (21%-34%)
Unpleasant taste, headache.
Occasional (4%-10%)
Somnolence, dry mouth, dyspepsia,
dizziness, nervousness, pain, nausea,
rash, pruritus, depression, diarrhea.
Rare (2%-3%)
Hallucinations, anxiety, confusion,
abnormal dreams, decreased
libido, neuralgia, dysmenorrhea,
gynecomastia.

SERIOUS REACTIONS
• Chest pain and peripheral edema
occur occasionally.

PRECAUTIONS & CONSIDERATIONS
Caution is warranted in patients
with clinical depression, drug abuse,

E

hepatic impairment, and compromised respiratory function. Abnormal thinking and behavioral changes may occur, so monitor. Amnesia, CNS depression, and hypersensitivity reactions can occur. Use cautiously in elderly patients and reduce dose. Safety and efficacy have not been evaluated in children. Avoid abrupt cessation of therapy to avoid withdrawal symptoms.

Administration

Take immediately before bedtime. Do not take with, or immediately following, a high-fat meal. Do not crush or break tablets. Patients should be able to devote time for a full night's rest.

Etanercept
e-tan′er-cept
(Enbrel)

CATEGORY AND SCHEDULE
Pregnancy Risk Category: B

Classification: Disease-modifying antirheumatic drugs, immunomodulators, tumor necrosis factor modulators.

MECHANISM OF ACTION
A protein that binds to tumor necrosis factor (TNF), blocking its interaction with cell surface receptors. Elevated levels of TNF, which is involved in inflammatory and immune responses, are found in the synovial fluid of rheumatoid arthritis patients. *Therapeutic Effect:* Relieves the symptoms of rheumatoid arthritis, psoriasis, and other inflammatory conditions.

PHARMACOKINETICS
Well absorbed after subcutaneous administration. *Half-life:* 115 h. Onset of action: 1-3 wks.

AVAILABILITY
Powder for Injection: 25 mg.
Prefilled Syringe: 50 mg/mL.

INDICATIONS AND DOSAGES
▸ **Rheumatoid arthritis, psoriatic arthritis, ankylosing spondylitis**
SUBCUTANEOUS
Adults, Elderly. 25 mg twice weekly given 72-96 h apart or 50 mg as one injection or two 25-mg injections on the same day.
▸ **Juvenile rheumatoid arthritis**
SUBCUTANEOUS
Children aged 2-17 yrs. 0.8 mg/kg/wk. Once-weekly dosing max 50 mg/dose or use twice weekly dosing 0.4 mg/kg (Maximum: 25 mg dose) twice weekly given 72-96 h apart.
▸ **Plaque psoriasis**
SUBCUTANEOUS
Adults, Elderly. 50 mg twice a week (give 3-4 days apart) for 3 mo. Maintenance: 50 mg/week given as once weekly 50 mg injection or as a 25 mg injection twice weekly 3-4 days apart.

CONTRAINDICATIONS
Serious active infection or sepsis, hypersensitivity to etanercept, significant hematologic abnormalities, latex hypersensitivity (auto-injection), benzyl alcohol hypersensitivity (diluent for powder for injection).

INTERACTIONS
Drug
Abatacept, anakinara: May increase the risk of infection.
Cyclophosphamide: Increase in risk for noncutaneous solid malignancies when used concurrently, avoid concomitant use.
Live vaccines: Secondary transmission of infection by the live vaccine may occur.

Herbal and Food
None known.

DIAGNOSTIC TEST EFFECTS
None known.

SIDE EFFECTS
Frequent (20%-37%)
Injection site erythema, pruritus, pain, and swelling; abdominal pain (children 19%), upper respiratory infection.
Occasional (4%-19%)
Headache, rhinitis, dizziness, pharyngitis, cough, asthenia, abdominal pain (adults 5%), stomatitis, dyspepsia, vomiting (more common in children than adults), rash, nausea.
Rare (< 3%)
Sinusitis, allergic reaction, lupus-like symptoms.

SERIOUS REACTIONS
• Infections (such as pyelonephritis, cellulitis, osteomyelitis, wound infection, leg ulcer, septic arthritis, diarrhea, bronchitis, and pneumonia) occur in 29%-38% of patients.
• Rare adverse effects include heart failure, hypertension, hypotension, pancreatitis, GI hemorrhage, and dyspnea. The patient also may develop autoimmune antibodies.
• Nervous system problems such as seizures, optic neuritis, weakness of arms or legs (rare).

PRECAUTIONS & CONSIDERATIONS
Serious infections (including bacterial sepsis and tuberculosis) leading to hospitalization or death have been observed in patients treated with etanercept. Screen patients for latent tuberculosis infection before beginning etanercept. Patients should be educated about the symptoms of infection and closely monitored for signs and symptoms of infection during and after treatment with the drug. Patients who develop an infection should be evaluated for appropriate antimicrobial treatment and, in patients who develop a serious infection, etanercept should be discontinued. Use with caution in patients with seizure disorders, multiple sclerosis, on pre-existing heart failure.

Caution is warranted in patients with history of recurrent infections and illnesses that predispose to infection, such as diabetes mellitus. It is unknown whether etanercept is excreted in breast milk. No age-related precautions have been noted in elderly patients or in children 4 yrs and older. Avoid receiving live-virus vaccines during treatment. Discontinue therapy and expect to treat with varicella-zoster immune globulin, as prescribed, if the patient experiences significant exposure to varicella virus during treatment.

Notify the physician of bleeding, bruising, pallor, or persistent fever. CBC and erythrocyte sedimentation rate or C-reactive protein level should be monitored. Signs of a therapeutic response, including improved grip strength, increased joint mobility, reduced joint tenderness, and relief of pain, stiffness, and swelling, should be assessed.

Storage
Refrigerate unopened vials and prefilled syringes. Do not freeze. Protect from light. Once reconstituted, the drug may be stored for up to 14 days in the refrigerator.

Administration
! Do not add other medications to the solution. Do not use a filter during reconstitution or administration. Allow to come to room temperature before administering prefilled syringes or autoinjector syringe.
! If using vials, reconstitute only with 1 mL sterile bacteriostatic water for injection (containing 0.9% benzyl

alcohol). Slowly inject the diluent into the vial. Some foaming will occur. To avoid excessive foaming, slowly swirl the contents until the powder is dissolved (< 5 min). The reconstituted solution normally appears clear and colorless. Discard the solution if it contains particles or becomes cloudy or discolored. Withdraw all the solution into the syringe. The final volume should be approximately 1 mL.

Subcutaneously inject into the abdomen, thigh, or upper arm. Rotate injection sites. Administer each new injection at least 1 in. from an old site, avoiding tender, bruised, hard, or red areas. Injection site reactions generally occur in the first month of treatment and decrease in frequency with continued etanercept therapy.

Ethambutol
e-tham′byoo-tole
(Etibi [CAN], Myambutol)
Do not confuse ethambutol or Myambutol with Nembutal.

CATEGORY AND SCHEDULE
Pregnancy Risk Category: C

Classification: Antimycobacterials

MECHANISM OF ACTION
An isonicotinic acid derivative that interferes with RNA synthesis. *Therapeutic Effect:* Suppresses the multiplication of mycobacteria.

PHARMACOKINETICS
Rapidly and well absorbed from the GI tract (80%). Protein binding: 20%-30%. Widely distributed.

Metabolized in the liver. Primarily excreted in urine. Removed by hemodialysis. *Half-life:* 3-4 h (increased in impaired renal function).

AVAILABILITY
Tablets: 100 mg, 400 mg.

INDICATIONS AND DOSAGES
▸ **Tuberculosis**
PO
Adults, Elderly, Adolescents 13 yr and older. 15-25 mg/kg/day as a single dose (maximum 1600 mg/dose) or 50 mg/kg 2 times/wk (maximum 4 g/dose). Consult recommended initial dosing and retreatment schedules, because treatment regimens can vary.
Children. 15-25 mg/kg/day as a single dose (maximum: 2.5 g/day).
▸ **Dosage in renal impairment**
Dosage interval is modified based on creatinine clearance.

Creatinine Clearance (mL/min)	Dosage Interval
10-50	q24-36h
< 10	q48h

OFF-LABEL USES
Treatment of atypical mycobacterial infections.

CONTRAINDICATIONS
Optic neuritis and patients who cannot report visual changes, hypersensitivity to ethambutol.

INTERACTIONS
Drug
Neurotoxic medications: May increase the risk of neurotoxicity.
Aluminum antacids: Decrease absorption of ethambutol, administer 4 h apart.
Herbal and Food
None known.

DIAGNOSTIC TEST EFFECTS
May increase serum uric acid levels, may elevate liver enzyme levels.

SIDE EFFECTS
Occasional
Acute gouty arthritis (chills, pain, swelling of joints with hot skin), confusion, abdominal pain, nausea, vomiting, anorexia, headache.
Rare
Rash, fever, blurred vision, eye pain, red-green color blindness.

SERIOUS REACTIONS
• Optic neuritis and sometimes irreversible blindness (more common with high-dosage or long-term ethambutol therapy), peripheral neuritis, liver toxicities, and an anaphylactoid reaction occur rarely.
• Thrombocytopenia.

PRECAUTIONS & CONSIDERATIONS
Caution is warranted in patients with cataracts, diabetic retinopathy, gout, recurrent ocular inflammatory conditions, and renal dysfunction. Ethambutol use is not recommended for children younger than 13 yrs of age. Be aware that ethambutol crosses the placenta and is excreted in breast milk. In elderly patients, age-related renal impairment may require dosage adjustment.

Initial complete blood count (CBC) and renal and liver function test results should be evaluated. Uric acid levels should be monitored and signs and symptoms of gout, including hot, painful, or swollen joints, especially in the ankle, big toe, or knee, should be assessed. Signs and symptoms of peripheral neuritis as evidenced by burning, numbness, or tingling of the extremities should also be assessed. Notify the physician if peripheral neuritis occurs. In addition, notify the physician immediately of any visual

problems. Monthly eye exams are advised. Visual effects are generally reversible after ethambutol is discontinued, but in rare cases visual problems may take up to a year to disappear or may be permanent.
Storage
Store at room temperature. Protect from light and moisture.
Administration
Administer daily doses at roughly the same time each day. Give with food to decrease GI upset. Do not skip drug doses and take ethambutol for the full length of therapy, which may be months or years.

Ethionamide
e-thye-on′am-ide
(Trecator)
Do not confuse with Tricor.

CATEGORY AND SCHEDULE
Pregnancy Risk Category: C

Classification:
Antimycobacterials

MECHANISM OF ACTION
An antitubercular agent that inhibits peptide synthesis. *Therapeutic Effect:* Suppresses mycobacterial multiplication. Bactericidal.

PHARMACOKINETICS
Rapidly absorbed from the GI tract. Widely distributed. Protein binding: 30%. Metabolized in liver. Primarily excreted in urine. Removed by hemodialysis. *Half-life:* 2-3 h (half-life is increased with impaired renal function).

AVAILABILITY
Tablets: 250 mg (Trecator).

E

INDICATIONS AND DOSAGES
▸ Tuberculosis
PO
Adults, Elderly. 15-20 mg/kg/day;
initiate dose at 250 mg/day for
1-2 days, then 250 mg twice daily
for 1-2 days; increase to highest
tolerated dose; average adult dose
750 mg/day. Maximum 1000 mg/day
in 3-4 divided doses.
Children. 10-20 mg/kg/day in 2 or 3
divided doses or 15 mg/kg once
daily. Maximum: 1 g/day.

OFF-LABEL USES
Treatment of atypical mycobacterial
infections.

CONTRAINDICATIONS
Severe hepatic impairment,
hypersensitivity to ethionamide.

INTERACTIONS
Drug
Cycloserine, isoniazid: May
increase the risk of toxicity.
Rifampin: May increase the risk of
hepatotoxicity.
Herbal
None known.
Food
Ethanol: Psychotic reaction has
occurred. Avoid alcoholic
beverages.

DIAGNOSTIC TEST EFFECTS
May increase ALT and AST, may
increase TSH.

SIDE EFFECTS
Occasional
Abdominal pain, nausea, vomiting,
weakness, postural hypotension,
psychiatric disturbances,
drowsiness, dizziness, headache,
confusion, anorexia, headache,
metallic taste, diarrhea, stomatitis,
peripheral neuritis, acne, alopecia,
photosensitivity, impotence.

Rare
Rash, fever, blurred vision, seizures,
hypothyroidism, hypoglycemia,
gynecomastia, thrombocytopenia,
jaundice, hypersensitivity reaction.

SERIOUS REACTIONS
• Peripheral neuropathy, anorexia,
seizures, and joint pain rarely occur.
• Optic neuritis, and loss of vision
may occur.

PRECAUTIONS & CONSIDERATIONS
Caution is warranted in patients
receiving cycloserine or isoniazid,
diabetics, patients with thyroid
disease, epileptics, and psychiatric
illness. Ethionamide crosses the
placenta and is excreted in breast
milk.
 In elderly patients, age-related
renal impairment may require dosage
adjustment.
 Stomach upset, loss of appetite,
metallic taste, burning, numbness,
tingling of the feet or hands, and
pain and swelling of joints should be
reported.
Administration
Take with food or at bedtime to
decrease GI upset.
! Expect use with pyridoxine to help
decrease neurotoxicity.

Ethosuximide
eth-oh-sux′i-mide
**Do not confuse with Zaroxolyn
or Neurontin.**

CATEGORY AND SCHEDULE
Pregnancy Risk Category: C

Classification: Anticonvulsants,
succinimides

MECHANISM OF ACTION

An anticonvulsant that increases the seizure threshold and suppresses paroxysmal spike-and-wave pattern in absence seizures; depresses nerve transmission in the motor cortex. *Therapeutic Effect:* Produces anticonvulsant activity.

PHARMACOKINETICS

Well absorbed from the GI tract. Metabolized in the liver. Excreted in urine. Removed by hemodialysis. *Half-life:* 50-60 h (in adults); 30 h (in children). Time to peak: 2-4 h (capsule), < 2-4h (syrup).

AVAILABILITY

Capsule: 250 mg.
Syrup: 250 mg/5 mL.

INDICATIONS AND DOSAGES
▶ **Absence seizures**
PO
Adults, Elderly, Children older than 6 yrs. Initially, 250-500 mg/day or 15 mg/kg/day in 2 divided doses. Maintenance: 15-40 mg/kg/day in 2 divided doses. Maximum: 1.5 g/day in 2 divided doses.
Children aged 3-6 yrs. Initially, 250 mg/day in 2 divided doses, increased by 250 mg as needed every 4-7 days. Maintenance: 20-40 mg/kg/day in 2 divided doses. Maximum: 1.5 g/day in 2 divided doses.

CONTRAINDICATIONS

Hypersensitivity to succinimides.

INTERACTIONS
Drug
Alcohol, central nervous system (CNS) depressants: May increase CNS depression.
Carbamazepine, phenobarbital, phenytoin, primidone, valproic acid, CYP3A4 inducers: May decrease ethosuximide blood concentration.

Azole antifungals, ciprofloxacin, clarithromycin, isoniazid, quinidine, protease inhibitors, verapamil, CYP3A4 inhibitors: May increase ethosuximide blood concentration.
Herbal
Evening primrose oil: May decrease effectiveness of ethosuximide.
Ginkgo: May decrease effectiveness of ethosuximide.
St. John's wort: May decrease ethosuximide blood concentrations.
Food
Ethanol: CNS depression; avoid use.

DIAGNOSTIC TEST EFFECTS

None known.

SIDE EFFECTS
Occasional
Dizziness, drowsiness, double vision, headache, ataxia, nausea, diarrhea, vomiting, somnolence, urticaria.
Rare
Agranulocytosis, gum hypertrophy, leukopenia, myopia, swelling of the tongue, systemic lupus erythematosus, vaginal bleeding, inability to concentrate.

SERIOUS REACTIONS

• Abrupt withdrawal may increase seizure frequency.
• Blood dyscrasias, Stevens-Johnson syndrome, systemic lupus erythematosus have been associated with succinimides.
• Overdosage results in nausea, vomiting, and CNS depression including coma with respiratory depression.

PRECAUTIONS & CONSIDERATIONS

Caution should be used with renal or hepatic function impairment. Ethosuximide should be used cautiously when given alone in mixed types of epilepsy. Alcohol and tasks that require mental alertness and motor skills should be avoided until response to the drug is established.

Toxic signs are evident as easy bruising, fever, joint pain, mouth ulcerations, sore throat, and unusual bleeding. Therapeutic serum level for ethosuximide is 40-100 mcg/mL, and the toxic serum level for ethosuximide is > 150 mcg/mL.

Administration
Take with meals to reduce risk of GI distress. When replacement by another anticonvulsant is necessary, plan to decrease ethosuximide gradually as therapy begins with a low replacement dose.

Etidronate
ee-tid′roe-nate
(Didronel)
Do not confuse etidronate with etidocaine or etomidate.

CATEGORY AND SCHEDULE
Pregnancy Risk Category: C

Classification: Bisphosphonates

MECHANISM OF ACTION
A bisphosphonate that decreases mineral release and matrix in bone and inhibits osteocytic osteolysis. *Therapeutic Effect:* Decreases bone resorption.

AVAILABILITY
Tablets: 200 mg, 400 mg.

INDICATIONS AND DOSAGES
▸ **Paget disease**
PO
Adults, Elderly. Initially, 5-10 mg/kg/day not to exceed 6 mo, or 11-20 mg/kg/day not to exceed 3 mo. Repeat only after drug-free period of at least 90 days.

▸ **Heterotopic ossification caused by spinal cord injury**
PO
Adult, Elderly. 20 mg/kg/day for 2 wks; then 10 mg/kg/day for 10 wks.
▸ **Heterotopic ossification complicating total hip replacement**
PO
Adults, Elderly. 20 mg/kg/day for 1 mo before surgery; then 20 mg/kg/day for 3 mo after surgery.
▸ **Hypercalcemia associated with malignancy**
PO
Adults, Elderly. 20 mg/kg/day for 30 days. If needed, maximum 90 days.

OFF-LABEL USES
Postmenopausal osteoporosis.

CONTRAINDICATIONS
Clinically overt osteomalacia, renal failure (SCr ≥5 mg/dL, hypersensitivity to etidronate or other bisphosphonates.

INTERACTIONS
Drug
Antacids containing aluminum, calcium, magnesium; calcium supplements, iron: May decrease the absorption of etidronate. Separate by at least 2 h.
Warfarin: Concurrent use may alter bleeding times.
Herbal
None known.
Food
Foods with calcium: May decrease the absorption of etidronate.

DIAGNOSTIC TEST EFFECTS
None known.

SIDE EFFECTS
Frequent
Nausea; diarrhea; continuing or more frequent bone pain in patients with Paget disease.

Occasional
Bone fractures, especially of the femur.
Metallic, altered taste.
Rare
Hypersensitivity reaction.

SERIOUS REACTIONS
• Nephrotoxicity, including hematuria, dysuria, and proteinuria, has occurred with parenteral route.
• Serious hypersensitivity (rare).
• Osteonecrosis of the jaw.

PRECAUTIONS & CONSIDERATIONS
Caution is warranted in patients with hyperphosphatemia, impaired renal function, and restricted calcium and vitamin D intake. Hyperphosphatemia may occur at doses of 10-20 mg/kg/day. Patients with Paget disease may be at increased risk for osteomalacia and fracture of long bones when used for periods > 6 mo. Adequate studies have not been done regarding the effect of oral etidronate use during pregnancy. Parenteral etidronate may cause skeletal malformations in the fetus. It is unknown whether etidronate is excreted in breast milk. Do not give to women who are breastfeeding. Safety and efficacy of etidronate have not been established in children.

Notify the physician of diarrhea. Serum electrolytes, BUN, fluid intake and output should be monitored.
Storage
Store at room temperature.
Administration
Take on an empty stomach. Take etidronate 2 h before antacids, food, or vitamins. The full therapeutic response may take up to 3 mo.

Etodolac
e-toe-doe′lak
(Apo-Etodolac [CAN], Ultradol [CAN])
Do not confuse Lodine with codeine or iodine.

E

CATEGORY AND SCHEDULE
Pregnancy Risk Category: C (D if used in third trimester or near delivery)

Classification: Analgesics, non-narcotic, nonsteroidal anti-inflammatory drugs

MECHANISM OF ACTION
An NSAID that produces analgesic and anti-inflammatory effects by inhibiting prostaglandin synthesis. *Therapeutic Effect:* Reduces the inflammatory response and intensity of pain.

PHARMACOKINETICS

Route	Onset	Peak	Duration
PO (analgesic)	30 min	N/A	4-12 h

Well absorbed from the GI tract. Protein binding: > 99%. Widely distributed. Metabolized in the liver. Primarily excreted in urine. Not removed by hemodialysis. *Half-life:* 6-7 h. Onset of analgesia: 2-4 h. Maximum anti-inflammatory: several days.

AVAILABILITY
Capsules: 200 mg, 300 mg.
Tablets: 400 mg, 500 mg.
Tablets (Extended-Release): 400 mg, 500 mg, 600 mg.

E

INDICATIONS AND DOSAGES
▸ **Osteoarthritis or rheumatoid arthritis**
PO (IMMEDIATE RELEASE)
Adults, Elderly. Initially, 300 mg 2-3 times a day or 400-500 mg twice daily. Maintenance: 600-1200 mg/day.
PO (EXTENDED RELEASE)
Adults, Elderly. Initially, 400 mg once daily. Maximum: 1000 mg once daily.
▸ **Analgesia**
PO (IMMEDIATE RELEASE)
Adults, Elderly. 200-400 mg q6-8h as needed. Maximum: 1200 mg/day.
▸ **Juvenile Rheumatoid arthritis**
PO
Children aged 6-16 yrs (Lodine XL).
20-30 kg: 400 mg once daily.
31-45 kg: 600 mg once daily.
46-60 kg: 800 mg once daily.
> 60 kg: 1000 mg once daily.

OFF-LABEL USES
Treatment of acute gouty arthritis, vascular headache.

CONTRAINDICATIONS
History of hypersensitivity to aspirin or NSAIDs, within 10-14 days of coronary artery bypass graft (CABG).

INTERACTIONS
Drug
ACE inhibitors, ARBs: May increase risk of renal dysfunction.
Antihypertensives, diuretics: May decrease the effects of these drugs.
Aspirin, antiplatelets, other salicylates, corticosteroids: May increase the risk of GI side effects such as bleeding.
Bisphosphonates: Increased risk for gastrointestinal ulceration.
Bone marrow depressants: May increase the risk of hematologic reactions.

Cyclosporine: Nephrotoxicity and cyclosporine levels may be increased.
Heparin, oral anticoagulants, thrombolytics: May increase the bleeding effects of these drugs.
Lithium: May increase the blood concentration and risk of toxicity of lithium.
Methotrexate: May increase the risk of methotrexate toxicity.
Pemetrexed: May increase levels and effects of pemetrexed. Avoid etodolac 2-5 days before pemetrexed and 2 days following.
Probenecid: May increase etodolac blood concentration.
Vancomycin: May increase level of vancomyin.
Herbal
Supplements with antiplatelet or anticoagulant effects (e.g., feverfew, garlic, ginger, ginkgo biloba, ginseng, red clover, sweet clover, white willow, etc.): May increase effects on platelets or risk of bleeding.
Food
None known.

DIAGNOSTIC TEST EFFECTS
May increase bleeding time, liver function test results, and serum creatinine level. May decrease serum uric acid level.

SIDE EFFECTS
Occasional (4%-9%)
Dizziness, headache, abdominal pain or cramps, bloated feeling, diarrhea, nausea, indigestion, flatulence, weakness.
Rare (1%-3%)
Constipation, rash, pruritus, visual disturbances, tinnitus, depression, nervousness.

SERIOUS REACTIONS
• Overdose may result in acute renal failure.

• Rare reactions with long-term use include peptic ulcer disease, GI bleeding, gastritis, severe hepatic reactions (jaundice), nephrotoxicity (hematuria, dysuria, proteinuria), and a severe hypersensitivity reaction (bronchospasm, angioedema).

• Hepatic and renal impairment have occurred.

PRECAUTIONS & CONSIDERATIONS

Caution is warranted in patients with hepatic or renal impairment, a predisposition to fluid retention, and history of GI tract disease such as active peptic ulcer disease, chronic inflammation of GI tract, GI bleeding or ulceration. Use the lowest effective dose for the shortest duration of time. Anaphylactoid reactions have occurred in patients with aspirin triad hypersensitivity. Do not use in patients with aspirin-sensitive asthma. Cardiovascular event risk may be increased with duration of use or preexisting cardiovascular risk factors or disease. Use caution in patients with fluid retention, heart failure, or hypertension. Concurrent administration of ibuprofen, and potentially other nonselective NSAIDs, may interfere with aspirin's cardioprotective effect. Use the lowest effective dose for the shortest duration. Discontinue at first sign of rash as NSAIDs have been associated with Stevens-Johnson syndrome. Risk of myocardial infarction and stroke may be increased following CABG surgery. Do not administer within 4-6 half-lives before surgical procedures. It is unknown whether etodolac crosses the placenta or is distributed in breast milk. Etodolac should not be used during the last trimester of pregnancy because it may cause adverse effects in the fetus, such as premature closure of the ductus arteriosus. Notify the physician if the patient is pregnant. The safety and efficacy of etodolac have not been established in children. In elderly paients, GI bleeding or ulceration is more likely to cause serious complications and age-related renal impairment may increase the risk of hepatotoxicity or renal toxicity; a decreased dosage is recommended. Avoid alcohol and aspirin during therapy because these substances increase the risk of GI bleeding. Tasks that require mental alertness or motor skills should be avoided until response to the drug has been established.

Notify the physician of edema, GI distress, headache, rash, signs of bleeding, or visual disturbances. CBC and blood chemistry studies should be monitored to assess hepatic and renal function. Therapeutic response, such as decreased pain, stiffness, swelling, or tenderness, improved grip strength, and increased joint mobility, should be evaluated.

Administration

Do not crush, open, or break capsules or extended-release tablets. Take etodolac with food or milk, or antacids if GI distress occurs.

Etoposide, VP-16

e-toe-poe'side

(Etopophos, Toposar)

Do not confuse VePesid with Pepcid or Versed. Do not confuse etoposide with Etopophos.

CATEGORY AND SCHEDULE

Pregnancy Risk Category: D

Classification: Antineoplastics, epipodophyllotoxins

E

MECHANISM OF ACTION

An epipodophyllotoxin that induces single- and double-stranded breaks in DNA. Cell cycle–dependent and phase-specific; most effective in the S and G_2 phases of cell division. *Therapeutic Effect:* Inhibits or alters DNA synthesis.

PHARMACOKINETICS

Variably absorbed from the GI tract (25%-75%). Rapidly distributed, low concentrations in cerebrospinal fluid (CSF). Protein binding: 97%. Metabolized in the liver. Etoposide phosphate rapidly converted to etoposide in plasma. Primarily excreted in urine. Not removed by hemodialysis. *Half-life:* 3-12 h, children 6-8 h.

AVAILABILITY

Capsules (VePesid): 50 mg.
Injection Solution (Toposar). 20 mg/mL.
Powder for Injection (water-soluble etoposide phosphate [Etopophos]). 100 mg vial.

INDICATIONS AND DOSAGES
▸ **Refractory testicular tumors**
IV
Adults. 50-100 mg/m^2/day on days 1-5, or 100 mg/m^2/day on days 1, 3, 5 (as combination therapy) every 3-4 wks.
▸ **Acute myelocytic leukemia**
IV
Children. Remission: 150 mg/m^2/day for 2-3 days and 2-3 cycles. Intensification or consolidation: 250 mg/m^2/day for 3 days courses 2-5.
▸ **Malignant glioma**
IV
Children. 150 mg/m^2/day on days 2 and 3 of treatment course.
▸ **Neuroblastoma**
IV
Children. 100 mg/m^2/day on days 1-5 of treatment course; repeated q4wk.

▸ **Small-cell lung carcinoma**
PO
Adults. Twice the IV dose rounded to nearest 50 mg. Give once a day for doses 400 mg or less or in divided doses for dosages > 400 mg.
IV
Adults. 35 mg/m^2/day for 4 consecutive days up to 50 mg/m^2/day for 5 consecutive days (as combination therapy) every 3-4 wks.
▸ **Dosage in renal impairment**
Creatinine clearance 15-50 mL/min. 75% of normal dose.
Creatinine clearance < 15 mL/min. 50% of normal dose.

OFF-LABEL USES

Treatment of acute myelocytic leukemia, AIDS-associated Kaposi sarcoma, Ewing sarcoma, Hodgkin's disease, non-Hodgkin's lymphoma, platinum-resistant ovarian cancer.

CONTRAINDICATIONS

Hypersensitivity.

INTERACTIONS
Drug
Bone marrow depressants: May increase myelosuppression.
Cyclosporine: High-dose cyclosporine has increased etoposide levels by 80%. Monitor for increased toxic effects of etoposide if cyclosporine is initiated, the dose is increased, or it has been recently discontinued.
Live-virus vaccines: May potentiate virus replication, increase vaccine side effects, and decrease the patient's antibody response to the vaccine.
Herbal and Food
None known.

DIAGNOSTIC TEST EFFECTS

Decreased platelet counts, WBC, RBC.

E.

ⓘ IV INCOMPATIBILITIES

VePesid: Cefepime (Maxipime), filgrastim (Neupogen), idarubicin (Idamycin), lansoprazole (Prevacid), pantoprazole (Protonix).
Etopophos: Allopurinol (Aloprim), amphotericin B (Fungizone), amphotericin B liposomal (Ambisome), cefepime (Maxipime), chlorpromazine (Thorazine), dantrolene, diazepam (Valium), imipenem/cilastatin (Primaxin), methylprednisolone sodium succinate (Solu-Medrol), mitomycin (Mutamycin), pantoprazole (Protonix), phenytoin, prochlorperazine (Compazine).

ⓘ IV COMPATIBILITIES

VePesid: Allopurinol (Aloprim), amifostine (Ethyol), amphotericin B liposomal (AmBisome), aztreonam (Azactam), bivalirudin (Angiomax), carboplatin (Paraplatin), caspofungin (Cancidas), cefepime (Maxipime), cisplatin (Platinol), cladribine (Leustatin), cyclophosphamide (Cytoxan), cytarabine (Cytosar), dactinomycin (Cosmegen), daptomycin (Cubicin), daunorubicin (Cerubidine), dexmedetomidine (Precedex), docetaxel (Taxotere), doxorubicin (Adriamycin), doxorubicin liposomal (Doxil), epirubicin (Ellence), ertapenem (Invanz), fenoldopam (Corlopam), fludarabine (Fludara), gemcitabine (Gemzar), granisetron (Kytril), ilfosfamide (Ifex), levofloxacin (Levaquin), magnesium sulfate, melphalan (Alkeran), meperidine (Demerol), methotrexate, micafungin (Mycamine), mitoxantrone (Novantrone), ondansetron (Zofran), oxaliplatin (Eloxatin), paclitaxel (Taxol), pemetrexed (Alimta), piperacillin/tazobactam (Zosyn), sargramostim (Leukine), sodium acetate, sodium bicarbonate,

teniposide (Vumon), thiotepa (Thioplex), tigecycline (Tygacil), tirofiban, topotecan (Hycamtim), vinblastine (Velban), vincristine (Vincasar), vinorelbine (Navelbine), voriconazole (Vfend).
Etopophos: Acyclovir (Zovirax), alfentanil (Alfenta), amifostine (Ethyol), amikacin (Amikar), aminophylline, ampicillin, ampicillin/sulbactam (Unasyn), anidulafungin (Eraxis), atracurium (Tracrium), aztreonam (Azactam), bivalirudin (Angiostat), bleomycin (Blenoxane), bumetanide (Bumex), buprenorphine (Buprenex), butorphanol (Stadol), calcium acetate, calcium chloride, calcium gluconate, carboplatin, carmustine (BiCNU), caspofungin (Cancidas), cefazolin, cefotaxime (Claforan), cefotetan, cefoxitin (Mefoxin), ceftazidime (Ceptaz, Fortaz, Tazicef, Tazidime), ceftizoxime (Cefizox), ceftriaxone (Rocephin), cefuroxime (Zinacef), chloramphenicol, cimetidine (Tagamet), ciprofloxacin (Cipro), cisplatin (Platinol), clindamycin (Cleocin), cyclophosphamide (Cytoxan), cyclosporine (Sandimmune), cytarabine (Cytosar), dacarbazine (DTIC-Dome), dactinomycin (Cosmegen), daunorubicin (Cerubidine), dexamethasone (Decadron), dexmedetomidine (Precedex), dexrazoxane (Zinecard), digoxin (Lanoxin), diltiazem, diphenhydramine (Benadryl), dobutamine, docetaxel (Taxotere), dopamine, doripenem (Doribax), doxorubicin (Adriamycin), enalaprilat, ephedrine, epinephrine, epirubicin (Ellence), ertapenem (Invanz), erythromycin lactobionate, esmolol (Brevibloc), famotidine (Pepcid), fenoldopam (Corlopam), fentanyl (Sublimaze), floxuridine (FUDR), fluconazole (Diflucan),

E

fludarabine (Fludara), fluorouracil, foscarnet (Foscavir), fosphenytoin (Cerebyx), furosemide (Lasix), ganciclovir (Cytovene), gemcitabine (Gemzar), gentamicin, granisetron (Kytril), haloperidol (Haldol), heparin, hydrocortisone sodium phosphate, hydrocortisone sodium succinate, hydromorphone (Dilaudid), hydroxyzine, idarubicin (Idamycin), ifosfamide (Ifex), insulin (regular, Humulin R, Novolin R), isoproternol (Isuprel), ketorolac, labetalol, leucovorin, levofloxacin (Levaquin), lidocaine, linezolid (Zyvox), lorazepam (Ativan), magnesium sulfate, mannitol, meperidine (Demerol), meropenem (Merrem), mesna (Mesnex), methotrexate, metoclopramide (Reglan), metronidazole (Flagyl), midazolam, minocycline (Minocin), mitoxantrone (Novantrone), morphine, nalbuphine (Nubain), naloxone (Narcan), nitroglycerin, nitroprusside sodium (Nitropress), norepinephrine (Levophed), ondansetron (Zofran), oxaliplatin (Eloxatin), paclitaxel (Taxol), palonosetron (Aloxi), pancuronium, pemetrexed (Alimta), pentobarbital, phenobarbital, piperacillin, piperacillin/tazobactam (Zosyn), potassium chloride, potassium phosphates, procainamide, promethazine, propranolol, ranitidine (Zantac), remifentanil (Ultiva), rituximab (Rituxan), rocuronium (Zemuron), sodium acetate, sodium bicarbonate, sodium phosphates, streptozocin, succinylcholine, sufentanil (Sufenta), sulfamethoxazole/trimethoprim, tacrolimus (Prograf), teniposide (Vumon), thiotepa (Thioplex), ticarcillin (Ticar), ticarcillin/clavulanate (Timentin), tigecycline (Tygacil), tirofibran, tobramycin, trastuzumab (Herceptin),

vancomycin, vecuronium (Norcuron), vinblastine (Velban), vincristine (Vincasar), vinorelbine (Navelbine), voriconazole (Vfend), zidovudine (Retrovir).

SIDE EFFECTS

Frequent (43%-66%)
Mild to moderate nausea and vomiting, alopecia, ovarian failure, amenorrhea.
Occasional (6%-13%)
Diarrhea, anorexia, stomatitis.
Rare (Up to 2%)
Hypotension (with rapid infusion), peripheral neuropathy.

SERIOUS REACTIONS

• Myelosuppression may result in hematologic toxicity, manifested as anemia, leukopenia (occurring 5-7 days after drug administration), thrombocytopenia (occurring 9-16 days after administration), anemia, and, to lesser extent, pancytopenia. Bone marrow recovery occurs by day 20-28.
• Hepatotoxicity occurs occasionally.
• Anaphylactic reaction to IV infusion.

PRECAUTIONS & CONSIDERATIONS

Caution is warranted with myelosuppression or hepatic or renal impairment. Because of the risk of fetal harm, pregnant women should not take etoposide, especially during the first trimester. Dose-limiting bone marrow suppression is the most significant toxicity associated with etoposide therapy. Treatment should be withheld for platelets < 50,000/mm^3 or absolute neutrophil count (ANC) < 500/mm^3. Use with caution and reduce dose in patients with hepatic or renal dysfunction. Breastfeeding women also should not take this drug. The safety and efficacy of etoposide have not been established in children. Preparations with polysorbate 80 should be avoided in neonates. Anaphylactic reactions have been reported in children. In elderly patients, age-related renal impairment may require dosage adjustment. Vaccinations and coming in contact with anyone who has recently received a live-virus vaccine should be avoided.

Notify the physician of easy bruising, fever, signs of local infection, sore throat, or unusual bleeding from any site. Hematology test results should be monitored before and frequently during etoposide therapy. WBC counts, hemoglobin and hematocrit levels, pattern of daily bowel activity and stool consistency, signs and symptoms of paresthesia and peripheral neuropathy, signs and symptoms of stomatitis should be assessed. Alopecia may occur and is reversible, but new hair growth may have a different color or texture.

Storage

Refrigerate gelatin capsules. Do not freeze.

Store most etoposide injections at room temperature before dilution. Reconstituted solution is stable at room temperature for up to 96 h at 0.2 mg/mL and 48 h at 0.4 mg/mL. Discard solution if crystallization occurs. Refrigerate Etopophos vials before reconstitution. Protect from light. After reconstitution, Etopophos is stable for up to 24 h at room temperature or refrigerated. Etoposide injection diluted for oral use to 10 mg/mL in NS may be stored at room temperature for 22 days. Mix with apple or orange juice to concentration < 0.4 mg/mL and use within 3 h.

Administration

! Etoposide dosage is individualized based on clinical response and tolerance of the drug's adverse effects. Treatment is repeated at 3- to 4-wks intervals. Administer parenteral etoposide by slow IV infusion. Wear gloves when preparing the solution. If the powder or solution comes in contact with skin, wash immediately and thoroughly with soap and water. Because etoposide may be carcinogenic, mutagenic, or teratogenic, handle it with extreme care during preparation and administration.

Etoposide solution concentrate for injection normally is clear and yellow. For IV use, dilute each 100 mg (5 mL) vial with at least 250 mL D5W or 0.9% NaCl to provide a concentration of 0.4 mg/mL (or 500 mL for a concentration of 0.2 mg/mL). Stability is concentration dependent and precipitates may occur > 0.4 mg/mL. Infuse slowly, over 30-60 min. Rapid IV infusion may produce marked hypotension. Monitor for an anaphylactic reaction manifested as back, chest, or throat pain; chills; diaphoresis; dyspnea; fever; lacrimation; and sneezing.

For Etopophos IV, reconstitute each 100 mg of Etopophos with 5-10 mL sterile water for injection, D5W, or 0.9% NaCl to provide a concentration of 20 mg/mL or 10 mg/mL, respectively. Etopophos may be given without further dilution or may be further diluted with 0.9% NaCl or D5W to a concentration as low as 0.1 mg/mL. Administer Etopophos over 5-10 min, as appropriate.

Exemestane
ex-uh-mess'tane
(Aromasin)

CATEGORY AND SCHEDULE
Pregnancy Risk Category: D

Classification: Antineoplastics, aromatase inhibitors, hormones/hormone modifiers

MECHANISM OF ACTION
Inactivates aromatase, the principal enzyme that converts androgens to estrogens in both premenopausal and postmenopausal women, thereby lowering the circulating estrogen level. *Therapeutic Effect:* Inhibits the growth of breast cancers that are stimulated by estrogens.

PHARMACOKINETICS
Rapidly absorbed after PO administration. Protein binding: 90%. Distributed extensively into tissues. Metabolized extensively in the liver; eliminated in urine and feces. *Half-life:* 24 h.

AVAILABILITY
Tablets: 25 mg.

INDICATIONS AND DOSAGES
▶ Breast cancer, advanced after tamoxifen therapy
PO
Adults, Elderly. 25 mg once a day after a meal.
If potent CYP3A4 inducer co-prescribed, give 50 mg once daily after a meal.

CONTRAINDICATIONS
Hypersensitivity to exemestane.

INTERACTIONS
Drug
CYP3A4 inducers: May decrease levels and effects of exemestane.
Herbal
St. John's wort: May decrease levels and effects of exemestane. Avoid use.
Food
None known.

DIAGNOSTIC TEST EFFECTS
May increase serum alkaline phosphatase, AST (SGOT), ALT (SGPT), creatinine, and bilirubin levels.

SIDE EFFECTS
Frequent (10%-22%)
Fatigue, nausea, depression, hypertension, alopecia, arthralgia, hot flashes, pain, insomnia, anxiety, dyspnea.
Occasional (5%-8%)
Headache, dizziness, vomiting, dermatitis, peripheral edema, abdominal pain, weight gain, anorexia, flu-like symptoms, diaphoresis, constipation, visual disturbances.
Rare (4%)
Diarrhea.

SERIOUS REACTIONS
• Myocardial infarction, angina, and thromboembolism have been reported.

PRECAUTIONS & CONSIDERATIONS
Exemestane is not for use in premenopausal women. Exemestane is indicated only for postmenopausal women. This drug is not used in children. No age-related precautions have been noted in elderly patients. Should not be used during pregnancy.

Potential side effects, including dizziness, headache, insomnia, depression, may occur. Notify the physician if hot flashes or nausea become unmanageable. Nausea and vomiting may be prevented or treated with an antiemetic. Baseline vital signs, especially BP, should be assessed because exemestane may cause hypertension.

Administration

Give oral exemestane after a meal.

Ezetimibe
eh-zet'eh-mibe
(Zetia)
Do not confuse with Zestril.

CATEGORY AND SCHEDULE
Pregnancy Risk Category: C

Classification:
Antihyperlipidemics

MECHANISM OF ACTION
An antihyperlipidemic that inhibits cholesterol absorption in the small intestine, leading to a decrease in the delivery of intestinal cholesterol to the liver. *Therapeutic Effect:* Reduces total serum cholesterol, LDL cholesterol, and triglyceride levels and increases HDL cholesterol concentration.

PHARMACOKINETICS
Variable absorption following oral administration. Protein binding: > 90%. Metabolized in the small intestine and liver. Excreted by the kidneys and bile. *Half-life:* 22 h.

AVAILABILITY
Tablets: 10 mg.

INDICATIONS AND DOSAGES
▶ **Hypercholesterolemia**
PO
Adults, Elderly, Children aged > 10 yrs. Initially, 10 mg once a day, given with or without food. If the patient is also receiving a bile acid sequestrant, give ezetimibe at least 2 h before or at least 4 h after the bile acid sequestrant.

CONTRAINDICATIONS
Hypersensitivity to ezetimibe. NOTE: If given with an HMG-CoA reductase inhibitor (atorvastatin, cerivastatin, fluvastatin, lovastatin, pravastatin, or simvastatin) follow statin contraindications. Patients with active hepatic disease or unexplained persistent elevations in serum transaminase levels, moderate or severe hepatic insufficiency, pregnancy, breast-feeding.

INTERACTIONS
Drug
Aluminum and magnesium-containing antacids: Decrease ezetimibe plasma concentration.
Cyclosporine: Increases ezetimibe concentration.
Fenofibrate, gemfibrozil: Increases ezetimibe plasma concentration. Fibrates may increase risk of cholelithiasis.
Cholestyramine: Decreases drug effectiveness. Administer 2 h before or 4 h after bile acid sequestrants.
Herbal and Food
None known.

DIAGNOSTIC TEST EFFECTS
May increase serum alkaline phosphatase, serum bilirubin, AST (SGOT), and ALT (SGPT) levels.

SIDE EFFECTS
Frequent (> 10%)
Upper respiratory tract infection.

Occasional (3%-9%)
Headache, back pain, diarrhea, myalgia, arthralgia, sinusitis, abdominal pain, chest pain.
Rare (2%)
Cough, pharyngitis, fatigue.

SERIOUS REACTIONS

• None known.

PRECAUTIONS & CONSIDERATIONS

Caution is warranted in patients with chronic renal failure, diabetes, hypothyroidism, liver function impairment, and obstructive liver disease. It is unknown whether ezetimibe crosses the placenta or is distributed in breast milk. Safety and efficacy of ezetimibe have not been established in children 10 yrs of age and younger. This drug is not recommended for use in patients with moderate or severe hepatic impairment. Concurrent use of fibric acid derivatives may increase the risk of cholelithiasis.

Notify the physician of any abdominal disturbances and back pain. Pattern of daily bowel activity and stool consistency should be assessed. Serum cholesterol and triglyceride levels should be checked at baseline and periodically thereafter.

Administration
Take ezetimibe without regard to food. Separate administration from that of bile sequestrants.

Factor IX Complex and Factor IX Concentrates
(AlphaNine SD, Bebulin VH, BeneFIX, Mononine, Profilnine)

CATEGORY AND SCHEDULE
Pregnancy Risk Category: C

Classification: Antihemophilic agents, blood clotting factors

MECHANISM OF ACTION
A blood modifier that raises the plasma levels of factor IX, restoring hemostasis in patients with factor IX deficiency. *Therapeutic Effect:* Increases blood clotting factor IX to restore hemostasis.

PHARMACOKINETICS
Mean half-time is 22 h (range, 11-36 h). Mean increase in circulating factor IX activity after infusion is 0.67-1.15 units/dL rise per units/kg body weight.

AVAILABILITY
Injection: Number of units is indicated on each vial.
AlphaNine SD: Contains factor IX; contains only low or nontherapeutic levels of factors II, VII, and X.
Mononine: Purified by monoclonal antibody process to isolate factor IX.
BeneFIX: Recombinant human factor IX.
Profilnine, Bebulin VH: Contains factor IX; also contains some factors, II, VII, and X and proteins S and C.

INDICATIONS AND DOSAGES
▶ **Bleeding caused by factor IX deficiency (hemophilia B, Christmas disease)**
IV INFUSION
Adults, Elderly, Children. Amount of factor IX required is individualized.

Dosage depends on degree of deficiency, level of each factor desired, patient's weight, and severity of bleeding.

OFF-LABEL USES
Emergency reversal of oral anticoagulant effects.

CONTRAINDICATIONS
Sensitivity to mouse protein (Mononine) or hamster protein (BeneFIX).

INTERACTIONS
Drug and Food
Aminocaproic acid: May increase the risk of thrombosis.
Herbal and Food
None known.

DIAGNOSTIC TEST EFFECTS
None known.

⊘ IV INCOMPATIBILITIES
Do not mix with other medications.

SIDE EFFECTS
Rare
Mild hypersensitivity reaction marked by fever, chills, change in BP and pulse rate, rash, and urticaria. Nausea, discomfort at IV site, altered taste, burning sensation in the jaw and skull, allergic rhinitis, light-headedness, headache, dizziness, chest tightness, phlebitis, or cellulitis at IV site. Rapid infusion rate: headache, flushing, changes in BP or pulse rate, transient fever, chills, tingling, urticaria, nausea, and vomiting may occur. Symptoms disappear promptly on discontinuation. Except in the most reactive individuals, the infusion may be resumed at a slower rate. Chills and fever (particularly when large doses are used).

SERIOUS REACTIONS
• There is a high risk of venous thrombosis during the postoperative period.
• Acute hypersensitivity reaction or anaphylactic reaction may occur.
• There is a risk of transmitting viral hepatitis and other viral diseases.
• High doses may be associated with myocardial infarction, disseminated intravascular coagulation, venous thrombosis, and pulmonary embolism.

PRECAUTIONS & CONSIDERATIONS
Caution is warranted with hepatic impairment, recent surgery, and sensitivity to factor IX. OTC medications should be avoided without physician approval. Efficacy and safety in children under age 6 yr have not been evaluated.

Notify the physician of abdominal or back pain, gingival bleeding, black or red stool, coffee-ground emesis, dark or red urine, or red-speckled mucus from cough. Intake and output and vital signs should be monitored. IV site should be assessed for oozing every 5-15 min for 1-2 h after administration.
Storage
AlphaNine SD: May also be stored at room temperature not to exceed 30° C (86° F) for up to 1 mo.

BeneFix: May also be stored at room temperature not to exceed 25° C (77° F) for up to 6 mo. Reconstituted solution at room temperature should be used within 3 h.

Mononine: May also be stored at room temperature not to exceed 25° C (77° F) for up to 1 mo.
Administration
Gently agitate vial until powder is completely dissolved so that the active components will not be removed when the solution is filtered during administration. Bring diluent and factors to room temperature

before combining. Filter before administration. Begin administration within 3 h of reconstitution. Administer by IV infusion. Infuse slowly, no faster than 2 mL/min (Bebulin and Mononine), 10 mL/min (Profilnine and AlphaNine), and over several minutes (BeneFix). Too rapid an IV infusion may produce a change in BP and pulse rate, headache, flushing, and a tingling sensation.

Famciclovir
fam-si´-klo-veer
(Famvir)
Do not confuse Famvir with Femhrt.

CATEGORY AND SCHEDULE
Pregnancy Risk Category: B

Classification: Antivirals

MECHANISM OF ACTION
A synthetic nucleoside that inhibits viral DNA synthesis. *Therapeutic Effect:* Suppresses replication of herpes simplex virus and varicella-zoster virus.

PHARMACOKINETICS
Rapidly and extensively absorbed after PO administration. Protein binding: 20%-25%. Rapidly metabolized to penciclovir by enzymes in the GI wall, liver, and plasma. Eliminated unchanged in urine. Removed by hemodialysis. *Half-life:* 2 h.

AVAILABILITY
Tablets: 125 mg, 250 mg, 500 mg.

INDICATIONS AND DOSAGES

▸ **Herpes zoster (shingles)**
PO
Adults. 500 mg q8h for 7 days.
Creatinine Clearance 40-59 mL/min:
Administer 500 mg every 12 h.
Creatinine Clearance 20-39 mL/min:
Administer 500 mg every 24 h.
Creatinine Clearance < 20 mL/min:
Administer 250 mg every 24 h.
Hemodialysis: Administer 250 mg
after each dialysis session.

▸ **Recurrent genital herpes**
PO
Adults. 1000 mg twice a day for
1 day within 6 h of symptom
onset.
Creatinine Clearance 40-59 mL/min:
Administer 500 mg every 12 h for
1 day.
Creatinine Clearance 20-39 mL/min:
Administer 500 mg as a single dose.
Creatinine Clearance < 20 mL/min:
Administer 250 mg as a single dose.
Hemodialysis: Administer 250 mg as
a single dose after dialysis session.

▸ **Suppression of recurrent genital herpes**
PO
Adults. 250 mg twice a day for up
to 1 yr.
Creatinine Clearance 20-39 mL/min:
Administer 125 mg every 12 h.
Creatinine Clearance < 20 mL/min:
Administer 125 mg every 24 h.
Hemodialysis: Administer 125 mg
after each dialysis session.

▸ **Recurrent herpes labialis (cold sores)**
PO
Adults. 1500 mg as a single dose
earliest sign or symptom of a cold
sore.
Creatinine Clearance 40-59 mL/min:
Administer 750 mg as a single dose.
Creatinine Clearance 20-39 mL/min:
Administer 500 mg as a single dose.
Creatinine Clearance < 20 mL/min:
Administer 250 mg as a single dose.

Hemodialysis: Administer 250 mg
as a single dose after dialysis session.

▸ **Recurrent orolabial or genital herpes simplex infection in patients with HIV infection**
PO
Adults. 500 mg twice a day for
7 days.
Cl_{cr} 20-39 mL/min: Administer
500 mg every 24 h.
Cl_{cr} < 20 mL/min: Administer 250 mg
every 24 h.
Hemodialysis: Administer 250 mg
after each dialysis session.

OFF-LABEL USES

Genital herpes simplex, hepatitis B.

CONTRAINDICATIONS

Hypersensitivity to famciclovir or
penciclovir.

INTERACTIONS

Drug
Probenecid: May inhibit active
tubular secretion and increase levels
of penciclovir.
Herbal
None known.
Food
None known.

DIAGNOSTIC TEST EFFECTS

Increases in AST, ALT. Decreases in
WBC.

SIDE EFFECTS

Frequent (> 10%)
Headache, nausea.
Occasional (2%-10%)
Diarrhea, abdominal pain,
dysmenorrhea, fatigue, vomiting,
pruritus, flatulence, paresthesia.
Rare (< 2%)
Insomnia, migraine.

SERIOUS REACTIONS

• Acute renal failure in patients with
underlying renal dysfunction.

F

F

PRECAUTIONS & CONSIDERATIONS

Caution is warranted in patients with renal impairment because acute renal failure may occur with inappropriately high doses. Dose adjustment is recommended for patients with CrCl < 60 mL/min. The safety and efficacy of famciclovir have not been established in children. The efficacy of famciclovir has not been established for initial-episode genital herpes infection, ophthalmic zoster, disseminated zoster, or in immunocompromised patients with herpes zoster. Famciclovir 125-, 250-, and 500-mg tablets contain lactose (26.9, 53.7, and 107.4 mg, respectively). Patients with rare hereditary problems of galactose intolerance, a severe lactase deficiency, or glucose-galactose malabsorption should not take famciclovir 125, 250, or 500 mg tablets. It is unknown whether famciclovir crosses the placenta or is distributed in breast milk. No age-related precautions have been noted in elderly patients.

Administration

May be taken without regard to meals.

Famotidine

fam-oh´-tah-deen
(Novo-Famotidine[CAN], Pepcid, Pepcid AC, Ulcidine[CAN])

CATEGORY AND SCHEDULE

Pregnancy Risk Category: B
RX (10-mg tablets, 20-mg tablets, 40-mg tablets, injection, orally dis-integrating tablets, oral suspension)
OTC (10-mg tablets, 20/mg tablets)

Classification: Histamine H₂-receptor antagonist

MECHANISM OF ACTION

An antiulcer agent and gastric acid secretion inhibitor that inhibits histamine action at H_2 receptors of parietal cells.
Therapeutic Effect: Inhibits gastric acid secretion when fasting, at night, or when stimulated by food, caffeine, or insulin.

PHARMACOKINETICS

Route	Onset	Peak	Duration
PO	1 h	1-4 h	10-12 h
IV	0.5-1 h	0.5-3 h	10-12 h

Rapidly, incompletely absorbed from the GI tract. Protein binding: 15%-20%. Partially metabolized in the liver. Primarily excreted in urine. Not removed by hemodialysis. *Half-life:* 2.5-3.5 h (increased with impaired renal function).

AVAILABILITY

Tablets (OTC): 10 mg, 20 mg.
Chewable tablets (OTC): 10 mg.
Gelcaps (OTC): 10 mg.
Tablets (Rx): 10 mg, 20 mg, 40 mg.
Orally disintegrating tablets (Rx): 20 mg, 40 mg.
Oral suspension (Rx): 40 mg/5 mL.
Injection (Rx): 10 mg/mL (1-mL, 2-mL, 4-mL, 20-mL, 50-mL vials; premixed 20 mg/50 mL).

INDICATIONS AND DOSAGES

▸ **Acute treatment of duodenal and gastric ulcers**
PO
Adults, Elderly, Children 17 yr and older. 40 mg/day at bedtime.
Children 1-16 yr. 0.5 mg/kg/day at bedtime. Maximum: 40 mg/day.

▸ **Duodenal ulcer maintenance**
PO
Adults, Elderly, Children 17 yr and older. 20 mg/day at bedtime.

▸ **Gastroesophageal reflux disease (GERD)**
PO
Adults, Elderly, Children 12 yr and older. 20 mg twice a day (maximum: 40 mg BID).
Children aged 1-11 yr. 1 mg/kg/day in 2 divided doses (maximum: 40 mg BID).
Children aged 3-12 mo. 0.5 mg/kg/dose twice a day.
Children younger than 3 mo. 0.5 mg/kg/dose once a day.
▸ **Esophagitis**
PO
Adults, Elderly, Children 12 yr and older. 20-40 mg twice a day.
▸ **Hypersecretory conditions**
PO
Adults, Elderly, Children 12 yr and older. Initially, 20 mg q6h. May increase up to 160 mg q6h.
▸ **Acid indigestion, heartburn (OTC)**
PO
Adults, Elderly, Children 12 yr and older. 10-20 mg 15-60 min before eating. Maximum: 2 doses per day.
▸ **Usual parenteral dosage**
IV
Adults, Elderly, Children 12 yr and older. 20 mg q12h.
Children 1-11 yr. 0.25-0.5 mg 1 kg q12h.
▸ **Dosage in renal impairment**
Dosing frequency is modified on the basis of creatinine clearance. May decrease dose by 50% or modify frequency, as follows:

Creatinine Clearance (mL/min)	Dosage Interval
10-50	q36-48h
< 10	q36-48h

OFF-LABEL USES
Urticaria, prevention of paclitaxel hypersensitivity reactions, stress ulcer prophylaxis in critically ill.

CONTRAINDICATIONS
Hypersensitivity to famotidine or other H_2 antagonists.

INTERACTIONS
Drug
Histamine H_2 antagonists: May decrease the absorption of azole antifungals (monitor), atazanavir (boost with ritonavir), cefpodoxime (separate oral doses by 2 h), cefuroxime (separate oral doses by 2 h), dasatinib (avoid), iron salts, saquinavir (monitor).
Cyclosporine: Histamine H_2 antagonists may increase the serum concentration of cyclosporine (monitor).
Herbal and Food
None known.

DIAGNOSTIC TEST EFFECTS
May rarely cause decreases in WBC counts.

⊘ IV INCOMPATIBILITIES
Amphotericin B cholesteryl sulfate complex (Amphotec), azathioprine, azithromycin (Zithromax), cefepime (Maxipime), dantrolene, diazepam (Valium), ganciclovir (Cytovene), lansoprazole (Prevacid), minocycline (Minocin), pantoprazole (Protonix), piperacillin/tazobactam (Zosyn), rocuronium (Zemuron), sulfamethoxazole/trimethoprim.

⊘ IV COMPATIBILITIES
Acyclovir (Zovirax), alfentanil (Alfenta), allopurinol (Aloprim), amifostine (Ethyol), aminophylline, amiodarone, anakinra (Kineret), anidulafungin (Eraxis), ascorbic acid, atracurium (Tracrium), atropine, aztreonam (Azactam), benztropine (Cogentin), bivalirudin (Angiomax), bretylium, bumetanide (Bumex), buprenorphine (Buprenex), butorphanol (Stadol), calcium chloride,

F

calcium gluconate, carboplatin, caspofungin (Cancidas), cefazolin, cefotaxime (Claforan), ceftazidime (Ceptaz, Fortaz, Tazicef, Tazidime), cefuroxime (Zinacef), chlorpromazine, cisatracurium (Nimbex), cisplatin, cladribine (Leustatin), clindamycin (Cleocin), cyclophosphamide (Cytoxan), cytarabine (Tarabine), dactinomycin (Cosmegen), daptomycin (Cubicin), dexamethasone sodium phosphate, dextran 40, digoxin (Lanoxin), diltiazem (Cardizem), diphenhydramine (Benadryl), dobutamine, docetaxel (Taxotere), dopamine, doripenem (Doribax), doxorubicin (Adriamycin), doxorubicin liposome (Doxil), droperidol (Inapsine), enalaprilat, epinephrine, epirubicin (Ellence), ertapenem (Invanz), erythromycin lactobionate, esmolol (Brevibloc), etoposide (VePesid), fenoldopam (Corlopam), fentanyl citrate (Sublimaze), filgrastim (Neupogen), fluconazole (Diflucan), fludarabine (Fludara), fluorouracil, folic acid, gemcitabine (Gemzar), gentamicin, granisetron (Kytril), heparin, hydrocortisone, hydrocortisone sodium succinate (Solu-Cortef), hydromorphone (Dilaudid), hydroxyzine, imipenem/cilastatin (Primaxin), isoproterenol (Isuprel), ketorolac, labetalol (Trandate), levofloxacin (Levaquin), lidocaine, linezolid (Zyvox), lorazepam (Ativan), magnesium sulfate, mannitol, melphalan (Alkeran), meperidine (Demerol), methotrexate, methylprednisolone sodium succinate (Solu-Medrol), metoclopramide (Reglan), metoprolol (Lopressor), metronidazole (Flagyl), midazolam, milrinone (Primacor), mitoxantrone (Novantrone), morphine, nafcillin, naloxone (Narcan), nicardipine (Cardene), nitroglycerin, norepinephrine (Levophed), ondansetron (Zofran), oxacillin, oxaliplatin (Eloxatin), oxytocin (Pitocin), paclitaxel (Taxol), palonosetron (Aloxi), pemetrexed (Alimta), penicillin G potassium, penicillin G sodium, phenylephrine (Neo-Synephrine), phytonadione, potassium chloride, potassium phosphates, procainamide, promethazine, propofol (Diprivan), propranolol (Inderal), protamine, ranitidine (Zantac), remifentanil (Ultiva), rituximab (Rituxan), sargramostim (Leukine), sodium acetate, sodium bicarbonate, sodium nitroprusside (Nitropress), succinylcholine (Anectine, Quelicin), sufentanil (Sufenta), tacrolimus (Prograf), teniposide (Vumon), theophylline, thiamine, thiotepa (Thioplex), ticarcillin (Ticar), ticarcillin/clavulanate potassium (Timentin), tigecycline (Tygacil), tirofiban (Aggrastat), tobramycin, trastuzumab (Herceptin), vecuronium (Norcuron), verapamil, vincristine (Vincasar), vinorelbine (Navelbine), voriconazole (Vfend).

SIDE EFFECTS
Occasional (2%-10%)
Headache.
Rare (1% or Less)
Constipation, diarrhea, dizziness.

SERIOUS REACTIONS
• Rare: agranulocytosis, parcytopenia, leukopenia, thrombocytopenia.

PRECAUTIONS & CONSIDERATIONS
Caution is warranted in patients with severe renal impairment because CNS adverse reactions may occur. Famotidine crosses the placenta and is distributed in breast milk. No age-related precautions have been noted in elderly patients. RPD and chewable tablets contain aspartame (caution: phenylketonuria).

Storage
Store tablets at controlled room temperature.

Solution is stable for 7 days at room temperature when added to or diluted with most commonly used IV solutions (e.g., water for injection, 0.9% sodium chloride injection, 5% or 10% dextrose injection, Ringer's lactate injection, 5% sodium bicarbonate injection). When added to or diluted with 5% sodium bicarbonate injection, a precipitate may form at higher concentrations of famotidine injection (more than 0.2 mg/mL). It is recommended that if not used immediately after preparation, diluted solutions of famotidine injection should be refrigerated and used within 48 h.

Store injection vials (non-premixed) at 2° to 8° C (36° to 46° F). Store premixed injection at room temperature (25° C; 77° F). If solution freezes, bring to room temperature; allow sufficient time to solubilize.

Administration
IV push: Dilute vial to total volume 5 or 10 mL and inject over not < 2 min.
IV infusion: Dilute with 100 mL of solution and administer over 15-30 min.

Felbamate
fel´-ba-mate
(Felbatol)

CATEGORY AND SCHEDULE
Pregnancy Risk Category: C

Classification: Anticonvulsant (carbamate derivative)

MECHANISM OF ACTION
An anticonvulsant, structurally similar to meprobamate, that weakly blocks repetitive, sustained firing of neurons by enhancing the ability of γ-aminobutyric acid (GABA) and antagonizes the strychnine-insensitive glycine recognition site of the *N*-methyl-D-aspartate receptor-ionophore complex. *Therapeutic Effect:* Decreases seizure activity.

PHARMACOKINETICS
Rapidly and almost completely absorbed after PO administration. Protein binding: 22%-25%, primarily to albumin. Partially excreted unchanged in the urine (40%-50% of absorbed dose). Unidentified metabolites and conjugates account for 40% of dose. *Half-life:* 20-23 h.

AVAILABILITY
Tablets: 400 mg, 600 mg.
Oral suspension: 600 mg/5mL (240 mL and 960 mL).

INDICATIONS AND DOSAGES
Not indicated as first-line antiepileptic treatment.
▶ **Monotherapy or adjunctive therapy in the treatment of partial seizures, with and without generalization**
PO
Adults, Children 14 yr and older. Initially, 1200 mg/day in divided doses 3-4 times a day. Increase the felbamate dosage by 600-mg increments every 2 wks to 2400 mg/day based on clinical response up to 3600 mg/day as clinically indicated. Reduce the dosage of other antiepileptic drugs (AEDs) by one third of their original dosage at initiation of felbamate. At wk 2, increase dose of felbamate to 2400 mg/day and reduce dose of other AEDs by an additional one third of their original dose.

At wk 3, increase the felbamate dosage up to 3600 mg/day and continue to reduce the dosage of other AEDs as clinically indicated.

▸ **Adjunctive therapy in the treatment of partial seizures, with and without generalization**

PO

Adults, Children 14 yr and older. Add 1200 mg/day in divided doses 3-4 times a day while reducing present AEDs by 20% in order-control plasma concentrations of concurrent phenytoin, valproic acid, and carbamazepine and its metabolites. Increase dosage by 1200 mg/day increments at weekly intervals to 3600 mg/day. Continual reduction of the other AEDs may be necessary to control side effects.

▸ **Lennox-Gastaut syndrome**

PO

Children 2-14 yr. Add felbamate at 15 mg/kg/day in divided doses 3-4 times a day while reducing present AEDs by 20% in order-control plasma concentrations of concurrent phenytoin, valproic acid, and carbamazepine and its metabolites. Increase the dosage of felbamate by 15 mg/kg/day increments at weekly intervals to 45 mg/kg/day. Continual reduction of the other AEDs may be necessary to control side effects.

▸ **Dosage in renal impairment**

Manufacturer recommends reducing usual dosages by 50%.

OFF-LABEL USES

None known.

CONTRAINDICATIONS

History of any blood dyscrasia or hepatic dysfunction, hypersensitivity to felbamate, its ingredients, or known sensitivity to other carbamates.

INTERACTIONS

Drug

Carbamazepine: Concentration of carbamazepine decreased, felbamate concenration decreased. Carbamazepine epoxide metabolite concentration increased.

CYP inducers and inhibitors: May affect felbamate concentrations.

Phenobarbital: Concentration of phenobarbital increased.

Phenytoin: Concentration of phenytoin increased, felbamate decreased (20% reduction in phenytoin dose resulted in phenytoin levels similar to baseline).

Valproate: Concentration of valproate increased.

Herbal and Food

None known.

DIAGNOSTIC TEST EFFECTS

Hemoglobin decreases. AST, ALT, GGT increases. Prothrombin increased or decreased.

SIDE EFFECTS

Frequent (> 10%)

Anorexia, vomiting, insomnia, nervousness, nausea, headache, dizziness, somnolence, dizziness, fatigue, constipation, dyspepsia, fever (children), upper respiratory infection.

Occasional (1%-10%)

Rhinitis, tremor, diplopia, taste perversion, abnormal vision, abnormal gait, abdominal pain, depression, anxiety, ataxia, parasthesia, rash, acne, intramenstrual bleeding, weight decrease, facial edema, myalgia, pharyngitis, chest pain, dry mouth, weight increase, palpitations, tachycardia, psychologic disturbance, aggressive reaction.

Rare (< 1%)

Anaphylactoid reaction, delusion, hallucinations, urinary retention, acute renal failure.

SERIOUS REACTIONS
Alert
! Aplastic anemia has been reported during felbamate therapy.
! Hepatic failure resulting in death has been reported.

PRECAUTIONS & CONSIDERATIONS
Lactation, warning of increased risk of aplastic anemia, hepatic failure; safety and efficacy in children with other types of seizures have not been established. Rapid withdrawal of antiepileptic drugs could result in rebound seizures. Should be used with caution in renal dysfunction.
Administration
Administer without regard to food. Shake suspension well before use.

Felodipine
fell-oh´-da-peen
(Plendil, Renedil[CAN])
Do not confuse Plendil with Pletal, or Renedil with Prinivil.

CATEGORY AND SCHEDULE
Pregnancy Risk Category: C

Classification: Calcium channel blockers, antihypertensive

MECHANISM OF ACTION
An antihypertensive and antianginal agent that inhibits calcium movement across cardiac and vascular smooth-muscle cell membranes. Potent peripheral vasodilator (does not depress SA or AV nodes) (dihydropyridine derivative).
Therapeutic Effect: Increases myocardial contractility, heart rate, and cardiac output; decreases peripheral vascular resistance and BP.

PHARMACOKINETICS

Route	Onset	Peak	Duration
PO	2-5 h	N/A	24 h

Rapidly, completely absorbed from the GI tract. Protein binding: > 99%. Undergoes first-pass metabolism in the liver (205%). Primarily excreted in urine. Not removed by hemodialysis. *Half-life:* 11-16 h.

AVAILABILITY
Tablets, Extended Release: 2.5 mg, 5 mg, 10 mg.

INDICATIONS AND DOSAGES
▸ **Hypertension**
PO
Adults. Initially, 5 mg/day as single dose. Adjust dosage at no < 2-wks intervals. Usual range: 2.5-10 mg/day.
Elderly, Patients with impaired hepatic function. Initially, 2.5 mg/day. Adjust dosage at no less than 2-wks intervals. Maintenance: 2.5-10 mg/day.

OFF-LABEL USES
Chronic angina pectoris, pediatric hypertension.

CONTRAIDICATIONS
Hypersensitivity, sick sinus syndrome, second- or third-degree heart block, SBP <90 mm Hg.

INTERACTIONS
Drug
Amiodarone: May result in bradycardia, atrioventricular block, and/or sinus arrest.
β blockers: Increased pharmacodynamic effects.
Carbamazepine, phenobarbital, phenytoin: Decreased felodipine concentration.

CYP inducers and inhibitors: May affect felodipine concentrations.
CYP2C8 substrates: Felodipine may inhibit metabolism of substrates.
Fentanyl: May result in severe hypotension.
Itraconazole (and other azole antifungals), erythromycin, cimetidine, cyclosporine: Increased felodipine concentration.
Nafcillin, rifampin: Decreased felodipine concentration.
NSAIDs: Decreased hypotensive effect or increased risk for GI complications.
Sildenafil, tadalafil, vardenafil: Additive hypotensive effects possible.
Tacrolimus: Concentration increased by felodipine.
Herbal
St. John's wort: May decrease felodipine levels.
Food
Grapefruit juice: Increases felodipine concentration.

SIDE EFFECTS

Frequent (> 10%)
Headache, peripheral edema.
Occasional (1%-10%)
Flushing, respiratory infection, dizziness, light-headedness, palpitations, dyspepsia, asthenia (loss of strength, weakness), constipation.
Rare
Paresthesia, abdominal discomfort, nervousness, muscle cramping, cough, diarrhea.

SERIOUS REACTIONS

• Overdose produces nausea, somnolence, confusion, slurred speech, hypotension, and bradycardia. Contact Poison Control Center if overdose suspected.
• Hypotension, syncope, reflex tachycardia. Arrhythmia, myocardial infarction.

Congestive heart failure, hypotension < 90 mm Hg systolic, hepatic injury/impairment, children, renal disease, elderly patients. It is unknown whether felodipine is distributed in breast milk, and it is not recommended for use.
Administration
Do not chew or crush tablets. Swallow whole. Administer with food or a light meal.

Fenofibrate
fee-no-fye´-brate
(Antara, Apo-Fenofibrate [CAN], Fenoglide, Lipofen, Lofibra, Tricor, Triglide)
Do not confuse Tricor with Tracleer.

CATEGORY AND SCHEDULE
Pregnancy Risk Category: C

Classification: Antihyperlipidemics, fibric acid derivatives

MECHANISM OF ACTION
An antihyperlipidemic that enhances synthesis of lipoprotein lipase and reduces triglyceride-rich lipoproteins and VLDLs. *Therapeutic Effect:* Increases VLDL catabolism and reduces total plasma triglyceride levels. Increases HDL levels.

PHARMACOKINETICS
Well absorbed from the GI tract. Micronized and nonmicronized forms are bioequivalent. Absorption increased when given with food. Protein binding: 99%. Rapidly metabolized in the liver to active metabolite. Excreted primarily in urine; lesser amount in feces. Not removed by hemodialysis. *Half-life:* 16-23 h.

AVAILABILITY

Tablets: 40 mg, 48 mg, 50 mg, 54 mg, 107 mg, 120 mg, 145 mg, 160 mg.
Capsules: 50 mg, 150 mg.
Capsules, Micronized Fenofibrate: 43 mg, 67 mg, 130 mg, 134 mg, 200 mg.

INDICATIONS AND DOSAGES
▸ **Hypertriglyceridemia**
PO
Adults, Elderly. Antara (micronized) capsule: Initially, 43-130 mg/day; may increase to 130 mg/day.
Fenoglide (nonmicronized) tablet: Initially, 40-120 mg/day; may increase to 120 mg/day.
Lipofen (nonmicronized) capsule: Initially, 50-150 mg/day; may increase to 150 mg/day.
Lofibra (micronized) capsule: Initially, 67-200 mg/day; may increase to 200 mg/day.
Lofibra (nonmicronized) tablet: Initially, 54-160 mg/day; may increase to 160 mg/day.
TriCor (nonmicronized) tablet: Initially, 48-145 mg/day; may increase to 145 mg/day.
Triglide (nonmicronized) tablet: Initially, 50-160 mg/day; may increase to 160 mg/day.
▸ **Dosage in renal impairment**
Antara (micronized) capsule: Initially, 43 mg/day.
Fenoglide (nonmicronized) tablet: CrCl 31-80 mL/min initially, 40 mg/day, CrCl < 30 mL/min contraindicated.
Lipofen (nonmicronized) capsule: Initially, 50 mg/day.
Lofibra (micronized) capsule: Initially, 67 mg/day.
Lofibra (nonmicronized) tablet: Initially, 54 mg/day.
TriCor (nonmicronized) tablet: CrCl 31-80 mL/min initially, 48 mg/day, CrCl < 30 mL/min contraindicated.
Triglide (nonmicronized) tablet: CrCl 11-49 mL/min initially,

50 mg/day. CrCl < 10 mL/min: Contraindicated.

OFF-LABEL USES
Hyperuricemia, gout, metabolic syndrome.

CONTRAINDICATIONS
Gallbladder disease, hypersensitivity to fenofibrate, severe renal or hepatic dysfunction (including primary biliary cirrhosis, unexplained persistent liver function abnormality).

INTERACTIONS
Drug
Bile acid sequestrants: Decrease absorption of fenofibrate (give fenofibrate 1 h before or 4-6 h after).
Cyclosporine: Concomitant use may lead to renal dysfunction.
Ezetimibe: Fenofibrate may increase concentrations.
HMG-CoA reductase inhibitors (atorvastatin, fluvastatin, lovastatin, pravastatin, rosuvastatin, simvastatin): May increase the risk of myopathy and rhabdomyolysis. Extreme caution is warranted if used concomitantly or avoid use. Monitor.
Sulfonylureas: Enhanced hypoglycemic effects.
Warfarin: May increase the anticoagulant effect of warfarin; monitor INR closely and adjust warfarin dose as needed.
Herbal
None known.
Food
None known.

DIAGNOSTIC TEST EFFECTS
Increased AST, ALT, CPK, creatinine, GGT.

SIDE EFFECTS
Occasional (1%-10%)
AST/ALT elevation, respiratory disorder, abdominal pain, back

F

pain, headache, flu symptoms, asthenia, nausea, vomiting, diarrhea, rhinitis, constipation, asthenia.

Rare (< 1%)

Anxiety, acne, anorexia, anemia, edema, arthralgia, insomnia, polyuria, cough, abnormal vision, eye floaters, earache.

SERIOUS REACTIONS

• Fenofibrate may increase excretion of cholesterol into bile, leading to cholelithiasis.

• Hypersensitivity reactions, pancreatitis, hepatitis, thrombocytopenia, and agranulocytosis occur rarely.

PRECAUTIONS & CONSIDERATIONS

Monitor liver function; may lead to cholelithiasis; can be associated with myositis, myopathy, or rhabdomyolysis; avoid if lactating; renal function impairment; safe use in children unknown; discontinue use if no response in 2 mo; base dose in elderly on renal function, monitor for adverse effects.

Administration

Fenoglide, Lofibra, Lipofen should be administered with meals.
Antara, Tricor may be administed with or without meals.
Triglide may be administered with or without meals.

Fenoprofen

fen-oh-proe fen
(Nalfon)
Do not confuse Nalfon with Naldecon.

CATEGORY AND SCHEDULE

Pregnancy Risk Category: B
(D if used in third trimester or near delivery)

Classification: Analgesics, nonnarcotic, nonsteroidal anti-inflammatory drugs

MECHANISM OF ACTION

An NSAID that produces analgesic, antipyretic, and anti-inflammatory effects by inhibiting prostaglandin synthesis. *Therapeutic Effect:* Reduces the inflammatory response, fever, and intensity of pain.

AVAILABILITY

Capsules: 200 mg, 300 mg.
Tablets: 600 mg.

INDICATIONS AND DOSAGES

▸ **Mild to moderate pain**
PO
Adults, Elderly. 200 mg q4-6h as needed.
▸ **Rheumatoid arthritis, osteoarthritis**
PO
Adults, Elderly. 300-600 mg 3-4 times a day. Total daily dose should not exceed 3200 mg.

OFF-LABEL USES

Treatment of ankylosing spondylitis, migraine, psoriatic arthritis, tendinitis, vascular headaches.

CONTRAINDICATIONS

Active peptic ulcer disease, chronic inflammation of GI tract,

GI bleeding or ulceration, history of hypersensitivity to aspirin or NSAIDs, significant renal impairment.

INTERACTIONS
Drug
SSRI, antidepressants: May increase antiplatelet effects.
Antihypertensives, diuretics: May decrease the effects of these drugs.
Aspirin, other salicylates: May increase the risk of GI side effects such as bleeding.
Bile acid sequestrants: May decrease absorption.
Bisphosphonates: May increase risk for GI ulceration with bisphosphonates.
Bone marrow depressants: May increase the risk of hematologic reactions.
Corticosteroids: May increase risk of GI ulceration.
Cyclosporine: May increase nephrotoxicity and serum levels of cyclosporine.
Heparin, oral anticoagulants, antiplatelets, thrombolytics: May increase the effects of these drugs.
Lithium: May increase the blood concentration and risk of toxicity of lithium.
Methotrexate: May increase the risk of methotrexate toxicity and methotrexate levels.
Probenecid: May increase fenoprofen blood concentration.
Vancomycin: May increase levels of vancomycin.
Herbal
Supplements with antiplatelet or anticoagulant effects (e.g., feverfew, garlic, ginger, ginkgo biloba, ginseng, red clover, sweet clover, white willow): May increase effects on platelets or risk of bleeding.
Food
None known.

DIAGNOSTIC TEST EFFECTS
May increase bleeding time, BUN and blood glucose levels, and serum protein, alkaline phosphatase, LDH, creatinine, AST (SGOT), and ALT (SGPT) levels.

SIDE EFFECTS
Frequent (3%-10%)
Headache, somnolence, dyspepsia, nausea, vomiting, constipation, dizziness, sweating, pruritus, rash, blurred vision.
Occasional (1%-2%)
Dizziness, nervousness, asthenia, diarrhea, abdominal cramps, flatulence, tinnitus, peripheral edema, tremor, confusion, and fluid retention.

SERIOUS REACTIONS
• Overdose may result in acute hypotension and tachycardia.
• Rare reactions with long-term use include peptic ulcer disease, GI bleeding, gastritis, severe hepatic reaction (jaundice), nephrotoxicity (hematuria, dysuria, proteinuria), and a severe hypersensitivity reaction (bronchospasm, angioedema).

PRECAUTIONS & CONSIDERATIONS
Caution is warranted with hepatic or renal impairment, a predisposition to fluid retention, and history of GI tract disease.

Clinical trials of several COX-2 selective and nonselective NSAIDs of up to 3-yr duration have shown an increased risk of serious cardiovascular (CV) thrombotic events, myocardial infarction, and stroke, which can be fatal. All NSAIDs, both COX-2 selective and nonselective, may present a similar risk. Patients with known CV disease or risk factors for CV disease may be at greater risk. To minimize the potential risk for an adverse CV event in patients treated with an NSAID, the lowest effective dose should be used for the shortest duration possible. Physicians and patients should remain alert for the development of such events, even in the absence of previous CV symptoms. Patients should be informed about the signs and/or symptoms of serious CV events and the steps to take if they occur.

Fenoprofen crosses the placenta and is distributed in breast milk. Fenoprofen should not be used during the last trimester of pregnancy because it may cause adverse effects in the fetus, such as premature closure of the ductus arteriosus. The safety and efficacy of fenoprofen have not been established in children. In elderly patients, GI bleeding or ulceration is more likely to cause serious complications and age-related renal impairment may increase the risk of hepatotoxicity or renal toxicity; a decreased drug dosage is recommended. Avoid alcohol and aspirin during therapy because these substances increase the risk of GI bleeding. Tasks that require mental alertness or motor skills should be avoided until response to the drug has been established.

Baseline bleeding time, BUN and blood glucose levels, serum alkaline phosphatase, LDH, creatinine, AST (SGOT) ALT (SGPT) levels, and urinary protein levels should be obtained at the beginning of therapy. Pattern of daily bowel activity and stool consistency should be assessed during fenoprofen use. Therapeutic response, such as decreased pain, stiffness, swelling, and tenderness, improved grip strength, and increased joint mobility, should be evaluated.

Administration
Swallow capsules whole; do not crush, open, or break capsules. Administer with food to decrease GI irritation.

Fentanyl
fen′ta-nil
(Actiq, Duragesic, Fentora, Ionsys, Sublimaze)
Do not confuse fentanyl with alfentanil, remifentanil, or sufentanil.

CATEGORY AND SCHEDULE
Pregnancy Risk Category: C (D if used for prolonged periods or at high dosages at term)
Controlled Substance Schedule: II

Classification: Analgesics, narcotic; anesthetics, general

MECHANISM OF ACTION
An opioid agonist that binds to opioid receptors in the CNS, reducing stimuli from sensory nerve endings and inhibiting ascending pain pathways. *Therapeutic Effect:* Alters pain reception and increases the pain threshold.

PHARMACOKINETICS

Route	Onset	Peak	Duration
IV	1-2 min	3-5 min	0.5-1 h
IM	7-15 min	20-30 min	1-2 h
Transder-mal	6-8 h	24 h	72 h
Transmu-cosal	5-15 min	20-30 min	1-2 h

Well absorbed after IM or topical administration. Transmucosal form absorbed through the buccal mucosa and GI tract. Protein binding: 80%-85%. Metabolized in the liver by CYP3A4. Primarily eliminated by biliary system. *Half-life:* 2-4 h IV; 17 h transdermal patch; 16 h transdermal iontophoretic system; 3.2-5.9 h transmucosal lozenge; 3-12 h buccal tablet.

AVAILABILITY

Injection (Sublimaze): 50 mcg/mL.
Transdermal Patch (Duragesic): 12.5 mcg/h, 25 mcg/h, 50 mcg/h, 75 mcg/h, 100 mcg/h.
Transdermal iontophoretic system (Ionsys): 40 mcg/dose.
Transmucosal Lozenges (Actiq): 200 mcg, 400 mcg, 600 mcg, 800 mcg, 1200 mcg, 1600 mcg.
Transmucosal Buccal Tablets: 100 mcg, 200 mcg, 400 mcg, 600 mcg, 800 mcg.

INDICATIONS AND DOSAGES
▸ **Premedication**
IV, IM
Adults, Elderly, Children 12 yr and older. 50-100 mcg/dose 30-60 min before surgery.
▸ **Adjunct to general anesthesia**
IV
Adults, Elderly, Children 12 yr and older. Low dose: 0.5-2 mcg/kg/dose; moderate dose: 2-20 mcg/kg/dose; high dose: 20-50 mcg/kg.
Children aged 2-12 yr. Induction and maintenance. 2-3 mcg/kg/dose.
▸ **Adjunct to regional anesthesia**
IV, IM
Adults, Elderly, Children 12 yr and older. 25-100 mcg over 1-2 min.
▸ **Postoperative pain**
IM
Adults, Elderly, Children 12 yr and older. 50-100 mcg every 1-2 h as needed.

TRANSDERMAL IONTOPHORETIC SYSTEM
Adults. To be used in hospital only. Each activation delivers 40 mcg. Six doses may be administered in 1 h. Each system operates for 24 h or until 80 doses have been administered, whichever occurs first. Maximum use 72 h.
▸ **Chronic pain management**
USUAL TRANSDERMAL DOSE
Adults, Elderly, Children 12 yr and older. Use dose conversion chart to convert patients from oral or IV opioids. May increase after 3 days and then every 6 days thereafter. Should not be used in opioid-naïve patients. Upon system removal, 17 h or more are required for a 50% decrease in serum fentanyl concentrations. Effects on respiratory system may persist for longer.
▸ **Breakthrough cancer pain**
USUAL TRANSMUCOSAL DOSE (LOZENGE)
Adults, Children. Initial 200 mcg. May start second unit 15 min after completing first if needed. If more than one lozenge is needed per episode for several episodes, consider prescribing next highest strength.
USUAL TRANSMUCOSAL DOSE (BUCCAL TABLET)
Adults, Children. Initial 100 mcg; redosing can occur 30 min after start of first tablet, if necessary. Dose titration should be done in 100-mcg increments up to 400 mcg. See prescribing information for converting from lozenge.
USUAL EPIDURAL DOSE
Adults, Elderly. Bolus dose of 100 mcg, followed by continuous infusion of 10 mcg/mL concentration at 4-12 mL/h.
▸ **Continuous analgesia**
IV
Adults, Elderly, Children aged 1-12 yr. Bolus dose of 1-2 mcg/kg,

F

followed by continuous infusion of 1 mcg/kg/h. Range: 1-5 mcg/kg/h. *Children younger than 1 yr.* Bolus dose of 1-2 mcg/kg, followed by continuous infusion of 0.5-1 mcg/kg/h.

▸ **Dosage in renal impairment**
Dosage is modified based on creatinine clearance.

Creatinine Clearance	Dosage
10-50 mL/min	75% of usual dose
< 10 mL/min	50% of usual dose

CONTRAINDICATIONS

Increased intracranial pressure, severe hepatic or renal impairment, severe respiratory depression, severe bronchial asthma, paralytic ileus. Hypersensitivity to fentanyl. Fentanyl lozenge, buccal tablet, and transdermal patch are contraindicated for acute or postoperative pain and opioid nontolerant patients.

INTERACTIONS

Drug
Amiodarone: Profound bradycardia, sinus arrest, and hypotension have occurred with coadministration.
Benzodiazepines, CNS depressants: May increase the risk of hypotension and respiratory depression, sedation.
Buprenorphine: May decrease the effects of fentanyl.
CYP3A4 inhibitors: May increase concentration of fentanyl. CYP3A4 inducers may decrease concentration of fentanyl.
MAOI: Should not be used.
Ritonavir: Increases fenanyl concentrations.
Herbal
St. John's wort: May decrease fentanyl levels.
Food
None known.

DIAGNOSTIC TEST EFFECTS

May increase serum amylase and lipase concentrations.

Ⓓ IV INCOMPATIBILITIES

Azithromycin (Zithromax), dantrolene, pantoprazole (Protonix), phenytoin (Dilantin), sulfamethoxazole/trimethoprim.

🔻 IV COMPATIBILITIES

Abciximab (Reopro), acyclovir (Zovirax), alfentanil (Alfenta), alprostadil (Prostin VR), amikacin (Amikin), aminophylline, amiodarone, amphotericin B cholesteryl complex (Amphotec), amphotericin B liposome (AmBisome), anidulafungin (Eraxis), argatroban, ascorbic acid, atracurium (Tracrium), atropine, azathioprine, aztreonam (Azactam), benztropine (Cogentin), bivalirudin (Angiomax), bretylium, bumetanide (Bumex), bupivacaine (Marcaine, Sensorcaine), buprenorphine (Buprenex), butorphanol (Stadol), caffeine citrate (Cafcit), calcium chloride, calcium gluconate, carboplatin, caspofungin (Cancidas), cefazolin, cefotaxime (Claforan), cefoxitin (Mefoxin), ceftazidime (Ceptaz, Fortaz, Tazicef, Tazidime), ceftizoxime (Cefizox), cefuroxime (Zinacef), chloramphenicol, chlorpromazine, cimetidine, cisatracurium (Nimbex), cisplatin, clindamycin (Cleocin), clonidine (Duraclon), cyanocobalamin, cyclophosphamide (Cytoxan), cyclosporine (Sandimmune), dactinomycin (Cosmegen), daptomycin (Cubicin), dexamethasone sodium phosphate, digoxin (Lanoxin), diltiazem (Cardizem), diphenhydramine (Benadryl), dobutamine (Dobutrex), docetaxel (Taxotere), dopamine (Intropin), doripenem (Doribax), doxorubicin (Adriamycin), droperidol (Inapsine), emolol (Brevibloc), enalaprilat, ephedrine, epinephrine, epirubicin (Ellence), epoetin alfa (Procrit), erythromycin lactobionate, etomidate (Amidate), etoposide phosphate (Etopophos), famotidine (Pepcid), fenoldopam (Corlopam), fluconazole (Diflucan), fludarabine (Fludara), folic acid, furosemide (Lasix), ganciclovir (Cytovene), gemcitabine (Gemzar), gentamicin, glycopyrrolate, granisetron (Kytril), heparin, hydrocortisone sodium succinate (Solu-Cortef), hydromorphone (Dilaudid), hydroxyzine, imipenem/ cliastatin (Primaxin), inamrinone, insulin (regular, Humulin R, Novolin R), isoproterenol (Isuprel), ketamine (Ketalar), ketorolac, labetalol, lansoprazole (Prevacid), levofloxacin (Levaquin), lidocaine, linezolid (Zyvox), lorazepam (Ativan), magnesium sulfate, mannitol, meperidine (Demerol), methicillin, methotrexate, methylprednisolone sodium succinate, metoclopramide (Reglan), metoprolol (Lopressor), metronidazole (Flagyl), midazolam, milrinone (Primacor), minocycline (Minocin), mitoxantron (Novantrone), mivacurium (Mivacron), morphine, nafcillin, nalbuphine (Nubain), naloxone (Narcan), nesiritide (Natrecor), nicardipine (Cardene), nitroglycerin, nitroprusside (Nitropress), norepinephrine (Levophed), ondansetron (Zofran), oxacillin, oxytocin (Pitocin), paclitaxel (Taxol), palonosetron (Aloxi), pancuronium, pemetrexed (Alimta), penicillin G potassium, penicillin G sodium, phenobarbital, phytonadione, piperacillin, piperacillin/tazobactam (Zosyn), potassium chloride, procainamide,

promethazine, propofol (Diprivan), propranolol (Inderal), protamine, pyridoxine, quinupristin/dalfopristin (Synercid), ranitidine (Zantac), remifentanil (Ultiva), rituximab (Rituxan), sargramostim (Leukine), scopolamine, sodium acetate, sodium bicarbonate, streptokinase, succinylcholine (Anectine, Quelicin), sufentanil (Sufenta), tacrolimus (Prograf), teniposide (Vumon), theophylline, thiamine, thiotepa (Thioplex), ticarcillin (Ticar), ticarcillin/clavulanate (Timentin), tigecycline (Tygacil), tirofiban (Aggrastat), tobramycin, trastuzumab (Herceptin), vancomyin, vecuronium (Norcuron), verapamil, vincristine (Vincasar), vinorelbine (Navelbine), voriconazole (Vfend).

SIDE EFFECTS
Frequent
IV: Postoperative drowsiness, nausea, vomiting, dizziness.
Transdermal (3%-10%): Headache, pruritus, nausea, vomiting, diaphoresis, dyspnea, confusion, dizziness, somnolence, diarrhea, constipation, decreased appetite.
Lozenge (> 10%): Nausea, dizziness, somnolence, vomiting, constipation.
Buccal tablet (> 10%): Dizziness, nausea, headache, somnolence, asthenia, constipation.
Occasional
IV: Postoperative confusion, blurred vision, chills, hypertension, orthostatic hypotension, constipation, difficulty urinating.
Transdermal (1%-3%): Chest pain, arrhythmias, erythema, pruritus, swelling of skin, syncope, agitation, tingling or burning of skin.
Lozenge (2%-10%): Asthenia, headache, confusion, constipation, dyspnea, anxiety, abnormal gait, nervousness, pruritus, rash, sweating, abnormal vision, vasodilation.

Buccal tablet (2%-10%):
Application-site reactions (pain, ulcer, irritation), vomiting, fatigue, confusion, depression, insomnia, abdominal pain, diarrhea, anorexia, weight decreased, arthralgia, back pain.

SERIOUS REACTIONS

• Respiratory depression, apnea, rigidity, and bradycardia are most common serious adverse reactions. If untreated, could lead to respiratory arrest, circulatory depression, or cardiac arrest.

• Overdose or too rapid IV administration may produce severe respiratory depression and skeletal and thoracic muscle rigidity (which may lead to apnea), laryngospasm, bronchospasm, cold and clammy skin, cyanosis, and coma.

• The patient who uses fentanyl repeatedly may develop a tolerance to the drug's analgesic effect.

PRECAUTIONS & CONSIDERATIONS

Caution is warranted with bradycardia; head injuries; altered level of consciousness; hepatic, renal, or respiratory disease; history of drug abuse; and concurrent use of MAOIs within 14 days of fentanyl administration. Fentanyl readily crosses the placenta; it is unknown whether fentanyl is distributed in breast milk. Fentanyl may prolong labor if administered in the latent phase of the first stage of labor or before the cervix has dilated 4-5 cm. Fentanyl may cause respiratory depression in the neonate if it is given to the mother during labor. The transdermal form of fentanyl is not recommended for children younger than 12 yr or children younger than 18 yr who weigh < 50 kg. Neonates and elderly patients are more susceptible to the drug's respiratory depressant effects. Age-related renal impairment may require a dosage adjustment in elderly patients. Abrupt discontinuation after prolonged use may result in withdrawal.

Dizziness and drowsiness may occur, so change positions slowly and avoid alcohol, CNS depressants, and tasks that require mental alertness or motor skills until response to the drug is established. BP, heart rate, respiratory rate, oxygen saturation, pattern of daily bowel activity and stool consistency, and clinical improvement of pain should be monitored.

Storage

Store the parenteral form at room temperature.

Administration

! Keep in mind that fentanyl may be combined with a local anesthetic, such as bupivacaine. Discontinue fentanyl slowly after long-term use.

For IV use, make sure resuscitative equipment and an opiate antagonist (naloxone 0.5 mcg/kg) are readily available before administering the drug. For initial anesthesia induction, give a small amount by tuberculin syringe, as prescribed. Give by slow IV push, over 1-2 min. A too-rapid IV infusion increases the risk of severe adverse reactions, such as anaphylaxis, bronchospasm, laryngospasm, peripheral circulatory collapse, cardiac arrest, and skeletal and thoracic muscle rigidity (which may result in apnea).

For transdermal patch use, clean the patch site before application; use only water, because soap and oils may irritate the skin. Allow the skin to dry. Apply the patch to a flat, unirritated, nonhairy (or clip hair; do not shave) area of intact skin on the upper torso, chest, back, flank, or upper arm. Apply immediately after removing from sealed package. Do not cut or alter patch. Press the patch onto the skin firmly and evenly for 30 s, ensuring that it comes in full contact with the skin, especially around the edges. Each patch should be worn continuously for 72 h. Rotate application sites. Patients must avoid exposing the patch to excessive heat, because this promotes the release of fentanyl from the patch and increases the absorption of fentanyl through the skin, which can result in fatal overdose. Monitor patients with a fever carefully. Carefully fold used patches so that they adhere to themselves, and discard them in the toilet. Patients should dispose of any patches remaining from a prescription as soon as they are no longer needed. Unused patches should be removed from their pouches, folded so that the adhesive side of the patch adheres to itself, and flushed down the toilet. If the gel from the drug reservoir accidentally contacts the skin of the patient or caregiver, the skin should be washed with copious amounts of water. Do not use soap, alcohol, or other solvents to remove the gel, because they may enhance the drug's ability to penetrate the skin. Keep out of the reach of children. Oral ingestion of gel from patches may cause fatality.

Transmucosal lozenge: Open the blister package with scissors immediately before product use. Place the unit in the patient's mouth between the cheek and lower gum, moving it from one side to the other, using the handle. Instruct the patient to suck, not chew, the lozenge for 15 min for optimal efficacy. If signs of excessive opioid effects appear before the unit is consumed, remove the drug matrix from the patient's mouth immediately and decrease future doses. Fentanyl lozenge contains medicine in an amount that could be fatal to a child. Dispose of units remaining from a prescription as soon as they are no longer needed. Dispose of all units immediately after use. Partially consumed units represent a special risk because they are no longer protected by the child-resistant pouch and yet may contain enough medicine to be fatal to a child. A temporary storage bottle is provided to be used in the event that a partially consumed unit cannot be disposed of promptly.

Transmucosal buccal tablet: Open the blister pack immediately before use. The blister backing should then be peeled back to expose the tablet. Patients should NOT attempt to push the tablet through the blister because to do so may cause damage to the tablet. The tablet should not be stored once it has been removed from the blister package because the tablet's integrity may be compromised and because this increases the risk of accidental exposure to the tablet. Remove the tablet from the blister unit and immediately place the entire fentanyl buccal tablet in the buccal cavity (above a rear molar, between the upper cheek and gum). Patients should not attempt to split the tablet. Do not suck, chew, or swallow tablet because to do so will result in lower plasma concentrations than when taken as directed. The fentanyl buccal tablet should be left between the cheek and gum until it has disintegrated, which usually takes approximately 14-25 min. After 30 min, if remnants from the fentanyl buccal tablet remain, they may be swallowed with a glass of water. Dispose of any remaining tablets immediately. May be fatal to a child.

Ferrous Salts

fer-rous

(Femiron, Feostat, Ferretts, Ferro-Sequels, Hemocyte, Nephro-Fer, Palafer [CAN]) (Apo-Ferrous Gluconate [CAN], Fergon) (Apo-Ferrous Sulfate [CAN], Fer-Gen-Sol, Fer-In-Sol, Fer-Iron, Ferro-Gradumet [AUS], Slow-Fe)

CATEGORY AND SCHEDULE

Pregnancy Risk Category: A
OTC

Classification: Hematinics

MECHANISM OF ACTION

An enzymatic mineral that is an essential component in the formation of hemoglobin, myoglobin, and enzymes. Promotes effective erythropoiesis and transport and utilization of oxygen (O_2).
Therapeutic Effect: Prevents and treats iron deficiency.

PHARMACOKINETICS

Absorbed in the duodenum and upper jejunum. Ten percent absorbed in patients with normal iron stores; increased to 20%-30% in those with inadequate iron stores. Bound primarily to serum transferrin. Excreted in urine, sweat, and sloughing of intestinal mucosa and by menses. *Half-life:* 6 h.

AVAILABILITY

Ferrous Fumarate
Tablets (Femiron): 63 mg (20 mg elemental iron).
Tablets (Ferretts): 325 mg (106 mg elemental iron).
Tablets (Hemocyte): 324 mg (106 mg elemental iron).
Tablets (Nephro-Fer): 350 mg (115 mg elemental iron).

Tablets (Chewable [Feostat]): 100 mg (33 mg elemental iron).
Tablet (Timed-Release [Ferro-Sequels]): 150 mg (50 mg elemental iron).
Ferrous Gluconate
Tablets: 325 mg (36 mg elemental iron).
Tablets (Fergon): 240 mg (27 mg elemental iron).
Ferrous Sulfate
Tablets: 325 mg (65 mg elemental iron).
Tablets, Exsiccated (Feosol): 200 mg (65 mg elemental iron).
Tablets (Timed-Release [Slow FE]): 160 mg (50 mg elemental iron).
Elixir: 220 mg/5 mL (44 mg elemental iron per 5 mL).
Oral Drops (Fer-Gen-Sol, Fer-In-Sol, Fer-Iron): 75 mg/0.6 mL (15 mg/0.6 mL elemental iron).

INDICATIONS AND DOSAGES
▸ **Iron deficiency anemia**
Dosage is expressed in terms of milligrams of elemental iron, degree of anemia, patient weight, and presence of any bleeding. Expect to use periodic hematologic determinations as guide to therapy.
PO
Adults, Elderly. Ferrous fumarate: 60-100 mg twice a day; ferrous gluconate: 60 mg 2-4 times a day; ferrous sulfate: 325 mg 2-4 times a day.
Children. Ferrous fumarate, ferrous gluconate, ferrous sulfate: 3-6 mg/kg/day in 2-3 divided doses.
▸ **Prevention of iron deficiency anemia**
PO
Adults, Elderly. Ferrous fumarate: 60-100 mg/day; ferrous gluconate: 60 mg/day; ferrous sulfate: 325 mg/day.
Children. Ferrous fumarate, ferrous gluconate, ferrous sulfate: 1-2 mg/kg/day, maximum 15 mg/day.

CONTRAINDICATIONS

Hemochromatosis, hemosiderosis, hemolytic anemias, peptic ulcer disease, regional enteritis, ulcerative colitis.

INTERACTIONS

Drug

Ascorbic acid: May increase absorption of iron by > 30%.

Antacids, H₂ antagonists, proton pump inhibitors, calcium supplements, pancreatin, pancrelipase: May decrease the absorption of ferrous fumarate, ferrous gluconate, and ferrous sulfate.

Etidronate, levodopa, levothyroxine, quinolones, tetracyclines: May decrease the absorption of etidronate, levodopa, levothyroxine, quinolones, and tetracyclines.

Herbal

None known.

Food

Eggs, dietary fiber, coffee, milk: Inhibit ferrous fumarate absorption.

DIAGNOSTIC TEST EFFECTS

May increase serum bilirubin level. May decrease serum calcium level. May obscure occult blood in stools.

SIDE EFFECTS

Occasional

Mild, transient nausea.

Rare

Heartburn, anorexia, constipation, diarrhea.

SERIOUS REACTIONS

• Large doses may aggravate existing GI tract disease, such as peptic ulcer disease, regional enteritis, and ulcerative colitis.

• Severe iron poisoning occurs most often in children and is manifested as vomiting, severe abdominal pain, diarrhea, and dehydration, followed by hyperventilation, pallor or cyanosis, and cardiovascular collapse. If accidental overdose occurs, contact the Poison Control Center immediately.

PRECAUTIONS & CONSIDERATIONS

Caution is warranted in patients with bronchial asthma and iron hypersensitivity. Ferrous fumarate, ferrous sulfate, and ferrous gluconate cross the placenta and are distributed in breast milk. No age-related precautions have been noted in children or elderly patients. Avoid taking the drug with milk or eggs.

Urine may darken in color. Hemoglobin, reticulocyte count, ferritin and serum iron levels, and total iron-binding capacity should be monitored. Daily bowel activity and stool consistency should be assessed. Clinical improvement should also be assessed, and relief of iron deficiency symptoms (fatigue, headache, irritability, pallor, and paresthesia of extremities) should be recorded.

Storage

Store all forms, including tablets, capsules, suspension, and drops, at room temperature and out of reach of children.

Administration

Take between meals with water unless GI discomfort occurs; if so, give with meals. Use dropper or calibrated oral syringe to administer the liquid preparation, and allow the drug solution to drop on the back of the patient's tongue to prevent mucous membrane and teeth staining. To avoid transient staining of mucous membranes and teeth, place liquid on back of tongue with a dropper or straw. Do not crush the sustained-release form. Avoid simultaneous administration of antacids.

Fexofenadine
fex-oh-fen′eh-deen
(Allegra, Telfast [AUS])

CATEGORY AND SCHEDULE
Pregnancy Risk Category: C

Classification: Antihistamines, H_1

MECHANISM OF ACTION
A piperidine that competes with histamine for H_1-receptor sites on effector cells. *Therapeutic Effect:* Relieves allergic rhinitis symptoms.

PHARMACOKINETICS
Rapidly absorbed after PO administration. Protein binding: 60%-70%. Does not cross the blood-brain barrier. Minimally metabolized. Eliminated in feces and urine. Not removed by hemodialysis. *Half-life:* 14.4 h (increased in renal impairment).

AVAILABILITY
Tablets: 30 mg, 60 mg, 180 mg.
Oral Disintegrating Tablets (ODT): 30 mg.
Oral Suspension: 30 mg/5 mL.

INDICATIONS AND DOSAGES
▶ **Allergic rhinitis, chronic idiopathic urticaria**
PO
Adults, Elderly, Children 12 yr and older. 60 mg twice a day or 180 mg once a day.
Children aged 6-11 yr. 30 mg twice a day.
▶ **Dosage in renal impairment**
Adults, Elderly, and Children 12 yr and older. Dosage is reduced to 60 mg once a day. For children aged 6-11 yr, dosage is reduced to 30 mg once a day.

▶ **Allergic rhinitis, chronic idiopathic urticaria**
PO
Children aged 2-11 yr. Oral suspension 30 mg twice a day. For children with renal dysfunction, dosage is reduced to 30 mg once daily.
▶ **Chronic idiopathic urticaria**
PO
Children aged 6 mo to 2 yr. Oral suspension 15 mg twice a day. For children with renal dysfunction, dosage is reduced to 15 mg once daily.

CONTRAINDICATIONS
Hypersensitivity.

INTERACTIONS
Drug
Antacids: May decrease fexofenadine absorption if given within 15 min of a fexofenadine dose.
Herbal
None known.
Food
Fruit juice.

DIAGNOSTIC TEST EFFECTS
May suppress wheal and flare reactions to antigen skin testing unless drug is discontinued at least 4 days before testing.

SIDE EFFECTS
Rare (< 2%)
Somnolence, headache, fatigue, nausea, vomiting, abdominal distress, dysmenorrhea.

SERIOUS REACTIONS
• Rare serious hypersensitivity reactions.

PRECAUTIONS & CONSIDERATIONS
ODTs contain phenylalanine (phenylketonuria).

Caution is warranted with severe renal impairment. It is unknown whether fexofenadine crosses the placenta or is distributed in breast milk. No age-related precautions have been noted in elderly patients. Avoid drinking alcoholic beverages and performing tasks that require alertness or motor skills until response to the drug is established.

Drowsiness may occur. Respiratory rate, depth, and rhythm; pulse rate and quality; BP; and therapeutic response should be monitored.

Administration
Take fexofenadine without regard to food. ODTs are designed to disintegrate on the tongue, followed by swallowing with or without water, and should be taken on an empty stomach. Do not chew ODT. Shake oral suspension well before each use.

Filgrastim
fil-gra′-stim
(Neupogen)
Do not confuse Neupogen with Epogen or Nutramigen.

CATEGORY AND SCHEDULE
Pregnancy Risk Category: C

Classification: Hematopoietic agents, recombinant DNA origin

MECHANISM OF ACTION
A biologic modifier that stimulates production, maturation, and activation of neutrophils to increase their migration and cytotoxicity. *Therapeutic Effect:* Increases neutrophil count and enhances count recovery. Decreases incidence of infection.

PHARMACOKINETICS
Readily absorbed after subcutaneous (SC) administration. Not removed by hemodialysis. *Half-life:* 3.5 h.

AVAILABILITY
Injection, Single-Dose Vials:
300 mcg/mL, 480 mcg/0.8 mL.
Prefilled Syringes (Single Ject):
300 mcg, 480 mcg.

INDICATIONS AND DOSAGES
▸ **Myelosuppression from chemotherapy**
IV OR SC INFUSION,
SC INJECTION
Adults, Elderly. Initially, 5 mcg/kg/day. May increase by 5 mcg/kg for each chemotherapy cycle based on duration or severity of absolute neutrophil count nadir. Administer daily for up to 2 wks until the ANC has reached 10,000/mm^3 following the expected chemotherapy-induced neutrophil nadir.
▸ **Bone marrow transplant**
IV OR SC INFUSION
Adults, Elderly. 10 mcg/kg/day given as an IV infusion of 4 or 24 h or as a continuous 24-h SC infusion. Adjust dosage daily during period of neutrophil recovery based on neutrophil response.
▸ **Mobilization progenitor cells**
SC INJECTION OR INFUSION
Adults. 10 mcg/kg/day beginning at least 4 days before first leukapheresis and continuing until last leukapheresis.
▸ **Chronic neutropenia, congenital neutropenia**
SC
Adults, Children. 6 mcg/kg/dose twice a day.
▸ **Idiopathic or cyclic neutropenia**
SC
Adults, Children. 5 mcg/kg/dose once a day.

OFF-LABEL USES

Treatment of AIDS-related neutropenia; drug-induced agranulocytosis; febrile neutropenia; myelodysplastic syndrome.

CONTRAINDICATIONS

Hypersensitivity to *Escherichia coli*–derived proteins; use within 24 h before or after cytotoxic chemotherapy.

INTERACTIONS

Drug

Lithium: May increase white blood cell count greater than expected.

Topotecan: May prolong the duration of neutropenia.

Herbal

None known.

Food

None known.

DIAGNOSTIC TEST EFFECTS

May increase LDH concentrations, leukocyte alkaline phosphatase (LAP) scores, and serum alkaline phosphatase and uric acid levels.

Ⓘ IV INCOMPATIBILITIES

Amphotericin (Fungizone), cefepime (Maxipime), cefotaxime (Claforan), cefoxitin (Mefoxin), ceftizoxime (Cefizox), ceftriaxone (Rocephin), cefuroxime (Zinacef), clindamycin (Cleocin), dactinomycin (Cosmegen), etoposide (VePesid), fluorouracil, furosemide (Lasix), heparin, mannitol, methylprednisolone (Solu-Medrol), metronidazole (Flagyl), mitomycin (Mutamycin), piperacillin, thiotepa (Thioplex), prochlorperazine (Compazine).

Ⓘ IV COMPATIBILITIES

Acyclovir (Zovirax), allopurinol (Aloprim), amikacin (Amikin), aminophylline, ampicillin, ampicillin-sulbactam (Unasyn), aztreonam (Azactam), bleomycin (Blenoxane), bumetanide (Bumex), buprenorphine (Buprenex), butorphanol (Stadol), calcium gluconate, carboplatin, carmustine (BiCNU), cefazolin, ceftazidime (Fortaz, Tazicef, Tazidime), chlorpromazine, cimetidine, cisplatin, cyclophosphamide (Cytoxan), cytarabine (Tarabine), dacarbazine (DTIC-Dome), daunorubicin (Cerubidine), dexamethasone sodium phosphate (Hexadrol), diphenhydramine (Benadryl), doxorubicin (Adriamycin), doxycycline (Doxy), enalaprilat, famotidine (Pepcid), floxuridine (FUDR), fluconazole (Diflucan), fludarabine (Fludara), ganciclovir (Cytovene), granisetron (Kytril), haloperidol (Haldol), hydrocortisone sodium phosphate, hydrocortisone sodium succinate (Solu-Cortef), hydromorphone (Dilaudid), hydroxyzine, idarubicin (Idamycin PFS), ifosfamide (Ifex), leucovorin, levofloxacin (Levaquin), lorazepam (Ativan), melphalan (Alkeran), mepiridine (Demerol), mesna (Mesnex), methotrexate, metoclopramide (Reglan), minocycline (Minocin), mitoxantrone (Novantrone), morphine, nalbuphine (Nubain), ondansetron (Zofran), potassium chloride, promethazine (Phenergan), ranitidine (Zantac), rituximab (Rituxan), sodium acetate, sodium bicarbonate, sulfamethoxazole-trimethoprim, ticarcillin (Ticar), ticarcillin-clavulanate (Timentin), tobramycin, trastuzumab (Herceptin), vancomycin, vinblastine (Velban), vincristine (Vincasar PFS), vinorelbine (Navelbine), zidovudine (Retrovir).

SIDE EFFECTS

Frequent

Nausea or vomiting (57%), mild to severe bone pain (22%) that occurs more frequently with high-dose IV form and less frequently with low-dose subcutaneous form; alopecia (18%), diarrhea (14%), fever (12%), fatigue (11%).

Occasional (5%-9%)

Anorexia, dyspnea, headache, cough, rash.

Rare (< 5%)

Psoriasis, hematuria or proteinuria, osteoporosis.

SERIOUS REACTIONS

• Long-term administration occasionally produces chronic neutropenia and splenomegaly.
• Splenic rupture, allergic-type reactions, and sickle cell crisis have occurred.
• Alveolar hemorrhage has occurred in healthy patients undergoing peripheral blood progenitor cell mobilization.
• Thrombocytopenia, myocardial infarction, and arrhythmias occur rarely.
• Adult respiratory distress syndrome may occur in patients with sepsis.

PRECAUTIONS & CONSIDERATIONS

Caution is warranted in patients with gout, malignancy with myeloid characteristics (because of the potential for granulocyte-colony-stimulating factor potential to act as a growth factor), preexisting cardiac conditions, and psoriasis. It is unknown whether filgrastim crosses the placenta or is distributed in breast milk. No age-related precautions have been noted in children or elderly patients. Avoid situations that might present risk for contracting an infectious disease, such as influenza.

Notify the physician of chest pain, chills, fever, palpitations, or severe bone pain. BP should be monitored for a transient decrease. Also, body temperature, hematocrit, CBC, and hepatic enzyme and serum uric acid levels should be assessed. CBC should be obtained before the start of filgrastim therapy and twice weekly thereafter. Those with preexisting cardiac conditions should be closely watched. Be alert for adult respiratory distress syndrome in those with sepsis.

Storage

Refrigerate vials for IV use. Filgrastim is stable for up to 24 h at room temperature, provided vial contents are clear and contain no particulate matter. The drug remains stable if accidentally exposed to freezing temperature. Store vials for SC use in refrigerator, but remove before use and allow to warm to room temperature.

Administration

! May be given by subcutaneous injection or short IV infusion (15-30 min) or by continuous IV infusion. Begin filgrastim therapy at least 24 h after last dose of chemotherapy; discontinue at least 24 h before next dose of chemotherapy. Begin therapy at least 24 h after bone marrow infusion.

For IV administration, use single-dose vial. Do not reenter vial. Do not shake. Dilute with 10-50 mL D5W to a concentration of 15 mcg/mL or higher. For a concentration from 5 to 14 mcg/mL, add 2 mL of 5% albumin to each 50 mL D5W to provide a final concentration of 2 mg/mL. Do not dilute to a final concentration of < 5 mcg/mL. For intermittent infusion (piggyback), infuse over 15-30 min. For continuous infusion, give single dose over 4-24 h. In all situations, flush

IV line with D5W before and after administration.

Finasteride
feen-as'ter-ide
(Propecia, Proscar)
Do not confuse Proscar with Posicor, ProSom, Prozac, or Psorcon.

CATEGORY AND SCHEDULE
Pregnancy Risk Category: X

Classification: 5-α-Reductase inhibitors, antiandrogens, hormones/hormone modifiers

MECHANISM OF ACTION
An androgen hormone inhibitor that inhibits 5-α-reductase, an intracellular enzyme that converts testosterone into dihydrotestosterone (DHT) in the prostate gland, resulting in a decreased serum DHT level. *Therapeutic Effect:* Reduces size of the prostate gland, decreases BPH symptoms, increases hair growth.

PHARMACOKINETICS

Route	Onset	Peak	Duration
PO	24 h	2-6 h	5-7 days

Rapidly absorbed from the GI tract. Protein binding: 90%. Widely distributed. Metabolized in the liver. *Half-life:* 6-8 h. Onset of clinical effect: 3-6 mo of continued therapy.

AVAILABILITY
Tablets (Propecia): 1 mg.
Tablets (Proscar): 5 mg.

INDICATIONS AND DOSAGES
▸ **Benign prostatic hyperplasia (BPH)**
PO
Adults, Elderly. 5 mg once a day (for a minimum of 6 mo).
▸ **Male-pattern hair loss**
PO
Adults. 1 mg/day (for a minimum of 3 mo).

OFF-LABEL USES
Adjuvant monotherapy after radical prostatectomy in treatment of prostate cancer, female hirsutism, prophylaxis of prostate cancer.

CONTRAINDICATIONS
Exposure to the patient's semen or handling of finasteride tablets or ingestion by those who are or may become pregnant.

INTERACTIONS
Drug
Androgens: Oppose finasteride.
Herbal
Saw palmetto: Effects may be additive on prostate tissue, but unstudied.
Food
None known.

DIAGNOSTIC TEST EFFECTS
Decreases (falsely) the serum prostate-specific antigen (PSA) level, even in patients with prostate cancer. After 6 mo of use, the PSA value should be doubled for comparison with normal levels in untreated men.

SIDE EFFECTS
Rare (1%-4%)
Gynecomastia, sexual dysfunction (impotence, decreased libido, decreased volume of ejaculate, ejaculation disorder), postural hypotension, weakness, dizziness.

SERIOUS REACTIONS

• Male breast neoplasia has been reported. High-grade prostate cancer has been reported.

PRECAUTIONS & CONSIDERATIONS

Caution is warranted in patients with hepatic impairment. Women who are or might be pregnant should not handle finasteride tablets because the drug may produce abnormal external genitalia in a male fetus. Finasteride is not indicated for use in children. The efficacy of this drug has not been established in elderly patients. It is unknown whether finasteride is excreted in breast milk, and it should not be taken by lactating women.

Finasteride may cause impotence and decrease ejaculate volume. Be aware that urinary flow might not improve, even if the prostate gland shrinks. Serum PSA determinations should be obtained before and periodically during therapy. Intake and output should also be monitored.

Administration

Do not break or crush film-coated tablets. Take finasteride without regard to food. Full therapeutic effect may take up to 6 mo.

Flavocoxid
fla-vo-cox′id
(Limbrel)
Do not confuse with Limbitrol.

CATEGORY AND SCHEDULE
Pregnancy Risk Category: Not classified.

Classification: Medical food, oral nutritional supplements

MECHANISM OF ACTION
An oral nutritional supplement that inhibits prostaglandin synthesis and arachidonic acid metabolism, reducing the production of leukotrienes. Also acts through an antioxidant mechanism. *Therapeutic Effect:* Produces anti-inflammatory and analgesic effects and increases mobility in osteoarthritis.

PHARMACOKINETICS
Undergoes hydrolysis at the gut mucosal border. Food decreases absorption. Little hepatic metabolism.

AVAILABILITY
Capsules: 250 mg, 500 mg.

INDICATIONS AND DOSAGES
▸ **Osteoarthritis**
PO
Adults 18 yr and older, Elderly.
250- or 500-mg capsule q12h.

CONTRAINDICATIONS
Hypersensitivity to flavocoxid and any component of flavocoxid.

INTERACTIONS
Drug
None known.
Herbal
None known.
Food
All foods: Decrease the absorption of flavocoxid.

DIAGNOSTIC TEST EFFECTS
None known.

SIDE EFFECTS
Rare (≥ 2%)
Increase in varicose veins, psoriasis, mild hypertension, fluid accumulation in knee, reduced flexibility.

SERIOUS REACTIONS
• GI bleeding, perforation, and ulceration occur rarely in patients currently or previously treated with NSAIDs or COX-2 inhibitors or with previous history of GI ulceration or bleeding.

F

PRECAUTIONS & CONSIDERATIONS
It is unknown whether flavocoxid crosses the placenta or is distributed in breast milk. Flavocoxid use is not recommended during pregnancy. The safety and efficacy of flavocoxid have not been established in children younger than 18 yr. No age-related precautions have been noted in elderly patients.

History of peptic ulcer: Therapeutic response, including improved grip strength, increased joint mobility, reduced joint tenderness, and relief of pain, stiffness, and swelling, should be assessed.

Administration
Do not take flavocoxid within 1 h of eating because food decreases the drug's absorption.

Flavoxate
fla-vox'ate
(Urispas)
Do not confuse Urispas with Urised.

CATEGORY AND SCHEDULE
Pregnancy Risk Category: B

Classification: Antispasmodic

MECHANISM OF ACTION
An anticholinergic that relaxes detrusor and other smooth muscles by cholinergic blockade, counteracting muscle spasm in the urinary tract. *Therapeutic Effect:* Produces anticholinergic, local anesthetic, and analgesic effects, relieving urinary symptoms.

AVAILABILITY
Tablets: 100 mg.

INDICATIONS AND DOSAGES
▸ **To relieve symptoms of nocturia, incontinence, suprapubic pain, dysuria, frequency and urgency associated with urologic conditions (symptomatic only).**
PO
Adults, Elderly, Adolescents.
100-200 mg 3-4 times a day.

CONTRAINDICATIONS
Duodenal or pyloric obstruction, GI hemorrhage or obstruction, ileus, lower urinary tract obstruction.

INTERACTIONS
Drug
Anticholingergic agents: May have additive effects.
Herbal
None known.
Food
None known.

DIAGNOSTIC TEST EFFECTS
None known.

SIDE EFFECTS
Frequent
Somnolence, dry mouth and throat.
Occasional
Constipation, difficult urination, blurred vision, dizziness, headache, increased light sensitivity, nausea, vomiting, abdominal pain.
Rare
Confusion (primarily in elderly), hypersensitivity, increased intraocular pressure, leukopenia.

SERIOUS REACTIONS

• Overdose may produce anticholinergic effects, including unsteadiness, severe dizziness, somnolence, fever, facial flushing, dyspnea, nervousness, and irritability.

PRECAUTIONS & CONSIDERATIONS

Caution is warranted in patients with glaucoma. Avoid tasks that require mental alertness and motor skills until response to the drug is established. Symptomatic relief should be assessed. Notify the physician of symptoms of flavoxate overdose, including unsteadiness, severe dizziness, drowsiness, fever, flushed face, shortness of breath, nervousness, and irritability.

Administration

Dosage of flavoxate should be reduced as symptoms improve. May administer with food if GI upset occurs.

Flecainide
fle´kah-nide
(Tambocor)

CATEGORY AND SCHEDULE
Pregnancy Risk Category: C

Classification: Antiarrhythmics, class IC

MECHANISM OF ACTION

An antiarrhythmic that slows atrial, AV, His-Purkinje, and intraventricular conduction. Decreases excitability, conduction velocity, and automaticity. *Therapeutic Effect:* Controls atrial, supraventricular, and ventricular arrhythmias.

AVAILABILITY

Tablets: 50 mg, 100 mg, 150 mg.

INDICATIONS AND DOSAGES
▶ **Life-threatening ventricular arrhythmias, sustained ventricular tachycardia**
PO
Adults, Elderly. Initially, 100 mg q12h, increased by 100 mg (50 mg twice a day) every 4 days until effective dose or maximum of 400 mg/day is attained. If CrCl 35 mL/min or less, initiate with 100 mg once daily or 50 mg twice daily.
▶ **Paroxysmal supraventricular tachycardia (PSVT), paroxysmal atrial fibrillation (PAF)**
PO
Adults, Elderly. Initially, 50 mg q12h, increased by 100 mg (50 mg twice a day) every 4 days until effective dose or maximum of 300 mg/day is attained.

CONTRAINDICATIONS

Cardiogenic shock, preexisting second- or third-degree AV block, right bundle-branch block (without presence of a pacemaker).

INTERACTIONS

Drug

Amiodarone: Decrease the usual flecainide dosage by 50%.
Antipsychotic agents, azoles, fluoroquinolones, macrolides, tricyclic antidepressants: May increase risk of cardiotoxicity, QT prolongation.
β blockers: May increase negative inotropic effects.
Bupropion, cinacalcet, quinidine, protease inhibitors: May increase flecainide concentrations.
Cimetidine: May increase flecainide concentrations.
Digoxin: May increase blood concentration of digoxin.
Other antiarrhythmics: May have additive effects.
Urinary acidifiers: May increase the excretion of flecainide.

F

Urinary alkalinizers: May decrease the excretion of flecainide.

Herbal

Black cohosh, gingko, ginseng: May increase flecainide concentrations.

Ephedra: May increase risk of cardiotoxicity.

Food

None known.

DIAGNOSTIC TEST EFFECTS

None significant.

SIDE EFFECTS

Frequent (10%-19%)

Dizziness, dyspnea, headache.

Occasional (4%-9%)

Nausea, fatigue, palpitations, chest pain, asthenia (loss of strength, energy), tremor, constipation.

SERIOUS REACTIONS

• Flecainide may worsen existing arrhythmias or produce new ones.

• Congestive heart failure (CHF) may occur, or existing CHF may worsen.

• Overdose may increase QRS duration, prolong QT interval, cause conduction disturbances, reduce myocardial contractility, and cause hypotension.

PRECAUTIONS & CONSIDERATIONS

Caution is warranted with CHF, recent MI, impaired myocardial function, second- and third-degree AV block (with pacemaker), and sick sinus syndrome. Be aware that therapeutic serum level is 0.2-1 mcg/mL. Nasal decongestant or OTC cold preparations should be avoided without physician approval.

SIDE EFFECTS

The side effects of flecainide therapy usually disappear with continued use or decreased dosage. Tasks that require mental alertness or motor skills should be avoided. Continuous cardiac monitoring should be given. ECG measurements, including QRS duration and QT interval, should be performed before and periodically during therapy. Pulmonary crackles, weight gain, intake and output, and dyspnea should be monitored in those with CHF.

Administration

Crush scored tablets as needed. May take without regard to food.

Fluconazole

floo-con′a-zole

(Apo-Fluconazole [CAN], Diflucan)

Do not confuse Diflucan with diclofenac.

CATEGORY AND SCHEDULE

Pregnancy Risk Category: C

Classification: Antifungals

MECHANISM OF ACTION

A fungistatic antifungal that interferes with cytochrome P-450, an enzyme necessary for ergosterol formation. *Therapeutic Effect:* Directly damages fungal membrane, altering its function.

PHARMACOKINETICS

Well absorbed from GI tract. Widely distributed, including to cerebrospinal fluid. Protein binding: 11%. Partially metabolized in the liver. Excreted unchanged, primarily in urine. Partially removed by hemodialysis. *Half-life:* 20-30 h (increased in impaired renal function).

AVAILABILITY

Tablets: 50 mg, 100 mg, 150 mg, 200 mg.

Powder for Oral Suspension:
10 mg/mL, 40 mg/mL.
Injection: 2 mg/mL (in 100- or
200-mL containers).

INDICATIONS AND DOSAGES
▸ **Oropharyngeal candidiasis**
PO, IV
Adults, Elderly. 200 mg once, then
100 mg/day for at least 14 days.
Children. 6 mg/kg/day once, then
3 mg/kg/day.
▸ **Esophageal candidiasis**
PO, IV
Adults, Elderly. 200 mg once, then
100 mg/day (up to 400 mg/day)
for 21 days and at least 14 days
following resolution of symptoms.
Children. 6 mg/kg/day once, then
3 mg/kg/day (up to 12 mg/kg/day)
for 21 days and at least 14 days
following resolution of symptoms.
▸ **Vaginal candidiasis**
PO
Adults. 150 mg once.
▸ **Prevention of candidiasis in
patients undergoing bone marrow
transplantation**
PO
Adults. 400 mg/day.
▸ **Systemic candidiasis**
PO, IV
Adults, Elderly. 400 mg once, then
200 mg/day (up to 400 mg/day) for
at least 28 days and at least 14 days
following resolution of symptoms.
Children. 6-12 mg/kg/day.
▸ **Cryptococcal meningitis**
PO, IV
Adults, Elderly. 400 mg once, then
200 mg/day (up to 800 mg/day) for
10-12 wks after cerebrospinal fluid
becomes negative (200 mg/day for
suppression of relapse in patients
with AIDS).
Children. 12 mg/kg/day once, then
6-12 mg/kg/day (6 mg/kg/day for
suppression of relapse in patients
with AIDS).

▸ **Onychomycosis**
PO
Adults. 150 mg/wk.
▸ **Dosage in renal impairment
(adults)**
After a loading dose of 400 mg, the
daily dosage is based on creatinine
clearance:

Creatinine Clearance	% of Recommended Dose
>50 mL/min	100
21-50 mL/min	50
11-20 mL/min	25
Dialysis	Dose after dialysis

OFF-LABEL USES
Treatment of coccidioidomycosis,
cryptococcosis, fungal pneumonia,
onychomycosis.

CONTRAINDICATIONS
None known.

INTERACTIONS
Drug
Cyclosporine: High fluconazole
doses increase cyclosporine blood
concentration.
Oral antidiabetics: May increase
blood concentration and effects of
oral antidiabetics.
Phenytoin, warfarin: May decrease
the metabolism of these drugs.
Rifampin: May increase fluconazole
metabolism.
Theophylline: May increase
theophylline concentrations.
Warfarin: Anticoagulant effect of
warfarin may be increased.
Herbal
None known.
Food
None known.

DIAGNOSTIC TEST EFFECTS
May increase serum alkaline
phosphatase, serum bilirubin, SGOT
(AST), and SGPT (ALT) levels.

Ⓘ IV INCOMPATIBILITIES

Amphotericin B (Fungizone), amphotericin B complex (Abelcet, AmBisome, Amphotec), ampicillin (Polycillin), calcium gluconate, cefotaxime (Claforan), ceftazidime (Fortaz), ceftriaxone (Rocephin), cefuroxime (Zinacef), chloramphenicol (Chloromycetin), clindamycin (Cleocin), co-trimoxazole (Bactrim), dantrolene (Dantrium), diazepam (Valium), digoxin (Lanoxin), erythromycin (Erythrocin), furosemide (Lasix), haloperidol (Haldol), hydroxyzine (Vistaril), imipenem and cilastatin (Primaxin), pantoprazole (Protonix), sulfamethoxazole and trimethoprim.

Ⓘ IV COMPATIBILITIES

Acyclovir, aldesleukin, alfentanil, allopurinol, amifostine, amikacin, aminophylline, amiodarone, ascorbic acid, atracurium, atropine, azathioprine, aztreonam, benztropine, bivalirudin, bretylium, bumetanide, buprenorphine, butorphanol, calcium chloride, carboplatin, cefamandole, cefazolin, cefepime, cefmetazole, cefonicid, cefoperazone, cefotetan, cefoxitin, ceftizoxime, cephalothin, chlorpromazine, cimetidine, cisatracurium, cisplatin, cyanocobalamin, cyclophosphamide, cyclosporine, dactinomycin, daptomycin, dexamethasone, Diltiazem (Cardizem), dimenhydrinate, diphenhydramine, dobutamine (Dobutrex), docetaxel, dopamine (Intropin), doripenem, doxacurium, doxycycline, droperidol, drotecogin alfa, enalaprilat, ephedrine sulfate, epinephrine, epirubicin, epoetin alfa, ertapenem, erythromycin lactobionate, esmolol, etoposide, famotidine, fenoldopam, fentanyl, filgrastim, fludarabine, fluorouracil, folic acid, foscarnet, furosemide, gallium nitrate, ganciclovir, gatifloxacin, gemcitabine, gentamicin, glycopyrrolate, granisetron, heparin, hetastarch 6% (Hextend), hydrocortisone sodium phosphate, hydrocortisone sodium succinate, hydromorphone, hydroxyzine, immune globulin, inamrinone lactate, indomethacin, insulin-regular, isoproterenol, ketorolac, labetolol, lactated Ringer's, lansoprazole, leucovorin, levofloxacin, lidocaine, linezolid, lorazepam (Ativan), magnesium sulfate, mannitol, meclorethamine, melphalan, meperidine, meropenem, metaraminol, methicillin, methoxamine, methyldopate, methylprednisolone, metoclopramide, metoprolol tartrate, metronidazole, mezlocillin, miconazole, midazolam (Versed), milrinone, minocycline, mitoxantrone, morphine sulfate, moxalactam, multiple vitamins, nafcillin, nalbuphine, naloxone, netilmicin, nitroglycerin, nitroprusside sodium, norepinephrine, ondansetron, oxacillin, paclitaxel, palonosetron, pancronium, pantoprazole, papaverine, pemetrexed, penicillin G potassium, penicillin G sodium, pentamidine, pentazocine, pentobarbital, phentolamine, phenylephrine, phytanadione, piperacillin and tazobactam, polymixin B, potassium chloride, procainamide, prochlorperazine, promethazine, propofol (Diprivan), propranolol, protamine sulfate, pyridooxine, quinidine, quinupristin and dalfopristin, ranitidine, remifentanil, ritodrine, rituximab, sargramostim, sodium acetate, sodium bicarbonate, streptokinase, succinylcholine, sufentanil, tacrolimus, teniposide, theophylline, thiotepa, ticarcillin, ticarcillin and clavulanate, tigecycline, tirofiban, tobramycin, tolazoline, trastuzumab, trimetaphan, urokinase, vancomycin, vasopressin, vecuronium, verapamil, vincristine, vinorelbine, voriconazole, zidovudine.

SIDE EFFECTS

Occasional (1%-4%)
Hypersensitivity reaction (including chills, fever, pruritus, and rash), dizziness, drowsiness, dyspepsia, headache, constipation, diarrhea, nausea, vomiting, abdominal pain, taste perversion.

SERIOUS REACTIONS

• Exfoliative skin disorders, serious hepatic effects, QT prolongation, torsade de pointes, seizures, and blood dyscrasias (such as eosinophilia, thrombocytopenia, anemia, and leukopenia) have been reported rarely.

PRECAUTIONS & CONSIDERATIONS

Caution is warranted in patients with liver or renal impairment; hypersensitivity to other triazoles, such as itraconazole or terconazole; or hypersensitivity to imidazoles, such as butoconazole and ketoconazole. Be aware that it is unknown whether fluconazole is excreted in breast milk. No age-related precautions have been noted in children. In elderly patients, age-related renal impairment may require dosage adjustment.

Expect to monitor the complete blood count (CBC), liver and renal function test results, platelet count, and serum potassium levels. Report any itching or rash promptly. Monitor the temperature daily. Assess the daily pattern of bowel activity and stool consistency. Evaluate for dizziness and provide assistance as needed; do not drive

or use machinery until response to the drug is established. If dark urine, pale stool, rash with or without itching, or yellow skin or eyes occur, notify the physician. Patients with oropharyngeal infections should be taught good oral hygiene. Administer with caution in patients with proarrhythmic conditions.

Storage
Store at room temperature.

Administration
Give oral fluconazole without regard to meals. Be aware that PO and IV therapy are equally effective and that IV therapy is for patients intolerant of the drug or unable to take it orally. Shake oral suspension well before each use.

For IV administration, do not remove from outer wrap until ready to use. Squeeze inner bag to check for leaks. Do not use parenteral form if the solution is cloudy, a precipitate forms, the seal is not intact, or it is discolored. Do not add another medication to the solution. Do not exceed maximum flow rate of 200 mg/h.

Flucytosine
floo-sye′toe-seen
(Ancobon)

CATEGORY AND SCHEDULE
Pregnancy Risk Category: C

Classification: Antifungals

MECHANISM OF ACTION

An antifungal that penetrates fungal cells and is converted to fluorouracil, which competes with uracil interfering with fungal RNA and protein synthesis. *Therapeutic Effect:* Damages fungal membrane.

PHARMACOKINETICS

Well absorbed from GI tract. Widely distributed, including cerebrospinal fluid. Protein binding: 2%-4%. Metabolized in liver. Partially removed by hemodialysis. *Half-life:* 3-8 h (half-life is increased with impaired renal function).

AVAILABILITY

Capsule: 250 mg, 500 mg.

INDICATIONS AND DOSAGES

▶ **Fungal infections, candidiasis, cryptococcosis**

PO

Adults, Elderly, Children.
50-150 mg/kg/day in equally divided doses q6h.

▶ **Dosage in renal function impairment**

Based on creatinine clearance:

Creatinine Clearance (mL/min)	Dosage Interval
20-40	q12h
10-20	q24h
0-10	q24-48h

CONTRAINDICATIONS

Hypersensitivity to flucytosine.

INTERACTIONS

Drug

Amphotericin B: May increase the effects of flucytosine.
Cytarabine: May decrease flucytosine efficacy.
Levomethadyl: May increase risk of cardiotoxicity.
Zidovudine: May increase the risk of hematologic toxicity.
Herbal
None known.
Food
None known.

DIAGNOSTIC TEST EFFECTS

May increase creatinine values if determined by the ektachem method.

SIDE EFFECTS

Occasional

Pruritus, rash, photosensitivity, dizziness, drowsiness, headache, diarrhea, nausea, vomiting, abdominal pain, increased liver enzymes, jaundice, increased BUN and creatinine, weakness, hearing loss.

SERIOUS REACTIONS

• Hepatic dysfunction and severe bone marrow suppression occur rarely.

PRECAUTIONS & CONSIDERATIONS

Caution is warranted in patients with liver or renal impairment, hematologic disease, or bone marrow suppression. Monotherapy should be avoided. It is unknown whether flucytosine is excreted in breast milk. No age-related precautions have been noted in children. In elderly patients, age-related renal impairment may require dosage adjustment.

Be alert to bone marrow suppressive symptoms. Unexplained fever, sore throat, rash or hives, trouble breathing, yellow skin or eyes, persistent chest pain, or bloody urine should be reported.

Blood concentrations, renal and hepatic function, and hematologic status should be monitored routinely.

Because of resistance, this medication should be used in combination with amphotericin B for treatment of systemic candidiasis and cryptococcosis.

Administration

To avoid GI upset, take a few capsules at a time over 15 min with food until full dose is taken. Flucytosine doses should be spaced evenly around the clock to promote less variation in peak and trough blood serum levels. Therapeutic blood serum level is 25-100 mcg/mL.

Peak should not exceed 100-120 mcg/mL to avoid bone marrow suppression.

Fludrocortisone
floo-droe-kor'ti-sone
(Florinef)
Do not confuse Florinef with Fioricet or Florinal.

CATEGORY AND SCHEDULE
Pregnancy Risk Category: C

Classification: Corticosteroid, mineralocorticoid

MECHANISM OF ACTION
A mineralocorticoid that acts at distal tubules. *Therapeutic Effect:* Increases potassium and hydrogen ion excretion. Replaces sodium loss and raises blood pressure (with low dosages). Inhibits endogenous adrenal cortical secretion, thymic activity, and secretion of corticotropin by pituitary gland (with higher dosages).

PHARMACOKINETICS
Well absorbed from the GI tract. Protein binding: 42%. Widely distributed. Metabolized in the liver and kidney. Primarily excreted in urine. *Half-life:* 3.5 h.

AVAILABILITY
Tablets: 0.1 mg.

INDICATIONS AND DOSAGES
▸ **Addison disease**
PO
Adults, Elderly. 0.05-0.1 mg/day. Range: 0.1 mg 3 times a wk to 0.2 mg/day. Administration with cortisone or hydrocortisone preferred.

▸ **Salt-losing adrenogenital syndrome**
PO
Adults, Elderly. 0.1-0.2 mg/day.
▸ **Usual pediatric dosage**
Children. 0.05-0.1 mg/day.

OFF-LABEL USES
Diagnosis of acidosis in renal tubular disorders, idiopathic orthostatic hypotension, congenital hypoaldosteronism, postoperative cerebral salt wasting syndrome.

CONTRAINDICATIONS
Systemic fungal infection.

INTERACTIONS
Drug
Antidiabetic agents (oral agents and insulin): Antidiabetic effect may be decreased. Monitor for signs of hyperglycemia; adjust dose if necessary.
Digoxin: May increase the risk of digoxin toxicity caused by hypokalemia.
Hepatic enzyme inducers (such as phenytoin): May increase the metabolism of fludrocortisone.
Hypokalemia-causing medications: May increase the effects of fludrocortisone.
Sodium-containing medications: May increase BP, incidence of edema, and serum sodium level.
Herbal and Food
None known.

DIAGNOSTIC TEST EFFECTS
May increase serum sodium level. May decrease Hct and serum potassium level.

SIDE EFFECTS
Frequent
Increased appetite, exaggerated sense of well-being, abdominal distention, weight gain, insomnia, mood swings.

F

High dosages, prolonged therapy, too rapid withdrawal: Increased susceptibility to infection with masked signs and symptoms, delayed wound healing, hypokalemia, hypocalcemia, GI distress, diarrhea or constipation, hypertension.

Occasional

Headache, dizziness, menstrual difficulty or amenorrhea, gastric ulcer development.

Rare

Hypersensitivity reaction.

SERIOUS REACTIONS

• Long-term therapy may cause muscle wasting (especially in the arms and legs), osteoporosis, spontaneous fractures, amenorrhea, cataracts, glaucoma, peptic ulcer disease, and congestive heart failure.

• Abruptly withdrawing the drug after long-term therapy may cause anorexia, nausea, fever, headache, joint pain, rebound inflammation, fatigue, weakness, lethargy, dizziness, and orthostatic hypotension.

PRECAUTIONS & CONSIDERATIONS

Caution is warranted with edema, hypertension, and impaired renal function. It is unknown whether fludrocortisone crosses the placenta or is distributed in breast milk. Fludrocortisone use in children may suppress growth and inhibit endogenous steroid production. Effects of fludrocortisone use in elderly patients are unknown.

Mood swings, ranging from euphoria to depression, may occur. Notify the physician of fever, muscle aches, sore throat, and sudden weight gain or swelling. Blood glucose level, serum renin, BP, serum electrolyte levels, height, and weight should be monitored before and during therapy. Be alert to signs and symptoms of infection caused by reduced immune response, including fever, sore throat, and vague symptoms.

Administration

Take fludrocortisone with food or milk. Taper the dosage slowly if fludrocortisone is to be discontinued. Expect to lower dosage if transient hypertension develops.

Flumazenil

flew-maz-ah-nil
(Anexate [CAN], Romazicon)

CATEGORY AND SCHEDULE

Pregnancy Risk Category: C

Classification: Antidotes

MECHANISM OF ACTION

An antidote that antagonizes the effect of benzodiazepines on the γ-aminobutyric acid receptor complex in the CNS. *Therapeutic Effect:* Reverses sedative effect of benzodiazepines.

PHARMACOKINETICS

Route	Onset	Peak	Duration
IV	1-2 min	6-10 min	< 1 h

Duration and degree of benzodiazepine reversal depend on dosage and plasma concentration. Protein binding: 50%. Metabolized by the liver; excreted in urine.

AVAILABILITY

Injection: 0.1 mg/mL.

INDICATIONS AND DOSAGES

▸ **Reversal of conscious sedation or general anesthesia**

IV

Adults, Elderly. Initially, 0.2 mg (2 mL) over 15 s; may repeat dose

in 45 s; then at 60-s intervals.
Maximum: 1 mg (10-mL) total
dose.
Children, Neonates. Initially,
0.01 mg/kg; may repeat in 45 s, then
at 60-s intervals. Maximum: 0.2-mg
single dose; 0.05-mg/kg or 1-mg
cumulative dose.
▸ **Benzodiazepine overdose**
IV
Adults, Elderly. Initially, 0.2 mg
(2 mL) over 30 s; if desired level of
consciousness is not achieved after
30 s, 0.3 mg (3 mL) may be given
over 30 s. Further doses of 0.5 mg
(5 mL) may be administered over
30 s at 60-s intervals. Maximum:
3 mg (30 mL) total dose. If
resedation occurs, may repeat
regimen in 20 min.
Children, Neonates. Initially,
0.01 mg/kg; may repeat in 45 s, then
at 60-s intervals. Maximum: 0.2-mg
single dose; 1-mg cumulative dose.

CONTRAINDICATIONS

Anticholinergic signs (such
as mydriasis, dry mucosa, and
hypoperistalsis), arrhythmias,
cardiovascular collapse,
history of hypersensitivity
to benzodiazepines, patients
with signs of serious cyclic
antidepressant overdose (such as
motor abnormalities), patients who
have been given a benzodiazepine
for control of a potentially life-
threatening condition (such as
control of status epilepticus or
increased intracranial pressure).

INTERACTIONS
Drug
Tricyclic antidepressants: May
produce seizures and arrhythmias
as flumazenil reverses the sedative
effects of tricyclic antidepressants.
Herbal and Food
None known.

DIAGNOSTIC TEST EFFECTS
None known.

IV INCOMPATIBILITIES
No information available for Y-site
administration.

IV COMPATIBILITIES
Heparin.

SIDE EFFECTS
Frequent (4%-11%)
Agitation, anxiety, dry mouth,
dyspnea, insomnia, palpitations,
tremors, headache, blurred vision,
dizziness, ataxia, nausea, vomiting,
pain at injection site, diaphoresis.
Occasional (1%-3%)
Fatigue, flushing, auditory
disturbances, thrombophlebitis, rash.
Rare (< 1%)
Urticaria, pruritus, hallucinations.

SERIOUS REACTIONS
• Toxic effects, such as seizures and
arrhythmias, of other drugs taken
in overdose, especially tricyclic
antidepressants; may emerge
with reversal of sedative effect of
benzodiazepines.
• Flumazenil may provoke a panic
attack in those with a history of
panic disorder.

PRECAUTIONS & CONSIDERATIONS
Caution is warranted with head
injury, impaired hepatic function,
alcoholism, or drug dependency. Be
aware that it is unknown whether
flumazenil crosses the placenta or
is distributed in breast milk. It is
not recommended during labor and
delivery. Be aware that flumazenil is
not approved for infants or neonates.
Be aware that benzodiazepine-
induced sedation tends to be deeper
and more prolonged, requiring
careful monitoring in elderly
patients. Be aware that flumazenil

may wear off before effects of benzodiazepines. Repeat dosing may be necessary. Obtain arterial blood gases before and at 30-min intervals during IV administration. Prepare to intervene in reestablishing airway, assisting ventilation. Tasks that require alertness or motor skills, ingestion of alcohol, or taking of nonprescription drugs should be avoided until at least 18-24 h after discharge.

Storage

Store parenteral form at room temperature. Discard after 24 h once medication is drawn into syringe, is mixed with any solutions, or if particulate or discoloration is noted.

Administration

Be aware that flumazenil is compatible with D5W, lactated Ringer's, or 0.9% NaCl. Be aware that if resedation occurs, dose should be repeated at 20-min intervals. Maximum: 1 mg (given as 0.2 mg/min) at any one time, 3 mg in any 1 h. Administer through freely running IV infusion into large vein (local injection produces pain, inflammation at injection site). For reversing conscious sedation or general anesthesia, administer over 15 s. For benzodiazepine overdose, administer over 30 s. Take care to avoid extravasation. Observe patient for at least 2 h for signs of resedation and hypoventilation.

Flunisolide

floo-niss'oh-lide
(AeroBid, Aerospan HFA, Nasalide, Nasarel, Rhinalar [CAN])
Do not confuse flunisolide with fluocinonide, or Nasalide with Nasalcrom.

CATEGORY AND SCHEDULE

Pregnancy Risk Category: C

Classification: Corticosteroids, inhalation

MECHANISM OF ACTION

An adrenocorticosteroid that controls the rate of protein synthesis, depresses migration of polymorphonuclear leukocytes, reverses capillary permeability, and stabilizes lysosomal membranes. *Therapeutic Effect:* Prevents or controls inflammation.

AVAILABILITY

Aerosol (AeroBid, Aerospan HFA): 250 mcg/activation, 80 mcg/activation.
Nasal Spray (Nasalide, Nasarel): 25 mcg/activation, 29 mcg/activation.

INDICATIONS AND DOSAGES

▸ **Long-term control of bronchial asthma, assists in reducing or discontinuing oral corticosteroid therapy**
INHALATION
Adults, Elderly. 2 inhalations twice a day, morning and evening. Maximum: 4 inhalations twice a day.
Children aged 6-15 yr. 2 inhalations twice a day.
▸ **Relief of symptoms of perennial and seasonal rhinitis**
INTRANASAL
Adults, Elderly. Initially, 2 sprays each nostril twice a day, may increase

at 4- to 7-day intervals to 2 sprays
3 times a day. Maximum: 8 sprays in
each nostril daily.
Children aged 6-14 yr. Initially,
1 spray 3 times a day or 2 sprays
twice a day. Maximum: 4 sprays
in each nostril daily. Maintenance:
1 spray into each nostril each day.

OFF-LABEL USES

To prevent recurrence of nasal
polyps after surgery,
bronchopulmonary dysplasia of
newborns, sinusitis.

CONTRAINDICATIONS

Hypersensitivity to any
corticosteroid, persistently positive
sputum cultures for *Candida
albicans,* primary treatment of
status asthmaticus, systemic fungal
infections, untreated local infection
(nasal).

INTERACTIONS

Drug
Bupropion: lowered seizure
threshold.
Herbal and Food
None known.

DIAGNOSTIC TEST EFFECTS

None known.

SIDE EFFECTS

Frequent
Inhalation (10%-25%):
Unpleasant taste, nausea, vomiting,
sore throat, diarrhea, upset stomach,
cold symptoms, nasal congestion.
Occasional
Inhalation (3%-9%): Dizziness,
irritability, nervousness, tremors,
abdominal pain, heartburn,
oropharynx candidiasis, edema.
Nasal: Mild nasopharyngeal
irritation or dryness, rebound
congestion, bronchial asthma,
rhinorrhea, altered taste.

SERIOUS REACTIONS

• An acute hypersensitivity reaction,
marked by urticaria, angioedema,
and severe bronchospasm, occurs
rarely.
• A transfer from systemic to
local steroid therapy may unmask
previously suppressed bronchial
asthma condition.
• Nasal septal perforation with
prolonged or inappropriate use of
nasal spray.

PRECAUTIONS & CONSIDERATIONS

Caution is warranted in patients with
adrenal insufficiency. Drink plenty
of fluids to decrease the thickness
of lung secretions. Pulse rate and
quality, ABG levels, and respiratory
rate, depth, rhythm, and type should
be monitored. Observe for cyanosis
manifested as lips and fingernails
with a blue or dusky color in light-
skinned patients; a gray color in
dark-skinned patients. Notify the
physician of nasal irritation or if
symptoms, such as sneezing, fail to
improve.
Administration
! Expect to see improvement of the
symptoms within a few days and
relief of symptoms within 3 wks.
Prepare to discontinue the drug after
3 wks if significant improvement
does not occur. Do not abruptly
discontinue or change the dosage
schedule. The dosage must be
tapered gradually under medical
supervision.
For inhalation, first shake the
container well. Exhale completely
and place the mouthpiece between
the lips. Inhale and hold breath for
as long as possible before exhaling.
Allow 1 min between inhalations
to promote deeper bronchial
penetration. Rinse mouth with water
immediately after inhalation to
prevent mouth and throat dryness

and oral candidiasis. If using a bronchodilator inhaler concomitantly with a steroid inhaler, use the bronchodilator several minutes before using the corticosteroid to help the steroid penetrate into the bronchial tree. Clear nasal passages before using flunisolide. This may require the use of a topical nasal decongestant 5-15 min before flunisolide use. Tilt head slightly forward. Insert spray tip up into the nostril, pointing toward inflamed nasal turbinates, away from the nasal septum. Spray the drug into the nostril while holding the other nostril closed, and at the same time inhale through the nose. Discard opened nasal solution after 3 mo.

Fluocinolone Acetonide
floo-oh-sin'oh-lone a-seat'oh-nide
(Capex, Derma-Smooth/FS, Fluoderm [CAN], Synalar, Tri-Luma)

CATEGORY AND SCHEDULE
Pregnancy Risk Category: C

Classification: Corticosteriods, topical, dermatologics

MECHANISM OF ACTION
A fluorinated topical corticosteroid that controls the rate of protein synthesis; depresses migration of polymorphonuclear leukocytes and fibroblasts; reduces capillary permeability; prevents or controls inflammation. *Therapeutic Effect:* Decreases tissue response to inflammatory process.

PHARMACOKINETICS
Use of occlusive dressings may increase percutaneous absorption. Protein binding: More than 90%. Excreted in urine. *Half-life:* Unknown.

AVAILABILITY
Cream: 0.01%, 0.025% (Synalar, Tri-Luma).
Oil: 0.01% (Derma-Smoothe/FS).
Ointment: 0.025% (Synalar).
Shampoo: 0.01% (Capex, FS).
Solution: 0.01% (Synalar).

INDICATIONS AND DOSAGES
▸ **Corticosteroid-responsive dermatoses**
TOPICAL
Adults, Elderly. Apply 3-4 times/day.
Children 2 yr and older. Apply 2 times/day.
▸ **Scalp psoriasis**
TOPICAL OIL
Adults, Elderly. Apply to damp or wet hair and leave on overnight or for at least 4 h. Remove by washing hair with shampoo.
▸ **Seborrheic dermatitis, scalp**
SHAMPOO
Adults, Elderly. Apply 1 OZ once daily. Allow to remain on scalp for at least 5 min.

CONTRAINDICATIONS
Hypersensitivity to fluocinolone or other corticosteroids.

INTERACTIONS
Drug, Herbal, and Food
None known.

DIAGNOSTIC TEST EFFECTS
None known.

SIDE EFFECTS

Occasional

Burning, dryness, itching, stinging.

Rare

Allergic contact dermatitis, purpura or blood-containing blisters, thinning of skin with easy bruising, telangiectasis or raised dark red spots on skin.

SERIOUS REACTIONS

• When taken in excessive quantities, systemic hypercorticism and adrenal suppression may occur.

PRECAUTIONS & CONSIDERATIONS

It is unknown whether fluocinolone crosses the placenta and is distributed in breast milk. Be aware that the safety and efficacy of fluocinolone have not been established in children younger than 2 yr. Be aware that children may absorb larger amounts of topical corticosteroids, which should be used sparingly. No age-related precautions have been noted in elderly patients. HPA axis suppression should be monitored by urinary free cortisol tests and an ACTH stimulation test.

Storage

Store at room temperature. Shampoo is stable for 3 mo after mixing by pharmacist.

Administration

Gently cleanse area before topical application. Use occlusive dressings only as ordered. Apply sparingly, and rub into area thoroughly. When using topical oil preparation on scalp, massage through dampened hair and scalp. Cover with shower cap. Leave on overnight or for at least 4 h. Remove by washing hair with shampoo. When using shampoo preparation, first shake well. Apply to wet hair, massage for 1 min, and allow to remain on scalp for 5 min. Rinse thoroughly.

Fluorescein
flure′e-seen
(AK-Fluor, Angiscein, Diofluor [CAN], Fluorescite, Fluorets, Fluor-I-Strip, Fluor-I-Strip-AT, Ful-Glo)
Do not confuse with fluoride.

CATEGORY AND SCHEDULE

Pregnancy Risk Category: X (parenteral), C (topical)

Classification: Diagnostics, nonradioactive, ophthalmic

MECHANISM OF ACTION

An indicator dye used as a diagnostic agent with a low molecular weight, high water solubility, and fluorescence that penetrates any break in epithelial barrier to permit rapid penetration. Emits light at a wavelength of 520-530 nm (green-yellow) when exposed to light in the blue wavelength (465-490 nm). *Therapeutic Effect:* Diagnosis of corneal and conjunctival abnormalities.

PHARMACOKINETICS

Rapidly absorbed. Protein binding: 85%. Widely distributed. Metabolized in liver to an active metabolite, fluorescein monoglucuronide. Primarily excreted in urine. *Half-life:* 24 min (parent compound), 4 h (metabolite).

AVAILABILITY

Injection, solution: 10% (AK-Fluor, Angiscein, Fluorescite), 25% (AK-Fluor, Fluorescite).
Strip, ophthalmic: 0.6 mg (Ful-Glo), 1 mg (Fluorets, Fluor-I-Strip-AT), 9 mg (Fluor-I-Strip).

INDICATIONS AND DOSAGES
▸ **Retinal angiography**
INJECTION
Adults, Elderly. Inject contents
(500 mg) of ampule or vial of
10% or 25% solution rapidly
into the antecubital vein. If laser
ophthalmoscope used, a reduced dose
of 200 mg may be appropriate.
Children. 7.7 mg/kg (actual body
weight) not to exceed 500 mg.
▸ **Applanation tonometry**
OPHTHLALMIC STRIPS
Adults, Elderly. Place strip, which
has been moistened with a drop of
sterile water, at the fornix in the lower
cul-de-sac close to the punctum.
Patient should close lid tightly over
strip until desired amount of staining
is observed or retract upper lid
and touch tip of strip to the bulbar
conjunctiva on the temporal side until
adequate staining is achieved.

CONTRAINDICATIONS
Concomitant soft contact lens use
(ophthalmic strips), hypersensitivity
to fluorescein or any component of
the formulation.

INTERACTIONS
Drug, Herbal, and Food
None known.

IV COMPATIBILITIES
Do not mix or dilute with other
solutions on drugs.

DIAGNOSTIC TEST EFFECTS
May interfere with digoxin assay
results.

SIDE EFFECTS
Occasional
Ophthalmic: Burning sensation in
the eye.
Injection: Stinging, bronchospasm,
generalized hives and itching,
hypersensitivity, headache,
gastrointestinal distress, nausea, strong
taste, vomiting, hypotension, syncope.
Rare
Injection: Anaphylaxis, basilar artery
ischemia, cardiac arrest, severe
shock, convulsions, thrombophlebitis
at injection site.

SERIOUS REACTIONS
• Anaphylactic reactions have
occurred, leading to laryngeal edema,
bronchospasm, shock, and even death.

PRECAUTIONS & CONSIDERATIONS
Injection preparation should be used
cautiously with bronchial asthma
or history of allergy. It is unknown
whether fluorescein crosses the
placenta or is distributed in breast
milk. Safety and efficacy have not
been established in children. No
age-related precautions have been
noted in elderly patients. Blockages
or leakage should be assessed on
map location for possible treatment.
Normal values will appear normal in
size. Skin and urine may temporarily
turn yellow. Abnormal results can
mean diabetic or other retinopathy,
macular degeneration, cancer, tumors,
circulatory problems, inflammation or
edema, microaneurysms, or swelling
of the optic disc.
Storage
Store at room temperature. Do not
freeze.
Administration
Allow a few seconds for staining
when using ophthalmic preparation.
Wash out excess with sterile water
or irrigating solution. Blink several
times after application of strip.
　For fluorescein injection, inject
rapidly into antecubital vein (5-10s).
　Flush IV cannula with saline flush
before and after use to prevent physical
incompatability with other drugs.

Fluoride, Sodium
(Fluor-A-Day, Fluorigard, Fluotic [CAN], Flura-Drops, Luride, NeutroGard, Pediaflor)
Do not confuse with Fludara.

CATEGORY AND SCHEDULE
Pregnancy Risk Category: N/A

Classification: Dental preparations, vitamins/minerals

MECHANISM OF ACTION
A trace element that increases tooth resistance to acid dissolution. *Therapeutic Effect:* Promotes remineralization of decalcified enamel, inhibits dental plaque bacteria, increases resistance to development of caries, maintains bone strength.

AVAILABILITY
Oral Solution Drops: 0.25 mg/mL, 0.5 mg/mL.
Tablets (Chewable): 0.25 mg, 0.5 mg, 1 mg.

INDICATIONS AND DOSAGES
▸ **Dietary supplement for prevention of dental caries in children**

Fluoride Level in Water (ppm)	Age	Oral Dosage (mg/day)
< 0.3	expressed as fluoride 6 mo to 2 yr	0.25
	3-5 yr	0.5
	6-16 yr	1
0.3-0.6	Younger than 2 yr	None
	3-5 yr	0.25
	6-16 yr	0.5

ppm, Parts per million.

CONTRAINDICATIONS
Arthralgia, GI ulceration, severe renal insufficiency (CrCl < 20 mL/min), areas where fluoride level in water exceeds 0.7 ppm.

INTERACTIONS
Drug
Aluminum hydroxide, calcium: May decrease the absorption of fluoride.
Herbal
None known.
Food
Dairy products: May decrease fluoride's absorption.

DIAGNOSTIC TEST EFFECTS
May increase serum alkaline phosphatase and AST (SGOT) levels.

SIDE EFFECTS
Rare
Oral mucous membrane ulceration.

SERIOUS REACTIONS
• Hypocalcemia, tetany, bone pain (especially in ankles and feet), electrolyte disturbances, and arrhythmias occur rarely.
• Fluoride use may cause skeletal fluorosis, osteomalacia, and osteosclerosis.

PRECAUTIONS & CONSIDERATIONS
Fluoride should not be taken with dairy products because they may decrease fluoride's absorption.
Administration
Chewable tablets should be chewed before swallowing. Oral drops can be given directly in mouth or mixed with cereal or fruit juice.

Administration at bedtime after brushing teeth is recommended for tablets.

There are many topical forms of fluoride for dental use. Always supervise young children. Avoid ingestion of any of these products.

F

F

Fluorouracil, 5FU
flure-oh-yoor´-ah-sill
(Adrucil, Carac, Efudex,
Efudix [AUS], Fluoroplex)
**Do not confuse Efudex with
Efidac.**

CATEGORY AND SCHEDULE
Pregnancy Risk Category: D

Classification: antineoplastic,
antimetabolite

MECHANISM OF ACTION
An antimetabolite that blocks
formation of thymidylic acid. Cell-
cycle–specific for S phase of cell
division. *Therapeutic Effect:* Inhibits
DNA and RNA synthesis. Topical
form destroys rapidly proliferating
cells.

PHARMACOKINETICS
Widely distributed. Crosses the
blood-brain barrier. Rapidly
metabolized in tissues to active
metabolite, which is localized
intracellularly. Primarily excreted by
lungs as carbon dioxide. Removed by
hemodialysis. *Half-life:* 20 h.

AVAILABILITY
Cream: 0.5%, 1%, 5%.
Solution, Topical: 2%, 5%.
Injection: 50 mg/mL.

INDICATIONS AND DOSAGES
▶**Carcinoma of breast, colon,
pancreas, rectum, and stomach; in
combination with levamisole after
surgical resection in patients with
Duke's stage C colon cancer**
IV
Adults, Elderly. Initially, 12 mg/kg/
day for 4-5 days. Maximum: 800
mg/day. followed by 6 mg/kg every
other day for 4 doses: Maintenance:

repeat initial dose every 30 days; or
10-15 mg/kg/wk as a single dose not
to exceed 1 g/wk.
! Note: After adult IV doses given,
lower dosages are recommended for
debilitated patients.
▶**Multiple actinic or solar keratoses**
TOPICAL 0.5% CREAM
Adults, Elderly. Apply once a day.
TOPICAL 1% & 5% CREAM, 2%
SOLUTION
Adults, Elderly. Apply twice a day.
▶**Basal cell carcinoma**
TOPICAL 5% SOLUTION
Adult, Elderly. Apply twice a day.

CONTRAINDICATIONS
Myelosuppression, poor nutritional
status, potentially serious infections,
hypersensitivity to fluorouracil or
product ingredients, dihydropyrmidine
dehydrogenase enzyme deficiency.

DRUG INTERACTIONS
**Leucovorin, levoleucovorin,
metronidazole, tinidazole:**
Increased fluorouracil toxicity.
Warfarin: Increased risk of bleeding.

⚘ IV INCOMPATIBILITIES
Cisplatin, cytarabine, diazepam,
doxorubicin, droperidol, filgrastim,
gallium nitrate, leucovorin,
levoleucovorin, methotrexate,
metoclopramide, morphine,
ondansetron, TPN, vinorelbine.

SIDE EFFECTS
Occasional
Parenteral: Anorexia, diarrhea,
minimal alopecia, fever, dry skin,
skin fissures, scaling, erythema.
Topical: Pain, pruritus,
hyperpigmentation, irritation,
inflammation, and burning at
application site; photosensitivity.
Rare
Nausea, vomiting, anemia, esophagitis,
proctitis, GI ulcer, confusion,

headache, lacrimation, visual disturbances, angina, allergic reactions.

SERIOUS REACTIONS

• The earliest sign of toxicity, which may occur 4-8 days after beginning therapy, is stomatitis (as evidenced by dry mouth, burning sensation, mucosal erythema, and ulceration at inner margin of lips).

• Hematologic toxicity may be manifested as leukopenia (generally within 9-14 days after drug administration, but possibly as late as the 25th day), thrombocytopenia (within 7-17 days after administration), pancytopenia, or agranulocytosis.

• The most common dermatologic toxicity is a pruritic rash on the extremities or, less frequently, the trunk.

PRECAUTIONS & CONSIDERATIONS

Patients should be hospitalized during the initial course of IV fluorouracil therapy. Use with caution in patients with a history of high-dose pelvic irradiation or previous use of alkylating agents, metastatic bone marrow involvement, or impaired hepatic or renal function. Discontinue therapy in patients developing stomatitis, leukopenia, intractable vomiting, diarrhea, GI ulceration or bleeding, thrombocytopenia, or hemorrhage from any site. Severe toxicity (abdominal pain, bloody diarrhea, neutropenia, neurotoxicity, chills, fever or vomiting) while receiving topical or systemic fluorouracil may occur in those with dipyrimidine dehydrogenase (DPD) deficiency; deficiency results in prolonged fluorouracil clearance. It is not known if fluorouracil is excreted in breast milk; avoid use. Safety and effectiveness of topical fluorouracil

have not been established in children. No age-related precautions have been observed in the elderly. Avoid application of topical fluorouracil to mucous membranes. Use with occlusive dressings cautiously; may increase penetration and incidence of inflammatory reactions in adjacent healthy skin. Avoid prolonged exposure to sunlight.

Storage
Injectable, topical cream and solution should be stored at room temperature.

Administration
Fluorouracil injection should be administered IV, either by slow IV push or IV infusion. Use care to avoid extravasation. No dilution is required.

Cleanse the affected area and wait 10 min before applying topical fluorouracil. Apply with fingertips and wash hands as soon as finish application. A moisturizer/sunscreen may be applied 2 h after fluorouracil.

Fluoxetine

floo-ox′e-teen
(Auscap [AUS], Fluohexal [AUS], Lovan [AUS], Novo-Fluoxetine [CAN], Prozac, Prozac Weekly, Sarafem, Zactin [AUS])
Do not confuse fluoxetine with fluvastatin; Prozac with Prilosec, Proscar, or ProSom; or Sarafem with Serophene.

CATEGORY AND SCHEDULE

Pregnancy Risk Category: C

Classification: Antidepressants, serotonin specific reuptake inhibitors

MECHANISM OF ACTION
A psychotherapeutic agent that selectively inhibits serotonin uptake in the CNS, enhancing serotonergic function. *Therapeutic Effect:* Relieves depression; reduces obsessive-compulsive and bulimic behavior.

PHARMACOKINETICS
Well absorbed from the GI tract. Crosses the blood-brain barrier. Protein binding: 94%. Metabolized in the liver to active metabolite. Primarily excreted in urine. Not removed by hemodialysis. *Half-life:* 2-3 days; metabolite 7-9 days.

AVAILABILITY
Capsules (Prozac): 10 mg, 20 mg, 40 mg.
Capsules (Sarafem): 10 mg, 20 mg.
Capsules (Enteric Coated [Prozac Weekly]): 90 mg.
Oral Solution (Prozac): 20 mg/5 mL.
Tablets (Prozac): 10 mg, 20 mg.
Tablets (Sarafem): 10 mg, 15 mg, 20 mg.

INDICATIONS AND DOSAGES
▸ **Depression, obsessive-compulsive disorder**
PO
Adults and Elderly. Initially, 20 mg each morning. If therapeutic improvement does not occur after 2 wks, gradually increase to maximum of 80 mg/day in 2 equally divided doses in morning and at noon. Prozac Weekly: 90 mg/wk, begin 7 days after last dose of 20 mg.
Children aged 8 yr and older for depression, 7 yr and older for OCD. Initially, 10-20 mg/day. Begin with 10 mg/day in lower weight or younger children. Usual dosage is 20 mg/day. Do not exceed 60 mg/day for OCD.
▸ **Panic disorder**
PO
Adults, Elderly. Initially, 10 mg/day. May increase to 20 mg/day after 1 wk. Maximum: 60 mg/day.

▸ **Bulimia nervosa**
PO
Adults. 60 mg each morning. May need to titrate up from lower dosage.
▸ **Premenstrual dysphoric disorder**
PO
Adults. 20 mg/day continuously, or 20 mg/day starting 14 days before the anticipated start of menstruation and continue through the first full day of menses.

OFF-LABEL USES
Treatment of hot flashes, fibromyalgia, posttraumatic stress disorder.

CONTRAINDICATIONS
Use within 14 days of MAOIs, hypersensitivity.

INTERACTIONS
Drug
Alcohol, other CNS depressants: May increase CNS depression.
Highly protein-bound medications (including oral anticoagulants): May increase adverse effects.
MAOIs: May produce serotonin syndrome and neuroleptic malignant syndrome. Contraindicated.
Phenytoin: May increase phenytoin blood concentration and risk of toxicity.
Serotonergic agents: Increased risk of serotonin syndrome.
Herbal
St. John's wort: May increase fluoxetine's pharmacologic effects and risk of toxicity.
Food
None known.

DIAGNOSTIC TEST EFFECTS
May increase liver enzymes.

SIDE EFFECTS
Frequent (> 10%)
Headache, asthenia, insomnia, anxiety, nervousness, somnolence, nausea, diarrhea, decreased appetite.

Occasional (2%-9%)
Dizziness, tremor, fatigue, vomiting, constipation, dry mouth, abdominal pain, nasal congestion, diaphoresis, rash.
Rare (< 2%)
Flushed skin, light-headedness, impaired concentration.

SERIOUS REACTIONS
• Overdose may produce seizures, nausea, vomiting, agitation, and restlessness (serotonin syndrome). As a result of long half-life, effects may be prolonged.

PRECAUTIONS & CONSIDERATIONS
Clinical worsening and suicidality have been noted with this class of agents.

Caution is warranted with cardiac dysfunction, diabetes, seizure disorder, and in those at high risk for suicide. It is unknown whether fluoxetine crosses the placenta or is distributed in breast milk. Children may be more sensitive to the drug's behavioral side effects, such as insomnia and restlessness. No age-related precautions have been noted in elderly patients.

Drowsiness and dizziness may occur, so avoid alcohol and tasks that require mental alertness or motor skills. CBC and liver and renal function tests should be performed before and periodically during long-term therapy. Assess pattern of daily bowel activity and stool consistency, skin for rash, and blood glucose level.
Administration
! Make sure that at least 14 days elapse between the use of MAOIs and fluoxetine. Expect to decrease dosage or frequency in elderly patients, in those with hepatic or renal impairment or a preexisting disease, and in those who take multiple medications.

Take fluoxetine with food or milk if GI distress occurs. Avoid administration at night. The therapeutic effects of fluoxetine will be noted within 1 to 4 wks. Do not abruptly discontinue fluoxetine. Divided doses can be given at morning and noon.

The full therapeutic effect may be delayed up to 5 wks of treatment or longer.

Prozac weekly: Swallow whole; do not crush or chew.

Fluoxymesterone
floo-ex-ih-mes-te-rone
(Androxy, Halotestin [CAN])

CATEGORY AND SCHEDULE
Pregnancy Risk Category: X
Controlled substance:
Schedule III

Classification: Androgens, hormones/hormone modifiers

MECHANISM OF ACTION
An androgen that suppresses gonadotropin-releasing hormone, LH, and FSH. *Therapeutic Effect:* Stimulates spermatogenesis, development of male secondary sex characteristics, and sexual maturation at puberty. Stimulates production of red blood cells (RBCs).

PHARMACOKINETICS
Rapidly absorbed from the GI tract. Protein binding: 98%. Metabolized in liver. Excreted in urine. *Half-life:* 9.2 h.

AVAILABILITY
Tablets: 10 mg.

INDICATIONS AND DOSAGES
▸ **Males (hypogonadism)**
PO
Adults. 5-20 mg/day.
▸ **Males (delayed puberty)**

PO
Adults. 2.5-10 mg/day for 4-6 mo.
Maximum: 20 mg/day.
▸**Females (inoperable breast cancer)**
PO
Adults. 10-40 mg/day in divided
doses for 1-3 mo.
Dosage must be strictly
individualized; suggested dose
for androgens varies, depending
on the age, sex, and diagnosis of the
patient. Dosage is adjusted according
to the patient's response and the
appearance of adverse reactions.

CONTRAINDICATIONS

Serious cardiac, renal, or hepatic
dysfunction, men with carcinomas of
the breast or prostate, hypersensitivity
to fluoxymesterone or any component
of the formulation including tartrazine,
known or suspected pregnancy,
breast-feeding.

INTERACTIONS

Drug
Cyclosporine: May increase the risk
of cyclosporine toxicity.
Hepatotoxic medications: May
increase the risk of hepatotoxicity.
Oral anticoagulants: May increase
the effect of these drugs.
Herbal
Chaparral, comfrey, eucalyptus,
germander, Jin Bu Huan, kava kava,
pennyroyal, skullcap, valerian:
May increase the risk of liver
damage.
Food
None known.

DIAGNOSTIC TEST EFFECTS

May decrease levels of thyroxine-
binding globulin, total T4 serum
levels, and resin uptake of T3 and T4.
May increase alkaline phosphatase,
SGOT (AST), bilirubin, calcium,
potassium, sodium, hemoglobin,
hematocrit, LDL. May decrease HDL.

SIDE EFFECTS

Frequent
Females: Amenorrhea, virilism
(e.g., acne, decreased breast size,
enlarged clitoris, male pattern
baldness), deepening voice.
Males: Urinary tract infection, breast
soreness, gynecomastia, priapism,
virilism (e.g., acne, early pubic hair
growth).
Occasional
Edema, nausea, vomiting, mild acne,
diarrhea, stomach pain.
Males: Impotence, testicular atrophy.

SERIOUS REACTIONS

• Peliosis hepatitis (liver, spleen
replaced with blood-filled
cysts), hepatic neoplasms, and
hepatocellular carcinoma have been
associated with prolonged high
dosage.

PRECAUTIONS & CONSIDERATIONS

Caution is warranted with impaired
renal or liver function, benign
prostate hypertrophy, hypercalcemia
(may be aggravated in patients with
metastatic breast cancer), history
of myocardial infarction, and
diabetes mellitus. Fluoxymesterone
use is contraindicated during
lactation. Safety and efficacy of
fluoxymesterone have not been
established in children, so use with
caution. Fluoxymesterone use in
elderly patients may increase the
risk of hyperplasia or stimulate
growth of occult prostate carcinoma.
Acne, nausea, pedal edema, or
vomiting should be reported to the
physician. In particular, female
patients should report deepening of
voice, hoarseness, and menstrual
irregularities; male patients should
report difficulty urinating, frequent
erections, and gynecomastia.
Patients should be monitored for
hypercalcemia.

Administration
Give with food to minimize GI upset.
May cut scored tablet to adjust dosage.

Fluphenazine
floo-fen′a-zeen
(Anatensol [AUS], Modecate [AUS],
Moditen [CAN], Permitil, Prolixin,
Prolixin Decanoate)
**Do not confuse Moditen with
Modane or Mobidin.**

CATEGORY AND SCHEDULE
Pregnancy Risk Category: C

Classification: Antipsychotics,
phenothiazines

MECHANISM OF ACTION
A phenothiazine that antagonizes
dopamine neurotransmission at
synapses by blocking postsynaptic
dopaminergic receptors in the brain.
Therapeutic Effect: Decreases
psychotic behavior. Also produces
weak anticholinergic, sedative,
and antiemetic effects and strong
extrapyramidal effects.

AVAILABILITY
Elixir (Prolixin): 2.5 mg/5 mL.
Tablets (Prolixin): 1 mg, 2.5 mg,
5 mg, 10 mg.
Injection (Prolixin): 2.5 mg/mL.
*Injection Suspension (Prolixin
Decanoate):* 25 mg/mL.

INDICATIONS AND DOSAGES
▸ **Psychosis**
PO
Adults, Elderly. 0.5-10 mg/day in
divided doses q6-8h. Doses above
20 mg/day are rarely needed.
IM
Adults, Elderly. Initially, 1.25-2.5 mg
IM q6-8 h. Usual effective dose:
1.5-10 mg/day. Divided doses q6-8h
or 12.5 mg (decanoate) q3 wks.

CONTRAINDICATIONS
Severe CNS depression, comatose
states, severe depression, subcortical
brain damage, presence of blood
dyscrasias or liver damage,
hypersensitivity to fluphenazine or
any component of the formulation
including tartrazine.

INTERACTIONS
Drug
Alcohol, other CNS depressants:
May increase hypotensive and CNS
and respiratory depressant effects.
Antithyroid agents: May increase
the risk of agranulocytosis.
**Extrapyramidal symptom-
producing medications:** May
increase extrapyramidal symptoms.
**Hypotension-producing
medications:** May increase
hypotension.
Levodopa: May decrease the effects
of this drug.
Lithium: May decrease the
absorption of fluphenazine and
produce adverse neurologic effects.
MAOIs, tricyclic antidepressants:
May increase anticholinergic and
sedative effects.
Herbal and Food
None known.

DIAGNOSTIC TEST EFFECTS
May produce false-positive pregnancy
and phenylketonuria test results. May
cause ECG changes, including Q- and
T-wave disturbances.

SIDE EFFECTS
Frequent
Hypotension, dizziness, and syncope
(occur frequently after first injection,
occasionally after subsequent
injections, and rarely with oral
doses).

Occasional
Somnolence (during early therapy), dry mouth, blurred vision, lethargy, constipation or diarrhea, nasal congestion, peripheral edema, urine retention.

Rare
Ocular changes, altered skin pigmentation (with prolonged use of high doses).

SERIOUS REACTIONS

• Extrapyramidal symptoms appear to be related to high dosages and are divided into three categories: akathisia (inability to sit still, tapping of feet), parkinsonian symptoms (such as hypersalivation, masklike facial expression, shuffling gait, and tremors), and acute dystonias (such as torticollis, opisthotonos, and oculogyric crisis).

• Tardive dyskinesia, manifested as tongue protrusion, puffing of the cheeks, and chewing or puckering of the mouth, occurs rarely but may be irreversible.

• Abrupt withdrawal after long-term therapy may precipitate dizziness, gastritis, nausea and vomiting, and tremors.

• Blood dyscrasias, particularly agranulocytosis and mild leukopenia, may occur.

• Fluphenazine use may lower the seizure threshold.

PRECAUTIONS & CONSIDERATIONS

Caution is warranted with Parkinson disease and seizures. Drowsiness may occur, so tasks that require mental alertness or motor skills should be avoided. Exposure to light and sunlight should also be avoided. Signs of tardive dyskinesia such as fine tongue movement and therapeutic response should be monitored. BP for hypotension, WBC for blood dyscrasias, and therapeutic response should be assessed during therapy. This medication is known to cross the placenta, and it is unknown if it appears in breast milk.

Administration
May take with food to decrease GI effects. Do not take antacids within 1 h of trifluoperazine. For IM use, administer deep injection in large muscle mass, keep patient recumbert for 30 min after injection to minimize hypotension.

Fluphenazine Decanoate

(Apo-Fluphenazine [CAN], Modecate [AUS], Prolixin); fluphenazine enanthate (Moditen [CAN], Prolixin); fluphenazine hydrochloride (Prolixin, Permitil)

CATEGORY AND SCHEDULE
Pregnancy Risk Category: C

Classification: Antipsychotics, phenothiazines

MECHANISM OF ACTION

A phenothiazine that blocks dopamine at postsynaptic receptor sites. Possesses weak anticholinergic, sedative, and entimetic effects and strong extrapyramidal activity. *Therapeutic Effect:* Decreases psychotic behavior.

PHARMACOKINETICS

Erratic and variable absorption from the GI tract. Widely distributed. Metabolized in liver. Primarily excreted in urine. *Half-life:* 163-232 h.

AVAILABILITY
Elixir, as Hydrochloride:
2.5 mg/5 mL (Prolixin).
Injection, as Decanoate: 25 mg/mL (Prolixin).
Injection, as Enanthate: 25 mg/mL (Prolixin).
Injection Solution, as Hydrochloride:
2.5 mg/mL (Prolixin).
Oral Solution, as Hydrochloride:
5 mg/mL (Prolixin).
Tablets, as Hydrochloride: 1 mg,
2.5 mg, 5 mg, 10 mg (Prolixin).

INDICATIONS AND DOSAGES
▶ **Psychotic disorders**
PO
Adults. Initially, 0.5-10 mg/day fluphenazine HCl in divided doses q6-8h. Increase gradually until therapeutic response is achieved (usually under 20 mg daily); decrease gradually to maintenance level (1-5 mg/day).
Elderly. Initially, 1-2.5 mg/day.
IM
Adults. Initially, 1.25 mg, followed by 2.5-10 mg/day in divided doses q6-8h.
▶ **Chronic schizophrenic disorder**
IM
*Adults.*Initially, 12.5-25 mg of fluphenazine decanoate q1-6wk, or 25 mg fluphenazine enanthate q2wk. Usual elderly dosage (nonpsychotic).
PO
Initially, 1-2.5 mg/day. May increase by 1-2.5 mg/day q4-7days.
Maximum: 20 mg/day.

OFF-LABEL USES
Treatment of neurogenic pain (adjunct to tricyclic antidepressants).

CONTRAINDICATIONS
Severe CNS depression, comatose states, severe depression, subcortical brain damage, presence of blood dyscrasias or liver damage, hypersensitivity to fluphenazine or any component of the formulation including tartrazine.

INTERACTIONS
Drug
Alcohol, CNS depressants: May increase respiratory depression and the hypotensive effects of fluphenazine.
Antithyroid agents: May increase the risk of agranulocytosis.
Extrapyramidal symptom (EPS)-producing medications: May increase EPSs.
Hypotensives: May increase hypotension.
Levodopa: May decrease the effects of levodopa.
Lithium: May decrease the absorption of fluphenazine and produce adverse neurologic effects.
MAOIs, tricyclic antidepressants: May increase the anticholinergic and sedative effects of fluphenazine.
Herbal
Dong quai, kava kava, gotu kola, St. John's wort, valerian: May increase risk of photosensitization or CNS depression.
Food
None known.

DIAGNOSTIC TEST EFFECTS
May produce false-positive pregnancy test, phenylketonuria. ECG changes may occur, including Q- and T-wave disturbances.

SIDE EFFECTS
Frequent
Hypotension, dizziness, and fainting occur frequently after first injection, occasionally after subsequent injections, and rarely with oral dosage.
Occasional
Drowsiness during early therapy, dry mouth, blurred vision, lethargy, constipation or diarrhea, nasal congestion, peripheral edema, urinary retention.

Rare
Ocular changes, skin pigmentation (those on high doses for prolonged periods).

SERIOUS REACTIONS

• Extrapyramidal symptoms appear dose related (particularly high dosage), divided into three categories: akathisia (inability to sit still, tapping of feet, urge to move around); parkinsonian symptoms (mask-like face, tremors, shuffling gait, hypersalivation); and acute dystonias: torticollis (neck muscle spasm), opisthotonos (rigidity of back muscles), and oculogyric crisis (rolling back of eyes).
• Dystonic reaction may also produce profuse sweating and pallor.
• Tardive dyskinesia (protrusion of tongue, puffing of cheeks, chewing/puckering of the mouth) occurs rarely (may be irreversible).
• Abrupt withdrawal after long-term therapy may precipitate nausea, vomiting, gastritis, dizziness, and tremors.
• Blood dyscrasias, particularly agranulocytosis, or mild leukopenia (sore mouth/gums/throat) may occur.
• May lower seizure threshold.

PRECAUTIONS & CONSIDERATIONS

Caution is warranted with impaired respiratory, hepatic, renal and cardiac function, alcohol withdrawal, history of seizures, urinary retention, glaucoma, prostatic hypertrophy, or hypocalcemia (increased susceptibility to dystonias). Withdrawal effects, including severe rhinorrhea, vomiting, respiratory distress, and extrapyramidal effects, have been reported in neonates. Its use should be avoided in pregnant women. Fluphenazine is distributed in breast milk. Children are more likely to develop neuromuscular

or extrapyramidal reactions, especially dystonias. Elderly patients may be more susceptible to orthostatic hypotension and exhibit an increased sensitivity to anticholinergic and sedative effects.

Visual disturbances should be reported immediately. Dry mouth, constipation, drowsiness, and dizziness are expected to occur. Avoid alcohol and tasks that require mental alertness or motor skills. Do not abruptly withdraw from long-term therapy.

Storage
Store at room temperature and protect from light.

Administration
Administer IM injection deep into gluteal area. The dosage may be gradually increased as needed and tolerated.

Be aware that the oral dose has been found to be approximately 2-3 times higher than the parenteral dose. Take with food or milk to reduce GI irritation.

Flurandrenolide
flure-an-dren′oh-lide
(Cordran, Cordran SP)

CATEGORY AND SCHEDULE
Pregnancy Risk Category: C

Classification: Corticosteroids, topical, dermatologics

MECHANISM OF ACTION

A fluorinated corticosteroid that decreases inflammation by suppression of the migration of polymorphonuclear leukocytes and reversal of increased capillary permeability. *Therapeutic Effect:* Decreases tissue response to inflammatory process. The amount of corticosteroid absorbed from the skin depends on the intrinsic properties of the drug, the vehicle used, the duration of exposure, the skin surface area, and the condition of the skin.

PHARMACOKINETICS

Repeated applications may lead to percutaneous absorption. Absorption is about 36% from scrotal area, 7% from forehead, 4% from scalp, and 1% from forearm. Metabolized in liver. Excreted in urine. *Half-life:* Unknown.

AVAILABILITY

Cream: 0.025%, 0.05% (Cordran SP).
Lotion: 0.05% (Cordran).
Ointment: 0.025%, 0.05% (Cordran).
Tape, Topical: 4 mcg/cm^2 (Cordran).

INDICATIONS AND DOSAGES

▸ **Anti-inflammatory, immunosuppressant, corticosteroid replacement therapy**
Topical
Adults, Elderly. Apply 2-3 times/day.
Children. Apply 1-2 times/day, once daily if tape used.

CONTRAINDICATIONS

Hypersensitivity to flurandrenolide or any component of the formulation; viral, fungal, or tubercular skin lesions.

INTERACTIONS

Drug
None known.
Herbal
None known.
Food
None known.

DIAGNOSTIC TEST EFFECTS

None known.

SIDE EFFECTS

Occasional
Itching, dry skin, folliculitis.
Rare
Intracranial hemorrhage, acne, striae, miliaria, allergic contact dermatitis, telangiectasis, or raised dark red spots on the skin.

SERIOUS REACTIONS

• When taken in excessive quantities, systemic hypercorticism and adrenal suppression may occur.

PRECAUTIONS & CONSIDERATIONS

Caution should be exercised when used over large areas of body, in denuded areas, for prolonged periods, with occlusive dressings, and in small children. It is unknown whether flurandrenolide crosses the placenta or is distributed in breast milk. Be aware that the safety and efficacy of flurandrenolide have not been established in children. Therefore, use the smallest dose necessary to achieve optimal results. Be aware that children are at an increased risk of systemic toxicity and side effects.

No age-related precautions have been noted in elderly patients. Urinary free cortisol test and ACTH stimulation test should be obtained for suspected HPA axis suppression.
Storage
Store at room temperature.
Administration
Avoid contact with eyes. Gently cleanse area before application. Use occlusive dressings only as ordered. Apply sparingly and rub into area thoroughly. Children using flurandrenolide tape should use it only once a day.

F

Flurazepam
flure-az′e-pam
(Apo-Flurazepam [CAN], Dalmane)
Do not confuse with Dialume.

CATEGORY AND SCHEDULE
Pregnancy Risk Category: X
Controlled Substance Schedule: IV

Classification: Benzodiazepines,
sedatives/hypnotics

MECHANISM OF ACTION
A benzodiazepine that enhances
the action of inhibitory
neurotransmitter gamma-
aminobutyric acid (GABA).
Therapeutic Effect: Produces
hypnotic effect due to central
nervous system (CNS)
depression.

PHARMACOKINETICS

Route	Onset	Peak	Duration
PO	15-20 min	3-6 h	7-8 h

Well absorbed from the GI tract.
Protein binding: 97%. Crosses
the blood-brain barrier. Widely
distributed. Metabolized in liver
to active metabolite. Primarily
excreted in urine. Not removed
by hemodialysis. *Half-life:* 2.3 h;
metabolite: 40-114 h.

AVAILABILITY
Capsules: 15 mg, 30 mg.

INDICATIONS AND DOSAGES
▸ **Insomnia**
PO
Adults. 15-30 mg at bedtime.
*Elderly, debilitated, liver disease, low
serum albumin, Children 15 yr and
older.* 15 mg at bedtime.

CONTRAINDICATIONS
Acute alcohol intoxication, acute
angle-closure glaucoma, pregnancy
or breastfeeding, sleep apnea.

INTERACTIONS
Drug
Alcohol, CNS depressants: May
increase CNS depression.
Digoxin: Increased digoxin serum
levels and toxicity may increase.
Herbal
**Dong quai, kava kava, magnolia,
passionflower, skullcap, valerian:**
May increase CNS depression.
St. John's wort: Decreased efficacy
of flurazepam.
Food
None known.

DIAGNOSTIC TEST EFFECTS
None known.

SIDE EFFECTS
Frequent
Drowsiness, dizziness, ataxia,
sedation.
Morning drowsiness may occur
initially.
Occasional
GI disturbances, nervousness,
blurred vision, dry mouth, headache,
confusion, skin rash, irritability,
slurred speech.
Rare
Paradoxical CNS excitement or
restlessness, particularly noted in
elderly or debilitated patients.

SERIOUS REACTIONS
• Abrupt or too-rapid withdrawal
after long-term use may result
in pronounced restlessness and
irritability, insomnia, hand tremors,
abdominal or muscle cramps,
vomiting, diaphoresis, and seizures.
• Overdose results in somnolence,
confusion, diminished reflexes, and
coma.

PRECAUTIONS & CONSIDERATIONS

Caution is warranted with impaired liver or renal function. Flurazepam crosses the placenta and may be distributed in breast milk. Chronic flurazepam ingestion during pregnancy may produce withdrawal symptoms and CNS depression in neonates. The safety and efficacy of flurazepam have not been established in children younger than 15 yr of age. Use small initial doses with gradual dose increases to avoid ataxia or excessive sedation in elderly patients. Avoid smoking, because it reduces the drug's effectiveness. Flurazepam may be habit-forming. Assess BP, pulse, and respirations immediately before beginning flurazepam administration. Disturbed sleep 1-2 nights after discontinuing the drug may occur.

Administration

Take flurazepam without regard to meals. If desired, empty capsules and mix with food. Do not abruptly withdraw the medication after long-term use.

Flurbiprofen

flure-bi´-proe-fen
(Ansaid, Froben [CAN], Ocufen, Strepfen [AUS])
Do not confuse Ocufen with Ocuflox.

CATEGORY AND SCHEDULE

Pregnancy Risk Category: B (D if used in third trimester or near delivery; C for ophthalmic solution)

Classification: Nonsteroidal antiinflammatory

MECHANISM OF ACTION

A phenylalkanoic acid that produces analgesic and antiinflammatory effect by inhibiting prostaglandin synthesis. Also relaxes the iris sphincter.
Therapeutic Effect: Reduces the inflammatory response and intensity of pain. Prevents or decreases miosis during cataract surgery.

PHARMACOKINETICS

Well absorbed from the GI tract; ophthalmic solution penetrates cornea after administration, and may be systemically absorbed. Protein binding: 99%. Widely distributed. Metabolized in the liver. Primarily excreted in urine. *Half-life:* 3–4 h.

AVAILABILITY

Tablets: 50 mg, 100 mg.
Ophthalmic Solution: 0.03%.

INDICATIONS AND DOSAGES
▸ **Rheumatoid arthritis, osteoarthritis**
PO
Adults, Elderly. 200–300 mg/day in 2-4 divided doses. Maximum: 100 mg/dose or 300 mg/day.
▸ **Dysmenorrhea, pain**
PO
Adults. 50 mg 4 times a day.
▸ **Intraoperative miosis**
OPHTHALMIC
Adults, Elderly, Children. Apply 1 drop q30min starting 2 h before surgery for total of 4 doses.

CONTRAINDICATIONS

Active peptic ulcer, chronic inflammation of GI tract, GI bleeding or ulceration, history of hypersensitivity to aspirin or NSAIDs; treatment of perioperative pain following CABG surgery.

DRUG INTERACTIONS

Aspirin, alcohol, corticosteroids: GI ulceration, bleeding.
Salicylates: Decreased action.
Oral anticoagulants, oral antidiabetics, lithium,

methotrexate : Risk of increased effects.
Diuretics: Decreased effects.
SSRIs, SNRIs: Increased risk GI bleeding.
Herbal
Herbs with antiplatelet effects (e.g., ginkgo, white willow): Increased risk of bleeding.

SIDE EFFECTS

Occasional
PO: Headache, abdominal pain, diarrhea, indigestion, nausea, fluid retention.
Ophthalmic: Burning or stinging on instillation, keratitis, elevated intraocular pressure.
Rare
PO: Blurred vision, flushed skin, dizziness, somnolence, nervousness, insomnia, unusual fatigue, constipation, decreased appetite, vomiting, confusion.

SERIOUS REACTIONS

• Overdose may result in acute renal failure.
• Rare reactions with long-term use include peptic ulcer disease, GI bleeding, gastritis, severe hepatic reaction (jaundice), nephrotoxicity (hematuria, dysuria, proteinuria), a severe hypersensitivity reaction (angioedema, bronchospasm), and cardiac arrhythmias.

PRECAUTIONS & CONSIDERATIONS

Use with caution in patients with CHF, hypertension, fluid retention, dehydration, history of GI disease (bleeding or ulcers), coagulation disorders, asthma, hepatic impairment, or renal impairment. Flurbiprofen should not be used in the third trimester of pregnancy as it may lead to premature closure of the ductus arteriosis. Flurbiprofen is excreted in breast milk; use in nursing mothers is not recommended. Safety and effectiveness have not been established in children. The elderly are at increased risk of adverse effects, particularly GI effects and renal toxicity.
Storage
Store at room temperature.
Administration
May be taken with food, milk, or antacid to reduce GI effects.

Flutamide
floo′ta-mide
(Euflex [CAN], Eulexin, Flugerel [AUS], Flutamin [AUS], Fugerel [AUS], Novo-Flutamide [CAN])
Do not confuse flutamide with Flumadine.

CATEGORY AND SCHEDULE
Pregnancy Risk Category: D

Classification: Antineoplastics, antiandrogens, hormones/hormone modifiers

MECHANISM OF ACTION
An antiandrogen hormone that inhibits androgen uptake and prevents androgen from binding to androgen receptors in target tissue. Used in conjuction with leuprolide to inhibit the stimulant effects of flutamide on serum testosterone levels. *Therapeutic Effect:* Suppresses testicular androgen production and decreases the growth of prostate carcinoma.

PHARMACOKINETICS
Completely absorbed from the GI tract. Protein binding: 94%-96%. Metabolized in the liver to active metabolite. Primarily excreted in urine. Not removed by hemodialysis.

Half-life: 6 h (increased in elderly patients).

AVAILABILITY
Capsules: 125 mg.

INDICATIONS AND DOSAGES
▶ **Prostatic carcinoma (in combination with leuprolide)**
PO
Adults, Elderly. 250 mg q8h.

CONTRAINDICATIONS
Severe hepatic impairment; pregnancy.

INTERACTIONS
Drug
Warfarin: May increase risk of bleeding.
Herbal
Chaparral, comfrey, eucalyptus, germander, Jin Bu Huan, kava kava, pennyroyal, skullcap, valerian: May increase risk of hepatotoxicity.
Food
None known.

DIAGNOSTIC TEST EFFECTS
May increase blood glucose level and serum estradiol, testosterone, bilirubin, creatinine, AST (SGOT), and ALT (SGPT) levels.

SIDE EFFECTS
Frequent
Hot flashes (50%); decreased libido, diarrhea (24%); generalized pain (23%); asthenia (17%); constipation (12%); nausea, nocturia (11%).
Occasional (6%-8%)
Dizziness, paresthesia, insomnia, impotence, peripheral edema, gynecomastia.
Rare (4%-5%)
Rash, diaphoresis, hypertension, hematuria, vomiting, urinary incontinence, headache, flulike symptoms, photosensitivity.

SERIOUS REACTIONS
• Hepatoxicity, including hepatic encephalopathy, and hemolytic anemia may be noted.

PRECAUTIONS & CONSIDERATIONS
Flutamide is not used in pregnant women or in children. No age-related precautions have been noted in elderly patients.

Clinical progression and drug therapy may be evaluated by PSA levels.

Overexposure to the sun or ultraviolet light should be avoided and protective clothing should be worn outdoors until tolerance of ultraviolet light is determined.

Urine may become amber or yellow-green during flutamide therapy. Liver function test results should be obtained before beginning drug therapy and periodically thereafter.
Storage
Store at room temperature.
Administration
Take oral flutamide without regard to food. Do not abruptly discontinue the drug.

Fluticasone
flu-tic′a-zone
(Cutivate, Flixotide Disks [AUS], Flixotide Inhaler [AUS], Flonase, Flovent, Flovent Diskus, Flovent HFA)

CATEGORY AND SCHEDULE
Pregnancy Risk Category: C

Classification: Corticosteroids, inhalation, topical, dermatologics

MECHANISM OF ACTION
A corticosteroid that controls the rate of protein synthesis, depresses migration of polymorphonuclear

leukocytes, reverses capillary permeability, and stabilizes lysosomal membranes. *Therapeutic Effect:* Prevents or controls inflammation.

PHARMACOKINETICS

Inhalation/intranasal: Protein binding: 91%. Undergoes extensive first-pass metabolism in liver. Excreted in urine. *Half-life:* 3-7.8 h. Topical: Amount absorbed depends on affected area and skin condition (absorption increased with fever, hydration, inflamed or denuded skin).

AVAILABILITY

Aerosol for Oral Inhalation (Flovent, Flovent HFA): 44 mcg/inhalation, 110 mcg/inhalation, 220 mcg/inhalation.
Powder for Oral Inhalation (Flovent Diskus): 50 mcg, 100 mcg, 250 mcg.
Intranasal Spray (Flonase): 50 mcg/inhalation.
Topical Cream (Cutivate): 0.05%.
Topical Ointment (Cutivate): 0.005%.

INDICATIONS AND DOSAGES
▸ **Allergic rhinitis**
INTRANASAL
Adults, Elderly. Initially, 200 mcg (2 sprays in each nostril once daily or 1 spray in each nostril q12h) for a few days. Maintenance: 1 spray in each nostril once daily. Maximum: 200 mcg/day.
Children older than 4 yr. Initially, 100 mcg (1 spray in each nostril once daily). Maximum: 200 mcg/day.
▸ **Relief of inflammation and pruritus associated with steroid-responsive disorders, such as contact dermatitis and eczema**
Topical
Adults, Elderly, Children older than 3 mo. Apply sparingly to affected area once or twice a day.

▸ **Maintenance treatment for asthma for those previously treated with bronchodilators**
INHALATION POWDER (FLOVENT DISKUS)
Adults, Elderly, Children 12 yr and older. Initially, 100 mcg q12h. Maximum: 500 mcg twice daily.
INHALATION (ORAL, FLOVENT)
Adults, Elderly, Children 12 yr and older. Initially, 88 mcg twice a day. Maximum: 440 mcg twice a day.
▸ **Maintenance treatment for asthma for those previously treated with inhaled steroids**
INHALATION POWDER (FLOVENT DISKUS)
Adults, Elderly, Children 12 yr and older. Initially, 100-250 mcg q12h. Maximum: 500 mcg q12h.
INHALATION, ORAL (FLOVENT)
Adults, Elderly, Children 12 yr and older. 88-220 mcg twice a day. Maximum: 440 mcg twice a day.
▸ **Maintenance treatment for asthma for those previously treated with oral steroids**
INHALATION POWDER (FLOVENT DISKUS)
Adults, Elderly, Children 12 yr and older. 500-1000 mcg twice a day.
INHALATION (ORAL, FLOVENT)
Adults, Elderly, Children 12 yr and older. 440-880 mcg twice a day.

CONTRAINDICATIONS

Primary treatment of status asthmaticus or other acute asthma episodes (inhalation); severe allergies to milk proteins (inhalation); untreated localized infection of nasal mucosa.

INTERACTIONS
Drug
Ketoconazole, protease inhibitors: May increase plasma fluticasone concentrations.

Herbal and Food
None known.

DIAGNOSTIC TEST EFFECTS
None known.

SIDE EFFECTS
Frequent
Inhalation: Throat irritation, hoarseness, dry mouth, cough, temporary wheezing, oropharyngeal candidiasis (particularly if the mouth is not rinsed with water after each administration).
Intranasal: Mild nasopharyngeal irritation; nasal burning, stinging, or dryness; rebound congestion; rhinorrhea; loss of taste.
Occasional
Inhalation: Oral candidiasis.
Intranasal: Nasal and pharyngeal candidiasis, headache.
Topical: Skin burning, pruritus.

SERIOUS REACTIONS
• Anaphylaxis, hypersensitivity reactions, and glaucoma occur rarely.
• Nasal septal perforation with prolonged innappropriate use.

PRECAUTIONS & CONSIDERATIONS
Caution is warranted with active or quiescent tuberculosis, ocular herpes simplex infection, and untreated systemic infections (including fungal, bacterial, or viral). It is unknown whether fluticasone crosses the placenta or is distributed in breast milk. The safety and efficacy of fluticasone have not been established in children younger than 4 yr. Children 4 yr and older may experience growth suppression with prolonged or high doses. No age-related precautions have been noted in elderly patients. Drink plenty of fluids to decrease the thickness of lung secretions. Pulse rate and quality, ABG levels, and respiratory rate, depth, rhythm, and type should be monitored. Notify the physician of nasal irritation or if symptoms, such as sneezing, fail to improve.
Administration
For inhalation, first shake the container well. Exhale completely and place the mouthpiece between the lips. Inhale and hold the breath for as long as possible before exhaling. Allow 1 min between inhalations to promote deeper bronchial penetration. Rinse mouth with water immediately after inhalation to prevent mouth and throat dryness and oral candidiasis. Clear the nasal passages before using nasal spray. May need to use a topical nasal decongestant 5-15 min before using fluticasone. Tilt head slightly forward. Insert spray tip up into the nostril, pointing toward the inflamed nasal turbinates, away from nasal septum. Spray the drug into the nostril while holding the other nostril closed, and at the same time inhale through the nose.

For topical fluticasone, rub a thin film gently on the affected area. Use the drug only on the prescribed area and for no longer than prescribed. Keep the preparation away from the eyes.

F

Fluvastatin
floo′va-sta-tin
(Lescol, Lescol XL, Vastin [AUS])
Do not confuse fluvastatin with fluoxetine.

CATEGORY AND SCHEDULE
Pregnancy Risk Category: X

Classification: Antihyper-lipidemics, HMG CoA reductase inhibitors

MECHANISM OF ACTION
An antihyperlipidemic that inhibits HMG-CoA reductase, the enzyme that catalyzes the early step in cholesterol synthesis. *Therapeutic Effect:* Decreases LDL cholesterol, VLDL, and plasma triglyceride levels. Slightly increases HDL cholesterol concentration.

PHARMACOKINETICS
Well absorbed from the GI tract and is unaffected by food. Does not cross the blood-brain barrier. Protein binding: > 98%. Primarily eliminated in feces. *Half-life:* 1.2 h.

AVAILABILITY
Capsules (Lescol): 20 mg, 40 mg.
Tablets (Extended-Release [Lescol XL]): 80 mg.

INDICATIONS AND DOSAGES
▸ **Hyperlipoproteinemia**
PO
Adults, Elderly. Initially, 20 mg/day (capsule) in the evening. May increase up to 40 mg/day. Maintenance: 20-40 mg/day in a single dose or divided doses. Patients requiring more than a 25% decrease in LDL cholesterol: 40-mg capsule 1-2 times a day or 80-mg extended-release tablet once a day.

▸ **Dosage in renal impairment**
Generally recommend not to exceed 40 mg/day.

CONTRAINDICATIONS
Active hepatic disease, unexplained increased serum transaminase levels, pregnancy, breast-feeding.

INTERACTIONS
Drug
Cyclosporine, fibrates, immunosuppressants, niacin: Increases the risk of acute renal failure and rhabdomyolysis with these drugs.
Bile acid seguestrant: Administer statin 2 h apart to avoid interaction.
Herbal and Food
None known.

DIAGNOSTIC TEST EFFECTS
May increase serum CK and transaminase concentrations.

SIDE EFFECTS
Frequent (5%-8%)
Headache, dyspepsia, back pain, myalgia, arthralgia, diarrhea, abdominal cramping, rhinitis.
Occasional (2%-4%)
Nausea, vomiting, insomnia, constipation, flatulence, rash, pruritus, fatigue, cough, dizziness.

SERIOUS REACTIONS
• Myositis (inflammation of voluntary muscle) with or without increased CK and muscle weakness occur rarely. These conditions may progress to frank rhabdomyolysis and renal impairment.

PRECAUTIONS & CONSIDERATIONS
Use fluvastatin cautiously in those who are receiving anticoagulant therapy, have a history of liver disease, or consume substantial amounts of alcohol. Caution is also warranted with hypotension, major

surgery, severe acute infection, renal failure secondary to rhabdomyolysis, uncontrolled seizures, and severe electrolyte, endocrine, and metabolic disorders. Expect to discontinue or withhold fluvastatin if these conditions appear. Fluvastatin use is contraindicated in pregnancy because the suppression of cholesterol biosynthesis may cause fetal toxicity. It is unknown whether fluvastatin is distributed in breast milk; therefore, it is contraindicated during lactation. Safety and efficacy of fluvastatin have not been established in children. No age-related precautions have been noted in elderly patients.

Notify the physician of any muscle pain and weakness, especially if accompanied by fever or malaise. Pattern of daily bowel activity and stool consistency should be assessed. Serum lipid cholesterol and triglyceride levels and hepatic function should be checked at baseline and periodically during treatment. Therapy with lipid-altering agents should be used in addition to a diet restricted in saturated fat and cholesterol.

Administration
Take fluvastatin without regard to food.

Fluvoxamine
floo-vox'a-meen
(Faverin [AUS], Luvox, Luvox CR)

CATEGORY AND SCHEDULE
Pregnancy Risk Category: C

Classification: Antidepressants, serotonin specific reuptake inhibitors

MECHANISM OF ACTION
An antidepressant and antiobsessive agent that selectively inhibits neuronal reuptake of serotonin. *Therapeutic*

Effect: Relieves anxiety and symptoms of obsessive-compulsive disorder.

AVAILABILITY
Tablets: 25 mg, 50 mg, 100 mg.
Extended-Release Capsule: 100 mg.

INDICATIONS AND DOSAGES
▸ **Obsessive-compulsive disorder**
PO
Adults. 50 mg at bedtime; may increase by 50 mg every 4-7 days. Dosages > 100 mg/day given in 2 divided doses. Maximum: 300 mg/day. Also may give as extended release, with target dose given once daily at bedtime. Maximum: 300 mg/day.
Children aged 8-17 yr. 25 mg at bedtime; may increase by 25 mg every 4-7 days. Dosages > 50 mg/day given in 2 divided doses. Maximum: 200 mg/day.
▸ **Social anxiety disorder**
PO (EXTENDED RELEASE)
Adults. 100 mg PO at bedtime. Titrate at 50 mg increments weekly as needed. Maximum: 300 mg/day.

OFF-LABEL USES
Treatment of depression, panic disorder, anxiety disorders in children.

CONTRAINDICATIONS
Use within 14 days of MAOIs.

INTERACTIONS
Drug
Benzodiazepines, carbamazepine, clozapine, theophylline: May increase the blood concentration and risk of toxicity of these drugs.
Lithium, tryptophan: May enhance fluvoxamine's serotonergic effects.
MAOIs: May produce excess serious reactions, including hyperthermia, rigidity, and myoclonus. Contraindicated.

Tricyclic antidepressants: May increase the fluvoxamine blood concentration.
Warfarin: May increase the effects of warfarin.
Herbal
St. John's wort: May increase fluvoxamine's pharmacologic effects and risk of toxicity.
Food
None known.

DIAGNOSTIC TEST EFFECTS
None known.

SIDE EFFECTS
Frequent
Nausea (40%); headache, somnolence, insomnia (21%-22%).
Occasional (8%-14%)
Nervousness, dizziness, diarrhea, dry mouth, asthenia, weakness, dyspepsia, constipation, abnormal ejaculation.
Rare (3%-6%)
Anorexia, anxiety, tremor, vomiting, flatulence, urinary frequency, sexual dysfunction, altered taste.

SERIOUS REACTIONS
• Overdose may produce seizures, nausea, vomiting, and extreme agitation and restlessness.

PRECAUTIONS & CONSIDERATIONS
Caution is warranted in patients with impaired hepatic or renal function and in elderly patients. Dizziness, somnolence, and dry mouth may occur. Avoid tasks requiring mental alertness or motor skills until response to the drug is established. Baseline blood chemistry tests to assess hepatic function should be performed.
Storage
Store at room temperature. Keep tightly closed.

Administration
! Expect to decrease the dosage for elderly patients and those with impaired hepatic function.
Do not abruptly discontinue the drug. Fluvoxamine's maximum therapeutic response may require 4 wks or more to appear.
Do not crush or chew extended-release capsules.

Folic Acid
foe'lik
(Apo-Folic [CAN], Folvite, Megafol [AUS]) (Folvite-parenteral)
Do not confuse Folvite with Florvite.

CATEGORY AND SCHEDULE
Pregnancy Risk Category: A (C if used in doses above the recommended daily allowance)
OTC (0.4-mg and 0.8-mg tablets only)

Classification: Hematinics, vitamins/minerals

MECHANISM OF ACTION
A coenzyme that stimulates production of platelets, RBCs, and WBCs. *Therapeutic Effect:* Essential for nucleoprotein synthesis and maintenance of normal erythropoiesis.

PHARMACOKINETICS
PO form almost completely absorbed from the GI tract (upper duodenum). Protein binding: High. Metabolized in the liver and plasma to active form. Excreted in urine. Removed by hemodialysis.

AVAILABILITY
Tablets: 0.4 mg, 0.8 mg, 1 mg.
Injection: 5 mg/mL.

INDICATIONS AND DOSAGES
▸ **Vitamin B₉ deficiency**
PO, IV, IM, SUBCUTANEOUS
Adults, Elderly, Children 12 yr and older. Initially, 1 mg/day.
Maintenance: 0.5 mg/day.
Children 1-11 yr. Initially 1 mg/day.
Maintenance: 0.1-0.4 mg/day.
Infants. 50 mcg/day.
▸ **Dietary supplement**
PO, IV, IM, SUBCUTANEOUS
Adults, Elderly, Children 4 yr and older. 0.4 mg/day.
Children 1-younger than 4 yr.
0.3 mg/day.
Children younger than 1 yr. 0.1 mg/day.
Pregnant women. 0.8 mg/day.

CONTRAINDICATIONS
Anemias (aplastic, normocytic, pernicious, refractory).

INTERACTIONS
Drug
Analgesics, carbamazepine, estrogens: May increase folic acid requirements.
Antacids, cholestyramine: May decrease the absorption of folic acid.
Hydantoin anticonvulsants: May decrease the effects of these drugs (rare).
Methotrexate, triamterene, trimethoprim: May antagonize the effects of folic acid.
Herbal and Food
None known.

DIAGNOSTIC TEST EFFECTS
May decrease vitamin B_{12} concentration.

SIDE EFFECTS
None known.

SERIOUS REACTIONS
• Allergic hypersensitivity occurs rarely with parenteral form. Oral folic acid is nontoxic.

PRECAUTIONS & CONSIDERATIONS
Folic acid is distributed in breast milk. No age-related precautions have been noted in children or elderly patients. Eating foods rich in folic acid, including fruits, vegetables, and organ meats, is encouraged.

Therapeutic improvement, including improved sense of well-being and relief from iron deficiency symptoms, such as fatigue, headache, pallor, dyspnea, and sore tongue, should be assessed. Pernicious anemia should be ruled out with a Schilling test and vitamin B_{12} blood level before beginning folic acid therapy, because the signs of pernicious anemia may be masked while irreversible neurologic damage progresses. Be aware that persons with alcoholism, decreased hematopoiesis, or deficiency of vitamin B_6, B_{12}, C, or E and those using antimetabolic drugs may develop a resistance to treatment.
Administration
! Parental folic acid is used in acutely ill patients, those receiving enternal or total parenteral nutrition, and patients with malabsorption syndrome who are unresponsive to the oral form. Folic acid dosages > 0.1 mg/day may conceal signs of pernicious anemia.

May give orally without regard to food.

F

Fomepizole
foe-mep′i-zoll
(Antizol)

CATEGORY AND SCHEDULE
Pregnancy Risk Category: C

Classification: Antidotes

F

MECHANISM OF ACTION

An alcohol dehydrogenase inhibitor that inhibits the enzyme that catalyzes the metabolism of ethanol, ethylene glycol, and methanol to their toxic metabolites. *Therapeutic Effect:* Inhibits conversion of ethylene glycol and methanol into toxic metabolites.

PHARMACOKINETICS

Protein binding: Low. Rapidly distributes to total body water after IV infusion. Extensively metabolized by the liver. Minimal excretion in the urine. Removed by hemodialysis. *Half-life:* 5 h.

AVAILABILITY

Solution for injection: 1 g/mL (Antizol).

INDICATIONS AND DOSAGES

▸ **Ethylene glycol or methanol intoxication**
IV INFUSION
Adults, Elderly. 15 mg/kg as loading dose, followed by 10 mg/kg q12h for four doses, then 15 mg/kg q12h until ethylene glycol or methanol concentrations are below 20 mg/dL. All doses should be administered as a slow IV infusion over 30 min.
▸ **Dosage in renal impairment**
During hemodialysis: 15 mg/kg as a loading dose, followed by 10 mg/kg q4h for 4 doses, then 15 mg/kg q4h until ethylene glycol or methanol concentrations are below 20 mg/dL.

After hemodialysis: If the time between the last dose and end of hemodialysis is < 1 h, do not give dose. If the time between is 1-3 h, give 50% of next scheduled dose. If time is > 3 h, give next scheduled dose.

OFF-LABEL USES

Butoxyethanol intoxication, diethylene glycol intoxication, ethanol sensitivity.

CONTRAINDICATIONS

Hypersensitivity to fomepizole or other pyrazoles.

INTERACTIONS

Drug
Alcohol: May reduce elimination of both drugs.
Herbal and Food
None known.

DIAGNOSTIC TEST EFFECTS

None known.

⊘ IV INCOMPATIBILITIES

No drug incompatibilities reported.

SIDE EFFECTS

Frequent
Hypertriglyceridemia, headache, nausea, dizziness.
Occasional
Abnormal sense of smell, nystagmus, visual disturbances, ringing in ears, agitation, seizures, anorexia, heartburn, anxiety, vertigo, light-headedness, altered sense of awareness.
Rare
Anuria, disseminated intravascular coagulopathy.

SERIOUS REACTIONS

• Mild allergic reactions including rash and eosinophilia occur rarely.
• Overdose may cause nausea, dizziness, and vertigo.

PRECAUTIONS & CONSIDERATIONS

Caution is warranted in patients with liver disease or renal impairment. Dialysis should be considered in addition to fomepizole in cases of renal failure. If < 6 h has passed since the last dose, do not give dose.

If more than 6 h has passed since the last dose, give the next scheduled dose. It is unknown whether fomepizole crosses the placenta or is distributed in breast milk. Safety and efficacy of fomepizole have not been established in children. Age-related renal impairment may require dosage adjustment in elderly patients.

This medication is given to treat antifreeze or windshield wiper fluid ingestion. If not treated, these poisons will cause kidney damage, eye damage, seizures, coma, and possibly death.

Storage

Do not freeze. Store unopened vial at room temperature.

Administration

Dilute in at least 100 mL of 0.9% NaCl or D5W. Administer fomepizole as a slow infusion over 30 min. Do not give undiluted or by bolus injection. Adjust dose if the person is receiving dialysis.

Fomivirsen
foh-mih-ver'sen
(Vitravene)
Discontinued in the United States

CATEGORY AND SCHEDULE
Pregnancy Risk Category: C

Classification: Antivirals, ophthalmics

MECHANISM OF ACTION
An antiviral that binds to messenger RNA, inhibiting the synthesis of viral proteins. *Therapeutic Effect:* Blocks replication of cytomegalovirus (CMV).

AVAILABILITY
Intravitreal Injection: 6.6 mg/mL.

INDICATIONS AND DOSAGES
▸ CMV retinitis
INTRAVITREAL INJECTION

Adults. 330 mcg (0.05 mL) every other week for 2 doses, then 330 mcg every 4 wks.

CONTRAINDICATIONS
Active retinal bleeding.

INTERACTIONS
None significant.

DIAGNOSTIC TEST EFFECTS
May alter liver function test results and serum alkaline phosphatase level. May decrease blood hemoglobin levels and neutrophil and platelet counts.

SIDE EFFECTS
Frequent (5%-10%)
Fever, headache, nausea, diarrhea, vomiting, abdominal pain, anemia, uveitis, abnormal vision.
Occasional (2%-5%)
Chest pain, confusion, dizziness, depression, neuropathy, anorexia, weight loss, pancreatitis, dyspnea, cough.

SERIOUS REACTIONS
• Thrombocytopenia may occur. Increased intraocular pressure has been reported.

PRECAUTIONS & CONSIDERATIONS
Caution is warranted with increased intraocular pressure. Be aware that fomivirsen use should be avoided in patients who have received cidofovir within 2-4 wks of fomivirsen therapy.

After fomivirsen injection, evaluate light perception, optic nerve head perfusion, and intraocular pressure. Signs and symptoms of extraocular CMV infection should be monitored, including pneumonitis and colitis.

Administration

Inject directly into eye (in the intravitreal space). Generally, it is administered once every other week for the first two treatments and then every 4 wks thereafter.

Fondaparinux
fawn-da-pear'ih-nux
(Arixtra)

CATEGORY AND SCHEDULE
Pregnancy Risk Category: B

Classification: Anticoagulants

MECHANISM OF ACTION
A factor Xa inhibitor and pentasaccharide that selectively binds to antithrombin and increases its affinity for factor Xa, thereby inhibiting factor Xa and stopping the blood coagulation cascade. *Therapeutic Effect:* Indirectly prevents formation of thrombin and subsequently the fibrin clot.

PHARMACOKINETICS
Well absorbed after subcutaneous administration. Undergoes minimal, if any, metabolism. Highly bound to antithrombin III. Distributed mainly in blood and to a minor extent in extravascular fluid. Excreted unchanged in urine. Removed by hemodialysis. *Half-life:* 17-21 h (prolonged in patients with impaired renal function).

AVAILABILITY
Injection: 2.5 mg/0.5 mL prefilled syringe.

INDICATIONS AND DOSAGES
▸ **Prevention of venous thromboembolism**
SUBCUTANEOUS
Adults. 2.5 mg once a day for 5-9 days after surgery. Initial dose should be given 6-8 h after surgery. Only approved for patients weighing 50 kg or more.

▸ **Treatment of pulmonary embolism or DVT in conjection with warfarin**
Adults. 5 mg SC once daily if < 50 kg, 50-100 kg, 7.5 mg SC once daily if > 100 kg. 10 mg SC once daily if usual duration 5-9 days; continue until warfarin treatment acheives INR 2-3.

CONTRAINDICATIONS
Active major bleeding, bacterial endocarditis, severe renal impairment (with creatinine clearance < 30 mL/ min), thrombocytopenia associated with antiplatelet antibody formation in the presence of fondaparinux.

INTERACTIONS
Drug
Anticoagulants, platelet inhibitors, thrombolytics: May increase bleeding.
Herbal
Ginger, gingko: May increase risk of bleeding.
Food
None known.

DIAGNOSTIC TEST EFFECTS
Increases reversible serum creatinine, AST (SGOT), and ALT (SGPT) levels. May decrease hemoglobin, hematocrit, and platelet count.

SIDE EFFECTS
Occasional (14%)
Fever.
Rare (1%-4%)
Injection site hematoma, nausea, peripheral edema.

SERIOUS REACTIONS
• Accidental overdose may lead to bleeding complications ranging from local ecchymoses to major hemorrhage.
• Thrombocytopenia occurs rarely.

PRECAUTIONS & CONSIDERATIONS
Caution is warranted in patients with conditions associated with increased

risk of hemorrhage, such as concurrent use of antiplatelet agents, GI ulceration, hemophilia, history of cerebrovascular accident, severe uncontrolled hypertension, history of heparin-induced thrombocytopenia, impaired renal function, indwelling epidural catheter or neuraxial anesthesia, and in elderly patients. Fondaparinux should be used with caution in pregnant women, particularly during the last trimester and immediately postpartum, because it increases the risk of maternal hemorrhage. It is unknown whether fondaparinux is excreted in breast milk. Safety and efficacy of fondaparinux have not been established in children. In elderly patients, age-related decreased renal function may increase the risk of bleeding. Women may experience heavier menstrual flow. Other medications, including OTC drugs, should be avoided. An electric razor and soft toothbrush should be used to prevent bleeding during therapy.

Notify the physician of bleeding from surgical site, chest pain, dyspnea, severe or sudden headache, swelling in the feet or hands, unusual back pain, bruising, weakness, black or red stool, coffee-ground vomitus, dark or red urine, or red-speckled mucus from cough. CBC, BUN and creatinine levels, BP, pulse, and stool of occult blood should be monitored. Be aware of signs of bleeding, including bleeding at injection or surgical sites or from gums, blood in stool, bruising, hematuria, and petechiae.

Storage
Store at room temperature. The parenteral form normally appears clear and colorless; discard if discoloration or particulate matter is noted.

Administration
Do not expel the air bubble from the prefilled syringe before injection to avoid expelling drug. Pinch a fold of the patient's skin at the injection site between the thumb and forefinger. Introduce the entire length of subcutaneous needle into the skinfold. Inject into fatty tissue between the left and right anterolateral or the left and right posterolateral abdominal wall. Rotate injection sites.

Formoterol
for-moe'ter-ol
(Foradil Aerolizer, Foradile [AUS], Oxis [AUS]), perforomist

CATEGORY AND SCHEDULE
Pregnancy Risk Category: C

Classification: Adrenergic agonists, bronchodilators, long-acting β-agonist

MECHANISM OF ACTION
A long-acting bronchodilator that stimulates β_2-adrenergic receptors in the lungs, resulting in relaxation of bronchial smooth muscle. Also inhibits release of mediators from various cells in the lungs, including mast cells, with little effect on heart rate. *Therapeutic Effect:* Relieves bronchospasm, reduces airway resistance. Improves bronchodilation, nighttime asthma control, and peak flow rates.

PHARMACOKINETICS

Route	Onset	Peak	Duration
Inhalation	1-3 min	0.5-1 h	12 h

Absorbed from bronchi after inhalation. Metabolized in the liver. Primarily excreted in urine. Unknown if removed by hemodialysis. *Half-life:* 10 h.

AVAILABILITY

Inhalation Powder in Capsules:
12 mcg.
Nebulizer Solution: 20 mcg/2 mL.

INDICATIONS AND DOSAGES
▸**Asthma, chronic obstructive pulmonary disease (COPD), exercise-induced bronchospasm**
INHALATION
Adults, Elderly, Children 5 yr and older. 12 mcg capsule q12h.
▸**Exercise-induced bronchospasm**
INHALATION
Adults, Elderly, Children 5 yr and older. 12 mcg capsule at least 15 min before exercise. Do not repeat for another 12 h.

CONTRAINDICATIONS
Status asthmaticus.

INTERACTIONS
Drug
β-blockers: May antagonize formoterol's bronchodilating effects.
Diuretics, steroids, xanthine derivatives: May increase the risk of hypokalemia.
Drugs that can prolong QT interval (including erythromycin, quinidine, and thioridazine), MAOIs, tricyclic antidepressants: May potentiate cardiovascular effects.
Herbal and Food
None known.

DIAGNOSTIC TEST EFFECTS
May decrease serum potassium level. May increase blood glucose level.

SIDE EFFECTS
Occasional
Tremor, muscle cramps, tachycardia, insomnia, headache, irritability, irritation of mouth or throat.

SERIOUS REACTIONS
• Excessive sympathomimetic stimulation may produce palpitations, extrasystole, and chest pain.

PRECAUTIONS & CONSIDERATIONS
Caution is warranted in patients with cardiovascular disease, hypertension, a seizure disorder, and thyrotoxicosis. It is unknown whether formoterol crosses the placenta or is distributed in breast milk. The safety and efficacy of formoterol have not been established in children younger than 5 yr. Elderly patients may be more prone to tachycardia and tremor because of increased sensitivity to sympathomimetics. Drink plenty of fluids to decrease the thickness of lung secretions. Avoid excessive use of caffeinated products, such as chocolate, cocoa, cola, coffee, and tea. Monotherapy with formoterol may increase risk of asthma-related events, such as hospitalization or mortality.

Pulse rate and quality, ECG, respiratory rate, depth, rhythm and type, ABG, and serum potassium levels should be monitored. Keep a log of measurements of peak flow readings.
Storage
Before dispensing, store in refrigerator. After dispensing, may be stored at room temperature until "use by" date.
Administration
Keep capsules in individual blister packs until immediately before use. Do not swallow the capsules. Do not use with a spacer. Pull off the aerolizer inhaler cover, twisting the mouthpiece in the direction of the arrow to open. Place the capsule in the chamber and twist the mouthpiece closed. Press both buttons on the side of the aerolizer only once. This action punctures the capsule. Exhale completely, then

place mouth on the mouthpiece and close the lips. Inhale quickly and deeply through the mouth, which causes the capsule to spin and dispense the drug. Hold breath for as long as possible before exhaling slowly. Check the capsule to make sure all the powder is gone. If not, inhale again to receive the rest of the dose. Rinse mouth with water immediately after inhalation to prevent mouth and throat dryness. Never swallow capsules orally. Never wash the Aerolizer inhaler.

Fosamprenavir
fos′am-pren-a-veer
(Lexiva)

CATEGORY AND SCHEDULE
Pregnancy Risk Category: C

Classification: Antivirals, protease inhibitors

MECHANISM OF ACTION
An antiretroviral that is rapidly converted to amprenavir, which inhibits HIV-1 protease by binding to the enzyme's active site, thus preventing the processing of viral precursors and resulting in the formation of immature, noninfectious viral particles. *Therapeutic Effect:* Impairs HIV replication and proliferation.

PHARMACOKINETICS
Rapidly absorbed after PO administration. Protein binding: 90%. Metabolized in the liver. Excreted in urine and feces. *Half-life:* 7.7 h.

AVAILABILITY
Tablets: 700 mg (equivalent to 600 mg amprenavir).

Oral Suspension: 50 mg/mL (equivalent to 43 mg/mL amprenavir).

INDICATIONS AND DOSAGES
▶**HIV infection in patients who have not had previous protease inhibitor therapy**
PO
Adults, Elderly. 1400 mg twice daily without ritonavir; or 1400 mg once daily plus ritonavir 200 mg once daily; or 1400 mg once daily plus ritonavir 100 mg once daily.
Children 6 yr and up. 30 mg/kg oral suspension twice daily (maximum 1400 mg twice daily) without ritonavir or 18 mg/kg [1400 mg] twice daily plus ritonavir 3 mg/kg [maximum: 100 mg] twice daily.
Children 2-5 yr. 30 mg/kg oral suspension twice daily without ritonavir (maximum 1400 mg twice daily).
▶**HIV infection in patients who have had previous protease inhibitor therapy**
PO
Adults, Elderly. 700 mg twice daily plus ritonavir 100 mg twice daily.
▶**Concurrent therapy with efavirenz**
PO
Adults, Elderly. In patients receiving fosamprenavir plus once-daily ritonavir with efavirenz, an additional 100 mg/day ritonavir (300 mg total/day) should be given.
▶**Dosage in hepatic impairment consult prescribing information**
Dosages must be adjusted in moderate and severe hepatic impairment.

CONTRAINDICATIONS
Concurrent use of amprenavir, cisapride, delarindia, dihydroergotamine, ergonovine, ergotamine, methylergonovine, pimozide, midazolam, triazolam lorastatin, simvastatin, or rifampin. If fosamprenavir is given concurrently with ritonavir,

flecainide and propafenone are also contraindicated.

Hypersensitivity to amprenavir or fosamprenavir.

INTERACTIONS
Drug

Amiodarone, bepridil, ergotamine, lidocaine, midazolam, oral contraceptives, quinidine, triazolam, tricyclic antidepressants: May interfere with the metabolism of these drugs.

Antacids, didanosine: May decrease the absorption of fosamprenavir.

Carbamazepine, phenobarbital, phenytoin, rifampin: May decrease the fosamprenavir blood concentration.

Clozapine, HMG-CoA reductase inhibitors (statins), warfarin: May increase the blood concentrations of these drugs.

PDES inhibitors (e.g., sildenafil): May increase risk for priapism, hypotension.

Herbal

St. John's wort: May decrease the fosamprenavir blood concentration. Avoid.

Oral suspension: Shake well before each use. Refrigeration may help palatability. Do not freeze.

Food

None known.

DIAGNOSTIC TEST EFFECTS
May increase serum lipase, triglyceride, AST (SGOT), and ALT (SGPT) levels.

SIDE EFFECTS
Frequent (35%-39%)
Nausea, rash, diarrhea.
Occasional (8%-19%)
Headache, vomiting, fatigue, depression.
Rare (2%-7%)
Pruritus, abdominal pain, perioral paresthesia.

SERIOUS REACTIONS
• Severe and possibly life-threatening dermatologic reactions occur rarely.

PRECAUTIONS & CONSIDERATIONS
Extreme caution should be used with liver impairment. Caution is also warranted in patients with diabetes mellitus, impaired renal function, or known sulfonamide allergy and in elderly patients. Fosamprenavir is not a cure for HIV infection, nor does it reduce risk of transmission to others.

Expect to obtain baseline lab values, including blood glucose levels, serum lipase, SGPT (ALT), SGOT (AST), and serum triglyceride levels. Find out which other drugs the person is taking, including ritonavir. Make sure the person is not also taking amprenavir because it is chemically similar to fosamprenavir. Report any side effects, including rash or diarrhea.

Administration

Do not chew, crush, or break film-coated tablets. May take without regard to food.

Foscarnet
foss-car′net
(Foscavir)

CATEGORY AND SCHEDULE
Pregnancy Risk Category: C

Classification: Antivirals

MECHANISM OF ACTION
An antiviral that selectively inhibits binding sites on virus-specific DNA polymerase and reverse transcriptase. *Therapeutic Effect:* Inhibits replication of herpes virus.

PHARMACOKINETICS
Sequestered into bone and cartilage. Protein binding: 14%-17%. Primarily

excreted unchanged in urine. Removed by hemodialysis. *Half-life:* 3.3-6.8 h (increased in impaired renal function).

AVAILABILITY
Injection: 24 mg/mL.

INDICATIONS AND DOSAGES
▸ **Cytomegalovirus (CMV) retinitis**
IV
Adults, Elderly. Initially, 60 mg/kg q8h or 100 mg/kg q12h for 2-3 wks. Maintenance: 90-120 mg/kg/day as a single IV infusion.
▸ **Herpes infection**
IV
Adults. 40 mg/kg q8-12h for 2-3 wks or until healed.
▸ **Dosage in renal impairment**
Dosages are individualized based on creatinine clearance. Refer to the dosing guide provided by the manufacturer.

CONTRAINDICATIONS
None known.

INTERACTIONS
Drug
Nephrotoxic medications: May increase the risk of nephrotoxicity.
Pentamidine (IV): May cause reversible hypocalcemia, hypomagnesemia, and nephrotoxicity.
Zidovudine (AZT): May increase the risk of anemia.
Herbal and Food
None known.

DIAGNOSTIC TEST EFFECTS
May increase serum alkaline phosphatase, bilirubin, creatinine, AST (SGOT), and ALT (SGPT) levels. May decrease serum magnesium and potassium levels. May alter serum calcium and phosphate concentrations.

ⓓ IV INCOMPATIBILITIES
Acyclovir (Zovirax), amphotericin B (Fungizone), co-trimoxazole (Bactrim), diazepam (Valium), digoxin (Lanoxin), diphenhydramine (Benadryl), dobutamine (Dobutrex), droperidol (Inapsine), ganciclovir (Cytovene), haloperidol (Haldol), leucovorin, midazolam (Versed), pentamidine (Pentam IV), prochlorperazine (Compazine), vancomycin (Vancocin). Also incompatible with any divalent cations, such as calcium or magnesium.

ⓓ IV COMPATIBILITIES
Dopamine (Intropin), heparin, hydromorphone (Dilaudid), lorazepam (Ativan), morphine, potassium chloride.

SIDE EFFECTS
Frequent
Fever (65%); nausea (47%); vomiting, diarrhea (30%).
Occasional (≥ 5%)
Anorexia, pain and inflammation at injection site, fever, rigors, malaise, headache, paresthesia, dizziness, rash, diaphoresis, abdominal pain.
Rare (1%-5%)
Back or chest pain, edema, flushing, pruritus, constipation, dry mouth.

SERIOUS REACTIONS
• Nephrotoxicity occurs to some extent in most patients.
• Seizures and serum mineral or electrolyte imbalances may be life threatening.

PRECAUTIONS & CONSIDERATIONS
Caution is warranted in patients with altered serum calcium or other serum electrolyte levels, a history of renal impairment, or cardiac or neurologic abnormalities. Be aware that it is unknown whether foscarnet is distributed in breast milk. Be

aware that the safety and efficacy of foscarnet have not been established in children. In elderly patients, age-related renal impairment may require dosage adjustment.

Renal impairment is reduced by ensuring sufficient fluid intake to promote diuresis before and during dosing. Signs and symptoms of anemia, such as bleeding, superinfections, and tremors, should be assessed. Institute safety measures for potential seizures. Report numbness in the extremities, paresthesias, or peri-oral tingling, during or after infusion, as this may indicate electrolyte abnormalities.

Storage

Store parenteral vials at room temperature. After dilution, foscarnet is stable for 24 h at room temperature. Do not use if foscarnet solution is discolored or contains particulate material.

Administration

Use the standard 24 mg/mL solution without diluting it when a central venous catheter is used for infusion; the 24 mg/mL solution must be diluted to 12 mg/mL when giving the drug through a peripheral vein catheter. Use only D5W or 0.9% NaCl solution for injection for dilution. Because foscarnet dosage is calculated on body weight, remove the unneeded quantity before the start of infusion to avoid overdosage. Use an IV infusion pump to administer foscarnet and prevent accidental overdose. Use aseptic technique and administer the solution within 24 h of the first entry into the sealed bottle.

!Do not give foscarnet as an IV injection or by rapid infusion because these routes increase the drug's toxicity. Administer foscarnet by IV infusion at a rate not faster than 1 h for doses up to 60 mg/kg and 2 h for doses > 60 mg/kg. To minimize the risk of phlebitis and toxicity, use central venous lines or veins with an adequate blood flow to permit rapid dilution and dissemination of foscarnet. Administer hydration fluid with each dose.

Fosfomycin
foss-fo-mye′sin
(Monurol)
Do not confuse Monurol with Monopril.

CATEGORY AND SCHEDULE
Pregnancy Risk Category: B

Classification: Antibiotics, miscellaneous, antiseptics, urinary tract

MECHANISM OF ACTION
An antibiotic that prevents bacterial cell wall formation by inhibiting the synthesis of peptidoglycan. *Therapeutic Effect:* Bactericidal.

AVAILABILITY
Powder for Oral Solution: 3 g.

INDICATIONS AND DOSAGES
▸**Uncomplicated urinary tract infection in females**
PO
Females. 3 g mixed in 4 oz water as a single dose.
▸**Uncomplicated urinary tract infection in males**
Males. 3 g/day for 2-3 days.

CONTRAINDICATIONS
Known hypersensitivity to fosfomysin.

INTERACTIONS
Drug
Metoclopramide: Lowers serum concentration and urinary excretion of fosfomycin.

Herbal and Food
None known.

DIAGNOSTIC TEST EFFECTS

May increase blood eosinophil count and serum alkaline phosphatase, bilirubin, AST (SGOT), and ALT (SGPT) levels. May alter platelet and WBC counts. May decrease blood hematocrit and hemoglobin levels.

SIDE EFFECTS

Occasional (3%-9%)
Diarrhea, nausea, headache, back pain.
Rare (< 2%)
Dysmenorrhea, pharyngitis, abdominal pain, rash.

SERIOUS REACTIONS

• Rare reports of serious hypersensitivity such as angioedema or hepatic reactions.

PRECAUTIONS & CONSIDERATIONS

Symptoms should improve 2-3 days after the initial dose of fosfomycin.
Administration
Take fosfomycin without regard to food. Always mix with 3-4 OZ of water before consuming. Do not use with hot water.

Fosinopril
fo-sin'o-pril
(Monopril)
Do not confuse Monopril with Monurol.

CATEGORY AND SCHEDULE

Pregnancy Risk Category: C (D if used in second or third trimester)

Classification: Angiotensin-converting enzyme inhibitors

MECHANISM OF ACTION

An ACE inhibitor that suppresses the renin-angiotensin-aldosterone system and prevents conversion of angiotensin I to angiotensin II, a potent vasoconstrictor; may also inhibit angiotensin II at local vascular and renal sites. Decreases plasma angiotensin II, increases plasma renin activity, and decreases aldosterone secretion. *Therapeutic Effect:* Reduces peripheral arterial resistance, pulmonary capillary wedge pressure; improves cardiac output, exercise tolerance.

PHARMACOKINETICS

Route	Onset	Peak	Duration
PO	1 h	2-6 h	24 h

Slowly absorbed from the GI tract. Protein binding: 97%-98%. Metabolized in the liver and GI mucosa to active metabolite. Primarily excreted in urine. Minimal removal by hemodialysis. *Half-life:* 11.5 h.

AVAILABILITY

Tablets: 10 mg, 20 mg, 40 mg.

INDICATIONS AND DOSAGES

▶ **Hypertension (monotherapy)**
PO
Adults, Elderly. Initially, 10 mg/day. Maintenance: 20-40 mg/day. Maximum: 80 mg/day.
▶ **Hypertension (with diuretic)**
PO
Adults, Elderly. Initially, 10 mg/day titrated to patient's needs.
▶ **Heart failure**
PO
Adults, Elderly. Initially, 10 mg. Once daily. Use 5 mg initially if patient has hypovolemia or moderate to severe renal impairment or is vigorously treated with diuretics. Maintenance: 20-40 mg/day. Target dose: 40 mg/day if tolerated.

OFF-LABEL USES

Treatment of diabetic and nondiabetic nephropathy, postmyocardial infarction, left ventricular dysfunction, renal crisis in scleroderma.

CONTRAINDICATIONS

History of angioedema from previous treatment with ACE inhibitors.

INTERACTIONS

Drug
Alcohol, antihypertensives, diuretics: May increase the effects of fosinopril.
Lithium: May increase lithium blood concentration and risk of lithium toxicity.
NSAIDs: May decrease the effects of fosinopril.
Potassium-sparing diuretics, potassium supplements: May cause hyperkalemia.
Herbal and Food
None known.

DIAGNOSTIC TEST EFFECTS

May increase BUN, serum alkaline phosphatase, serum bilirubin, serum creatinine, serum potassium, AST (SGOT), and ALT (SGPT) levels. May decrease serum sodium levels. May cause positive antinuclear antibody titer.

SIDE EFFECTS

Frequent (9%-12%)
Dizziness, cough.
Occasional (2%-4%)
Hypotension, nausea, vomiting, upper respiratory tract infection.

SERIOUS REACTIONS

• Excessive hypotension (first-dose syncope) may occur in patients with congestive heart failure and in those who are severely salt and volume depleted.
• Angioedema (swelling of face and lips) and hyperkalemia occur rarely.
• Agranulocytosis and neutropenia may be noted in those with collagen vascular disease, including scleroderma and systemic lupus erythematosus, and impaired renal function.
• Nephrotic syndrome may be noted in those with history of renal disease.

PRECAUTIONS & CONSIDERATIONS

Caution is warranted with cerebrovascular and coronary insufficiency, hypovolemia, renal impairment, sodium depletion, and those on dialysis or receiving diuretics. Fosinopril crosses the placenta, is distributed in breast milk, and may cause fetal or neonatal morbidity or mortality. Safety and efficacy of fosinopril have not been established in children. Neonates and infants may be at increased risk for neurologic abnormalities and oliguria. Elderly patients may be more sensitive to the hypotensive effects of fosinopril.

Dizziness may occur. BP should be obtained immediately before giving each fosinopril dose, in addition to regular monitoring. Be alert to fluctuations in BP. If an excessive reduction in BP occurs, place the person in the supine position with legs elevated. CBC and blood chemistry should be obtained before beginning fosinopril therapy, then every 2 wks for the next 3 mo, and periodically thereafter in patients with autoimmune disease or renal impairment, and in those who are taking drugs that affect immune response or leukocyte count. BUN, serum creatinine, and serum potassium should also be monitored in those who are receiving a diuretic. Crackles and wheezes should be assessed for in persons with congestive heart failure.
Storage
Store at room temperature.
Administration
! Expect to discontinue diuretics 2-3 days before beginning fosinopril therapy (for hypertension).

Take fosinopril without regard to food. Crush tablets if necessary.

Fosphenytoin
fos-fen′i-toyn
(Cerebyx)
Do not confuse Cerebyx with Celebrex or Celexa.

CATEGORY AND SCHEDULE
Pregnancy Risk Category: D

Classification: Anticonvulsants, hydantoins

MECHANISM OF ACTION
A hydantoin anticonvulsant that stabilizes neuronal membranes by decreasing sodium and calcium ion influx into the neurons. Also decreases post-tetanic potentiation and repetitive discharge. *Therapeutic Effect:* Decreases seizure activity.

PHARMACOKINETICS
Completely absorbed after IM administration. Protein binding: 95%-99%. Rapidly and completely hydrolyzed to phenytoin after IM or IV administration. Time of complete conversion to phenytoin: 4 h after IM injection; 2 h after IV infusion. *Half-life:* 8-15 min (for conversion to phenytoin).

AVAILABILITY
Injection: 75 mg/mL (equivalent to 50 mg/mL phenytoin).

INDICATIONS AND DOSAGES
▸ **Status epilepticus**
IV
Adults. Loading dose: 15-20 mg phenytoin equivalent (PE)/kg infused at rate of 100-150 mg PE/min.
▸ **Nonemergent seizures**
IV, IM
Adults. Loading dose: 10-20 mg PE/kg. Maintenance: 4-6 mg PE/kg/day.

▸ **Short term substitution for oral phenytoin**
IM, IV
Adults. May substitute for oral phenytoin at same total daily dose of phenytoin equivalent (PE).

CONTRAINDICATIONS
Adams-Stokes syndrome, hypersensitivity to fosphenytoin or phenytoin, second- or third-degree AV block, severe bradycardia, sinoatrial block.

INTERACTIONS
Drug
Alcohol, other CNS depressants: May increase CNS depression.
Amiodarone, anticoagulants, cimetidine, disulfiram, fluoxetine, isoniazid, sulfonamides: May increase fosphenytoin blood concentration, effects, and risk of toxicity.
Antacids: May decrease fosphenytoin absorption.
Fluconazole, ketoconazole, miconazole: May increase fosphenytoin blood concentration.
Glucocorticoids: May decrease the effects of glucocorticoids.
Lidocaine, propranolol: May increase cardiac depressant effects.
Valproic acid: May increase the blood concentration and decrease the metabolism of fosphenytoin.
Xanthines: May increase the metabolism of xanthines.
Herbal and Food
None known.

DIAGNOSTIC TEST EFFECTS
May increase blood glucose, serum GGT, and serum alkaline phosphatase levels.

⊘ IV INCOMPATIBILITIES
Midazolam (Versed).

⊜ IV COMPATIBILITIES
Lorazepam (Ativan), phenobarbital, potassium chloride.

SIDE EFFECTS
Frequent
Dizziness, paresthesia, tinnitus, pruritus, headache, somnolence.
Occasional
Morbilliform rash.

SERIOUS REACTIONS
• An elevated fosphenytoin blood concentration may produce ataxia, nystagmus, diplopia, lethargy, slurred speech, nausea, vomiting, and hypotension. As the drug level increases, extreme lethargy may progress to coma.

PRECAUTIONS & CONSIDERATIONS
Caution is warranted with hypoalbuminemia, hypotension, hepatic and renal disease, porphyria, and severe myocardial insufficiency. Fosphenytoin use during pregnancy may increase the frequency of seizures in the mother and the risk of congenital malformations in the fetus. It is unknown whether fosphenytoin is excreted in breast milk. The safety of this drug has not been established in children. A lower fosphenytoin dosage is recommended for elderly patients.

Drowsiness and dizziness may occur, so alcohol and tasks that require mental alertness or motor skills should be avoided. Assess history of the seizure disorder, including the duration, frequency, and intensity of seizures. BP, ECG, and cardiac and respiratory function should be monitored during and for 10-20 min after infusion. Blood level of fosphenytoin should be assessed 2 h after IV infusion or 4 h after IM injection.
Storage
Refrigerate unopened vials. Do not store the drug at room temperature for longer than 48 h; discard vials that contain particulate matter. After dilution, the solution is stable for 8 h at room temperature or 24 h if refrigerated.

Administration
! Always confirm dosage and injection amount before administration to avoid overdose.
! Know that 150 mg fosphenytoin yields 100 mg phenytoin and that the dose, concentration solution, and infusion rate of fosphenytoin are expressed in terms of phenytoin equivalents (PEs). Keep in mind that elderly patients may require lower, less frequent dosing and that the drug is not approved for use in children.

For IV use, dilute the drug in D5W or 0.9% NaCl to a concentration of 1.5-25 mg PE/mL. Administer at < 150 mg PE/min to decrease the risk of hypotension and arrhythmias. May also be given IM.

Frovatriptan
fro-va-trip´-tan
(Frovan)

CATEGORY AND SCHEDULE
Pregnancy Risk Category: C

Classification: Antimigraine agent; 5HT$_1$-receptor agonist

MECHANISM OF ACTION
A serotonin receptor agonist that binds selectively to vascular receptors, producing a vasoconstrictive effect on cranial blood vessels. *Therapeutic Effect:* Relieves migraine headache.

PHARMACOKINETICS
Well absorbed after PO administration. Metabolized by the liver to inactive metabolite. Eliminated in urine. *Half-life:* 26 h (increased in hepatic impairment).

AVAILABILITY
Tablets: 2.5 mg.

INDICATIONS AND DOSAGES
▸ **Acute Migraine Attack**
PO
Adults, Elderly. Initially 2.5 mg. If headache improves but then returns, dose may be repeated after 2 h. Maximum: 7.5 mg/day.

CONTRAINDICATIONS
Basilar or hemiplegic migraine, cerebrovascular or peripheral vascular disease, coronary artery disease, ischemic heart disease (including angina pectoris, history of myocardial infarction, silent ischemia, and Prinzmetal's angina), uncontrolled hypertension, use within 24 h of ergotamine-containing preparations or another serotonin receptor agonist.

DRUG INTERACTIONS
SSRIs, SNRIs, sibutramine, linezolid: Increased risk of serotonin syndrome.
Ergot-containing drugs (avoid use within 24 h of taking this drug): Potential serotonin crisis. Contraindicated.

SIDE EFFECTS
Occasional
Dizziness, paresthesia, fatigue, flushing.
Rare
Hot or cold sensation, dry mouth, dyspepsia.

SERIOUS REACTIONS
Cardiac reactions (including ischemia, coronary artery vasospasm, and MI), and noncardiac vasospasm-related reactions (such as hemorrhage and CVA), occur rarely, particularly in patients with hypertension, diabetes, or a strong family history of coronary artery disease; obese patients; smokers; males older than 40 yrs; and postmenopausal women.

PRECAUTIONS & CONSIDERATIONS
Avoid use in patients with risk factors for heart disease unless receive a satisfactory cardiovascular evaluation. Reassess cardiovascular status periodically in all patients receiving frovatriptan. It is unknown if frovatriptan is excreted in breast milk. Safety and effectiveness have not been established in children. No age-related precautions have been identified in the elderly; however, frovatriptan blood concentrations are increased 1.5- to 2 times in the elderly compared with younger adults.
Storage
Store at room temperature.
Administration
Swallow tablets with liquid.

Fulvestrant
full'veh-strant
(Faslodex)
Do not confuse with Fosamax.

CATEGORY AND SCHEDULE
Pregnancy Risk Category: D

Classification: Antineoplastics, antiestrogens, hormones/hormone modifiers

MECHANISM OF ACTION
An estrogen antagonist that competes with endogenous estrogen at estrogen receptor binding sites. *Therapeutic Effect:* Inhibits tumor growth.

PHARMACOKINETICS
Extensively and rapidly distributed after IM administration. Protein binding: 99%. Metabolized in the liver. Eliminated by hepatobiliary route; excreted in feces. *Half-life:* 40 days in postmenopausal women. Peak serum levels occur in 7-9 days.

AVAILABILITY
Prefilled Syringe: 50 mg/mL in 2.5-mL and 5-mL syringes.

INDICATIONS AND DOSAGES
▸ **Breast cancer**
IM
Adults, Elderly. 250 mg given once monthly.

CONTRAINDICATIONS
Known or suspected pregnancy, intravenous use, breast-feeding.

INTERACTIONS
Drug, Herbal, and Food
None known.

DIAGNOSTIC TEST EFFECTS
None known.

SIDE EFFECTS
Frequent (13%-26%)
Nausea, hot flashes, pharyngitis, asthenia, vomiting, vasodilation, headache.
Occasional (5%-12%)
Injection site pain, constipation, diarrhea, abdominal pain, anorexia, dizziness, insomnia, paresthesia, bone or back pain, depression, anxiety, peripheral edema, rash, diaphoresis, fever.
Rare (1%-2%)
Vertigo, weight gain.

SERIOUS REACTIONS
• Urinary tract infections, vaginitis, anemia, thromboembolic phenomena, and leukopenia occur rarely.

PRECAUTIONS & CONSIDERATIONS
Caution should be used in those receiving anticoagulant therapy and in those with bleeding diathesis, estrogen receptor-negative breast cancer, hepatic disease or reduced hepatic flow, and thrombocytopenia. Do not administer fulvestrant to pregnant women. It is unknown whether fulvestrant is excreted in breast milk. Fulvestrant is not for use in children. No age-related precautions have been noted in elderly patients.

Notify the physician if weakness, hot flashes, or nausea becomes unmanageable. An estrogen receptor assay test should be performed before therapy, and a computed tomography scan should be performed before and periodically thereafter fulvestrant therapy. Blood chemistry and plasma lipid levels should also be monitored.
Storage
Store unopened syringes in original packaging in the refrigerator. Do not freeze.
Administration
For IM use, administer the drug slowly into the buttock as a single 5-mL injection or two concurrent 2.5-mL injections at separate sites.

Furosemide
fur-oh′se-mide
(Apo-Furosemide [CAN], Frusehexal [AUS], Frusid [AUS], Lasix, Uremide [AUS], Urex-M [AUS])
Do not confuse Lasix with Lidex, Luvox, or Luxiq, or furosemide with Torsemide.

CATEGORY AND SCHEDULE
Pregnancy Risk Category: C (D if used in pregnancy-induced hypertension)

Classification: Diuretics, loop

MECHANISM OF ACTION
A loop diuretic that enhances excretion of sodium, chloride, and potassium by direct action at the ascending limb of the loop of Henle. *Therapeutic Effect:* Produces diuresis and lowers BP.

PHARMACOKINETICS

Route	Onset (min)	Peak	Duration (h)
PO	30-60	1-2 h	6-8
IV	5	20-60 min	2
IM	30	N/A	N/A

Well absorbed from the GI tract. Protein binding: 91%-97%. Partially metabolized in the liver. Primarily excreted in urine (nonrenal clearance increases in severe renal impairment). Not removed by hemodialysis. *Half-life:* 30-90 min (increased in renal or hepatic impairment, and in neonates).

AVAILABILITY

Oral Solution: 10 mg/mL.
Tablets: 20 mg, 40 mg, 80 mg.
Injection: 10 mg/mL.

INDICATIONS AND DOSAGES
▸ **Edema, hypertension**
PO
Adults, Elderly. Initially, 20-80 mg/dose; may increase by 20-40 mg/dose q6-8h. May titrate up to 600 mg/day in severe edematous states.
Children. 1-6 mg/kg/day in divided doses q6-12h.
IV, IM
Adults, Elderly. 20-40 mg/dose; may increase by 20 mg/dose q1-2h. Once desired dosage confirmed, give once or twice daily to maintain effect. Maximum: 80 mg/dose. Usual initial dose for pulmonary edema is 40 mg.
Children. 1-2 mg/kg/dose q6-12h. Maximum: 6 mg/kg/day.
Neonates. 1-2 mg/kg/dose q12-24h. Maximum: 1 mg/kg/day if premature.
IV INFUSION
Adults, Elderly. Bolus of 0.1 mg/kg, followed by infusion of 0.1 mg/kg/h; may double q2h. Maximum: 0.4 mg/kg/h.
Children. 0.05 mg/kg/h; titrate to desired effect.

OFF-LABEL USES
Hypercalcemia.

CONTRAINDICATIONS
Anuria, hepatic coma, severe electrolyte depletion, hypersensitivity to furosemide.

INTERACTIONS
Drug
Amphotericin B, nephrotoxic and ototoxic medications: May increase the risk of nephrotoxicity and ototoxicity.
Lithium: May increase the risk of lithium toxicity.
Other hypokalemia-causing medications: May increase the risk of hypokalemia.
Herbal and Food
None known.

DIAGNOSTIC TEST EFFECTS
May increase blood glucose, BUN, and serum uric acid levels. May decrease serum calcium, chloride, magnesium, potassium, and sodium levels.

ⓘ IV INCOMPATIBILITIES
Cimetidine, Ciprofloxacin (Cipro), diltiazem (Cardizem), dobutamine (Dobutrex), dopamine (Intropin), doxorubicin (Adriamycin), droperidol (Inapsine), esmolol (Brevibloc), famotidine (Pepcid), filgrastim (Neupogen), fluconazole (Diflucan), gemcitabine (Gemzar), gentamicin (Garamycin), idarubicin (Idamycin), Inamrinone, labetalol (Trandate), meperidine (Demerol), metoclopramide (Reglan), midazolam (Versed), milrinone (Primacor), nicardipine (Cardene), ondansetron (Zofran), quinidine, thiopental (Pentothal), vecuronium (Norcuron), vinblastine (Velban), vincristine (Oncovin), vinorelbine (Navelbine).

F

🖥 IV COMPATIBILITIES

Aminophylline, bumetanide (Bumex), calcium gluconate, heparin, hydromorphone (Dilaudid), lidocaine, nitroglycerin, potassium chloride, propofol (Diprivan).

SIDE EFFECTS

Expected
Increased urinary frequency and urine volume.
Frequent
Nausea, dyspepsia, abdominal cramps, diarrhea or constipation, electrolyte disturbances.
Occasional
Dizziness, light-headedness, headache, blurred vision, paresthesia, photosensitivity, rash, fatigue, bladder spasm, restlessness, diaphoresis.
Rare
Flank pain.

SERIOUS REACTIONS

• Vigorous diuresis may lead to profound water loss and electrolyte depletion, resulting in hypokalemia, hyponatremia, and dehydration.
• Sudden volume depletion may result in increased risk of thrombosis, circulatory collapse, and sudden death.
• Acute hypotensive episodes may occur, sometimes several days after beginning therapy.
• Ototoxicity—manifested as deafness, vertigo, or tinnitus—may occur, especially in patients with severe renal impairment.
• Furosemide use can exacerbate diabetes mellitus, systemic lupus erythematosus, gout, and pancreatitis.
• Blood dyscrasias have been reported.

PRECAUTIONS & CONSIDERATIONS

Caution is warranted in patients with hepatic cirrhosis. Furosemide crosses the placenta and is distributed in breast milk. Neonates may require an increased dosage interval because the drug's half-life is increased in this age-group. Elderly patients may be more sensitive to the drug's electrolyte and hypotensive effects and are at increased risk for circulatory collapse and thromboembolic effects. Age-related renal impairment may require a dosage adjustment in elderly patients. Consuming foods high in potassium, such as apricots; bananas; legumes; meat; orange juice; raisins; whole grains, including cereals; and white and sweet potatoes, is encouraged. Avoid prolonged exposure to sunlight.

An increase in the frequency and volume of urination and hearing abnormalities, such as a sense of fullness or ringing in the ears, may occur. BP, vital signs, electrolytes, intake and output, and weight should be monitored before and during treatment. Be aware of signs of electrolyte disturbances such as hypokalemia or hyponatremia. Hypokalemia may cause arrhythmias, altered mental status, muscle cramps, asthenia, and tremor. Hyponatremia may result in cold and clammy skin, confusion, and thirst.

Administration
Take furosemide with food to avoid GI upset, preferably with breakfast to help prevent nocturia.

The solution for injection normally appears clear and colorless. Discard yellow solutions. Furosemide is compatible with D5W, 0.9% NaCl, and lactated Ringer's solution, but it may also be given undiluted. Administer each 20-40 mg or less by IV push over 1-2 min. Do not exceed an infusion administration rate of 4 mg/min in adults or 0.5 mg/kg/min in children.

After IM use, monitor for temporary pain at the injection site.

INDIVIDUAL DRUG MONOGRAPHS

Gabapentin
ga′ba-pen-tin
(Gantin [AUS], Neurontin)
Do not confuse Neurontin with Noroxin.

CATEGORY AND SCHEDULE
Pregnancy Risk Category: C

Classification: Anticonvulsants, GABA analog

MECHANISM OF ACTION
An anticonvulsant and antineuralgic agent whose exact mechanism is unknown. May increase the synthesis or accumulation of γ-aminobutyric acid by binding to as-yet-undefined receptor sites in brain tissue.
Therapeutic Effect: Reduces seizure activity and neuropathic pain.

PHARMACOKINETICS
Well absorbed from the GI tract (not affected by food). Protein binding: < 5%. Widely distributed. Crosses the blood-brain barrier. Primarily excreted unchanged in urine. Removed by hemodialysis.
Half-life: 5-7 h (increased in patients with impaired renal function and in elderly patients).

AVAILABILITY
Capsules: 100 mg, 300 mg, 400 mg.
Oral Solution: 250 mg/5 mL.
Tablets: 100 mg, 300 mg, 400 mg, 600 mg, 800 mg.

INDICATIONS AND DOSAGES
▸ **Adjunctive therapy for seizure control**
PO
Adults, Elderly, Children 12 yr and older. Initially, 300 mg 3 times a day. May titrate dosage. Range: 900-1800 mg/day in 3 divided doses. Maximum: 3600 mg/day.
Children 3-12 yr. Initially, 10-15 mg/kg/day in 3 divided doses. May titrate up to 25-35 mg/kg/day (for children 5-12 yr) and 40 mg/kg/day (for children 3-4 yr) Maximum: 50 mg/kg/day.
▸ **Postherpetic neuralgia**
PO
Adults, Elderly. 300 mg on day 1, 300 mg twice a day on day 2, and 300 mg 3 times a day on day 3. Titrate up to 1800 mg/day.
▸ **Dosage in renal impairment**
Adults, Children 12 yr and older. Dosage and frequency are modified based on creatinine clearance: An example is given below. See manufacturer prescribing information for full table.

CrCl (mL/min)	Dosage
60 or higher	400 mg q8h
30-59	300 mg q12h
16-29	300 mg daily
< 16	300 mg every other day
Hemodialysis	200-300 mg after each 4-h hemodialysis session

OFF-LABEL USES
Treatment of essential tremor, hot flashes, diabetic neuropathy.

CONTRAINDICATIONS
Hypersensitivity to gabapentin.

INTERACTIONS
Drug
Antacids: May decrease gabapentin effectiveness.
Hydrocodone: Gabapentin may decrease hydrocodone concentrations.

Morphine: May increase plasma concentrations of gabapentin.
Herbal
Evening primrose oil, ginkgo: May decrease anticonvulsant effectiveness.
Food
None known.

DIAGNOSTIC TEST EFFECTS
May decrease serum WBC count.

SIDE EFFECTS
Frequent (10%-19%)
Fatigue, somnolence, dizziness, ataxia.
Occasional (3%-8%)
Nystagmus, tremor, diplopia, rhinitis, weight gain.
Rare (< 2%)
Nervousness, dysarthria, memory loss, dyspepsia, pharyngitis, myalgia.

SERIOUS REACTIONS
• Abrupt withdrawal may increase seizure frequency.
• Overdosage may result in diplopia, slurred speech, drowsiness, lethargy, and diarrhea.

PRECAUTIONS & CONSIDERATIONS
Caution is warranted in patients with renal impairment. It is unknown whether gabapentin is distributed in breast milk. The safety and efficacy of this drug have not been established in children 3 yr and younger. In elderly patients, age-related renal impairment may require dosage adjustment. Alcohol and tasks requiring mental alertness or motor skills should be avoided.

Seizure disorder, including the onset, duration, frequency, intensity, and type of seizures, should be assessed before and during treatment. Weight, renal function, and behavior should also be monitored.

Storage
Store capsules and tablets at room temperature. Store oral solution in refrigerator. Do not freeze.
Administration
! The interval between drug doses should not exceed 12 h.

Gabapentin may be taken with food to reduce GI upset. If gabapentin treatment will be discontinued or another anticonvulsant added to the treatment regimen, expect to make the changes gradually over at least 1 wk to prevent loss of seizure control.

Galantamine
ga-lan′ta-mene
(Razadyne)
Do not confuse Razadyne with Rozerem or Reyataz.

CATEGORY AND SCHEDULE
Pregnancy Risk Category: B

Classification: Cholinesterase inhibitors

MECHANISM OF ACTION
A cholinesterase inhibitor that inhibits the enzyme acetylcholinesterase, thus increasing the concentration of acetylcholine at cholinergic synapses and enhancing cholinergic function in the CNS. *Therapeutic Effect:* Slows the progression of Alzheimer disease.

PHARMACOKINETICS
Rapidly absorbed from the GI tract. Protein binding: 18%. Distributed to blood cells; binds to plasma proteins, mainly albumin. Metabolized in the liver. Excreted in urine.
Half-life: 7 h.

AVAILABILITY

Capsule (Extended Release): 8 mg, 16 mg, 24 mg.
Oral Solution: 4 mg/mL.
Tablets (Immediate Release): 4 mg, 8 mg, 12 mg.

INDICATIONS AND DOSAGES

▸ **Alzheimer disease**
PO
Adults, Elderly. Initially, 4 mg twice a day (8 mg/day) of the immediate release tablets or 8 mg once daily of the extended-release capsules. After a minimum of 4 wks (if well tolerated), may increase to 8 mg twice a day (16 mg/day) of the immediate-release tablets or 16 mg once daily of the extended-release capsules. After another 4 wks, may increase to 12 mg twice daily (24 mg/day) of the immediate-release tablets or 24 mg once daily of the extended release capsules. Range: 16-24 mg/day in 2 divided doses for the immediate-release tablets or once daily for the extended-release capsules.

▸ **Dosage in renal impairment**
For moderate impairment, maximum dosage is 16 mg/day. Drug is not recommended for patients with severe impairment (CrCl < 9 mL/min).

CONTRAINDICATIONS

Severe hepatic or renal impairment.

INTERACTIONS

Drug
Anticholinergics: May oppose effects of galantamine.
Bethanechol, succinylcholine: May interfere with the effects of these drugs.
Cimetidine, erythromycin, ketoconazole, paroxetine: May increase the galantamine blood concentration.

Herbal and Food
None known.

DIAGNOSTIC TEST EFFECTS

None known.

SIDE EFFECTS

Frequent (5%-17%)
Nausea, vomiting, diarrhea, anorexia, weight loss.
Occasional (4%-9%)
Abdominal pain, insomnia, depression, headache, dizziness, fatigue, rhinitis.
Rare (< 3%)
Tremors, constipation, confusion, cough, anxiety, urinary incontinence.

SERIOUS REACTIONS

• Overdose may cause cholinergic crisis, characterized by increased salivation, lacrimation, severe nausea and vomiting, bradycardia, respiratory depression, hypotension, and increased muscle weakness. Treatment usually consists of supportive measures and an anticholinergic such as atropine.

PRECAUTIONS & CONSIDERATIONS
Caution is warranted in patients with asthma, bladder outflow obstruction, chronic obstructive pulmonary disease (COPD), peptic ulcer disease, a history of seizures, moderate hepatic or renal impairment, supraventricular conduction disturbances, and concurrent use of NSAIDs. It is unknown whether galantamine crosses the placenta or is distributed in breast milk. Galantamine is not prescribed for children. No age-related precautions have been noted in elderly patients, but galantamine is not recommended for those with severe hepatic or renal impairment (creatinine clearance of < 9 mL/min). Be aware that galantamine is not

a cure for Alzheimer disease, but it might slow the progression of its symptoms.

Notify the physician if the patient experiences excessive sweating, tearing, or salivation, depression, dizziness, excessive fatigue, muscle weakness, insomnia, weight loss, or persistent GI disturbances. A 12-lead ECG and rhythm strips should be performed periodically. Liver and renal function test results should also be assessed.

Administration

! If galantamine therapy is interrupted for several days or longer, reinstitute therapy as prescribed.

Take immediate-release galantamine with morning and evening meals, and take the extended-release capsule with morning meals.

Ganciclovir

gan-sy′clo-ver
(Cymevene [AUS], Cytovene, Vitrasert)
Do not confuse Cytovene with Cytosar.

CATEGORY AND SCHEDULE
Pregnancy Risk Category: C

Classification: Antivirals, nucleoside analogue

MECHANISM OF ACTION
This synthetic nucleoside competes with viral DNA polymerase and is incorporated into growing viral DNA chains. *Therapeutic Effect:* Interferes with synthesis and replication of viral DNA.

PHARMACOKINETICS
Widely distributed. Protein binding: 1%-2%. Undergoes minimal metabolism. Excreted unchanged primarily in urine. Removed by hemodialysis. *Half-life:* 2.5-3.6 h (increased in patients with impaired renal function).

AVAILABILITY
Capsules (Cytovene): 250 mg, 500 mg.
Powder for Injection (Cytovene): 500 mg.
Implant (Vitrasert): 4.5 mg.

INDICATIONS AND DOSAGES
▸ **Cytomegalovirus (CMV) retinitis**
IV
Adults, Children 3 mo and older. 10 mg/kg/day in divided doses q12h for 14-21 days, then 5 mg/kg/day as a single daily dose 7 days/wk or 6 mg/kg/day as a single daily dose 5 days/wk.
▸ **Prevention of CMV disease in transplant patients**
IV
Adults, Children. 10 mg/kg/day in divided doses q12h for 7-14 days, then 5 mg/kg/day as a single daily dose 7 days/wk or 6 mg/kg/day as a single daily dose 5 days/wk.
ORAL
Adults. 1000 mg three times daily; continue for 14 wks.
▸ **Other CMV infections**
IV
Adults. Initially, 10 mg/kg/day in divided doses q12h for 14-21 days, then 5 mg/kg/day as a single daily dose 7 days/wk or 6 mg/kg/day as a single daily dose 5 days/wk. Maintenance: 1000 mg orally 3 times a day or 500 mg q3h (6 times a day) after IV regimen.
Children. Initially, 10 mg/kg/day in divided doses q12h for 14-21 days, then 5 mg/kg/day as a single daily dose 7 days/wk or 6 mg/kg/day as a single daily dose 5 days/wk. Maintenance: 30 mg/kg/dose q8h. PO.

▶ **Intravitreal implant**
Adults. 1 implant q6-9mo plus oral ganciclovir (1-1.5 g 3 times daily). *Children 9 yr and older.* 1 implant q6-9mo plus oral ganciclovir (30 mg/dose q8h).
▶ **Adult dosage in renal impairment**
Dosage and frequency are modified based on CrCl.

CrCl (mL/ min)	IV Induction Dosage	IV Maintenance Dosage	Oral
50-69	2.5 mg/kg q12h	2.5 mg/kg q24h	1500 mg/day
25-49 daily	2.5 mg/kg q24h	1.25 mg/kg q24h	1000 mg/day
10-24	1.25 mg/kg q24h	0.625 mg/kg q24h	500 mg/day
< 10	1.25 mg/kg 3 times/ wk	0.625 mg/kg 3 times/wk	500 mg 3 times/ wk

CrCl, Creatinine clearance.

OFF-LABEL USES
Treatment of other CMV infections, such as gastroenteritis, hepatitis, and pneumonitis.

CONTRAINDICATIONS
Absolute neutrophil count < 500/mm^3, platelet count < 25,000/mm^3, hypersensitivity to acyclovir or ganciclovir, immunocompetent patients, patients with congenital or neonatal CMV disease.

INTERACTIONS
Drug
Bone marrow depressants: May increase bone marrow depression.
Didanosine: May increase ganciclovir levels.
Imipenem and cilastatin: May increase the risk of seizures.
Nephrotoxic agents: May cause added risk of nephrotoxicity.
Probenecid: May decrease the clearance of ganciclovir.
Zidovudine (AZT): May increase the risk of hepatotoxicity.
Herbal and Food
None known.

DIAGNOSTIC TEST EFFECTS
May increase serum alkaline phosphatase, bilirubin, AST (SGOT), and ALT (SGPT) levels.

Ⓓ IV INCOMPATIBILITIES
Aldesleukin (Proleukin), amifostine (Ethyol), amikacin (Amikin), aminophylline, amphotericin B colloidal (Amphotec), ampicillin (Polycillin), ampicillin and sulbactam (Unasyn), amsacrine (Amsa P-D), ascorbic acid, atracurium (Tracrium), azathioprine (Imuran), aztreonam (Azactam), benztropine (Cogentin), bumetanide (Bumex), buprenorphine (Buprenex), butorphanol (Stadol), calcium chloride, cefamandole (Mandol), cefazolin (Ancef), cefepime (Maxipime), cefmetazole (Zefazone), cefonicid (Monocid), cefoperazone (Cefobid), cefotaxime (Claforan), cefotetan (Cefotan), cefoxitin (Mefixitin), ceftazidime (Fortaz), ceftizoxime (Cefizox), ceftriaxone (Rocephin), cefuroxime (Zinacef), cephalothin (Keflin), cephapirin (Cefadyl), chloramphenicol (Chloromycetin), chlorpromazine (Thorazine), cimetidine (Tagamet), cisatracurium (Nimbex), clindamycin (Cleocin), cytarabine (ARA-C), dantrolene (Dantrium), diazepam (Valium), diazoxide (Proglycem), diltiazem (Cardizem), diphenhydramine (Benadryl), dobutamine (Dobutrex), dopamine (Intropin), doxorubicin (Adriamycin), doxycycline (Vibramycin), ephedrine, epinephrine, epirubicin (Ellence), erythromycin lactobionate

G

(Erythrocin), esmolol (BreviBloc), famotidine (Pepcid), fenoldopam (Corlopam), fludarabine (Fludara), foscarnet (Foscavir), gemcitabine (Gemzar), gentamicin (Garamycin), haloperidol (Haldol), hydralazine (Apresoline), hydrocortisone sodium succinate (Solu Cortef), inamrinone (Inocor), isoproterenol (Isuprel), ketorolac (Toradol), levofloxacin (Levofloxacin), lidocaine, magnesium sulfate, meperidine (Demerol), metaraminol (Aramine), methicillin (Staphcillin), methoxamine (Vasoxyl), methyldopate (Aldomet), methylprednisolone (Solu-Medrol), metoclopramide (Reglan), metronidazole (Flagyl), mezlocillin (Mezlin), midazolam (Versed), minocycline (Minocin), morphine sulfate (Avinza, Kadian, Robinul), moxalactam (Moxam), multiple vitamins, nalbuphine (Nubain), netilmicin (Netromycin), norepinephrine (Levophed), ondansetron (Zofran), oxacillin (Bactocil), palonosetron (Aloxi), papaverine, penicillin G potassium (Pfizerpen), penicillin G sodium, pentamidine (Pentam), pentazocine (Talwin), phentolamine (Regitine), phenylephrine, phenytoin (Dilantin), piperacillin (Piperacil), piperacillin and tazobactam (Zosyn), procainamide (Pronestyl), prochlorperazine (Compazine), promethazine (Phenergan), pyridoxine, quinidine, quinupristin and dalfopristin (Synercid), sargramostim (Leukine), sodium bicarbonate, streptokinase (Streptase), succinylcholine (Anectine), sulfamethoxazole and trimethoprim (Bactrim), tacrolimus (Prograf), theophylline (Theodur), thiamine, ticarcillin (Ticar), ticarcillin and clavulanate (Timentin), tobramycin (Nebcin),

tolazoline (Tolazolin), urokinase (Abbokinase), vancomycin (Vancocin), verapamil (Calan), vinorelbine (Navelbine).

⬛ IV COMPATIBILITIES

Alfentanil (Alfenta), allopurinol (Alloprim), amphotericin B cholesteryl (Amphotec), anidulafungin (Eraxis), atropine, bivalirudin (Angiomax), bretylium (Bretylol), calcium gluconate, carboplatin (Paraplatin), caspofungin (Cancidas), cisplatin (Platinol-AQ), cyanocobalamin, cyclophosphamide (Cytoxan), cyclosporine (Gengraf, Neoral, Sandimmune), dactinomycin (Cosmegen), dexamethasone (Decadron), dexmedetomidine (Precedex), digoxin (Lanoxin), docetaxel (Taxotere), doxacurium (Nuromax), enalaprilat (Vasotec), epoetin alfa (Epogen, Procrit), ertapenem (Invanz), etoposide (VePesid), fentanyl (Sublimaze), filgrastim (Neupogen), fluconazole (Diflucan), fluorouracil (Efurix), folic acid, furosemide (Lasix), gatifloxacin (Tequin), glycopyrrolate (Robinul), granisetron (Kytril), heparin, hetastarch 6% (Hextend), hydromorphone (Dilaudid), hydroxyzine (Vistaril), imipenem and cilastatin (Primaxin), indomethacin (Indocen), insulin (regular), labetalol (Normodyne, Trandate), lactated Ringer's, lansoprazole (Prevacid), linezolid (Zyvox), lorazepam (Ativan), mannitol, mechlorethamine (Mustargen), melphalan (Alkeran), methotrexate, metoprolol (Lopressor), miconazole (Monistat), milrinone (Primacor), mitoxantrone (Novantrone), nafcillin (Unipen), naloxone (Narcan), nitroglycerin (NitroBid), nitroprusside (Nitropress), oxytocin (Pitocin), paclitaxel (Taxol), pantoprazole (Protonix), pemetrexed

(Alimta), pentobarbital (Nembutal), phenobarbital, phytonadione, polymyxin B (Aerosporin), potassium chloride, propofol (Diprivan), propranolol (Inderal), protamine, ranitidine (Zantac), remifentanil (Ultiva), Ringer's, ritodrine (Yutopar), rituximab (Rituxan), sodium acetate, sufentanil (Sufenta), teniposide (Vumon), thiotepa (Thioplex), tigecycline (Tygacil), tirofiban (Aggrastat), trastuzumab (Herceptin), trimetaphan (Camsylate), vasopressin (Pitressin), vincristine (Oncovin), voriconazole (Vfend).

SIDE EFFECTS
Frequent
Diarrhea (41%), fever (40%), nausea (25%), abdominal pain (17%), vomiting (13%).
Occasional (6%-11%)
Diaphoresis, infection, paresthesia, flatulence, pruritus.
Rare (2%-4%)
Headache, stomatitis, dyspepsia, phlebitis.

SERIOUS REACTIONS
• Hematologic toxicity occurs commonly: Leukopenia in 29%-41% of patients and anemia in 19%-25%.
• Intraocular insertion occasionally results in visual acuity loss, vitreous hemorrhage, and retinal detachment.
• GI hemorrhage occurs rarely.
• Aspermatogenesis.

PRECAUTIONS & CONSIDERATIONS
Caution should be used in pediatric patients. The long-term safety of this drug has not been determined because of the potential for long-term adverse reproductive and carcinogenic effects. Caution is warranted with impaired renal function, neutropenia, and thrombocytopenia. Be aware that ganciclovir should not be used during pregnancy and that breastfeeding should be discontinued during ganciclovir use. Breastfeeding may be resumed no sooner than 72 h after the last dose of ganciclovir. Be aware that effective contraception should be used during ganciclovir therapy. Be aware that the safety and efficacy of ganciclovir have not been established in children younger than 12 yr of age. In elderly patients, age-related renal impairment may require dosage adjustment. Ganciclovir may temporarily or permanently inhibit sperm production in males and suppress fertility in females. Barrier contraception should be used during ganciclovir administration and for 90 days after therapy because of mutagenic potential.

Specimens (blood, feces, throat culture, urine) should be obtained for culture and sensitivity testing, as ordered, before giving the drug. Keep in mind that test results are needed to support the differential diagnosis and rule out retinal infection as the result of hematogenous dissemination. Intake and output should be monitored as well as adequate hydration (minimum 1500 mL/24 h). Hematology reports for decreased platelets, neutropenia, and thrombocytopenia should be evaluated. Altered vision, complications, and therapeutic improvement should be assessed.
Storage
Store vials at room temperature. Do not refrigerate. Reconstituted solution in vial is stable for 12 h at room temperature. After dilution, refrigerate and use within 24 h. Discard the solution if precipitate forms or discoloration occurs.
Administration
Give ganciclovir with food.

Avoid inhaling the solution. Also avoid solution exposure to the eyes, mucous membranes, and skin. Use latex gloves and safety glasses during the preparation and handling of ganciclovir solution. If the solution comes in contact with mucous membranes or the skin, wash the affected area thoroughly with soap and water; rinse the eyes thoroughly with plain water.

Reconstitute 500-mg vial with 10 mL sterile water for injection to provide a concentration of 50 mg/mL; do not use bacteriostatic water, which contains parabens and is therefore incompatible with ganciclovir. Further dilute with 100 mL D5W, 0.9% NaCl, lactated Ringer's, or any combination thereof, to provide a concentration of 5 mg/mL. Do not give by IV push or rapid IV infusion because these routes increase the risk of ganciclovir toxicity. Administer only by IV infusion over 1 h. Protect from infiltration because the high pH of this drug causes severe tissue irritation. Use large veins to permit rapid dilution and dissemination of ganciclovir and to minimize the risk of phlebitis. Keep in mind that central venous ports tunneled under subcutaneous tissue may reduce catheter-associated infection.

Gatifloxacin
gah-tee-floks′a-sin
(Zymar)

CATEGORY AND SCHEDULE
Pregnancy Risk Category: C

Classification: Antibiotics, quinolones, ophthalmic

MECHANISM OF ACTION
A fluoroquinolone that inhibits two enzymes, topoisomerase II and IV, in susceptible microorganisms. *Therapeutic Effect:* Interferes with bacterial DNA replication. Prevents or delays resistance emergence. Bactericidal.

AVAILABILITY
Ophthalmic Solution (Zymar): 0.3%.

INDICATIONS AND DOSAGES
▸ **Bacterial conjunctivitis**
Adults, Elderly, Children 1 yr and older. 1 drop q2h while awake for 2 days, then 1 drop up to 4 times/day for days 3-7.

CONTRAINDICATIONS
Hypersensitivity to quinolones.

INTERACTIONS
Drug
None known.
Herbal
None known.
Food
None known.

DIAGNOSTIC TEST EFFECTS
None known.

SIDE EFFECTS
Occasional (5%-10%)
Ophthalmic: Conjunctival irritation, increased tearing, corneal inflammation.
Rare (0.1%-3%)
Ophthalmic: Corneal swelling, dry eye, eye pain, eyelid swelling, headache, red eye, reduced visual acuity, altered taste.

SERIOUS REACTIONS
Conjunctival hemorrhage has been reported.

PRECAUTIONS & CONSIDERATIONS

Patients should be advised to avoid contact lens use while they have signs and symptoms of bacterial conjunctivitis. It is unknown if gatifloxacin is distributed in breast milk. The safety and efficacy of gatifloxacin have not been established in children < 1 yr. History of hypersensitivity to gatifloxacin and other quinolones should be determined before therapy.

Administration

Tilt head backward and look up. Gently pull the lower eyelid down until a pocket is formed. Hold the dropper above the pocket, and without touching the eyelid or conjunctival sac, place drops into the center of the pocket. Close the eye, and then apply gentle digital pressure to the lacrimal sac at the inner canthus. Remove excess solution around the eye with a tissue.

Gefitinib

ge-fi´tye-nib
(Iressa)

CATEGORY AND SCHEDULE

Pregnancy Risk Category: D

Classification: Antineoplastic, miscellaneous; epidermal growth factor receptor inhibitor

MECHANISM OF ACTION

Blocks the signaling pathway that binds to the epidermal growth factor receptor (EGFR) on the surface of normal and cancer cells. EGFR activates the enzyme tyrosine kinase, which sends signals instructing the cells to grow. *Therapeutic Effect:* Inhibits the growth of cancer cells.

PHARMACOKINETICS

Slowly absorbed and extensively distributed throughout the body. Protein binding: 90%. Undergoes extensive metabolism in the liver. Excreted in the feces. *Half-life:* 48 h.

AVAILABILITY

Tablets: 250 mg.

INDICATIONS AND DOSAGES

▶ **Non–small cell lung cancer**

PO

Adults, Elderly. 250 mg/day; may increase to 500 mg/day for patients receiving drugs that may decrease gefitinib blood concentrations (CYP3A4 inducers), such as rifampin and phenytoin.

CONTRAINDICATIONS

None known.

INTERACTIONS

Drug

CYP3A4 inducers (e.g., rifamycins, phenytoin): Reduce gefitinib concentrations. Dosage adjustment and careful monitoring recommended.

Erythromycin, fluconazole, itraconazole, ketoconazole, and CYP3A4 inhibitors: May increase gefitinib blood concentration and toxicity.

Hz antagonists (e.g., cimetidine, ranitidine): Decrease absorption of gefitinib.

Vinorelbine: Increased risk of neutropenia.

Warfarin: Increases the risk of bleeding.

Herbal

St. John's wort: May reduce gefitinib concentrations. Avoid.

Food
None known.

DIAGNOSTIC TEST EFFECTS
May increase serum alkaline phosphatase, bilirubin, AST (SGOT), and ALT (SGPT) levels.

SIDE EFFECTS
Frequent (25%-48%)
Diarrhea, rash, acne.
Occasional (8%-13%)
Dry skin, nausea, vomiting, pruritus.
Rare (2%-7%)
Anorexia, asthenia, weight loss, peripheral edema, eye pain.

SERIOUS REACTIONS
• Pancreatitis and ocular hemorrhage occur rarely.
• Hypersensitivity reaction produces angioedema and urticaria. Interstitial lung disease has been reported and if it occurs, requires discontinuation of the drug.

PRECAUTIONS & CONSIDERATIONS
Caution is warranted in patients with hepatic impairment and severe renal impairment. Gefitinib may cause fetal harm and result in termination of pregnancy. Pregnant or breastfeeding women should not receive this drug. Pregnancy should be avoided during therapy, and contraceptive methods should be used during treatment and for up to 12 mo afterward. The safety and efficacy of gefitinib have not been established in children. No age-related precautions have been noted in elderly patients. Vaccinations without the physician's approval and crowds and people with known infections should be avoided.

Notify the physician of anorexia, nausea, vomiting, persistent or severe diarrhea, and signs and symptoms of infection, including fever and flu-like symptoms.

Adequate hydration should be maintained. Bowel sounds for hyperactivity and pattern of daily bowel activity and stool consistency should be assessed. Antidiarrheals and antiemetics should be ordered to help prevent and treat diarrhea, nausea, and vomiting. For those who cannot tolerate diarrhea, expect to interrupt gefitinib therapy for up to 14 days. If dyspnea, cough or other pulmonary symptoms occur, interrupt therapy until cause is determined.
Administration
Take gefitinib without regard to food. For patients who have difficulty swallowing, the tablets may be dropped in a half glass of noncarbonated drinking water and stirred to dissolve (approximately 10 min); then drink the liquid immediately. Rinse the glass with half a glass of water and drink that as well. The liquid may also be given via nasogastric tube.

Gemfibrozil
gem-fi′broe-zil
(Apo-Gemfibrozil [CAN], Ausgem [AUS], Gemfibromax [AUS], Jezil [AUS], Lipazil [AUS], Lopid, Novo-Gemfibrozil [CAN])
Do not confuse with Lorabid or Levbid.

CATEGORY AND SCHEDULE
Pregnancy Risk Category: C

Classification: Antihyperlipidemics, fibric acid derivatives

MECHANISM OF ACTION
A fibric acid derivative that inhibits lipolysis of fat in adipose tissue, decreases liver uptake of free fatty acids, and reduces hepatic triglyceride

production. Inhibits synthesis of VLDL carrier apolipoprotein B. *Therapeutic Effect:* Lowers serum cholesterol and triglycerides (decreases VLDL, LDL; increases HDL).

PHARMACOKINETICS

Well absorbed from the GI tract. Protein binding: 99%. Metabolized in liver. Primarily excreted in urine. Not removed by hemodialysis. *Half-life:* 1.5 h.

AVAILABILITY

Tablets: 600 mg.

INDICATIONS AND DOSAGES

▶ **Hyperlipidemia, hypertriglyceridemia**
PO
Adults, Elderly. 1200 mg/day in 2 divided doses 30 min before breakfast and dinner.

CONTRAINDICATIONS

Hypersensitivity, liver dysfunction (including primary biliary cirrhosis), preexisting gallbladder disease, severe renal dysfunction, administration with cerivastatin.

INTERACTIONS

Drug
Cyclosporine: May potentiate renal problems.
HMG CoA reductase inhibitors, especially cerivastatin, lovastatin: May increase risk of rhabdomyolysis, leading to acute renal failure.
Pioglitazone, repaglinide, warfarin: May increase the effect of these drugs.
Herbal
None known.
Food
None known.

DIAGNOSTIC TEST EFFECTS

May increase serum alkaline phosphatase, serum bilirubin, serum creatinine kinase, serum LDH concentrations, and SGOT (AST) and SGPT (ALT) levels. May decrease blood hemoglobin and hematocrit levels, leukocyte counts, and serum potassium levels.

SIDE EFFECTS

Frequent (20%)
Dyspepsia.
Occasional (2%-10%)
Abdominal pain, diarrhea, nausea, vomiting, fatigue.
Rare (< 2%)
Constipation, acute appendicitis, vertigo, headache, rash, pruritus, altered taste.

SERIOUS REACTIONS

• Cholelithiasis, cholecystitis, acute appendicitis, pancreatitis, and malignancy occur rarely.

PRECAUTIONS & CONSIDERATIONS

Caution is warranted in patients with diabetes mellitus, receiving estrogen or anticoagulant therapy, and with hypothyroidism. Be aware that it is unknown whether gemfibrozil crosses the placenta or is distributed in breast milk. Also know that the decision to discontinue breastfeeding or gemfibrozil should be based on the potential for serious adverse effects to the infant. Be aware that gemfibrozil use is not recommended in children younger than 2 yr of age because cholesterol is necessary for normal development in this age group. In elderly patients, age-related renal impairment may require dosage adjustment.

Notify the physician of any abdominal pain, diarrhea, dizziness, nausea, or vomiting. Pattern of daily bowel activity and stool consistency should be assessed. Serum LDL, VLDL, triglyceride, and cholesterol levels should be checked at baseline and periodically during treatment. Hematology and liver function test results should also be assessed. Blood glucose should be monitored in those receiving insulin or oral antihyperglycemics.

Be aware of the increased risk of developing rhabdomyolysis when coadministered with a statin. Lovastatin should be limited to a maximum of 20 mg/day if given concomitantly with gemfibrozil.

Administration
Take gemfibrozil 30 min before morning and evening meals.

Gemifloxacin
gem-ih-flocks′ah-sin
(Factive)

CATEGORY AND SCHEDULE
Pregnancy Risk Category: C

Classification: Antibiotics, quinolones

MECHANISM OF ACTION
A fluoroquinolone that inhibits the enzyme DNA gyrase in susceptible microorganisms, interfering with bacterial cell replication and repair. *Therapeutic Effect:* Bactericidal.

PHARMACOKINETICS
Rapidly and well absorbed from the GI tract. Protein binding: 70%. Widely distributed. Penetrates well into lung tissue and fluid. Undergoes limited metabolism in the liver. Primarily excreted in feces; lesser amount eliminated in urine. Partially removed by hemodialysis. *Half-life:* 4-12 h.

AVAILABILITY
Tablets: 320 mg.

INDICATIONS AND DOSAGES
▸ **Acute bacterial exacerbation of chronic bronchitis**
PO
Adults, Elderly. 320 mg once a day for 5 days.
▸ **Community-acquired pneumonia**
PO
Adults, Elderly. 320 mg once a day for 7 days.
▸ **Dosage in renal impairment**
Dosage and frequency are modified based on creatinine clearance.

Creatinine Clearance (mL/min)	Dosage
> 40	320 mg once a day
≤ 40	160 mg once a day

CONTRAINDICATIONS
Concurrent use of amiodarone, quinidine, procainamide, or sotalol; history of prolonged QTC interval; hypersensitivity to fluoroquinolones; uncorrected electrolyte disorders (such as hypokalemia and hypomagnesemia).

INTERACTIONS
Drug
Aluminum and magnesium-containing antacids, bismuth subsalicylate, didanosine, iron preparations and other metals, sucralfate, zinc preparations: May decrease the absorption of gemifloxacin. Avoid administration within 3 h before or 2 h after gemifloxacin.
Antipsychotics, class 1A and class III antiarrhythmics, erythromycin, tricyclic antidepressants: May increase the risk of prolonged QTC interval and life-threatening arrhythmias.
Corticosteroids: May increase risk of tendon rupture, especially in elderly patients.
Cyclosporine: Increases the risk of nephrotoxicity.

Probenecid: Increases gemifloxacin serum concentration.

Warfarin: May increase the effect of warfarin.

Herbal and Food

None known.

DIAGNOSTIC TEST EFFECTS

May increase BUN and serum alkaline phosphatase, bilirubin, LDH, creatinine, AST (SGOT), and ALT (SGPT) levels.

SIDE EFFECTS

Occasional (2%-4%)

Diarrhea, rash, nausea.

Rare (≥ 1%)

Headache, abdominal pain, dizziness.

SERIOUS REACTIONS

• Antibiotic-associated colitis may result from altered bacterial balance.

• Hypersensitivity reactions, including photosensitivity (as evidenced by rash, pruritus, blisters, edema, and burning skin), have occurred in patients receiving fluoroquinolones. With gemifloxacin, serious rashes occur more frequently in women under 40 and women of any age receiving hormone replacement therapy.

• Tendon ruptures and peripheral neuropathy have been reported.

PRECAUTIONS & CONSIDERATIONS

Caution is warranted in patients with acute myocardial ischemia, clinically significant bradycardia, or impaired hepatic or renal function. Gemifloxacin may be teratogenic. Substitute formula feedings for breastfeeding. The safety and efficacy of gemifloxacin have not been established in children 18 yr of age and younger. Age-related renal impairment may require a dosage adjustment in elderly patients.

Dizziness, headache, nausea, signs of infection, and skin for rash should be evaluated. Pattern of daily bowel activity and stool consistency should be assessed. Liver function and white blood cell (WBC) count should be monitored. QT and QTC intervals should be checked for prolongation. History of hypersensitivity to gemifloxacin and other quinolones should be determined before therapy.

Fluoroquinolone use has been associated with hypoglycemia in patients with and without diabetes. Patients with diabetes should be monitored frequently while taking gemifloxacin.

Administration

Take gemifloxacin without regard to food. Do not crush or break tablets. Take 2 h before giving antacids, buffered tablets or solutions, ferrous sulfate, or multivitamins with minerals.

Gemtuzumab Ozogamicin

gem-too′-ze-mab
(Mylotarg)

CATEGORY AND SCHEDULE

Pregnancy Risk Category: D

Classification: Antineoplastics, monoclonal antibodies.

MECHANISM OF ACTION

Binds to an antigen on the surface of leukemic blast cells, resulting in the formation of a complex that leads to the release of the antibiotic inside the myeloid cells. The antibiotic then binds to DNA, resulting in DNA double-strand breaks and cell death. *Therapeutic Effect:* Inhibits colony formation in cultures of adult leukemic bone marrow cells.

PHARMACOKINETICS
Elimination Half-life: 45 h after first infusion; 60 h after second infusion.

AVAILABILITY
Powder for Injection: 5 mg.

INDICATIONS AND DOSAGES
▸ CD33-positive acute myeloid leukemia
IV INFUSION
Adults 60 yr and older. 9 mg/m^2 repeated in 14 days for a total of 2 doses.

CONTRAINDICATIONS
Patients with anti-CD33, antibody, previous hypersensitivity is the major toxicity.

INTERACTIONS
Drug
Abciximab, monoclonal antibodies: May increase the risk of hypersensitivity and thrombocytopenia.
Herbal
None known.
Food
None known.

DIAGNOSTIC TEST EFFECTS
May increase serum bilirubin, AST (SGOT), and ALT (SGPT) levels. May decrease blood hemoglobin and hematocrit levels, platelet count, WBC count, and serum magnesium and potassium levels.

✪ IV INCOMPATIBILITIES
Do not mix gemtuzumab with any other medications.

SIDE EFFECTS
! Most patients experience a postinfusion symptom complex of fever (85%), chills (73%), nausea (70%), and vomiting (63%) that resolves within 2-4 h with supportive therapy
Frequent (31%-44%)
Asthenia, diarrhea, abdominal pain, headache, stomatitis, dyspnea, epistaxis.
Occasional (15%-25%)
Constipation, neutropenic fever, nonspecific rash, herpes simplex infection, hypertension, hypotension, petechiae, peripheral edema, dizziness, insomnia, back pain.
Rare (10%-14%)
Pharyngitis, ecchymosis, dyspepsia, tachycardia, hematuria, rhinitis.

SERIOUS REACTIONS
• Severe myelosuppression, characterized by neutropenia, anemia, and thrombocytopenia, occurs in 98% of all patients.
• Sepsis occurs in 25% of patients.
• Hepatotoxicity also may occur.
• Serious bleeding may occur (1%).

PRECAUTIONS & CONSIDERATIONS
Caution is warranted in patients with hepatic impairment. Pregnant women should not receive gemtuzumab because it may cause fetal harm. It is unknown whether gemtuzumab is excreted in breast milk; however, women receiving this drug should not breastfeed. The safety and efficacy of gemtuzumab have not been established in children. No age-related precautions have been noted in elderly patients. Vaccinations without the physician's approval and crowds and people with known infections should be avoided. Patients with pulmonary disease may be at risk for pulmonary reactions during infusion.

Notify the physician of bruising, fever, signs of local infection, sore throat, or unusual bleeding from any site. Baseline serum chemistry levels, CBC (to monitor for myelosuppression), BP, and liver function test results should be obtained before and during therapy. Signs and symptoms for stomatitis (burning or erythema of oral mucosa, ulceration, sore throat, difficulty swallowing), anemia (excessive fatigue and weakness), and myelosuppression (ecchymosis, fever, signs of local infection, sore throat, and unusual bleeding from any site) should be assessed.

Storage

Protect the drug from direct and indirect sunlight and unshielded fluorescent light during preparation and administration. Refrigerate—do not freeze—the powder for injection. After reconstitution, protect the solution from light. The solution is stable for up to 8 h if refrigerated.

Administration

! Give diphenhydramine 50 mg and acetaminophen 650-1000 mg 1 h before administering gemtuzumab, as prescribed. Follow with acetaminophen 650-1000 mg every 4 h for 2 doses, then every 4 h as prescribed and as needed. Full recovery from hematologic toxicities is not a requirement for giving the second gemtuzumab dose. Corticosteroids may also be prescribed to pre-medicate.

Use strict aseptic technique in preparing the drug to protect the patient from infection. Prepare the drug in a biologic safety hood with the fluorescent light off. Before reconstitution, let the vials come to room temperature. Using sterile syringes, reconstitute each vial with 5 mL sterile water for injection to provide a concentration of 1 mg/mL. Gently swirl the vial;

then inspect for particulate matter or discoloration. Withdraw the desired volume from each vial, and inject into an IV bag containing 100 mL 0.9% NaCl; place the IV bag into an ultraviolet protectant bag. Administer the solution as soon as it has been diluted in 100 mL 0.9% NaCl. Infuse the drug over 2 h, using a separate peripheral or central line equipped with a low-protein-binding 1.2-micron filter. Do not give by IV push or bolus.

G

Gentamicin

jen-ta-mye′sin
(Alcomicin [CAN], Cidomycin [CAN], Garamycin, Genoptic, Gentacidin, Gentak)

CATEGORY AND SCHEDULE

Pregnancy Risk Category: C

Classification: Anti-infectives, ophthalmic, topical, antibiotics, aminoglycosides, dermatologics

MECHANISM OF ACTION

An aminoglycoside antibiotic that irreversibly binds to the protein of bacterial ribosomes. *Therapeutic Effect:* Interferes with protein synthesis of susceptible microorganisms. Bactericidal.

PHARMACOKINETICS

Rapid, complete absorption after IM administration. Protein binding: < 30%. Widely distributed (does not cross the blood-brain barrier, low concentrations in CSF). Excreted unchanged in urine. Removed by hemodialysis. *Half-life:* 2-4 h (increased in impaired renal function and neonates; decreased in cystic fibrosis and burn or febrile patients).

AVAILABILITY

Injection (Garamycin): 10 mg/mL, 40 mg/mL.
Ophthalmic Solution (Gentacidin, Genoptic, Gentak): 0.3%.
Ophthalmic Ointment (Gentak): 0.3%.
Cream (Garamycin): 0.1%.
Ointment: 0.1%.

INDICATIONS AND DOSAGES

▸ **Acute pelvic, bone, intra-abdominal, joint, respiratory tract, burn wound, postoperative, and skin or skin-structure infections; complicated urinary tract infection; septicemia; meningitis**
IV, IM
Adults, Elderly. Usual dosage, 3-6 mg/kg/day in divided doses q8h or 4-7 mg/kg once a day.
Children 5-12 yr. Usual dosage 2-2.5 mg/kg/dose q8h.
Children younger than 5 yr. Usual dosage, 2.5 mg/kg/dose q8h.
Neonates. Usual dosage 2.5-3.5 mg/kg/dose q8-12h.

▸ **Hemodialysis**
IV, IM
Adults, Elderly. 1-1.7 mg/kg after dialysis.
Children. 1-1.7 mg/kg/dose after dialysis.

▸ **Intrathecal (preservative-free injection only)**
Adults. 4-8 mg/day.
Children 3 mo to 12 yr. 1-2 mg/day.
Neonates. 1 mg/day.

▸ **Superficial eye infections**
OPHTHALMIC OINTMENT
Adults, Elderly. Usual dosage, apply thin strip to conjunctiva 2-3 times a day.
OPHTHALMIC SOLUTION
Adults, Elderly, Children.
Usual dosage, 1-2 drops q2-4h up to 2 drops/h.

▸ **Superficial skin infections**
TOPICAL
Adults, Elderly. Usual dosage, apply 3-4 times/day.

▸ **Dosage in renal impairment (adults)**
For traditional dosing regimens.
Creatinine clearance 40-60 mL/min. Dosage interval q12h.
Creatinine clearance 20-40 mL/min. Dosage interval q24h.
Creatinine clearance < 20 mL/min. Monitor levels to determine dosage interval.

CONTRAINDICATIONS

Hypersensitivity to gentamicin, other aminoglycosides (cross-sensitivity), or their components. Sulfite sensitivity may result in anaphylaxis, especially in asthmatic patients.

INTERACTIONS

Drug
Nephrotoxic medications, other aminoglycosides, ototoxic medications: May increase the risk of nephrotoxicity or ototoxicity.
Neuromuscular blockers: May increase neuromuscular blockade.
Herbal
None known.
Food
None known.

DIAGNOSTIC TEST EFFECTS

May increase serum creatinine, serum bilirubin, BUN, serum LDH, SGOT (AST), and SGPT (ALT) levels. May decrease serum calcium, magnesium, potassium, and sodium concentrations. In traditional dose regimens, the therapeutic peak serum level is 6-10 mcg/mL and trough is 0.5-2 mcg/mL. For all regimens, toxic trough level is > 2 mcg/mL.

ⓘ IV INCOMPATIBILITIES

Allopurinol (Aloprim), amphotericin B complex (Abelcet, AmBisome, Amphotec), ampicillin (Polycillin), cefamandole (Mandol), cefepime (Maxipime), cefotaxime (Claforan), cefotetan (Cefotan), cefuroxime (Ancef), clindamycin (Cleocin), cytarabine (Cytosar), dopamine (Intropin), filgrastim (Neupogen), furosemide (Lasix), heparin, hetastarch (Hespan), idarubicin (Idamycin), indomethacin (Indocin), nafcillin (Unipen), phenytoin (Dilantin), propofol (Diprivan), ticarcillin (Ticar), warfarin (Coumadin).

ⓘ IV COMPATIBILITIES

Acyclovir (Zovirax), alatrofloxacin (Trovan), amifostine (Ethyol), amiodarone (Cordarone), amsacrine (AMSA), atracurium (Tracrium), aztreonam (Azactam), bleomycin (Blenoxane), cefoxitin (Mefixitin), cimetidine (Tagamet), ciprofloxacin (Cipro), cisatracurium (Nimbex), clarithromycin (Biaxin), cyclophosphamide (Cytoxan), diltiazem (Cardizem), enalaprilat (Vasotec), esmolol (BreviBloc), etoposide (VePesid), famotidine (Pepcid), fluconazole (Diflucan), fludarabine (Fludara), foscarnet (Foscavir), gatifloxacin (Tequin), gemcitabine (Gemzar), granisetron (Kytril), hydromorphone (Dilaudid), insulin, labetolol (Normodyne, Trandate), levofloxacin (Levaquin), lidocaine (Xylocaine), linezolid (Zyvox), lorazepam (Ativan), magnesium sulfate, melphalan (Alkeran), meperidine (Demerol), meropenem (Merrem), metronidazole (Flagyl), midazolam (Versed), morphine, multivitamins, ondansetron (Zofran), paclitaxel (Taxol), pancuronium (Pavulon), perphenazine (Trilafon), ranitidine (Zantac), remifentanil (Ultiva), sargramostim (Leukine), tacrolimus (Prograf), teniposide (Vumon), theophylline (Theodur), thiotepa (Thioplex), tolazone (Tolazolin), vecuronium (Norcuron), verapamil (Calan), vinorelbine (Navelbine), vitamin B complex with C, zidovudine (Retrovir).

SIDE EFFECTS

Occasional
IM: Pain, induration.
IV: Phlebitis, thrombophlebitis, hypersensitivity reactions (fever, pruritus, rash, urticaria).
Ophthalmic: Burning, tearing, itching, blurred vision.
Topical: Redness, itching.
Rare
Alopecia, hypertension, weakness.

SERIOUS REACTIONS

• Nephrotoxicity (as evidenced by increased BUN and serum creatinine levels and decreased creatinine clearance) may be reversible if the drug is stopped at the first sign of symptoms.
• Irreversible ototoxicity (manifested as tinnitus, dizziness, ringing or roaring in the ears, and diminished hearing) and neurotoxicity (as evidenced by headache, dizziness, lethargy, tremor, and visual disturbances) occur occasionally. The risk of these effects increases with higher dosages or prolonged therapy and when the solution is applied directly to the mucosa.
• Superinfections, particularly with fungal infections, may result from bacterial imbalance no matter which administration route is used.
• Ophthalmic application may cause paresthesia of conjunctiva or mydriasis.

G

G

PRECAUTIONS & CONSIDERATIONS

! Cumulative gentamicin effects may occur with concurrent systemic administration and topical application to large areas. Caution is warranted with neuromuscular disorders because of the potential for respiratory depression, prior hearing loss, renal impairment, and vertigo and in elderly and neonatal patients because of age-related renal insufficiency or immaturity. Gentamicin readily crosses the placenta; it is unknown whether it is distributed in breast milk. Age-related renal impairment may require a dosage adjustment in elderly patients.

Before giving gentamicin, determine whether the patient has a history of allergies, especially to aminoglycosides, sulfites, and parabens (for topical and ophthalmic forms). Expect to correct dehydration before beginning parenteral therapy. Establish baseline hearing acuity before starting therapy. Intake and output and urinalysis results should be monitored as well as casts, RBCs, WBCs, and decreased specific gravity. Drink fluids to maintain adequate hydration. Monitor urinalysis results for casts, RBCs, WBCs, and decreased specific gravity. Be alert for ototoxic and neurotoxic side effects. If giving ophthalmic gentamicin, monitor the patient's eye for burning, itching, redness, and tearing. If giving topical gentamicin, monitor for itching and redness. Be alert for signs and symptoms of superinfection, particularly changes in the oral mucosa, diarrhea, and genital or anal pruritus. Monitor peak and trough serum drug levels.

Storage

Store ophthalmic preparations and solution vials for injection at room temperature. The solution normally appears clear or slightly yellow. Intermittent IV infusion or IV piggyback solution is stable for 24 h at room temperature. Discard the IV solution if a precipitate forms.

Administration

! Space parenteral doses evenly around the clock. Gentamicin dosage is based on ideal body weight. As ordered, monitor peak and trough serum drug levels periodically to maintain the desired serum concentrations and to minimize the risk of toxicity. The therapeutic peak serum level is 6-10 mcg/mL, and the therapeutic trough level is 0.5-2 mcg/mL. The toxic trough level is > 2 mcg/mL.

For IV administration, dilute with 50-200 mL of D5W or 0.9% NaCl. The amount of diluent for infants and children depends on individual needs. Infuse over 30-60 min for adults and older children. Infuse over 60-120 min for infants and young children.

Administer the IM injection slowly and deep in the gluteus maximus rather than the lateral aspect of the thigh to minimize injection site pain.

For intrathecal administration, use only 2 mg/mL of the intrathecal preparation without preservative. Mix with 10% of the estimated cerebrospinal fluid volume or NaCl. Use the intrathecal form immediately after preparation. Discard any unused portion. Give over 3-5 min.

For ophthalmic use, place a gloved finger on the lower eyelid and pull it out until a pocket is formed between the eye and lower lid. Hold the dropper above the pocket, and place the correct number of drops (or ¼ to ½ inch of ointment) into the pocket. Close the eye gently. After administering ophthalmic solution, apply digital pressure to the lacrimal sac for 1-2 min to minimize drainage into the nose and throat, thereby reducing the risk of systemic effects. After applying ophthalmic ointment, close the patient's eye for 1-2 min. Roll the eyeball to increase the drug's contact with the eye. Use tissue to remove excess solution or ointment around the eye.

Glatiramer
gla-teer′a-mer
(Copaxone)
Do not confuse Copaxone with Compazine.

CATEGORY AND SCHEDULE
Pregnancy Risk Category: B

Classification:
Immunosuppressives

MECHANISM OF ACTION
An immunosuppressive whose exact mechanism is unknown. May act by modifying immune processes thought to be responsible for the pathogenesis of multiple sclerosis (MS). *Therapeutic Effect:* Slows progression of MS.

PHARMACOKINETICS
Substantial fraction of glatiramer is hydrolyzed locally. Some fraction of injected material enters the lymphatic circulation, reaching regional lymph nodes; some may enter systemic circulation intact.

AVAILABILITY
Injection: 20 mg/mL in prefilled syringes.

INDICATIONS AND DOSAGES
▸ **MS**
SUBCUTANEOUS
Adults, Elderly. 20 mg once a day.

CONTRAINDICATIONS
Hypersensitivity to glatiramer or mannitol.

INTERACTIONS
Drug
None known.
Herbal
None known.
Food
None known.

DIAGNOSTIC TEST EFFECTS
None known.

SIDE EFFECTS
Expected (40%-73%)
Pain, erythema, inflammation, or pruritus at injection site; asthenia.
Frequent (18%-27%)
Arthralgia, vasodilation, anxiety, hypertonia, nausea, transient chest pain, dyspnea, flu-like symptoms, rash, pruritus.
Occasional (10%-17%)
Palpitations, back pain, diaphoresis, rhinitis, diarrhea, urinary urgency.
Rare (6%-8%)
Anorexia, fever, neck pain, peripheral edema, ear pain, facial edema, vertigo, vomiting.

SERIOUS REACTIONS
• Infection is a common effect.
• Lymphadenopathy occurs occasionally.
• Hypertension may occur.
• Transient eosinophilia may occur.

PRECAUTIONS & CONSIDERATIONS
Caution is warranted with an immediate post-injection reaction, including anxiety, chest pain, dyspnea, flushing, palpitations, and

G

urticaria. This reaction is usually transient and self-limiting. Pregnancy should be avoided during therapy. It is unknown whether glatiramer is distributed in breast milk. The safety and efficacy of glatiramer have not been established in children. No information is available on glatiramer use in elderly patients.

Notify the physician of rash, weakness, difficulty breathing or swallowing, or itching or swelling of the legs. Vital signs, including temperature, should be obtained at baseline.

Storage

Refrigerate syringes. Do not freeze.

Administration

Administer as subcutaneous injection in the arms, abdomen, thighs, or hips. Bring to room temperature before administering.

Glimepiride

gly-mep'er-ide
(Amaryl)
Do not confuse glimepiride with glipizide or glyburide.

CATEGORY AND SCHEDULE
Pregnancy Risk Category: C

Classification: Antidiabetic agents, sulfonylureas, second generation

MECHANISM OF ACTION
A second-generation sulfonylurea that promotes release of insulin from β cells of the pancreas and increases insulin sensitivity at peripheral sites. *Therapeutic Effect:* Lowers blood glucose concentration.

PHARMACOKINETICS

Route	Onset	Peak	Duration
PO	N/A	2-3 h	24 h

Completely absorbed from the GI tract. Protein binding: > 99%. Metabolized in the liver. Excreted in urine and eliminated in feces. *Half-life:* 5-9.2 h.

AVAILABILITY
Tablets: 1 mg, 2 mg, 4 mg.

INDICATIONS AND DOSAGES
▸ **Diabetes mellitus**
PO
Adults, Elderly. Initially, 1-2 mg once a day, with breakfast or first main meal. Maintenance: 1-4 mg once a day. After dose of 2 mg/day is reached, dosage should be increased in increments of up to 2 mg q1-2wk, based on blood glucose response. Maximum: 8 mg/day.
▸ **Dosage in renal impairment**
PO
Adults. Initially, 1 mg once a day. Titrate with care.

CONTRAINDICATIONS
Diabetic complications, such as ketosis, acidosis, and diabetic coma; monotherapy for type 1 diabetes mellitus.

INTERACTIONS
Drug
β-Blockers: May increase the hypoglycemic effect of glimepiride and mask signs of hypoglycemia. **Cimetidine, ciprofloxacin, fluconazole, MAOIs, quinidine, ranitidine, tricyclic antidepressant agents, large doses of salicylates:** May increase the effects of glimepiride. **Corticosteroids, lithium, thiazide diuretics:** May decrease the effects of glimepiride.

Cyclosporine: Sulfonylureas may increase cyclosporine levels.
Oral anticoagulants: May increase the effects of oral anticoagulants.
Herbal
Alfalfa, aloe, bilberry, bitter melon, burdock, celery, damiana, fenugreek, garcinia, garlic, ginger, ginseng (American), gymnema, marshmallow, stinging nettle: May enhance the hypoglycemic effects of glimepiride.
Food
Hypoglycemia is more likely to occur if alcohol is ingested.

DIAGNOSTIC TEST EFFECTS

May increase BUN and LDH concentrations and serum alkaline phosphatase, creatinine, and AST (SGOT) levels.

SIDE EFFECTS

Frequent
Altered taste sensation, dizziness, somnolence, weight gain, constipation, diarrhea, heartburn, nausea, vomiting, stomach fullness, headache.
Occasional
Increased sensitivity of skin to sunlight, peeling of skin, itching, rash.

SERIOUS REACTIONS

• Overdose or insufficient food intake may produce hypoglycemia, especially with increased glucose demands.
• GI hemorrhage, cholestatic hepatic jaundice, leukopenia, thrombocytopenia, pancytopenia, agranulocytosis, and aplastic or hemolytic anemia occur rarely.

PRECAUTIONS & CONSIDERATIONS

Caution is warranted in patients with adrenal insufficiency, debilitation, hepatic disease, impaired renal or hepatic function, intestinal obstruction, malnutrition, pituitary insufficiency, prolonged vomiting, severe diarrhea, sulfonamide allergy, uncontrolled hyperthyroidism, and stress situations (including severe infection, trauma, surgery). Be alert to conditions that alter blood glucose requirements, such as fever, increased activity, stress, or a surgical procedure. Glimepiride use is not recommended during pregnancy. It is unknown whether glimepiride is distributed in breast milk. Safety and efficacy of glimepiride have not been established in children. Hypoglycemia may be difficult to recognize in elderly patients. Also, age-related renal impairment may increase sensitivity to glucose-lowering effect. Wear sunscreen and protective eyewear to prevent the effects of light sensitivity.

Food intake and blood glucose should be monitored before and during therapy. Be aware of signs and symptoms of hypoglycemia (anxiety, cool wet skin, diplopia, dizziness, headache, hunger, numbness in the mouth, tachycardia, tremors), or hyperglycemia (deep rapid breathing, dim vision, fatigue, nausea, polydipsia, polyphagia, polyuria, vomiting); carry candy, sugar packets, or other sugar supplements for immediate response to hypoglycemia. Consult the physician when glucose demands are altered (such as with fever, heavy physical activity, infection, stress, trauma). Exercise, good personal hygiene (including foot care), not smoking, and weight control are essential parts of therapy.

Hypoglycemic agents may be associated with increased cardiovascular mortality.
Storage
Store at room temperature.
Administration
Take glimepiride with breakfast or the first main meal.

G

Glipizide
glip′i-zide
(Glucotrol, Glucotrol XL,
Melizide [AUS], Minidiab [AUS])
**Do not confuse glipizide with
glimepiride or glyburide.**

CATEGORY AND SCHEDULE
Pregnancy Risk Category: C

Classification: Antidiabetic agents,
sulfonylureas, second generation

MECHANISM OF ACTION
A second-generation sulfonylurea
that promotes the release of insulin
from β cells of the pancreas and
increases insulin sensitivity at
peripheral sites. *Therapeutic Effect:*
Lowers blood glucose concentration.

PHARMACOKINETICS

Route	Onset	Peak	Duration
PO	15-30 min	2-3 h	12-24 h
Extended-release	2-3 h	6-12 h	24 h

Well absorbed from the GI tract.
Protein binding: 99%. Metabolized
in the liver. Excreted in urine.
Half-life: 2-4 h.

AVAILABILITY
Tablets (Glucotrol): 5 mg, 10 mg.
*Tablets (Extended-Release [Glucotrol
XL]):* 2.5 mg, 5 mg, 10 mg.

INDICATIONS AND DOSAGES
▶ **Diabetes mellitus**
PO
Adults. Initially, 5 mg/day or 2.5 mg
in elderly patients or in those with
hepatic disease. Adjust dosage in
2.5- to 5-mg increments at intervals
of several days. Maximum single

dose: 15 mg. Maximum dose:
40 mg/day (rarely needed).
Maintenance (extended-release
tablet): Usually 5-20 mg once daily.
Elderly. Initially, 2.5-5 mg/day.
May increase by 2.5-5 mg/day
q1-2wk, according to adult dosage
recommendations.
Patients with hepatic impairment:
Begin at 2.5 mg once daily; titrate
cautiously.

CONTRAINDICATIONS
Diabetic ketoacidosis with or without
coma, type 1 diabetes mellitus,
hypersensitivity.

INTERACTIONS
Drug
β-Blockers: May increase the
hypoglycemic effect of glipizide and
mask signs of hypoglycemia.
**Cimetidine, ciprofloxacin,
fluconazole, MAOIs, quinidine,
ranitidine, large doses of salicylates:**
May increase the effects of glipizide.
**Corticosteroids, lithium, thiazide
diuretics:** May decrease the effects
of glipizide.
Cyclosporine: Sulfonylureas may
increase cyclosporine levels.
Oral anticoagulants: May increase
the effects of oral anticoagulants.
Herbal
**Alfalfa, aloe, bilberry, bitter melon,
burdock, celery, damiana, fenugreek,
garcinia, garlic, ginger, ginseng
(American), gymnema, marshmallow,
stinging nettle:** May enhance the
hypoglycemic effects of glipizide.
Food
Alcohol: Hypoglycemia is more
likely to occur if alcohol is ingested.

DIAGNOSTIC TEST EFFECTS
May increase BUN and LDH
concentrations and serum alkaline
phosphatase, creatinine, and AST
(SGOT) levels.

G

SIDE EFFECTS

Frequent

Altered taste sensation, dizziness, somnolence, weight gain, constipation, diarrhea, heartburn, nausea, vomiting, stomach fullness, headache.

Occasional

Increased sensitivity of skin to sunlight, peeling of skin, itching, rash.

SERIOUS REACTIONS

• Overdose or insufficient food intake may produce hypoglycemia, especially with increased glucose demands.

• GI hemorrhage, cholestatic hepatic jaundice, leukopenia, thrombocytopenia, pancytopenia, agranulocytosis, and aplastic or hemolytic anemia occur rarely.

PRECAUTIONS & CONSIDERATIONS

Caution is warranted with adrenal or pituitary insufficiency, hypoglycemic reactions, and impaired hepatic or renal function. Be alert to conditions that alter blood glucose requirements, such as fever, increased activity, stress, or a surgical procedure. Insulin is the drug of choice during pregnancy. Glipizide given within 1 mo of delivery may produce neonatal hypoglycemia. Glipizide crosses the placenta and is distributed in breast milk. Safety and efficacy of glipizide have not been established in children. Hypoglycemia may be difficult to recognize in elderly patients. Also, age-related renal impairment may increase sensitivity to the glucose-lowering effect. Wear sunscreen and protective eyewear to prevent the effects of light sensitivity.

Food intake and blood glucose should be monitored before and during therapy. Be aware of signs and symptoms of hypoglycemia (anxiety, cool wet skin, diplopia, dizziness, headache, hunger, numbness in mouth, tachycardia, tremors) or hyperglycemia (deep rapid breathing, dim vision, fatigue, nausea, polydipsia, polyphagia, polyuria, vomiting); carry candy, sugar packets, or other sugar supplements for immediate response to hypoglycemia. Consult the physician when glucose demands are altered (such as with fever, heavy physical activity, infection, stress, trauma). Exercise, good personal hygiene (including foot care), not smoking, and weight control are essential parts of therapy.

Hypoglycemic agents may be associated with increased cardiovascular mortality.

Administration

Take glipizide 30 min before a meal; the extended-release tablets should be taken before breakfast. Do not crush extended-release tablets.

Glucagon Hydrochloride

gloo′ka-gon

(GlucaGen, GlucaGen Diagnostic Kit, Glucagen [AUS], Glucagon, Glucagon Diagnostic Kit, Glucagon Emergency Kit)

Do not confuse glucagon with Glaucon.

CATEGORY AND SCHEDULE

Pregnancy Risk Category: B

Classification: Antihypoglycemics, hormones/hormone modifiers

MECHANISM OF ACTION

A glucose-elevating agent that promotes hepatic glycogenolysis, gluconeogenesis. Stimulates the production of cyclic adenosine monophosphate (cAMP), which results in increased plasma glucose concentration, smooth muscle relaxation, and an inotropic myocardial effect. *Therapeutic Effect:* Increases plasma glucose level.

AVAILABILITY

Powder for Injection: 1 mg.

INDICATIONS AND DOSAGES

▸ **Hypoglycemia**
IV, IM, SUBCUTANEOUS
Adults, Elderly, Children weighing more than 20 kg. 0.5-1 mg. May give 1 or 2 additional doses if response is delayed.
Children weighing 20 kg or less. 0.5 mg.
▸ **Diagnostic aid**
IV, IM
Adults, Elderly. 0.25-2 mg 10 min before procedure.

OFF-LABEL USES

Treatment of esophageal obstruction by solid food (food impaction), toxicity associated with β-blockers or calcium channel blockers.

CONTRAINDICATIONS

Hypersensitivity to glucagon or beef or pork proteins, known pheochromocytoma or insulinoma.

INTERACTIONS

Drug
Anticoagulants: May increase the effects of these drugs.
Herbal and Food
None known.

DIAGNOSTIC TEST EFFECTS

May decrease serum potassium level.

🥄 IV INCOMPATIBILITIES

Do not mix glucagon with any other medications.

SIDE EFFECTS

Occasional
Nausea, vomiting.
Rare
Allergic reaction, such as urticaria, respiratory distress, and hypotension.

SERIOUS REACTIONS

• Overdose may produce persistent nausea and vomiting and hypokalemia, marked by severe weakness, decreased appetite, irregular heartbeat, and muscle cramps.
• Serious allergic reactions are rare.

PRECAUTIONS & CONSIDERATIONS

Caution is warranted in patients with a history suggestive of insulinoma or pheochromocytoma. Be aware of how to recognize symptoms of hypoglycemia, including anxiety, increased sweating, difficulty concentrating, headache, hunger, nausea, nervousness, pale and cool skin, shakiness, unusual fatigue, weakness, and unconsciousness. Treat early signs of hypoglycemia with a simple sugar first, such as hard candy, honey, orange juice, sugar cubes, or table sugar dissolved in water or juice, followed by a protein source, such as cheese and crackers, half a sandwich, or a glass of milk.
Storage
Store vials at room temperature. After reconstitution, the solution is stable for 48 h if refrigerated. If reconstituted with sterile water for injection, use it immediately. Do not use glucagon solution unless it is clear.

Administration
! Place the patient on his or her side to avoid aspiration because glucagon (as well as hypoglycemia) may produce nausea and vomiting.
! If patient fails to respond in 15 min, get emergency assistance.
  Administer IV dextrose if the patient fails to respond to glucagon.
  Reconstitute the powder with the diluent supplied by the manufacturer when preparing doses of 2 mg or less. For doses > 2 mg, dilute with sterile water for injection. To provide 1 mg glucagon/mL, reconstitute the 1-mg vial with 1 mL diluent. The patient will usually awaken in 5-20 min. If the patient fails to respond after 1 or 2 additional doses, give IV dextrose as prescribed. When the patient awakens, give oral carbohydrates to restore hepatic glycogen stores and prevent secondary hypoglycemia.

Glyburide
glye'byoor-ide
(Daonil [CAN], DiaBeta, Euglucon [CAN], Glimel [AUS], Glynase, Micronase, Semi-Daonil [AUS], Semi-Euglucon [AUS])
Do not confuse glyburide with glimepiride or glipizide, or Micronase with Micro-K, Micronor.

CATEGORY AND SCHEDULE
Pregnancy Risk Category: C

Classification: Antidiabetic agents, sulfonylureas, second generation

MECHANISM OF ACTION
A second-generation sulfonylurea that promotes the release of insulin from β cells of the pancreas and increases insulin sensitivity at peripheral sites. *Therapeutic Effect:* Lowers blood glucose concentration.

PHARMACOKINETICS

Route	Onset	Peak	Duration
PO	0.25-1 h	1-2 h	12-24 h

Well absorbed from the GI tract. Protein binding: 99%. Metabolized in the liver to weakly active metabolite. Primarily excreted in urine. Not removed by hemodialysis. *Half-life:* 1.4-1.8 h.

AVAILABILITY
Tablets (DiaBeta, Micronase): 1.25 mg, 2.5 mg, 5 mg.
Tablets (Glynase): 1.5 mg, 3 mg, 6 mg.

INDICATIONS AND DOSAGES
▸ **Diabetes mellitus**
PO
Adults. Initially 2.5-5 mg. May increase by 2.5 mg/day at weekly intervals. Maintenance: 1.25-20 mg/day. Maximum: 20 mg/day.
Elderly. Initially, 1.25-2.5 mg/day. May increase by 1.25-2.5 mg/day at 1- to 3-wks intervals.
PO (MICRONIZED TABLETS [GLYNASE])
Adults, Elderly. Initially, 0.75-3 mg/day. May increase by 1.5 mg/day at weekly intervals. Maintenance: 0.75-12 mg/day as a single dose or in divided doses.
▸ **Dosage in renal impairment**
Glyburide is not recommended in patients with creatinine clearance < 50 mL/min.

CONTRAINDICATIONS
Diabetic ketoacidosis with or without coma, monotherapy for type 1

G

diabetes mellitus, hypersensitivity to drug, concurrent use with bosentan.

INTERACTIONS

Drug

β-Blockers: May increase the hypoglycemic effect of glyburide and mask signs of hypoglycemia.

Bosentan: May increase the risk of hepatotoxicity. Concurrent use may increase the metabolism of both agents.

Cimetidine, ciprofloxacin, fluconazole, MAOIs, quinidine, ranitidine, tricyclic antide-pressant agents, large doses of salicylates: May increase the effects of glyburide.

Corticosteroids, lithium, thiazide diuretics: May decrease the effects of glyburide.

Oral anticoagulants: May increase the effects of oral anticoagulants.

Herbal

Alfalfa, aloe, bilberry, bitter melon, burdock, celery, damiana, fenugreek, garcinia, garlic, ginger, ginseng (American), gymnema, marshmallow, stinging nettle: May increase the risk of hypoglycemia.

Food

Alcohol: Hypoglycemia is more likely to occur if alcohol is ingested.

DIAGNOSTIC TEST EFFECTS

May increase BUN and LDH concentrations and serum alkaline phosphatase, creatinine, and AST (SGOT) levels.

SIDE EFFECTS

Frequent

Altered taste sensation, dizziness, somnolence, weight gain, constipation, diarrhea, heartburn, nausea, vomiting, stomach fullness, headache.

Occasional

Increased sensitivity of skin to sunlight, peeling of skin, itching, rash.

SERIOUS REACTIONS

• Overdose or insufficient food intake may produce hypoglycemia, especially in patients with increased glucose demands.

• Cholestatic jaundice, leukopenia, thrombocytopenia, pancytopenia, agranulocytosis, and aplastic or hemolytic anemia occur rarely.

PRECAUTIONS & CONSIDERATIONS

Caution is warranted in patients with adrenal or pituitary insufficiency, hypoglycemic reactions sulfonamide hypersensitivity, and impaired hepatic or renal function. Be alert to conditions that alter blood glucose requirements, such as fever, increased activity, stress, or a surgical procedure. Insulin is the drug of choice during pregnancy. Glyburide crosses the placenta and is distributed in breast milk. Glyburide use within 2 wks of delivery may produce neonatal hypoglycemia. Safety and efficacy of glyburide have not been established in children. Hypoglycemia may be difficult to recognize in elderly patients. Also, age-related renal impairment may increase sensitivity to the glucose-lowering effect. Wear sunscreen and protective eyewear to prevent the effects of light sensitivity.

Food intake and blood glucose should be monitored before and during therapy. Be aware of signs and symptoms of hypoglycemia (anxiety, cool wet skin, diplopia, dizziness, headache, hunger, numbness in the mouth, tachycardia, tremors) or hyperglycemia (deep rapid breathing, dim vision, fatigue, nausea, polydipsia, polyphagia, polyuria, vomiting); carry candy, sugar packets, or other sugar supplements for immediate response to hypoglycemia. Consult the physician when glucose demands are altered (such as with fever, heavy physical activity, infection, stress, trauma). Exercise, good personal hygiene (including foot care), not smoking, and weight control are essential parts of therapy.

Hypoglycemic agents have been associated with increased cardiovascular mortality.

Storage
Store at room temperature in a tightly closed container.

Administration
Take glyburide with food to reduce GI symptoms.

Glycerin
gli´ser-in
(Bausch & Lomb Computer Eye Drops, Fleet Babylax, Fleet Liquid Glycerin Suppositories for Adults and Children, Fleet Glycerin Suppositories for Adults, Fleet Glycerin Suppositories for Children, Fleet Maximum-Strength Glycerin Suppositories, Glyrol, Osmoglyn, Sani-Supp)

CATEGORY AND SCHEDULE
Pregnancy Risk Category: B
OTC (suppositories)

Classification: Osmotic diuretic, antiglaucoma, laxative

MECHANISM OF ACTION
An osmotic dehydrating agent that increases osmotic pressure and draws fluid into the colon and stimulates evacuation of inspissated feces. Lowers both intraocular and intracranial pressure by osmotic dehydrating effects. Increases blood flow to ischemic areas, decreases serum free fatty acids, and increases synthesis of glycerides in the brain. *Therapeutic Effect:* Aids in fecal evacuation.

PHARMACOKINETICS
Well absorbed after PO administration but poorly absorbed after rectal administration. Widely distributed to extracellular space. Rapidly metabolized in liver. Primarily excreted in urine. *Half-life:* 30-45 min.

AVAILABILITY
Ophthalmic Solution: 1% (Bausch & Lomb Computer Eye Drops).
Oral Solution: 50% (Osmoglyn).
Rectal Solution: 2.3 g (Fleet Babylax), 5.6 g (Fleet Liquid Glycerin Suppositories).
Suppositories: 1 g (Fleet Glycerin Suppositories for Children), 2 g (Fleet Glycerin Suppositories), 3 g (Fleet Maximum-Strength Glycerin Suppositories), 82.5% (Sani-Supp).

INDICATIONS AND DOSAGES
▸ **Constipation**
RECTAL
Adults, Elderly, Children 6 yr and older. 3 g/day.
Children younger than 6 yr. 1-1.5 g/day.
▸ **Ophthalmologic procedures**
OPHTHALMIC
Adults, Elderly, Children. 1 or 2 drops prior to examination q3-4h.

▸ **Reduction of intraocular pressure**
PO
Adults, Elderly. 1-1.5 g/kg.
Maximum reduction in IOP occurs in
1 h and lasts approximately 5 h. May
give twice to four times a day.

OFF-LABEL USES
Viral meningoencephalitis.

CONTRAINDICATIONS
Hypersensitivity to any component
in the preparation, well-established
anuria, severe dehydration, frank
or impending acute pulmonary
edema, severe cardiac
decompensation.

INTERACTIONS
Drug
PO medications: May decrease
transit time of concurrently
administered oral medication,
decreasing absorption.
Herbal
Licorice: May increase risk of
hypokalemia.
Food
None known.

DIAGNOSTIC TEST EFFECTS
May suppress wheal and flare
reactions to antigen skin testing
unless antihistamines are
discontinued 4 days before testing.

SIDE EFFECTS
Frequent
Oral: Nausea, headache, vomiting.
Rectal: Some degree of abdominal
discomfort, nausea, mild cramps,
headache, vomiting.
Occasional
Oral: Diarrhea, dizziness, dry mouth
or increased thirst.
Ophthalmic: Pain and irritation may
occur upon instillation.
Rectal: Faintness, weakness,
abdominal pain, bloating.

SERIOUS REACTIONS
• Laxative abuse includes symptoms
of abdominal pain, weakness,
fatigue, thirst, vomiting, edema, bone
pain, fluid and electrolyte imbalance,
hypoalbuminemia, and syndromes
that mimic colitis.

PRECAUTIONS & CONSIDERATIONS
Caution is warranted in patients with
diabetes mellitus because product
orally will increase blood sugar and
osmotic load. Hemolytic anemia;
altered hydration; cardiac, renal,
or hepatic disease. It is unknown
whether glycerin crosses the
placenta or is excreted in breast
milk. No age-related precautions
have been noted in children. Be
aware that glycerin may increase
the risk of dehydration in elderly
patients because it reduces the water
in the body. Unrelieved constipation,
dizziness, muscle cramps or pain,
rectal bleeding, confusion, irregular
heartbeat, and weakness should be
reported.
Storage
Discard ophthalmic preparation
6 mo after dropper is first placed
in drug solution. Store at room
temperature away from damp
places like the bathroom or near
the kitchen sink as well as heat and
direct light because it may cause the
medicine to break down. Refrigerate
suppositories.
Administration
Instill ophthalmic drops of solution
in each lower conjunctival sac.
Gently massage the closed eyelids
to help spread the solution to all
areas of the conjunctiva. Gently
wipe away excess solution from the
eyelids and surrounding skin with
sterile cotton.
　　Mix oral glycerin unflavored 50%
oral solution with orange juice.
Pour solution over crushed ice and

drink through a straw to improve palatability. Have patient drink over 5-10 min to reduce vomiting risk. May administer doses at 5-h intervals for the reduction of intraocular pressure. Tell the patient to lie down after oral solution to minimize risk of developing headache.

If rectal suppository is too soft, chill for 30 min in refrigerator or run cold water over foil wrapper. Remove wrapper and moisten suppository with cold water before inserting well into rectum. Lie on the left side. Insert suppository high in rectum and retain for 15 min. If administering liquid glycerin rectally, gently insert stem with steady pressure at tip pointing toward the navel and squeeze unit until almost all the liquid has been delivered. A small amount of liquid will remain. Withdraw unit.

Increase fluid intake, exercise, and eat a high-fiber diet to promote defecation.

Warn the patient to notify the physician if he or she experiences unrelieved constipation, dizziness, muscle cramps or pain, rectal bleeding, confusion, irregular heartbeat, and weakness.

Glycopyrrolate
glye-koe-pye′roe-late
(Robinul, Robinul Forte, Robinul Injection [AUS])
Do not confuse with Reminyl.

CATEGORY AND SCHEDULE
Pregnancy Risk Category: B

Classification: Anticholinergics, gastrointestinals

MECHANISM OF ACTION
A quaternary anticholinergic that inhibits the action of acetylcholine at postganglionic parasympathetic sites in smooth muscle, secretory glands, and the central nervous system (CNS). *Therapeutic Effect:* Reduces salivation and excessive secretions of respiratory tract; reduces gastric secretions and acidity.

PHARMACOKINETICS
Poorly and irregularly absorbed from GI tract after oral administration. Metabolized in the liver. Primarily excreted in urine. *Half-life:* 1.7 h.

AVAILABILITY
Injection: 0.2 mg/mL.
Tablets: 1 mg, 2 mg.

INDICATIONS AND DOSAGES
▸ **Preoperative inhibition of salivation and excessive respiratory tract secretions**
IM
Adults, Elderly. 4 mcg/kg 30-60 min before procedure.
Children 2 yr and older. 4 mcg/kg.
Children younger than 2 yr.
4-9 mcg/kg. Do not use in neonates (< 1 mo).
▸ **To block the effects of anticholinesterase agents**
IV
Adults, Elderly, Children. 0.2 mg for each 1 mg neostigmine or 5 mg pyridostigmine.
▸ **Peptic ulcer disease, adjunct**
IV, IM
Adults, Elderly. 0.1 mg IV or IM 3-4 times a day.
PO
Adults, Elderly. 1-2 mg 2-3 times a day. Maximum: 8 mg/day.

CONTRAINDICATIONS
Acute hemorrhage, myasthenia gravis, narrow-angle glaucoma,

obstructive uropathy, paralytic ileus, tachycardia, ulcerative colitis, obstructive diseases of the GI tract, neonates.

INTERACTIONS
Drug
Antacids, antidiarrheals:
May decrease the absorption of glycopyrrolate.
Ketoconazole: May decrease the absorption of ketoconazole.
Other anticholinergics:
May increase the effects of glycopyrrolate.
Potassium chloride: May increase the severity of GI lesions with the wax matrix formulation of potassium chloride.
Pramlinitide: May increase anticholinergic effects.
Herbal
None known.
Food
None known.

DIAGNOSTIC TEST EFFECTS
May decrease serum uric acid levels.

ⓘ IV INCOMPATIBILITIES
Chloramphenicol, dexamethasone sodium phosphate (Decadron), diazepam (Valium), dimenhydrinate (Dramamine), methohexital (Brevital), methylprednisolone sodium succinate (Solu-Medrol), pentazocine (Talwin), pentobarbital (Nembutal), secobarbital (Seconal), sodium bicarbonate, thiopental (Pentothal).

ⓘ IV COMPATIBILITIES
Atropine, buprenorphine (Buprenex), butorphanol (Stadol), chlorpromazine (Thorazine), cimetidine (Tagamet), codeine, diphenhydramine (Benadryl), droperidol (Inapsine),

hydromorphone (Dilaudid), hydroxyzine (Vistaril), levorphanol (Levo-Dromoran), lidocaine, meperidine (Demerol), midazolam (Versed), morphine, nalbuphine (Nubain), neostigmine, ondansetron (Zofran), oxymorphone (Opana), physostigmine, procaine (Pronestyl), prochlorperazine (Compazine), promazine (Sparine), promethazine (Phenergan), propofol (Diprivan), pyridostigmine (Mestinon), ranitidine (Zantac), scopolamine, triflupromazine (Vesprin), trimethobenzamide (Tigan).

SIDE EFFECTS
Frequent
Dry mouth, decreased sweating, constipation.
Occasional
Blurred vision, gastric bloating, urinary hesitancy, somnolence (with high dosage), headache, intolerance to light, loss of taste, nervousness, flushing, insomnia, impotence, mental confusion or excitement (particularly in the elderly and children), temporary light-headedness (with parenteral form), local irritation (with parenteral form).
Rare
Dizziness, faintness.

SERIOUS REACTIONS
• Overdose may produce temporary paralysis of the ciliary muscle; pupillary dilation; tachycardia; palpitations; hot, dry, or flushed skin; absence of bowel sounds; hyperthermia; increased respiratory rate; ECG abnormalities; nausea; vomiting; rash over face or upper trunk; CNS stimulation; and psychosis (marked by agitation, restlessness, rambling speech, visual hallucinations, paranoid behavior, and delusions, followed by depression).

Caution is warranted with congestive heart failure, diarrhea, fever, GI infections, hepatic or renal disease, hypothyroidism, and reflux esophagitis. Avoid hot baths, saunas, and becoming overheated while exercising in hot weather because they may cause heat stroke. Tasks that require mental alertness or motor skills should also be avoided until response to the drug has been established. Antacids or antidiarrheals should not be taken within 1 h of taking glycopyrrolate because they will decrease glycopyrrolate's effectiveness.

Dry mouth may occur. BP, body temperature, heart rate, pattern of daily bowel activity and stool consistency, and urine output should be monitored. The person should void before giving the drug to reduce the risk of urine retention.

Administration
For direct injection, administer undiluted through the tubing of a free-flowing compatible IV solution, over 1-2 min.

For IM use, administer undiluted or diluted with D5W, $D_{10}W$, or 0.9% NaCl.

Take oral tablets 30-60 min before meals.

Gold Sodium Thiomalate
gold so′dee-um thye-oh-mah′late
(Myochrysine, Myocrisin [AUS])

CATEGORY AND SCHEDULE
Pregnancy Risk Category: C

Classification: Disease-modifying antirheumatic drugs, gold compounds

MECHANISM OF ACTION
A gold compound whose mechanism of action is unknown. May decrease prostaglandin synthesis or alter cellular mechanisms by inhibiting sulfhydryl systems. *Therapeutic Effect:* Decreases synovial inflammation, retards cartilage and bone destruction, suppresses or prevents—but does not cure—arthritis and synovitis.

AVAILABILITY
Injection: 50 mg/mL.

INDICATIONS AND DOSAGES
▸ **Rheumatoid arthritis**
IM
Adults, Elderly. Initially, 10 mg, followed by 25 mg for second dose, then 25-50 mg/wk until improvement noted or total of 1 g has been administered. Maintenance: 25-50 mg q2wk for 2-20 wks; if stable, may increase intervals to q3-4wk. Maximum: 100 mg/dose.
▸ **JRA (JIA)**
Children. Initially, 10 mg, then 1 mg/kg/wk up to a maximum single dose of 50 mg. Maintenance: 1 mg/kg/dose q2-4wk.
▸ **Dosage in renal impairment**
Dosage is modified based on creatinine clearance.

CrCL (mL/min)	Dosage
50-80	50% of usual dose
< 50	Not recom-mended

OFF-LABEL USES
Treatment of psoriatic arthritis.

CONTRAINDICATIONS
Colitis; concurrent use of antimalarials, immunosuppressive agents, penicillamine, or phenylbutazone; congestive heart failure; exfoliative dermatitis; history of blood dyscrasias; severe hepatic

or renal impairment; systemic lupus erythematosus, hypersensitivity to the drug or benzyl alcohol.

INTERACTIONS

Drug

ACE inhibitors: May increase toxic effects of gold sodium thiomalate.
Bone marrow depressants, hepatotoxic and nephrotoxic medications: May increase the risk of toxicity.
Penicillamine: May increase the risk of adverse hematologic or renal effects.
Herbal and Food
None known.

DIAGNOSTIC TEST EFFECTS

May decrease hemoglobin level, hematocrit, and WBC and platelet counts. May increase urine protein level. May alter liver function test results.

SIDE EFFECTS

Frequent
Pruritic dermatitis, stomatitis, diarrhea, abdominal pain, nausea.
Occasional
Vomiting, anorexia, flatulence, dyspepsia, conjunctivitis, photosensitivity.
Rare
Constipation, urticaria, rash.

SERIOUS REACTIONS

• Signs and symptoms of gold toxicity include decreased hemoglobin level, decreased granulocyte count ($< 150,000/mm^3$), proteinuria, hematuria, blood dyscrasias (anemia, leukopenia [WBC < 4000 mm^3], thrombocytopenia, and eosinophilia), glomerulonephritis, nephrotic syndrome, and cholestatic jaundice.

PRECAUTIONS & CONSIDERATIONS

Avoid exposure to sunlight, which may turn skin gray or blue. Oral hygiene should be diligently maintained to help prevent stomatitis. Gold appears in breast milk; discontinue breast-feeding during treatment. Gold therapy is avoided during pregnancy.

Pattern of daily bowel activity and stool consistency, urine for hematuria and proteinuria, CBC (particularly hemoglobin level, hematocrit, and WBC and platelet counts), renal and liver function tests (especially BUN level and serum alkaline phosphatase, creatinine, AST [SGOT], and ALT [SGPT] levels), skin for rash, and oral mucous membranes for stomatitis should be monitored. Therapeutic response, including improved grip strength, increased joint mobility, reduced joint tenderness, and relief of pain, stiffness, and swelling, should also be assessed.

Storage
Store at room temperature. Protect from light. Solution should be clear or pale yellow.

Administration
! Give gold sodium thiomalate IM only, as prescribed.

Full therapeutic effect may take 6 mo or longer to appear.

Inject intrasluteally with patient lying down; keep recumbent for 10 min after injection.

Gonadorelin Acetate/Gonadorelin Hydrochloride

goe-nad-oh-rell′-in
(Factrel), Lutrepulse
Discontinued in the United States

CATEGORY AND SCHEDULE

Pregnancy Risk Category: B

Classification: Hormones/hormone modifiers, stimulants, ovarian

MECHANISM OF ACTION

A synthetic luteinizing hormone that binds to specific transmembrane glycoprotein receptors on gonadotropic cells of the anterior pituitary, which then stimulates the synthesis and secretion of gonadotropins through mobilization of intracellular calcium, activation of protein kinase C, and gene transcription. *Therapeutic Effect:* Stimulates synthesis, release of luteinizing hormone (LH), follicle-stimulating hormone (FSH) from anterior pituitary. Stimulates release of gonadotropin-releasing hormone from hypothalamus.

PHARMACOKINETICS

Maximal LH release occurs within 20 min. Metabolized in plasma. Excreted in urine as inactive metabolites. *Half-life:* 4 min.

AVAILABILITY

Powder for Reconstitution, as Hydrochloride: 100 mcg (Factrel).

INDICATIONS AND DOSAGES

▸ **Gonadotropin function evaluation**
IV/SUBCUTANEOUS FACTREL (HCl FORM)
Adults. 100 mcg. In women, perform test in early follicular phase of menstrual cycle.

CONTRAINDICATIONS

Any condition exacerbated by pregnancy, patients with ovarian cysts or causes of anovulation other than hypothalamic origin, the presence of a hormonally dependent tumor, any conditions worsened by an increase of reproductive hormones, hypersensitivity to gonadorelin acetate or gonadorelin hydrochloride.

SIDE EFFECTS

Occasional
Swelling, pain, or itching at injection site with subcutanous administration, local or generalized skin rash with chronic subcutaneous administration.
Rare
Headache, nausea, light-headedness, abdominal discomfort, hypersensitivity reactions (bronchospasm, tachycardia, flushing, urticaria), induration at injection site.

SERIOUS REACTIONS

• Anaphylactic reaction occurs rarely.

PRECAUTIONS & CONSIDERATIONS

Caution is warranted in patients with pregnancy because gonadorelin could worsen preexisting conditions such as pituitary prolactinemia. Caution should also be used with the concurrent use of drugs that directly affect the pituitary secretion of gonadotropin, including androgens, estrogens, progestins, glucocorticoids, spironolactone, levodopa, oral contraceptives, digoxin, phenothiazines, and dopamine antagonists, which would affect a rise in prolactin. It is unknown whether gonadorelin crosses the placenta or is distributed in breast milk. Safety and efficacy have not been established in children. No age-related precautions have been noted in elderly patients. Patients should be told that multiple pregnancy is possible.
Storage
Store at room temperature. Discard reconstituted product after 24 h.
Administration
For gonadorelin HCl, using standard aseptic technique, add 1 mL of diluent provided to the 100-mcg vial or 2 mL of diluent to the 500-mcg vial. Administer within the early follicular phase of the menstrual cycle if it can be determined. The solution should be made immediately before use. Unused reconstituted solution and diluent should be discarded.

Goserelin
go′seh-rel-in
(Zoladex, Zoladex Implant [AUS], Zoladex LA)

CATEGORY AND SCHEDULE
Pregnancy Risk Category: D (advanced breast cancer), X (endometriosis, endometrial thinning)

Classification: Antineoplastics, hormones/hormone modifiers, gonadotropin-releasing hormone analogues

MECHANISM OF ACTION
A gonadotropin-releasing hormone analogue and antineoplastic agent that stimulates the release of luteinizing hormone (LH) and follicle-stimulating hormone (FSH) from the anterior pituitary gland. In men, it increases testosterone concentrations initially, then suppresses secretion of LH and FSH, resulting in decreased testosterone levels. *Therapeutic Effect:* In females, it causes a reduction in ovarian size and function, a reduction in uterine and mammary gland size, and regression of sex-hormone-responsive tumors. In men, it produces pharmacologic castration and decreases the growth of abnormal prostate tissue.

AVAILABILITY
Implant: 3.6 mg, (monthly).
Implant: 10.8 mg (83 mo).

INDICATIONS AND DOSAGES
▸ **Prostatic carcinoma**
IMPLANT
Adult Males. 3.6 mg every 28 days or 10.8 mg q12wk subcutaneously into upper abdominal wall.

▸ **Breast carcinoma, endometriosis**
IMPLANT
Adult Females. 3.6 mg every 28 days subcutaneously into upper abdominal wall. Do not use 10.8 mg implant in females.

OFF-LABEL USES
Uterine fibroids, endometrial thinning before ablation procedure.

CONTRAINDICATIONS
Pregnancy; hypersensitivity to goserelin products, luteinizing hormone-releasing hormone (LHRH), or LHRH analogues; breastfeeding.

INTERACTIONS
Drug, Herbal, and Food
None known.

DIAGNOSTIC TEST EFFECTS
May increase serum prostatic acid phosphatase and testosterone levels.

SIDE EFFECTS
Frequent
Headache (60%), hot flashes (55%), depression (54%), diaphoresis (45%), sexual dysfunction (21%), decreased erection (18%), lower urinary tract symptoms (13%).
Occasional (5%-10%)
Pain, lethargy, dizziness, insomnia, anorexia, nausea, rash, upper respiratory tract infection, hirsutism, abdominal pain.
Rare
Pruritus.

SERIOUS REACTIONS
• Arrhythmias, congestive heart failure, and hypertension occur rarely.
• Ureteral obstruction and spinal cord compression have been

observed. An immediate orchiectomy may be necessary if these conditions occur.

• Deep vein thrombosis has been reported.

• Decreased bone mineral density/osteoporosis with long-term use/fractures.

PRECAUTIONS & CONSIDERATIONS

Goserelin crosses the placenta and may cause fetal harm. Women who are or may be pregnant should not use this drug. Pregnancy status should be determined before beginning therapy. Women should use nonhormonal contraceptive measures during therapy. It is unknown whether goserelin is excreted in breast milk. The safety and efficacy of goserelin have not been established in children. No age-related precautions have been noted in elderly patients.

Women should notify the physician if regular menstruation persists or if they become pregnant. Breakthrough bleeding may occur if a goserelin dose is missed. Signs and symptoms of worsening of prostatic cancer, especially in the first month, should be monitored. Decreased bone mineral density secondary to this medication may be irreversible. Caution should be used if other risk factors are present.

Administration

For implant, inspect the package for damage before opening. If the package is damaged, do not use the syringe. Remove the sterile syringe from the package immediately before use. Examine the syringe for damage, and check that goserelin is visible in the translucent chamber. Clean an area of skin on the upper abdominal wall with an alcohol swab. Grasp the safety clip tab, pull it out and away from the needle, and discard it immediately. Then remove the needle cover. Using aseptic technique, stretch or pinch the patient's skin with one hand and grip the syringe barrel. Insert the needle into the subcutaneous tissue.

! The goserelin syringe should not be used for aspiration. If the needle penetrates a large vessel, you will see blood instantly in the syringe chamber. If a vessel is penetrated, withdraw the needle and use a new syringe elsewhere.

! Confirm Implant dosage against patient prescription before insertion.

Direct the needle so that it parallels the abdominal wall. Push the needle in until the barrel hub touches the patient's skin. Withdraw the needle 1 cm to create a space to discharge goserelin. Fully depress the plunger to discharge the drug. Withdraw the needle. Then bandage the site. Confirm the discharge of goserelin by ensuring that the tip of the plunger is visible within the tip of the needle. Dispose of the used needle and syringe in a safe manner.

Granisetron
gra-ni′se-tron
(Kytril)

CATEGORY AND SCHEDULE
Pregnancy Risk Category: B

Classification: Antiemetics/antivertigo, serotonin receptor antagonists

MECHANISM OF ACTION
A 5-HT$_3$ receptor antagonist that acts centrally in the chemoreceptor trigger zone or peripherally at the vagal

nerve terminals. *Therapeutic Effect:* Prevents nausea and vomiting.

PHARMACOKINETICS

Route	Onset	Peak	Duration
IV	1-3 min	N/A	24 h

Rapidly and widely distributed to tissues. Protein binding: 65%. Metabolized in the liver to active metabolite. Eliminated in urine and feces. *Half-life:* 10-12 h (increased in the elderly).

AVAILABILITY

Oral Solution: 1 mg/5 mL.
Tablets: 1 mg.
Injection: 1 mg/mL, 0.1 mg/mL.

INDICATIONS AND DOSAGES
▸ **Prevention of chemotherapy-induced nausea and vomiting**
PO
Adults, Elderly, Children 2 yr and older. 2 mg once a day up to 1 h before chemotherapy or 1 mg twice a day, with first dose 1 h before chemotherapy.
IV
Adults, Elderly, Children 2 yr and older. 10 mcg/kg/dose (or 1 mg/dose) within 30 min of chemotherapy.
▸ **Prevention of radiation-induced nausea and vomiting**
PO
Adults, Elderly. 2 mg once a day given 1 h before radiation therapy.
▸ **Postoperative nausea or vomiting**
IV
Adults, Elderly. 1 mg as a single postoperative dose.

CONTRAINDICATIONS
Hypersensitivity to drug or similar agents. (use caution.)

Hypersensitivity to benzyl alcohol (IV form).

INTERACTIONS
Drug
Apomorphine: May cause significant hypotension.
Hepatic enzyme inducers: May decrease the effects of granisetron.
Herbal
St. John's wort: May decrease levels of granisetron.
Food
None known.

DIAGNOSTIC TEST EFFECTS
May increase AST (SGOT) and ALT (SGPT) levels.

ⓘ IV INCOMPATIBILITIES
Amphotericin B (Fungizone), diazepam, lansoprazole, phenytoin.

ⓘ IV COMPATIBILITIES
Acyclovir (Zovirax), allopurinol (Aloprim), amifostine (Ethyol), amikacin (Amikin), aminophylline, amphotericin B cholesteryl sulfate complex (Amphotec), ampicillin (Polycillin), ampicillin and sulbactam (Unasyn), amsacrine (Amsa), aztreonam (Azactam), bleomycin (Blenoxane), bumetanide (Bumex), buprenorphine (Buprenex), butorphanol (Stadol), calcium gluconate, carboplatin (Paraplatin), carmustine (BiCNU), cefazolin (Ancef), cefepime (Maxipime), cefoperazone (Cefobid), cefotaxime (Claforan), cefotetan (Cefotan), cefoxitin (Mefixitin), ceftazidime (Fortaz), ceftizoxime (Cefizox), ceftriaxone (Rocephin), cefuroxime (Zinacef), chlorpromazine (Thorazine), cimetidine (Tagamet), ciprofloxacin (Cipro), cisplatin (Platinol), cladribine (Leustatin), clindamycin (Cleocin),

co-trimoxazole (Bactrim),
cyclophosphamide (Cytoxan),
cytarabine (Ara-C), dacarbazine
(DTIC-Dome), dactinomycin
(Cosmegen), daunorubicin
(Cerubidine), dexamethasone
(Decadron), diphenhydramine
(Benadryl), docetaxel (Taxotere),
dopamine (Intropin), doxorubicin
(Adriamycin), doxycycline
(Vibramycin), droperidol
(Inapsine), enalaprilat (Vasotec),
etoposide (VePesid), famotidine
(Pepcid), filgrastim (Neupogen),
floxuridine (FUDR), fluconazole
(Diflucan), fludarabine (Fludara),
fluorouracil (Efurix), furosemide
(Lasix), ganciclovir (Cytovene),
gatifloxacin (Tequin), gemcitabine
(Gemzar), gentamicin (Garamycin),
haloperidol (Haldol), heparin,
hydrocortisone sodium phosphate,
hydrocortisone sodium succinate
(Solu-Cortef), hydromorphone
(Dilaudid), hydroxyzine
(Vistaril), idarubicin (Idamycin),
ifosfamide (Ifex), imipenem
and cilastatin (Primaxin),
leucovorin, linezolid (Zyvox),
lorazepam (Ativan), magnesium,
mechlorethamine (Mustargen),
melphalan (Alkeran), meperidine
(Demerol), mesna (Mesnex),
methotrexate, methylprednisolone
sodium succinate (Solu-Medrol),
metoclopramide (Reglan),
metronidazole (Flagyl),
minocycline (Minocin), mitomycin
(Mutamycin), mitoxantrone
(Novantrone), morphine (Avinza,
Kadian, Roxanol), nalbuphine
(Nubain), netilmicin (Netromycin),
ofloxacin (Floxin), paclitaxel
(Taxol), piperacillin (Piperacil),
piperacillin and tazobactam
(Zosyn), plicamycin (Mithracin),
potassium, prochlorperazine
(Compazine), promethazine
(Phenergan), propofol (Diprivan),
ranitidine (Zantac), sargramostim
(Leukine), sodium bicarbonate,
streptozocin (Zanosar), teniposide
(Vumon), thiotepa (Thioplex),
ticarcillin (Ticar), ticarcillin and
clavulanate (Timentin), tobramycin
(Nebcin), topotecan (Hycamtin),
vancomycin (Vancocin), vinblastine
(Velban), vincristine (Oncovin),
vinorelbine (Navelbine), zidovudine
(Retrovir).

SIDE EFFECTS
Frequent (14%-21%)
Headache, constipation, asthenia.
Occasional (6%-8%)
Diarrhea, abdominal pain.
Rare (< 2%)
Altered taste, hypersensitivity
reaction.

SERIOUS REACTIONS
• Serious hypersensitivity and
anaphylaxis are rare.

PRECAUTIONS & CONSIDERATIONS
It is unknown whether granisetron is
distributed in breast milk. The safety
and efficacy of granisetron have not
been established in children younger
than 2 yr. No age-related precautions
have been noted in elderly patients.
Use this medication cautiously with
other medications that may prolong
the QT interval.

The drug may affect the sense
of taste temporarily. Notify the
physician if headache occurs. The
pattern of daily bowel activity and
stool consistency should be assessed.
Storage
Keep the bottle of oral solution
tightly closed. Protect the bottle
from light and store it in an
upright position. Store vials for
IV use at room temperature; the
solution normally appears clear and
colorless; inspect it for particles and
discoloration. After dilution, the

solution for injection is stable for at least 24 h at room temperature.

Administration

! Administer only on days of chemotherapy, as prescribed. Administer oral granisetron within 1 h and the IV form within 30 min before starting chemotherapy.

For IV use, administer granisetron undiluted or dilute it with 20-50 mL 0.9% NaCl or D5W. Do not mix it with other medications. Administer the undiluted drug by IV push over 30 s. For IV piggyback, infuse over 5-20 min, depending on the volume of diluent used.

Griseofulvin
griz-ee-oh-full'vin
(Grifulvin V, Gris-PEG, Grisovin [AUS])

CATEGORY AND SCHEDULE
Pregnancy Risk Category: C

Classification: Antifungals

MECHANISM OF ACTION
An antifungal that inhibits fungal cell mitosis by disrupting mitotic spindle structure. *Therapeutic Effect:* Fungistatic.

AVAILABILITY
Oral Suspension (Grifulvin V): 125 mg/5 mL.
Tablets (Microsize [Grifulvin V]): 500 mg.
Tablets (Ultramicrosize [Gris-PEG]): 125 mg, 250 mg.

INDICATIONS AND DOSAGES
▶ **Tinea capitis, tinea corporis, tinea cruris, tinea pedis, tinea unguium**

MICROSIZE TABLETS, ORAL SUSPENSION
Adults. Usually, 500 mg once daily or in 2 divided doses.
Children 2 yr and older. Usual dosage, 10-20 mg/kg/day in 1 or 2 divided doses.
ULTRAMICROSIZE TABLETS
Adults. Usual dosage, 300-750 mg/day as a single dose or in divided doses.
Children 2 yr and older.
5-10 mg/kg/day.

CONTRAINDICATIONS
Hepatocellular failure, porphyria, pregnancy.

INTERACTIONS
Drug
Barbiturates: May decrease the effects of griseofulvin.
Cyclosporine: Cyclosporine levels may be decreased.
Oral contraceptives, warfarin: May decrease the effects of these drugs.
Herbal
None known.
Food
Alcohol: May cause disulfiram-like reaction.

DIAGNOSTIC TEST EFFECTS
None known.

SIDE EFFECTS
Occasional
Hypersensitivity reaction (including pruritus, rash, and urticaria), headache, nausea, diarrhea, excessive thirst, flatulence, oral thrush, dizziness, insomnia.
Rare
Paresthesia of hands or feet, proteinuria, photosensitivity reaction.

SERIOUS REACTIONS
• Granulocytopenia occurs rarely.
• Hepatotoxicity.

PRECAUTIONS & CONSIDERATIONS

Caution is warranted with hypersensitivity to penicillins or in those who are exposed to sun or ultraviolet light because photosensitivity may develop. Determine any history of allergies, especially to griseofulvin and penicillins, before giving the drug. Avoid alcohol and exposure to sunlight. Maintain good hygiene to help prevent superinfection. Separate personal items that come in direct contact with affected areas.

! Monitor the granulocyte count as appropriate. If granulocytopenia develops, notify the physician and expect to discontinue the drug. If headache occurs, establish and document the headache's location, onset, and type. Assess for dizziness. Evaluate skin for rash and therapeutic response to the drug. Assess daily pattern of bowel activity and stool consistency.

Storage
Store at room temperature; protect from light.

Administration
! The duration of treatment depends on the site of infection. Take oral griseofulvin with foods high in fat, such as milk or ice cream, to reduce GI upset and assist in drug absorption. Shake oral suspension well before each use. Keep affected areas dry and wear light clothing for ventilation.

Guaifenesin
gwye-fen′e-sin
(Allfen, Balminil [CAN], Benylin E [CAN], Diabetic Tussin, Fenesin, Ganidin, Guiatuss, Humibid LA, Mucinex, Organidin, Phanasin, Refenesen, Robitussin, Scot-tussin, Siltussin, Tussin, XPECT)
Do not confuse guaifenesin with guanfacine.

CATEGORY AND SCHEDULE
Pregnancy Risk Category: C
OTC

Classification: Expectorants

MECHANISM OF ACTION
An expectorant that stimulates respiratory tract secretions by decreasing the adhesiveness and viscosity of phlegm. *Therapeutic Effect:* Promotes removal of viscous mucus.

PHARMACOKINETICS
Well absorbed from the GI tract. Metabolized in the liver. Excreted in urine.

AVAILABILITY
Caplets (Fenesin, Refenesen): 400 mg.
Granules (Mucinex): 50 mg/packet, 100 mg/packet.
Tablets (Allfen, Organidin, Refenesen, XPECT): 200 mg, 400 mg.
Tablets (Extended-Release [Humibid LA, Mucinex]): 600 mg, 1200 mg.
Syrup (Guiatuss, Robitussin, Tussin): 100 mg/5 mL.

INDICATIONS AND DOSAGES
▶ **Expectorant**
PO
Adults, Elderly, Children older than 12 yr. 200-400 mg q4h.

Children 6-12 yr. 100-200 mg q4h.
Maximum: 1.2 g/day.
Children 2-5 yr. 50-100 mg q4h.
Children younger than 2 yr.
12 mg/kg/day in 6 divided
doses.
PO (EXTENDED-RELEASE)
*Adults, Elderly, Children older
than 12 yr.* 600-1200 mg q12h.
Maximum: 2.4 g/day.
Children 2-5 yr. 600 mg
q12h. Maximum: 600 mg/day.

CONTRAINDICATIONS
None known.

INTERACTIONS
Drug
None known.
Herbal
None known.
Food
None known.

DIAGNOSTIC TEST EFFECTS
None known.

SIDE EFFECTS
Rare
Dizziness, headache, rash,
diarrhea, nausea, vomiting,
abdominal pain.

SERIOUS REACTIONS
• Overdose may produce nausea and
vomiting.

PRECAUTIONS & CONSIDERATIONS
It is unknown whether guaifenesin
crosses the placenta or is distributed
in breast milk. No age-related
precautions have been noted in
children or in elderly patients. Use
guaifenesin cautiously in children
younger than 2 yr with a persistent
cough. Avoid tasks that require
mental alertness or motor skills
until response to the drug has
been established. Fluid intake and

environmental humidity should be
increased to lower the viscosity of
secretions.

Notify the physician of cough
that persists or is accompanied by
fever, rash, headache, or sore throat.
Clinical improvement should be
assessed.
Storage
Store syrup, liquid, and capsules at
room temperature.
Administration
! Take extended-release capsules at
12-h intervals, as prescribed.

Take guaifenesin without regard
to food. Do not crush or break
extended-release capsules. Contents
may be sprinkled on soft food and
then swallowed without chewing or
crushing. Do not take for chronic
cough.

Maintain adequate fluid intake to
aid expectoration.

Guanabenz
gwan′a-benz
(Wytensin)
Do not confuse with Guanfacine.

CATEGORY AND SCHEDULE
Pregnancy Risk Category: C

Classification: Antiadrenergics,
centrally acting or central;
antihypertensive

MECHANISM OF ACTION
An α-adrenergic agonist that
stimulates α_2-adrenergic receptors.
Inhibits sympathetic cardioaccelerator
and vasoconstrictor center to heart,
kidneys, peripheral vasculature.
Therapeutic Effect: Decreases systolic,
diastolic BP. Chronic use decreases
peripheral vascular resistance.

PHARMACOKINETICS

Well absorbed from GI tract. Widely distributed. Protein binding: 90%. Metabolized in liver. Excreted in urine and feces. Not removed by hemodialysis. *Half-life:* 6 h.

AVAILABILITY

Tablets (Wytensin): 4 mg, 8 mg.

INDICATIONS AND DOSAGES
▸ **Hypertension**
PO
Adults. Initially, 4 mg 2 times/day. Increase by 4-8 mg at 1- to 2-wks intervals. Usual effective range is 8-32 mg/day.
Elderly. Initially, 4 mg/day. May increase q1-2wk. Maintenance: 8-16 mg/day. Maximum: 32 mg/day.

CONTRAINDICATIONS

History of hypersensitivity to guanabenz or any component of the formulation.

INTERACTIONS

Drug
β-Blockers, hypotensive-producing medications: May increase antihypertensive effect.
Nitroprusside: May cause additive hypotension.
Noncardioselective β-blockers: May exacerbate rebound hypertension.
Tricyclic antidepressant agents: May decrease effects of guanabenz.
Herbal
Licorice, yohimbine: May decrease guanabenz effectiveness.
Food
None known.

DIAGNOSTIC TEST EFFECTS

May decrease cholesterol, total triglyceride concentrations.

SIDE EFFECTS

Frequent
Drowsiness, dry mouth, dizziness.
Occasional
Weakness, headache, nausea, decreased sexual ability.
Rare
Ataxia, sleep disturbances, rash, itching, diarrhea, constipation, altered taste, muscle aches.

SERIOUS REACTIONS

• Abrupt withdrawal may result in rebound hypertension manifested as nervousness, agitation, anxiety, insomnia, hand tingling, tremor, flushing, and sweating.
• Overdosage produces hypotension, somnolence, lethargy, irritability, bradycardia, and miosis (pupillary constriction).

PRECAUTIONS & CONSIDERATIONS

Caution is warranted in patients with severe coronary insufficiency, recent myocardial infarction, cerebrovascular disease, severe hepatic or renal failure. It is unknown whether guanabenz crosses the placenta or is distributed in breast milk. Safety and efficacy of guanabenz have not been established in children. No age-related precautions have been noted in elderly patients. Diabetic patients should be educated that this medication may mask symptoms of hypoglycemia.

Side effects such as dry mouth, drowsiness, dizziness, headache, decreased sexual ability, and GI upset may occur during the first 2 wks of therapy but generally diminish during continued therapy. If increased or decreased heartbeat or swollen ankles or feet occur, notify the physician. Avoid alcohol, and caution should be used driving or operating machinery until tolerance to medication is established.

G

Storage
Store at room temperature and protect from light.
Administration
Give with or without food.

Avoid skipping doses or voluntarily discontinuing drug because it may produce severe, rebound hypertension.

Guanfacine
gwan'fa-seen
(Tenex)
Do not confuse with Guanabenz.

CATEGORY AND SCHEDULE
Pregnancy Risk Category: B

Classification: Antiadrenergics, central; antihypertensive

MECHANISM OF ACTION
An α-adrenergic agonist that stimulates $α_2$-adrenergic receptors and inhibits sympathetic cardioaccelerator and vasoconstrictor center to heart, kidneys, peripheral vasculature. *Therapeutic Effect:* Decreases systolic, diastolic BP. Chronic use decreases peripheral vascular resistance.

PHARMACOKINETICS
Well absorbed from GI tract. Widely distributed. Protein binding: 71%. Metabolized in liver. Excreted in urine and feces. Not removed by hemodialysis. *Half-life:* 17 h.

AVAILABILITY
Tablets (Tenex): 1 mg, 2 mg.

INDICATIONS AND DOSAGES
▸ **Hypertension**
PO

Adults, Elderly. Initially, 1 mg/day. Increase by 1 mg/day at intervals of 3-4 wks up to 3 mg/day in single or divided doses.

OFF-LABEL USES
Attention deficit hyperactivity disorder (ADHD).

CONTRAINDICATIONS
History of hypersensitivity to guanfacine or any component of the formulation.

INTERACTIONS
Drug
β-Blockers, hypotensive-producing medications: May increase antihypertensive effect.
Bupropion: May increase risk of seizure activity.
Nitroprusside: May have additive hypotensive effects.
Noncardioselective β-blockers: May exacerbate rebound hypertension when guanfacine is withdrawn.
Tricyclic antidepressant agents: May decrease the hypotensive effects of guanfacine.
Herbal
Licorice, yohimbine: May decrease guanfacine effectiveness.
Ma huang: May increase BP.
Food
None known.

DIAGNOSTIC TEST EFFECTS
May increase growth hormone concentration. May decrease urinary catecholamine and VMA excretion.

SIDE EFFECTS
Frequent
Dry mouth, somnolence.
Occasional
Fatigue, headache, asthenia (loss of strength, energy), dizziness.

SERIOUS REACTIONS

• Overdosage may produce difficult breathing, dizziness, faintness, severe drowsiness, bradycardia.

PRECAUTIONS & CONSIDERATIONS

Caution should be used with impaired renal function. It is unknown if guanfacine crosses the placenta or is distributed in breast milk. Be aware that guanfacine is not recommended in treatment of acute hypertension associated with preeclampsia. Safety and efficacy of guanfacine have not been established in children. There are no age-related precautions noted in the elderly. Diabetic patients should be educated that this medication may mask symptoms of hypoglycemia.

Therapeutic effect may take 1 wk and peak effect should be noted in 1-3 mo. Avoid alcohol, and caution should be used driving or operating machinery.

Storage

Store at room temperature and protect from light.

Administration

Give guanfacine at bedtime.

Avoid skipping doses or voluntarily discontinuing drug, which may produce severe, rebound hypertension.

G

Halcinonide
hal-sin'o-nide
(Halog, Halog-E)

CATEGORY AND SCHEDULE
Pregnancy Risk Category: C

Classification: Corticosteroids, topical, dermatologics, anti-inflammatory

MECHANISM OF ACTION
A topical high-potency corticosteroid that has anti-inflammatory, antipruritic, and vasoconstrictive properties. The exact mechanism of the anti-inflammatory process is unclear. *Therapeutic Effect:* Reduces or prevents tissue response to the inflammatory process.

PHARMACOKINETICS
Well absorbed systemically. Large variation in absorption among sites. Protein binding: Varies. Metabolized in liver. Primarily excreted in urine.

AVAILABILITY
Cream: 0.1% (Halog).
Cream (Emollient Base): 0.1% (Halog-E).
Ointment: 0.1% (Halog).
Solution: 0.1% (Halog).

INDICATIONS AND DOSAGES
▸ **Corticosteroid-responsive dermatoses**
Topical
Adults, Elderly. Apply sparingly 1-3 times/day.

CONTRAINDICATIONS
History of hypersensitivity to halcinonide or other corticosteroids; viral, fungal, or tubercular skin lesions.

INTERACTIONS
Drug
None known.
Herbal
None known.
Food
None known.

DIAGNOSTIC TEST EFFECTS
None known.

SIDE EFFECTS
Occasional
Itching, redness, irritation, burning at site of application, dryness, folliculitis, acneiform eruptions, hypopigmentation.
Rare
Allergic contact dermatitis, maceration of the skin, secondary infection, skin atrophy.

SERIOUS REACTIONS
• The serious reactions of long-term therapy and the addition of occlusive dressings are reversible hypothalamic-pituitary-adrenal (HPA) axis suppression, manifestations of Cushing syndrome, hyperglycemia, and glucosuria.

PRECAUTIONS & CONSIDERATIONS
Caution should be used over large surface areas and with prolonged use. It is unknown whether halcinonide is excreted in breast milk. Halcinonide should not be used during pregnancy because it may cause harmful effects in the fetus. Absorption is more likely with occlusive dressings or extensive application in young children.
Administration
Gently cleanse area before application preferably after bath or shower for best absorption. Use occlusive dressings only as directed. Apply sparingly. Rub into area gently and thoroughly.

Halobetasol
hal-oh-be′ta-sol
(Ultravate)

CATEGORY AND SCHEDULE
Pregnancy Risk Category: C

Classification: Corticosteroids, topical, dermatologics

MECHANISM OF ACTION
A very-high-potency corticosteroid that inhibits accumulation of inflammatory cells at inflammation sites, phagocytosis, lysosomal enzyme release, and synthesis or release of mediators of inflammation. *Therapeutic Effect:* Decreases or prevents tissue response to inflammatory process.

PHARMACOKINETICS
Variation in absorption among individuals and sites: scrotum 36%, forehead 7%, scalp 4%, forearm 1%.

AVAILABILITY
Cream: 0.05% (Ultravate).
Ointment: 0.05% (Ultravate).

INDICATIONS AND DOSAGES
▶ **Dermatoses, corticosteroid-responsive**
Topical
Adults, Elderly, Children 12 yr and older. Apply 1-2 times/day. Maximum: 50 g/wk for no more than 2 wks.

CONTRAINDICATIONS
Hypersensitivity to halobetasol or other corticosteroids; viral, fungal, or tubercular skin lesions.

INTERACTIONS
Drug
None known.

Herbal
None known.
Food
None known.

DIAGNOSTIC TEST EFFECTS
None known.

SIDE EFFECTS
Frequent
Burning, stinging, pruritus.
Rare
Cushing syndrome, hyperglycemia, glucosuria, HPA axis suppression.

SERIOUS REACTIONS
• Overdosage can occur from topically applied halobetasol absorbed in sufficient amounts to produce systemic effects producing reversible adrenal suppression, manifestations of Cushing syndrome, hyperglycemia, and glucosuria in some patients.

PRECAUTIONS & CONSIDERATIONS
Occlusive dressings should be avoided. It is unknown whether halobetasol crosses the placenta or is distributed in the breast milk. Safety and efficacy have not been established in children. No age-related precautions have been noted in elderly patients.
Administration
Avoid the use of occlusive dressings unless otherwise directed by a physician. Apply sparingly to the skin or scalp and rub into area thoroughly. Administer for no longer than 2 wks. Only small areas should be treated at one time. Discontinue treatment when control is achieved. Do not apply on face, groin, or axillae. Avoid contact with eyes.

H

Haloperidol
ha-loe-per′idole
(Apo-Haloperidol [CAN], Haldol, Haldol Decanoate, Novoperidol [CAN], Peridol [CAN], Serenace [AUS])
Do not confuse Haldol with Halcion, Halog, or Stadol.

CATEGORY AND SCHEDULE
Pregnancy Risk Category: C

Classification: Antipsychotics, butyrophenone

MECHANISM OF ACTION
An antipsychotic, antiemetic, and antidyskinetic agent that competitively blocks postsynaptic dopamine receptors, interrupts nerve impulse movement, and increases turnover of dopamine in the brain. Has strong extrapyramidal and antiemetic effects, weak anticholinergic and sedative effects. *Therapeutic Effect:* Produces tranquilizing effect.

PHARMACOKINETICS
Readily absorbed from the GI tract. Protein binding: 92%. Extensively metabolized in the liver. Primarily excreted in urine. Not removed by hemodialysis. *Half-life:* 12-37 h PO; 10-19 h IV; 17-25 h IM.

AVAILABILITY
Oral Concentrate: 2 mg/mL.
Tablets: 0.5 mg, 1 mg, 2 mg, 5 mg, 10 mg, 20 mg.
Injection (Lactate): 5 mg/mL.
Injection (Decanoate): 50 mg/mL, 100 mg/mL.

INDICATIONS AND DOSAGES
▸ **Treatment of psychotic disorders**
PO
Adults, Children 12 yr and older. Initially, 0.5-5 mg 2-3 times/day.

Dosage gradually adjusted as needed.
Elderly. 0.5-2 mg 2-3 times/day.
Dosage gradually adjusted as needed.
Children 3-12 yr or weighing 15-40 kg. Initially, 0.05 mg/kg/day in 2-3 divided doses. May increase by 0.5-mg increments at 5- to 7-day intervals. Maximum: 0.15 mg/kg/day in divided doses.
IM (LACTATE)
Adults, Elderly, Children 12 yr and older. Initially, 2-5. May repeat at 1-h intervals as needed. Convert to oral treatment as soon as possible.
IM (DECANOATE)
Adults, Elderly, Children 12 yr and older. Initially, 10-15 times previous daily oral dose up to maximum initial dose of 100 mg. Injections are given once every 28 days. Maximum: 300 mg/mo.
▸ **Treatment of nonpsychotic disorders, Tourette syndrome**
PO
Children 3-12 yr or weighing 15-40 kg. Initially, 0.05 mg/kg/day in 2-3 divided doses. May increase by 0.5 mg at 5- to 7-day intervals. Maximum: 0.075 mg/kg/day.

OFF-LABEL USES
Treatment of nausea or vomiting associated with cancer chemotherapy, used IV off-label for agitation in hospitalized patients.

CONTRAINDICATIONS
Angle-closure glaucoma, severe central nervous system (CNS) depression, Parkinson's disease, coma, hypersensitiviy.

INTERACTIONS
Drug
Alcohol, other CNS depressants: May increase CNS depression.
Amphetamines, selected β-blockers, dextromethorphan,

fluoxetine, lidocaine, mirtazapine, nefazodone, paroxetine, risperidone, ritonavir, thioridazine, tricyclic antidepressants, venlafaxine, and other CYP2D6 substrates: May increase the levels of haloperidol.

Antihypertensives: May cause additive hypotension.

Azole antifungals, clarithromycin, diclofenac, doxycycline, erythromycin, imatinib, isoniazid, nefazodone, nicardipine, propofol, protease inhibitors, quinidine, telithromycin, verapamil, and other CYP3A4 inhibitors: May increase the effects of haloperidol.

Carbamazepine, nafcillin, nevirapine, phenobarbital, phenytoin, rifamycins, and other CYP3A4 inducers: May decrease the effects of haloperidol.

Chlorpromazine, delavirdine, fluoxetine, miconazole, paroxetine, pergolide, quinidine, quinine, ritonavir, ropinirole, and other CYP2D6 inhibitors: May increase the levels of haloperidol.

Epinephrine: May block α-adrenergic effects.

Extrapyramidal symptom-producing medications: May increase extrapyramidal symptoms.

Lithium: May increase neurologic toxicity.

QT prolonging medications: May increase the risk of QT prolongation.

SSRIs: May increase the risk of extrapyramidal symptoms.

Tricyclic antidepressants: May cause increased toxicity.

Herbal

Valerian, St. John's wort, kava kava, gotu kola: May increase CNS depression.

Food

Alcohol: May increase CNS depression.

DIAGNOSTIC TEST EFFECTS

None known. Therapeutic serum drug level is 0.2-1 mcg/mL; toxic serum drug level is > 1 mcg/mL.

💉 IV INCOMPATIBILITIES

Allopurinol (Aloprim), amphotericin B complex (Abelcet, AmBisome, Amphotec), cefepime (Maxipime), diphenhydramine (Benadryl), fluconazole (Diflucan), foscarnet (Foscavir), heparin, hydroxyzine (Vistaril), ketorolac (Toradol), nitroprusside (Nipride), piperacillin, and tazobactam (Zosyn).

💉 IV COMPATIBILITIES

Amifostine (Ethyol), amsacrine (Amsa), aztreonam (Azactam), cimetidine (Tagamet), cisatracurium (Nimbex), cladribine (Leustatin), dobutamine (Dobutrex), docetaxel (Taxotere), dopamine (Intropin), doxorubicin (Rubex), etoposide (VePesid), famotidine (Pepcid), fentanyl (Sublimaze), filgrastim (Neupogen), fludarabine (Fludara), gatifloxacin (Tequin), gemcitabine (Gemzar), granisetron (Kytril), hydromorphone (Dilaudid), lidocaine, linezolid (Zyvox), lorazepam (Ativan), midazolam (Versed), morphine, nitroglycerin, norepinephrine (Levophed), ondansetron (Zofran), paclitaxel (Taxol), phenylephrine, propofol (Diprivan), remifentanil (Ultiva), sufentanil (Sufenta), tacrolimus (Prograf), teniposide (Vumon), theophylline (Theodur), thiotepa (Thioplex), vinorelbine (Navelbine).

SIDE EFFECTS

Frequent

Blurred vision, constipation, orthostatic hypotension, dry mouth, swelling or soreness of female breasts, peripheral edema.

H

Occasional
Allergic reaction, difficulty urinating, decreased thirst, dizziness, decreased sexual function, drowsiness, nausea, vomiting, photosensitivity, lethargy.

SERIOUS REACTIONS

• Extrapyramidal symptoms appear to be dose related and typically occur in the first few days of therapy. Marked drowsiness and lethargy, excessive salivation, and fixed stare occur frequently. Less common reactions include severe akathisia (motor restlessness) and acute dystonias (such as torticollis, opisthotonos, and oculogyric crisis).

• Tardive dyskinesia (tongue protrusion, puffing of the cheeks, chewing or puckering of the mouth) may occur during long-term therapy or after discontinuing the drug and may be irreversible. Elderly women have a greater risk of developing this reaction.

PRECAUTIONS & CONSIDERATIONS

Caution is warranted in patients with cardiovascular disease, hepatic or renal dysfunction, a history of seizures, and with concurrent use with medications that may prolong the QT interval. Haloperidol crosses the placenta and is distributed in breast milk. Children are more susceptible to dystonias. Haloperidol use is not recommended for children younger than 3 yr. A decreased dosage is recommended for elderly patients, who are more susceptible to extrapyramidal and anticholinergic effects, orthostatic hypotension, and sedation. Exposure to sunlight and any conditions that may cause dehydration or overheating should be avoided because they may increase the risk of heat stroke.

Drowsiness may occur but generally subsides with continued therapy. Alcohol and tasks that require mental alertness or motor skills should be avoided. Notify the physician if muscle stiffness occurs. Fine tongue movement, masklike facial expression, rigidity, and tremor should be assessed if they occur.

Storage
Store vials at room temperature. Protect them from freezing and light. Discard the solution if it becomes discolored or contains precipitate.

Administration
! Only haloperidol lactate is given IV. Know that the therapeutic serum level for haloperidol is 0.2-1 mcg/mL, and the toxic serum level is > 1 mcg/mL.

Widely accepted practice but not FDA approved: Off-label, haloperidol may be given undiluted by IV push. Flush with at least 2 mL 0.9% NaCl before and after administration. To dilute, add the drug to 30-50 mL of most solutions; D5W is preferred. Give IV push at a 5 mg/min. Infuse IV piggyback over 30 min. For IV infusion, administer up to 25 mg/h, titrating dosage to patient response.

Prepare haloperidol decanoate IM injection using a 21-gauge needle. Do not exceed 3 mL per IM injection site. Slowly inject the drug deep into the upper outer quadrant of the gluteus maximus. Keep recumbent (head low and legs raised) for 30-60 min after administration to minimize hypotensive effects.

Take oral haloperidol without regard to food. Crush scored tablets as needed. Full therapeutic effect may take up to 6 wks to appear. Do not abruptly discontinue the drug after long-term use.

Heparin
hep′a-rin
(Hepalean [CAN], Heparin injection
B.P. [AUS], Heparin Leo, Uniparin
[AUS])
**Do not confuse heparin with
Hespan.**

CATEGORY AND SCHEDULE
Pregnancy Risk Category: C

Classification: Anticoagulants

MECHANISM OF ACTION
A blood modifier that interferes
with blood coagulation by blocking
the conversion of prothrombin to
thrombin and fibrinogen to fibrin.
Therapeutic Effect: Prevents further
extension of existing thrombi or
new clot formation. Has no effect on
existing clots.

PHARMACOKINETICS
Well absorbed following
subcutaneous administration. Protein
binding: Very high. Metabolized
in the liver. Removed from the
circulation via uptake by the
reticuloendothelial system. Primarily
excreted in urine. Not removed by
hemodialysis. *Half-life:* 1-6 h.

AVAILABILITY
Injection: 10 units/mL, 100 units/mL,
1000 units/mL, 2500 units/mL,
5000 units/mL, 7500 units/mL,
10,000 units/mL, 20,000 units/mL,
25,000 units/500 mL infusion.

INDICATIONS AND DOSAGES
▶ **Line flushing**
IV
Adults, Elderly, Children. 100 units
q6-8h.
Infants weighing < 10 kg.
10 units q6-8h. Caution: Always
verify strength of solution
before giving heparin flush to
infants.
▶ **Treatment of venous thrombosis,
pulmonary embolism, peripheral
arterial embolism, atrial fibrillation
with embolism**
INTERMITTENT IV
Adults, Elderly. Initially,
10,000 units, then 50-70 units/kg
(5000-10,000 units) q4-6h, adjust to
a PTT.
Children 1 yr and older. Initially,
50-100 units/kg, then 50-100 units
q4h, adjust to a PTT.
IV INFUSION
Adults, Elderly. Loading dose:
80 units/kg, then 18 units/kg/h, with
adjustments based on a PTT. Range:
10-30 units/kg/h.
Children 1 yr and older. Loading
dose: 75 units/kg, then 20 units/kg/h
with adjustments based on a PTT.
Children younger than 1 yr. Loading
dose: 75 units/kg, then 28 units/kg/h,
adjust to a PTT.
▶ **Prevention of venous thrombosis,
pulmonary embolism, peripheral
arterial embolism, atrial fibrillation
with embolism**
SUBCUTANEOUS
Adult, Elderly. 5000 units q8-12h.

CONTRAINDICATIONS
Intracranial hemorrhage,
severe hypotension, severe
thrombocytopenia, subacute
bacterial endocarditis, uncontrolled
bleeding, history of heparin-induced
thrombocytopenia (HIT).

INTERACTIONS
Drug
**Antithyroid medications,
cefoperazone, cefotetan,
valproic acid:** May cause
hypoprothrombinemia.
**Other anticoagulants, platelet
aggregation inhibitors,**

H

thrombolytics: May increase the risk of bleeding.

Probenecid: May increase the effects of heparin.

Herbal

Cat's claw, dong quai, evening primrose, feverfew, red clover, horse chestnut, garlic, green tea, ginseng, ginkgo: May have an additive effect.

Food

None known.

DIAGNOSTIC TEST EFFECTS

May increase free fatty acid, AST (SGOT), and ALT (SGPT) levels. May decrease serum cholesterol and triglyceride levels.

ⓘ IV INCOMPATIBILITIES

Alatrofloxacin (Trovan), alteplase (Activase), amikacin (Amikin), amiodarone (Cordarone), amphotericin B complex (Abelcet, AmBisome, Amphotec), amsacrine (Amsa), atracurium (Tracrium), chlorpromazine (Thorazine), ciprofloxacin (Cipro), clarithromycin (Biaxin), cytarabine (Cytosar), dacarbazine (DTIC), daunorubicin (Cerubidine), diazepam (Valium), dobutamine (Dobutrex), doxorubicin (Adriamycin), doxycycline (Vibramycin), droperidol (Inapsine), erythromycin (Erythrocin), filgrastim (Neupogen), gatifloxacin (Tequin), gentamicin (Garamycin), haloperidol (Haldol), idarubicin (Idamycin), isosorbide dinitrate, kanamycin (Kantrex), labetalol (Trandate), levofloxacin (Levaquin), levorphanol (Levo-Dromoran), meperidine (Demerol), morphine (Avinza, Kadian, Roxanol), nicardipine (Cardene), phenytoin (Dilantin), promethazine (Phenergan), quinidine, tobramycin (Nebcin), vancomycin (Vancocin), warfarin (Coumadin).

ⓘ IV COMPATIBILITIES

Acyclovir (Zovirax), aldesleukin (Proleukin), allopurinol (Alloprim), amifostine (Ethyol), aminophylline, ampicillin (Polycillin), ampicillin/ sulbactam (Unasyn), ascorbic acid, atropine, aztreonam (Azactam), betamethasone sodium phosphate (Celestone), bleomycin (Blenoxane), calcium gluconate, cefamandole (Mandol), cefazolin (Ancef), cefepime (Maxipime), cefoperazone (Cefobid), cefotaxime (Claforan), cefotetan (Cefotan), cefoxitin (Mefixitin), ceftazidime (Fortaz), ceftriaxone (Rocephin), chloramphenicol (Chloromycetin), chlordiazepoxide (Librium), cimetidine (Tagamet), cisplatin (Platinol-AQ), cladribine (Leustatin), clindamycin (Cleocin), cyanocobalamin, cyclophosphamide (Cytoxan), cytarabine (Cytosar), dexamethasone sodium phosphate (Decadron), digoxin (Lanoxin), diltiazem (Cardizem), diphenhydramine (Benadryl), docetaxel (Taxotere), dopamine (Intropin), doxorubicin (Rubex), edrophonium (Tensilon), enalapril (Vasotec), epinephrine, erythromycin lactobionate (Erythrocin), esmolol (BreviBloc), estrogens (conjugated), ethacrynate (Edecrin), etoposide (VePesid), famotidine (Pepcid), fentanyl (Sublimaze), fluconazole (Diflucan), fludarabine (Fludara), fluorouracil (Efurix), foscarnet (Foscavir), furosemide (Lasix), gemcitabine (Gemzar), granisetron (Kytril), hydralazine (Apresoline), hydrocortisone sodium succinate (Solu-Cortef), hydromorphone (Dilaudid), insulin, isoproterenol (Isuprel), leucovorin, lidocaine, linezolid (Zyvox), lorazepam (Ativan), magnesium sulfate, methotrexate, methylprednisolone (Solu-Medrol), metoclopramide (Reglan), metronidazole (Flagyl),

H

midazolam (Versed), milrinone (Primacor), minocycline (Minocin), mitomycin (Mutamycin), nafcillin (Unipen), neostigmine, nitroglycerin, norepinephrine (Levophed), ondansetron (Zofran), oxacillin (Bactocil), oxytocin (Pitocin), paclitaxel (Taxol), pancuronium (Pavulon), penicillin G potassium (Pfizerpen), pentazocine (Talwin), phytonadione, piperacillin (Piperacil), piperacillin/tazobactam (Zosyn), potassium chloride, procainamide (Pronestyl), propofol (Diprivan), propranolol (Inderal), pyridostigmine (Mestinon), ranitidine (Zantac), remifentanil (Ultiva), sargramostim (Leukine), scopolamine, sodium bicarbonate, sodium nitroprusside (Nitropress), streptokinase (Streptase), succinylcholine (Anectine), tacrolimus (Prograf), theophylline (Theodur), thiopental (Pentothal), thiotepa (Thioplex), ticarcillin (Ticar), ticarcillin/clavulanate potassium (Timentin), tirofiban (Aggrastat), trimethaphan camsylate (Arfonad), trimethobenzamide (Tigan), trimethoprim/sulfamethoxazole (Bactrim), vecuronium (Norcuron), vinblastine (Velban), vincristine (Oncovin), zidovudine (Retrovir).

SIDE EFFECTS
Occasional
Itching, burning (particularly on soles of feet) caused by vasospastic reaction.
Rare
Pain, cyanosis of extremity 6-10 days after initial therapy lasting 4-6 h; hypersensitivity reaction, including chills, fever, pruritus, urticaria, asthma, rhinitis, lacrimation, and headache.

SERIOUS REACTIONS
• Bleeding complications ranging from local ecchymoses to major hemorrhage occur more frequently in

high-dose therapy, in intermittent IV infusion, and in women 60 yr of age and older.
• Antidote: Protamine sulfate 1-1.5 mg, IV, for every 100 units heparin subcutaneous within 30 min of overdose, 0.5-0.75 mg for every 100 units heparin subcutaneous if within 30-60 min of overdose, 0.25-0.375 mg for every 100 units heparin subcutaneous if 2 h have elapsed since overdose, 25-50 mg if heparin was given by IV infusion.

PRECAUTIONS & CONSIDERATIONS
Caution should be used during menstruation in persons receiving IM injections and in those with peptic ulcer disease, recent invasive or surgical procedures, and severe hepatic or renal disease. Heparin should be used with caution in pregnant women, particularly during the last trimester and immediately postpartum, because it increases the risk of maternal hemorrhage. Heparin does not cross the placenta and is not distributed in breast milk. No age-related precautions have been noted in children. The benzyl alcohol preservative may cause gasping syndrome in infants. Elderly patients are more susceptible to hemorrhage, and age-related decreased renal function may increase the risk of bleeding. Other medications, including OTC drugs, should be avoided. An electric razor and soft toothbrush should be used to prevent bleeding during therapy.
Notify the physician of bleeding from surgical site, chest pain, dyspnea, severe or sudden headache, swelling in the feet or hands, unusual back pain, bruising, weakness, black or red stool, coffee-ground vomitus, dark or red urine, or red-speckled mucus from cough. CBC, BUN and creatinine levels, BP, pulse, potassium, and stool for occult blood should be monitored.

Be aware of signs of bleeding, including bleeding at injection or surgical sites or from gums, blood in stool, bruising, hematuria, and petechiae.

Storage

Store at room temperature.

Administration

! Do not give by IM injection because it may cause pain, hematoma, ulceration, and erythema. The subcutaneous route is used for low-dose therapy.

! Always confirm the choice of correct heparin vial or solution before administration. Fatal medication errors may occur with incorrect selections.

For subcutaneous use, after withdrawing heparin from the vial, change the needle before injection to prevent leakage along the needle track. Inject the heparin dose above the iliac crest or in the abdominal fat layer. Do not inject within 2 in. of umbilicus or scar tissue.

For IV use, dilute IV infusion in isotonic sterile saline, D5W, or lactated Ringer's solution. Invert IV bag at least 6 times to ensure mixing and to prevent pooling of the medication. Use constant-rate IV infusion pump.

Hepatitis B Immune Globulin (Human)

hep-ah-tie'tis B ih-mewn' glah'byew-lin

(Bayhep B, H-B-Vax II [AUS], Nabi-HB)

CATEGORY AND SCHEDULE

Pregnancy Risk Category: C

Classification: Immune globulins, vaccine

MECHANISM OF ACTION

An immune globulin of inactivated hepatitis B virus that provides passive immunity against hepatitis B virus.

AVAILABILITY

Injection: 0.5-mL, 1-mL, 5-mL vials.

INDICATIONS AND DOSAGES

▸ **Prevention of hepatitis B infection**

IM

Adults, Elderly. Usual 0.06 mL/kg; for acute exposure 3-5 mL. Repeat 28-30 days after exposure.

▸ **Perinatal exposure of infants born to HBsAg-positive mothers**

Infants. 0.5 mL IM after stable after birth, preferably within 12 h of birth.

CONTRAINDICATIONS

Allergies to gamma globulin or thimerosal, IgA deficiency, IM injection in patients with coagulation disorders or thrombocytopenia.

INTERACTIONS

Drug

Live virus vaccines: May decrease immune response.

Herbal and Food

None known.

DIAGNOSTIC TEST EFFECTS

None known.

SIDE EFFECTS

Frequent

Headache (26%), injection site pain (12%).

OCCASIONAL (5%)

Malaise, nausea, myalgia.

SERIOUS REACTIONS

• None known.

PRECAUTIONS & CONSIDERATIONS

Caution is warranted in patients with coagulation disorders; thrombocytopenia; IgA deficiency;

and allergies to gamma globulin, eggs, chicken, or thimerosal. Notify the physician of any side effects, including headache or injection site pain. Baseline and periodic liver function studies and hepatitis B antibody levels should be obtained. Live vaccine administration should be deferred for 3 mo after immune globulin.

Storage
Refrigerate this drug; do not freeze it.

Administration
! Avoid giving IM injections to patients with coagulation disorders or thrombocytopenia. This drug is for IM injection only.

In adults, administer by IM injection only in the gluteal or deltoid area. Complete full course of immunization.

For infants, administer IM in the anterolateral muscles of the thigh.

Hetastarch
het′ah-starch
(Hespan, Hextend)

CATEGORY AND SCHEDULE
Pregnancy Risk Category: C

Classification: Plasma expanders

MECHANISM OF ACTION
A plasma volume expander that exerts osmotic pull on tissue fluids. *Therapeutic Effect:* Reduces hemoconcentration and blood viscosity; increases circulating blood volume.

PHARMACOKINETICS
Smaller molecules: < 50,000 molecular weight, rapidly excreted by kidneys; larger molecules: 50,000 molecular weight and greater, slowly degraded to smaller-sized molecules, then excreted. *Half-life:* 17 days.

AVAILABILITY
Injection: 6 g/100 mL 0.9% NaCl (500 mL infusion container).

INDICATIONS AND DOSAGES
▸ **Plasma volume expansion**
IV
Adults, Elderly. 500-1000 mL/day up to 1500 mL/day (20 mg/kg) at a rate up to 20 mL/kg/h in hemorrhagic shock and at a slower rate in burns and septic shock.
▸ **Leukapheresis**
IV
Adults, Elderly. 250-700 mL infused at a constant rate, usually 1:8 to venous whole blood.

CONTRAINDICATIONS
Anuria, oliguria, severe bleeding disorders, severe congestive heart failure.

INTERACTIONS
Drug
None significant.
Herbal and Food
None known.

DIAGNOSTIC TEST EFFECTS
May prolong bleeding, and clotting times, PTT, and PT. May decrease Hct concentration.

⊘ IV INCOMPATIBILITIES
Amikacin (Amikin), amphotericin B (Fungizone), ampicillin (Polycillin), cefamandole (Mandol), cefazolin (Ancef, Kefzol), cefoperazone (Cefobid), cefotaxime (Claforan), cefoxitin (Mefoxin), diazepam (Valium), gentamicin (Garamycin), ranitidine (Zantac), sodium

H

bicarbonate, theophylline (Theodur), tobramycin (Nebcin).

⚕ IV COMPATIBILITIES

Alatrofloxacin (Trovan), alfentanil (Alfenta), aminophylline, amiodarone (Cordarone), ampicillin (Polycillin), ampicillin-sulbactam (Unasyn), atracurium (Tracrium), azithromycin (Zithromax), bumetanide (Bumex), butorphanol (Stadol), calcium gluconate, cefepime (Maxipime), cefotaxime (Claforan), cefotetan (Cefotan), ceftazidime (Fortaz), ceftizoxime (Cefizox), ceftriaxone (Rocephin), cefuroxime (Zinacef), chlorpromazine (Thorazine), cimetidine (Tagamet), ciprofloxacin (Cipro), cisatracurium (Nimbex), clindamycin (Cleocin), dexamethasone (Decadron), digoxin (Lanoxin), diltiazem (Cardizem), diphenhydramine (Benadryl), dobutamine (Dobutrex), dolasetron (Anzemet), dopamine (Intropin), doxycycline (Vibramycin), droperidol (Inapsine), enalaprilat (Vasotec), ephedrine, epinephrine, erythromycin (Erythrocin), esmolol (BreviBloc), famotidine (Pepcid), fentanyl (Sublimaze), fluconazole (Diflucan), furosemide (Lasix), granisetron (Kytril), haloperidol (Haldol), heparin, hydrocortisone (Solu-Cortef), hydromorphone (Dilaudid), hydroxyzine (Vistaril), inamrinone (Inocor), isoproterenol (Isuprel), ketorolac (Toradol), labetalol (Normodyne, Trandate), levofloxacin (Levaquin), lidocaine (Xylocaine), lorazepam (Ativan), magnesium, mannitol, meperidine (Demerol), methylprednisolone (Solu-Medrol), metoclopramide (Reglan), metronidazole (Flagyl), midazolam (Versed), milrinone (Primacor), mivacurium (Mivacron), morphine (Avinza, Kadian, Roxanol), nalbuphine (Nubain), nitroglycerin (Nitrobid), norepinephrine (Levophed), ofloxacin (Floxin), ondansetron (Zofran), pancuronium (Pavulon), phenylephrine, piperacillin (Piperacil), piperacillin-tazobactam (Zosyn), potassium chloride, procainamide (Pronestyl), prochlorperazine (Compazine), promethazine (Phenergan), rocuronium (Zemuron), sodium nitroprusside (Nitropress), succinylcholine (Anectine), sufentanil (Sufenta), thiopental (Pentothal), ticarcillin (Ticar), ticarcillin-clavulanate (Timentin), tobramycin (Nebcin), trimethoprim-sulfamethoxazole (Bactrim), vancomycin (Vancocin), vecuronium (Norcuron), verapamil (Calan).

SIDE EFFECTS

Rare

Allergic reaction resulting in vomiting, mild temperature elevation, chills, itching, submaxillary and parotid gland enlargement, peripheral edema of lower extremities, mild flulike symptoms, headache, muscle aches.

SERIOUS REACTIONS

• Fluid overload may occur marked by increased BP and distended neck veins. Neurologic changes that may occur include headache, weakness, blurred vision, behavioral changes, incoordination, and isolated muscle twitching. Pulmonary edema may also occur, manifested by rapid breathing, crackles, wheezing, and coughing.

• Anaphylactic reaction, including periorbital edema, urticaria, and wheezing, may occur.

PRECAUTIONS & CONSIDERATIONS

Caution is warranted with congestive heart failure, hepatic disease, pulmonary edema, sodium-restricted diets, thrombocytopenia, and in elderly patients or children. An electric razor and soft toothbrush should be used to prevent bleeding during dextran therapy.

Notify the physician of bleeding from the surgical site, wheezing, itching, rash, black or red stool, coffee-ground emesis, dark or red urine, or red-speckled mucus from cough. Urine output, vital signs, and laboratory tests, including coagulation studies and CBC, should be monitored. Central venous pressure (CVP) should also be monitored to detect blood volume overexpansion. Be aware of signs and symptoms of fluid overload, such as peripheral or pulmonary edema, and impending congestive heart failure.

Storage

Store solution at room temperature. Solution normally appears clear, pale yellow to amber. Do not use if discolored a deep turbid brown or if precipitate forms.

Administration

Administer only by IV infusion. Do not add drugs to IV line or mix with other IV fluids. In acute hemorrhagic shock, administer at a rate approaching 1.2 g/kg/h (20 mL/kg/h), as prescribed. Expect to use slower rates in burns and septic shock. Monitor CVP when giving by rapid infusion. If CVP rises precipitously, immediately discontinue the drug, as prescribed, to prevent blood volume overexpansion.

Hyaluronan
(Euflexxa, Hyalgan, Orthovisc, Supartz, Synvisc Injection)

CATEGORY AND SCHEDULE
Pregnancy Risk Category: NR

Classification: Hyaluronic acid derivatives

H

MECHANISM OF ACTION
A natural complex sugar of the glycosaminoglycan family that enhances viscoelastic properties of synovial fluid. *Therapeutic Effect:* Produces lubrication for knee joint and relieves pain and increases mobility.

PHARMACOKINETICS
Not known.

AVAILABILITY
Prefilled Syringe: 8 mg/1 mL (Synvisc), 10 mg/1 mL (Euflexxa, Hyalgan, Supartz), 15 mg/1 mL (Orthovisc).

INDICATIONS AND DOSAGES
▶ **Knee osteoarthritis**
PO
Adults, Elderly. Euflexxa: inject 20 mg into one knee weekly for 3 wks; Hyalagan: inject 20 mg into one knee weekly for 3-5 wks; Orthovisc: inject 30 mg into one knee weekly for 3 or 4 wks; Supartz: inject 25 mg into one knee weekly for 5 wks; Synvisc: inject 16 mg into one knee weekly for 3 wks.

OFF-LABEL USES
Treatment of psoriatic arthritis.

CONTRAINDICATIONS
Allergies to avian or avian-derived products (including eggs, feathers, or poultry), skin disease or infection in

area of injection site, hypersensitivity to hyaluronate preparations or any one of its components, including preservatives.

INTERACTIONS
Drug
Anticoagulants or antiplatelet agents: May increase the risk of injection site bleeding.
Herbal
None known.
Food
None known.

DIAGNOSTIC TEST EFFECTS
None known.

SIDE EFFECTS
Occasional
Arthralgia, back pain, pain at injection site.
Rare
Joint stiffness, swelling.

SERIOUS REACTIONS
• Transient increases in inflammation in the injected knee following hyaluronan injection have been reported in some patients with OA.
• Rare allergic reactions.

PRECAUTIONS & CONSIDERATIONS
Be aware that the safety and effectiveness of hyaluronan have not been established in joints other than the knee. Be aware that use of disinfectants containing quartenary ammonium salts for skin preparation as hyaluronic acid can precipitate in their presence. Safety and efficacy of this drug have not been tested in pregnant, nursing women, or children. No age-related precautions have been noted in elderly patients. Strenuous activity or weight-bearing activities should be avoided within 48 h following injection.

Storage
Store syringes at room temperature. Do not freeze.
Administration
Be aware that the prefilled syringe is for single use only. Discard syringe after administering. Remove the protective rubber cap on the tip of the syringe, and attach small-gauge needle (18-21-gauge) to the tip. Inject full contents of syringe into one knee. If treatment is bilateral, use a separate syringe for each knee.

Hydralazine
hye-dral′a-zeen
(Alphapress [AUS], Apresoline, Novohylazin [CAN])
Do not confuse hydralazine with hydroxyzine.

CATEGORY AND SCHEDULE
Pregnancy Risk Category: C

Classification: Vasodilators, antihypertensive

MECHANISM OF ACTION
An antihypertensive with direct vasodilating effects on arterioles. *Therapeutic Effect:* Decreases BP and systemic resistance.

PHARMACOKINETICS

Route	Onset (min)	Peak	Duration
PO	20-30	N/A	2-4 h
IV	5-20	N/A	2-6 h

Well absorbed from the GI tract. Widely distributed. Protein binding: 85%-90%. Metabolized in the liver to active metabolite. Primarily excreted in urine. Not removed by hemodialysis. *Half-life:* 3-7 h (increased with impaired renal function).

AVAILABILITY
Tablets: 10 mg, 25 mg, 50 mg, 100 mg.
Injection: 20 mg/mL.

INDICATIONS AND DOSAGES
▸ **Moderate to severe hypertension**
PO
Adults. Initially, 10 mg 4 times a day. May increase by 10-25 mg/dose q2-5 days. Maximum: 300 mg/day.
Children. Initially, 0.75-1 mg/kg/day in 2-4 divided doses, not to exceed 25 mg/dose. May increase over 3-4 wks. Maximum: 7.5 mg/kg/day (5 mg/kg/day in infants).
IV, IM
Adults, Elderly. Initially, 10-20 mg/dose q4-6h. Maximum: 20 mg per dose IV, 50 mg IM.
Children. Initially, 0.1-0.2 mg/kg/dose (maximum: 20 mg) q4-6h, as needed, up to 1.7-3.5 mg/kg/day in divided doses q4-6h.
▸ **Dosage in renal impairment**
Dosage interval is based on creatinine clearance.

CrCl (mL/min)	Dosage Interval
10-50	q8h
< 10	q8-24h

OFF-LABEL USES
Treatment of congestive heart failure, hypertension secondary to eclampsia and preeclampsia, primary pulmonary hypertension.

CONTRAINDICATIONS
Coronary artery disease, lupus erythematosus, rheumatic heart disease.

INTERACTIONS
Drug
Diuretics, other antihypertensives: May increase hypotensive effect.
Herbal
Licorice, ma huang, yohimbine: May decrease the effectiveness of hydralazine.
Food
None known.

DIAGNOSTIC TEST EFFECTS
May produce positive direct Coombs' test.

ⓦ IV INCOMPATIBILITIES
Aminophylline, ampicillin (Polycillin), chlorothiazide (Diuril), edetate calcium disodium, ethacrynate (Edecrin), furosemide (Lasix), hydrocortisone sodium succinate (Solu-Cortef), methohexital (Brevital), nitroglycerin (Nitrobid), phenobarbital, verapamil (Calan).

ⓦ IV COMPATIBILITIES
Dobutamine (Dobutrex), heparin, potassium.

SIDE EFFECTS
Frequent
Headache, palpitations, tachycardia (generally disappears in 7-10 days).
Occasional
GI disturbance (nausea, vomiting, diarrhea), paresthesia, fluid retention, peripheral edema, dizziness, flushed face, nasal congestion.

SERIOUS REACTIONS
• High dosage may produce lupus erythematosus-like reaction, including fever, facial rash, muscle and joint aches, and splenomegaly.
• Severe orthostatic hypotension, skin flushing, severe headache, myocardial ischemia, and cardiac arrhythmias may develop.

• Profound shock may occur with severe overdosage.

PRECAUTIONS & CONSIDERATIONS
Caution is warranted with cerebrovascular disease, pulmonary hypertension, and impaired renal function. Hydralazine crosses the placenta; it is unknown whether it is distributed in breast milk. Hematomas, leukopenia, petechial bleeding, and thrombocytopenia have occurred in newborns; these conditions resolve within 1-3 wks. No age-related precautions have been noted in children. Elderly patients are more sensitive to the drug's hypotensive effects. In elderly patients, age-related renal impairment may require dosage adjustment.

Dizziness and light-headedness may occur. Rise slowly from a lying to a sitting position, and permit legs to dangle from the bed momentarily before standing to reduce the hypotensive effect of hydralazine. Those receiving high doses of hydralazine should notify the physician if fever (lupus-like reaction) or joint and muscle aches occur. Also, notify the physician if headache, palpitations, tachycardia, or peripheral edema of the hands and feet occurs. BP and pulse should be obtained immediately before each hydralazine dose, in addition to regular BP monitoring. Be alert for BP fluctuations. Daily bowel activity and stool consistency should also be monitored.

Storage
Store drug at room temperature.

Administration
Hydralazine is best given with food or regularly spaced meals. Crush tablets if necessary.

For IV use, give undiluted. Do not add to infusion solutions. Give single dose over 1 min.

Hydrochlorothiazide
hye-droe-klor-oh-thye′a-zide
(Apo-Hydro [CAN], Dichlotride [AUS], Dithiazide [AUS], Esidrix, Microzide, Oretic)

CATEGORY AND SCHEDULE
Pregnancy Risk Category: B (D if used in pregnancy-induced hypertension)

Classification: Diuretics, thiazide and derivatives

MECHANISM OF ACTION
A sulfonamide derivative that acts as a thiazide diuretic, and antihypertensive. As a diuretic, blocks reabsorption of water, sodium, and potassium at the cortical diluting segment of the distal tubule. As an antihypertensive, reduces plasma, extracellular fluid volume, and peripheral vascular resistance by direct effect on blood vessels. *Therapeutic Effect:* Promotes diuresis; reduces BP.

PHARMACOKINETICS

Route	Onset	Peak	Duration
PO (diuretic)	2 h	4-6 h	6-12 h

Variably absorbed from the GI tract. Primarily excreted unchanged in urine. Not removed by hemodialysis. *Half-life:* 5.6-14.8 h.

AVAILABILITY
Capsules (Microzide): 12.5 mg.
Oral Solution: 50 mg/5 mL.
Tablets (Esidrix, Oretic): 12.5 mg, 25 mg, 50 mg,

INDICATIONS AND DOSAGES
▸ **Edema, hypertension**
PO
Adults. 12.5-100 mg/day. Maximum: 200 mg/day.

▶ **Usual pediatric dosage**
PO
Children 6 mo to 12 yr. 2 mg/kg/day in 2 divided doses. Maximum for children aged 2-12 yr: 100 mg/day. Maximum for children up to 2 yr: 12.5-37.5 mg/day.
Infants younger than 6 mo. 2-3 mg/kg/day in 2 divided doses. Maximum: 12.5-37.5 mg/day.

OFF-LABEL USES
Treatment of diabetes insipidus, prevention of calcium-containing renal calculi.

CONTRAINDICATIONS
Anuria, history of hypersensitivity to sulfonamides or thiazide diuretics, renal decompensation, pregnancy.

INTERACTIONS
Drug
β-Blockers: May increase hyperglycemic effects in type 2 diabetics.
Cholestyramine, colestipol: May decrease the absorption and effects of hydrochlorothiazide.
Cyclosporine: Concurrent use with hydrochlorothiazide may increase the risk of gout or renal toxicity.
Digitalis glycosides: May increase the risk of digitalis toxicity.
Digoxin: May increase the risk of digoxin toxicity associated with hydrochlorothiazide-induced hypokalemia.
Lithium: May increase the risk of lithium toxicity.
Neuromuscular blocking agents: May prolong blockade.
Herbal
Ephedra, ginseng, ma huang, yohimbine: May reduce hypotensive effect of hydrochlorothiazide.
Garlic: May have additive hypotensive effects.
Ginkgo biloba: May increase BP.
Licorice: May increase risk of hypokalemia and reduce the effectiveness of hydrochlorothiazide.
Food
None known.

DIAGNOSTIC TEST EFFECTS
May increase blood glucose and serum cholesterol, LDL, bilirubin, calcium, creatinine, uric acid, and triglyceride levels. May decrease urinary calcium levels and serum magnesium, potassium, and sodium levels.

SIDE EFFECTS
Expected
Increase in urinary frequency and urine volume.
Frequent
Potassium depletion.
Occasional
Orthostatic hypotension, headache, GI disturbances, photosensitivity.

SERIOUS REACTIONS
• Vigorous diuresis may lead to profound water and electrolyte depletion, resulting in hypokalemia, hyponatremia, and dehydration.
• Acute hypotensive episodes may occur.
• Hyperglycemia may occur during prolonged therapy.
• Pancreatitis, blood dyscrasias, pulmonary edema, allergic pneumonitis, and dermatologic reactions occur rarely.
• Overdose can lead to lethargy and coma without changes in electrolytes or hydration.

PRECAUTIONS & CONSIDERATIONS
Caution is warranted in patients with diabetes mellitus, thyroid disorders, hepatic impairment, severe renal disease, and in elderly patients and debilitated patients.

Hydrochlorothiazide crosses the placenta, and a small amount is distributed in breast milk. Breastfeeding is not recommended. No age-related precautions have been noted in children, except that jaundiced infants may be at risk for hyperbilirubinemia. Elderly patients may be more sensitive to the drug's electrolyte and hypotensive effects. Age-related renal impairment may require cautious use in elderly patients. Consuming foods high in potassium such as apricots, bananas, legumes, meat, orange juice, raisins, whole grains, including cereals, and white and sweet potatoes, is encouraged. Avoid prolonged exposure to sunlight and ultraviolet rays because a photosensitivity reaction may occur.

Dizziness or light-headedness may occur, so change positions slowly and let legs dangle momentarily before standing. An increase in the frequency and volume of urination may also occur. BP, vital signs, electrolytes, intake and output, and weight should be monitored before and during treatment. Be aware of signs of electrolyte disturbances such as hypokalemia or hyponatremia. Hypokalemia may cause arrhythmias, altered mental status, muscle cramps, asthenia, and tremor. Hyponatremia may result in cold and clammy skin, confusion, and thirst.

Administration
Take hydrochlorothiazide with food or milk if GI upset occurs, preferably with breakfast to help prevent nocturia. Tablets may be crushed and mixed with fluid, if necessary.

Hydrocodone
hye-droe-koe′done
Hydrocodone and acetaminophen, (Anexsia, Bancap HC, Ceta-Plus, Co-Gesic, Hycet, Hydrocet, Hydrogesic, Lorcet 10/650, Lorcet-HD, Lorcet Plus, Lortab, Margesic H, Maxidone, Norco, Stagesic, Vicodin, Vicodin ES, Vicodin HP, Zydone); hydrocodone and aspirin (Azdone, Vicoprin); hydrocodone and chlorpheniramine (Tussionex); hydrocodone and guaifenesin (Codiclear DH, Extendryl, Hycosin, Hycotuss, Kwelcof, Pneumotussin, Vicodin Tuss, Vitussin, Xpect); hydrocodone and homatropine (Hycodan, and Hydromet, Hydropane, Tussigon); hydrocodone and ibuprofen, (Reprexain, Vicoprofen); hydrocodone and pseudoephedrine (Coldcough, Detussin, Histussin D, Pancof, P-V Tussin, SymTan); hydrocodone, chlorpheniramine, phenylephrine, acetaminophen, and caffeine (Hycomine Compound).

CATEGORY AND SCHEDULE
Pregnancy Risk Category: C, D if used for prolonged periods, high dosages at term
Controlled substance: Schedule III

Classification: Antitussive, narcotic analgesic, opiate derivative, phenanthrene derivative

MECHANISM OF ACTION
Hydrocodone blocks pain perception in the cerebral cortex by binding to specific opiate receptors (μ and κ) neuronal membranes of synapses. This binding results in a decreased

synaptic chemical transmission throughout the central nervous system (CNS), thus inhibiting the flow of pain sensations into the higher centers and causing analgesia. *Therapeutic Effect:* Alters perception of pain and produces analgesic effect.

PHARMACOKINETICS

Well absorbed. Metabolized in liver. Excreted in urine. *Half-life:* 3.3-3.4 h.

AVAILABILITY

Hydrocodone and Acetaminophen
Capsules: Hydrocodone bitartrate 5 mg and acetaminophen 500 mg (Bancap HC, Ceta-Plus, Hydrocet, Hydrogesic, Lorcet-HD, Margesic H, Stagesic).
Elixir: Hydrocodone bitartrate 7.5 mg and acetaminophen 500 mg/15 mL (Lortab).
Solution, Oral: Hydrocodone bitartrate 7.5 mg and acetaminophen 325 mg/15 mL (Hycet).
Tablets: Hydrocodone bitartrate 2.5 mg and acetaminophen 500 mg (Lortab), hydrocodone bitartrate 5 mg and acetaminophen 325 mg (Norco), hydrocodone bitartrate 5 mg and acetaminophen 400 mg (Zydone), hydrocodone bitartrate 5 mg and acetaminophen 500 mg (Anexsia, Co-Gesic, Lortab 5/500, Vicodin), hydrocodone bitartrate 7.5 mg and acetaminophen 325 mg (Norco), hydrocodone bitartrate 5 mg and acetaminophen 400 mg (Zydone), hydrocodone bitartrate 7.5 mg and acetaminophen 500 mg (Lortab 7.5/500), hydrocodone bitartrate 7.5 mg and acetaminophen 650 mg (Anexsia, Lorcet Plus), hydrocodone bitartrate 7.5 mg and acetaminophen 750 mg (Vicodin ES), hydrocodone bitartrate 10 mg and acetaminophen 325 mg (Norco), hydrocodone bitartrate 5 mg and acetaminophen 400 mg (Zydone),

hydrocodone bitartrate 10 mg and acetaminophen 500 mg (Lortab 10/500), hydrocodone bitartrate 10 mg and acetaminophen 650 mg (Lorcet 10/650), hydrocodone bitartrate 10 mg and acetaminophen 660 mg (Vicodin HP), hydrocodone bitartrate 10 mg and acetaminophen 750 mg (Maxidone).
Hydrocodone and Aspirin
Tablets: Hydrocodone bitartrate 5 mg and aspirin 500 mg (Azdone, Vicoprin).
Hydrocodone and Chlorpheniramine
Syrup, Extended Release: Hydrocodone polistirex 10 mg and chlorpheniramine polistirex 8 mg/5 mL (Tussionex).
Hydrocodone and Guaifenesin
Liquid: Hydrocodone bitartrate 2.5 mg and guaifenesin 200 mg/ 5 mL (Pneumotussin), hydrocodone bitartrate 5 mg and guaifenesin 100 mg/5 mL (Codiclear DH, Hycosin, Hycotuss, Kwelcof, Vicoden Tuss, Vitussin).
Tablets: Hydrocodone bitartrate 2.5 mg and guaifenesin 300 mg (Pneumotussin), hydrocodone bitartrate 2.5 mg and guaifenesin 1000 mg (Extendryl HC), hydrocodone bitartrate 5 mg and guaifenesin 575 mg (Touro HC), hydrocodone bitartrate 5 mg and guaifenesin 600 mg (Xpect HC).
Hydrocodone and Homatropine
Syrup: Hydrocodone bitartrate 5 mg and homatropine methylbromide 1.5 mg/5 mL (Hycodan, Hydromet, Hydropane).
Tablets: Hydrocodone bitartrate 5 mg and homatropine methylbromide 1.5 mg (Hycodan, Tussigon).
Hydrocodone and Ibuprofen
Tablets: Hydrocodone bitartrate 5 mg and ibuprofen 200 mg (Reprexain), hydrocodone bitartrate 7.5 mg and ibuprofen 200 mg (Vicoprofen).

H

Hydrocodone and Pseudoephedrine
Liquid: Hydrocodone bitartrate 3 mg and pseudoephedrine 15 mg/5 mL (Coldcough, Pancof), hydrocodone bitartrate 5 mg and pseudoephedrine 60 mg/5 mL (Detussin, Histussin D), hydrocodone bitartrate 10 mg and pseudoephedrine 45 mg/5 mL (SymTan).

Tablets: Hydrocodone bitartrate 5 mg and pseudoephedrine 60 mg (P-V Tussin).

Hydrocodone, chlorpheniramine, phenylephrine, acetaminophen, and caffeine.
Tablets: Hydrocodone bitartrate 5 mg, chlorpheniramine maleate 2 mg, phenylephrine hydrochloride 10 mg, acetaminophen 250 mg, and caffeine 30 mg (Hycomine Compound).

INDICATIONS AND DOSAGES
Hydrocodone and acetaminophen
▸ **Analgesia**
PO (DOSAGE GIVEN AS HYDROCODONE)
Adults, Children older than 13 yr or > 50 kg. 2.5-10 mg q4-6h. Maximum: 60 mg/day hydrocodone. Maximum dose of acetaminophen: 4 g/day.
Elderly. 2.5-5 mg hydrocodone q4-6h. Titrate dose to appropriate analgesic effect. Maximum: 4 g/day acetaminophen.
Children 2-13 yr or < 50 kg. 0.135 mg/kg/dose hydrocodone q4-6h. Maximum: 6 doses/day of hydrocodone or maximum recommended dose of acetaminophen. See weight-based dosage chart in manufacturer's prescribing information for liquid dosage forms.
▸ **Hydrocodone and aspirin**
PO
Adults. 2.5-10 mg q4-6h. Maximum: 60 mg/day hydrocodone.

Elderly. 2.5-5 mg hydrocodone q4-6h. Titrate dose to appropriate analgesic effect.
Children 2-13 yr or < 50 kg. 0.135 mg/kg/dose hydrocodone q4-6h.
▸ **Hydrocodone and chlorpheniramine**
Adults, Elderly, Children 12 yr and older. 5 mL q12h. Maximum: 10 mL/24h.
Children 6-12 yr. 2.5 mL q12h. Maximum: 5 mL/24h.
▸ **Hydrocodone and guaifenesin**
Adults, Elderly, Children 12 yr and older. 5 mL q4h. Maximum: 30 mL/24h.
Children 2-12 yr. 2.5 mL q4h.
Children < 2 yr. 0.3 mg/kg/day (hydrocodone) in 4 divided doses.
▸ **Hydrocodone and homatropine**
Adults, Elderly. 10 mg (hydrocodone) q4-6h. A single dose should not exceed 15 mg and not more frequently than q4h.
Children. 0.6 mg/kg/day (hydrocodone) in 3-4 divided doses. Do not administer more frequently than q4h.
▸ **Hydrocodone and ibuprofen**
Adults. 7.5-15 mg (hydrocodone) q4-6h as needed for pain. Maximum: 5 tablets/day.
▸ **Hydrocodone and pseudoephedrine**
Adults, Elderly. 5 mL 4 times/day.
▸ **Hydrocodone, chlorpheniramine, phenylephrine, acetaminophen, and caffeine**
Adults, Elderly. 1 tablet q4h up to 4 times/day.

CONTRAINDICATIONS
Central nervous system (CNS) depression, severe respiratory depression, hypersensitivity to hydrocodone or to any component of the formulation.

INTERACTIONS
Drug
Alcohol, CNS depressants: May increase hypotension

and CNS or respiratory depression.

CYP2D6 inhibitors (e.g., chlorpromazine): May decrease the effects of hydrocodone.

Hepatotoxic medications (e.g., phenytoin), liver enzyme inducers (e.g., cimetidine): May increase the risk of hepatotoxicity associated with acetaminophen with prolonged high dose or single toxic dose.

MAOIs, tricyclic antidepressants: May increase effects of MAOIs and TCAs and hydrocodone.

Warfarin: May increase the risk of bleeding with regular use.

Herbal
Valerian, St. John's wort, SAMe, kava kava: May increase sedative effects.

Food
None known.

DIAGNOSTIC TEST EFFECTS

None known.

SIDE EFFECTS

Frequent
Dizziness, sedation, drowsiness, bradycardia.

Occasional
Anxiety, dysphoria, euphoria, fear, lethargy, light-headedness, malaise, mental clouding, mental impairment, mood changes, physiologic dependence, sedation, somnolence, constipation, bradycardia, heartburn, nausea, vomiting.

Rare
Hypersensitivity reaction, rash.

SERIOUS REACTIONS

• Cardiac arrest, circulatory collapse, coma, hypotension, hypoglycemic coma, ureteral spasm, urinary retention, vesical sphincter spasm, agranulocytosis, bleeding time prolonged, hemolytic anemia, iron deficiency anemia, occult blood loss

thrombocytopenia, hepatic necrosis, hepatits, skeletal muscle rigidity, renal toxicity, and renal tubular necrosis have been reported.

• Hearing impairment or loss has been reported with chronic overdose.

• Acute airway obstruction, apnea, dyspnea, and respiratory depression occur rarely and are usually dose related.

PRECAUTIONS & CONSIDERATIONS

Caution is warranted with hypersensitivity reactions to other phenanthrene derivative opioid agonists (morphine, hydrocodone, hydromorphone, levorphanol, oxycodone, oxymorphone). Be aware that tablets with metabisulfite may cause allergic reactions. Information is not available for hydrocodone during pregnancy. The manufacturers recommend discontinuing the medication or to discontinue nursing during therapy. Be aware that hydrocodone should be used cautiously in children and elderly patients.

Drug dependence or tolerance may occur with prolonged use of high dosages. Avoid alcohol and tasks that require mental alertness or motor skills. Change positions slowly to avoid orthostatic hypotension.

Storage
Store at room temperature.

Administration
Be aware that ambulatory persons and those not in severe pain may experience dizziness, hypotension, nausea, and vomiting more frequently than patients in the supine position or with severe pain. Be aware to expect to reduce the initial dosage in those with concurrent central nervous system (CNS) depressants, elderly, and debilitated. Shake any oral liquid or suspension well before use to avoid improper dosing.

Take without regard to meals.

Hydrocodone (combinations)

high-drough-koe′doan
(Hycodan [CAN], Robidone [CAN])

CATEGORY AND SCHEDULE

Pregnancy Risk Category: C (D if used for prolonged periods or at high dosages at term)
Controlled Substance Schedule: III

Classification: Narcotic (opioid), analgesic

MECHANISM OF ACTION

A narcotic analgesic and antitussive that binds with opioid receptors in the CNS. *Therapeutic Effect:* Alters the perception of and emotional response to pain; suppresses cough reflex.

PHARMACOKINETICS

Route	Onset	Peak	Duration
PO (analgesic)	10-20 min	30-60 min	4-6 h
PO (antitussive)	N/A	N/A	4-6 h

Well absorbed from the GI tract. Metabolized in the liver. Primarily excreted in urine. *Half-life:* 3.8 h (increased in elderly).

INDICATIONS AND DOSAGES

▸ **Analgesia**
PO
Adults, Children older than 12 yr. 5-10 mg q4-6h.
Elderly. 2.5-5 mg q4-6h.
▸ **Cough**
PO
Adults. 5-10 mg q4-6h as needed. Maximum: 15 mg/dose.
Children. 0.6 mg/kg/day in 3-4 divided doses at intervals of at least 4 h. Maximum single dose: 5 mg (children 2-12 yr), 1.25 mg (children younger than 2 yr).
PO (EXTENDED-RELEASE)
Adults. 10 mg q12h.
Children 6-12 yr. 5 mg q12h.

CONTRAINDICATIONS

Children < 6 yr old.

INTERACTIONS

Drug
Alcohol, other CNS depressants: May increase CNS or respiratory depression and hypotension.
MAOIs: May produce a severe, sometimes fatal reaction; plan to administer one quarter of the usual hydrocodone dose.
Herbal
Valerian, St. John's wort, SAMe, kava kava: May increase sedative effects.
Food
None known.

DIAGNOSTIC TEST EFFECTS

May increase serum amylase and lipase levels.

SIDE EFFECTS

Frequent
Sedation, hypotension, diaphoresis, facial flushing, dizziness, somnolence.
Occasional
Urine retention, blurred vision, constipation, dry mouth, headache, nausea, vomiting, difficult or painful urination, euphoria, dysphoria.

SERIOUS REACTIONS

• Overdose results in respiratory depression, skeletal muscle flaccidity, cold or clammy skin, cyanosis, and extreme somnolence progressing to seizures, stupor, and coma.

• The patient who uses hydrocodone repeatedly may develop a tolerance to the drug's analgesic effect as well as physical dependence.

• The drug may have a prolonged duration of action and cumulative effect in patients with hepatic or renal impairment.

PRECAUTIONS & CONSIDERATIONS

Extreme caution should be used with acute alcoholism, anoxia, CNS depression, hypercapnia, respiratory depression or dysfunction, seizures, shock, and untreated myxedema. Caution is also warranted with acute abdominal conditions, Addison disease, chronic obstructive pulmonary disease (COPD), hypothyroidism, hepatic impairment, increased intracranial pressure, benign prostatic hyperplasia, and urethral stricture. Hydrocodone readily crosses the placenta and is distributed in breast milk. Regular use of hydrocodone during pregnancy may produce withdrawal symptoms in the neonate, including irritability, excessive crying, tremors, hyperactive reflexes, fever, vomiting, diarrhea, yawning, sneezing, and seizures. Hydrocodone use may prolong labor if administered in the latent phase of the first stage of labor or before the cervix has dilated 4-5 cm. The neonate may develop respiratory depression if the mother receives hydrocodone during labor. Children younger than 2 yr may be more susceptible to respiratory depression. Elderly patients may be more susceptible to respiration depression and paradoxical excitement. In elderly patients, age-related renal impairment, benign prostatic hyperplasia, or obstruction may increase the risk of urine retention. A dosage adjustment is recommended.

Dizziness and drowsiness may occur, so change positions slowly and avoid alcohol, CNS depressants, and tasks that require mental alertness or motor skills until response to the drug is established. Notify the physician if constipation, difficulty breathing, nausea, or vomiting occurs during therapy. Vital signs, pattern of daily bowel activity and stool consistency, and clinical improvement of pain should be monitored. The bladder should be palpated for urine retention.

Administration

! Ambulatory patients and those not in severe pain may be more prone to dizziness, hypotension, nausea, and vomiting than patients in the supine position and those in severe pain.

Take hydrocodone orally without regard to food. Crush tablets if needed.

Hydrocortisone

hye-dro-kor'ti-sone
(A-HydroCort, Anusol-HC, Cortaid, Cortef cream [AUS], Cortic cream [AUS], Cortic DS [AUS], Cortifoam [AUS], Cortizone-5, Cortizone-10, Dermaid [AUS], Derm-Aid cream [AUS], Dermaid soft cream [AUS], Egocort cream [AUS], Emcort, Hycor [AUS], Hycor eye ointment [AUS], Hysone [AUS], Hytone, Locoid, Nupercainal Hydrocortisone Cream, Preparation H Hydrocortisone, Protocort, Siquent Hycor [AUS], Solu-Cortef, Squibb HC [AUS], WestCort).

CATEGORY AND SCHEDULE

Pregnancy Risk Category: C (D if used in first trimester)
OTC (Hydrocortisone 0.5% and 1% Cream, Gel, and Ointment)

Classification: Corticosteroids, topical, dermatologics, anti-inflammatory

MECHANISM OF ACTION

An adrenocortical steroid that inhibits the accumulation of inflammatory cells at inflammation sites, phagocytosis, lysosomal enzyme release, and synthesis and release of mediators of inflammation. *Therapeutic Effect:* Prevents or suppresses cell-mediated immune reactions. Decreases or prevents tissue response to inflammatory process.

PHARMACOKINETICS

Route	Onset	Peak	Duration
IV	N/A	4-6 h	8-12 h

Well absorbed after IM administration. Widely distributed. Metabolized in the liver. *Half-life:* Plasma, 1.5-2 h; biologic, 8-12 h.

AVAILABILITY

Tablet (Cortef): 5 mg, 10 mg, 20 mg.
Cream (Rectal [Nupercainal Hydrocortisone Cream, Cortizone-10, Preparation H Hydrocortisone]): 1%.
Cream (Topical [Cortizone-5]): 0.5%.
Cream (Topical [Caldecort, Cortizone-10]): 1%.
Cream (Topical [Hytone]): 2.5%.
Ointment (Topical [Locoid]): 0.1%.
Ointment (Topical [Westcort]): 0.2%.
Ointment (Topical [Cortizone-5]): 0.5%.
Ointment (Topical [Anusol-HC, Cortaid, Cortizone-10]): 1%.
Ointment (Topical [Hytone]): 2.5%.
Suppositories (Anusol-HC): 25 mg.
Suppositories (Emcort, Protocort): 30 mg.
Injection (A-hydro-Cort, Solu-Cortef): 100 mg, 250 mg, 500 mg, 1 g.

INDICATIONS AND DOSAGES
▸ **Acute adrenal insufficiency**
IV
Adults, Elderly. 100 mg IV bolus; then 300 mg/day in divided doses q8h.

Children. 1-2 mg/kg IV bolus; then 150-250 mg/day in divided doses q6-8h.
Infants. 1-2 mg/kg/dose IV bolus; then 25-150 mg/day in divided doses q6-8h.
▸ **Anti-inflammation, immunosuppression**
IV, IM
Adults, Elderly. 15-240 mg q12h.
Children. 1-5 mg/kg/day in divided doses q12h.
▸ **Physiologic replacement**
PO
Children. 0.5-0.75 mg/kg/day in divided doses q8h.
IM
Children. 0.25-0.35 mg/kg/day as a single dose.
▸ **Status asthmaticus**
IV
Adults, Elderly. 100-500 mg q6h.
Children. 2 mg/kg/dose q6h.
▸ **Shock**
IV
Adults, Elderly, Children. 12 yr and older. 100-500 mg q6h.
Children younger than 12 yr. 50 mg/kg. May repeat in 4 h, then q24h as needed.
▸ **Adjunctive treatment of ulcerative colitis**
RECTAL (RETENTION ENEMA)
Adults, Elderly. 100 mg at bedtime for 21 nights or until clinical and proctologic remission occurs (may require 2-3 mo of therapy).
RECTAL SUPPOSITORIES
Adults. Suppository 2-3 times/day. Usually for 2 wks.
RECTAL (CORTIFOAM)
Adults, Elderly. 1 applicator 1-2 times a day for 2-3 wks, then every second day until therapy ends.
▸ **Hemmorhoidal irritation**
TOPICAL
Adults, Elderly. Apply sparingly 2-4 times a day.

CONTRAINDICATIONS

Fungal, tuberculosis, or viral skin lesions; serious infections.

INTERACTIONS
Drug
Amphotericin: May increase hypokalemia.

Cyclosporine: May increase the effects of cyclosporine.

Digoxin: May increase the risk of digoxin toxicity caused by hypokalemia.

Diuretics, insulin, oral hypoglycemics, potassium supplements: May decrease the effects of these drugs.

Hepatic enzyme inducers: May decrease the effects of hydrocortisone.

Live virus vaccines: May decrease the patient's antibody response to vaccine, increase vaccine side effects, and potentiate virus replication.

Herbal
Cat's claw, echinacea: Avoid use because of its immunostimulant properties.

St. John's wort: May decrease hydrocortisone levels.

Food
Calcium: May interfere with calcium absorption.

DIAGNOSTIC TEST EFFECTS
May increase blood glucose and serum lipid, amylase, and sodium levels. May decrease serum calcium, potassium, and thyroxine levels.

🚫 IV INCOMPATIBILITIES
Bleomycin (Blenoxane), ciprofloxacin (Cipro), diazepam (Valium), doxapram (Dopram), ephedrine, hydralazine (Apresoline), idarubicin (Idamycin), midazolam (Versed), nafcillin (Unipen), pentobarbital (Nembutal), phenobarbital, phenytoin (Dilantin), prochlorperazine (Compazine), promethazine (Phenergan), sargramostim (Leukine).

💧 IV COMPATIBILITIES
Acyclovir (Zovirax), allopurinol (Alloprim), amikacin (Amikin), amifostine (Ethyol), aminophylline, amphotericin, ampicillin (Polycillin), amsacrine (Amsa), atracurium (Tracrium), atropine, aztreonam (Azactam), betamethasone sodium phosphate (Celestone), calcium gluconate, cefepime (Maxipime), chloramphenicol (Chloromycetin), chlordiazepoxide (Librium), chlorpromazine (Thorazine), cisatracurium (Nimbex), cladribine (Leustatin), clindamycin (Cleocin), corticotropin, cyanocobalamin, cytarabine (Cytosar), daunorubicin (Cerubidine), dexamethasone sodium phosphate (Decadron), digoxin (Lanoxin), diltiazem (Cardizem), diphenhydramine (Benadryl), docetaxel (Taxotere), dopamine (Intropin), doxorubicin (Rubex), droperidol (Inapsine), edrophonium (Tensilon), enalaprilat (Vasotec), epinephrine, erythromycin (Erythrocin), esmolol (BreviBloc), estrogens (conjugated), ethacrynate sodium (edecrin), etoposide (VePesid), famotidine (Pepcid), fentanyl (Sublimaze), filgrastim (Neupogen), fludarabine (Fludara), fluorouracil (Efurix), foscarnet (Foscavir), furosemide (Lasix), gatifloxacin (Tequin), gemcitabine (Gemzar), granisetron (Kytril), heparin, inamrinone (Inocor), insulin, isoproterenol (Isuprel), kanamycin (Kantrex), lidocaine, linezolid (Zyvox), lorazepam (Ativan), magnesium sulfate, meperidine (Demerol), metronidazole (Flagyl), metoclopramide (Reglan), methoxamine (Vasoxyl), methylergonovine (Methergine), minocycline (Minocin),

H

mitomycin (Mutamycin), mitoxantrone (Novantrone), morphine, neostigmine, norepinephrine (Levophed), ondansetron (Zofran), oxacillin (Floxin), oxytocin (Pitocin), paclitaxel (Taxol), pancuronium (Pavulon), penicillin G potassium (Pfizerpen), pentazocine (Talwin), phytonadione, piperacillin/ tazobactam (Zosyn), potassium chloride, procainamide (Pronestyl), propofol (Diprivan), propranolol (Inderal), pyridostigmine, remifentanil (Ultiva), scopolamine, sodium bicarbonate, succinylcholine (Anectine), tacrolimus (Prograf), teniposide (Vumon), theophylline (Theodur), thiopental (Pentothal), thiotepa (Thioplex), trimethaphan camsylate (Arfonad), trimethobenzamide (Tigan), vancomycin (Vancocin), vecuronium (Norcuron), verapamil (Calan), vinorelbine (Navelbine).

SIDE EFFECTS

Frequent
Insomnia, heartburn, nervousness, abdominal distention, diaphoresis, acne, mood swings, increased appetite, facial flushing, delayed wound healing, increased susceptibility to infection, diarrhea, or constipation.
Occasional
Headache, edema, change in skin color, frequent urination.
Topical: Itching, redness, irritation.
Rare
Tachycardia, allergic reaction (such as rash and hives), psychologic changes, hallucinations, depression.
Topical: Allergic contact dermatitis, purpura.
Systemic: Absorption more likely with use of occlusive dressings or extensive application in young children.

SERIOUS REACTIONS

• Long-term therapy may cause hypocalcemia, hypokalemia, muscle wasting (especially in arms and legs), osteoporosis, spontaneous fractures, amenorrhea, cataracts, glaucoma, peptic ulcer disease, and congestive heart failure.
• Abruptly withdrawing the drug after long-term therapy may cause anorexia, nausea, fever, headache, sudden severe joint pain, rebound inflammation, fatigue, weakness, lethargy, dizziness, and orthostatic hypotension.

PRECAUTIONS & CONSIDERATIONS

Caution is warranted in patients with cirrhosis, congestive heart failure, diabetes mellitus, hypertension, hyperthyroidism, osteoporosis, peptic ulcer disease, seizure disorders, thromboembolic tendencies, thrombophlebitis, and ulcerative colitis. Hydrocortisone crosses the placenta and is distributed in breast milk. Persons taking hydrocortisone should not breastfeed. Prolonged hydrocortisone use during the first trimester of pregnancy may produce cleft palate in the neonate. Prolonged treatment or high dosages may decrease the cortisol secretion and short-term growth rate in children. Elderly patients may be more susceptible to developing hypertension or osteoporosis. Dentist and other physicians should be informed of hydrocortisone therapy if taken within the past 12 mo. Consult with the physician before taking aspirin or other medications. Avoid alcohol, and limit caffeine intake. Hydrocortisone should not be overused for symptomatic relief.

Mood swings, ranging from euphoria to depression, may occur.

Notify the physician of fever, muscle aches, sore throat, and sudden weight gain or swelling. Blood glucose level, intake and output, BP, serum electrolyte levels, height, and weight should be monitored before and during therapy. Be alert to signs and symptoms of infection caused by reduced immune response, including fever, sore throat, and vague symptoms. In long-term therapy, signs and symptoms of hypocalcemia (such as muscle twitching, cramps, and positive Chvostek's or Trousseau's signs) or hypokalemia (such as ECG changes, nausea and vomiting, irritability, weakness and muscle cramps, and numbness or tingling, especially in the lower extremities) should be assessed.

Storage

Store at room temperature. After reconstitution, store hydrocortisone sodium succinate solution at room temperature and use within 72 h.

Administration

For IV administration, use immediately if further diluted with D5W, 0.9% NaCl, or other compatible diluent. For hydrocortisone sodium succinate IV push, dilute to 50 mg/mL; for intermittent infusion, dilute to 1 mg/mL. Administer hydrocortisone sodium succinate solution IV push over 3-5 min. Give intermittent infusion over 20-30 min.

For topical use, gently cleanse area before applying drug; apply topical hydrocortisone valerate after bath or shower for best absorption. Apply sparingly, and rub into area thoroughly. Use occlusive dressings only as ordered. Avoid contact with eyes.

For rectal use, shake homogeneous suspension well. Lie on the left side with left leg extended and right leg flexed. Gently insert applicator tip into rectum, pointed slightly toward umbilicus, and slowly instill medication.

Hydromorphone

hye-droe-mor'fone
(Dilaudid, Dilaudid HP, Hydro-morph Contin [CAN], Palladone)
Do not confuse with morphine or Dilantin.

CATEGORY AND SCHEDULE

Pregnancy Risk Category: C (D if used for prolonged periods or at high dosages at term)
Controlled Substance Schedule: II

Classification: Analgesics, narcotic

MECHANISM OF ACTION

An opioid agonist that binds to opioid receptors in the CNS, reducing the intensity of pain stimuli from sensory nerve endings. *Therapeutic Effect:* Alters the perception of and emotional response to pain; suppresses cough reflex.

PHARMACOKINETICS

Route	Onset (min)	Peak (min)	Duration (h)
PO	30	90-120	4
IV	10-15	15-30	2-3
IM	15	30-60	4-5
Subcuta-neous	15	30-90	4
Rectal	15-30	N/A	N/A

Well absorbed from the GI tract after IM administration. Widely distributed. Metabolized in the liver. Excreted in urine. *Half-life:* 1-3 h.

AVAILABILITY
Liquid (Dilaudid): 5 mg/5 mL.
Capsules (Extended-Release).
Tablets (Dilaudid): 2 mg, 4 mg, 8 mg.
Injection (Dilaudid): 1 mg/mL,
2 mg/mL, 4 mg/mL.
Injection (Dilaudid HP): 10 mg/mL.
Suppository (Dilaudid): 3 mg.

INDICATIONS AND DOSAGES
▸ **Analgesia**
PO
*Adults, Elderly, Children weighing
50 kg and more.* 2-4 mg q3-4h.
Range: 2-8 mg/dose.
*Children older than 6 mo and
weighing < 50 kg.* 0.03-0.08 mg/kg/
dose q3-4h.
IV
*Adults, Elderly, Children weighing
more than 50 kg.* 0.2-0.6 mg q2-3h.
Children weighing 50 kg or less.
0.015 mg/kg/dose q3-6h as needed.
RECTAL
Adults, Elderly. 3 mg q6-8h.
▸ **Patient-controlled analgesia (PCA)**
IV
Adults, Elderly. 0.05-0.5 mg at
5-15 min lockout. Maximum (4-h):
4-6 mg.
EPIDURAL
Adults, Elderly. Bolus dose of
1-1.5 mg at rate of 0.04-0.4 mg/h.
Demand dose of 0.15 mg at 30-min
lockout.

CONTRAINDICATIONS
Respiratory depression in the
absence of resuscitative equipment,
status asthmatics, depressed
ventilatory function, obstetric
anesthesia, severe CNS depression,
pregnancy.

INTERACTIONS
Drug
Alcohol, other CNS depressants:
May increase CNS or respiratory
depression and hypotension.

MAOIs: May produce a severe,
sometimes fatal, reaction; plan to
administer one quarter of the usual
hydromorphone dose.
**Selective serotonin reuptake
inhibitors (SSRIs):** May cause
additive serotonergic symptoms
leading to serotonin syndrome.
Herbal
**Gotu kola, kava kava, St. John's
wort, valerian:** May cause additive
sedative effects.
Food
None known.

DIAGNOSTIC TEST EFFECTS
May increase serum amylase and
lipase concentrations.

🚫 IV INCOMPATIBILITIES
Amphotericin B complex (Abelcet,
AmBisome, Amphotec), ampicillin
(Polycillin), cefazolin (Ancef,
Kefzol), diazepam (Valium),
hyaluronidase (Wydase), minocycline
(Minocin), phenobarbital, phenytoin
(Dilantin), sargramostim (Leukine),
sodium bicarbonate, tetracycline
(Sumycin), thiopental (Pentothal).

💉 IV COMPATIBILITIES
Acyclovir (Zovirax), albuterol
(Ventolin), allopurinol (Alloprim),
amifostine (Ethyol), amikacin
(Amikin), amsacrine (Amsa),
atropine, aztreonam (Azactam),
bupivacaine (Marcaine),
cefamandole (Mandol), cefepime
(Maxipime), cefoperazone (Cefobid),
cefotaxime (Claforan), cefoxitin
(Mefixitin), ceftazidime (Fortaz),
ceftizoxime (Cefizox), cefuroxime
(Zinacef), chloramphenicol
(Chloromycetin), chlorpromazine
(Thorazine), cimetidine (Tagamet),
cisatracurium (Nimbex), cisplatin
(Platinol-AQ), cladribine
(Leustatin), clindamycin (Cleocin),
cyclophosphamide (Cytoxan),

cytarabine (Cytosar), diltiazem (Cardizem), dimenhydrinate (Dramamine), diphenhydramine (Benadryl), dobutamine (Dobutrex), docetaxel (Taxotere), dopamine (Intropin), doxorubicin (Rubex), doxycycline (Vibramycin), epinephrine, erythromycin lactobionate (Erythrocin), etoposide (VePesid), famotidine (Pepcid), fentanyl (Sublimaze), filgrastim (Neupogen), fludarabine (Fludara), fluorouracil (Efurix), foscarnet (Foscavir), furosemide (Lasix), gatifloxacin (Tequin), gemcitabine (Gemzar), gentamicin (Garamycin), glycopyrrolate (Robinul), granisetron (Kytril), haloperidol (Haldol), heparin, hydroxyzine (Vistaril), kanamycin (Kantrex), labetalol (Normodyne, Trandate), linezolid (Zyvox), lorazepam (Ativan), magnesium sulfate, melphalan (Alkeran), methotrexate, metoclopramide (Reglan), metronidazole (Flagyl), midazolam (Versed), milrinone (Primacor), morphine, nafcillin (Unipen), nicardipine (Cardene), nitroglycerin (Nitrobid), norepinephrine (Levophed), ondansetron (Zofran), oxacillin (Bactocil), paclitaxel (Taxol), penicillin G potassium (Pfizerpen), pentazocine (Talwin), pentobarbital (Nembutal), piperacillin (Piperacil), piperacillin/tazobactam (Zosyn), prochlorperazine (Compazine), promethazine (Phenergan), propofol (Diprivan), ranitidine (Zantac), remifentanil (Ultiva), tacrolimus (Prograf), teniposide (Vumon), thiotepa (Thioplex), ticarcillin (Ticar), tobramycin (Nebcin), trimethobenzamide (Tigan), trimethoprim/sulfamethoxazole (Bactrim), vancomycin (Vancocin), vecuronium (Norcuron), verapamil (Calan), vinorelbine (Navelbine).

SIDE EFFECTS
Frequent
Somnolence, dizziness, hypotension (including orthostatic hypotension), decreased appetite.
Occasional
Confusion, diaphoresis, facial flushing, urine retention, constipation, dry mouth, nausea, vomiting, headache, pain at injection site.
Rare
Allergic reaction, depression.

SERIOUS REACTIONS
• Overdose results in respiratory depression, skeletal muscle flaccidity, cold or clammy skin, cyanosis, and extreme somnolence progressing to seizures, stupor, and coma.
• The patient who uses hydromorphone repeatedly may develop a tolerance to the drug's analgesic effect as well as physical dependence.
• This drug may have a prolonged duration of action and cumulative effect in patients with hepatic or renal impairment.

PRECAUTIONS & CONSIDERATIONS
Extreme caution should be used in patients with acute alcoholism, anoxia, CNS depression, hypercapnia, respiratory depression or dysfunction, seizures, shock, and untreated myxedema. Caution is also warranted in patients with acute abdominal conditions, Addison disease, COPD, hypotension, hypothyroidism, hepatic impairment, increased intracranial pressure, benign prostatic hyperplasia, and urethral stricture. Hydromorphone readily crosses the placenta; it is unknown whether it is distributed in breast milk. Regular use of opioids during pregnancy may produce withdrawal symptoms in the neonate, including diarrhea, excessive

crying, fever, hyperactive reflexes, irritability, seizures, sneezing, tremors, vomiting, and yawning. Hydromorphone use may prolong labor if administered in the latent phase of the first stage of labor or before cervical dilation of 4-5 cm. The neonate may develop respiratory depression if the mother receives hydromorphone during labor. Children younger than 2 yr may be more susceptible to respiratory depression. Elderly patients may be more susceptible to respiratory depression and paradoxical excitement. In elderly patients, age-related benign prostatic hyperplasia, obstruction, or renal impairment may increase the risk of urine retention; a dosage adjustment is recommended.

Dizziness and drowsiness may occur, so change positions slowly and avoid alcohol, CNS depressants, and tasks that require mental alertness or motor skills until response to the drug is established. Vital signs, pattern of daily bowel activity and stool consistency, and clinical improvement of pain should be monitored. The drug should be held and the physician should be notified if the respiratory rate is 12 breaths/min or less in an adult or 20 breaths/min or less in a child.

Storage

Store vials at room temperature; protect from light. A slight yellow discoloration of the parenteral form does not indicate a loss of potency. Refrigerate suppositories.

Administration

! Ambulatory patients and those not in severe pain may be more prone to dizziness, hypotension, nausea, and vomiting than patients in the supine position and those in severe pain.

Take oral hydromorphone without regard to food. Crush tablets as needed.

! Be aware that a high concentration injection (10 mg/mL) should be used only in patients currently receiving high doses of another opioid agonist for severe, chronic pain caused by cancer or those who have developed a tolerance to high doses of other opioids.

For IV use, hydromorphone may be given undiluted as IV push over 2-5 min, or it may be further diluted with 5 mL sterile water for injection or 0.9% NaCl. Be aware that rapid IV administration increases the risk of a severe anaphylactic reaction, marked by apnea, cardiac arrest, and circulatory collapse.

For IM and subcutaneous administration, use a short 25- to 30-gauge needle for subcutaneous injection. Administer the drug slowly; rotate injection sites. Know that those with circulatory impairment are at increased risk for overdose because of delayed absorption of repeated injections.

For rectal use, moisten the suppository with cold water before inserting it well into the rectum.

Hydroquinone

hye-droe-kwin′one

(Alphaquin HP, Alustra, Claripel,
Eldopaque, Eldopaque Forte,
Eldoquin, EpiQuin Micro, Esoterica
Regular, Glyquin, Lustra, Lustra-
AF, Melanex, Melpaque HP,
Melquin-3, Melquin HP, NeoStrata
AHA, Nuquin HP, Neostrata HQ,
Palmer's Skin Success Fade Cream,
Solaquin, Solaquin Forte)

CATEGORY AND SCHEDULE

Pregnancy Risk Category: C

Classification: Depigmenting
agents, dermatologics

MECHANISM OF ACTION

A depigmenting agent that
suppresses melanocyte metabolic
processes of the skin. Inhibits the
enzymatic oxidation of tyrosine to
DOPA (3,4-dihydroxyphenylalanine).
Sun exposure reverses this effect and
causes repigmentation. *Therapeutic
Effect:* Lighten hyperpigmented
areas.

PHARMACOKINETICS

Onset and duration of
depigmentation vary among
individuals. About 35% is absorbed.

AVAILABILITY

Cream: 2% (Eldopaque, Esoterica
Regular, Palmer's Skin Success Fade
Cream), 4% (Alphaquin HP, Alustra,
EpiQuin Micro, Lustra, Melquin HP,
Nuquin HP).
Cream, with Sunscreen: 2%
(Solaquin), 4% (Claripel, Glyquin,
Solaquin, Solaquin Forte, Lustra-AF,
Melpaque HP).
Gel: 2% (NeoStrata AHA).
Gel, with Sunscreen: 4% (Nuquin
HP, Solaquin Forte)

Solution, Topical: 3% (Melanex,
Melquin-3)

INDICATIONS AND DOSAGES
▸ **Hyperpigmentation, melanin**
TOPICAL
*Adults, Elderly, Children 12 yr and
older.* Apply twice daily.

OFF-LABEL USES

None known.

CONTRAINDICATIONS

Hypersensitivity to hydroquinone,
sulfites, or any other component of
its formulation.

INTERACTIONS

Drug
None known.
Herbal
None known.
Food
None known.

DIAGNOSTIC TEST EFFECTS

None known.

ⓦ IV INCOMPATIBILITIES

None known.

🖫 IV COMPATIBILITIES

None known.

SIDE EFFECTS

Occasional
Burning, itching, stinging,
erythema, such as localized
contact dermatitis.
Rare
Conjunctival changes, fingernail
staining.

SERIOUS REACTIONS

• Gradual blue-black darkening of
skin has been reported.
• Occasional cutaneous
hypersensitivity (localized contact
dermatitis) may occur.

PRECAUTIONS & CONSIDERATIONS

It is unknown whether hydroquinone crosses the placenta or is distributed in breast milk. Caution should be used in pregnant women. Therapeutic effect may take several weeks.

Be aware that safety and efficacy of hydroquinone have not been established in children younger than 12 yr. No age-related precautions have been noted in elderly patients. Sun exposure should be avoided. Protective sunscreen or clothing to cover the skin should be used if sun is unavoidable.

Administration

Hydroquinone is for external use only. It is recommended to try a test response in a small area of skin and monitor for irritation or blistering over 24 h before using on a larger skin surface. Gently cleanse the area before application. Limit to small areas of the body at one time. Apply sparingly on skin spots and rub into area thoroughly. Avoid contact with eyes.

Hydroxocobalamin (Vitamin B$_{12}$)

hye-drox'oh-co-bal'a-min
(Cyanokit)

CATEGORY AND SCHEDULE

Pregnancy Risk Category: C

Classification: Vitamins/minerals

MECHANISM OF ACTION

A coenzyme for metabolic functions, including fat and carbohydrate metabolism and protein synthesis. *Therapeutic Effect:* Necessary for growth, cell replication, hematopoiesis, and myelin synthesis.

PHARMACOKINETICS

Rapidly absorbed after IM administration. Protein binding: High. Primarily excreted in urine. Metabolized in liver. *Half-life:* 6 days.

AVAILABILITY

Injection: 5 g/200 mL.

INDICATIONS AND DOSAGES

▸ **Schilling test**
IM
1000 mcg IM.
▸ **Vitamin B$_{12}$ deficiency**
IM
Adults, Elderly. 30-100 mcg/day for 5-10 days, then 100-200 mcg monthly.
Children. 1-5 mg divided over a period of 2 or more wks in doses of 100 mcg. Then 30-50 mcg monthly.

CONTRAINDICATIONS

Folate deficient anemia, hereditary optic nerve atrophy, hypersensitivity to cobalt, hypersensitivity to hydroxocobalamin or any component of the formulation.

OFF-LABEL USES

Cyanide toxicity, homocystinuria.

INTERACTIONS

Drug
Chloramphenicol: May interface with hydroxocobalamine response.
Herbal
None known.
Food
None known.

DIAGNOSTIC TEST EFFECTS

None known.

SIDE EFFECTS

Occasional
Diarrhea, itching, pain at injection site.

SERIOUS REACTIONS
• Rare allergic reaction generally due to impurities in preparation, may occur.
• May produce peripheral vascular thrombosis, pulmonary edema, hypokalemia, and congestive heart failure (CHF).

PRECAUTIONS & CONSIDERATIONS
Hydroxocobalamin crosses the placenta and is excreted in breast milk. No age-related precautions have been noted in children or elderly patients. Be aware that injection formulations contain benzoyl alcohol and should be avoided in premature infants. Signs and symptoms of congestive heart failure and hypokalemia, especially in those receiving hydroxocobalamin by IM route, and pulmonary edema should be assessed. Foods rich in vitamin B_{12} including clams, dairy products, egg yolks, fermented cheese, herring, muscle meats, organ meats, oysters, and red snapper should be suggested.

Reversal of deficiency symptoms including anorexia, ataxia, fatigue, hyporeflexia, insomnia, irritability, loss of positional sense, pallor, and palpitations on exertion should be evaluated. Serum potassium levels, which normally range between 3.5-5 mEq/L, and serum B_{12} levels, which normally range between 200 and 800 mcg/mL, should be monitored. Also monitor for a rise in the blood reticulocyte count, which peaks in 5-8 days.
Storage
Store at room temperature.
Administration
Administer IM only. May require coadministration of folic acid.

Hydroxychloroquine
hye-drox-ee-klor'oh-kwin
(Apo-Hydroxyquine [CAN], Plaquenil)
Do not confuse hydroxychloroquine with hydrocortisone or hydroxyzine.

CATEGORY AND SCHEDULE
Pregnancy Risk Category: C

Classification: Antiprotozoals, disease modifying antirheumatic drugs, antimalarial

MECHANISM OF ACTION
An antimalarial and antirheumatic that concentrates in parasite acid vesicles, increasing the pH of the vesicles and interfering with parasite protein synthesis. Antirheumatic action may involve suppressing formation of antigens responsible for hypersensitivity reactions.
Therapeutic Effect: Inhibits parasite growth.

PHARMACOKINETICS
PO: Peak 1-2 h. *Half-life:* 3-5 days; metabolized in liver; excreted in urine, feces, breast milk; crosses placenta.

AVAILABILITY
Tablets: 200 mg (155 mg base).

INDICATIONS AND DOSAGES
▸ **Treatment of acute attack of malaria (dosage in mg base)**
PO

Dose	Times	Adults (mg)	Children (mg/kg)
Initial	Day 1	620	10
Second	6 h later	310	5
Third	Day 2	310	5
Fourth	Day 3	310	5

▶ **Suppression of malaria**
PO
Adults. 400 mg (310 mg base)
weekly on same day each week,
beginning 2 wks before entering an
endemic area and continuing for
4-6 wks after leaving the area.
If therapy is not begun before
exposure, administer a loading dose
of 800 mg (620 mg base), then begin
the usual suppressive dose.
Children. 5 mg base/kg/wk, beginning
2 wks before entering an endemic
area and continuing for 4-6 wks after
leaving the area. If therapy is not
begun before exposure, administer
a loading dose of 10 mg base/kg in
2 equally divided doses 6 h apart,
followed by the usual dosage regimen.
▶ **Rheumatoid arthritis**
PO
Adults. Initially, 400-600 mg
(310-465 mg base) daily for
5-10 days; gradually increased to
optimum response level. Maintenance
(usually within 4-12 wks): Dosage
decreased by 50% and then continued
at maintenance dose of
200-400 mg/day. Maximum effect
may not be seen for several months.
▶ **Lupus erythematosus**
PO
Adults. Initially, 400 mg once or twice
a day for several weeks or months.
Maintenance: 200-400 mg/day.

OFF-LABEL USES
Sarcoidosis.

CONTRAINDICATIONS
Long-term therapy for children,
hypersensitivity, to 4-aminoquinolines,
retinal or visual field changes
attributable to 4-aminoquinolines.

INTERACTIONS
Drug
Aurothioglucose: May increase the
risk of blood dyscrasias.

Cimetidine: May increase levels of
hydroxychloroquine.
Digoxin: May increase serum
digoxin concentrations.
Penicillamine: May increase blood
penicillamine concentration and the
risk of hematologic, renal, or severe
skin reactions.
Herbal
None known.
Food
None known.

DIAGNOSTIC TEST EFFECTS
None known.

SIDE EFFECTS
Frequent
Mild, transient headache; anorexia;
nausea; vomiting.
Occasional
Visual disturbances, nervousness,
fatigue, pruritus (especially of
palms, soles, and scalp), irritability,
personality changes, diarrhea.
Rare
Stomatitis, dermatitis, impaired
hearing.

SERIOUS REACTIONS
• Ocular toxicity, especially
retinopathy, may occur and
may progress even after drug is
discontinued.
• Prolonged therapy may result in
peripheral neuritis, neuromyopathy,
hypotension, ECG changes,
agranulocytosis, aplastic anemia,
thrombocytopenia, seizures, and
psychosis.
• Overdosage may result in
headache, vomiting, visual
disturbances, drowsiness, seizures,
and hypokalemia followed by
cardiovascular collapse and death.

PRECAUTIONS & CONSIDERATIONS
Caution is warranted in patients with
glucose-6-phosphate dehydrogenase

deficiency, hepatic disease, alcoholism, and a history of alcohol abuse. May precipitate attacks in patients with porphyria. Be aware that children are especially susceptible to hydroxychloroquine's fatal effects.

Report decreased hearing, tinnitus, visual difficulties, muscle weakness, or any other new symptoms. Visual disturbances, impaired hearing, and GI distress should be monitored. Liver function should be assessed. The buccal mucosa and skin should be checked for pruritus.

Administration

! Be aware that 200 mg hydroxychloroquine equals 155 mg of base. Take the drug dose with food or milk to limit GI effects.

Hydroxyprogesterone
(progestin derivative, antineoplastic, progestin)
(Gestrol LA)
Discontinued in the United States

CATEGORY AND SCHEDULE
Pregnancy Risk Category: D

Classification: Antineoplastic, progestin, progestin derivative

MECHANISM OF ACTION
A hormone that influences proliferative endometrium and transforms into secretory endometrium. Secretion of pituitary gonadotropins is inhibited, which prevents follicular maturation and ovulation. *Therapeutic Effect:* Facilitates ureteral dilation associated with hydronephrosis of pregnancy.

AVAILABILITY
Injection: 250 mg/mL (Gestrol LA).

INDICATIONS AND DOSAGES
▸ **Amenorrhea**
IM
Adults. 375 mg given at any point in the menstrual cycle.
▸ **Endogenous estrogen production**
IM
Adults. 125-250 mg beginning on the 10th day of cycle and repeated every 7 days until suppression is no longer desired.
▸ **Endometrial carcinoma**
IM
Adults. 1000 mg 1 or more times weekly.
▸ **Abnormal uterine bleeding**
IM
Adults. 5-10 mg for 6 days. When estrogen is given concomitantly, begin progesterone after 2 wks of estrogen therapy; discontinue when menstrual flow begins.
▸ **Prevention of endometrial hyperplasia**
IM
Adults. 200 mg in evening for 12 days per 28-day cycle in combination with daily conjugated estrogen.
▸ **Premature labor**
IM
Adults. 250-500 mg once weekly.

OFF-LABEL USES
Alopecia, stress incontinence, menopausal symptoms, preterm delivery, treatment of prostatic hyperplasia, seborrhea, ureteral stones.

CONTRAINDICATIONS
Breast cancer, cerebral apoplexy or history of these conditions, missed abortion, severe liver dysfunction, thromboembolic disorders, thrombophlebitis, undiagnosed vaginal bleeding, genital malignancy, used as a diagnostic test for pregnancy.

H

H

INTERACTIONS
Drug
Bromocriptine: May interfere with
the effects of bromocriptine.
Herbal
None known.
Food
None known.

DIAGNOSTIC TEST EFFECTS
May increase LDL concentrations
and serum alkaline phosphatase
levels. May decrease glucose
tolerance and HDL concentrations.
May cause abnormal thyroid,
metapyrone, liver, and endocrine
function tests.

SIDE EFFECTS
Frequent
Breakthrough bleeding or spotting
at beginning of therapy, amenorrhea,
change in menstrual flow, breast
tenderness.
Occasional
Edema, weight gain or loss, rash,
pruritus, photosensitivity, skin
pigmentation.
Rare
Pain or swelling at injection site,
acne, mental depression, alopecia,
hirsutism.

SERIOUS REACTIONS
• Thrombophlebitis, cerebrovascular
disorders, retinal thrombosis, and
pulmonary embolism rarely occur.

PRECAUTIONS & CONSIDERATIONS
Caution is warranted with conditions
aggravated by fluid retention,
asthma, epilepsy, diabetes mellitus,
cardiac or renal dysfunction, or
a history of mental depression.
Pain, redness, swelling, or warmth
in the calf, chest pain, migraine
headache, peripheral paresthesia,
sudden decrease in vision, and
sudden shortness of breath should

be reported immediately. Smoking
should be avoided during therapy.
Administration
Rotate the vial to disperse drug in
solution. Give deep IM injection into
the gluteus maximus.

Hydroxyzine
hye-drox′i-zeen
(Apo-Hydroxyzine [CAN], Atarax,
Novohydroxyzin [CAN], Vistaril)
**Do not confuse hydroxyzine with
hydralazine or hydroxyurea.**

CATEGORY AND SCHEDULE
Pregnancy Risk Category: C

Classification: Antiemetics/
antivertigo, antihistamines, H₁
anxiolytics, sedatives/hypnotics

MECHANISM OF ACTION
A piperazine derivative that competes
with histamine for receptor sites
in the GI tract, blood vessels, and
respiratory tract. May exert CNS
depressant activity in subcortical
areas. Diminishes vestibular
stimulation and depresses labyrinthine
function. *Therapeutic Effect:*
Produces anxiolytic, anticholinergic,
antihistaminic, and analgesic effects;
relaxes skeletal muscle; controls
nausea and vomiting.

PHARMACOKINETICS

Route	Onset	Peak	Duration
PO	15-30 min	N/A	4-6 h

Well absorbed from the GI
tract and after parenteral
administration. Metabolized in the
liver. Primarily excreted in urine. Not

removed by hemodialysis.
Half-life: 20-25 h (increased in elderly patients).

AVAILABILITY
Capsules (Vistaril): 25 mg, 50 mg, 100 mg.
Oral Suspension (Vistaril): 25 mg/5 mL.
Syrup (Atarax): 10 mg/5 mL.
Tablets (Atarax): 10 mg, 25 mg, 50 mg.
Injection (Vistaril): 25 mg/mL, 50 mg/mL.

INDICATIONS AND DOSAGES
▸ **Anxiety**
PO
Adults, Elderly. 25-100 mg 4 times a day. Maximum: 400 mg/day.
▸ **Nausea and vomiting**
IM
Adults, Elderly. 25-100 mg/dose q4-6hr.
▸ **Pruritus**
PO
Adults, Elderly. 25 mg 3-4 times a day.
▸ **Preoperative sedation**
PO
Adults, Elderly. 50-100 mg.
IM
Adults, Elderly. 25-100 mg.
▸ **Usual pediatric dosage**
PO
Children. 2 mg/kg/day in divided doses q6-8h.
IM
Children. 0.5-1 mg/kg/dose q4-6h.

CONTRAINDICATIONS
Early pregnancy.

INTERACTIONS
Drug
Alcohol, other CNS depressants: May increase CNS depressant effects.
MAOIs: May increase anticholinergic and CNS depressant effects.

Herbal
Gotu kola, kava kava, St. John's wort, valerian: May cause additive CNS depressant effects.
Food
None known.

DIAGNOSTIC TEST EFFECTS
May cause false-positive urine 17-hydroxycorticosteroid determinations.

SIDE EFFECTS
Side effects are generally mild and transient.
Frequent
Somnolence, dry mouth, marked discomfort with IM injection.
Occasional
Dizziness, ataxia, asthenia, slurred speech, headache, agitation, increased anxiety.
Rare
Paradoxical CNS reactions, such as hyperactivity or nervousness in children and excitement or restlessness in elderly or debilitated patients (generally noted during first 2 wks of therapy, particularly in presence of uncontrolled pain).

SERIOUS REACTIONS
• A hypersensitivity reaction, including wheezing, dyspnea, and chest tightness, may occur.

PRECAUTIONS & CONSIDERATIONS
Caution is warranted in patients with asthma, bladder neck obstruction, COPD, angle-closure glaucoma, and benign prostatic hyperplasia. It is unknown whether hydroxyzine crosses the placenta or is distributed in breast milk. Hydroxyzine use is not recommended for neonates or premature infants because they are at increased risk for anticholinergic

effects. Children may experience paradoxical excitement. Elderly patients are at increased risk for confusion, dizziness, sedation, hypotension, and hyperexcitability. Be aware of dehydration, which can occur with severe vomiting.

Drowsiness and dizziness may occur. Change positions slowly from recumbent to sitting before standing to prevent dizziness. Alcohol, caffeine, and tasks that require mental alertness or motor skills should also be avoided. Autonomic responses, such as cold, clammy hands and diaphoresis, and motor responses, such as agitation, trembling, and tension, should be assessed. CBC and blood chemistry tests should be performed periodically in long-term therapy. Breath sounds, electrolyte levels, and CNS reactions should also be assessed.

Administration

Crush scored tablets as needed, but do not crush or break capsules. Shake the oral suspension thoroughly.

! Do not give hydroxyzine by the subcutaneous intra-arterial or IV route because doing so can cause significant tissue damage, thrombosis, and gangrene.

The IM form may be given undiluted. Inject the drug deep into the gluteus maximus or midlateral thigh in adults and the midlateral thigh in children. Use the Z-track technique of injection to prevent subcutaneous infiltration. IM injection may cause marked discomfort.

Hyoscyamine
hye-oh-sye′a-meen
(Anaspaz, Buscopan [CAN], Cystospaz, Cystospaz-M, Hyosine, Levbid, Levsin, Levsinex, Levsin/SL, NuLev, Spacol, Spacol T/S, Symax SL, Symax SR)
Do not confuse Anaspaz with Anaprox.

CATEGORY AND SCHEDULE
Pregnancy Risk Category: C

Classification: Anticholinergics, gastrointestinals

MECHANISM OF ACTION
A GI antispasmodic and anticholinergic agent that inhibits the action of acetylcholine at post-ganglionic (muscarinic) receptor sites. *Therapeutic Effect:* Decreases secretions (bronchial, salivary, sweat gland) and gastric juices and reduces motility of GI and urinary tract.

AVAILABILITY
Tablets (Anaspaz, Cystospaz, Levsin, Spacol): 0.125 mg, 0.15 mg.
Tablets (Oral-Disintegrating [NuLev]): 0.125 mg.
Tablets (Sublingual [Levsin S/L, Symax SL]): 0.125 mg.
Tablets (Extended-Release [Levbid, Spacol T/S, Symax SR]): 0.375 mg.
Capsules (Extended-Release [Cystospaz-M, Levsinex]): 0.375 mg.
Liquid (Hyoscine, Spacol): 0.125 mg/5 mL.
Oral Solution (Hyoscine, Levsin): 0.125 mg/5 mL.
Oral Solution Drops (Hyoscine, Levsin): 0.125 mg/1 mL.
Injection (Levsin): 0.5 mg/mL.

INDICATIONS AND DOSAGES

▸ **GI tract disorders**

PO or SL

Adults, Elderly, Children 12 yr and older. 0.125-0.25 mg q4h as needed. Extended-release: 0.375-0.75 mg q12h. Maximum: 1.5 mg/day.

Children 2-11 yr. 0.0625-0.125 mg q4h as needed. Maximum: 0.75 mg/day.

IM, IV

Adults, Elderly, Children 12 yr and older. 0.25-0.5 mg q4h for 1-4 doses.

▸ **Hypermotility of lower urinary tract**

PO, SUBLINGUAL

Adults, Elderly. 0.15-0.3 mg 4 times a day; or extended-release 0.375 mg q12h.

▸ **Infant colic**

PO

Infants. Individualized drops dosed q4h as needed. See manufacturer-provided weight-based dosing.

CONTRAINDICATIONS

GI or genitourinary obstruction, myasthenia gravis, narrow-angle glaucoma, paralytic ileus, severe ulcerative colitis, intestinal atony of elderly or debilitated patients, toxic megacolon complicating ulcerative colitis, unstable cardiovascular status in acute hemorrhage, myocardial ischemia.

INTERACTIONS

Drug

Antacids, antidiarrheals: May decrease the absorption of hyoscyamine.

Haloperidol, phenothiazines, tricyclic antidepressants: May have additive adverse effects.

Ketoconazole: May decrease the absorption of this drug.

Other anticholinergics: May increase the effects of hyoscyamine.

Potassium chloride: May increase the severity of GI lesions with the matrix formulation of potassium chloride.

Herbal

None known.

Food

None known.

DIAGNOSTIC TEST EFFECTS

None known.

SIDE EFFECTS

Frequent

Dry mouth (sometimes severe), decreased sweating, constipation.

Occasional

Blurred vision, bloated feeling, urinary hesitancy, somnolence (with high dosage), headache, intolerance to light, loss of taste, nervousness, flushing, insomnia, impotence, mental confusion or excitement (particularly in elderly patients and children; temporary light-headedness (with parenteral form), local irritation (with parenteral form).

Rare

Dizziness, faintness.

SERIOUS REACTIONS

• Overdose may produce temporary paralysis of ciliary muscle; pupillary dilation; tachycardia; palpitations; hot, dry, or flushed skin; absence of bowel sounds; hyperthermia; increased respiratory rate; ECG abnormalities; nausea; vomiting; rash over face or upper trunk; CNS stimulation; and psychosis (marked by agitation, restlessness, rambling speech, visual hallucinations, paranoid behavior, and delusions, followed by depression).

PRECAUTIONS & CONSIDERATIONS

Caution is warranted with cardiac arrhythmias, congestive heart failure, chronic lung disease, hyperthyroidism, neuropathy, and prostatic hyperplasia. Avoid hot baths, saunas, and becoming overheated while exercising in hot weather because they may cause heat stroke. Tasks that require mental alertness or motor skills should also be avoided until response to the drug has been established.

Dry mouth may occur, so good oral hygiene should be maintained because the lack of saliva may increase the risk of cavities. Notify the physician of constipation, difficulty urinating, eye pain, or rash. BP, body temperature, heart rate, pattern of daily bowel activity and stool consistency, and urine output should be monitored. The person should void before giving the drug to reduce the risk of urine retention.

Administration

Give oral hyoscyamine without regard to meals. Crush or have patient chew tablets. Extended-release capsule should be swallowed whole. Orally disintegrating tablets may be placed on tongue; dissolve. May be taken with or without water.

For parenteral use, hyoscyamine may be given undiluted. If given IV, inject slowly.

Ibandronate
eye-band'droh-nate
(Boniva)

CATEGORY AND SCHEDULE
Pregnancy Risk Category: C

Classification: Bisphosphonates

MECHANISM OF ACTION
A bisphosphonate that binds to bone hydroxyapatite (part of the mineral matrix of bone) and inhibits osteoclast activity. *Therapeutic Effect:* Reduces rate of bone turnover and bone resorption, resulting in a net gain in bone mass.

PHARMACOKINETICS
Absorbed in the upper GI tract. Extent of absorption impaired by food or beverages (other than plain water). Rapidly binds to bone. Unabsorbed portion is eliminated in urine. Protein binding: 90%. *Half-life:* 10-60 h.

AVAILABILITY
Tablets: 2.5 mg, 150 mg.
Injection: 3 mg/3 mL.

INDICATIONS AND DOSAGES
▸ Osteoporosis
PO
Adults, Elderly. Oral: 2.5 mg daily or 150 mg once a month.
IV
Adults, Elderly. 3 mg every 3 mo.

CONTRAINDICATIONS
Hypersensitivity to other bisphosphonates, including alendronate, etidronate, pamidronate, risedronate, and tiludronate; inability to stand or sit upright for at least 60 min; severe renal impairment with creatinine clearance < 30 mL/min; uncorrected hypocalcemia.

INTERACTIONS
Drug
Antacids containing aluminum, calcium, magnesium; vitamin D: Decrease the absorption of ibandronate.
Herbal
None known.
Food
Beverages other than plain water, dietary supplements, food: Interfere with the absorption of ibandronate.

DIAGNOSTIC TEST EFFECTS
May decrease serum alkaline phosphatase level. May increase blood cholesterol level.
May cause transient decrease in serum calcium (IV).

SIDE EFFECTS
Frequent (6%-13%)
Back pain; dyspepsia, including epigastric distress and heartburn; peripheral discomfort; diarrhea; headache; myalgia.
Occasional (3%-4%)
Dizziness, arthralgia, asthenia.
Rare (2% or Less)
Vomiting, hypersensitivity reaction.

SERIOUS REACTIONS
• Upper respiratory tract infection occurs occasionally.
• Overdose causes hypocalcemia, hypophosphatemia, and significant GI disturbances.
• Osteonecrosis of the jaw.

PRECAUTIONS & CONSIDERATIONS
Caution is warranted with GI diseases, including duodenitis, dysphagia, esophagitis, gastritis, ulcers, and mild to moderate renal impairment. Bone, joint, and muscle pain have been reported with ibandronate therapy. Osteonecrosis of the jaw has also been reported with

ibandronate therapy and has been associated more commonly in cancer patients and in those with preexisting dental disease. Ibandronate may have teratogenic effects. It is unknown whether ibandronate is excreted in breast milk. Breastfeeding is not recommended for women taking ibandronate. The safety and efficacy of ibandronate have not been established in children. No age-related precautions have been noted in elderly patients. Consider beginning weight-bearing exercises, reduce alcohol consumption, and stop cigarette smoking.

Hypocalcemia and vitamin D deficiencies, if present, should be corrected before beginning ibandronate therapy. BUN, creatinine levels, and serum electrolytes, especially calcium and serum alkaline phosphatase levels, should be monitored during therapy.

ADMINISTRATION

Expect patients to receive calcium and vitamin D during bisphosphonate treatment. Take ibandronate on an empty stomach with 6-8 oz of plain water 60 min before the patient receives his or her first food or beverage of the day. Avoid taking ibandronate with coffee, mineral water, and orange juice because they significantly reduce the absorption of the drug. Stay in an upright position while standing or sitting; do not lie down for 60 min after drug administration. Do not chew or suck the tablet because of the potential for oropharyngeal ulceration. Give once-monthly dose on the same date of the month. Give injection IV only over 15-30 sec. Do not mix with calcium-containing solutions or any other drugs. Do not administer paravenously or intra-arterially because this may cause tissue damage.

Ibuprofen
eye-byoo′pro-fen
(Act-3 [AUS], Advil, Apo-Ibuprofen, Brufen [AUS], Codral Period Pain [AUS], Motrin, Neoprofen, Novoprofen [CAN], Nurofen [AUS], Rafen [AUS])

CATEGORY AND SCHEDULE

Pregnancy Risk Category: B (D if used in third trimester or near delivery)
OTC (Tablets: 200 mg, Oral Suspension: 100 mg/5 mL Oral drops: 40 mg/mL)

Classification: Analgesics, non-narcotic, antipyretics, nonsteroidal anti-inflammatory drug (NSAID)

MECHANISM OF ACTION

An NSAID that inhibits prostaglandin synthesis. Also produces vasodilation by acting centrally on the heat-regulating center of the hypothalamus. *Therapeutic Effect:* Produces analgesic and anti-inflammatory effects and decreases fever.

PHARMACOKINETICS

Route	Onset	Peak	Duration
PO (anal-gesic)	0.5 h	N/A	4-6 h
PO (anti-rheumatic)	2 days	1-2 wks	NA

Rapidly absorbed from the GI tract. Protein binding: > 90%. Metabolized in the liver. Primarily excreted in urine. Not removed by hemodialysis. *Half-life:* 2-4 h.

AVAILABILITY

Caplets (Advil, Menadol, Motrin): 100 mg, 200 mg.

Capsules (Advil, Advil Migraine):
200 mg.
Gelcaps (Advil, Motrin IB): 200 mg.
Tablets (Advil, Motrin IB): 200 mg.
Tablets (Motin): 400 mg, 600 mg,
800 mg.
*Tablets (Chewable [Children's Advil,
Children's Motrin]):* 50 mg.
*Tablets (Chewable [Junior Advil,
Junior Strength Motrin]):* 100 mg.
*Oral Suspension (Children's Advil,
Children's Motrin):* 100 mg/5 mL.
*Oral Drops (Infant Advil, Infant
Motrin):* 40 mg/mL.

INDICATIONS AND DOSAGES

▸ **Acute or chronic rheumatoid
arthritis, osteoarthritis, migraine
pain, gouty arthritis**
PO
Adults, Elderly. 300-800 mg
3-4 times a day. Maximum:
3.2 g/day.
▸ **Mild to moderate pain, primary
dysmenorrhea**
PO
Adults, Elderly. 200-400 mg q4-6h as
needed. Maximum: 1.6 g/day.
▸ **Fever, minor aches or pain**
PO
Adults, Elderly. 200-400 mg q4-6h.
Maximum: 1.6 g/day.
Children, Infants 6 mo and older.
5-10 mg/kg/dose q6-8h.
Maximum: 40 mg/kg/day. OTC:
7.5 mg/kg/dose q6-8h. Maximum:
30 mg/kg/day.
▸ **Juvenile arthritis**
PO
Children. 30-40 mg/kg/day in 3-4
divided doses. Maximum: 400 mg/day
in children weighing < 20 kg,
600 mg/day in children weighing
20-30 kg, 800 mg/day in children
weighing > 30-40 kg.

OFF-LABEL USES

Treatment of psoriatic arthritis,
vascular headaches.

CONTRAINDICATIONS

Active peptic ulcer, chronic
inflammation of GI tract, GI bleeding
disorders or ulceration, history
of hypersensitivity to aspirin or
NSAIDs within 14 days of
coronary artery bypass graft
surgery.

INTERACTIONS

Drug
Antihypertensives, diuretics: May
decrease the effects of these drugs.
Aspirin, other salicylates: May
increase the risk of GI side effects
such as bleeding.
Bile acid sequestrants: May
decrease the absorption of NSAIDs.
Separate administration by at least 2 h.
Bone marrow depressants: May
increase the risk of hematologic
reactions.
Corticosteroids: May increase risk
of GI ulceration.
**Heparin, oral anticoagulants,
thrombolytics:** May increase the
effects of these drugs.
Lithium: May increase the blood
concentration and risk of toxicity of
lithium.
Methotrexate: May increase the risk
of methotrexate toxicity.
Probenecid: May increase the
ibuprofen blood concentration.
Herbal
Feverfew: May decrease the effects
of feverfew.
**Alfalfa, anise, bilberry,
bladderwrack, bromelain, cat's
claw, celery, chamomile, coleus,
cordyceps, dong quai, evening
primrose, fenugreek, feverfew,
garlic, ginger, ginkgo biloba,
ginseng (American, Panax,
Siberian), grapeseed, green tea,
guggul, horse chestnut seed,
horseradish, licorice, prickly
ash, red clover, reishi, SAMe
(S-adenosylmethionine), sweet**

I

clover, turmeric, white willow: May increase the risk of bleeding.
Food
None known.

DIAGNOSTIC TEST EFFECTS

May prolong bleeding time. May alter blood glucose level. May increase BUN level, and serum creatinine, potassium, AST (SGOT), and ALT (SGPT) levels. May decrease blood hemoglobin and hematocrit.

SIDE EFFECTS

Occasional (3%-9%)
Nausea with or without vomiting, dyspepsia, dizziness, rash.
Rare (< 3%)
Diarrhea or constipation, flatulence, abdominal cramps or pain, pruritus.

SERIOUS REACTIONS

• Acute overdose may result in metabolic acidosis.
• Rare reactions with long-term use include peptic ulcer disease, GI bleeding, gastritis, a severe hepatic reaction (cholestasis, jaundice), nephrotoxicity (dysuria, hematuria, proteinuria, nephrotic syndrome), and a severe hypersensitivity reaction (particularly in patients with systemic lupus erythematosus or other collagen diseases).

PRECAUTIONS & CONSIDERATIONS

NSAIDs may increase the risk of cardiovascular events. Caution is warranted with congestive heart failure, hypertension, dehydration, GI disease (such as GI bleeding or ulcers), hepatic or renal impairment, and concurrent anticoagulant use. The lowest effective dose should be used for the shortest duration of time possible. It is unknown whether ibuprofen crosses the placenta or is distributed in breast milk. Ibuprofen

should not be used during the third trimester of pregnancy because it may cause adverse effects in the fetus, such as premature closure of the ductus arteriosus. The safety and efficacy of this drug have not been established in children younger than 6 mo. In elderly patients, GI bleeding or ulceration is more likely to cause serious complications and age-related renal impairment may increase the risk of hepatotoxicity or renal toxicity; a reduced dosage is recommended. Avoid alcohol and aspirin during therapy because these substances increase the risk of GI bleeding. Tasks that require mental alertness or motor skills should be avoided.

CBC, platelet count, serum alkaline phosphatase, bilirubin, creatinine, AST (SGOT), ALT (SGPT) levels, pattern of daily bowel activity and stool consistency, and skin for rash should be monitored. Therapeutic response, such as decreased pain, stiffness, swelling, and tenderness, improved grip strength, and increased joint mobility, should be evaluated.
Administration
Do not crush or break enteric-coated tablets. Take ibuprofen with food, milk, or antacids.

Shake suspensions well before each use, including infant drops. Take care to measure accurate dosage.

Ibutilide
eye-byoo'ti-lide
(Corvert)

CATEGORY AND SCHEDULE
Pregnancy Risk Category: C

Classification: Antiarrhythmics, class III

MECHANISM OF ACTION
An antiarrhythmic that prolongs both atrial and ventricular action potential duration and increases the atrial and ventricular refractory period. Activates slow, inward current (mostly of sodium); produces mild slowing of sinus node rate and AV conduction; and causes dose-related prolongation of QT interval. *Therapeutic Effect:* Converts arrhythmias to sinus rhythm.

PHARMACOKINETICS
After IV administration, highly distributed1, rapidly cleared. Protein binding: 40%. Primarily excreted in urine as metabolite. *Half-life:* 2-12 h (average: 6 h).

AVAILABILITY
Injection: 0.1 mg/mL solution.

INDICATIONS AND DOSAGES
▸ **Rapid conversion of atrial fibrillation or flutter of recent onset to normal sinus rhythm**
IV INFUSION
Adults, Elderly weighing 60 kg or more. One vial (1 mg) given over 10 min. If arrhythmia does not stop within 10 min after the end of initial infusion, a second 1 mg/10-min infusion may be given.
Adults, elderly weighing < 60 kg. 0.01 mg/kg given over 10 min. If arrhythmia does not stop within 10 min after end of initial infusion, a second 0.01 mg/kg, 10-min infusion may be given.

CONTRAINDICATIONS
QTc interval > 440msec, hypersensitivity.

INTERACTIONS
Drug
Class IA antiarrhythmics (disopyramide, moricizine, procainamide, quinidine), class III antiarrhythmics (amiodarone, bretylium, sotalol): Do not give ibutilide with these drugs or give these drugs within 4 h after infusing ibutilide.
Digoxin: Signs of digoxin toxicity may be masked with coadministration.
H₁ receptor antagonists, phenothiazines, tricyclic and tetracyclic antidepressants: May prolong QT interval.
Herbal
None known.
Food
None known.

DIAGNOSTIC TEST EFFECTS
None known.

ⓘ IV INCOMPATIBILITIES
No information is available for Y-site administration.

SIDE EFFECTS
Ibutilide is generally well tolerated.
Occasional
Ventricular extrasystoles (5.1%), ventricular tachycardia (4.9%), headache (3.6%), hypotension, orthostatic hypotension (2%).
Rare
Bundle-branch block, AV block, bradycardia, hypertension.

SERIOUS REACTIONS
• Sustained polymorphic ventricular tachycardia, occasionally with QT prolongation (torsade de pointes) occurs rarely.
• Overdose results in central nervous system (CNS) toxicity, including CNS depression, rapid gasping breathing, and seizures.
• Expect prolongation of repolarization may be exaggerated.
• Existing arrhythmias may worsen or new arrhythmias may develop.

Caution is warranted with abnormal hepatic function or heart block. Avoid coadministration with other medications that may prolong the QT interval. Because ibutilide is embryocidal and teratogenic in animals, breastfeeding is not recommended during ibutilide therapy. Safety and efficacy of ibutilide have not been established in children. No age-related precautions have been noted in elderly patients.

Notify the physician if palpitations or other adverse reactions occur. BP and ECG should be continuously monitored during therapy. Serum electrolyte levels, especially magnesium and potassium, should be monitored, and arrhythmias requiring overdrive cardiac pacing, electrical cardioversion, or defibrillation should be surveyed. Patients with atrial fibrillation lasting more than 3 days should be given an anticoagulant for at least 2 wks before ibutilide therapy is started. Proarrhythmias may develop.

Storage
Store unopened vials at room temperature in carton. Admixtures with diluent are stable at room temperature for up to 24 h or up to 48 h if refrigerated.

Administration
Have advanced cardiac life-support equipment, medications, and trained personnel on hand during and after ibutilide administration. Ibutilide is compatible with D5W and 0.9% NaCl. It is also compatible with polyvinyl chloride plastic and polyolefin bag admixtures. Give undiluted or may dilute in 50 mL 0.9% NaCl or dextrose 5%. Give IV over 10 min.

Iloprost
eye'low-prost
(Ventavis)

CATEGORY AND SCHEDULE
Pregnancy Risk Category: C

Classification: Miscellaneous respiratory agents, antihypertensive

MECHANISM OF ACTION
A prostaglandin that dilates systemic and pulmonary arterial vascular beds, alters pulmonary vascular resistance, and suppresses vascular smooth muscle proliferation. *Therapeutic Effect:* Improves symptoms and exercise tolerance in patients with pulmonary hypertension; delays deterioration of condition.

AVAILABILITY
Solution for Oral Inhalation: 10 mcg/ mL (2-mL ampule or 1-mL ampule).

INDICATIONS AND DOSAGES
▸ **Pulmonary hypertension in patients with New York Heart Association (NYHA) class III or IV symptoms**
ORAL INHALATION
Adults. Initially, 2.5 mcg/dose; if tolerated, increased to 5 mcg/dose. Administer 6-9 times a day at intervals of 2 h or longer while patient is awake. Maintenance: 5 mcg/dose. Maximum daily dose: 45 mcg (5 mcg given 9 times/day).

CONTRAINDICATIONS
None known.

INTERACTIONS
Drug
Antihypertensives, other vasodilators: May increase the hypotensive effects of iloprost.

Herbal
None known.
Food
None known.

DIAGNOSTIC TEST EFFECTS
May increase serum alkaline phosphatase and GGT levels.

SIDE EFFECTS
Frequent (27%-39%)
Increased cough, headache, flushing.
Occasional (11%-13%)
Flu-like symptoms, nausea, lockjaw, jaw pain, hypotension.
Rare (2%-8%)
Insomnia, syncope, palpitations, vomiting, back pain, muscle cramps.

SERIOUS REACTIONS
• Hemoptysis and pneumonia occur occasionally.
• Congestive heart failure, renal failure, dyspnea, and chest pain occur rarely.

PRECAUTIONS & CONSIDERATIONS
Caution is warranted with renal and hepatic impairment and in those who are concurrently taking medications that may increase the risk of syncope. Discontinue therapy immediately if pulmonary edema occurs.
Administration
Iloprost is administered by inhalation only, using the Prodose ADD or the I-neb AAD systems. Transfer the entire contents of the ampule into the medication chamber. Ampule size used (e.g., 1 or 2 mL) is system dependent. After use, discard any unused portion from the system's medication chamber.
! Do not give doses more frequently than every 2 h, even though the clinical effect of the medication may not last the full 2 h.

Imatinib
im′a-tin-ib
(Gleevec, Glivec [AUS])

CATEGORY AND SCHEDULE
Pregnancy Risk Category: D

Classification: Antineoplastics, signal transduction inhibitors

MECHANISM OF ACTION
Inhibits Bcr-Abl tyrosine kinase, an enzyme created by the Philadelphia chromosome abnormality found in patients with chronic myeloid leukemia (CML). *Therapeutic Effect:* Suppresses tumor growth during the three stages of CML: blast crisis, accelerated phase, and chronic phase.

PHARMACOKINETICS
Well absorbed after PO administration. Binds to plasma proteins, particularly albumin. Metabolized in the liver. Eliminated mainly in the feces as metabolites. *Half-life:* 18 h.

AVAILABILITY
Tablets: 100 mg, 400 mg.

INDICATIONS AND DOSAGES
▸ **Ph and CML**
PO
Adults, Elderly. 400 mg/day for patients in chronic-phase CML; 600 mg/day for patients in accelerated phase or blast crisis. May increase dosage from 400 to 600 mg/day for patients in chronic phase or from 600 to 800 mg (given as 300-400 mg twice a day) for patients in accelerated phase or blast crisis in the absence of a severe drug reaction or severe neutropenia or thrombocytopenia in the following circumstances: progression of

the disease, failure to achieve a satisfactory hematologic response after 3 mo or more of treatment, or loss of a previously achieved hematologic response.
Children 2 yr and older. Newly diagnosed CML: 340 mg/m^2/day (maximum: 600 mg). Chronic phase: 260 mg/m^2 a day as a single daily dose or in 2 divided doses.

▸ **Dosage adjustments**

Dosage adjustments are recommended for hepatic dysfunction and hematologic toxicity. See manufacturer's information.

CONTRAINDICATIONS

Known hypersensitivity to imatinib.

INTERACTIONS

Drug

Carbamazepine, dexamethasone, phenobarbital, phenytoin, rifampicin: Decrease imatinib plasma concentration.

Clarithromycin, erythromycin, itraconazole, ketoconazole: Increase imatinib plasma concentration.

Cyclosporine, pimozide: May alter the therapeutic effects of these drugs.

Dihydropyridine calcium channel blockers, simvastatin, triazolo-benzodiazepines: May increase the blood concentration of these drugs.

Digoxin: Imatinib may decrease the absorption of digoxin.

HMG CoA reductase inhibitors: Imatinib may inhibit the metabolism of HMG CoA reductase inhibitors.

Lansoprazole: May increase dermatological side effects of imatinib.

Live-virus vaccines: May potentiate viral replication, and decrease the patient's antibody response to the vaccine.

Warfarin: Reduces the effect of warfarin. Use heparin or low-molecular-weight heparin instead during treatment.

Herbal

St. John's wort: Decreases imatinib concentration. Avoid.

Food

Grapefruit juice: Increases imatinib concentration. Avoid.

DIAGNOSTIC TEST EFFECTS

May increase serum bilirubin, AST (SGOT), and ALT (SGPT) levels. May decrease platelet count, WBC count, and serum potassium level.

SIDE EFFECTS

Frequent (24%-68%)

Nausea, diarrhea, vomiting, headache, fluid retention (periorbital, lower extremities), rash, musculoskeletal pain, muscle cramps, arthralgia.

Occasional (10%-23%)

Abdominal pain, cough, myalgia, fatigue, fever, anorexia, dyspepsia, constipation, night sweats, pruritus.

Rare (< 10%)

Nasopharyngitis, petechiae, asthenia, epistaxis, infection.

SERIOUS REACTIONS

• Severe fluid retention (manifested as pleural effusion, pericardial effusion, pulmonary edema, and ascites) and hepatotoxicity occur rarely.

• Neutropenia and thrombocytopenia are expected responses to the drug; bleeding may occur.

• Respiratory toxicity, manifested as dyspnea and pneumonia, may occur.

• Stevens-Johnson syndrome and other bullous skin reactions.

PRECAUTIONS & CONSIDERATIONS

Caution is warranted in patients with hepatic and renal impairment and in patients with congestive heart failure or pulmonary disease. Severe dermatologic reactions, including Stevens-Johnson syndrome, have been reported with imatinib. Because imatinib may cause severe teratogenic effects, women should avoid becoming pregnant and avoid breastfeeding while taking this drug. The safety and efficacy of imatinib have not been established in children. Elderly patients are at increased risk for fluid retention. Vaccinations without the physician's approval, crowds, and contact with people with known infections should be avoided.

Notify the physician of rapid weight gain, fluid retention, nausea, and vomiting. Antiemetics should be ordered to control nausea and vomiting. Pattern of daily bowel activity and stool consistency should be monitored. CBC for evidence of neutropenia and thrombocytopenia and liver function test results for evidence of hepatotoxicity should be assessed. Neutropenia and thrombocytopenia usually last 2-4 wks.

Administration
Give oral imatinib with a meal and a large glass of water.

Imiglucerase
im-i-gloo'-ser-ase
(Cerezyme)
Do not confuse Cerezyme with Cerebyx or Ceredase.

CATEGORY AND SCHEDULE
Pregnancy Risk Category: C

Classification: Enzymes, metabolic, recombinant DNA origin

MECHANISM OF ACTION
An enzyme analogue of the enzyme β-glucocerebrosidase, which catalyzes hydrolysis of the glycolipid glucocerebroside to glucose and ceramide. *Therapeutic Effect:* Minimizes conditions associated with Gaucher disease, such as anemia and bone disease.

AVAILABILITY
Powder for Injection: 212 units (equivalent to a reconstituted withdrawal dose of 200 units), 424 units (equivalent to a reconstituted withdrawal dose of 400 units).

INDICATIONS AND DOSAGES
▸ **Gaucher disease**
IV
Adults, Elderly, Children. Initially, 2.5 units/kg infused over 1-2 h 3 times a week up to 60 units/kg/wk. Maintenance: Progressive reduction in dosage while monitoring patient response.

CONTRAINDICATIONS
None known. If serious hypersensitivity occurs, re-evaluate continued treatment.

INTERACTIONS
None known.

DIAGNOSTIC TEST EFFECTS
None known.

ⓘ IV INCOMPATIBILITIES
Do not mix imiglucerase with any solution other than 0.9% NaCl.

SIDE EFFECTS
Frequent (3%)
Headache.
Occasional (< 3% to 1%)
Nausea, abdominal discomfort, dizziness, pruritus, rash, small decrease in BP, urinary frequency.

PRECAUTIONS & CONSIDERATIONS
CBC, platelet count, and liver function test results should be monitored. Notify the physician of headache.
Storage
Refrigerate vials. The reconstituted solution is stable for 24 h if

refrigerated or 12 h at room temperature.

Administration
For IV use, reconstitute the 200-unit vial with 5.1 mL sterile water (or the 400-unit vial with 10.2 mL) to provide a concentration of 40 units/mL. Further dilute with 100-200 mL 0.9% NaCl. Infuse the solution over 1-2 h.

Imipenem-Cilastatin
i-me-pen'em
(Primaxin, Primaxin IM)

CATEGORY AND SCHEDULE
Pregnancy Risk Category: C

Classification: Antibiotics, carbapenems

MECHANISM OF ACTION
A fixed-combination carbapenem. Imipenem penetrates the bacterial cell membrane and binds to penicillin-binding proteins, inhibiting cell wall synthesis. Cilastatin competitively inhibits the enzyme dehydropeptidase, preventing renal metabolism of imipenem. *Therapeutic Effect:* Produces bacterial cell death.

PHARMACOKINETICS
Readily absorbed after IM administration. Protein binding: 13%-21%.Widely distributed. Metabolized in the kidneys. Primarily excreted in urine. Removed by hemodialysis. *Half-life:* 1 h (increased in impaired renal function).

AVAILABILITY
IV Injection: 250 mg, 500 mg.
IM Injection: 500 mg, powder for suspension.

INDICATIONS AND DOSAGES
▸ **Serious respiratory tract, skin and skin-structure, gynecologic, bone, joint, intra-abdominal, nosocomial, and polymicrobic infections; UTIs; endocarditis; septicemia**
IV
Adults, Elderly. 2-4 g/day in divided doses q6h.
▸ **Mild to moderate respiratory tract, skin and skin-structure, gynecologic, bone, joint, intra-abdominal, and polymicrobic infections; urinary tract infection; endocarditis; septicemia**
IV
Adults, Elderly. 1-2 g/day in divided doses q6-8h.
Children older than 3 mo to 12 yr. 60-100 mg/kg/day in divided doses q6h. Maximum: 4 g/day.
Children 1-3 mo. 100 mg/kg/day in divided doses q6h.
Children younger than 1 mo. 20-25 mg/kg/dose q8-24h.
IM (ONLY FOR SKIN, LOWER RESPIRATORY SYSTEM, OR ABDOMINAL INFECTIONS)
Adults, Elderly. 500-750 mg q12h.
▸ **Dosage in renal impairment**
Dosage and frequency must be based on creatinine clearance, patient weight, and the severity of the infection. The manufacturer provides detailed and specific tables for dosage adjustments. See prescribing information. Do not give to children with impaired renal function.

CONTRAINDICATIONS
Hypersensitivity to amide anesthetics; severe shock or heart block, (IM, since diluted with lidocaine). All dosage forms: Hypersensitivity to primaxin or serious previous hypersensitivity with other β-lactams, such as penicillins or cephalosporins.

INTERACTIONS
Drug
Cyclosporine: May increase neurotoxicity of imipenem; may cause increased levels of cyclosporine.
Ganciclovir: May increase risk of seizures.
Valproic acid: May decrease levels of valproic acid.
Herbal and Food
None known.

DIAGNOSTIC TEST EFFECTS
May increase BUN level and serum alkaline phosphatase, bilirubin, creatinine, LDH, AST (SGOT) and ALT (SGPT) levels. May decrease blood hematocrit and hemoglobin levels.

IV INCOMPATIBILITIES
Allopurinol (Aloprim), amphotericin B complex (Abelcet, AmBisome, Amphotec), etoposide (VePesid), fluconazole (Diflucan), gemcitabine (Gemzar), lorazepam (Ativan), meperidine (Demerol), midazolam (Versed), sargramostim (Leukine), sodium bicarbonate.

IV COMPATIBILITIES
Acyclovir (Valtrex), amifostine (Ethyol), aztreonam (Azactam), cefepime (Maxipime), cisatracurium (Nimbex), diltiazem (Cardizem), docetaxel (Taxotere), famotidine (Pepcid), fludarabine (Fludara), foscarnet (Foscavir), gatifloxacin (Tequin), granisetron (Kytril), idarubicin (Idamycin), insulin, linezolid (Zyvox), melphalan (Alkeran), methotrexate, ondansetron (Zofran), propofol (Diprivan), remifentanil (Ultiva), tacrolimus (Prograf), teniposide (Vumon), thiotepa (Thioplex), vinorelbine (Navelbine), zidovudine (Retrovir).

SIDE EFFECTS
Occasional (2%-3%)
Diarrhea, nausea, vomiting, pruritus, urticaria.
Rare (1%-2%)
Rash.

SERIOUS REACTIONS
• Antibiotic-associated colitis and other superinfections may occur.
• Anaphylactic reactions have been reported, serious skin reactions.
• Seizures, especially with high doses in presence of renal insufficiency.

PRECAUTIONS & CONSIDERATIONS
Caution is warranted with a history of seizures, renal impairment, and sensitivity to penicillins. Superinfection may occur with prolonged use. Be aware that imipenem crosses the placenta and is distributed in amniotic fluid, breast milk, and cord blood. This drug may be used safely in children younger than 12 yr, but the IM form should not be used. Do not give to children with renal impairment. In elderly patients, age-related renal function impairment may require dosage adjustment. Notify the physician if severe diarrhea occurs, but avoid taking antidiarrheals.

Notify the physician of the onset of troublesome or serious adverse reactions, including infusion site pain, redness, or swelling, nausea or vomiting, or skin rash or itching. History of allergies, particularly to β-lactams, cephalosporins, and penicillins should be determined before beginning drug therapy.
Storage
IM suspension will be light tan once reconstituted. IV solution normally appears colorless to yellow; discard if solution turns brown. IV infusion (piggyback) is stable for 4 h at room temperature, 24 h if refrigerated. Discard if precipitate forms.

Administration

For IM use, prepare primaxin IM with 1% lidocaine without epinephrine, as prescribed; 500-mg vial with 2 mL, 750-mg vial with 3 mL lidocaine HCl. Administer suspension within 1 h of preparation. Do not mix the suspension with any other medications. Give deep IM injections slowly into a large muscle to minimize patient discomfort. To further minimize discomfort, administer IM injections into the gluteus maximus instead of the lateral aspect of the thigh. Be sure to aspirate with the syringe before injecting the drug to decrease risk of injection into a blood vessel.

For IV use, dilute each 250- or 500-mg vial with 100 mL D5W or 0.9% NaCl. Give by intermittent IV infusion (piggyback). Do not give IV push. Infuse over 20-30 min (1-g dose longer than 40-60 min). Observe the patient during the first 30 min of the infusion for possible hypersensitivity reaction. Infusions can be slowed if patient complains of nausea. Doses > 500 mg in children should be given over 40-60 min.

Imipramine
ih-mih'prah-meen
(Apo-Imipramine [CAN], Melipramine [AUS], Tofranil, Tofranil-PM)
Do not confuse imipramine with desipramine.

CATEGORY AND SCHEDULE
Pregnancy Risk Category: D

Classification: Antidepressants, tricyclic

MECHANISM OF ACTION

A tricyclic antidepressant, antibulimic, anticataplectic, antinarcoleptic, antineuralgic, antineuritic, and antipanic agent that blocks the reuptake of neurotransmitters, such as norepinephrine and serotonin, at presynaptic membranes, increasing their concentration at postsynaptic receptor sites. *Therapeutic Effect:* Relieves depression and controls nocturnal enuresis.

AVAILABILITY

Tablets: 10 mg, 25 mg, 50 mg.
Capsules: 75 mg, 100 mg, 125 mg, 150 mg.

INDICATIONS AND DOSAGES
▶ **Depression**
PO
Adults. Initially, 75-100 mg/day. May gradually increase to 300 mg/day for hospitalized patients, or 200 mg/day for outpatients; then reduce dosage to effective maintenance level, 50-150 mg/day.
Elderly, Adolescents. Initially, 30-40 mg/day at bedtime. May increase by 10-25 mg every 3-7 days. Range: 50-100 mg/day.
Children older than 6 yr. 1.5 mg/kg/day. May increase by 1 mg/kg every 3-4 days. Maximum: 2.5 mg/kg/day.
▶ **Enuresis**
PO
Children older than 6 yr. Initially, 10-25 mg at bedtime. May increase by 25 mg/day. Maximum: 50 mg if under 12 yr, 75 mg if over 12 yr; do not exceed 2.5 mg/kg/day.

OFF-LABEL USES

Treatment of attention-deficit hyperactivity disorder, cataplexy associated with narcolepsy, neurogenic pain, panic disorder.

CONTRAINDICATIONS

Acute recovery period after myocardial infarction, use within 14 days of MAOIs, pregnancy, hypersensitivity.

INTERACTIONS

Drug

Alcohol, other central nervous system (CNS) depressants: May increase the hypotensive effects and CNS and respiratory depression caused by imipramine.

Anticholinergic agents: May have additive adverse effects.

β-agonists: May increase risk of arrhythmias.

Bile acid sequestrants: May bind to and decrease levels of tricyclic antidepressants.

Carbamazepine: May increase carbamazepine levels.

CYPZD6 inhibitors (e.g., SSRIs, quinidine, and cimetidine): May increase imipramine blood concentration and risk of toxicity.

Clonidine, guanadrel: May decrease the effects of these drugs.

Linezolid: Serotonin syndrome may occur. Avoid this combination.

MAOIs: May increase the risk of neuroleptic malignant syndrome, hyperpyrexia, hypertensive crisis, and seizures. Contraindicated.

Methylphenidate: May inhibit imipramine metabolism.

Phenothiazines: May increase the anticholinergic and sedative effects of imipramine.

Phenytoin: May decrease the imipramine blood concentration.

Sympathomimetics: May increase the risk of cardiac effects.

Valproic acid: May increase adverse effects.

Herbal

Ginkgo biloba: May decrease seizure threshold.

Kava kava, SAMe, valerian: May increase risk of serotonin syndrome and excessive sedation.

St. John's wort: May increase imipramine's pharmacologic effects and risk of toxicity.

Food

None known.

DIAGNOSTIC TEST EFFECTS

May alter blood glucose levels and ECG readings. Therapeutic serum drug level is 225-300 ng/mL; toxic serum drug level is > 500 ng/mL.

SIDE EFFECTS

Frequent

Somnolence, fatigue, dry mouth, blurred vision, constipation, delayed micturition, orthostatic hypotension, diaphoresis, impaired concentration, increased appetite, urine retention, photosensitivity.

Occasional

GI disturbances (nausea, metallic taste).

Rare

Paradoxical reactions (agitation, restlessness, nightmares, insomnia), extrapyramidal symptoms (particularly fine hand tremor).

SERIOUS REACTIONS

• Overdose may produce seizures; cardiovascular effects, such as severe orthostatic hypotension, dizziness, tachycardia, palpitations, and arrhythmias; and altered temperature regulation, including hyperpyrexia or hypothermia.

• Antidepressants have been associated with an increased risk of suicidality in adolescents and young adults. Patients should be monitored closely for 1-2 mo after initiation and dosage changes.

• Abrupt discontinuation after prolonged therapy may produce headache, malaise, nausea, vomiting, and vivid dreams.

PRECAUTIONS & CONSIDERATIONS

Caution is warranted with cardiac disease, diabetes mellitus, glaucoma, hiatal hernia, history of seizures, history of urinary obstruction or retention, hyperthyroidism, increased intraocular pressure, benign prostatic hyperplasia, renal or hepatic disease, and schizophrenia. Imipramine is minimally distributed in breast milk. Imipramine use is not recommended for children younger than 6 yr. Expect to administer a lower dosage to elderly patients because they are at increased risk for drug toxicity.

Anticholinergic, sedative, and hypotensive effects may occur during early therapy, but tolerance to these effects usually develops. Because dizziness may occur, change positions slowly and avoid alcohol and tasks that require mental alertness or motor skills. Assess pattern of daily bowel activity, bladder for urine retention, BP and pulse rate to detect hypotension and arrhythmias, CBC and blood serum chemistry tests to monitor blood glucose level, and liver and renal function tests.

Administration

! Make sure at least 14 days elapse between the use of MAOIs and imipramine. Be aware that the therapeutic serum level for imipramine is 225-300 ng/mL; the toxic serum level is > 500 ng/mL.

Take imipramine with food or milk if GI distress occurs. Do not crush or break film-coated tablets. Improvement may occur 2-5 days after starting therapy but the full therapeutic effect will likely occur within 2-3 wks. Do not abruptly discontinue imipramine.

Imiquimod
im-ick'wih-mod
(Aldara)

CATEGORY AND SCHEDULE
Pregnancy Risk Category: C

Classification: Dermatologics, immunomodulators, keratolytic agent

MECHANISM OF ACTION
An immune response modifier whose mechanism of action is uknown. *Therapeutic Effect:* Reduces genital and perianal warts.

PHARMACOKINETICS
Minimal absorption after topical administration. Minimal excretion in urine and feces.

AVAILABILITY
Cream: 5% (Aldara).

INDICATIONS AND DOSAGES
▸ **Condyloma acuminata/genital and perianal warts**
TOPICAL
Adults, Elderly, Children 12 yr and older. Apply 3 times/wk before normal sleeping hours; leave on skin 6-10 h. Remove following treatment period. Continue therapy for maximum of 16 wks.
▸ **Actinic keratosis**
Adults. Apply to defined treatment area of face or scalp 2 times/wk (e.g., Monday and Thursday) for 16 wks at bedtime. Leave on skin approximately 8 h before washing.
▸ **Superficial Basal cell carcinoma**
Adults. Apply 5 times/wk before bedtime for a full 6 wks. Leave on skin 8 h, then wash.

CONTRAINDICATIONS
History of hypersensitivity to imiquimod.

INTERACTIONS
None known.

DIAGNOSTIC TEST EFFECTS
None known.

SIDE EFFECTS
Frequent
Local skin reactions: erythema, itching, burning, erosion, excoriation/flaking, fungal infections (women).
Occasional
Pain, induration, ulceration, scabbing, soreness, headache, flulike symptoms.

SERIOUS REACTIONS
• If local reactions are intense, continue rest periods from treatment.
• Skin color change (hyperpigmentation or hypopigmentation) may occur. Some changes may be permanent.

PRECAUTIONS & CONSIDERATIONS
Caution should be used with inflammatory conditions of the skin. Be aware that safety and efficacy have not been established for basal cell nevus syndrome or xeroderma pigmentosum. It is unknown whether imiquimod crosses the placenta or is distributed in breast milk. Safety and efficacy of imiquimod have not been established in children younger than 12 yr. No age-related precautions have been noted in elderly patients.

If severe local skin reaction occurs, the cream should be removed by washing the treatment area and may be resumed after the reaction has subsided.
Storage
Store at room temperature.
Administration
Wash application site with soap and water 6-10 h after applying. Apply a thin layer to affected area. Avoid contact with eyes, lips, and nostrils. Wash hands after application.
Discard any partially used packets.

Immune Globulin IV (IGIV)
(Baygam [CAN], Carimune, Flebogamma, Gamimune N, Gammagard S/D, Gammar-P-IV, Gamunex, Iveegam EN, Octagam, Panglobulin, Polygam S/D, Privigen, Sandoglobulin [AUS])
Do not confuse Sandoglobulin with Sandimmune or Sandostatin.

CATEGORY AND SCHEDULE
Pregnancy Risk Category: C

Classification: Immune globulins

MECHANISM OF ACTION
An immune serum that increases antibody titer and antigen-antibody reaction. *Therapeutic Effect:* Provides passive immunity against infection; induces rapid increase in platelet count; produces anti-inflammatory effect.

PHARMACOKINETICS
Evenly distributed between intravascular and extravascular space. *Half-life:* 21-23 days.

AVAILABILITY
Injection Solution (Gamimune N, Gamunex, Privigen): 10%.
Injection Solution (Flebogamma, Octagam): 5%.
Injection Powder for Reconstitution (Carimune, Panglobulin): 3 g, 6 g, 12 g.
Injection Powder for Reconstitution (Gammagard S/D, Polygam S/D): 2.5 g, 5 g, 10 g.

Injection Powder for Reconstitution (Gammar-P-IV): 5 g, 10 g.
Injection Powder for Reconstitution (Iveegam EN): 0.5 g, 1 g, 2.5 g, 5 g.

INDICATIONS AND DOSAGES
▸ **Primary immunodeficiency syndrome**
IV
Adults, Elderly, Children.
200-800 mg/kg once monthly.
▸ **Idiopathic thrombocytopenic purpura (ITP)**
IV
Adults, Elderly, Children.
400-1000 mg/kg/day for 2-5 days.
▸ **Kawasaki disease**
IV
Adults, Elderly, Children. 2 g/kg as a single dose; 400 mg/kg/day for 4 days has also been used.
▸ **Chronic lymphocytic leukemia**
IV
Adults, Elderly, Children. 400 mg/kg q3-4wk.
▸ **Bone marrow transplant**
IV
Adults, Elderly, Children.
400-500 mg/kg/dose every week for 12 wks, then every month.

OFF-LABEL USES
Control and prevention of infections in infants and children with immunosuppression from AIDS or AIDS-related complex; prevention of acute infections in immunosuppressed patients; prevention and treatment of infections in high-risk, preterm, low-birth-weight neonates; treatment of chronic inflammatory demyelinating polyneuropathies and multiple sclerosis.

CONTRAINDICATIONS
Allergies to γ-globulin, thimerosal, or anti-IgA antibodies; isolated IgA deficiency; hyperprolinemia.

INTERACTIONS
Drug
Live-virus vaccines: IVIG contains antibodies that may interfere with proper response to the vaccine.
Herbal and Food
None known.

DIAGNOSTIC TEST EFFECTS
None known.

▣ IV COMPATIBILITIES
Fluconazole (Diflucan), sargramostim (Leukine).

SIDE EFFECTS
Frequent
Tachycardia, backache, headache, arthralgia, myalgia.
Occasional
Fatigue, wheezing, injection site rash or pain, leg cramps, urticaria, bluish lips and nailbeds, lightheadedness.

SERIOUS REACTIONS
• Anaphylactic reactions are rare, but the incidence increases with repeated injections of IGIV. Keep epinephrine readily available.
• Renal dysfunction/failure (especially with sucrose-containing products) as a result of osmotic nephrosis.
• Overdose may produce chest tightness, chills, diaphoresis, dizziness, facial flushing, nausea, vomiting, fever, and hypotension.

PRECAUTIONS & CONSIDERATIONS
Caution is warranted with cardiovascular disease, diabetes mellitus, a history of thrombosis, impaired renal function, sepsis, or volume depletion and concurrent use of nephrotoxic drugs. It is unknown whether IGIV crosses the placenta or is distributed in breast milk. No age-related precautions have been noted in children or elderly patients.

Adequate hydration should be maintained before giving IGIV. Notify the physician if dyspnea, decreased urine output, fluid retention, edema, or sudden weight gain occurs. Vital signs and platelet count should be monitored.

Storage

Refer to individual IV preparations for storage requirements and information about stability after reconstitution.

Administration

Reconstitute IGIV only with the diluent provided by the manufacturer. Discard partially used or turbid preparations. Administer IGIV by infusion only through separate tubing. Avoid mixing IGIV with other medications or IV infusion fluids. The infusion rate varies among products. Control the infusion rate carefully. A too-rapid infusion increases the risk of a precipitous drop in BP and an anaphylactic reaction, marked by chest tightness, chills, diaphoresis, facial flushing, fever, nausea, and vomiting. Monitor BP and vital signs diligently during and immediately after IV administration. Stop the infusion immediately if a suspected anaphylactic reaction occurs or with signs of infusion reaction (fever, chills, nausea, vomiting, shock). Keep epinephrine readily available. A rapid response occurs to therapy lasting 1-3 mo.

Inamrinone Lactate
in-am′ri-nohn
(Inamrinone)
Do not confuse with Amiodarone.

CATEGORY AND SCHEDULE
Pregnancy Risk Category: C

Classification: Inotropes, vasodilators

MECHANISM OF ACTION
A positive inotropic agent that inhibits myocardial cyclic adenosine monophosphate (cAMP) phosphodiesterase activity and directly stimulates cardiac contractility. Peripheral vasodilation reduces both preload and afterload. *Therapeutic Effect:* Reduces preload and afterload; increases cardiac output.

PHARMACOKINETICS
After IV administration, rapidly absorbed from the GI tract. Protein binding: 10%-49%. Partially metabolized in liver. Excreted in urine as both inamrinone and its metabolites. *Half-life:* 3-6 h (half-life increased with congestive heart failure).

AVAILABILITY
Injection: 5 mg/mL (Inamrinone).

INDICATIONS AND DOSAGES
▶ **Short-term management of intractable heart failure**
IV INFUSION (CONTINUOUS)
Adults. Initially, 0.75 mg/kg loading dose over 2-3 min followed by a maintenance infusion of 5-10 mcg/kg/min. A repeat bolus dose of 0.75 mg/kg may be given 30 min after the initiation of therapy. Maximum: 10 mg/kg/day.

CONTRAINDICATIONS
Severe aortic or pulmonic valvular disease; hypersensitivity to inamrinone or bisulfites.

INTERACTIONS
Drug
Anagrelide: Additive cAMP effects.
Digitalis: May increase the inotropic effects.
Diuretics: May cause hypovolemia and decrease filling pressure.
Dysopyramide: May cause hypotension.

Herbal and Food
None known.

DIAGNOSTIC TEST EFFECTS

Elevated AST or ALT, decreased platelets.

ⓘ IV INCOMPATIBILITIES

Furosemide (Lasix), sodium bicarbonate, amphotericin B, ampicillin, aztreonam, calcium gluconate, all cephalosporins, clindamycin, esmolol, imipenem-cilastin, insulin, levofloxacin, many penicillins, vancomycin.

ⓘ IV COMPATIBILITIES

Atropine, calcium chloride, cisatracurium (Nimbex), digoxin (Lanoxin), labetalol, lidocaine (Xylocaine), metaraminol (Aramine), nitroprusside (Nitropress), propafenone (Rhythmol), propofol (Diprivan), propranolol (Inderal), remifentanil (Ultiva), verapamil (Calan).

SIDE EFFECTS

Occasional
Arrhythmia, nausea, hypotension, thrombocytopenia.
Rare
Fever, vomiting, abdominal pain, anorexia, chest pain, decreased tear production hepatotoxicity, and burning at the site of injection, hypersensitivity to inamrinone.

SERIOUS REACTIONS

• Overdose may cause severe hypotension.
• Improved diuresis may cause fluid or electrolyte imbalance.
• If thrombocytopenia is persistant, may require discontinuation of drug.

PRECAUTIONS & CONSIDERATIONS

BP and pulse should be obtained immediately before each inamrinone dose, in addition to regular BP monitoring. Be alert for BP fluctuations. Elderly patients are more sensitive to the drug's hypotensive effects, and age-related renal impairment may require dosage adjustment. Caution should be used in children and elderly patients. Cardiac index, stroke volume, systemic vascular resistance, and pulmonary vascular resistance, BP, heart rate, platelet count, fluid status, and liver and renal function should be monitored.

Storage
Store at room temperature. Store unopened vial at room temperature. Do not freeze. Protect from light.
Administration
Give IV bolus dose undiluted over 2-3 min. Reconstituted solutions should be used within 24 h. Dosage is based on clinical response. Do not dilute with solutions containing dextrose. Do not administer furosemide in intravenous lines containing inamrinone. Inamrinone is for short-term therapy; use infusions within 24 h of preparation. To make recommended 2.5 mg/mL concentration for infusion, mix inamrinone solution with an equal volume of 0.9% or 0.45% NaCl.

Indapamide
in-dap′a-mide
(Dapa-tabs [AUS], Indahexal [AUS], Insig [AUS], Lozide [CAN], Lozol, Natrilix [AUS], Natrilix SR [AUS])
Do not confuse indapamide with iodamide or iopamidol.

CATEGORY AND SCHEDULE
Pregnancy Risk Category: B
(D if used in pregnancy-induced hypertension)

Classification: Diuretics, thiazide and derivatives

MECHANISM OF ACTION
A thiazide-like diuretic that blocks the reabsorption of water, sodium, and potassium at the cortical diluting segment of the distal tubule; also reduces plasma and extracellular fluid volume and peripheral vascular resistance by direct effect on blood vessels. *Therapeutic Effect:* Promotes diuresis and reduces BP.

AVAILABILITY
Tablets: 1.25 mg, 2.5 mg.

INDICATIONS AND DOSAGES
▸ **Edema**
PO
Adults. Initially, 2.5 mg/day, may increase to 5 mg/day after 1 wk.
▸ **Hypertension**
PO
Adults, Elderly. Initially, 1.25 mg, may increase to 2.5 mg/day after 4 wks or 5 mg/day after additional 4 wks.

CONTRAINDICATIONS
Hypersensitivity to sulfonamide-derived drugs; anuria; renal decompensation; pregnancy.

INTERACTIONS
Drug
β-blockers: May increase hyperglycemic effects in type 2 diabetic patients.
Cyclosporine: May increase risk of gout or renal toxicity.
Digoxin: May increase the risk of digoxin toxicity associated with indapamide-induced hypokalemia.
Lithium: May increase the risk of lithium toxicity.
Herbal
Ephedra, ginseng, yohimbe: May cause hypertension.
Food
None known.

DIAGNOSTIC TEST EFFECTS
May increase plasma renin activity. May decrease protein-bound iodine and serum calcium, potassium, and sodium levels.

SIDE EFFECTS
Frequent (≥ 5%)
Fatigue, numbness of extremities, tension, irritability, agitation, headache, dizziness, light-headedness, insomnia, muscle cramps.
Occasional (< 5%)
Tingling of extremities, urinary frequency, urticaria, rhinorrhea, flushing, weight loss, orthostatic hypotension, depression, blurred vision, nausea, vomiting, diarrhea or constipation, dry mouth, impotence, rash, pruritus.

SERIOUS REACTIONS
• Vigorous diuresis may lead to profound water and electrolyte depletion, resulting in hypokalemia, hyponatremia, and dehydration.
• Acute hypotensive episodes may occur.
• Hyperglycemia may occur during prolonged therapy.
• Pancreatitis, blood dyscrasias, pulmonary edema, allergic pneumonitis, and dermatologic reactions occur rarely.
• Overdose can lead to lethargy and coma without changes in electrolytes or hydration.

PRECAUTIONS & CONSIDERATIONS
Caution is warranted in patient with anuria, diabetes mellitus, a history of hypersensitivity to sulfonamides or thiazide diuretics, hepatic impairment, severe renal disease, thyroid disorders, and in elderly patients and debilitated. Consuming foods high in potassium, such as apricots, bananas, legumes, meat, orange juice, raisins, whole grains, including cereals,

and white and sweet potatoes, is encouraged.

Dizziness or lightheadedness may occur, so change positions slowly and let legs dangle momentarily before standing. An increase in the frequency and volume of urination may occur. BP, vital signs, electrolytes, intake and output, and weight should be monitored before and during treatment. Be aware of signs of electrolyte disturbances such as hypokalemia or hyponatremia. Hypokalemia may cause arrhythmias, altered mental status, muscle cramps, asthenia, and tremor. Hyponatremia may result in cold and clammy skin, confusion, and thirst.

Administration
Take indapamide with food or milk if GI upset occurs, preferably with breakfast to help prevent nocturia. Do not crush or break tablets.

Indinavir
in-din′ah-veer
(Crixivan)
Do not confuse indinavir with Denavir.

CATEGORY AND SCHEDULE
Pregnancy Risk Category: C

Classification: Antivirals, protease inhibitors

MECHANISM OF ACTION
A protease inhibitor that suppresses HIV protease, an enzyme necessary for splitting viral polyprotein precursors into mature and infectious viral particles. *Therapeutic Effect:* Interrupts HIV replication, slowing the progression of HIV infection.

PHARMACOKINETICS
Rapidly absorbed after PO administration. Protein binding: 60%.

Metabolized in the liver. Primarily excreted in urine. Unknown if removed by hemodialysis. *Half-life:* 1.8 h (increased in impaired hepatic function).

AVAILABILITY
Capsules: 100 mg, 200 mg, 333 mg, 400 mg.

INDICATIONS AND DOSAGES
▸ **HIV infection (in combination with other antiretrovirals)**
PO
Adults. 800 mg (two 400-mg capsules) q8h; 400 mg twice daily when used with ritonavir 400 mg twice daily *or* 800 mg twice daily when used with ritonavir 100-200 mg twice daily.
▸ **HIV infection in patients with hepatic insufficiency**
PO
Adults. 600 mg q8h (when used without ritonavir).

OFF-LABEL USES
Prophylaxis following occupational exposure to HIV.

CONTRAINDICATIONS
Hypersensitivity to indinavir; concurrent use of alprazolam, amiodarone, cisapride, triazolam, midazolam, pimozide, or ergot alkaloids.

INTERACTIONS
Drug
Amiodarone: May increase amiodarone levels. Contraindicated.
Antacids: May decrease absorption of indinavir.
Anticonvulsants, venlafaxine: May decrease levels of indinavir.
Antifungal agents, delavirdine, NNRTIs: May increase levels of indinavir.
Atazanavir: Increases blood bilirubin.
Calcium channel blockers: Indinavir may increase concentrations of calcium channel blockers.

Clarithromycin: May increase levels of clarithromycin.
CYP3A4 inducers: May decrease effects of indinavir.
CYP3A4 inhibitors: May increase effects of indinavir.
CYP3A4 substrates: Levels of CYP3A4 substrates may be increased by indinavir. Contraindicated with cisapride and pimozide.
Didanosine: Separate administration by at least 1 h.
Ergot alkaloids: Effects of ergot alkaloids may be increased. Contraindicated.
Fentanyl: Effects of fentanyl may be increased.
HMG CoA reductase inhibitors, lidocaine: Indinavir may increase effects. Use not recommended with lovastatin, simvastatin, and rosuvastatin.
Immunosuppressants, Sildenafil, vandenafil, tadalafil, phosphodiesterase inhibitors: Levels may be increased by indinavir.
Alprazolam, midazolam, triazolam: Increases the risk of arrhythmias and prolonged sedation. Contraindicated.
Rifamycins: Decrease indinavir concentrations. Avoid.
Herbal
St. John's wort: May decrease indinavir blood concentration and effect. Avoid.
Food
Grapefruit juice: May decrease indinavir blood concentration and effect. Avoid.
High-fat, high-calorie, and high-protein meals: May decrease indinavir blood concentration.

DIAGNOSTIC TEST EFFECTS

May increase serum bilirubin (in 10% of patients), AST (SGOT), and ALT (SGPT) levels.

SIDE EFFECTS

Frequent
Nausea (12%), abdominal pain (9%), headache (6%), diarrhea (5%).
Occasional
Vomiting, asthenia, fatigue (4%); insomnia; accumulation of fat in waist, abdomen, or back of neck.
Rare
Abnormal taste sensation, heartburn, symptomatic urinary tract disease, tubulointerstitial nephritis, transient renal dysfunction, hyperglycemia.

SERIOUS REACTIONS

• Nephrolithiasis (flank pain with or without hematuria) occurs in 4% of patients, 24% in children.
• Indinavir should be discontinued if hemolytic anemia develops.
• Hepatitis/liver failure.

PRECAUTIONS & CONSIDERATIONS

Caution is warranted in patients with renal or liver function impairment. Be aware that it is unknown whether indinavir is excreted in breast milk. Breastfeeding is not recommended in this population because of the possibility of HIV transmission. Be aware that the safety and efficacy of this drug have not been established in children; Children have increased risk of nephrolithiasis. No information on the effects of this drug's use in elderly patients is available. Avoid St. John's wort and grapefruit or grapefruit juice because they will lower indinavir levels.
! Monitor for signs and symptoms of nephrolithiasis as evidenced by flank pain and hematuria, and notify the physician if symptoms occur. If nephrolithiasis occurs, expect therapy to be interrupted for 1-3 days. Establish baseline lab values and monitor renal function before and during therapy; in particular evaluate

the results of the serum creatinine and urinalysis tests. Maintain adequate hydration and drink 48 oz (1.5 L) of liquid over each 24-h period during therapy. Assess the pattern of daily bowel activity and stool consistency. Evaluate for abdominal discomfort or headache.

Storage

Store drug at room temperature, keep it in the original bottle, and protect it from moisture. Keep in mind that indinavir capsules are sensitive to moisture. Leave the desiccant in the bottle.

Administration

For optimal drug absorption, take indinavir with water only and without food 1 h before or 2 h after a meal. May take indinavir with coffee, juice, skim milk, tea, or water and with a light meal (e.g., dry toast with jelly). Do not take indinavir with meals high in fat, calories, and protein. If indinavir and didanosine are given concurrently, give the drugs at least 1 h apart on an empty stomach. If a dose is missed, take the next dose at the regularly scheduled time; do not double the dose.

Indomethacin

in-doe-meth′a-sin
(Apo-Indomethacin [CAN], Arthrexin [AUS], Indocid [CAN], Indocin, Indocin IV, Indocin-SR, Novomethacin [CAN])
Do not confuse with Imodium or Vicodin.

CATEGORY AND SCHEDULE

Pregnancy Risk Category: B (D if used after 34 wks' gestation, close to delivery, or for longer than 48 h)

Classification: Analgesics, non-narcotic, nonsteroidal anti-inflammatory drugs, antipyretic

MECHANISM OF ACTION

An NSAID that produces analgesic and anti-inflammatory effects by inhibiting prostaglandin synthesis. Also increases the sensitivity of the premature ductus to the dilating effects of prostaglandins. *Therapeutic Effect:* Reduces the inflammatory response and intensity of pain. Closure of the patent ductus arteriosus.

PHARMACOKINETICS

PO: Onset 1-2 h, peak 3 h, duration 4-6 h; 99% plasma-protein binding; metabolized in liver, kidneys; excreted in urine, bile, feces, breast milk; crosses placenta.

AVAILABILITY

Capsules (Indocin): 25 mg, 50 mg.
Capsules (Sustained-Release [Indocin-SR]): 75 mg.
Oral Suspension (Indocin): 25 mg/5 mL.
Powder for Injection (Indocin IV): 1 mg.
Suppository: 50 mg.

INDICATIONS AND DOSAGES

▸ **Moderate to severe rheumatoid arthritis, osteoarthritis, ankylosing spondylitis**
PO
Adults, Elderly. Initially, 25 mg 2-3 times a day; increased by 25-50 mg/wk up to 150-200 mg/day. Or 75 mg/day (extended-release) up to 75 mg twice a day.
Children. 1-2 mg/kg/day. Maximum: 3 mg/kg/day (or 150-200 mg/day). Do not use extended release.
▸ **Acute gouty arthritis**
PO
Adults, Elderly. 50 mg 3 times a day until pain decreases. For short-term use.
▸ **Acute shoulder pain, bursitis, tendinitis**
PO
Adults, Elderly. 75-150 mg/day in

3-4 divided doses. Usually no more than 7-14 days.

▸ **Usual rectal dosage**
Adults, Elderly. 50 mg 4 times a day. Maximum: 200 mg/day.
Children. Initially, 1.5-2.5 mg/kg/day, increased up to 4 mg/kg/day. Maximum: 150-200 mg/day.

▸ **Patent ductus arteriosus**
IV
Neonates. Initially, 0.2 mg/kg. Subsequent doses are based on age, as follows and are given at 12-24 h intervals.
Neonates older than 7 days. 0.25 mg/kg for second and third doses.
Neonates 2-7 days. 0.2 mg/kg for second and third doses.
Neonates < 48 h. 0.1 mg/kg for second and third doses.
If ductus arteriosis reopens, a second course may be given (not necessary if ductus closes or significantly reduces within 48 h of first course).

OFF-LABEL USES
Treatment of fever from malignancy, pericarditis, psoriatic arthritis, rheumatic complications associated with Paget disease of bone, vascular headache.

CONTRAINDICATIONS
Active GI bleeding or ulcerations; history of proctitis or recent rectal bleeding, hypersensitivity to aspirin, indomethacin, or other NSAIDs; renal impairment, thrombocytopenia; perioperative pain in the setting of coronary artery bypass graft surgery (use within 14 days of surgery).
For IV in neonates, active bleeding, thrombocytopenia, coagulation problems, necrotizing enterocolitis, severe renal dusfunction, if patency ductus arteriosis necessary for blood flow.

INTERACTIONS
Drug
Aminoglycosides: May increase the blood concentration of these drugs in neonates.
Antihypertensives, diuretics: May decrease the effects of these drugs.
Aspirin, other salicylates: May increase the risk of GI side effects such as bleeding.
Bile acid sequestrants: May decrease absorption of NSAIDs.
Bone marrow depressants: May increase the risk of hematologic reactions.
Corticosteroids: May increase risk of GI ulceration.
Heparin, oral anticoagulants, thrombolytics: May increase the effects of these drugs.
Lithium: May increase the blood concentration and risk of toxicity of lithium.
Methotrexate: May increase the risk of methotrexate toxicity.
Probenecid: May increase the indomethacin blood concentration.
Quinolone antibiotics: May increase seizure potential.
Triamterene: May potentiate acute renal failure. Do not give concurrently.
Herbal
Alfalfa, anise, bilberry, bladderwrack, bromelain, cat's claw, celery, chamomile, coleus, cordyceps, dong quai, evening primrose, fenugreek, feverfew, garlic, ginger, ginkgo biloba, ginseng (American, Panax, Siberian), grapeseed, green tea, guggul, horse chestnut seed, horseradish, licorice, prickly ash, red clover, reishi, SAMe (S-adenosylmethionine), sweet clover, turmeric, white willow: May increase the risk of bleeding.
Feverfew: May decrease the effects of feverfew.

Food
None known.

DIAGNOSTIC TEST EFFECTS
May prolong bleeding time. May alter blood glucose level. May increase BUN level, and serum creatinine, potassium, AST (SGOT), and ALT (SGPT) levels. May decrease serum sodium level and platelet count.

🔘 IV INCOMPATIBILITIES
Amino acid injection, calcium gluconate, cimetidine (Tagamet), dobutamine (Dobutrex), dopamine (Intropin), gentamicin (Garamycin), levofloxacin (Levaquin), tobramycin (Nebcin).

🔘 IV COMPATIBILITIES
Furosemide (Lasix), insulin, potassium, sodium bicarbonate, sodium nitroprusside (Nitropress).

SIDE EFFECTS
Frequent (3%-11%)
Headache, nausea, vomiting, dyspepsia, dizziness.
Occasional (< 3%)
Depression, tinnitus, diaphoresis, somnolence, constipation, diarrhea, bleeding disturbances in patent ductus arteriosus.
Rare
Hypertension, confusion, urticaria, pruritus, rash, blurred vision.

SERIOUS REACTIONS
• Paralytic ileus and ulceration of the esophagus, stomach, duodenum, or small intestine may occur.
• Patients with impaired renal function may develop hyperkalemia and worsening of renal impairment.
• Indomethacin use may aggravate epilepsy, parkinsonism, and depression or other psychiatric disturbances.

• Nephrotoxicity, including dysuria, hematuria, proteinuria, and nephrotic syndrome, occurs rarely.
• Metabolic acidosis or alkalosis, apnea, and bradycardia occur rarely in patients with patent ductus arteriosus.

PRECAUTIONS & CONSIDERATIONS
Caution is warranted in patients with cardiac dysfunction, hypertension, epilepsy, hepatic or renal impairment, and in those receiving anticoagulant therapy concurrently. Use of the lowest effective dose for the shortest duration is recommended. Avoid alcohol and aspirin during therapy because these substances increase the risk of GI bleeding. Tasks that require mental alertness or motor skills should be avoided.

BUN, serum alkaline phosphatase, bilirubin, creatinine, potassium, AST (SGOT), ALT (SGPT) levels, BP, ECG, heart rate, platelet count, serum sodium, blood glucose levels, and urine output should be monitored. Therapeutic response, such as decreased pain, stiffness, swelling, and tenderness, improved grip strength, and increased joint mobility, should be evaluated.
Storage
Store at room temperature below 86° F. Do not freeze. Protect injection from light.
Administration
Take oral indomethacin after meals or with food or antacids. Don't crush extended-release capsules. Shake oral suspension well before each use. ! IV injection is the preferred route for neonates with patent ductus arteriosus. The drug may also be given orally, by nasogastric tube, or rectally. Administer no more than 3 doses at 12- to 24-h intervals.

For IV use, reconstitute by adding only 1 or 2 mL preservative-free sterile water for injection or 0.9% NaCl to the 1-mg vial to provide a concentration of 1 mg or 0.5 mg/mL, respectively. Do not dilute the solution any further. Administer the IV immediately after reconstitution. The solution normally appears clear; discard if it becomes cloudy or contains precipitate; discard any unused portion. Administer the drug over 20-30 min. Restrict fluid intake, as ordered. Take care to avoid extravasation.

For rectal use, if suppository is too soft, refrigerate it for 30 min or run cold water over the foil wrapper. Moisten the suppository with cold water before inserting it into the rectum.

Infliximab
in-flicks'ih-mab
(Remicade)
Do not confuse Remicade with Reminyl.

CATEGORY AND SCHEDULE
Pregnancy Risk Category: C

Classification: Disease modifying antirheumatic drugs, gastrointestinals, immunomodulators, monoclonal antibodies, tumor necrosis factor modulators

MECHANISM OF ACTION
A monoclonal antibody that binds to tumor necrosis factor (TNF), inhibiting functional activity of TNF. Reduces infiltration of inflammatory cells. *Therapeutic Effect:* Decreases inflamed areas of the intestine, decreases synovitis and joint erosion.

PHARMACOKINETICS

Route	Onset	Peak	Duration
IV	1-2 wks	N/A	8-48 wks (Crohn disease)
IV	3-7 days	N/A	6-12 wks (rheumatoid arthritis[RA])

Absorbed into the GI tissue; primarily distributed in the vascular compartment. *Half-life:* 9.5 days.

AVAILABILITY
Powder for Injection: 100 mg.

INDICATIONS AND DOSAGES
▸ **Moderate to severe Crohn disease and fistulizing Crohn disease**
IV INFUSION
Adults, Elderly, Children aged 6 yr and older. Initially, 5 mg/kg followed by additional 5-mg/kg doses at 2 and 6 wks after first infusion. Maintenance: 5 mg/kg q8wk.
▸ **RA**
IV INFUSION
Adults, Elderly. 3 mg/kg; followed by additional doses at 2 and 6 wks after first infusion. Maintenance: 3 mg/kg q8wk.
▸ **Ankylosing spondylitis, prosiatic arthritis, plaque psoriasis, and moderate to severe ulcerative colitis**
IV INFUSION
Adults, Elderly. Initially, 5 mg/kg at wks 0, 2 and 6. Maintenance: 5 mg/kg q8wk.

CONTRAINDICATIONS
Sensitivity to infliximab or murine proteins, sepsis, serious active infection, doses > 5 mg/kg in patients with moderate or severe congestive heart failure.

INTERACTIONS
Drug
Abatacept, rilonacept, anakinra:
May increase adverse effects such as
infection risk.
Immunosuppressants: May reduce
frequency of infusion reactions
and antibodies to infliximab. May
increase risk of serious infection.
Live vaccines: May decrease
immune response to vaccine.
Herbal
Echinacea: May decrease effect of
infliximab.
Food
None known.

DIAGNOSTIC TEST EFFECTS
None known.

⊘ IV INCOMPATIBILITIES
Do not infuse infliximab in the same
IV line with other agents.

SIDE EFFECTS
Frequent (10%-22%)
Headache, nausea, fatigue, fever.
Occasional (5%-9%)
Fever or chills during infusion,
pharyngitis, vomiting, pain, dizziness,
bronchitis, rash, rhinitis, cough,
pruritus, sinusitis, myalgia, back pain.
Rare (1%-4%)
Hypotension or hypertension,
paresthesia, anxiety, depression,
insomnia, diarrhea, urinary tract
infection.

SERIOUS REACTIONS
• Hypersensitivity reaction, serum-
sickness–like illness, and lupus-like
syndrome may occur. Most occur
within 2 h of infusion.
• Severe hepatic reactions and
reactivation of hepatitis B have been
reported with therapy.
• Lymphoma has been reported in
adolescents and young adults with
Crohn disease.

• New or worsening heart failure.
• Reactivation of latent tuberculosis
has occurred; other serious infections.

PRECAUTIONS & CONSIDERATIONS
Caution is warranted in patients
with a history of recurrent infections
and in patients on concomitant
immunosuppressant agents. It is
unknown whether infliximab is
distributed in breast milk. Safety
and efficacy of infliximab have not
been established in children for JRA;
trials failed to establish effectiveness.
Use infliximab cautiously in elderly
patients because of a higher rate of
infection in this population.
    Follow-up tests, such as ESR,
C-reactive protein measurement,
and urinalysis, should be obtained.
Notify the physician of signs of
infection, such as fever. Persons with
rheumatoid arthritis should report
increase in pain, stiffness, or swelling
of joints. Persons with Crohn disease
should report changes in stool color,
consistency, or elimination pattern.
Hydration status should be assessed
before and during therapy.
Storage
Refrigerate vials.
Administration
Reconstitute each vial with 10 mL
sterile water for injection, using
21-gauge or smaller needle. Direct
the stream of sterile water to the
glass wall of the vial. Swirl the vial
gently to dissolve the contents. Do
not shake. Allow the solution to
stand for 5 min. Because infliximab
is a protein, the solution may develop
a few translucent particles; do not
use if particles are opaque or foreign
particles are present. The solution
normally appears colorless to light
yellow and opalescent; do not use
if discolored. Withdraw and waste a
volume of 0.9% NaCl from a 250-
mL bag that is equal to the volume of

reconstituted solution to be injected into the 250-mL bag (approximately 10 mL). Total dose to be infused should equal 250-mL. Slowly add the reconstituted infliximab solution to the 250-mL infusion bag. Gently mix. Infusion concentration should range between 0.4 and 4 mg/mL. Begin infusion within 3 h of reconstitution. Administer IV infusion over 2 h, using set with a low-protein-binding filter.

Insulin

in′sull-in

Rapid acting: Insulin Lispro (Humalog), Insulin Aspart (NovoLog, Novorapid [AUS]), Regular Insulin (Actrapid [AUS], Humulin R, Novolin R, Regular Iletin II), Intermediate acting: NPH (Humulin N, Novolin N, Pork), Lente: (Humulin L, Lente Iletin II, Monotard [AUS], Novolin L) NPH/regular mixture (70%/30%): Humulin 70/30, Novolin 70/30 NPH/regular mixture (50%/50%): Humulin 50/50 NPH/Lispro mixture (75%/25%): Humalog Mix 75/25, NovoLog Mix 70/30 Long acting: Insulin Glargine (Lantus)

CATEGORY AND SCHEDULE

Pregnancy Risk Category: B
OTC

Classification: Antidiabetic agents

MECHANISM OF ACTION

An exogenous insulin that facilitates passage of glucose, potassium, and magnesium across the cellular membranes of skeletal and cardiac muscle and adipose tissue. Controls storage and metabolism of carbohydrates, protein, and fats. Promotes conversion of glucose to glycogen in the liver. *Therapeutic Effect:* Controls glucose levels in diabetic patients.

PHARMACOKINETICS

Drug	Onset (h)	Peak (h)	Duration Form (h)
Insulin Lispro	0.25	0.5-1.5	4-5
Insulin Aspart	1/6	1-3	3-5
Regular	0.5-1	2-4	5-7
NPH	1-2	6-14	24+
Lente	1-3	6-14	24+
Insulin Glargine	N/A	N/A	24

AVAILABILITY

All insulins are available as 100 units/mL concentrations.
Rapid Acting: Humulin R, Novolin R, Novolog, Humalog.
Intermediate Acting: Humulin N, Novolin N.
Long Acting: Lantus.
Combinations: NovoLog Mix 70/30, Humalog Mix 50/50, Humalog Mix 75/25, Humulin 70/30, Novolin 70/30.

INDICATIONS AND DOSAGES

▸ **Treatment of insulin-dependent type 1 diabetes mellitus and non-insulin-dependent type 2 diabetes mellitus when diet or weight control has failed to maintain satisfactory blood glucose levels or in event of fever, infection, pregnancy, surgery, or trauma, or severe endocrine, hepatic or renal dysfunction; emergency treatment of ketoacidosis (regular insulin); to promote passage of glucose across cell membrane in hyperalimentation**

(regular insulin): to facilitate intracellular shift of potassium in hyperkalemia (regular insulin)
SUBCUTANEOUS
Adults, Elderly, Children.
0.5-1 unit/kg/day.
Adolescents (during growth spurt).
0.8-1.2 unit/kg/day.

CONTRAINDICATIONS

Hypersensitivity or insulin resistance may require change of type or species' source of insulin.

INTERACTIONS

Drug
Alcohol: May increase the effects of insulin.
β-adrenergic blockers: May increase the risk of hyperglycemia or hypoglycemia; may mask signs and prolong periods of hypoglycemia.
Glucocorticoids, thiazide diuretics: May increase blood glucose level.
Herbal
Chromium, garlic, gymnema : May increase hypoglycemic effects.
Food
None known.

DIAGNOSTIC TEST EFFECTS

May decrease serum magnesium, phosphate, and potassium concentrations.

IV INCOMPATIBILITIES

Regular insulin only: Diltiazem (Cardizem), dopamine (Intropin), nafcillin (Nafcil).

IV COMPATIBILITIES

Regular insulin only: Amiodarone (Cordarone), ampicillin/sulbactam (Unasyn), cefazolin (Ancef), cimetidine (Tagamet), digoxin (Lanoxin), dobutamine (Dobutrex), famotidine (Pepcid), gentamicin, heparin, magnesium sulfate, metoclopramide (Reglan), midazolam (Versed), milrinone (Primacor), morphine, nitroglycerin, potassium chloride, propofol (Diprivan), vancomycin (Vancocin).

SIDE EFFECTS

Occasional
Localized redness, swelling, and itching caused by improper injection technique or allergy to cleansing solution or insulin.
Infrequent
Somogyi effect, including rebound hyperglycemia with chronically excessive insulin dosages: systemic allergic reaction, marked by rash, angioedema, and anaphylaxis; lipodystrophy or depression at injection site from breakdown of adipose tissue; lipohypertrophy or accumulation of subcutaneous tissue at injection site from inadequate site rotation.
Rare
Insulin resistance.

SERIOUS REACTIONS

• Severe hypoglycemia caused by hyperinsulinism may occur with insulin overdose, decrease or delay of food intake, or excessive exercise and in those with brittle diabetes.
• Diabetic ketoacidosis may result from stress, illness, omission of insulin dose, or long-term poor insulin control.

PRECAUTIONS & CONSIDERATIONS

Dose adjustments may be necessary in renal and hepatic dysfunction. Insulin is the drug of choice for treating diabetes mellitus during pregnancy, but close medical supervision is needed. Insulin needs may drop for 24-72 h postpartum, then rise to prepregnancy levels. Insulin is not secreted in breast milk. Lactation may decrease insulin requirements. No age-related precautions have been noted in children. Decreased vision and shakiness in elderly patients may lead to inaccurate insulin self-dosing. Be alert to conditions that alter blood glucose requirements, such as fever, increased activity, stress, or a surgical procedure.

Food intake and blood glucose should be monitored before and during therapy. Be aware of signs and symptoms of hypoglycemia (anxiety, cool wet skin, diplopia, dizziness, headache, hunger, numbness in mouth, tachycardia, tremors) or hyperglycemia (deep rapid breathing, dim vision, fatigue, nausea, polydipsia, polyphagia, polyuria, vomiting); carry candy, sugar packets, or other sugar supplements for immediate response to hypoglycemia. Consult the physician when glucose demands are altered (such as with fever, heavy physical activity, infection, stress, trauma). Exercise, good personal hygiene (including foot care), not smoking, and weight control are essential parts of therapy.

Storage

Store currently used insulin at room temperature; avoid extreme temperatures and direct sunlight. Store extra unopened vials in refrigerator. Discard open vials after 28 days. For home situations, prefilled syringes are stable for 1 wk when refrigerated, including mixtures once they have stabilized; for example NPH/Regular stabilizes after 15 min and Lente/Regular stabilizes after 24 h. Prefilled pens and syringes should be stored in the vertical or oblique position to avoid plugging.

Administration

! Insulin dosages are individualized and monitored. Adjust dosage, as prescribed, to achieve premeal and bedtime glucose levels of 80-140 mg/dL (100-200 mg/dL in children younger than 5 yr).

Give subcutaneous only. Regular insulin is the only insulin that may be given IV or IM for ketoacidosis or other specific situations. Warm the drug to room temperature; do not give cold insulin. Roll the drug vial gently between hands; do not shake. Regular insulin normally appears clear. Administer insulin approximately 30 min before a meal. Insulin Lispro may be given up to 15 min before meals. Check blood glucose concentration before administration. Insulin dosages are highly individualized. Always draw regular insulin first when insulin is mixed. Mixtures must be administered at once because binding can occur within 5 min. Humalog may be mixed with Humulin N and Humulin L. Give subcutaneous injections in the abdomen, buttocks, thigh, upper arm, or upper back if there is adequate adipose tissue. Maintain a careful record of rotated injection sites.

To use prefilled syringes, the plunger should be pulled back slightly and the syringe rocked to remix the solution before injection.

For IV administration, use insulin regular and only if solution is clear. May give undiluted. An infusion can be prepared by adding 100 units of regular insulin (only) to 100 mL of 0.9% NaCl. Administration rate must be individualized. Initial rates are typically 0.1 unit/kg/h. Use with controlled infusion device.

Insulin Glulisine
in´sull-in
(Apidra)

CATEGORY AND SCHEDULE
Pregnancy Risk Category: C

Classification: Antidiabetic agents, insulins

MECHANISM OF ACTION

A recombinant, rapid-acting insulin analog that facilitates passage of glucose, potassium, magnesium across cellular membranes of skeletal and cardiac muscle, adipose tissue; controls storage and metabolism of carbohydrates, protein, fats. Promotes conversion of glucose to glycogen in liver. *Therapeutic Effect:* Controls glucose levels in diabetic patients.

PHARMACOKINETICS

Drug	Onset (min)	Peak (min)	Dura-tion	Form
Insulin	20	55 min	5 h	Gluli-sine

AVAILABILITY

Injection: 100 IU/mL (Apidra).

INDICATIONS AND DOSAGES

▶ **Diabetes mellitus (type 1 and type 2)**
SC INFUSION PUMP
Adults, Elderly, Children.
Individualize per patient needs.

CONTRAINDICATIONS

Current hypoglycemic episode, hypersensitivity, or insulin resistance may require a change of type or species' source of insulin.

INTERACTIONS

Drug
Alcohol: May increase the effects of insulin glulisine.
β-adrenergic blockers: May increase the risk of hyperglycemia or hypoglycemia, mask signs of hypoglycemia, and prolong the period of hypoglycemia.
Glucocorticoids, thiazide diuretics: May increase blood glucose.
Herbal
Chromium, garlic, gymnema : May increase hypoglycemic effects.

Food
None known.

DIAGNOSTIC TEST EFFECTS

May decrease serum magnesium, phosphate, and potassium concentrations.

SIDE EFFECTS

Occasional
Local redness, swelling, itching, caused by improper injection technique or allergy to cleansing solution or insulin.
Infrequent
Somogyi effect, including rebound hyperglycemia with chronically excessive insulin doses. Systemic allergic reaction, marked by rash, angioedema, and anaphylaxis, lipodystrophy or depression at injection site due to breakdown of adipose tissue, lipohypertrophy or accumulation of subcutaneous tissue at injection site because of lack of adequate site rotation.
Rare
Insulin resistance.

SERIOUS REACTIONS

• Severe hypoglycemia caused by hyperinsulinism may occur in overdose of insulin, decrease or delay of food intake, excessive exercise, or those with brittle diabetes.
• Diabetic ketoacidosis may result from stress, illness, omission of insulin dose, or long-term poor insulin control.

PRECAUTIONS & CONSIDERATIONS

Dosage adjustments may be necessary in renal and hepatic dysfunction. Insulin is the drug of choice for treating diabetes mellitus during pregnancy, but close medical supervision is needed. Following delivery, insulin needs may drop for 24-72 h, then rise to pre-pregnancy levels. Be aware that insulin is not secreted in breast milk and that lactation may decrease insulin requirements. Be aware that no age-related precautions have been noted in children. Be aware that in elderly patients, decreased vision and shakiness may lead to inaccurate dosage administration.

Hypoglycemia, including anxiety, cool, wet skin, diplopia, dizziness, headache, hunger, numbness in mouth, tachycardia, and tremors, or hyperglycemia, including deep, rapid breathing, dim vision, fatigue, nausea, polydipsia, polyphagia, polyuria, and vomiting may occur.

Be alert to conditions that alter blood glucose requirements, such as fever, increased activity, stress, or a surgical procedure.

Storage
Store currently used insulin at room temperature, avoiding extreme temperatures and direct sunlight. Store extra vials in refrigerator. Discard unused vials if not used for several weeks. No insulin should have precipitate or discoloration. Candy, sugar packets, or other sugar supplements should be carried at all times for immediate response to hypoglycemia.

Administration
Know that insulin dosages are individualized and monitored. Adjust dosage, as prescribed, to achieve premeal and bedtime glucose level of 80-140 mg/dL in adults and 100-200 mg/dL in children younger than 5 yr.

Give subcutaneous only. Warm the drug to room temperature; do not give cold insulin. Roll the drug vial gently between hands; do not shake. Regular insulin normally appears clear. No insulin should have precipitate or discoloration. Administer insulin approximately

15 min before a meal. Give subcutaneous injections in the abdomen, buttocks, thigh, upper arm, or upper back if there is adequate adipose tissue. Maintain a careful record of rotated injection sites. If insulin glulisine is mixed with NPH insulin, insulin glulisine should be drawn into the syringe first.

Interferon Alfa-2a
inn-ter-fear′on
(Roferon-A)
Do not confuse interferon alfa-2a with interferon alfa-2b.

CATEGORY AND SCHEDULE
Pregnancy Risk Category: C

Classification: Immunologic agents; biologic response modifier

MECHANISM OF ACTION
A biological response modifier that inhibits viral replication in virus-infected cells, suppresses cell proliferation, increases phagocytic action of macrophage, and augments specific lymphocytic cell toxicity. *Therapeutic Effect:* Prevents rapid growth of malignant cells; inhibits hepatitis virus.

PHARMACOKINETICS
Well absorbed after IM and subcutaneous (SC) administration. Undergoes proteolytic degradation during reabsorption in kidneys. *Half-life:* 2 h (IM); 3 h (subcutaneous).

AVAILABILITY
Injection (Prefilled Syringe): 3 million units/0.5 mL, 6 million units/0.5 mL, 9 million units/0.5 mL.

INDICATIONS AND DOSAGES
▶ **Hairy cell leukemia**
IM, SC
Adults. Initially, 3 million units/day
for 16-24 wks. Maintenance:
3 million units 3 times a wk. Do not
use 36-million-unit vial.
▶ **Chronic myelocytic leukemia**
IM, SC
Adults. 9 million units/day.
▶ **Melanoma**
IM, SC
Adults, Elderly. 12 million units/m^2
3 times a week for 3 mo.
▶ **AIDS-related Kaposi sarcoma**
IM, SC
Adults. Initially, 36 million units/day
for 10-12 wks, may give 3 million
units on day 1, 9 million units on day
2, 18 million units on day 3, then
36 million units/day for remaining of
10-12 wks. Maintenance: 36 million
units/day 3 times a wk.
▶ **Chronic hepatitis C**
IM, SC
Adults, Elderly. 6 million units
3 times a week for 3 mo, then
3 million units 3 times a week for
9 mo.

OFF-LABEL USES
Treatment of active, chronic
hepatitis; bladder or renal carcinoma;
malignant melanoma; multiple
myeloma; mycosis fungoides; non-
Hodgkin lymphoma.

CONTRAINDICATIONS
Autoimmune hepatitis; hepatic
decompensation interactions.
Drug
Bone marrow depressants: May
have increased myelosuppression.
Ribavirin: May increase risk of
hemolytic anemia.
Theophylline: May increase levels
of theophylline.
Zidovudine: May increase levels of
zidovudine.

Herbal and Food
None known.

DIAGNOSTIC TEST EFFECTS
May increase serum LDH, alkaline
phosphatase, AST (SGOT), and
ALT (SGPT) levels. May decrease
hematocrit, blood hemoglobin level,
and leukocyte and platelet counts.

SIDE EFFECTS
Frequent (> 20%)
Flulike symptoms, nausea, vomiting,
cough, dyspnea, hypotension,
edema, chest pain, dizziness,
diarrhea, weight loss, altered taste,
abdominal discomfort, confusion,
paresthesia, depression, visual and
sleep disturbances, diaphoresis,
lethargy.
Occasional (5%-20%)
Alopecia (partial), rash, dry
throat or skin, pruritus, flatulence,
constipation, hypertension,
palpitations, sinusitis.
Rare (< 5%)
Hot flashes, hypermotility, Raynaud
syndrome, bronchospasm, earache,
ecchymosis.

SERIOUS REACTIONS
• Arrhythmias, cerebrovascular
accident, transient ischemic attacks,
congestive heart failure, pulmonary
edema, and myocardial infarction
occur rarely.
• Cytopenias including aplastic
anemia may occur. Use with caution
in patients with myelosuppression.
• May cause severe psychiatric adverse
events in patients with or without
previous psychiatric symptoms.

PRECAUTIONS & CONSIDERATIONS
Caution is warranted with
cardiac diseases or abnormalities,
compromised CNS function,
hepatic or renal impairment,
myelosuppression, and seizure

disorders. Interferon alfa-2a should not be used by pregnant or breastfeeding women. An effective contraceptive method should be used during therapy, and the physician should be notified if the woman becomes or may be pregnant. The safety and efficacy of interferon alfa-2a have not been established in children. Elderly patients are more prone to cardiotoxicity and neurotoxicity. Age-related renal impairment may require cautious use of interferon alfa-2a in elderly patients. Avoid tasks that require mental alertness or motor skills until response to the drug has been established.

Flulike symptoms may occur but tend to diminish with continued therapy. Notify the physician if nausea and vomiting continues at home. Vital signs, including temperature, should be obtained at baseline. Adequate hydration should be maintained, particularly during early therapy.

Storage
Refrigerate the drug.

Administration
! Subcutaneous administration is preferred for thrombocytopenic patients and other patients at risk for bleeding. Dosage is individualized based on clinical response and tolerance of the drug's adverse effects. When used in combination therapy, expect to consult specific protocols for optimum dosage and sequence of drug administration. If severe adverse reactions occur, modify the dosage or temporarily discontinue the drug, as prescribed. Do not shake the vial.

Administer as IM or SC injection. The solution normally appears colorless; do not use it if it contains precipitate or becomes discolored. Therapeutic effects may take 1-3 mo to appear.

Interferon Alfa-2a/2b
inn-ter-fear'on
(Roferon-A)/(Intron-A)

CATEGORY AND SCHEDULE
Pregnancy Risk Category: C

Classification: Immunologic agents; biologic response modifier

MECHANISM OF ACTION
A biologic response modifier that inhibits viral replication in virus-infected cells. *Therapeutic Effect:* Suppresses cell proliferation; increases phagocytic action of macrophages; augments specific lymphocytic cell toxicity.

PHARMACOKINETICS
Interferon Alfa-2a
Well absorbed after IM, SC administration. Undergoes proteolytic degradation during reabsorption in kidney. *Half-life:* IM: 2 h; Subcutaneous: 3 h.
Interferon Alfa-2b
Well absorbed after IM, SC administration. Undergoes proteolytic degradation during reabsorption in kidney. *Half-life:* 2-3 h.

AVAILABILITY
Interferon Alfa-2a
Injection: 3 million units, 6 million units, 9 million units, (Roferon-A).
Interferon Alfa-2b,
Injection Powder for Reconstitution: 10 million units, 18 million units, 25 million units, 50 million units (Intron-A).
Injection, Prefilled Syringes: 3 million units, 5 million units, 6 million units, 10 million units, 18 million units, 25 million units, 50 million units (Intron-A).

INDICATIONS AND DOSAGES

▸ **Hairy cell leukemia**
Interferon Alfa-2a
SC/IM
Adults. Initially, 3 million units/day for 16-24 wks. Maintenance: 3 million units 3 times/wk. Do not use 36-million-unit vial.
Interferon Alfa-2b
SUBCUTANEOUS/IM
Adults. 2 million units/m^2 3 times/wk. If severe adverse reactions occur, modify dose or temporarily discontinue.

▸ **Chronic myelocytic leukemia (CML)**
Interferon Alfa-2a
SC/IM
Adults. 9 million units daily.

▸ **Condylomata acuminata**
Interferon Alfa-2b
INTRALESIONAL
Adults. 1 million units/lesion 3 times/wk for 3 wks. Use only 10-million-unit vial, reconstitute with no more than 1 mL diluent. Use tuberculin (TB) syringe with 25- or 26-gauge needle. Give in evening with acetaminophen, which alleviates side effects.

▸ **Melanoma**
Interferon Alfa-2a
SC/IM
Adults, Elderly. 12 million units/m^2 3 times/wk for 3 mo.
Interferon Alfa-2b
IV
Adults. Initially, 20 million units/m^2 5 times/wk for 4 wks. Maintenance: 10 million units IM/Subcutaneous for 48 wks.

▸ **AIDS-related Kaposi's sarcoma**
Interferon Alfa-2a
SC/IM
Adults. Initially, 36 million units/day for 10-12 wks, may give 3 million units on day 1; 9 million units on day 2; 18 million units on day 3; then begin 36 million units/day for remainder of 10-12 wks. Maintenance: 36 million units/day 3 times/wk.

Interferon Alfa-2b
SC/IM
Adults. 30 million units/m^2 3 times/wk. Use only 50-million-unit vials. If severe adverse reactions occur, modify dose or temporarily discontinue.

▸ **Chronic hepatitis B**
Interferon Alfa-2b
SC/IM
Adults. 30-35 million units/wk, 5 million units/day, or 10 million units 3 times/wk.

▸ **Chronic hepatitis C**
Interferon Alfa-2a
SC/IM
Adults. Initially, 6 million units once a day for 3 wks, then 3 million units 3 times/wk for 6 mo.
Interferon Alfa-2b
SC/IM
Adults. 3 million units 3 times/wk for up to 6 mo, for up to 18-24 mo for chronic hepatitis C.

OFF-LABEL USES

Interferon Alfa-2a
Treatment of active, chronic hepatitis, bladder or renal carcinoma, malignant melanoma, multiple myeloma, mycosis fungoides, non-Hodgkin lymphoma.
Interferon Alfa-2b
Treatment of bladder, cervical, renal carcinoma, chronic myelocytic leukemia, laryngeal papillomatosis, multiple myeloma, mycosis fungoides.

CONTRAINDICATIONS

Hypersensitivity to any component of the formulations, autoimmune hepatitis, hepatic decompensation.

INTERACTIONS

Drug
Bone marrow depressants: May have additive effect.
Ribavirin: May increase risk of hemolytic anemia.

Theophylline: May increase levels of theophylline.

Zidovudine: May increase levels of zidovudine.

Herbal and Food

None known.

DIAGNOSTIC TEST EFFECTS

May increase LDH concentration, serum alkaline phosphatase, SGOT (AST), and SGPT (ALT) levels. May decrease blood hemoglobin and hematocrit, and leukocyte and platelet counts.

ⓘ IV INCOMPATIBILITIES

No information available. Do not mix with other medications via Y-site administration.

SIDE EFFECTS

Frequent

INTERFERON ALFA-2A

Flulike symptoms, including fever, fatigue, headache, aches, pains, anorexia, nausea, vomiting, coughing, dyspnea, hypotension, edema, chest pain, dizziness, diarrhea, weight loss, taste change, abdominal discomfort, confusion, paresthesia, depression, visual and sleep disturbances, diaphoresis, lethargy.

INTERFERON ALFA-2B

Flulike symptoms, including fever, fatigue, headache, aches, pains, anorexia, and chills, rash with hairy cell leukemia (Kaposi sarcoma only).

Kaposi sarcoma: All previously mentioned side effects plus depression, dyspepsia, dry mouth or thirst, alopecia, rigors.

Occasional

INTERFERON ALFA-2A

Partial alopecia, rash, dry throat or skin, pruritus, flatulence, constipation, hypertension, palpitations, sinusitis.

INTERFERON ALFA-2B

Dizziness, pruritus, dry skin, dermatitis, alteration in taste.

Rare

INTERFERON ALFA-2A

Hot flashes, hypermotility, Raynaud syndrome, bronchospasm, earache, ecchymosis.

INTERFERON ALFA-2B

Confusion, leg cramps, back pain, gingivitis, flushing, tremor, nervousness, eye pain.

SERIOUS REACTIONS

• Arrhythmias, stroke, transient ischemic attacks, congestive heart failure (CHF), pulmonary edema, and myocardial infarction (MI) occur rarely with interferon alfa-2a.

• Hypersensitivity reaction occurs rarely with interferon alfa-2b.

• Severe adverse reactions of flulike symptoms appear dose-related with interferon alfa-2b.

• Cytopenias including aplastic anemia may occur. Use with caution in patients with myelosuppression.

• May cause severe psychiatric adverse events in patients with or without previous psychiatric symptoms.

PRECAUTIONS & CONSIDERATIONS

Caution is warranted with cardiac diseases, compromised central nervous system (CNS) function, history of cardiac abnormalities, liver or renal impairment, myelosuppression, and seizure disorders. Be aware that interferon alfa-2a and -2b use should be avoided during pregnancy. Breastfeeding is not recommended in this patient population. Safety and efficacy of interferon alfa-2a and -2b have not been established in children. Be aware that in elderly patients, cardiotoxicity and neurotoxicity may occur more frequently. Age-related renal impairment may require cautious use of interferon alfa-2a and -2b in elderly patients.

Clinical response may take 1-3 mo to appear. Flulike symptoms tend to diminish with continued therapy. Alcohol and tasks that require mental alertness or motor skills should be avoided during drug therapy. Women should use contraception and notify the physician if she suspects pregnancy.

Storage

Refrigerate interferon alfa-2a. Stable for 7 days at room temperature. Prepare immediately before use.

Administration

Know that the drug dosage is individualized based on the patient's clinical response and tolerance of the drug's adverse effects. When used in combination therapy, consult specific protocols for optimum dosage and sequence of drug administration, as prescribed. Remember that side effects are dose related. Be aware that the SC route of administration is preferred for thrombocytopenic patients and other patients at risk for bleeding. Remember that the drug dosage is individualized based on the patient's clinical response and tolerance of the drug's adverse effects. When used in combination therapy, expect to consult specific protocols for optimum dosage and sequence of drug administration. If severe adverse reactions occur, modify the drug dosage or temporarily discontinue the medication, as prescribed.

Do not shake the vial. Do not use if precipitate or discoloration occurs; solution normally appears colorless. Give as subcutaneous or IM injection.

Do not give interferon alfa-2b intramuscularly if the platelet count is < 50,000/m³; instead give subcutaneously.

For hairy cell leukemia, reconstitute each 3-million-unit vial of interferon alfa-2b with 1 mL bacteriostatic water for injection to provide concentration of 3 million units/mL, 1-mL to 5-million-unit vial; 2-mL to 10-million-unit vial;

5-mL to 25-million-unit vial provides concentration of 5 million units/mL.

For condylomata acuminata, reconstitute each 10-million-unit vial of interferon alfa-2b with 1 mL bacteriostatic water for injection to provide concentration of 10 million units/mL.

For acquired immune deficiency syndrome (AIDS)-related Kaposi sarcoma patients, reconstitute 50-million-unit vial interferon alfa-2b with 1 mL bacteriostatic water for injection to provide concentration of 50 million units/mL.

Agitate the vial gently and withdraw solution with sterile syringe.

For IV use, reconstitute interferon alfa-2b with diluent provided by manufacturer. Withdraw desired dose and further dilute with 100 mL 0.9% NaCl to provide final concentration at least 10 million units/100 mL. Administer over 20 min.

Interferon Alfa-2b

inn-ter-fear′on
(Intron-A)
Do not confuse interferon alfa-2b with interferon alfa-2a.

CATEGORY AND SCHEDULE

Pregnancy Risk Category: C

Classification: Immunologic agents

MECHANISM OF ACTION

A biological response modifier that inhibits viral replication in virus-infected cells, suppresses cell proliferation, increases phagocytic action of macrophages, and augments specific cytotoxicity of lymphocytes for target cells. *Therapeutic Effect:* Prevents rapid growth of malignant cells; inhibits hepatitis virus.

PHARMACOKINETICS

Well absorbed after IM and SC administration. Undergoes proteolytic degradation during reabsorption in kidneys. *Half-life:* 2-3 h.

AVAILABILITY

Injection (Multidose Vial): 6 million units/mL, 10 million units/mL.
Injection (Single-Dose Vial): 10 million units/mL.
Injection (Prefilled Solution): 3 million units/0.2 mL, 5 million units/0.2 mL, 10 million units/0.2 mL.
Injection (Powder for Reconstitution): 10 million units, 18 million units, 50 million units.

INDICATIONS AND DOSAGES
▸ **Hairy cell leukemia**
IM, SC
Adults. 2 million units/m^2 3 times a week. If severe adverse reactions occur, modify dose or temporarily discontinue drug.
▸ **Condyloma acuminatum**
INTRALESIONAL
Adults. 1 million units/lesion 3 times a week for 3 wks. Use only 10-million-unit vial, and reconstitute with no more than 1 mL diluent.
▸ **AIDS-related Kaposi sarcoma**
IM, SC
Adults. 30 million units/m^2 3 times a week. Use only 50-million-unit vials. If severe adverse reactions occur, modify dose or temporarily discontinue drug.
▸ **Chronic hepatitis C**
IM, SC
Adults. 3 million units 3 times a week for up to 6 mo. For patients who tolerate therapy and whose ALT (SGPT) level normalizes within 16 wks, therapy may be extended for up to 18-24 mo.
▸ **Chronic hepatitis B**
IM, SC
Adults. 30-35 million units weekly, either as 5 million units/day or 10 million units 3 times a week.
▸ **Malignant melanoma**
IV
Adults. Initially, 20 million units/m^2 5 times a week for 4 wks. Maintenance: 10 million units IM or subcutaneously 3 times a week for 48 wks.
▸ **Follicular lymphoma**
SC
Adults. 5 million units 3 times a week for up to 18 mo.

OFF-LABEL USES

Treatment of bladder, cervical, or renal carcinoma; chronic myelocytic leukemia; laryngeal papillomatosis; multiple myeloma; mycosis fungoides.

CONTRAINDICATIONS

Decompensated liver disease; autoimmune hepatitis interactions, hypersensitivity to interferon alfa-2b, *E.coli* proteins, albumin.
Drug
Bone marrow depressants: May increase myelosuppression.
Ribavirin: May increase risk of hemolytic anemia.
Theophylline: May increase levels of theophylline.
Zidovudine: May increase levels of zidovudine.
Herbal and Food
None known.

DIAGNOSTIC TEST EFFECTS

May increase PT, aPTT, and serum LDH, alkaline phosphatase, AST (SGOT), and ALT (SGPT) levels. May decrease blood hemoglobin level, hematocrit, and leukocyte and platelet counts.

ⓘ IV INCOMPATIBILITIES

No information available. Do not mix with other medications for Y-site administration.

SIDE EFFECTS

Frequent

Flulike symptoms, rash (only in patients with hairy cell leukemia Kaposi sarcoma).

Patients with Kaposi sarcoma: All previously mentioned side effects plus depression, dyspepsia, dry mouth or thirst, alopecia, rigors.

Occasional

Dizziness, pruritus, dry skin, dermatitis, altered taste.

Rare

Confusion, leg cramps, back pain, gingivitis, flushing, tremor, nervousness, eye pain.

SERIOUS REACTIONS

• Hypersensitivity reactions occur rarely.

• Severe flulike symptoms may occur at higher doses.

• May cause severe psychiatric adverse events in patients with or without previous psychiatric symptoms.

PRECAUTIONS & CONSIDERATIONS

Caution is warranted in patients with cardiac diseases or abnormalities, compromised CNS function, hepatic or renal impairment, myelosuppression, and seizure disorders. Interferon alfa-2b should not be used by pregnant or breastfeeding women. Effective contraceptive measures should be used during therapy, and the physician should be notified if the woman is or might be pregnant. The safety and efficacy of interferon alfa-2b have not been established in children. Elderly patients are more prone to cardiotoxicity and neurotoxicity. Age-related renal impairment may require cautious use of interferon alfa-2b in elderly patients. Avoid receiving immunizations without the physician's approval and coming in contact with people who have recently received a live-virus vaccine because interferon alfa-2b lowers the body's resistance. Also, avoid tasks that require mental alertness or motor skills until response to the drug has been established.

Flulike symptoms may occur but may be minimized by taking the drug at bedtime and tend to diminish with continued therapy. Urinalysis, CBC, platelet count, BUN level, serum alkaline phosphatase, creatinine, AST (SGOT), and ALT (SGPT) levels should be obtained before and routinely during therapy.

Storage

Refrigerate unopened vials and multi-dose pens; however, the drug remains stable for 7 days at room temperature.

Administration

❗ Dosage is individualized based on clinical response and tolerance of the drug's adverse effects. When used in combination therapy, consult specific protocols for optimum dosage and sequence of drug administration, as prescribed. Remember that side effects are dose related. The drug's therapeutic effect may take 1-3 mo to appear.

❗ For most uses, give the drug in the evening with acetaminophen, which alleviates side effects.

For IV use, prepare the solution immediately before use. Reconstitute with the diluent provided by the manufacturer. Withdraw the desired dose and further dilute with 100 mL 0.9% NaCl to provide final concentration at least 10 million units/100 mL. Administer the drug over 20 min.

Do not administer interferon alfa-2b by IM injection if platelet count is < 50,000/m^3; instead give it subcutaneously.

For hairy cell leukemia, reconstitute as follows: add 1 mL bacteriostatic water for injection to each 3-million-unit vial to provide a concentration of 3 million units/mL, or add 1 mL to each 5-million-unit vial, 2 mL to each 10-million-unit vial, or 5 mL to each 25-million-unit vial to provide a concentration of 5 million units/mL.

For condylomata acuminata, (intralesional use), reconstitute each 10-million-unit vial with 1 mL bacteriostatic water for injection to provide a concentration of 10 million units/mL. Use a tuberculin syringe with a 25- or 26-gauge needle.

For AIDS-related Kaposi sarcoma, reconstitute each 50-million-unit vial with 1 mL bacteriostatic water for injection to provide a concentration of 50 million units/mL. Agitate the vial gently and withdraw the solution with a sterile syringe.

For hepatitis indications, multidose pens are available for ease of chronic treatment. See specialized literature for appropriate use.

Interferon Alfa-n3
in-ter-fear'on
(human leukocyte interferon, antiviral)
(Alferon N)

CATEGORY AND SCHEDULE
Pregnancy Risk Category: C

Classification: Immunologic agents; biologic response modifier, interferons

MECHANISM OF ACTION
A biological response modifier that inhibits viral replication in virus-infected cells, suppresses cell proliferation, increases phagocytic action of macrophages, and augments the specific cytotoxicity of lymphocytes for target cells. *Therapeutic Effect:* Inhibits viral growth in condylomata acuminatum.

PHARMACOKINETICS
Plasma levels below detectable limits.

AVAILABILITY
Injection: 5 million International Units/mL.

INDICATIONS AND DOSAGES
▸ **Condyloma acuminatum**
INTRALESIONAL
Adults, Children 18 yr and older.
0.05 mL (250,000 International Units) per wart twice a week up to 8 wks. Maximum dose/treatment session: 0.5 mL (2.5 million International Units). Do not repeat for 3 mo after initial 8-wks course unless warts enlarge or new warts appear.

CONTRAINDICATIONS
Previous history of anaphylactic reaction to egg protein, murine proteins, or neomycin (trace).

INTERACTIONS
Drug
ACE inhibitors: May increase risk of granulocytopenia.
Bone marrow depressants: May increase myelosuppression.
Prednisone: May decrease effects of interferon.
Theophylline: May increase levels of theophylline.
Warfarin: May increase anticoagulant effects.
Zidovudine: May increase levels of zidovudine.
Herbal and Food
None known.

DIAGNOSTIC TEST EFFECTS

May increase serum LDH, alkaline phosphatase, AST (SGOT), and ALT (SGPT) levels. May decrease blood hemoglobin level, hematocrit, and leukocyte and platelet counts.

SIDE EFFECTS

Frequent
Flulike symptoms.
Occasional
Dizziness, pruritus, dry skin, dermatitis, altered taste.
Rare
Confusion, leg cramps, back pain, gingivitis, flushing, tremor, nervousness, eye pain.

SERIOUS REACTIONS

• Hypersensitivity reaction occurs rarely.
• Severe flulike symptoms may occur at higher doses.

PRECAUTIONS & CONSIDERATIONS

Caution is warranted with diabetes mellitus and ketoacidosis, hemophilia, pulmonary embolism, seizure disorders, severe myelosuppression, severe pulmonary disease, thrombophlebitis, uncontrolled congestive heart failure, and unstable angina.

Flulike symptoms may occur but may be minimized by taking the drug at bedtime and tend to diminish with continued therapy. Diagnostic tests, such as CBC, should be obtained before and routinely during therapy.
Storage
Refrigerate vials. Do not freeze or shake them.
Administration
Using a 30-gauge needle, inject 0.05 mL into the base of each wart. Used intralesionally only.

Interferon Alfacon-1

in-ter-fear′on
(Infergen)

CATEGORY AND SCHEDULE

Pregnancy Risk Category: C

Classification: Immunologic agents; biologic response modifier, interferons

MECHANISM OF ACTION

A biological response modifier that stimulates the immune system. *Therapeutic Effect:* Inhibits hepatitis C virus.

AVAILABILITY

Injection: 15 mcg/0.5 mL.

INDICATIONS AND DOSAGES
▸ **Chronic hepatitis C**
SC
Adults. 9 mcg 3 times a week for 24 wks. May increase to 15 mcg 3 times a week in patients who tolerate but fail to respond to 9-mcg dose, for up to 48 wks.

CONTRAINDICATIONS

History of autoimmune hepatitis or hepatic decompensation, hypersensitivity to any drug or component of the product.

SIDE EFFECTS

Frequent (> 50%)
Headache, fatigue, fever, depression.

SERIOUS REACTIONS

• Bone marrow suppression (rare).
• Cardiac effects, hypertension.
• Hypersensitivity.
• Psychiatric disturbances.

PRECAUTIONS & CONSIDERATIONS

Caution is warranted in patients with a history of autoimmune disease, cardiac disease, depression, endocrine disorders, hepatic disorders, myelosuppression, and renal dysfunction. May cause severe psychiatric adverse events in patients with or without previous psychiatric symptoms. Notify the physician of side effects, including headache or injection site pain, as soon as possible. Serum alkaline phosphatase, AST (SGOT), ALT (SGPT), hepatitis C virus (HCV) antibody, and HCV-RNA levels should be obtained before and during therapy.

Storage

Refrigerate unopened vials; do not freeze. Warm to room temperature before administration.

Administration

! Make sure at least 48 h elapse between doses of interferon alfacon-1.

Administer as SC injection.

Sometimes, doses are reduced in 1.5 or 3 mcg increments to help tolerance. The lowest effective dose is 7.5 mcg (0.25 mL).

Interferon Beta-1a

in-ter-fear'-on

(Avonex, Rebif)

Do not confuse interferon beta-1a with interferon beta-1b or Avonex with Avelox.

CATEGORY AND SCHEDULE

Pregnancy Risk Category: C

Classification: Immunologic agents; biologic response modifier

MECHANISM OF ACTION

A biological response modifier that interacts with specific cell receptors found on the surface of human cells. *Therapeutic Effect:* Produces antiviral and immunoregulatory effects.

PHARMACOKINETICS

Peak serum levels attained 3-15 h after IM administration. Biological markers increase within 12 h and remain elevated for 4 days. *Half-life:* 10 h (Avonex); 69 h (Rebif).

AVAILABILITY

Injection Solution (Prefilled Syringe [Avonex]): 30 mcg/0.5 mL.
Injection Solution (Prefilled Syringe [Rebif]): 22 mcg/0.5 mL, 44 mcg/0.5 mL.
Rebif Titration Pack (Pre-Filled Syringes): 8.8 mcg/0.2 mL and 22 mcg/0.5 mL.

INDICATIONS AND DOSAGES

▸ **Relapsing-remitting multiple sclerosis**

IM (AVONEX)

Adults. 30 mcg once weekly.

SC (REBIF)

Adults. Initially 8.8 mcg 3 times a week; may increase to 44 mcg 3 times a week over 4-6 wks.

OFF-LABEL USES

Treatment of AIDS, AIDS-related Kaposi sarcoma, malignant melanoma, renal cell carcinoma.

CONTRAINDICATIONS

Hypersensitivity to albumin or interferon.

INTERACTIONS

Drug

Hepatotoxic agents: May increase risk of hepatotoxicity.
Theophylline: May increase levels of theophylline.
Warfarin: May increase anticoagulant effects.
Telbivudine: May increase neuropathy.
Zidovudine: May increase effects of zidovudine.
Herbal
None known.

Food
Ethanol: Limit or avoid because may increase risk of hepatic adverse effects.

DIAGNOSTIC TEST EFFECTS

May increase blood glucose and BUN levels and serum alkaline phosphatase, bilirubin, calcium, AST (SGOT), and ALT (SGPT) levels. May decrease blood hemoglobin level and neutrophil, platelet, and WBC counts.

SIDE EFFECTS
Frequent
Headache (67%), flulike symptoms (61%), myalgia (34%), upper respiratory tract infection (31%), generalized pain (24%), asthenia, chills (21%), sinusitis (18%), infection (11%).
Occasional
Abdominal pain, arthralgia (9%), chest pain, dyspnea (6%), malaise, syncope (4%).
Rare
Injection site reaction, hypersensitivity reaction (3%).

SERIOUS REACTIONS
• Anemia occurs in 8% of patients.

PRECAUTIONS & CONSIDERATIONS
Caution is warranted with chronic, progressive multiple sclerosis and in children younger than 18 yr. May cause severe psychiatric adverse events in patients with or without previous psychiatric symptoms. Interferon beta-1a may cause spontaneous abortion. It is unknown whether interferon beta-1a is distributed in breast milk. Interferon beta-1a should be used cautiously in children because its safety and efficacy have not been established in this age group. No information is available on the use of interferon beta-1a in elderly patients.

Notify the physician of flulike symptoms, headache, or muscle pain or weakness. CBC and serum alkaline phosphatase, AST (SGOT), and ALT (SGPT) levels should be obtained before and during therapy.
Storage
Refrigerate unopened vials of Avonex prefilled syringes; warm vials to room temperature before use; if the drug is not used immediately after reconstitution, refrigerate it and use it within 6 h; after 6 h discard any unused portion because the drug contains no preservative. Use Avonex prefilled syringe within 12 h after removal from refrigerator. Refrigerate Rebif prefilled syringes; if refrigeration is unavailable, the drug may be stored at room temperature, away from heat, and light, up to 30 days.
Administration
For IM use (Avonex powder for injection), reconstitute 30 mcg MicroPin (6.6-million-unit) vial with 1.1 mL of the diluent, provided by the manufacturer. Discard it if it becomes discolored or contains a precipitate.
! Gently swirl do not shake the vial to dissolve the drug.

For IM use (Avonex prefilled syringes), allow the drug to warm to room temperature prior to use. Administer on the same day each week.

For subcutaneous use (Rebif prefilled syringes), administer the drug at the same time of day 3 days each week. Separate doses by at least 48 h.

Interferon Beta-1a/b
inn-ter-fear´on
(Avonex, Rebif); (Betaferon, Betaseron)

CATEGORY AND SCHEDULE
Pregnancy Risk Category: C

Classification: Immunologic agents; biologic response modifier

MECHANISM OF ACTION

A biologic response modifier that interacts with specific cell receptors found on surface of human cells. *Therapeutic Effect:* Possesses antiviral and immunoregulatory activities.

PHARMACOKINETICS

Interferon Beta-1a

After IM administration, peak serum levels attained in 3-15 h. Biologic markers increase within 12 h and remain elevated for 4 days. *Half-life:* 10 h (IM).

Interferon Beta-1b

Half-life: 8 min to 4.3 h.

AVAILABILITY

Interferon Beta-1a

Prefilled Syringes Powder for Injection: 22 mcg (Rebif), 30 mcg (Avonex), 44 mcg (Rebif).

Interferon Beta-1b

Powder for Injection: 0. 3 mg (9.6 million units) (Betaseron).

INDICATIONS AND DOSAGES

▸ **Relapsing-remitting multiple sclerosis**

Interferon Beta-1a

IM

Adults. 30 mcg Avonex once weekly.

SC

Adults. Initially 8.8 mcg Rebif 3 times/wks, may increase over 4-6 wks to 44 mcg Rebif 3 times/wk.

Interferon Beta-1b

SC

Adults. 0.25 mg (8 million units) every other day.

OFF-LABEL USES

Treatment of acquired immune deficiency syndrome (AIDS), AIDS-related Kaposi sarcoma, malignant melanoma, renal cell carcinoma.

CONTRAINDICATIONS

Hypersensitivity to albumin, interferon.

INTERACTIONS

Drug

ACE inhibitors: May increase risk of granulocytosis.

Hepatotoxic agents: May increase risk of hepatotoxicity.

Theophylline: May increase levels of theophylline.

Warfarin: May increase anticoagulant effects.

Zidovudine: May increase effects of zidovudine.

Herbal

None known.

Food

None known.

DIAGNOSTIC TEST EFFECTS

May increase blood glucose levels, BUN, serum alkaline phosphatase, bilirubin, calcium, SGOT (AST), and SGPT (ALT) levels. May decrease blood hemoglobin, neutrophil, platelet, and white blood cell (WBC) counts.

SIDE EFFECTS

Frequent

Interferon beta-1a: Headache (67%), flu-like symptoms (61%), myalgia (34%), upper respiratory infection (31%), pain (24%), asthenia, chills (21%), sinusitis (18%), infection (11%). Interferon beta-1a: Injection site reaction (85%), headache (84%), flu-like symptoms (76%), fever (59%), pain (52%), asthenia (49%), myalgia (44%), sinusitis (36%), diarrhea, dizziness (35%), mental status changes (29%), constipation (24%), diaphoresis (23%), vomiting (21%).

Occasional

Interferon beta-1a: Abdominal pain, arthralgia (9%), chest pain, dyspnea (6%), malaise, syncope (4%). Interferon beta-1b: Malaise (15%), somnolence (6%), alopecia (4%).

Rare

Interferon beta-1a: Injection site reaction, hypersensitivity reaction (3%).

SERIOUS REACTIONS

• Anemia occurs in 8% of patients taking interferon beta-1a.
• May cause severe psychiatric adverse events in patients with or without previous psychiatric symptoms.
• Seizures occur rarely in patients taking interferon beta-1b.

PRECAUTIONS & CONSIDERATIONS

Caution is warranted with children younger than 18 yr and in patients with chronic progressive multiple sclerosis. Be aware that interferon beta-1a has abortifacient potential. Be aware that it is unknown whether interferon beta-1a is distributed in breast milk. Be aware that the safety and efficacy of interferon beta-1a have not been established in children. Be aware that there is no information on interferon beta-1a use in elderly patients. Be aware that it is unknown whether interferon beta-1b is distributed in breast milk. Be aware that the safety and efficacy of interferon beta-1b have not been established in children. Be aware that there is no information available on interferon beta-1b use in elderly patients.

Dispose of needles and syringes in the provided puncture-resistant container. Document the type and severity of any injection-site reactions; these reactions will not require discontinuation of therapy. Immediately notify the physician if depression or suicidal ideation occurs.

Storage

Refrigerate vials of interferon beta-1a. Following reconstitution of interferon beta-1a, use within 6 h if refrigerated. Discard if discolored or contains a precipitate.

Store interferon beta-1b vials at room temperature. After reconstitution the solution of interferon beta-1b is stable for 3 h if refrigerated. Use within 3 h of reconstitution. Discard the solution if it is discolored or contains a precipitate.

Administration

For IM use of interferon beta-1a, reconstitute 33-mcg (6.6-million-unit) vial with 1.1 mL diluent, which is supplied by the manufacturer. Gently swirl to dissolve medication; do not shake. Discard unused portion because it contains no preservative. For SC use of interferon beta-1a, administer drug at the same time of day 3 days each week. Doses should be separated by at least 48 h.

For SC use of interferon beta-1b, reconstitute 0.3-mg (9.6-million-unit) vial with 1.2 mL diluent, which is supplied by manufacturer, to provide concentration of 0.25 mg/mL (8 million units/mL). Gently swirl to dissolve medication; do not shake. Withdraw 1 mL solution and inject subcutaneously into the patient's abdomen, arms, hips, or thighs using a 27-gauge needle. Discard unused portion because it contains no preservative.

Interferon Beta-1b

in-ter-fear'-on
(Betaseron)
Do not confuse interferon beta-1b with interferon beta-1a.

CATEGORY AND SCHEDULE

Pregnancy Risk Category: C

Classification: Immunologic agents; biologic response modifier

MECHANISM OF ACTION

A biological response modifier that interacts with specific cell receptors found on the surface of human cells. *Therapeutic Effect:* Produces antiviral and immunoregulatory effects.

PHARMACOKINETICS
Half-life: 8 min-4.3 h.

AVAILABILITY
Powder for Injection: 0.3 mg (9.6 million units).

INDICATIONS AND DOSAGES
▶ **Relapsing-remitting multiple sclerosis**
SC
Adults. Target dose is: 0.25 mg (8 million units) every other day. Start with 62.5 mcg SC every other day and increase to 125 mcg every other day after 2 wks, etc.

CONTRAINDICATIONS
Hypersensitivity to albumin or interferon.

INTERACTIONS
Drug
Theophylline: May increase levels of theophylline.
Herbal and Food
None known.

DIAGNOSTIC TEST EFFECTS
May increase blood glucose and BUN levels and serum alkaline phosphatase, bilirubin, calcium, AST (SGOT), and ALT (SGPT) levels. May decrease blood hemoglobin level and neutrophil, platelet, and WBC counts.

SIDE EFFECTS
Frequent
Injection site reaction (85%), headache (84%), flulike symptoms (76%), fever (59%), asthenia (49%), myalgia (44%), sinusitis (36%), diarrhea, dizziness (35%), mental status changes (29%), constipation (24%), diaphoresis (23%), vomiting (21%).
Occasional
Malaise (15%), somnolence (6%), alopecia (4%).

SERIOUS REACTIONS
• Seizures occur rarely.
• May cause severe psychiatric adverse events in patients with or without previous psychiatric symptoms.
• Injection site necrosis.
• Rare serious hypersensitivity.

PRECAUTIONS & CONSIDERATIONS
Caution is warranted with chronic, progressive multiple sclerosis and in children younger than 18 yr. Pregnancy should be avoided. It is unknown whether interferon beta-1b is distributed in breast milk. The safety and efficacy of interferon beta-1b have not been established in children. No information is available on the use of interferon beta-1b in elderly patients. Sunscreen and protective clothing should be worn when exposed to sunlight or ultraviolet light until the extent of photosensitivity has been determined.

Notify the physician of flulike symptoms, headache, or muscle pain or weakness. CBC and serum alkaline phosphatase, AST (SGOT), and ALT (SGPT) levels should be obtained before and during therapy. Pattern of daily bowel activity and stool consistency and food intake should be monitored.
Storage
Store vials at room temperature. After reconstitution, the solution is stable for 3 h if refrigerated. Use the solution within 3 h of reconstitution.
Administration
! Gently swirl do not shake the vial to dissolve the drug.

For subcutaneous injection, reconstitute the 0.3-mg (9.6-million-unit) vial with 1.2 mL of the diluent, supplied by the manufacturer to provide a concentration of 0.25 mg/mL (8 million units/mL). Using a 27-gauge needle, inject the appropriate dose of the solution subcutaneously into the abdomen, arms, hips, or thighs. Discard the solution if it becomes discolored or contains a precipitate. Discard any unused portion because the solution contains no preservative.

Interferon Gamma-1b

in-ter-fear'on
(Actimmune, Imukin [AUS])

CATEGORY AND SCHEDULE
Pregnancy Risk Category: C

Classification: Immunologic agents; biologic response modifier

MECHANISM OF ACTION
A biological-response modifier that induces the activation of macrophages in blood monocytes to phagocytes, which is necessary in the body's cellular immune response to intracellular and extracellular pathogens. Enhances phagocytic function and antimicrobial activity of monocytes. *Therapeutic Effect:* Decreases signs and symptoms of serious infections in chronic granulomatous disease.

PHARMACOKINETICS
Slowly absorbed after subcutaneous administration.

AVAILABILITY
Injection: 100 mcg (2 million units).

INDICATIONS AND DOSAGES
▸ **Chronic granulomatous disease; severe, malignant osteopetrosis**
SC
Adults, Children older than 1 yr.
50 mcg/m^2 (1.5 million units/m^2) in patients with body surface area (BSA) > 0.5 m^2; 1.5 mcg/kg/dose

in patients with BSA 0.5 m^2 or less. Give 3 times a week.

CONTRAINDICATIONS
Hypersensitivity to *Escherichia coli*–derived products, mannitol, ortho drug.

INTERACTIONS
Drug
Bone marrow depressants: May increase myelosuppression.
Theophylline: May increase levels of theophylline.
Herbal and Food
None known.

DIAGNOSTIC TEST EFFECTS
May elevate AST or ALT.

SIDE EFFECTS
Frequent
Fever (52%); headache (33%); rash (17%); chills, fatigue, diarrhea (14%).
Occasional (10%-13%)
Vomiting, nausea.
Rare (3%-6%)
Weight loss, myalgia, anorexia.

SERIOUS REACTIONS
• Interferon gamma-1b may exacerbate preexisting central nervous system (CNS) disturbances, including decreased mental status, seizures, gait disturbance, and dizziness, as well as cardiac disorders.
• Neutropenia or thrombocytopenia.

PRECAUTIONS & CONSIDERATIONS
Caution is warranted with compromised CNS function, myelosuppression, preexisting cardiac disorders (including arrhythmias, congestive heart failure, and myocardial ischemia), and seizure disorders. It is unknown whether interferon gamma-1b crosses the placenta or is distributed in breast milk. The safety and efficacy of

interferon gamma-1b have not been established in children younger than 1 yr. Children are more likely to experience flulike symptoms. No information is available on the use of interferon gamma-1b in elderly patients. Avoid performing tasks that require mental alertness or motor skills until response to the drug has been established.

Notify the physician of flulike symptoms or rash. CBC, urinalysis, BUN level and serum alkaline phosphatase, creatinine, AST (SGOT), and ALT (SGPT) levels should be obtained before and every 3 mo during therapy.

Storage
Refrigerate unopened vials; do not freeze them. Discard vials kept at room temperature for longer than 12 h.

Administration
! Avoid excessive agitation of the vial; do not shake it.

Vials come in single doses; discard any unused portion. The solution normally appears clear and colorless. Do not use it if it becomes discolored or contains a precipitate. Administer the drug subcutaneously 3 times a week. Rotate injection sites.

Interleukin-2 (Aldesleukin)
al-des-loo′kin
(IL-2, Proleukin)
Do not confuse interleukin-2 with interferons.

CATEGORY AND SCHEDULE
Pregnancy Risk Category: C

Classification: Antineoplastics, biological response modifiers, recombinant DNA origin, interleukins

MECHANISM OF ACTION
A biological response modifier that acts like human recombinant interleukin-2, promoting proliferation, differentiation, and recruitment of T and B cells, lymphokine-activated and natural cells, and thymocytes. *Therapeutic Effect:* Enhances cytolytic activity in lymphocytes.

PHARMACOKINETICS
Primarily distributed into plasma, lymphocytes, lungs, liver, kidney, and spleen. Metabolized to amino acids in the cells lining the kidneys. *Half-life:* 85 min.

AVAILABILITY
Powder for Injection: 22 million units (1.3 mg).

INDICATIONS AND DOSAGES
▶ **Metastatic melanoma, metastatic renal cell carcinoma**
IV
Adults. 600,000 units/kg q8h for 14 doses, followed by 9 days of rest, then another 14 doses for a total of 28 doses per course. Course may be repeated after rest period of at least 7 wks from date of hospital discharge.

OFF-LABEL USES
Treatment of non-Hodgkin's lymphoma, acute myelogenous leukemia.

CONTRAINDICATIONS
Hypersensitivity to the drug or mannitol, abnormal pulmonary function or thallium stress test results, bowel ischemia or perforation, coma or toxic psychosis lasting longer than 48 h, GI bleeding requiring surgery, intubation lasting more than 72 h, organ allografts, pericardial tamponade, renal dysfunction requiring dialysis

for longer than 72 h, repetitive or difficult-to-control seizures. Retreatment in those who experience any of the following toxicities: angina, MI, recurrent chest pain with EKG changes, sustained ventricular tachycardia, uncontrolled or unresponsive cardiac rhythm disturbances.

INTERACTIONS
Drug
Antihypertensives: May increase hypotensive effect.
Cardiotoxic, hepatotoxic, myelotoxic, or nephrotoxic medications: May increase the risk of toxicity.
Glucocorticoids: May decrease the effects of interleukin.
Herbal
None known.
Food
None known.

DIAGNOSTIC TEST EFFECTS
May increase BUN and serum alkaline phosphatase, bilirubin, creatinine, AST (SGOT), and ALT (SGPT) levels. May decrease serum calcium, magnesium, phosphorus, potassium, and sodium levels.

ⓘ IV INCOMPATIBILITIES
Ganciclovir (Cytovene), lorazepam (Ativan), pentamidine (Pentam), prochlorperazine (Compazine), promethazine (Phenergan).

ⓘ IV COMPATIBILITIES
Amikacin (Amikin), amphotericin B (Abelcet, AmBisome, Amphotec), calcium gluconate, co-trimoxazole (Bactrim), diphenhydramine (Benadryl), dopamine (Intropin), fat emulsion 10%, fluconazole (Diflucan), foscarnet (Foscavir), gentamicin (Garamycin), heparin, lorazepam (Ativan), magnesium,

metoclopramide (Reglan), morphine (Avinza, Kadian, Roxanol), ondansetron (Zofran), piperacillin (Piperacil), potassium, ranitidine (Zantac), thiethylperazine, ticarcillin (Ticar), tobramycin (Nebcin).

SIDE EFFECTS
Side effects are generally self-limiting and reversible within 2-3 days after discontinuing therapy.
Frequent (48%-89%)
Fever, chills, nausea, vomiting, hypotension, diarrhea, oliguria or anuria, mental status changes, irritability, confusion, depression, sinus tachycardia, pain (abdominal, chest, back), fatigue, dyspnea, pruritus.
Occasional (17%-47%)
Edema, erythema, rash, stomatitis, anorexia, weight gain, infection (urinary tract infection, injection site, catheter tip), dizziness.
Rare (4%-15%)
Dry skin, sensory disorders (vision, speech, taste), dermatitis, headache, arthralgia, myalgia, weight loss, hematuria, conjunctivitis, proteinuria.

SERIOUS REACTIONS
• Anemia, thrombocytopenia, and leukopenia occur commonly.
• GI bleeding and pulmonary edema occur occasionally.
• Capillary leak syndrome results in hypotension (systolic pressure < 90 mm Hg or a 20 mm Hg drop from baseline systolic pressure), extravasation of plasma proteins and fluid into extravascular space, and loss of vascular tone. It may result in cardiac arrhythmias, angina, myocardial infarction, and respiratory insufficiency.
• Other rare reactions include fatal malignant hyperthermia, cardiac arrest, cerebrovascular

accident, pulmonary emboli, bowel perforation, gangrene, and severe depression leading to suicide.

PRECAUTIONS & CONSIDERATIONS

Extreme caution should be used with a history of cardiac or pulmonary disease, even if they have normal thallium stress and pulmonary function test results. Also use the drug cautiously with fixed requirements for large volumes of fluid (such as those with hypercalcemia) or a history of seizures. Interleukin use should be avoided in patients of either sex who do not practice effective contraception. The safety and efficacy of interleukin have not been established in children. Elderly patients may require cautious use of the drug because of age-related renal impairment. They are also less able to tolerate drug-related toxicities.

Notify the physician of difficulty urinating, black tarry stools, pinpoint red spots on the skin, bruising, fever, signs of local infection, sore throat, or unusual bleeding from any site. Treat persons with bacterial infection and those with indwelling central lines with antibiotic therapy before beginning interleukin therapy. A negative CT scan must be obtained before beginning therapy. Immediately report any symptoms of depression or suicidal ideation. CBC, electrolytes, liver and renal function, amylase concentration, BP, mental status, intake and output, extravascular fluid accumulation, platelet count, pulse oximetry values, and weight should be assessed.

Storage
Refrigerate-do not freeze-unopened vials. The reconstituted solution is stable for 48 h at room temperature or refrigerated (refrigerated is preferred) because of lack of preservative.

Administration
! Withhold the drug in patients who exhibit moderate to severe lethargy or somnolence because continued administration may result in coma. Restrict interleukin therapy to patients with normal cardiac and pulmonary function as determined by thallium stress testing and pulmonary function testing. Dosage is individualized based on clinical response and tolerance of the drug's adverse effects.

For IV use, reconstitute the 22-million-unit vial with 1.2 mL sterile water for injection to provide a concentration of 18 million units/mL. Do not use bacteriostatic water for injection or 0.9% NaCl. During reconstitution, direct the diluent at the side of the vial. Swirl the contents gently-do not shake-to avoid foaming. Further dilute the appropriate dose in 50 mL D5W and infuse over 15 min. Do not use an in-line filter. Warm the solution to room temperature before infusion. Closely monitor the patient for a drop in mean arterial BP, a sign of capillary leak syndrome. Continued treatment may result in edema, pleural effusion, mental status changes, and significant hypotension (systolic pressure < 90 mm Hg or a 20 mm Hg drop from baseline systolic pressure).

Iodoquinol
eye-oh-do-kwin'ole
(Yodoxin, Diodoquin [CAN])

CATEGORY AND SCHEDULE
Pregnancy Risk Category: C

Classification: Antiprotozoals, amebicide

MECHANISM OF ACTION
An antibacterial, antifungal, and antitrichomonal agent that works in the intestinal lumen by an unknown mechanism. *Therapeutic Effect:* Amebicidal.

PHARMACOKINETICS
Partially and irregularly absorbed from the GI tract. Metabolized in liver. Primarily excreted in feces.

AVAILABILITY
Tablets: 210 mg, 650 mg (Yodoxin).

INDICATIONS AND DOSAGES
▸ **Intestinal amebiasis**
PO
Adults, Elderly. 650 mg 3 times a day for 20 days.
Children. 30-40 mg/kg in 3 divided doses for 20 days. Maximum: 650 mg/dose.

CONTRAINDICATIONS
Hepatic impairment, hypersensitivity to iodine and 8-hydroxyquinolones.

INTERACTIONS
Drug, Herbal, and Food
None known.

DIAGNOSTIC TEST EFFECTS
May result in false-positive ferric chloride test for phenylketonuria. May increase protein-bound serum iodine concentrations reflecting a decrease in I^{131} uptake.

SIDE EFFECTS
Occasional
Fever, chills, headache, nausea, vomiting, diarrhea, cramps, urticaria, pruritus.

SERIOUS REACTIONS
• Optic neuritis, atrophy, and peripheral neuropathy have been reported with high dosages and long-term use.

PRECAUTIONS & CONSIDERATIONS
Caution should be used in patients with thyroid disease and neurologic disorders. It is unknown whether iodoquinol is distributed in breast milk. No age-related precautions have been noted in children. Age-related renal impairment may limit the use of iodoquinol in elderly patients.

Nausea, diarrhea, or GI upset may occur. Be aware that iodoquinol may temporarily stain skin, hair, and clothing a yellow-brown color.
Administration
Give after meals. May crush tablets and mix with applesauce. Avoid long-term use.

Ipratropium
eye-pra-troep'ee-um
(Apo-Ipravent [CAN], Aproven [AUS], Atrovent, Atrovent Aerosol [AUS], Atrovent Nasal [AUS], Novo-Ipramide [CAN], Nu-Ipratropium [CAN], PMS-Ipratropium [CAN])
Do not confuse Atrovent with Alupent.

CATEGORY AND SCHEDULE
Pregnancy Risk Category: B

Classification: Anticholinergics, bronchodilators

MECHANISM OF ACTION
An anticholinergic that blocks the action of acetylcholine at parasympathetic sites in bronchial smooth muscle. *Therapeutic Effect:* Causes bronchodilation and inhibits nasal secretions.

PHARMACOKINETICS

Route	Onset	Peak	Duration
Inhalation	1-3 min	1-2 h	4-6 h

Minimal systemic absorption after inhalation. Metabolized in the liver (systemic absorption). Primarily eliminated in feces. *Half-life:* 1.5-4 h.

AVAILABILITY

Oral Inhalation: 17 mcg/actuation.
Nebulizer Solution for Inhalation: 0.02%.
Nasal Spray: 0.03%, 0.06%.

INDICATIONS AND DOSAGES

▸ **Bronchospasm, acute treatment, adjunctive**
INHALATION
Adults, Elderly, Children. 2-3 puffs q6h initially.
NEBULIZATION
Adults, Elderly, Children 12 yr and older. 500 mcg q30min for 3 doses, then q2-4h as needed.
Children younger than 12 yr.
250 mcg q20min for 3 doses, then q2-4h as needed.
▸ **Bronchospasm, maintenance treatment, associated with COPD**
INHALATION
Adults, Elderly. 2-3 puffs q6h.
NEBULIZATION
Adults, Elderly. 500 mcg q6-8h.
▸ **Rhinorrhea, common cold**
INTRANASAL
Adults, Children older than 12 yr.
2 sprays per nostril of 0.06% solution 3-4 times a day for up to 4 days.
▸ **Rhinorrhea, allergic or non-allergic perennial**
Adults, Children 6 yr and older.
2 sprays of (0.03%) solution 2-3 times a day per nostril.
Usually used for up to 4 days.

CONTRAINDICATIONS

History of hypersensitivity to atropine.

INTERACTIONS

Drug
Anticholinergic agents: May increase risk of adverse events.

Cromolyn inhalation solution:
Avoid mixing these drugs because they form a precipitate.
Herbal and Food
None known.

DIAGNOSTIC TEST EFFECTS

None known.

SIDE EFFECTS

Frequent
Inhalation (3%-6%): Cough, dry mouth, headache, nausea.
Nasal: Dry nose and mouth, headache, nasal irritation.
Occasional
Inhalation (2%): Dizziness, transient increased bronchospasm.
Rare (< 1%)
Inhalation: Hypotension, insomnia, metallic or unpleasant taste, palpitations, urine retention.
Nasal: Diarrhea or constipation, dry throat, abdominal pain, stuffy nose.

SERIOUS REACTIONS

• Worsening of angle-closure glaucoma, acute eye pain, and hypotension occur rarely.

PRECAUTIONS & CONSIDERATIONS

Caution is warranted in patients with bladder neck obstruction, angle-closure glaucoma, and benign prostatic hyperplasia. It is unknown whether ipratropium is distributed in breast milk. No age-related precautions have been noted in children or elderly patients. Drink plenty of fluids to decrease the thickness of lung secretions. Avoid excessive use of caffeinated products, such as chocolate, cocoa, cola, coffee, and tea.

Pulse rate and quality, respiratory rate, depth, rhythm and type, ABG levels, and serum potassium levels should be monitored. Lips and fingernails should be examined for a blue or gray color in light-skinned patients and a gray color in dark-skinned patients, which are signs of hypoxemia. Clinical improvement, such as cessation of retractions, quieter and slower respirations, and a relaxed facial expression should also be evaluated.

Administration

Shake the HFA container well. Exhale completely through mouth; then place the mouthpiece into the mouth and close lips, holding the inhaler upright. Inhale deeply through the mouth while fully depressing the top of the canister. Hold breath for as long as possible before exhaling slowly. Wait 2 min before inhaling the second dose to allow for deeper bronchial penetration. Rinse mouth with water immediately after inhalation to prevent mouth and throat dryness. Do not take more than 2 inhalations at a time because excessive use decreases the drug's effectiveness or produces paradoxical bronchoconstriction.

Nasal spray: Before using first time, prime unit with 7 sprays; if unit not used for 24 h, prime with 2 sprays, away from body. Blow nose gently to clear before use. Close one nostril, bend head slightly forward, insert nasal tip into open nostril. Point to back and outer wall of nose. Spray and sniff deeply. Repeat then repeat with other nostril (2 sprays per nostril).

Irbesartan

erb′ba-sar-tan
(Avapro, Karvea [AUS])

CATEGORY AND SCHEDULE

Pregnancy Risk Category: C (D if used in second or third trimester)

Classification: Angiotensin II receptor antagonists; antihypertensive

MECHANISM OF ACTION

An angiotensin II receptor, type AT_1, antagonist that blocks the vasoconstrictor and aldosterone-secreting effects of angiotensin II, inhibiting the binding of angiotensin II to the AT_1 receptors. *Therapeutic Effect:* Causes vasodilation, decreases peripheral resistance, and decreases BP.

PHARMACOKINETICS

Rapidly and completely absorbed after PO administration. Protein binding: 90%. Undergoes hepatic metabolism to inactive metabolite. Recovered primarily in feces and, to a lesser extent, in urine. Not removed by hemodialysis. *Half-life:* 11-15 h.

AVAILABILITY

Tablets: 75 mg, 150 mg, 300 mg.

INDICATIONS AND DOSAGES

▸ **Hypertension alone or in combination with other antihypertensives**
PO
Adults, Elderly. Initially, 150 mg/day. May increase to 300 mg/day. Use lower 75 mg/day initial dose if volume-depleted.

▸ **Diabetic nephropathy**
PO
Adults, Elderly. Target dose of 300 mg/day.

OFF-LABEL USES

Treatment of heart failure.

CONTRAINDICATIONS

Hypersensitivity to irbesartan.

INTERACTIONS

Drug

CYP2C9 Substrates: May increase levels of CYP2C9 substrates.
Hydrochlorothiazide: Further reduces BP.

NSAIDs: May decrease efficacy of irbesartan.
Potassium sparing diuretics: May increase risk of hyperkalemia.
Herbal
Ephedra, ginseng, yohimbe: May increase blood pressure.
Food
None known.

DIAGNOSTIC TEST EFFECTS
May slightly increase BUN and serum creatinine levels. May decrease blood hemoglobin level.

SIDE EFFECTS
Occasional (3%-9%)
Upper respiratory tract infection, fatigue, diarrhea, cough.
Rare (1%-2%)
Heartburn, dizziness, headache, nausea, rash.

SERIOUS REACTIONS
• Overdosage may manifest as hypotension and tachycardia. Bradycardia occurs less often.
• Rare serious hypersensitivity reactions.

PRECAUTIONS & CONSIDERATIONS
Caution is warranted in patients with congestive heart failure, coronary artery disease, mild to moderate hepatic dysfunction, sodium and water depletion, renal dysfunction and unilateral renal artery stenosis. It is unknown whether irbesartan is distributed in breast milk. Irbesartan may cause fetal or neonatal morbidity or mortality. Safety and efficacy of irbesartan have not been established in children. In clinical studies, irbesartan did not effectively lower blood pressure in hypertensive children. No age-related precautions have been noted in elderly patients. Sodium consumption and alcohol should be avoided.

Apical pulse and BP should be assessed immediately before each irbesartan dose and regularly throughout therapy. Be alert to fluctuations in apical pulse and BP. If an excessive reduction in BP occurs, place the person in the supine position with feet slightly elevated, and notify the physician. Tasks that require mental alertness or motor skills should be avoided. BUN, serum electrolytes, serum creatinine levels, heart rate for tachycardia, and urinalysis results should be obtained before and during therapy. Maintain adequate hydration; exercising outside during hot weather should be avoided to decrease the risk of dehydration and hypotension.
Administration
! Irbesartan may be given concurrently with other antihypertensives; if BP is not controlled by irbesartan alone, a diuretic may also be prescribed.
Take irbesartan without regard to meals.

Irinotecan
eye-ri-noe-tee′kan
(Camptosar)

CATEGORY AND SCHEDULE
Pregnancy Risk Category: D

Classification: Antineoplastics, topoisomerase inhibitors

MECHANISM OF ACTION
A DNA topoisomerase inhibitor that inhibits the action of topoisomerase I, an enzyme that allows DNA replication by producing reversible single-strand breaks in DNA that relieve torsional strain. Irinotecan prevents religation of the DNA strand, resulting in damage to

double-strand DNA and cell death. *Therapeutic Effect:* Kills cancer cells.

PHARMACOKINETICS

Metabolized to active metabolite in the liver after IV administration. Protein binding: 95% (metabolite). Excreted in urine and eliminated by biliary route. *Half-life:* 6 h; metabolite 10 h.

AVAILABILITY

Injection: 20 mg/mL.

INDICATIONS AND DOSAGES

▸ **Carcinoma of the colon or rectum that has progressed**
IV INFUSION
Adults, Elderly. Initially, 125 mg/m^2 once weekly for 4 wks, followed by a rest period of 2 wks. Additional courses may be repeated q6wk. Dosage may be adjusted in 25-50 mg/m^2 increments to as high as 150 mg/m^2 or as low as 50 mg/m^2.

CONTRAINDICATIONS

Concurrent use of ketoconazole or St. John's wort.

INTERACTIONS

Drug
Anticonvulsants: May decrease effects of irinotecan.
Atazanavir: May increase levels of irinotecan.
Bevacizumab: May increase adverse effects of irinotecan.
CYP2B6 inducers: May decrease levels of irinotecan.
CYP2B6 inhibitors: May increase levels of irinotecan.
CYP3A4 inducers: May decrease levels of irinotecan.
CYP3A4 inhibitors: May increase levels of irinotecan.
Diuretics: May increase the risk of dehydration from vomiting and diarrhea.

Ketoconazole: Increases levels of irinotecan and the active metabolite.
Laxatives: May increase the severity of diarrhea.
Live-virus vaccines: May potentiate virus replication, increase vaccine side effects, and decrease the patient's antibody response to the vaccine.
Other bone marrow depressants: May increase the risk of myelosuppression.
Prochlorperazine: May increase akathisia.
Herbal
St. John's wort: Decreases therapeutic effect of irinotecan.
Food
None known.

DIAGNOSTIC TEST EFFECTS

May increase serum alkaline phosphatase and AST (SGOT) levels.

Ⓘ IV INCOMPATIBILITIES

Epirubicin, gemcitabine (Gemzar), methylprednisolone sodium succinate (Solu-Medrol), pemetrexed, trastuzumab.

SIDE EFFECTS

Expected
Nausea (64%), alopecia (49%), vomiting (45%), diarrhea (32%).
Frequent
Constipation, fatigue (29%); fever (28%); asthenia (25%); skeletal pain (23%); abdominal pain, dyspnea (22%).
Occasional
Anorexia (19%); headache, stomatitis (18%); rash (16%).

SERIOUS REACTIONS

• Myelosuppression characterized as neutropenia occurs in 97% of patients; severe neutropenia, a neutrophil count < 50/mm^3-occurs in 78% of patients.
• Thrombocytopenia, anemia, and sepsis are common reactions.

PRECAUTIONS & CONSIDERATIONS

Caution is warranted in those who have previously received abdominal or pelvic irradiation because these patients are at increased risk for myelosuppression, patients with renal dysfunction, and elderly patients. Because of the risk of fetal harm, pregnant women should not take irinotecan, especially in the first trimester. It is unknown whether irinotecan is distributed in breast milk; however, breastfeeding is not recommended for patients taking this drug. The safety and efficacy of irinotecan have not been established in children. Elderly patients are at increased risk for diarrhea. Use the drug cautiously in patients older than 65 yr. Vaccinations and coming in contact with crowds, people with known infections, and anyone who has recently received a live-virus vaccine should be avoided.

Notify the physician if diarrhea, rash, or inflammation at the infusion site occurs. Hemoglobin levels, CBC, serum electrolytes, and hydration status should be monitored. Hair loss may occur and is reversible, but new hair may have a different color or texture.

Storage

Store vials at room temperature, and protect them from light. If the solution is reconstituted in D5W, it remains stable for up to 24 h at room temperature or 48 h if refrigerated. However, because the drug contains no preservative, it should be used within 6 h if kept at room temperature or within 24 h if refrigerated. Do not refrigerate the solution if it is diluted with 0.9% NaCl.

Administration

! As prescribed, begin a new irinotecan course when the patient's granulocyte count recovers to at least 1500/mm^3, platelet count recovers to at least 100,000/mm^3, and treatment-related diarrhea fully resolves.

Dilute the drug in D5W (the preferred diluent) or 0.9% NaCl to a concentration of 0.12-2.8 mg/mL. Infusion volume is usually 250-500 mL. Administer all doses by IV infusion over 90 min. Assess the patient for signs and symptoms of extravasation. If extravasation occurs, flush the site with sterile water and apply ice.

Iron Dextran

iron dex'tran

(Dexferrum, Dexiron [CAN], Infed, Infufer [CAN])

CATEGORY AND SCHEDULE

Pregnancy Risk Category: C

Classification: Hematinics, vitamins/minerals

MECHANISM OF ACTION

A trace element and essential component in the formation of hemoglobin. Necessary for effective erythropoiesis and transport and utilization of oxygen. Serves as cofactor of several essential enzymes. *Therapeutic Effect:* Replenishes hemoglobin and depleted iron stores.

PHARMACOKINETICS

Readily absorbed after IM administration. Most absorption occurs within 72 h; remainder within 3-4 wks. Bound to protein to form hemosiderin, ferritin, or transferrin. No physiologic system of elimination. Small amounts lost daily in shedding of skin, hair, and nails and in feces, urine, and perspiration. *Half-life:* 5-20 h.

AVAILABILITY
Injection: 50 mg/mL.

INDICATIONS AND DOSAGES
▸ **Iron deficiency anemia (no blood loss)**
IV, IM
Adults, Elderly. DOSE (mL) = 0.0442 (desired Hb - observed Hb) × LBW + (0.26 × LBW) (Lean body weight for males = 50 kg + 2.3 kg for each inch over 5 ft.
Lean body weight for females = 45.5 kg + 2.3 kg for each inch over 5 ft). Maximum: 100 mg/day.
▸ **Iron replacement secondary to blood loss**
IM, IV
Adults, Elderly. Replacement iron (mg) = blood loss (mL) times hematocrit.
▸ **Maximum daily dosage**
Adults weighing more than 50 kg. 100 mg.
Children weighing 10-50 kg. 100 mg.
Children weighing 5-9 kg. 50 mg.
Infants weighing < 5 kg. 25 mg.

CONTRAINDICATIONS
Hypersensitivity to the product. All anemias except iron deficiency anemia, including pernicious, aplastic, normocytic, and refractory; hemochromatosis; hemolytic anemia.

INTERACTIONS
Drug
Chloramphenicol: May decrease effect of iron dextran.
Herbal and Food
None known.

DIAGNOSTIC TEST EFFECTS
None known.

ⓦ IV INCOMPATIBILITIES
No information available via Y-site administration.

SIDE EFFECTS
Frequent
Allergic reaction (such as rash and itching), backache, myalgia, chills, dizziness, headache, fever, nausea, vomiting, flushed skin, pain or redness at injection site, brown discoloration of skin, metallic taste.

SERIOUS REACTIONS
• Anaphylaxis has occurred during the first few minutes after injection, causing death rarely.
• Leukocytosis and lymphadenopathy occur rarely.

PRECAUTIONS & CONSIDERATIONS
Extreme caution should be used with serious hepatic impairment. Caution is warranted with bronchial asthma, a history of allergies, and rheumatoid arthritis. Iron dextran may cross the placenta in some form and trace amounts of the drug are distributed in breast milk. No age-related precautions have been noted in children and elderly patients. Avoid taking oral iron while receiving iron injections.

Stools may become black during iron therapy, but this side effect is harmless unless accompanied by abdominal cramping, pain, or red streaking or sticky consistency of stool. Notify the physician of abdominal cramping or pain, back pain, fever, headache, or red streaking or sticky consistency of stool. Be alert for acute exacerbation of joint pain and swelling in persons with rheumatoid arthritis and iron deficiency anemia.
Storage
Store at room temperature.
Administration
! Plan to discontinue oral iron before administering iron dextran because excessive iron intake may

produce excessive iron storage
(hemosiderosis). Know that a test
dose is generally given before the
full dose; stay with the patient for
several minutes after injection of the
test dose because of the potential for
anaphylactic reaction.
! Before giving a therapeutic dose,
it is customary to give a test dose
of 25 mg. The patient is usually
observed for 1 h before commencing
therapeutic treatment.
   For IV use, may give undiluted or
dilute in 0.9% NaCl for infusion.
Do not exceed an administration
rate of 50 mg/min (1 mL/min).
A too-rapid IV rate may produce
flushing, chest pain, shock,
hypotension, and tachycardia. The
patient should stay recumbent for
30-45 min after IV administration to
minimize orthostatic hypotension.
   For IM use, draw up medication
with one needle; use new needle for
injection to minimize skin staining.
Use Z-tract technique by displacing
subcutaneous tissue lateral to
injection site before inserting
needle to minimize skin staining.
Administer deep into upper outer
quadrant of buttock only.

Iron Sucrose
iron su′crose
(Venofer)

CATEGORY AND SCHEDULE
Pregnancy Risk Category: B

Classification: Hematinics,
vitamins/minerals

MECHANISM OF ACTION
A trace element that is an
essential component in the
formation of hemoglobin.
It is necessary for effective
erythropoiesis and oxygen
transport capacity of blood,
and transport and utilization of
oxygen, and it serves as cofactor
of several essential enzymes.
Therapeutic Effect: Replenishes
body iron stores in patients on
long-term hemodialysis who have
iron deficiency anemia and are
receiving erythropoietin.

AVAILABILITY
Injection: 20 mg/mL or 100 mg
elemental iron in 5-mL single-dose
vial.

INDICATIONS AND DOSAGES
▸ **Iron deficiency anemia in patients
on chronic hemodialysis!**
Dosage is expressed in terms of
milligrams of elemental iron.
IV
Adults, Elderly. 5 mL iron sucrose,
or 100 mg elemental iron, delivered
during dialysis; administer 1-3 times
a wk to total dose of 1000 mg in
10 doses. Give no more than 3 times
weekly.
NOTE: Other dose regimens are
approved for patients receiving
peritoneal dialysis and who
are nondialysis dependent. See
manufacturer's literature.

CONTRAINDICATIONS
Hypersensitivity to iron sucrose;
all anemias except iron deficiency
anemia, including pernicious,
aplastic, normocytic, and refractory
anemia; evidence of iron overload.

INTERACTIONS
Drug
Dimercaprol: May increase
nephrotoxicity.
Oral iron preparations: Iron
sucrose may decrease absorption of
oral agents.

Herbal and Food
None known.

DIAGNOSTIC TEST EFFECTS
Increases hemoglobin and hematocrit, serum ferritin level, and serum transferrin saturation.

🚫 IV INCOMPATIBILITIES
Do not mix with other medications or add to parenteral nutrition solution for IV infusion.

SIDE EFFECTS
Frequent (23%-36%)
Hypotension, leg cramps, diarrhea.

SERIOUS REACTIONS
• Too rapid IV administration may produce severe hypotension, headache, vomiting, nausea, dizziness, paresthesia, abdominal and muscle pain, edema, and cardiovascular collapse.
• Hypersensitivity reaction occurs rarely.

PRECAUTIONS & CONSIDERATIONS
Caution is warranted in patients with cardiac dysfunction, bronchial asthma, history of allergies, and hepatic or renal impairment. Notify the physician of leg cramps or diarrhea. Initially, hematocrit, hemoglobin, serum ferritin, and serum transferrin levels should be obtained monthly, then every 2-3 mo as determined by the physician. Serum levels should be obtained 48 h after iron sucrose Administration. Monitor closely for hypotension.
Storage
Store at room temperature.
Administration
! Administer directly into dialysis line during hemodialysis, as prescribed.
   Can be given as undiluted, slow IV injection. For IV infusion, dilute each vial in maximum of 100 mL 0.9%

NaCl immediately before infusion. For IV injection, administer into the dialysis line at a rate of 1 mL, or 20 mg iron, undiluted solution per minute. Allow 5 min per vial; do not exceed 1 vial per injection. For IV infusion, administer into dialysis line at a rate of 100 mg iron over at least 15 min, to reduce the risk of hypotensive episodes. Expect to monitor the results of treatment.

Isocarboxazid
eye-soe-kar-box'a-zid
(Marplan)

CATEGORY AND SCHEDULE
Pregnancy Risk Category: C

Classification: Antidepressants, monoamine oxidase inhibitors

MECHANISM OF ACTION
An antidepressant that inhibits the MAO enzyme system at central nervous system (CNS) storage sites. The reduced MAO activity causes an increased concentration in epinephrine, norepinephrine, serotonin, and dopamine at neuron receptor sites. *Therapeutic Effect:* Produces antidepressant effect.

PHARMACOKINETICS
PO: Good absorption; maximum MAO inhibition 5-10 days, duration up to 2 wks; metabolized by liver; excreted by kidneys.

AVAILABILITY
Tablets: 10 mg (Marplan).

INDICATIONS AND DOSAGES
▸ **Depression refractory to other antidepressants or electroconvulsive therapy**

PO
Adults, Elderly. Initially, 10 mg
3 times/day. May increase to
60 mg/day.

OFF-LABEL USES

Treatment of panic disorder, vascular
or tension headaches.

CONTRAINDICATIONS

Cardiovascular disease (CVD),
cerebrovascular disease, liver
impairment, pheochromocytoma.
NOTE: Many drugs are contraindicated
for use within 14 days of MAOI use.

INTERACTIONS

Drug

Alcohol, CNS depressants: May
increase CNS depressant effects.

Bupropion: May increase neurotoxic
effects.

Buspirone: May increase BP.

Caffeine-containing medications:
May increase cardiac arrhythmias
and hypertension.

**Carbamazepine, cyclobenzaprine,
maprotiline, other MAOIs:** May
precipitate hypertensive crises.

CNS depressants: May increase
adverse effects.

CNS stimulants: Isocarboxazid may
increase hypertensive effects.

COMT inhibitors: May increase
adverse effects of isocarboxacid.

**Dextromethorphan, trazodone,
SSRIs, tricyclic antidepressants:**
May cause serotonin syndrome.
Contraindicated.

Insulin, oral hypoglycemics: May
increase effects of insulin and oral
hypoglycemics.

Linezolid: Additive MAOI actions.
Contraindicated.

Lithium: May increase adverse
effects of lithium.

**Meperidine, other opioid
analgesics:** May produce coma,
convulsions, death, diaphoresis,
immediate excitation, rigidity,
severe hypertension or hypotension,
severe respiratory distress, or
vascular collapse. Meperidine is
contraindicated.

Methylphenidate: May increase
the CNS stimulant effects of
methylphenidate.

Sympathomimetics: May
increase the cardiac stimulant and
vasopressor effects of isocarboxazid.
Contraindicated.

Tramadol: May increase risk of
seizures.

Tyramine: May cause severe,
sudden hypertension.

Herbal
None known.

Food
Foods high in tyramine: May cause
hypertensive crisis.

DIAGNOSTIC TEST EFFECTS

None known.

SIDE EFFECTS

Frequent (>10%)
Postural hypotension, drowsiness,
decreased sexual ability, weakness,
trembling, visual disturbances.

Occasional (1%-10%)
Tachycardia, peripheral
edema, nervousness, chills,
diarrhea, anorexia, constipation,
xerostomia.

Rare (< 1%)
Hepatitis, leukopenia, parkinsonian
syndrome.

SERIOUS REACTIONS

• Hypertensive crisis, marked
by severe hypertension, occipital
headache radiating frontally, neck
stiffness or soreness, nausea,
vomiting, sweating, fever or
chilliness, clammy skin, dilated
pupils, palpitations, tachycardia or
bradycardia, and constricting chest
pain.

PRECAUTIONS & CONSIDERATIONS

Caution is warranted in patients with asthma, bronchitis, bipolar disorder, cardiac arrhythmias, cardiovascular disease, diabetes mellitus, epilepsy, headaches, hepatic function impairment, hypertension, hyperthyroidism, Parkinson disease, renal function impairment, schizophrenia, and those with suicidal tendencies. Foods that require bacteria or molds for their preparation or preservation or containing tyramine, including avocados, bananas, beer, broad beans, cheese, figs, meat tenderizers, papaya, raisins, sour cream, soy sauce, wine, yeast extracts, yogurt, or excessive amounts of caffeine, such as chocolate, coffee, and tea should be avoided. It is unknown whether isocarboxazid crosses the placenta or is distributed in breast milk. Safety and efficacy have not been established in children or elderly patients.

Blurred vision, drowsiness, increased sweating, decreased sexual ability, and dizziness may be experienced while taking isocarboxazid. Headache, neck soreness or stiffness should be reported.

Administration
Use the lowest effective dose. Take with or without meals.

Isoetharine Hydrochloride/ Isoetharine Mesylate

eye-soe-eth′a-reen
(β-2)
Discontinued in the United States

CATEGORY AND SCHEDULE

Pregnancy Risk Category: C

Classification: Adrenergic agonists, bronchodilators

MECHANISM OF ACTION

A sympathomimetic (adrenergic agonist) that stimulates β_2-adrenergic receptors in the lungs, resulting in relaxation of bronchial smooth muscle. *Therapeutic Effect:* Relieves bronchospasm, reduces airway resistance.

PHARMACOKINETICS

Rapidly, well absorbed from the GI tract. Extensive metabolism in GI tract. Unknown extent metabolized in liver and lungs. Excreted in urine. *Half-life:* 4 h.

AVAILABILITY

Solution for Inhalation: 1%.

INDICATIONS AND DOSAGES

▸ **Bronchospasm**
HAND-BULB NEBULIZER
Adults, Elderly. 4 inhalations (range: 3-7 inhalations) undiluted. May be repeated up to 5 times/day.
▸ **IPPB, Oxygen Aerolization**
Adults, Elderly. 0.5 mL of a 1% solution diluted 1:3.

CONTRAINDICATIONS

History of hypersensitivity to sympathomimetics.

INTERACTIONS

Drug
β-adrenergic blocking agents (β-blockers): Antagonizes effects of isoetharine.
Digoxin: May increase risk of arrhythmias with digoxin.
MAOIs, tricyclic antidepressants: May potentiate cardiovascular effects.
Herbal and Food
None known.

DIAGNOSTIC TEST EFFECTS

May decrease serum potassium levels.

SIDE EFFECTS

Occasional

Tremor, nausea, nervousness, palpitations, tachycardia, peripheral vasodilation, dryness of mouth, throat, dizziness, vomiting, headache, increased BP, insomnia.

SERIOUS REACTIONS

• Excessive sympathomimetic stimulation may produce palpitations, extrasystoles, tachycardia, chest pain, slight increase in BP followed by a substantial decrease, chills, sweating, and blanching of skin.

• Too frequent or excessive use may lead to loss of bronchodilating effectiveness and severe and paradoxical bronchoconstriction.

PRECAUTIONS & CONSIDERATIONS

Caution is warranted in patients with cardiovascular disease, diabetes mellitus, hypertension, and hyperthyroidism. It is unknown whether isoetharine crosses the placenta or is distributed in breast milk. Safety and efficacy have not been established in children. Elderly patients may be more likely to develop tremors or tachycardia because of the age-related increased sympathetic sensitivity.

Avoid excessive use of caffeine derivatives, such as chocolate, cocoa, coffee, cola, and tea.

Storage

Store at room temperature.

Administration

For inhalation use, shake container well and exhale completely through the mouth. Place the mouthpiece into the mouth and close the lips while holding the inhaler upright. Inhale deeply through the mouth while fully depressing the top of the canister, and hold breath as long as possible before exhaling slowly. Wait 1 min before inhaling the second dose because this allows for deeper bronchial penetration. Rinse mouth with water immediately after inhalation to prevent mouth and throat dryness.

For nebulizer use, administer undiluted. May repeat up to 5 times daily.

For oxygen aerolization, administer over 15-20 min. Oxygen flow is usually adjusted to 4-6 L/min. Treatments are usually not repeated more than every 4 h.

Isoniazid (INH)

eye-soe-nye′a-zid

(INH, Isotamine [CAN], Nydrazid, PMS Isoniazid [CAN])

CATEGORY AND SCHEDULE

Pregnancy Risk Category: C

Classification:

Antimycobacterials; antitubercular

MECHANISM OF ACTION

An isonicotinic acid derivative that inhibits mycolic acid synthesis and causes disruption of the bacterial cell wall and loss of acid-fast properties in susceptible mycobacteria. Active only during bacterial cell division. *Therapeutic Effect:* Bactericidal against actively growing intracellular and extracellular susceptible mycobacteria.

PHARMACOKINETICS

Readily absorbed from the GI tract. Protein binding: 10%-15%. Widely distributed (including to the cerebrospinal fluid). Metabolized in the liver. Primarily excreted in urine. Removed by hemodialysis. *Half-life:* 0.5-5 h.

AVAILABILITY
Tablets: 100 mg, 300 mg.
Syrup: 50 mg/5 mL.
Injection: 100 mg/mL.

INDICATIONS AND DOSAGES
▸ **Tuberculosis (in combination with one or more antituberculars)**
PO, IM
Adults, Elderly. 5 mg/kg/day as a single dose. Maximum 300 mg/day.
Children. 10-15 mg/kg/day as a single dose. Maximum 300 mg/day.
▸ **Prevention of tuberculosis**
PO, IM
Adults, Elderly. 300 mg/day as a single dose.
Children. 10 mg/kg/day as a single dose. Maximum 300 mg/day.

CONTRAINDICATIONS
Acute hepatic disease, history of hypersensitivity reactions or hepatic injury with previous isoniazid therapy.

INTERACTIONS
Drug
Acetaminophen: May potentiate adverse effects of acetaminophen.
Alcohol: May increase isoniazid metabolism and the risk of hepatotoxicity.
Antacids: May decrease absorption of isoniazid.
Benzodiazepines: May decrease metabolism of benzodiazepines.
Carbamazepine, phenytoin, valproic acid: May increase the toxicity of these drugs.
Corticosteroids: May decrease concentrations of isoniazid.
CYP2C19 substrates: May increase levels of CYP2C19 substrates.
CYP2E1 substrates: May decrease levels of CYP2E1 substrates.
CYP3A4 substrates: May increase levels of CYP3A4 substrates.

Disulfiram: May increase central nervous system (CNS) effects.
Hepatotoxic medications: May increase the risk of hepatotoxicity.
Ketoconazole: May decrease ketoconazole blood concentration when INH given with rifampin.
Herbal
None known.
Food
All foods: Significantly reduce INH bioavailability.
Tyramine-containing foods: May cause a hypertensive crisis.

DIAGNOSTIC TEST EFFECTS
May increase serum bilirubin, AST (SGOT), and ALT (SGPT) levels.

SIDE EFFECTS
Frequent
Nausea, vomiting, diarrhea, abdominal pain.
Rare
Pain at injection site, hypersensitivity reaction.

SERIOUS REACTIONS
• Rare reactions include neurotoxicity (as evidenced by ataxia and paresthesia), optic neuritis, and hepatotoxicity.

PRECAUTIONS & CONSIDERATIONS
Caution should be used with alcoholic patients or those with chronic liver disease or severe renal impairment because it is more likely cross sensitivity to nicotinic acid or other chemically related medications will occur. Be aware that prophylactic use of isoniazid is usually postponed until after childbirth. Be aware that isoniazid crosses the placenta and is distributed in breast milk. No age-related precautions have been noted in children. Elderly patients are more susceptible to developing hepatitis.

Avoid consuming alcohol during treatment and taking any other medications without first notifying the physician, including antacids. Avoid foods containing tyramine, including aged cheeses, sauerkraut, smoked fish, and tuna because these foods may cause a reaction such as headache, a hot or clammy feeling, lightheadedness, pounding heartbeat, and red or itching skin.

! Determine whether the patient has any history of hypersensitivity reactions or liver injury from isoniazid as well as sensitivity to nicotinic acid or chemically related medications before starting drug therapy. Monitor the patient's liver function test results, and assess the patient for signs and symptoms of hepatitis as evidenced by anorexia, dark urine, fatigue, jaundice, nausea, vomiting, and weakness. If hepatitis is suspected, withhold the drug and notify the physician promptly. In addition, assess for burning, numbness, and tingling of the extremities. People at risk for neuropathy, such as alcoholics, those with chronic liver disease, diabetics, elderly patients, and malnourished individuals, may receive pyridoxine prophylactically.

Administration

Give 1 h before or 2 h after meals. Do not give with food. Administer at least 1 h before antacids, especially those containing aluminum. Do not skip doses and continue taking isoniazid for the full length of therapy (6-24 mo).

Isoproterenol
eye-soe-proe-ter´e-nole
(Isuprel)

CATEGORY AND SCHEDULE
Pregnancy Risk Category: C

Classification: Adrenergic agonists, bronchodilators

MECHANISM OF ACTION
A sympathomimetic (adrenergic agonist) that stimulates β_1-adrenergic receptors. *Therapeutic Effect:* Increases myocardial contractility, stroke volume, cardiac output.

PHARMACOKINETICS
Readily absorbed. Metabolized in liver. Primarily excreted in urine. *Half-life:* 2.5-5 min.

AVAILABILITY
Injection: 0.02 mg/mL, 0.2 mg/mL (Isuprel).

INDICATIONS AND DOSAGES
▶ **Arrhythmias**
IV BOLUS
Adults, Elderly. Initially, 0.02-0.06 mg (1-3 mL of diluted solution). Subsequent dose range: 0.01-0.2 mg (0.5-10 mL of diluted solution).
IV INFUSION
Adults, Elderly. Initially, 5 mcg/min (1.25 mL/min of diluted solution). Subsequent dose range: 2-20 mcg/min. *Children.* Initially, 0.1 mcg/kg per min. Range: 0.1-1 mcg/kg/min.
▶ **Shock and hypoperfusion**
IV INFUSION
Adults, Elderly. Rate of 0.5-5 mcg/min (0.25-2.5 mL of 1:500,000 dilution); rate of infusion based on clinical response (heart rate, central venous pressure, systemic BP, urine flow measurements).

CONTRAINDICATIONS

Tachycardia resulting from digitalis toxicity, preexisting arrhythmias, angina, precordial distress, hypersensitivity to isoproterenol, other sympathomimetic amines, or any component of the formulation.

INTERACTIONS

Drug

β-blockers: May antagonize the effects of isoproterenol.

Digoxin: May increase the risk of arrhythmias.

General anesthetics: May increase risk of arrhythmias.

Tricyclic antidepressants: May increase cardiovascular effects.

Sympathomimetic agents: May increase adverse effects.

Herbal

Ephedra, ma huang, yohimbe: May increase CNS stimulation.

Food

None known.

DIAGNOSTIC TEST EFFECTS

Decreases serum potassium levels.

ⓘ IV INCOMPATIBILITIES

Aminophylline, furosemide (Lasix), sbicarbonate.

ⓘ IV COMPATIBILITIES

Amiodarone (Cordarone), atracurium (Tracrium), bretylium (Bretylol), calcium chloride, cimetidine (Tagamet), cisatracurium (Nimbex), dobutamine (Dobutrex), famotidine (Pepcid), heparin, hydrocortisone sodium succinate (Solu-Cortef), inamrinone (Inocor), levofloxacin (Levaquin), magnesium sulfate, milrinone (Primacor), pancuronium (Panvulon), potassium chloride, propofol (Diprivan), ranitidine (Zantac), remifentanil (Ultiva), succinylcholine

(Anectine), tacrolimus (Prograf), vecuronium (Norcuron), verapamil (Calan), vitamin B complex with C.

SIDE EFFECTS

Frequent

Palpitations, tachycardia, restlessness, nervousness, tremor, insomnia, anxiety.

Occasional

Increased sweating, headache, nausea, flushed skin, dizziness, coughing.

SERIOUS REACTIONS

• Excessive sympathomimetic stimulation may cause palpitations, extrasystoles, tachycardia, chest pain, slight increase in BP followed by a substantial decrease, chills, sweating, and blanching of skin.

• Ventricular arrhythmias may occur if heart rate is above 130 beats/min.

• Parotid gland swelling may occur with prolonged use.

PRECAUTIONS & CONSIDERATIONS

Caution is warranted with hypersensitivity to sulfite, elderly or debilitated, hypertension, cardiovascular disease, impaired renal function, hyperthyroidism, diabetes mellitus, prostatic hypertrophy, seizure disorder, glaucoma. It is unknown whether isoproterenol crosses the placenta or is distributed in breast milk, so it is not administered to pregnant women. Safety and efficacy have not been established in children. Be aware that elderly patients may exhibit decreased therapeutic response (decreased heart rate, peripheral vascular response).

If chest pain or palpitations occur, notify the physician.

Storage

Store solution at room temperature. Do not use if the solution is pink to brown, contains a precipitate, or appears cloudy. Stability of parenteral admixture at room temperature or at refrigeration is 24 h.

Administration

Reconstitutite for IV push by diluting 0.2 mg (1 mL) of 1:5000 solution to a volume of 10 mL 0.9% NaCl or D5W. Give IV push at rate of 1 mL/min.

For IV infusion, dilute 0.2-2 mg (1-10 mL) of 1:5000 solution in 500 mL D5W to provide a solution of 0.4-4 mcg/mL. Rate of IV infusion determined by the person's heart rate, central venous pressure, systemic BP, and urine flow measurements. Use microdrip (60 drops/mL) or infusion pump to administer drug.

Regulate by ECG monitoring. If ECG changes occur, heart rate exceeds 110 beats/min, or premature beats occur, consider reducing rate of infusion or temporarily stopping infusion.

Isosorbide Dinitrate/ Mononitrate

(Apo-ISDN [CAN], Cedocard [CAN], Dilatrate, Isogen [AUS], Isordil, Sorbidin [AUS])(Duride [AUS], Imdur, Imtrate [AUS], ISMO, Monodur Durules [AUS], Monoket)

Do not confuse Isordil with Isuprel or Plendil, or Imdur with Inderal or K-Dur.

CATEGORY AND SCHEDULE

Pregnancy Risk Category: C

Classification: Vasodilators; nitrate antianginal

MECHANISM OF ACTION

A nitrate that stimulates intracellular cyclic guanosine monophosphate. *Therapeutic Effect:* Relaxes vascular smooth muscle of both arterial and venous vasculature. Decreases preload and afterload.

Dinitrate poorly absorbed and metabolized in the liver to its active metabolite isosorbide mononitrate. Mononitrate well absorbed after PO administration. Excreted in urine and feces. *Half-life:* Dinitrate, 1-4 h; mononitrate, 4 h.

AVAILABILITY

Capsules (Sustained Release [Dilatrate]): 40 mg.
Tablets (Isordil): 5 mg, 10 mg, 20 mg, 30 mg, 40 mg.
Tablets (ISMO, Monoket): 10 mg, 20 mg.
Tablets (Chewable): 5 mg, 10 mg.
Tablets (Extended Release [Imdur]): 30 mg, 60 mg, 120 mg.
Tablets (Sublingual [Isordil]): 2.5 mg, 5 mg, 10 mg.

INDICATIONS AND DOSAGES
▶ **Angina**
PO (ISOSORBIDE DINITRATE)
Adults, Elderly. 5-40 mg 4 times a day. Sustained-release: 40 mg q8-12h.
PO (ISOSORBIDE MONONITRATE)
Adults, Elderly. 5-10 mg twice a day given 7 h apart. Sustained-release: Initially, 30-60 mg/day in morning as a single dose. May increase dose at 3-day intervals. Maximum: 240 mg/day.

OFF-LABEL USES

Congestive heart failure, dysphagia, pain relief, relief of esophageal spasm with gastroesophageal reflux.

CONTRAINDICATIONS

Closed-angle glaucoma, GI hypermotility or malabsorption

(extended-release tablets), head trauma, hypersensitivity to nitrates, increased intracranial pressure, orthostatic hypotension, severe anemia (extended-release tablets).

INTERACTIONS

Drug

Antihypertensives, vasodilators: May increase risk of orthostatic hypotension.

CYP3A4 inducers: May decrease levels of isosorbide.

CYP3A4 inhibitors: May increase levels of isosorbide.

Sildenafil, tadalafil, vardenafil: May significantly decrease blood pressure. Concurrent use is contraindicated.

Herbal

None known.

Food

Alcohol: May increase risk of orthostatic hypotension.

DIAGNOSTIC TEST EFFECTS

May increase urine catecholamine and urine vanillylmandelic acid levels.

SIDE EFFECTS

Frequent

Burning and tingling at the oral point of dissolution (sublingual), headache (possibly severe) occurs mostly in early therapy, diminishes rapidly in intensity, and usually disappears during continued treatment, transient flushing of face and neck, dizziness (especially if the patient is standing immobile or is in a warm environment), weakness, orthostatic hypotension, nausea, vomiting, restlessness.

Occasional

GI upset, blurred vision, dry mouth.

SERIOUS REACTIONS

• Blurred vision or dry mouth

may occur (drug should be discontinued).

• Isosorbide administration may cause severe orthostatic hypotension manifested by fainting, pulselessness, cold or clammy skin, and diaphoresis.

• Tolerance may occur with repeated, prolonged therapy but may not occur with the extended-release form. Minor tolerance may be seen with intermittent use of sublingual tablets.

• High dosage tends to produce severe headache.

PRECAUTIONS & CONSIDERATIONS

Caution is warranted with acute MI, blood volume depletion from therapy, glaucoma (contraindicated in closed-angle glaucoma), hepatic or renal disease, and systolic BP < 90 mm Hg. It is unknown if isosorbide crosses the placenta or is distributed in breast milk. The safety and efficacy of isosorbide have not been established in children. Elderly patients may be more sensitive to the drug's hypotensive effects. In elderly patients, age-related decreased renal function may require cautious use. Alcohol should be avoided because it intensifies the drug's hypotensive effect. If alcohol is ingested soon after taking nitrates, an acute hypotensive episode marked by pallor, vertigo, and a drop in BP may occur.

Dizziness, lightheadedness, and headache may occur. Notify the physician of facial or neck flushing. The onset, type (sharp, dull, or squeezing), radiation, location, intensity, and duration of anginal pain and its precipitating factors, such as exertion and emotional stress, should be recorded before therapy begins.

Administration

Best if taken on an empty stomach; however, take oral isosorbide with meals if the headache occurs. Oral tablets, except the extended-release form, may be crushed. Do not crush or break the extended-release form. Do not crush the chewable form before administering.

For sublingual use, do not crush or chew tablets. Dissolve tablets under tongue without swallowing. Isosorbide should be taken at the first sign or symptom of angina. If angina is not relieved within 5 min, dissolve a second tablet under the tongue and then repeat the dosage 5 min later if there is no relief. Do not take more than 3 tablets within 15-30 min.

Isotretinoin
eye-soe-tret′i-noyn
(Accutane, Amnesteem, Claravis, Isotrex [CAN], Sotret)
Do not confuse Accutane with Accupril or Accurbron.

CATEGORY AND SCHEDULE
Pregnancy Risk Category: X

Classification: Retinoids; vitamin A derivative

MECHANISM OF ACTION
Reduces the size of sebaceous glands and inhibits their activity. *Therapeutic Effect:* Decreases sebum production; produces antikeratinizing and anti-inflammatory effects.

PHARMACOKINETICS
Metabolized in the liver; major metabolite active. Eliminated in urine and feces. *Half-life:* 21 h; metabolite, 21-24 h.

AVAILABILITY
Capsules: 10 mg, 20 mg, 30 mg, 40 mg.

INDICATIONS AND DOSAGES
▶ **Recalcitrant cystic acne that is unresponsive to conventional acne therapies**
PO
Adults, Children 12 yr of age and older. Initially, 0.5-1 mg/kg/day, divided into 2 doses for 15-20 wks. May repeat after at least 2 mo off therapy. Severe acne may require 2 mg/kg/day.

OFF-LABEL USES
Treatment of gram-negative folliculitis, severe keratinization disorders, severe rosacea.

CONTRAINDICATIONS
Hypersensitivity to isotretinoin or parabens (component of capsules); pregnancy.

INTERACTIONS
Drug
Carbamazepine: May decrease levels of carbamazepine.
Etretinate, tretinoin, vitamin A: May increase toxic effects.
Oral contraceptives: May decrease efficacy of oral contraceptives.
Tetracycline: May increase the risk of pseudotumor cerebri.
Tigecycline: May cause pseudotumor cerebri.
Herbal
Dong quai, St John's wort: May cause photosensitization.
Food
Milk: May increase bioavailability of isotretinoin.

DIAGNOSTIC TEST EFFECTS
May increase serum alkaline phosphatase, total cholesterol, LDH, triglyceride, ALT (SGPT), and AST (SGOT) levels; urine uric acid level; erythrocyte sedimentation rate; and fasting blood glucose level. May decrease HDL level.

SIDE EFFECTS
Frequent (20%-90%)
Cheilitis (inflammation of lips), dry skin and mucous membranes, skin fragility, pruritus, epistaxis, dry nose and mouth, conjunctivitis, hypertriglyceridemia, nausea, vomiting, abdominal pain.
Occasional (5%-16%)
Musculoskeletal symptoms (including bone pain, arthralgia, generalized myalgia), photosensitivity.
Rare
Decreased night vision, depression.

SERIOUS REACTIONS
• Inflammatory bowel disease and pseudotumor cerebri (benign intracranial hypertension) have been associated with isotretinoin therapy.
• Hearing impairment may occur and may continue after isotretinoin is discontinued.

PRECAUTIONS & CONSIDERATIONS
Caution should be used in patients with renal or hepatic dysfunction. Depression, psychosis, aggressive behavior, and suicide have been reported with this medication. Be aware that isotretinoin is contraindicated in pregnancy. Patients, prescribers, wholesalers, and dispensing pharmacists must register with the iPledge program. There is an extremely high risk of major deformities in infants if pregnancy occurs while taking any amount of isotretinoin, even for short periods. The person must be capable of understanding and carrying out instructions and of complying with mandatory contraception (two forms). Be aware that excretion in milk is unknown; due to potential for serious adverse effects, it is not recommended during nursing. No age-related precautions have been noted in children or elderly patients.

Women must have two negative serum pregnancy tests within 2 wks before starting therapy; therapy will begin on the second or third day of the next normal menstrual period. Effective contraception (using 2 reliable forms of contraception simultaneously) must be used for at least 1 mo before, during, and for at least 1 mo after therapy. Give both oral and written warnings, with the patient acknowledging in writing that she understands the warnings and consents to treatment. Prescriptions may only be written for 30 days and pregnancy testing and counseling should be repeated monthly.

Isotretinoin may have decreased tolerance to contact lenses during and after therapy. Notify the physician immediately if abdominal pain, severe diarrhea, rectal bleeding (possible inflammatory bowel disease), or headache, nausea and vomiting, visual disturbances (possible pseudotumor cerebri) occur.
Storage
Store at room temperature and protect from light.
Administration
Give isotretinoin with food and a full glass of liquid to reduce esophogeal irritation. Patients should receive and read a Med Guide with each prescription and refill.

Isradipine
is-rad´-ih-peen
(DynaCirc, DynaCirc CR)
**Do not confuse DynaCirc with
Dynabac or Dynacin.**

CATEGORY AND SCHEDULE
Pregnancy Risk Category: C

Classification: Calcium channel
blockers

MECHANISM OF ACTION
An antihypertensive that inhibits
calcium movement across cardiac
and vascular smooth-muscle cell
membranes. Potent peripheral
vasodilator that does not depress SA
or AV nodes. *Therapeutic Effect:*
Produces relaxation of coronary
vascular smooth muscle and
coronary vasodilation. Increases
myocardial oxygen delivery to those
with vasospastic angina.

PHARMACOKINETICS

Route	Onset	Peak	Duration
PO	2-3 h	2-4 wks (with multiple doses)	NA
		8-16 h (with single dose)	
PO (controlled release)	2 h	8-10 h	NA

Well absorbed from the GI tract.
Protein binding: 95%. Metabolized
in the liver (undergoes first-pass
effect). Primarily excreted in urine.
Not removed by hemodialysis.
Half-life: 8 h.

AVAILABILITY
Capsules (DynaCirc): 2.5 mg, 5 mg.
*Capsules (Controlled-Release
[DynaCirc CR]):* 5 mg, 10 mg.

INDICATIONS AND DOSAGES
▸ **Hypertension**
PO (IMMEDIATE RELEASE)
Adults, Elderly. Initially 2.5 mg twice
a day. May increase by 2.5 mg at
2- to 4-wks intervals. Range:
5-20 mg/day in divided doses
twice daily.
PO (EXTENDED RELEASE)
Initially, 5 mg once daily. Usual
dose 5-10 mg/day. Maximum:
20 mg/day.

OFF-LABEL USES
Treatment of chronic angina pectoris,
Raynaud's phenomenon.

CONTRAINDICATIONS
Cardiogenic shock, congestive heart
failure, heart block, hypotension, sinus
bradycardia, ventricular tachycardia.

INTERACTIONS
Drug
β-blockers: May have additive
effect.
Carbamazepine: May increase the
effect of carbamazepine.
**Indomethacin, possibly other
NSAIDs, phenobarbital:** May
decrease effect.
**Parenteral and inhalation general
anesthetics, hypotensive agents,
itraconazole:** Possible increased
effect.
Herbal
None known.
Food
Grapefruit, grapefruit juice: May
increase the absorption of isradipine.
Avoid.

DIAGNOSTIC TEST EFFECTS
None known.

SIDE EFFECTS

Frequent (4%-7%)
Peripheral edema, palpitations (higher frequency in female patients).
Occasional (3%)
Facial flushing, cough.
Rare (1%-2%)
Angina, tachycardia, rash, pruritus.

SERIOUS REACTIONS

• Overdose produces nausea, drowsiness, confusion, and slurred speech.
• Congestive heart failure occurs rarely.
Caution
Congestive heart failure, hypotension, hepatic disease, lactation, children, renal disease, elderly patients.

PRECAUTIONS & CONSIDERATIONS

Caution is warranted in patients with edema, hepatic disease, severe left ventricular dysfunction, sick sinus syndrome, and in those concurrently receiving β-blockers or digoxin. It is unknown whether isradipine crosses the placenta or is distributed in breast milk. The safety and efficacy of isradipine have not been established in children. In elderly patients, age-related renal impairment may require cautious use. Grapefruit juice, which may increase isradipine blood concentration, should be avoided. Tasks that require alertness and motor skills should also be avoided.

Avoid using sodium-containing products, such as IV saline fluids, for patients with a dietary salt restriction. Patients should be assessed for stress-induced angina episodes, which may occur during isradipine therapy.

Notify the physician if irregular heartbeat, nausea, pronounced dizziness, or shortness of breath

occurs. Rise slowly from a lying to a sitting position and wait momentarily before standing to avoid isradipine's hypotensive effect. Apical pulse and BP should be assessed immediately before beginning isradipine administration. If the pulse rate is 60 beats/min or lower or systolic BP is < 90 mm Hg, withhold the medication and contact the physician. Liver function tests should also be performed before and during therapy. Skin should be assessed for flushing and peripheral edema, especially behind the medial malleolus and the sacral area. Blood dyscrasias may occur in patients on chronic isradipine therapy, which may include signs of infection, bleeding, and poor healing.
Administration
Do not crush, open, or break extended-release capsules. Do not abruptly discontinue isradipine. Compliance is essential to control hypertension. May take without regard to food.

Itraconazole

it-ra-con′a-zol
(Sporanox)
Do not confuse Sporanox with Suprax.

CATEGORY AND SCHEDULE

Pregnancy Risk Category: C

Classification: Systemic triazole antifungal

MECHANISM OF ACTION

A fungistatic antifungal that inhibits the synthesis of ergosterol, a vital component of fungal cell formation. *Therapeutic Effect:* Damages the fungal cell membrane, altering its function.

PHARMACOKINETICS

Moderately absorbed from the GI tract. Absorption is increased if the drug is taken with food. Protein binding: 99%. Widely distributed, primarily in the fatty tissue, liver, and kidneys. Metabolized in the liver to active metabolite. Primarily excreted in urine. Not removed by hemodialysis. *Half-life:* 21 h; metabolite, 12 h.

AVAILABILITY

Capsules: 100 mg.
Oral Solution: 10 mg/mL.
Injection: 10 mg/mL (25-mL ampule).

INDICATIONS AND DOSAGES

▸ **Blastomycosis, histoplasmosis, and aspergillosis**
PO
Adults, Elderly. Initially, 200 mg once a day. Maximum: 400 mg/day in 2 divided doses.
IV INFUSION
Adults, Elderly. 200 mg twice a day for 4 doses, then 200 mg once a day.
▸ **Life-threatening fungal infections**
PO
Adults, Elderly. 600 mg/day in 3 divided doses for 3-4 days, then 200-400 mg/day in 2 divided doses.
IV
Adults, Elderly. 200 mg twice a day for 4 doses, then 200 mg once a day.
▸ **Esophageal candidiasis**
PO (ORAL SOLUTION ONLY)
Adults, Elderly. Swish 10 mL in mouth for several seconds, then swallow. Maximum: 200 mg/day.
▸ **Oropharyngeal candidiasis**
PO (ORAL SOLUTION ONLY)
Adults, Elderly. Vigorously swish 10 mL in the mouth for several seconds and then swallow (20 mL total daily dose) once a day. Usually given 1-2 wks.

▸ **Dosage in renal impairment**
Do not use itraconazole IV if CrCl < 30 mL/min.
▸ **Onychomycosis of toenails**
PO
Adults. 200 mg once daily for 12 wks.
▸ **Onychomycosis of fingernails**
PO
Adults. Give 200 mg twice daily for 1 wk; rest for 3 wks; then give 200 mg twice daily for 1 wk.

OFF-LABEL USES

Suppression of histoplasmosis; treatment of disseminated sporotrichosis, fungal pneumonia and septicemia, or ringworm of the hand.

CONTRAINDICATIONS

Hypersensitivity to itraconazole, fluconazole, ketoconazole, or miconazole. Do not use itraconazole for treatment of onychomycosis if patient has CHF. Coadministration with cisapride, pimozide, quinidine, dofetilide, levomethadyl, lovastatin, simvastatin, and ergot alkaloids is contraindicated.

INTERACTIONS

Drug
Antacids, didanosine, H₂ antagonists: May decrease itraconazole absorption; take itraconazole 2 h before taking antacids, didanosine or H₂ antagonists.
Buspirone, cyclosporine, digoxin, midazolam, triazolam, allopurinol, felodipine: May increase blood concentration of these drugs.
Carbamazepine, phenobarbital: May increase metabolism of itraconazole.
Cyclosporine, protease inhibitors, nisoldipine, haloperidol, carbamazepine, erythromycin, clarithromycin, azithromycin, alfentanil, corticosteroids, zolpidem: May increase plasma level of these drugs.

HMG-CoA reductase inhibitors (statins): May increase side effects and plasma levels of statins; either avoid using itraconazole with statins or lower their dosages when using itraconazole to limit the risk of rhabdomyolysis. Lovastatin and simvastatin are contraindicated.

Oral anticoagulants, warfarin: May inhibit warfarin metabolism; may increase the effect of oral anticoagulants generally.

Oral antidiabetic agents: May increase the risk of hypoglycemia developing.

Phenytoin, rifampin: May decrease itraconazole blood concentration.

Herbal
None known.

Food

Cola products: May increase plasma levels of itraconazole.

Grapefruit juice: May decrease itraconazole absorption.

DIAGNOSTIC TEST EFFECTS

May increase serum LDH, serum alkaline phosphatase, serum bilirubin, SGOT (AST), and SGPT (ALT) levels. May decrease serum potassium level.

Ⓓ IV INCOMPATIBILITIES

! Dilution compatibilities of itraconazole with any solution other than 0.9% NaCl is unknown. Don't mix with D5W or lactated Ringer's solution. Not for IV bolus administration. Do not administer any medication in same bag or through same IV line as itraconazole.

SIDE EFFECTS

Frequent (9%-11%)
Nausea, rash.

Occasional (3%-5%)
Vomiting, headache, diarrhea, hypertension, peripheral edema, fatigue, fever.

Rare (2% or less)
Abdominal pain, dizziness, anorexia, pruritus.

SERIOUS REACTIONS

• Hepatitis (as evidenced by anorexia, abdominal pain, unusual fatigue or weakness, jaundiced skin or sclera, and dark urine) occurs rarely.

• May cause new or worsened heart failure.

PRECAUTIONS & CONSIDERATIONS

Caution is warranted in patients with achlorhydria, hepatitis, HIV infection, hypochlorhydria, or impaired liver function, or patients with heart failure on risk factors for cardiac compromise. Be aware that itraconazole is distributed in breast milk. Be aware that the safety and efficacy of itraconazole have not been established in children. In elderly patients, age-related renal impairment may require dosage adjustment. Carefully assess potential serious drug interactions.

Obtain the baseline temperature, check the liver-function test results, as appropriate, and determine whether there is a history of allergies before giving the drug. Assess for signs and symptoms of liver dysfunction. Report any anorexia, dark urine, nausea, pale stool, unusual fatigue, yellow skin, or vomiting to the physician. Development of hepatic problems may require durg discontinuation. Avoid grapefruits and grapefruit juice because they can alter itraconazole absorption. Therapy will continue for at least 3 mo and until lab tests and overall condition indicate that the infection is controlled. Be aware that itraconazole has a tendency to create GI side effects; telling the patient to remain in semisupine position while reclining will reduce these effects. Capsules should be taken with food to avoid GI effects.

Storage

Store oral formulations and solutions for injection at room temperature. Do not freeze.

Administration

! Doses larger than 200 mg should be given in 2 divided doses. Give capsules with food to increase absorption. Give solution on an empty stomach.

For IV administration, use only components provided by the manufacturer. Do not dilute with any other diluent. Add full contents of amp (250 mg/10 mL) to infusion bag provided (50 mL 0.9% NaCl) and mix gently.

! Then withdraw 15 mL of the solution from the bag before administering to patient; otherwise, patient will receive overdosage. Infuse over 60 min using the extension line and infusion set provided. After administration, flush infusion set with 15-20 mL 0.9% NaCl over 30 s to 15 min, and discard entire infusion line.

Ivermectin (Systemic)

eye-ver-mek′tin
(Stromectol, Mectizan [CAN])

CATEGORY AND SCHEDULE

Pregnancy Risk Category: C

Classification: Antihelmintics, systemic

MECHANISM OF ACTION

Selectively binds to chloride ion channels in invertebrate nerve/muscle cells, increasing permeability to chloride ions. In general, the following organisms are susceptible to ivermectin: *Onchocerca volvulus,* pediculosis capitis, *Strongyloides stercoralis, Sarcoptes scabiei,* and *Wuchereria bancrofti. Therapeutic Effects:* Causes paralysis/death of parasites.

PHARMACOKINETICS

Does not readily cross the blood-brain barrier. Metabolized in the liver. Excreted in the feces. *Half-life:* 4 h. Well absorbed with plasma concentrations proportional to the dose.

AVAILABILITY

Tablets: 3 mg.

INDICATIONS AND DOSAGES
▸ **Strongyloidiasis**
PO
Adults, Elderly, Children weighing < 3 lb. 200 mcg/kg as a single dose.
▸ **Onchocerciasis (river blindness)**
PO
Adults, Elderly, Children weighing more than33 lbs. 150 mcg/kg as a single dose at 3-12-mo intervals (12 mo is most common).
▸ **Scabies**
PO
Adults. 200 mcg/kg as a single dose and repeat 2 wks later.
▸ **Norwegian scabies (crusted scabies infection), superinfected scabies, or resistant scabies**
PO
Adults. 200 mcg/kg with repeated treatments or combined with a topical scabicide.
▸ **Pediculosis (resistant cases)**
PO
Adults. A regimen of 2 doses of 200 mcg/kg with each dose separated by 10 days.

OFF-LABEL USES

Cutaneous larva migrans, filariasis, pediculosis, scabies, *Wuchereria bancrofti* (Bancroft's filariasis).

CONTRAINDICATIONS

Hypersensitivity to ivermectin or to any one of its components. Should not be used in women who are pregnant, in infants or children under 33 lb.

INTERACTIONS

Drug
Carbamazepine: May decrease the concentration of ivermectin.
Corticosteroids: May have a synergistic effect with ivermectin reducing inflammation caused by river blindness infestation.
CYP3A4 inducers: Decrease the levels of ivermectin.
CYP3A4 inhibitors: Increase the levels of ivermectin.
Warfarin: Reports of increased INR.
Herbal
None known.
Food
None known.

DIAGNOSTIC TEST EFFECTS

May increase SGOT (AST), SGPT (ALT), alkaline phosphatase, BUN, eosinophil count.
May decrease WBC.

SIDE EFFECTS

Occasional
Abdominal pain, anorexia, arthralgia, constipation, diarrhea, dizziness, drowsiness, edema, fatigue, fever, lymphadenopathy, maculopapular or unspecified rash, nausea, vomiting, orthostatic hypotension, pruritus, Stevens-Johnson syndrome, toxic epidermal necrolysis, tremor, urticaria, vertigo, visual impairment, weakness.
Less Common
Eye or eyelid irritation, pain, redness, swelling, headache, swelling of the face, arms, feet or legs.
Rare
Orthostatic hypotension, loss of appetite, shaking or trembling, sleepiness.

PRECAUTIONS & CONSIDERATIONS

Caution is warranted in patients with bronchial asthma. Treating *Loa loa* infection with ivermectin may result in encephalopathy. It is unknown whether ivermectin crosses the placenta and should be avoided during pregnancy. Ivermectin is distributed into breast milk; however, it is not reported to cause problems in nursing babies. Safety and efficacy have not been established in children under 33 pounds or in elderly patients.

Lightheadedness may occur. Tasks that require mental alertness or motor skills should be avoided. Joint or muscle pain, fever, pain and tender glands in neck, armpits or groin, skin rash or rapid heartbeat may also occur (primarily during onchocerciasis therapy).

Follow-up medical examination schedules should be adhered to; additional treatment may be required in intervals of 3-12 mo.
Administration
Take as a single dose with a full glass of water 1 h before breakfast.

Kanamycin Sulfate
kan-a-mye′sin suhl-feyt
(Kantrex)

CATEGORY AND SCHEDULE
Pregnancy Risk Category
(injectible): D

Classification: Antibiotics,
aminoglycosides

MECHANISM OF ACTION
An aminoglycoside antibiotic
that irreversibly binds to
protein on bacterial ribosomes.
Therapeutic Effect: Interferes with
protein synthesis of susceptible
microorganisms.

PHARMACOKINETICS
Rapidly absorbed after IM injection;
poorly absorbed from GI tract
(orally). Little if any metabolic
transformation occurs; excreted
unchanged through urine and feces.
Half-life: 2 h.

AVAILABILITY
Injection: 333 mg/mL.

INDICATIONS AND DOSAGES
▸ **Topical wound and surgical site
irrigation**
Adults, Elderly. 0.25% solution to
irrigate pleural space, ventricular or
abscess cavities, wounds, or surgical
sites.
▸ **Infection**
IM/IV
Adults, Elderly, Children.
15 mg/kg/day in 2-4 divided doses
not to exceed 1.5 g daily.
▸ **Tuberculosis**
IM/IV
Adults, Elderly, Children.
15-30 mg/kg/day not to exceed
1 g/day.

▸ **Dosage in renal impairment**
Extend IV or IM dosage interval to
q18h or q24h depending on degree of
impairment; guide further doses by
peak and trough concentration.

CONTRAINDICATIONS
Hypersensitivity to kanamycin, other
aminoglycosides (cross-sensitivity),
or their components.
Pregnancy: Teratogenic.
Caution
Renal impairment, severe burn wounds.

INTERACTIONS
Drug
**Amphotericin, cephalosporins,
enflurane, methoxyflurane,
vancomycin:** May increase the risk
of nephrotoxicity.
Loop diuretics: May increase risk of
ototoxicity.
**Other aminoglycosides
(concurrent use):** Increased
risk of nephrotoxicity, ototoxicity
and neuromuscular
blockade.
Herbal
None significant.
Food
None significant.

DIAGNOSTIC TEST EFFECTS
May increase BUN/Scr. Peak serum
concentrations > 35 mcg/mL and
trough concentrations > 10 mcg/mL
should be avoided.

SIDE EFFECTS
Occasional
Hypersensitivity reactions (fever,
pruritus, rash, urticaria).
Rare
Headache.

SERIOUS REACTIONS
• Hearing loss with high dose or
prolonged use.
• Renal impairment.

PRECAUTIONS & CONSIDERATIONS

No information is available regarding pregnancy for irrigating solution. Teratogenic in pregnancy, excreted in breast milk (IM, IV). Use cautiously in premature infants and newborns because of their renal immaturity. No age-related precautions have been noted in children or in elderly patients. Assess for hypersensitivity to kanamycin or other aminoglycosides before beginning therapy.

In severely burned patients, half-life may significantly decrease. Dose adjustment is required in patients with renal function impairment to avoid increased risk of ototoxicity developing.

May manifest both auditory and vestibular ototoxicity, which occurs most often in patients with renal damage who are undergoing prolonged therapy. Partial or total irreversible deafness may continue to develop after drug therapy is stopped.

Advise the patient that ringing in the ears, hearing impairment, rash, difficulty urinating, and dizziness should be reported to the health care provider for further evaluation and possible medication change.

Storage
Darkening of solution over time does not affect potency. Store at room temperature.

Administration
Irrigating solution is administered topically and into body cavities.

For IV administration, dilute each 500 mg with 100-200 mL or more of 0.9% NaCl or D5W. Give slowly over 30-60 min.

IM injection should be given deeply into upper outer quadrant of gluteal muscle.

Ketamine Hydrochloride
kee-ta-meen high-droh-klor-ide
(Ketalar)

CATEGORY AND SCHEDULE
Pregnancy Risk Category: B

Classification: Anesthetics, general

MECHANISM OF ACTION
A rapidly acting general anesthetic that selectively blocks afferent impulses and interacts with central nervous system (CNS) transmitter systems. *Therapeutic Effect:* Produces an anesthetic state characterized by profound analgesia and normal pharyngeal-laryngeal reflexes.

PHARMACOKINETICS

Route	Onset	Peak	Duration
IM (anesthetic)	3-4 min	N/A	12-25 min
IM (analgesic)	30 min	N/A	15-30 min
IV (anesthetic)	30 s	N/A	5-10 min
IV (analgesic)	10-15 min	N/A	NA

Rapidly distributed. Metabolized in the liver. Primarily excreted in urine. *Half-life:* Distribution: 10-15 min, elimination: 2-3 h.

AVAILABILITY
Injection: 10 mg/mL, 50 mg/mL, 100 mg/mL.

INDICATIONS AND DOSAGES
▸ **Sole anesthetic for short diagnostic and surgical procedures that do not require skeletal muscle relaxation, induction of anesthesia**

before administering other general anesthetics, supplement to low-potency agents
IM
Adults, Elderly. 3-8 mg/kg.
Children. 3-7 mg/kg.
IV
Adults, Elderly. 1-4.5 mg/kg.
Children. 0.5-2 mg/kg.

CONTRAINDICATIONS

Known hypersensitivity, aneurysms, angina, congestive heart failure, elevated intracranial pressure, hypertension, thyrotoxicosis.

INTERACTIONS

Drug
All CNS depressants and nondepolarizing muscle relaxants: May increase the risk of hypotension and prolonged respiratory depression.
Herbal and Food
None known.

DIAGNOSTIC TEST EFFECTS

May increase intraocular pressure.

⊘ IV INCOMPATIBILITIES

No information available for Y-site administration.

⬗ IV COMPATIBILITIES

Bupivacaine (Marcaine), clonidine (Duraclon), fentanyl (Sublimaze), lidocaine, morphine, propofol (Diprivan).

SIDE EFFECTS

Frequent
Increased BP and pulse rate; emergence reaction (marked by dreamlike state, delirium, hallucinations, and vivid imagery and occasionally accompanied by confusion, excitement, and irrational behavior; lasts from few hours to 24 h after ketamine administration).

Occasional
Pain at injection site.
Rare
Rash.

SERIOUS REACTIONS

• Continuous or repeated intermittent infusion may result in extreme somnolence and circulatory or respiratory depression.
• Too-rapid IV administration of ketamine may produce severe hypotension, respiratory depression, and irregular muscle movements.
• Psychiatric effects: hallucinations, emergence delirium.

PRECAUTIONS & CONSIDERATIONS

Caution is warranted with intoxication, chronic alcoholism, a full stomach, gastroesophageal reflux disease, and hepatic impairment. Ketamine is not recommended for pregnant or breastfeeding women. No age-related precautions have been noted in children or in elderly patients. Avoid tasks requiring mental alertness or motor skills until 24 h after anesthesia has been discontinued.

Patients must be continually monitored and facilities for maintenance of patent airway, ventilatory support, oxygen supplementation, and circulatory resuscitation should be immediately available.

Strict aseptic techniques must be followed in handling ketamine HCl.

Vital signs should be monitored before and every 3-5 min during and after ketamine administration until the patient has recovered. A barbiturate or hypnotic should be administered in an emergence reaction. Verbal, tactile, and visual stimulation should be minimized during the recovery period. Advise the patient to avoid performing tasks requiring mental alertness or motor skills for 24 h after

K

anesthesia has been discontinued. A responsible person must drive patient home after recovery.

Storage
Store unopened vials at room temperature. Protect from light.

Administration
Give ketamine by IV push over 60 sec when it is used to induce anesthesia. Dilute the 100 mg/mL vial of ketamine with an equal volume of sterile water for injection, D5W, or 0.9% NaCl. For a maintenance IV infusion, dilute the 50-mg/mL vial (10 mL) or 100-mg/mL vial (5 mL) of ketamine with 250-500 mL D5W or 0.9% NaCl to provide a concentration of 1-2 mg/mL. Administer maintenance dose by IV push slowly at a rate of 0.5 mg/kg/min over 60 s. A too-rapid IV administration may result in severe hypotension and respiratory depression.

For IM administration, use the 10-mg/mL vial of ketamine. Do not dilute the 10-mg/mL vial.

Ketoconazole
kee-toe-koe′na-zole
(Apo-Ketocomazole [CAN], Nizoral, Nizoral AD, Sebizole [AUS])
Do not confuse Nizoral with Nasarel.

CATEGORY AND SCHEDULE
Pregnancy Risk Category: C
OTC (1% shampoo only)

Classification: Imidazole antifungal

MECHANISM OF ACTION
A fungistatic antifungal that inhibits the synthesis of ergosterol, a vital component of fungal cell formation. *Therapeutic Effect:* Damages the fungal cell membrane, altering its function.

PHARMACOKINETICS
PO: Peak serum concentrations achieved in 1-2 h; Highly protein bound. Metabolized in liver, excreted in bile, feces. Requires acidic pH for absorption; distributed poorly to cerebrospinal fluid (CSF). *Half-life:* 2 h; terminal half-life: 8 h.

AVAILABILITY
Tablets (Nizoral): 200 mg.
Cream (Nizoral): 2%.
Shampoo (Nizoral AD): 1%.

INDICATIONS AND DOSAGES
▸ **Histoplasmosis, blastomycosis, systemic candidiasis, chronic mucocutaneous candidiasis, coccidioidomycosis, paracoccidioidomycosis, chromomycosis, seborrheic dermatitis, tinea corporis, tinea capitis, tinea manus, tinea cruris, tinea pedis, tinea unguium (onychomycosis), oral thrush, candiduria**
PO
Adults, Elderly. 200-400 mg/day. Maximum: 800 mg/day in 2 divided doses.
Children 2 yr of age and older. 3.3-6.6 mg/kg/day.
Topical
Adults, Elderly. Apply to affected area 1-2 times a day for 2-4 wks.
Shampoo
Adults, Elderly. Use twice weekly for 4 wks, allowing at least 3 days between shampooing. Use intermittently to maintain control.

OFF-LABEL USES
Systemic: Treatment of fungal pneumonia.

CONTRAINDICATIONS
Hypersensitivity, lactation, fungal meningitis.
Systemic coadministration with cisapride, pimozide, quinidine, dofetilide, lovastatin, simvastatin, ergot alkaloids, terfenadine, astemizole, and triazolam is contraindicated.

INTERACTIONS
Drug
Alcohol, acetaminophen (high-dose, long-term use); carbamazepine, sulfonamides, and other hepatotoxic medications: May increase hepatotoxicity of ketoconazole.
Antacids, anticholinergics, didanosine, H_2 antagonists, proton-pump inhibitors (omeprazole): May decrease ketoconazole absorption; take 2 h after ketoconazole dose.
Benzodiazepines (midazolam, triazolam), warfarin: May inhibit metabolism of these drugs.
Cyclosporine, HMG-CoA reductase inhibitors (statins): May increase blood concentration and risk of hepatotoxicity of these drugs. Contraindicated with lovastatin and simvastatin.
Buspirone, carbamazepine, corticosteroids, haloperidol, Indinavir, nisoldipine, ritonavir, saquinavir, tricyclic antidepressants, zolpidem: May increase levels of these drugs.
Isoniazid, rifampin: May decrease blood concentration of ketoconazole.
Tacrolimus: May cause leukocytic disorders.
Systemic coadministration with cisapride, pimozide, quinidine, dofetilide, lovastatin, simvastin, ergot alkaloids, terfenadine, astemizole, and triazolam: Contraindicated; do not use.
Herbal
Echinacea: May have additive hepatotoxic effects.
Food
None known.

DIAGNOSTIC TEST EFFECTS
May increase serum alkaline phosphatase, serum bilirubin, SGOT (AST), and SGPT (ALT) levels. May decrease serum corticosteroid and testosterone concentrations.

SIDE EFFECTS
Occasional (3%-10%)
Nausea, vomiting.
Rare (< 2%)
Abdominal pain, diarrhea, headache, dizziness, photophobia, pruritus.
Topical: itching, burning, irritation.

SERIOUS REACTIONS
• Hematologic toxicity (as evidenced by thrombocytopenia, hemolytic anemia, and leukopenia) occurs occasionally.
• Hepatotoxicity may occur within 1 wk to several months after starting therapy.
• Anaphylaxis occurs rarely.

PRECAUTIONS & CONSIDERATIONS
Caution is warranted with liver impairment. Use with care in lactation, pregnancy, children, elderly with renal impairment.
Confirm that a culture or histologic test was done for accurate diagnosis; therapy may begin before results are known.
Expect to monitor liver function test results. Be alert for signs and symptoms of hepatotoxicity, including anorexia, dark urine, fatigue, nausea, pale stools, and vomiting, that are unrelieved by giving the medication

with food. Monitor complete blood count (CBC) for evidence of hematologic toxicity. Assess the daily pattern of bowel activity and stool consistency. Assess for dizziness, provide assistance as needed, and institute safety precautions. Evaluate skin for itching, rash, and urticaria.

Prolonged therapy over weeks or months is usually necessary. Do not miss a dose, and continue therapy for as long as directed. Avoid alcohol to avoid potential liver toxicity. Avoid tasks that require mental alertness or motor skills until response to the drug is established.

If dark urine, increased irritation in topical use, onset of other new symptoms, pale stool, or yellow skin or eyes develop, notify the physician.

In dermatologic treatment, separate personal items that come in direct contact with the affected area.

Administration
Give oral ketoconazole with food to minimize GI irritation. Tablets may be crushed. Ketoconazole requires acidity for absorption in the GI tract; give didanosine, antacids, anticholinergics, H$_2$ blockers, and proton-pump inhibitors (all) at least 2 h after dosing.

Apply ketoconazole shampoo to wet hair, massage for 1 min, rinse thoroughly, reapply for 3 min, then rinse. Use initially twice weekly for 4 wks with at least 3 days between shampooing. Further shampooing will be based on the response to the initial treatment.

Apply topical ketoconazole sparingly and rub gently into the affected and surrounding area. Avoid drug contact with the eyes, keep the skin clean and dry, and wear light clothing for ventilation.

Ketoprofen
kee-toe-proe′fen
(Apo-Keto [CAN], Novo-Keto-EC, Orudis [AUS], Orudis KT [CAN], Orudis SR [AUS], Oruvail, Oruvail SR [AUS], Rhodis [CAN])

CATEGORY AND SCHEDULE
Pregnancy Risk Category: B (D if used in third trimester or near delivery)
OTC (tablets)

Classification: Analgesics, nonsteroidal anti-inflammatory drug

MECHANISM OF ACTION
An NSAID that produces analgesic and anti-inflammatory effects by inhibiting prostaglandin synthesis. *Therapeutic Effect:* Reduces the inflammatory response and intensity of pain.

PHARMACOKINETICS
PO: Peak levels achieved in 2 h. 99% plasma protein binding. Metabolized in liver, excreted in urine and breast milk as metabolites. *Half-life:* 3-3.5 h.

AVAILABILITY
Capsules: 50 mg, 75 mg.
Capsules (Extended-Release [Oruvail]): 100 mg, 150 mg, 200 mg.
Tablets (Orudis KT): 12.5 mg (OTC).

INDICATIONS AND DOSAGES
▸ **Acute or chronic rheumatoid arthritis and osteoarthritis**
PO (CAPSULES)
Adults. Initially, 75 mg 3 times a day or 50 mg 4 times a day.
Elderly. Initially, 25-50 mg 3-4 times a day. Maintenance: 150-300 mg/day in 3-4 divided doses.

PO (EXTENDED-RELEASE)
Adults, Elderly. 100-200 mg once a day.
▶ **Mild to moderate pain, dysmenorrhea**
PO
Adults, Elderly. 25-50 mg q6-8h. Maximum: 300 mg/day.
▶ **Over-the-counter (OTC) dosage**
PO
Adults, Elderly. 12.5 mg q4-6h. Maximum: 6 tablets/day.
▶ **Dosage in renal impairment**
Mild: 150 mg/day maximum.
Severe: 100 mg/day maximum.

OFF-LABEL USES

Treatment of acute gouty arthritis, psoriatic arthritis, ankylosing spondylitis, vascular headache.

CONTRAINDICATIONS

Active peptic ulcer disease, chronic inflammation of the GI tract, GI bleeding or ulceration, history of hypersensitivity to aspirin or NSAIDs; use within 14 days of CABG surgery.

INTERACTIONS

Drug
Acetaminophen (long-term or chronic use): Increased risk of nephrotoxicity, hepatotoxicity.
Antihypertensives, diuretics: May decrease the effects of these drugs.
Aspirin, other NSAIDs, corticosteroids, alcohol, or other salicylates: May increase the risk of GI side effects such as bleeding.
Bone marrow depressants: May increase the risk of hematologic reactions.
Cyclosporine: Possible decreased renal function.
Diuretics: May decrease diuretic effect.
First time users of SSRIs: May have a higher risk of GI side effects.

Heparin, oral anticoagulants, thrombolytics, oral antidiabetic agents: May increase the effects of these drugs.
Lithium: May increase the blood concentration and risk of toxicity of lithium.
Methotrexate: May increase the risk of methotrexate toxicity.
Probenecid: May increase the ketoprofen blood concentration.
Tetracycline: Possible increased photosensitivity.
Herbal
Feverfew: May decrease the effects of feverfew.
Ginkgo biloba: May increase the risk of bleeding.
Food
None known.

DIAGNOSTIC TEST EFFECTS

May prolong bleeding time. May increase serum alkaline phosphatase levels and liver function test results. May decrease hematocrit, blood hemoglobin, and serum sodium levels.

SIDE EFFECTS

Frequent (11%)
Dyspepsia.
Occasional (> 3%)
Nausea, diarrhea or constipation, flatulence, abdominal cramps, headache.
Rare (< 2%)
Anorexia, vomiting, visual disturbances, fluid retention.

SERIOUS REACTIONS

• Rare reactions with long-term use include peptic ulcer disease, GI bleeding, gastritis, and severe hepatic reactions (cholestasis, jaundice), nephrotoxicity (dysuria, hematuria, proteinuria, nephrotic syndrome), and severe hypersensitivity reaction (bronchospasm, angioedema).

K

PRECAUTIONS & CONSIDERATIONS

Caution is warranted with a history of GI tract disease, hepatic or renal impairment, and a predisposition to fluid retention. Avoid alcohol and aspirin during therapy because these substances increase the risk of GI bleeding. Drug is excreted in breast milk as metabolite; caution is warranted in lactation. It is not known whether drug crosses placenta; use with caution in pregnancy. No age-related precautions are noted except in cases of impaired renal function where dose adjustment may be required or in individuals age 75 or older.

CBC, blood chemistry studies, PT, aPTT, and renal and liver function tests should be obtained at the beginning and throughout therapy. Therapeutic response, such as improved grip strength, increased mobility, improved range of motion, and decreased pain, tenderness, stiffness, and swelling, should be assessed.

Because of possible increased photosensitivity attributed to NSAIDs, patients should be advised to wear a sunscreen with SPF 15 while in sunlight or high sunlight reflectivity (e.g., snow, water) environments.

Storage

Store at room temperature. Protect from light and moisture.

Administration

! Do not exceed a ketoprofen dosage of 300 mg/day. Oruvail is not recommended as initial therapy for those older than 75 yr or those with renal impairment.

Take ketoprofen with food, a full glass (8 oz) of water, or milk to minimize GI distress. Do not break, open, or chew extended-release capsules.

Ketorolac Tromethamine

kee-tor-oh-lak tro-meth-ay-meen
(Acular, Acular LS, Acular PF, Toradol)

Do not confuse Acular with Acthar or Ocular.

CATEGORY AND SCHEDULE

Pregnancy Risk Category: C (D if used in third trimester)

Classification: Nonsteroidal anti-inflammatory drugs, ophthalmics

MECHANISM OF ACTION

An NSAID that inhibits prostaglandin synthesis and reduces prostaglandin levels in the aqueous humor and body. *Therapeutic Effect:* Relieves pain stimulus and reduces intraocular inflammation.

PHARMACOKINETICS

Route	Onset	Peak	Duration
PO	30-60 min	1.5-4 h	4-6 h
IV/IM	30 min	1-2 h	4-6 h

Readily absorbed from the GI tract, after IM administration. Protein binding: 99%. Largely metabolized in the liver. Primarily excreted in urine. Not removed by hemodialysis. *Half-life:* 3.8-6.3 h (increased with impaired renal function and in elderly patients).

AVAILABILITY

Tablets (Toradol): 10 mg.
Injection (Toradol): 15 mg/mL, 30 mg/mL.
Ophthalmic Solution (Acular): 0.5%.
Ophthalmic Solution (Acular LS): 0.4%.

Ophthalmic Solution (Acular PF):
0.5%.

INDICATIONS AND DOSAGES
▸ **Short-term relief of mild to moderate pain (multiple doses)**
PO
Adults, Elderly. 10 mg q4-6h.
Maximum: 40 mg/24 h.
IV/IM
Adults younger than 65 yr. 30 mg q6h. Maximum: 120 mg/24 h.
Elderly 65 yr and older, Adults with renal impairment or weighing < 50 kg. 15 mg q6h. Maximum: 60 mg/24 h.
▸ **Short-term relief of mild to moderate pain (single dose)**
IV
Adults younger than 65 yr, Adolescents 17 yr and older weighing more than 50 kg: 30 mg.
Elderly 65 yr and older, Adults with renal impairment or weighing < 50 kg. 15 mg.
Children 2-16 yr. 0.5 mg/kg. Maximum: 15 mg.
IM
Adults younger than 65 yr, Children 17 yr and older, weighing more than 50 kg. 60 mg.
Elderly 65 yr and older, Adults with renal impairment or weighing < 50 kg. 30 mg.
Children 2-16 yr. 1 mg/kg. Maximum: 30 mg.
▸ **Allergic conjunctivitis**
OPHTHALMIC (ACULAR)
Adults, Elderly, Children 3 yr and older. 1 drop 4 times a day.
▸ **Cataract extraction**
OPHTHALMIC
Adults, Elderly. 1 drop 4 times a day. Begin 24 h after surgery and continue for 2 wks.
▸ **Refractive surgery**
OPHTHALMIC (ACULAR
LS OR ACULAR PF)
Adults, Elderly. 1 drop 4 times a day

for 4 days for Acular LS, 3 days for Acular PF.

OFF-LABEL USES
Prevention or treatment of ocular inflammation (ophthalmic form).

CONTRAINDICATIONS
Active peptic ulcer disease, chronic inflammation of the GI tract, GI bleeding or ulceration, history of hypersensitivity to aspirin or NSAIDs, use with 14 days of CABG surgery, advanced renal failure, labor and delivery, breast-feeding, cerebrovascular bleeding and other serious bleeding or risk for such bleeding, use with probenecid or pentoxifylline, use with aspirin or other NSAIDs.

INTERACTIONS
Drug
Aspirin, other salicylates, other NSAIDs, alcohol, corticosteroids: May increase the risk of GI side effects such as bleeding.
β-Blockers, ACE inhibitors, diuretics: May decrease the antihypertensive effects of these.
Bone marrow depressants: May increase the risk of hematologic reactions.
Cyclosporine: Possible decreased renal function.
First time users of SSRIs: May have a higher risk of GI side effects.
Heparin, oral anticoagulants, thrombolytics: May increase the effects of these drugs.
Lithium: May increase the blood concentration and risk of toxicity of lithium.
Methotrexate: May increase the risk of methotrexate toxicity.
Other NSAIDs: Contraindicated for concurrent use.
Pentoxifylline: Contraindicated for concurrent use.

K

Probenecid: May increase ketorolac blood concentration to dangerous levels; contraindicated; do not use.
Herbal
Feverfew: May decrease the effects of feverfew.
Ginkgo biloba: May increase the risk of bleeding.
Food
None known.

DIAGNOSTIC TEST EFFECTS

May prolong bleeding time. May increase liver function test results.

Ⓘ IV INCOMPATIBILITIES

Promethazine (Phenergan).

Ⓘ IV COMPATIBILITIES

Fentanyl (Sublimaze), hydromorphone (Dilaudid), morphine, nalbuphine (Nubain).

SIDE EFFECTS

Frequent (12%-17%)
Headache, nausea, abdominal cramps or pain, dyspepsia.
Occasional (3%-9%)
Diarrhea.
Ophthalmic: Transient stinging and burning.
Rare (1%-3%)
Constipation, vomiting, flatulence, stomatitis, dizziness.
Ophthalmic: Ocular irritation, allergic reactions, superficial ocular infection, keratitis.

SERIOUS REACTIONS

• Rare reactions with long-term use include peptic ulcer disease, GI bleeding, gastritis, severe hepatic reactions (cholestasis, jaundice), nephrotoxicity (glomerular nephritis, interstitial nephritis, nephrotic syndrome), and an acute hypersensitivity reaction (including fever, chills, and joint pain).

• Hemmorrhage.
• Hypersensitivity.

PRECAUTIONS & CONSIDERATIONS

Caution is warranted with a history of GI tract disease, hepatic or renal impairment, and a predisposition to fluid retention. It is unknown whether ketorolac is excreted in breast milk. Ketorolac should not be used during the third trimester of pregnancy because it can cause adverse effects in the fetus, such as premature closure of the ductus arteriosus. Notify the physician if pregnant. The safety and efficacy of ketorolac have not been established in children, for continued use; a single-dose regimen should be adhered to.

GI bleeding or ulceration is more likely to cause serious complications, and age-related renal impairment may increase the risk of hepatotoxicity or renal toxicity; a decreased dosage is recommended. Avoid alcohol and aspirin during therapy because these substances increase the risk of GI bleeding. Tasks that require mental alertness or motor skills should also be avoided.

CBC, liver and renal function test results, urine output, BUN level, serum alkaline phosphatase, bilirubin, and creatinine levels should be assessed. Be alert for signs of bleeding, which may also occur with ophthalmic use if systemic absorption occurs. Therapeutic response, such as decreased pain, stiffness, swelling, and tenderness; improved grip strength; and increased joint mobility, should be evaluated.
Administration
! Ketorolac should not be administered by any route or combination of routes for more than 5 days. This drug may be given as a

single dose, on a schedule, or on an as-needed basis, as prescribed.

Take oral ketorolac with food, milk, or antacids if GI distress occurs. Oral dosing is usually preceded by IM injection. Oral medication should not be taken for more than 5 consecutive days.

For IV use, administer ketorolac undiluted by IV push over at least 15 s.

For IM use, slowly inject the drug deeply into a large muscle mass.

For ophthalmic use, place a finger on lower eyelid, and pull it out until a pocket is formed between the eye and lower lid. Hold the dropper above the pocket, and place the prescribed number of drops in the pocket. Gently close eye and apply digital pressure to the lacrimal sac for 1-2 min to minimize drainage into the nose and throat, reducing the risk of systemic effects. Remove excess solution with a tissue.

K

Labetalol Hydrochloride

la-bet'a-lole high-droh-klor-ide
(Normodyne, Presolol [AUS],
Trandate)
**Do not confuse Trandate with
tramadol or Trental.**

CATEGORY AND SCHEDULE

Pregnancy Risk Category: C (D if
used in second or third trimester)

Classification: Nonselective
adrenergic β-blocker and selective
α_1-blocker; antihypertensive

MECHANISM OF ACTION

An antihypertensive that blocks
α_1-, β_1-, and β_2- (large doses)
adrenergic receptor sites. Large
doses increase airway resistance.
Therapeutic Effect: Slows sinus
heart rate; decreases peripheral
vascular resistance, cardiac output,
and BP.

PHARMACOKINETICS

Route	Onset	Peak	Duration (h)
PO	0.5-2 h	2-4 h	8-12 h
IV	2-5 min	5-15 min	2-4 h

Completely absorbed from the
GI tract. Protein binding: 50%.
Undergoes first-pass metabolism.
Metabolized in the liver. Primarily
excreted in urine. Not removed by
hemodialysis. *Half-life:* PO, 6-8 h;
IV, 5.5 h.

AVAILABILITY

Tablets (Normodyne, Trandate):
100 mg, 200 mg, 300 mg.
Injection (Trandate): 5 mg/mL.

INDICATIONS AND DOSAGES

▶ **Hypertension**
PO
Adults. Initially, 100 mg twice a day
adjusted in increments of 100 mg
twice a day q2-3 days. Maintenance:
200-400 mg twice a day. Maximum:
2.4 g/day.
Elderly. Initially, 100 mg 1-2 times
a day. May increase as needed.
▶ **Severe hypertension, hypertensive
emergency**
IV
Adults. Initially, 20 mg. Additional
doses of 20-80 mg may be given at
10-min intervals, up to total dose of
300 mg.
IV INFUSION
Adults. Initially, 2 mg/min up to total
dose of 300 mg.
PO (AFTER IV THERAPY)
Adults. Initially, 200 mg; then,
200-400 mg in 6-12 h. Increase dose
at 1-day intervals to desired level.

OFF-LABEL USES

Control of hypotension during
surgery, treatment of chronic angina
pectoris.

CONTRAINDICATIONS

Bronchial asthma, cardiogenic
shock, second- or third-degree
heart block, severe bradycardia,
uncontrolled congestive heart failure,
hypersensitivity.

INTERACTIONS

Drug
Diphenhydramine: May increase
plasma level.
Diuretics, other antihypertensives:
May increase hypotensive effect.
**Hydrocarbon inhalation
anesthetics:** May increase risk
of hypotension or myocardial
depression.
Indomethacin, NSAIDs: May
decrease hypotensive effect.

Insulin, oral hypoglycemics: May mask symptoms of hypoglycemia and prolong hypoglycemic effect of these drugs.
Lidocaine: May result in decreased metabolism of labetalol.
MAOIs: May produce hypertension.
Sympathomimetics, xanthines: May mutually inhibit effects.
Herbal
None known.
Food
None known.

DIAGNOSTIC TEST EFFECTS

May increase serum antinuclear antibody titer and BUN, serum LDH, lipoprotein, alkaline phosphatase, bilirubin, creatinine, potassium, triglyceride, uric acid, AST (SGOT), and ALT (SGPT) levels.

ⓘ IV INCOMPATIBILITIES

Amphotericin B complex (Abelcet, AmBisome, Amphotec), ceftriaxone (Rocephin), furosemide (Lasix), heparin, nafcillin (Nafcil), thiopental, sodium bicarbonate solutions.

ⓘ IV COMPATIBILITIES

Aminophylline, amiodarone (Cordarone), calcium gluconate, diltiazem (Cardizem), dobutamine (Dobutrex), dopamine (Intropin), enalapril (Vasotec), fentanyl (Sublimaze), hydromorphone (Dilaudid), lidocaine, lorazepam (Ativan), magnesium sulfate, midazolam (Versed), milrinone (Primacor), morphine, nitroglycerin, norepinephrine (Levophed), potassium chloride, potassium phosphate, propofol (Diprivan).

SIDE EFFECTS

Frequent
Drowsiness, difficulty sleeping, unusual fatigue or weakness, diminished sexual ability, transient scalp tingling.
Occasional
Dizziness, dyspnea, peripheral edema, depression, anxiety, constipation, diarrhea, nasal congestion, nausea, vomiting, abdominal discomfort.
Rare
Altered taste, dry eyes, increased urination, paresthesia.

SERIOUS REACTIONS

• Labetolol administration may precipitate or aggravate congestive heart failure (CHF) because of decreased myocardial stimulation.
• Abrupt withdrawal may precipitate ischemic heart disease, producing sweating, palpitations, headache, and tremor.
• May mask signs and symptoms of acute hypoglycemia (tachycardia, BP changes) in patients with diabetes.
• Hepatic injury, necrosis (rare).

PRECAUTIONS & CONSIDERATIONS

Caution is warranted in patients with diabetes mellitus, medication-controlled CHF, impaired cardiac or hepatic function, nonallergic bronchospastic disease, including chronic bronchitis and emphysema. Patient with pheochromocytoma may require higher doses or closer monitoring to avoid paradoxical hypertension. Labetalol crosses the placenta and is distributed in small amounts in breast milk. The safety and efficacy of labetalol have not been established in children. In elderly patients, age-related peripheral vascular disease may increase susceptibility to decreased peripheral circulation. Be aware that salt and alcohol intake should be restricted. Nasal decongestants or OTC cold preparations (stimulants) should not be used without physician approval.

Notify the physician of excessive fatigue, headache, prolonged dizziness, shortness of breath, or weight gain. BP for hypotension, respiratory status for shortness of breath, pattern of daily bowel activity and stool consistency, ECG for arrhythmias, and pulse for quality, rate, and rhythm should be monitored during treatment. If pulse rate is 60 beats/min or lower or systolic BP is < 90 mm Hg, withhold the medication and contact the physician. Signs and symptoms of CHF, such as decreased urine output, distended neck veins, dyspnea (particularly on exertion or lying down), night cough, peripheral edema, and weight gain should also be assessed.

Storage

Store at room temperature. After dilution, IV solution is stable for 24 h.

Administration

Labetalol may be taken without regard to meals. Crush tablets if necessary. Do not abruptly discontinue the drug.

! Place the patient in a supine position for IV administration and for 3 h after receiving the medication. Expect a substantial drop in BP if the patient stands within 3 h following drug administration.

The solution for injection normally appears clear and colorless to light yellow; discard the solution if precipitate forms or discoloration occurs. For IV infusion, dilute 200 mg in 160 mL dextrose 5% in water, 0.9% NaCl, lactated Ringer's solution, or any combination of these solutions to provide a concentration of 1 mg/mL. For IV push, give slowly over 2 min at 10-min intervals. For IV infusion, administer at a rate of 2 mg/min (2 mL/min) initially. Adjust the rate according to the patient's BP. Monitor the patient's BP immediately before and every 5-10 min during IV administration. Maximum effect occurs within 5 min of any IV push injection.

Lactulose
lak′tyoo-lose
(Apo-Lactulose[CAN], Cholac, Constilac, Constulose, Duphalac [CAN], Enulose, Generlac, Genlac [AUS], PMS-Lactulose[CAN], RatioLactulose [CAN]).
Do not confuse Cholac with diclofenac or lactulose with lactose.

CATEGORY AND SCHEDULE
Pregnancy Risk Category: B

Classification: Hyperosmotic agent

MECHANISM OF ACTION
A lactose derivative that retains ammonia in the colon and decreases serum ammonia concentration, producing an osmotic effect. *Therapeutic Effect:* Promotes increased peristalsis and bowel evacuation, which expels ammonia from the colon.

PHARMACOKINETICS

Route	Onset	Peak	Duration
PO	24-48 h	NA	NA
Rectal	30-60 min	NA	NA

Poorly absorbed from the GI tract. Acts in the colon. Primarily excreted in feces.

AVAILABILITY
Syrup: 10 g/15 mL.
Packets: 10 g, 20 g.

INDICATIONS AND DOSAGES
▸ **Constipation (Chronulac, Constilac, Duphalac, Constulose)**
PO
Adults, Elderly. 15-30 mL(10-20 g lactulose)/day, up to 60 mL (40 g)/day.

Children. 7.5 mL (5 g)/day after breakfast.

▸ **Portal-systemic encephalopathy (Cephalac, Cholac, Enulose)**
PO
Adults, Elderly. Initially, 30-45 mL every 3-4 h/day. Then 30-45 mL (20-30 g) 3-4 times a day. Adjust dose q1-2 days to produce 2-3 soft stools a day. Hourly doses of 30-45 mL may be used for rapid laxation initially; then it may be reduced to recommended daily dose levels.
Children. 40-90 mL/day in divided doses to produce 2-3 soft stools/day.
Infants. 2.5-10 mL/day in divided doses to produce 2-3 soft stools/day.
RECTAL (AS RETENTION ENEMA)
Adults, Elderly. 300 mL with 700 mL water or saline solution; patient should retain 30-60 min. Repeat q4-6h. If evacuation occurs too promptly, repeat immediately.

CONTRAINDICATIONS

Abdominal pain, appendicitis, nausea, patients on a galactose-free diet, vomiting.
Other laxatives: Do not use concomitantly.

INTERACTIONS

Drug
Neomycin, other anti-infectives: May interfere with degradation of lactulose and prevent acidification of colonic contents.
Nonabsorbable antacids: May inhibit colonic acidification.
Oral medication: May decrease transit time of concurrently administered oral medications, decreasing lactulose absorption.
Herbal and Food
None known.

DIAGNOSTIC TEST EFFECTS

None well documented.

SIDE EFFECTS

Occasional
Abdominal cramping, flatulence, increased thirst, abdominal discomfort.
Rare
Nausea, vomiting.

SERIOUS REACTIONS

• Diarrhea indicates overdose; adjust dosage downward.
• Long-term use may result in laxative dependence, chronic constipation, and loss of normal bowel function.

PRECAUTIONS & CONSIDERATIONS

Caution is warranted in patients with diabetes mellitus. It is unknown whether lactulose crosses the placenta or is distributed in breast milk. Lactulose use should be avoided in children younger than 6 yr of age as the child may develop hyponatremia and dehydration. No age-related precautions have been noted in elderly patients, but extended use (> 6 mo) may increase risk of dehydration and electrolyte imbalance.
    Maintain adequate fluid intake. Electrolyte levels and pattern of daily bowel activity and stool consistency should be monitored. Periodic serum ammonia levels should be obtained. Mix with fruit juice, water, or milk to make oral solution more palatable.
Storage
Store solution at room temperature.
Administration
Oral solution normally appears pale yellow to yellow and viscous in consistency. However, cloudy, darkened solution does not indicate potency loss. Evacuation occurs in 24-48 h of the initial drug dose. To promote defecation, increase fluid intake, exercise, and eat a high-fiber diet. Some patients find liquid more palatable when mixed with fruit juice, water, or milk.

L

The powder for oral solution (10- or 20-g packet) should be dissolved in at least 4 oz of water.

For rectal use, lubricate anus with petroleum jelly before applicator insertion. Insert applicator carefully, to prevent damage to the rectal wall, with nozzle toward navel. Squeeze container until entire dose has been expelled. Retain liquid until definite lower abdominal cramping is felt. Evacuation occurs in 24-48 h of the initial drug dose.

Lamivudine (3TC)

la-miv'yoo-deen
(Epivir, Epivir-HBV, Heptovir [CAN], Zeffix [AUS])
Do not confuse lamivudine with lamotrigine.

CATEGORY AND SCHEDULE

Pregnancy Risk Category: C

Classification: Antiretrovirals, nucleoside reverse transcriptase inhibitors

MECHANISM OF ACTION

An antiviral that inhibits HIV reverse transcriptase by viral DNA chain termination. Also inhibits RNA- and DNA-dependent DNA polymerase, an enzyme necessary for HIV replication. *Therapeutic Effect:* Interrupts HIV replication, slowing the progression of HIV infection.

PHARMACOKINETICS

Rapidly and completely absorbed from the GI tract. Protein binding: 36%. Widely distributed (crosses the blood-brain barrier). Primarily excreted unchanged in urine. Not removed by hemodialysis or peritoneal dialysis. *Half-life:* 11-15 h

(intracellular), 2-11 h (serum, adults), 1.7-2 h (serum, children) (increased in impaired renal function).

AVAILABILITY

Oral Solution: (Epivir): 10 mg/mL; (Epivir-HBV): 5 mg/mL.
Tablets: (Epivir): 150 mg, 300 mg; (Epivir-HBV): 100 mg.

INDICATIONS AND DOSAGES
▸ **HIV infection (in combination with other antiretrovirals)**
PO
Adults, Children aged 12-16 yr weighing more than 50 kg (100 lb). 150 mg twice a day or 300 mg once a day.
Children 3 mo to 11 yr. 4 mg/kg twice a day (up to 150 mg/dose).
▸ **Chronic hepatitis B**
PO
Adults, Children 17 yr and older. 100 mg/day.
Children younger than 17 yr. 3 mg/kg/day. Maximum: 100 mg/day.
▸ **Dosage in renal impairment (adult and adolescent)**
Dosage and frequency are modified based on creatinine clearance.

CrCl (mL/ min)	HIV Dosage	Hepatitis B dosage
≥ 60	150 mg twice a day	100 mg once a day
30-49	150 mg once a day	100 mg first dose, then 50 mg once a day
15-29	150 mg first dose, then 100 mg once a day	100 mg first dose, then 25 mg once a day
5-14	150 mg first dose, then 50 mg once a day	35 mg first dose, then 15 mg once a day
< 5	50 mg first dose, then 25 mg once a day	35 mg first dose, then 10 mg once a day

OFF-LABEL USES
Prophylaxis in health care workers at risk of acquiring HIV after occupational exposure.

CONTRAINDICATIONS
Hypersensitivity, history of pancreatitis as a child.
Caution
Reduce dose in renal disease, lactation.

INTERACTIONS
Drug
Co-trimoxazole: Increases lamivudine blood concentration.
Herbal
St. John's wort: May decrease lamivudine blood concentration and effect.
Zalcitabine: May inhibit intracellular phosphorylation when used concomitantly.
Food
None known.

DIAGNOSTIC TEST EFFECTS
May increase blood hemoglobin values, neutrophil count, and serum amylase, AST (SGOT), and ALT (SGPT) levels.

SIDE EFFECTS
Frequent
Headache (35%), nausea (33%), malaise and fatigue (27%), nasal disturbances (20%), diarrhea, cough (18%), musculoskeletal pain, neuropathy (12%), insomnia (11%), anorexia, dizziness, fever, or chills (10%).
Occasional
Depression (9%), myalgia (8%), abdominal cramps (6%), dyspepsia, arthralgia (5%).

SERIOUS REACTIONS
• Pancreatitis occurs in 13% of pediatric patients.
• Anemia, neutropenia, and thrombocytopenia occur rarely.

• Lactic acidosis.
• Severe hepatomegaly with steatosis.

PRECAUTIONS & CONSIDERATIONS
Caution is warranted in patients with impaired renal function, a history of pancreatitis, and a history of peripheral neuropathy and in young children. Be aware that lamivudine crosses the placenta, and it is unknown whether lamivudine is distributed in breast milk. Breastfeeding is not recommended in this population because of the possibility of HIV transmission. Be aware that the safety and efficacy of this drug have not been established in children younger than 3 mo. In elderly patients, age-related renal impairment may require dosage adjustment. Lamivudine is not a cure for HIV, and the patient may continue to experience illnesses, including opportunistic infections.

Before starting drug therapy, check the baseline lab values, especially renal function. Expect to monitor the serum amylase, BUN, and serum creatinine levels. Assess for altered sleep patterns, cough, dizziness, headache, nausea, and pattern of daily bowel activity and stool consistency. Avoid activities that require mental acuity if dizziness occurs. Modify diet or administer a laxative, if ordered, as needed. Closely monitor children for symptoms of pancreatitis, manifested as clammy skin, hypotension, nausea, severe and steady abdominal pain often radiating to the back, and vomiting accompanying abdominal pain. If pancreatitis occurs in a child, help the child to sit up or flex at the waist to relieve abdominal pain aggravated by movement.
Administration
Give without regard to meals. Take lamivudine for the full length of treatment and evenly space drug doses around the clock.

Lamotrigine

la-moe-trih′jeen
(Lamictal,
Apo-Lamotrigine [CAN], Lamictal
cD)
**Do not confuse lamotrigine with
lamivudine.**

CATEGORY AND SCHEDULE
Pregnancy Risk Category: C

Classification: Antiepileptic

MECHANISM OF ACTION
An anticonvulsant whose exact
mechanism is unknown. May block
voltage-sensitive sodium channels,
thus stabilizing neuronal membranes
and regulating presynaptic
transmitter release of excitatory
amino acids. *Therapeutic Effect:*
Reduces seizure activity.

PHARMACOKINETICS
Rapidly absorbed from the GI tract.
Protein binding: 55%. Metabolized
primarily by glucuronic acid
conjugation. Excreted in the urine.
Half-life: 13-30 h.

AVAILABILITY
Tablets: 25 mg, 100 mg, 150 mg,
200 mg.
Tablets (Chewable): 2 mg, 5 mg,
25 mg.

INDICATIONS AND DOSAGES
▸ **Seizure control in patients receiving
enzyme-inducing antiepileptic drug
(EIAEDs) but not valproic acid**
PO
*Adults, Elderly, Children 12 yr and
older.* Recommended as add-on
therapy: 50 mg once a day for 2 wks,
followed by 100 mg/day in 2 divided
doses for 2 wks. Maintenance:
Dosage may be increased by

100 mg/day every week, up to
300-500 mg/day in 2 divided doses.
Children aged 2-12 yr.
0.6 mg/kg/day in 2 divided doses
for 2 wks, then 1.2 mg/kg/day in
2 divided doses for wks 3 and 4.
Maintenance: 5-15 mg/kg/day.
Maximum: 400 mg/day.
▸ **Seizure control in patients
receiving combination therapy
of EIAEDs and valproic acid**
PO
*Adults, Elderly, Children 12 yr and
older.* 25 mg every other day for 2 wks,
followed by 25 mg once a day for
2 wks. Maintenance: Dosage may be
increased by 25-50 mg/day q1-2wk,
up to 150 mg/day in 2 divided doses.
Children aged 2-12 yr. 0.15 mg/kg/
day in 2 divided doses for 2 wks, then
0.3 mg/kg/day in 2 divided doses for
wks 3 and 4. Maintenance: 1-5 mg/
kg/day in 2 divided doses. Maximum:
200 mg/day.
▸ **Conversion to monotherapy in
patients receiving EIAEDs**
PO
*Adults, Elderly, Children 16 yr and
older.* Add lamotrigine 50 mg/day in
divided doses for 2 wks; then titrate
to the desired dose while maintaining
EIAED at a fixed level until
maintenance dosage is achieved.
Gradually discontinue other EIAEDs
by 20% each week over 4 wks once
maintenance dose is achieved.
▸ **Conversion to monotherapy in
patients receiving valproic acid**
PO
*Adults, Elderly, Children 16 yr. and
older.* Titrate lamotrigine to 200 kg/day,
maintaining valproic acid dose. Maintain
lamotrigine dose and decrease valproic
acid to 500 mg/day not to exceed
500 mg/day/wk, then maintain
500 mg/day for 1 wk. Increase
lamotrigine to 300 mg/day, and decrease
valproic acid to 250 mg/day and
maintain for 1 wk. Then discontinue

valproic acid and increase lamotrigine by 100 mg/day each week until maintenance dose of 500 mg/day is reached.

▸ **Bipolar disorder in patients receiving EIAEDs**
PO
Adults, Elderly. 50 mg/day for 2 wks, then 100 mg/day for 2 wks, then 200 mg/day for 1 wk, then 300 mg/day for 1 wk. Then increase to usual maintenance dose of 400 mg/day in divided doses.

▸ **Bipolar disorder in patients receiving valproic acid**
PO
Adults, Elderly. 25 mg/day every other day for 2 wks, then 25 mg/day for 2 wks, then 50 mg/day for 1 wk, then 100 mg/day. Usual maintenance dose with valproic acid: 100 mg/day.

▸ **Discontinuation therapy**
Adults, Children older than 16 yr. A dosage reduction of approximately 50% per week over at least 2 wks is recommended.

▸ **General recommendations for patients with hepatic impairment**
For initial dosing, decrease normal initial dose by 25% for moderate to severe impairment; up to 50% if ascites is present. Escalate and adjust to clinical response.

CONTRAINDICATIONS

Previous hypersensitivity or drug-induced rash from lamotrigine.

INTERACTIONS

Drug
Acetaminophen (long-term, high dose 900 mg 3times/day): Possible increased excretion of lamotrigine.
Carbamazepine, phenobarbital, phenytoin, primidone: Decrease lamotrigine blood concentration.
Valproic acid: Doubles lamotrigine concentration.
Oral hormonal contraceptives: May increase CNS side effects; May decrease effectiveness of lamotrigine or oral contraceptive.
Herbal and Food
None known.

DIAGNOSTIC TEST EFFECTS

None known.

SIDE EFFECTS

Frequent
Dizziness (38%), diplopia (28%), headache (29%), ataxia (22%), nausea (19%), blurred vision (16%), somnolence, rhinitis (14%).
Occasional (5%-10%)
Rash, pharyngitis, vomiting, cough, flulike symptoms, diarrhea, dysmenorrhea, fever, insomnia, dyspepsia.
Rare
Constipation, tremor, anxiety, pruritus, vaginitis, hypersensitivity reaction.

SERIOUS REACTIONS

• Abrupt withdrawal may increase seizure frequency.
• Serious rashes including Stevens-Johnson syndrome, requiring hospitalization and discontinuation of treatment, have been reported; can be life-threatening.

PRECAUTIONS & CONSIDERATIONS

Caution is warranted in patients with cardiac, hepatic, and renal impairment. Exposure to sunlight and artificial light should be avoided.

Drowsiness and dizziness may occur, so alcohol and tasks requiring mental alertness or motor skills should be avoided. Notify the physician if fever, rash, or swollen glands occur. If rash suspected to be drug-related, discontinuation of lamotrigine is recommended. Seizure disorder, including the onset, duration, frequency, intensity, and type of seizures, should be assessed before and during treatment. Changes

L

in frequency or characterization of seizures should be reported to the health care provider immediately.

Administration

! If the patient is currently taking valproic acid, expect to reduce the lamotrigine dosage to less than half the normal dosage.

Take lamotrigine without regard to food. Do not discontinue the drug abruptly after long-term therapy. Strict maintenance of drug therapy is essential for seizure control.

Lamotrigine regular tablets should be swallowed whole because of their bitter taste. The chewable-dispersable tablets may be chewed or dissolved in a small amount of liquid (5 mL) in a spoon, then swallowed.

Lansoprazole
lan-soe'pray-zole
(Prevacid, Prevacid IV, Prevacid Solu-Tab, Zoton [AUS])
Do not confuse Prevacid with Pepcid, Pravachol, or Prevpac.

CATEGORY AND SCHEDULE
Pregnancy Risk Category: B

Classification: Antisecretory, proton pump inhibitors

MECHANISM OF ACTION
A proton-pump inhibitor that selectively inhibits the parietal cell membrane enzyme system (hydrogen-potassium adenosine triphosphatase) or proton pump. *Therapeutic Effect:* Suppresses gastric acid secretion.

PHARMACOKINETICS

Route	Onset	Peak	Duration
PO (15 mg)	2-3 h	NA	8-24 h
PO (30 mg)	1-2 h	NA	Longer than 24 h

Rapid and complete absorption (food may decrease absorption) once the drug has left the stomach. Protein binding: 97%. Distributed primarily to gastric parietal cells and converted to two active metabolites. Extensively metabolized in the liver. Eliminated in bile and urine. Not removed by hemodialysis. *Half-life:* 1.5 h (increased in elderly patients and in those with hepatic impairment).

AVAILABILITY
Capsules (Extended-Release [Prevacid]): 15 mg, 30 mg.
Granules for Oral Suspension (Delayed-Release Granules) (Prevacid): 15 mg/pack; 30 mg/pack.
Injection Powder for Reconstitution (Prevacid IV): 30 mg.
Oral-Disintegrating Tablets (Prevacid Solu-Tab): 15 mg, 30 mg.

INDICATIONS AND DOSAGES
▸ **Duodenal ulcer**
PO
Adults, Elderly. 15 mg/day, before eating, preferably in the morning, for up to 4 wks.
▸ **Erosive esophagitis**
PO
Adults, Elderly. 30 mg/day, before eating, for up to 8 wks. If healing does not occur within 8 wks (in 5%-10% of cases), may give for additional 8 wks. Maintenance: 15 mg/day.
IV
Adults, Elderly. 30 mg once a day for up to 7 days. Switch to oral lansoprazole therapy as soon as the patient can tolerate the oral route.
▸ **Gastric ulcer**
PO
Adults. 30 mg/day for up to 8 wks.
▸ **NSAID gastric ulcer**
PO
Adults, Elderly. (Healing): 30 mg/day for up to 8 wks. (Prevention): 15 mg/day for up to 12 wks.

▸ **Healed duodenal ulcer, gastroesophageal reflux disease (GERD)**

PO

Adults. 15 mg/day.

▸ **Usual pediatric dosage**

Children 3 mo to 14 yr, weighing more than 20 kg. 30 mg once daily.
Children 3 mo to 14 yr, weighing 10-20 kg. 15 mg once daily.
Children 3 mo to 14 yr, weighing < 10 kg. 7.5 mg once daily.

▸ *Helicobacter pylori* **infection**

PO

Adults. 30 mg twice a day for 10 days (with amoxicillin and clarithromycin).

▸ **Pathologic hypersecretory conditions (including Zollinger-Ellison syndrome)**

PO

Adults, Elderly. 60 mg/day. Individualize dosage according to patient needs and for as long as clinically indicated. May increase to 120 mg/day in divided doses.

▸ **Severe hepatic disease**

Consider dosage reduction.

CONTRAINDICATIONS

Hypersensitivity to lansoprazole or any of its components.

INTERACTIONS

Drug

Ampicillin, digoxin, iron salts, ketoconazole: May interfere with the absorption of ampicillin, digoxin, iron salts, and ketoconazole.
Sucralfate: May delay the absorption of lansoprazole.
Atazanavir: Do not give PPI with atazanavir because effectiveness against HIV will be diminished.
Herbal and Food
None known.

DIAGNOSTIC TEST EFFECTS

May increase LDH, serum alkaline phosphatase, bilirubin, cholesterol, creatinine, AST (SGOT), ALT (SGPT), triglyceride, and uric acid levels. May produce abnormal albumin/globulin ratio, electrolyte balance, and platelet, RBC, and WBC counts. May increase hemoglobin and hematocrit levels.

Ⓡ IV INCOMPATIBILITIES

Do not administer with other drugs via Y-site.

SIDE EFFECTS

Occasional (2%-3%)
Diarrhea, abdominal pain, rash, pruritus, altered appetite.
Rare (1%)
Nausea, headache.

SERIOUS REATIONS

• Bilirubinemia, eosinophilia, and hyperlipemia occur rarely.
• Serious hypersensitivity-dermatologic reactions (rare).

L

PRECAUTIONS & CONSIDERATIONS

Caution is warranted in impaired hepatic function. It is unknown whether lansoprazole is distributed in breast milk; caution is warranted in pregancy and lactation. Safety and efficacy of lansoprazole have not been established in children. No age-related precautions have been noted in elderly patients, but doses larger than 30 mg are not recommended. Laboratory values, including CBC and blood chemistry, should be obtained before and periodically during therapy. Some gastric disruption, such as loose stool or flatulence, is common, especially early in therapy.
Storage
Store the drug at room temperature.
Administration
Take lansoprazole capsules while fasting or before meals, because food diminishes absorption. Do not chew or crush delayed-release capsules. May open capsules and sprinkle granules on 1 tbsp of applesauce; swallow immediately. May also sprinkle in 2 oz

of apple, orange, or tomato juice. Take lansoprazole 30 min before sucralfate because sucralfate may delay lansoprazole absorption.

May give solu-tabs with oral syringe or NG tube. May dissolve in 4 mL water (15 mg) or 10 mL water (30 mg). Shake gently.

Delayed-release oral suspension: Mix packet with 30 mL of water only. Stir well and drink immediately. Oral suspension not for use with nasogastric tube.

For IV use, infuse over 30 min. The IV vial must only be reconstituted with 5 mL of sterile water for injection. Mix gently. Then add dose to either 50 mL of 0.9% NaCl or Dextrose 5% injection. Must use provided m-line filter (1.2 μm) to deliver. Flush administration port before and after administration.

Lanthanum Carbonate
lan-than'um car-bo'nate
(Fosrenol)

CATEGORY AND SCHEDULE
Pregnancy Risk Category: C

Classification: Chelators

MECHANISM OF ACTION
A phosphate regulator that dissociates in the acidic environment of the upper GI tract to lanthanum ions, which bind to dietary phosphate released from food during digestion, forming highly insoluble lanthanum phosphate complexes. *Therapeutic Effect:* Reduces phosphate absorption.

PHARMACOKINETICS
Phosphate complexes are eliminated in urine.

AVAILABILITY
Tablets (Chewable): 250 mg, 500 mg.

INDICATIONS AND DOSAGES
▸ **Reduce serum phosphate in end-stage renal disease**
PO
Adults, Elderly. 750-1500 mg in divided doses, taken with or immediately after a meal. Dosage may be titrated in 750-mg increments q2-3wk based on serum phosphate levels. Most patients require 1500-3000 mg/day.

CONTRAINDICATIONS
None known.

INTERACTIONS
Drug
Antacids: Interact with lanthanum; separate administration by 2 h.
Herbal and Food
None known.

DIAGNOSTIC TEST EFFECTS
During abdominal X-ray studies, drug may show up similar to a radio opaque imaging agent.

SIDE EFFECTS
Frequent
Nausea (11%), vomiting (9%), dialysis graft occlusion (8%), abdominal pain (5%).

SERIOUS REACTIONS
• None known.

PRECAUTIONS & CONSIDERATIONS
Caution is warranted in patients with acute peptic ulcer disease, bowel obstruction, Crohn disease, and ulcerative colitis. Side effects of nausea and vomiting should decrease over time.
Storage
Store at room temperature. Protect from moisture.

Administration
Chew the tablets thoroughly before swallowing. Take the drug with or immediately after a meal. Take lanthanum 2 h before or after antacids.

Leflunomide
le-flu′na-mide
(Arava)

CATEGORY AND SCHEDULE
Pregnancy Risk Category: X

Classification:
Disease-modifying antirheumatic drugs, immunosuppressives

MECHANISM OF ACTION
An immunomodulatory agent that inhibits dihydroorotate dehydrogenase, the enzyme involved in autoimmune process that leads to rheumatoid arthritis. *Therapeutic Effect:* Reduces signs and symptoms of rheumatoid arthritis and slows structural damage.

PHARMACOKINETICS
Well absorbed after PO administration. Protein binding: > 99%. Metabolized to active metabolite in the GI wall and liver. Excreted through both renal and biliary systems. Not removed by hemodialysis. *Half-life:* 16 days.

AVAILABILITY
Tablets: 10 mg, 20 mg.

INDICATIONS AND DOSAGES
▸ **Rheumatoid arthritis**
PO
Adults, Elderly. Initially, 100 mg/day for 3 days, then 10-20 mg/day. May eliminate loading dose if patient is at risk for hematologic or hepatic toxicity, such as receiving concurrent methotrexate.

CONTRAINDICATIONS
Pregnancy or plans to become pregnant, known hypersensitivity to the drug.

INTERACTIONS
Drug
Activated charcoal and cholestyramine: Rapidly decrease concentration of leflunomide's active metabolite.
Hepatotoxic medications: May increase risk of liver toxicity.
Rifampin: Increases the blood concentration of leflunomide's active metabolite; use is generally contraindicated.
Warfarin: May increase the effects of warfarin.
Herbal and Food
None known.

DIAGNOSTIC TEST EFFECTS
May increase hepatic enzyme levels, especially AST (SGOT) and ALT (SGPT).

SIDE EFFECTS
Frequent (10%-20%)
Diarrhea, respiratory tract infection, alopecia, rash, nausea.

SERIOUS REACTIONS
• Transient thrombocytopenia and leukopenia occur rarely.
• Hypersensitivity.
• Hepatic injury.
! NOTE: If any serious toxicity occurs, a drug-elimination procedure, using cholestyramine or activated charcoal, must be given because of the long half-life of the drug.

PRECAUTIONS & CONSIDERATIONS
Caution is warranted in patients with immunodeficiency, bone marrow dysplasia, impaired hepatic or renal function, and positive serology for hepatitis B or C. Leflunomide may cause fetal harm. Avoid becoming

pregnant. Although it is not known whether leflunomide is excreted in breast milk, the drug is not recommended for breastfeeding women. The safety and efficacy of leflunomide have not been established in children younger than 18 yr. No age-related precautions have been noted in elderly patients, although decreased renal function or hepatic disease may require decreased dosage or total discontinuation of drug.

Liver function test results should be monitored. Symptomatic relief of rheumatoid arthritis, including relief of pain and improved range of motion, grip strength, and mobility, should be assessed.

Administration

Take leflunomide without regard to food. Therapeutic effect may take longer than 8 wks to appear.

Lepirudin
leh-peer′u-din
(Refludan)

CATEGORY AND SCHEDULE
Pregnancy Risk Category: B

Classification: Anticoagulants, thrombin inhibitors, hirudin, recombinant

MECHANISM OF ACTION
An anticoagulant that inhibits thrombogenic action of thrombin (independent of antithrombin II and not inhibited by platelet factor 4). One molecule of lepirudin binds to one molecule of thrombin. *Therapeutic Effect:* Produces dose-dependent increases in aPTT.

PHARMACOKINETICS
Distributed primarily in extracellular fluid. Primarily eliminated by the kidneys. *Half-life:* 1.3 h (increased in impaired renal function).

AVAILABILITY
Powder for Injection: 50 mg.

INDICATIONS AND DOSAGES
▸ **Heparin-induced thrombocytopenia and associated thromboembolic disease to prevent further thromboembolic complications**
IV, IV INFUSION
Adults, Elderly. 0.4 mg/kg IV slowly over 15-20 s, followed by IV infusion of 0.15 mg/kg/h for 2-10 days or longer. For patients weighing more than 110 kg, the maximum initial dose is 44 mg, with maximum rate of 16.5 mg/h.
▸ **Dosage in renal impairment**
Initial dose is decreased to 0.2 mg/kg, with infusion rate adjusted based on creatinine clearance.

Creatinine Clearance (mL/min)	Percentage of Standard Infusion Rate (mL/min)	Infusion Rate (mg/kg/h)
45-60	50%	0.075
30-44	30%	0.045
15-29	15%	0.0225
<15	Do not use	

CONTRAINDICATIONS
Hypersensitivity to drug or to components of injection, such as mannitol; avoid use or stop use if CrCl < 15 mL/min.

INTERACTIONS
Drug
Platelet aggregation inhibitors, thrombolytics, NSAIDs, aspirin and other salicylates, warfarin: May increase the risk of bleeding complications.
Herbal
Ginkgo biloba: May increase the risk of bleeding.

Food
None known.

DIAGNOSTIC TEST EFFECTS
Increases aPTT and thrombin time; assess aPPT, PT, and INR.

Ⓘ IV INCOMPATIBILITIES
Do not mix with other medications.

SIDE EFFECTS
Frequent (5%-14%)
Bleeding from gums, puncture sites, or wounds; hematuria; fever; GI and rectal bleeding.
Occasional (1%-3%)
Epistaxis; allergic reaction, such as rash and pruritus; vaginal bleeding.

SERIOUS REACTIONS
• Overdose is characterized by excessively high aPTT.
• Intracranial bleeding occurs rarely.
• Abnormal hepatic function occurs in 6% of patients.

PRECAUTIONS & CONSIDERATIONS
Caution is warranted in conditions associated with increased risk of bleeding, such as bacterial endocarditis, cerebrovascular accident, hemorrhagic diathesis, intracerebral surgery, recent major bleeding, recent major surgery, severe hypertension, severe hepatic or renal impairment, and stroke. Overdose is indicated by an excessively high aPPT. It is unknown whether lepirudin crosses the placenta or is distributed in breast milk. Safety and efficacy of lepirudin have not been established in children. In elderly patients, age-related renal impairment may require dosage adjustment. Female patients may experience a heavier menstrual flow. Other medications, including OTC drugs, should be avoided. An electric razor and soft toothbrush should

be used to prevent bleeding during therapy.

Notify the physician of bleeding, breathing difficulty, bruising, dizziness, edema, fever, itching, light-headedness, rash, black or red stool, coffee-ground vomitus, dark or red urine, or red-speckled mucus from cough. CBC, BP, pulse rate, hematocrit, platelet count, renal function, BUN, serum creatinine, AST and ALT levels, and stool and urine specimen for occult blood should be monitored before and during therapy. Be aware of signs of bleeding, including bleeding at injection or surgical sites or from gums, blood in stool, bruising, hematuria, and petechiae.
Storage
Store unreconstituted vials at room temperature. Reconstituted solution should be used immediately, but the IV infusion is stable for up to 24 h at room temperature.
Administration
❗ Give initial dose as soon as possible after surgery but not more than 24 h after surgery. Dosage adjusted according to aPTT ratio with target range of 1.5-2.5 normal.

To reconstitute, add 1 mL sterile water for injection or 0.9% NaCl to 50-mg vial and shake gently. Be aware that reconstitution normally produces a clear, colorless solution; do not use if solution is cloudy. For IV push, further dilute by transferring to syringe and adding sufficient sterile water for injection, 0.9% NaCl, or D5W to produce a concentration of 5 mg/mL. For IV infusion, add the contents of 2 vials (100 mg) to 250 or 500 mL 0.9% NaCl or D5W, providing a concentration of 0.4 or 0.2 mg/mL, respectively. Give the IV push over 15-20 s. Expect to adjust IV infusion based on aPTT.
❗ Do not start if baseline aPTT ratio is 2.5 or greater.

L

Letrozole
le′tro-zole
(Femara)
Do not confuse with Femhrt.

CATEGORY AND SCHEDULE
Pregnancy Risk Category: D

Classification: Antineoplastics, aromatase inhibitors

MECHANISM OF ACTION
Decreases the level of circulating estrogen by inhibiting aromatase, an enzyme that catalyzes the final step in estrogen production. *Therapeutic Effect:* Inhibits the growth of breast cancers that are stimulated by estrogens.

PHARMACOKINETICS
Rapidly and completely absorbed. Metabolized in the liver. Primarily eliminated by the kidneys. Unknown if removed by hemodialysis. *Half-life:* Approximately 2 days.

AVAILABILITY
Tablets: 2.5 mg.

INDICATIONS AND DOSAGES
Breast Cancer, hormone-replacement
PO
Adults, Elderly. 2.5 mg/day. Continue until tumor progression is evident.
▸ **Dosage in severe hepatic impairment**
Give 2.5 mg every other day.

CONTRAINDICATIONS
Hypersensitivity to letrozole or any of its components, pregnancy, pre-menopausal women.

INTERACTIONS
Drug
Estrogens: Oppose actions of letrozole.
Herbal
None known.
Food
None known.

DIAGNOSTIC TEST EFFECTS
May increase serum calcium, cholesterol, GGT, AST (SGOT), and ALT (SGPT) levels.

SIDE EFFECTS
Frequent (9%-21%)
Musculoskeletal pain (back, arm, leg), nausea, headache.
Occasional (5%-8%)
Constipation, arthralgia, fatigue, vomiting, hot flashes, diarrhea, abdominal pain, cough, rash, anorexia, hypertension, peripheral edema.
Rare (1%-4%)
Asthenia, somnolence, dyspepsia, weight gain, pruritus.

SERIOUS REACTIONS
• May decrease bone mineral density with long-term use.
• Peripheral thrombotic events.

PRECAUTIONS & CONSIDERATIONS
Caution is warranted in patients with hepatic and renal impairment. Women who are or may be pregnant should not use this drug. Pregnancy should be determined before beginning therapy. It is unknown whether letrozole is distributed in breast milk. The safety and efficacy of letrozole have not been established in children. No age-related precautions have been noted in elderly patients.
　Potential side effects, including asthenia, dizziness, headache, nausea, vomiting, and

musculoskeletal pain, may occur. Notify the physician if weakness, hot flashes, or nausea become unmanageable. Vital signs, especially BP, should be assessed before therapy begins because letrozole may cause hypertension. CBC, serum electrolyte levels, thyroid function, and liver and renal function tests should be monitored during therapy. Signs of infection or blood dyscrasias should be reported to healthcare provider immediately.

Storage

Store at a controlled room temperature.

Administration

Take oral letrozole without regard to food.

Leucovorin Calcium (Folinic Acid, Citrovorum Factor)

loo-koe-vor'in kal-see-um
(Calcium Leucovorin [AUS], Wellcovorin)

Do not confuse Wellcovorin with Wellbutrin or Wellferon. Do not confuse folinic acid with folic acid.

It is recommended always to use leucovorin as the drug name to avoid drug errors.

CATEGORY AND SCHEDULE

Pregnancy Risk Category: C

Classification: Folic acid antagonist, antineoplastic adjunct.

MECHANISM OF ACTION

An antidote to folic acid antagonists that may limit methotrexate action on normal cells by competing with methotrexate for the same transport processes into the cells. *Therapeutic*

Effect: Reverses toxic effects of folic acid antagonists. Reverses folic acid deficiency.

PHARMACOKINETICS

Readily absorbed from the GI tract. Widely distributed. Primarily concentrated in the liver. Metabolized in the liver and intestinal mucosa to active metabolite. Primarily excreted in urine. *Half-life:* 15 min; metabolite, 30-35 min.

AVAILABILITY

Tablets: 5 mg, 10 mg, 15 mg, 25 mg.
Injection: 10 mg/mL.
Powder for Injection: 50 mg, 100 mg, 200 mg, 350 mg.

INDICATIONS AND DOSAGES

▸ **Conventional rescue dosage in high-dose methotrexate therapy**
PO, IV, IM
Adults, Elderly, Children. 10 mg/m^2 IM or IV one time, then PO q6h until serum methotrexate level is $< 10^{-8}$ M. If 24-h serum creatinine level increases by 50% or greater over baseline or methotrexate level exceeds 5×10^{-6} M or 48-h level exceeds 9×10^{-7} M, increase to 100 mg/m^2 IV q3h until methotrexate level is $< 10^{-8}$ M.

▸ **Folic acid antagonist overdose**
PO/IM
Adults, Elderly, Children. 2-15 mg/day for 3 days or 5 mg every 3 days.

▸ **Megaloblastic anemia, congenital**
IM
Adults, Elderly, Children. 3-6 mg/day.

▸ **Megaloblastic anemia secondary to folate deficiency**
IM/IV
Adults, Elderly, Children. 1 mg/day.

▸ **Prevention of hematologic toxicity (for toxoplasmosis) with sulfadiazine**
PO, IV
Adults, Elderly, Children. 5-10 mg/day, repeat every 3 days.

L

▸**Prevention of hematologic toxicity with pyrimethamine, PCP**
PO, IV
Adults, Children. 25 mg once weekly
Regimens may vary depending on other medications used.

OTHER USES
Used with 5-FU in standard approved regimens for colorectal cancer.

CONTRAINDICATIONS
Pernicious anemia, other megaloblastic anemias secondary to vitamin B_{12} deficiency.

INTERACTIONS
Drug
Anticonvulsants: May decrease the effects of anticonvulsants.
Chemotherapeutic agents: May increase the effects and toxicity of these drugs when taken in combination.
Herbal and Food
None known.

DIAGNOSTIC TEST EFFECTS
None known.

ⓥ IV INCOMPATIBILITIES
Amphotericin B complex (Abelcet, AmBisome, Amphotec), droperidol (Inapsine), foscarnet (Foscavir).

ⓥ IV COMPATIBILITIES
Cisplatin (Platinol AQ), cyclophosphamide (Cytoxan), doxorubicin (Adriamycin), etoposide (VePesid), filgrastim (Neupogen), 5-fluorouracil, gemcitabine (Gemzar), granisetron (Kytril), heparin, methotrexate, metoclopramide (Reglan), mitomycin (Mutamycin), piperacillin and tazobactam (Zosyn), vinblastine (Velban), vincristine (Oncovin).

SIDE EFFECTS
Frequent
When combined with chemotherapeutic agents: Diarrhea, stomatitis, nausea, vomiting, lethargy or malaise or fatigue, alopecia, anorexia.
Occasional
Urticaria, dermatitis.

SERIOUS REACTIONS
• Excessive dosage may negate chemotherapeutic effects of folic acid antagonists.
• Anaphylaxis occurs rarely.
• Diarrhea may cause rapid clinical deterioration.

PRECAUTIONS & CONSIDERATIONS
Caution is warranted in patients with bronchial asthma and a history of allergies. Caution should also be used with 5-fluorouracil in persons with GI toxicities. It is unknown whether leucovorin crosses the placenta or is distributed in breast milk. Leucovorin use in children may increase the risk of seizures by counteracting the anticonvulsant effects of barbiturates and hydantoins. Age-related renal impairment may require a dosage adjustment for elderly patients receiving drug for rescue from effects of high-dose methotrexate therapy. Consuming foods with folic acid, including dried beans, meat proteins, and green leafy vegetables, is encouraged in those with folic acid deficiency.
Caution in individuals with severe anemia or those receiving cancer chemotherapy. Report development of infection immediately.
CBC, BUN, and serum creatinine levels (important in leucovorin rescue) should be monitored. Electrolyte levels and liver function test results in those receiving chemotherapeutic agents in combination with leucovorin should be assessed. For treatment of accidental overdosage of folic acid

antagonists, leucovorin should be given as soon as possible (preferably within 1 h), as prescribed.

Storage
Store vials for parenteral use at room temperature. Use the solution immediately if reconstituted with sterile water for injection and within 7 days if reconstituted with bacteriostatic water for injection.

Administration
Scored tablets may be crushed.

The injection solution normally appears clear and yellowish. Reconstitute each 50-mg vial with 5 mL sterile water for injection or bacteriostatic water for injection (containing benzyl alcohol) to provide a concentration of 10 mg/mL. Reconstitute doses >10 mg/m² with sterile water for injection. Further dilute with D5W or 0.9% NaCl. Do not exceed an infusion rate of 160 mg/min (because of the drug's calcium content).
! Never administer intrathecally. Do not mix in same infusion as 5-FU.

Leuprolide Acetate
loo´proe-lide ass-eh-tayte
(Eligard, Lucrin [AUS], Lucrin Depot Inj [AUS], Lupron, Lupron Depot, Lupron Depot Ped, Viadur)
Do not confuse leuprolide or Lupron with Lopurin or Nuprin.

CATEGORY AND SCHEDULE
Pregnancy Risk Category: X

Classification: Antineoplastics, hormones, gonadotropin-releasing hormone analog

MECHANISM OF ACTION
A gonadotropin-releasing hormone analogue and antineoplastic agent that stimulates the release of luteinizing hormone (LH) and follicle-stimulating hormone (FSH) from the anterior pituitary gland. *Therapeutic Effect:* Produces pharmacologic castration and decreases the growth of abnormal prostate tissue in males, causes endometrial tissue to become inactive and atrophic in females, and decreases the rate of pubertal development in children with central precocious puberty.

PHARMACOKINETICS
Rapidly and well absorbed after SC administration. Absorbed slowly after IM administration. Protein binding: 43%-49%. *Half-life:* 3-4 h.

AVAILABILITY
Implant (Viadur): 65 mg.
Injection Depot Formulation (Eligard): 7.5 mg, 22.5 mg, 30 mg.
Injection Depot Formulation (Leupron Depot): 3.75 mg, 7.5 mg, 11.25 mg, 22.5 mg, 30 mg.
Injection Depot Formulation (Lupron Depot-Ped): 7.5 mg, 11.25 mg, 15 mg.
Injection Solution (Lupron): 5 mg/mL.

INDICATIONS AND DOSAGES
▶ **Advanced prostatic carcinoma**
IM
Adults, Elderly. Lupron Depot: 7.5 mg/mo or 22.5 mg every 3 mo or 30 mg every 4 mo.
SC
Adults, Elderly. Eligard: 7.5 mg every month or 22.5 mg every 3 mo or 30 mg every 4 mo. Lupron: 1 mg/day. Viadur: 65 mg implanted every 12 mo.
▶ **Endometriosis**
IM
Adults, Elderly. Lupron Depot: 3.75 mg/mo for up to 6 mo or 11.25 mg every 3 mo for up to 2 doses.

▸ **Uterine leiomyomata**
IM (WITH IRON)
Adults, Elderly. Lupron Depot:
3.75 mg/mo for up to 3 mo or
11.25 mg as a single injection.
▸ **Precocious puberty**
IM
Children. Lupron Depot:
0.3 mg/kg/dose every 28 days.
Minimum: 7.5 mg. If downregulation
is not achieved, titrate upward in
3.75-mg increments q4wk.
SC
Children. Lupron: 20-45 mcg/kg/day.
Titrate upward by 10 mcg/kg/day if
downregulation is not achieved.

CONTRAINDICATIONS
Pregnancy, breast-feeding,
hypersensitivity to drug or
GnRH analogs.

INTERACTIONS
Drug, Herbal, and Food
None known.

DIAGNOSTIC TEST EFFECTS
May increase serum prostatic acid
phosphatase (PAP) levels. Initially
increases, then decreases, serum
testosterone concentration.

SIDE EFFECTS
Frequent
Hot flashes (ranging from mild
flushing to diaphoresis).
Females: Amenorrhea, spotting.
Occasional
Arrhythmias; palpitations; blurred
vision; dizziness; edema; headache;
burning, itching, or swelling at
injection site; nausea; insomnia;
weight gain.
Females: Deepening voice, hirsutism,
decreased libido, increased breast
tenderness, vaginitis, altered mood.
Males: Constipation, decreased
testicle size, gynecomastia,
impotence, decreased appetite, angina.

Rare
Males: Thrombophlebitis.

SERIOUS REACTIONS
• Signs and symptoms of metastatic
prostatic carcinoma (such as bone
pain, dysuria or hematuria, and
weakness or paresthesia of the lower
extremities) occasionally worsen
1-2 wks after the initial dose but then
subside with continued therapy.
• Pulmonary embolism and MI occur
rarely.

PRECAUTIONS & CONSIDERATIONS
Caution is warranted when
administered to children receiving
long-term therapy. Leuprolide use
is contraindicated in pregnancy
because the drug may cause
spontaneous abortion. Pregnancy
should be determined before therapy.
Nonhormonal contraceptives should
be used during leuprolide use. The
long-term safety of leuprolide in
children has not been established. No
age-related precautions have been
noted in elderly patients.
    Potential side effects, including
dizziness, nausea, and vomiting,
may occur. Females should notify
the physician if regular menstruation
persists or pregnancy occurs. The
patient should be assessed for
peripheral edema, arrhythmias and
palpitations, sleep-pattern changes,
and visual difficulties. Serum
testosterone and PAP levels should
be obtained periodically during
leuprolide therapy. Be aware that
serum testosterone and PAP levels
should increase during the first week
of therapy. The testosterone level
should decrease to baseline level or
less within 2 wks, and the PAP level
should decrease within 4 wks.
Storage
Refrigerate Lupron vials. Store
Lupron Depot at room temperature; do

not freeze and protect from light and heat. Store Eligard in the refrigerator.
Administration
! Because leuprolide may be carcinogenic, mutagenic, or teratogenic, handle it with extreme care during preparation and administration.

For SC (Lupron) use, the injection should appear clear and colorless. Discard the solution if it appears discolored or contains precipitate. Administer the drug undiluted into the abdomen, anterior thigh, or deltoid muscle.

For IM (Lupron Depot) use, reconstitute only with the diluent provided. Follow mixing instructions provided by the manufacturer. Use the reconstituted solution immediately. Do not use needles smaller than 22 gauge; use syringes provided by the manufacturer (0.5-mL low-dose insulin syringes may be used as an alternative).

For IM (Eligard) use, allow drug to warm to room temperature before reconstitution. Follow mixing instructions provided by the manufacturer. Administer the drug within 30 min after reconstitution.

Viadur implant: Implanted SC in inner aspect of upper arm. Removed after 12 mo.

Levalbuterol
lee-val-byoo′ter-ole
(Xopenex)
Do not confuse Xopenex with Xanax.

CATEGORY AND SCHEDULE
Pregnancy Risk Category: C

Classification: Bronchodilators

MECHANISM OF ACTION
A sympathomimetic that stimulates β_2-adrenergic receptors in the lungs resulting in relaxation of bronchial smooth muscle. *Therapeutic Effect:* Relieves bronchospasm and reduces airway resistance.

PHARMACOKINETICS

Route	Onset	Peak	Duration
Inhalation	10-17 min	1.5 h	5-6 h

Metabolized in the liver to inactive metabolite. *Half-life:* 3.3-4 h.

AVAILABILITY
Solution for Nebulization: 0.31 mg in 3-mL vials, 0.63 mg in 3-mL vials, 1.25 mg in 3-mL vials.

INDICATIONS AND DOSAGES
▸ **Treatment and prevention of bronchospasm**
NEBULIZATION
Adults, Elderly, Children 12 yr and older. Initially, 0.63 mg 3 times a day 6-8 h apart. May increase to 1.25 mg 3 times a day with dose monitoring. *Children aged 3-11 yr.* Initially 0.31 mg 3 times a day. Maximum: 0.63 mg 3 times a day.

CONTRAINDICATIONS
History of hypersensitivity to sympathomimetics.
Caution
Paradoxic bronchospasm, cardiovascular disorders, seizures, diabetes, hyperthyroidism, coronary insufficiency, cardiac arrhythmias, hypertension, -adrenergic blockers, MAOIs, tricyclic antidepressants, lactation, children younger than 12 yr.

INTERACTIONS
Drug
Aspirin, vasoconstrictors: Can exacerbate asthma.

β-Adrenergic blockers: Antagonize the effects of levalbuterol.

Digoxin: May increase the risk of arrhythmias.

MAOIs, tricyclic antidepressants, methylxanthines: May potentiate cardiovascular effects.

Herbal
None known.

Food
Sulfite preservatives: Can exacerbate asthma.

DIAGNOSTIC TEST EFFECTS
May increase serum potassium level.

SIDE EFFECTS
Frequent
Tremor, nervousness, headache, throat dryness and irritation.
Occasional
Cough, bronchial irritation.
Rare
Somnolence, diarrhea, dry mouth, flushing, diaphoresis, anorexia.

SERIOUS REACTIONS
• Excessive sympathomimetic stimulation may produce palpitations, extrasystoles, tachycardia, chest pain, a slight increase in BP followed by a substantial decrease, chills, diaphoresis, and blanching of skin.
• Too-frequent or excessive use may lead to decreased bronchodilating effectiveness and severe, paradoxical bronchoconstriction.

PRECAUTIONS & CONSIDERATIONS
Caution is warranted in patients with cardiovascular disorders (such as arrhythmias), diabetes mellitus, hypertension, and seizures. Levalbuterol crosses the placenta. It is unknown whether the drug is distributed in breast milk. The safety and efficacy of levalbuterol have not been established in children younger than 12 yr. A lower initial dosage is recommended for elderly patients. Drink plenty of fluids to decrease the thickness of lung secretions. Avoid excessive use of caffeinated products, such as chocolate, cocoa, cola, coffee, and tea.

Pulse rate and quality, respiratory rate, depth, rhythm and type, ECG, ABG levels, and serum potassium levels should be monitored.

Acute asthma episodes can be addressed with rapid acting sympathomimetic inhalants.

Storage
Protect the solution from light and excessive heat. Store it at room temperature.

Administration
For nebulization, use the solution within 2 wks of opening the foil. Discard the solution if it is not colorless. Do not dilute the solution. Do not mix levalbuterol with other medications. Administer levalbuterol over 5-15 min.

Levetiracetam
leva-tir-ass′eh-tam
(Keppra, Keppra XR)
Do not confuse Keppra with Kaletra.

CATEGORY AND SCHEDULE
Pregnancy Risk Category: C

Classification: Anticonvulsants

MECHANISM OF ACTION
An anticonvulsant that inhibits burst firing without affecting normal neuronal excitability. *Therapeutic Effect:* Prevents seizure activity.

PHARMACOKINETICS
Bioavailability is 100%. Onset 1 h, peak plasma levels attained in 20 min to 2 h. < 10% plasma protein bound;

limited hepatic metabolism and renal excretion (66%). *Half-life:* 6-8 h.

AVAILABILITY
Extended-Release Tablets: 500 mg.
Liquid: 100 mg/mL.
Tablets: 250 mg, 500 mg, 750 mg.
Injection: 100 mg/mL.

INDICATIONS AND DOSAGES
▶ **Partial-onset seizures**
PO
Adults, Elderly. Initially, 500 mg q12h. May increase by 1000 mg/day q2wk. Maximum: 3000 mg/day.
Children aged 4-16 yr.
10-20 mg/kg/day in 2 divided doses. May increase at weekly intervals by 10-20 mg/kg. Maximum: 60 mg/kg.
▶ **Dosage in renal impairment**
Dosage is modified based on creatinine clearance.

Creatinine Clearance (mL/min)	Adult Dosage (mg q12h)
>80	500-1500
50-80	500-1000
30-50	250-750
< 30 mL/min	250-500
End-stage renal disease using dialysis	500-1000 every 24 h
After dialysis, supplemental dose is recommended	250-500

CONTRAINDICATIONS
Hypersensitivity reaction.

INTERACTIONS
Drug
None known.
Herbal
None known.
Food
None significant.

DIAGNOSTIC TEST EFFECTS
Minor decreases in blood hemoglobin level, hematocrit, and RBC and WBC counts.

IV COMPATIBILITIES
Lorazepam, diazepam, valproate sodium.

SIDE EFFECTS
Frequent (10%-15%)
Somnolence, asthenia, headache, infection.
Occasional (4%-9%)
Dizziness, pharyngitis, pain, depression, nervousness, vertigo, rhinitis, anorexia.
Rare (< 3%)
Amnesia, anxiety, emotional lability, cough, sinusitis, anorexia, diplopia, neutropenia (mild).

SERIOUS REACTIONS
• Psychotic reactions (rare).

PRECAUTIONS & CONSIDERATIONS
Caution is warranted in patients with renal impairment. Drowsiness and dizziness may occur, so alcohol and tasks requiring mental alertness or motor skills should be avoided. Seizure disorder, including the onset, duration, frequency, intensity, and type of seizures, should be assessed before and during treatment.
Report symptoms of blood dyscrasias or infection immediately to healthcare provider.
Administration
Take levetiracetam without regard to food. Because of bitter taste, do not cut tablets; administer whole. Do not crush, cut or chew extended-release tablets. IV must be diluted before use with 100 mL of 0.9% NaCl or Dextrose 5% injection. Give *over* 15 min. Do not discontinue the drug abruptly after long-term therapy. Strict maintenance of drug therapy is essential for seizure control. Use caution in lactation, children, and blood dyscrasias.

L

Levodopa

lev-oh-dope-ah
(Dopar, Larodopa)

Discontinued in the United states

CATEGORY AND SCHEDULE

Pregnancy Risk Category: C

Classification: Antiparkinson agents, dopaminergics

MECHANISM OF ACTION

A dopamine prodrug that is converted to dopamine in basal ganglia. Increases dopamine concentrations in the brain, inhibiting hyperactive cholinergic activity. *Therapeutic Effect:* Decreases signs and symptoms of Parkinson disease.

PHARMACOKINETICS

About 30% absorbed. May be reduced with high-protein meal. Protein binding: Minimal. Crosses the blood-brain barrier. Converted to dopamine. Eliminated primarily in urine and to a lesser amount in feces and expired air. Not removed by hemodialysis. *Half-life:* 0.75-1.5 h.

AVAILABILITY

Capsules: 100 mg, 250 mg, 500 mg (Dopar).
Tablets: 100 mg, 250 mg, 500 mg (Larodopa).

INDICATIONS AND DOSAGES

▸ **Parkinsonism**
PO
Adults, Elderly. Initially, 0.5-1 g 2-4 times/day. May increase in increments not exceeding 0.75 g every 3-7 days, up to a maximum of 8 g/day.

CONTRAINDICATIONS

Nonselective MAOI therapy, hypersensitivity to levodopa or any component of its formulation.
Caution
Renal disease, cardiac disease, hepatic disease, respiratory disease, myocardial infarction without dysrhythmia, convulsions, peptic ulcer, asthma, endocrine disease, affective disorders, psychosis, lactation, children younger than 12 yr.

INTERACTIONS

Drug
Alcohol: May increase the risk of CNS depression.
Antichloinergics: May decrease absorption of drug.
Anticonvulsants, benzodiazepines, bromperidol, droperidol, haloperidol, phenothiazines, pyroxidine (vitamin B_6), tricyclic antidepressants: May decrease the therapeutic effects of levodopa.
Bupropion: May increase risk of nausea, vomiting, excitation, restlessness, and postural tremor.
Cisapride: May increase risk of levodopa adverse effects.
Ferric ammonium citrate: May decrease the effects of levodopa.
Indinavir: May increase dyskinesias.
Iron: May decrease the effects of levodopa.
Isoniazid: May increase symptomatic deterioration of Parkinson disease.
MAOIs: May increase risk of hypertensive crises.
Metoclopramide: May increase bioavailability and increase incidence of extrapyramidal symptoms.
Phenytoin: May decrease the effects of levodopa.
Selegiline: May increase dyskinesias, nausea, orthostatic hypotension, confusion, hallucinations.
Herbal
Kava kava: May decrease the effects of levodopa.

Pyridoxine: May decrease the effects of levodopa.
Food
High-protein meals: May decrease peak levodopa concentrations.

DIAGNOSTIC TEST EFFECTS
May increase BUN, LDH concentrations, serum alkaline phosphatase and bilirubin, SGOT (AST), and SGPT (ALT) levels. May falsely increase acetaminophen levels. May result in false-positive urine glucose measurements.

SIDE EFFECTS
Frequent
Uncontrolled body movements of the face, tongue, arms, and upper body; nausea and vomiting, anorexia.
Occasional
Depression, anxiety, confusion, nervousness, difficulty urinating, irregular heartbeats, hiccoughs, dizziness, light-headedness, decreased appetite, blurred vision, constipation, dry mouth, flushed skin, headache, insomnia, diarrhea, unusual tiredness, darkening of urine, discolored sweat.
Rare
Hypertension, ulcer, hemolytic anemia, marked by tiredness or weakness.

SERIOUS REACTIONS
• High incidence of involuntary dystonic and dyskinetic movements may be noted in patients on long-term therapy.
• Mental changes, such as paranoid ideation, psychotic episodes, and depression, may be noted.
• Numerous mild to severe central nervous system (CNS) psychiatric disturbances may include reduced attention span, anxiety, nightmares, daytime somnolence, euphoria, fatigue, paranoia, and hallucinations.

PRECAUTIONS & CONSIDERATIONS
Caution is warranted in patients with active peptic ulcer; underlying depression or psychosis; asthma; history of melanoma; concurrent pyridoxine use; diabetes mellitus; history of myocardial infarction (MI); severe cardiac, liver, pulmonary, and renal impairment; and treated open-angle glaucoma. It is unknown whether levodopa crosses the placenta or is distributed in breast milk. Know that levodopa may inhibit lactation. Do not breastfeed while taking this drug. Be aware that the safety and efficacy of levodopa have not been established in children younger than 18 yr. Elderly patients are more sensitive to the effects of levodopa and may require lower doses. Alcohol and tasks that require mental alertness or motor skills should be avoided. High-protein meals may delay the effects of levodopa.

Clinical reversal of symptoms, such as improvement of masklike facial expression, muscular rigidity, shuffling gait, and resting tremors of hands and head, should be assessed. Difficulty urinating; irregular heartbeats; mental changes; severe nausea or vomiting; or uncontrolled movement of arms, eyelids, face, hands, mouth, legs, or tongue should be reported.
Administration
Levodopa should be given with a dopa decarboxylase inhibitor such as carbidopa. In rare cases when the patient is intolerant to carbidopa, levodopa monotherapy is given. May be given with meals if GI upset occurs, but it is preferred to be taken on an empty stomach for best absorption. When discontinuing levodopa therapy, gradually taper dose to prevent the occurrence of a condition resembling neuroleptic malignant syndrome.

L

Levofloxacin
levo-flox'a-sin
(Iquix, Levaquin, Quixin)

CATEGORY AND SCHEDULE
Pregnancy Risk Category: C

Classification: Fluoroquinolone
anti-infectives

MECHANISM OF ACTION
A fluoroquinolone that inhibits the
enzyme DNA gyrase in susceptible
microorganisms, interfering with
bacterial cell replication and repair.
Therapeutic Effect: Bactericidal.

PHARMACOKINETICS
Well absorbed after both PO and IV
administration. Protein binding:
8%-24%. Penetrates rapidly and
extensively into leukocytes, epithelial
cells, and macrophages. Lung
concentrations are 2-5 times higher
than those of plasma. Eliminated
unchanged in the urine. Partially
removed by hemodialysis.
Half-life: 8 h.

AVAILABILITY
Tablets (Levaquin): 250 mg, 500 mg,
750 mg.
Oral solution: 25 mg/mL.
Injection (Levaquin): 500-mg/20-mL
vials.
Premixed IV Solution (Levaquin):
250 mg/50 mL, 500 mg/100 mL,
750 mg/150 mL.
Ophthalmic Solution (Quixin): 1.5%.
Ophthalmic Solution (Iquix): 0.5%.

INDICATIONS AND DOSAGES
▶ **Bronchitis**
PO, IV
Adults, Elderly. 500 mg q24h
for 7 days.

▶ **Community-acquired pneumonia**
PO
Adults, Elderly. 750 mg/day for 5 days.
▶ **Pneumonia**
PO, IV
Adults, Elderly. 500 mg q24h for
7-14 days.
▶ **Acute maxillary sinusitis**
PO, IV
Adults, Elderly. 500 mg q24h for
10-14 days.
▶ **Skin and skin-structure infections**
PO, IV
Adults, Elderly. 500 mg q24h for
7-10 days.
▶ **Urinary tract infection, acute
pyelonephritis**
PO, IV
Adults, Elderly. 250 mg q24h for
10 days.
▶ **Bacterial conjunctivitis**
OPHTHALMIC
*Adults, Elderly, Children 1 yr and
older.* 1-2 drops q2h for 2 days (up
to 8 times a day), then 1-2 drops q4h
for 5 days.
▶ **Corneal ulcer**
OPHTHALMIC
*Adults, Elderly, Children older than
5 yr.* Days 1-3: Instill 1-2 drops q30min
to 2 h while awake and 4-6 h after
retiring. Days 4 through completion:
1-2 drops q1-4h while awake.
▶ **Dosage in renal impairment**
For bronchitis, pneumonia, sinusitis,
and skin and skin-structure infections,
dosage and frequency are modified
based on creatinine clearance.

Creatinine Clearance (mL/min)	Adult Dosage
50-80	No change
20-49	500 mg initially, then 250 mg q24h
10-19	500 mg initially, then 250 mg q48h
Dialysis	500 mg initially, then 250 mg q48h

For UTIs and pyelonephritis, dosage and frequency are modified based on creatinine clearance.

Creatinine Clearance (mL/min)	Dosage
20	No change
10-19	250 mg initially, then 250 mg q48h

CONTRAINDICATIONS

Hypersensitivity to levofloxacin, other fluoroquinolones, or nalidixic acid.
Caution
Children younger than 18 yr; seizure disorders; renal insufficiency; excessive exposure to sunlight; alterations in blood glucose (diabetes); lactation; drinking fluids liberally; tendon rupture in shoulder, hand, or Achilles tendon.

INTERACTIONS

Drug
Antacids, iron preparations, sucralfate, zinc: Decrease levofloxacin absorption.
NSAIDs: May increase the risk of central nervous system (CNS) stimulation or seizures.
Warfarin: May increase risk of bleeding.
Herbal
None known.
Food
None known.

DIAGNOSTIC TEST EFFECTS

May alter blood glucose levels.

IV INCOMPATIBILITIES

Furosemide (Lasix), heparin, insulin, nitroglycerin, propofol (Diprivan).

IV COMPATIBILITIES

Aminophylline, dobutamine (Dobutrex), dopamine (Intron), fentanyl (Sublimaze), lidocaine, lorazepam (Ativan), morphine.

SIDE EFFECTS

Occasional (1%-3%)
Diarrhea, nausea, abdominal pain, dizziness, drowsiness, headache, light-headedness.
Ophthalmic: Local burning or discomfort, margin crusting, crystals or scales, foreign body sensation, ocular itching, altered taste.
Rare (< 1%)
Flatulence; altered taste; pain; inflammation or swelling in calves, hands, or shoulder; chest pain; difficulty breathing; palpitations; edema; tendon pain.
Ophthalmic: Corneal staining, keratitis, allergic reaction, eyelid swelling, tearing, reduced visual acuity.

SERIOUS REACTIONS

• Antibiotic-associated colitis and other superinfections may occur from altered bacterial balance.
• Hypersensitivity reactions, including photosensitivity (as evidenced by rash, pruritus, blisters, edema, and burning skin) have occurred in patients receiving fluoroquinolones.

PRECAUTIONS & CONSIDERATIONS

Caution is warranted with bradycardia, cardiomyopathy, hypokalemia, hypomagnesemia, impaired renal function, seizure disorders, or suspected CNS disorder. Levofloxacin is excreted in breast milk and should be avoided during pregnancy. The safety and efficacy of levofloxacin have not been established in children younger than 18 yr. Age-related renal impairment may require a dosage adjustment in elderly patients.

Chest pain, difficulty breathing, palpitations, edema, tendon pain, as well as hypersensitivity reactions, including photosensitivity, pruritus, skin rash, and urticaria, should be reported immediately. Be alert for signs and symptoms of superinfection, such as moderate to severe diarrhea, new or increased fever, and ulceration or changes in the oral mucosa. Symptomatic relief should be provided for nausea. Blood glucose levels, liver and renal function, and white blood cell (WBC) count should be monitored. History of hypersensitivity to levofloxacin and other quinolones should be determined before therapy.

Discontinue treatment if patient experiences pain or inflammation of a tendon; seek medical consultation, rest and refrain from exercise.

Administration

Take levofloxacin tablets without regard to food. Oral solution should be given 1 h before or 2 h after food. Do not take antacids (containing aluminum or magnesium), sucralfate, iron preparations, or multivitamins containing zinc within 2 h of levofloxacin because these drugs significantly reduce levofloxacin absorption.

For IV use, levofloxacin is available in single-dose 20-mL (500-mg) vials and as a premixed (with D5W), ready-to-infuse solution. For infusion using the single-dose vial, withdraw the desired amount (10 mL for 250 mg, 20 mL for 500 mg). Dilute each 10 mL (250 mg) with at least 40 mL 0.9% NaCl or D5W. Administer the drug slowly, over not < 60 min.

For ophthalmic use, place a gloved finger on the lower eyelid, and pull it out until a pocket is formed between the eye and lower lid. Hold the dropper above the pocket, and place the correct number of drops into the pocket. Close the eye gently. Apply digital pressure to the lacrimal sac for 1-2 min to minimize drainage of the medication into the patient's nose and throat, reducing the risk of systemic effects.

Levonorgestrel

lee-voe-nor-jes'truhl

(Ange 28 [JAPAN], Duofem [GERMANY], ECEEZ [INDIA], Levonelle [NEW ZEALAND], Microlut [COLOMBIA], Microval [COLOMBIA], Mirena [CHINA, COLOMBIA, GERMANY, HONG KONG, ISRAEL, KOREA, PHILIPPINES, SOUTH AFRICA, THAILAND], Norlevo [FRANCE, SOUTH AFRICA], Norplant System, Norplant 36 [ISRAEL], Plan B, Postinor-2 [ISRAEL, NEW ZEALAND, SINGAPORE], Vikela [FRANCE])

CATEGORY AND SCHEDULE

Pregnancy Risk Category: X

Classification: Contraceptives, hormones, progestins

MECHANISM OF ACTION

A contraceptive hormone that causes thickening of cervical mucus, inhibition of ovulation, and inhibition of implantation. *Therapeutic Effect:* Prevents ovulation or fertilization.

PHARMACOKINETICS

Levonorgestrel is rapidly and completely absorbed after oral administration. Maximum serum concentrations of approximately 15 mg/mL occur at an average of 2 h. Does not appear to be extensively metabolized by the liver. Protein binding: 97.5%. Primarily excreted in the urine, with smaller amounts recovered in the feces.

AVAILABILITY
Tablets: 0.75 mg.
IUD, Intrauterine: 52 mg in T-shaped unit.

INDICATIONS AND DOSAGES
▶ **Long-term prevention of pregnancy**
INTRAUTERINE
Adults, Elderly. Insert 1 system into uterine cavity within 7 days of onset of menstruation or immediately after first trimester abortion. Replace after 5 yr.
▶ **Emergency contraception**
PO (PLAN B)
Adults, Elderly. One 0.75-mg tablet as soon as possible within 72 h of unprotected sexual intercourse. A second 0.75-mg tablet 12 h after the first dose.

CONTRAINDICATIONS
INTRAUTERINE SYSTEM
History of congenital or acquired uterine anomaly, acute pelvic inflammatory disease (PID) or history of PID unless subsequent intrauterine pregnancy, postpartum endometrosis or infected abortion in prior 3 mo, cervical vaginitis, bacterial vaginosis, or other lower genital tract infection unless controlled.
PO (PLAN B)
Known pregnancy.

INTERACTIONS
Drug
CYP3A4 inducers: (e.g., Rifampin): May decrease efficacy of levonorgestrel through increased metabolism.
Herbal
St. John's wort: May decrease levonorgestrel serum levels.

Food
None known.

DIAGNOSTIC TEST EFFECTS
Decreased concentrations of sex hormone-binding globulin; decreased thyroxine concentrations; increased triiodothyronine uptake.

SIDE EFFECTS
Occasional
Hypertension, headache, depression, nervousness, breast pain, dysmenorrhea, decreased libido, abdominal pain, nausea, weight gain, leukorrhea, vaginitis.
Rare
Alopecia, anemia, cervicitis, dyspareunia, eczema, failed insertion, migraine, sepsis, vomiting.

SERIOUS REACTIONS
• IUD: Syncope during insertion, uterine rupture, ectopic pregnancy, pelvic inflammatory disease.
PO (Plan B): Serious side effects uncommon.

PRECAUTIONS & CONSIDERATIONS
Caution is necessary in patients with coagulopathy or concomitant anticoagulant use, vaginitis or cervicitis, valvular or congenital heart disease and surgically constructed systemic-pulmonary shunts, conditions aggravated by fluid retention, diabetes mellitus, and a history of mental depression. Levonorgestrel is contraindicated in pregnancy and is in breast milk and may be harmful to fetus. Levonorgestrel should not be used during breastfeeding. Safety and efficacy of this drug have not been established in children. No

age-related precautions have been noted in elderly patients. Avoid smoking while taking levonorgestrel. Encourage low-fat, low-cholesterol diet because of possible cardiovascular effects.

Menstrual spotting may occur between periods. Pain, redness, swelling, or warmth in the calf; chest pain; migraine headache; peripheral paresthesia; jaundice; fluid retention; depression; vision changes; weight gain; a sudden decrease in vision; and sudden shortness of breath should be reported immediately. Overdose is indicated by fluid retention and uterine bleeding irregularities.

Storage
Store at room temerapture away from heat and moisture.

Administration
As postcoital contraception, take tablets as soon as possible within 72 h after unprotected intercourse. The second dose must be taken 12 h later.

Do not insert intrauterine device until 6 wks postpartum or until involution of the uterus is complete.

Levorphanol
lee-vor′fa-nole
(Levo-Dromoran)

CATEGORY AND SCHEDULE
Pregnancy Risk Category: C
Controlled substance: Schedule II

Classification: Analgesics, narcotic

MECHANISM OF ACTION
An opioid agonist that binds at opiate receptor sites in central nervous system (CNS). *Therapeutic Effect:* Reduced intensity of pain stimuli incoming from sensory nerve endings, altering pain perception and emotional response to pain.

PHARMACOKINETICS
Rapidly absorbed after oral administration; onset of effect within 15-30 min after IM administration. Protein binding: 40%-50%. Extensively distributed. Metabolized in liver. Excreted in urine. Steady-state plasma levels attained by third day of dosing.
Half-life: 11 h.

AVAILABILITY
Tablets: 2 mg (Levo-Dromoran).
Injection: 2 mg/mL (Levo-Dromoran).

INDICATIONS AND DOSAGES
▸ **Pain**
PO
Adults, Elderly. 2 mg. May be increased to 3 mg, if needed and may increase dose to 3 mg every 6-8 h. Not to exceed 6-12 mg/day.
IM/SC
Adults, Elderly. 1-2 mg as a single dose. May repeat in 6-8 h as needed. Maximum: 3-8 mg/day.
IV
Adults. Up to 1 mg injection in divided doses by slow injection. May repeat in 3-6 h as needed. Maximum: 4-8 mg/day.
▸ **Preoperative**
IM/SC
Adults, Elderly. 1-2 mg as a single dose 60-90 min before surgery. Adjustment may be needed in elderly patients.
▸ **Perioperative**
IM/SC
Adults, Elderly. Dosing based on age, weight, physical status, underlying pathology, and other anesthetic being used during procedure.

CONTRAINDICATIONS

Hypersensitivity to levorphanol or any component of the formulation.

Caution

Respiratory function impairment in adults may require dosage reduction of ≥50%.

Elderly, debilitated, severe renal or hepatic impairment, hypothyroidism, Addison disease, toxic psychosis, benign prostatic hypertrophy, urethral stricture, acute alcoholism, delerium tremens.

INTERACTIONS

Drug

Alcohol, barbiturates, general anesthetics, hypnotics, other opioids, phenothiazines, sedatives, skeletal muscle relaxants, tranquilizers, tricyclic antidepressants and other central nervous system (CNS) depressants: May increase CNS or respiratory depression, profound sedation and coma, hypotension.

MAOIs: May produce severe, fatal reaction.

Herbal

None known.

Food

None known.

DIAGNOSTIC TEST EFFECTS

May increase serum amylase and lipase levels.

🚫 IV INCOMPATIBILITIES

Do not mix with aminophylline, ammonium dichloride, amobarbital, chlorothiazide, dietholamine, heparin, methicillin, nitrofurantoin, novobiocin, pentobarbital, perphenazine, phenobarbital, phenytoin, secobarbital, sodium bicarbonate, sodium iodide, sulfadiazine, sulfasoxazole, thiopental.

SIDE EFFECTS

Effects are dependent on dosage amount, route of administration. Ambulatory patients and those not in severe pain may experience dizziness, nausea, vomiting, or hypotension more frequently than those in supine position or having severe pain.

Frequent

Dizziness, drowsiness, hypotension, nausea, vomiting.

Occasional

Shortness of breath, confusion, decreased urination, stomach cramps, altered vision, constipation, dry mouth, headache, difficult or painful urination.

Rare

Allergic reaction (rash, itching), histamine reaction (decreased BP, increased sweating, flushed face, wheezing).

SERIOUS REACTIONS

• Overdosage results in respiratory depression, skeletal muscle flaccidity, cold clammy skin, cyanosis, extreme somnolence progressing to convulsions, stupor, coma, hypotension, respiratory depression, and death.
• Tolerance to analgesic effect, physical dependence may occur with repeated use.
• Paralytic ileus may occur with prolonged use.

PRECAUTIONS & CONSIDERATIONS

Extreme caution should be used in patients with acute alcoholism, anoxia, CNS depression, hypercapnia, respiratory depression, respiratory dysfunction, seizures, shock, and untreated myxedema. Caution is also warranted with acute abdominal conditions, Addison's disease, chronic obstructive pulmonary disease

(COPD), hypothyroidism, impaired renal or liver function, increased intracranial pressure, benign prostatic hypertrophy, and urethral stricture; expect to reduce the initial dosage in these conditions. Safety and efficacy in children are not established. Unknown if excreted in breast milk; caution warranted in pregnancy and lactation.

Vital signs should be taken before giving medication. If respirations are 12/min or lower (20/min or lower in children), withhold medication and contact the physician. Vital signs should be monitored after administration as well.

Be aware that ambulatory persons and those not in severe pain may experience dizziness, hypotension, nausea, and vomiting more frequently than persons in the supine position or with severe pain. Avoid alcohol and tasks that require mental alertness or motor skills. Change positions slowly to avoid orthostatic hypotension.

Drug has abuse potential. Caution warranted in patients with addictive disorders.

May cause serious or potentially fatal respiratory depression if given in excessive dose, given too frequently, or given in full dose to compromised patients. Discontinuing after chronic use may result in withdrawal syndrome.

Any of the follwing symptoms should be reported immediately to health care providers: dizziness, light-headedness, sleepiness, drowsiness, difficulty urinating, fainting, shallow breathing, excessive sleepiness.

Storage
Store at room temperature.
Administration
Dosage should be individualized based on degree of pain and physical condition of the person. Administration may be IV, IM, or SC. Give by slow IV injection.

Levothyroxine
lee-voe-thye-rox′een
(Droxine [AUS], Eltroxin [CAN], Eutroxsig [AUS], Levothroid, Levoxyl, Novothyrox [CAN], Oroxine [AUS], Synthroid, Unithroid)
Do not confuse levothyroxine with liothyronine.

CATEGORY AND SCHEDULE
Pregnancy Risk Category: A

Classification: Thyroid hormone

MECHANISM OF ACTION
A synthetic isomer of thyroxine involved in normal metabolism, growth, and development, especially of the CNS in infants. Possesses catabolic and anabolic effects. *Therapeutic Effect:* Increases basal metabolic rate, enhances gluconeogenesis, and stimulates protein synthesis.

PHARMACOKINETICS
Variable, incomplete absorption from the GI tract. Protein binding: 99%. Widely distributed. Deiodinated in peripheral tissues, minimal metabolism in the liver. Eliminated by biliary excretion.
Half-life: 6-7 days.

AVAILABILITY
Tablets (Levo-T, Levothroid, Levoxyl, Synthroid, Unithroid): 0.025 mg, 0.05 mg, 0.075 mg, 0.088 mg, 0.1 mg, 0.112 mg, 0.125 mg, 0.137 mg, 0.15 mg, 0.175 mg, 0.2 mg, 0.3 mg.
Injection (Synthroid): 500 mcg.

INDICATIONS AND DOSAGES
▸ **Hypothyroidism**
PO
Adults, Elderly. Initially, 12.5-50 mcg.
May increase by 25-50 mcg/day
q2-4wk. Maintenance:
100-200 mcg/day.
Children 13 yr and older. 150 mcg/day.
Children aged 6-12 yr.
100-125 mcg/day.
Children aged 1-5 yr. 75-100 mcg/day.
Children 7-11 mo. 50-75 mcg/day.
Children 3-6 mo. 25-50 mcg/day.
Children 3 mo and younger.
10-15 mcg/day.
▸ **Thyroid-suppression therapy**
PO
Adults, Elderly. 2-6 mcg/kg/day for
7-10 days.
▸ **Thyroid-stimulating hormone suppression in thyroid cancer, nodules, euthyroid**
PO
Adults, Elderly. 2-6 mcg/kg/day for
7-10 days.
▸ **Usual Dosage**
IV
Adults, Elderly, Children. Initial
dosage approximately half the
previously established oral
dosage.

CONTRAINDICATIONS
Hypersensitivity to tablet
components, such as tartrazine;
allergy to aspirin; lactose
intolerance; myocardial infarction,
and thyrotoxicosis uncomplicated
by hypothyroidism; treatment of
obesity.

INTERACTIONS
Drug
Cholestyramine, colestipol, enteral feedings, antacids, calcium and iron supplements: May decrease the
absorption of levothyroxine.
Oral anticoagulants: May alter the
effects of oral anticoagulants.

Sympathomimetics: May increase
the risk of coronary insufficiency and
the effects of levothyroxine.
Herbal
None known.
Food
Coffee, dairy foods: May decrease
absorption.

DIAGNOSTIC TEST EFFECTS
None known. Dose is adjusted based
on monitoring of TSH Response.

Ⓓ IV INCOMPATIBILITIES
Do not use or mix with other IV
solutions.

SIDE EFFECTS
Occasional
Reversible hair loss at the start of
therapy (in children).
Rare
Dry skin, GI intolerance, rash, hives,
pseudotumor cerebri, or severe
headache in children.

SERIOUS REACTIONS
• Excessive dosage produces signs
and symptoms of hyperthyroidism,
including weight loss, palpitations,
increased appetite, tremors,
nervousness, tachycardia,
hypertension, headache, insomnia,
and menstrual irregularities.
• Cardiac arrhythmias occur rarely.

PRECAUTIONS & CONSIDERATIONS
Caution is warranted in patients
with angina pectoris, hypertension,
other cardiovascular disease, and
in elderly patients. Levothyroxine
does not cross the placenta and
is minimally excreted in breast
milk. No age-related precautions
have been noted in children. Use
caution in interpreting thyroid
function tests in neonates. Elderly
patients may be more sensitive
to thyroid effects. Individualized

dosages are recommended for this population. Increased nervousness, excitability, sweating, or tachycardia indicates possible uncontrolled hyperthyroidism or overdosage.

Reversible hair loss or increased aggressiveness may occur during the first few months of therapy. Notify the physician of chest pain, insomnia, nervousness, tremors, weight loss, or a pulse rate of 100 beats/min or more. Weight and vital signs, especially pulse rate and rhythm, should be monitored. Keep in mind that levothyroxine may intensify the signs and symptoms of adrenal insufficiency, diabetes insipidus, diabetes mellitus, and hypopituitarism. Also, know that adrenocortical steroids should be prescribed before thyroid therapy in persons with coexisting hypoadrenalism and hypothyroidism.

Storage
Store vials at room temperature.

Administration
! Do not use different brands of levothyroxine interchangeably, although problems with bioequivalence among manufacturers are minimized with today's manufacturing process; it is better for patients to use same product throughout treatment or be carefully monitored during product switches. Begin therapy with small doses and increase the dosage gradually, as prescribed.

Take oral levothyroxine at same time each day to maintain hormone levels. Take before breakfast or at bed time on empty stomach and without other medications or foods. Take with plenty of water. Full therapeutic effect of the drug may take 1-3 wks to appear. Crush tablets as needed. Do not discontinue

this drug; replacement therapy for hypothyroidism is lifelong.

For IV use, reconstitute 500-mcg vial with 5 mL 0.9% NaCl to provide a concentration of 100 mcg/mL; shake until clear. Use immediately, and discard unused portion. Give each 100 mcg or less over 1 min.

Lidocaine Hydrochloride

lye'doe-kane high-droh-klor-ide
(Lidoderm, Lignocaine Gel [AUS], Xylocaine, Xylocaine Aerosol [AUS], Xylocaine Ointment [AUS], Xylocaine Viscous Topical Solution [AUS], Xylocard [CAN], Zilactin-L [CAN])

CATEGORY AND SCHEDULE
Pregnancy Risk Category: B

Classification:
Antidysrhythmics class IB

MECHANISM OF ACTION
An amide anesthetic that inhibits the conduction of nerve impulses. *Therapeutic Effect:* Causes temporary loss of feeling and sensation. Also an antiarrhythmic that decreases depolarization, automaticity, excitability of the ventricle during diastole by direct action. *Therapeutic Effect:* Inhibits ventricular arrhythmias.

PHARMACOKINETICS

Route	Onset	Peak	Duration
IV	30-90 s	NA	10-20 min
Local	2.5 min	NA	30-60 min anesthetic

Completely absorbed after IM administration. Protein binding: 60%-80%. Widely distributed. Metabolized in the liver. Primarily excreted in urine. Minimally removed by hemodialysis. *Half-life:* 1-2 h.

AVAILABILITY

IM Injection: 300 mg/3 mL.
Direct IV Injection: 10 mg/mL, 20 mg/mL.
IV Admixture Injection: 40 mg/mL, 100 mg/mL, 200 mg/mL.
IV Infusion: 2 mg/mL, 4 mg/mL, 8 mg/mL.
Injection (Anesthesia): 0.5%, 1%, 1.5%, 2%, 4%.
Liquid: 2.5%, 5%.
Ointment: 2.5%, 5%.
Cream: 0.5%.
Gel: 0.5%, 2.5%.
Topical Spray: 0.5%.
Topical Solution: 2%, 4%.
Topical Jelly: 2%.
Dermal Patch (Lidoderm): 5%.

INDICATIONS AND DOSAGES

▶ **Rapid control of acute ventricular arrhythmias after myocardial infarction, cardiac catheterization, cardiac surgery, or digitalis-induced ventricular arrhythmias**
IM
Adults, Elderly. 300 mg (or 4.3 mg/kg). May repeat in 60-90 min.
IV
Adults, Elderly. Initially, 50-100 mg (1 mg/kg) IV bolus at rate of 25-50 mg/min. May repeat in 5 min. Give no more than 200-300 mg in 1 h. Maintenance: 20-50 mcg/kg/min (1-4 mg/min) as IV infusion.
Children, Infants. Initially, 0.5-1 mg/kg IV bolus; may repeat but total dose not to exceed 3-5 mg/kg. Maintenance: 10-50 mcg/kg/min as IV infusion.

▶ **Dental or surgical procedures, childbirth**
INFILTRATION OR NERVE BLOCK
Adults. Local anesthetic dosage varies with the procedure, degree of anesthesia, vascularity, duration. Maximum dose: 4.5 mg/kg. Do not repeat within 2 h.

▶ **Local skin disorders (minor burns, insect bites, prickly heat, skin manifestations of chickenpox, abrasions), and mucous membrane disorders (local anesthesia of oral, nasal, and laryngeal mucous membranes; local anesthesia of respiratory, urinary tract; relief of discomfort of pruritus ani, hemorrhoids, pruritus vulvae)**
TOPICAL
Adults, Elderly. Apply to affected areas as needed.

▶ **Treatment of shingles-related skin pain**
TOPICAL (DERMAL PATCH)
Adults, Elderly. Apply to intact skin over most painful area (up to 3 patches once for up to 12 h in a 24-h period).

CONTRAINDICATIONS

Adams-Stokes syndrome, hypersensitivity to amide-type local anesthetics, septicemia (spinal anesthesia), supraventricular arrhythmias, Wolff-Parkinson-White syndrome.
Caution
Lactation, children, renal disease, liver disease, congestive heart failure, respiratory depression, malignant hyperthermia (questionable), elderly.

INTERACTIONS

Drug
Anticonvulsants: May increase cardiac depressant effects.
β-Adrenergic blockers: May increase risk of toxicity.

Other antiarrhythmics: May increase cardiac effects.
Herbal
None known.
Food
None known.

DIAGNOSTIC TEST EFFECTS

IM lidocaine may increase creatine kinase level (used to diagnose acute myocardial infarction). Therapeutic blood level is 1.5-6 mcg/mL; toxic blood level is >6 mcg/mL. Monitor ECG.

ⓘ IV INCOMPATIBILITIES

Amphotericin B complex (Abelcet, AmBisome, Amphotec), thiopental.

ⓘ IV COMPATIBILITIES

Aminophylline, amiodarone (Cordarone), calcium gluconate, digoxin (Lanoxin), diltiazem (Cardizem), dobutamine (Dobutrex), dopamine (Intropin), enalapril (Vasotec), furosemide (Lasix), heparin, insulin, nitroglycerin, potassium chloride.

SIDE EFFECTS

Central nervous system (CNS) effects are generally dose-related and of short duration.
Occasional
IM: Pain at injection site.
Topical: Burning, stinging, tenderness at application site.
Rare
Generally with high dose: Drowsiness; dizziness; disorientation; light-headedness; tremors; apprehension; euphoria; sensation of heat, cold, or numbness; blurred or double vision; ringing or roaring in ears (tinnitus); nausea.

SERIOUS REACTIONS

• Although serious adverse reactions to lidocaine are uncommon, high dosage by any route may produce cardiovascular depression, bradycardia, hypotension, arrhythmias, heart block, cardiovascular collapse, and cardiac arrest.
• Potential for malignant hyperthermia.
• CNS toxicity may occur, especially with regional anesthesia use, progressing rapidly from mild side effects to tremors, somnolence, seizures, vomiting, and respiratory depression.
• Methemoglobinemia (evidenced by cyanosis) has occurred following topical application of lidocaine for teething discomfort and laryngeal anesthetic spray.

PRECAUTIONS & CONSIDERATIONS

Caution is warranted in patients with atrial fibrillation, bradycardia, heart block, hypovolemia, liver disease, marked hypoxia, and severe respiratory depression. Be aware that lidocaine crosses the placenta and is distributed in breast milk. No age-related precautions have been noted in children. Elderly patients are more sensitive to the adverse effects of lidocaine. Lidocaine dose and rate of infusion should be reduced in elderly patients. In elderly patients, age-related renal impairment may require dosage adjustment. Chewing gum, drinking, or eating for 1 h after oral mucous membrane lidocaine application should be avoided; the swallowing reflex may be impaired, increasing risk of aspiration, and numbness of tongue or buccal mucosa may lead to trauma.

A loss of feeling or sensation will occur, and patients will need protection from trauma until anesthetic wears off. Hypersensitivity to amide anesthetics and lidocaine should be determined before beginning drug therapy. BP, pulse, respirations, ECG, and serum electrolytes should be obtained at baseline and periodically thereafter.

Storage

Store at room temperature.

Administration

! Keep resuscitative equipment and drugs, including O$_2$, readily available when administering lidocaine by any route. Know that lidocaine's therapeutic serum level is 1.5-6 mcg/mL and the toxic serum level is >6 mcg/mL.

For IM administration, use 10% (100 mg/mL) and clearly identify the lidocaine preparation. Give injection in deltoid muscle because the blood level will be significantly higher than if the injection is given in gluteus muscle or lateral thigh. For transdermal use, may cut patch to size before removing adhesive backing. ! Use only lidocaine without preservative, clearly marked for IV use.

For IV infusion, prepare solution by adding 1 g to 1 L D5W to provide concentration of 1 mg/mL (0.1%). Know that commercially available preparations of 0.2%, 0.4%, and 0.8% may be used for IV infusion. Be aware that the maximum concentration is 4 g/250 mL. For IV push, use 1% (10 mg/mL) or 2% (20 mg/mL). Administer IV push at rate of 25-50 mg/min. Administer for IV infusion at rate of 1-4 mg/min (1-4 mL) and use a volume control IV set.

For topical use, be aware that this form is not for ophthalmic use. For skin disorders, apply directly to affected area or put on a gauze or bandage, which is then applied to the skin. For mucous membrane use, apply to desired area as per manufacturer's insert. Administer the lowest dosage possible that still provides anesthesia. Dermal patches may be cut to fit area.

Lindane (Gamma Benzene Hexachloride)

lin'dane

(Lindane, Hexit [CAN], PMS-Lindane [CAN])

Do not confuse lindane with lidocaine.

CATEGORY AND SCHEDULE

Pregnancy Risk Category: B

Classification: Anti-infectives, topical, dermatologics, scabicides/pediculicides

MECHANISM OF ACTION

A scabicidal agent that is directly absorbed by parasites and ova through the exoskeleton. *Therapeutic Effect:* Stimulates the nervous system resulting in seizures and death of parasitic arthropods.

PHARMACOKINETICS

May be absorbed systemically. Metabolized in liver. Excreted in the urine and feces. *Half-life:* 17-22 h.

AVAILABILITY

Lotion: 1% (Lindane).
Shampoo: 1% (Lindane).

INDICATIONS AND DOSAGES

▸ **Treatment of scabies**

TOPICAL

Adults, Elderly, Children weighing 110 lb (50 kg) or more. Apply thin layer. Massage on skin from neck to the toes. Bathe and remove drug after 8-12 h.

▸ **Head lice, crab lice**

TOPICAL

Adults, Elderly, Children. weighing 110 lb (50 kg) or more. Apply about 30 mL of shampoo to dry

hair and massage into hair for
4 min. Add small amounts of water
to hair until lather forms, then rinse
hair thoroughly and comb with a
fine-tooth comb to remove nits.
Maximum: 60 mL of shampoo.

CONTRAINDICATIONS

Hypersensitivity to lindane or any
component of the formulation,
uncontrolled seizure disorders,
crusted (Norwegian) scabies, acutely
inflamed skin or raw, weeping
surfaces, or other skin conditions
that might increase systemic
absorption.

INTERACTIONS
Drug
None known.
Herbal
None known.
Food
None known.

DIAGNOSTIC TEST EFFECTS
None known.

SIDE EFFECTS
Rare (< 1%)
Burning, stinging, cardiac
arrhythmia, ataxia, dizziness,
headache, restlessness, seizures, pain,
alopecia, contact dermatitis, skin and
adipose tissue may act as repositories,
eczematous eruptions, pruritus,
urticaria, nausea, vomiting, aplastic
anemia, hepatitis, paresthesias,
hematuria, pulmonary edema.

SERIOUS REACTIONS
• Seizures.

PRECAUTIONS & CONSIDERATIONS
Lindane is second-line choice
because of the potential for systemic
absorption and CNS side effects,
especially in children. Do not use in
children < 50 kg. Caution should be

used in people taking medications
for seizures. It is unknown whether
lindane is excreted in breast milk.
Avoid using on infants. No age-
related precautions have been noted
in elderly patients. Clothing and
bedding should be washed in hot
water or by dry cleaning to kill the
scabies mite.
Administration
! Never apply more than 2 oz of
lotion! Wait at least 1 h after bathing
or showering to apply. Skin should be
clean and free of any lotions, creams,
or oils before lindane application.
Apply a thin layer and massage onto
clean, dry skin from the neck to
the toes. Wait at least 8-12 h after
bathing or showering. Avoid contact
with eyes or face.

Apply shampoo to clean, dry hair.
Wait at least 1 h after washing hair
before applying lindane shampoo.
Hair should be washed with a
shampoo that does not contain
conditioner. Hair should be free of
any lotions, oils, or creams before
lindane application.

Linezolid
li-nee′zoh-lid
(Zyvox, Zyvoxam)
**Do not confuse Zyvox with
Zovirax or Vioxx.**

CATEGORY AND SCHEDULE
Pregnancy Risk Category: C

Classification: Antibiotics,
oxazolidinone derivative

MECHANISM OF ACTION
An oxazolidinone anti-infective
that binds to a site on bacterial
23S ribosomal RNA, preventing
the formation of a complex that is

essential for bacterial translation. *Therapeutic Effect:* Bacteriostatic against enterococci and staphylococci; bactericidal against streptococci.

PHARMACOKINETICS

Rapidly and extensively absorbed after PO administration. Protein binding: 31%. Metabolized in the liver by oxidation. Excreted in urine. *Half-life:* 4-5.4 h.

AVAILABILITY

Powder for Oral Suspension: 100 mg/5 mL.
Tablets: 400 mg, 600 mg.
Injection: 2 mg/mL in 100-mL, 200-mL, 300-mL bags.

INDICATIONS AND DOSAGES
▸ **Vancomycin-resistant infections (VRE, VR-MSRA)**
PO, IV
Adults, Elderly, Children older than 11 yr. 600 mg q12h for 14-28 days.
▸ **Pneumonia, complicated skin and skin-structure infections**
PO, IV
Adults, Elderly, Children older than 11 yr. 600 mg q12h for 10-14 days.
▸ **Uncomplicated skin and skin-structure infections**
PO
Adults, Elderly. 400 mg q12h for 10-14 days.
▸ **Usual Pediatric dosage**
Children older than 11 yr. 600 mg q12h.
Children aged 5-11 yr. 10 mg/kg/dose q8-12h.
▸ **Usual neonate dosage**
PO, IV
Neonates. 10 mg/kg/dose q8-12h.

CONTRAINDICATIONS
Hypersensitivity to oxazolidinones or any of their components. Use within 14 days of an MAOI, uncontrolled hypertension.

INTERACTIONS
Drug
Adrenergic agents (indirect-acting sympathomimetics) and vasopressors (dopaminergic drugs, phenylephrine, pseudoephedrine, epinephrine): May increase pressor effects.
MAOIs: Additive side effects. Contraindicated.
SSRI antidepressants and other serotonergic drugs: Occasional reports of serotonin syndrome with co-use. Avoid use if possible.
Herbal
None known.
Food
Tyramine-containing foods and beverages: Excessive amounts may cause hypertension.

DIAGNOSTIC TEST EFFECTS
May decrease blood hemoglobin, platelet count, WBC count, and ALT (SGPT) levels; monitor platelet counts and CBC in patients at risk for bleeding.

Ⓜ IV INCOMPATIBILITIES
Amphotericin B complex (Abelcet, AmBisome, Amphotec), chlorpromazine (Thorazine), co-trimoxazole (Bactrim), diazepam (Valium), erythromycin (Erythrocin), pentamidine (Pentam IV), phenytoin (Dilantin).

SIDE EFFECTS
Occasional (2%-5%)
Diarrhea, nausea, headache.
Rare (< 2%)
Altered taste, vaginal candidiasis, fungal infection, dizziness, tongue discoloration.

SERIOUS REACTIONS
• Thrombocytopenia and myelosuppression occur rarely.

• Antibiotic-associated colitis and other superinfections may result from altered bacterial balance.
• Serotonin syndrome or hypertension with serotonergic or pressor agents (rare).

PRECAUTIONS & CONSIDERATIONS

Caution is warranted in patients with carcinoid syndrome, pheochromocytoma, severe renal or hepatic impairment, uncontrolled hypertension, or untreated hyperthyroidism. It is unknown whether linezolid is distributed in breast milk. The safety and efficacy of linezolid have not been established in children. No age-related precautions have been noted in elderly patients. Avoid excessive amounts of tyramine-containing foods (such as aged cheese and red wine) because these foods may cause severe reactions and increased hypertension, including diaphoresis, neck stiffness, palpitations, and severe headache. May promote overgrowth of nonsusceptible bacterial strains; monitor platelet counts in patients at risk for bleeding.

Mild GI effects may be tolerable, but severe symptoms may indicate the onset of antibiotic-associated colitis. Pattern of daily bowel activity and stool consistency should be monitored. Be alert for signs and symptoms of superinfection, including abdominal pain, moderate to severe diarrhea, severe anal or genital pruritus, fever or fatigue, and severe mouth soreness. CBC should be monitored weekly.

Storage
Use the oral suspension within 21 days of reconstitution. Store the drug at room temperature and protect it from light. A yellow color does not affect potency.

Administration
Take oral linezolid without regard to food. May take with food or milk if GI upset occurs. Space drug doses evenly around the clock, and continue linezolid therapy for the full course of treatment.
! Do not mix linezolid for IV use with other medications. If the same line is used to administer another drug, flush it with a compatible fluid (D5W, 0.9% NaCl, lactated Ringer's). Infuse the drug over 30-120 min.

Liothyronine T₃
lye-oh-thye'roe-neen
(Cytomel, Tertroxin [AUS], Triostat)
Do not confuse liothyronine with levothyroxine.

CATEGORY AND SCHEDULE
Pregnancy Risk Category: A

Classification: Thyroid hormone

MECHANISM OF ACTION
A synthetic form of triiodothyronine (T_3), a thyroid hormone involved in normal metabolism, growth, and development, especially of the central nervous system in infants. Possesses catabolic and anabolic effects. *Therapeutic Effect:* Increases basal metabolic rate, enhances gluconeogenesis, and stimulates protein synthesis.

PHARMACOKINETICS
PO: Peak 12-48 h. *Half-life:* 0.6-1.4 days.

AVAILABILITY
Tablets (Cytomel): 5 mcg, 25 mcg, 50 mcg.
Injection (Triostat): 10 mcg/mL.

INDICATIONS AND DOSAGES
▶ **Hypothyroidism**
PO
Adults, Elderly. Initially, 25 mcg/day.
May increase in increments of
12.5-25 mcg/day q1-2wk. Maximum:
100 mcg/day.
Children. Initially, 5 mcg/day. May
increase by 5 mcg/day q3-4wk.
Maintenance: 100 mcg/day (children
older than 3 yr); 50 mcg/day
(children 1-3 yr); 20 mcg/day
(infants).
▶ **Myxedema**
PO
Adults, Elderly. Initially, 5 mcg/day.
Increase by 5-10 mcg q1-2wk (after
25 mcg/day has been reached, may
increase in 12.5-mcg increments).
Maintenance: 50-100 mcg/day.
▶ **Nontoxic goiter**
PO
Adults, Elderly. Initially, 5 mcg/day.
Increase by 5-10 mcg/day q1-2wk.
When 25 mcg/day has been reached,
may increase by 12.5-25 mcg/day
q1-2wk. Maintenance: 75 mcg/day.
Children. 5 mcg/day. May increase
by 5 mcg q1-2wk. Maintenance:
15-20 mcg/day.
▶ **Congenital hypothyroidism**
PO
Children. Initially, 5 mcg/day.
Increase by 5 mcg/day q3-4 days.
Maintenance: Full adult dosage
(children older than 3 yr);
50 mcg/day (children 1-3 yr);
20 mcg/day (infants).
▶ **T$_3$ suppression test**
PO
Adults, Elderly. 75-100 mcg/day
for 7 days; then repeat ^{131}I thyroid
uptake test.
▶ **Myxedema coma, precoma**
IV
Adults, Elderly. Initially, 25-50 mcg
(10-20 mcg in patients with cardi-
ovascular disease). Total dose at least
65 mcg/day.

CONTRAINDICATIONS
Myocardial infarction and
thyrotoxicosis uncomplicated by
hypothyroidism; obesity.
Caution
Hypoadrenalism, diabetes insipidus,
diabetes mellitus, hypopituitarism.

INTERACTIONS
Drug
Cholestyramine, colestipol: May
decrease the absorption of
liothyronine.
Oral anticoagulants: May alter the
effects of these drugs.
Sympathomimetics: May increase
the risk of coronary insufficiency and
the effects of liothyronine.
Herbal
None known.
Food
None known.

DIAGNOSTIC TEST EFFECTS
None known.

SIDE EFFECTS
Occasional
Reversible hair loss at start of
therapy (in children).
Rare
Dry skin, GI intolerance, rash,
hives, pseudotumor cerebri or severe
headache in children.

SERIOUS REACTIONS
• Excessive dosage produces signs
and symptoms of hyperthyroidism,
including weight loss, palpitations,
increased appetite, tremors,
nervousness, tachycardia,
hypertension, headache, insomnia,
and menstrual irregularities.
• Cardiac arrhythmias occur rarely.

PRECAUTIONS & CONSIDERATIONS
Signs of excessive overdose should
be reported immediately and
include signs and symptoms of

hyperthyroidism, including weight loss, palpitations, increased appetite, tremors, nervousness, tachycardia, hypertension, headache, insomnia, and menstrual irregularities.

Caution is warranted in patients with adrenal insufficiency, cardiovascular disease, coronary artery disease, diabetes insipidus, and diabetes mellitus. Liothyronine does not cross the placenta and is minimally excreted in breast milk. No age-related precautions have been noted in children. Use caution in interpreting thyroid function test results in neonates. Elderly patients may be more sensitive to thyroid effects. Individualized dosages are recommended for this population.

Reversible hair loss or increased aggressiveness may occur during the first few months of therapy. Notify the physician of chest pain, insomnia, nervousness, tremors, weight loss, or a pulse rate of 100 beats/min or more. Weight and vital signs, especially pulse rate and rhythm, should be monitored. Keep in mind that liothyronine may intensify the signs and symptoms of adrenal insufficiency, diabetes insipidus, diabetes mellitus, and hypopituitarism.

Also, know that adrenocortical steroids should be prescribed before thyroid therapy in persons with coexisting hypoadrenalism and hypothyroidism.

Administration
! Initial and subsequent dosages are based on the clinical status and response. Do not use different brands of liothyronine interchangeably because of problems with bioequivalence among manufacturers.

Take at the same time each day, preferably in the morning.

Do not abruptly discontinue the drug; replacement therapy for hypothyroidism is lifelong.

Administer IV dose over 4 h but no longer than 12 h apart.

Lisinopril
ly-sin'oh-pril
(Apo-Lisinopril [CAN], Fibsol [AUS], Lisodur [AUS], Prinivil, Zestril)
Do not confuse Prinivil with Desyrel, fosinopril, or Plendil; Fibsol with Lioresal; or Zestril with Zostrix. Do not confuse lisinopril's combination form Zestoretic with Prilosec.

CATEGORY AND SCHEDULE
Pregnancy Risk Category: C (D if used in second or third trimester)

Classification: Angiotensin converting enzyme inhibitors (ACE)

MECHANISM OF ACTION
This ACE inhibitor suppresses the renin-angiotensin-aldosterone system and prevents the conversion of angiotensin I to angiotensin II, a potent vasoconstrictor; may also inhibit angiotensin II at local vascular and renal sites. Decreases plasma angiotensin II, increases plasma renin activity, and decreases aldosterone secretion. *Therapeutic Effect:* Reduces peripheral arterial resistance, BP, afterload, pulmonary capillary wedge pressure (preload), pulmonary vascular resistance. In those with heart failure, also decreases heart size, increases

cardiac output, and increases exercise tolerance time.

PHARMACOKINETICS

Route	Onset	Peak	Duration
PO	1 h	6 h	24 h

Incompletely absorbed from the GI tract. Protein binding: 25%. Primarily excreted unchanged in urine. Removed by hemodialysis. *Half-life:* 12 h (half-life is prolonged in those with impaired renal function).

AVAILABILITY

Tablets (Prinivil, Zestril): 2.5 mg, 5 mg, 10 mg, 20 mg, 30 mg, 40 mg.

INDICATIONS AND DOSAGES

▶ **Hypertension (used alone)**
PO
Adults. Initially, 10 mg/day. May increase by 5-10 mg/day at 1- to 2-wks intervals. Maximum: 40 mg/day.
Elderly. Initially, 2.5-5 mg/day. May increase by 2.5-5 mg/day at 1- to 2-wks intervals. Maximum: 40 mg/day.
▶ **Hypertension (used in combination with other hypertensives)**
PO
Adults. Initially, 2.5-5 mg/day titrated to patient's needs.
▶ **Adjunctive therapy for management of heart failure**
PO
Adults, Elderly. Initially, 2.5-5 mg/day. May increase by no more than 10 mg/day at intervals of at least 2 wks. Maintenance: 5-40 mg/day.
▶ **Improve survival in patients after myocardial infarction (MI)**
PO
Adults, Elderly. Initially, 5 mg, then 5 mg after 24 h, 10 mg after 48 h, then 10 mg/day for 6 wks. For patients with low systolic BP, give 2.5 mg/day for 3 days, then 2.5-5 mg/day.

▶ **Dosage in renal impairment**
Titrate to patient's needs after giving the following initial dose:

Creatinine Clearance (mL/min)	% Normal Dose
10-50	50-75
< 10	25-50

OFF-LABEL USES

Treatment of hypertension or renal crises with scleroderma.

CONTRAINDICATIONS

History of angioedema from previous treatment with ACE inhibitors.
Caution
Lactation, pregnancy, children.

INTERACTIONS

Drug
Alcohol, phenothiazines, diuretics, hypotensive agents: May increase hypotensive effects.
Lithium: May increase lithium blood concentration and risk of toxicity.
NSAIDs, indomethacin, sympathomimetics: May decrease hypotensive effects.
Potassium-sparing diuretics, potassium supplements: May cause hyperkalemia.
Salicylates: May reduce hypotensive and vasodilator effects.
Herbal
None known.
Food
None known.

DIAGNOSTIC TEST EFFECTS

May increase BUN, serum alkaline phosphatase, serum bilirubin, serum creatinine, serum potassium, SGOT (AST), and SGPT (ALT) levels. May decrease serum sodium levels. May cause positive ANA titer. Monitor BP before, at initiation of therapy, and periodically thereafter.

SIDE EFFECTS

Frequent (5%-12%)
Headache, dizziness, postural hypotension.
Occasional (2%-4%)
Chest discomfort, fatigue, rash, abdominal pain, nausea, diarrhea, upper respiratory infection.
Rare (≤ 1%)
Palpitations, tachycardia, peripheral edema, insomnia, paresthesia, confusion, constipation, dry mouth, muscle cramps.

SERIOUS REACTIONS

• Excessive hypotension ("first-dose syncope") may occur in patients with congestive heart failure (CHF) and severe salt and volume depletion.
• Angioedema (swelling of face and lips) and hyperkalemia occur rarely.
• Agranulocytosis and neutropenia may be noted in patients with collagen vascular disease, including scleroderma and systemic lupus erythematosus, and impaired renal function.
• Nephrotic syndrome may be noted in patients with history of renal disease.

PRECAUTIONS & CONSIDERATIONS

Caution is warranted in patients with cerebrovascular and coronary insufficiency, hypovolemia, renal impairment, sodium depletion, and those on dialysis or receiving diuretics. Be aware that lisinopril crosses the placenta and that it is unknown whether lisinopril is distributed in breast milk; caution is warranted in lactation. Lisinopril has caused fetal or neonatal morbidity or mortality. Be aware that the safety and efficacy of lisinopril have not been established in children. Elderly patients may be more sensitive to the hypotensive effects of lisinopril.

First-dose syncope may occur in patients with congestive heart failure and severe salt and fluid depletion. Nephrotic syndrome may occur in patients with impaired renal function.

Dizziness may occur. BP should be obtained immediately before giving each lisinopril dose, in addition to regular monitoring. Be alert to fluctuations in BP since orthostatic hypotension may occur; avoid rapid postural changes.

CBC and blood chemistry should be obtained before beginning lisinopril therapy, then every 2 wks for the next 3 mo, and periodically thereafter in patients with autoimmune disease or renal impairment and in those who are taking drugs that affect immune response or leukocyte count. BUN, serum creatinine, serum potassium, renal function, and WBC should also be monitored. Lungs should be auscultated for rales. Pattern of daily bowel activity and stool consistency should be assessed.

Administration
Take lisinopril without regard to food. Crush tablets if necessary.

Lithium Carbonate/ Lithium Citrate

lith´ee-um kahr-buh-neyt/sit-rayte
Lithium Carbonate (Duralith [CAN], Eskalith, Lithicarb [AUS], Lithobid, Quilonum SR [AUS])
Lithium Citrate (Cibalith-S)
Do not confuse Lithobid with Levbid, Lithostat, or Lithotabs.

CATEGORY AND SCHEDULE

Pregnancy Risk Category: D

Classification: Antimanic, inorganic salt.

MECHANISM OF ACTION

A psychotherapeutic agent that affects the storage, release, and reuptake of neurotransmitters. Antimanic effect may result from increased norepinephrine reuptake and serotonin receptor sensitivity. *Therapeutic Effect:* Produces antimanic and antidepressant effects.

PHARMACOKINETICS

Rapidly and completely absorbed from the GI tract. Primarily excreted unchanged in urine. Removed by hemodialysis. *Half-life:* 18-24 h (increased in elderly).

AVAILABILITY

Capsules: 150 mg, 300 mg, 600 mg.
Syrup: 300 mg/mL.
Tablets: 300 mg.
Tablets (Controlled Release): 450 mg.
Tablets (Slow Release): 300 mg.

INDICATIONS AND DOSAGES
ALERT

During acute phase, a therapeutic serum lithium concentration of 1-1.4 mEq/L is required. For long-term control, the desired level is 0.5-1.3 mEq/L. Monitor serum drug concentration and clinical response to determine proper dosage.

▸ **Prevention or treatment of acute mania, manic phase of bipolar disorder (manic-depressive illness)**
PO
Adults. 300 mg 3-4 times a day or 450-900 mg slow-release form twice a day. Maximum: 2.4 g/day.
Elderly. 300 mg twice a day. May increase by 300 mg/day q1wk. Maintenance: 900-1200 mg/day.
Children 12 yr and older. 600-1800 mg/day in 3-4 divided doses (2 doses/day for slow-release).
Children younger than 12 yr. 15-60 mg/kg/day in 3-4 divided doses.

OFF-LABEL USES

Prevention of vascular headache; treatment of depression, neutropenia.

CONTRAINDICATIONS

Debilitated patients, severe cardiovascular disease, severe dehydration, severe renal disease, severe sodium depletion.
Caution
Elderly, thyroid disease, seizure disorders, diabetes mellitus, systemic infection, urinary retention.

INTERACTIONS
Drug
Aspirin, indomethacin, other NSAIDs, metronidazole, carbamazepine: May increase risk of toxicity developing.
Antithyroid medications, iodinated glycerol, potassium iodide: May increase the effects of these drugs.
Diuretics, NSAIDs: May increase lithium serum concentration and risk of toxicity.
Haloperidol: May increase extrapyramidal symptoms and the risk of neurologic toxicity.
Molindone: May increase the risk of neurotoxicity.
Neuromuscular blocking agents: May increase effects of these drugs.
Phenothiazines: May decrease the absorption of phenothiazines, increase the intracellular concentration and renal excretion of lithium, and increase delirium and extrapyramidal symptoms. Antiemetic effect of some phenothiazines may mask early signs of lithium toxicity.
Herbal
None known.
Food
None known.

DIAGNOSTIC TEST EFFECTS

May increase blood glucose, immunoreactive parathyroid hormone, and serum calcium levels.

Therapeutic lithium serum level is 0.6-1.2 mEq/L; toxic serum level is >1.5 mEq/L.

SIDE EFFECTS
! Side effects are dose related and seldom occur at lithium serum levels < 1.5 mEq/L.
Occasional
Fine hand tremor, polydipsia, polyuria, mild nausea.
Rare
Weight gain, bradycardia or tachycardia, acne, rash, muscle twitching, cold and cyanotic extremities, pseudotumor cerebri (eye pain, headache, tinnitus, vision disturbances).

SERIOUS REACTIONS
• A lithium serum concentration of 1.5-2.0 mEq/L may produce vomiting, diarrhea, drowsiness, confusion, incoordination, coarse hand tremor, muscle twitching, and T-wave depression on ECG.
• A lithium serum concentration of 2.0-2.5 mEq/L may result in ataxia, giddiness, tinnitus, blurred vision, clonic movements, and severe hypotension.
• Acute toxicity may be characterized by seizures, oliguria, circulatory failure, coma, and death.

PRECAUTIONS & CONSIDERATIONS
Caution is warranted in patients with thyroid disease, renal impairment, or cardiovascular disease as well as those receiving medications that alter sodium such as diuretics, ACE inhibitors, and NSAIDs. Caution should also be used if there is a risk of suicide. Lithium crosses the placenta and is excreted in breast milk. Children and elderly are more sensitive to an increased drug dosage and have a higher risk for toxicity. Steady salt and fluid intake should

be maintained, especially during summer months.
Acute toxicity is characterized by seizures, oliguria, circulatory failure, coma and death; indications of any of these symptoms should be immediately reported to the health care provider.
Lithium concentrations should be monitored. Therapeutic serum levels are 0.6-1.2 mEq/mL. The toxic serum level for lithium is >1.5 mEq/mL. Adverse effects are seen at levels about 1.5 mEq/mL. Serum lithium should be monitored every 4-5 days during initial therapy, then every 1-3 mo when stable. Draw lithium serum concentrations 8-12 h after dose. Closely supervise patients at risk for committing suicide during early therapy.
Administration
Take with food or milk if GI distress occurs. Slow-release tablets must be swallowed whole. Do not crush or chew. Drink 2-3 L of water daily.

Lodoxamide Tromethamine
loe-dox′a-mide troh-meth-aye-meen
(Alomide)

CATEGORY AND SCHEDULE
Pregnancy Risk Category: B

Classification: Mast cell stabilizers, ophthalmics

MECHANISM OF ACTION
A mast cell stabilizer that prevents an increase in cutaneous vascular permeability and antigen-stimulated histamine release and that may prevent calcium influx into mast cells.

Therapeutic Effect: Inhibits sensitivity reaction.

PHARMACOKINETICS
Nondetectable absorption. *Half-life:* 8.5 h.

AVAILABILITY
Ophthalmic Solution: 0.1% (Alomide).

INDICATIONS AND DOSAGES
▶ **Treatment of vernal keratoconjunctivitis, conjunctivitis, keratitis**
OPHTHALMIC
Adults, Elderly, Children 2 yr or older. 1-2 drops 4 times/day, for up to 3 mo.

CONTRAINDICATIONS
Wearing soft contact lenses (product contains benzalkonium chloride) or hypersensitivity to lodoxamide tromethamine or any component of the formulation.
Caution
Children younger than 2 yr, lactation.

INTERACTIONS
Drug
None known.
Herbal
None known.
Food
None known.

DIAGNOSTIC TEST EFFECTS
None known.

SIDE EFFECTS
Frequent
Transient stinging, burning, instillation discomfort.
Occasional
Ocular itching, blurred vision, dry eye, tearing/discharge/foreign body sensation, headache.

Rare
Scales on lid or lash, ocular swelling, sticky sensation, dizziness, somnolence, nausea, sneezing, dry nose, rash.

SERIOUS REACTIONS
• None reported.

PRECAUTIONS & CONSIDERATIONS
Be aware that lodoxamide tromethamine is for ophthalmic use only. Not for injection. It is unknown whether lodoxamide tromethamine crosses the placenta or is distributed in breast milk. Be aware that the safety and efficacy of lodoxamide tromethamine have not been established in children younger than 2 yr. No age-related precautions have been noted in elderly patients. Continual use for longer than 2 wks could result in dry mouth.
Storage
Store at room temperature.
Administration
Tilt the patient's head back; place solution in conjunctival sac. Close eyes, then press gently on the lacrimal sac for 1 min. Do not wear soft contact lenses during therapy. Therapy may last up to 3 mo.

Loperamide
loe-per'a-mide
(Apo-Loperamide [CAN],
Gastro-Stop [AUS], Imodium [AUS],
Imodium A-D, Loperacap [CAN],
Novo-Loperamide [CAN])
**Do not confuse Imodium with
Indocin or Ionamin.**

CATEGORY AND SCHEDULE
Pregnancy Risk Category: B
OTC liquid, tablets

Classification: Antidiarrheals,
opioids

MECHANISM OF ACTION
An antidiarrheal that directly
affects the intestinal wall muscles.
Therapeutic Effect: Slows intestinal
motility and prolongs transit time of
intestinal contents by reducing fecal
volume, diminishing loss of fluid and
electrolytes, and increasing viscosity
and bulk of stool.

PHARMACOKINETICS
Poorly absorbed from the GI tract.
Protein binding: 97%. Metabolized
in the liver. Eliminated in feces and
excreted in urine. Not removed by
hemodialysis. *Half-life:* 9.1-14.4 h.

AVAILABILITY
Capsules: 2 mg.
Liquid: 1 mg/5 mL (OTC).
Tablets: 2 mg (OTC).

INDICATIONS AND DOSAGES
▸ **Acute diarrhea**
PO (CAPSULES)
Adults, Elderly. Initially, 4 mg; then
2 mg after each unformed stool.
Maximum: 16 mg/day.
*Children aged 9-12 yr, weighing
more than 30 kg.* Initially, 2 mg
3 times a day for 24 h.

*Children aged 6-8 yr, weighing
20-30 kg.* Initially, 2 mg twice a day
for 24 h.
*Children aged 2-5 yr, weighing
13-20 kg.* Initially, 1 mg 3 times/day
for 24 h. Maintenance: 1 mg/10 kg
only after loose stool.
▸ **Chronic diarrhea**
PO
Adults, Elderly. Initially, 4 mg; then
2 mg after each unformed stool until
diarrhea is controlled.
Children. 0.08-0.24 mg/kg/day in 2-3
divided doses. Maximum: 2 mg/dose.
▸ **Traveler's diarrhea**
PO
Adults, Elderly. Initially, 4 mg; then
2 mg after each loose bowel
movement (LBM). Maximum:
8 mg/day for 2 days.
Children 9-11 yr. Initially, 2 mg;
then 1 mg after each LBM.
Maximum: 6 mg/day for 2 days.
Children 6-8 yr. Initially, 1 mg; then
1 mg after each LBM. Maximum:
4 mg/day for 2 days.

CONTRAINDICATIONS
Acute ulcerative colitis (may
produce toxic megacolon), diarrhea
associated with pseudomembranous
enterocolitis from broad-spectrum
antibiotics or to organisms that
invade intestinal mucosa (such
as *Escherichia coli,* shigella, and
salmonella), patients who must avoid
constipation.
Caution
Lactation, children younger than
2 yr, liver disease, dehydration,
bacterial disease, bloody diarrhea,
temperature over 101° F.

INTERACTIONS
Drug
Opioid (narcotic) analgesics: May
increase the risk of constipation.
Herbal
None known.

Food
None known.

DIAGNOSTIC TEST EFFECTS
None known.

SIDE EFFECTS
Rare
Dry mouth, somnolence, abdominal discomfort, allergic reaction (such as rash and itching).

SERIOUS REACTIONS
• Toxicity results in constipation, GI irritation, including nausea and vomiting, and central nervous system (CNS) depression. Activated charcoal is used to treat loperamide toxicity.

PRECAUTIONS & CONSIDERATIONS
Caution is warranted in patients with fluid and electrolyte depletion and hepatic impairment. It is unknown whether loperamide crosses the placenta or is distributed in breast milk. Loperamide use is not recommended in children younger than 6 yr. Infants younger than 3 mo are more susceptible to CNS effects. Loperamide use in elderly patients may mask dehydration and electrolyte depletion. Tasks that require mental alertness or motor skills should be avoided until response to the drug has been established. Alcohol should also be avoided during drug therapy.

Dry mouth may occur. Notify the physician if abdominal distention and pain, diarrhea that does not stop within 3 days, or fever occurs. Pattern of daily bowel activity and stool consistency and hydration status should be monitored.
Administration
Do not give if bloody diarrhea is present or temperature is >101° F. When administering the oral liquid to children, use the accompanying plastic dropper to measure the liquid.

Lopinavir/Ritonavir
lop-in'a-veer/rit-on'a-veer
(Kaletra)
Do not confuse Kaletra with Keppra.

CATEGORY AND SCHEDULE
Pregnancy Risk Category: C

Classification: Antivirals, protease inhibitors

MECHANISM OF ACTION
A protease inhibitor combination drug in which lopinavir inhibits the activity of the enzyme protease late in the HIV replication process and ritonavir increases plasma levels of lopinavir. *Therapeutic Effect:* Formation of immature, noninfectious viral particles.

PHARMACOKINETICS
Readily absorbed after PO administration (absorption increased when taken with food). Protein binding: 98%-99%. Metabolized in the liver. Eliminated primarily in feces. Not removed by hemodialysis. *Half-life:* 5-6 h.

AVAILABILITY
Capsules: 133.3 mg lopinavir/33.3 mg ritonavir.
Oral Solution: 80 mg/mL lopinavir/20 mg/mL ritonavir.

INDICATIONS AND DOSAGES
▸ **HIV infection (monotherapy)**
PO
Adults. 3 capsules (400 mg lopinavir/100 mg ritonavir) or 5 mL

twice a day. Increase to 4 capsules (533 mg lopinavir/133 mg ritonavir) or 6.5 mL when taken with efavirenz or nevirapine.

Children aged 6 mo to 12 yr.
General: Dose based on lopinavir component of combination:

Children weighing more than 40 kg who are not taking amprenavir, efavirenz, or nevirapine. PO adult dose.

Children weighing 15-40 kg who are not taking efavirenz or nevirapine. 10 mg/kg twice a day.

Children weighing 7-14 kg who are not taking alprenavir, efavirenz, nelfinavir, or nevirapine. 12 mg/kg twice a day.

▸ **HIV infection concomitant therapy with amprenavir, efavirenz, or nevirapine**
PO

Adults. 3 capsules (400 mg lopinavir/100 mg ritonavir) or 5 mL twice a day. Increase to 4 capsules (533 mg lopinavir/133 mg ritonavir) or 6.5 mL when taken with efavirenz or nevirapine.

Children aged 6 mo to 12 yr. General: Dose based on lopinavir component of combination:

Children weighing 15-40 kg who are taking efavirenz or nevirapine. 11 mg/kg twice a day.

Children weighing 7-14 kg who are taking amprenavir, efavirenz, or nevirapine. 13 mg/kg twice a day.

Children weighing more than 45 kg who are taking amprenavir, efavirenz, or nevirapine. PO adult dose.

▸ **HIV infection in therapy-naïve patients**
PO

Adults. 400/100 mg twice daily or 800/200 mg once daily.

▸ **HIV infection in therapy-experienced patients**
PO

Adults. 400/100 mg twice daily.

▸ **HIV infection concomitant therapy with amprenavir, efavirenz, nelfinavir, nevirapine**
PO

Adults. A dose increase in lopinavir/ritonavir to 533/133 mg 2×/day with food is recommended when combined.

CONTRAINDICATIONS

Coadministration with drugs that are highly dependent on CYP3A4 for clearance and for which elevated plasma levels are associated with serious and or life-threatening reactions (astemizole, cisapride, conivaptan, dihydroergotamine, ergonovine, ergotamine, methylergonovine, midazolam, pimozide, ranolazine, sulfasalazine, terfenadine, triazolam).

Hypersensitivity to lopinavir or ritonavir or any of its components, breast-feeding.

Caution

Pregnancy, children younger than 6 mo; elderly with or without impaired cardiac, hepatic, or renal function; hemophilia; immune reconstitution syndrome; pancreatitis.

INTERACTIONS

Drug

Abacavir, amprenavir, atovaquone, lamotrigine, methadone, oral contraceptives, phenytoin, zidovudine: May reduce serum levels of these drugs, decreasing efficacy.

Antiarrhythmic agents (amiodarone, bepridil, lidocaine systemic, quinidine), antifungal agents (itraconazole, ketoconazole), atorvastatin, buspirone, calcium channel blockers (amiodipine, diltiazem, felodipine, nicardipine, nifedepine), cetirizine, clarithromycin, cyclosporine, dihydropyridine, fexofenadine,

fluticasone, phosphodiesterase type 5 inhibitors (sildenafil, tadalafil, vardenafil), protease inhibitors (amprenavir, indinavir, nelfinavir, saquinavir), rifabutin, tacrolimus, tenofovir, trazodone: May increase levels of these drugs, increasing adverse pharmacologic and adverse reactions.

Astemizole, cisapride, conivaptanm ergot derivatives (dihydroergotamine, ergonovine, ergotamine, methylergonovine), HMG-CoA reductase inhibitors (lovastatin, simvastatin), midazolam, pimozide, ranolazine, rifampin, sulfasalazine, terfenadine, triazolam: Contraindicated due to potentially life-threatening reactions.

Carbamazepine, dexamethasone, NNRTIs (efavirenz, nevirapine), phenobarbital, pheytoin, protease inhibitors (amprenavir, fosamprenavir, nelfinavir), rifampin: May reduce lopinavir concentrations, decreasing efficacy.

Delavirdine, ritonavir: May elevate lopinavir concentrations, increasing efficacy and adverse effects.

Didanosine: Must be given 1 h before or 2 h after lopinavir/ritonavir capsules or oral solution.

Disulfiram, Metronidazole: May produce a disulfiram-like reaction when administered with the oral solution which contains alcohol.

Oral contraceptives: May decrease efficacy; advise patient to use alternative nonhormonal contraception during therapy.

Warfarin: May affect efficacy; monitor INR levels.

Herbal
St. John's wort: May decrease blood concentration and effects of lopinavir and ritonavir. Avoid.

Food
None known.

DIAGNOSTIC TEST EFFECTS

May increase blood glucose, GGT, total cholesterol, total bilirubin, total cholesterol, and serum uric acid (at least 2%), AST (SGOT), ALT (SGPT), and triglyceride levels, INR.

SIDE EFFECTS

Frequent (14%)
Mild to moderate diarrhea.
Occasional (2%-6%)
Nausea, asthenia, abdominal pain, headache, vomiting.
Rare (< 2%)
Insomnia, rash.

SERIOUS REACTIONS

• Anemia, leukopenia, lymphad-enopathy, deep vein thrombosis, Cushing syndrome, pancreatitis, and hemorrhagic colitis occur rarely.

PRECAUTIONS & CONSIDERATIONS

! High-doses of itraconazole or ketoconazole are not recommended in persons taking lopinavir/ritonavir. Lopinavir/ritonavir oral solution contains alcohol and should not be given to those receiving metronidazole because this combination may cause a disulfiram-type reaction. Caution is warranted with hepatitis B or C or impaired liver function and pancreatitis where fatalites have been reported. Be aware that it is unknown whether lopinavir/ritonavir is excreted in breast milk. Breastfeeding is not recommended in this population because of the possibility of HIV transmission. Be aware that the safety and efficacy of lopinavir/ritonavir have not been established in children younger than 6 mo. In elderly patients, age-related cardiac function, renal, or liver impairment requires caution. Lopinavir/ritonavir is not a cure for HIV infection, nor does it reduce risk of transmission to others.

Alcohol-related toxicity may occur because of the 42.5% alcohol content of the oral solution; caution warranted in using this product or any other alcohol-containing product or beverage.

Advise patient that caution is necessary when taking sildenafil, tadalafil, or vardenafil, which may cause low BP, sustained erection, or visual changes; any symptoms should be reported to the health care provider immediately; priapism must be treated immediately. Women should be advised to use another nonhormonal-based contraceptive while taking this medication.

Expect to establish baseline values for CBC, renal and liver function tests, and weight. Assess for nausea and vomiting, pattern of daily bowel activity and stool consistency, and signs and symptoms of pancreatitis as evidenced by abdominal pain, nausea, and vomiting. Eat small, frequent meals to offset nausea or vomiting. Evaluate for signs and symptoms of opportunistic infections as evidenced by cough, onset of fever, oral mucosal changes, or other respiratory symptoms. Check the weight at least twice a week.

Storage

Refrigerate until dispensed, and avoid exposure to excessive heat. If stored at room temperature, use within 2 mo.

Administration

Take with food. Do not administer lopinavir/ritonavir as a once-daily regimen in combination with amprenavir, efavirenz, nelfinavir, or nevirapine; once-daily administration of lopinavir/ritonavir is not recommended in therapy-experienced patients.

Loratadine

loer-at'ah-deen
(Alavert, Claritin, Claritin RediTab, Dimetapp, Tavist ND)

CATEGORY AND SCHEDULE

Pregnancy Risk Category: B

Classification: OTC
Antihistamines, H_1 histamine antagonist

MECHANISM OF ACTION

A long-acting antihistamine that competes with histamine for H_1 receptor sites on effector cells. *Therapeutic Effect:* Prevents allergic responses mediated by histamine, such as rhinitis, urticaria, and pruritus.

PHARMACOKINETICS

Route	Onset	Peak	Duration
PO	1-3 h	8-12 h	Longer than 24 h

Rapidly and almost completely absorbed from the GI tract. Protein binding, 97%; metabolite, 73%-77%. Distributed mainly to the liver, lungs, GI tract, and bile. Metabolized in the liver to active metabolite; undergoes extensive first-pass metabolism. Eliminated in urine and feces. Not removed by hemodialysis. *Half-life:* 8.4 h; metabolite, 28 h (increased in elderly and hepatic impairment).

AVAILABILITY

Syrup (Claritin): 10 mg/10 mL.
Tablets (Alavert, Claritin, Tavist ND): 10 mg.
Tablets (Rapid-Disintegrating [Alavert, Claritin RediTab]): 10 mg.

INDICATIONS AND DOSAGES

▶ **Allergic rhinitis, urticaria**
PO
Adults, Elderly, Children 6 yr and older. 10 mg once a day.
Children 2-5 yr. 5 mg once a day.
▶ **Dosage in hepatic impairment**
For adults, elderly, and children 6 yr and older, dosage is reduced to 10 mg every other day.

CONTRAINDICATIONS

Hypersensitivity to loratadine or its ingredients.
Caution
Increased intraocular pressure, bronchial asthma, patients at risk for syncope or drowsiness, renal impairment.

INTERACTIONS

Drug
All central nervous system (CNS) depressants, alcohol: May increase CNS depressive effects.
Anticholinergics, antihistamines, antiparkinsonian drugs: May increase anticholinergic effects.
Clarithromycin, erythromycin, fluconazole, ketoconazole: May increase the loratadine blood concentration.
Conscious sedation drugs: May cause synergistic sedative activity.
Herbal
None known.
Food
All foods: Delay the absorption of loratadine.

DIAGNOSTIC TEST EFFECTS

May suppress wheal and flare reactions to antigen skin testing unless the drug is discontinued 4 days before testing.

SIDE EFFECTS

Frequent (8%-12%)
Headache, fatigue, somnolence.

Occasional (3%)
Dry mouth, nose, or throat.
Rare
Photosensitivity.

SERIOUS REACTIONS

• None known.

PRECAUTIONS & CONSIDERATIONS

Caution should be used in breastfeeding women, children, and those with hepatic impairment. Loratadine is excreted in breast milk. Children and elderly patients are more sensitive to the drug's anticholinergic effects, such as dry mouth, nose, and throat. Avoid exposure to sunlight, drinking alcoholic beverages, and tasks that require alertness or motor skills until response to the drug is established.

Drowsiness and dry mouth may occur. Respiratory rate, depth, and rhythm; pulse rate and quality; BP; and therapeutic response should be monitored.
Administration
Take loratadine on an empty stomach because food delays its absorption.

Lorazepam

lor-a′ze-pam
(Apo-Lorazepam [CAN], Ativan, Lorazepam Intensol, Novolorazepam [CAN])
Do not confuse lorazepam with alprazolam.

CATEGORY AND SCHEDULE

Pregnancy Risk Category: D
Controlled Substance Schedule: IV

Classification: Anxiolytics, benzodiazepines

MECHANISM OF ACTION

A benzodiazepine that enhances the action of the inhibitory neurotransmitter -aminobutyric acid in the CNS, affecting memory, as well as motor, sensory, and cognitive function. *Therapeutic Effect:* Produces anxiolytic, anticonvulsant, sedative, muscle relaxant, and antiemetic effects.

PHARMACOKINETICS

Route	Onset (min)	Peak	Duration (h)
PO	60	NA	8-12
IV	15-30	NA	8-12
IM	30-60	NA	8-12

Well absorbed after PO and IM administration. Protein binding: 85%. Widely distributed. Metabolized in the liver. Primarily excreted in urine. Not removed by hemodialysis. *Half-life:* 10-20 h.

AVAILABILITY

Tablets (Ativan): 0.5 mg, 1 mg, 2 mg.
Injection (Ativan): 2 mg/mL, 4 mg/mL.
Oral Solution (Lorazepam Intensol): 2 mg/mL.

INDICATIONS AND DOSAGES
▸ **Anxiety**
PO
Adults. 1-10 mg/day in 2-3 divided doses. Average: 2-6 mg/day.
Elderly. Initially, 0.5-1 mg/day. May increase gradually. Range: 0.5-4 mg.
IV
Adults, Elderly. 0.02-0.06 mg/kg q2-6h.
IV INFUSION
Adults, Elderly. 0.01-0.1 mg/kg/h.
PO, IV
Children. 0.05 mg/kg/dose q4-8h. Range: 0.02-0.1 mg/kg. Maximum: 2 mg/dose.

▸ **Insomnia due to anxiety**
PO
Adults. 2-4 mg at bedtime.
Elderly. 0.5-1 mg at bedtime.
▸ **Preoperative sedation**
IV
Adults, Elderly. 0.044 mg/kg 15-20 min before surgery. Maximum total dose: 2 mg.
IM
Adults, Elderly. 0.05 mg/kg 2 h before procedure. Maximum total dose: 4 mg.
▸ **Status epilepticus**
IV
Adults, Elderly. 4 mg over 2-5 min. May repeat in 10-15 min. Maximum: 8 mg in 12-h period.
Children. 0.1 mg/kg over 2-5 min. May give second dose of 0.05 mg/kg in 15-20 min. Maximum: 4 mg.
Neonates. 0.05 mg/kg. May repeat in 10-15 min.

OFF-LABEL USES

Treatment of alcohol withdrawal, panic disorders, skeletal muscle spasms, chemotherapy-induced nausea or vomiting, tension headache, tremors; adjunctive treatment before endoscopic procedures (diminishes patient recall).

CONTRAINDICATIONS

Angle-closure glaucoma; pre-existing CNS depression; severe hypotension; severe uncontrolled pain.
Caution
Elderly, debilitated patients, hepatic disease, renal disease, myasthenia gravis.

INTERACTIONS
Drug
Alcohol, other CNS depressants, probenecid: May increase CNS depression.

Opioid analgesics: Increases CNS effects; reduce dosage by a third in elderly patients.

Scopolamine: Possible increased sedation, hallucination.

Herbal

Kava kava, valerian: May increase CNS depression.

Food

None known.

DIAGNOSTIC TEST EFFECTS

None known. Therapeutic serum drug level is 50-240 mg/mL; toxic serum drug level is unknown.

🔘 IV INCOMPATIBILITIES

Aldesleukin (Proleukin), aztreonam (Azactam), idarubicin (Idamycin), ondansetron (Zofran), sufentanil (Sufenta).

🔘 IV COMPATIBILITIES

Bumetanide (Bumex), cefepime (Maxipime), diltiazem (Cardizem), dobutamine (Dobutrex), dopamine (Intropin), heparin, labetalol (Normodyne, Trandate), milrinone (Primacor), norepinephrine (Levophed), piperacillin and tazobactam (Zosyn), potassium, propofol (Diprivan).

SIDE EFFECTS

Frequent

Somnolence (initially in the morning), ataxia, confusion.

Occasional

Blurred vision, slurred speech, hypotension, headache.

Rare

Paradoxical CNS restlessness or excitement in elderly or debilitated.

SERIOUS REACTIONS

• Abrupt or too-rapid withdrawal may result in pronounced restlessness, irritability, insomnia, hand tremor, abdominal or muscle cramps, diaphoresis, vomiting, and seizures.

• Overdose results in somnolence, confusion, diminished reflexes, and coma.

PRECAUTIONS & CONSIDERATIONS

Caution is warranted in patients with pulmonary, hepatic, and renal impairment and in those using other CNS depressants concurrently. Lorazepam may cross the placenta and be distributed in breast milk. Lorazepam may increase the risk of fetal abnormalities if administered during the first trimester of pregnancy. Women on long-term therapy should use effective contraception during therapy and notify the physician immediately if they become or might be pregnant. Chronic lorazepam use during pregnancy may produce withdrawal symptoms in the patient and CNS depression in the neonate. The safety and efficacy of this drug have not been established in children younger than 12 yr. In elderly patients, expect to give small doses initially and to increase dosage gradually to avoid ataxia and excessive sedation.

Lorazepam may be abused by those with addictive propensities; psychologic and physical dependence may occur with chronic administration.

Elderly persons are more prone to orthostatic hypotension and anticholinergic and sedative effects; it may be advisable to reduce their dosages.

Drowsiness and dizziness may occur. Change positions slowly from recumbent, to sitting, before standing to prevent dizziness or orthostatic hypotension from developing. Alcohol, caffeine, and tasks that require mental alertness or motor skills should also be avoided. BP, heart rate, respiratory rate, CBC with differential, and hepatic and renal function should be monitored.

Storage

Refrigerate—do not freeze—parenteral form.

Administration

Take oral lorazepam with food. Crush tablets as needed.

Do not use the solution for injection if it appears discolored or contains a precipitate. Dilute with an equal volume of sterile water for injection, 0.9% NaCl, or D5W. To dilute a prefilled syringe, remove air from a half-filled syringe, aspirate an equal volume of diluent, pull the plunger back slightly to allow for mixing, and gently invert the syringe several times—do not shake vigorously. Give by IV push into the tubing of a free-flowing IV infusion of 0.9% NaCl or D5W at a rate not exceeding 2 mg/min. Stay recumbent for up to 8 h after parenteral administration to reduce the drug's hypotensive effect. The therapeutic serum level for lorazepam is 50-240 mg/mL; the toxic serum level is unknown.

For IM use, inject the drug deep into a large muscle mass, such as the gluteus maximus.

Losartan

lo-sar′tan

(Cozaar)

Do not confuse Cozaar with Zocor.

CATEGORY AND SCHEDULE

Pregnancy Risk Category: C (D if used in second or third trimesters)

Classification: Angiotensin II receptor antagonists

MECHANISM OF ACTION

An angiotensin II receptor, type AT_1, antagonist that blocks vasoconstrictor and aldosterone-secreting effects of angiotensin II, inhibiting the binding of angiotensin II to the AT_1 receptors. *Therapeutic Effect:* Causes vasodilation, decreases peripheral resistance, and decreases BP.

PHARMACOKINETICS

Route	Onset	Peak	Duration
PO	N/A	6 h	24 h

Well absorbed after PO administration. Protein binding: 98%. Undergoes first-pass metabolism in the liver to active metabolites. Excreted in urine and via the biliary system. Not removed by hemodialysis. *Half-life:* 2 h, metabolite: 6-9 h.

AVAILABILITY

Tablets: 25 mg, 50 mg, 100 mg.

INDICATIONS AND DOSAGES
▸ **Hypertension**

PO

Adults, Elderly. Initially, 50 mg once a day. Maximum: May be given once or twice a day, with total daily doses ranging from 25 to 100 mg.

▸ **Nephropathy**

PO

Adults, Elderly. Initially, 50 mg/day. May increase to 100 mg/day based on BP response.

▸ **Stroke reduction**

PO

Adults, Elderly. 50 mg/day. Maximum: 100 mg/day.

▸ **Hypertension in patients with impaired hepatic function**

PO

Adults, Elderly. Initially, 25 mg/day.

CONTRAINDICATIONS
Hypersensitivity, second or third trimester of pregnancy.
Caution
Lactation, children, sodium- and volume-depleted patients, renal impairment.

INTERACTIONS
Drug
Cimetidine: May increase the effects of losartan.
Fluconazole, ketoconazole, troleandomycin: Suspected increase in antihypertensive effects; monitor BP if used concurrently.
General anesthetics: May increase risk of hypotensive episode.
Lithium: May increase lithium blood concentration and risk of lithium toxicity.
Other hypotensive drugs and sedatives: May increase hypotensive effects.
Phenobarbital, rifampin: May decrease hypotensive effects of losartan.
Herbal
None known.
Food
Grapefruit juice: May alter the absorption of losartan.

DIAGNOSTIC TEST EFFECTS
May increase BUN, serum alkaline phosphatase, serum bilirubin, serum creatinine, AST (SGOT), and ALT (SGPT) levels. May decrease blood hemoglobin and hematocrit levels.

SIDE EFFECTS
Frequent (8%)
Upper respiratory tract infection.
Occasional (2%-4%)
Dizziness, diarrhea, cough.
Rare (≤ 1%)
Insomnia, dyspepsia, heartburn, back and leg pain, muscle cramps, myalgia, nasal congestion, sinusitis.

SERIOUS REACTIONS
• Overdosage may manifest as hypotension and tachycardia. Bradycardia occurs less often.

PRECAUTIONS & CONSIDERATIONS
Caution is warranted in patients with hepatic and renal impairment and renal arterial stenosis. Losartan has caused fetal or neonatal morbidity or mortality and may adversely affect the breastfed infant. Patients should not breastfeed while taking losartan. Safety and efficacy of losartan have not been established in children. No age-related precautions have been noted in elderly patients.

Apical pulse and BP should be assessed immediately before each losartan dose and regularly throughout therapy. Be alert to fluctuations in apical pulse and BP. If an excessive reduction in BP occurs, place the person in the supine position with feet slightly elevated and notify the physician. Tasks that require mental alertness or motor skills should be avoided. BUN, serum electrolytes, serum creatinine levels, heart rate, urinalysis, and pattern of daily bowel activity and stool consistency should be assessed. Maintain adequate hydration; exercising outside during hot weather should be avoided to decrease the risk of dehydration and hypotension.
Administration
Take losartan without regard to food. Do not crush or break tablets.

L

Lovastatin

lo'va-sta-tin

(Altoprev, Lotrel, Mevacor)

Do not confuse with Leustatin, Livostin, or Mivacron.

CATEGORY AND SCHEDULE

Pregnancy Risk Category: X

Classification:

Antihyperlipidemics, HMG CoA reductase inhibitors

MECHANISM OF ACTION

An antihyperlipidemic that inhibits HMG-CoA reductase, the enzyme that catalyzes the early step in cholesterol synthesis. *Therapeutic Effect:* Decreases LDL cholesterol, VLDL cholesterol, plasma triglycerides; increases HDL cholesterol.

PHARMACOKINETICS

Route	Onset	Peak	Duration
PO	3 days	4-6 wks	NA

Incompletely absorbed from the GI tract (increased on empty stomach). Protein binding: 95%. Hydrolyzed in the liver to active metabolite. Primarily eliminated in feces. Not removed by hemodialysis. *Half-life:* 1.1-1.7 h.

AVAILABILITY

Tablets (Mevacor): 10 mg, 20 mg, 40 mg.
Tablets (Extended-Release [Altoprev]): 20 mg, 40 mg, 60 mg.

INDICATIONS AND DOSAGES

▸ **Hyperlipoproteinemia, primary prevention of coronary artery disease**
PO

Adults, Elderly. Initially, 20-40 mg/day with evening meal. Increase at 4-wks intervals up to maximum of 80 mg/day.

Maintenance: 20-80 mg/day in single or divided doses.
PO (EXTENDED RELEASE)
Adults, Elderly. Initially, 20 mg/day. May increase at 4-wks intervals up to 60 mg/day.
Children 10-17 yr. 10-40 mg/day with evening meal.

▸ **Heterozygous familial hypercholesterolemia**
PO
Children aged 10-17 yr. Initially, 10 mg/day. May increase to 20 mg/day after 8 wks and 40 mg/day after 16 wks if needed.

CONTRAINDICATIONS

Hypersensitivity, active liver disease, pregnancy, unexplained elevated liver function tests. See Drug Interactions for contraindicated drugs.

INTERACTIONS

Drug

Amiodarone, verapamil: Do not exceed lovastatin 40 mg/day.
Cyclosporine, gemfibrozil, other fibrates, danazol, niacin: Increases the risk of acute renal failure, myalgia, and rhabdomyolysis. Do not exceed lovastatin 20 mg/day.
Erythromycin, itraconazole, clarithromycin, HIV protease inhibitors, ergot alkaloids, nefazodone, ketoconazole: Contraindicated.
Herbal
None known.
Food
Grapefruit juice: Large amounts of grapefruit juice may increase risk of side effects, such as myalgia and weakness.

DIAGNOSTIC TEST EFFECTS

May increase serum creatinine kinase and serum transaminase concentrations.

SIDE EFFECTS

Generally well tolerated. Side effects usually mild and transient.

Frequent (5%-9%)

Headache, flatulence, diarrhea, abdominal pain or cramps, rash and pruritus.

Occasional (3%-4%)

Nausea, vomiting, constipation, dyspepsia.

Rare (1%-2%)

Dizziness, heartburn, myalgia, blurred vision, eye irritation.

SERIOUS REACTIONS

• There is a potential for cataract development.

PRECAUTIONS & CONSIDERATIONS

Caution is warranted in patients with history of heavy or chronic alcohol use, renal impairment, and those who use cyclosporine, fibrates, and niacin. Be aware that lovastatin use is contraindicated in pregnancy because the suppression of cholesterol biosynthesis may cause fetal toxicity and in lactation because it is unknown whether lovastatin is distributed in breast milk. Be aware that the safety and efficacy of lovastatin have not been established in children. No age-related precautions have been noted in elderly patients. Be aware that grapefruit juice should be avoided.

It should be noted that there is a potential for cataract development over time with lovastatin therapy.

Notify the physician of changes in the color of stool or urine, muscle weakness, myalgia, severe gastric upset, rash, unusual bruising, vision changes, or yellowing of eyes or skin. Pattern of daily bowel activity and stool consistency should be assessed. Serum lipid cholesterol and triglyceride levels and hepatic function should be checked at baseline and periodically during treatment.

Storage

Lovastatin should be kept at room temperature in a container with low light exposure.

Administration

Take lovastatin with meals.

Loxapine

lox′a-peen

(Apo-Loxapine [CAN], Loxapac [CAN], Loxitane)

CATEGORY AND SCHEDULE

Pregnancy Risk Category: C

Classification: Antipsychotics

MECHANISM OF ACTION

A dibenzodiazepine derivative that interferes with the binding of dopamine at postsynaptic receptor sites in the brain. Strong anticholinergic effects. *Therapeutic Effect:* Suppresses locomotor activity, produces tranquilization.

PHARMACOKINETICS

Onset of action occurs within 1 h. Metabolized to active metabolites 8-hydroxyloxapine, 7-hydroxyloxapine, and 8-hydroxyamoxapine. Excreted in urine. *Half-life:* 4 h.

AVAILABILITY

Capsules: 5 mg, 10 mg, 25 mg, 50 mg (Loxitane).

INDICATIONS AND DOSAGES
▸ **Psychotic disorders**

PO

Adults. 10 mg 2 times/day. Increase dosage rapidly during first week to 50 mg, if needed. Usual therapeutic, maintenance range: 60-100 mg daily in 2-4 divided doses. Maximum: 250 mg/day.

CONTRAINDICATIONS

Severe central nervous system (CNS) depression, comatose states, hypersensivitiy to loxapine or any component of the formulation.

Caution

Lactation, seizure disorders, hepatic disease, cardiac disease, benign prostatic hypertrophy, cardiac conditions, children younger than 16 yr.

INTERACTIONS

Drug

Alcohol, all CNS depressants: May increase CNS depressant effects.
Antacids, antidiarrheals: May decrease absorption of loxapine.
Anticholinergics: May increase effects of both drugs.
Extrapyramidal symptom (EPS)-producing medications: May increase risk of EPS.
Sympathomimetics, carbamazepine: May decrease effect of these drugs.

Herbal

None known.

Food

None known.

DIAGNOSTIC TEST EFFECTS

None known.

SIDE EFFECTS

Frequent

Blurred vision, confusion, drowsiness, dry mouth, dizziness, light-headedness.

Occasional

Allergic reaction (rash, itching), decreased urination, constipation, decreased sexual ability, enlarged breasts, headache, photosensitivity, nausea, vomiting, insomnia, weight gain.

SERIOUS REACTIONS

• Extrapyramidal symptoms frequently noted are akathisia (motor restlessness, anxiety). Less frequently noted are akinesia (rigidity, tremor, salivation, masklike facial expression, reduced voluntary movements). Infrequently noted dystonias: torticollis (neck muscle spasm), opisthotonos (rigidity of back muscles), and oculogyric crisis (rolling back of eyes). Tardive dyskinesia (protrusion of tongue, puffing of cheeks, chewing/puckering of mouth) occurs rarely but may be irreversible. Risk is greater in elderly women.
• Seizures.

PRECAUTIONS & CONSIDERATIONS

Extreme caution should be used in patients with a history of seizures. Caution is also warranted with cardiovascular disease, glaucoma, history of seizures, prostatic hypertrophy, and urinary retention. It is unknown whether loxapine crosses the placenta or is distributed in breast milk. Safety and efficacy of loxapine have not been established in children. Elderly patients are more susceptible to anticholinergic effects and sedation, increased risk for extrapyramidal effects, and orthostatic hypotension. A decreased dosage is recommended in elderly patients. Avoid alcohol and tasks that require mental alertness or motor skills.

Assess for presence of extrapyramidal motor symptoms, such as tardive dyskinesia and akathisia.

Storage

Store at room temperature.

Administration

Give loxapine with food or a full glass of water or milk to decrease GI irritation. The full therapeutic effect may take up to 6 wks. Do not abruptly discontinue loxapine.

Lymphocyte Immune Globulin N
lym′phow-site
(Atgam)
Do not confuse Atgam with Ativan.

CATEGORY AND SCHEDULE
Pregnancy Risk Category: C

Classification: Immune globulins

MECHANISM OF ACTION
A biological response modifier that acts as a lymphocyte selective immunosuppressant, reducing the number and altering the function of T lymphocytes, which are responsible for cell-mediated and humoral immunity. Lymphocyte immune globulin N also stimulates the release of hematopoietic growth factors.
Therapeutic Effect: Prevents allograft rejection; treats aplastic anemia.

PHARMACOLOGY
Onset rapid, absorption T_{max} is 5 days. Elimination mean half-life is 5.7 days.
Half-life: 2.7-8.7 days.

AVAILABILITY
Injection: 250 mg/5 mL.

INDICATIONS AND DOSAGES
▶ **To delay onset of renal graft allograft rejection**
IV
Adults, Elderly, Children.
15 mg/kg/day for 14 days, then every other day for 14 days. First dose within 24 h before or after transplantation.
▶ **Treatment of renal allograft rejection**
IV
Adults, Elderly, Children. First dose can be delayed until the diagnosis of the first rejection episode. Then give 10-15 mg/kg/day for 14 days, then every other day for 14 more days. Maximum: 21 doses.
▶ **Renal allograft recipients**
IV
Adults, Elderly. 10-30 mg/kg/day.
Children. 5-25 mg/kg/day.
▶ **Aplastic anemia**
IV
Adults, Elderly, Children. 10-20 mg/kg once a day for 8-14 days, then every other day. Maximum: 21 doses.

OFF-LABEL USES
Immunosuppressant in bone marrow, heart, and liver transplants, treatment of pure red cell aplasia, multiple sclerosis, myasthenia gravis, and scleroderma.

CONTRAINDICATIONS
Systemic hypersensitivity reaction to previous injection of lymphocyte immune globulin N or other equine gamma globulin preparations.
Caution
Lactation, pregnancy.

INTERACTIONS
Drug
Immunosuppressants: May increase risk of infection developing.
Herbal
None known.
Food
None known.

DIAGNOSTIC TEST EFFECTS
May alter renal function test results.

Ⓘ IV INCOMPATIBILITIES
No information is available for Y-site administration.

SIDE EFFECTS
Frequent
Fever (51%), thrombocytopenia (30%), rash (2%), chills (16%), leukopenia (14%), systemic infection (13%).

Occasional (5%-10%)
Serum sickness-like reaction, dyspnea, apnea, arthralgia, chest pain, back pain, flank pain, nausea, vomiting, diarrhea, phlebitis.

SERIOUS REACTIONS

• Thrombocytopenia may occur but is generally transient.
• A severe hypersensitivity reaction, including anaphylaxis, occurs rarely.

PRECAUTIONS & CONSIDERATIONS

! Lymphocyte immune globulin should be administered by physicians experienced in immunosuppressive treatment of renal transplant or aplastic anemia. Adequate laboratory and support equipment should be available.

Although rare, there is a risk of transmitting human and equine blood-based infections, particularly Creutzfeld-Jakob disease.

Caution is warranted with concurrent immunosuppressive therapy. Immediately notify the physician of chest pain, rapid or irregular heartbeat, shortness of breath, wheezing, or swelling of the face or throat, which may occur during the IV infusion. Avoid exposure to people with colds or infections, and notify the physician as soon as signs or symptoms of infection, thrombocytopenia, or leukopenia develop. Dosage adjustments should be considered in patients with profound bone marrow suppression.

Although risk of hypersensitivity is rare, hypersensitivity can occur at any time during therapy. Serum sickness, although rare, could occur within the first 6-18 days of therapy.

Experience with children is limited; it has been administered safely to a small number of renal allograft pediatric recipients and aplastic anemia pediatric patients at dosages comparable to those used in adults.

Before administration, test the patient with an intradermal injection of 0.1 mL of a freshly prepared 1:1000 dilution of lymphocyte immune globulin in normal saline and a contralateral NaCl injection as control.

Storage
Keep the drug refrigerated before and after dilution. Discard the diluted solution after 24 h. Protect from freezing.

Administration
Do not use intradermally, subcutaneously, intramuscularly, intra-arterially, or by IV bolus.

For IV use, dilute the total daily dose with 0.9% NaCl, as prescribed, to a final concentration of no more than 4 mg/mL. Gently rotate the diluted solution; avoid shaking it. Use a 0.2- to 1-micron filter, and infuse the total dose over at least 4 h. To prevent chemical phlebitis, avoid using a peripheral vein for IV infusion. Instead, expect to use a central venous catheter, a Groshong catheter, or a peripherally inserted central catheter. Avoid contact of the undiluted lymphocyte immune globulin with air. Expect to monitor frequently for chills, fever, erythema, and pruritus. An order for prophylactic antihistamines or corticosteroids should be obtained to treat these potential side effects.

Lyrica (pregabalin)
lear-reek-a (pre-gab-a-lyn)
(Lyrica)
**Do not confuse Lyrica with
Cymbalta or pregabalin with
gabapentin.**

CATEGORY AND SCHEDULE
Pregnancy Risk Category: C

Classification: Anticonvulsant

MECHANISM OF ACTION
Exact mechanism of pregabalin's
antinociceptive and antiseizure action
is unknown. Effects may be related to
high-affinity binding to α_2-delta site,
an auxiliary subunit of voltage-gated
calcium channels in CNS tissue.
Therapeutic Effect: Alleviation of
fibromyalgia, postherpetic neuralgia,
and partial-onset seizure symptoms.

PHARMACOLOGY
Well absorbed after oral
administration; bioavailability is more
than 90%. Steady state achieved within
24-48 h. Distributed across the blood-
brain barrier; negligible metabolism.
Largely eliminated through renal
excretion, 90% unchanged. *Half-life:*
6 h. In renal impairment, clearance is
proportional to CrCl.

AVAILABILITY
Capsules: 25 mg, 50 mg, 75 mg,
100 mg, 150 mg, 200 mg, 225 mg,
300 mg.

INDICATIONS AND DOSAGES
▸ **Neuropathic pain associated with
diabetic peripheral neuropathy**
PO
Adults, Elderly. Initially, 50 mg 3 times/
day increasing to 100 mg 3 times/day
within 1 wk based on efficacy and
tolerability. Not to exceed 300 mg/day.

▸ **Partial-onset seizures**
PO
Adults, Elderly. Initially, 75 mg
2 times/day or 50 mg 3 times/day
increased to a maximum dose of 300
mg 2 times/day or 200 mg 3 times/day.

▸ **Postherpetic neuralgia**
PO
Adults, Elderly. Initially, 75 mg
2 times/day or 50 mg 3 times/day,
increasing to 300 mg/day within 1 wk
based on efficacy and tolerability.
Dosage may be increased to 300 mg
2 times/day or 200 mg 3 times/day
not to exceed 600 mg/day.

▸ **Fibromyalgia**
PO
Adults, Elderly. Initially, 75 mg 2 times/
day increasing to 150 mg 2 times/day
within 1 wk based on efficacy and
tolerability. May further increase dose
to 225 mg 2 times/day not to exceed
450 mg/day.

▸ **Treatment requiring dosage
adjustment for renal function
impairment**
PO
Adults, Elderly. For
CrCl > 60 mL/min: total daily dose
range 150-600 mg/day, administered
2 or 3 times/day.
For CrCl 30-60 mL/min: total daily
dose range 75-300 mg 2 times/day or
3 times/day.
For CrCl 15-30 mL/min: total daily
dose range 25-150 mg 1×/day or
2 times/day.
For CrCl <15 mL/min: total daily
dose range 25-75 mg once daily.

▸ **Treatment for patients on
hemodialysis**
PO
Adults, Elderly. Maintenance based
on CrCl as recommended plus
supplemental posthemodialysis
dose administered after each 4 h of
hemodialysis as follows:
If maintenance dose is 25 mg/day,
postdialysis dose is 25-50 mg.

L

If maintenance dose is 25-50 mg/day, postdialysis dose is 50-75 mg.
If maintenance dose is 50-75 mg/day, postdialysis dose is 75-100 mg.
If maintenance dose is 75 mg/day, postdialysis dose is 100-150 mg.

OFF-LABEL USES

Treatment of generalized anxiety disorder.

CONTRAINDICATIONS

Alcohol, hypersensitivity to pregabalin or any of its components.
Caution
Lactation, pregnancy.

INTERACTIONS

Drug
All CNS depressants, alcohol, lorazepam, oxycodone, and other opiates: May have additive cognitive and gross motor function effects; may increase CNS depressant effects.
Immunosuppressants: May increase risk of infection developing.
Thiazolidinedione antidiabetic agents: May cause peripheral edema; use caution in concurrent use.
Herbal
None known.
Food
None known.

DIAGNOSTIC TEST EFFECTS

May increase creatinine kinase levels; significant decreases (20% or below baseline and <150 × 103 mcL) are documented. Check ECG PR interval prolongation (3-6 msec) with an increased risk of PR of more than 25% from baseline, on-treatment PR > 200 msec, or increased 2nd or 3rd degree AV block.

SIDE EFFECTS

Frequent
Dizziness, somnolence, ataxia, headache, tremor, blurred vision, peripheral edema, weight gain.

Occasional
Abnormal gait, fatigue, asthenia, confusion, euphoria, increased appetite, speech disorder, vertigo, myoclonus, anxiety, depression, disorientation, lethargy, nervousness, dry mouth, constipation, increased appetite, GI effects.

SERIOUS REACTIONS

• Unexplained muscle pain, tenderness, weakness, especially if accompanied by general body discomfort or fever.
• A severe hypersensitivity reaction, including anaphylaxis, occurs rarely.

PRECAUTIONS & CONSIDERATIONS

No gender- or race-related precautions have been noted.

Drug should be discontinued by tapering down the dose over a 1-wk period. Where antiepileptic drug withdrawal is needed, withdraw gradually over at least 1 wk to minimize potential of increased seizure frequency in seizure disorder patients.

It is unknown whether pregabalin crosses the placenta or is excreted in breast milk; caution in pregnancy and lactation is warranted. Safety and efficacy are not established in children. Because of possible renal function impairment, dosage adjustment may be needed. Caution warranted in patients with New York Heart Association class III or IV cardiac status.

Drug may cause drowsiness and dizziness; use caution when driving or performing other activities that require mental or physical acuity.

Reductions in visual acuity, visual field changes, and funduscopic changes are noted; weight gain is possible.

Symptoms of unexplained muscle pain, tenderness, or weakness, especially if accompanied by general body discomfort or fever, should be reported immediately.

Storage

Ambient conditions.

Administration

Drug may be taken without regard to food; however, if GI effects occur, it can be taken with a meal. Advise the patient to take medication as directed; if medication needs to be discontinued, it should be withdrawn over a 1-wk period unless safety concerns (hypersensitivity, rash) dictate a more rapid withdrawal. Patients taking antiepileptic medications should continue to take these medications unless otherwise advised by their healthcare practitioner.

L

Mafenide
Mafenide
ma′fe-nide
(Sulfamylon)

CATEGORY AND SCHEDULE
Pregnancy Risk Category: C

Classification: Anti-infectives, topical, dermatologics, sulfonamides

MECHANISM OF ACTION
A topical anti-infective that decreases number of bacteria avascular tissue of second- and third-degree burns. *Therapeutic Effect:* Bacteriostatic. Promotes spontaneous healing of deep partial-thickness burns.

PHARMACOKINETICS
Absorbed through devascularized areas into systemic circulation following topical administration. Excreted in the form of its metabolite rho-carboxybenzenesulfonamide.

AVAILABILITY
Cream: 85 mg base/g (Sulfamylon).

INDICATIONS AND DOSAGES
▸ **Burns**
TOPICAL
Adults, Elderly, Children. Apply 1-2 times/day.

CONTRAINDICATIONS
Hypersensitivity to mafenide or sulfonamides or any other component of the formulation.

INTERACTIONS
Drug
None known.
Herbal
None known.
Food
None known.

DIAGNOSTIC TEST EFFECTS
None known.

SIDE EFFECTS
Difficult to distinguish side effects and effects of severe burn.
Frequent
Pain, burning upon application.
Occasional
Allergic reaction (usually 10-14 days after initiation): itching, rash, facial edema, swelling; unexplained syndrome of marked hyperventilation with respiratory alkalosis.
Rare
Delay in eschar separation, excoriation of new skin.

SERIOUS REACTIONS
• Hemolytic anemia, porphyria, bone marrow depression, superinfections (especially with fungi), metabolic acidosis occur rarely.

PRECAUTIONS & CONSIDERATIONS
Caution is warranted with impaired renal function because of the risk of metabolic acidosis. Be aware that cross-sensitivity to sulfonamides is not certain. It is unknown whether mafenide crosses the placenta or is distributed in breast milk. Be aware that mafenide is not recommended in newborn infants because sulfonamides may cause kernicterus. No age-related precautions have been noted in elderly patients.

Signs and symptoms of metabolic acidosis should be monitored, such as Kussmaul's respirations, nausea, vomiting, diarrhea, headache, tremors, weakness, and cardiac arrhythmias (caused by associated hyperkalemia), sensorium changes, decreased Pco_2, blood pH, and Hco_3. Caution is warranted regarding the patient's stress tolerance because of possible cardiovascular effects from injury.

Storage
Store at room temperature.

Administration
Mafenide is for external use only. Apply mafenide with gloved hands. Burned area should be kept covered with mafenide at all times. Apply to thickness of around 16 mm.

Magaldrate
(Iosopan Plus, Lowsium Plus, Riopan Plus)

CATEGORY AND SCHEDULE
Pregnancy Risk Category: C

Classification: Antacid/ aluminum/magnesium hydroxide

MECHANISM OF ACTION
An antacid that causes less hydrogen ion available for diffusion thru the GI mucosa. *Therapeutic Effect:* Reduces and neutralizes gastric acid.

PHARMACOKINETICS
Onset 10-15 min; duration longer than 3 h. *Half-life:* Unreported.

AVAILABILITY
Suspension: Magaldrate 540 mg and simethicone 20 mg/5 mL, magaldrate 540 mg and simethicone 40 mg/5 mL, magaldrate 1080 mg and simethicone 40 mg/5 mL.
Tablets (Chewable): magaldrate 540 mg and simethicone 20 mg, magaldrate 1080 mg and simethicone 20 mg.

INDICATIONS AND DOSAGES
▸ **Hyperacidity and gas**

PO
Adults, Elde.
between meal

CONTRAINDICATIONS
Hypersensitivity to mag. colostomy or ileosv, appendicitis, ulcerativecolitis, diverticulitis.
Caution
Elderly, fluid restriction, decreased GI motility, GI obstruction, dehydration, nal disease, sodium-restricted ets, colitis, gastric outlet obstruction syndrome, colostomy.

INTERACTIONS
Drug
Anticholinergics, corticosteroids, sodium fluoride, chlordiazepoxide, metronidazole: May interfere with absorption of these medications.
Fluoroquinolones: May decrease the absorption of fluoroquinolones.
Ketoconazole, methenamine: May decrease the absorption of ketoconazole or methenamine.
Tetracyclines: May decrease the absorption of tetracyclines.
Herbal
None known.
Food
None known.

SIDE EFFECTS
Rare
Constipation, diarrhea, fluid retention, dizziness or lightheadedness, continuing discomfort, irregular heartbeat, loss of appetite, mood or mental changes, muscle weakness, unusual tiredness or weakness, weight loss, chalky taste.

SERIOUS REACTIONS
• None known.

M

...RECTIONS & CO...
...aut...hould be us...
...with...gestive hea... Caution
Dia...a should be ...that can
re...ng any medi...es; patients
ex...bate GI dis...e NSAIDs
s...d be advise... speaking with a
...spirin only ...care pr...ti...er familiar with
...eir medical st.... Patients should
...be divsed t...che in a semisupine
po...ition if ...disurbances are
s...gnificant.
Administ...tio...
Drink sev...al glasses of water a day
to help r...duce possible constipation.
Take oth...r medications at least
2 h befo...e ...r after taking with
magaldrate

Magnesium
(Mag-Delay SR, Slow-Mag)
(Citrate of Magnesia, Citro-Mag
[CAN]) (Phillips Milk of Magnesia)
(Mag-Ox 400, Uro-Mag)
**Do not confuse magnesium
sulfate with manganese sulfate.**

CATEGORY AND SCHEDULE
Pregnancy Risk Category: B

Classification: Anticonvulsant

MECHANISM OF ACTION
An antacid, laxative, electrolyte,
and anticonvulsant. As an antacid,
it acts in the stomach to neutralize
gastric acid. *Therapeutic Effect:*
Increases pH. As a laxative has
an osmotic effect, primarily in the
small intestine, and draws water
into the intestinal lumen, thereby
increasing intraluminal pressure.
Therapeutic Effect: Produces
distention and promotes peristalsis
and bowel evacuation. As a systemic
dietary supplement and electrolyte
replacement, it is found primarily
in intracellular fluids and is
essential for enzyme activity, nerve
conduction, and muscle contraction.
As an anticonvulsant, it blocks
neuromuscular transmission and the
amount of acetylcholine released
at the motor endplate. *Therapeutic
Effect:* Controls seizure. Maintains
and restores magnesium levels.

PHARMACOKINETICS
Antacid, laxative: Minimal
absorption through the intestine.
Absorbed dose primarily excreted in
urine. Systemic: Widely distributed.
Excreted primarily in urine.

AVAILABILITY
Magnesium Chloride
Tablets (Slo-Mag, Mag Delay SR):
64 mg.
Magnesium Citrate
Oral Solution (Citrate of Magnesia):
290 mg/5 mL.
Magnesium Hydroxide
*Oral Liquid (Phillips Milk of
Magnesia):* 400 mg/5 mL,
800 mg/5 mL.
*Chewable Tablets (Phillips Milk of
Magnesia):* 311 mg.
Magnesium Oxide
Tablets (Mag-Ox 400): 400 mg.
Capsules (Uro-Mag): 140 mg.
Magnesium Sulfate
Premix Infusion Solution: 10 mg/mL,
20 mg/mL, 40 mg/mL, 80 mg/mL.
Injection: 4% (0.325 mEq/mL), 8%
(0.65 mEq/mL), 12.5% (1 mEq/mL),
50% (4 mEq/mL).

INDICATIONS AND DOSAGES
▸ **Mild hypomagnesemia (magnesium
sulfate)**
PO
Adults, Elderly. 3 g q6h for 4 doses
as needed.

stress tolerance because of possible cardiovascular effects from injury.

Storage
Store at room temperature.

Administration
Mafenide is for external use only. Apply mafenide with gloved hands. Burned area should be kept covered with mafenide at all times. Apply to thickness of around 16 mm.

Magaldrate
(Iosopan Plus, Lowsium Plus, Riopan Plus)

CATEGORY AND SCHEDULE
Pregnancy Risk Category: C

Classification: Antacid/ aluminum/magnesium hydroxide

MECHANISM OF ACTION
An antacid that causes less hydrogen ion available for diffusion thru the GI mucosa. *Therapeutic Effect:* Reduces and neutralizes gastric acid.

PHARMACOKINETICS
Onset 10-15 min; duration longer than 3 h. *Half-life:* Unreported.

AVAILABILITY
Suspension: Magaldrate 540 mg and simethicone 20 mg/5 mL, magaldrate 540 mg and simethicone 40 mg/5 mL, magaldrate 1080 mg and simethicone 40 mg/5 mL.
Tablets (Chewable): magaldrate 540 mg and simethicone 20 mg, magaldrate 1080 mg and simethicone 20 mg.

INDICATIONS AND DOSAGES
▶ **Hyperacidity and gas**

PO
Adults, Elderly. 540-1080 mg between meals and at bedtime.

CONTRAINDICATIONS
Hypersensitivity to magaldrate, colostomy or ileostomy, appendicitis, ulcerative colitis, diverticulitis.
Caution
Elderly, fluid restriction, decreased GI motility, GI obstruction, dehydration, renal disease, sodium-restricted diets, colitis, gastric outlet obstruction syndrome, colostomy.

INTERACTIONS
Drug
Anticholinergics, corticosteroids, sodium fluoride, chlordiazepoxide, metronidazole: May interfere with absorption of these medications.
Fluoroquinolones: May decrease the absorption of fluoroquinolones.
Ketoconazole, methenamine: May decrease the absorption of ketoconazole or methenamine.
Tetracyclines: May decrease the absorption of tetracyclines.
Herbal
None known.
Food
None known.

SIDE EFFECTS
Rare
Constipation, diarrhea, fluid retention, dizziness or lightheadedness, continuing discomfort, irregular heartbeat, loss of appetite, mood or mental changes, muscle weakness, unusual tiredness or weakness, weight loss, chalky taste.

SERIOUS REACTIONS
• None known.

PRECAUTIONS & CONSIDERATIONS

Caution should be used in patients with congestive heart failure. Diarrhea should be reported. Caution regarding any medications that can exacerbate GI disturbances; patients should be advised to use NSAIDs or aspirin only after speaking with a health care practitioner familiar with their medical history. Patients should be adivsed to recline in a semisupine position if GI disturbances are significant.

Administration

Drink several glasses of water a day to help reduce possible constipation. Take other medications at least 2 h before or after taking with magaldrate.

Magnesium

(Mag-Delay SR, Slow-Mag)
(Citrate of Magnesia, Citro-Mag [CAN]) (Phillips Milk of Magnesia) (Mag-Ox 400, Uro-Mag)
Do not confuse magnesium sulfate with manganese sulfate.

CATEGORY AND SCHEDULE

Pregnancy Risk Category: B

Classification: Anticonvulsant

MECHANISM OF ACTION

An antacid, laxative, electrolyte, and anticonvulsant. As an antacid, it acts in the stomach to neutralize gastric acid. *Therapeutic Effect:* Increases pH. As a laxative has an osmotic effect, primarily in the small intestine, and draws water into the intestinal lumen, thereby increasing intraluminal pressure. *Therapeutic Effect:* Produces distention and promotes peristalsis

and bowel evacuation. As a systemic dietary supplement and electrolyte replacement, it is found primarily in intracellular fluids and is essential for enzyme activity, nerve conduction, and muscle contraction. As an anticonvulsant, it blocks neuromuscular transmission and the amount of acetylcholine released at the motor endplate. *Therapeutic Effect:* Controls seizure. Maintains and restores magnesium levels.

PHARMACOKINETICS

Antacid, laxative: Minimal absorption through the intestine. Absorbed dose primarily excreted in urine. Systemic: Widely distributed. Excreted primarily in urine.

AVAILABILITY

Magnesium Chloride
Tablets (Slo-Mag, Mag Delay SR): 64 mg.
Magnesium Citrate
Oral Solution (Citrate of Magnesia): 290 mg/5 mL.
Magnesium Hydroxide
Oral Liquid (Phillips Milk of Magnesia): 400 mg/5 mL, 800 mg/5 mL.
Chewable Tablets (Phillips Milk of Magnesia): 311 mg.
Magnesium Oxide
Tablets (Mag-Ox 400): 400 mg.
Capsules (Uro-Mag): 140 mg.
Magnesium Sulfate
Premix Infusion Solution: 10 mg/mL, 20 mg/mL, 40 mg/mL, 80 mg/mL.
Injection: 4% (0.325 mEq/mL), 8% (0.65 mEq/mL), 12.5% (1 mEq/mL), 50% (4 mEq/mL).

INDICATIONS AND DOSAGES
▸ **Mild hypomagnesemia (magnesium sulfate)**
PO
Adults, Elderly. 3 g q6h for 4 doses as needed.

IV, IM
Adults, Elderly. 1 g/day equivalent to 8.12 mEq magnesium (2 mL 50% solution) q6h for 4 doses, equivalent to 32.5 mEq/24 h, in divided doses.
Children. 25-50 mg/kg/dose q4-6h for 3-4 doses. Maintenance: 30-60 mg/kg/day.

▶ **Severe hypomagnesemia (magnesium sulfate)**
IV
Adults, Elderly. 250 mg/kg q4h, or 5 g (40 mEq) added to 1 L dextrose 5%, or 0.9% NaCl for slow IV infusion over 3 h.

▶ **Eclampsia (magnesium sulfate)**
IV/IM
Adults, Elderly. 10-14 g magnesium sulfate in combination mixture of IM and IV administration appropriately diluted.

▶ **Hypertension, seizures (magnesium sulfate)**
IV, IM
Children. 20-100 mg/kg/dose q4-6h as needed.
IV
Adults. Initially, 4 g then 1-4 g/h by continuous infusion.

▶ **Arrhythmias (magnesium sulfate)**
IV
Adults, Elderly. Initially, 1-2 g then infusion of 1-2 g/h.

▶ **Constipation (magnesium sulfate)**
PO
Adults, Elderly, Children older than 11 yrs. 10-30 g/day in divided doses.
Children 6-11 yrs. 5-10 g/day in divided doses.
Children 2-5 yrs. 2.5-5 g/kg/day in divided doses.

▶ **Constipation (magnesium hydroxide)**
PO
Adults, Elderly, Children older than 11 yrs. 6-8 tablets or 30-60 mL/day.
Children 6-11 yrs. 3-4 tablets or 7.5-15 mL/day.

Children 2-5 yrs. 1-2 tablets or 2.5-7.5 mL/day.

▶ **Hyperacidity (magnesium hydroxide)**
PO
Adults, Elderly. 2-4 tablets or 5-15 mL as needed up to 4 times a day.
Children 7-14 yrs. 1 tablet or 2.5-5 mL as needed up to 4 times a day.

▶ **Magnesium deficiency (magnesium oxide)**
PO
Adults, Elderly. 1-2 tablets 2-3 times/day.

▶ **Dietary supplement (magnesium chloride)**
PO
Adults, Elderly. 54-483 mg/day in 2-4 divided doses.

▶ **Hyperalimentation (magnesium sulfate or magnesium chloride)**
TPN
Adults, Elderly. Maintenance dose 8-24 mEq (1-3 g) daily.
Infants. 2-10 mEq (0.25-1.25 mEq) daily.

▶ **Cathartic (magnesium citrate)**
PO
Adults, Elderly, Children 12 yrs and older. 120-300 mL.
Children 6-11 yrs. 100-150 mL.
Children younger than 6 yrs. 0.5 mL/kg up to maximum of 200 mL.

CONTRAINDICATIONS

Antacid: Appendicitis or symptoms of appendicitis, ileostomy, intestinal obstruction, severe renal impairment.
Laxative: Appendicitis, congestive heart failure, colostomy, hypersensitivity, ileostomy, intestinal obstruction, undiagnosed rectal bleeding.
Systemic: Heart block, myocardial damage, renal failure, toxemia of

pregnancy during 2 h preceding delivery.

INTERACTIONS
Drug
ANTACID
Ketoconazole, tetracyclines: May decrease the absorption of ketoconazole and tetracyclines.
Methenamine: May decrease the effects of methenamine.
Nitrofurantoin: May decrease absorption.
Penicillinamine: May reduce effects of penicillinamine.
ANTACID, LAXATIVE
Digoxin, oral anticoagulants, phenothiazines: May decrease the effects of these drugs or cause heart block when administered with calcium.
Tetracyclines: May form nonabsorbable complex with tetracyclines.
SYSTEMIC (DIETARY SUPPLEMENT, ELECTROLYTE REPLACEMENT)
Calcium: May reverse the effects of magnesium.
Central nervous system (CNS) depression-producing medications: May increase CNS depression.
Digoxin: May cause changes in cardiac conduction or heart block with digoxin.
Herbal
None known.
Food
None known.

DIAGNOSTIC TEST EFFECTS
Antacid: May increase gastrin production and pH.
Laxative: May decrease serum potassium level.
Systemic (dietary supplement, electrolyte replacement): None known.

IV INCOMPATIBILITIES
Amphotericin B complex (Abelcet, AmBisome, Amphotec), cefepime (Maxipime).

IV COMPATIBILITIES
Amikacin (Amikin), cefazolin (Ancef), ciprofloxacin (Cipro), dobutamine (Dobutrex), enalapril (Vasotec), gentamicin, heparin, hydromorphone (Dilaudid), insulin, milrinone (Primacor), morphine, piperacillin/tazobactam (Zosyn), potassium chloride, propofol (Diprivan), tobramycin (Nebcin), vancomycin (Vancocin).

SIDE EFFECTS
Frequent
Antacid: Chalky taste, diarrhea, laxative effect.
Occasional
Antacid: Nausea, vomiting, stomach cramps.
Antacid, laxative: With prolonged use or large doses in renal impairment, possible hypermagnesemia, marked by dizziness, irregular heartbeat, mental changes, fatigue, and weakness.
Laxative: Cramping, diarrhea, increased thirst, flatulence.
Systemic (dietary supplement, electrolyte replacement): Reduced respiratory rate, decreased reflexes, flushing, hypotension, decreased heart rate.

SERIOUS REACTIONS
• Magnesium as an antacid or laxative has no known serious reactions.
• Systemic use of magnesium may produce prolonged PR interval and widening of QRS interval.
• Magnesium toxicity may cause loss of deep tendon reflexes, heart block, respiratory paralysis, and cardiac

M

arrest. The antidote for toxicity is 10-20 mL 10% calcium gluconate (5-10 mEq of calcium).

PRECAUTIONS & CONSIDERATIONS

Magnesium antacids should be used cautiously with chronic diarrhea, colostomy, diverticulitis, ulcerative colitis, and undiagnosed GI and rectal bleeding. The laxative form should be used cautiously with diabetes mellitus and in those on a low-salt diet because some magnesium supplements contain sugar or sodium. When magnesium is given for systemic use, it should be used cautiously in severe renal impairment. It is unknown whether antacid forms of magnesium are distributed in breast milk. Parenteral magnesium readily crosses the placenta and is distributed in breast milk for 24 h after therapy has been discontinued. Continuous IV infusion of magnesium increases the risk of magnesium toxicity in the neonate. Magnesium should not be administered IV during the 2 h preceding delivery. Magnesium should be used cautiously in children younger than 6 yrs because safety is unknown. Elderly patients are at increased risk for developing magnesium deficiency because of decreased magnesium absorption, other medications they may be taking, and poor diet.

Adequate hydration should be maintained. Notify the physician if signs and symptoms of hypermagnesemia occur, including confusion, cramping, dizziness, irregular heartbeat, lightheadedness, or unusual fatigue or weakness. ECG, BUN, serum creatinine, and magnesium levels should be monitored in those receiving systemic form. Patellar reflexes

should be tested before giving repeat parenteral doses of systemic magnesium to assess for CNS depression. Know that suppressed reflexes may indicate impending respiratory arrest. Patellar reflexes should be present, and respiratory rate should be > 16 breaths/min before each parenteral dose.

Report any unrelieved constipation, rectal bleeding, symptoms of electrolyte imbalance, particularly muscle cramps, pain, weakness, and dizziness immediately.

Storage
Refrigerate citrate of magnesia to retain potency and improve palatability. Store parenteral formulation at room temperature. Discard if any particulate matter appears in injectible solutions, is cloudy or discolored. In oral forms, if any degradation of tablets or nonmiscibility of suspension appeears, discard.

Administration
! Keep in mind that antacids may be given up to 4 times a day.

When using antacids, shake suspension well before use. Make sure that chewable tablets are chewed thoroughly before swallowing and are followed by a full glass of water. Take magnesium antacids at least 2 h before or 2 h after other medications. Do not take magnesium antacids for longer than 2 wks, unless directed by the physician. Those with peptic ulcer disease should take magnesium antacids 1 and 3 h after meals and at bedtime for 4-6 wks.

When using laxatives, drink a full glass of liquid (8 oz) with each dose to prevent dehydration. Follow dose with citrus carbonated beverage or fruit juice to improve flavor. Magnesium laxatives are for short-term use only.

For IV use, the solution must be diluted. For infusion, do not exceed magnesium sulfate concentration of 200 mg/mL (20%). Do not exceed infusion rate of 150 mg/min. Do not mix with other IV drugs unless compatibility is established.

For IM use, for adults and elderly patients, use 250 mg/mL (25%) or 500 mg/mL (50%) magnesium sulfate concentration (undiluted) deep into a large muscle mass, as prescribed. For children and infants, do not exceed 200 mg/mL (20%) as prescribed.

M

Magnesium Salicylate
Mag-nee-see-um sal-e-sigh-late
OTC
(Backache Relief, Doan's Extra Strength)
RX
Trisilate, Malsalate, Novasal

CATEGORY AND SCHEDULE
Pregnancy Risk Category: NR
OTC

Classification: Analgesics, non-narcotic, salicylates, platelet aggregation inhibitors

MECHANISM OF ACTION
A nonsteroidal anti-inflammatory that inhibits cyclooxygenase and suppresses prostaglandin synthesis. *Therapeutic Effect:* Produces analgesic and anti-inflammatory effect.

PHARMACOKINETICS
Rapidly absorbed from the GI tract. Widely distributed. Protein binding: 80%-90%. Metabolized in the liver. Excreted primarily in urine. Removed by hemodialysis. *Half-life:* 2-3 h.

AVAILABILITY
Tablets (OTC). 580 mg.
Tablets (RX). 600 mg.

INDICATIONS AND DOSAGES
▸ **Arthritis, inflammation, musculoskeletal disorders (backache)**
PO
Adults, Elderly. 580-600 mg PO q4-6h. Maximum: 4.8q/day. (RX use) or 3.5q/day (OTC use).

CONTRAINDICATIONS
Severe renal impairment, hypersensitivity to magnesium salicylate or any component of the formulation.

Severe hypersensitivity to aspirin, other salicylates, or NSAIDS.

INTERACTIONS
Drug
Antidiabetics, oral: May increase antidiabetic effects.
Ciprofloxacin, enoxacin, itraconazole, ketoconazole, norfloxacin, ofloxacin, tetracyclines: May interfere with absorption and activity of these drugs.
Heparin, oral anticoagulants, thrombolytics, carbenicillin IM, cefmandole, sulfinpyrazone, dipyramidole, divalproex, heparin, pentoxyfilline, pilcamycin, ticarcillin, valproic acid: May increase the risk of bleeding.

Probenecid: May increase magnesium salicylate blood concentration; may increase gout symptoms.
Urinary alkalizers (acetazolamide, dichlorphenamide, methazolamide): May increase excretion and lower efficacy of salicylates.
Varicella virus vaccine: May increase risk of developing Reye syndrome.
Herbal
Tamarind: May increase salicylate toxicity.
Tan-shen: May increase salicylate concentrations and decrease tan-shen concentrations.
Food
None known.

DIAGNOSTIC TEST EFFECTS

May cause false increases in acetaminophen levels, urinary and blood pH, blood glucose levels.

SIDE EFFECTS

Occasional
Gastric mucosal irritation, bleeding.

SERIOUS REACTIONS

• Overdosage may cause tinnitus.
• Toxic levels may be reached quickly in dehydrated, febrile children. Marked toxicity is manifested as hyperthermia, restlessness, abnormal breathing patterns, convulsions, respiratory failure, and coma.

PRECAUTIONS & CONSIDERATIONS

Caution is warranted in patients with acute or chronic renal or hepatic insufficiency, gastritis, peptic ulcer disease, and chronic alcoholism. It is unknown whether magnesium salicylate crosses the placenta or is distributed in breast milk; generally, salicylates pass into breast milk, so

caution is warranted in lactation. Be aware that magnesium salicylate use should be avoided during the last trimester of pregnancy because the drug may adversely affect the fetal cardiovascular system, causing premature closure of ductus arteriosus as well as increase and prolong labor or cause severe bleeding prenatally and postnatally. Use caution in giving this drug to children with acute febrile viral (flu, chickenpox) illness because this increases the risk of developing Reye syndrome. Magnesium salicylate should not be given to children or teenagers who have the chickenpox or flu because to do so would increase the risk of developing Reye syndrome. Be aware that lower aspirin dosages are recommended in elderly patients because this age group may be more susceptible to toxicity. Report immediately any symptoms of tinnitus, fever, headache, skin rash, nausea, vomiting. Do not use 5 days before any surgical procedure unless otherwise advised by a medical practitioner.
Storage
Store at room temperature. Do not use if a vinegar smell is present.
Administration
May give with food, milk, or antacids if GI distress occurs. Do not lie down for 15-30 min after swallowing the medication. If pain is not relieved within 10 days, fever within 3 days, or sore throat within 2 days, notify the physician.

Mannitol
man´i-tall
(Osmitrol)

CATEGORY AND SCHEDULE
Pregnancy Risk Category: C

Classification: Diuretics, osmotic

MECHANISM OF ACTION
An osmotic diuretic, antiglaucoma, and antihemolytic agent that elevates osmotic pressure of the glomerular filtrate, inhibiting tubular reabsorption of water and electrolytes, resulting in increased flow of water into interstitial fluid and plasma. *Therapeutic Effect:* Produces diuresis; reduces intraocular pressure (IOP); reduces intracranial pressure (ICP) and cerebral edema.

PHARMACOKINETICS

Route	Onset (min)	Peak	Duration (h)
IV (diuresis)	15-30	N/A	2-8
IV (Reduced ICP)	15-30	N/A	3-8
IV (Reduced IOP)	N/A	30-60 min	4-8

Remains in extracellular fluid. Primarily excreted in urine. Removed by hemodialysis. *Half-life:* 100 min.

AVAILABILITY
Injection: 5%, 10%, 15%, 20%, 25%.

INDICATIONS AND DOSAGES
▸ **Prevention and treatment of oliguric phase of acute renal failure, to promote urinary excretion of toxic substances (such as aspirin, barbiturates, bromides, and imipramine); to reduce increased ICP due to cerebral edema or edema of injured spinal cord; to reduce increased IOP due to acute glaucoma**
IV
Adults, Elderly, Children. Initially, 0.5-1 g/kg, then 0.25-0.5 g/kg q4-6h.

CONTRAINDICATIONS
Severe dehydration, active intracranial bleeding (except during craniotomy), severe pulmonary edema and congestion, severe renal disease (well established anuria), progressive renal damage or dysfunction after receiving mannitol, including increasing oliguria and azotemia, progressive heart failure. Hypersensitivity to mannitol.

INTERACTIONS
Drug
Digoxin: May increase the risk of digoxin toxicity associated with mannitol-induced hypokalemia.
Herbal
None known.
Food
None known.

DIAGNOSTIC TEST EFFECTS
May decrease serum phosphate, potassium, and sodium levels; measure glomerular filtration rate (GFR).

Ⓘ IV INCOMPATIBILITIES
Cefepime (Maxipime), doxorubicin liposomal (Doxil), filgrastim (Neupogen), whole blood for transfusion.

🔟 IV COMPATIBILITIES

Cisplatin (Platinol), ondansetron (Zofran), propofol (Diprivan).

SIDE EFFECTS

Frequent
Dry mouth, thirst.
Occasional
Blurred vision, increased urinary frequency and urine volume, headache, arm pain, backache, nausea, vomiting, urticaria, dizziness, hypotension or hypertension, tachycardia, fever, angina-like chest pain.

SERIOUS REACTIONS

• Fluid and electrolyte imbalance may occur from rapid administration of large doses or inadequate urine output resulting in overexpansion of extracellular fluid.
• Circulatory overload may produce pulmonary edema and congestive heart failure.
• Excessive diuresis may produce hypokalemia and hyponatremia.
• Fluid loss in excess of electrolyte excretion may produce hypernatremia and hyperkalemia.

PRECAUTIONS & CONSIDERATIONS

It is unknown whether mannitol crosses the placenta or is distributed in breast milk. The safety and efficacy of mannitol have not been established in children younger than 12 yrs. Age-related renal impairment may require cautious use in elderly patients.

Dry mouth and an increase in the frequency and volume of urination may occur. BP, BUN, liver function test results, electrolytes, and urine output should be assessed before and during treatment. Weight should be monitored daily. Be aware of signs of electrolyte disturbances such as hypokalemia or hyponatremia. Hypokalemia may cause arrhythmias, altered mental status, muscle cramps, asthenia, and tremor. Hyponatremia may result in cold and clammy skin, confusion, and thirst.

May increase cerebral blood flow and worsen intracranial hypertension in chldren who develop generalized cerebral hyperemia 24-48 h post injury.
Storage
Store the drug at room temperature. Do not use if container is damaged or solution is not clear. Do not use if crystals are visible; brief storage in a warmer (<40° C) may help redispense crystals.
Administration
! Assess the IV site for patency before administering each dose. Pain and thrombosis are noted with extravasation. With suspected renal insufficiency or marked oliguria, a test dose should be given. The test dose is 12.5 g for adults (200 mg/kg for children) over 3-5 min to produce a urine flow of at least 30-50 mL/h (1 mL/kg/h for children) over 2-3 h.

If the solution crystallizes, warm the bottle in hot water and shake it vigorously at intervals. Do not use the solution if crystals remain after the warming procedure. Cool the solution to body temperature before administration. Use an in-line filter (< 5 μm) for drug concentrations > 20%. The test dose for oliguria is IV push over 3-5 min. The test dose for cerebral edema or elevated ICP

M

is IV over 20-30 min. Maximum concentration is 25%. Do not add potassium chloride or sodium chloride to mannitol with a concentration of 20% or greater. Do not add mannitol to whole blood for transfusion conjointly. If it is necessary to co-administer whole blood, use at least 20 mEq NaCl added to each L of mannitol solution to prevent pseudoagglutineation.

Do not put into PVC bags for administration.

Maprotiline
mah-pro′tih-leen
(Ludiomil)

CATEGORY AND SCHEDULE
Pregnancy Risk Category: B

Classification: Antidepressants, tetracyclic

MECHANISM OF ACTION
A tetracyclic compound that blocks reuptake norepinephrine by central nervous system (CNS) presynaptic neuronal membranes, increasing availability at postsynaptic neuronal receptor sites, and enhances synaptic activity. *Therapeutic Effect:* Produces antidepressant effect, with prominent sedative effects and low anticholinergic activity.

PHARMACOKINETICS
Slowly and completely absorbed after PO administration. Protein binding: 88%. Metabolized in the liver by hydroxylation and oxidative modification. Excreted in urine. Unknown whether removed by hemodialysis. *Half-life:* 27-58 h.

AVAILABILITY
Tablets: 25 mg, 50 mg, 75 mg (Ludiomil).

INDICATIONS AND DOSAGES
▸ **Mild to moderate depression**
PO
Adults. 75 mg/day to start, in 1-3 divided doses.
Elderly. Initially, 25 mg at bedtime. In 1 wk, increase dosage gradually in 25-mg increments until therapeutic response is achieved. Reduce to lowest effective maintenance level. Usual dose 50-75 mg/day.
▸ **Severe depression**
PO
Adults. 100-150 mg/day in 1-3 divided doses. May increase gradually to maximum 225 mg/day.

CONTRAINDICATIONS
Acute recovery period following myocardial infarction (MI), within 14 days of MAOI ingestion, known or suspected seizure disorder, hypersensitivity to maprotiline or any component of the formulation.
Caution
Suicidal patients, severe depression, increased intraocular pressure, narrow-angle glaucoma, urinary retention, cardiac disease, hepatic or renal disease, hypothyroidism, hyperthyroidism, electroshock therapy, elective surgery, elderly, lactation, benign prostatic hypertrophy, schizophrenia, MAOIs.

INTERACTIONS

Drug

Alcohol, all CNS depressants:
Potential risk of increased CNS depression.

Clonidine, guanadrel, guanethidine: May decrease antihypertensive effect.

Direct acting sympathomimetics (epinephrine): May increase cardiovascular effects (arrhythmias, tachycardias, severe hypertension).

MAOIs: May increase risk of hypertensive crisis and severe convulsions. Contraindicated.

Herbal

None known.

Food

None known.

DIAGNOSTIC TEST EFFECTS

None known.

SIDE EFFECTS

Frequent

Drowsiness, fatigue, dry mouth, blurred vision, constipation, delayed micturition, postural hypotension, excessive sweating, disturbed concentration, increased appetite, urinary retention.

Occasional

GI disturbances (nausea, GI distress, metallic taste sensation), photosensitivity.

Rare

Paradoxical reaction (agitation, restlessness, nightmares, insomnia), extrapyramidal symptoms (particularly fine hand tremor).

SERIOUS REACTIONS

• Higher incidence of seizures than with tricyclic antidepressants, especially in those with no previous history of seizures.

• High dosage may produce cardiovascular effects, such as severe postural hypotension, dizziness, tachycardia, palpitations, and arrhythmias.

• May also result in altered temperature regulation (hyperpyrexia or hypothermia).

• Abrupt withdrawal from prolonged therapy may produce headache, malaise, nausea, vomiting, and vivid dreams.

PRECAUTIONS & CONSIDERATIONS

Caution is warranted in patients with prostatic hypertrophy, history of urinary retention or obstruction, glaucoma, diabetes mellitus, history of seizures, hyperthyroidism, cardiac/hepatic/renal disease, schizophrenia, increased intraocular pressure, and hiatal hernia. Be aware that maprotiline is distributed in breast milk. Be aware that the safety and efficacy of this drug have not been established in children. In elderly patients, age-related renal impairment may require cautious use.

Tolerance usually develops to postural hypotension, sedative, and anticholinergic effects. Avoid alcohol and tasks that require mental alertness and motor skills. Visual disturbances should be reported immediately as well as any indications of blood dyscrasias (infection, poor healing, bleeding). Xerostomic effects should also be reported, including sore tongue, problems eating or swallowing, so medication changes can be considered.

Storage

Store at room temperature.

Administration

Take maprotiline without food. Be aware to make sure at least 14 days elapse between discontinuing MAOIs and instituting maprotiline therapy. Also, plan to allow at least 14 days to pass after discontinuing maprotiline and instituting MAOI therapy.

Mebendazole
meh-ben'dah-zole
(Vermox)

CATEGORY AND SCHEDULE
Pregnancy Risk Category: C

Classification: Antihelmintics, carbamate

M

MECHANISM OF ACTION
A synthetic benzimidazole derivative that degrades parasite cytoplasmic microtubules and irreversibly blocks glucose uptake in helminthes and larvae. Vermicidal. *Therapeutic Effect:* depletes glycogen, decreases ATP, causes helminth death.

PHARMACOKINETICS
Poorly absorbed from GI tract (absorption increases with food). Metabolized in liver. Primarily eliminated in feces. *Half-life:* 2.5-9 h (half life increased with impaired renal function).

AVAILABILITY
Tablets, Chewable: 100 mg (Vermox).

INDICATIONS AND DOSAGES
▶ **Trichuriasis, ascariasis, hookworm**
PO
Adults, Elderly, Children older than 2 yrs. 1 tablet in morning and at bedtime for 3 days.
▶ **Enterobiasis**
PO
Adults, Elderly, Children older than 2 yrs. 1 tablet one time.

OFF-LABEL USES
Ancylostoma duodenale or Necator americanus.

CONTRAINDICATIONS
Hypersensitivity to mebendazole or any component of the formulation.
Caution
Pregnancy, lactation.

INTERACTIONS
Drug
Carbamazepine: May decrease concentrations of mebendazole.
Herbal
None known.
Food
None known.

DIAGNOSTIC TEST EFFECTS
May increase SGOT (AST), SGPT (ALT), alkaline phosphatase, BUN. May decrease hemoglobin.

SIDE EFFECTS
Occasional
Nausea, vomiting, headache, dizziness, transient abdominal pain, diarrhea with massive infection and expulsion of helminthes.
Rare
Fever.

SERIOUS REACTIONS
• High dosage may produce reversible myelosuppression (granulocytopenia, leukopenia, neutropenia).

Be aware that mebendazole is ineffective in hydatid disease. It is unknown whether mebendazole crosses the placenta or is distributed in breast milk; caution is warranted in lactation. Safety and efficacy have not been established in children 2 yrs and younger. No age-related precautions have been noted in elderly patients.

Avoid walking barefoot (larval entry into system). Change and launder underclothing, pajamas, bedding, towels, and washcloths daily. Because of the high transmission of pinworm infections, all family members should be treated simultaneously; the infected person should sleep alone and shower frequently.

Storage
Store at room temperature.

Administration
For high dosages, take with food. Tablets may be crushed, swallowed, or mixed with food. Take and continue iron supplements as long as ordered (may be 6 mo after treatment) for anemia associated with whipworm and hookworm.

Mecamylamine
mek-a-mil'a-meen hye-droe-klor-ide
(Inversine)

CATEGORY AND SCHEDULE
Pregnancy Risk Category: C

Classification: Antiadrenergics, peripheral

MECHANISM OF ACTION
A ganglionic blocker that inhibits acetylcholine at the autonomic ganglia. Blocks central nicotinic cholinergic receptors, which inhibits effects of nicotine. *Therapeutic Effect:* Reduces BP; decreases desire to smoke.

PHARMACOKINETICS
Completely absorbed following PO administration. Widely distributed. Excreted in urine. *Half-life:* 24 h.

AVAILABILITY
Tablets: 2.5 mg (Inversine).

INDICATIONS AND DOSAGES
▸ **Hypertension**
PO
Adults. Initially, 2.5 mg q12h for 2 days, then increase by 2.5 mg increments at more than 2 day intervals until desired BP is achieved. The average daily dose is 25 mg/day in 3 divided doses.
▸ **Smoking cessation**
PO
Adults. Initially, 2.5 mg q12h for 2 days; then increase by 2.5-mg increments during the first week of therapy. Range: 10-20 mg/day in divided doses.

OFF-LABEL USES
Tourette syndrome.

CONTRAINDICATIONS
Coronary insufficiency, pyloric stenosis, glaucoma, uremia, recent myocardial infarction, unreliable patients.

INTERACTIONS
Drug
Sulfonamides, antibiotics: May increase the effect of mecamylamine.

M

Herbal
None known.
Food
None known.

DIAGNOSTIC TEST EFFECTS
None known.

SIDE EFFECTS
Occasional
Nausea, diarrhea, orthostatic hypotension, tachycardia, drowsiness, urinary retention, blurred vision, dilated pupils, confusion, mental depression, decreased sexual ability, loss of appetite.
Rare
Pulmonary edema, pulmonary fibrosis, paresthesias.

SERIOUS REACTIONS
• Overdosage includes symptoms such as hypotension, nausea, vomiting, urinary retention, and constipation.

PRECAUTIONS & CONSIDERATIONS
Caution should be used in elderly patients and with renal impairment. Caution is also warranted in patients with central nervous system (CNS) abnormalities, prostatic hyperplasia, bladder obstruction or urethral strictive, as well as patients under general anesthesia. It is unknown whether mecamylamine crosses the placenta or is distributed in breast milk; therefore, caution is warranted in lactation. Safety and efficacy of mecamylamine have not been established in children. BP should be taken immediately before each mecamylamine dose and regularly monitor throughout therapy. Be alert to fluctuations in BP. For use in pregnancy, the benefits of using this medication for smoking cessation should outweigh any risks to the mother or fetus.
Administration
Administer with meals. Do not abruptly discontinue mecamylamine.

Meclizine Hydrochloride
mek′li-zeen high-droh-klor-ide
(Antivert, Bonamine [CAN], Bonine)
Do not confuse with Axert.

CATEGORY AND SCHEDULE
Pregnancy Risk Category: B

Classification: Antihistamines

MECHANISM OF ACTION
An anticholinergic that reduces labyrinthine excitability and diminishes vestibular stimulation of the labyrinth, affecting the chemoreceptor trigger zone. *Therapeutic Effect:* Reduces nausea, vomiting, and vertigo.

PHARMACOKINETICS

Route	Onset	Peak	Duration
PO	30-60 min	N/A	12-24 h

Well absorbed from the GI tract. Widely distributed. Metabolized in the liver. Primarily excreted in urine. *Half-life:* 6 h.

AVAILABILITY
Tablets (Antivert): 12.5 mg, 25 mg, 50 mg.
Tablets, Chewable (Bonine): 25 mg.

INDICATIONS AND DOSAGES
▸ **Motion sickness**
PO
Adults, Elderly, Children 12 yrs and older. 25-50 mg 1 h before travel. May repeat 24 h. May require a dose of 50 mg.
▸ **Vertigo**
PO
Adults, Elderly, Children 12 yrs and older. 25-100 mg/day in divided doses, as needed.

CONTRAINDICATIONS
Hypersensitivity to cyclizines.

INTERACTIONS
Drug
Alcohol, CNS depressants:
May increase CNS depressant effect.
Herbal
None known.
Food
None known.

DIAGNOSTIC TEST EFFECTS
May produce false-negative results in antigen skin testing unless meclizine is discontinued 4 days before testing.

SIDE EFFECTS
Frequent
Drowsiness.
Occasional
Blurred vision; dry mouth, nose, or throat.

SERIOUS REACTIONS
• A hypersensitivity reaction, marked by eczema, pruritus, rash, cardiac disturbances, and photosensitivity may occur.
• Overdose may produce CNS depression (manifested as sedation, apnea, cardiovascular collapse, or death) or severe paradoxical reactions (such as hallucinations, tremor, and seizures).

• Children may experience paradoxical reactions, including restlessness, insomnia, euphoria, nervousness, and tremors.
• Overdose in children may result in hallucinations, seizures, and death.

PRECAUTIONS & CONSIDERATIONS
Caution is warranted in patients with asthma, prostate enlargement, angle-closure glaucoma and obstructive diseases of the GI or genitourinary tract. It is unknown whether meclizine crosses the placenta or is distributed in breast milk. Meclizine use may produce irritability in breastfeeding infants. Safety and efficacy in children under age 12 are not established. Children and elderly patients may be more sensitive to the drug's anticholinergic effects, such as dry mouth. Alcohol and tasks that require mental alertness or motor skills should be avoided.

Dizziness, drowsiness, and dry mouth may occur. BP, electrolytes, and skin should be assessed.
Administration
! Elderly patients (older than 60 yrs) are at increased risk for developing agitation, disorientation, dizziness, sedation, hypotension, confusion, and psychotic-like symptoms.

Take meclizine orally without regard to food. Crush scored tablets if needed.

M

Meclofenamate Sodium

me′kloe-fen′a-mate soe-dee-um
(Meclomen [CAN])
Do not confuse meclofenamate or meclomen with meclizine.

CATEGORY AND SCHEDULE
Pregnancy Risk Category: B
(D if used in third trimester or near delivery)

Classification: Analgesics, non-narcotic, nonsteroidal anti-inflammatory drugs

MECHANISM OF ACTION
A nonsteroidal anti-inflammatory drug (NSAID) that inhibits prostaglandin synthesis by decreasing activity of the enzyme, cyclooxygenase, which results in decreased formation of prostaglandin precursors. *Therapeutic Effect:* Reduces inflammatory response and intensity of pain stimulus reaching sensory nerve endings.

PHARMACOKINETICS
PO route, onset 15 min, peak 0.5-1.5 h, duration 2-4 h. Completely absorbed from the GI tract. Widely distributed. Protein binding: > 99%. Metabolized in the liver. Excreted primarily in urine and feces as metabolites. Not removed by hemodialysis. *Half-life:* 2-3.3 h.

AVAILABILITY
Capsules: 50 mg, 100 mg.

INDICATIONS AND DOSAGES
▸ **Mild to moderate pain**
PO
Adults, Elderly. 50 mg q 4-6h as needed. May increase to 100 mg/dose if needed; use lowest effective dose. Maximum: 400 mg/day.
▸ **Excessive menstrual blood loss and primary dysmenorrhea**
PO
Adults, Elderly. 100 mg 3 times/day for 6 days, starting at the onset of menstrual flow.
▸ **Rheumatoid arthritis, osteoarthritis**
PO
Adults. 200-400 mg/day given in 3-4 divided dose. Maximum: 400 mg/day. Use lower starting doses in the elderly.

CONTRAINDICATIONS
Active peptic ulcer disease, chronic inflammation of GI tract, GI bleeding disorders, GI ulceration, history of hypersensitivity to aspirin or NSAIDs, use with 14 days of CABG.
Caution
Lactation, children under 14 yrs., bleeding disorders, upper GI disorders, cardiac disorders, hypersensitivity to other NSAIDs and salicylates.

INTERACTIONS
Drug
Antihypertensives, diuretics: May decrease the effects of antihypertensives and diuretics.
Anticoagulants, aspirin, salicylates: May increase the risk of GI bleeding and side effects.
Bone marrow depressants: May increase the risk of hematologic reactions.
Cyclosporine: May increase nephrotoxicity.
Heparin, oral anticoagulants, thrombolytics: May increase the effects of heparin, oral anticoagulants, and thrombolytics.
Lithium: May increase the blood concentration and risk of toxicity of lithium.

Methotrexate: May increase the risk of toxicity with methotrexate.

Probenecid: May increase meclofenamate blood concentration.

Herbal

Feverfew: May increase the risk of bleeding.

Ginkgo biloba: May increase the risk of bleeding.

Food

None known.

DIAGNOSTIC TEST EFFECTS

May increase chloride and sodium test results. May increase BUN; serum LDH concentration; serum alkaline phosphatase, serum creatinine, potassium, and transaminase levels; and urine protein levels. May decrease serum uric acid levels.

SIDE EFFECTS

Frequent (10%-33%)
Diarrhea, nausea, abdominal cramping/pain, dyspepsia (heartburn, indigestion, epigastric pain).

Occasional (1%-9%)
Flatulence, rash, dizziness.

Rare (< 1%)
Constipation, anorexia, stomatitis, headache, ringing in the ears, rash.

SERIOUS REACTIONS

• Overdosage may result in headache, seizure, vomiting, and cerebral edema.

• Peptic ulcer disease, GI bleeding, gastritis, severe hepatic reactions, such as jaundice, nephrotoxicity marked by hematuria, dysuria, proteinuria, and severe hypersensitivity reaction, including bronchospasm, and facial edema occur rarely.

PRECAUTIONS & CONSIDERATIONS

Caution is warranted in patients with a history of GI tract disease, impaired liver or renal function, and predisposition to fluid retention. Pregnancy should be reported immediately. It is unknown whether meclofenamate crosses the placenta or is distributed in breast milk. Meclofenamate use should be avoided during the last trimester of pregnancy because the drug may adversely affect the fetal cardiovascular system. Safety and efficacy have not been established in children. GI bleeding and ulceration are more likely to cause serious adverse effects in elderly patients. Age-related renal impairment may increase risk of liver or renal toxicity, and a decreased dosage is recommended. If taken for heavy menstruation, advise the patient to report any between-cycle bleeding or worsening of flow immediately as this indicates the drug therapy is not appropriate.

Administration

Do not crush, open, or break capsules. May give with antacids, food, or milk if the patient starting dose experiences GI distress. Starting dose should be reduced in elderly patients.

M

Medroxyproges-terone Acetate

me-drox'ee-proe-jess'te-rone
ass-e-tayte
(Depo-Provera, Depo-Provera
Contraceptive, Novo-Medrone
[CAN], Provera, Ralovera [AUS])
Do not confuse medroxypro-gesterone with hydroxyproges-terone, methylprednisolone, or methyltestosterone.

CATEGORY AND SCHEDULE
Pregnancy Risk Category: X

Classification: Progestogen

MECHANISM OF ACTION
A hormone that transforms
endometrium from proliferative to
secretory in an estrogen-primed
endometrium. Inhibits secretion of
pituitary gonadotropins. *Therapeutic
Effect:* Prevents follicular maturation
and ovulation. Stimulates the growth
of mammary alveolar tissue and
relaxes uterine smooth muscle.
Corrects hormonal imbalance.

PHARMACOKINETICS
Slowly absorbed after IM
administration. Protein binding: 90%.
Metabolized in the liver. Excreted
primarily in urine. *Half-life:* 30 days.

AVAILABILITY
Tablets (Provera): 2.5 mg, 5 mg,
10 mg.
*Injection (Depo-Provera
Contraceptive):* 150 mg/mL.
Injection (Depo-Provera): 400 mg/mL.

INDICATIONS AND DOSAGES
▸ **Endometrial hyperplasia**
PO
Adults. 2.5-10 mg/day for 14 days.

▸ **Secondary amenorrhea**
PO
Adults. 5-10 mg/day for 5-10 days,
beginning at any time during
menstrual cycle or 2.5 mg/day.
▸ **Abnormal uterine bleeding**
PO
Adults. 5-10 mg/day for
5-10 days, beginning on calculated
day 16 or day 21 of menstrual cycle.
▸ **Endometrial, renal carcinoma**
IM
Adults, Elderly. Initially,
400-1000 mg; repeat at 1-wk
intervals. If improvement occurs
and disease is stabilized, begin
maintenance with as little as
400 mg/mo.
▸ **Prevention of pregnancy**
IM (DEPO-PROVERA 150)
Adults. 150 mg q3mo. Do not use for
> 2 years unless necessary.

OTHER USES
Endometriosis (Depo-sub Q provera
104).

CONTRAINDICATIONS
Carcinoma of breast;
hormone-dependent neoplasm;
history of or active thrombotic
disorders, such as cerebral
apoplexy, thrombophlebitis,
or thromboembolic disorders;
hypersensitivity to progestins;
known or suspected pregnancy;
missed abortion; severe hepatic
dysfunction; undiagnosed abnormal
genital bleeding; use as pregnancy
test.
Caution
Lactation, hypertension, asthma,
blood dyscrasias, gallbladder disease,
congestive heart failure, diabetes
mellitus, bone disease, depression,
migraine headache, convulsive
disorders, hepatic disease, renal
disease, family history of breast or
reproductive tract cancers.

INTERACTIONS
Drug
Bromocriptine: May interfere with the effects of bromocriptine.
Herbal
None known.
Food
None known.

DIAGNOSTIC TEST EFFECTS
May alter results for serum thyroid and liver function tests, prothrombin time, and metapyrone test.

SIDE EFFECTS
Frequent
Transient menstrual abnormalities (including spotting, change in menstrual flow or cervical secretions, and amenorrhea) at initiation of therapy.
Occasional
Edema, weight change, breast tenderness, nervousness, insomnia, fatigue, dizziness.
Rare
Alopecia, depression, dermatologic changes, headache, fever, nausea.

SERIOUS REACTIONS
• Thrombophlebitis, pulmonary or cerebral embolism, and retinal thrombosis occur rarely.
• Lowered Bone mineral density with use > 2 yr; may be nonreversible.

PRECAUTIONS & CONSIDERATIONS
Caution is warranted in patients with conditions aggravated by fluid retention, including asthma, seizures, migraine, cardiac or renal dysfunction, and in those with diabetes mellitus or history of depression. Medroxyprogesterone use should be avoided during pregnancy, especially in the first 4 mo because the drug may cause congenital heart and limb-reduction defects in the neonate.

Medroxyprogesterone is distributed in breast milk; caution in lactation is warranted. Safety and efficacy of medroxyprogesterone have not been established in children. No age-related precautions have been noted in elderly patients. Avoid smoking because of the increased risk of blood clot formation and myocardial infarction.

Notify the physician of chest pain, blood-tinged expectorants, hemoptysis, numbness in the arm or leg, severe headache, severe pain or swelling in the calf, severe abdominal pain or tenderness, sudden loss of vision, or unusually heavy vaginal bleeding. BP, weight, blood glucose, hepatic enzyme, and serum calcium levels should be monitored.
Administration
Take oral medroxyprogesterone without regard to meals.

For IM use, shake vial immediately before administering to ensure complete suspension. Inject IM only in upper arm or upper outer aspect of buttock. Rarely, a residual lump, change in skin color, or sterile abscess occurs at injection site.

M

Mefenamic Acid
me-fe-nam′ik ass-id
(Apo-Mefenamic [CAN],
Nu-Mefenamic [CAN],
PMS-Mefenamic Acid [CAN],
Ponstan [CAN], Ponstel)

CATEGORY AND SCHEDULE
Pregnancy Risk Category: C (D if used in third trimester or near delivery)

Classification: Nonsteroidal anti-inflammatory drugs

MECHANISM OF ACTION

A nonsteroidal anti-inflammatory drug (NSAID) that produces analgesic and anti-inflammatory effect by inhibiting prostaglandin synthesis. *Therapeutic Effect:* Reduces inflammatory response and intensity of pain stimulus reaching sensory nerve endings.

PHARMACOKINETICS

Rapidly absorbed from the GI tract. Protein binding: High. Metabolized in liver. Partially excreted in urine and partially in the feces. Not removed by hemodialysis. *Half-life:* 3.5 h.

AVAILABILITY

Capsules: 250 mg (Ponstel).

INDICATIONS AND DOSAGES

▸ **Mild to moderate pain, lower back pain, dysmenorrhea**
PO
Adults, Elderly, Children 14 yrs and older. Initially, 500 mg to start, then 250 mg q4h as needed. Maximum: 1 wk of therapy.

CONTRAINDICATIONS

History of hypersensitivity to aspirin or NSAIDs, pregnancy; use within 14 days of CABG.
Caution
Lactation, children, bleeding disorders, GI disorders, cardiac disorders, hypersensitivity to NSAIDs and other salicylates.

INTERACTIONS

Drug
Acetaminophen (prolonged use, high dose): May increase risk of nephrotoxicity and hepatotoxicity.
Antihypertensives, diuretics: May decrease the effects of antihypertensives and diuretics.

Aspirin, alcohol, corticosteroids, or other salicylates: May increase the risk of GI bleeding and side effects.
Bone marrow depressants: May increase the risk of hematologic reactions.
Cyclosporine: May increase risk of decreased renal function.
Diuretics: May decrease diuretic effects.
First-time users of SSRIs who are also taking NSAIDs: May have a higher incidence of GI side effects.
Heparin, oral anticoagulants, thrombolytics: May increase the effects of heparin, oral anticoagulants, and thrombolytics.
Lithium: May increase the blood concentration and risk of toxicity of lithium.
Methotrexate: May increase the risk of toxicity of methotrexate.
Probenecid: May increase mefenamic acid blood concentration.

DIAGNOSTIC TEST EFFECTS

May increase chloride and sodium levels. May prolong bleeding time. May increase liver function tests.

SIDE EFFECTS

Occasional (1%-10%)
Dyspepsia, including heartburn, indigestion, flatulence, abdominal cramping, constipation, nausea, diarrhea, epigastric pain, vomiting, headache, nervousness, dizziness, bleeding, elevated liver function tests, tinnitus.
Rare (< 1%)
Fluid retention, arrhythmias, tachycardia, confusion, drowsiness, rash, dry eyes, blurred vision, hot flashes.

SERIOUS REACTIONS

• Peptic ulcer, GI bleeding, gastritis, and severe hepatic reaction, such as cholestasis and jaundice, occur rarely.

• Nephrotoxicity, including dysuria, hematuria, proteinuria, and nephrotic syndrome and severe hypersensitivity reaction, marked by bronchospasm, and angioedema occur rarely.

PRECAUTIONS & CONSIDERATIONS

Caution is warranted in patients with asthma, congestive heart failure (CHF), dehydration, hemostatic disease, history of GI disease, such as ulcers, hypertension, impaired liver or renal function, as well as concurrent use of anticoagulants. Report pregnancy or suspicion of pregnancy; do not use in last trimester of pregnancy. Mefenamic acid is excreted in breast milk; caution is warranted in lactation. Safety and efficacy of mefenamic acid have not been established in children younger than 14 yrs. In elderly patients, age-related renal impairment may require dosage adjustment. Be aware that elderly patients are more susceptible to GI toxicity and a lower dosage of the drug is recommended for this patient population. Alcohol and aspirin should be avoided during therapy because of an increased risk of GI bleeding. Avoid use when possible in patients who have a higher risk for thromboembolism.

Administration

Take mefenamic acid with regard to meals. Do not to chew or crush capsules. Antacids, food, or milk may be taken if GI distress occurs.

Mefloquine
me'flow-quine
(Lariam)
Do not confuse with Librium.

CATEGORY AND SCHEDULE
Pregnancy Risk Category: C

Classification: Antimalarial

MECHANISM OF ACTION
A quinolone-methanol compound structurally similar to quinine that destroys the asexual blood forms of malarial pathogens, *Plasmodium falciparum, P. vivax, P. malariae, and P. ovale. Therapeutic Effect:* Inhibits parasite growth.

PHARMACOKINETICS
Well absorbed from the GI tract. Protein binding: 98%. Widely distributed, including cerebrospinal fluid (CSF). Metabolized in liver. Primarily excreted in urine. *Half-life:* 21-22 days.

AVAILABILITY
Tablets: 250 mg.

INDICATIONS AND DOSAGES
▸ **Suppression of malaria**
PO
Adults. 250 mg base weekly starting 1 wk before travel, continuing weekly during travel and for 4 wks after leaving endemic area.
Children weighing more than 45 kg. 250 mg weekly starting 1 wk before travel, continuing weekly during travel and for 4 wks after leaving the endemic area.
Children weighing 45-31 kg. 187.5 mg (¾ tablet) weekly starting 1 wk before travel, continuing weekly during travel, and for 4 wks after leaving the endemic area.

M

Children weighing 30-20 kg. 125 mg (½ tablet) weekly starting 1 wk before travel, continuing weekly during travel, and for 4 wks after leaving the endemic area.
Children weighing 19-15 kg. 62.5 mg (¼ tablet) weekly starting 1 wk before travel, continuing weekly during travel, and for 4 wks after leaving the endemic area.

▸ **Treatment of malaria**
PO
Adults. 1250 mg as a single dose.
Children. 15-25 mg/kg in a single dose. Maximum: 1250 mg.

CONTRAINDICATIONS
Cardiac abnormalities, severe psychiatric disorders, epilepsy, history of hypersensitivity to mefloquine, quinine or quinidine, use with halofantrine.

INTERACTIONS
Drug
Anticonvulsants: May decrease the effect of anticonvulsants.
Cytochrome P450 effect: Inhibits CYP 3A4.
β-Blockers: May increase bradycardia with β-blockers.
Chloroquine, quinine, quinidine: May increase the risk of toxicity with these drug (seizures or ECG changes).
Halofantrine: Risk of fatal QT prolongation; do not use.
Herbal
None known.
Food
None known.

DIAGNOSTIC TEST EFFECTS
None known.

SIDE EFFECTS
Occasional
Mild transient headache, difficulty concentrating, insomnia, lightheadedness, vertigo, diarrhea, nausea, vomiting, visual disturbances, tinnitus.
Rare
Aggressive behavior, anxiety, bradycardia, depression, hallucinations, hypotension, panic attacks, paranoia, psychosis, syncope, tremor.

SERIOUS REACTIONS
• Prolonged therapy may result in peripheral neuritis, neuromyopathy, hypotension, ECG changes, agranulocytosis, aplastic anemia, thrombocytopenia, seizures, and psychosis.
• Overdosage may result in headache, vomiting, visual disturbance, drowsiness, and seizures.
• Acute hypersensitivity.

PRECAUTIONS & CONSIDERATIONS
Caution is warranted in patients with history of depression, liver disease, and people who pilot airplanes and operate machines because dizziness and disturbed sense of balance are side effects. It is unknown whether mefloquine crosses the placenta or is excreted in breast milk. Advise female patients to use adequate contraception during the period of prophylaxis. No age-related precautions have been noted in children or elderly patients. Determine the patient's tolerance for NSAIDs and aspirin therapy and predisposition to GI distress when using these medications.

Any new symptoms of anxiety, confusion, depression, restlessness, tinnitus, and visual difficulties should be reported.
Administration
Begin therapy before and continue after trip. Take mefloquine with food and at least 8 oz. of water. Tablets may be crushed and mixed with water or sugar water for oral administration. Continue taking mefloquine for the full length of treatment.

M

Megestrol Acetate
me-jess'trole ass-ee-tayte
(Apo-Megestrol [CAN], Megace,
Megostat [AUS])

CATEGORY AND SCHEDULE
Pregnancy Risk Category: X (for
suspension), D (for tablets)

Classification: Progestin
derivative

MECHANISM OF ACTION
A hormone and antineoplastic
agent that suppresses the release
of luteinizing hormone from the
anterior pituitary gland by inhibiting
pituitary function. *Therapeutic
Effect:* Shrinks tumors. Also
increases appetite by an unknown
mechanism.

PHARMACOKINETICS
Well absorbed from the GI tract.
Metabolized in the liver; excreted
in urine.

AVAILABILITY
Tablets: 20 mg, 40 mg.
Suspension: 40 mg/mL, 125 mg/mL.

INDICATIONS AND DOSAGES
▸ **Palliative treatment of advanced
breast cancer**
PO
Adults, Elderly. 160 mg/day in
4 equally divided doses.
▸ **Palliative treatment of advanced
endometrial carcinoma**
PO
Adults, Elderly. 40-320 mg/day in
divided doses. Maximum:
800 mg/day in 1-4 divided doses.
▸ **Anorexia, cachexia, weight loss**
PO (MEGACE)
Adults, Elderly. 800 mg
(20 mL)/day.

PO (MEGACE ES)
Adults, Elderly: 625 mg (5 mL) once
daily.

OFF-LABEL USES
Appetite stimulant, treatment of
hormone-dependent or advanced
prostate carcinoma (palliative).

CONTRAINDICATIONS
Hypersensitivity to megestrol acetate
or any of its components.

INTERACTIONS
Drug
None known.
Herbal
None known.
Food
None known.

DIAGNOSTIC TEST EFFECTS
May increase blood glucose level.

M

SIDE EFFECTS
Frequent
Weight gain secondary to increased
appetite.
Occasional
Nausea, breakthrough bleeding,
backache, headache, breast
tenderness, carpal tunnel syndrome.
Rare
Feeling of coldness.

SERIOUS REACTIONS
• Thrombophlebitis and pulmonary
embolism occur rarely.

PRECAUTIONS & CONSIDERATIONS
Caution is warranted in patients
with a history of thrombophlebitis.
Megestrol use should be avoided
during pregnancy, if possible,
especially in the first 4 mo.
Pregnancy should be determined
before initiating megestrol therapy.
Megestrol has a pregnancy risk
category of X in suspension form

and D in tablet form. Contraception is imperative during therapy. Breastfeeding is not recommended for patients taking this drug. The safety and efficacy of megestrol have not been established in children. No age-related precautions have been noted in elderly patients.

Potential side effects, including backache, breast tenderness, headache, nausea, and vomiting, may occur. Notify the physician if calf pain, difficulty breathing, or vaginal bleeding develops.

Patients receiving chemotherapy may require palliative treatment for stomatitis.

Administration

Shake suspension well before using. Note difference in dosage of megace and megace ES suspensions.

Meloxicam

mel-oks′i-kam
(Mobic)

CATEGORY AND SCHEDULE

Pregnancy Risk Category: C (D if used in third trimester or near delivery)

Classification: Nonsteroidal anti-inflammatory drugs

MECHANISM OF ACTION

An NSAID that produces analgesic and anti-inflammatory effects by inhibiting prostaglandin synthesis. *Therapeutic Effect:* Reduces the inflammatory response and intensity of pain.

PHARMACOKINETICS

Route	Onset	Peak	Duration
PO (anal-gesic)	30 min	4-5 h	NA

Well absorbed after PO administration. Protein binding: 99%. Metabolized in the liver. Eliminated in urine and feces. Not removed by hemodialysis. *Half-life:* 15-20 h.

AVAILABILITY

Tablets: 7.5 mg, 15 mg.

INDICATIONS AND DOSAGES
▶ **Osteoarthritis, rheumatoid arthritis**
PO
Adults. Initially, 7.5 mg/day. Maximum: 15 mg/day.

CONTRAINDICATIONS

Hypersensitivity to meloxicam, other NSAIDs, or aspirin. Use within 14 days of CABG.

INTERACTIONS

Drug

Aspirin (except low dose form), other NSAIDs, other salicylates, oral glucocorticoids, alcoholism, smoking, older age, generally poor health: May increase the risk of epigastric distress, such as heartburn and indigestion.
First-time users of SSRIs also using NSAIDs: May have a higher risk of GI side effects.
Furosemide, other loop diuretics: May reduce natriuretic effects.
Lithium: May increase the plasma concentration and risk of toxicity of lithium.
Herbal
Ginkgo biloba: May increase the risk of bleeding.
Food
None known.

DIAGNOSTIC TEST EFFECTS

May increase serum creatinine, AST (SGOT), and ALT (SGPT) levels.

SIDE EFFECTS
Frequent (7%-9%)
Dyspepsia, headache, diarrhea, nausea.
Occasional (3%-4%)
Dizziness, insomnia, rash, pruritus, flatulence, constipation, vomiting.
Rare (< 2%)
Somnolence, urticaria, photosensitivity, tinnitus.

SERIOUS REACTIONS
• Rare reactions with long-term use include peptic ulcer disease, GI bleeding, gastritis, severe hepatic reaction (jaundice), nephrotoxicity (hematuria, dysuria, proteinuria), and a severe hypersensitivity reaction (bronchospasm, angioedema).

PRECAUTIONS & CONSIDERATIONS
Caution is warranted in patients with asthma, congestive heart failure, hypertension, dehydration, hemostatic disease, hepatic or renal impairment, a history of GI disorders (such as ulcers), and concurrent anticoagulant use. Meloxicam should not be used during pregnancy because it can cause fetal harm. Meloxicam is excreted in breast milk; caution is advisable in lactation. The safety and efficacy of meloxicam have not been established in children. Elderly patients require a dosage adjustment because of age-related renal impairment and increased susceptibility to GI toxicity. Avoid alcohol and aspirin during therapy because these substances increase the risk of GI bleeding. Tasks that require mental alertness or motor skills should also be avoided.

Notify the physician if chest pain, difficulty breathing, palpitations, peripheral edema, persistent abdominal cramps or pain, rash, ringing in the ears, severe nausea or vomiting, or unusual bleeding or ecchymosis occurs. CBC, BUN level, and serum alkaline phosphatase, bilirubin, creatinine, AST (SGOT), and ALT (SGPT) levels should be assessed during therapy. Therapeutic response, such as decreased pain, stiffness, swelling, and tenderness, improved grip strength, and increased joint mobility, should be evaluated. Avoid using in patients with predisposition to thromboembolism. Report any indications of infection, bleeding, or poor healing to the health care provider. Consider a semisupine reclining position for patients experiencing GI side effects when resting is desired.
Administration
Take meloxicam without regard to food.

M

Memantine hydrochloride
meh-man'teen high-droh-klor-ide
(Namenda)

CATEGORY AND SCHEDULE
Pregnancy Risk Category: B

Classification: NMDA receptor antagonists

MECHANISM OF ACTION
A neurotransmitter inhibitor that decreases the effects of glutamate, the principal excitatory neurotransmitter in the brain. Persistent central nervous system (CNS) excitation by glutamate is thought to cause the symptoms of

Alzheimer's disease. *Therapeutic Effect:* May reduce clinical deterioration in moderate to severe Alzheimer disease.

PHARMACOKINETICS

Rapidly and completely absorbed after PO administration. Protein binding: 45%. Undergoes little metabolism; most of the dose is excreted unchanged in urine. *Half-life:* 60-80 h.

AVAILABILITY

Tablets: 5 mg, 10 mg.

INDICATIONS AND DOSAGES
▸ **Alzheimer disease**
PO
Adults, Elderly. Initially, 5 mg once a day. May increase dosage at intervals of at least 1 wk in 5-mg increments to 10 mg/day (5 mg twice a day), then 15 mg/day (5 mg and 10 mg as separate doses), and finally 20 mg/day (10 mg twice a day). Target dose: 20 mg/day.
▸ **Dosage in renal impairment (CrCl < 30 mL/min)**
Initially, 5 mg once daily. Target dose is 5 mg twice daily.

CONTRAINDICATIONS

Hypersensitivity to the drug, administration with dofetilide.

INTERACTIONS
Drug
Carbonic anhydrase inhibitors, sodium bicarbonate: May decrease the renal elimination of memantine.
Dofetilide: Competes for renal tubular excretion; contraindicated.
Metformin: Competes for renal tubular excretion and may increase risk of lactic acidosis.
Herbal
None known.
Food
None known.

DIAGNOSTIC TEST EFFECTS
None known.

SIDE EFFECTS
Occasional (4%-7%)
Dizziness, headache, confusion, constipation, hypertension, cough.
Rare (2%-3%)
Back pain, nausea, fatigue, anxiety, peripheral edema, arthralgia, insomnia.

SERIOUS REACTIONS
• Atrioventricular block.

PRECAUTIONS & CONSIDERATIONS
Caution is warranted in patients with moderate renal impairment. It is unknown whether memantine crosses the placenta or is distributed in breast milk. Memantine is not prescribed for use in children. No age-related precautions have been noted in elderly patients. Be aware that memantine is not a cure for Alzheimer disease but may slow the progression of its symptoms.

Adequate fluid intake should be maintained. Renal function and urine pH should be monitored; alkaline urine may lead to an accumulation of the drug and a possible increase in side effects.
Administration
Take memantine without regard to food. Do not abruptly discontinue or adjust the drug dosage. If therapy is interrupted for several days, restart the drug at the lowest dose and increase the dosage at intervals of at least 1 wk to the most recent dose, as prescribed.

Menotropins

men-oh-troe′-pins
(Humegon, Pergonal, Repronex, Menopur)

CATEGORY AND SCHEDULE

Pregnancy Risk Category: X

Classification: Ovarian stimulant

MECHANISM OF ACTION

A mixture of equal activity of follicle stimulating hormone (FSH) and lutenizing hormone (LH) isolated from the urine of postmenopausal women and necessary for the development, maturation, and release of ova from ovaries and for spermatogenesis in the testes. *Therapeutic Effect:* Promotes ovulation and pregnancy in infertile women.

PHARMACOKINETICS

Not absorbed from the GI tract. Cleared from the circulation by glomerular filtration. Degraded in proximal tubule or excreted unchanged in urine. *Half-life:* 2.2-2.9 h.

AVAILABILITY

Injection: 75 units FSH activity and 75 or 150 units LH activity/ 2 mL ampule (Humegon,Menopur, Pergonal, Repronex), 75 or 150 units FSH activity, and 75 or 150 units LH activity/2 mL ampule (Humegon, Pergonal, Repronex).

INDICATIONS AND DOSAGES

▸Follicle maturation, ovulation and pregnancy induction
SC (MENOPUR ONLY)
Adults. 225 International Units (IU) daily. Adjust dose by 150 IU/day every 2 days based on clinical response. Maximum: 450 IU/day; do not exceed 20 days. Continue until follicular development is adequate. Give hCG 1 day after last dose of Menopur in preparation for oocyte retrieval.
▸Follicle maturation, ovulation, and pregnancy induction
IM OR SC (REPRONEX ONLY)
Adults. 225 International units (IU) daily. Adjust dose by 75-150 IU/day every 2 days based on clinical response. May divide daily dose and give twice a day, Maximum 450 IU/ day; do not exceed 12 days. Continue until follicular development is adequate. Give hCG 1 day after last dose of Repronex in preparation for oocyte retrieval.
▸Stimulation of spermatogenesis
IM
Adults. Pretreatment with 5000 units hCG 3 times weekly is required before initiating concomitant therapy with menotropins. Continue pretreatment until serum testosterone levels are in the normal range and masculinization is reached (may require 4-6 mo); then initiate therapy with menotropins 75 IU 3 times weekly and 2000 units hCG twice weekly for a minimum of 4 mo. If the patient has not responded after 4 mo, continue treatment with 75 IU menotropins 3 times weekly or increase dose to 150 IU 3 times weekly, keeping the dose for hCG the same.

CONTRAINDICATIONS

Prior hypersensitivity to menotropins.
    Women: Known or suspected pregnancy, high FSH level indicating primary ovarian failure, abnormal bleeding of undetermined origin, an organic intracranial lesion such as a pituitary tumor, elevated

M

gonadotropin levels indicating primary testicular failure, the presence of any cause of infertility other than anovulation, unless they are candidates for in vitro fertilization, ovarian cysts or enlargement not due to polycystic ovary syndrome, uncontrolled thyroid and adrenal dysfunction.

Sex hormone–dependent tumors of reproductive tract and accessory organs (Menopur only).

Men: Infertility disorders other than hypogonadotropic hypogonadism, normal gonadotropin levels indicating normal pituitary function.

INTERACTIONS
Drug
None known.
Herbal
None known.
Food
None known.

DIAGNOSTIC TEST EFFECTS
None known.

ⓘ IV INCOMPATIBILITIES
None known.

ⓘ IV COMPATIBILITIES
None known.

SIDE EFFECTS
Occasional
Women: Abdominal pain, bloating, diarrhea, nausea, vomiting, body rash, dizziness, dyspnea, tachypnea, ovarian cysts, ovarian enlargement, pain, rash, swelling at injection site, tachycardia.
Men: Gynecomastia.

SERIOUS REACTIONS
• Acute respiratory distress syndrome, atelectasis, pulmonary embolism, pulmonary infarction, arterial occlusion, cerebral vascular occlusion, venous thrombophlebitis, congenital abnormalities, ectopic pregnancy, and ovarian hyperstimulation syndrome have been reported.

PRECAUTIONS & CONSIDERATIONS
Be aware that menotropins should be discontinued if the ovaries become enlarged or abdominal pain occurs. Be aware that multiple births can occur with menotropin use for ovulation induction. Be aware that menotropins are contraindicated in pregnancy, and whether it is distributed in breast milk is not known. Be aware that the safety and efficacy of this drug have not been established in children and elderly patients. Overdose evidenced by ovarian hyperstimulation.

Thorough gynecologic and endocrine evaluation is necessary before starting therapy to assess for excessive ovarian stimulation (abdominal pain, distress, diarrhea, dyspnea, nausea, oliguria, rapid weight gain, severe pelvic pain, vomiting), and thromboembolic events. Once therapy is initiated, must report signs of ovarian hyperstimulation immediately to health care practitioners.
Storage
Lyophilized powder may be refrigerated or stored at room temperature. After reconstitution, inject immediately. Discard any unused portion. Protect from light.
Administration
Be aware that doses to produce maturation of the follicle must be individualized for each person. Single courses of therapy in women should not exceed 12-20 days.

Be aware that hCG should be withheld if the ovaries are abnormally enlarged on the last day of menotropins therapy. Stop administration of menotropins if the ovaries become abnormally enlarged or abdominal pain occurs.

Be aware that the couple should have intercourse daily, beginning on the day before the administration of hCG until ovulation becomes apparent.

Repronex may be administered IM or SC. Administer Menopur subcutaneously only. Administer in the lower abdomen, alternating sides, for administration.

Menopur is given subcutaneously.

Meperidine Hydrochloride

me-per′i-deen high-droh-klor-ide
(Demerol, Pethidine Injection [AUS])
Do not confuse Demerol with Demulen or Dymelor.

CATEGORY AND SCHEDULE

Pregnancy Risk Category: B (D if used for prolonged periods or at high dosages at term)
Controlled Substance Schedule: II

Classification: Analgesics, narcotic, preanesthetics, synthetic narcotic analgesic

MECHANISM OF ACTION

An opioid agonist that binds to opioid receptors in the central nervous system (CNS). *Therapeutic Effect:* Alters the perception of and emotional response to pain.

PHARMACOKINETICS

Route	Onset (min)	Peak (min)	Duration (h)
PO	15	60	2-4
IV	< 5	5-7	2-3
IM	10-15	30-50	2-4
Subcuta-neous	10-15	30-50	2-4

Variably absorbed from the GI tract; well absorbed after IM administration. Protein binding: 60%-80%. Widely distributed. Metabolized in the liver to active metabolite. Excreted primarily in urine. Not removed by hemodialysis. *Half-life:* 2.4-4 h; metabolite 8-16 h (increased in hepatic impairment and disease).

AVAILABILITY

Syrup: 50 mg/5 mL.
Tablets: 50 mg, 100 mg.
Injection: 25 mg/mL, 50 mg/mL, 75 mg/mL, 100 mg/mL.

INDICATIONS AND DOSAGES
▸ **Analgesia**
PO, IM, SC
Adults, Elderly. 25-150 mg q3-4h.
Children. 1.1-1.5 mg/kg q3-4h. Do not exceed single dose of 100 mg.
▸ **Patient-controlled analgesia (PCA)**
IV
Adults. Loading dose: 50-100 mg. Intermittent bolus: 5-30 mg. Lockout interval: 10-20 min. Continuous infusion: 5-40 mg/h. Maximum (4-h): 200-300 mg.
▸ **Dosage in renal impairment**
Dosage is based on creatinine clearance.

Creatinine Clearance (mL/min)	Dosage
10-50	75% of usual dose
< 10	50% of usual dose

M

CONTRAINDICATIONS

Hypersensitivity to meperidine, use within 14 days of MAOIs.

INTERACTIONS

Drug

Alcohol, other CNS depressants, alcohol, neuromuscular blocking agents: May increase CNS or respiratory depression and hypotension.

Anticholinergics: Increased anticholinergic effects.

Antihypertensive drugs: May increase risk of hypotension.

MAOIs: May produce a severe, sometimes fatal reaction. Meperidine use is contraindicated.

Ritonavir: Suspected increase in meperidine levels.

Sibutramine: Meperidine use is contraindicated.

Herbal

Valerian: May increase CNS depression.

Food

None known.

DIAGNOSTIC TEST EFFECTS

May increase serum amylase and lipase levels. Therapeutic serum level is 100-550 ng/mL; toxic serum level is > 1000 ng/mL.

ⓘ IV INCOMPATIBILITIES

Allopurinol (Aloprim), amphotericin B complex (Abelcet, AmBisome, Amphotec), cefepime (Maxipime), cefoperazone (Cefobid), doxorubicin liposomal (Doxil), furosemide (Lasix), idarubicin (Idamycin), nafcillin (Nafcil), *all* barbiturates.

ⓘ IV COMPATIBILITIES

Bumetanide (Bumex), diltiazem (Cardizem), dobutamine (Dobutrex), dopamine (Intropin), heparin, insulin, lidocaine, magnesium, oxytocin (Pitocin), potassium.

SIDE EFFECTS

Frequent

Sedation, hypotension (including orthostatic hypotension), diaphoresis, facial flushing, dizziness, nausea, vomiting, constipation.

Occasional

Confusion, arrhythmias, tremors, urine retention, abdominal pain, dry mouth, headache, irritation at injection site, euphoria, dysphoria.

Rare

Allergic reaction (rash, pruritus), insomnia.

SERIOUS REACTIONS

• Overdose results in respiratory depression, skeletal muscle flaccidity, cold or clammy skin, cyanosis, and extreme somnolence progressing to seizures, stupor, and coma. The antidote is 0.4 mg naloxone.

• The patient who uses meperidine repeatedly may develop a tolerance to the drug's analgesic effect and physical dependence.

PRECAUTIONS & CONSIDERATIONS

Caution is warranted in patients with acute abdominal conditions, cor pulmonale, history of seizures, increased intracranial pressure, hepatic or renal impairment, respiratory abnormalities, supraventricular tachycardia, and in debilitated or elderly patients. Be aware that with renal impairment, meperidine's metabolite may increase and cause seizures, tremors, and twitching. Meperidine crosses the placenta and is distributed in breast milk. Regular use of opiates during pregnancy may produce withdrawal symptoms in the neonate, such as diarrhea, excessive crying, fever, hyperactive reflexes, irritability, seizures, sneezing, tremors, vomiting, and yawning. The neonate may develop respiratory depression if the mother receives meperidine during labor. Children are more prone to develop paradoxical excitement. Children younger than 2 yrs and elderly patients are more susceptible to the drug's respiratory depressant effects. In elderly patients, age-related renal impairment may increase the risk of urine retention. Be aware that drug dependence and tolerance may occur with prolonged use of high doses.

Dizziness and drowsiness may occur, so change positions slowly and avoid alcohol, CNS depressants, and tasks that require mental alertness or motor skills until response to the drug is established. Vital signs, pattern of daily bowel activity and stool consistency, and clinical improvement of pain should be monitored. The drug should be withheld and the physician should be notified if the respiratory rate is 12 breaths/min or less in an adult, or 20 breaths/min or less in a child. Vital signs should be monitored for 15-30 min after an IM or SC dose and for 5-10 min after an IV dose. Be alert for decreased BP as well as a change in quality and rate of pulse. Psychological and physical dependence may occur with chronic administration; drug has an abuse potential in predisposed individuals.
Storage
Store vials at room temperature.
Administration
! Be aware that meperidine's side effects are dependent on the dosage and route of administration. Know that ambulatory patients and those not in severe pain may be more prone to dizziness, nausea, and vomiting than those in the supine position and those in severe pain.

Take oral meperidine without regard to food. Dilute the syrup in a half-glass of water to prevent an anesthetic effect on mucous membranes.
! Give meperidine by slow IV push or IV infusion. Know that therapeutic serum drug level is 100-550 ng/mL; toxic serum drug level is > 1000 ng/mL.

Meperidine may be given undiluted or may be diluted in D5W, Ringer's solution, lactated Ringer's solution, a dextrose-saline combination (such as 2.5%, 5%, or 10% dextrose and 0.45% or 0.9% NaCl), or Molar (M/6) Sodium Lactate Injection for IV injection or infusion. Place the patient in a recumbent position before administering parenteral meperidine. Administer IV push very slowly, over 2-3 min. Rapid IV administration increases the risk of a severe anaphylactic reaction, marked by apnea, cardiac arrest, and circulatory collapse.
! The IM route is preferred over the SC route because it can produce induration, local irritation, and pain.

For IM use, inject the drug slowly. Know that patients with circulatory impairment are at increased risk for overdose because of delayed absorption of repeated injections.

M

Mephobarbital
me′foe-bar′bi-tal
(Mebaral)

CATEGORY AND SCHEDULE
Controlled substance: Schedule IV

Classification: Barbiturate anticonvulsant

MECHANISM OF ACTION
A barbiturate that increases seizure threshold in the motor cortex.

Therapeutic Effect: Depresses monosynaptic and polysynaptic transmission in the central nervous system (CNS).

PHARMACOKINETICS

PO route onset 20-60 min, peak not applicable, duration 6-8 h. Well absorbed after PO administration. Widely distributed. Metabolized in liver to active metabolite, a form of phenobarbital. Minimally excreted in urine. Removed by hemodialysis. *Half-life:* 34 h.

AVAILABILITY

Tablets: 32 mg, 50 mg, 100 mg (Mebaral).

INDICATIONS AND DOSAGES

▸ **Epilepsy**
PO
Adults, Elderly. 400-600 mg/day in divided doses or at bedtime.
Children older than 5 yrs. 32-64 mg 3 or 4 times/day.
Children younger than 5 yrs. 16-32 mg 3 or 4 times/day.
▸ **Sedation**
PO
Adults, Elderly. Usually 50 mg 3-4 times/day.
Children > 5 years. 16-32 mg 3-4 times daily.

CONTRAINDICATIONS

Porphyria, history of hypersensitivity to mephobarbital or other barbiturates.

INTERACTIONS

Drug
Alcohol, all CNS depressants: May increase the effects of mephobarbital.
Barbiturates: May induce liver microsomal enzymes, which may alter the metabolism of this and other drugs.
Carbamazepine: May increase the metabolism of carbamazepine.
Corticosteroids, digoxin, doxycycline, glucocorticoids, metronidazole, oral anticoagulants, quinidine, tricyclic antidepressants: May decrease the effects of these medications.
Phenothiazines: May lower seizure threshold.
Pyridoxine: May decrease the effectiveness of mephobarbital.
Valproic acid: Decreases the metabolism and increases the concentration and risk of toxicity of mephobarbital.
Warfarin: May decrease effectiveness of warfarin.
Herbal
Catnip oil, kava kava, passion flower, valerian: May increase the CNS effects of mephobarbital.
Eucalyptol: May decrease the effectiveness of mephobarbital.
Evening primrose oil, ginkgo biloba: May decrease the anticonvulsant effectiveness of mephobarbital.
St. John's wort: May decrease CNS depressive effects of mephobarbital.
Food
None known.

DIAGNOSTIC TEST EFFECTS

None reported.

SIDE EFFECTS

Frequent
Dizziness, lightheadedness, somnolence.
Occasional
Confusion, headache, insomnia, mental depression, nervousness, nightmares, unusual excitement.
Rare
Rash, paradoxical CNS hyperactivity or nervousness

in children, excitement or restlessness in elderly, generally noted during first 2 wks of therapy, particularly noted in the presence of uncontrolled pain.

SERIOUS REACTIONS

• Abrupt withdrawal after prolonged therapy may produce effects including markedly increased dreaming, nightmares or insomnia, tremor, sweating, vomiting, hallucinations, delirium, seizures, and status epilepticus.
• Skin eruptions appear as hypersensitivity reaction.
• Blood dyscrasias, liver disease, and hypocalcemia occur rarely.
• Overdosage produces cold or clammy skin, hypothermia, severe CNS depression, cyanosis, rapid pulse, and Cheyne-Stokes respirations.
• Toxicity may result in severe renal impairment.

PRECAUTIONS & CONSIDERATIONS

Caution should be used in patients with liver or renal impairment. Mephobarbital readily crosses the placenta and is distributed in breast milk; caution in lactation is warranted. Withdrawal symptoms may appear in neonates born to women receiving barbiturates during the last trimester of pregnancy. Mephobarbital use may cause paradoxical excitement in children. Elderly patients may exhibit confusion, excitement, and mental depression while taking mephobarbital. Alcohol should be avoided and caffeine intake should be limited. Tasks that require mental alertness or motor skills should be avoided because mephobarbital may cause dizziness and drowsiness. Ensure that the patient continues to take antiseizure medication(s) as prescribed. Must evaluate type of epilepsy, seizure frequency, and quality of control before using this medication. Evaluate patient for stress tolerance.

Administration

Take mephobarbital without regard to meals. Crush tablets as needed. Do not discontinue the drug abruptly.

Meprobamate
me-proe′ba-mate
(Miltown, Novo-Mepro [CAN])

CATEGORY AND SCHEDULE
Pregnancy Risk Category: D

Classification: Anxiolytics, sedative-hypnotic

MECHANISM OF ACTION
A carbamate derivative that affects the thalamus and limbic system. Appears to inhibit multineuronal spinal reflexes. *Therapeutic Effect:* Anxiolytic and sedative activity.

PHARMACOKINETICS
Slowly absorbed from the GI tract. Protein binding: 0%-30%. Metabolized in liver. Excreted in urine and feces. Moderately dialyzable. *Half-life:* 10 h.

AVAILABILITY
Tablets: 200 mg, 400 mg, (Miltown).

INDICATIONS AND DOSAGES
▸ **Anxiety disorders**
PO
Adults, Children 12 yrs and older. 400 mg 3-4 times/day. Maximum: 2400 mg/day.

M

Children aged 6-12 yrs. 100-200 mg 2-3 times/day. Maximum: 600 mg/day.
Elderly. Use lowest effective dose. Maximum: 200 mg 2-3 times/day.

▸**Dosage in Renal Impairment**

Creatinine Clearance (mL/min)	Dosage Interval (h)
10-50	Every 9-12 h
< 10	Every 12-18 h

OFF-LABEL USES
Muscle contraction, headache, premenstrual tension, external sphincter spasticity, muscle rigidity, opisthotonos associated with tetanus.

CONTRAINDICATIONS
Acute intermittent porphyria, hypersensitivity to meprobamate or related compounds, such as carisoprodol.
Caution
Suicidal patients, severe depression, renal disease, hepatic disease, elderly, patients with addictive personality disorder.

INTERACTIONS
Drug
Alcohol, all central nervous system (CNS) depressants: May increase CNS depression.
Herbal
Gotu kola, kava kava, St. John's wort: May increase CNS depression.
Food
None known.

DIAGNOSTIC TEST EFFECTS
None known.

SIDE EFFECTS
Frequent
Drowsiness, dizziness.
Occasional
Tachycardia, palpitations, headache, lightheadedness, dermatitis, diarrhea, nausea, vomiting, dyspnea, rash, weakness, blurred vision, wheezing.

SERIOUS REACTIONS
• Agranulocytosis, aplastic anemia, leukopenia, anaphylaxis, cardiac arrhythmias, hypotensive crisis, syncope, Stevens-Johnson syndrome and bullous dermatitis have been reported.
• Overdose may cause CNS depression, ataxia, coma, shock, hypotension, and death.

PRECAUTIONS & CONSIDERATIONS
Caution is warranted with elderly patients as well as those with liver or renal impairment and those who use alcohol, psychotropic drugs, or other CNS depressants. Prolonged use of meprobamate may produce dependence. Meprobamate crosses the placenta and is distributed in breast milk. Be aware that the safety and efficacy of meprobamate have not been established in children younger than 6 yrs. In elderly patients, there is an increased risk of CNS toxicity, manifested as confusion, hallucinations, mental depression, and sedation. Age-related renal impairment may require a decreased dosage in elderly patients.

Complete blood count (CBC), renal function tests, BUN, serum creatinine, liver function tests including aspartate amino transferase (AST) and alanine amino transferase (ALT) and alkaline phosphatase should be monitored as well as blood concentrations of meprobamate. Therapeutic levels range between 6 and 12 ng/mL. Toxic signs are CNS manifestations (drowsiness, lethargy, coma, shock) and cardiovascular disturbances (arrhythmias, tachycardia, bradycardia, persistent and profound hypotension).

Dizziness and drowsiness are expected side effects with meprobamate. Avoid alcohol and sudden changes in posture to help prevent hypotensive effects. Evaluate the patient's tolerance to stress from possible cardiovascular events while on therapy. Psychologic and physical dependence may occur with chronic administration.

Administration

May give without regard to meals. Give last dose at bedtime. Avoid abrupt discontinuation in patients with prolonged use of meprobamate.

Meropenem
mear-ro-pen'em
(Merrem IV)

CATEGORY AND SCHEDULE
Pregnancy Risk Category: B

Classification: Antiinfective, miscellaneous, carbapenem

MECHANISM OF ACTION
A carbapenem that binds to penicillin-binding proteins and inhibits bacterial cell wall synthesis. *Therapeutic Effect:* Produces bacterial cell death.

PHARMACOKINETICS
After IV administration, widely distributed into tissues and body fluids, including cerebrospinal fluid (CSF). Protein binding: 2%. Primarily excreted unchanged in urine. Removed by hemodialysis. *Half-life:* 1 h.

AVAILABILITY
Powder for Injection: 500 mg, 1 g.

INDICATIONS AND DOSAGES
▶ **Skin, skin structure, and intra-abdominal**
IV
Adults, Elderly. 0.5-1 g q8h.
Children 3 mo and older. 10-20 mg/kg/dose q8h.
Children younger than 3 mo. 10-20 mg/kg/dose q8-12h.
▶ **Meningitis**
IV
Adults, Elderly. Children weighing 50 kg or more. 2 g q8h.
Children 3 mo and older weighing < 50 kg. 40 mg/kg q8h. Maximum: 2 g/dose.
▶ **Dosage in renal impairment**
Dosage and frequency are modified based on creatinine clearance.

Creatinine Clearance (mL/min)	Dosage Interval
26-49	Recommended dose q 12 h
10-25	½ of Recommended dose q 12 h
< 10	½ of Recommended dose q 24 h

OFF-LABEL USES
Lower respiratory tract infections, febrile neutropenia, gynecologic and obstetric infections, sepsis.

CONTRAINDICATIONS
Hypersensitivity to the drug or other carbapenems; use caution in patients with immediate hypersensitivity to other β-lactams.

INTERACTIONS
Drug
Probenecid: Reduces renal excretion of meropenem.
Herbal
None known.
Food
None known.

M

DIAGNOSTIC TEST EFFECTS

May increase BUN level and serum alkaline phosphatase, bilirubin, creatinine, LDH, AST (SGOT), and ALT (SGPT) levels. May decrease blood hematocrit and hemoglobin levels and serum potassium levels.

ⓘ IV INCOMPATIBILITIES

According to manufacturer, do not mix with or add to solutions containing other drugs. Acyclovir (Zovirax), amphotericin B (Fungizone), diazepam (Valium), doxycycline (Vibramycin), metronidazole (Flagyl), ondansetron (Zofran).

ⓘ IV COMPATIBILITIES

Dobutamine (Dobutrex), dopamine (Intropin), heparin, magnesium.

SIDE EFFECTS

Frequent (3%-5%)
Diarrhea, nausea, vomiting, headache, inflammation at injection site.
Occasional (2%)
Oral candidiasis, rash, pruritus.
Rare (< 2%)
Constipation, glossitis.

SERIOUS REACTIONS

• Antibiotic-associated colitis and other superinfections may occur.
• Anaphylactic reactions have been reported.
• Seizures may occur in those with CNS disorders (including brain lesions and a history of seizures), bacterial meningitis, or impaired renal function.

PRECAUTIONS & CONSIDERATIONS

Caution is warranted in patients with CNS disorders (particularly a history of seizures); hypersensitivity to cephalosporins, penicillins, or other β-lactams; and renal function impairment. Assess penicillin and cephalosporin sensitivity before dosing. Be aware that it is unknown whether meropenem is distributed in breast milk; caution is warranted in lactation. Be aware that the safety and efficacy of meropenem have not been established in children younger than 3 mo. In elderly patients, age-related renal impairment may require dosage adjustment. Notify the physician if severe diarrhea occurs, but avoid taking antidiarrheals.

Notify the physician of the onset of troublesome or serious adverse reactions, including infusion-site pain, redness, or swelling, nausea or vomiting, or skin rash or itching. Electrolytes (especially potassium), intake and output, and renal function test results should be monitored. BP, temperature, and mental status should be monitored. Examine the patient periodically for opportunistic secondary infection. Report any oral soreness, lesions, or bleeding. Drug is to be administered only in a hospital or outpatient institutional setting.

Storage

Store vials at room temperature. After reconstitution with 0.9% NaCl, infusion is stable for 2 h at room temperature, 18 h if refrigerated (with D5W, stable for 1 h at room temperature, 8 h if refrigerated).

Administration

! Space drug doses evenly around the clock.

For IV use, reconstitute each 500 mg with 10 mL sterile water for injection to provide a concentration of 50 mg/mL. Shake to dissolve until clear. May further dilute with 100 mL 0.9% NaCl or D5W. May give by IV push or IV intermittent infusion (piggyback). If administering as IV intermittent infusion (piggyback), give over 15-30 min; if administered by IV push (5-20 mL), give over 3-5 min.

Mesalamine/ 5 Aminosalicylic Acid (5-ASA)

mez-al'a-meen/ 5- am-ee-no-sal-ee-sil-ic ass-id
(Apriso, Asacol, Fiv-Canasa, Mesasal [CAN], Pentasa, Rowasa, Salofalk [CAN])
Do not confuse Asacol with Os-Cal.

CATEGORY AND SCHEDULE
Pregnancy Risk Category: B

Classification: Anti-inflammatory, Gastrointestinal, 5-aminosalicylate.

MECHANISM OF ACTION
A salicylic acid derivative that locally inhibits arachidonic acid metabolite production, which is increased in patients with chronic inflammatory bowel disease. *Therapeutic Effect:* Blocks prostaglandin production and diminishes inflammation in the colon.

PHARMACOKINETICS
Poorly absorbed from the colon. Moderately absorbed from the GI tract. Metabolized in the liver to active metabolite. Unabsorbed portion eliminated in feces; absorbed portion excreted in urine. Unknown whether removed by hemodialysis. *Half-life:* 0.5-1.5 h; metabolite, 5-10 h.

AVAILABILITY
Tablets (Delayed-Release [Asacol]): 400 mg.
Capsules (Controlled-Release [Pentasa]): 250 mg.
Rectal Suspension (Rowasa): 4 g/60 mL.
Suppositories (Canasa): 500 mg.
Capsules (Extended-Release [Apriso]). 0.375 g.

INDICATIONS AND DOSAGES
▸ **Ulcerative colitis, proctosigmoiditis, proctitis**
PO (ASACOL)
Adults, Elderly. 800 mg 3 times a day for 6 wks.
Children. 50 mg/kg/day q8-12h.
PO (PENTASA)
Adults, Elderly. 1 g 4 times a day for 8 wks.
Children. 50 mg/kg/day q6-12h.
RECTAL (RETENTION ENEMA)
Adults, Elderly. 60 mL (4 g) at bedtime; retain overnight (about 8 h) for 3-6 wks.
RECTAL (SUPPOSITORY)
Adults, Elderly. 1 suppository (500 mg) twice a day, retain 1-3 h for 3-6 wks.
▸ **Maintenance of remission in ulcerative colitis**
PO (ASACOL)
Adults, Elderly. 1.6 g/day in divided doses.
PO (PENTASA)
Adults, Elderly. 1 g 4 times a day.
PO (APRISO)
Adults. 1.5 g PO once daily.

CONTRAINDICATIONS
Hypersensitivity to drug or other 5-aminosalicylates or salicylates.

INTERACTIONS
Drug
Antacids: Do not administer Apriso capsules with antacids.
Azathioprine, mercaptopurine: May increase side effects of these antineoplastics.
Herbal
None known.
Food
None known.

M

DIAGNOSTIC TEST EFFECTS

May increase BUN, serum alkaline phosphatase, creatinine, AST (SGOT), and ALT (SGPT) levels.

SIDE EFFECTS

Mesalamine is generally well tolerated, with only mild and transient effects.

Frequent (> 6%)

PO: Abdominal cramps or pain, diarrhea, dizziness, headache, nausea, vomiting, rhinitis, unusual fatigue.

Rectal: Abdominal or stomach cramps, flatulence, headache, nausea.

Occasional (2%-6%)

PO: Hair loss, decreased appetite, back or joint pain, flatulence, acne.

Rectal: Hair loss.

Rare (< 2%)

Rectal: Anal irritation.

SERIOUS REACTIONS

• Acute intolerance syndrome may occur in susceptible patients, manifested by cramping, headache, diarrhea, fever, rash, hives, itching, and wheezing. Discontinue drug immediately.

• Hepatitis, pancreatitis, and pericarditis occur rarely with oral forms.

• Interstitial nephritis (rare).

PRECAUTIONS & CONSIDERATIONS

Caution is warranted in patients with preexisting renal disease and sulfasalazine sensitivity. It is unknown whether mesalamine crosses the placenta or is distributed in breast milk; caution is warranted in lactation. Safety and efficacy of mesalamine have not been established in children. In elderly patients, age-related renal impairment may require cautious use. Avoid tasks that require mental alertness or motor skills until response to the drug has been established.

Be aware that mesalamine use may discolor urine yellow-brown; mesalamine suppositories stain fabrics. Adequate fluid intake should be maintained. Daily bowel activity and stool consistency and skin for rash should be assessed. Mesalamine should be discontinued if cramping, diarrhea, fever, or rash occurs. To avoid the possibility of pseudomembranous colitis developing, medical consultation is warranted before selecting an antibiotic for infection.

Storage

Store rectal suspension, suppositories, and oral forms at room temperature.

Administration

For tablet, use, do not break outer coating of tablet; swallow whole. Take mesalamine without regard to food. Extended and delayed-release capsules should be swallowed whole.

For rectal use, shake bottle well. Lie on the left side with the lower leg extended, upper leg flexed forward, or to assume the knee-chest position. Insert applicator tip into rectum, pointing toward umbilicus. Squeeze bottle steadily until contents are emptied. Retain the enema for as long as tolerable, preferably for a minimum of 8 h.

Metaproterenol Sulfate

met-a-proe-ter′e-nole sull-feyt
(Alupent)
Do not confuse metaproterenol with metipranolol or metoprolol, or Alupent with Atrovent.

CATEGORY AND SCHEDULE

Pregnancy Risk Category: C

Classification: Selective β_2-agonist

MECHANISM OF ACTION

A sympathomimetic that stimulates β_2-adrenergic receptors, resulting in relaxation of bronchial smooth muscle. *Therapeutic Effect:* Relieves bronchospasm and reduces airway resistance.

PHARMACOKINETICS

3% absorbed through lungs after inhalation. Primarily metabolized in the GI tract. Duration 1-5 h following a single dose (reduced to 1-2.5 h after repetitive dosing).

AVAILABILITY

Solution: 10 mg/5 mL.
Tablets: 10 mg, 20 mg.
Solution for Nebulization: 0.4%, 0.6%.

INDICATIONS AND DOSAGES

▶ **Treatment of bronchospasm**
PO
Adults, Children older than 9 yr and > 27 kg 20 mg 3-4 times a day.
Elderly. 10 mg 3-4 times a day. May increase to 20 mg/dose.
Children aged 6-9 yr or > 27 kg. 10 mg 3-4 times a day.
Children aged 2-5 yrs. 1.3-2.6 mg/kg/day in 3-4 divided doses.
NEBULIZATION
Adults, Elderly, Children 12 yrs and older. 10-15 mg (0.2-0.3 mL) q4-6h.

CONTRAINDICATIONS

Preexisting arrhythmias associated with tachycardia, hypersensitivity to drug or product components.
Caution
Cardiac disorders, hyperthyroidism, diabetes mellitus, benign prostatic hypertrophy.

INTERACTIONS

Drug
Aspirin, sulfite preservatives: May exacerbate asthma conditions.
β-Blockers: May decrease the effects of β-blockers.
Digoxin, other sympathomimetics, central nervous system (CNS) stimulants: May increase the risk of arrhythmias.
Halogenated hydrocarbon anesthetics: Increased risk of dysrhythmias.
MAOIs: May increase the risk of hypertensive crisis.
Tricyclic antidepressants: May increase cardiovascular effects.
Herbal
None known.
Food
None known.

DIAGNOSTIC TEST EFFECTS

May decrease serum potassium level.

SIDE EFFECTS

Frequent (>10%)
Rigors, tremors, anxiety, nausea, dry mouth.
Occasional (1%-9%)
Dizziness, vertigo, asthenia, headache, GI distress, vomiting, cough, dry throat.
Rare (< 1%)
Somnolence, diarrhea, altered taste.

SERIOUS REACTIONS

• Excessive sympathomimetic stimulation may cause palpitations, extrasystoles, tachycardia, chest pain, a slight increase in BP followed by a substantial decrease, chills, diaphoresis, and blanching of skin.
• Too-frequent or excessive use may lead to decreased drug effectiveness and severe, paradoxical bronchoconstriction.

PRECAUTIONS & CONSIDERATIONS

Caution is warranted in patients with arrhythmias, congestive heart

M

failure (CHF), ischemic heart disease, diabetes mellitus, hypertension, hyperthyroidism, and a seizure disorder. Drink plenty of fluids to decrease the thickness of lung secretions. Avoid excessive use of caffeinated products, such as chocolate, cocoa, cola, coffee, and tea.

Anxiety, insomnia, and restlessness may occur. Notify the physician of chest pain, difficulty breathing, dizziness, flushing, headache, palpitations, tachycardia, or tremors. Pulse rate and quality, respiratory rate, depth, rhythm and type, ECG, ABG levels, pulmonary function, and clinical improvement should be monitored. Evidence of cyanosis, a blue or a dusky color in light-skinned patients and a gray color in dark-skinned patients, should also be assessed. Sympathomimetic inhalants should be available for emergency use or acute asthma episodes.

Storage
Store at room temperature keep nebulizer solution in foil pouch protected from light until time of use.

Administration
Do not exceed the recommended dosage.

May take orally without regard to food.

Nebulizer solutions of 0.4% and 0.6% may go into apparatus without further dilution.

Metaraminol
met-ar-am′e-nol
(Aramine)
Discontinued in the United States

CATEGORY AND SCHEDULE
Pregnancy Risk Category: D

Classification: Adrenergic agonists

MECHANISM OF ACTION
An α-adrenergic receptor agonist that causes vasoconstriction, reflex bradycardia, inhibits GI smooth muscle and vascular smooth muscle supplying skeletal muscle; increases heart rate and force of heart muscle contraction. *Therapeutic Effect:* Increases both systolic and diastolic pressure.

PHARMACOKINETICS

Route	Onset (min)	Peak	Duration
IM (pressor effect)	10	NA	20-60 min
IV	1-2	NA	
SC	5-20	NA	

Metabolized in the liver. Excreted in the urine and the bile.

AVAILABILITY
Injection: 10 mg/mL (Aramine).

INDICATIONS AND DOSAGES
▶ **Prevention of hypotension**
IM/SC
Adults, Elderly. 2-10 mg as a single dose.
Children. 0.01 mg/kg as a single dose.
▶ **Adjunctive treatment of hypotension**
IV INFUSION
Adults, Elderly. 15-100 mg IV infusion, administered at a rate to maintain the desired BP.
▶ **Severe shock**
IV
Adults, Elderly. 0.5-5 mg direct IV injection followed by 15-100 mg IV infusion in 250-500 mL fluid for control of BP.

CONTRAINDICATIONS
Cyclopropane or halothane anesthesia, use of MAOIs, pregnancy, hypersensitivity to metaraminol.

INTERACTIONS
Drug
Cyclopropane, halothane, MAOIs, digoxin, oxytocin, reserpine: May increase the risk of metaraminol toxicity.
Halogenated hydrocarbon anesthetics: Increased risk of arrhythmia.
Tricyclic antidepressants: May decrease the effect of metaraminol.
Herbal
None known.
Food
None known.

DIAGNOSTIC TEST EFFECTS
None known.

IV INCOMPATIBILITIES
Amphotericin B, dexamethasone, erythromycin, hydrocortisone, methicillin, penicillin G, prednisolone, thiopental (Pentothal).

IV COMPATIBILITIES
Amikacin (Amikin), amiodarone (Cordarone), cephalothin (Ceporacin), cephapirin (Cefadyl), chloramphenicol, cimetidine (Tagamet), cyanocobalamin, dexamethasone, dobutamine (Dobutrex), ephedrine, hydrocortisone, inamrinone, lidocaine, oxytocin (Pitocin), potassium, procainamide, promazine (Sparine), secobarbital (Seconal), sodium bicarbonate, sulfisoxazole (Gantrisin), tetracycline, verapamil.

SIDE EFFECTS
Occasional
Tachycardia, hypertension, cardiac arrhythmias, flushing, palpitations, hypotension, angina, tremors, nervousness, headache, dizziness, weakness, sloughing of skin, nausea, abscess formation, diaphoresis.

SERIOUS REACTIONS
• Overdosage produces hypertension, cerebral hemorrhage, cardiac arrest, and seizures.

PRECAUTIONS & CONSIDERATIONS
! This drug should be used only in hospitals or emergency departments for selected hypotensive episodes.

Caution should be used with previous myocardial infarction, hypertension, and hyperthyroidism. Metaraminol crosses the placenta and is distributed in breast milk. Use metaraminol with caution in children. In elderly patients, age-related renal impairment may require dosage adjustment. Increased heart rate or palpitations should be reported.
Administration
For IM and SC injection, to prevent necrosis, infiltrate area with 10-15 mL of saline containing 5-10 mg of phentolamine.

For IV injection, as adjunctive treatment of hypotension or severe shock, mix 15-100 mg in 250-500 mL NS or D5W. For severe shock, metaraminol may also be administered endotracheally. Prolonged use may produce cumulative effects.

Metaxalone
me-tax′a-lone
(Skelaxin)

CATEGORY AND SCHEDULE
Pregnancy Risk Category: C

Classification: Muscle relaxant

MECHANISM OF ACTION
A central depressant whose exact mechanism is unknown. Many

effects due to its central depressant actions. *Therapeutic Effect:* Relieves pain or muscle spasms.

PHARMACOKINETICS

PO route onset 1 h, peak 3 h, duration 4-6 h. Well absorbed from the GI tract. Metabolized in the liver. Excreted primarily in urine. *Half-life:* 9 h.

AVAILABILITY

Tablets: 400 mg, 800 mg (Skelaxin).

INDICATIONS AND DOSAGES

▸ **Muscle relaxant**
PO
Adults, Elderly, Children older than 12 yrs. 800 mg 3-4 times/day.

CONTRAINDICATIONS

Significantly impaired renal or hepatic function, history of drug-induced hemolytic anemias or other anemias, history of hypersensitivity to metaxalone.

INTERACTIONS

Drug
Alcohol, central nervous system (CNS) depression-producing medications, tricyclic antidepressants: May increase CNS depression.
Herbal
None known.
Food
None known.

DIAGNOSTIC TEST EFFECTS

May give false-positive Benedict's test.

SIDE EFFECTS

Occasional
Drowsiness, headache, lightheadedness, dermatitis, nausea, vomiting, stomach cramps, dyspnea.

SERIOUS REACTIONS

• Overdose may cause CNS depression, coma, shock, and respiratory depression.
• Hemolytic anemia (rare)
• Jaundice
• Rare reports of anaphylaxis

PRECAUTIONS & CONSIDERATIONS

Caution should be used in patient with impaired liver or renal function. It is unknown whether metaxalone crosses the placenta or is distributed in breast milk. Safety and efficacy of metaxalone have not been established in children younger than 12 yrs. In elderly patients, there is an increased risk of CNS toxicity, manifested as confusion, hallucinations, mental depression, and sedation. Age-related renal impairment may require a decreased dosage in elderly patients. Alcohol as well as tasks that require mental alertness or motor skills should be avoided during therapy.
Administration
Take metaxalone without regard to food.

Metformin Hydrochloride

met-for′min high-droh-klor-ide (Fortamet, Glucophage, Glucophage XL, Glycon [CAN], Novo-Metformin [CAN], Riomet)

CATEGORY AND SCHEDULE

Pregnancy Risk Category: B

Classification: Biguanide derivative, oral antihyperglycemic

MECHANISM OF ACTION

An antihyperglycemic that decreases hepatic production of glucose. Decreases absorption of glucose and improves insulin sensitivity. *Therapeutic Effect:* Improves glycemic control, stabilizes or decreases body weight, and improves lipid profile.

PHARMACOKINETICS

Slowly, incompletely absorbed after oral administration. Food delays or decreases the extent of absorption. Protein binding: Negligible. Distributed primarily to intestinal mucosa and salivary glands. Primarily excreted unchanged in urine. Removed by hemodialysis. *Half-life:* 3-6 h.

AVAILABILITY

Oral Solution (Riomet): 100 mg/mL.
Tablets (Glucophage): 500 mg, 850 mg, 1000 mg.
Tablets (Extended-Release [Glucophage XL]): 500 mg, 750 mg.
Tablets (Extended-Release [Fortamet]): 500 mg, 1000 mg.

INDICATIONS AND DOSAGES
▸ **Diabetes mellitus**
PO (500-MG, 1000-MG TABLET)
Adults, Elderly. Initially, 500 mg twice a day, with morning and evening meals. May increase in 500-mg increments every week in divided doses. May give twice a day up to 2000 mg/day (for example, 1000 mg twice a day [with morning and evening meals]). If 2500 mg/day is required, give 3 times a day with meals. Maximum: 2500 mg/day.
Children 10-16 yrs. Initially, 500 mg twice a day. May increase by 500 mg/day at weekly intervals. Maximum: 2000 mg/day.

PO (850-MG TABLET)
Adults, Elderly. Initially, 850 mg/day, with morning meal. May increase dosage in 850-mg increments every other week, in divided doses. Maintenance: 850 mg twice a day, with morning and evening meals. Maximum: 2550 mg/day (850 mg 3 times a day).
PO (EXTENDED-RELEASE TABLETS)
Adults, Elderly. Initially, 500 mg once a day. May increase by 500 mg/day at weekly intervals. Maximum: 2000 mg once a day.
▸ **Adjunct to insulin therapy**
PO
Adults, Elderly. Initially, 500 mg/day. May increase by 500 mg at 7-day intervals. Maximum: 2500 mg/day (2000 mg/day for extended-release form).

OFF-LABEL USES

Treatment of metabolic complications of AIDS, prediabetes, polycystic ovary syndrome.

CONTRAINDICATIONS

Acute diabetic ketoacidosis, myocardial infarction (MI), cardiovascular collapse, renal disease or dysfunction (defined as SCr > 1.4 mg/dL for females, SCr > 1.5 mg/dL for males), respiratory failure, septicemia, lactic acidosis.

Do not use in patients > 80 yr of age unless normal renal function is documented, use with dofetilide, hepatic disease.

INTERACTIONS
Drug
Alcohol, amiloride, cimetidine, digoxin, furosemide, morphine, nifedipine, procainamide, quinidine, quinine, ranitidine, triamterene, trimethoprim, vancomycin: May increase metformin blood concentration.

M

Dofetilide: Decreases excretion of dofetilide. Contraindicated.

Furosemide, hypoglycemia-causing medications: May require a decrease in metformin dosage.

Iodinated contrast studies: May cause acute renal failure and increased risk of lactic acidosis. Discontinue metformin before such tests and for 48 h after the procedure.

Herbal

None known.

Food

None known.

DIAGNOSTIC TEST EFFECTS

None known.

SIDE EFFECTS

Occasional (> 3%)

GI disturbances (including diarrhea, nausea, vomiting, abdominal bloating, flatulence, and anorexia) that are transient and resolve spontaneously during therapy.

Rare (1%-3%)

Unpleasant or metallic taste that resolves spontaneously during therapy.

SERIOUS REACTIONS

• Lactic acidosis occurs rarely but is a fatal complication in 50% of cases. Lactic acidosis is characterized by an increase in blood lactate levels (> 5 mmol/L), a decrease in blood pH, and electrolyte disturbances. Signs and symptoms of lactic acidosis include unexplained hyperventilation, myalgia, malaise, and somnolence, which may advance to cardiovascular collapse (shock), acute CHF, acute MI, and prerenal azotemia.

PRECAUTIONS & CONSIDERATIONS

Caution is warranted in patients with CHF, chronic respiratory difficulty, and uncontrolled hyperthyroidism or hypothyroidism, concurrent use of drugs that affect renal function, conditions that cause hyperglycemia

or hypoglycemia or delay food absorption (such as diarrhea, high fever, malnutrition, gastroparesis, and vomiting), and in elderly patients, debilitated, or malnourished with renal impairment. Caution should also be used in those who consume excessive amounts of alcohol; alcohol should be avoided during therapy. Insulin is the drug of choice during pregnancy. Metformin is distributed in breast milk in animals. Safety and efficacy of metformin have not been established in children. In elderly patients, age-related renal impairment or peripheral vascular disease may require dosage adjustment or discontinuation of drug; in general, do not titrate up to adult maximum doses.

Notify the physician of diarrhea, easy bleeding or bruising, change in color of stool or urine, headache, nausea, persistent rash, and vomiting. Hemoglobin and hematocrit, RBC count, and serum creatinine level should be obtained before beginning metformin therapy and annually thereafter. Food intake, blood glucose level, glycosylated hemoglobin, folic acid level, and renal function should also be monitored. Be aware of signs and symptoms of hypoglycemia (anxiety, cool wet skin, diplopia, dizziness, headache, hunger, numbness in mouth, tachycardia, tremors) or hyperglycemia (deep rapid breathing, dim vision, fatigue, nausea, polydipsia, polyphagia, polyuria, vomiting), especially in persons also taking oral sulfonylureas; carry candy, sugar packets, or other sugar supplements for immediate response to hypoglycemia. Consult the physician when glucose demands are altered (such as with fever, heavy physical activity, infection, stress, trauma). Exercise, good personal hygiene (including foot care), not smoking, and weight control are essential parts of therapy.

Notify the physician immediately if any of the following symptoms occur, evidencing lactic acidosis: myalgia, respiratory distress, weakness, diarrhea, malaise, muscle creamps, somnolence. Surgical procedures may warrant stopping metformin therapy or adjustment in dose.

Administration

! Lactic acidosis is a rare but potentially severe consequence of metformin therapy. Expect to withhold metformin in patients with conditions that may predispose to lactic acidosis, such as dehydration, hypoperfusion, hypoxemia, and sepsis, radiographic tests using contrast.

Take metformin orally with meals. Do not crush film-coated tablets or extended-release tablets. Once-daily extended-release tablets usually given with evening meal or with a full glass of water.

Methacholine
meth-a-ko′leen
(Provocholine)

CATEGORY AND SCHEDULE
Pregnancy Risk Category: C

Classification: Cholinergics, diagnostics, nonradioactive

MECHANISM OF ACTION
A cholinergic, parasympathomimetic, synthetic analogue of acetylcholine that stimulates muscarinic, postganglionic parasympathetic receptors. *Therapeutic Effect:* Results in smooth muscle contraction of the airways and increased tracheobronchial secretions.

PHARMACOKINETICS
PO route onset rapid, peak 1-4 min, duration 15-75 min or 5 min if methacholine challenge is followed with a β-agonist agent. Undergoes rapid hydrolysis in the plasma by acetylcholinesterase.

AVAILABILITY
Powder for Oral Inhalation:
100-mg/5 mL (Provocholine).

INDICATIONS AND DOSAGES
Asthma diagnosis
INHALATION

Challenge test: Before inhalation challenge, perform baseline pulmonary function tests; the patient must have an FEV_1 of at least 70% of the predicted value. The following is a suggested schedule for administration of methacholine challenge. Calculate cumulative units by multiplying the number of breaths by the concentration given. Total cumulative units are the sum of cumulative units for each concentration given.

VIAL E
• Serial concentration: 0.025 mg/mL.
• No. of breaths: 5.
• Cumulative units per concentration: 0.125.
• Total cumulative units: 0.125.

VIAL D
• Serial concentration: 0.25 mg/mL.
• No. of breaths: 5.
• Cumulative units per concentration: 1.25.
• Total cumulative units: 1.375.

VIAL C
• Serial concentration: 2.5 mg/mL.
• No. of breaths: 5.
• Cumulative units per concentration: 12.5.
• Total cumulative units: 13.88.

VIAL B:
• Serial concentration: 10 mg/mL.
• No. of breaths: 5.
• Cumulative units per concentration: 50.
• Total cumulative units: 63.88.

VIAL A
• Serial concentration: 25 mg/mL.
• No. of breaths: 5.
• Cumulative units per concentration: 125.
• Total cumulative units: 188.88.

M

Determine FEV1 within 5 min of challenge, a positive challenge is a 20% reduction in FEV_1.

OFF-LABEL USES
Adie syndrome diagnosis, familial dysautonomia diagnosis.

CONTRAINDICATIONS
Asthma, wheezing, or very low baseline pulmonary function tests, concomitant use of β-blockers, hypersensitivity to the drug; because of the potential for severe bronchoconstriction.

INTERACTIONS
Drug
β-Blockers: May increase risk of prolonged bronchoconstriction.
Herbal
None known.
Food
None known.

DIAGNOSTIC TEST EFFECTS
None known.

SIDE EFFECTS
Occasional
Headache, lightheadedness, itching, throat irritation, wheezing.

SERIOUS REACTIONS
• Severe bronchoconstriction and reduction in respiratory function can result. Patients with severe hyper-reactivity of the airways can experience bronchoconstriction at a dosage as low as 0.025 mg/mL (0.125 cumulative units). If severe bronchoconstriction occurs, reverse immediately by administration of a rapid-acting inhaled bronchodilator (β-agonist).

PRECAUTIONS & CONSIDERATIONS
Caution is warranted in patients with liver function impairment,

pulmonary disease, and significant cardiovascular disease. Safety and efficacy of methacholine have not been established in children. Chest, dyspnea, coughing, and wheezing indicate a positive response. Rapid acting β-agonist inhaler should be available for emergency rescue inhalation.

Administration
The following are guidelines for reconstitution and further dilution of methacholine chloride powder for a single-patient testing:

All dilutions should be made with 0.9% NaCl injection containing 0.4% phenol (pH 7). Add 4 mL of 0.9% NaCl injection to the 5-mL vial containing 100 mg of methacholine chloride (vial A). The final concentration will be 25 mg/mL (vial A). Remove 1 mL of solution from vial A and add 1.5 mL of 0.9% NaCl injection (vial B). The final concentration will be 10 mg/mL. Remove 1 mL of solution from vial A and transfer to another vial with an additional 9 mL of 0.9% NaCl injection. The final concentration will be 2.5 mg/mL (vial C). Remove 1 mL of solution from vial C and transfer to another vial with an additional 9 mL of 0.9% NaCl injection. The final concentration will be 0.25 mg/mL (vial D). Remove 1 mL of solution from vial D and transfer to another vial with an additional 9 mL of 0.9% NaCl injection. The final concentration will be 0.025 mg/mL (vial E). A 0.22-μm filter should be used when transferring the solutions from each vial to a nebulizer.

The solutions in vials A through D may be refrigerated for a maximum of 2 wks. Vial E must be prepared on the day of challenge.

Methadone Hydrochloride
meth′a-done high-droh-klor-ide
(Dolophine, Metadol [CAN],
Methadone Intensol, Methadose,
Physeptone [AUS])

CATEGORY AND SCHEDULE
Pregnancy Risk Category: B (D if
used for prolonged periods or at
high dosages at term)
Controlled Substance Schedule: II

Classification: Synthetic
narcotic analgesic

MECHANISM OF ACTION
An opioid agonist that binds with
opioid receptors in the central
nervous system (CNS). *Therapeutic
Effect:* Alters the perception of and
emotional response to pain; reduces
withdrawal symptoms from other
opioid drugs.

PHARMACOKINETICS

Route	Onset	Peak
Oral	0.5-1 h 1.5-2 h	6-8 h
IM	10-20 min 1-2 h	4-5 h
IV	NA	15-30 min

Well absorbed after IM injection.
Protein binding: 80%-85%.
Metabolized in the liver. Primarily
excreted in urine. Not removed by
hemodialysis. *Half-life:* 8-59 h.

AVAILABILITY
*Oral Concentrate (Methadone
Intensol, Methadose):* 10 mg/mL.
Oral Solution: 5 mg/5 mL,
10 mg/5 mL.
Tablets (Dolophine, Methadose):
5 mg, 10 mg.
Tablets (Dispersible [Methadose]):
40 mg.
Injection (Dolophine): 10 mg/mL.

INDICATIONS AND DOSAGES
▸ **Analgesia**
PO, IV, IM, SC
Adults. 2.5-10 mg q3-8h as needed
up to 5-20 mg q6-8h.
Elderly. 2.5 mg q8-12h.
Children. Initially, 0.1 mg/kg/dose
q4h for 2-3 doses, then q6-12h.
Maximum: 10 mg/dose.
▸ **Detoxification**
PO
Adults, Elderly. 15-40 mg/day.
▸ **Temporary maintenance treatment
of narcotic abstinence syndrome**
PO
Adults, Elderly. 20-120 mg/day.

CONTRAINDICATIONS
Hypersensitivity to methadone,
respiratory depression in absence of
monitored setting, acute bronchial
asthma, hypercarbia.

INTERACTIONS
Drug
**Alcohol, narcotics, sedative-
hypnotics, skeletal muscle
relaxants, benzodiazepines, other
CNS depressants:** May increase
CNS or respiratory depression and
hypotension.
Anticholinergics: Increased effects
of anticholinergics.
CYP3A4 or CYP2D6 inducers:
May decrease methadone effect or
precipitate withdrawal.
CYP3A4 or CYP2D6 inhibitors:
May increase methadone
concentrations.
MAOIs: May produce a severe,
sometimes fatal reaction; expect
to begin methadone at smaller
incremental doses.
Nevirapine, efavirenz, ritonavir: May
decrease methadone concentrations.

M

Herbal
Valerian: May increase CNS depression.
Food
None known.

DIAGNOSTIC TEST EFFECTS

May increase serum amylase and lipase levels.

SIDE EFFECTS

Frequent
Sedation, decreased BP (including orthostatic hypotension), diaphoresis, facial flushing, constipation, dizziness, nausea, vomiting.
Occasional
Confusion, urine retention, palpitations, abdominal cramps, visual changes, dry mouth, headache, decreased appetite, anxiety, insomnia.
Rare
Allergic reaction (rash, pruritus).

SERIOUS REACTIONS

• Overdose results in respiratory depression, skeletal muscle flaccidity, cold or clammy skin, cyanosis, and extreme somnolence progressing to seizures, stupor, and coma. The antidote is 0.4 mg naloxone.
• The patient who uses methadone long-term may develop a tolerance to the drug's analgesic effect and physical dependence.

PRECAUTIONS & CONSIDERATIONS

Caution is warranted with acute abdominal conditions, cor pulmonale, history of seizures, impaired hepatic or renal function, increased intracranial pressure, respiratory abnormalities, supraventricular tachycardia, and in debilitated or elderly patients. Methadone crosses the placenta and is distributed in breast milk. Regular use of opioids during pregnancy may produce withdrawal symptoms in the neonate, such as diarrhea, excessive crying, fever, hyperactive reflexes, irritability, seizures, sneezing, tremors, vomiting, and yawning. The neonate may develop respiratory depression if the mother receives methadone during labor. Children are more prone to experience paradoxical excitement. Children younger than 2 yrs and elderly patients are more susceptible to the drug's respiratory depressant effects. Age-related renal impairment may increase the risk of urine retention in elderly patients.

Dizziness and drowsiness may occur, so change positions slowly and avoid alcohol, CNS depressants, and tasks that require mental alertness or motor skills until response to the drug is established. Vital signs should be monitored for 15-30 min after an IM or SC dose and for 5-10 min after an IV dose. Clinical improvement should be monitored. The drug should be withheld and the physician should be notified if the respiratory rate is 12 breaths/min or less in an adult or 20 breaths/minute or less in a child. Overdose is treated with 0.4 mg naloxone. Psychologic and physical dependence may occur with chronic administration. In opioid- dependent patients, NSAIDs are the drugs of choice for post-treatment pain control.

Patients in the methadone maintenance program should not receive additional opioids or other controlled substances without a consultation.
Storage
Store all dosage forms at room temperature.
Administration
Know that oral methadone is one-half as potent as parenteral methadone. Take methadone without regard to food. Dilute the concentrate

in a 3-4 oz of water or citrus fruit juice to prevent an anesthetic effect on mucous membranes.

Dispersable tablets are placed in 3-4 oz of water, orange juice, citrus tang, or citrus-flavoured Kool-Aid and allowed to disperse (1 min). Drink entire dose after stirring well. ! Be aware that the IM route is preferred over the subcutaneous route because the subcutaneous route may produce induration, local irritation, and pain.

For IM and subcutaneous, do not use the solution if it appears cloudy or contains a precipitate. Place the patient in the recumbent position before giving parenteral methadone. Inject the drug slowly. Know that patients with circulatory impairment are at increased risk for overdose because of delayed absorption of repeated injections.

Methamphetamine
meth-am-fet′a-meen
(Desoxyn)
Do not confuse with Desoxyn with Dextran, dextromethorphan, or Excedrin.

CATEGORY AND SCHEDULE
Pregnancy Risk Category: C
Controlled substance: Schedule II

Classification: Amphetamine, anorexient

MECHANISM OF ACTION
A sympathomimetic amine related to amphetamine and ephedrine that enhances central nervous system (CNS) stimulant activity. Peripheral actions include elevation of systolic and diastolic BP and weak bronchodilator and respiratory stimulant action.

Therapeutic Effect: Increases motor activity, mental alertness; decreases drowsiness, fatigue.

PHARMACOKINETICS
Rapidly absorbed from the GI tract. Metabolized in liver. Excreted primarily in the urine. Unknown if removed by hemodialysis. *Half-life:* 4-5 h.

AVAILABILITY
Tablets: 5 mg.

INDICATIONS AND DOSAGES
▶ **Attention deficit hyperactivity disorder (ADHD)**
PO
Adults, Children 6 yrs and older. Initially, 5 mg 1-2 times/day. Increase by 5 mg/day at weekly intervals until therapeutic response is achieved. Usual effective dose is 10 mg-12.5 mg twice daily.
▶ **Appetite suppressant**
PO
Adults, Children 12 yrs and older. 5 mg daily, given 30 min before meals. Give only for a few weeks.

OFF-LABEL USES
Narcolepsy.

CONTRAINDICATIONS
Advanced arteriosclerosis, agitated states, glaucoma, history of drug abuse, history of hypersensitivity to sympathomimetic amines, hyperthyroidism, moderate to severe hypertension, symptomatic cardiovascular disease, within 14 days following discontinuation of an MAOI, sibutramine use.

INTERACTIONS
Drug
β-**Blockers:** May increase risk of bradycardia, heart block, and hypertension.

M

CNS stimulants, sympathomimetics: May increase the effects of methamphetamine. Contraindicated with sibutramine.

Digoxin: May increase the risk of arrhythmias with this drug.

Haloperidol, sedative-hypnotics: Decreased effects of both drugs.

Inhalation anesthetics: May cause ventricular dysrhythmias.

MAOIs: May prolong and intensify the effects of methamphetamine. Contraindicated.

Meperidine: May increase the risk of hypotension, respiratory depression, seizures, and vascular collapse.

Tricyclic antidepressants: May increase cardiovascular effects.

Herbal

Ephedra: May cause arrhythmias and hypertension.

Food

None known.

DIAGNOSTIC TEST EFFECTS

May increase plasma corticosteroid concentrations.

SIDE EFFECTS

Frequent

Irregular pulse, increased motor activity, talkativeness, nervousness, mild euphoria, insomnia.

Occasional

Headache, chills, dry mouth, GI distress, worsening depression in patients who are clinically depressed or having tachycardia, palpitations, chest pain.

SERIOUS REACTIONS

• Overdose may produce skin pallor, flushing, arrhythmias, and psychosis.
• Abrupt withdrawal following prolonged administration of high dosage may produce lethargy that can last for weeks.

• Prolonged administration to children with ADHD may produce a temporary suppression of normal weight and height patterns.
• Methamphetamine is a highly-sought street drugs. Be alert to the potential diversion for nontherapeutic use.

PRECAUTIONS & CONSIDERATIONS

Caution is warranted in patients with bipolar disorder, diabetes mellitus, cardiovascular disease, seizure disorders, insomnia, or mild hypertension. It is unknown whether methamphetamine crosses the placenta or is excreted in breast milk. Children may be more susceptible to develop abdominal pain, anorexia, decreased weight, and insomnia. Chronic methamphetamine use may inhibit growth in children. No age-related precautions have been noted in elderly patients.

Decreased appetite, dizziness, dry mouth, or pronounced nervousness may occur and should be reported to the physician. Report sore tongue, problems eating or swallowing to health care practitioners immediately. Overdose may cause skin pallor, flushing, arrhythmias and psychosis.

Administration

Do not take methamphetamine in late evening because the drug can cause insomnia. Take dose 30 min before meals when used for obesity. Do not abruptly discontinue methamphetamine in patients who have received the drug for prolonged periods.

Methazolamide
meth-ah-zole′ah-mide
(Apo-Methazolamide [CAN],
Glauctabs, Neptazane)
Do not confuse with nefazodone.

CATEGORY AND SCHEDULE
Pregnancy Risk Category: C

Classification: Carbonic
anhydrase inhibitors

MECHANISM OF ACTION
A noncompetitive inhibitor of
carbonic anhydrase that inhibits
the enzyme at the luminal border
of cells of the proximal tubule.
Increases urine volume and changes
to an alkaline pH with subsequent
decreases in the excretion of
titratable acid and ammonia.
Therapeutic Effect: Produces a
diuretic and antiglaucoma effect.

PHARMACOKINETICS
PO route onset 2-4 h, peak 6-8 h,
duration 10-18 h. Well absorbed
slowly from the GI tract. Protein
binding: 55%. Distributed into the
tissues (including CSF). Metabolized
slowly from the GI tract. Excreted
primarily in urine. Not removed by
hemodialysis. *Half-life:* 14 h.

AVAILABILITY
Tablets: 25 mg, 50 mg.

INDICATIONS AND DOSAGES
▶Glaucoma
PO
Adults, Elderly. 50-100 mg/day
2-3 times/day.

OFF-LABEL USES
Prevention of altitude sickness,
essential tremor.

CONTRAINDICATIONS
Hypersensitivity to methazolamide,
severe kidney or liver disease, failure
of adrenal glands, hypechloremic
acidosis.

INTERACTIONS
Drug
**Amphetamines, quinidine,
procainamide, methenamine,
phenobarbital, salicylates (high
doses):** May increase the excretion
of these drugs.
**Aspirin and other salicylates (high
doses):** May increase the risk for
anorexia, tachypnea, lethargy, coma,
and death have been reported when
receiving high-dose aspirin and
methazolamide concomitantly.
**Corticosteroids (systemic use),
diuretics:** May cause hypokalemia.
Lithium: May increase the excretion
of lithium.
Memantine: May decrease the
clearance of memantine.
Steroids: May increase the risk of
hypokalemia.
Topiramate: May increase the risk
of nephrolithiasis.
Herbal
None known.
Food
None known.

DIAGNOSTIC TEST EFFECTS
Monitor complete blood count,
for blood dyscrasias. May cause
hypokalemic.

SIDE EFFECTS
Occasional
Paresthesias, hearing dysfunction
or tinnitus, fatigue, malaise, loss of
appetite, taste alteration, nausea,
vomiting, diarrhea, polyuria,
drowsiness, confusion, hypokalemia.
Rare
Metabolic acidosis, electrolyte
imbalance, transient myopia,

M

urticaria, melena, hematuria, glycosuria, hepatic insufficiency, flaccid paralysis, photosensitivity, convulsions, and rarely crystalluria, renal calculi.

SERIOUS REACTIONS
• Malaise and complaints of tiredness and myalgia are signs of excessive dosing and acidosis in elderly patients.
• Stevens-Johnson syndrome, toxic epidermal necrolysis, fulminant hepatic necrosis, agranulocytosis, aplastic anemia, and other blood dyscrasias have been reported and have caused fatalities.
• Nephrolithiasis.

PRECAUTIONS & CONSIDERATIONS
Caution should be used in patients with allergies to sulfonamides, sulfonylureas, carbonic anhydrase inhibitors, thiazides, and loop diuretics (except ethacrynic acid) because of a risk of cross-reaction. Anorexia, tachypnea, lethargy, coma, and death have been reported with concomitant use of high-dose aspirin and methazolamide. Caution is also warranted with respiratory acidosis, diabetes mellitus, or mental impairment. It is unknown whether methazolamide crosses the placenta and is excreted in breast milk. Safety and efficacy of this drug have not been established in children. Elderly patients may be at an increased risk for developing hypokalemia.

Hypokalemia may result in cardiac arrhythmias, changes in mental status and muscle strength, muscle cramps, and tremor. In patients with cirrhosis or serious hepatic insufficiency, hepatic coma may be precipitated. Potassium should be assessed before and during treatment. Frequency and volume of urination are expected to increase.

Administration
Take methazolamide with food to avoid GI upset. Maintain adequate hydration.

Methenamine
(Dehydral [CAN], Hiprex, Hip-Rex [CAN], Urasal [CAN], Urex)

CATEGORY AND SCHEDULE
Pregnancy Risk Category: C

Classification: Anti-infectives, urinary

MECHANISM OF ACTION
A hippuric acid salt that hydrolyzes to formaldehyde and ammonia in acidic urine. *Therapeutic Effect:* Formaldehyde has antibacterial action. Bacteriocidal.

PHARMACOKINETICS
Readily absorbed from the GI tract. Partially metabolized by hydrolysis (unless protected by enteric coating) and partially by the liver. Primarily excreted in urine. *Half-life:* 3-6 h.

AVAILABILITY
Tablets, as Hippurate: 1 g (Urex, Hiprex).

INDICATIONS AND DOSAGES
▸ **Suppressive therapy for frequently recurring urinary tract infection (UTI)**
PO
Adults, Elderly. 1 g 2 times/day (as hippurate).
Children 6-12 yrs. 25-50 mg/kg/day q12h (as hippurate).

OFF-LABEL USES
Hyperhidrosis.

CONTRAINDICATIONS
Moderate to severe renal impairment, hepatic impairment (hippurate salt),

tartrazine sensitivity (Hiprex contains tartrazine), hypersensitivity to methenamine or any of its components.

INTERACTIONS
Drug
Acetazolamide, antacids, methazolamide, sodium bicarbonate: May decrease effect secondary to alkalinization of urine.
Dichlorphenamide: May inhibit the action of methenamine to alkalinize the urine.
Sulfonamides: May increase the risk of crystalluria. Avoid.
Herbal
None known.
Food
None known.

DIAGNOSTIC TEST EFFECTS
Formaldehyde, the active form of methenamine, interferes with fluorometric procedures for the determination of urinary catecholamines and vanillylmandelic acid (VMA), causing false high results.

SIDE EFFECTS
Occasional
Rash, nausea, dyspepsia, difficulty urinating.
Rare
Bladder irritation, increased liver enzymes.

SERIOUS REACTIONS
• Crystalluria can occur when there is low urinary output.

PRECAUTIONS & CONSIDERATIONS
Caution should be used in patients with hepatic impairment. Be aware that Hiprex contains tartrazine. It is unknown whether methenamine crosses the placenta and is excreted in breast milk; caution is warranted in lactation. No age-related precautions have been noted in children older than 6 yrs of age. Avoid using in elderly patients with age-related renal impairment. Antacids should be avoided. Sun and ultraviolet light should be avoided. If it is not avoidable, sunscreens and protective clothing should be worn. Urine pH should be monitored.
Administration
Take methenamine with food or milk to reduce GI upset. Usually taken with cranberry juice or ascorbic acid to acidify urine. Maintain adequate hydration. Not to be used as primary treatment of UTI.

Methimazole
meth-im′a-zole
(Tapazole)

M

CATEGORY AND SCHEDULE
Pregnancy Risk Category: D

Classification: Thyroid hormone antagonist

MECHANISM OF ACTION
A thiomidazole derivative that inhibits synthesis of thyroid hormone by interfering with the incorporation of iodine into tyrosyl residues. *Therapeutic Effect:* Effectively treats hyperthyroidism by decreasing thyroid hormone levels.

PHARMACOKINETICS
High bioavailability in oral administration (80%-95%). Excreted in breast milk. High transplacental passage. 0% protein bonding. Rapidly metabolized; < 10% eliminated in urine. *Half-life:* 6-13 h.

AVAILABILITY
Tablets: 5 mg, 10 mg.

INDICATIONS AND DOSAGES
▶ **Hyperthyroidism**
PO
Adults, Elderly. Initially, 15-60 mg/day in 3 divided doses. Maintenance: 5-15 mg/day in 3 divided doses. Generally avoid doses > 40 mg/day because of increased risk of blood dyscrasias.
Children. Initially, 0.4 mg/kg/day in 3 divided doses. Maintenance: ½ the initial dose, or alternately: 0.5-0.7 mg/kg/day in 3 divided doses initially and ½ initial dose for maintenance.

CONTRAINDICATIONS
Hypersensitivity, to the drug, breast-feeding agranulocytosis.

INTERACTIONS
Drug
Anticholinergics and sympathomimetics: May increase cardiovascular side effects in uncontrolled patients.
Amiodarone, iodinated glycerol, iodine, potassium iodide: May decrease response to methimazole.
β-Blockers: May increase effect and toxicity as patient becomes euthyroid.
Central nervous system (CNS) depressants: May have increased response to these drugs in uncontrolled patients.
Digoxin: May increase the blood concentration of digoxin as patient becomes euthyroid.
I^{131}: May decrease thyroid uptake of I^{131}.
Oral anticoagulants: May decrease the effects of oral anticoagulants.
Theophylline: May alter theophylline clearance in hyperthyroid or hypothyroid patients.
Vasoconstrictors: Uncontrolled hypothyroid patients are at higher risk when using methimazole.

Herbal
None known.
Food
None known.

DIAGNOSTIC TEST EFFECTS
May increase LDH, serum alkaline phosphatase, bilirubin, AST (SGOT), and ALT (SGPT) levels and prothrombin time. May decrease prothrombin level and WBC count.

SIDE EFFECTS
Frequent (4%-5%)
Fever, rash, pruritus.
Occasional (1%-3%)
Dizziness, loss of taste, nausea, vomiting, stomach pain, peripheral neuropathy or numbness in fingers, toes, face.
Rare (< 1%)
Swollen lymph nodes or salivary glands.

SERIOUS REACTIONS
• Agranulocytosis as long as 4 mo after therapy, pancytopenia, and hepatitis have occurred.

PRECAUTIONS & CONSIDERATIONS
Caution is warranted in patients with concurrent use of other agranulocytosis-inducing drugs, impaired hepatic function, and in persons older than 40 yrs. Methimazole is excreted in breast milk should be avoided during breastfeeding. Methimazole is not the agent of choice in pregnancy because it crosses the placenta. Restrict the consumption of iodine products and seafood. Uncontrolled hyperthyroid patients should not engage in any surgical procedures until blood levels are established.

Notify the physician of illness, unusual bleeding or bruising, burning, fever, infection, jaundice, or rash. Weight, pulse, CBC, prothrombin time, thyroid function, and serum hepatic enzymes should be monitored. Overdose is evidenced by nausea, vomiting, epigastric distress, headache, fever, arthralgia, pruritis, edema, pancytopenia, agranulocytosis, exfoliative dermatitis, hepatitis, neuropathies, CNS stimulation, or depression. Drug may cause drowsiness; driving or performing tasks requiring mental alertness should be avoided until blood levels are established and control attained.

Storage

Store at room temperature in a light-resistant container.

Administration

Take with food if GI symptoms occur. Space doses evenly around the clock.

Methocarbamol

meth-oh-kar′ba-mole
(Carbacot, Robaxin)

CATEGORY AND SCHEDULE

Pregnancy Risk Category: C

Classification: Skeletal muscle relaxant

MECHANISM OF ACTION

A carbamate derivative of guaifenesin that causes skeletal muscle relaxation by general central nervous system (CNS) depression. *Therapeutic Effect:* Relieves muscle spasticity.

PHARMACOKINETICS

Rapidly and almost completely absorbed from the GI tract. Protein binding: 46%-50%. Metabolized in liver by dealkylation and hydroxylation. Primarily excreted in urine as metabolites. *Half-life:* 1-2 h.

AVAILABILITY

Injection: 100 mg/mL (Robaxin).
Tablets: 325 mg, 500 mg (Carbacot, Robaxin), 750 mg (Carbacot).

INDICATIONS AND DOSAGES

▸ **Musculoskeletal spasm**

IM/IV

Adults, Children 16 yrs and older. 1 g q8h for no more than 3 consecutive days. May repeat course of therapy after a drug-free interval of 48 h.

PO

Adults, Children 16 yrs and older. 1.5 g 4 times/day for 2-3 days (up to 8 g/day may be given in severe conditions). Decrease to 4 g/day in 3-6 divided doses.

Elderly. Initially, 500 mg 4 times a day. May gradually increase dosage.

▸ **Tetanus spasm**

IV, FOLLOWED BY NASOGAS-TRIC ADMINISTRATION OF ORAL TABLETS

Adults. 1-3 g q6h until oral dosing is possible. Injection should be used no more than 3 consecutive days. Oral dosage in tetanus can require up to 24 g/day in divided doses q6h.

Children. 15 mg/kg/dose or 500 mg/m^2/dose q6h as needed. Maximum: 1.8 g/m^2/day for 3 days only.

CONTRAINDICATIONS

Hypersensitivity to methocarbamol or any component of the formulation, renal impairment (injection formulation).

INTERACTIONS

Drug

CNS depressants, including alcohol, narcotics, sedative-hypnotics: May potentiate effects when used with other CNS depressants, including alcohol.

Herbal

Gotu kola, kava kava, St. John's wort: May increase CNS depression.

Food
None known.

DIAGNOSTIC TEST EFFECTS
None known.

SIDE EFFECTS
Frequent
Transient drowsiness, weakness, dizziness, lightheadedness, nausea, vomiting.
Occasional
Headache, constipation, anorexia, hypotension, confusion, blurred vision, vertigo, facial flushing, rash.
Rare
Paradoxical CNS excitement and restlessness, slurred speech, tremor, dry mouth, diarrhea, nocturia, impotence, bradycardia, hypotension, syncope.

SERIOUS REACTIONS
• Anaphylactoid reactions, leukopenia, and seizures (IV form) have been reported.
• Methocarbamol overdosage results in cardiac arrhythmias, nausea, vomiting, drowsiness, and coma.

PRECAUTIONS & CONSIDERATIONS
Caution is necessary in patients with oral formulation with renal or hepatic impairment. Due to polyethylene glycol 3000, NF in injection, do not use injection in renal impairment. Use injectable formulation cautiously in patients with a history of seizures or hepatic impairment. It is unknown whether methocarbamol crosses the placenta or is distributed in breast milk. Be aware that the safety and efficacy of methocarbamol have not been established in children younger than 16 yrs. In elderly patients, there is an increased risk of CNS toxicity, manifested as confusion, hallucinations, mental depression, and sedation.

Age-related renal impairment may necessitate a decreased dosage in elderly patients. Symptoms of overdosage indicated as arrhythmia, nausea, vomiting, drowsiness, and coma should be reported immediately.
Administration
Maximum of 5 mL can be administered into each gluteal region with IM injection.
! Take care with IV use because pain and sloughing may occur.

IV injection may be administered undiluted as a direct IV bolus at a maximum rate of 3 mL/min. Solution is hypertonic. May dilute 1 g of methocarbamol to no more than 250 mL with 0.9% NaCl or dextrose 5% injection. Do not use for more than 3 consecutive days. Except in tetanus, total parenteral dosage will not exceed 3 vials (30 mL) a day by any route. Administer IV while in recumbent position. Maintain position for 15-30 min following infusion.

Give oral formulation without regard to meals. Tablets may be crushed and mixed with food or liquid if needed. May crush tablets and give by nasogastric (NG) tube if necessary (often necessary in tetanus treatment).

Methotrexate sodium
meth-oh-trex´-ate soe´-dee-um
(Apo-Methotrexate[CAN], Ledertrexate[AUS], Methoblastin[AUS], Rheumatrex, Trexall)
Do not confuse Trexall with Trexan.

CATEGORY AND SCHEDULE
Pregnancy Risk Category: D (X for patients with psoriasis or rheumatoid arthritis)

Classification: Folic acid antagonist, antineoplastic

MECHANISM OF ACTION

An antimetabolite that competes with enzymes necessary to reduce folic acid to tetrahydrofolic acid, a component essential to DNA, RNA, and protein synthesis. This action inhibits DNA, RNA, and protein synthesis. *Therapeutic Effect:* Causes death of cancer cells.

PHARMACOKINETICS

Variably absorbed from the GI tract. Completely absorbed after IM administration. Protein binding: 50%-60%. Widely distributed. Metabolized intracellularly in the liver. Excreted primarily in urine. Removed by hemodialysis but not by peritoneal dialysis. *Half-life:* 8-12 h (large doses, 8–15 h).

AVAILABILITY

Tablets: 2.5 mg, 5 mg, 7.5 mg, 10 mg, 15 mg.
Injection Solution: 25 mg/mL.
Injection, lyophilized Powder: 1g.

INDICATIONS AND DOSAGES

▸ **Head and neck cancer**
PO, IV, IM
Adults, Elderly. 25-50 mg/m^2 once weekly.
▸ **Choriocarcinoma, chorioadenoma destruens, hydatidiform mole, trophoblastic neoplasms**
PO, IM
Adults, Elderly. 15-30 mg/day for 5 days; repeat 3-5 times with 1-2 wks between courses.
▸ **Breast cancer**
IV
Adults, Elderly. 30-60 mg/m^2 days 1 and 8 q3-4wk.
▸ **ALL**
PO, IV, IM
Adults, Elderly. Induction: 3.3 mg/m^2/day in combination with other chemotherapeutic agents. Maintenance: 30 mg/m^2/wk PO or IM in divided doses or 2.5 mg/kg IV every 14 days.
▸ **Burkitt's lymphoma**
PO
Adults. 10-25 mg/day for 4-8 days; repeat with 7- to 10-day rest between courses.
▸ **Lymphosarcoma**
PO
Adults, Elderly. 0.625-2.5 mg/kg/day.
▸ **Mycosis fungoides**
PO
Adults, Elderly. 5-50 mg once weekly or 15-37.5 mg twice weekly.
▸ **Rheumatoid arthritis**
PO
Adults, Elderly. 7.5 mg once a wk or 2.5 mg q12h for 3 doses once a wk. Maximum: 20 mg/wk.
▸ **Juvenile rheumatoid arthritis**
PO, IM, SC
Children. 5-15 mg/m^2/wk as a single dose or in 3 divided doses given q12h.
▸ **Psoriasis**
PO
Adults, Elderly. 10-25 mg once a wk or 2.5-5 mg q12h for 3 doses once a wk.
IM
Adults, Elderly. 10-25 mg once a wk.
▸ **Antineoplastic dosage for children**
PO, IM
Children. 7.5-30 mg/m^2/wk or q2wk.
▸ **Dosage in renal impairment**
Creatinine clearance 61-80 mL/min. Reduce dose by 25%.
Creatinine clearance 51-60 mL/min. Reduce dose by 33%.
Creatinine clearance 10-50 mL/min. Reduce dose by 50%-70%.

CONTRAINDICATIONS

Contraindicated in nursing mothers and those with hypersensitivity to the drug. In patients with psoriasis or rheumatoid arthritis also contraindicated if pregnant, alcoholic, or have alcoholic liver

M

disease, chronic liver disease, immunodeficiency syndromes, or preexisting blood dyscrasias.

INTERACTIONS
Drug
Amoxicillin, tetracycline, doxycycline: Suspected increase in methotrexate toxicity.
Aspirin, alcohol, NSAIDs: Increased toxicity.
Cyclosporine: Increased levels of both, increased toxicity.
NSAIDs, high-dose IV methotrexate: Possible fatal interactions.
Sulfonamides, co-trimoxazole, trimethoprim: Increased hematologic toxicity.

ⓘ IV INCOMPATIBILITIES
Droperidol, idarubicin, propofol

SIDE EFFECTS
Frequent
Nausea, vomiting, stomatitis; burning and erythema at psoriatic site (in patients with psoriasis).
Occasional
Diarrhea, rash, dermatitis, pruritus, alopecia, dizziness, anorexia, malaise, headache, drowsiness, blurred vision.

SERIOUS REACTIONS
• GI toxicity may produce gingivitis, glossitis, pharyngitis, stomatitis, enteritis, and hematemesis.
• Hepatotoxicity is more likely to occur with frequent small doses than with large intermittent doses.
• Pulmonary toxicity may be characterized by interstitial pneumonitis.
• Hematologic toxicity, which may develop rapidly from marked myelosuppression, may be manifested as leukopenia, thrombocytopenia, anemia, and hemorrhage.
• Dermatologic toxicity may produce a rash, pruritus, urticaria, pigmentation, photosensitivity, petechiae, ecchymosis, and pustules.
• Severe nephrotoxicity may produce azotemia, hematuria, and renal failure.

PRECAUTIONS & CONSIDERATIONS
Use with caution in patients with renal or hepatic impairment, ascites, pleural effusions, debility, peptic ulcer disease, ulcerative colitis, active infection. Ensure adequate hydration and monitoring of renal function. Monitor liver function tests; periodic liver biopsies recommended for patients with psoriasis receiving long-term treatment.
Storage
Store tablets and injectable at room temperature. Injection solution diluted for administration in D5W or NS is stable for up to 24 h at room temperature.
Administration
Formulations containing preservatives must not be used for intrathecal or high-dose therapy. May be administered IV as slow push, short bolus infusion or 24- to 42-h continuous infusion.
! For oral use, always check dosage against indication for use. Dosages for ambulatory conditions, such as rheumatoid arthritis, are usually once weekly and do not exceed 20-30 mg/wk maximum. Medication errors that occur can be fatal or cause significant morbidity.

Methoxsalen

meth-ox′a-len
(8-MOP, Oxsoralen, Oxsoralen-Ultra, Psoralen, Ultramop [CAN], Uvadex)
Do not confuse methoxsalen with methsuximide or methotrexate or Psoralen with Psorcon, Uvadex with Urotraxal, Ultramop with Ultram.

CATEGORY AND SCHEDULE

Pregnancy Risk Category: C
(8-MOP, Oxsoralen-Ultra, Psoralen)
Pregnancy Risk Category: D
(Uvadex)

Classification: Photosensitizers, psoralens

MECHANISM OF ACTION

A member of the family of psoralens that induces an augmented sunburn reaction followed by hyperpigmentation in the presence of long-wave ultraviolet radiation. Bonds covalently to pyrimidine bases in DNA, inhibits the synthesis of DNA, and suppresses cell division. The augmented sunburn reaction involves excitation of the methoxsalen molecule by radiation in the long-wave ultraviolet light (UVA), resulting in transference of energy to the methoxsalen molecule, producing an excited state or "triplet electronic state." The molecule, in this "triplet state," then reacts with cutaneous DNA. ***Therapeutic Effect:*** Results in symptomatic control of severe, recalcitrant disabling psoriasis, repigmentation of idiopathic vitiligo, palliative treatment of skin manifestations of cutaneous T-cell lymphoma (CTCL), repigmentation of idiopathic vitiligo, and palliative treatment of skin manifestations of CTCL.

PHARMACOKINETICS

Absorption varies. Food increases peak serum levels. Reversibly bound to albumin. Metabolized rapidly in the liver. Excreted in the urine.
Half-life: 1.5-2.1 h, depending on form.

AVAILABILITY

Capsule: 10 mg (8-MOP).
Gelcap: 10 mg (Oxsoralen-Ultra).
Lotion: 1% (Oxsoralen).
Extracorporeal Solution: 20 mcg/mL (Uvadex).

INDICATIONS AND DOSAGES
▶ **Psoriasis**
PO
Adults, Elderly. 10-70 mg given 1.5-2 h before exposure to UVA light, repeated 2-3 times/wk. Give at least 48 h apart. Dosage is based on patient's body weight and skin type: < 30 kg, 10 mg; 30-50 kg, 20 mg; 51-65 kg, 30 mg; 66-80 kg, 40 mg; 81-90 kg, 50 mg; 91-115 kg, 60 mg; more than 115 kg, 70 mg.
▶ **Vitiligo**
PO
Adults, Elderly, Children older than 12 yrs. 20 mg 2-4 h before exposure to UVA light, 2-3 times/wk. Give at least 48 h apart.
▶ **Topical**
Adults, Elderly, Children older than 12 yrs. Apply 1-2 h. before exposure to UVA light, no more than once weekly, for 6-9 mo.
▶ **Continuous T-cell lymphoma (CTCL)**
EXTRACORPOREAL (WITH UVAR PHOTOPHERESIS SYSTEM ONLY)
Adults, Elderly. Inject 200 mcg into the photoactivation bag during the collection cycle using the UVAR photopheresis system, 2 consecutive days every 4 wks, for a minimum of 7 treatment cycles (6 mo).

M

OFF-LABEL USES

Dermographism, eczema, hypereosinophilic syndrome, hypopigmented sarcoidosis, ichthyosis linearis circumflexa, lymphomatoid papulosis, mycosis fungoides, palmoplantar pustulosis, pruritus, scleromyxedema, systemic sclerosis.

DIAGNOSTIC TEST EFFECTS

Hematocrit, CBC with differential, plateleet, serum bilirubin, SGOT, AST, LDH, uric acid, BUN, SCr, and ANA.

CONTRAINDICATIONS

Cataract, invasive squamous cell cancer, aphakia, melanoma, pregnancy (Uvadex), diseases associated with photosensitivity, hypersensitivity to methoxsalen (psoralens) or any component of the formulation.
Caution
Known photosensitizers (anthralin, coal tar and derivatives, fluoroquinolones, griseofulvin, halogenated salicylanilides, nalidixic acid, organic staining dyes, phenothiazines, sulfonamides, tetracyclines, thiazide diuretics).

INTERACTIONS

Drug
Phenytoin, fosphenytoin: May decrease the effectiveness of methoxsalen.
Photosensitizing drugs: May increase risk of untoward photoreaction.
Herbal
None known.
Food
Figs, parsley, parsnip, mustard, carrot, celery: May increase response to UVA and sun exposure.

SIDE EFFECTS

Occasional
Nausea, pruritus, edema, hypotension, nervousness, vertigo, depression, dizziness, headache, malaise, painful blistering, burning, rash, urticaria, loss of muscle coordination, leg cramps.

SERIOUS REACTIONS

• Hypersensitivity reaction, such as nausea and severe burns, may occur.

PRECAUTIONS & CONSIDERATIONS

Caution should be used in patients with renal disease and with other agents that may cause photosensitivity. Methoxsalen crosses the placenta, but it is unknown whether it is excreted in breast milk. Safety and efficacy have not been determined in children younger than 12 yrs. No age-related precautions in elderly patients have been noted. Hematocrit, white blood cell count differential, platelets, serum bilirubin, SGOT, alkaline phosphatase, LDH, uric acid, BUN, serum creatinine, ANA, and urinalysis should be monitored at 6 mo, 1 yr, and yearly thereafter. Ophthalmologic evaluation should be given at 6 mo, 1 yr, and yearly thereafter. Histopathologic exams should be performed for any skin lesion suspected of being malignant at any time during therapy. Risk of squamous cell carcinoma among PUVA-treated patients is increased; also with ionizing radiation and arsenic exposures.

Burning or blistering or intractable pruritus must be reported. Direct and indirect sunlight should be avoided for 8 h after oral and 12-48 h after topical therapy. If sunlight cannot be avoided, protective clothing and/or sunscreens should be worn. Sunbathing should be avoided for at least 24 h before therapy or 48 h after PUVA therapy.
Administration
Take oral methoxsalen with food or milk.

Hands and fingers of the person applying the lotion should be protected to prevent possible photosensitization and burns. Administer in conjunction with scheduled controlled doses of UVA radiation.

Methscopolamine Bromide
meth-scoe-pol-a-meen bro-myde
(Pamine, Pamine Forte)

CATEGORY AND SCHEDULE
Pregnancy Risk Category: C

Classification: Anticholinergics, gastrointestinals

MECHANISM OF ACTION
A peripheral anticholinergic agent that has limited ability to cross the blood-brain barrier and provides a peripheral blockade of muscarinic receptors. *Therapeutic Effect:* Reduces the volume and the total acid content of gastric secretions, inhibits salivation, and reduces GII motility.

PHARMACOKINETICS
Poorly and unreliably absorbed from the GI tract. Limited ability to cross the blood-brain barrier. Excreted primarily in the urine and the bile. The effects of methscopolamine appear to occur within 1 h and last for 4-6 h. Primarily excreted in urine. *Half-life:* Unknown.

AVAILABILITY
Tablets: 2.5 mg (Pamine), 5 mg (Pamine Forte).

INDICATIONS AND DOSAGES
▸ **Peptic ulcer**
Adults, Elderly. Initially, 2.5 mg 30 min before meals and 2.5-5 mg at bedtime. Starting dose 12.5 mg/day is most effective. May increase dose to 5 mg every 12 h. Can start with 20 mg/day in 5-mg doses, each half an hour before meals and at bedtime in severe GI distress.

OFF-LABEL USES
Gastrointestinal spasm.

CONTRAINDICATIONS
Reflux esophagitis, glaucoma, obstructed uropathy, obstructed disease of the GI tract (pyloroduodenal stenosis), paralytic ileus, intestinal atony of elderly or debilitated individuals, unstable cardiovascular status in acute hemorrhage, severe ulcerative colitis, toxic megacolon, complicated ulcerative colitis, myasthenia gravis, hypersensitivity to methscopolamine, any component of the formulation, or related drugs.

INTERACTIONS
Drug
Antacids: May decrease absorption of methscopolamine.
Antipsychotic agents: May produce additive anticholinergic effects.
Tricyclic antidepressants, anticholinergics: May produce additive anticholinergic effects.
Herbal
None known.
Food
None known.

DIAGNOSTIC TEST EFFECTS
None known.

SIDE EFFECTS
Occasional
Dry mouth, throat, and nose, urinary hesitancy and/or retention, constipation, tachycardia, palpitations, headache, insomnia, dry skin, urticaria, weakness.

M

SERIOUS REACTIONS
• Overdosage may vary from central nervous system (CNS) depression, including sedation, apnea, hypotension, cardiovascular collapse, or death to severe paradoxical reaction (such as hallucinations, tremor, and seizures).

PRECAUTIONS & CONSIDERATIONS
Caution is necessary in patients with diarrhea because it may be an early symptom of incomplete intestinal obstruction. Large doses should be used cautiously because methscopolamine may suppress intestinal motility, causing paralytic ileus and precipitate, or aggravate toxic megacolon. Caution is also warranted in patients with autonomic neuropathy, benign prostatic hyperplasia, hyperthyroidism, ulcerative colitis, hepatic or renal dysfunction, arrhythmias, cardiovascular disease, congestive heart failure, hypertension, or in elderly patients. Elderly patients are at an increased risk of developing confusion, dizziness, hyperexcitability, hypotension, and sedation. It is unknown whether methscopolamine crosses the placenta or is excreted in breast milk; caution warranted in lactation. Safety and efficacy have not been established in children. Peptic ulcers should be monitored while under treatment of methscopolamine by upper GI contrast radiology or endoscopy to ensure healing.

Expected responses to the drug include dizziness, drowsiness, and dry mouth. Tasks that require mental alertness or motor skills should be avoided. Blood in stool should be reported to the physician. Overdose includes CNS disturbances, circulatory changes, respiratory failure, paralysis, and coma. Any of these responses should be immediately reported.

Administration
Take methscopolamine 30 min before food and at bedtime.

Methsuximide
meth-sux′i-mide
(Celontin)
Do not confuse with methoxsalen.

CATEGORY AND SCHEDULE
Pregnancy Risk Category: C

Classification: Anticonvulsants, Succinimides

MECHANISM OF ACTION
A succinimide anticonvulsant agent that increases the seizure threshold, suppresses paroxysmal spike-and-wave pattern in absence seizures and depresses nerve transmission in the motor cortex. *Therapeutic Effect:* Controls absence (petit mal) seizures.

PHARMACOKINETICS
Rapidly metabolized in liver to active metabolite, *N*-desmethylmethsuximide. Excreted primarily in urine. Unknown whether it is removed by hemodialysis. *Half-life:* 1.4 h.

AVAILABILITY
Capsules: 150 mg, 300 mg (Celontin).

INDICATIONS AND DOSAGES
▸ **Absence seizures**
PO
Adults, Elderly. Initially, 300 mg/day for the first week. Increase dosage by 300 mg/day at weekly intervals until response is attained. Maintenance: 1200 mg/day divided 2-4 times/day. Do not exceed 1000 mg/day in children 12-15 yrs, 1200 mg/day in patients older than 15 yrs.

Children. Initially, 10-15 mg/kg/day 3-4 times/day. Increase at weekly intervals. Maximum: 30 mg/kg/day.

OFF-LABEL USES
Partial complex (psychomotor) seizures.

CONTRAINDICATIONS
Hypersensitivity to succinimides or any component of the formulation.

INTERACTIONS
Drug
Alcohol, benzodiazepines, barbiturates, and other CNS depressants: May cause increased sedative effects.
Anticonvulsants: May increase plasma concentrations of other anticonvulsants.
Cyclosporine: May decrease cyclosporine blood levels by increasing its metabolism.
Haloperidol: May cause change in frequency and pattern of seizures.
Phenothiazines, thioxanthenes, barbiturates: May cause decreased effects of these drugs.
Herbal
Evening primrose oil: May decrease the effects of methsuximide.
Ginkgo biloba: May decrease the effects of methsuximide.
Food
None known.

DIAGNOSTIC TEST EFFECTS
None known.

SIDE EFFECTS
Frequent
Drowsiness, dizziness, nausea, vomiting.
Occasional
Visual abnormalities, such as spots before eyes, difficulty focusing, blurred vision, dry mouth or pharynx, tongue irritation, nervousness, insomnia, headache, constipation or diarrhea, rash, weight loss, proteinuria, edema.
Rare
Systemic lupus-like syndrome.

SERIOUS REACTIONS
• Toxic reactions appear as blood dyscrasias, including aplastic anemia, agranulocytosis, thrombocytopenia, leukopenia, leukocytosis, eosinophilia.
• Dermatologic effects, such as rash, urticaria, pruritus, photosensitivity, Stevens-Johnson syndrome.
• Abrupt withdrawal may precipitate status epilepticus.

PRECAUTIONS & CONSIDERATIONS
Caution is warranted with impaired cardiac, liver, or renal function. Caution should be used in any seizure type. Methsuximide is not first-line therapy. It is unknown if methsuximide crosses the placenta and is distributed in breast milk. Behavioral changes are more likely to occur in children taking methsuximide. Elderly patients are more susceptible to agitation, atrioventricular (AV) block, bradycardia, and confusion. Blood tests should be repeated frequently during first 3 mo of therapy and at monthly intervals thereafter for 2-3 yrs. Assess patients for stress tolerance to avoid changes in seizure frequency and frequency of seizure control adjustments being needed.

Drowsiness usually disappears during therapy. Tasks that require mental alertness and motor skills should be avoided.
Storage
Keep at controlled room temperature. Heat of 104° F or higher will melt the drug.
Administration
Take with meals to reduce risk of GI distress. Be aware when replacement

M

by another anticonvulsant is necessary, plan to decrease methsuximide gradually as therapy begins with a low replacement dose. Abrupt withdrawal of the drug may precipitate absence status. Methsuximide must be used in combination with other anticonvulsants in patients with both absence and tonic-clonic seizures.

Methyclothiazide
meth-i-kloe-thye'ah-zide
(Aquatensen, Enduron)

CATEGORY AND SCHEDULE
Pregnancy Risk Category: B
(D if used in pregnancy-induced hypertension)

Classification: Diuretics, thiazide and derivatives

MECHANISM OF ACTION
A sulfonamide derivative that acts as a thiazide diuretic and antihypertensive. As a diuretic it blocks the reabsorption of water, sodium, and potassium at cortical diluting segment of distal tubule. As an antihypertensive it reduces plasma and extracellular fluid volume and decreases peripheral vascular resistance (PVR) by direct effect on blood vessels. *Therapeutic Effect:* Promotes diuresis, reduces BP.

PHARMACOKINETICS
Variably absorbed from the GI tract. Excreted unchanged primarily in urine. Not removed by hemodialysis. *Half-life:* 24 h.

AVAILABILITY
Tablets: 2.5 mg, 5 mg (Aquatensen, Enduron).

INDICATIONS AND DOSAGES
▶ **Edema**
PO
Adults. 2.5-10 mg/day; may also give dose every other day or 3-5 times/wk to control symptoms.
▶ **Hypertension**
PO
Adults. 2.5-5 mg/day.

OFF-LABEL USES
Treatment of diabetes insipidus, prevention of calcium-containing renal stones.

CONTRAINDICATIONS
Anuria, history of hypersensitivity to sulfonamides or thiazide diuretics.

INTERACTIONS
Drug
ACE inhibitors: May increase the risk of postural hypotension.
β-Blockers: May increase hyperglycemic effects in patients with type 2 diabetes mellitus.
Cylosporine, other thiazides: May increase the risk of gout or renal toxicity.
Cholestyramine, colestipol: May decrease the absorption and effects of methyclothiazide.
Digoxin: May increase the risk of toxicity of digoxin caused by hypokalemia.
Lithium: May increase the risk of toxicity of lithium.
Neuromuscular blocking agents: May prolong neuromuscular blockade.
NSAIDs: May decrease the effects of methychlothiazide.
Herbal
Dong quai, St. John's wort: May cause photosensitization.
Ephedra, ginseng, yohimbine: May decrease the effects of methyclothiazide.
Garlic: May increase antihypertensive effect.

Ginkgo biloba: May increase BP.
Gossypol: May increase the risk of hypokalemia.
Licorice: May increase the risk of hypokalemia and/or reduce effectiveness of methychlorthiazide.
Ma Huang: May decrease hypotensive effect of methyclothiazide.
Food
None known.

DIAGNOSTIC TEST EFFECTS

May increase blood glucose levels, serum cholesterol, LDL, bilirubin, calcium, creatinine, uric acid, and triglyceride levels. May decrease urinary calcium, and serum magnesium, potassium, and sodium levels.

SIDE EFFECTS

Expected
Increase in urinary frequency and volume.
Frequent
Potassium depletion.
Occasional
Postural hypotension, headache, GI disturbances, photosensitivity reaction, anorexia.

SERIOUS REACTIONS

• Vigorous diuresis may lead to profound water loss and electrolyte depletion, leading to hypokalemia, hyponatremia, and dehydration.
• Acute hypotensive episodes may occur.
• Hyperglycemia may be noted during prolonged therapy.
• GI upset, pancreatitis, dizziness, paresthesias, headache, blood dyscrasias, pulmonary edema, allergic pneumonitis, and dermatologic reactions occur rarely.
• Overdosage can lead to lethargy and coma without changes in electrolytes or hydration.

PRECAUTIONS & CONSIDERATIONS

Caution is necessary with debilitated and elderly persons. Caution is warranted with diabetes mellitus, impaired liver function, severe renal disease, electrolyte disturbances, history of gout, and thyroid disorders. Methyclothiazide crosses the placenta, and a small amount is distributed in breast milk. No age-related precautions have been noted in children, except that jaundiced infants may be at risk for hyperbilirubinemia. Be aware that elderly patients may be more sensitive to the drug's electrolyte and hypotensive effects. In elderly patients, age-related renal impairment may require dosage adjustment.

Frequency and volume of urination are expected to increase. Be aware that methyclothiazide may aggravate digitalis toxicity. Be aware that sensitivity reactions may occur with or without a history of allergy or asthma. Skin should be protected from sunlight.

Hypokalemia may result in change in mental status, muscle cramps, nausea, tachycardia, tremor, vomiting, and weakness. Hyponatremia may result in clammy and cold skin, confusion, and thirst. Be especially alert for potassium depletion in persons taking digoxin, such as cardiac arrhythmias. Foods high in potassium, such as apricots, bananas, legumes, meat, orange juice, white and sweet potatoes, raisins, and whole grains, such as cereals, should be eaten during treatment.

Administration
May give methyclothiazide with food or milk if GI upset occurs, preferably with breakfast to help prevent nocturia. Tablets may be crushed for patients with difficulty swallowing.

M

Methylcellulose
meth-ill-cell'you-los
(Citrucel, Cologel)
Do not confuse Citrucel with Citracal

CATEGORY AND SCHEDULE
Pregnancy Risk Category: C
OTC

Classification: Laxatives, bulk-forming

MECHANISM OF ACTION
A bulk-forming laxative that dissolves and expands in water. *Therapeutic Effect:* Provides increased bulk and moisture content in stool, increasing peristalsis and bowel motility.

PHARMACOKINETICS

Route	Onset	Peak	Duration
PO	12-24 h	NA	NA

Acts in small and large intestines. Full effect may not be evident for 2-3 days.

AVAILABILITY
Powder for oral solution or suspension (citrucel)
Caplets. 500 mg.
Soft chews: 500 mg per chew.

INDICATIONS AND DOSAGES
▶ **Constipation**
PO (POWDER)
Adults, Elderly. 1 tbsp (15 mL) in 8 oz water 1-3 times a day.
Children 6-12 yrs. 1 tsp (5 mL) in 4 oz water 3-4 times a day.
PO (CAPLETS)
Adults. 2 caplets up to 6 times/day.
PO (CHEWS)
Adults. 2-4 chews up to 3 times/day.

CONTRAINDICATIONS
Abdominal pain, dysphagia, nausea, partial bowel obstruction, symptoms of appendicitis, vomiting or difficulty swallowing.
Caution
Children under 6 yrs., elderly, ileostomy, colostomy, type 2 diabetes (due to increasing levels of sugars in these products), heart disease, kidney disease.

INTERACTIONS
Drug
Ciprofloxacin, etidronate, sodium polystyrene sulfate, tetracyclines: May prevent drug from working because it may interfere with absorption.
Digoxin, oral anticoagulants, salicylates: May decrease the effects of digoxin, oral anticoagulants, and salicylates by decreasing absorption of these drugs.
Potassium-sparing diuretics, potassium supplements: May interfere with the effects of potassium-sparing diuretics and potassium supplements.
Herbal
None known.
Food
None known.

DIAGNOSTIC TEST EFFECTS
May increase blood glucose level. May decrease serum potassium level.

SIDE EFFECTS
Rare
Some degree of abdominal discomfort, nausea, mild cramps, griping, faintness.

SERIOUS REACTIONS
• Esophageal or bowel obstruction may occur if administered with < 250 mL or 1 full glass of liquid.

PRECAUTIONS & CONSIDERATIONS

Methylcellulose can be used safely in pregnancy. Safety and efficacy of methylcellulose have not been established in children younger than 6 yrs. Methylcellulose use is not recommended in this age group. No age-related precautions have been noted in elderly patients. Pattern of daily bowel activity and stool consistency and serum electrolyte levels should be monitored. Caution is warranted in individuals who have difficulty swallowing, ileostomy, colostomy and diabetes type 2.

Administration

Drink 6-8 glasses of water a day to aid in stool softening. Powder should not be swallowed in dry form but should be mixed with at least 1 full glass (8 oz) of liquid. For all products, a full glass of water should be taken with each dose; an inadequate amount of fluid may cause choking or swelling in the throat. To promote defecation, increase fluid intake, exercise, and eat a high-fiber diet.

Methyldopa

meth-ill-doe′pa
(Aldomet, Apo-Methyldopa [CAN], Hydopa [AUS], Novomedopa [CAN], Nudopa [AUS])
Do not confuse Aldomet with Anzemet.

CATEGORY AND SCHEDULE

Pregnancy Risk Category: B

Classification: Centrally acting antihypertensive

MECHANISM OF ACTION

An antihypertensive agent that stimulates central inhibitory alpha-adrenergic receptors, lowers arterial pressure, and reduces plasma renin activity. *Therapeutic Effect:* Reduces BP.

PHARMACOKINETICS

PO: Peak 4-6 h, duration 12-24 h. IV: Peak 2 h, duration 10-16 h. Metabolized by liver, excreted in urine.

AVAILABILITY

Tablets: 250 mg, 500 mg.
Injection: 50 mg/mL.

INDICATIONS AND DOSAGES
▸ **Moderate to severe hypertension**
PO
Adults. Initially, 250 mg 2-3 times a day for 2 days. Adjust dosage at intervals of 2 days (minimum).
Elderly. Initially, 125 mg 1-2 times a day. May increase by 125 mg q2-3 days. Maintenance: 500 mg to 2 g/day in 2-4 divided doses.
Children. Initially, 10 mg/kg/day given in 2-4 divided doses. Maximum: 65 mg/kg/day or 3 g/day, whichever is less.
IV
Adults. 250-1000 mg q6-8h. Maximum: 4 g/day.
Children. Initially, 20-40 mg/kg/day in divided doses q6h. Maximum: 65 mg/kg/day or 3 g/day, whichever is less.

ⓘ IV INCOMPATIBILITIES

Diazepam, furosamide, imipenem-cilastin, phenobarbital, phenytoin.

CONTRAINDICATIONS

Hepatic disease, pheochromocytoma, previous liver problems with methyldopa, hypersensitivity, treatment with MAO Inhibitors.

INTERACTIONS

Drug
Epinephrine and other sympathomimetics: May increase pressor response.

M

General anesthetics: May increase hypotensive action of these drugs.
Haloperidol, alcohol and other central nervous system (CNS) depressants: May increase sedative effects of these drugs.
Hypotensive-producing medications, such as antihypertensives and diuretics: May increase the effects of methyldopa.
Indomethacin and other NSAIDs: May decrease effects of methyldopa.
Iron supplements: Decrease oral absorption of methyldopa.
Lithium: May increase the risk of lithium toxicity.
MAOIs: May cause hyperexcitability. Contraindicated.
NSAIDs, tricyclic antidepressants: May decrease the effects of methyldopa.
Herbal
None known.
Food
None known.

DIAGNOSTIC TEST EFFECTS

May increase BUN and serum prolactin, alkaline phosphatase, bilirubin, creatinine, potassium, sodium, uric acid, AST (SGOT), and ALT (SGPT) levels. May produce positive Coombs' test and prolong prothrombin time.

SIDE EFFECTS

Frequent
Peripheral edema, somnolence, headache, dry mouth.
Occasional
Mental changes (such as anxiety, depression), decreased sexual function or libido, diarrhea, swelling of breasts, nausea, vomiting, lightheadedness, paraesthesia, rhinitis.

SERIOUS REACTIONS

• Hepatotoxicity (abnormal liver function test results, jaundice, hepatitis), hemolytic anemia, unexplained fever, and flulike symptoms may occur. If these conditions appear, discontinue the medication and contact the physician.
• Granulocytopenia.

PRECAUTIONS & CONSIDERATIONS

Caution is warranted in patients with renal impairment. Dizziness, drowsiness, and lightheadedness may occur. Tasks requiring mental alertness and motor skills should be avoided. BP, pulse, weight, and liver function tests should be monitored before and during therapy. BP and pulse should be monitored every 30 min until stabilized. Chronic use may cause infection, bleeding, or poor healing, and these symptoms should be reported so medication changes can be considered. Orthostatic hypotension may result with rapid positional changes; caution is warranted.

Administration
Inspect the drug vial for particulate matter and discoloration and discard if present. For IV infusion, add the prescribed dose to 100 mL D5W and infuse over 30-60 min. Alternatively, add the prescribed dose to D5W to make a final concentration of 100 mg/10 mL and infuse over 30-60 min.

Orally may give without regard to food. Do not give at the same time as iron supplements.

Methylergonovine
meth-ill-er-goe-noe'veen
(Methergine)

CATEGORY AND SCHEDULE
Pregnancy Risk Category: C

Classification: Oxytocics

MECHANISM OF ACTION

An ergot alkaloid that stimulates α-adrenergic and serotonin receptors, producing arterial vasoconstriction. Causes vasospasm of coronary arteries and directly stimulates uterine muscle. *Therapeutic Effect:* Increases strength and frequency of uterine contractions. Decreases uterine bleeding.

PHARMACOKINETICS

Route	Onset	Peak	Duration
PO	5-10 min	NA	NA
IV	Immediate	NA	3 h
IM	2-5 min	NA	NA

Rapidly absorbed from the GI tract after IM administration. Distributed rapidly to plasma, extracellular fluid, and tissues. Metabolized in the liver and undergoes first-pass effect. Excreted in urine. *Half-life:* IV (alpha phase), 2-3 min or less; IV (beta phase), 20-30 min or longer.

AVAILABILITY

Tablets: 0.2 mg.
Injection: 0.2 mg/mL.

INDICATIONS AND DOSAGES

▸ **Prevention and treatment of postpartum and postabortion hemorrhage due to atony or involution**
PO
Adults. 0.2 mg 3-4 times a day. Continue for up to 7 days, but 48 h of use is usually sufficient.
IV, IM
Adults. Initially, 0.2 mg. May repeat q 2-4 h for no more than a total of 5 doses.

OFF-LABEL USES

Treatment of incomplete abortion.

CONTRAINDICATIONS

Hypertension, pregnancy, toxemia, untreated hypocalcemia.

INTERACTIONS

Drug
Vasoconstrictors, vasopressors: May increase the effects of methylergonovine.
Protease inhibitors, clarithromycin, erythromycin, itraconazole, ketoconazole: Increase risk of ergot toxicity. Generally contraindicated.
Sympathomimetics: May increase effects.
Herbal
None known.
Food
None known.

DIAGNOSTIC TEST EFFECTS

May decrease serum prolactin concentration.

Ⓜ IV INCOMPATIBILITIES

No information available for Y-site administration.

🍶 IV COMPATIBILITIES

Heparin, potassium.

SIDE EFFECTS

Frequent
Nausea, uterine cramping, vomiting.
Occasional
Abdominal pain, diarrhea, dizziness, diaphoresis, tinnitus, bradycardia, chest pain.
Rare
Allergic reaction, such as rash and itching; dyspnea; severe or sudden hypertension.

SERIOUS REACTIONS

• Severe hypertensive episodes may result in cerebrovascular accident, serious arrhythmias, and seizures. Hypertensive effects are more frequent with patient susceptibility, rapid IV administration, and concurrent use of regional anesthesia or vasoconstrictors.

M

• Peripheral ischemia may lead to gangrene.

PRECAUTIONS & CONSIDERATIONS
! Drug is not intended for use in any location other than a hosptial setting.
! Methyl ergonovine should never be used for induction or augmentation of labor.

Caution is warranted with in patients with coronary artery disease, hepatic or renal impairment, occlusive peripheral vascular disease, and sepsis. Methylergonovine use is contraindicated during pregnancy. Small amounts of the drug are distributed in breast milk; caution is warranted in lactation. Safety and efficacy of methylergonovine use in children or elderly patients are unknown. Avoid smoking because of added effects of vasoconstriction.

Notify the physician of chest pain, increased bleeding, cold or pale feet or hands, cramping, or foul-smelling lochia. Be aware that the drug may diminish circulation. BP, pulse rate, and uterine tone should be monitored every 15 min until stable for 1-2 h.
Storage
Refrigerate vials. Protect from light.
Administration
! Methylergonovine should never be used for induction or augmentation of labor.

Administration may be PO, IV, or IM. Initial dose may be given parenterally, followed by an oral regimen.

Use IV route in life-threatening situations only, as prescribed. Dilute drug with 0.9% NaCl to a volume of 5 mL. Give over at least 1 min, carefully monitoring BP.

Methylphenidate Hydrochloride
meth-ill-fen'i-date high-droh-klor-ide
(Attenta [AUS], Concerta, Metadate CD, Metadate ER, Methylin, Methylin ER, PMS-Methylphenidate [CAN], Riphenidate [CAN], Ritalin, Ritalin LA, Ritalin SR)
Do not confuse Ritalin with Rifadin.

CATEGORY AND SCHEDULE
Pregnancy Risk Category: C
Controlled Substance Schedule: II

Classification: Central nervous system (CNS) stimulant related to amphetamine

MECHANISM OF ACTION
A CNS stimulant that blocks the reuptake of norepinephrine and dopamine into presynaptic neurons. *Therapeutic Effect:* Decreases motor restlessness and fatigue; increases motor activity, attention span, and mental alertness; produces mild euphoria.

PHARMACOKINETICS

Onset	Peak	Duration
Immediate- release	2 h	3-5 h
Sustained release	4-7 h	3-8 h
Extended release	N/A	8-12 h

Slowly and incompletely absorbed from the GI tract. Protein binding: 15%. Metabolized in the liver. Eliminated in urine and in feces by biliary system. Unknown whether it is removed by hemodialysis. *Half-life:* 2-4 h.

AVAILABILITY
Capsules (Extended-Release [Metadate CD]): 10 mg, 20 mg, 30 mg.

Capsules (Extended-Release [Ritalin LA]): 20 mg, 30 mg, 40 mg.
Tablets (Ritalin): 5 mg, 10 mg, 20 mg.
Tablets (Extended-Release [Mentadate ER, Methylin ER]): 10 mg, 20 mg.
Tablets (Extended-Release [Concerta]): 18 mg, 27 mg, 36 mg, 54 mg.
Tablets (Sustained-Release [Ritalin SR]): 20 mg.
Tablets (Chewable [Methylin]): 2.5 mg, 5 mg, 10 mg.
Oral Solution (Methylin): 5 mg/5 mL, 10 mg/5 mL.

INDICATIONS AND DOSAGES
▸ **Attention deficit hyperactivity disorder (ADHD)**
PO
Children 6 yrs and older. Immediate release: Initially, 2.5-5 mg before breakfast and lunch. May increase by 5-10 mg/day at weekly intervals. Maximum: 60 mg/day.
PO (CONCERTA)
Children 6 yrs and older. Initially, 18 mg once a day; may increase by 18 mg/day at weekly intervals. Maximum: 54-72 mg/day.
PO (METADATE CD)
Children 6 yrs and older. Initially, 20 mg/day. May increase by 20 mg/day at weekly intervals. Maximum: 60 mg/day.
PO (RITALIN LA)
Children 6 yrs and older. Initially, 20 mg/day. May increase by 10 mg/day at weekly intervals. Maximum: 60 mg/day.
▸ **Narcolepsy**
PO
Adults, Elderly. 10 mg 2-3 times a day. Range: 10-60 mg/day.

OFF-LABEL USES
Treatment of refractory mental depression.

CONTRAINDICATIONS
Do not use within 14 days of MAOIs, marked agitation, glaucoma, Tourette's or tics, known serious cardiac abnormalities or serious heart rhythmic problems.

INTERACTIONS
Drug
MAOIs: May increase the effects of methylphenidate. Contraindicated.
Other CNS stimulants, tricyclic antidepressants, SSRIs, sympathomimetics: May have an additive effect.
Herbal and Food
None known.

DIAGNOSTIC TEST EFFECTS
None known.

SIDE EFFECTS
Frequent
Anxiety, insomnia, anorexia.
Occasional
Dizziness, drowsiness, headache, nausea, abdominal pain, fever, rash, arthralgia, vomiting.
Rare
Blurred vision, Tourette syndrome (marked by uncontrolled vocal outbursts, repetitive body movements, and tics), palpitations.

SERIOUS REACTIONS
• Prolonged administration to children with ADHD may delay growth.
• Overdose may produce tachycardia, palpitations, arrhythmias, chest pain, psychotic episode, seizures, and coma.
• Hypersensitivity reactions and blood dyscrasias occur rarely.

PRECAUTIONS & CONSIDERATIONS
Caution is warranted in patients with hypertension, seizures, acute stress reaction, emotional instability, and

M

a history of drug dependence. It is unknown whether methylphenidate crosses the placenta or is distributed in breast milk; therefore, caution is warranted in lactation. Children are more prone to develop abdominal pain, anorexia, weight loss, and insomnia. Long-term methylphenidate use may inhibit growth in children. No age-related precautions have been noted in elderly patients. Caffeinated beverages should be avoided during therapy.

Tasks that require mental alertness and motor skills should be avoided until response to the drug is established. Notify the physician if fever, anxiety, palpitations, a rash, vomiting or, for those with a seizure disorder, an increase in the number of seizures, occurs. CBC, WBC count with differential, and platelet should be monitored. Baseline height and weight should be obtained at the beginning and periodically throughout therapy.

Administration

! Sustained- and extended-release tablets may be given in place of regular tablets once the daily dose is titrated using regular tablets and if the titrated dosage corresponds to the sustained- or extended-release tablet strength.

Take methylphenidate 30-45 min before meals (usually before breakfast and lunch). Take the last dose before 6:00 PM to help prevent insomnia. Crush tablets as needed, but do not eat, crush or chew extended-release tablets or capsules. Open the Metadate CD or Ritalin-LA or capsule and sprinkle the pellets on applesauce, if desired. Do not chew.

Methylprednisolone

meth-il-pred-niss'oh-lone
(Medrol) (Depo-Medrol,
Depo-Nisolone [AUS])
(A-Methapred, Solu-Medrol)
**Do not confuse methylpredniso-
lone with medroxyprogesterone
or Medrol with Mebaral.**

CATEGORY AND SCHEDULE
Pregnancy Risk Category: C

Classification: Glucocorticoid, immediate acting

MECHANISM OF ACTION
An adrenocortical steroid that suppresses the migration of polymorphonuclear leukocytes and reverses increased capillary permeability. *Therapeutic Effect:* Decreases inflammation.

PHARMACOKINETICS

Route	Onset	Peak	Duration
PO	NA	1-2 h	30-36 h
IM	NA	4-8 days	1-4 wks

Well absorbed from the GI tract after IM administration. Widely distributed. Metabolized in the liver. Excreted in urine. Removed by hemodialysis. *Half-life:* 3.5 h.

AVAILABILITY
Tablets (Medrol): 2 mg, 4 mg, 8 mg, 16 mg, 32 mg.
Injection Powder for Reconstitution (A-Methapred, Solu-Medrol): 40 mg, 125 mg, 500 mg, 1 g.
Injection Suspension (Depo-Medrol): 20 mg/mL, 40 mg/mL, 80 mg/mL.

INDICATIONS AND DOSAGES
▸ **Substitution therapy for deficiency states: acute or chronic adrenal**

insufficiency, adrenal insufficiency secondary to pituitary insufficiency, and congenital adrenal hyperplasia; nonendocrine disorders: allergic, collagen, hepatic, intestinal tract, ocular, renal, and skin diseases; arthritis, bronchial asthma; cerebral edema; malignancies; rhematoid carditis

PO
Adults, Elderly. Usual range: 4-60 mg/day, given in 4 divided doses.
IV (METHYLPREDNISOLONE SODIUM SUCCINATE)
Adults, Elderly. 40-250 mg q 4-6 h. High dosage: 30 mg/kg over at least 30 min. Repeat q 4-6 h for 48-72 h.
▸ **Spinal cord injury**
IV BOLUS AND INFUSION
Adults, Elderly. 30 mg/kg over 15 min. Maintenance dose: 5.4 mg/kg/h for 23 h, to be given within 45 min of bolus dose.
▸ **Usual IM dosage**
IM (METHYLPREDNISOLONE ACETATE)
Adults, Elderly. 10-80 mg. Frequency of repeat doses dependent on condition being treated.
INTRA-ARTICULAR, INTRALESIONAL
Adults, Elderly. 4-40 mg, up to 80 mg q1-5wk.
▸ **Usual pediatric dose:**
PO/IM/IV
Pediatric. 0.5-1.7 mg/kg/day or 5-25 mg/m²/day in 2-4 divided doses.

CONTRAINDICATIONS

Hypersensitivity to product, systemic fungal infections; some injections contain benzyl alcohol and are not for use in neonates.

INTERACTIONS

Drug
Acetaminophen (chronic, high dose): May increase risk of hepatotoxicity.

Alcohol, salicylates, NSAIDs: Possible increase in GI effects.
Amphotericin: May increase hypokalemia.
Barbiturates, rifampin, rfabutin: Possible decreased action.
Digoxin: May increase the risk of digoxin toxicity caused by hypokalemia.
Diuretics, insulin, oral hypoglycemics, potassium supplements: May decrease the effects of these drugs.
Hepatic enzyme inducers: May decrease the effects of methylprednisolone.
Keotoconazole, macrolide antibiotics: Possible increased activity.
Live virus vaccines: May decrease the patient's antibody response to vaccine, increase vaccine side effects, and potentiate virus replication.
Herbal and Food
None known.

DIAGNOSTIC TEST EFFECTS

May increase blood cholesterol, glucose and serum lipid, amylase, and sodium levels. May decrease serum calcium, potassium, and thyroxine levels.

⊘ IV INCOMPATIBILITIES

Ciprofloxacin (Cipro), diltiazem (Cardizem), docetaxel (Taxotere), etoposide (VePesid), filgrastim (Neupogen), gemcitabine (Gemzar), paclitaxel (Taxol), potassium chloride, propofol (Diprivan), vinorelbine (Navelbine).

⊜ IV COMPATIBILITIES

Dopamine (Intropin), heparin, midazolam (Versed), theophylline.

SIDE EFFECTS

Frequent
Insomnia, heartburn, anxiety, abdominal distention, diaphoresis,

acne, mood swings, increased appetite, facial flushing, GI distress, delayed wound healing, increased susceptibility to infection, diarrhea, or constipation.

Occasional

Headache, edema, tachycardia, change in skin color, frequent urination, depression.

Rare

Psychosis, increased blood coagulability, hallucinations.

SERIOUS REACTIONS

• Long-term therapy may cause hypocalcemia, hypokalemia, muscle wasting (especially in arms and legs), osteoporosis, spontaneous fractures, amenorrhea, cataracts, glaucoma, peptic ulcer disease, and congestive heart failure (CHF).

• Abruptly withdrawing the drug after long-term therapy may cause anorexia, nausea, fever, headache, sudden severe myalgia, rebound inflammation, fatigue, weakness, lethargy, dizziness, and orthostatic hypotension.

PRECAUTIONS & CONSIDERATIONS

Caution is warranted with cirrhosis, CHF, diabetes mellitus, hypertension, hypothyroidism, thromboembolic disorders, and ulcerative colitis. Methyl-prednisolone crosses the placenta and is distributed in breast milk. Women taking methylprednisolone should not breastfeed. Prolonged methylprednisolone use in the first trimester of pregnancy may cause cleft palate in the neonate. Prolonged treatment or high dosages may decrease cortisol secretion and short-term growth rate in children. No age-related precautions have been noted in elderly patients. Severe stress, including serious infection, surgery, or trauma, may require an increase in methylprednisolone dosage.

Dentist or another physician should be informed of methylprednisolone therapy if taken within the past 12 mo.

Mood swings, ranging from euphoria to depression, may occur. Notify the physician of fever, muscle aches, sore throat, and sudden weight gain or swelling. Blood glucose level, intake and output, BP, serum electrolyte levels, pattern of daily bowel activity, height, and weight should be monitored before and during therapy. Be alert to signs and symptoms of infection caused by reduced immune response, including fever, sore throat, and vague symptoms. In long-term therapy, signs and symptoms of hypocalcemia (such as muscle twitching, cramps, and positive Chvostek's or Trousseau's signs) or hypokalemia (such as ECG changes, nausea and vomiting, irritability, weakness and muscle cramps, and numbness or tingling, especially in the lower extremities) should be reported to health care providers immediately.

Storage

Store vials for injection at room temperature.

Administration

! Individualize dosage based on the disease, person, and response.

Take oral methylprednisolone with food or milk. Take single doses before 9:00 AM; give multiple doses at evenly spaced intervals. Do not abruptly discontinue the drug or change the dosage or schedule; the drug must be withdrawn gradually under medical supervision.

For IV use, follow directions with Mix-o-vial. For infusion, add to D5W or 0.9% NaCl. Give IV push over 2-3 min. Give IV piggyback over 10-20 min. Do not give methylprednisolone acetate suspension IV.

For IM use, methylprednisolone acetate should not be further diluted.

Give deep IM injection into gluteus maximus. Methylprednisolone acetate may be given locally as an intra-articular injection.

Methyltestosterone

meth-il-tes-tos′te-rone
(Android, Android-10, Android-25, Oreton Methyl, Testred, Virilon)
Do not confuse with methylprednisolone.

CATEGORY AND SCHEDULE
Pregnancy Risk Category: X
Controlled substance: Schedule III

Classification: Androgens, hormones/hormone modifiers

MECHANISM OF ACTION
A synthetic testosterone derivative with androgen activity that promotes growth and development of male sex organs and maintains secondary sex characteristics in androgen-deficient males. *Therapeutic Effect:* Treats hypogonadism and delayed puberty in males.

PHARMACOKINETICS
Well absorbed from the GI tract. Protein binding: 98%. Metabolized in liver. Primarily excreted in urine. Unknown whether it is removed by hemodialysis. *Half-life:* 10-100 min.

AVAILABILITY
Capsules: 10 mg (Android, Testred, Virilon).
Tablets: 10 mg (Android-10, Oreton Methyl), 25 mg (Android-25).

INDICATIONS AND DOSAGES
▸ **Breast cancer, palliative**
PO
Adults, Elderly. 50-200 mg/day.

▸ **Delayed puberty**
PO
Adolescents. 5-25 mg/day for 4-6 mo.
▸ **Hypogonadism**
PO
Adults. 10-50 mg/day.

OFF-LABEL USES
Hereditary angiodema.

CONTRAINDICATIONS
Pregnancy, prostatic or breast cancer in males, hypersensitivity to methyltestosterone or any other component of its formulation.

INTERACTIONS
Drug
ACTH, Corticosteroids: Possible increased edema risk.
Bupropion: May increase the risk of seizures by decreasing seizure threshold.
Cyclosporine: May increase risk of cyclosporine toxicity.
Liver toxic medications: May increase liver toxicity.
Oral anticoagulants: May increase the effects of oral anticoagulants.
Herbal
None known.
Food
None known.

DIAGNOSTIC TEST EFFECTS
May increase blood hemoglobin and hematocrit, LDL concentrations, serum alkaline phosphatase, bilirubin, calcium, potassium, SGOT (AST) levels, and sodium levels. May decrease HDL concentrations.

SIDE EFFECTS
Frequent
Gynecomastia, acne, amenorrhea or other menstrual irregularities. Females: Hirsutism, deepening of voice, clitoral enlargement that

M

may not be reversible when drug is discontinued.

Occasional

Edema, nausea, insomnia, oligospermia, priapism, male pattern of baldness, bladder irritability, hypercalcemia in immobilized patients or those with breast cancer, hypercholesterolemia.

Rare

Polycythemia.

SERIOUS REACTIONS

• Cholestatic jaundice, hepatocellular neoplasms, peliosis hepatitis, edema with or without CHF and suppression of clotting factors II, V, VII, and X have been reported.

• Priapism.

PRECAUTIONS & CONSIDERATIONS

Caution is warranted in patients with diabetes, CHF of preexisting cardiac, liver or renal disease, epilepsy, history of migraine, other conditions that may be aggravated by fluid retention, and hypertension due to the risk of increased BP. Methyltestosterone should not be used during lactation. Safety and efficacy of methyltestosterone have not been established in prepubertal children, so use with caution. Be aware that methyltestosterone use in elderly patients may increase the risk of hyperplasia or stimulate the growth of occult prostate carcinoma. Adequate calories and protein should be consumed.

Acne, nausea, pedal edema, or vomiting may occur. Women should report deepening of voice, hoarseness, and menstrual irregularities. Men should report difficulty urinating, frequent erections, and gynecomastia. Weight should be obtained each day. Weekly weight gains of more than 5 lb should be reported.

Storage

Store at room temperature.

Administration

Give methyltestosterone with meals.

Metipranolol Hydrochloride

met-ee-pran´-oh-lol high-droh-klor´-ide

(OptiPranolol)

Do not confuse with metoprolol or propranolol.

CATEGORY AND SCHEDULE

Pregnancy Risk Category: C

Classification: Antiglaucoma agent (ophthalmic)

MECHANISM OF ACTION

An antiglaucoma agent that nonselectively blocks β-adrenergic receptors. Reduces aqueous humor production. *Therapeutic Effect:* Reduces intraocular pressure (IOP).

PHARMACOKINETICS

Route	Onset	Peak	Duration
Eye drops	0.5-3 h	2-7 h	≥24 h

Systemic absorption may occur.

AVAILABILITY

Ophthalmic solution: 0.3%.

INDICATIONS AND DOSAGES

▸ **Glaucoma, ocular hypertension**

OPHTHALMIC

Adults, Elderly. Instill 1 drop 2 times a day.

CONTRAINDICATIONS

Bronchial asthma or chronic obstructive pulmonary disease,

cardiogenic shock, overt cardiac failure, second- or third- degree heart atrioventricular block, severe sinus bradycardia, hypersensitivity to metipranolol or any component of the formulation.

DRUG INTERACTIONS
Oral β-blockers: Additive systemic effects.
Calcium channel blockers: Hypotension.

SIDE EFFECTS
Frequent
Eye burning/stinging, hyperemia, blurred vision, headache, fatigue.
Occasional
Sensitivity to light, dizziness, hypotension.
Rare
Dry eye, conjunctivitis, eye pain, rash, muscle pain.

SERIOUS REACTIONS
• Ophthalmic overdosage may produce bradycardia, hypotension, bronchospasm, and acute cardiac failure.
• Arrhythmias and myocardial infarction have been reported.

PRECAUTIONS & CONSIDERATIONS
Caution in patients with hyperthyroidism, diabetes, cerebrovascular insufficiency, and depression. Safety and efficacy not established in children. No unique precautions in elderly.
Storage
Store at room temperature.
Administration
Use nasolacrimal occlusion after administration to reduce systemic absorption.

Metoclopramide
met′oh-kloe-pra′mide
(Apo-Metoclop [CAN], Maxolon [AUS], Pramin [AUS], Reglan)
Do not confuse Reglan with Renagel.

CATEGORY AND SCHEDULE
Pregnancy Risk Category: B

Classification: Centrally acting dopamine receptor antagonist

MECHANISM OF ACTION
A dopamine receptor antagonist that stimulates motility of the upper GI tract and decreases reflux into the esophagus. Also raises the threshold of activity in the chemoreceptor trigger zone. *Therapeutic Effect:* Accelerates intestinal transit and gastric emptying; relieves nausea and vomiting.

PHARMACOKINETICS

Route	Onset (min)	Peak	Duration
PO	30-60	NA	NA
IV	1-3	NA	NA
IM	10-15	NA	NA

Well absorbed from the GI tract. Metabolized in the liver. Protein binding: 30%. Primarily excreted in urine. Not removed by hemodialysis. *Half-life:* 4-6 h.

AVAILABILITY
Syrup: 5 mg/5 mL.
Tablets: 5 mg, 10 mg.
Injection: 5 mg/mL.

INDICATIONS AND DOSAGES
▸ **Prevention of chemotherapy-induced nausea and vomiting**

IV

Adults, Elderly, Children. 1-2 mg/kg 30 min before chemotherapy; repeat q2h for 2 doses, then q3h as needed.

▸**Postoperative nausea and vomiting**
IV

Adults, Elderly, Children 15 yrs and older. 10 mg; repeat q6-8h as needed.
Children 14 yrs and younger.
0.1-0.2 mg/kg/dose; repeat q6-8h as needed.

▸**Diabetic gastroparesis**
PO, IV

Adults. 10 mg 30 min before meals and at bedtime for 2-8 wks.
PO

Elderly. Initially, 5 mg 30 min before meals and at bedtime. May increase to 10 mg.
IV

Elderly. 5 mg over 1-2 min. May increase to 10 mg.

▸**Symptomatic gastroesophageal reflux**
PO

Adults. 10-15 mg up to 4 times a day or single doses up to 20 mg as needed.
Elderly. Initially, 5 mg 4 times a day. May increase to 10 mg.
Children. 0.4-0.8 mg/kg/day in 4 divided doses.

▸**To facilitate small bowel intubation (single dose)**
IV

Adults, Elderly. 10 mg as a single dose.
Children 6-14 yrs. 2.5-5 mg as a single dose.
Children younger than 6 yrs.
0.1 mg/kg as a single dose.

▸**Dosage in renal impairment**
Initial dosage is modified based on creatinine clearance.

Creatinine Clearance (mL/min)	Initial % of Normal Dose
< 40 mL/min	50

May be increased or decreased to clinical effect.

OFF-LABEL USES
Prevention of aspiration pneumonia; persistent hiccups, slow gastric emptying, vascular headaches to offset nausea from ergot alkaloids.

CONTRAINDICATIONS
Concurrent use of medications likely to produce extrapyramidal reactions, GI hemorrhage, GI obstruction or perforation, history of seizure disorders, pheochromocytoma, hypersensitivity to metoclopramide.

INTERACTIONS
Drug
Alcohol, other central nervous system (CNS) suppressants: May increase CNS depressant effect.
Anticholintergics, opioids:
Decreased GI action.
MAOIs: Use cautiously; may increase risk of hypertension.
Herbal
None known.
Food
None known.

DIAGNOSTIC TEST EFFECTS
May increase serum aldosterone and prolactin concentrations.

ⓦ IV INCOMPATIBILITIES
Allopurinol (Aloprim), cefepime, cephalothin, (Maxipime), doxorubicin liposomal (Doxil), furosemide (Lasix), propofol (Diprivan), sodium bicarbonate.

⛫ IV COMPATIBILITIES
Dexamethasone, diltiazem (Cardizem), diphenhydramine (Benadryl), fentanyl (Sublimaze), heparin, hydromorphone (Dilaudid), morphine, potassium chloride.

SIDE EFFECTS
Frequent (10%)
Somnolence, restlessness, fatigue, lethargy.

Occasional (3%)
Dizziness, anxiety, headache, insomnia, breast tenderness, altered menstruation, constipation, rash, dry mouth, galactorrhea, gynecomastia.
Rare (< 3%)
Hypotension or hypertension, tachycardia.

SERIOUS REACTIONS

• Extrapyramidal reactions occur most commonly in children and young adults (18-30 yrs) receiving large doses (2 mg/kg) during chemotherapy and are usually limited to akathisia (involuntary limb movement and facial grimacing).
• Neuroleptic malignant syndrome.

PRECAUTIONS & CONSIDERATIONS

Caution is warranted in patients with cirrhosis, CHF, and renal impairment. Metoclopramide crosses the placenta and is distributed in breast milk; therefore, caution is warranted in lactation. Children and young adults (aged 18-30 yrs) are more susceptible to dystonic reactions at larger doses during chemotherapy and are usually evidenced by akathisia of the face and limbs. Elderly patients are more likely to have parkinsonian reactions and dyskinesias after long-term therapy. Alcohol and tasks that require mental alertness or motor skills should be avoided.

Dizziness, drowsiness, and dry mouth may occur. Notify the physician if involuntary eye, facial, or limb movement occurs. BP, heart rate, renal function, skin for rash, and pattern of daily bowel activity and stool consistency should be monitored.
Storage
Store vials at room temperature. After dilution, IV piggyback infusion is stable for 48 h.

Administration
! Metoclopramide may be given by PO and IM routes and by IV push or IV infusion. Doses of 2 mg/kg or more or prolonged therapy may increase the incidence of side effects.

Take oral metoclopramide 30 min before meals and at bedtime. Crush tablets as needed.

For IV use, dilute doses > 10 mg in 50 mL, 0.9% NaCl (preferred), or Dextrose 5%, lactated Ringer's solution. Infuse over 15 min. Give slow IV push of 10 mg over 1-2 min. Too-rapid IV injection may produce intense anxiety or restlessness, followed by drowsiness.

Metolazone
met-tole′a-zone
(Mykrox, Zaroxolyn)
Do not confuse metolazone with metaxalone, methazolamide, or metoprolol; or Zaroxolyn with Zarontin.

CATEGORY AND SCHEDULE
Pregnancy Risk Category: B, D if used in pregnancy-induced hypertension

Classification: Diuretics, thiazide-like effects

MECHANISM OF ACTION
A thiazide-like diuretic and antihypertensive. As a diuretic, blocks reabsorption of sodium, potassium, and chloride at the distal convoluted tubule, increasing renal excretion of sodium and water. As an antihypertensive, reduces plasma and extracellular fluid volume and peripheral vascular resistance. *Therapeutic Effect:* Promotes diuresis and reduces BP.

PHARMACOKINETICS

Route	Onset	Peak	Duration
PO (diuretic)	1 h	2 h	12-24 h

Incompletely absorbed from the GI tract. Protein binding: 95%. Primarily excreted unchanged in urine. Not removed by hemodialysis. *Half-life:* 14 h.

AVAILABILITY

Tablets (Prompt-Release [Mykrox]): 0.5 mg.
Tablets (Extended-Release [Zaroxolyn]): 2.5 mg, 5 mg, 10 mg.

INDICATIONS AND DOSAGES

▸ **Edema**
PO (ZAROXOLYN)
Adults, Elderly. 5-10 mg/day. May increase to 20 mg/day in edema associated with renal disease or heart failure.
Children. 0.2-0.4 mg/kg/day in 1-2 divided doses.
▸ **Hypertension**
PO (ZAROXOLYN)
Adults, Elderly. 2.4-5 mg/day.
PO (MYDROX)
Adults, Elderly. Initially, 0.5 mg/day. May increase up to 1 mg/day.
PO
Elderly. Initially, 2.5 mg/day or every other day.

CONTRAINDICATIONS

Anuria, hepatic coma or precoma, history of hypersensitivity to sulfonamides or thiazide diuretics.

INTERACTIONS

Drug
Cholestyramine, colestipol: May decrease the absorption and effects of metolazone.
Digoxin: May increase the risk of digoxin toxicity associated with metolazone-induced hypokalemia.

Indomethacin and other NSAIDs: May have decreased hypotensive response.
Lithium: May increase the risk of lithium toxicity.
Tetracyclines: May increase risk of photosentization.
Herbal
None known.
Food
None known.

DIAGNOSTIC TEST EFFECTS

May increase blood glucose and serum cholesterol, LDL, bilirubin, calcium, creatinine, uric acid, and triglyceride levels. May decrease urinary calcium, and serum magnesium, potassium, and sodium levels.

SIDE EFFECTS

Expected
Increase in urinary frequency and urine volume.
Frequent (9%-10%)
Dizziness, lightheadedness, headache.
Occasional (4%-6%)
Muscle cramps and spasm, fatigue, lethargy.
Rare (< 2%)
Asthenia, palpitations, depression, nausea, vomiting, abdominal bloating, constipation, diarrhea, urticaria.

SERIOUS REACTIONS

• Vigorous diuresis may lead to profound water and electrolyte depletion, resulting in hypokalemia, hyponatremia, and dehydration.
• Acute hypotensive episodes may occur.
• Hyperglycemia may occur during prolonged therapy.
• Pancreatitis, paresthesia, blood dyscrasias, pulmonary edema, allergic pneumonitis, and dermatologic reactions occur rarely.

• Overdose can lead to lethargy and coma without changes in electrolytes or hydration.

with breakfast to help prevent nocturia.

PRECAUTIONS & CONSIDERATIONS

Caution is warranted in patients with diabetes, elevated cholesterol and triglyceride levels, gout, hepatic impairment, lupus erythematosus, and severe renal disease. Metolazone crosses the placenta, and a small amount is distributed in breast milk. Breastfeeding is not recommended for patients taking this drug. No age-related precautions have been noted in children. Elderly patients may be more sensitive to the drug's electrolyte and hypotensive effects. Age-related renal impairment may require cautious use in elderly patients. Consuming foods high in potassium, such as apricots, bananas, legumes, meat, orange juice, raisins, whole grains, including cereals, and white and sweet potatoes, is encouraged. Patient should be advised about limiting salt intake and sodium-containing products.

An increase in the frequency and volume of urination may occur. BP, vital signs, electrolytes, intake and output, and weight should be monitored before and during treatment. Be aware of signs of electrolyte disturbances such as hypokalemia or hyponatremia. Hypokalemia may cause arrhythmias, altered mental status, muscle cramps, asthenia, and tremor. Hyponatremia may result in cold and clammy skin, confusion, and thirst. Any of these indicators should be reported immediately. Because of the possible cardiovascular effects, patients should be evaluated for stress tolerance during therapy.

Administration

Take metolazone with food or milk if GI upset occurs, preferably

Metoprolol tartrate

me-toe′pro-lole tar-tray-te
(Apo-Metoprolol [CAN], Betaloc [CAN], Lopresor [AUS], Lopressor, Metohexal [AUS], Metolol [AUS], Minax [AUS], Nu-Metop [CAN], PMS-Metoprolol [CAN], Toprol XL)

Do not confuse metoprolol with metaproterenol or metolazone. Do not confuse Toprol XL with Topamax.

CATEGORY AND SCHEDULE

Pregnancy Risk Category: C (D if used in second or third trimester)

Classification: Antihypertensive, selective β1-blocker

MECHANISM OF ACTION

An antianginal, antihypertensive, and myocardial infarction (MI) adjunct that selectively blocks β_1-adrenergic receptors; high dosages may block β_2-adrenergic receptors. Decreases oxygen requirements. Large doses increase airway resistance. *Therapeutic Effect:* Slows sinus node heart rate, decreases cardiac output, and reduces BP. Also decreases myocardial ischemia severity.

PHARMACOKINETICS

Route	Onset	Peak	Duration
PO	10-15 min	1 h	6 h
PO (extended release)	N/A	6-12 h	24 h
IV	Immediate	20 min	5-8 h

M

Well absorbed from the GI tract. Protein binding: 12%. Widely distributed. Metabolized in the liver (undergoes significant first-pass metabolism). Primarily excreted in urine. Removed by hemodialysis. *Half-life:* 3-7 h.

AVAILABILITY

Tablets (Lopressor): 25 mg, 50 mg, 100 mg.
Tablets (Extended-Release [Toprol XL]): 25 mg, 50 mg, 100 mg, 200 mg.
Injection (Lopressor): 1 mg/mL.

INDICATIONS AND DOSAGES
▸ **Mild to moderate hypertension**
PO
Adults. Initially, 100 mg/day as single or divided dose. Increase at weekly (or longer) intervals. Maintenance: 100-450 mg/day.
Elderly. Initially, 25 mg/day. Range: 25-300 mg/day.
PO (EXTENDED-RELEASE TABLETS)
Adults. 50-100 mg/day as single dose. May increase at least at weekly intervals until optimum BP attained. Maximum: 200 mg/day.
▸ **Chronic, stable angina pectoris**
PO
Adults. Initially, 100 mg/day as single or divided dose. Increase at weekly (or longer) intervals. Maintenance: 100-450 mg/day.
PO (EXTENDED-RELEASE TABLETS)
Adults. Initially, 100 mg/day as single dose. May increase at least at weekly intervals until optimum clinical response achieved. Maximum: 200 mg/day.
▸ **Congestive heart failure (CHF)**
PO (EXTENDED-RELEASE TABLETS)
Adults. Initially, 25 mg/day. May double dose q 2 wk. Maximum: 200 mg/day.
▸ **Early treatment of MI**
IV
Adults. 5 mg q2min for 3 doses, followed by 50 mg orally q6h for 48 h. Begin oral dose 15 min after last IV dose. Or, in patients who do not tolerate full IV dose, give 25-50 mg orally q6h, 15 min after last IV dose.
▸ **Late treatment and maintenance after an MI**
PO
Adults. Target dose: 100 mg twice a day for at least 3 mo.

OFF-LABEL USES

To increase survival rate in diabetic patients with coronary artery disease (CAD); treatment or prevention of anxiety; cardiac arrhythmias; hypertrophic cardiomyopathy; mitral valve prolapse syndrome; pheochromocytoma; tremors; thyrotoxicosis; vascular headache.

CONTRAINDICATIONS

Cardiogenic shock, MI with a heart rate < 45 beats/min or systolic BP < 100 mm Hg, overt heart failure, second- or third-degree heart block, sinus bradycardia.

INTERACTIONS
Drug
Cimetidine: May increase metoprolol blood concentration.
Didanosine: May decrease effects.
Diphenhydramine: May increase plasma concentrations.
Diuretics, other antihypertensives: May increase hypotensive effect.
Epinephrine, levonordefrin, isoproterenol, other sympathomimetics: May decrease β-blocking, β-adrenergic effects.
Fentanyl derivatives, inhalation anesthetics: Possible increased hypotension and bradycardia.

Indomethacin and other NSAIDs, sympathomimetics: Possible decreased antihypertensive effects.

Insulin, oral hypoglycemics: May mask symptoms of hypoglycemia and prolong hypoglycemic effect of these drugs.

Lidocaine: May slow metabolism of lidocaine.

NSAIDs: May decrease antihypertensive effect.

Sympathomimetics, xanthines: May mutually inhibit effects.

Herbal
None known.

Food
None known.

DIAGNOSTIC TEST EFFECTS

May increase serum antinuclear antibody titer and BUN, serum lipoprotein, serum LDH, serum alkaline phosphatase, serum bilirubin, serum creatinine, serum potassium, serum uric acid, AST (SGOT), ALT (SGPT), and serum triglyceride levels.

⊘ IV INCOMPATIBILITIES

Amphotericin B complex (Abelcet, AmBisome, Amphotec), diazepam, pantoprazole, phenytoin.

⬩ IV COMPATIBILITIES

Alteplase (Activase), morphine.

SIDE EFFECTS

Metoprolol is generally well tolerated, with transient and mild side effects.

Frequent
Diminished sexual function, drowsiness, insomnia, unusual fatigue or weakness.

Occasional
Anxiety, nervousness, diarrhea, constipation, nausea, vomiting, nasal congestion, abdominal discomfort,

dizziness, difficulty breathing, cold hands or feet.

Rare
Altered taste, dry eyes, nightmares, paraesthesia, allergic reaction (rash, pruritus).

SERIOUS REACTIONS

• Overdose may produce profound bradycardia, hypotension, and bronchospasm.

• Abrupt withdrawal of metoprolol may result in diaphoresis, palpitations, headache, tremulousness, exacerbation of angina, MI, and ventricular arrhythmias.

• Metoprolol administration may precipitate CHF and MI in patients with heart disease; thyroid storm in those with thyrotoxicosis; and peripheral ischemia in those with existing peripheral vascular disease.

• Hypoglycemia may occur in patients with previously controlled diabetes.

PRECAUTIONS & CONSIDERATIONS

Caution is warranted with bronchospastic disease, diabetes, hyperthyroidism, impaired renal function, inadequate cardiac function, and peripheral vascular disease. Metoprolol crosses the placenta and is distributed in breast milk; therefore, care in lactation is warranted. Metoprolol use should be avoided in pregnant women after the first trimester because it may result in low-birth-weight infants. The drug may also produce apnea, bradycardia, hypoglycemia, or hypothermia during childbirth. The safety and efficacy of metoprolol have not been established in children. In elderly patients, age-related peripheral vascular disease may increase susceptibility to decreased peripheral circulation. Be aware that

M

salt and alcohol intake should be restricted. Nasal decongestants or OTC cold preparations (stimulants) should not be used without physician approval.

Notify the physician of excessive fatigue, headache, prolonged dizziness, shortness of breath, or weight gain. BP for hypotension, respiratory status for shortness of breath, pattern of daily bowel activity and stool consistency, ECG for arrhythmias, and pulse for quality, rate, and rhythm should be monitored during treatment. If pulse rate is 60 beats/min or lower or systolic BP is < 90 mm Hg, withhold the medication and contact the physician. In those receiving metoprolol for treatment of angina, the onset, type (sharp, dull, squeezing), radiation, location, intensity, and duration of anginal pain and its precipitating factors, including exertion and emotional stress should be recorded. Signs and symptoms of CHF, such as decreased urine output, distended neck veins, dyspnea (particularly on exertion or lying down), night cough, peripheral edema, and weight gain should also be assessed. Do not abruptly discontinue metoprolol; may result in symptoms of diaphoresis, palpitations, headache, tremors, angina, MI, and ventricular arrhythmias.

Storage
Store at room temperature.

Administration
Crush tablets if necessary; do not crush or break extended-release tablets. Take at same time each day. Take with or immediately after meals to enhance absorption.

For IV use, give undiluted as necessary. Administer IV injection over 1 min. Monitor the patient's ECG and BP during administration.

Metronidazole Hydrochloride

me-troe-ni′da-zole high-droh-klor-ide

(Apo-Metronidazole [CAN], Flagyl, Flagyl ER, MetroCream, MetroGel, Metrogyl [AUS], MetroLotion, Metronidazole IV [AUS], Metronide [AUS], NidaGel [CAN], Noritate, Novonidazol [CAN], Rozex [AUS])

CATEGORY AND SCHEDULE
Pregnancy Risk Category: B

Classification: Trichomonacide, amebicide, antiinfective

MECHANISM OF ACTION
A nitroimidazole derivative that disrupts bacterial and protozoal DNA, inhibiting nucleic acid synthesis. *Therapeutic Effect:* Produces bactericidal, antiprotozoal, amebicidal, and trichomonacidal effects. Produces anti-inflammatory and immunosuppressive effects when applied topically.

PHARMACOKINETICS
Well absorbed from the GI tract; minimally absorbed after topical application. Protein binding: < 20%. Widely distributed; crosses blood-brain barrier. Metabolized in the liver to active metabolite. Primarily excreted in urine; partially eliminated in feces. Removed by hemodialysis. *Half-life:* 8 h (increased in alcoholic hepatic disease and in neonates).

AVAILABILITY
Capsules (Flagyl): 375 mg.
Tablets (Flagyl): 250 mg, 500 mg.

Tablets (Extended-Release [Flagyl ER]): 750 mg.
Injection (Infusion): 500 mg/100 mL.
Lotion: 0.75%.
Topical Gel (MetroGel): 0.75%.
Topical Cream (MetroCream): 0.75%.
Topical Cream (Noritate): 1%.
Vaginal Gel (MetroGel-Vaginal): 0.75%.

INDICATIONS AND DOSAGES
▸ **Amebiasis**
PO
Adults, Elderly. 500-750 mg q8h.
Children. 35-50 mg/kg/day in divided doses q8h.
▸ **Trichomoniasis**
PO
Adults, Elderly. 250 mg q8h or 2 g as a single dose.
Children. 15-30 mg/kg/day in divided doses q8h.
▸ **Anaerobic skin and skin-structure infection, cns, lower respiratory tract, bone, joint, intra-abdominal, gynelogic infections; endocarditis; septicemia.**
PO, IV
Adults, Elderly, Children.
Generally, 7.5 mg/kg/dose q6h.
Maximum: 4 g/day.
▸ **Antibiotic-associated pseudomembranous colitis**
PO
Adults, Elderly. 250-500 mg 3-4 times a day for 10-14 days.
Children. 30 mg/kg/day in divided doses q6h for 7-10 days.
▸ **Helicobacter pylori infections**
PO
Adults, Elderly. 250-500 mg 3 times a day (in combination).
Children. 15-20 mg/kg/day in 2 divided doses.
▸ **Bacterial vaginosis**
PO
Adults. 750 mg at bedtime for 7 days.

INTRAVAGINAL
Adults. One full applicator twice a day or once a day at bedtime for 5 days.
▸ **Rosacea**
TOPICAL
Adults. Apply thin layer of lotion or gel to affected area twice a day or cream once a day.

OFF-LABEL USES
Treatment of grade III-IV decubitus ulcers with anaerobic infection, inflammatory bowel disease.

CONTRAINDICATIONS
Hypersensitivity to metronidazole or other nitroimidazole derivatives (also parabens with topical application).
    Alcohol and alcohol-containing foods and products.
    Refrain from sexual intercourse during therapy for trichomoniasis.

INTERACTIONS
Drug
Alcohol and alcohol-containing products: May cause a disulfiram-type reaction. Generally, do not ingest during treatment and for 3 days after treatment.
Disulfiram: May increase the risk of toxicity.
Oral anticoagulants: May increase the effects of these drugs.
Phenobarbital: Possible decreased action.
Tacrolimus: Possible increased levels of tacrolimus.
Warfarin, carbamazepine: Possible increased effects of these drugs.
Herbal
None known.
Food
Ethanol: (See Alcohol above).

DIAGNOSTIC TEST EFFECTS
May increase serum LDH, AST (SGOT), and ALT (SGPT) levels.

M

ⓦ IV INCOMPATIBILITIES

Amphotericin B complex (Abelcet, AmBisome, Amphotec), filgrastim (Neupogen).

ⓦ IV COMPATIBILITIES

Diltiazem (Cardizem), dopamine (Intropin), heparin, hydromorphone (Dilaudid), lorazepam (Ativan), magnesium sulfate, midazolam (Versed), morphine.

SIDE EFFECTS

Frequent
Systemic: Anorexia, nausea, dry mouth, metallic taste.
Vaginal: Symptomatic cervicitis and vaginitis, abdominal cramps, uterine pain.
Occasional
Systemic: Diarrhea or constipation, vomiting, dizziness, erythematous rash, urticaria, reddish brown urine.
Topical: Transient erythema, mild dryness, burning, irritation, stinging, tearing when applied too close to eyes.
Vaginal: Vaginal, perineal, or vulvar itching; vulvar swelling.
Rare
Mild, transient leukopenia; thrombophlebitis with IV therapy, visual impairment.

SERIOUS REACTIONS

• Oral therapy may result in furry tongue, glossitis, cystitis, dysuria, pancreatitis, and flattening of T waves on ECG readings.
• Peripheral neuropathy, manifested as numbness and tingling in hands or feet, is usually reversible if treatment is stopped immediately after neurologic symptoms appear.
• Seizures occur occasionally.

PRECAUTIONS & CONSIDERATIONS

Caution is warranted with blood dyscrasias, central nervous system (CNS) disorders, severe hepatic dysfunction, predisposition to edema, and in those receiving corticosteroid therapy concurrently. Metronidazole readily crosses the placenta and is distributed in breast milk; caution warranted in lactation. Metronidazole use is contraindicated during the first trimester of pregnancy in women with trichomoniasis. Topical use during pregnancy or breastfeeding is discouraged. No age-related precautions have been noted in children; however, the safety and efficacy of topical administration in those younger than 21 yrs have not been established. Age-related hepatic impairment may require a dosage adjustment in elderly patients. Prolonged indwelling catheters should be avoided. Avoid alcohol and alcohol-containing preparations (such as cough syrups and elixirs) during and for at least 3 days post therapy, excessive sunlight, exposure to very hot and cold temperatures, and hot and spicy foods while taking metronidazole. Avoid sexual intercourse, if taking metronidazole for trichomoniasis, until the full treatment is completed.

Urine may become reddish brown during therapy. Skin should be examined for rash and urticaria. Pattern of daily bowel activity and stool consistency should be monitored; document the number and characteristics of stools in those with amebiasis. Be alert for signs and symptoms of superinfection, including abdominal pain, moderate to severe diarrhea, severe anal or genital pruritus, and severe mouth soreness. In addition, be alert for neurologic symptoms such as dizziness and paresthesia. Any of these symptoms should be reported to a health care provider immediately for re-evaluation of medical choice. Avoid tasks requiring mental alertness or motor skills until the drug is established. Metronidazole acts on papules, pustules, and erythema but has no effect on ocular problems (conjunctivitis, keratitis, blepharitis), rhinophyma (hypertrophy of nose), or telangiectasia.

Storage
Store ready-to-use infusion bags at room temperature.

Administration
Take oral metronidazole without regard to food. However, give it with food if GI upset occurs.

For IV use, infuse metronidazole over 30-60 min. Do not give as an IV bolus injection.

Metyrosine
me-tye'roe-seen
(Demser)

CATEGORY AND SCHEDULE
Pregnancy Risk Category: C

Classification: Antihypertensives

MECHANISM OF ACTION
A tyrosine hydroxylase inhibitor that blocks conversion of tyrosine to dihydroxyphenylalanine, the rate-limiting step in the biosynthetic pathway of catecholamines. *Therapeutic Effect:* Reduces levels of endogenous catecholamines.

PHARMACOKINETICS
Well absorbed from the GI tract. Metabolized in the liver. Excreted primarily in the urine. *Half-life:* 7.2 h.

AVAILABILITY
Capsules: 250 mg (Demser).

INDICATIONS AND DOSAGES
▸ **Pheochomocytoma**
PO
Adults, Elderly, Children 12 yr and older. Initially, 250 mg 4 times/day. Increase by 250-500 mg/day up to 4 g/day. Maintenance: 2-4 g/day in 4 divided doses.

CONTRAINDICATIONS
Hypertension of unknown etiology, hypersensitivity to metyrosine or any component of the formulation.

INTERACTIONS
Drug
Alcohol and CNS depressants: May increase CNS depressant effects.
Phenothiazines, haloperidol: May potentiate extrapyramidal symptoms (EPS).
Herbal
None known.
Food
None known.

DIAGNOSTIC TEST EFFECTS
None known.

SIDE EFFECTS
Frequent
Drowsiness, extrapyramidal symptoms, diarrhea.
Occasional
Galactorrhea, edema of the breasts, nausea, vomiting, dry mouth, impotence, nasal congestion.
Rare
Lower extremity edema, urinary problems, urticaria, anemia,

M

depression, disorientation, crystalluria.

SERIOUS REACTIONS
• Serious or life-threatening allergic reaction characterized hallucinations, hematuria, hyperstimulation after withdrawal, severe lower-extremity edema, and parkinsonism.

PRECAUTIONS & CONSIDERATIONS
❗ Medication may be given in advance of adrenal tumor removal, usually 5-7 days before surgery.

Caution should be used with impaired liver or renal function. It is unknown whether metyrosine is distributed in breast milk; caution in lactation is warranted. Safety and efficacy of metyrosine have not been established in children younger than 12 yrs old. Elderly patients with impaired renal function may need dose adjustment. Alcoholic beverages should be avoided during therapy.

Trismus may indicate overdosage and needs to be reported.

Administration
Take without regard to food. Maintain adequate fluid intake.

Mexiletine Hydrochloride
mex-il′e-teen high-droh-klor-ide (Mexitil)

CATEGORY AND SCHEDULE
Pregnancy Risk Category: C

Classification: Antiarrhythmics (class IB, lidocaine analogue)

MECHANISM OF ACTION
An antiarrhythmic that shortens duration of action potential and decreases effective refractory period in the His-Purkinje system of the myocardium by blocking sodium transport across myocardial cell membranes. *Therapeutic Effect:* Suppresses ventricular arrhythmias.

PHARMACOKINETICS
PO: Peak 2-3 h. Metabolized by the liver; excreted unchanged by kidneys (10%); excreted in breast milk. *Half-life:* 12 h.

AVAILABILITY
Capsules: 150 mg, 200 mg, 250 mg.

INDICATIONS AND DOSAGES
▸ **Arrhythmias**
PO
Adults, Elderly. Initially, 200 mg q8h. Adjust dosage by 50-100 mg at 2- to 3-day intervals. Maximum: 1200 mg/day, in divided doses q8h.

OFF-LABEL USES
Treatment of diabetic neuropathy.

CONTRAINDICATIONS
Cardiogenic shock, preexisting second- or third-degree AV block, right bundle-branch block without presence of pacemaker.

INTERACTIONS
Drug
Anesthetics, vasoconstrictors, anticholinergics: No specific interactions are noted; however, these drugs should be used in the lowest effective dose to avoid affecting the cardiac activity of mexilitine.
Cimetidine: May increase mexiletine blood concentration.

CYP2D6 inhibitors: Would be expected to increase mexiletine concentrations.

Metoclopramide: May increase mexiletine absorption.

Phenobarbital, phenytoin, rifampin: May decrease mexiletine blood concentration.

Herbal
None known.

Food
None known.

DIAGNOSTIC TEST EFFECTS

May increase liver enzymes, such as ALT and AST. May decrease WBCs and thrombocytes.

SIDE EFFECTS

Frequent (> 10%)
GI distress, including nausea, vomiting, and heartburn; dizziness; lightheadedness; tremor.

Occasional (1%-10%)
Nervousness, change in sleep habits, headache, visual disturbances, paresthesia, diarrhea or constipation, palpitations, chest pain, rash, respiratory difficulty, edema.

SERIOUS REACTIONS

• Mexiletine has the ability to worsen existing arrhythmias or produce new ones.
• CHF may occur, and existing CHF may worsen.

PRECAUTIONS & CONSIDERATIONS

Caution is warranted with CHF, impaired myocardial function, second- and third-degree AV block, with pacemaker, and sick-sinus syndrome. Nasal decongestants and OTC cold preparations should be avoided without physician approval. Alcohol and salt intake should be restricted.

Notify the physician if dark urine, cough, generalized fatigue, nausea, pale stools, severe or persistent abdominal pain, shortness of breath, unexplained sore throat or fever, vomiting, or yellowing of the eyes or skin occurs. ECG and vital signs should be monitored before and during therapy. Pulse for irregular rate and quality, GI disturbances, pattern of daily bowel activity and stool consistency, dizziness and syncope, hand movement for evidence of tremor, and signs and symptoms of CHF should be assessed.

Administration
If 300 mg every 8 h or less controls arrhythmias, the same total daily dose may be divided and given q12h. Do not crush, open, or break capsules. Take with food or antacid.

M

Miconazole
mih-kon′ah-zole
(Femizol-M, Micatin, Micozole
[CAN], Monistat [CAN],
Monistat-3, Monistat-7,
Monistat-Derm, Zeasorb AF)

CATEGORY AND SCHEDULE
Pregnancy Risk Category: C

Classification: Antifungals,
Imidazole

MECHANISM OF ACTION
An imidazole derivative that
inhibits synthesis of ergosterol (vital
component of fungal cell formation),
damaging cell membrane. *Therapeutic
Effect:* Fungistatic; may be fungicidal,
depending on concentration.

PHARMACOKINETICS
Parenteral: Widely distributed
in tissues. Metabolized in liver.
Primarily excreted in urine.
Half-life: 24 h. Topical: No
systemic absorption following
application to intact skin.
Intravaginally: Small amount
absorbed systemically.

AVAILABILITY
Vaginal Suppository: 100 mg
(Monistat-7), 200 mg
(Monistat-3).
Topical Cream: 2% (Micatin,
Monistat-Derm).
Vaginal Cream: 2% (Femizol-M).
Topical Powder: 2% (Micatin).
Topical Spray: 2% (Lotrimin-AF).
Topical Gel: 2% (Zeasorb AF).

INDICATIONS AND DOSAGES
▸ **Vulvovaginal candidiasis**
INTRAVAGINALLY
Adults, Elderly. One 200 mg
suppository at bedtime for
3 days; one 100-mg suppository
or one applicatorful at bedtime for
7 days.
▸ **Topical fungal infections,
cutaneous candidiasis**
TOPICAL
*Adults, Elderly, Children 2 yrs and
older.* Apply liberally 2 times/day,
morning, and evening. Usually for
2-4 wks.

CONTRAINDICATIONS
Hypersensitivity to miconazole or
any component of the formulation.
Topically: Children younger than
2 yrs old.

INTERACTIONS
Drug
**Oral anticoagulants, oral
hypoglycemics, warfarin:** May
increase effects of these drugs, even
with nonsystemic use (e.g., vaginal
use).
Herbal
None known.
Food
None known.

DIAGNOSTIC TEST EFFECTS
None known.

SIDE EFFECTS
Frequent
Phlebitis, fever, chills, rash, itching,
nausea, vomiting.
Occasional
Dizziness, drowsiness, headache,
flushed face, abdominal pain,
constipation, diarrhea, decreased
appetite.
Topical: Itching, burning, stinging,
erythema, urticaria.
Vaginal: Vulvovaginal burning,
itching, irritation, headache, skin rash.

SERIOUS REACTIONS
• Anemia, thrombocytopenia, and
liver toxicity occur rarely.

PRECAUTIONS & CONSIDERATIONS

Caution should be used with liver impairment. It is unknown whether miconazole crosses the placenta or is excreted in breast milk; therefore, caution warranted in pregnancy and lactation.

No age-related precautions have been noted in children or elderly patients. Medical consultation is necessary before administering antibiotics because of the propensity of antibiotic therapy to evoke a vaginal yeast infection.

Storage

Store at room temperature.

Administration

For intravaginal use, insert high in vagina. Be aware that the base in the vaginal preparation interacts with certain latex products such as contraceptive diaphragm.

For topical administration, wash and dry area before applying medication. Apply a thin layer on affected area. Avoid contact with eyes. Keep areas clean, dry; wear light clothing for ventilation. Separate personal items in contact with affected areas.

M

Midazolam Hydrochloride

mid-az′zoe-lam high-droh-klor-ide
(Apo-Midazolam [CAN], Hypnovel
[AUS], Versed)
**Do not confuse Versed with
VePesid.**

CATEGORY AND SCHEDULE

Pregnancy Risk Category: D
Controlled Substance: Schedule
IV

Classification: Benzodiazepines,
preanesthetics, sedatives adjunct

MECHANISM OF ACTION

A benzodiazepine that enhances
the action of γ-aminobutyric
acid, one of the major inhibitory
neurotransmitters in the brain.
Therapeutic Effect: Produces
anxiolytic, hypnotic, anticonvulsant,
muscle relaxant, and amnestic
effects.

PHARMACOKINETICS

Route	Onset (min)	Peak (min)	Duration
PO	10-20	NA	N/A
IV	1-5	5-7	20-30 min
IM	5-15	15-60	2-6 h

Well absorbed after IM
administration. Protein binding:
97%. Metabolized in the liver
to active metabolite. Primarily
excreted in urine. Not removed by
hemodialysis. *Half-life:* 1-5 h.

AVAILABILITY

Syrup: 2 mg/mL.
Injection: 1 mg/mL, 5 mg/mL.

INDICATIONS AND DOSAGES
▸ **Preoperative sedation**

PO
Children. 0.25-0.5 mg/kg.
Maximum: 20 mg.
IV
Children 6-12 yrs. 0.025-0.05 mg/kg.
Usual maximum: 10 mg.
Children 6 mo to 5 yrs. 0.05-0.1 mg/kg.
Usual maximum: 6 mg.
IM
Adults, Elderly. 0.07-0.08 mg/kg
30-60 min before surgery.
Children. 0.1-0.15 mg/kg 30-60 min
before surgery. Maximum: 10 mg.
▸ **Conscious sedation for diagnostic,
therapeutic, and endoscopic
procedures**
IV
Adults, Elderly. 1-2.5 mg over 2 min.
Titrate as needed. Maximum total
dose: 2.5-5 mg.
▸ **Conscious sedation during
mechanical ventilation**
IV
Adults, Elderly. 0.01-0.05 mg/kg;
may repeat q10-15min until
adequately sedated. Then continuous
infusion at initial rate of
0.02-0.1 mg/kg/h (1-7 mg/h).
Children older than 32 wks. Initially,
1 mcg/kg/min as continuous
infusion.
Children 32 wks and younger.
Initially, 0.5 mcg/kg/min as
continuous infusion.
▸ **Status epilepticus**
IV
Children older than 2 mo. Loading
dose of 0.15 mg/kg followed by
continuous infusion of 1 mcg/kg/min.
Titrate as needed. Range:
1-18 mcg/kg/min.

CONTRAINDICATIONS

Acute alcohol intoxication, acute
angle-closure glaucoma, coma, shock,
hypersensitivity to drug, cherries (PO
syrup), or other components.
 Nelfinavir, ritonavir, indinavir,
saquinavir: Contraindicated use.

Caution
Congestive heart failure (CHF), chronic obstructive pulmonary disease (COPD), chronic renal failure, chills, elderly, debilitated, children younger than 18 yrs.

To be used only by health care professionals skilled in airway maintenance and ventilation and resuscitation techniques.

INTERACTIONS
Drug
Alcohol, other CNS depressants: May increase CNS and respiratory depression and hypotensive effects of midazolam.
Erythromycin, clarithromycin, ketoconazole, itraconazole, fluconazole, miconazole (systemic), dilitiazem, fluvoxamine: Likely increased serum levels and prolonged effect of benzodiazepines.
Hypotension-producing medications: May increase hypotensive effects of midazolam.
Protease inhibitors: Increase midazolam concentrations. Generally contraindicated.
Herbal
Kava kava, valerian: May increase CNS depression.
Food
Grapefruit juice: Increases the oral absorption and systemic availability of midazolam.

DIAGNOSTIC TEST EFFECTS
None known.

⊘ IV INCOMPATIBILITIES
Albumin, ampicillin and sulbactam (Unasyn), amphotericin B complex (Abelcet, AmBisome, Amphotec), ampicillin (Polycillin), bumetanide (Bumex), co-trimoxazole (Bactrim), dexamethasone (Decadron), fosphenytoin (Cerebyx), furosemide (Lasix),

hydrocortisone (Solu-Cortef), methotrexate, nafcillin (Nafcil), sodium bicarbonate, sodium pentothal (Thiopental).

⬗ IV COMPATIBILITIES
Amiodarone (Cordarone), calcium gluconate, diltiazem (Cardizem), dobutamine (Dobutrex), dopamine (Intropin), etomidate (Amidate), fentanyl (Sublimaze), heparin, hydromorphone (Dilaudid), insulin, lorazepam (Ativan), milrinone (Primacor), morphine, nitroglycerin, norepinephrine (Levophed), potassium chloride, propofol (Diprivan).

SIDE EFFECTS
Frequent (4%-10%)
Decreased respiratory rate, tenderness at IM or IV injection site, pain during injection, oxygen desaturation, hiccups.
Occasional (2%-3%)
Hypotension, paradoxical CNS reaction.
Rare (< 2%)
Nausea, vomiting, headache, coughing.

SERIOUS REACTIONS
• Inadequate or excessive dosage or improper administration may result in cerebral hypoxia, agitation, involuntary movements, hyperactivity, and combativeness.
• A too-rapid IV rate, excessive doses, or a single large dose increases the risk of respiratory depression or arrest.
• Respiratory depression or apnea may produce hypoxia and cardiac arrest.

PRECAUTIONS & CONSIDERATIONS
Caution is warranted in patients with acute illness, CHF, pulmonary, renal, or hepatic impairment, severe fluid and electrolyte imbalance, and

M

treated angle-closure glaucoma. Midazolam crosses the placenta; it is unknown whether midazolam is distributed in breast milk; caution in lactation is warranted. Women on long-term therapy should use effective contraception during therapy. Notify the physician immediately if she becomes or might be pregnant. Neonates are more likely to experience respiratory depression. In elderly patients, age-related renal impairment may require dosage adjustment.

! Respiratory depression or apnea may produce hypoxia and cardiac arrest. Flumazenil would be reversal agent. Oral drug is not for chronic or home administration. Only give if patient is under direct observation of a health care professional.

Midazolam produces an amnesic effect. Vital signs should be obtained before and after administering midazolam. Respiratory rate and oxygen saturation should be monitored continuously during parenteral administration to detect apnea and respiratory depression. Sedation should be assessed every 3-5 min.

! All doses of midazolam must be reduced when used in combination with any CNS depressant; serious respiratory and cardiovascular depression, including death, has occurred when midazolam is used in combination with other CNS depressants or is given too rapidly. Medically compromised and elderly patients are at the greatest risk for this effect.

Storage
Store vials at room temperature.

Administration
! Midazolam dosage is individualized based on age, underlying disease, and medications and on the desired effect.

Midazolam may be given undiluted or as an infusion. Ensure that resuscitative supplies, such as endotracheal tubes, suction equipment, and oxygen, are readily available. Administer the drug by slow IV injection in incremental doses. Give each incremental dose over 2 min or more and wait at least 2 min between doses. Reduce the IV rate in patients older than 60 yrs, debilitated patients, and those with chronic diseases or impaired pulmonary function. A too-rapid IV rate, excessive doses, or a single large dose increases the risk of respiratory depression or arrest.

For IM use, inject the drug deep into a large muscle mass, such as the gluteus maximus.

Midodrine
mid′o-dreen
(Amatine, ProAmatine)
Do not confuse ProAmantine with Amantadine or protamine.

CATEGORY AND SCHEDULE
Pregnancy Risk Category: C

Classification: Vasopresor; orthostatic hypotension adjunct

MECHANISM OF ACTION
A vasopressor that forms the active metabolite desglymidodrine, an alpha$_1$-agonist, activating alpha receptors of the arteriolar and venous vasculature. *Therapeutic Effect:* Increases vascular tone and BP.

PHARMACOKINETICS
Peak: 1-2 h. Bioavailability 90%. *Half-life:* 3-4 h.

AVAILABILITY
Tablets: 2.5 mg, 5 mg, 10 mg.

INDICATIONS AND DOSAGES
▶ **Orthostatic hypotension**
PO
Adults, Elderly. 10 mg 3 times
a day. Give during the day
when patient is upright, such as
upon arising, midday, and late
afternoon. Do not give later than
6:00 PM.
▶ **Dosage in renal impairment**
For adults and elderly patients,
give 2.5 mg 3 times a day; increase
gradually, as tolerated.

CONTRAINDICATIONS
Acute renal function impairment,
persistent hypertension,
pheochromocytoma, severe cardiac
disease, thyrotoxicosis, urine retention.

INTERACTIONS
Drug
α-Adrenergic agonists: Increased
risk of pressor effects.
Digoxin: May have additive
bradycardia effects.
**Sodium-retaining steroids (such
as fludrocortisone):** May increase
sodium retention.
Vasoconstrictors: May have an
additive vasoconstricting effect.
Herbal
None known.
Food
None known.

DIAGNOSTIC TEST EFFECTS
None known.

SIDE EFFECTS
Frequent (7%-20%)
Paresthesia, piloerection, pruritus,
dysuria, supine hypertension.
Occasional (< 1%-7%)
Pain, rash, chills, headache, facial
flushing, confusion, dry mouth, anxiety.

SERIOUS REACTIONS
• None known.

PRECAUTIONS & CONSIDERATIONS
Caution is warranted with a history
of vision problems and renal and
hepatic impairment. BP and liver and
renal function test results should be
monitored. OTC medications, such
as cough, cold, and diet preparations
should be avoided because they may
affect BP.
Administration
Do not take the last dose of the
day after the evening meal or
< 4 h before bedtime. Do not
take the medication while lying
down. Caution warranted with
position changes due to possible
development of orthostatic
hypotension. Use cough, cold, and
diet aids cautiously because of their
effect on BP.

M

Mifepristone
miff-eh-pris′tone
(Mifeprex)
**Do not confuse Mifeprex with
Mirapex or mifepristone with
misoprostol.**

CATEGORY AND SCHEDULE
Pregnancy Risk Category: X

Classification: Abortifacients,
oxazolidinediones, stimulants,
uterine

MECHANISM OF ACTION
An abortifacient that has
antiprogestational activity resulting
from competitive interaction
with progesterone. Inhibits
the activity of endogenous or
exogenous progesterone. Also
has antiglucocorticoid and weak

antiandrogenic activity. *Therapeutic Effect:* Terminates pregnancy.

PHARMACOKINETICS
Rapidly absorbed; absolute bioavailability (20 mg oral dose) is 90%, 98% protein bound; nonlinear kinetics. Metabolized in liver by CYP 450 3A4 hepatic enzymes. Eliminated in feces and urine. *Half-life:* 18 h.

AVAILABILITY
Tablets: 200 mg.

INDICATIONS AND DOSAGES
▸ **Termination of pregnancy**
PO
Adults. Day 1: 600 mg as single dose. Day 3: 400 mcg misoprostol. Day 14: Post-treatment examination.

OFF-LABEL USES
Cushing syndrome, endometriosis, intrauterine fetal death or nonviable early pregnancy, postcoital contraception, refractory hormone-responsive breast cancer.

CONTRAINDICATIONS
Chronic adrenal failure, concurrent long-term steroid or anticoagulant therapy, confirmed or suspected ectopic pregnancy, intrauterine device (IUD) in place, hemorrhagic disorders, inherited porphyria.

INTERACTIONS
Drug
Carbamazepine, phenobarbital, phenytoin, rifampin: May increase the metabolism of mifepristone.
Erythromycin, dexamethasone, itraconazole, ketoconazole: May induce the CYP metabolism of mifepristone.
Herbal
St. John's wort: May increase the metabolism of mifepristone.

Food
Grapefruit: May inhibit the metabolism of mifepristone.

DIAGNOSTIC TEST EFFECTS
May decrease hemoglobin level and hematocrit and RBC count.

SIDE EFFECTS
Frequent (> 10%)
Headache, dizziness, abdominal pain, nausea, vomiting, diarrhea, fatigue.
Occasional (3%-10%)
Uterine hemorrhage, insomnia, vaginitis, dyspepsia, back pain, fever, viral infections, rigors.
Rare (1%-2%)
Anxiety, syncope, anemia, asthenia, leg pain, sinusitis, leucorrhea.

SERIOUS REACTIONS
• None known.

PRECAUTIONS & CONSIDERATIONS
Caution is warranted with cardiovascular disease, diabetes, hepatic or renal impairment, hypertension, severe anemia, and in persons older than 35 yrs of age or who smoke more than 10 cigarettes a day. Be aware that anticonvulsants, erythromycin, itraconazole, ketoconazole, and rifampin may inhibit the metabolism of mifepristone. Uterine cramping and vaginal bleeding may occur. Hemoglobin level and hematocrit should be monitored. An IUD, if in place, should be removed before therapy begins.
! Sometimes serious or fatal infection and bleeding occur very rapidly following spontaneous, surgical and medical abortions, including the use of mifepristone. Immediately report sustained fever > 100.4° F, severe abdominal pain, prolonged heavy bleeding, syncope.

! Health care provider must supervise administration of mifepristone. Clinical examination is necessary to confirm complete termination of pregnancy 14 days post treatment. Overdose is evidenced by adrenal failure. Bleeding for 9-16 days is not unexpected; heavy bleeding must be reported immediately.

Storage
Refrigerate ampoules.

Administration
! Treatment with mifepristone and misoprostol requires three office visits; only distributed to registered prescribers in the United States.

Miglitol
mig-lee′tall
(Glyset)

CATEGORY AND SCHEDULE
Pregnancy Risk Category: B

Classification: Oligosaccharide, glucosidase enzyme inhibitor, Antidiabetic agents

MECHANISM OF ACTION
An α-glucosidase inhibitor that delays the digestion of ingested carbohydrates into simple sugars such as glucose. *Therapeutic Effect:* Produces smaller rise in blood glucose concentration after meals.

PHARMACOKINETICS
PO: Peak plasma levels 2-3 h; negligible plasma protein binding, not metabolized, urinary excretion.

AVAILABILITY
Tablets: 25 mg, 50 mg, 100 mg.

INDICATIONS AND DOSAGES
▸ **Diabetes mellitus**
PO
Adults, Elderly. Initially, 25 mg 3 times a day with first bite of each main meal. Maintenance: 50 mg 3 times a day. Maximum: 100 mg 3 times a day.

CONTRAINDICATIONS
Colonic ulceration, diabetic ketoacidosis, hypersensitivity to miglitol, inflammatory bowel disease, partial intestinal obstruction.

INTERACTIONS
Drug
Digoxin, propranolol, ranitidine: May decrease the blood concentrations and effects of these drugs.
Herbal
None known.
Food
None known.

DIAGNOSTIC TEST EFFECTS
None known.

SIDE EFFECTS
Frequent (10%-40%)
Flatulence, loose stools, diarrhea, abdominal pain.
Occasional (5%)
Rash.

PRECAUTIONS & CONSIDERATIONS
Caution is warranted in patients with renal impairment. Adequate studies have not been done in pregnant women. Miglitol is distributed to a very low amount in breast milk; caution warranted in lactation. Safety and efficacy have not been established in children.

Food intake and blood glucose should be monitored before and during therapy. Be aware of signs

M

and symptoms of hypoglycemia (anxiety, cool wet skin, diplopia, dizziness, headache, hunger, numbness in mouth, tachycardia, tremors) or hyperglycemia (deep rapid breathing, dim vision, fatigue, nausea, polydipsia, polyphagia, polyuria, vomiting); carry glucose-based supplement for immediate response to hypoglycemia. Consult the physician when glucose demands are altered (such as with fever, heavy physical activity, infection, stress, trauma). Exercise, good personal hygiene (including foot care), not smoking, and weight control are essential parts of therapy. Type 2 diabetic patients may be using insulin concomitantly; if symptomatic hypoglycemia occurs while taking miglitol, use glucose rather than sucrose to reverse hypoglycemic effect owing to interference with sucrose metabolism.

Administration
Take with the first bite of each main meal. If a meal is skipped, do not give that dose.

Miglustat
mig-lew′stat
(Zavesca)

CATEGORY AND SCHEDULE
Pregnancy Risk Category: X

Classification: Enzyme inhibitor

MECHANISM OF ACTION
A Gaucher disease agent that inhibits the enzyme, glucosylceramide synthase, reducing the rate of synthesis of most glycosphingolipids. Allows the residual activity of the deficient enzyme, glucocerebrosidase, to be more effective in degrading lysosomal storage within tissues. *Therapeutic Effect*: Minimizes conditions associated with Gaucher disease, such as anemia and bone disease.

PHARMACOKINETICS
PO: Maximum plasma levels attained in 2-2.5 h; oral bioavailability 97%, no plasma protein binding. Excreted unchanged in the urine. *Half-life:* Approximately 6-7 h.

AVAILABILITY
Capsules: 100 mg.

INDICATIONS AND DOSAGES
▸ **Gaucher disease**
PO
Adults, Elderly. One 100-mg capsule 3 times a day at regular intervals.
▸ **Dosage in renal impairment**
For patients with creatinine clearance of 50-70 mL/min, dosage is reduced to 100 mg twice a day.
For patients with creatinine clearance of 30-49 mL/min dosage is 100 mg once a day. If CrCl < 30 mL/min, use is not recommended.

CONTRAINDICATIONS
Women who are or may become pregnant, severe renal impairment, hypersensitivity.

INTERACTIONS
Drug
Aspirin, NSAIDs, other salicylates: May decrease platelet aggregation.
Imiglucerase: May decrease the effects of imiglucerase.
Herbal
None known.

Food
None known.

DIAGNOSTIC TEST EFFECTS
None known but should provide pretreatment neurologic evaluation.

SIDE EFFECTS
Expected (65%-89%)
Diarrhea, weight loss.
Frequent (11%-39%)
Hand tremor, flatulence, headache, abdominal pain, nausea.
Occasional (4%-7%)
Paresthesia, anorexia, dyspepsia, leg cramps, vomiting, neuropathy.

SERIOUS REACTIONS
• Thrombocytopenia occurs in 7% of patients.
• Overdose produces dizziness and neutropenia.

PRECAUTIONS & CONSIDERATIONS
Caution is warranted in patients with impaired fertility and renal function. Reliable contraceptive methods are necessary during miglustat treatment and for 3 mo afterward. Notify the physician and plan to stop miglustat therapy before trying to conceive. Avoid high-carbohydrate foods during miglustat treatment if diarrhea occurs. Contraindicated in pregnancy; extreme caution is warranted in lactation.

Notify the physician of hand tremor. Adequate hydration should be maintained. Baseline neurologic evaluation should be performed, with follow-up evaluations every 6 mo throughout treatment. Pattern of daily bowel activity and stool consistency and weight should be monitored.

Administration
Take miglustat without regard to food. Do not open, crush, or break capsules.

Milrinone Lactate
mill're-none lack-tayte
(Primacor)

CATEGORY AND SCHEDULE
Pregnancy Risk Category: C

Classification: Inotropes

MECHANISM OF ACTION
A cardiac inotropic agent that inhibits phosphodiesterase, which increases cyclic adenosine monophosphate and potentiates the delivery of calcium to myocardial contractile systems. *Therapeutic Effect:* Relaxes vascular muscle, causing vasodilation. Increases cardiac output; decreases pulmonary capillary wedge pressure and vascular resistance.

PHARMACOKINETICS

Route	Onset	Peak	Duration
IV	5-15 min	NA	NA

Protein binding: 70%. Primarily excreted unchanged in urine. *Half-life:* 2.4 h.

AVAILABILITY
Injection: 1 mg/mL, 10-mL single-dose vial, 20-mg single-dose vial, 50-mL single-dose vial, 5-mL sterile cartridge unit.
Injection (Premix): 200 mcg/mL.

INDICATIONS AND DOSAGES
▸ **Short-term management of congestive heart failure (CHF)**
IV INFUSION
Adults. Initially, 50 mcg/kg over 10 min. Continue with maintenance infusion rate of 0.375-0.75 mcg/kg/min based on hemodynamic and clinical

response. Total daily dosage:
0.59-1.13 mg/kg/day.
▸**Dosage in renal impairment**
For patients with severe renal
impairment, reduce initial dosage
to 0.2-0.43 mcg/kg/min.
Maximum: 0.75 mcg/kg/min.

CONTRAINDICATIONS

Hypersensitivity, severe obstructive
aortic or pulmonic vascular disease
(untreated).

INTERACTIONS

Drug
Other cardiac glycosides: Produces
additive inotropic effects.
Herbal
None known.
Food
None known.

DIAGNOSTIC TEST EFFECTS

None known.

⃠ IV INCOMPATIBILITIES

Furosemide (Lasix).

▽ IV COMPATIBILITIES

Calcium gluconate, digoxin
(Lanoxin), diltiazem (Cardizem),
dobutamine (Dobutrex), dopamine
(Intropin), heparin, lidocaine,
magnesium, midazolam (Versed),
nitroglycerin, potassium, propofol
(Diprivan).

SIDE EFFECTS

Occasional (1%-3%)
Headache, hypotension.
Rare (< 1%)
Angina, chest pain.

SERIOUS REACTIONS

• Supraventricular and ventricular
arrhythmias (12%), nonsustained
ventricular tachycardia (2%), and
sustained ventricular tachycardia
(1%) may occur.

PRECAUTIONS & CONSIDERATIONS

Caution is warranted in patients with
atrial fibrillation or flutter, history
of ventricular arrhythmias, impaired
renal function, and severe obstructive
aortic or pulmonic valvular disease.
It is unknown whether milrinone
crosses the placenta or is distributed
in breast milk; therefore, caution is
warranted in lactation. The safety
and efficacy of milrinone have not
been established in children. In
elderly patients, age-related renal
impairment may require dosage
adjustment.

Notify the physician if palpitations
or chest pain occurs. Cardiac output,
heart rate, BP, renal function, and
serum potassium levels should be
assessed before beginning treatment
and during IV therapy. Breath sounds
for crackles and rhonchi and skin
for edema should also be assessed.
Headache, tremors should be
reported immediately; should not use
for more than 5 days concurrently.
Storage
Store at room temperature. Do not
freeze.
Administration
For IV infusion, dilute 20-mg
(20-mL) vial with 80 or 180 mL
diluent (0.9% NaCl, D5W) or 10-mg
(10-mL) vial with 40 or 90 mL
diluent to provide concentration of
200 or 100 mcg/mL, respectively.
Maximum concentration:
100 mg/250 mL. For a loading-
dose IV injection, administer
milrinone undiluted slowly over
10 min. Monitor for arrhythmias
and hypotension during IV therapy.
If one or both of these conditions
occur, reduce or temporarily
discontinue infusion until condition
stabilizes.

Minocycline Hydrochloride

mi-noe-sye'kleen high-droh-klor-ide
(Arestin, Akamin [AUS], Dynacin, Minocin, Minomycin [AUS], Myrac, Novo Minocycline [CAN])

Do not confuse Dynacin with Dynabac or Minocin with Mithracin or niacin, or Akamin with Amikacin.

CATEGORY AND SCHEDULE

Pregnancy Risk Category: D

Classification: Tetracycline anti-infective

MECHANISM OF ACTION

A tetracycline antibiotic that inhibits bacterial protein synthesis by binding to ribosomes. *Therapeutic Effects:* Bacteriostatic.

PHARMACOKINETICS

PO: Peak 2-3 h. 55%-88% protein bound; Excreted in urine, feces, breast milk; crosses placenta.
Half-life: 11-17 h.

AVAILABILITY

Capsules (Dynacin, Minocin): 50 mg, 75 mg, 100 mg.
Capsules, Pellet-Filled (Minocin): 50 mg, 100 mg.
Tablets (Minocin, Myrac): 50 mg, 75 mg, 100 mg.
Microspheres for Peridontal Use: 1 mg (Arestin).

INDICATIONS AND DOSAGES

▸ **Mild, moderate or severe prostate, urinary tract, central nervous system (CNS) infections (excluding meningitis); uncomplicated gonorrhea; inflammatory acne; brucellosis; skin granulomas;**
cholera; trachoma; nocardiasis; yaws; syphillis when penicillins are contraindicated
PO
Adults, Elderly. Initially, 100-200 mg, then 100 mg q12h or 50 mg q6h.
PO
Children older than 8 yrs. Initially, 4 mg/kg, then 2 mg/kg q12h.
▸ **Periodontitis**
Adults. 1 unit dose cartridge (1 mg) per periodontal pocket.

CONTRAINDICATIONS

Children younger than 8 yrs, hypersensitivity to tetracyclines, last half of pregnancy.

INTERACTIONS

Drug
Carbamazepine, phenytoin: May decrease minocycline blood concentration.
Cholestyramine, colestipol: May decrease minocycline absorption.
Isotretinoin: Contraindicated use.
Oral contraceptives: May decrease the effects of oral contraceptives.
Herbal
St. John's wort: May increase the risk of photosensitivity.
Food
Antacids; milk; other magnesium-, iron-, calcium-, and aluminum-containing products: Decreased antiinfective effect. Separate times of administration.

DIAGNOSTIC TEST EFFECTS

May increase serum alkaline phosphatase, amylase, bilirubin, AST (SGOT), and ALT (SGPT) levels.

May increase eosinophil counts; check CBC with differential; SCr and CrCl periodically during therapy.

M

SIDE EFFECTS

Frequent

Dizziness, lightheadedness, diarrhea, nausea, vomiting, abdominal cramps, possibly severe photosensitivity, drowsiness, vertigo.

Occasional

Altered pigmentation of skin or mucous membranes, rectal or genital pruritus, stomatitis, eosinophilia.

SERIOUS REACTIONS

• Superinfection (especially fungal), anaphylaxis, and benign intracranial hypertension may occur.

• Bulging fontanelles occur rarely in infants.

• Pseudomembranous colitis from *Clostridium difficile* infection may occur during treatment or at any time several mo after therapy is discontinued.

PRECAUTIONS & CONSIDERATIONS

Caution is warranted in patients with renal impairment and in those who cannot avoid sun or ultraviolet exposure because such exposure may produce a severe photosensitivity reaction.

History of allergies, especially to tetracyclines or sulfites, should be determined before drug therapy. Dizziness, drowsiness, and vertigo may occur while taking minocycline. Avoid tasks that require mental alertness or motor skills until response to the drug is established. Pattern of daily bowel activity, stool consistency, food intake and tolerance, renal function, skin for rash should be assessed. Be alert for signs and symptoms of superinfection, such as anal or genital pruritus, diarrhea, sore tongue, fever, fatigue and ulceration or changes of the oral mucosa or tongue; report symptoms to health care provider immediately. BP and level of consciousness should be monitored because of the potential for increased intracranial pressure. Do not use in patients under 8 yrs or in pregnancy because of the likelihood of permanent intrinsic staining in erupted permanent teeth not associated with the calcification stage. Advise patient to report any signs or symptoms associated with frequent loose stools or bloody diarrhea, both of which could indicate pseudomembranous colitis or *C. difficile* infection. Advise patient to maintain compliance with oral contraceptive medications while using an additional nonhormonal form of contraception throughout the duration of therapy.

Storage

Store the oral drug at room temperature.

Administration

Take capsules and tablets with a full glass of water. Space drug doses evenly around the clock.

Microspheres for periodontal use are administered by the periodontist.

Minoxidil
min-nox′i-dill
(Apo-Gain [CAN], Loniten, Milnox [CAN], Regaine [AUS], Rogaine, Rogaine Extra Strength)
Do not confuse Loniten with Lotensin.

CATEGORY AND SCHEDULE
Pregnancy Risk Category: C
OTC (topical solution)

Classification: Antihypertensives

MECHANISM OF ACTION
An antihypertensive and hair growth stimulant that has direct action on vascular smooth muscle, producing vasodilation of arterioles. *Therapeutic Effect:* Decreases peripheral vascular resistance and BP; increases cutaneous blood flow; stimulates hair follicle epithelium and hair follicle growth.

PHARMACOKINETICS

Route	Onset	Peak	Duration
PO	0.5 h	2-8 h	2-5 days

Well absorbed from the GI tract; minimal absorption after topical application. Protein binding: None. Widely distributed. Metabolized in the liver to active metabolite. Primarily excreted in urine. Removed by hemodialysis. *Half-life:* 4.2 h.

AVAILABILITY
Tablets (Loniten): 2.5 mg, 10 mg.
Topical Solution (Rogaine): 2% (20 mg/mL).
Topical Solution (Rogaine Extra Strength): 5% (50 mg/mL).
Topical Foam. 5%

INDICATIONS AND DOSAGES
▸ **Severe symptomatic hypertension, hypertension associated with organ damage; hypertension that has failed to respond to maximal therapeutic dosages of a diuretic or two other antihypertensives**
PO
Adults, Children 12 yr and older. Initially, 5 mg/day. Increase with at least 3-day intervals to 10 mg, then 20 mg, then up to 40 mg/day in 1-2 doses. Maximum: 100 mg/day.
Elderly. Initially, 2.5 mg/day. May increase gradually. Maintenance: 10-40 mg/day. Maximum: 100 mg/day.
Children under 12 yr of age. Initially, 0.1-0.2 mg/kg (5-mg maximum) daily. Gradually increase at minimum 3-day intervals. Maintenance: 0.25-1 mg/kg/day divided in 1-2 doses. Maximum: 50 mg/day.
▸ **Hair regrowth**
TOPICAL
Adults. 1 mL to affected areas of scalp 2 times a day. Total daily dose not to exceed 2 mL.

CONTRAINDICATIONS
Pheochromocytoma, hypersensitivity.
Caution
Lactation, children, renal disease, coronary artery disease (CAD), congestive heart failure (CHF).

INTERACTIONS
Drug
Central nervous system (CNS) depressants used in conscious sedation technique: May increase hypotensive effect.
Parenteral antihypertensives: May increase hypotensive effect.
NSAIDs, indomethacin, sympathomimetics: May decrease the hypotensive effects of minoxidil.

M

Herbal
None known.
Food
None known.

DIAGNOSTIC TEST EFFECTS
May increase plasma renin activity and BUN, serum alkaline phosphatase, serum creatinine, and serum sodium levels. May decrease blood hemoglobin and hematocrit levels and erythrocyte count.

SIDE EFFECTS
Frequent
PO: Edema with concurrent weight gain, hypertrichosis (elongation, thickening, increased pigmentation of fine body hair; develops in 80% of patients within 3-6 wks after beginning therapy).
Occasional
PO: T-wave changes (usually revert to pretreatment state with continued therapy or drug withdrawal).
Topical: Pruritus, rash, dry or flaking skin, erythema.
Rare
PO: Breast tenderness, headache, photosensitivity reaction.
Topical: Allergic reaction, alopecia, burning sensation at scalp, soreness at hair root, headache, visual disturbances.

SERIOUS REACTIONS
• Tachycardia and angina pectoris may occur because of increased oxygen demands associated with increased heart rate and cardiac output.
• Fluid and electrolyte imbalance and CHF may occur, especially if a diuretic is not given concurrently with minoxidil.
• Too rapid reduction in BP may result in syncope, cerebrovascular accident (CVA), myocardial infarction (MI), and ocular or vestibular ischemia.

• Pericardial effusion and tamponade may be seen in patients with impaired renal function who are not on dialysis.

PRECAUTIONS & CONSIDERATIONS
Caution is warranted with chronic CHF, coronary artery disease, recent MI (within 1 mo), and severe renal impairment. Minoxidil crosses the placenta and is distributed in breast milk; caution in lactation is warranted. No age-related precautions have been noted in children, but dosages must be carefully titrated. Elderly patients are more sensitive to the drug's hypotensive effects. In elderly patients, age-related renal impairment may require dosage adjustment. Exposure to sunlight and artificial light sources should be avoided.

BP should be assessed on both arms. Take the patient's pulse for 1 full minute immediately before giving the medication. If pulse rate increases 20 beats/min or more over baseline, or systolic or diastolic BP decreases more than 20 mm Hg, withhold minoxidil and contact the physician. Weight and electrolytes should also be monitored during therapy. Women of childbearing age should be careful and avoid handling the pills unnecessarily because of a possible birth defect that could occur. Because of the cardiovascular effects of this medication, patients should be assessed for stress tolerance before initiating therapy. Postural changes should be made slowly in consideration of possible orthostatic hypotension developing.
Administration
Take oral minoxidil without regard to food. Can take with food if GI upset occurs. Crush tablets if necessary.

Maximum BP response occurs 3-7 days after initiation of minoxidil therapy, and reversible growth of fine body hair may begin 3-6 wks after the start of treatment.

For topical use, shampoo and dry hair before applying medication. Wash hands immediately after application. Do not use a hair dryer to dry the hair after application (reduces effectiveness). Treatment must continue on a permanent basis and any cessation of treatment will reverse new hair growth.

Mirtazapine

mir-taz′a-peen
(Avanza [AUS], Remeron, Remeron Soltab)
Do not confuse Remeron with Premarin.

CATEGORY AND SCHEDULE
Pregnancy Risk Category: C

Classification: Antidepressants, tetracyclic

MECHANISM OF ACTION
A tetracyclic compound that acts as an antagonist at presynaptic α_2-adrenergic receptors, increasing both norepinephrine and serotonin neurotransmission. Has low anticholinergic activity. *Therapeutic Effect:* Relieves depression and produces sedative effects.

PHARMACOKINETICS
Rapidly and completely absorbed after PO administration; absorption not affected by food. Protein binding: 85%. Metabolized in the liver. Primarily excreted in urine. Unknown if removed by hemodialysis. *Half-life:* 20-40 h (longer in males [37 h] than females [26 h]).

AVAILABILITY
Tablets: 7.5 mg, 15 mg, 30 mg, 45 mg.
Tablets (Disintegrating): 15 mg, 30 mg, 45 mg.

INDICATIONS AND DOSAGES
▸ **Depression**
PO
Adults. Initially, 15 mg at bedtime. May increase by 15 mg/day q1-2wk. Maximum: 45 mg/day.
Elderly. Initially, 7.5 mg at bedtime. May increase by 7.5-15 mg/day q1-2wk. Maximum: 45 mg/day.

OFF LABEL USES
Essential tremor, intractable pruritus.

CONTRAINDICATIONS
Do not use within 14 days of MAOIs, hypersensitivity.

INTERACTIONS
Drug
Alcohol, diazepam and other benzodiazepines: May increase impairment of cognition and motor skills.
MAOIs: May increase the risk of neuroleptic malignant syndrome, hypertensive crisis, and severe seizures. Do not use together.
Opioid anlagesics: May impair cognitive or motor performance.
Herbal
None known.
Food
None known.

DIAGNOSTIC TEST EFFECTS
May increase serum cholesterol, triglyceride, AST (SGOT), and ALT (SGPT) levels.

M

SIDE EFFECTS

Frequent

Somnolence (54%), dry mouth (25%), increased appetite (17%), constipation (13%), weight gain (12%).

Occasional

Asthenia (8%), dizziness (7%), flu-like symptoms (5%), abnormal dreams (4%).

Rare

Abdominal discomfort, vasodilation, paresthesia, acne, dry skin, thirst, arthralgia.

SERIOUS REACTIONS

• Mirtazapine poses a higher risk of seizures than tricyclic antidepressants, especially in those with no previous history of seizures.

• Overdose may produce cardiovascular effects, such as severe orthostatic hypotension, dizziness, tachycardia, palpitations, and arrhythmias.

• Abrupt discontinuation after prolonged therapy may produce headache, malaise, nausea, vomiting, and vivid dreams.

• Agranulocytosis occurs rarely.

PRECAUTIONS & CONSIDERATIONS

Caution is warranted with cardiovascular disorders, GI disorders, angle-closure glaucoma, benign prostatic hyperplasia, hepatic or renal impairment, and urine retention. It is unknown whether mirtazapine is distributed in breast milk; caution is warranted in lactation. The safety and efficacy of this drug have not been established in children. In elderly patients, age-related renal impairment may require cautious use.

Drowsiness and dizziness may occur, so avoid alcohol and tasks that require mental alertness or motor skills. CBC, serum alkaline phosphatase, bilirubin, AST (SGOT), and ALT (SGPT) levels should be assessed before and periodically during therapy to assess hepatic and renal function in patients on long-term therapy. ECG should also be performed to assess for arrhythmias. Abrupt discontinuation after long-term therapy may produce headache, nausea, malaise, vomiting and vivid dreams; use caution in surgery with sedation or general anesthesia because of the greater risk of hypotensive episode.

Storage

Store at room temperature. Keep disintegrating tablets in blister pack until time of use.

Administration

! Make sure at least 14 days elapse between the use of MAOIs and mirtazapine.

Take mirtazapine at bedtime without regard to food. Scored tablets may be crushed or broken if needed.

Orally disintegrating tablets may be placed on tongue to dissolve. No water is necessary.

Misoprostol

mis-oh-pros-toll
(Cytotec)
Do not confuse with Cytomel.

CATEGORY AND SCHEDULE

Pregnancy Risk Category: X

Classification: Gastic mucosa protectant

MECHANISM OF ACTION

A prostaglandin that inhibits basal, nocturnal gastric acid secretion via direct action on parietal cells.

Therapeutic Effect: Increases production of protective gastric mucus.

PHARMACOKINETICS

Rapidly absorbed from the GI tract. Rapidly converted to active metabolite. Primarily excreted in urine. *Half-life:* 20-40 min.

AVAILABILITY

Tablets: 100 mcg, 200 mcg (Cytotec).

INDICATIONS AND DOSAGES
▸ **Prevention of NSAID-induced gastric ulcer**
PO
Adults. 200 mcg 4 times/day with food (last dose at bedtime). Continue for duration of NSAID therapy. May reduce dosage to 100 mcg if 200-mcg dose is not tolerable.
Elderly. 100-200 mcg 4 times/day with food.

OFF-LABEL USES

Treatment of gastric ulcer, used with mifepristone for termination of pregnancy, also used in low-dose intravaginal protocols for cervical ripening.

CONTRAINDICATIONS

Pregnancy (produces uterine contractions), hypersensitivity to misoprostol or any component of the formulation.

INTERACTIONS
Drug
Antacids: May decrease misoprostol effectiveness.
NSAIDs: May increase upper GI distress or cause ulceration.
Phenylbutazone: May increase neurosensory effects (headache, dizziness, ataxia).

Herbal
None known.
Food
None known.

DIAGNOSTIC TEST EFFECTS
None known.

SIDE EFFECTS
Frequent
Abdominal pain, diarrhea.
Occasional
Nausea, flatulence, dyspepsia, headache.
Rare
Vomiting, constipation.

SERIOUS REACTIONS
• Overdosage may produce sedation, tremor, convulsions, dyspnea, palpitations, hypotension, and bradycardia.
• Hyperstimulation of uterus and possible uterine rupture (use during labor).

PRECAUTIONS & CONSIDERATIONS
Caution is warranted in patients with renal impairment and women of childbearing age. Be aware that misoprostol is contraindicated in pregnancy and will produce uterine contractions, uterine bleeding, and expulsion of products of conception. Be aware that it is unknown whether misoprostol is distributed in breast milk; caution is warranted in lactation. Safety and efficacy of the drug have not been established in children. No age-related precautions have been noted in elderly patients.
Storage
Store at room temperature in a dry area.
Administration
Take with or after meals to minimize diarrhea. The last dose of the day is taken at bedtime.

M

Mitotane
mye'toe-tane
(Lysodren)

CATEGORY AND SCHEDULE
Pregnancy Risk Category: C

Classification: Antineoplastics

MECHANISM OF ACTION
A hormonal agent that inhibits activity of the adrenal cortex. *Therapeutic Effect:* Suppresses functional and nonfunctional adrenocortical neoplasms by direct cytoxic effect.

PHARMACOKINETICS
Adequately absorbed orally (40%). Hepatic metabolism; excreted in urine, bile. *Half-life:* 18-19 days.

AVAILABILITY
Tablets: 500 mg.

INDICATIONS AND DOSAGES
▶ **Adrenocortical carcinomas**
PO
Adults, Elderly. Initially, 2-6 g/day in 3-4 divided doses. Increase by 2-4 g/day every 3-7 days up to 9-10 g/day. Range: 2-16 g/day.

OFF-LABEL USES
Treatment of Cushing syndrome.

CONTRAINDICATIONS
Known hypersensitivity to mitotane.

INTERACTIONS
Drug
All central nervous system (CNS) depressants: May increase CNS depression.
Corticosteroids: Decreased effects; use hydrocortisone instead.
Warfarin: Accelerates warfarin metabolism, monitor INR.

Herbal
None known.
Food
None known.

DIAGNOSTIC TEST EFFECTS
May decrease levels of plasma cortisol, urinary 17-hydroxycorticosteroids, protein-bound iodine, and serum uric acid.

SIDE EFFECTS
Frequent (> 15%)
Anorexia, nausea, vomiting, diarrhea, lethargy, somnolence, adrenocortical insufficiency, dizziness, vertigo, maculopapular rash, hypouricemia.
Occasional (< 15%)
Blurred or double vision, retinopathy, hearing loss, excessive salivation, urine abnormalities (hematuria, cystitis, albuminuria), hypertension, orthostatic hypotension, flushing, wheezing, dyspnea, generalized aching, fever.

SERIOUS REACTIONS
• Brain damage and functional impairment may occur with long-term, high-dosage therapy.
• Adrenal insufficiency may require adrenal steroid replacement.

PRECAUTIONS & CONSIDERATIONS
! Brain damage and functional impairment may occur with long-term, high-dose therapy. Drug may cause adrenal hypofunction; administer hydrocorticose or mineralocorticoid as needed after evaluation and monitoring.

Caution is warranted with impaired hepatic function. Vaccinations and coming in contact with crowds, people with known infections, and anyone who has recently received a live-virus vaccine should be avoided.

Dizziness and drowsiness may occur; tasks that require mental alertness or motor skills should be avoided. Notify the physician if darkening of the skin, diarrhea, depression, loss of appetite, nausea and vomiting, or rash occurs. Adequate hydration should be maintained to prevent urinary side effects. The drug should be discontinued immediately after shock or trauma, as prescribed, because it produces adrenal suppression. Liver function test results, serum uric acid levels, and urine tests, including urine chemistry and urinalysis should be assessed. Be aware that neurologic and behavioral assessments are performed periodically on those receiving prolonged therapy (> 2 yrs).

Administration

! Mitotane may be carcinogenic, mutagenic, or teratogenic; handle it with extreme care during administration; wear impervious gloves.

Mitoxantrone
mye-toe-zan'trone
(Novantrone, Onkotrone [AUS])

CATEGORY AND SCHEDULE
Pregnancy Risk Category: D

Classification: Antineoplastics, antiinfective, immunomodulator; synthetic anthraquinone

---

MECHANISM OF ACTION
An anthracenedione that inhibits B-cell, T-cell, and macrophage proliferation and DNA and RNA synthesis. Active throughout the entire cell cycle. *Therapeutic Effect:* Causes cell death.

PHARMACOKINETICS
Protein binding: 78%. Widely distributed. Metabolized in the liver. Primarily eliminated in feces by the biliary system. Not removed by hemodialysis. *Half-life:* 2.3-13 days.

AVAILABILITY
Injection: 2 mg/mL.

INDICATIONS AND DOSAGES
▸ **AML**
IV
Adults, Elderly, Children 2 yrs and older. 12 mg/m^2 once a day on days 1-3 is a common first-cycle regimen. *Children younger than 2 yrs.* 0.4 mg/kg once a day for 3-5 days.
▸ **AML in relapse**
IV
Adults, Elderly, Children older than 2 yrs. 12 mg/m^2 once a day for 3-5 days are common regimens.
▸ **Prostate cancer**
IV
Adults, Elderly. 12-14 mg/m^2 every 21 days.
▸ **Multiple sclerosis**
IV
Adults, Elderly. 12 mg/m^2/dose q3mo.

OFF-LABEL USES
Treatment of breast or hepatic carcinoma, non-Hodgkin's lymphoma.

CONTRAINDICATIONS
Baseline left ventricular ejection fraction < 50%, cumulative lifetime mitoxantrone dose of 140 mg/m^2 or more hypersensitivity.

INTERACTIONS
Drug
Aspirin, other salicylates, NSAIDs: Avoid use.

M

Antigout medications: May decrease the effects of these drugs.
Bone marrow depressants: May increase myelosuppression.
Live-virus vaccines: May potentiate virus replication, increase vaccine side effects, and decrease the patient's antibody response to the vaccine.
Herbal and Food
None known.

DIAGNOSTIC TEST EFFECTS

May increase serum bilirubin and uric acid, AST (SGOT), and ALT (SGPT) levels.

⊘ IV INCOMPATIBILITIES

Heparin, paclitaxel (Taxol), piperacillin and tazobactam (Zosyn).

⦿ IV COMPATIBILITIES

Allopurinol (Aloprim), etoposide (VePesid), gemcitabine (Gemzar), granisetron (Kytril), ondansetron (Zofran), potassium chloride.

SIDE EFFECTS

Frequent (> 10%)
Nausea, vomiting, diarrhea, cough, headache, stomatitis, abdominal discomfort, fever, alopecia.
Occasional (4%-9%)
Ecchymosis, fungal infection, conjunctivitis, urinary tract infection.
Rare (3%)
Arrhythmias.

SERIOUS REACTIONS

• Myelosuppression may be severe, resulting in GI bleeding, hematologic toxicity, sepsis, and pneumonia.
• Renal failure, seizures and jaundice may occur.
• Extravasation can cause serious pain, discoloration, skin necrosis.
• Cardiac arrhythmias, ECG changes, heart failure. Decreased ejection fraction may be permanent.
• Anaphylaxis (rare).

PRECAUTIONS & CONSIDERATIONS

Caution is warranted with impaired hepatobiliary function and preexisting myelosuppression and in those who have previously been treated with cardiotoxic medications. Patients with hepatic impairment have higher mitoxantrone exposure because of reduced clearance. Mitoxantrone use should be avoided during pregnancy, especially during the first trimester, because it can cause fetal harm. Contraceptive measures should be used during mitoxantrone therapy. Breastfeeding also is not recommended. The safety and efficacy of mitoxantrone have not been established in children. No age-related precautions have been noted in elderly patients. Vaccinations and coming in contact with crowds and people with known infections should be avoided.

Urine will appear blue or green and sclera may have a blue tint for 24 h after mitoxantrone administration. Notify the physician if fever, signs of local infection, unusual bleeding from any site, blush skin, burning or erythema of oral mucosa, difficulty swallowing, oral ulcerations, or sore throat occurs. Adequate hydration should be maintained to protect against renal impairment. Hematologic status and liver, renal, and pulmonary function test.
Storage
Store vials at room temperature. Do not freeze.
Administration
! Because mitoxantrone may be carcinogenic, mutagenic, or teratogenic, handle the drug with extreme care during preparation and administration.
! Must be diluted before use. Dilute with at least 50 mL D5W or 0.9% NaCl. Do not administer

by subcutaneous, IM, intrathecal, or intra-arterial injection. Do not give IV push over < 3 min. Give IV bolus over at least 3 min or intermittent IV infusion over 15-60 min into the tubing of a freely running IV infusion of 0.9% NaCl or dextrose 5% injection. Administer continuous IV infusion of 0.02-0.5 mg/mL in D5W or 0.9% NaCl.

Take care to avoid extravasation.

Modafinil
mode-ah-feen'awl
(Alertec [CAN], Provigil)

CATEGORY AND SCHEDULE
Pregnancy Risk Category: C

Classification: Central nervous system (CNS) stimulants

MECHANISM OF ACTION
An α_1-agonist that may bind to dopamine reuptake carrier sites, increasing α activity and decreasing Θ, T, and β brain wave activity. *Therapeutic Effect:* Reduces the number of sleep episodes and total daytime sleep.

PHARMACOKINETICS
Well absorbed. Protein binding: 60%. Widely distributed. Metabolized in the liver. Excreted by the kidneys. Unknown if removed by hemodialysis. *Half-life:* 8-10 h.

AVAILABILITY
Tablets: 100 mg, 200 mg.

INDICATIONS AND DOSAGES
▶ **Narcolepsy, other Sleep disorders.**
PO
Adults, Elderly, Adolescents 16 yrs and older. 200-400 mg/day.
▶ **Dosage in hepatic impairment**
Reduce normal dosage by 50% in those with moderate to severe liver disease.

CONTRAINDICATIONS
Hypersensitivity to modafinil or armodafinil.

INTERACTIONS
Drug
Antifungals, erythromycins, other CYP 450 isoenzyme inhibitors: Could result increased modafinil concentrations.
Cyclosporine, oral contraceptives, theophylline: May decrease plasma concentrations of these drugs.
Diazepam, phenytoin, propranolol, tricyclic antidepressants, warfarin; and other CYPZC19 and CYPZC9 substrates: May increase plasma concentrations of these drugs.
Other CNS stimulants: May increase CNS stimulation.
Herbal
None known.
Food
None known.

DIAGNOSTIC TEST EFFECTS
None known.

SIDE EFFECTS
Frequent
Anxiety, insomnia, nausea, nervousness.
Occasional
Anorexia, diarrhea, dizziness, dry mouth or skin, muscle stiffness, polydipsia, rhinitis, paraesthesia, tremor, headache, vomiting.

M

SERIOUS REACTIONS
• Agitation, excitation, hypertension, and insomnia may occur.
• Serious rash, including Stevens-Johnson syndrome, TEN, and eosinophilia.
• Serious hypersensitivity with angioedema (rare).

PRECAUTIONS & CONSIDERATIONS
Caution is warranted in patients with hepatic impairment or a history of clinically significant mitral valve prolapse, left ventricular hypertrophy, and seizures. Nonhormonal contraceptive methods should be used during modafinil therapy and 1 mo afterward because modafinil decreases the effectiveness of hormonal contraceptives. It is unknown whether modafinil is excreted in breast milk; caution warranted in lactation. Use caution when giving modafinil to pregnant women. The safety and efficacy of this drug have not been established in children younger than 16 yrs. Age-related hepatic or renal impairment may require decreased dosage in elderly patients.

Dizziness may occur, so tasks that require mental alertness and motor skills should be avoided until response to the drug is established. Sleep pattern should be assessed throughout therapy. Should only be used in patients with a diagnosis of narcolepsy, obstructive sleep apnea-hypopnea syndrome, or shift work sleep disorder.

Administration
Take modafinil without regard to food. If treating narcolepsy, dose is taken as single dose in the morning. In patients with shift-work sleep disorder, the drug is taken 1 h before the start of the work shift.

Moexipril hydrochloride
moe-ex′a-prile high-droh-klor-ide
(Univasc)

CATEGORY AND SCHEDULE
Pregnancy Risk Category: C (D if used in second or third trimesters)

Classification: Angiotensin converting enzyme (ACE) inhibitors

MECHANISM OF ACTION
An ACE inhibitor that suppresses the renin-angiotensin-aldosterone system and prevents conversion of angiotensin I to angiotensin II, a potent vasoconstrictor; may also inhibit angiotensin II at local vascular and renal sites. *Therapeutic Effect:* Reduces peripheral arterial resistance and lowers BP.

PHARMACOKINETICS

Route	Onset	Peak	Duration
PO	1 h	3-6 h	24 h

Incompletely absorbed from the GI tract. Food decreases drug absorption. Rapidly converted to active metabolite. Protein binding: 50%. Primarily recovered in feces, partially excreted in urine. Unknown whether removed by dialysis. *Half-life:* 1 h, metabolite 2-9 h.

AVAILABILITY
Tablets: 7.5 mg, 15 mg.

INDICATIONS AND DOSAGES
▸ **Hypertension**
PO
Adults, Elderly. For patients not receiving diuretics, initial dose is

7.5 mg once a day 1 h before meals. Adjust according to BP effect. Maintenance: 7.5-30 mg a day in 1-2 divided doses 1 h before meals.

▶ **Hypertension in patients with impaired renal function**
PO
Adults, Elderly. 3.75 mg once a day in patients with creatinine clearance of 40 mL/min or less. Maximum: May titrate up to 15 mg/day.

CONTRAINDICATIONS

History of angioedema from previous treatment with ACE inhibitors.

INTERACTIONS

Drug
Alcohol, antihypertensives, diuretics phenothiazines: May increase hypotensive effects.
Indomethacin, other NSAIDs, sympathomimetics: May decrease hypotensive effects.
Lithium: May increase lithium blood concentration and risk of lithium toxicity.
NSAIDs: May decrease the effects of moexipril.
Potassium-sparing diuretics, potassium supplements: May cause hyperkalemia.
Salicylates: May reduce antihypertensive and vasodilator effects if used concurrently with moexepril.
Herbal
None known.
Food
None specified, however, although food may interfere with absorption of moexepril.

DIAGNOSTIC TEST EFFECTS

May increase BUN, serum alkaline phosphatase, serum bilirubin, serum creatinine, serum potassium, AST (SGOT), and ALT (SGPT) levels. May decrease serum sodium levels. May cause positive serum antinuclear antibody titer.

SIDE EFFECTS

Occasional
Cough, headache (6%); dizziness (4%); fatigue (3%).
Rare
Flushing, rash, myalgia, nausea, vomiting.

SERIOUS REACTIONS

• Excessive hypotension (first-dose syncope) may occur in patients with CHF and in those who are severely salt or volume depleted.
• Angioedema (swelling of face and lips) and hyperkalemia occur rarely.
• Agranulocytosis and neutropenia may be noted in those with collagen vascular disease, including scleroderma and SLE, and impaired renal function.
• Nephrotic syndrome may be noted in those with history of renal disease.

PRECAUTIONS & CONSIDERATIONS

Caution is warranted with angina, aortic stenosis, cerebrovascular disease, cerebrovascular and coronary insufficiency, hypovolemia, ischemic heart disease, renal impairment, severe CHF, sodium depletion, and those on dialysis and/or receiving diuretics. Moexipril crosses the placenta and it is unknown whether it is distributed in breast milk; caution is warranted in lactation and pregnancy. Moexipril has caused fetal or neonatal morbidity or mortality. Safety and efficacy of moexipril have not been established in children. In elderly patients, age-related renal

M

impairment may require cautious use of moexipril.

Dizziness may occur. Notify the physician if chest pain, cough, difficulty breathing, fever, sore throat, or swelling of the eyes, face, feet, hands, lips, or tongue occurs. BP should be obtained immediately before giving each moexipril dose, in addition to regular monitoring. Be alert to fluctuations in BP. If an excessive reduction in BP occurs, place the patient in the supine position with legs elevated. CBC and blood chemistry should be obtained before beginning moexipril therapy, then every 2 wks for the next 3 mo, and periodically thereafter in patients with autoimmune disease or renal impairment and in those who are taking drugs that affect immune response or leukocyte count. BUN, serum creatinine, serum potassium, renal function, and white blood cell count (WBC) should also be monitored. Lungs should be auscultated for rales. Heart rate for irregularities should be assessed.

Administration

! To reduce the risk of hypotension, expect to discontinue diuretics 2-3 days before initiating moexipril therapy. If BP is not controlled, resume diuretic as ordered. If diuretic cannot be discontinued, prepare to give a lowered initial dose of moexipril.

Take moexipril 1 h before meals. Crush tablets if necessary.

Molindone
moe-lin′done
(Moban)
Do not confuse with Mobic.

CATEGORY AND SCHEDULE
Pregnancy Risk Category: C

Classification: Antipsychotics

MECHANISM OF ACTION
An indole derivative of dihydroindole compounds that reduces spontaneous locomotion and aggressiveness. *Therapeutic Effect:* Suppresses behavioral response in psychosis.

PHARMACOKINETICS
Rapidly absorbed from the GI tract. Metabolized in liver. Excreted feces and a small amount excreted via lungs as carbon dioxide. Not removed by dialysis. *Half-life:* Unknown.

AVAILABILITY
Oral Solutions: 20 mg/mL (Moban).
Tablets: 5 mg, 10 mg, 25 mg, 50 mg, 100 mg (Moban).

INDICATIONS AND DOSAGES
▸ **Schizophrenia**
PO
Adults, Children 12 yrs and older.
Initially, 50-75 mg/day, increased to 100 mg/day in 3-4 days.
Maintenance: 5-15 mg 3-4 times/day (mild psychosis). Maintenance: 10-25 mg 3-4 times/day (moderate psychosis). Maintenance: 225 mg/day maximum in divided doses (severe psychosis).
Elderly. Start at a lower dose.

CONTRAINDICATIONS
Coma or severe central nervous system (CNS) depression,

hypersensitivity to molindone or any component of the formulation.

INTERACTIONS
Drug
Alcohol, CNS depressants: May increase CNS and respiratory depression of molindone.
Anticholinergics, antihistamines: May increase anticholinergic effects.
Lithium: May produce adverse neurologic effects.
Herbal
Betel nut: May increase extrapyramidal side effects of molindone.
Kava kava: May add to dopamine antagonist effects.
Food
None known.

DIAGNOSTIC TEST EFFECTS
None known.

SIDE EFFECTS
Frequent
Blurred vision, constipation, drowsiness, headache, extrapyramidal symptoms.
Occasional
Mental depression.
Rare
Skin rash, hot and dry skin, inability to sweat, muscle weakness, confusion, jaundice, convulsions.

SERIOUS REACTIONS
• Neuroleptic malignant syndrome or tardive dyskinesia has been reported.

PRECAUTIONS & CONSIDERATIONS
Caution should be used in persons allergic to sulfites (oral concentrate contains sodium metabisulfite); who have a history of breast cancer, brain tumor, or intestinal obstruction; who have a history of BPH, urinary retention, glaucoma, or liver impairment. Be aware that neuroleptic agents should not be reintroduced to persons with a history of neuroleptic malignant syndrome; however, in some cases neuroleptic agents have been reintroduced safely, without recurrence of this syndrome. It is unknown whether molindone crosses the placenta or is distributed in breast milk; caution is warranted in pregnancy and lactation. Safety and efficacy of molindone have not been established in children younger than 12 yrs. No age-related precautions have been noted in elderly patients.

If high fever, muscle stiffness, fast or irregular heartbeat, unexplained weakness or tiredness, muscle spasms, twitching, or uncontrolled tongue occurs, notify the physician. Avoid alcohol or other CNS depressants during molindone therapy.
Storage
Store at room temperature.
Administration
Take with or without food.

M

Mometasone Furoate
mo-met′a-sone fur-oh-ate
mon-o-high-drate
(Allermax Aqueous [AUS], Elocon
Cream [AUS], Asmanex Twisthaler,
Elocon Ointment [AUS], Nasonex,
Nasonex Nasal Spray [AUS],
Novasone Cream [AUS], Novasone
Lotion [AUS], Novasone Ointment
[AUS])

CATEGORY AND SCHEDULE
Pregnancy Risk Category: C

Classification: Synthetic
corticosteroids

MECHANISM OF ACTION
An adrenocorticosteroid that
inhibits the release of inflammatory
cells, preventing early activation of
the allergic reaction. *Therapeutic
Effect:* Decreases response to
seasonal and perennial rhinitis,
stabilizes asthma.

PHARMACOKINETICS
Undetectable in plasma.
Protein binding: 98%-99%. The
swallowed portion undergoes
extensive metabolism. Excreted
primarily through bile and, to a
lesser extent, urine. *Half-life:* 5.8 h
(nasal).

AVAILABILITY
Nasal Spray: 50 mcg/spray.
Topical Cream. 0.1%.
Topical Ointment. 0.1%.
Topical lotion: 0.1%.
Oral Inhalation: 110 mcg/actuation,
220 mcg/actuation (Asmanex
Twisthaler).

INDICATIONS AND DOSAGES
▸ **Allergic Rhinitis**

NASAL SPRAY
*Adults, Elderly, Children 12 yrs and
older.* 2 sprays in each nostril once
a day.
Children 2-11 yrs. 1 spray in each
nostril once a day.
▸ **Asthma**
INHALATION
*Adults, Elderly, Children 12 yrs
and older.* Initially inhale 220 mcg
(1 puff) once a day; Maximum:
880 mcg once a day.
Children 4-11 yr. Initially, 110 mcg
once daily.
▸ **Corticosteroid-responsive
dermatoses**
TOPICAL
*Adults, Elderly, Children 12 yrs
and older.* Apply cream, lotion or
ointment to affected area once
a day.
▸ **Nasal polyp**
NASAL SPRAY
Adults, Elderly. 2 sprays in each
nostril 2x/day.

CONTRAINDICATIONS
Hypersensitivity to any
corticosteroid, persistently positive
sputum cultures for *Candida
albicans,* systemic fungal infections,
untreated localized infection
involving nasal mucosa.

INTERACTIONS
Drug
None known.
Herbal
None known.
Food
None known.

DIAGNOSTIC TEST EFFECTS
None known.

SIDE EFFECTS
Occasional
Nasal irritation, stinging, sore throat,
headache.

Rare
Nasal or pharyngeal candidiasis, sinus infection, HPA-axis suppression.

SERIOUS REACTIONS
• An acute hypersensitivity reaction, including urticaria, angioedema, and severe bronchospasm, occurs rarely.
• Transfer from systemic to local steroid therapy may unmask previously suppressed bronchial asthma condition.
• Nasal septum perforation with prolonged improper use of nasal spray.
• Adrenal insufficiency.

PRECAUTIONS & CONSIDERATIONS
Caution is warranted with adrenal insufficiency, cirrhosis, glaucoma, hypothyroidism, osteoporosis, tuberculosis, and untreated infection. It is unknown whether mometasone crosses the placenta or is distributed in breast milk; caution warranted in lactation and pregnancy. In children, prolonged treatment and high dosages may decrease cortisol secretion and short-term growth rate. No age-related precautions have been noted in elderly patients.

Pulse rate and quality, ABG levels, and respiratory rate, depth, rhythm and type should be monitored. Symptoms should start to improve within 2 days of the first dose, but the drug's maximum benefit may take up to 2 wks to appear. Notify the physician if symptoms fail to improve.
Administration
For inhalation, see instructions for use of the Twisthaler. Exhale completely and place the mouthpiece between the lips. Inhale and hold breath for as long as possible before exhaling. Allow 1 min between inhalations to promote deeper bronchial penetration. Rinse mouth with water immediately after inhalation to prevent mouth and throat dryness and oral candidiasis. Once-daily inhalation doses are administered in the evening.

Clear the nasal passages before using mometasone. May need to use a topical nasal decongestant 5-15 min before using mometasone. Tilt head slightly forward. Insert spray tip up into the nostril, pointing toward the inflamed nasal turbinates, away from nasal septum. Spray the drug into the nostril while holding the other nostril closed, and at the same time inhale through the nose.

Monobenzone
mon-oh-benz-one
(Benoquin)

CATEGORY AND SCHEDULE
Pregnancy Risk Category: C

Classification: Dermatologics

MECHANISM OF ACTION
The mechanism of action is not fully understood. Monobenzone may be converted to hydroquinone, which inhibits the enzymatic oxidation of tyrosine to DOPA; it may have a direct action on tyrosinase; or it may act as an antioxidant to prevent SH-group oxidation so that more SH groups are available to inhibit tyrosinase. *Therapeutic Effect:* Depigmentation in extensive vitiligo.

PHARMACOKINETICS
Not fully understood. Initial response occurs in 1-4 mo.

AVAILABILITY
Cream: 20% (Benoquin).

INDICATIONS AND DOSAGES
▸ **Vitiligo**
TOPICAL
Adults, Elderly. Apply 2-3 times/day
to affected area.

CONTRAINDICATIONS
History of hypersensitivity
to monobenzone or any of its
components.
Use in any other condition other than
disseminated vitiligo.

INTERACTIONS
Drug
None known.
Herbal
None known.
Food
None known.

DIAGNOSTIC TEST EFFECTS
None known.

SIDE EFFECTS
Occasional
Irritation, burning sensation,
dermatitis.

SERIOUS REACTIONS
• None known.

PRECAUTIONS & CONSIDERATIONS
Caution should be used with
hyperpigmentation because of
photosensitization. It is unknown
whether monobenzone is excreted
in breast milk; caution warranted
in lactation. Safety and efficacy
of monobenzone have not been
established in children. No age-related
precautions have been noted in elderly
patients. Sunlight should be avoided.
If exposure cannot be avoided, wear
clothing that covers the skin.
Monobenzone is a potent
dipigmenting agent, not a mild
cosmetic bleach. Irritation or burning
should be reported.

Administration
Monobenzone is for external use
only. Depigmentation is usually
observed after 1-4 mo of therapy.
Treatment should be discontinued
if satisfactory results have not been
obtained within four mo. Apply and
rub gently into the pigmented area.
After use, the patient's skin will
be sun-sensitive for life. Counsel
regarding sun protective clothing and
regular use of sunscreen.

Montelukast
mon-te′loo-kast
(Singulair)

CATEGORY AND SCHEDULE
Pregnancy Risk Category: B

Classification: Selective leukotriene receptor antagonists/inhibi-
tors

MECHANISM OF ACTION
An antiasthmatic that binds to
cysteinyl leukotriene receptors,
inhibiting the effects of leukotrienes
on bronchial smooth muscle.
Therapeutic Effect: Decreases
bronchoconstriction, vascular
permeability, mucosal edema, and
mucus production.

PHARMACOKINETICS

Route	Onset	Peak	Duration
PO	NA	N/A	24 h
PO (chewable)	NA	N/A	24 h

Rapidly absorbed from the GI tract.
Protein binding: 99%. Extensively
metabolized in the liver. Excreted

almost exclusively in feces. *Half-life:* 2.7-5.5 h (slightly longer in elderly patients).

AVAILABILITY
Oral Granules: 4 mg/packet.
Tablets: 10 mg.
Tablets (Chewable): 4 mg, 5 mg.

INDICATIONS AND DOSAGES
▶ **Bronchial asthma and seasonal and perennial allergic rhinitis**
PO
Adults, Elderly, Adolescents older than 14 yrs. One 10-mg tablet a day, taken in the evening.
Children 6-14 yrs. One 5-mg chewable tablet a day, taken in the evening.
Children 2-5 yrs. One 4-mg chewable tablet a day, taken in the evening or 1 packet of 4-mg oral granules.
Children, Infants age 6-23 mo. 1 packet 4-mg oral granules daily, in the evening.

CONTRAINDICATIONS
Hypersensitivity.
Not for acute asthma attacks.

INTERACTIONS
Drug
Phenobarbital, rifampin: May decrease montelukast's duration of action.
Herbal
None known.
Food
None known.

DIAGNOSTIC TEST EFFECTS
May increase AST (SGOT) and ALT (SGPT) levels.

SIDE EFFECTS
Adults, adolescents older than 14 yrs.
Frequent (18%)
Headache.

Occasional (4%)
Influenza.
Rare (2%-3%)
Abdominal pain, cough, dyspepsia, dizziness, fatigue, dental pain.
Children 6-14 yrs.
Rare (< 2%)
Diarrhea, laryngitis, pharyngitis, nausea, otitis media, sinusitis, viral infection.

SERIOUS REACTIONS
• Systemic eosinophilia, Churg-Strauss syndrome, vasulitis.

PRECAUTIONS & CONSIDERATIONS
Caution is warranted in patients with hepatic impairment and in those who are tapering systemic corticosteroid dosage during montelukast therapy. Use montelukast during pregnancy only if necessary. It is unknown whether montelukast is excreted in breast milk. No age-related precautions have been noted in children older than 6 yrs or in elderly patients. Parents of children with phenylketonuria should be informed that montelukast chewable tablets contain phenylalanine, a component of aspartame. Be aware montelukast is not intended to treat acute asthma attacks. Drink plenty of fluids to decrease the thickness of lung secretions. Avoid aspirin and NSAIDs while taking montelukast.

Pulse rate and quality as well as respiratory depth, rate, rhythm, and type should be monitored. Fingernails and lips should also be assessed for a blue or dusky color in light-skinned patients and a gray color in dark-skinned patients, which may be signs of hypoxemia.
Administration
Take montelukast tablets in the evening without regard to food. Do not abruptly substitute montelukast for inhaled or oral corticosteroids.

M

Take montelukast as prescribed, even during symptom-free periods and exacerbations. Do not alter the dosage or abruptly discontinue other asthma medications.

Chewable tablets should be chewed thoroughly before swallowing. For oral granules, may administer directly in mouth; dissolved in 1 tsp (5 mL) of cold or room-temperature formula or breast milk or mixed with a spoonful of cold food such as applesauce, carrots, rice or ice cream.

Moricizine Hydrochloride
mor-iss′i-zeen high-droh-klor-ide
(Ethmozine)

CATEGORY AND SCHEDULE
Pregnancy Risk Category: B

Classification:
Antiarrhythmics, Class IA

MECHANISM OF ACTION
An antiarrhythmic that prevents sodium current across myocardial cell membranes. Has potent local anesthetic activity and membrane stabilizing effects. Slows AV and His-Purkinje conduction and decreases action potential duration and effective refractory period. *Therapeutic Effect:* Suppresses ventricular arrhythmias.

PHARMACOKINETICS
Peak 0.5-2.2 h. Protein binding > 90%; metabolized in the liver; metabolites excreted in urine, feces. *Half-life:* 1.5-3.5 h.

AVAILABILITY
Tablets: 200 mg, 250 mg, 300 mg.

INDICATIONS AND DOSAGES
▸ **Ventricular arrhythmias**
PO
Adults, Elderly. 200-300 mg q8h. May increase by 150 mg/day at no < 3-day intervals.
Usual dose is 600-900 mg/day, given in 3 divided doses q8h. Patients with hepatic or renal impairment should be started at 600 mg/day or lower in divided doses.

OFF-LABEL USES
Atrial arrhythmias, complete and non-sustained ventricular arrhythmias, premature ventricular contractions (PVCs).

CONTRAINDICATIONS
Cardiogenic shock, preexisting second- or third-degree AV block or right bundle-branch block without pacemaker, known hypersensitivity.

INTERACTIONS
Drug
Cimetidine: May increase blood concentration of moricizine.
Theophylline: May decrease blood concentrations of theophylline.
Herbal
None known.
Food
None known.

DIAGNOSTIC TEST EFFECTS
May cause ECG changes, such as prolonged PR and QT intervals.

SIDE EFFECTS
Frequent (6%-15%)
Dizziness, nausea, headache, fatigue, dyspnea, GI upset.
Occasional (2%-5%)
Nervousness, paresthesia, sleep disturbances, dyspepsia, vomiting, diarrhea.

SERIOUS REACTIONS

• Moricizine may worsen existing arrhythmias or produce new ones.
• Jaundice with hepatitis occurs rarely.
• Overdosage produces vomiting, lethargy, syncope, hypotension, conduction disturbances, exacerbation of CHF, myocardial infarction, and sinus arrest.

PRECAUTIONS & CONSIDERATIONS

Caution is warranted with CHF, electrolyte imbalance, impaired hepatic or renal function, and sick sinus syndrome.

Dizziness, GI upset, headache, and nausea may occur. Notify the physician if chest pain or irregular heartbeat occurs. ECG for changes, especially increase in PR and QRS intervals, should be monitored before and during therapy. Pulse rate, electrolyte levels, intake and output, and liver and renal function should also be assessed.

Administration

Moricizine may be taken without regard to food, but give with food if GI upset occurs.

Once well stabilized on a q8h regimen, some patients can be transferred to q12h dosing at same daily dose.

Morphine

mor'feen

(Anamorph [AUS], Astramorph, Avinza, DepoDur, Duramorph, Infumorph, Kadian, Kapanol [AUS], M-Eslon, Morphine Mixtures [AUS], MS Contin, MSIR, MS Mono [AUS], Oramorph SR, RMS, Roxanol, Statex [CAN])

Do not confuse morphine with hydromorphone or Roxanol with Roxicet.

CATEGORY AND SCHEDULE

Pregnancy Risk Category: C (D if used for prolonged periods or at high dosages at term)
Controlled Substance Schedule: II

Classification: Opioid analgesic, narcotic

MECHANISM OF ACTION

An opioid agonist that binds with opioid receptors in the central nervous system (CNS). *Therapeutic Effect:* Alters the perception of and emotional response to pain; produces generalized CNS depression.

PHARMACOKINETICS

Route	Onset	Peak (h)	Duration (h)
Oral solution	NA	1	3-5
Tablets	NA	1	3-5
Tablets (ER)	NA	3-4	8-12
IV	Rapid	0.3	3-5
IM	5-30 min	0.5-1	3-5
Epidural	NA	1	12-20
Subcutaneous	NA	1.1-5	3-5
Rectal	NA	0.5-1	3-7

Variably absorbed from the GI tract. Readily absorbed after IM or SC administration. Protein binding: 20%-35%. Widely distributed. Metabolized in the liver. Primarily excreted in urine. Removed by hemodialysis. *Half-life:* 2-3 h. (increased in patients with hepatic disease).

AVAILABILITY

Capsules (Extended-Release [Kadian]): 20 mg, 30 mg, 50 mg, 60 mg, 100 mg.
Capsules (Extended-Release [Avinza]): 30 mg, 60 mg, 90 mg, 120 mg.
Solution for Injection: 0.5 mg/mL, 1 mg/mL, 2 mg/mL, 4 mg/mL, 5 mg/mL, 8 mg/mL, 10 mg/mL, 15 mg/mL, 25 mg/mL, 50 mg/mL.
Solution for Injection (Preservative-Free): 0.5 mg/mL, 1 mg/mL, 10 mg/mL, 25 mg/mL, 50 mg/mL.
Epidural and Intrathecal via Infusion Device (Infumorph): 10 mg/mL, 25 mg/mL.
Epidural, Intrathecal, IV Infusion (Astramorph, Duramorph): 0.5 mg/mL, 1 mg/mL, 4 mg/mL.
IV Infusion (Via Patient-Controlled Analgesia [PCA]): 1 mg/mL, 5 mg/mL.
Oral Solution (Roxanol): 10 mg/5 mL, 20 mg/5 mL, 20 mg/mL, 100 mg/5 mg.
Suppository (RMS): 5 mg, 10 mg, 20 mg, 30 mg.
Tablets (MSIR): 15 mg/30 mg.
Tablets (Extended-Release [MS Contin, Oramorph SR]): 15 mg, 30 mg, 60 mg, 100 mg, 200 mg.
Liposomal Injection (DepoDur): 10 mg/mL, 15 mg/1.5 mL, 20 mg/2 mL.

INDICATIONS AND DOSAGES
Alert

! Dosage should be titrated to desired effect.

▶ **Analgesia**
PO (PROMPT-RELEASE)
Adults, Elderly. 10-30 mg q3-4h as needed.
Children. 0.15-0.3 mg/kg q3-4h as needed.
! For the Kadian dosage information below, be aware that this drug is to be administered q12h or once a day only.
! Be aware that pediatric dosages of extended-release preparations Kadian and Avinza have not been established.
! For the MSContin and Oramorph SR dosage information below, be aware that the daily dosage is divided and given q 8 h or q 12 h.
PO (EXTENDED-RELEASE [AVINZA])
Adults, Elderly. Dosage requirement should be established using prompt-release formulations and is based on total daily dose (one-half the dose is given q12h or one-third the dose is given q8h).
PO (EXTENDED-RELEASE [KADIAN])
Adults, Elderly. Dosage requirement should be established using prompt-release formulations and is based on total daily dose. Dose is given once a day or divided and given q12h.
PO (EXTENDED-RELEASE [MSCONTIN, ORAMORPH SR]
Adults, Elderly. Dosage requirement should be established using prompt-release formulations and is based on total daily dose. Daily dose is divided and given q8h or q12h.
Children. 0.3-0.6 mg/kg/dose q12h.
IM
Adults, Elderly. 5-10 mg q3-4h as needed.
Children. 0.1 mg/kg q3-4 h as needed.

IV
Adults, Elderly. 2.5-5 mg q3-4h
as needed. **Note:** Repeated doses
(e.g., 1-2 mg) may be given more
frequently (e.g., every hour) if
needed.
Children. 0.05-0.1 mg/kg q3-4h
as needed.
IV CONTINUOUS INFUSION
Adults, Elderly. 0.8-10 mg/h. Range:
Up to 80 mg/h.
Children. 10-30 mcg/kg/h.
EPIDURAL
Adults, Elderly. Initially, 1-6 mg
bolus, infusion rate: 0.1-1 mg/h.
Maximum: 10 mg/24 h.
INTRATHECAL (UNPRESERVED,
E.G., DURAMORPH)
Adults, Elderly. One tenth of the
epidural dose: 0.2-1 mg/dose.
▶ PCA
IV
Adults, Elderly. Loading dose:
5-10 mg. Intermittent bolus:
0.5-3 mg. Lockout interval:
5-12 min. Continuous infusion:
1-10 mg/h. 4-h limit: 20-30 mg.

CONTRAINDICATIONS

Hypersensitivity, acute or severe
asthma, GI obstruction, severe
hepatic or renal impairment, severe
respiratory depression, asthma,
severe liver or renal impairment.
Caution
Addictive personality disorder,
lactation, myocardial infarction
(acute), severe heart disease, elderly,
respiratory depression, hepatic
disease, renal disease, children
younger than 18 yrs.

INTERACTIONS

Drug
Alcohol, other CNS depressants:
May increase CNS or respiratory
depression and hypotension.
Anticholinergics: May increase
anticholinergic effects.

MAOIs: May produce a severe,
sometimes fatal reaction; expect
to administer one-quarter of usual
morphine dose.
Herbal
None known.
Food
None known.

DIAGNOSTIC TEST EFFECTS

May increase serum amylase and
lipase levels.

🚫 IV INCOMPATIBILITIES

Amphotericin B complex (Abelcet,
AmBisome, Amphotec), cefepime
(Maxipime), doxorubicin liposomal
(Doxil), thiopental.

💉 IV COMPATIBILITIES

Amiodarone (Cordarone), bumetanide
(Bumex), bupivacaine (Marcaine,
Sensorcaine), diltiazem (Cardizem),
dobutamine (Dobutrex), dopamine
(Intropin), heparin, lidocaine,
lorazepam (Ativan), magnesium,
midazolam (Versed), milrinone
(Primacor), nitroglycerin, potassium,
propofol (Diprivan).

SIDE EFFECTS

Frequent
Sedation, decreased BP (including
orthostatic hypotension), diaphoresis,
facial flushing, constipation, dizziness,
somnolence, nausea, vomiting.
Occasional
Allergic reaction (rash, pruritus),
dyspnea, confusion, palpitations,
tremors, urine retention, abdominal
cramps, vision changes, dry mouth,
headache, decreased appetite, pain or
burning at injection site.
Rare
Paralytic ileus.

SERIOUS REACTIONS

• Overdose results in respiratory
depression, skeletal muscle flaccidity,

M

cold or clammy skin, cyanosis, and extreme somnolence progressing to seizures, stupor, and coma.

• The patient who uses morphine repeatedly may develop a tolerance to the drug's analgesic effect and physical dependence.

• The drug may have a prolonged duration of action and cumulative effect in those with hepatic and renal impairment.

PRECAUTIONS & CONSIDERATIONS

Extreme caution should be used with chronic obstructive pulmonary disease (COPD), cor pulmonale, head injury, hypoxia, hypercapnia, increased intracranial pressure, preexisting respiratory depression, and severe hypotension. Caution is also warranted with Addison disease, alcoholism, biliary tract disease, CNS depression, hypothyroidism, pancreatitis, benign prostatic hyperplasia, seizure disorders, toxic psychosis, urethral stricture, and in elderly or debilitated patients. Morphine crosses the placenta and is distributed in breast milk; caution in pregnancy and lactation is warranted. Regular use of opioids during pregnancy may produce withdrawal symptoms in the neonate, such as diarrhea, excessive crying, fever, hyperactive reflexes, irritability, seizures, sneezing, tremors, vomiting, and yawning. Morphine may prolong labor if administered in the latent phase of the first stage of labor or before the cervix is dilated 4-5 cm. The neonate may develop respiratory depression if the mother receives morphine during labor. Children and elderly patients are more prone to experience paradoxical excitement. Children younger than 2 yrs and elderly patients are more

susceptible to the drug's respiratory depressant effects. Age-related renal impairment may increase the risk of urine retention in elderly patients.

Dizziness and drowsiness may occur, so change positions slowly and avoid alcohol, CNS depressants, and tasks that require mental alertness or motor skills until response to the drug is established. Pattern of daily bowel activity and clinical improvement should be monitored. Vital signs should be monitored for 5-10 min after IV administration and 15-30 min after IM or SC injection. Be alert for bradycardia and hypotension. The drug should be held and the physician should be notified if the respiratory rate is 12 breaths/min or less in an adult or 20 breaths/min or less in a child.

Storage
Store vials at room temperature.
Administration
! Expect to reduce morphine dosage for debilitated and elderly patients and those using CNS depressants concurrently. Titrate dosage to desired effect, as prescribed. Morphine's side effects are dependent on the dosage and route of administration. Ambulatory patients and those not in severe pain are more prone to experience dizziness, nausea, and vomiting than those in the supine position and those in severe pain.

For oral use, mix the liquid form with fruit juice to improve the taste. Do not crush, open, or break extended-release capsules. Kadian (extended-release capsules) may be mixed with applesauce just before administration.

Morphine may be given undiluted as IV push. For IV injection, 2.5-15 mg morphine may be diluted in 4-5 mL sterile water for injection. For continuous IV infusion, dilute to a concentration of 0.1-1 mg/mL in D5W and administer through a controlled infusion device. Place the patient in the recumbent position before giving parenteral morphine. Always administer IV morphine very slowly because rapid IV administration increases the risk of a severe anaphylactic reaction, marked by apnea, cardiac arrest, and circulatory collapse.

For IM and SC administration, inject the drug slowly; rotate injection sites. Know that patients with circulatory impairment are at increased risk for overdose because of delayed absorption of repeated injections.

For rectal use, if the suppository is too soft, refrigerate it for 30 min or run cold water over the foil wrapper. Remove the foil wrapper; remove and moisten the suppository with cold water before inserting it well into the rectum.

Intrathecal: Only select injections are preservative free and suitable for intrathecal use. Pay close attention to dose limits.

Moxifloxacin Hydrochloride

moks-i-floks′a-sin high-droh-klor-ide

(Avelox, Avelox IV, Vigamox)
Do not confuse Avelox with Avonex or moxifloxacin with minoxidil.

CATEGORY AND SCHEDULE
Pregnancy Risk Category: C

Classification: Fluoroquinolone antiinfective, ophthalmics, systemic

MECHANISM OF ACTION
A fluoroquinolone that inhibits two enzymes, topoisomerase II and IV, in susceptible microorganisms. *Therapeutic Effect:* Interferes with bacterial DNA replication. Prevents or delays emergence of resistant organisms. Bactericidal.

PHARMACOKINETICS
Well absorbed from the GI tract after PO administration. Protein binding: 50%. Widely distributed throughout body with tissue concentration often exceeding plasma concentration. Metabolized in liver. Primarily excreted in urine with a lesser amount in feces. *Half-life:* 10.7-13.3 h.

AVAILABILITY
Tablets (Avelox): 400 mg.
Injection (Avelox IV): 400 mg.
Ophthalmic Solution (Vigamox): 0.5%.

INDICATIONS AND DOSAGES
▸ **Acute bacterial sinusitis, community-acquired pneumonia, complicated intra-abdominal infection**
IV/PO
Adults, Elderly. 400 mg q24h for 10 days (sinusitis); 7-14 days (pneumonia or intra-abdominal infusion).
▸ **Acute bacterial exacerbation of chronic bronchitis.**
IV/PO
Adults, Elderly. 400 mg q24h for 5 days.
▸ **Skin and skin-structure infection**
IV/PO
Adults, Elderly. 400 mg once a day for 7 days (uncomplicated), up to 21 days if complicated.
▸ **Topical treatment of bacterial conjunctivitis caused by susceptible strains of bacteria**

OPHTHALMIC
Adults, Elderly, Children older than 1 yr. 1 drop 3 times/day for 7 days.

CONTRAINDICATIONS
Hypersensitivity to quinolones.

INTERACTIONS
Drug
Antacids, didanosine chewable, buffered tablets or pediatric powder for oral solution, iron preparations, sucralfate, zinc preparations: May decrease moxifloxacin absorption.
Erythromycin, tricyclic antidepressants: Possible risk of QT interval elongation.
NSAIDs: Increased risk of central nervous system (CNS) stimulation and seizures.
Procainamide: Increased risk of life-threatening arrhythmias.
Herbal and Food
None known.

DIAGNOSTIC TEST EFFECTS
None known.

ⓘ IV INCOMPATIBILITIES
Do not add or infuse other drugs simultaneously through the same IV line. Flush line before and after use if same IV line is used with other medications.

SIDE EFFECTS
Frequent (6%-8%)
Nausea, diarrhea.
Occasional (2%-3%)
Dizziness, headache, abdominal pain, vomiting.
Ophthalmic (1%-6%): conjunctival irritation, reduced visual acuity, dry eye, keratitis, eye pain, ocular itching, swelling of tissue around cornea, eye discharge, fever, cough, pharyngitis, rash, rhinitis.

Rare (1%)
Change in sense of taste, dyspepsia (heartburn, indigestion), photosensitivity.

SERIOUS REACTIONS
• Pseudomembranous colitis as evidenced by fever, severe abdominal cramps or pain, and severe watery diarrhea may occur.
• Superinfection manifested as anal or genital pruritus, moderate to severe diarrhea, and stomatitis may occur.
• Tendonopathy and tendon rupture.
• QT prolongation.
• Seizures (rare).
• Serious hypersensitivity reaction.

PRECAUTIONS & CONSIDERATIONS
Caution is warranted in patients with cerebral arthrosclerosis, CNS disorders, liver or renal impairment; seizures, those with a prolonged QT interval, uncorrected hypokalemia, and those receiving amiodarone, procainamide, quinidine, and sotalol. Be aware that moxifloxacin may be distributed in breast milk and may produce teratogenic effects. Be aware that the safety and efficacy of moxifloxacin have not been established in children. No age-related precautions have been noted in elderly patients.

Avoid exposure to sunlight and ultraviolet light, and wear sunscreen and protective clothing if photosensitivity develops.

Abdominal pain, altered sense of taste, dyspepsia (heartburn, indigestion), headache, vomiting, and signs and symptoms of infections should be assessed. Pattern of daily bowel activity, stool consistency, and WBC count should be monitored. History of hypersensitivity to moxifloxacin and other quinolones should be determined before therapy.

Storage
Store at room temperature. Do not refrigerate.
Administration
Take oral moxifloxacin without regard to meals. Take 4 h before or 8 h after antacids, didanosine chewable, buffered tablets or pediatric powder for oral solution, iron preparations, multivitamins with minerals, or sucralfate. Take full course of therapy.

For ophthalmic use, tilt the head back, and look up. With a gloved finger, gently pull the lower eyelid down until a pocket is formed. Hold the dropper above the pocket and, without touching the eyelid or conjunctival sac, place drops into the center of the pocket. Close the eye gently, and apply gentle finger pressure to the lacrimal sac at the inner canthus. Remove excess solution around the eye with a tissue.
! Infuse IV over 60 min or longer. IV formulation is available in ready-to-use containers. Give by IV infusion only. Avoid rapid or bolus IV infusion.

Mupirocin
mew-peer′oh-sin
(Bactroban)
Do not confuse Bactroban with Bactrim or Bacitracin

CATEGORY AND SCHEDULE
Pregnancy Risk Category: B

Classification: Topical antiinfective, pseudomonic acid A

MECHANISM OF ACTION
An antibacterial agent that inhibits bacterial protein, RNA synthesis.

Less effective on DNA synthesis. Nasal: Eradicates nasal colonization of MRSA. *Therapeutic Effect:* Prevents bacterial growth and replication. Bacteriostatic.

PHARMACOKINETICS
Metabolized in skin to inactive metabolite. Transported to skin surface; removed by normal skin desquamation.

AVAILABILITY
Ointment: 2% (Bactroban).
Nasal Ointment: 2% (Bactroban).

INDICATIONS AND DOSAGES
▶ **Impetigo, infected traumatic skin lesions**
TOPICAL
Adults, Elderly, Children. Apply 3 times/day (may cover w/gauze).
▶ **Nasal colonization of resistant Staphylococcus aureus.**
INTRANASAL
Adults, Elderly, Children 12 yrs and older. Apply 2 times/day for 5 days.
▶ **Nasal colonization of resistant Staphylococcus aureus.**
INTRANASAL
Adults, Elderly, Children age 12 or older. Apply twice a day for 5 days.

OFF-LABEL USES
Treatment of infected eczema, folliculitis, minor bacterial skin infections.

CONTRAINDICATIONS
Hypersensitivity to mupirocin or any component of the formulation.
Caution
Lactation.

INTERACTIONS
Drug
None known.
Herbal
None known.

M

Food
None known.

DIAGNOSTIC TEST EFFECTS
None known.

SIDE EFFECTS
Frequent
Nasal: Headache, rhinitis, upper respiratory congestion, pharyngitis, altered taste.
Occasional
Nasal: Burning, stinging, cough.
Topical: Pain, burning, stinging, itching.
Rare
Nasal: Pruritis, diarrhea, dry mouth, epistaxis, nausea, rash.
Topical: Rash, nausea, dry skin, contact dermatitis.

SERIOUS REACTIONS
• Superinfection may result in bacterial or fungal infections, especially with prolonged or repeated therapy.

PRECAUTIONS & CONSIDERATIONS
Caution should be used in patients with impaired renal function. It is unknown whether mupirocin crosses the placenta or is distributed in breast milk. Use with caution. Safety and efficacy of nasal preparation have not been established in children younger than 12 yrs. No age-related precautions have been noted in children or elderly patients. Neonates or persons with poor hygiene should be kept isolated.
Storage
Store at room temperature.
Administration
Gown and gloves are to be worn until 24 h after therapy is effective. Disease is spread by direct contact with moist discharges. Apply small amount to affected areas. Cover affected areas with gauze dressing if desired.
    Discard single-use tubes immediately after use.

Muromonab-CD3
mur-oo-mon′ab
(Orthoclone, OKT3)

CATEGORY AND SCHEDULE
Pregnancy Risk Category: C

Classification: Immunosuppressives, monoclonal antibodies, recombinant DNA Origin

MECHANISM OF ACTION
A monoclonal antibody derived from purified IgG_2 that reacts with a T-3 (CD3) antigen of human T-cell membranes, blocking the production and function of T cells, which play a major role in acute organ rejection. *Therapeutic Effect:* Reverses organ rejection.

PHARMACOKINETICS
Steady state achieved in 3 days. Onset minutes after administration. Duration of activity: approximately 1 wk. *Half-life:* unknown.

AVAILABILITY
Injection: 1 mg/mL (5 mL).

INDICATIONS AND DOSAGES
▸ **Treatment of acute organ rejection**
IV
Adults, Elderly, Children weighing > 30 kg. 5 mg/day for 10-14 days, beginning as soon as acute rejection is diagnosed.
Children 30 kg or less: 2.5 mg/day. 10-14 days, beginning as soon as acute rejection is diagnosed.

CONTRAINDICATIONS
History of hypersensitivity to muromonab-CD3 or any murine-derived product, fluid overload (as evidenced by chest X-ray or weight gain of more than 3%) in the week before initial treatment.

INTERACTIONS
Drug
Indomethacin: Increased risk of encephalopathy, CNS effects.
Live-virus vaccines: May potentiate virus replication, increase the vaccine's side effects, and decrease the patient's response to the vaccine.
Other immunosuppressants: May increase the risk of infection or lymphoproliferative disorders; may cause psychosis, infection, malignancies, seizures or thrombotic events.
Herbal
Echinacea: May decrease the effects of muromonab.
Food
None known.

DIAGNOSTIC TEST EFFECTS
None known.

⊘ IV INCOMPATIBILITIES
Do not mix muromonab with any other medications.

SIDE EFFECTS
Frequent
Fever, chills, dyspnea, malaise (first-dose reaction occurring 30 min to 6 h after first dose reaction that diminishes after the 2nd day of treatment).
Occasional
Chest pain, nausea, vomiting, diarrhea, tremor.

SERIOUS REACTIONS
• Symptoms of cytokine release syndrome, a common reaction, may range from mild flulike symptoms to a life-threatening, shocklike reaction.
• Infection caused by immunosuppression generally occurs within 45 days after initial treatment. Cytomegalovirus occurs in 19% of patients, and herpes simplex occurs in 27% of patients. A severe, life-threatening infection occurs in fewer than 5% of patients.
• Severe pulmonary edema occurs in fewer than 2% of patients.
• Fatal hypersensitivity reactions occur occasionally.

PRECAUTIONS & CONSIDERATIONS
Caution is warranted in patients with impaired cardiac, hepatic, or renal function. Avoid receiving immunizations and coming in contact with crowds and people with known infections during muromonab therapy.

A chest radiogram should be obtained within 24 h of beginning muromonab therapy to ensure that the lungs are free of fluid. Fluid overload should be checked before beginning muromonab treatment to decrease the risk of pulmonary edema. Immunologic test results (including plasma drug levels and quantitative T-lymphocyte surface phenotyping), liver and renal function test results, intake and output, pattern of daily bowel activity and stool consistency, and WBC count should be obtained before and during therapy.
Storage
Refrigerate ampules. Do not use the drug if it has been left out of the refrigerator for longer than 4 h. Do not freeze or shake.
Administration
Do not shake the ampule before using. The solution may develop fine translucent particles, which

M

will not affect potency. Draw the solution into the syringe through a 0.22-μm filter. Discard the filter; use a new needle for IV administration. Administer by IV push over < 1 min. Give 1 mg/kg methylprednisolone 1-4 h before and 100 mg hydrocortisone 30 min after the first dose of muromonab, as prescribed, to decrease the risk and severity of cytokine release syndrome. Expect a first-dose reaction, including chest tightness, chills, fever, diarrhea, nausea, vomiting, and wheezing.

Mycophenolate Mofetil

my-co-fen′o-late moff-ee-till
(CellCept)

M

CATEGORY AND SCHEDULE
Pregnancy Risk Category: C

Classification:
Immunosuppressives

MECHANISM OF ACTION
An immunologic agent that suppresses the immunologically mediated inflammatory response by inhibiting inosine monophosphate dehydrogenase, an enzyme that deprives lymphocytes of nucleotides necessary for DNA and RNA synthesis, thus inhibiting the proliferation of T and B lymphocytes. *Therapeutic Effect:* Prevents transplant rejection.

PHARMACOKINETICS
Rapidly and extensively absorbed after PO administration (food decreases drug plasma concentration but does not affect absorption). Protein binding: 97%. Completely hydrolyzed

to active metabolite mycophenolic acid. Primarily excreted in urine. Not removed by hemodialysis. *Half-life:* 17.9 h.

AVAILABILITY
Capsules: 250 mg.
Oral Suspension: 200 mg/mL once reconstituted.
Tablets: 500 mg.
Injection: 500 mg.

INDICATIONS AND DOSAGES
▸ **Prevention of renal transplant rejection**
PO, IV
Adults, Elderly. 1 g twice a day.
PO
Children 3 mos-18 years. $600/m^2$ twice daily (maximum: 2 g/day).
▸ **Prevention of heart transplant rejection**
PO, IV
Adults, Elderly. 1.5 g twice a day.
▸ **Prevention of liver transplant rejection**
PO
Adults, Elderly. 1.5 g twice a day.
IV
Adults, Elderly. 1 g twice a day.
▸ **Usual pediatric dosage**
PO
Children. 600 mg/m^2/dose twice a day. Maximum: 2 g/dose.

OFF-LABEL USES
Treatment of transplantation rejection, graft-versus-host disease.

CONTRAINDICATIONS
Hypersensitivity to mycophenolic acid.

INTERACTIONS
Drug
Acyclovir, ganciclovir: May increase plasma concentrations of both drugs in patients with renal impairment.

Antacids (aluminum and magnesium-containing), cholestyramine: May decrease the absorption of mycophenolate.

Live-virus vaccines: May potentiate virus replication, increase vaccine side effects, and decrease the patient's antibody response to the vaccine.

Other immunosuppressants: May increase the risk of infection or lymphomas.

Probenecid: May increase mycophenolate plasma concentration.

Norfloxacin, metronidazole, rifampin: Lower mycophenolate concentrations. Avoid co-use.

Herbal

Echinacea: May decrease the effects of mycophenolate.

Food

All foods: May decrease mycophenolate plasma concentration.

DIAGNOSTIC TEST EFFECTS

May increase serum cholesterol, alkaline phosphatase, creatinine, AST (SGOT), and ALT (SGPT) levels. May increase or decrease blood glucose as well as serum lipid, calcium, potassium, phosphate, and uric acid levels.

⊘ IV INCOMPATIBILITIES

Mycophenolate is compatible only with D5W. Do not infuse it concurrently with other drugs or IV solutions.

SIDE EFFECTS

Frequent (20%-37%)

Urinary tract infection, hypertension, peripheral edema, diarrhea, constipation, fever, headache, nausea.

Occasional (10%-18%)

Dyspepsia; dyspnea; cough; hematuria; asthenia; vomiting; edema; tremors; abdominal, chest, or back pain; oral candidiasis; acne.

Rare (6%-9%)

Insomnia, respiratory tract infection, rash, dizziness.

SERIOUS REACTIONS

• Significant anemia, leukopenia, thrombocytopenia, neutropenia, and leukocytosis may occur, particularly in those undergoing renal transplant rejection.

• Sepsis and infection occur occasionally.

• GI tract hemorrhage occurs rarely.

• Patients receiving mycophenolate have an increased risk of developing neoplasms.

PRECAUTIONS & CONSIDERATIONS

Caution is warranted with active serious digestive disease, neutropenia, renal impairment, and in women of childbearing potential. Women (except those who had a hysterectomy) should use effective contraception before, during, and for 6 wks after discontinuing mycophenolate therapy, even if she has had a history of infertility. Two forms of contraception should be used concurrently (e.g. hormonal [oral] and nonhormonal) unless patient will remain abstinent. It is unknown whether mycophenolate crosses the placenta or is distributed in breast milk; caution is warranted in pregnancy and lactation. Women taking this drug should avoid breastfeeding. The safety and efficacy of mycophenolate have not been established in children. Age-related renal impairment may require a dosage adjustment in elderly patients.

Notify the physician of abdominal pain, fever, sore throat, or unusual bleeding or bruising. A pregnancy test should be performed before

M

therapy. CBC should be obtained weekly during the first month of therapy, twice monthly during the second and third month, then monthly for the rest of the first year. The dosage should be reduced or discontinue if a rapid fall in WBC count occurs.

Storage

Store the reconstituted suspension in the refrigerator or at room temperature. It remains stable for 60 days after reconstitution. Store vials at room temperature. Do not freeze.

Administration

Give oral mycophenolate on an empty stomach. Do not open or crush capsules. Avoid inhaling the powder in capsules, and keep the powder away from the skin and mucous membranes. If contact occurs, wash thoroughly with soap and water, and rinse the eyes profusely with plain water. The suspension can be administered orally or by nasogastric tube (minimum size: 8 French). Shake well before each use.

For IV use, reconstitute each 500-mg vial with 14 mL D5W. Gently agitate the vial. For a 1-g dose, further dilute with 140 mL D5W; for a 1.5-g dose, further dilute with 210 mL D5W to provide a concentration of 6 mg/mL. Infuse the drug over at least 2 h.

M

Nabumetone
na-byu′me-tone
(Apo-Nabumetone, Relafen)

CATEGORY AND SCHEDULE
Pregnancy Risk Category: C (D if used in third trimester or near delivery)

Classification: Nonsteroidal anti-inflammatory drugs (NSAIDs)

MECHANISM OF ACTION
An NSAID that produces analgesic and anti-inflammatory effects by inhibiting prostaglandin synthesis. *Therapeutic Effect:* Reduces the inflammatory response and intensity of pain.

PHARMACOKINETICS
Readily absorbed from the GI tract. Protein binding: 99%. Widely distributed. Metabolized in the liver to active metabolite. Excreted primarily in urine. Not removed by hemodialysis. *Half-life:* 22-30 h.

AVAILABILITY
Tablets: 500 mg, 750 mg.

INDICATIONS AND DOSAGES
▸ **Acute or chronic rheumatoid and osteoarthritis**
PO
Adults, Elderly. Initially, 1000 mg as a single dose or in 2 divided doses. May increase up to 2000 mg/day as a single or in 2 divided doses. If patient < 50 kg, usual maximum is 1000 mg/day.

CONTRAINDICATIONS
Active peptic ulcer disease, chronic inflammation of GI tract, GI bleeding or ulceration, history of hypersensitivity to aspirin or NSAIDs, significant renal impairment, use within 14 days of coronary artery bypass graft surgery. **Caution**
Lactation, children, bleeding disorders, GI disorders, cardiac disorders, renal disorders, hepatic dysfunction, elderly patients, and patients at increased risk of thromboembolism.

INTERACTIONS
Drug
Antihypertensives, diuretics: May decrease the effects of these drugs.
Aspirin, other salicylates, alcohol, corticosteroids: May increase the risk of GI side effects such as bleeding.
Bone marrow depressants: May increase the risk of hematologic reactions.
Cyclosporine: May decrease renal function.
First-time users of SSRIs also taking NSAIDs, nabumetone: May have a higher risk of GI side effects.
Heparin, oral anticoagulants, thrombolytics: May increase the effects of these drugs.
Lithium: May increase the blood concentration and risk of toxicity of lithium.
Methotrexate: May increase the risk of methotrexate toxicity.
Probenecid: May increase the nabumetone blood concentration.
Herbal
Feverfew: May decrease the effects of feverfew.
Ginkgo biloba: May increase the risk of bleeding.
Food
None known.

DIAGNOSTIC TEST EFFECTS
May increase BUN level; urine protein levels; and serum LDH,

alkaline phosphatase, creatinine, potassium, AST (SGOT), and ALT (SGPT) levels. May decrease serum uric acid level.

SIDE EFFECTS

Frequent (12%-14%)
Diarrhea, abdominal cramps or pain, dyspepsia.
Occasional (4%-9%)
Nausea, constipation, flatulence, dizziness, headache.
Rare (1%-3%)
Vomiting, stomatitis, confusion.

SERIOUS REACTIONS

• Overdose may result in acute hypotension and tachycardia.
• Rare reactions with long-term use include peptic ulcer disease, GI bleeding, gastritis, nephrotoxicity (dysuria, cystitis, hematuria, proteinuria, nephrotic syndrome), severe hepatic reactions (cholestasis, jaundice), and severe hypersensitivity reactions (bronchospasm, angioedema).

PRECAUTIONS & CONSIDERATIONS

Caution is warranted in patients with congestive heart failure (CHF), hypertension, hepatic or renal impairment, and in those using anticoagulants concurrently. Nabumetone is distributed in low concentrations in breast milk; caution is warranted in lactation. Nabumetone should not be used during the last trimester of pregnancy because it can cause adverse effects in the fetus, such as premature closing of the ductus arteriosus. The safety and efficacy of this drug have not been established in children. In elderly patients, GI bleeding or ulceration is more likely to cause serious complications, and age-related renal impairment may increase

the risk of hepatotoxicity or renal toxicity; a reduced drug dosage is recommended. Avoid alcohol and aspirin during therapy because these substances increase the risk of GI bleeding. Tasks that require mental alertness or motor skills should also be avoided. Caution should be exercised in patients at risk for thromboembolism because of the greater possible risk of adverse cardiovascular events occuring while on nabumetone therapy.

Blood chemistry studies, renal and liver function studies, and pattern of daily bowel activity and stool consistency should be assessed before and during therapy. Therapeutic response, such as decreased pain, stiffness, swelling, and tenderness, improved grip strength, and increased joint mobility, should be evaluated. Overdose manifests as acute hypotension and tachyardia.
Storage
Store at room temperature.
Administration
Swallow tablets whole. Take nabumetone with food, milk, or antacids if GI distress occurs.

Nadolol
nay-doe′lole
(Apo-Nadol [CAN], Corgard,
Novo-Nadolol [CAN])

CATEGORY AND SCHEDULE
Pregnancy Risk Category: C (D if
used in second or third trimester)

Classification: Antiadrenergics,
β-blocking

MECHANISM OF ACTION
A nonselective β-blocker that
blocks β_1- and β_2-adrenergic
receptors. Large doses increase
airway resistance. *Therapeutic
Effect:* Slows sinus heart rate,
decreases cardiac output and BP.
Decreases myocardial ischemia
severity by decreasing oxygen
requirements.

PHARMACOKINETICS
PO: Onset variable, peak 3-4 h,
duration 17-24 h. Not metabolized;
excreted unchanged in urine, bile,
and breast milk. *Half-life:* 16-24 h.

AVAILABILITY
Tablets: 20 mg, 40 mg, 80 mg,
120 mg, 160 mg.

INDICATIONS AND DOSAGES
▶ **Mild to moderate hypertension
and angina**
PO
Adults, Elderly. Initially, 40 mg/day.
May increase by 40-80 mg at
intervals of 3-7 days. Maximum:
240 mg/day for angina, 320 mg/day
for hypertension.
▶ **Dosage in renal impairment**
Dosage is modified based on
creatinine clearance.

Creatinine Clearance (mL/min)	Dosage Interval
31-50	24-36 h
10-30	24-48 h
< 10	40-60 h

OFF-LABEL USES
Treatment of atrial fibrillation
hypertrophic cardiomyopathy,
pheochromocytoma, essential tremor,
thyrotoxicosis, vascular headache
prophylaxis.

CONTRAINDICATIONS
Bronchial asthma, cardiogenic
shock, second- or third-degree heart
block, sinus bradycardia, overt
cardiac failure.
Caution
Diabetes mellitus, renal disease,
lactation, hyperthyroidism,
peripheral vascular disease,
myasthenia gravis.

INTERACTIONS
Drug
Cimetidine: May increase nadolol
blood concentration.
Diuretics, other antihypertensives:
May increase hypotensive effect.
**Fentanyl, hydrocarbon inhalation
anesthetics:** May increase
hypotension, myocardial depression.
Indomethacin, other NSAIDs: May
decrease hypotensive effects.
Insulin, oral hypoglycemics: May
mask symptoms of hypoglycemia
and prolong the hypoglycemic
effect of insulin and oral
hypoglycemics.
Lidocaine: Slows metabolism of
nadolol.
NSAIDs: May decrease
antihypertensive effect.
**Sympathomimetics (epinephrine,
norepinephrine, isoproterenol),
xanthines:** May mutually inhibit
effects.

N

Herbal
None known.
Food
None known.

DIAGNOSTIC TEST EFFECTS

May increase serum antinuclear antibody titer and BUN, serum LDH, serum lipoprotein, serum alkaline phosphatase, serum bilirubin, serum creatinine, serum potassium, serum uric acid, AST (SGOT), ALT (SGPT), and serum triglyceride levels.

SIDE EFFECTS

Nadolol is generally well tolerated, with transient and mild side effects.
Frequent
Diminished sexual ability, drowsiness, unusual fatigue or weakness.
Occasional
Bradycardia, difficulty breathing, depression, cold hands or feet, diarrhea, constipation, anxiety, nasal congestion, nausea, vomiting.
Rare
Altered taste, dry eyes, itching.

SERIOUS REACTIONS

• Overdose may produce profound bradycardia and hypotension.
• Abrupt withdrawal of nadolol may result in diaphoresis, palpitations, headache, tremulousness, exacerbation of angina, MI, and ventricular arrhythmias.
• Nadolol administration may precipitate CHF and MI in patients with cardiac disease; thyroid storm in those with thyrotoxicosis; and peripheral ischemia in those with existing peripheral vascular disease.
• Hypoglycemia may occur in patients with previously controlled diabetes.

PRECAUTIONS & CONSIDERATIONS

Caution is warranted in patients with diabetes mellitus, hyperthyroidism, chronic bronchitis or asthma, impaired hepatic and renal function, and inadequate cardiac function. Be aware that salt and alcohol intake should be restricted. Nasal decongestants or OTC cold preparations (stimulants) should not be used without physician approval. Tasks that require mental alertness or motor skills should be avoided. Caution with postural changes resulting from increased risk of orthostatic hypotension developing.

Notify the physician of confusion, depression, difficulty breathing, dizziness, fever, night cough, rash, slow pulse, sore throat, swelling of arms and legs, or unusual bleeding or bruising. BP for hypotension; respiratory status for shortness of breath; pattern of daily bowel activity and stool consistency; ECG for arrhythmias; and pulse for quality, rate, and rhythm should be monitored during treatment. If pulse rate is ≤60 beats/min or systolic BP ≤90 mm Hg, withhold the medication and contact the physician. In those receiving nadolol for treatment of angina, the onset, type (sharp, dull, squeezing), radiation, location, intensity, and duration of anginal pain and its precipitating factors, including exertion and emotional stress, should be recorded. Signs and symptoms of CHF, such as decreased urine output, distended neck veins, dyspnea (particularly on exertion or lying down), night cough, peripheral edema, and weight gain should also be assessed.

Storage
Store at room temperature.
Administration
Take nadolol without regard to meals. Tablets may be crushed.

Nafarelin
naf-ah-rell-in
(Synarel)

CATEGORY AND SCHEDULE
Pregnancy Risk Category: X

Classification: Gonadotropin, analogue of gonadotropin-releasing hormone (GnRH)

MECHANISM OF ACTION
A gonadotropin inhibitor that initially stimulates the release of the pituitary gonadotropins, luteinizing hormone and follicle-stimulating hormone, then decreases secretion of gonadal steroids. *Therapeutic Effect:* Temporarily increases ovarian steroidogenesis, abolishes the stimulatory effect on the pituitary gland, and decreases secretion of gonadal steroids.

PHARMACOKINETICS
Rapidly absorbed after nasal administration. Protein binding: 78%-84%, binds primarily to albumin. Metabolism: Unknown. Excreted in urine. *Half-life:* 3 h.

AVAILABILITY
Nasal Spray: 2 mg/mL (Synarel).

INDICATIONS AND DOSAGES
▸ **Endometriosis**
INTRANASAL
Adults. 400 mcg/day: 200 mcg (1 spray) into 1 nostril in morning, 1 spray into other nostril in evening. For patients with persistent regular menstruation after months of treatment, increase dose to 800 mcg/day (1 spray into each nostril in morning and evening).

▸ **Central precocious puberty**
INTRANASAL
Children. 1600 mcg/day: 400 mcg (2 sprays into each nostril in morning and evening; total 8 sprays). May increase up to 1800 mcg/day (3 sprays into alternating nostrils 3 times/day).

CONTRAINDICATIONS
Pregnancy, undiagnosed abnormal vaginal bleeding, hypersensitivity to nafarelin or any component of the formulation or other GnRH-related drugs, breast-feeding.

INTERACTIONS
Drug
None known.
Herbal
None known.
Food
None known.

DIAGNOSTIC TEST EFFECTS
None known.

SIDE EFFECTS
Frequent
Hot flashes, muscle pain, decreased breast size, myalgia.
Occasional
Nasal irritation, decreased libido, vaginal dryness, headache, emotional lability, acne, transient increase in pubic hair.
Rare
Insomnia, edema, weight gain, seborrhea, depression.

SERIOUS REACTIONS
• None reported.

PRECAUTIONS & CONSIDERATIONS
Caution is warranted in patients with a history of osteoporosis, chronic alcohol or tobacco use, and intercurrent rhinitis. Be aware that nafarelin is contraindicated in

N

pregnancy and is distributed in breast milk, warranting caution in lactation. Be aware that safety and efficacy have not been established in children younger than 18 yr. No age-related precautions have been noted in elderly patients.

Nonhormonal contraception should be used during nafarelin therapy. Do not take nafarelin if pregnancy is suspected (risk to fetus).

Storage

Store at room temperature.

Administration

Nafarelin is for nasal use only. In women, initiate treatment between days 2 and 4 of menstrual cycle. Duration of therapy is 6 mo.

For children, treatment is continued until onset of puberty is desired.

Remove spray cap; prime before first use with 7-10 pumps away from the body. Gently blow nose before use. Tilt head back slightly. Insert tip gently and aim toward back and outer side of nose. Close nostril with one finger. Pump sprayer and sniff gently.

Nafcillin Sodium

naph-sil′in so-dee-um
(Nafcil, Nallpen, Unipen)

CATEGORY AND SCHEDULE

Pregnancy Risk Category: B

Classification: Antibiotics, penicill nose-resistant penicillin

MECHANISM OF ACTION

A penicillin that acts as a bactericidal in susceptible penicillinase-producing staphlococcal microorganisms. *Therapeutic Effect:* Inhibits bacterial cell wall synthesis. Bactericidal.

PHARMACOKINETICS

Poorly absorbed from the GI tract. Protein binding: 87%-90%. Widely distributed in bile, pleural, amniotic, synovial fluids. Metabolized in liver. Excreted 30% unchanged primarily in urine. High cerebrospinal fluid penetration. Not removed by hemodialysis. *Half-life:* 0.5-1 h (half-life increased with impaired renal function, neonates).

AVAILABILITY

Powder for Injection: 1 g, 2 g (as base), 10 g (Nafcil, Nallpen, Unipen).

INDICATIONS AND DOSAGES

▶ **Staphylococcal infections**
IV
Adults, Elderly. 500 mg q4h or 1 g q4h (severe infection), infused over 30-60 min.
Not approved for IV use in neonates or children.

OFF-LABEL USES

Surgical prophylaxis.

CONTRAINDICATIONS

Hypersensitivity to any penicillin or cephalosporins; IV use in neonates or children.

INTERACTIONS

Drug
Probenecid: May increase nafcillin blood concentration and risk for nafcillin toxicity.
Herbal
None known.
Food
None known.

DIAGNOSTIC TEST EFFECTS

May cause positive Coombs' test.
May cause false-positive test for
urine protein when sulfosalicylic
acid test is used.

🔄 IV INCOMPATIBILITIES

Ditiazem (Cardizem), droperidol
(Inapsine), fentanyl, insulin, labetalol
(Normodyne, Trandate), midazolam
(Versed), nalbuphine (Nubain),
vancomycin (Vancocin), verapamil
(Isoptin).

🔄 IV COMPATIBILITIES

None known.

SIDE EFFECTS

Frequent
Mild hypersensitivity reaction (fever,
rash, pruritus); GI effects (nausea,
vomiting, diarrhea), which are more
frequent with oral administration.
Occasional
Hypokalemia with high IV doses,
phlebitis, thrombophlebitis (more
common in elderly).
Rare
Extravasation with IV administration.

SERIOUS REACTIONS

• Superinfections, potentially
fatal antibiotic-associated colitis
may result from altered bacterial
balance.
• Hematologic effects (especially
involving platelets, WBCs), severe
hypersensitivity reactions, and
anaphylaxis occur rarely.
• Thrombophlebitis.
• Neurotoxic reactions (rare).

PRECAUTIONS & CONSIDERATIONS

Caution should be used in patients
with antibiotic-associated colitis
or a history of allergies, especially
to cephalosporins. Be aware that
amoxicillin crosses the placenta and
is distributed in breast milk in low

concentrations, warranting caution
in lactation. Not approved for IV
use in neonates or children. Delayed
excretion may occur in neonates or
infants. Age-related renal impairment
may require dosage adjustment in
elderly patients. Report itching, rash,
hives, difficulty breathing, diarrhea,
loose foul-smellng stools, and
injection site reactions for medical
assessment immediately.
Storage
Reconstituted parenteral solution is
stable for 3 days at room temperature
and 7 days when refrigerated or
12 wks when frozen. For IV infusion
in 0.9% NaCl or D5W, solution is
stable for 72 h at room temperature
and 21 days when refrigerated (41° F).
Administration
Be certain to space doses evenly
around the clock.
  Limit IV therapy to < 48 h, if
possible. Stop infusion if patient
complains of pain. Because of
potential for hypersensitivity or
anaphylaxis, start the initial dose at
a few drops per minute and increase
slowly to the ordered rate; stay with
the patient on the first 10-15 min,
then check every 10 min. Doses
are diluted in 50-100 mL of either
0.9% NaCl or dextrose 5% injection.
Infuse over 30-60 min.

N

Naftifine
naf-ti-feen
(Naftin)
**Do not confuse naftifine with
nafcillin or nafarelin.**

CATEGORY AND SCHEDULE
Pregnancy Risk Category: B

Classification: Antifungals,
topical, dermatologics

MECHANISM OF ACTION
An antifungal that selectively
inhibits the enzyme squalene
epoxidase in a dose-dependent
manner, which results in the primary
sterol, ergosterol, within the fungal
membrane not being synthesized.
Therapeutic Effect: Results in
fungal cell death. Fungistatic and
fungicidal.

PHARMACOKINETICS
Minimal systemic absorption.
Metabolized in the liver. Excreted
in the urine as well as the feces and
bile. *Half-life:* 48-72 h.

AVAILABILITY
Gel: 1% (Naftin).
Cream: 1% (Naftin).

INDICATIONS AND DOSAGES
▸ **Tinea pedis, tinea cruris, tinea
corporis**
TOPICAL
*Adults, Elderly, Children 12 yr and
older.* Apply cream 1 time a day for
4 wks or until signs and symptoms
significantly improve. Apply gel
2 times a day for 4 wks or until
signs and symptoms significantly
improve.

OFF-LABEL USES
Trichomycosis.

CONTRAINDICATIONS
Hypersensitivity to naftifine or any
of its components.

INTERACTIONS
Drug
None known.
Herbal
None known.
Food
None known.

DIAGNOSTIC TEST EFFECTS
None known.

SIDE EFFECTS
Frequent
Burning, stinging.
Occasional
Erythema, itching, dryness, irritation.

SERIOUS REACTIONS
• Excessive irritation may indicate
hypersensitivity reaction.

PRECAUTIONS & CONSIDERATIONS
Occlusive dressings should be
avoided. It is unknown whether
naftifine is distributed in breast milk,
warranting caution in lactation.
Safety and efficacy of naftifine have
not been established in children.
Use in pregnancy only aftter
determination that benefits outweigh
possible risks. No age-related
precautions have been noted in
elderly patients.
Administration
Naftifine is for external use only.
Topical therapy should not exceed
4 wks. Avoid getting the topical form
in contact with the eyes, mouth,
nose, or other mucous membranes.
Wash hands after application.

N

Nalbuphine Hydrochloride

nal'byoo-feen high-droh-klor-ide
(Nubain)
**Do not confuse Nubain with
Navane.**

CATEGORY AND SCHEDULE

Pregnancy Risk Category: B (D if
used for prolonged periods or at
high dosages at term)

Classification: Narcotic
agonist-antagonist analgesic

MECHANISM OF ACTION

A narcotic agonist-antagonist that
binds with opioid receptors in the
central nervous system (CNS).
May displace opioid agonists
and competitively inhibit their
action; may precipitate withdrawal
symptoms. *Therapeutic Effect:* Alters
the perception of and emotional
response to pain.

PHARMACOKINETICS

Route	Onset (min)	Peak (min)	Duration (h)
IV	2-3	30	3-6
IM	< 15	60	3-6
SC	< 15	NA	3-6

Well absorbed after IM or SC
administration. Protein binding: 50%.
Metabolized in the liver. Eliminated
primarily in feces by biliary
secretion. Crosses the placenta.
Duration 3-6 h. *Half-life:* 3.5-5 h.

AVAILABILITY

Injection: 10 mg/mL, 20 mg/mL.

INDICATIONS AND DOSAGES

▸ **Analgesia (moderate to severe
pain, obstetric)**

IV, IM, SC
Adults, Elderly. 10 mg q3-6h as
needed. Do not exceed maximum
single dose of 20 mg or daily dose
of 160 mg. For patients receiving
long-term narcotic analgesics of
similar duration of action, give 25%
of usual dose.
Children. 0.1 mg/kg q3-6h as
needed.
▸ **Supplement to anesthesia**
IV
Adults, Elderly. Induction: 0.3-3 mg/kg
over 10-15 min. Maintenance:
0.25-0.5 mg/kg as needed.

CONTRAINDICATIONS

Hypersensitivity to nalbuphine.
Caution
Renal function impairment, hepatic
function impairment, impaired
respiration, head injury, increasing
intracranial pressure, myocardial
infarction (MI) with nausea or
vomiting, patient undergoing biliary
tract surgery.

INTERACTIONS

Drug
**Alcohol, other CNS depressants,
barbiturates:** May increase CNS
or respiratory depression and
hypotension.
Buprenorphine: May decrease the
effects of nalbuphine.
MAOIs: May produce a severe,
possibly fatal reaction; plan to
administer 25% of the usual
nalbuphine dose.
Nafcillin, ketorolac:
Contraindicated use.
Nalbuphine: Can precipitate
withdrawal.
Herbal
None known.
Food
Sulfites: May cause anaphylactic
symptoms or life threatening
asthma.

N

DIAGNOSTIC TEST EFFECTS

May increase serum amylase and lipase levels.

May interfere with enzymatic methods to detect opioids.

Ⓓ IV INCOMPATIBILITIES

Amphotericin B complex (Abelcet, AmBisome, Amphotec), cefepime (Maxipime), docetaxel (Doxil), methotrexate, nafcillin (Nafcil), piperacillin and tazobactam (Zosyn), sargramostim (Leukine, Prokine), sodium bicarbonate.

🛡 IV COMPATIBILITIES

Diphenhydramine (Benadryl), droperidol (Inapsine), glycopyrrolate (Robinul), hydroxyzine (Vistaril), ketorolac (Toradol), lidocaine, midazolam (Versed), propofol (Diprivan).

SIDE EFFECTS

Frequent (35%)
Sedation.
Occasional (3%-9%)
Diaphoresis, cold and clammy skin, nausea, vomiting, dizziness, vertigo, dry mouth, headache.
Rare (< 1%)
Restlessness, emotional lability, paresthesia, flushing, paradoxical reaction.

SERIOUS REACTIONS

• Abrupt withdrawal after prolonged use may produce symptoms of narcotic withdrawal, such as abdominal cramping, rhinorrhea, lacrimation, anxiety, fever, and piloerection (goose bumps).
• Overdose results in severe respiratory depression, skeletal muscle flaccidity, cyanosis, and extreme somnolence progressing to seizures, stupor, and coma.
• Repeated use may result in drug tolerance and physical dependence.

PRECAUTIONS & CONSIDERATIONS

Caution is warranted in pregnancy and in patients who are opioid dependent or have head trauma, increased intracranial pressure, hepatic or renal impairment, recent MI, respiratory depression, and those about to undergo biliary tract surgery. Nalbuphine readily crosses the placenta and is distributed in breast milk, but the amount is low; use caution. Children may experience paradoxical excitement; not approved for children < 18 yr. Children younger than 2 yr and elderly patients are more likely to develop respiratory depression. In elderly patients, age-related renal impairment may increase the risk of urine retention. Overdose is evidenced by respiratory depression, hypoxemia, sedation.

Low abuse potential but withdrawal symptoms on discontinuation after long-term use; can be abused by patients with narcotic abuse potential. Ensure naloxone, oxygen, resuscitation and intubation equipment are available if needed.

Dizziness and drowsiness may occur, so change positions slowly and avoid alcohol, CNS depressants, and tasks that require mental alertness or motor skills until response to the drug is established. BP, pulse rate and quality, respirations, pattern of daily bowel activity and stool consistency, and clinical improvement of pain should be monitored.

Storage
Store at room temperature. Do not administer if particulate matter is present or solution is discolored.

Administration
! Keep in mind that nalbuphine dosage is based on the person's physical condition, the severity of pain, and concurrent use of other drugs.

For IV use, nalbuphine may be given undiluted. For IV push, administer each 10 mg over 3-5 min.

For IM use, rotate IM injection sites.

Nalmefene Hydrochloride
nal'meh-feen high-droh-klor-ide
(Revex)
Discontinued in the United States

CATEGORY AND SCHEDULE
Pregnancy Risk Category: B

Classification: Opioid antagonist

MECHANISM OF ACTION
A narcotic antagonist that binds to opioid receptors. *Therapeutic Effect:* Prevents and reverses effects of opioids (respiratory depression, sedation, hypotenstion).

PHARMACOKINETICS
Well absorbed. Protein binding: 45%. Metabolized primarily via glucuronidation. Excreted in urine and feces. *Half-life:* 8.5-10.8 h.

AVAILABILITY
Solution for Injection: 100 mcg/mL ([blue label] Revex), 1000 mcg/mL ([green label] Revex).

INDICATIONS AND DOSAGES
▸ **Reversal of opioid depression use only**
Solution for Injection: 100 mcg/mL ([blue label] Revex).
IV
Adults. Initially, 0.25 mcg/kg, followed by additional 0.25 mcg doses at 2-5 min intervals until desired response. Cumulative doses

> 1 mcg/kg do not provide additional therapeutic effect; titrate all doses as follows:

Body Weight (kg)	Solution (mL of 100 mcg/mL)
50	0.125
60	0.150
70	0.175
80	0.200
90	0.225
100	0.250

▸ **Known or suspected opioid overdose**
IV (USING 1000 mcg/mL [GREEN LABEL] CONCENTRATION)
Adults. Initially, 0.5 mg/70 kg. May give 1 mg/70 kg 2-5 min later. If physical opioid dependence is suspected, the initial dose is 0.1 mg/70 kg. Additional doses > 1.5 mg/70 kg are unlikely to be beneficial.

CONTRAINDICATIONS
Hypersensitivity to nalmefene; use in newborns.
Caution
Nursing mothers, children, withdrawal in symptoms in opioid addicts, renal impairment.

INTERACTIONS
Drug
None known.
Herbal
None known.
Food
None known.

DIAGNOSTIC TEST EFFECTS
None known.

ⓦ IV INCOMPATIBILITIES
None known.

▨ IV COMPATIBILITIES
None known.

SIDE EFFECTS

Oral: Dry mouth.
Central nervous system (CNS):
Dizziness, headache, dysphoria,
perception of pain, nervousness.
Cardiovascular: Tachycardia,
hypertension, dysrhythmia,
hypotension.
GI: Nausea, abdominal cramps,
vomiting, diarrhea.
Respiratory: Pharyngitis, pulmonary
edema.
Genitourinary: Urinary retention.
Integumentary system: Pruritus.
Multiple sclerosis: Myalgia, joint
pains.
Miscellaneous: Chills.

SERIOUS REACTIONS

• Precipitation of acute withdrawal
syndrome in opioid-dependent
persons indicated by stuffy or runny
nose; tearing; yawning; sweating;
tremor; vomiting; piloerection;
feeling of temperature change; joint,
bone, or muscle pain; abdominal
cramps, and feeling of skin crawling.

PRECAUTIONS & CONSIDERATIONS

❗ Drug is intended only for acute
use. A risk of seizures has been
reported in animal studies; be aware
of this possibility. Buprenorphine
depression may not be completely
reversed.

Caution should be used in
patients with active liver disease or
cardiovascular disease or who have
received potentially cardiotoxic
drugs or who have physical
dependence on narcotic or narcotic-
like agents. Be aware that nalmefene
should not be used as primary
treatment for ventilatory failure.
Be aware that nalmefene might not
reverse buprenorphine-induced
respiratory depression completely.
Be aware that nalmefene, particularly
in higher doses (1 or 2 mg), may

produce long-lasting antianalgesia
effects when used to reverse opioid
effects in postoperative patients or
in outpatients undergoing surgical
procedures. It is unknown whether
nalmefene crosses the placenta
or is distributed in breast milk,
warranting caution in lactation. Be
aware that nalmefene should be
avoided in newborns. No age-related
precautions have been noted in
children or elderly patients.

Heroin or other opiates will
have no effect during nalmefene
therapy. Any attempt to overcome
nalmefene's prolonged 24- to 72-h
blockade of opioid effects by taking
large amount of opioids is very
dangerous and may result in coma,
serious injury, or fatal overdose.
Notify the physician of abdominal
pain that lasts longer than 3 days,
dark-colored urine, white bowel
movements, or yellow of the whites
of the eyes.

Storage
Store at room temperature.

Administration
❗ Be aware that nalmefene is
supplied in 2 concentrations.
Labeling is color-coded.
Postoperative reversal—blue.
Overdose management—green.
Be aware that if recurrence of
respiratory depression occurs, dose
may again be titrated to clinical
effect using incremental doses.

Administer IV push. Dilute drug
1:1 with diluent 0.9% NaCl or sterile
water for injection and use smaller
incremental doses in patients known
to be at increased cardiovascular risk.
For overdose, administration may
be IM or SC if venous access is not
available. Single dose is usually
effective 5-15 min after IM/SC doses
of 1 mg.

Naloxone Hydrochloride

nal-oks′one high-droh-klor-ide
(Narcan)
**Do not confuse naloxone
with naltrexone, Narcan with
Norcuron.**

CATEGORY AND SCHEDULE
Pregnancy Risk Category: B

Classification: Narcotic
antagonist

MECHANISM OF ACTION
A narcotic antagonist that displaces
opioids at opioid-occupied receptor
sites in the central nervous system
(CNS). *Therapeutic Effect:* Reverses
opioid-induced sleep or sedation,
increases respiratory rate, raises BP
to normal range.

PHARMACOKINETICS

Route	Onset (min)	Peak	Duration (min)
IV	1-2	NA	20-60
IM	2-5	NA	20-60
SC	2-5	NA	20-60

Well absorbed after IM or SC
administration. Metabolized in the
liver. Excreted primarily in urine.
Half-life: 60-100 min.

AVAILABILITY
Injection: 0.02 mg/mL (neonatal
injection), 0.4 mg/mL, 1 mg/mL.

INDICATIONS AND DOSAGES
▶ Opioid toxicity
IV, IM, SC
Adults, Elderly. 0.4-2 mg q2-3min as
needed. May repeat q20-60min.

*Children 5 yr and older and
weighing ≥ 22 kg.* 2 mg/dose; if no
response, may repeat q2-3 min. May
need to repeat q20-60 min.
*Children and Infants younger than
5 yr and weighing < 22 kg.* 0.1 mg/
kg; if no response, repeat q 2-3 min.
May need to repeat q20-60 min.
▶ Postanesthesia narcotic reversal
IV
Children. 0.01 mg/kg; may repeat
q2-3 min.

CONTRAINDICATIONS
Hypersensitivity to naloxone.

INTERACTIONS
Drug
**Butorphanol, nalbuphine, opioid
agonist analgesics, pentazocine:**
Reverses the analgesic and adverse
effects of these drugs and may
precipitate withdrawal symptoms.
Herbal
None known.
Food
None known.

DIAGNOSTIC TEST EFFECTS
None known.

⊘ IV INCOMPATIBILITIES
Amphotericin B complex (Abelcet,
AmBisome, Amphotec).

⊍ IV COMPATIBILITIES
Heparin, ondansetron (Zofran),
propofol (Diprivan).

SIDE EFFECTS
None known; little or no
pharmacologic effect in absence of
narcotics.

SERIOUS REACTIONS
• Too-rapid reversal of narcotic-
induced respiratory depression may
result in nausea, vomiting, tremors,
increased BP, and tachycardia.

N

• Excessive dosage in postoperative patients may produce significant excitement, tremors, and reversal of analgesia.
• Patients with cardiovascular disease may experience hypotension or hypertension, ventricular tachycardia and fibrillation, and pulmonary edema.

PRECAUTIONS & CONSIDERATIONS

! Drug is intended for acute use only. Risk of seizures reported in animal studies; be aware of this possibility. Buprenorphine depression may not be completely reversed.

Caution is warranted in patients with chronic cardiovascular or pulmonary disease, postoperative patients (to avoid cardiovascular complications), and those suspected of having opioid dependence. It is unknown whether naloxone crosses the placenta or is distributed in breast milk. No age-related precautions have been noted in children or elderly patients. Notify the physician of pain or increased sedation. Vital signs, especially respiratory rate and rhythm, should be monitored. Serious cardiovascular events have been associated with opioid reversal in postoperative patients; doses should be carefully titrated to reduce these events.

Storage

Store the parenteral form at room temperature and protect it from light. The reconstituted solution remains stable in D5W or 0.9% NaCl at 4 mcg/mL for 24 h; discard any unused solution.

Administration

! The American Academy of Pediatrics recommends an initial dose of 0.1 mg/kg for infants and children younger than 5 yr and weighing < 20 kg and an initial dose of 2 mg for children 5 yr and older and weighing > 20 kg. Obtain body weight of children to calculate the drug dosage.

For continuous IV infusion, dilute each 2 mg of naloxone with 500 mL D5W or 0.9% NaCl to provide a concentration of 0.004 mg/mL.

Naloxone may also be administered undiluted. Give each 0.4 mg as IV push over 15 s. Use the 0.4-mg/mL and 1-mg/mL vials for adults and the 0.02-mg/mL concentration for neonates.

For IM use, inject naloxone in a large muscle mass.

Naltrexone Hydrochloride

nal-trex′one high-droh-klor-ide
(ReVia, Vivitrol)

CATEGORY AND SCHEDULE
Pregnancy Risk Category: C

Classification: Narcotic antagonist

MECHANISM OF ACTION
A narcotic antagonist that displaces opioids at opioid-occupied receptor sites in the central nervous system (CNS). *Therapeutic Effect:* Blocks physical effects of opioid analgesics; decreases craving for alcohol and relapse rate in alcoholism.

PHARMACOKINETICS
Rapidly and nearly completely absorbed from GI tract. Peak 2 hr followed by second peak 2-3 days later. IM exposure greater than oral. Low plasma protein binding (20%). Eliminated through urine; undergoes enterohepatic recirculation. *Half-life:* 5-10 days.

AVAILABILITY
Tablets: 50 mg. (ReVia).
Injection for Suspension: 380 mg/vial (Vivitrol).

INDICATIONS AND DOSAGES
▸ **Naloxone challenge test to determine whether patient is opioid dependent**
! Expect to perform the naloxone challenge test if there is any question that the patient is opioid dependent. Do not administer naltrexone until the naloxone challenge test is negative.
IV NALOXONE
Adults, Elderly. Draw 2 mL (0.8 mg) of naloxone into syringe. Inject

0.5 mL (0.2 mg); while needle is still in the vein, observe the patient for 30 s for withdrawal signs or symptoms. If no evidence of withdrawal, inject remaining 1.5 mL (0.6 mg); observe patient for additional 20 min for withdrawal signs or symptoms.
SC
Adults, Elderly. Inject 2 mL (0.8 mg) of naloxone; observe patient for 45 min for withdrawal signs or symptoms.
▸ **Treatment of opioid dependence in patients who have been opioid free for at least 7-10 days**
PO
Adults, Elderly. Initially, 25 mg. Observe patient for 1 h. If no withdrawal signs or symptoms appear, give another 25 mg. If a total of 50 mg does not elicit withdrawal, give 50-150 mg/day. Other common regimens are 100 mg every other day or 150 mg every 3 days.
▸ **Adjunctive treatment of alcohol dependence**
PO OR IM
Adults, Elderly. 50 mg once a day for 12 wks or 380 mg IM every 4 wks.

CONTRAINDICATIONS
Acute opioid withdrawal, failed naloxone challenge test, history of hypersensitivity to naltrexone, opioid dependence, positive urine screen for opioids; acute hepatitis or liver failure. Do not use vivitrol for opioid withdrawal.

INTERACTIONS
Drug
Disulfuram: May increase hepatotoxicity.
Opioid-containing products (including analgesics, antidiarrheals, and antitussives): Blocks the therapeutic effects of these drugs. The concurrent use of

N

any opioid, including methadone, is contraindicated.

Thioridazine: May produce lethargy and somnolence.

Herbal

None known.

Food

None known.

DIAGNOSTIC TEST EFFECTS

May increase AST (SGOT) and ALT (SGPT) levels, bilirubin.

SIDE EFFECTS

Frequent

Alcoholism (7%-10%): Nausea, headache, depression.

Narcotic addiction (5%-10%): Insomnia, anxiety, nervousness, headache, low energy, abdominal cramps, nausea, vomiting, arthralgia, myalgia.

Occasional

Alcoholism (2%-4%): Dizziness, nervousness, fatigue, insomnia, vomiting, anxiety, suicidal ideation.

Narcotic addiction (2%-5%): Irritability, increased energy, dizziness, anorexia, diarrhea or constipation, rash, chills, increased thirst.

SERIOUS REACTIONS

• Signs and symptoms of opioid withdrawal include stuffy or runny nose, tearing, yawning, diaphoresis, tremor, vomiting, piloerection, feeling of temperature change, bone pain, arthralgia, myalgia, abdominal cramps, and feeling of skin crawling.

• Accidental naltrexone overdose produces withdrawal symptoms within 5 min of ingestion that may last for up to 48 h. Symptoms include confusion, visual hallucinations, somnolence, and significant vomiting and diarrhea.

• Hepatocellular injury may occur with large doses.

PRECAUTIONS & CONSIDERATIONS

! May cause hepatocelular injury when given in excessive doses.

Caution is warranted in patients with active hepatic disease. Before treatment, baseline laboratory tests, including creatinine clearance, serum bilirubin, AST (SGOT), and ALT (SGPT) levels, should be obtained. Liver function should be monitored throughout therapy.

Unknown whether excreted in breast milk; warrants caution in lactation. Safety and efficacy in children are not established. Taking opioids while on naltrexone may lead to fatal overdose or coma. Not safe for use in rapid opioid withdrawal procedures.

Be aware that opioid-containing drugs used during naltrexone therapy will have no effect. Any attempt to overcome naltrexone's prolonged 24- to 72-h blockade of opioid effects by taking large amounts of opioids may result in coma, serious injury, or death. Notify the physician if abdominal pain lasts longer than 3 days or if dark urine, white stools, or yellowing of the whites of the eyes occurs. Overdose is evidenced by abdominal pain, dizziness, nausea, and somnolence.

Storage

Store the tablets form at room temperature and protect from light.

Injection form should be stored in the refrigerator. After reconstitution the IM suspension will be milky white without clumps. Use immediately.

Administration

Take oral naltrexone with antacids, after meals, or with food to avoid adverse GI effects. Give IM injection deep into gluteal muscle. Do not administer intravenously. Use only diluent provided.

Nandrolone Decanoate

nan′droe-lone deh-kan-oh-ate
(Deca-Durabolin, Durabolin [CAN])
Do not confuse with testolactone.

CATEGORY AND SCHEDULE

Pregnancy Risk Category: X
Controlled Substance: Schedule III

Classification: Anabolic
steroids, hormones/hormone
modifiers

MECHANISM OF ACTION

An anabolic steroid that promotes
tissue-building processes, increases
production of erythropoietin,
causes protein anabolism, and
increases hemoglobin and red blood
cell volume. *Therapeutic Effect:*
Controls metastatic breast cancer
and helps manage anemia of renal
insufficiency.

PHARMACOKINETICS

Well absorbed after IM
administration (about 77%).
Metabolized in liver. Excreted
primarily in urine. *Half-life:*
6-8 days.

AVAILABILITY

Injection, as decanoate (in sesame
oil): 100 mg/mL, 200 mg/mL (Deca-
Durabolin).

INDICATIONS AND DOSAGES

▸ **Breast cancer in females,
disseminated**
IM
Adults, Elderly. 50-100 mg/wk.
▸ **Anemia of renal insufficiency**
IM
Adults, Elderly (men).
100-200 mg/wk for 6 mo; if no
improvement, then discontinue.

Adults, Elderly (women).
50-100 mg/wk for 6 mo; if no
improvement, then discontinue.
Children, 2-13 yr. 25-50 mg every
3-4 wks.

OFF-LABEL USES

AIDS-associated wasting syndrome,
dialysis patients with cachexia.

CONTRAINDICATIONS

Nephrosis, pregnancy, carcinoma
of breast or prostate, not for
use in infants, patients with
hypersensitivity to nandrolone or
any component of the formulation,
such as sesame oil; pregnancy,
nephrotic phase of nephritis.

INTERACTIONS

Drug
Adrenal steroids: May increase the
effects of adrenal steroids.
Insulin, oral hypoglycemic agents:
May increase the effects of insulin
and hypoglycemic agents.
Oral anticoagulants: May increase
the effects of oral anticoagulants.
Herbal
Chaparral: May increase liver
enzymes.
Comfrey: May increase liver
enzymes.
Eucalyptus: May increase risk of
heptotoxicity.
Germander: May increase liver
enzymes.
Jin bu huan: May increase liver
enzymes.
Kava kava: May increase risk of
liver damage.
Pennyroyal: May increase liver
enzymes.
Skullcap: May increase the risk of
liver damage.
Valerian: May increase the risk of
heptotoxicity.
Food
None known.

DIAGNOSTIC TEST EFFECTS

May decrease thyroxine binding globulin decreasing T4 level and increasing resin uptake of T3 and T4.

Assess hematocrit, hemoglobin, AST, SGOT, ALP, PSA, LDL, HDL-C, blood glucose, serum and urine calcium.

SIDE EFFECTS

Frequent

Male, postpubertal: Gynecomastia, acne, bladder irritability, priapism. Male, prepubertal: Acne, virilism. Females: Virilism.

Occasional

Male, postpubertal/prepubertal: Insomnia, chills, decreased libido, hepatic dysfunction, nausea, diarrhea, prostatic hyperplasia (elderly), iron-deficiency anemia, suppression of clotting factors. Male, prepubertal: Chills, insomnia, hyperpigmentation, diarrhea, nausea, iron deficiency anemia, suppression of clotting factors. Female: Chills, insomnia, hypercalcemia, nausea, diarrhea, iron deficiency anemia, suppression of clotting factors, hepatic dysfunction.

Rare

Hepatic necrosis, heptocellular carcinoma. Atherosclerosis.

SERIOUS REACTIONS

• Peliosis hepatitis of liver, spleen replaced with blood-filled cysts, hepatic neoplasms and hepatocellular carcinoma have been associated with prolonged high-dosage, anaphylactic reactions.
• Malignant liver cell tumors can occur that usually disappear with discontinuation of therapy.
• Cholestatic jaundice.
• Children: Compromised adult stature.
• Priapism (rare).

PRECAUTIONS & CONSIDERATIONS

Caution is warranted in patients with diabetes, epilepsy, or liver or renal impairment. Breast-feeding is recommended to be discontinued during use. Nandrolone use in elderly patients may increase the risk of hyperplasia or stimulate growth of occult prostate carcinoma. Adequate calories and protein should be consumed. Do not use in infants; rarely used in children.

Acne, nausea, pedal edema, or vomiting may occur. Women should report deepening of voice, hoarseness, and menstrual irregularities. Men should report difficulty urinating, frequent erections, and gynecomastia. Weight should be obtained each day. Weekly weight gains of more than 5 lb should be reported.

Administration

Give IM injection deep in gluteal muscle. Do not give as IV injection and rotate injection sites. Do not give if particulate matter is seen or if cloudy or discolored.

Naphazoline
naf-az'oh-leen
(AK-Con, Albalon Liquifilm [AUS], Clear Eyes [AUS], Naphcon, Privine, Vasocon)

CATEGORY AND SCHEDULE
Pregnancy Risk Category: C

Classification: Ophthalmic and nasal vasoconstrictor, decongestant

MECHANISM OF ACTION
A sympathomimetic that directly acts on α-adrenergic receptors in conjunctival arterioles and nasal blood vessels. *Therapeutic Effect:* Causes vasoconstriction, resulting in decreased congestion.

PHARMACOKINETICS
Instillation: Duration 2-3 h.

AVAILABILITY
Ophthalmic Solution: 0.012%, 0.1%.
Nasal Drops: 0.05%.
Nasal Spray: 0.05%.

INDICATIONS AND DOSAGES
▸ **Nasal congestion from acute or chronic rhinitis, common cold, hay fever, or other allergies**
INTRANASAL
Adults, Elderly, Children older than 12 yr. 1-2 drops or sprays in each nostril q3-6h.
Children aged 6-12 yr. 1 spray or drop in each nostril q6h as needed.
▸ **Control of hyperemia in patients with superficial corneal vascularity; relief of congestion and inflammation; for use during ocular diagnostic procedures**
OPHTHALMIC
Adults, Elderly, Children older than 6 yr. 1-2 drops in affected eye q3-4h for 3-4 days.

CONTRAINDICATIONS
Angle-closure glaucoma, before peripheral iridectomy, patients with a narrow angle who do not have glaucoma.
Caution
Hypertension, hyperthroidism, elderly, severe arteriosclerosis, cardiac disease.

INTERACTIONS
Drug
Maprotiline, MAOIs, tricyclic antidepressants: May increase pressor effects.
Herbal
None known.
Food
None known.

DIAGNOSTIC TEST EFFECTS
None known.

SIDE EFFECTS
Occasional
Nasal: Burning, stinging, or drying of nasal mucosa; sneezing; rebound congestion.
Ophthalmic: Blurred vision, dilated pupils, increased eye irritation.

SERIOUS REACTIONS
• If naphazoline is systemically absorbed, the patient may experience tachycardia, palpitations, headache, insomnia, lightheadedness, nausea, nervousness, and tremor.
• Large doses may produce tachycardia, palpitations, lightheadedness, nausea, and vomiting.
• Overdose in patients older than 60 yr may produce hallucinations, CNS depression, and seizures.

PRECAUTIONS & CONSIDERATIONS
Caution is warranted in patients with cerebral arteriosclerosis,

N

diabetes, heart disease (including coronary artery disease), hypertension, hypertensive cardiovascular disease, hyperthyroidism, and longstanding bronchial asthma. Avoid performing tasks that require visual acuity in those using ophthalmic naphazoline. BP should be monitored for increases. Tell the physician if taking tricyclic antidpressants.

Storage
Store nasal and ophthalmic drugs in a tightly closed container. Do not freeze.

Administration
Whenever possible, place oneself in the upright position to instill nasal spray. To minimize the risk of systemic absorption, tilt head slightly downward and avoid directing the spray toward the nasopharynx. Do not use naphazoline for more than 72 h without consulting a physician because too-frequent use may cause rebound congestion. Discontinue the drug and contact the physician if acute eye redness or eye pain, floating spots, vision changes, headache, dizziness, insomnia, irregular heartbeat, tremor, or weakness occurs.

Naproxen Naproxen Sodium

na-prox′en

(Crysanal [AUS], EC-Naprosyn, Inza [AUS], Naprelan, Naprosyn) (Aleve, Anaprox, Anaprox DS, Apo-Naprosyn [CAN], Naprogesic [AUS], Novo-Naprox [CAN], Nu-Naprox [CAN], Pamprin)
Do not confuse Aleve with Alesse, Anaspaz.

CATEGORY AND SCHEDULE
Pregnancy Risk Category: B (D if used in third trimester or near delivery)
OTC (220-mg gelcaps, 220-mg tablets)

Classification: Nonsteroidal anti-inflammatory drugs (NSAIDs)

MECHANISM OF ACTION
An NSAID that produces analgesic and anti-inflammatory effects by inhibiting prostaglandin synthesis. *Therapeutic Effect:* Reduces the inflammatory response and intensity of pain.

PHARMACOKINETICS

Route	Onset	Peak	Duration
PO	< 1 h	NA	≤ 7 h
PO (anti-rheumatic)	< 14 day	2-4 wks	NA

Completely absorbed from the GI tract. Protein binding: 99%. Metabolized in the liver. Primarily excreted in urine. Not removed by hemodialysis. *Half-life:* 13 h.

AVAILABILITY
Gelcaps (Aleve): 220 mg naproxen sodium (equivalent to 200 mg naproxen) (OTC).

Oral Suspension (Naprosyn):
125 mg/5 mL naproxen.
Tablets (Aleve): 220 mg naproxen
(OTC).
Tablets (Anaprox): 275 mg naproxen
sodium (equivalent to 250 mg
naproxen).
Tablets (Anaprox DS): 550 mg
naproxen sodium (equivalent to
500 mg naproxen).
*Tablets (Controlled-Release
[EC-Naprosyn]):* 375 mg naproxen,
500 mg naproxen.
*Tablets (Controlled-Release
[Naprelan]):* 421 mg naproxen,
550 mg naproxen sodium (equivalent
to 500 mg naproxen).

INDICATIONS AND DOSAGES
▸ **Rheumatoid arthritis, osteoarthritis,
ankylosing spondylitis**
PO
Adults, Elderly. 250-500 mg
naproxen (275-550 mg naproxen
sodium) twice a day or 250 mg
naproxen (275 mg naproxen sodium)
in morning and 500 mg naproxen
(550 mg naproxen sodium) in
evening. Naprelan: 750-1000 mg
once a day.
▸ **Acute gouty arthritis**
PO
Adults, Elderly. Initially, 750 mg
naproxen (825 mg naproxen sodium),
then 250 mg naproxen (275 mg
naproxen sodium) q8h until attack
subsides. Naprelan: Initially,
1000-1500 mg, then 1000 mg once a
day until attack subsides.
▸ **Mild to moderate pain,
dysmenorrhea, bursitis, tendinitis**
PO
Adults, Elderly. Initially, 500 mg
naproxen (550 mg naproxen sodium),
then 250 mg naparoxen (275 mg
naproxen sodium) q6-8h as needed.
Maximum: 1.25 g/day naproxen
(1.375 g/day naproxen sodium).
Naprelan: 1000 mg once a day.

▸ **Juvenile rheumatoid arthritis**
PO (NAPROXEN ONLY)
Children. 10-15 mg/kg/day in
2 divided doses. Maximum:
1000 mg/day.

OFF-LABEL USES
Treatment of vascular headaches.

CONTRAINDICATIONS
Hypersensitivity to aspirin, naproxen,
or other NSAIDs; use within 14 days
of coronary artery bypass graft
surgery.
Caution
Lactation, children, bleeding
disorders, GI disorders, cardiac
disorders, hypersensitivity to
other NSAIDs, elderly, more than
2 alcohol drinks per day.

INTERACTIONS
Drug
Antihypertensives, diuretics:
May decrease the effects of these
drugs.
**Aspirin, alcohol, other salicylates,
corticosteroids:** May increase
the risk of GI side effects such as
bleeding.
**β-Adrenergic blockers, diuretics,
ACE inhibitors:** Possible decreased
antihypertensive effects.
Bone marrow depressants:
May increase the risk of hematologic
reactions.
Cyclosporine: Possible risk of
decreased renal function.
**First-time users of SSRIs also
using NSAIDs:** May have a higher
risk of GI side effects.
**Heparin, oral anticoagulants,
thrombolytics:** May increase the
effects of these drugs.
Lithium: May increase the blood
concentration and risk of toxicity of
lithium.
Methotrexate: May increase the risk
of methotrexate toxicity.

N

Oral anticoagulants, oral antidiabetics, thium, methotrexate: Risk of increased effects.

Probenecid: May increase the naproxen blood concentration.

Tetracyclines: May increase risk of photosensitization.

Herbal

Feverfew: May decrease the effects of feverfew.

Ginkgo biloba: May increase the risk of bleeding.

Food

None known.

DIAGNOSTIC TEST EFFECTS

May prolong bleeding time and alter blood glucose level. May increase serum hepatic function test results. May decrease serum sodium and uric acid levels.

SIDE EFFECTS

Frequent (4%-9%)

Nausea, constipation, abdominal cramps or pain, heartburn, dizziness, headache, somnolence.

Occasional (1%-3%)

Stomatitis, diarrhea, indigestion.

Rare (< 1%)

Vomiting, confusion.

SERIOUS REACTIONS

• Rare reactions with long-term use include peptic ulcer disease, GI bleeding, gastritis, severe hepatic reactions (cholestasis, jaundice), nephrotoxicity (dysuria, hematuria, proteinuria, nephrotic syndrome), and a severe hypersensitivity reaction (fever, chills, bronchospasm).

PRECAUTIONS & CONSIDERATIONS

❗ Possible increased cardiovascular events in patients at risk for thromboembolism. Caution is warranted in patients with cardiac disease, GI disease, impaired hepatic or renal function and those using anticoagulants concurrently. Naproxen crosses the placenta and is distributed in breast milk, warranting caution in lactation. Naproxen should not be used during the third trimester of pregnancy because it may cause adverse effects in the fetus, such as premature closing of the ductus arteriosus. The safety and efficacy of naproxen have not been established in children younger than 2 yr. Children older than 2 yr are at an increased risk for developing a rash during naproxen therapy. In elderly patients, GI bleeding or ulceration is more likely to cause serious complications, and age-related renal impairment may increase the risk of hepatotoxicity and renal toxicity; a reduced dosage is recommended. Avoid alcohol and aspirin during therapy because these substances increase the risk of GI bleeding. Tasks that require mental alertness or motor skills should also be avoided.

Notify the physician if black or tarry stools, persistent headache, rash, visual disturbances, or weight gain occurs. CBC (particularly hemoglobin, hematocrit, and platelet count), BUN level, serum alkaline phosphatase, bilirubin, creatinine, AST (SGOT), and ALT (SGPT) levels to assess hepatic and renal function, and pattern of daily bowel activity and stool consistency should be assessed during therapy. Therapeutic response, such as decreased pain, stiffness, swelling and tenderness, improved grip strength, and increased joint mobility, should be evaluated.

Administration
! Be aware that each 275- or 550-mg tablet of naproxen sodium equals 250 or 500 mg of naproxen, respectively.

Swallow enteric-coated tablets whole; scored tablets may be broken or crushed. Take naproxen with food, milk, or antacids if GI distress occurs. Shake oral suspension well before each use.

Naratriptan
nare-a-trip′tan
(Amerge, Naramig [AUS])
Do not confuse Amerge with Amaryl.

CATEGORY AND SCHEDULE
Pregnancy Risk Category: C

Classification: Serotonin agonists

MECHANISM OF ACTION
A serotonin receptor agonist that binds selectively to vascular receptors, producing a vasoconstrictive effect on cranial blood vessels. *Therapeutic Effect:* Relieves migraine headache.

PHARMACOKINETICS
Well absorbed after PO administration. Protein binding: 28%-31%. Metabolized by the liver to inactive metabolite. Eliminated primarily in urine and, to a lesser extent, in feces. *Half-life:* 6 h (increased in hepatic or renal impairment).

AVAILABILITY
Tablets: 1 mg, 2.5 mg.

INDICATIONS AND DOSAGES
▸ **Acute migraine attack**
PO
Adults. 1 mg or 2.5 mg. If headache improves but then returns, dose may be repeated after 4 h. Maximum: 5 mg/24 h.
▸ **Dosage in mild to moderate renal or hepatic impairment**
A lower starting dose is recommended. Do not exceed 2.5 mg/24 h.

CONTRAINDICATIONS
Basilar or hemiplegic migraine, cerebrovascular or peripheral vascular disease, coronary artery disease, ischemic heart disease (including angina pectoris, history of myocardial infarction (MI), silent ischemia, and Prinzmetal angina), severe hepatic impairment—(Child-Pugh grade C), severe renal impairment (serum creatinine < 15 mL/min), uncontrolled hypertension, use within 24 h of ergotamine-containing preparations or another serotonin receptor agonist, use within 14 days of MAOIs.

INTERACTIONS
Drug
5 HT1 agonists: Do not use within 24 h.
Ergotamine-containing medications: May produce a vasospastic reaction. Contraindicated within 24 h.
Fluoxetine, fluvoxamine, paroxetine, sertraline: May produce hyperreflexia, incoordination, and weakness (serotonin syndrome).
MAOIs: Contraindicated.
Oral contraceptives: Decrease naratriptan clearance and volume of distribution.
Herbal
None known.

N

Food
None known.

DIAGNOSTIC TEST EFFECTS
None known.

SIDE EFFECTS
Occasional (5%)
Nausea.
Rare (2%)
Paresthesia; dizziness; fatigue; somnolence; jaw, neck, or throat pressure.

SERIOUS REACTIONS
• Corneal opacities and other ocular defects may occur.
• Cardiac reactions (including ischemia, coronary artery vasospasm, and MI) and noncardiac vasospasm-related reactions (such as hemorrhage or cerebrovascular accident) occur rarely, particularly in patients with hypertension, diabetes, or a strong family history of coronary artery disease; obese patients; smokers; men older than 40 yr; and postmenopausal women.

PRECAUTIONS & CONSIDERATIONS
Caution is warranted with mild to moderate hepatic or renal impairment and cardiovascular risk factors. It is unknown whether naratriptan is excreted in breast milk, warranting caution in lactation. The safety and efficacy of naratriptan have not been established in children. Naratriptan is not recommended for elderly patients. Tasks that require mental alertness or motor skills should be avoided.

Notify the physician immediately if anxiety, chest pain, palpitations, or tightness in the throat occurs. Migraines and associated symptoms, including nausea and vomiting, photophobia, and phonophobia (sound sensitivity), should be assessed before and during treatment.
Administration
Take naratriptan without regard to food. Swallow tablets whole; do not crush them. Take another dose of naratriptan, if needed, 4 h after the first dose for a maximum of 5 mg/24 h in adults.

Natalizumab
nat-ah-lih′zoo-mab
(Tysabri)

CATEGORY AND SCHEDULE
Pregnancy Risk Category: C

Classification: Immunologic agents, monoclonal antibodies

MECHANISM OF ACTION
A monoclonal antibody that binds to the surface of leukocytes, inhibiting their adhesion to the vascular endothelial cells of the GI tract and preventing them from migrating across the endothelium into inflamed parenchymal tissue. *Therapeutic Effect:* Decreases clinical exacerbations of multiple sclerosis.

PHARMACOKINETICS
Half-life: 11 days.

AVAILABILITY
Injection Solution: 300 mg/15 mL concentrate.

INDICATIONS AND DOSAGES
▸ **Relapses of multiple sclerosis**

IV INFUSION
Adults 18 yr and older, Elderly.
300 mg infused over 1 h every
4 wks.

CONTRAINDICATIONS
Multifocal leukoencephalopathy,
hypersensitivity to product or murine
proteins.

INTERACTIONS
Drug
Antineoplastic, corticosteroid,
immunosuppressant,
immodulating agents: May cause
increase in infection.
Herbal
None known.
Food
None known.

DIAGNOSTIC TEST EFFECTS
Increases basophil, eosinophil,
lymphocyte, monocyte, and RBC
counts (increases are reversible,
usually within 16 wks after last
natalizumab dose). May alter
liver function test results. Monitor
patient at 3 mo, 6 mo, after
first infusion, and every 6 mo
thereafter.

Ⓘ IV INCOMPATIBILITIES
Do not mix natalizumab with any
other medication or with any diluent
other than 0.9% NaCl.

SIDE EFFECTS
Frequent (15%-35%)
Headache, fatigue, depression,
arthralgia.
Occasional (5%-10%)
Abdominal discomfort, rash, urinary
frequency or urgency, menstrual
irregularities, dysmenorrhea,
dermatitis.
Rare (2%-4%)
Pruritus, chest discomfort, local
bleeding, rigors, tremor, syncope.

SERIOUS REACTIONS
• Urinary tract infection, lower
respiratory tract infection,
gastroenteritis, vaginitis, allergic
reaction, and tonsillitis occur
occasionally.
• Progressive multifocal
leukoencephalopathy.

PRECAUTIONS & CONSIDERATIONS
Increased risk of progressive
multifocal leukoencephalopathy
that can lead to death or disability.
Patients receiving natalizumab must
be enrolled and meet conditions of
special distribution and registration
program (TOUCH program).
   Caution is warranted in patients
with chronic progressive multiple
sclerosis and in children younger
than 18 yr. It is unknown whether
natalizumab crosses the placenta
or is distributed in breast milk,
warranting caution in lactation. The
safety and efficacy of natalizumab
have not been established in children
younger than 18 yr. No age-related
precautions have been noted for
elderly patients.
   Notify the physician of arthralgia,
rash, depression, menstrual
irregularities, or urinary changes.
CBC and liver function test results
should be monitored.
Storage
Protect natalizumab vials from
light. Do not freeze them. After
reconstitution, the solution is stable
for 8 h if refrigerated.
Administration
To reconstitute, withdraw 15 mL
(300 mg) natalizumab from the vial
and inject it into 100 mL 0.9%
NaCl. Invert the bag to mix the
solution completely. Do not shake
it. Inspect the solution for particles.
Discard it if it contains particles
or becomes discolored. Infuse
natalizumab over 1 h. Following the

N

infusion, flush the IV line with 0.9% NaCl. Observe patient for 1 h after infusion.

Natamycin
na-ta-mye′sin
(Natacyn)
Do not confuse with naproxen.

CATEGORY AND SCHEDULE
Pregnancy Risk Category: C

Classification: Antifungals, ophthalmics

MECHANISM OF ACTION
A polyene antifungal agent that increases cell membrane permeability in susceptible fungi. *Therapeutic Effect:* Fungicidal.

PHARMACOKINETICS
Minimal systemic absorption. Adheres to cornea and retained in conjunctival fornices.

AVAILABILITY
Ophthalmic Suspension: 5% (Natacyn).

INDICATIONS AND DOSAGES
▸ **Fungal keratitis, ophthalmic fungal infections**
OPHTHALMIC
Adults, Elderly. Instill 1 drop in conjunctival sac every 1-2 h. After 3-4 days, reduce to 1 drop 6-8 times daily. Usual course of therapy is 2-3 wks or until the fungal infection is resolved. If limited to blepharitis or conjunctivitis, application 4-6 times/day may be sufficient.

CONTRAINDICATIONS
Hypersensitivity to natamycin or any component of the formulation.

INTERACTIONS
Drug
Topical corticosteroids: May increase risk of toxicity. Concomitant use is contraindicated.
Herbal
None known.
Food
None known.

DIAGNOSTIC TEST EFFECTS
None known.

SIDE EFFECTS
Occasional (3%-10%)
Blurred vision, eye irritation, eye pain, photophobia.

SERIOUS REACTIONS
• Vomiting and diarrhea have occurred with large doses in the treatment of systemic mycoses.

PRECAUTIONS & CONSIDERATIONS
If symptoms do not improve within 7-10 days, or become worse, notify the physician. It is unknown whether natamycin is excreted in breast milk, warranting caution in lactation. Safety and efficacy of natamycin have not been established in children. No age-related precautions have been noted in elderly patients.
Administration
Shake ophthalmic suspension before using. Do not touch dropper to eye. Gently clean eye of any exudate before instilling medication. Form a slight pouch and instill medication into the pouch; close the eye and allow the medication to cover the eye before reopening. Wipe gently any extra medication.

Nateglinide
na-teg'lin-ide
(Starlix)

CATEGORY AND SCHEDULE
Pregnancy Risk Category: C

Classification: Antidiabetic agents, meglitinide class

MECHANISM OF ACTION
An antihyperglycemic that stimulates the release of insulin from β-cells of the pancreas by depolarizing β-cells, leading to an opening of calcium channels. Resulting calcium influx induces insulin secretion. *Therapeutic Effect:* Lowers blood glucose concentration.

PHARMACOKINETICS
PO: Rapid absorption; peak plasma levels in 1 h; bioavailability 73%. Plasma protein binding 98%, hepatic metabolism by CYP450 A29 isoenzyme (70%) and CYP450 3A4 isoenzyme (30%); excretion in urine and feces.

AVAILABILITY
Tablets: 60 mg, 120 mg.

INDICATIONS AND DOSAGES
▶ **Diabetes mellitus**
PO
Adult, Elderly. 120 mg 3 times a day before meals. Initially, 60 mg/dose may be given in patients close to goal HbA1C.

CONTRAINDICATIONS
Diabetic ketoacidosis, type 1 diabetes mellitus, hypersensitivity.
Caution
Hypoglycemia (geriatric, malnourished adrenal insufficiency, or pituitary insufficiency more susceptible to hypoglycemia); β-blocker may mask hypoglycemia, administer before meals, infection, hepatic dysfunction, lactation, children.

INTERACTIONS
Drug
β-Blockers, MAOIs, NSAIDs, salicylates: May increase hypoglycemic effect of nateglinide. **Corticosteroids, thiazide diuretics, thyroid medication, sympathomimetics:** May decrease hypoglycemic effect of nateglinide.
Herbal
None known.
Food
Liquid meal: Peak plasma levels may be significantly reduced if administered 10 min before a liquid meal.

DIAGNOSTIC TEST EFFECTS
None known.

SIDE EFFECTS
Frequent (10%)
Upper respiratory tract infection.
Occasional (3%-4%)
Back pain, flu symptoms, dizziness, arthropathy, diarrhea.
Rare (2%)
Bronchitis, cough.

SERIOUS REACTIONS
• Hypoglycemia occurs in < 2% of patients.

PRECAUTIONS & CONSIDERATIONS
Caution is warranted with hepatic or renal impairment. Food intake and blood glucose should be monitored before and during therapy. Be aware of signs and symptoms of hypoglycemia (anxiety, cool wet skin, diplopia, dizziness, headache, hunger, numbness in mouth, tachycardia, tremors) or

N

hyperglycemia (deep rapid breathing, dim vision, fatigue, nausea, polydipsia, polyphagia, polyuria, vomiting); carry candy, sugar packets, or other sugar supplements for immediate response to hypoglycemia. Consult the physician when glucose demands are altered (such as with fever, heavy physical activity, infection, stress, trauma). Exercise, good personal hygiene (including foot care), not smoking, and weight control are essential parts of therapy.

Administration

Ideally, take within 15 min of a meal; however, may take immediately to as long as 30 min before a meal. Allow at least 1 wk to elapse to assess the response to the drug before new dose adjustment is made.

Nedocromil Sodium

ned-oh-crow′mil so-dee-um
(Alocril, Mireze [CAN], Tilade)

CATEGORY AND SCHEDULE

Pregnancy Risk Category: B

Classification: Antiasthmatic, mast cell stabilizers

MECHANISM OF ACTION

A mast cell stabilizer that prevents the activation and release of inflammatory mediators, such as histamine, leukotrienes, mast cells, eosinophils, and monocytes. *Therapeutic Effect:* Prevents both early and late asthmatic responses.

PHARMACOKINETICS

Inhalation: Peak 15 min, duration 4-6 h. *Half-life:* 80 min; excreted unchanged in feces.

AVAILABILITY

Aerosol for Inhalation (Tilade): 1.75 mg/activation.
Ophthalmic Solution (Alocril): 2%.

INDICATIONS AND DOSAGES

▶ **Mild to moderate asthma**
ORAL INHALATION
Adults, Elderly, Children 6 yr and older. 2 inhalations 4 times a day. May decrease to 3 times a day, then twice a day as asthma becomes controlled.
▶ **Allergic conjunctivitis**
OPHTHALMIC
Adults, Elderly, Children 3 yr and older. 1-2 drops in each eye twice a day.

OFF-LABEL USES

Prevention of bronchospasm in patients with reversible obstructive airway disease.

CONTRAINDICATIONS

Hypersensitivity to this drug or lactose, status asthmaticus.
Caution
Lactation, renal disease, hepatic disease, safety and efficacy of inhalation in children younger than 6 yr or ophthalmic solution in children younger than 3 yr not established.

INTERACTIONS

Drug
Aspirin or vasoconstrictor drugs: Can exacerbate asthma.
Herbal
None known.
Food
Sulfite preservatives: May exacerbate asthma.

DIAGNOSTIC TEST EFFECTS

None known.

SIDE EFFECTS

Frequent (6%-10%)
Cough, pharyngitis, bronchospasm, headache, altered taste.

Occasional (1%-5%)
Rhinitis, upper respiratory tract
infection, abdominal pain, fatigue.
Rare (< 1%)
Diarrhea, dizziness.

SERIOUS REACTIONS
• None known.

PRECAUTIONS & CONSIDERATIONS
Nedocromil is not used to reverse
acute bronchospasm. Drink
plenty of fluids to decrease the
thickness of lung secretions.
Therapeutic response, such as
less frequent or severe asthmatic
attacks or reduced dependence
on antihistamines, should be
monitored. A log of peak flow
meter values should be kept.
Storage
Protect the drug from direct exposure
to light.
Administration
For oral inhalation, shake the
container well before each use.
Administer nedocromil at regular
intervals, even when symptom free,
to achieve optimal results. Rinse
mouth with water immediately after
inhalation to help relieve unpleasant
taste.

For ophthalmic administration,
wash hands before and after. Tilt
head back slightly, look up, and pull
lower eyelid down to form a pouch.
Squeeze drop(s) into pouch then
close eye gently. Do not touch bottle
tip with eye, eyelid, or fingers.

Nefazodone Hydrochloride
neh-faz'oh-doan high-droh-klor-
ide
(Serzone)
Do not confuse with Seroquel.

CATEGORY AND SCHEDULE
Pregnancy Risk Category: C

Classification: Antidepressants,
miscellaneous

MECHANISM OF ACTION
Exact mechanism is unknown.
Appears to inhibit neuronal uptake
of serotonin and norepinephrine
and to antagonize α_1-adrenergic
receptors. *Therapeutic Effect:*
Relieves depression.

PHARMACOKINETICS
Rapidly and completely absorbed
from the GI tract; food delays
absorption. Protein binding: 99%.
Widely distributed in body tissues,
including the central nervous system
(CNS). Extensively metabolized to
active metabolites. Excreted in urine
and eliminated in feces. Unknown
whether removed by hemodialysis.
Half-life: 2-4 h.

AVAILABILITY
Tablets: 50 mg, 100 mg, 150 mg,
200 mg, 250 mg.

INDICATIONS AND DOSAGES
▶ **Depression, prevention of relapse
in acute depressive episode**
PO
Adults. Initially, 200 mg/day in
2 divided doses. Gradually increase
by 100-200 mg/day at intervals of at
least 1 wk. Range: 300-600 mg/day.
Elderly. Initially, 100 mg/day in
2 divided doses. Subsequent dosage

titration based on clinical response.
Range: 200-400 mg/day.
Children. 300-400 mg/day.

CONTRAINDICATIONS

Do not use within 14 days of
MAOIs, previous history of liver
problems from nefazodone, or other
hypersensitivity.
Coadministration of terfenadine,
cisapride, astemizole, pimozide,
carbamazepine or triazolam is
contraindicated.

INTERACTIONS

Drug
**Alprazolam, alcohol or alcohol-
containing products:** May increase
the blood concentration and risk of
toxicity of these drugs.
Carbamazepine: Reduces
nefazodone concentrations
significantly.
Isoenzymes CYP 3A4: May risk
interaction with drugs metabolized
with CYP 3A4.
MAOIs: May produce severe
reactions if used concurrently
with or within 14 days of MAOI
discontinuation.
Triazolam: Increases triazolam
concentration by 75%. Try to avoid,
or greatly reduce triazolam dose.
Herbal
St. John's wort: May increase the
risk of adverse effects.
Food
None known.

DIAGNOSTIC TEST EFFECTS

None known.

SIDE EFFECTS

Frequent
Headache (36%); dry mouth,
somnolence (25%); nausea (22%);
dizziness (17%); constipation (14%);
insomnia, asthenia, lightheadedness
(10%).

Occasional
Dyspepsia, blurred vision (9%);
diarrhea, infection (8%); confusion,
abnormal vision (7%); pharyngitis
(6%); increased appetite (5%);
orthostatic hypotension, flushing,
feeling of warmth (4%); peripheral
edema, cough, flulike symptoms (3%).

SERIOUS REACTIONS

• Serious reactions, such as
hyperthermia, rigidity, myoclonus,
extreme agitation, delirium, and coma,
will occur if the patient takes an MAOI
concurrently or fails to let enough time
elapse when switching from an MAOI
to nefazodone or vice versa.

PRECAUTIONS & CONSIDERATIONS

Caution is warranted in patients with
cerebrovascular or cardiovascular
disease, recent myocardial infarction,
dehydration, hypovolemia, cirrhosis,
a history of hypomania or mania, and
a history of seizures. It is unknown
whether nefazodone crosses the
placenta or is distributed in breast
milk, warranting caution in lactation.
The safety and efficacy of this drug
have not been established in children.
Elderly and debilitated patients are
more susceptible to side effects.
Lower dosages are recommended
for elderly patients, although no age-
related precautions have been noted
for this age group.
   Drowsiness, dizziness, and
lightheadedness may occur, so avoid
alcohol and tasks that require mental
alertness or motor skills. BP and
pulse rate should be assessed during
therapy. Caution is warranted in
postural changes because of possible
orthostatic hypotension developing.
Administration
! Allow at least 14 days to elapse
before switching the patient from
an MAOI to nefazodone and at least
7 days to elapse before switching

the patient from nefazodone to an MAOI.

Take nefazodone without regard to food.

Nelfinavir
nel-fin'eh-veer
(Viracept)

CATEGORY AND SCHEDULE
Pregnancy Risk Category: B

Classification: Antivirals, protease inhibitors

MECHANISM OF ACTION
Inhibits the activity of HIV-1 protease, the enzyme necessary for the formation of infectious HIV. *Therapeutic Effect:* Formation of immature noninfectious viral particles rather than HIV replication.

PHARMACOKINETICS
Well absorbed after PO administration (absorption increased with food). Protein binding: 98%. Metabolized in the liver. Highly bound to plasma proteins. Eliminated primarily in feces. Unknown if removed by hemodialysis. *Half-life:* 3.5-5 h.

AVAILABILITY
Powder for Oral Suspension: 50 mg/g.
Tablets: 250 mg, 625 mg.

INDICATIONS AND DOSAGES
▶ **HIV infection**
PO
Adults. 750 mg (three 250-mg tablets) 3 times a day or 1250 mg twice a day in combination with nucleoside analogues (enhances antiviral activity).

Children aged 2-13 yr.
25-35 mg/kg/dose 3 times a day.
Maximum: 750 mg q8h.

CONTRAINDICATIONS
Hypersensitivity; co-administration with: amiodarone, quinidine, ergot alkaloids, pimozide, triazolam, midazolam, rifampin, St. John's wort, and proton pump inhibitors; moderate on severe liver dysfunction.
Caution
Pediatric use, phenylketonuria (powder contains phenylalanine), diabetes mellitus, hyperglycemia, hepatic impairment, development of resistance, hemophilia, lactation, children younger than 2 yr, inhibitor of CYP 450 3A4 isoenzymes; use with caution with drugs that are inducers of CYP3A4 or CYP2C19 isoenzymes.

INTERACTIONS
Drug
Alcohol, psychoactive drugs: May produce additive central nervous system (CNS) effects.
Anticonvulsants, rifabutin, rifampin: Decrease nelfinavir plasma concentration.
Erythromycin, ketoconazole: May increase plasma levels.
Fentanyl: May increase plasma concentrations of fentanyl.
Indinavir, saquinavir: Increases plasma concentration of these drugs.
Oral contraceptives: Decreases the effects of these drugs.
Rifampin: Decreases nelfinavir concentrations.
Ritonavir: Increases nelfinavir plasma concentration.
Triazolam, midazolam and other drugs dependent on CYP 3A4 for metabolism: Contraindicated use.
Herbal
St. John's wort: May decrease plasma concentration and effects of nelfinavir.

N

Food
All foods: Increase nelfinavir plasma concentration. Take with food.

DIAGNOSTIC TEST EFFECTS
May decrease hemoglobin values and neutrophil and WBC counts. May increase serum CK, AST (SGOT), and ALT (SGPT) levels.

SIDE EFFECTS
Frequent (20%)
Diarrhea.
Occasional (3%-7%)
Nausea, rash.
Rare (1%-2%)
Flatulence, asthenia.

SERIOUS REACTIONS
• None known.

PRECAUTIONS & CONSIDERATIONS
Caution is warranted with mild liver function impairment. Be aware that it is unknown whether nelfinavir is distributed in breast milk, warranting caution in lactation. No age-related precautions have been noted in children older than 2 yr. No information is available on the effects of this drug's use in elderly patients. Nelfinavir is not a cure for HIV infection, nor does it reduce the risk of transmitting HIV to others. Illnesses associated with advanced HIV infection, including opportunistic infections, may occur. ! Monitor the patient for signs and symptoms of opportunistic infections as evidenced by chills, cough, fever, and myalgia. Expect to check hematology and liver function tests to establish an accurate baseline before beginning drug therapy. Assess the pattern of daily bowel activity and stool consistency.

Patient should be advised to remain compliant with oral contraceptive regimen and add another nonhormonal form of contraception through the duration of therapy.
Administration
Take with food, a light meal, or snack. Mix oral powder with a small amount of dietary supplement, formula, milk, soy formula, soy milk or dairy food such as pudding or ice cream. The entire contents must be consumed to ingest a full dose. Do not mix with acidic food, such as apple juice, applesauce, or orange juice, or with water in its original container. Take the medication every day as prescribed, and evenly space drug doses around the clock.

Neomycin Sulfate
nee-oh-mye′sin sull-fate
(Myciguent, NeoFradin, Neosulf [AUS])

CATEGORY AND SCHEDULE
Pregnancy Risk Category: C
OTC (topical ointment 0.5% only)

Classification: Antibiotics, aminoglycosides

MECHANISM OF ACTION
An aminoglycoside antibiotic that binds to bacterial microorganisms. *Therapeutic Effect:* Interferes with bacterial protein synthesis.

PHARMACOKINETICS
Poorly absorbed from the GI tract. Rapidly distributed to tissues. Removed by dialysis. 97% eliminated through feces.

AVAILABILITY
Tablets: 500 mg.
Ointment: 0.5% (Myciguent).
Oral Solution: 125 mg/5 mL (Neo-Fradin).

INDICATIONS AND DOSAGES
▶ **Preoperative bowel antisepsis prophylaxis**
PO
Adults, Elderly. 1 g neomycin plus 1 g erythromycin on day prior to surgery at 1:00 PM, 2:00 PM, and 11:00 PM.
Children. 90 mg/kg/day in divided doses or 25 mg/kg at 1 PM, 2 PM, and 11 PM on day before surgery.
▶ **Hepatic encephalopathy**
PO
Adults, Elderly. 4-12 g/day in divided doses q4-6h.
Children. 2.5-7 g/m^2/day in divided doses q4-6h.
▶ **Diarrhea caused by**
Escherichia coli
PO
Adults, Elderly. 3 g/day in divided doses q6h.
Children. 50 mg/kg/day in divided doses q6h.
▶ **Minor skin infections**
TOPICAL
Adults, Elderly, Children. Usual dosage, apply to affected area 1-3 times/day.

CONTRAINDICATIONS
Hypersensitivity to neomycin, other aminoglycosides (cross-sensitivity), or their components; patients with intestinal stricture, any inflammatory or ulcerative GI disease.

INTERACTIONS
Drug
Anticoagulants: May increase anticoagulant effect and lower vitamin K availability.
Digoxin, fluorouracil, methotrexate, penicillin V, vitamin B$_{12}$: May inhibit absorption of these drugs.
Nephrotoxic medications, other aminoglycosides, ototoxic, neurotoxic or nephrotoxic medications: May increase nephrotoxicity and ototoxicity if significant systemic absorption occurs.
Potent diuretics (ethacrynic acid, furosemide): May increase neomycin toxicity (IV).
Herbal
None known.
Food
None known.

DIAGNOSTIC TEST EFFECTS
None known.

SIDE EFFECTS
Frequent
Systemic: Nausea, vomiting, diarrhea, irritation of mouth or rectal area.
Topical: Itching, redness, swelling, rash.
Rare
Systemic: Malabsorption syndrome, neuromuscular blockade (difficulty breathing, drowsiness, weakness).

SERIOUS REACTIONS
• Nephrotoxicity (as evidenced by increased BUN and serum creatinine levels and decreased creatinine clearance) may be reversible if the drug is stopped at the first sign of nephrotoxic symptoms.
• Irreversible ototoxicity (manifested as tinnitus, dizziness, and impaired hearing) and neurotoxicity (as evidenced by headache, dizziness, lethargy, tremor, and visual disturbances) occur occasionally.
• Severe respiratory depression and anaphylaxis occur rarely.
• Superinfections, particularly fungal infections, may occur.

PRECAUTIONS & CONSIDERATIONS
! Systemic absorption may occur after oral administration, increasing the risk of toxicity, neuromuscular blockade, respiratory paralysis, and increased dehydration.

N

Caution is warranted in elderly patients, infants, and other patients with renal insufficiency or immaturity as well as those with neuromuscular disorders, hearing loss, or vertigo.

Expect to correct dehydration before beginning neomycin therapy. Establish the patient's baseline hearing acuity before beginning therapy. Signs and symptoms of hypersensitivity reaction should be monitored. With topical application, symptoms may include a rash, redness, or itching. If dizziness, impaired hearing, or ringing in the ears occurs, notify the physician.

May cause malabsorption (oral) of fat, nitrogen, cholesterol, carotene, glucose, xylose, lactose, sodium, calcium, cyanocobalamin, iron.

Report diarrhea with blood or pus, hearing loss, tinnitus, vestibular symptoms, muscle twitch, numbness, skin tingling, loose or foul-smelling stools.

Administration
Continue taking neomycin for the full course of treatment, and space doses evenly around the clock.

Clean the affected area gently before applying the topical preparation.

Neostigmine
nee-oh-stig′meen
(Prostigmin)
Do not confuse neostigmine with physostigmine.

CATEGORY AND SCHEDULE
Pregnancy Risk Category: C

Classification: Cholinesterase inhibitors

MECHANISM OF ACTION
A cholinergic that prevents destruction of acetylcholine by inhibiting the enzyme acetylcholinesterase, thus enhancing impulse transmission across the myoneural junction. *Therapeutic Effect:* Improves intestinal and skeletal muscle tone; stimulates salivary and sweat gland secretions.

PHARMACOKINETICS
PO: Onset 45-75 min, duration 2.5-4 h.
IM/SC: Onset 10-30 min, duration 2.5-4 h.
IV: Onset 4-8 min, duration 2-4 h.
Metabolized in the liver, excreted in urine.

AVAILABILITY
Tablets: 15 mg.
Injection: 0.5 mg/mL, 1 mg/mL.

INDICATIONS AND DOSAGES
▸ **Myasthenia gravis**
PO
Adults, Elderly. Initially, 15-30 mg 3-4 times a day. Increase as necessary. Maintenance: 150 mg/day (range of 15-375 mg).
Children. 2 mg/kg/day or 60 mg/m^2/day divided q3-4hr.
IV, IM, SC
Adults. 0.5-2.5 mg as needed.
Children. 0.01-0.04 mg/kg q2-4h.
▸ **Diagnosis of myasthenia gravis**
IM
Adults, Elderly. 0.022 mg/kg. If cholinergic reaction occurs, discontinue tests and administer 0.4-0.6 mg or more atropine sulfate intravenously.
Children. 0.025-0.04 mg/kg preceded by atropine sulfate 0.011 mg/kg subcutaneously.
▸ **Prevention of postoperative urinary retention**
IM, SC
Adults, Elderly. 0.25 mg q4-6h for 2-3 days.
▸ **Postoperative abdominal distention and urine retention**

IM, SC
Adults, Elderly. 0.5-1 mg. Catheterize
patient if voiding does not occur
within 1 h. After voiding, administer
0.5 mg q3h for 5 injections.
▸ **Reversal of neuromuscular
blockade**
IV
Adults, Elderly. 0.5-2.5 mg given
slowly.
Children. 0.025-0.08 mg/kg/dose.
Infants. 0.025-0.1 mg/kg/dose.

CONTRAINDICATIONS
GI or genitourinary obstruction,
peritonitis.
Caution
Bradycardia, hypotension, seizure
disorders, bronchial asthma,
coronary occlusion, hyperthyroidism,
dysrhythmias, peptic ulcer, megacolon,
poor GI motility, lactation, children.

INTERACTIONS
Drug
Anticholinergics: Reverse or
prevent the effects of neostigmine;
may be contraindicated.
Cholinesterase inhibitors: May
increase the risk of toxicity.
Ester-type local anesthetics: May
increase risk of toxicity.
**Hydrocarbon inhalation
anesthetics, corticosteroids:**
Decreased action.
Neuromuscular blockers:
Antagonizes the effects of these
drugs.
Procainamide, quinidine: May
antagonize the action of neostigmine.
Succinylcholine: May increase
activity.
Herbal
None known.
Food
None known.

DIAGNOSTIC TEST EFFECTS
None known.

🔵 IV INCOMPATIBILITIES
None known.

🟦 IV COMPATIBILITIES
Glycopyrrolate (Robinul), heparin,
ondansetron (Zofran), potassium
chloride, thiopental (Pentothal).

SIDE EFFECTS
Frequent
Muscarinic effects (diarrhea,
diaphoresis, increased salivation,
nausea, vomiting, abdominal cramps
or pain).
Occasional
Muscarinic effects (urinary urgency
or frequency, increased bronchial
secretions, miosis, lacrimation).

SERIOUS REACTIONS
• Overdose produces a cholinergic
crisis manifested as abdominal
discomfort or cramps, nausea,
vomiting, diarrhea, flushing, facial
warmth, excessive salivation,
diaphoresis, lacrimation, pallor,
bradycardia or tachycardia,
hypotension, bronchospasm, urinary
urgency, blurred vision, miosis, and
fasciculation (involuntary muscular
contractions visible under the skin).

PRECAUTIONS & CONSIDERATIONS
Caution is warranted with
arrhythmias, asthma, bradycardia,
epilepsy, hyperthyroidism, peptic
ulcer disease, and recent coronary
occlusion.
   Notify the physician of diarrhea,
difficulty breathing, increased
salivation, irregular heartbeat,
muscle weakness, nausea and
vomiting, severe abdominal
pain, or increased sweating.
Vital signs, muscle strength, and
fluid intake and output should be
monitored. Therapeutic response
to the drug, including decreased
fatigue, improved chewing and

N

swallowing, and increased muscle strength, should also be assessed. Overdosage evidenced by a cholinergic crisis.

Administration

! Discontinue all anticholinesterase therapy at least 8 h before testing, as prescribed. Plan to give 0.011 mg/kg atropine sulfate IV simultaneously with neostigmine or IM 30 min before administering neostigmine to prevent adverse effects.

Expect to give larger doses when the patient is most tired.

Nesiritide
neh-sir'i-tide
(Natrecor)

CATEGORY AND SCHEDULE
Pregnancy Risk Category: C

Classification: Brain natriuetic peptide; endogenous hormone

MECHANISM OF ACTION
A brain natriuretic peptide that facilitates cardiovascular homeostasis and fluid status through counterregulation of the renin-angiotensin-aldosterone system, stimulating cyclic guanosine monophosphate, thereby leading to smooth muscle cell relaxation. *Therapeutic Effect:* Promotes vasodilation, natriuresis, and diuresis, correcting congestive heart failure (CHF).

PHARMACOKINETICS

Route	Onset	Peak	Duration
IV	15-30 min	1-2 h	4 h

Excreted primarily in the heart by the left ventricle. Metabolized by the natriuretic neutral

endopeptidase enzymes on the vascular luminal surface. *Half-life:* 18-23 min.

AVAILABILITY
Injection Powder for Reconstitution: 1.5 mg/5-mL vial.

INDICATIONS AND DOSAGES
▸ **Treatment of acutely decompensated CHF in patients with dypsnea at rest or with minimal activity**
IV BOLUS
Adults, Elderly. 2 mcg/kg followed by a continuous IV infusion of 0.01 mcg/kg/min. May be incrementally increased q3h to a maximum of 0.03 mcg/kg/min.

CONTRAINDICATIONS
Cardiogenic shock, systolic BP < 90 mm Hg, hypersensitivity, low cardiac filling pressures.

INTERACTIONS
Drug
ACE inhibitors, IV nitroglycerin, milrinone, nitroprusside: May increase risk of hypotension.
Herbal
None known.
Food
None known.

DIAGNOSTIC TEST EFFECTS
None known.

ⓘ IV INCOMPATIBILITIES
Manufacturer states not to mix or infuse with any other medications. Sodium metabisulfite, bumetanide (Bumex), enalapril (Vasotec), ethacrynic acid (Edecrin), furosemide (Lasix), heparin, hydralazine (Apresoline), insulin.

SIDE EFFECTS
Frequent (11%)
Hypotension.

Occasional (3%-8%)
Headache, nausea, bradycardia,
azotemia.
Rare (≤ 1%)
Confusion, paresthesia, somnolence,
tremor.

SERIOUS REACTIONS
• Ventricular arrhythmias, including
ventricular tachycardia, atrial
fibrillation, AV node conduction
abnormalities, and angina pectoris
occur rarely.
• Hypotension requiring medical
intervention.

PRECAUTIONS & CONSIDERATIONS
❗ Drug is intended for acute use in
hospitals or emergency rooms.
  Caution is warranted in
patients with atrial conduction
defects, constrictive pericarditis,
hypotension, hepatic impairment,
pericardial tamponade, renal
impairment, restrictive or obstructive
cardiomyopathy, significant valvular
stenosis, suspected low cardiac
filling pressures, and ventricular
conduction defects. It is unknown
whether nesiritide crosses the
placenta or is distributed in breast
milk, warranting caution in lactation.
The safety and efficacy of nesiritide
have not been established in children.
No age-related precautions have been
noted for elderly patients.
  BP should be obtained
immediately before each nesiritide
dose, in addition to regular
monitoring. Be alert to BP
fluctuations. Place the patient in the
supine position with legs elevated
unless an excessive reduction in BP
occurs. Intake and output records
should be maintained. Notify the
physician of chest pain, palpitations,
cardiac arrhythmias, decreased urine
output, or severe decrease in BP or
heart rate.

Storage
Store vial at room temperature.
Once reconstituted, store at room
temperature or refrigerate; use
within 24 h.
Administration
❗ Do not mix with other injections or
infusions. Do not give IM.
  Reconstitute one 1.5-mg vial with
5 mL D5W, 0.9% NaCl, 0.2% NaCl,
or any combination thereof. Swirl
or rock gently, and add to 250-mL
bag D5W, 0.9% NaCl, 0.2% NaCl, or
any combination thereof yielding a
solution of 6 mcg/mL. Give initially as
an IV bolus over approximately 60 s,
followed by continuous IV infusion.
The bolus dose is drawn from the
infusion bag. Titrate infusion rate up
no more frequently than every 3 h.

Nevirapine
neh-veer′a-peen
(Viramune)

N

CATEGORY AND SCHEDULE
Pregnancy Risk Category: C

Classification: Antiretrovirals,
non-nucleoside reverse transcriptase
inhibitors (NNRTI)

MECHANISM OF ACTION
A nonnucleoside reverse transcriptase
inhibitor that binds directly to HIV-1
reverse transcriptase, thus changing
the shape of this enzyme and
blocking RNA- and DNA-dependent
polymerase activity. *Therapeutic
Effect:* Interferes with HIV
replication, slowing the progression
of HIV infection.

PHARMACOKINETICS
Readily absorbed after PO
administration. Protein binding:
60%. Widely distributed. Extensively

metabolized in the liver. Excreted primarily in urine. *Half-life:* 45 h (single dose), 25-30 h (multiple doses).

AVAILABILITY

Tablets: 200 mg.
Oral Suspension: 50 mg/5 mL.

INDICATIONS AND DOSAGES
▸ **HIV infection**
PO
Adults. 200 mg once a day for 14 days (to reduce the risk of rash). Maintenance: 200 mg twice a day in combination with nucleoside analogues.
Children 15 days old and older. 150 mg/m^2 once daily for 14 days, followed by 150 mg/m^2 twice daily. Do not exceed 400 mg/day.

OFF-LABEL USES

To reduce the risk of transmitting HIV from infected mother to newborn.

CONTRAINDICATIONS

Hypersensitivity, moderate to severe hepatic impairment.

INTERACTIONS
Drug
Clarithromycin: May decrease activity of clarithromycin.
Efavirenz, methadone: May decrease concentrations of these drugs.
Fluconazone: May increase concentration of nevirapine.
Ketoconazole: Contraindicated; nevirapine negates ketoconazole effectiveness.
Oral contraceptives: May reduce effectiveness of oral contraception.
Rifabutin: May increase concentration.
Rifampin, Rifabutin: may decrease nevirapine levels. Avoid.
Warfarin and other related anticoagualants: May increase INR.

Herbal
St. John's wort: May decrease blood concentration and effects of nevirapine. Avoid.
Food
None known.

DIAGNOSTIC TEST EFFECTS
May significantly increase serum bilirubin, GGT, AST (SGOT), and ALT (SGPT) levels. May significantly decrease hemoglobin level and neutrophil and platelet counts.

SIDE EFFECTS
Frequent (3%-8%)
Rash, fever, headache, nausea, fatigue, myalgia, granulocytopenia (more common in children).
Occasional (1%-3%)
Stomatitis (burning, erythema, or ulceration of the oral mucosa; dysphagia).
Rare (< 1%)
Paresthesia, abdominal pain.

SERIOUS REACTIONS
• Hepatitis and rash may become severe and life threatening.

PRECAUTIONS & CONSIDERATIONS
Caution is warranted in elderly patients, infants, and other patients with renal insufficiency or immaturity as well as those with neuromuscular disorders, hearing loss, or vertigo.
❗ 14-day dosing regimen must be strictly followed, with 18 mo of patient monitoring for skin and hepatic issues.
❗ Severe life-threatening and sometimes fatal, fulminant and cholestatic hepatic necrosis and failure is reported with this drug.

Drug is excreted in breast milk; breastfeeding is contraindicated. Nevirapine interferes with oral contraceptives; advise patient to remain compliant with oral regimen while adding another nonhormonal form of contraception for the duration of therapy.

Administration

Continue taking nevirapine for the full course of treatment. May take without regard to food.

The suspension should be shaken gently before each use.

Niacin (Vitamin B₃; Nicotinic Acid)

nye'a-sin

(Niacor, Niaspan, Nicotinex, Slo-Niacin)

Do not confuse niacin, Niacor, or Niaspan with minocin, Nitro-Bid.

OTC

CATEGORY AND SCHEDULE

Pregnancy Risk Category: A (C if used at dosages above the recommended daily allowance)

Classification: Vitamin B₃

MECHANISM OF ACTION

An antihyperlipidemic, water-soluble vitamin that is a component of two coenzymes needed for tissue respiration, lipid metabolism, and glycogenolysis. Inhibits synthesis of VLDLs. *Therapeutic Effect:* Reduces total, LDL, and VLDL cholesterol levels and triglyceride levels; increases HDL cholesterol concentration.

PHARMACOKINETICS

Readily absorbed from the GI tract. Widely distributed. Metabolized in the liver. Primarily excreted in urine. *Half-life:* 45 min.

AVAILABILITY

Capsules (Timed-Release): 125 mg, 250 mg, 400 mg, 500 mg.

Tablets (Niacor): 50 mg, 100 mg, 250 mg, 500 mg.
Tablets (Timed-Release [Slo-Niacin]): 250 mg, 500 mg, 750 mg.
Tablets (Timed-Release [Niaspan]): 500 mg, 750 mg, 1000 mg.
Elixir (Nicotinex): 50 mg/5 mL.

INDICATIONS AND DOSAGES

▸ Hyperlipidemia

PO (IMMEDIATE-RELEASE)
Adults, Elderly. Initially, 50-100 mg twice a day for 7 days. Increase gradually by doubling dose weekly up to 1-1.5 g/day in 2-3 doses. Maximum: 3 g/day.
Children. Initially, 100-250 mg/day (maximum: 10 mg/kg/day) in 3 divided doses. May increase by 100 mg/wk or 250 mg q2-3wk. Maximum: 2250 mg/day.
PO (TIMED-RELEASE)
Adults, Elderly. Initially, 500 mg/day in 2 divided doses for 1 wk; then increase to 500 mg twice a day. Maintenance: 2 g/day.

▸ Nutritional supplement

PO (IMMEDIATE RELEASE)
Adults, Elderly. 10-20 mg/day. Maximum: 100 mg/day.

▸ Pellegra

PO (IMMEDIATE RELEASE)
Adults, Elderly. 50-100 mg 3-4 times a day. Maximum: 500 mg/day.
Children. 50-100 mg 3 times a day.

CONTRAINDICATIONS

Active peptic ulcer disease, arterial hemorrhaging, significant hepatic dysfunction, hypersensitivity to niacin or tartrazine (frequently seen in patients sensitive to aspirin).

INTERACTIONS

Drug
Lovastatin, pravastatin, simvastatin and other

N

HMG-CoA reductase inhibitors:
May increase the risk of myalgia and
rhabdomyolysis.
Herbal
None known.
Food
Alcohol and hotdrinks: May
increase risk of niacin side effects,
such as flushing.

DIAGNOSTIC TEST EFFECTS
May increase serum uric acid level.

SIDE EFFECTS
Frequent
Flushing (especially of the face
and neck) occurring within 20 min
of drug administration and lasting
for 30-60 min, GI upset, pruritus.
Flushing will decrease with continued
therapy.
Occasional
Dizziness, hypotension, headache,
blurred vision, burning or tingling
of skin, flatulence, nausea, vomiting,
diarrhea.
Rare
Hyperglycemia, glycosuria, rash,
hyperpigmentation, dry skin.

SERIOUS REACTIONS
• Arrhythmias occur rarely.
• Hepatic toxicity, necrosis (rare, but
more common with sustained-release
dosage forms).

PRECAUTIONS & CONSIDERATIONS

Caution is warranted with diabetes
mellitus, gallbladder disease, gout,
and a history of hepatic disease or
jaundice. Niacin is not recommended
for use during pregnancy and
lactation. Niacin is distributed in
breast milk and is not recommended
during lactation. No age-related
precautions have been noted in
children or elderly patients. Niacin
use is not recommended for children
younger than 2 yr.

Be aware that itching, flushing
of the skin, sensation of warmth,
and tingling may occur. Notify the
physician of dark urine, dizziness,
loss of appetite, nausea, vomiting,
weakness, yellowing of the skin,
blurred vision, or headache. Pattern
of daily bowel activity and stool
consistency should be assessed.
Blood glucose level, serum
cholesterol and triglyceride levels,
and hepatic function test results
should be checked at baseline and
periodically during treatment.
Administration
Avoid administration with alcohol
or hot liquids to reduce incidence of
flushing.
  Pretreatment with aspirin
or NSAIDs can minimize skin
flushing (if patient not allergic).
Administration with food can lessen
GI distress and pruritus.

Nicardipine Hydrochloride
nye-card′i-peen high-droh-klor-ide
(Cardene, Cardene IV, Cardene
SR)
**Do not confuse nicardipine
with nifedipine, Cardene with
codeine, or Cardene SR with
Cardizem SR or codeine.**

CATEGORY AND SCHEDULE
Pregnancy Risk Category: C

Classification: Calcium channel
blockers (dihydropyridine group)

MECHANISM OF ACTION
An antianginal and antihypertensive
agent that inhibits calcium ion
movement across cell membranes,
depressing contraction of cardiac and
vascular smooth muscle. *Therapeutic
Effect:* Increases heart rate and

cardiac output. Decreases systemic vascular resistance and BP.

PHARMACOKINETICS

Route	Onset	Peak	Duration
PO	NA	1-2 h	8 h

Rapidly, completely absorbed from the GI tract. Protein binding: 95%. Undergoes first-pass metabolism in the liver. Primarily excreted in urine. Not removed by hemodialysis. *Half-life:* 2-4 h.

AVAILABILITY

Capsules (Cardene): 20 mg, 30 mg.
Capsules, (Sustained-Release [Cardene SR]): 30 mg, 45 mg, 60 mg.
Injection (Cardene IV): 2.5 mg/mL.
Premixed Infusion Bags: 20 mg/ 200 mL, 40 mg/200 mL.

INDICATIONS AND DOSAGES
▸ **Chronic stable (effort-associated) angina**
PO
Adults, Elderly. Initially, 20 mg 3 times a day. Range: 20-40 mg 3 times a day.
▸ **Essential hypertension**
PO
Adults, Elderly. Initially, 20 mg 3 times a day. Range: 20-40 mg 3 times a day.
PO (SUSTAINED-RELEASE)
Adults, Elderly. Initially, 30 mg twice a day. Range: 30-60 mg twice a day.
▸ **Short-term treatment of hypertension when oral therapy is not feasible or desirable (substitute for oral nicardipine)**
IV
Adults, Elderly. 0.5 mg/h (for patient receiving 20 mg PO q8h); 1.2 mg/h (for patient receiving 30 mg PO q8h); 2.2 mg/h (for patient receiving 40 mg PO q8h).
▸ **Patients not already receiving nicardipine**
IV
Adults, Elderly (gradual BP decrease).

Initially, 5 mg/h. May increase by 2.5 mg/h q15min. After BP goal is achieved, decrease rate to 3 mg/h.
Adults, Elderly (rapid BP decrease).
Initially, 5 mg/h. May increase by 2.5 mg/h q5min. Maximum: 15 mg/h until desired BP is attained. After BP goal is achieved, decrease rate to 3 mg/h.
▸ **Changing from IV to oral antihypertensive therapy**
Adults, Elderly. Begin antihypertensives other than nicardipine when IV has been discontinued; for nicardipine, give first dose 1 h before discontinuing IV.
▸ **Dosage in hepatic impairment**
ORAL
For adults and elderly patients, initially give 20 mg twice a day; then titrate.
▸ **Dosage in renal impairment**
ORAL
For adults and elderly patients, initially give 20 mg q8h (30 mg twice a day [sustained-release capsules]); then titrate.

OFF-LABEL USES

Diabetic nephropathy, hypertensive urgency, postoperative hypertension.

CONTRAINDICATIONS

Atrial fibrillation or flutter associated with accessory conduction pathways, cardiogenic shock, congestive heart failure (CHF), second- or third-degree heart block, severe hypotension, sinus bradycardia, ventricular tachycardia, advanced aortic stenosis.

INTERACTIONS
Drug
β-Blockers: May have additive effect.
Carbamazepine: May increase effect of carbamazepine.

Digoxin: May have additive heart effects, monitor digoxin levels.

Erythromycin, ketoconazole, cimetidine, other CYP 3A4 inhibitors: May increase plasma levels requiring patient monitoring.

Hypokalemia-producing agents (such as furosemide and certain other diuretics): May increase risk of arrhythmias.

Cyclosporine: May increase cyclosporine levels.

Indomethacin, possibly other NSAIDs, phenobarbital: May decrease effect of nicardipine.

Parenteral and inhalational general anesthetics or other drugs with hypotensive effects: May increase effects of these drugs.

Herbal

St. John's wort: May decrease effect of nicardipine.

Food

Grapefruit, grapefruit juice: May alter absorption of nicardipine and increase serum concentrations.

DIAGNOSTIC TEST EFFECTS
None known.

🚫 IV INCOMPATIBILITIES
Furosemide (Lasix), heparin, thiopental (Pentothal).

🦺 IV COMPATIBILITIES
Diltiazem (Cardizem), dobutamine (Dobutrex), dopamine (Intropin), epinephrine, hydromorphone (Dilaudid), labetalol (Trandate), lorazepam (Ativan), midazolam (Versed), milrinone (Primacor), morphine, nitroglycerin, norepinephrine (Levophed).

SIDE EFFECTS
Frequent (7%-10%)
Headache, facial flushing, peripheral edema, lightheadedness, dizziness.

Occasional (3%-6%)
Asthenia (loss of strength, energy), palpitations, angina, tachycardia.
Rare (< 2%)
Nausea, abdominal cramps, dyspepsia, dry mouth, rash.

SERIOUS REACTIONS
• Overdose produces confusion, slurred speech, somnolence, marked hypotension, and bradycardia.

PRECAUTIONS & CONSIDERATIONS
Caution is warranted in patients with cardiomyopathy, edema, hepatic or renal impairment, severe left ventricular dysfunction, sick sinus syndrome, and in those concurrently receiving β-blockers or digoxin. It is unclear whether nicardipine crosses the placenta. It should be administered only when the benefit to the mother exceeds the risk to the fetus. It is unknown whether nicardipine is distributed in breast milk, warranting caution in lactation. The safety and efficacy of nicardipine have not been established in children. In elderly patients, age-related renal impairment may require cautious use. Alcohol and caffeine should be limited while taking nicardipine. Patient should be advised to remain compliant with salt and chloride dietary restrictions.

Notify the physician if anginal pain is not relieved by the medication and if constipation, dizziness, irregular heartbeat, nausea, shortness of breath, swelling, or symptoms of hypotension such as lightheadedness occur. BP for hypotension, skin for dermatitis, facial flushing and rash, liver function test results, ECG and pulse for tachycardia should be assessed. The onset, type (sharp, dull, or squeezing), radiation, location, intensity, and duration of anginal pain and its precipitating factors, such as exertion and emotional stress should

N

be recorded. Be aware that concurrent administration of sublingual nitroglycerin therapy may be used for relief of anginal pain. Caution with postural changes to avoid orthostatic hypotension from developing.

Storage
Store at room temperature. Store diluted IV solution for up to 24 h at room temperature.

Administration
Do not crush, open, or break sustained-release capsules. Take oral nicardipine without regard to food.

For IV use, dilute each 25-mg ampoule with 250 mL D5W, 0.9% NaCl, 0.45% NaCl, or any combination thereof to provide a concentration of 1 mg/10 mL. Maximum concentration is 4 mg/10 mL. Give by slow IV infusion. Change IV site every 12 h if drug is administered by a peripheral rather than a central venous catheter line.

Nicotine
nik'o-teen
(Commit, Habitrol [CAN], NicoDerm [CAN], NicoDerm CQ, Nicorette, Nicorette Plus [CAN], Nicotrol, Nicotrol NS, Nicotrol Patch [CAN])
Do not confuse nicotine with Nicoderm with Nitroderm.

CATEGORY AND SCHEDULE
Pregnancy Risk Category: C (chewing gum), D (transdermal) OTC (Nicoderm transdermal patch, Nicotrol transdermal patch, Nicorette chewing gum)

Classification: Smoking deterrent

MECHANISM OF ACTION
A cholinergic-receptor agonist binds to acetylcholine receptors, producing both stimulating and depressant effects on the peripheral and central nervous systems. *Therapeutic Effect:* Provides a source of nicotine during nicotine withdrawal and reduces withdrawal symptoms.

PHARMACOKINETICS
Absorbed slowly after transdermal administration. Protein binding: 5%. Metabolized in the liver. Excreted primarily in urine. *Half-life:* 4 h.

AVAILABILITY
Chewing Gum (Nicorette, OTC): 2 mg, 4 mg.
Lozenge (Commit): 2 mg, 4 mg.
Transdermal Patch (NicoDerm CQ, Nicotrol): 7 mg, 14 mg, 21 mg.
Nasal Spray (Nicotrol NS): 0.5 mg/spray.
Inhalation (Nicotrol Inhaler): 10 mg cartridge.

INDICATIONS AND DOSAGES
▸ **Smoking cessation aid to relieve nicotine withdrawal symptoms**
PO (CHEWING GUM)
Adults, Elderly. Usually, 10-12 pieces/day. Maximum: 30 pieces/day.
PO (LOZENGE)
! For those who smoke the first cigarette within 30 min of waking, administer the 4-mg lozenge; otherwise, administer the 2-mg lozenge.
Adults, Elderly. One 4-mg or 2-mg lozenge q1-2h for the first 6 wks; one lozenge q2-4h for wks 7-9; and one lozenge q4-8h for wks 10-12. Maximum: one lozenge at a time, 5 lozenges/6 h, 20 lozenges/day.
TRANSDERMAL
Adults, Elderly who smoke 10 cigarettes or more per day. Follow the guidelines below:
Step 1: 21 mg/day for 4-6 wks.

N

Step 2: 14 mg/day for 2 wks.
Step 3: 7 mg/day for 2 wks.
*Adults, Elderly who smoke < 10
cigarettes per day. Follow the
guidelines below:*
Step 1: 14 mg/day for 6 wks.
Step 2: 7 mg/day for 2 wks.
P*atients weighing < 100 lb, patients
with a history of cardiovascular
disease.* Initially, 14 mg/day for
4-6 wks, then 7 mg/day for 2-4 wks.
TRANSDERMAL (NICOTROL)
Adults, Elderly. One patch a day for
6 wks.
NASAL
Adults, Elderly. 1-2 doses/h (1 dose =
2 sprays [1 in each nostril] = 1 mg).
Maximum. 5 doses (5 mg)/h;
40 doses (40 mg)/day.
INHALER (NICOTROL)
Adults, Elderly. Puff on nicotine
cartridge mouthpiece for about
20 min as needed.

CONTRAINDICATIONS
Immediate post myocardial infarction
(MI) period, life-threatening
arrhythmias, severe or worsening
angina.
    Skin disease, angina pectoris,
MI, renal or hepatic insufficiency,
peptic ulcer, serious cardiac
dysrhythmias, hyperthyroidism,
pheochromocytoma, insulin-
dependent diabetes, elderly.

INTERACTIONS
Drug
**Acetaminophen, caffeine,
oxazepam, pentazocine,
theophylline, β-adrenergic
blockers, insulin:** Increased effects
of these drugs as smoking ceases.
Expect a need to decrease dose as
smoking ceases.
Herbal
None known.
Food
None known.

DIAGNOSTIC TEST EFFECTS
None known.

SIDE EFFECTS
Frequent
All forms: Hiccups, nausea.
Gum: Mouth or throat soreness,
nausea, hiccups.
Transdermal: Erythema, pruritus, or
burning at application site.
Occasional
All forms: Eructation, GI upset,
dry mouth, insomnia, diaphoresis,
irritability.
Gum: Hiccups, hoarseness.
Inhaler: Mouth or throat irritation,
cough.
Rare
All forms: Dizziness, myalgia,
arthralgia.

SERIOUS REACTIONS
• Overdose produces palpitations,
tachyarrhythmias, seizures,
depression, confusion, diaphoresis,
hypotension, rapid or weak pulse,
and dyspnea. Lethal dose for adults
is 40-60 mg. Death results from
respiratory paralysis.

PRECAUTIONS & CONSIDERATIONS
Caution is warranted in patients with
eczematous dermatitis, esophagitis,
hyperthyroidism, insulin-dependent
diabetes mellitus, oral or pharyngeal
inflammation, peptic ulcer disease,
pheochromocytoma, or severe renal
impairment. Nicotine passes freely into
breast milk, and smoking and nicotine
gum are associated with a decrease
in fetal breathing movements. The
use of nicotine is not recommended
for breastfeeding women. Nicotine
use is not recommended for children.
In elderly patients, an age-related
decrease in cardiac function may
require cautious use.
    Notify the physician of itching or a
persistent rash during treatment with

the transdermal patch. Vital signs, including BP and pulse rate, should be obtained before and during treatment. A baseline ECG should be performed.

Administration

! Expect to individualize nicotine dosage and to administer the drug when the patient plans to stop smoking.

Chew 1 piece of gum slowly and intermittently for 30 min when there is an urge to smoke. Chew until the distinctive peppery nicotine taste or slight tingling in mouth occurs. When the tingling is almost gone, after approximately 1 min, repeat the chewing procedure to allow constant, slow buccal absorption. Do not chew too rapidly because this may cause excessive release of nicotine, resulting in adverse effects similar to those of oversmoking, such as nausea and throat irritation. Do not swallow the gum.

! For transdermal use, decrease the dosage, as prescribed, for persons taking more than 600 mg cimetidine (Tagamet) daily.

Apply the patch as soon as it has been removed from the protective pouch. This wrapping prevents evaporation and loss of nicotine. Use only an intact pouch. Do not cut the patch. Apply the patch only once daily to a hairless, clean, dry area on the upper body or outer arm. Rotate application sites; do not use the same site for 7 days or the same patch for longer than 24 h. Wash hands with water alone after applying the patch because soap may increase nicotine absorption. To discard a used patch, fold it in half with the sticky sides together, place it in the pouch of the new patch, and discard it in a receptacle that is not accessible to children or pets. Do not smoke while wearing the patch.

To use the inhaler, insert the cartridge into mouthpiece and puff vigorously for 20 min.

Nifedipine
nye-fed′i-peen
(Adalat 5 [AUS], Adalat 10 [AUS], Adalat 20 [AUS], Adalat CC, Adalat Oros [AUS], Apo-Nifed [CAN], Nifecard [AUS], Nifedicol XL, Nifehexal [AUS], Novo-Nifedin [CAN], Nyefax [AUS], Procardia, Procardia XL)

Do not confuse nifedipine with nicardipine or nimodipine.

CATEGORY AND SCHEDULE
Pregnancy Risk Category: C

Classification: Calcium channel blockers (dihydropyridine group)

MECHANISM OF ACTION
An antianginal and antihypertensive agent that inhibits calcium ion movement across cell membranes, depressing contraction of cardiac and vascular smooth muscle. *Therapeutic Effect:* Increases heart rate and cardiac output. Decreases systemic vascular resistance and BP.

PHARMACOKINETICS

Route	Onset	Peak	Duration
Sublingual	1-5 min	NA	N/A
PO	20-30 min	NA	4-8 h
PO (extended release)	2 h	NA	24 h

Rapidly, completely absorbed from the GI tract. Protein binding: 92%-98%. Undergoes first-pass metabolism in the liver. Excreted primarily in urine. Not removed by hemodialysis. *Half-life:* 2-5 h.

AVAILABILITY
Capsules (Procardia): 10 mg.
Tablets (Extended-Release [Adalat CC, Procardia XL]): 30 mg, 60 mg, 90 mg.

Tablets (Extended-Release [Nifedical XL]): 30 mg, 60 mg.

INDICATIONS AND DOSAGES
▶ **Prinzmetal's variant angina, chronic stable (effort associated) angina**
PO
Adults, Elderly. Initially, 10 mg 3 times a day. Increase at 7- to 14-day intervals. Maintenance: 10 mg 3 times a day up to 30 mg 4 times a day.
PO (EXTENDED-RELEASE)
Adults, Elderly. Initially, 30-60 mg/day. Maintenance: Up to 120 mg/day.
▶ **Essential hypertension**
PO (EXTENDED-RELEASE)
Adults, Elderly. Initially, 30-60 mg/day. Maintenance: Up to 120 mg/day.

OFF-LABEL USES
Premature labor.

CONTRAINDICATIONS
Hypersensitivity, advanced aortic stenosis, severe hypotension.
Caution
Congestive heart failure (CHF), hypotension, sick sinus syndrome, second- or third- degree heart block, hypotension < 90 mm Hg systolic, hepatic injury, lactation, children, renal disease.

INTERACTIONS
Drug
β-Blockers: May have additive effect.
Carbamazepine: May increase effects of carbamazepine.
Digoxin: May increase digoxin blood concentration.
Hypokalemia-producing agents (such as furosemide and certain other diuretics): May increase risk of arrhythmias.
Indomethacin, other NSAIDs, phenobarbital: May decrease effect of these drugs.

Inhibitors of CYP 3A4 isoenzymes: May increase effects of nifedipine.
Parenteral and inhalational general anesthetics or other drugs with hypotensive actions: May increase these effects.
Herbal
None known.
Food
Grapefruit, grapefruit juice: May increase nifedipine plasma concentration. Avoid.

DIAGNOSTIC TEST EFFECTS
May cause positive ANA and direct Coombs' test.

SIDE EFFECTS
Frequent (11%-30%)
Peripheral edema, headache, flushed skin, dizziness.
Occasional (6%-12%)
Nausea, shakiness, muscle cramps and pain, somnolence, palpitations, nasal congestion, cough, dyspnea, wheezing.
Rare (3%-5%)
Hypotension, rash, pruritus, urticaria, constipation, abdominal discomfort, flatulence, sexual difficulties.

SERIOUS REACTIONS
• Nifedipine may precipitate CHF and myocardial infarction (MI) in patients with cardiac disease and peripheral ischemia.
• Overdose produces nausea, somnolence, confusion, and slurred speech.
• When given via the sublingual method for rapid control of hypertension, may cause profound hypotension, acute MI, or death. Do not use nifedipine for this purpose.

PRECAUTIONS & CONSIDERATIONS
Caution is warranted in patients with impaired hepatic and renal function. It is unclear whether nifedipine

crosses the placenta. It should be administered only when the benefit to the mother outweighs the risk to the fetus. An insignificant amount of nifedipine is distributed in breast milk. The safety and efficacy of nifedipine have not been established in children. In elderly patients, age-related renal impairment may require cautious use. Grapefruit juice, which may increase nifedipine blood concentration, should be avoided. Alcohol and tasks that require alertness and motor skills should also be avoided. Patients should be advised to remain compliant with dietary salt restrictions.

Dizziness or lightheadedness may occur. Notify the physician if irregular heartbeat, prolonged dizziness, nausea, or shortness of breath occurs. BP and liver function should be monitored. Skin should be assessed for flushing and peripheral edema, especially behind the medial malleolus and the sacral area. The onset, type (sharp, dull, or squeezing), radiation, location, intensity, and duration of anginal pain and its precipitating factors, such as exertion and emotional stress, should be recorded. Be aware that concurrent administration of sublingual nitroglycerin therapy may be used for relief of anginal pain. Overdose produces nausea, somnolence, confusion, and slurred speech.

Storage
Store at room temperature. Store diluted IV solution for up to 24 h at room temperature.

Administration
Do not crush or break extended-release tablets. Take oral nifedipine without regard to meals.

Avoid co-administration with grapefruit juice.

Nilutamide
nih-lute′ah-myd
(Anandron [CAN], Nilandron)

CATEGORY AND SCHEDULE
Pregnancy Risk Category: C

Classification: Hormone; antineoplastic

MECHANISM OF ACTION
An antiandrogen hormone and antineoplastic agent that competitively inhibits androgen action by binding to androgen receptors in target tissue. *Therapeutic Effect:* Decreases growth of abnormal prostate tissue.

PHARMACOKINETICS
Rapidly and completely absorbed; excreted in urine and feces as metabolites.

AVAILABILITY
Tablets: 150 mg.

INDICATIONS AND DOSAGES
▸ **Prostatic carcinoma**
PO
Adults, Elderly. 300 mg once a day for 30 days, then 150 mg once a day. Begin on day of, or day after, surgical castration.

CONTRAINDICATIONS
Severe hepatic impairment, severe respiratory insufficiency, hypersensitivity.

INTERACTIONS
Drug
Avoid drugs that may aggravate urinary retention when symptoms are present.
Herbal
None known.

Food
None known.

DIAGNOSTIC TEST EFFECTS

May increase serum bilirubin, creatinine, AST (SGOT), and ALT (SGPT) levels.

SIDE EFFECTS

Frequent (> 10%)
Hot flashes, delay in recovering vision after bright illumination (such as sun, television, bright lights), decreased libido, diminished sexual function, mild nausea, gynecomastia, alcohol intolerance.
Occasional (< 10%)
Constipation, hypertension, dizziness, dyspnea, urinary tract infection.

SERIOUS REACTIONS

• Interstitial pneumonitis occurs rarely.
• Hepatitis, severe liver injury.

PRECAUTIONS & CONSIDERATIONS

Caution is warranted in patients with hepatitis and markedly increased serum hepatic function test results. Avoid driving at night. Tinted glasses are recommended to help decrease the visual effect of bright headlights and streetlights. Caution is warranted with drugs that may need to be metabolized by CYP 3A4 isoenzymes as nilutamide inhibits CYP 3A4 isoenzyme.

Notify the physician if signs of hepatotoxicity occur, such as abdominal pain, dark urine, fatigue, and jaundice. A baseline chest radiogram and liver function test results should be obtained before therapy and periodically during long-term therapy.
Administration
Take oral nilutamide with or without food.

Nimodipine

nye-mode′i-peen
(Nimotop)
Do not confuse nimodipine with nifedipine.

CATEGORY AND SCHEDULE

Pregnancy Risk Category: C

Classification: Calcium channel blockers

MECHANISM OF ACTION

A cerebral vasospasm agent that inhibits movement of calcium ions across vascular smooth-muscle cell membranes. *Therapeutic Effect:* Produces favorable effect on severity of neurologic deficits due to cerebral vasospasm. Exerts greatest effect on cerebral arteries; may prevent cerebral spasm.

PHARMACOKINETICS

Rapidly absorbed from the GI tract. Protein binding: 95%. Metabolized in the liver. Excreted in urine; eliminated in feces. Not removed by hemodialysis. *Half-life:* terminal, 3 h.

AVAILABILITY

Capsules: 30 mg.

INDICATIONS AND DOSAGES

▸ **Improvement in neurologic deficits after subarachnoid hemorrhage from ruptured congenital aneurysms**
PO
Adults, Elderly. 60 mg q4h for 21 days. Begin within 96 h of subarachnoid hemorrhage.
▸ **Dosage in hepatic impairment (cirrhosis)**
PO
Adults. 30 mg q4h for 21 days; closely monitor BP and heart rate.

CONTRAINDICATIONS
Hypersensitivity.

INTERACTIONS
Drug
Anesthetics, other antihypertensive medications: May increase risk of hypotension.
β-Blockers: May prolong SA and AV conduction, which may lead to severe hypotension, bradycardia, and cardiac failure.
Cimetidine: Increases nimodipine concentrations.
Erythromycin, itraconazole, ketoconazole, protease inhibitors: May inhibit the metabolism of nimodipine.
Indomethacin and possibly other NSAIDs: May antagonize antihypertensive effect.
Rifabutin, rifampin: May increase the metabolism of nimodipine.
Sympathomimetics: May reduce antihypertensive effects.
Herbal
Garlic: May increase antihypertensive effect.
Ginseng, yohimbe: May worsen hypertension.
Food
Grapefruit juice: May increase nimodipine blood concentration and risk of toxicity.

DIAGNOSTIC TEST EFFECTS
None known.

SIDE EFFECTS
Occasional (2%-6%)
Hypotension, peripheral edema, diarrhea, headache.
Rare (< 2%)
Allergic reaction (rash, hives), tachycardia, flushing of skin.

SERIOUS REACTIONS
• Overdose produces nausea, weakness, dizziness, somnolence, confusion, and slurred speech.

PRECAUTIONS & CONSIDERATIONS
Caution is warranted in patients with impaired hepatic and renal function. It is unknown whether nimodipine crosses the placenta or is distributed in breast milk; caution is warranted in lactation. The safety and efficacy of nimodipine have not been established in children. In elderly patients, age-related renal impairment may require cautious use. Elderly patients may also experience greater hypotensive response and constipation.
Notify the physician if constipation, dizziness, irregular heartbeat, nausea, shortness of breath, or swelling occurs. Liver function, neurologic response, BP, and heart rate should be assessed before and during therapy. If the pulse rate is 60 beats/min or lower or systolic BP is < 90 mm Hg, withhold the medication and contact the physician.
Administration
If unable to swallow, place a hole in both ends of a capsule with an 18-gauge needle to extract contents into a syringe. Empty contents of syringe into an nasogastric (NG) tube; flush tube with 30 mL normal saline.
! Do not administer contents of capsules IV. Fatal medication errors have occurred.

N

Nisoldipine
nye-soul-dih-peen
(Sular)
Do not confuse nisoldipine with nicardipine.

CATEGORY AND SCHEDULE
Pregnancy Risk Category: C

Classification: Calcium channel antagonist (dihydropyridine group)

MECHANISM OF ACTION
A calcium channel blocker that inhibits calcium ion movement across cell membrane, depressing contraction of cardiac and vascular smooth muscle. *Therapeutic Effect:* Increases heart rate and cardiac output. Decreases systemic vascular resistance and BP.

PHARMACOKINETICS
Poor absorption from the GI tract. Food increases bioavailability. Protein binding: > 99%. Metabolism occurs in the gut wall. Primarily excreted in urine. Not removed by hemodialysis. *Half-life:* 7-12 h.

AVAILABILITY
Tablets (Extended-Release): 8.5 mg, 17 mg, 25.5 mg, 34 mg (Sular).

INDICATIONS AND DOSAGES
▸ **Hypertension**
PO
Adults. Initially, 17 mg once daily; then increase by 8.5 mg/wk or longer intervals until therapeutic BP response is attained. In the elderly or in those with impaired liver function, start 8.5 mg once daily. Increase by 8.5 mg/wk to therapeutic response. Maintenance: 17.34 mg once daily.

OFF-LABEL USES
Stable angina pectoris.

CONTRAINDICATIONS
Sick-sinus syndrome/second- or third-degree AV block (except in presence of pacemaker), hypersensitivity to nisoldipine or any component of the formulation.
Caution
Avoid high-fat meals, severe coronary artery disease, monitor BP, CHF, severe hepatic impairment, do not break or crush tablets, lactation, geriatric patients.

INTERACTIONS
Drug
Amiodarone: May increase risk of bradycardia, atrioventricular block, or sinus arrest.
β-Blockers: May have additive effect.
Delavirdine, ketoconazole, voriconazole: May increase serum nisoldipine concentrations.
Digoxin: May increase digoxin blood concentration.
Epirubicin: May increase risk of heart failure.
Fentanyl: May increase risk of severe hypotension.
Phenytoin, fosphenytoin: May decrease nisoldipine concentrations.
NSAIDs, oral anticoagulants: May increase risk of gastrointestinal hemorrhage and/or antagonism of hypotensive effect.
Quinidine: May increase risk of quinidine toxicity.
Quinupristin/dalfopristin, saquinavir: May increase risk of nisoldipine toxicity.
Rifampin: May decrease nisoldipine efficacy.
Herbal
Licorice, Ma huang, peppermint oil, yohimbine: May decrease effectiveness of nisoldipine.

St. John's wort: May decrease bioavailability of nisoldipine.
Food
Grapefruit and grapefruit juice, or high-fat meal: May increase nisoldipine plasma concentration.

DIAGNOSTIC TEST EFFECTS
None known.

SIDE EFFECTS
Frequent
Giddiness, dizziness, lightheadedness, peripheral edema, headache, flushing, weakness, nausea.
Occasional
Transient hypotension, heartburn, muscle cramps, nasal congestion, cough, wheezing, sore throat, palpitations, nervousness, mood changes.
Rare
Increase in frequency, intensity, duration of anginal attack during initial therapy.

SERIOUS REACTIONS
• May precipitate CHF and myocardial infarction (MI) in patients with cardiac disease and peripheral ischemia.
• Overdose produces nausea, drowsiness, confusion, and slurred speech.

PRECAUTIONS & CONSIDERATIONS
Caution is warranted in patients with impaired liver or renal function, aortic stenosis, or cirrhosis. It is unknown whether nisoldipine crosses the placenta or is distributed in breast milk, warranting caution in lactation. Safety and efficacy of nisoldipine have not been established in children. Age-related renal impairment may require cautious use in elderly patients. Avoid high-fat meals and grapefruit juice after taking medication because it may alter

absorption. May cause CHF or MI in patients with cardiac disease and peripheral ischemia. Overdose causes nausea, drowsiness, confusion, and slurred speech.

Rise slowly from lying to sitting position and permit legs to dangle from bed momentarily before standing to reduce hypotensive effect. Contact physician if irregular heartbeat, shortness of breath, pronounced dizziness, or nausea occurs.
Storage
Store at room temperature. Protect from light and moisture.
Administration
Swallow capsule whole. Do not chew, divide, or crush. Take at the same time each day to ensure minimal fluctuation of serum levels. Do not administer with grapefruit juice. Take on an empty stomach 1 h before on 2 h after a meal.

N

Nitazoxanide
nigh-tazz-oks'ah-nide
(Alinia)

CATEGORY AND SCHEDULE
Pregnancy Risk Category: B

Classification: Antiprotozoals

MECHANISM OF ACTION
An antiparasitic that interferes with the body's reaction to pyruvate ferredoxin oxidoreductase, an enzyme essential for anaerobic energy metabolism. *Therapeutic Effect:* Produces antiprotozoal activity, reducing or terminating diarrheal episodes.

PHARMACOKINETICS
Rapidly hydrolyzed to an active metabolite. Protein binding: 99%. Excreted in the urine, bile, and feces. *Half-life:* 2-4 h.

AVAILABILITY
Powder for Oral Suspension: 100 mg/5 mL.
Tablet: 500 mg.

INDICATIONS AND DOSAGES
▸ **Diarrhea**
PO
Adults, Children aged 12 yr and older. 500 mg q12h for 3 days.
Children 4-11 yr. 200 mg (10 mL) q12h for 3 days.
Children aged 12-47 mo. 100 mg (5 mL) q12h for 3 days.

CONTRAINDICATIONS
History of sensitivity to the drug.

INTERACTIONS
Drug
None known.
Herbal
None known.
Food
None known.

DIAGNOSTIC TEST EFFECTS
May increase serum creatinine and ALT (SGPT) levels.

SIDE EFFECTS
Occasional (8%)
Abdominal pain.
Rare (1%-2%)
Diarrhea, vomiting, headache.

SERIOUS REACTIONS
• None known.

PRECAUTIONS & CONSIDERATIONS
! This drug is intended for acute use. Caution is warranted with biliary or hepatic disease, GI disorders, and renal impairment. It is unknown if nitazoxanide is distributed in breast milk, warranting cautious use in lactation. The safety and efficacy of nitazoxanide have not been established in children older than 11 yr of age. Nitazoxanide is not indicated for use in elderly patients. Pattern of daily bowel activity and stool consistency, electrolytes, and hydration status should be monitored. Patients should be cautioned to maintain hydration and electrolyte levels following recovery.
Storage
Store unreconstituted powder at room temperature. Reconstituted solution is stable for 7 days at room temperature.
Administration
Reconstitute oral suspension with 48 mL water to provide a concentration of 100 mg/5 mL. Shake vigorously to suspend powder. Be aware that the oral suspension of nitazoxanide contains 1.48 g of sucrose per 5 mL. Shake well before use. Take all dosage forms with food.

Nitrofurantoin
nye-troe-fyoor'an-toyn
(Apo-Nitrofurantoin [CAN], Furadantin, Macrobid, Macrodantin, Novo-Furan [CAN], Ralodantin [AUS])

CATEGORY AND SCHEDULE
Pregnancy Risk Category: B

Classification: Antibiotics, nitrofurans

MECHANISM OF ACTION
An antibacterial urinary tract infection (UTI) agent that inhibits the synthesis of bacterial DNA, RNA,

proteins, and cell walls by altering or inactivating ribosomal proteins. *Therapeutic Effect:* Bacteriostatic (bactericidal at high concentrations).

PHARMACOKINETICS

Microcrystalline form rapidly and completely absorbed; macrocrystalline form more slowly absorbed. Food increases absorption. Protein binding: 40%. Primarily concentrated in urine and kidneys. Metabolized in most body tissues. Primarily excreted in urine. Removed by hemodialysis. *Half-life:* 20-60 min.

AVAILABILITY

Capsules (Macrobid [Macrocrystalline]): 100 mg.
Capsules (Macrodantin [Macrocrystalline]): 25 mg, 50 mg, 100 mg.
Oral Suspension (Furadantin [Microcrystalline]): 25 mg/5 mL.

INDICATIONS AND DOSAGES
▸ **Urinary tract infections (UTIs)**
PO
Adults, Elderly, Children older than 12 yr. (Furadantin, Macrodantin): 50-100 mg q6h with food for 7 days and 3 days thereafter until sterile urine is obtained. (Macrobid): 100 mg 2 times/day. Maximum: 400 mg/day for 7 days.
Children older than 1 mo and younger than 12 yr. (Furadantin, Macrodantin): 5-7 mg/kg/day in divided doses q6h with food for 7 days and 3 days thereafter until sterile urine is obtained. Maximum: 400 mg/day.
▸ **Long-term prevention of UTIs**
PO
Adults, Elderly. 50-100 mg at bedtime.
Children. 1-2 mg/kg/day as a single dose or in 2 divided doses not to exceed maximum: 100 mg/day.

OFF-LABEL USES
Prevention of bacterial UTIs.

CONTRAINDICATIONS
Anuria, oliguria, substantial renal impairment (creatinine clearance < 60 mL/min); infants younger than 1 mo old because of the risk of hemolytic anemia.

INTERACTIONS
Drug
Anticholinergic drugs: May increase absorption of nitrofurantoin.
Hemolytics: May increase the risk of nitrofurantoin toxicity.
Magnesium salts: May decrease absorption and antiinfective activity of nitrofurantoin.
Neurotoxic medications: May increase the risk of neurotoxicity.
Probenecid: May increase blood concentration and toxicity of nitrofurantoin.
Herbal
None known.
Food
None known.

DIAGNOSTIC TEST EFFECTS
Urinary creatine elevation and false positive glucose determination with Benedict reagent.

SIDE EFFECTS
Frequent
Anorexia, nausea, vomiting, dark urine.
Occasional
Abdominal pain, diarrhea, rash, pruritus, urticaria, hypertension, headache, dizziness, drowsiness.
Rare
Photosensitivity, transient alopecia, asthmatic exacerbation in those with history of asthma.

N

SERIOUS REACTIONS
• Superinfection, hepatotoxicity, peripheral neuropathy (may be irreversible), Stevens-Johnson syndrome, permanent pulmonary function impairment, and anaphylaxis occur rarely.
• Hemolytic anemia.

PRECAUTIONS & CONSIDERATIONS
Caution is warranted with debilitated patients (greater risk of peripheral neuropathy) and in patients with anemia, diabetes mellitus, electrolyte imbalance, glucose-6-phosphate dehydrogenase (G6PD) deficiency (greater risk of hemolytic anemia), renal impairment, or vitamin B deficiency. Nitrofurantoin readily crosses the placenta and is distributed in breast milk. Nitrofurantoin use is contraindicated at term and during breastfeeding if the infant is suspected of having G6PD deficiency. No age-related precautions have been noted in children older than 1 month. Elderly patients are more likely to develop acute pneumonitis and peripheral neuropathy and may require a dosage adjustment because of age-related renal impairment. Avoid sun and ultraviolet light.

Urine may turn dark yellow, orange, or brown. Hair loss may occur but is only temporary. Notify the physician if chest pain, cough, difficult breathing, fever, or numbness and tingling occur. Intake and output, renal function, bowel activity, skin for rash, and breathing should be monitored.

Do not give to any person who has pulmonary reaction to nitrofurantoin. Overdosage is manifested by vomiting.

Administration
Take nitrofurantoin with food or milk to enhance absorption and reduce GI upset.

Shake suspension well before each use.

Nitrofurazone
nye-troe-fyoor′a-zone
(Furacin)
Do not confuse nitrofurazone with nitrofurantoin.

CATEGORY AND SCHEDULE
Pregnancy Risk Category: C
OTC (ointment)

Classification: Coronary vasodilator, antianginal, nitrate

MECHANISM OF ACTION
A synthetic nitrofuran that inhibits bacterial enzymes involved in carbohydrate metabolism. *Therapeutic Effect:* Inhibits a variety of enzymes. Bactericidal.

PHARMACOKINETICS
Not known.

AVAILABILITY
Cream: 0.2% (Furacin).
Ointment: 0.2% (Furacin).
Solution: 0.2% (Furacin).

INDICATIONS AND DOSAGES
▶ **Burns, catheter-related urinary tract infections, skin grafts**
TOPICAL
Adults. Apply directly on lesion with spatula or place on a piece of gauze first. Use of a bandage is optional. Preparation should remain on lesion for at least 24 h. Dressing may be changed several times daily or left on the lesion for a longer period.

CONTRAINDICATIONS
Hypersensitivity to nitrofurazone or any of its components.

INTERACTIONS
Drug
None known.
Herbal
None known.
Food
None known.

DIAGNOSTIC TEST EFFECTS
None known.

SIDE EFFECTS
Occasional
Itching, rash, swelling.

SERIOUS REACTIONS
• Use of nitrofurazone may result
in bacterial or fungal overgrowth of
nonsusceptible pathogens, which
may lead to secondary infection.

PRECAUTIONS & CONSIDERATIONS
Caution should be used with renal
impairment and G6PD deficiency. It
is unknown whether nitrofurazone
is distributed in breast milk; caution
warranted with lactation. Safety
and efficacy of nitrofurazone have
not been established in children.
Irritation, inflammation, or rash
should be reported. Watch for signs
of infection or fungal overgrowth and
report any symptoms immediately.
Administration
Apply topical formulation directly
on the lesion with a spatula or first
place on a piece of gauze. Use of a
bandage is optional. The preparation
should remain on the lesion for at
least 24 h.

Nitroglycerin
nye-troe-gli′ser-in
(Anginine [AUS], Minitran,
Nitradisc [AUS], Nitrek, Nitro-Bid,
Nitro-Dur, Nitrogard, Nitroject
[CAN], Nitrolingual, Nitrong-SR,
NitroQuick, Nitrostat, Nitro-Tab,
Rectogesic [AUS], Transiderm
Nitro [AUS], Trinipatch [CAN])
**Do not confuse nitroglycerin
with nitroprusside; Nitro-Bid
with Nicobid; Nitro-Dur with
Nicoderm; Nitrostat with
Hyperstat, Nilstat, or Nystatin;
or Nitrong-SR with Nizoral.**

CATEGORY AND SCHEDULE
Pregnancy Risk Category: B

Classification: Vasodilators

MECHANISM OF ACTION
A nitrate that decreases myocardial
oxygen demand. Reduces left
ventricular preload and afterload.
Therapeutic Effect: Dilates coronary
arteries and improves collateral
blood flow to ischemic areas within
myocardium. IV form produces
peripheral vasodilation.

PHARMACOKINETICS

Route	Onset (min)	Peak (min)	Duration
Sublingual	1-3	4-8	30-60 min
Translingual spray	2	4-10	30-60 min
Buccal tablet	2-5	4-10	2 hr
PO (extended-release)	20-45	45-120	4-8 h
Topical	15-60	30-120	2-12 h
Transdermal patch	40-60	60-180	18-24 h
IV	Immediate	1-2	3-5 min

Well absorbed after PO, sublingual, and topical administration. Undergoes extensive first-pass metabolism. Metabolized in the liver and by enzymes in the bloodstream. Primarily excreted in urine. Not removed by hemodialysis. *Half-life:* 1-4 min.

AVAILABILITY

Capsules (Extended-Release [NitroBid]): 2.5 mg, 6.5 mg, 9 mg.
Tablets (Buccal [Nitrogard]): 2 mg, 3 mg.
Tablets (Sublingual [NitroQuick, Nitrostat, Nitro-Tab]): 0.4 mg, 0.6 mg.
Spray (Translingual [Nitrolingual]): 0.4 mg/spray.
Infusion Solution: 0.1 mg/mL, 0.2 mg/mL, 0.4 mg/mL.
Topical Ointment (Nitro-Bid, Nitrol): 2%.
Transdermal Patch (Minitran): 0.1 mg/h, 0.2 mg/h, 0.3 mg/h, 0.4 mg/h.
Transdermal Patch (NitroDur): 0.1 mg/h, 0.2 mg/hr, 0.3 mg/h, 0.4 mg/h, 0.6 mg/h, 0.8 mg/h.
Transdermal Patch (Nitrek): 0.2 mg/h, 0.4 mg/h, 0.6 mg/h.

INDICATIONS AND DOSAGES
▸ **Acute relief of angina pectoris, acute prophylaxis**
LINGUAL SPRAY
Adults, Elderly. 1 spray onto or under tongue q3-5min until relief is noted (no more than 3 sprays in 15-min period).
SUBLINGUAL
Adults, Elderly. 0.4 mg q5min until relief is noted (no more than 3 doses in 15-min period). Use prophylactically 5-10 min before activities that may cause an acute attack.
▸ **Long-term prophylaxis of angina**
PO (EXTENDED-RELEASE)
Adults, Elderly. 2.5-9 mg q8-12h.

TOPICAL
Adults, Elderly. Initially, ½ inch q8h. Increase by ½ inch with each application. Range: 1-2 inches q8h up to 4-5 inches q4h.
TRANSDERMAL PATCH
Adults, Elderly. Initially, 0.2-0.4 mg/h. Maintenance: 0.4-0.8 mg/h. Consider patch on for 12-14 h, patch off for 10-12 h (prevents tolerance).
▸ **Congestive heart failure (CHF) associated with acute myocardial infarction (MI)**
IV
Adults, Elderly. Initially, 5 mcg/min via infusion pump. Increase in 5-mcg/min increments at 3- to 5-min intervals until BP response is noted or until dosage reaches 20 mcg/min; then increase as needed by 10 mcg/min. Dosage may be further titrated according to clinical, therapeutic response up to 200 mcg/min.
Children. Initially, 0.25-0.5 mcg/kg/min; titrate by 0.5-1 mcg/kg/min up to 20 mcg/kg/min.

CONTRAINDICATIONS
Allergy to adhesives (transdermal), closed-angle glaucoma, constrictive pericarditis (IV), early MI (sublingual), GI hypermotility or malabsorption (extended-release), head trauma, hypotension (IV), inadequate cerebral circulation (IV), increased intracranial pressure, nitrates, orthostatic hypotension, pericardial tamponade (IV), severe anemia, uncorrected hypovolemia (IV).
Caution
Postural hypotension, lactation, nitroglycerin.

INTERACTIONS
Drug
Alcohol, opioids, benzodiazepines, phenthiazines, other drugs used

in conscious sedation techniques: May increase hypotensive effects.

Nitroglycerin: should be discontinued if blurred vision or dry mouth occurs.

Other antihypertensives, vasodilators: May increase risk of orthostatic hypotension.

Sildenafil, tadalafil, vardenafil: Concurrent use of these drugs produces significant hypotension.

Herbal
None known.

Food
Alcohol: May increase risk of orthostatic hypotension.

DIAGNOSTIC TEST EFFECTS

May increase blood methemoglobin, urine catecholamine, and urine vanillylmandelic acid concentrations.

ⓘ IV INCOMPATIBILITIES
Alteplase (Activase).

ⓘ IV COMPATIBILITIES

Amiodarone (Cordarone), diltiazem (Cardizem), dobutamine (Dobutrex), dopamine (Intropin), epinephrine, famotidine (Pepcid), fentanyl (Sublimaze), furosemide (Lasix), heparin, hydromorphone (Dilaudid), insulin, labetalol (Trandate), lidocaine, lorazepam (Ativan), midazolam (Versed), milrinone (Primacor), morphine, nicardipine (Cardene), nitroprusside (Nipride), norepinephrine (Levophed), propofol (Diprivan).

SIDE EFFECTS

Frequent
Headache (possibly severe; occurs mostly in early therapy, diminishes rapidly in intensity, and usually disappears during continued treatment), transient flushing of face and neck, dizziness (especially if patient is standing immobile or is in a warm environment), weakness, orthostatic hypotension.
Sublingual: Burning, tingling sensation at oral point of dissolution.
Ointment: Erythema, pruritus.
Occasional
GI upset.
Transdermal: Contact dermatitis.

SERIOUS REACTIONS

• Nitroglycerin should be discontinued if blurred vision or dry mouth occurs.
• Severe orthostatic hypotension may occur, manifested by fainting, pulselessness, cold or clammy skin, and diaphoresis.
• Tolerance may occur with repeated, prolonged therapy; minor tolerance may occur with intermittent use of sublingual tablets.
• High doses of nitroglycerin tend to produce severe headache.

PRECAUTIONS & CONSIDERATIONS

Caution is warranted with acute MI, blood volume depletion from therapy, glaucoma (contraindicated in closed-angle glaucoma), hepatic or renal disease, and systolic BP < 90 mm Hg. It is unknown whether nitroglycerin crosses the placenta or is distributed in breast milk, warranting caution in lactation. The safety and efficacy of nitroglycerin have not been established in children. Elderly patients are more susceptible to the hypotensive effects of nitroglycerin. In elderly patients, age-related renal impairment may require cautious use. Alcohol should be avoided because it intensifies the drug's hypotensive effect. If alcohol is ingested soon after taking nitrates, an acute hypotensive episode marked by pallor, vertigo, and a drop in BP may occur.

Dizziness, lightheadedness, and headache may occur. Rise slowly from a lying to a sitting position and dangle legs momentarily before standing to avoid the drug's hypotensive effect. Notify the physician of facial or neck flushing. The onset, type (sharp, dull, or squeezing), radiation, location, intensity, and duration of anginal pain and its precipitating factors, such as exertion and emotional stress, should be recorded before therapy begins. Apical pulse and BP should be determined before administration and periodically after the dose has been given. ECG should be closely monitored during IV administration.

Storage
Keep sublingual tablets in their original container. Store solution for injection at room temperature. Keep away from heat and moisture.

Administration
! The cardioverter or defibrillator must not be discharged through a paddle electrode overlying a nitroglycerin system because to do so may cause burns to the patient or damage the paddle via arching. Do not give nitrates if the patient has recently taken Cialis, Levitra, or Viagra.

Swallow extended-release capsules whole; capsules should not be chewed or crushed. Take nitroglycerin, preferably on an empty stomach; take the medication with meals if headache occurs during therapy.

Do not shake aerosol canister before lingual spraying. Use the translingual spray only when lying down. Spray under the tongue and avoid inhaling or swallowing lingual spray.

For sublingual use, dissolve under the tongue and avoid swallowing. Administer while seated. To lessen the burning sensation under the tongue, place the tablet in the buccal pouch. Take sublingual tablets at the first sign of angina. If anginal pain is not relieved within 5 min of the first dose, seek emergency assistance and dissolve a second tablet under the tongue. If the second dose does not relieve anginal pain within 5 min, dissolve a third tablet under the tongue.

For topical use, spread a thin layer on clean, dry, hairless skin of the upper arm or body, not below the knee or elbow, using the applicator or dose-measuring papers. Do not use fingers; do not rub or massage into skin.

! Transdermal patch should be removed before cardioversion or defibrillation because the electrical current may cause arching which can burn the person and damage the paddles.

For transdermal use, apply patch on clean, dry, hairless skin of the upper arm or body, not below the knee or elbow.

The IV form is available in ready-to-use injectable containers. To use, dilute vials in 250 or 500 mL D5W or 0.9% NaCl to a maximum concentration of 250 mg/250 mL. Use microdrop or infusion pump.

Nitroprusside
nye-troe-pruss′ide
(Nipride [CAN], Nitropress)
Do not confuse nitroprusside with nitroglycerin or Nitrostat.

CATEGORY AND SCHEDULE
Pregnancy Risk Category: C

Classification: Vasodilators

MECHANISM OF ACTION

A potent vasodilator used to treat emergent hypertensive conditions; acts directly on arterial and venous smooth muscle. Decreases peripheral vascular resistance, preload and afterload; improves cardiac output. *Therapeutic Effect:* Dilates coronary arteries, decreases oxygen consumption, and relieves persistent chest pain.

PHARMACOKINETICS

Route	Onset	Peak	Duration
IV	1-10 min	Dependent on infusion rate	Dissipates rapidly after stopping IV

Reacts with hemoglobin in erythrocytes, producing cyanmethemoglobin, and cyanide ions. Excreted primarily in urine. *Half-life:* < 10 min.

AVAILABILITY

Injection: 25 mg/mL.

INDICATIONS AND DOSAGES

▶ **Immediate reduction of BP in hypertensive crisis; to produce controlled hypotension in surgical procedures to reduce bleeding; treatment of acute congestive heart failure (CHF)**
IV
Adults, Elderly, Children. Initially, 0.3 mcg/kg/min. Range: 0.5-10 mcg/kg/min. Do not exceed 10 mcg/kg/min (risk of precipitous drop in BP).

OFF-LABEL USES

Control of paroxysmal hypertension before and during surgery for pheochromocytoma, peripheral vasospasm caused by ergot alkaloid overdose, treatment adjunct with dopamine for acute myocardial infarction (MI), valvular regurgitation.

CONTRAINDICATIONS

Compensatory hypertension (atrioventricular [AV] shunt or coarctation of aorta), inadequate cerebral circulation, moribund patients (ASA Class 5E), congenital Leber's optic atrophy, tobacco amblyopia, acute CHF with reduced peripheral vascular resistance.

INTERACTIONS

Drug
Antihypertensives, ganglionic blockers, volatile anesthetics: May increase hypotensive effect.
Dobutamine: May increase cardiac output and decrease pulmonary wedge pressure.
Herbal
None known.
Food
None known.

DIAGNOSTIC TEST EFFECTS

None known.

ⓘ IV INCOMPATIBILITIES

Cisatracurium (Nimbex).

ⓘ IV COMPATIBILITIES

Diltiazem (Cardizem), dobutamine (Dobutrex), dopamine (Intropin), enalapril (Vasotec), heparin, insulin, labetalol (Normodyne, Trandate), lidocaine, midazolam (Versed), milrinone (Primacor), nitroglycerin, propofol (Diprivan).

SIDE EFFECTS

Occasional
Flushing of skin, increased intracranial pressure, rash, pain or redness at injection site.

SERIOUS REACTIONS

• A too rapid IV infusion rate reduces BP too quickly.

N

• Nausea, vomiting, diaphoresis, apprehension, headache, restlessness, muscle twitching, dizziness, palpitations, retrosternal pain, and abdominal pain may occur. Symptoms disappear rapidly if rate of administration is slowed or drug is temporarily discontinued.
• Overdose produces metabolic acidosis and cyanide toxicity (rare).

PRECAUTIONS & CONSIDERATIONS

Caution is warranted in patients with hyponatremia, hypothyroidism, severe hepatic or renal impairment, and in elderly patients. It is unknown whether nitroprusside crosses the placenta or is distributed in breast milk, warranting caution in lactation. The safety and efficacy of nitroprusside have not been established in children. Elderly patients are more sensitive to the drug's hypotensive effect. In elderly patients, age-related renal impairment may require cautious use. Be aware of signs and symptoms of metabolic acidosis, including disorientation, headache, hyperventilation, nausea, vomiting, and weakness. Alcohol should be avoided because it intensifies the drug's hypotensive effect. If alcohol is ingested soon after taking nitrates, an acute hypotensive episode marked by pallor, vertigo, and a drop in BP may occur.

Notify the physician of pain, redness, or swelling at the IV insertion, dizziness, headache, nausea, palpitations, or other unusual signs or symptoms. Desired BP levels should be determined with the physician before treatment; it is normally maintained at about 30% to 40% below pretreatment levels. BP and ECG should be monitored before and during treatment. Acid-base balance, electrolyte levels, intake and output, and laboratory results should also be assessed. Nitroprusside should be discontinued if the therapeutic response is not achieved within 10 min after IV infusion at 10 mcg/kg/min is initiated.
! Overdose evidenced by severe hypotension, dyspnea, loss of consciousness, metabolic lactic acidosis, headache, and death. Report symptoms of rare cyanide toxicity from drug metabolism evidenced by venous hyperoxemia with bright red venous blood, lactic acidosis, air hunger, confusion, or death.
Storage
Protect solution from light. Use only freshly prepared solution. Once the solution has been prepared, it must be used within 24 h; do not keep it for longer than 24 h. Discard unused portion.
! Do not infuse any other medication with nitroprusside.
Administration
Inspect IV solution, which normally appears faint brown. A color change from brown to blue, green, or dark red indicates drug deterioration. Use only freshly prepared solution. Once the solution has been prepared, it must be used within 24 h; do not keep it longer than 24 h. Discard unused portion. Further dilute with 250-500 mL D5W to provide a concentration of 200 mcg/mL to 50 mcg/mL, respectively, up to a maximum concentration of 200 mg/250 mL. Wrap infusion bottle in aluminum foil immediately after mixing. Give by IV infusion only using infusion rate chart provided by manufacturer or facility protocol. Administer using IV infusion pump and lock in the rate. The rate of infusion should be monitored frequently. Be alert

for extravasation, which produces severe pain and sloughing.

Nizatidine
ni-za′ti-deen
(Axid, Axid AR, Tazac [AUS])

CATEGORY AND SCHEDULE
Pregnancy Risk Category: B
OTC Capsules: 75 mg

Classification: Antihistamines, H2 receptor antagonist

MECHANISM OF ACTION
An antiulcer agent and gastric acid secretion inhibitor that inhibits histamine action at H_2 receptors of parietal cells. *Therapeutic Effect:* Inhibits basal and nocturnal gastric acid secretion.

PHARMACOKINETICS
Rapidly, well absorbed from the GI tract. Protein binding: 35%. Metabolized in the liver. Excreted primarily in urine. Not removed by hemodialysis. *Half-life:* 1-2 h (increased with impaired renal function).

AVAILABILITY
Capsules: 75 mg (OTC), 150 mg, 300 mg.
Oral solution.

INDICATIONS AND DOSAGES
▶ **Active duodenal ulcer**
PO
Adults, Elderly. 300 mg at bedtime or 150 mg twice a day.
▶ **Prevention of duodenal ulcer recurrence**
PO
Adults, Elderly. 150 mg at bedtime.

▶ **Gastroesophageal reflux disease (GERD)**
PO
Adults, Elderly. 150 mg twice a day.
▶ **Active benign gastric ulcer**
PO
Adults, Elderly. 150 mg twice a day or 300 mg at bedtime.
▶ **Dyspepsia**
PO (OTC)
Adults, Elderly. 75 mg 30-60 min before meals; no more than 2 tablets a day.
▶ **Dosage in renal impairment**
Dosage adjustment is based on creatinine clearance.

Creatinine Clearance (mL/min)	Active Ulcer Disease	Maintenance Therapy
20-50	150 mg every bedtime	150 mg every other day
< 20	150 mg every other day	150 mg every 3 days

OFF-LABEL USES
Gastric hypersecretory conditions, multiple endocrine adenoma, Zollinger-Ellison syndrome.

CONTRAINDICATIONS
Hypersensitivity to other H_2 antagonists.
Caution
Hepatic disease, renal disease, lactation, children under 16 yr.

INTERACTIONS
Drug
Antacids: May decrease the absorption of nizatidine.
Aspirin: May increase serum salicylate levels with high doses of aspirin.

Ketoconazole: May decrease the absorption of ketoconazole; take 2 h before or after nizatidine.
Herbal
None known.
Food
None known.

DIAGNOSTIC TEST EFFECTS

Interferes with skin tests using allergen extracts. May increase serum alkaline phosphatase, AST (SGOT), and ALT (SGPT) levels.

SIDE EFFECTS

Occasional (2%)
Somnolence, fatigue.
Rare (1%)
Diaphoresis, rash.

SERIOUS REACTIONS

• Asymptomatic ventricular tachycardia, hyperuricemia not associated with gout, and nephrolithiasis occur rarely.

PRECAUTIONS & CONSIDERATIONS

Caution is warranted in patients with impaired hepatic or renal function. It is unknown whether nizatidine crosses the placenta or is distributed in breast milk, warranting caution in pregnancy and lactation. The safety and efficacy of nizatidine have not been established in children younger than 16 yr of age. No age-related precautions have been noted in elderly patients. Tasks that require mental alertness or motor skills should be avoided until response to the drug has been established. Also, avoid alcohol, aspirin, and coffee, all of which may cause GI distress, during nizatidine therapy.

Notify the physician if acid indigestion, gastric distress, or heartburn occurs after 2 wks of continuous nizatidine therapy. Blood chemistry laboratory test results, including BUN, serum alkaline phosphatase, bilirubin, creatinine, AST (SGOT), and ALT (SGPT) levels, to assess hepatic and renal function should be obtained before and during therapy.

Administration
Take nizatidine without regard to meals; however, it is best given after meals or at bedtime. Take right before eating for heartburn prevention. Do not administer within 1 h of magnesium- or aluminum-containing antacids because it can decrease the absorption of nizatidine.

Norepinephrine Bitartrate

nor-ep-i-nef′rin bye-tar-trayte
(Levophed)
Do not confuse Levophed with Levid or Levbid, Levothyroxine or Levaquin, or norepinephrine with epinephrine or norethindrone.

CATEGORY AND SCHEDULE

Pregnancy Risk Category: C

Classification: Adrenergic catecholamine

MECHANISM OF ACTION

A sympathomimetic that stimulates β_1-adrenergic receptors and α-adrenergic receptors, increasing peripheral resistance. Enhances contractile myocardial force, increases cardiac output. Constricts resistance and capacitance vessels. *Therapeutic Effect:* Increases systemic BP and coronary blood flow.

PHARMACOKINETICS

Route	Onset	Peak	Duration
IV	Rapid	1-2 min	NA

Localized in sympathetic tissue. Metabolized in the liver. Primarily excreted in urine.

AVAILABILITY

Injection: 1-mg/mL ampules.

INDICATIONS AND DOSAGES

▸ **Acute hypotension unresponsive to fluid volume replacement**
IV
Adults, Elderly. Initially, administer at 0.5-1 mcg/min. Adjust rate of flow to establish and maintain desired BP. Average maintenance dose: 2-4 mcg/min. Maximum: 30 mcg/min.
Children. Initially, 0.05-0.1 mcg/kg/min; titrate to desired effect. Maximum: 1-2 mcg/kg/min. Range: 0.5-3 mcg/min.

CONTRAINDICATIONS

Hypovolemic states (unless as an emergency measure), mesenteric or peripheral vascular thrombosis, profound hypoxia.

INTERACTIONS

Drug
β-Blockers: May have mutually inhibitory effects.
Digoxin: May increase risk of arrhythmias.
Ergonovine, oxytocin: May increase vasoconstriction.
Halogenated hydrocarbon anesthetics: May increase risk of arrhythmias.
Maprotiline, tricyclic antidepressants, oxytocin, guanethidine: Increased risk of severe hypotension.

Methyldopa: May decrease the effects of methyldopa.
Herbal
None known.
Food
None known.

DIAGNOSTIC TEST EFFECTS

None known.

Ⓓ IV INCOMPATIBILITIES

Regular insulin.

◎ IV COMPATIBILITIES

Amiodarone (Cordarone), calcium gluconate, diltiazem (Cardizem), dobutamine (Dobutrex), dopamine (Intropin), epinephrine, esmolol (Brevibloc), fentanyl (Sublimaze), furosemide (Lasix), haloperidol (Haldol), heparin, hydromorphone (Dilaudid), labetalol (Trandate), lorazepam (Ativan), magnesium, midazolam (Versed), milrinone (Primacor), morphine, nicardipine (Cardene), nitroglycerin, potassium chloride, propofol (Diprivan).

SIDE EFFECTS

Norepinephrine produces less pronounced and less frequent side effects than epinephrine.
Occasional (3%-5%)
Anxiety, bradycardia, palpitations.
Rare (1%-2%)
Nausea, anginal pain, shortness of breath, fever.

SERIOUS REACTIONS

• Extravasation may produce tissue necrosis and sloughing.
• Overdose is manifested as severe hypertension with violent headache (which may be the first clinical sign of overdose), arrhythmias, photophobia, retrosternal or pharyngeal pain, pallor, excessive sweating, and vomiting.

N

• Prolonged therapy may result in plasma volume depletion. Hypotension may recur if plasma volume is not restored.

PRECAUTIONS & CONSIDERATIONS

❗ This drug is used in acute settings in hospitals or emergencies for selected hypotensive episodes.

Caution is warranted in patients with hypertension, hypothyroidism, severe cardiac disease, and concurrent MAOI therapy. Norepinephrine readily crosses the placenta and may produce fetal anoxia as a result of constriction of uterine blood vessels and uterine contraction. Use in pregnancy is contraindicated unless the benefits of therapy clearly outweigh potential risks to the mother and fetus. No age-related precautions have been noted in children or elderly patients.

BP and ECG should be monitored continuously. Be alert to precipitous drops in BP. Intake and output should be assessed hourly or as ordered. If urine output is < 30 mL/h, the infusion should be stopped unless the systolic BP falls below 80 mm Hg. Prolonged therapy may result in plasma volume depleting, causing hypotension to persist or not return to normal levels.

Storage
Store ampules at room temperature.
Administration
❗ Expect to restore blood and fluid volume before administering norepinephrine.

Do not use if solution is brown or contains precipitate. Add 4 mL (4 mg) to 1 L of D5W for a 4-mcg/mL solution. Maximum concentration: 32 mcg/mL. Administer infusion through a central venous catheter, if available, to avoid extravasation. Closely monitor the infusion flow rate with a microdrip or infusion pump.

Monitor the BP every 2 min during the infusion until desired therapeutic response is achieved, then every 5 min during the remainder of the infusion. Never leave unattended during the infusion. Be alert to any complaint of headache. Plan to maintain BP at 80-100 mm Hg in previously normotensive patients. Reduce the infusion gradually, as prescribed. Avoid abrupt withdrawal. Check the peripherally inserted catheter IV site frequently for signs of extravasation, including blanching, coldness, hardness, and pallor to the extremity. If extravasation occurs, expect to infiltrate the affected area with 10-15 mL sterile saline containing 5-10 mg phentolamine. Know that phentolamine does not alter the pressor effects of norepinephrine.

Norethindrone
nor-eth′in-drone
(Aygestin, Camilla, Errin, Jolivette, Micronor, Nora-BE, Nor-QD, Norlutate [CAN])

CATEGORY AND SCHEDULE
Pregnancy Risk Category: X

Classification: Progesterone derivative

MECHANISM OF ACTION
A synthetic progestin that is used as a single agent or in combination with estrogens for the treatment of gynecological disorders. It inhibits secretion of pituitary gonadotropin (LH), which prevents follicular maturation and ovulation.

Therapeutic Effect: Transforms endometrium from proliferative to secretory in an estrogen-primed endometrium, promotes mammary gland development, relaxes uterine smooth muscle.

PHARMACOKINETICS

Rapidly absorbed from the GI tract. Widely distributed. Protein binding: 61%. Metabolized in liver. Excreted in urine and feces. *Half-life:* 4-13 h.

AVAILABILITY

Contraceptive Tablets: 0.35 mg (Camila, Errin, Jolivette, Micronor, Nora-BE, Nor-QD).
Tablets, as Norethindrone Acetate: 5 mg (Aygestin).

INDICATIONS AND DOSAGES

▶ **Contraception**
PO
Adults. 1 tablet/day.
▶ **Amenorrhea and abnormal uterine bleeding**
PO
Adults. 5-20 mg/day cyclically (21 days on; 7 days off or continuously) or for acetate salt formulation, 2.5-10 mg cyclically.
▶ **Endometriosis**
PO
Adults. 10 mg/day for 2 wks, increase at increments of 5 mg/day every 2 wks until 30 mg/day; continue for 6-9 mo or until breakthrough bleeding demands temporary termination. For acetate salt formulation, 5 mg/day for 14 days, increase at increments of 2.5 mg/day every 2 wks up to 15 mg/day continue for 6-9 mo or until breakthrough bleeding demands temporary termination.

OFF-LABEL USES

Treatment of corpus luteum dysfunction.

CONTRAINDICATIONS

Acute liver disease, benign or malignant liver tumors, hypersensitivity to norethindrone and any component of the formulation, known or suspected carcinoma of the breast, known or suspected pregnancy, undiagnosed abnormal genital bleeding.
Caution
Lactation, hypertension, asthma, blood dyscrasias, gallbladder disease, congestive heart failure, diabetes mellitus, bone disease, depression, migraine headache, convulsive disorders, hepatic disease, renal disease, family history of breast or reproductive tract cancers.

INTERACTIONS

Drug
Antibiotics such as the penicillins and erythromycin, barbiturates: May decrease effectiveness of norethindrone.
Amprenavir, nelfinavir, nevirapine, ritonavir: May decrease norethindrone concentrations.
Aprepitant: May decrease the effects of both drugs.
Atorvastatin, rosuvastatin: May increase concentrations of norethindrone.
Benzodiazepines: May increase risk of benzodiazepine toxicity.
Cyclosporine: May increase risk of cyclosporine toxicity.
CYP3A4 inducers (carbamazepine, phenobarbital, phenytoin, rifampin, rifabutin): May decrease the levels and/or effects of norethindrone.
Corticosteroids: May prolong the effects of cortisones.
Fluconazole: May increase risk of adverse effects of norethindrone.
Griseofulvin, modafinil, primidone: May decrease effectiveness of norethindrone.

N

Lamotrigine: May increase or decrease plasma lamotrigine concentrations.
Selegiline: May increase the risk of adverse effects of selegiline.
Theophylline: May increase the risk of theophylline toxicity.
Thiazolidinediones: May decrease the effects of norethindrone.
Warfarin: May increase or decrease anticoagulant effects.
Zolmitriptan: May increase risk of adverse effects of zolmitriptan.
Herbal
Licorice: May increase risk of fluid retention and elevated blood pressure.
Red clover: May alter effectiveness of norethindrone or increase side effects.
St. John's wort: May decrease plasma concentrations of norethindrone.
Vitamin C (at high doses, more than 1 g/day): May increase adverse effects of norethindrone.
Food
Caffeine: May increase CNS stimulation.

DIAGNOSTIC TEST EFFECTS
May increase LDL concentrations and serum alkaline phosphatase levels. May decrease glucose tolerance and HDL concentrations. May cause abnormal thyroid, metapyrone, liver, and endocrine function tests.

SIDE EFFECTS
Occasional
Breast tenderness, dizziness, headache, breakthrough bleeding, amenorrhea, menstrual irregularity, nausea, weakness.
Rare
Mental depression, fever, insomnia, rash, acne, increased breast tenderness, weight gain/loss, changes in cervical erosion and secretions, cholestatic jaundice.

SERIOUS REACTIONS
• Thrombophlebitis, cerebrovascular disorders, retinal thrombosis, cholestatic jaundice, and pulmonary embolism occur rarely.

PRECAUTIONS & CONSIDERATIONS
Caution is warranted in patients with conditions aggravated by fluid retention, delayed follicular atresia or ovarian cysts, asthma, cardiac dysfunction, epilepsy, migraine headache, renal insufficiency, diabetes mellitus, and a history of mental depression. Norethindrone is distributed in breast milk and may be harmful to fetus and is contraindicated in pregnancy. Patient's pregnancy status should be assessed before beginning therapy. If pregnancy is suspected, notify physician immediately. Norethindrone should not be used during breastfeeding. Safety and efficacy of this drug have not been established in children. No age-related precautions have been noted in elderly patients. Avoid smoking while taking norethindrone.

Menstrual spotting may occur between periods. Pain, redness, swelling, or warmth in the calf; chest pain; migraine headache; peripheral paresthesia; sudden decrease in vision; and sudden shortness of breath should be reported immediately. Patient should be advised to use an additional nonhormonal form of birth control during therapy if antibiotics or anti-infectives are prescribed while remaining compliant with the oral contraceptive therapy schedule.
Administration
For oral contraception to be effective, take norethindrone at the same time each day. Do not take a break between packs. Do not skip doses.

Norfloxacin
nor-flox′a-sin
(Apo-Norflox [CAN], Insensye
[AUS], Norfloxacine [CAN],
Noroxin, Novo-Norfloxacin [CAN],
PMS-Norfloxacin [CAN], Roxin
[AUS])

CATEGORY AND SCHEDULE
Pregnancy Risk Category: C

Classification: Fluoroquinolone
anti-infective

MECHANISM OF ACTION
A quinolone that inhibits
DNA gyrase in susceptible
microorganisms, interfering with
bacterial cell replication and repair.
Therapeutic Effect: Bactericidal.

PHARMACOKINETICS
PO: Peak 1 h, steady state in 2 days.
Excreted in urine as active drug and
metabolites. *Half-life:* 3-4 h.

AVAILABILITY
Tablets: 400 mg.
Ophthalmic Solution (Chibroxin):
0.3%.

INDICATIONS AND DOSAGES
▸ **Bacterial conjunctivitis**
OPHTHALMIC
Adults, Children 1 yr and older. 1 or
2 drops 4 times/day for up to 7 days.
First day of therapy may be 1 or 2
drops every 2 h during the waking
hours.
▸ **Urinary tract infections (UTIs)**
PO
Adults, Elderly. 400 mg twice a day
for 7-21 days.
▸ **Prostatitis**
PO
Adults. 400 mg twice a day for 28 days.

▸ **Uncomplicated gonococcal
infections**
PO
Adults. 800 mg as a single dose.
▸ **Dosage in renal impairment**
Dosage and frequency are modified
based on creatinine clearance.

Creatinine Clearance (mL/min)	Adult Dosage (mg)
≥ 30	400 twice a day
< 30	400 once a day

CONTRAINDICATIONS
Children younger than 18 yr
because of risk arthropathy
(systemic use). Hypersensitivity to
norfloxacin, other quinolones, or
their components.

INTERACTIONS
Drug
**Antacids, sucralfate, iron
supplements, multivitamins with
minerals, zinc, didanozine:** May
decrease norfloxacin absorption.
Cyclosporine: May increase
cyclosporine concentrations.
Oral anticoagulants: May increase
effects of oral anticoagulants.
Theophylline: Decreases clearance
and may increase blood concentration
and risk of toxicity of theophylline.
Herbal
None known.
Food
Dairy products: May decrease
nonfloxacin absorbtion.

DIAGNOSTIC TEST EFFECTS
May increase BUN level and serum
alkaline phosphatase, bilirubin,
creatinine, LDH, AST (SGOT), and
ALT (SGPT) levels.

SIDE EFFECTS
Burning or discomfort. Other
reactions were conjunctival
hypermia, chemosis, corneal

N

deposits, photophobia, and a bitter taste following installations.
Frequent
Nausea, headache, dizziness.
Rare
Vomiting, diarrhea, dry mouth, bitter taste, nervousness, drowsiness, insomnia, photosensitivity, tinnitus, crystalluria, rash, fever, seizures.

SERIOUS REACTIONS
• Superinfection, anaphylaxis, Stevens-Johnson syndrome, and arthropathy occur rarely.
• Hypersensitivity reactions, including photosensitivity (as evidenced by rash, pruritus, blisters, edema, and burning skin), have occurred in patients receiving fluoroquinolones.
• Tendonitis and terdon rupture.

PRECAUTIONS & CONSIDERATIONS
Caution is warranted in patients with impaired renal function and a predisposition to seizures. Dizziness, headache, nausea, signs of infection, and vaginitis should be evaluated. Food tolerance should be assessed. Patients should be cautioned to watch for pain, swelling, or tenderness in any tendon or ligament in the shoulder, hand, or Achilles tendon, and report any of these symptoms for evaluation by a healthcare practitioner.
Administration
Take norfloxacin with 8 oz of water 1 h before or 2 h after a meal and consume several glasses of water between meals. Do not take antacids divalent cations, dairy products, or didanosine, within 2 h of norfloxacin.

Norgestrel
nor-jes'trel
(Ovrette)
Discontinued in the United States

CATEGORY AND SCHEDULE
Pregnancy Risk Category: X

Classification: Progesterone derivative

MECHANISM OF ACTION
A progestin that inhibits secretion of pituitary gonadotropin (LH), which prevents follicular maturation and ovulation. *Therapeutic Effect:* Transforms endometrium from proliferative to secretory in an estrogen-primed endometrium, promotes mammary gland development, relaxes uterine smooth muscle.

PHARMACOKINETICS
Well absorbed from the GI tract. Widely distributed. Protein binding: 97%. Metabolized in liver via reduction and conjugation. Primarily excreted in urine. *Half-life:* 20 h.

AVAILABILITY
Tablets: 0.075 mg (Ovrette).

INDICATIONS AND DOSAGES
▸ **Contraception, female**
PO
Adults. 0.075 mg/day.

OFF-LABEL USES
Endometrial protection, endometriosis, menorrhagia.

CONTRAINDICATIONS
Hypersensitivity to norgestrel or any component of the

formulation or to tartrazine. Thromboembolic disorders, severe hepatic disease, breast cancer; undiagnosed vaginal bleeding, pregnancy.

Caution

Lactation, hypertension, asthma, blood dyscrasias, gallbladder disease, congestive heart failure, diabetes mellitus, bone disease, depression, migraine headache, convulsive disorders, hepatic disease, renal disease, family history of breast or reproductive tract cancers.

INTERACTIONS

Drug

Antibiotics, such as the penicillins, barbiturates: May decrease contraceptive efficacy.

Amprenavir, nevirapine, ritonavir: May decrease contraceptive efficacy.

Aprepitant: May reduce efficacy of norgestrel.

Bromocriptine: May interfere with the effects of bromocriptine.

Caffeine: May increase the effects of caffeine.

Fluconazole: May increase risk of norgestrel adverse effects.

Griseofulvin, phenobarbital, phenytoin, pioglitazone, rifampin, troglitazone: May decrease contraceptive effectiveness.

Rosuvastatin: May increase plasma concentrations of norgestrel.

Warfarin: May decrease or increase anticoagulant effects.

Herbal

St. John's wort: May decrease levels of St. John's wort.

Dong quai, black cohosh: May add estrogen activity.

Saw palmetto, red clover, ginseng: May alter contraceptive effectiveness or increase side effects.

Food

None known.

DIAGNOSTIC TEST EFFECTS

None known.

SIDE EFFECTS

Frequent

Breakthrough bleeding or spotting at beginning of therapy, amenorrhea, change in menstrual flow, breast tenderness.

Occasional

Edema, weight gain or loss, rash, pruritus, photosensitivity, skin pigmentation.

Rare

Pain or swelling at injection site, acne, mental depression, alopecia, hirsutism.

SERIOUS REACTIONS

• Thrombophlebitis, cerebrovascular disorders, retinal thrombosis, and pulmonary embolism occur rarely.

PRECAUTIONS & CONSIDERATIONS

Caution is necessary with conditions aggravated by fluid retention, diabetes mellitus, and a history of mental depression. Norgestrel is distributed in breast milk and may be harmful to fetus. Norgestrel should not be used during breastfeeding. Safety and efficacy of this drug have not been established in children. No age-related precautions have been noted in elderly patients. Avoid smoking while taking norgestrel.

Menstrual spotting may occur between periods. Pain, redness, swelling, or warmth in the calf; chest pain; migraine headache; peripheral paresthesia; sudden decrease in vision; and sudden shortness

N

of breath should be reported immediately.
Administration
Take at same time daily, every day, to maintain contraceptive effectiveness.

Nortriptyline Hydrochloride
nor-trip'ti-leen high-droh-klor-ide
(Allegron [AUS], Aventyl, Norventyl, Pamelor)
Do not confuse nortriptyline with amitriptyline, or Aventyl with Ambenyl or Bentyl.

CATEGORY AND SCHEDULE
Pregnancy Risk Category: D

Classification: Antidepressants, tricyclic

MECHANISM OF ACTION
A tricyclic antidepressant that blocks reuptake of the neurotransmitters norepinephrine and serotonin at neuronal presynaptic membranes, increasing their availability at postsynaptic receptor sites. *Therapeutic Effect:* Relieves depression.

PHARMACOKINETICS
Well absorbed from the GI tract. Protein binding: 86%-95%. Metabolized in the liver. Primarily excreted in the urine. *Half-life:* 17.6 r.

AVAILABILITY
Capsules (Aventyl): 10 mg, 25 mg.
Capsules (Pamelor): 10 mg, 25 mg, 75 mg.

Oral Solution (Aventyl, Pamelor): 10 mg/5 mL.

INDICATIONS AND DOSAGES
▸ **Depression**
PO
Adults. Initially 25-50 mg/day. Usual dose is 75-100 mg/day in 1-4 divided doses. Reduce dosage gradually to effective maintenance level. Maximum: 150 mg/day.
Elderly. Initially, 10-25 mg at bedtime. May increase by 25 mg every 3-7 days. Maximum: 150 mg/day.
Children 12 yr and older. 30-50 mg/day in 3-4 divided doses.
▸ **Enuresis**
PO
Children 12 yr and older. 25-35 mg/day.
Children aged 8-11 yr. 10-20 mg/day.
Children aged 6-7 yr. 10 mg/day.

OFF-LABEL USES
Treatment of neurogenic pain, panic disorder; prevention of migraine headache, enuresis.

CONTRAINDICATIONS
Acute recovery period after myocardial infarction (MI), use within 14 days of MAOIs.
Caution
Suicidal patients, severe depression, increased intraocular pressure (IOP), narrow-angle glaucoma, urinary retention, cardiac disease, hepatic disease, hyperthyroidism, electroshock therapy, elective surgery, MAOIs.

INTERACTIONS
Drug
Alcohol, other central nervous system (CNS) depressants, barbiturates, benzodiazepines: May increase CNS and respiratory depression and the hypotensive effects of nortriptyline.

Antihistamines, phenothiazines, muscarinic blockers: May increase anticholinergic effects.
Antithyroid agents: May increase the risk of agranulocytosis.
Cimetidine: May increase the blood concentration and risk of toxicity of nortriptyline.
Clonidine, guanadre, guanethidine: May decrease the effects of these drugs.
MAOIs: May increase the risk of neuroleptic malignant syndrome, seizures, hyperpyrexia, and hypertensive crisis.
Phenothiazines: May increase the anticholinergic and sedative effects of nortriptyline.
Sympathomimetics, epinephrine, levonordefrin: May increase the risk of cardiac effects.
Herbal
St. John's wort: Avoid concurrent use with St. John's wort.
Food
None known.

DIAGNOSTIC TEST EFFECTS

May alter blood glucose level and ECG readings. The therapeutic peak serum level is 6-10 mcg/mL; the therapeutic trough serum level is 0.5-2 mcg/mL. The toxic peak serum level is > 12 mcg/mL; the toxic trough serum level is > 2 mcg/mL.

SIDE EFFECTS

Frequent
Somnolence, fatigue, dry mouth, blurred vision, constipation, delayed micturition, orthostatic hypotension, diaphoresis, impaired concentration, increased appetite, urine retention.
Occasional
GI disturbances (nausea, GI distress, metallic taste), photosensitivity.
Rare
Paradoxical reactions (agitation, restlessness, nightmares, insomnia),
extrapyramidal symptoms (particularly fine hand tremor).

SERIOUS REACTIONS

• Overdose may produce seizures; cardiovascular effects, such as severe orthostatic hypotension, dizziness, tachycardia, palpitations, and arrhythmias; and altered temperature regulation, such as hyperpyrexia or hypothermia.
• Abrupt discontinuation after prolonged therapy may produce headache, malaise, nausea, vomiting, and vivid dreams.

PRECAUTIONS & CONSIDERATIONS

Caution is warranted in patients with cardiac disease, diabetes mellitus, glaucoma, hiatal hernia, history of seizures, history of urinary obstruction or urine retention, hyperthyroidism, increased IOP, prostatic hypertrophy, hepatic or renal disease, and schizophrenia. Sunscreens and protective clothing should be worn because the drug may cause photosensitivity to sunlight.

Anticholinergic, sedative, and hypotensive effects may occur, but tolerance usually develops. Because dizziness may occur, change positions slowly, avoid alcohol and tasks that require alertness or motor skills. Pattern of daily bowel activity and stool consistency, bladder for urine retention, BP and pulse rate, and ECG should be assessed during therapy. Patient should report xerostomic effects, such as sore tongue or problems with eating or swallowing so that a medication change can be considered.
Administration
! Make sure at least 14 days elapse between the use of MAOIs and nortriptyline. Be aware that nortriptyline's therapeutic peak serum level is 6-10 mcg/mL and therapeutic trough serum level is

0.5-2 mcg/mL; nortriptyline's toxic peak serum level is > 12 mcg/mL and toxic trough serum level is > 2 mcg/mL.

Take nortriptyline with food or milk if GI distress occurs. Nortriptyline's therapeutic effect may be noted in 2 wks or longer.

Nystatin
nye-stat′in
(Mycostatin, Nilstat [CAN], Nyaderm, Nystop)
Do not confuse nystatin or mycostatin with Nitrostat.

CATEGORY AND SCHEDULE
Pregnancy Risk Category: C

Classification: Antifungals

MECHANISM OF ACTION
A fungistatic antifungal that binds to sterols in the fungal cell membrane. *Therapeutic Effect:* Increases fungal cell-membrane permeability, allowing loss of potassium and other cellular components.

PHARMACOKINETICS
PO: Poorly absorbed from the GI tract. Eliminated unchanged in feces. Topical: Not absorbed systemically from intact skin.

AVAILABILITY
Oral Suspension (Mycostatin): 100,000 units/mL.
Tablets (Mycostatin): 500,000 units.
Vaginal Tablets: 100,000 units.

Cream (Mycostatin): 100,000 units/g.
Ointment: 100,000 units/g.
Topical Powder (Mycostatin, Nystop): 100,000 units/g.

INDICATIONS AND DOSAGES
▸ **Intestinal infections**
PO
Adults, Elderly. 500,000-1,000,000 units q8h.
▸ **Oral candidiasis**
PO
Adults, Elderly, Children. 400,000-600,000 units swished and swallowed 4 times/day.
Infants. 200,000 units 4 times/day.
▸ **Vaginal infections**
VAGINAL
Adults, Elderly, Adolescents. 1 tablet/day at bedtime for 14 days.
▸ **Cutaneous candidal infections**
TOPICAL
Adults, Elderly, Children. Apply 2-4 times/day.

OFF-LABEL USES
Prophylaxis and treatment of oropharyngeal candidiasis.

CONTRAINDICATIONS
Hypersensitivity to nystatin or any of its components in formulation.
Caution
Broad-spectrum antibiotic therapy and *Candida* infection.

INTERACTIONS
Drug
Broad-spectrum antibiotic may exacerbate *Candida* infection, which it may be treating.
Herbal
None known.
Food
None known.

DIAGNOSTIC TEST EFFECTS
None known.

SIDE EFFECTS

Occasional
PO: None known.
Topical: Skin irritation.
Vaginal: Vaginal irritation.

SERIOUS REACTIONS

• High dosages of oral form may produce nausea, vomiting, diarrhea, and GI distress.

PRECAUTIONS & CONSIDERATIONS

It is unknown whether nystatin is distributed in breast milk, warranting caution in lactation. During pregnancy, vaginal applicators may be contraindicated, requiring manual insertion of tablets. No age-related precautions have been noted for suspension or topical use in children. Be aware that lozenges are not recommended for use in children 5 yr old or younger. No age-related precautions have been noted in elderly patients.

Confirm that cultures or histologic tests were done for accurate diagnosis before giving the drug. Assess for increased irritation with topical application or increased vaginal discharge with vaginal application. Separate personal items that come in contact with affected areas. Notify the physician if diarrhea, nausea, stomach pain, or vomiting develops.

Overdosage is indicated by nausea, vomiting, diarrhea, and GI distress, which should be reported immediately. Consider using condoms during therapy and sexual intercourse.

Administration
Shake suspension well before administration. Place and hold the suspension in the mouth or swish throughout the mouth as long as possible before swallowing. In infants, place half of dose in each cheek/side of mouth.

Use nystatin cream or powder sparingly on erythematous areas. Rub the topical form well into affected areas, keep affected areas clean and dry, and wear light clothing for ventilation. Avoid contact with eyes.

Insert the vaginal form high into the vagina at bedtime. Vaginal use should be continued during menses.

Octreotide

Octreotide acetate

ok-tree'oh-tide ass-ih-tayte

(Sandostatin, Sandostatin LAR)

Do not confuse octreotide with OctreoScan or Sandostatin with Sandimmune or Sandoglobulin.

CATEGORY AND SCHEDULE

Pregnancy Risk Category: B

Classification: Secretory inhibitor, growth hormone suppressant

MECHANISM OF ACTION

An antidiarrheal and growth hormone suppressant that suppresses the secretion of serotonin and gastroenteropancreatic peptides and enhances fluid and electrolyte absorption from the GI tract. *Therapeutic Effect*: Prolongs intestinal transit time by decreasing secretions and decreasing splanchnic blood flow.

PHARMACOKINETICS

Route	Onset	Peak	Duration
SC	NA	NA	Up to 12 h

Rapidly and completely absorbed from injection site. Excreted in urine. Removed by hemodialysis. *Half-life:* 1.5 h.

AVAILABILITY

Injection (Sandostatin): 0.05 mg/mL, 0.1 mg/mL, 0.2 mg/mL, 0.5 mg/mL, 1 mg/mL.

Suspension for Depot Injection (Sandostatin LAR): 10-mg, 20-mg, 30-mg vials.

INDICATIONS AND DOSAGES

▸ **Diarrhea**

IV (SANDOSTATIN)

Adults, Elderly. Initially, 50-100 mcg q8h. May increase by 100 mcg/dose q48h. Maximum: 500 mcg q8h.

SC (SANDOSTATIN)

Adults, Elderly. 50 mcg 1-2 times a day.

IV, SC (SANDOSTATIN)

Children. 1-10 mcg/kg q12h.

▸ **Carcinoid tumors**

IV, SC (SANDOSTATIN)

Adults, Elderly. 100-600 mcg/day in 2-4 divided doses.

IM (SANDOSTATIN LAR)

Adults, Elderly. 20 mg q4wk.

▸ **Vipomas**

IV, SC (SANDOSTATIN)

Adults, Elderly. 200-300 mcg/day in 2-4 divided doses.

IM (SANDOSTATIN LAR)

Adults, Elderly. 20 mg q4wk.

▸ **Esophageal varices**

IV (SANDOSTATIN)

Adults, Elderly. Bolus of 25-50 mcg followed by IV infusion of 25-50 mcg/h.

▸ **Acromegaly**

IV, SC (SANDOSTATIN)

Adults, Elderly. 50 mcg 3 times a day. Increase as needed. Maximum: 500 mcg 3 times a day.

IM (SANDOSTATIN LAR)

Adults, Elderly. 20 mg q4wk for 3 mo. Maximum: 40 mg q4wk.

⊚ IV INCOMPATIBILITIES

Diazepam, pantoprazole, phenytoin.

OFF-LABEL USES

Treatment of AIDS-associated secretory diarrhea, chemotherapy-induced diarrhea, insulinomas, small-bowel fistulas, control of bleeding esophageal varices.

CONTRAINDICATIONS

Sensitivity to the drug or product components.

(IV) IV INCOMPATIBILITIES

Not compatible in TPN. Other incompatibilities include diazepam, micafungin, pantoprazole, phenytoin.

INTERACTIONS

Drug
Glucagon, growth hormone, insulin, oral antidiabetics: May alter glucose concentrations.
Vitamin B_{12}: May cause a decrease in Vitamin B_{12} levels.
Herbal
None known.
Food
None known.

DIAGNOSTIC TEST EFFECTS

May decrease serum thyroxine (T_4) concentration. May increase or decrease blood glucose.

SIDE EFFECTS

Frequent (6%-10%, 30%-35% in Acromegaly Patients)
Diarrhea, nausea, abdominal discomfort, headache, injection site pain.
Occasional (1%-5%)
Vomiting, flatulence, constipation, alopecia, facial flushing, pruritus, dizziness, fatigue, arrhythmias, ecchymosis, blurred vision.
Rare (< 1%)
Depression, diminished libido, vertigo, palpitations, dyspnea.

SERIOUS REACTIONS

• Patients using octreotide may develop cholelithiasis or, with prolonged high dosages, hypothyroidism.
• GI bleeding, hepatitis, pancreatitis and seizures occur rarely.
Caution
Insulin-dependent diabetes, renal failure, pregnancy, lactation.

PRECAUTIONS & CONSIDERATIONS

Caution is warranted in patients with insulin-dependent diabetes and renal failure. It is unknown whether octreotide is excreted in breast milk; therefore, caution is warranted in lactation. The children's dosage has not been established. No age-related precautions have been noted in elderly patients.

Notify the physician of unusual signs or symptoms, such as palpitations or unusual bleeding. Blood glucose levels, BP, pulse rate, respiratory rate, weight, growth hormone, pattern of daily bowel activity and stool consistency, fecal fat, fluid and electrolyte balance, and thyroid function test results should be monitored. Be alert for decreased urine output and peripheral edema, especially of the ankles. Take care in making abrupt postural changes because of the possible risk of orthostatic hypotension developing. Any signs of infection should be reported immediately.

Storage
Store injection solution and depot suspension under refrigeration and protect from light. At room temperature, the injection solution is stable for 14 days if protected from light.

Administration
! Sandostatin administration may be IV or SC. Sandostatin LAR administration may be only IM.

Do not use solution if it becomes discolored or contains particulates.

Inject Sandostatin LAR depot in a large muscle mass at 4-wk intervals. Avoid deltoid injections.

Sandostatin injection solution is usually administered as an SC injection. Avoid multiple injections at the same site within a short period. If injection solution is given IV, it may be diluted in 0.9% NaCl or 5% dextrose injection 50-200 mL and infused over 15-30 min or administered by IV push over 3-5 min. Infusions are stable for 24 h.

O

Ofloxacin
o-flox′a-sin
(Apo-Oflox [CAN], Floxin, Floxin Otic, Ocuflox)
Do not confuse Floxin with Flexeril or Flexon, or Ocuflox with Ocufen.

CATEGORY AND SCHEDULE
Pregnancy Risk Category: C

Classification: Anti-infectives, fluoroquinolones

MECHANISM OF ACTION
A fluoroquinolone antibiotic that inhibits DNA gyrase in susceptible microorganisms, interfering with bacterial cell replication and repair. *Therapeutic Effect*: Bactericidal.

PHARMACOKINETICS
Rapidly and well absorbed from the GI tract. Protein binding: 20%-25%. Widely distributed (including to the cerebrospinal fluid [CSF]). Metabolized in the liver. Primarily excreted in urine. Removed by hemodialysis. *Half-life:* 4.7-7 h (increased in impaired renal function, cirrhosis, and elderly patients).

AVAILABILITY
Tablets (Floxin): 200 mg, 300 mg, 400 mg.
Ophthalmic Solution (Ocuflox): 0.3%.
Otic Solution (Floxin): 0.3%.

INDICATIONS AND DOSAGES
▸ **Urinary tract infection (UTIs)**
PO
Adults, Elderly. 200 mg q12h for 3-10 days.
▸ **Pelvic inflammatory disease (PID)**
PO
Adults, Elderly. 400 mg q12h for 10-14 days.

▸ **Lower respiratory tract, skin, and skin-structure infections**
PO
Adults, Elderly. 400 mg q12h for 10 days.
▸ **Prostatitis, sexually transmitted diseases (cervicitis, urethritis)**
PO
Adults, Elderly. 300 mg q12h for 7days or for 6 wks for prostatitis.
▸ **Acute, uncomplicated gonorrhea**
PO
Adults, Elderly. 400 mg 1 time.
▸ **Bacterial conjunctivitis**
OPHTHALMIC
Adults, Elderly. 1-2 drops q2-4h for 2 days, then 4 times a day for 5 days.
▸ **Corneal ulcers, bacterial**
OPHTHALMIC
Adults. 1-2 drops q30min while awake for 2 days, then q60min while awake for 5-7 days, then 4 times a day.
▸ **Acute otitis media with typanostomy tubes**
OTIC
Children aged 1-12 yr. 5 drops into the affected ear 2 times/day for 10 days.
▸ **Otitis externa**
OTIC
Adults, Elderly, Children 12 yr and older. 10 drops into the affected ear once a day for 7 days.
Children aged 6 mo to 11 yr. 5 drops into the affected ear once a day for 7 days.
▸ **Dosage in hepatic impairment (Adults)**
Do not exceed 400 mg/day.
▸ **Dosage in renal impairment**
After a normal initial dose, dosage and frequency are based on creatinine clearance (systemic).

Creatinine Clearance (mL/min)	Adjusted Dose	Dosage Interval (h)
> 50	None	q12
20-50	None	q24
< 20	1/2	q24

CONTRAINDICATIONS

Hypersensitivity to any quinolones.
Caution
Lactation, children under age 18 yr, elderly patients, renal disease, seizure disorders, excessive sunlight, tendon rupture in shoulder, hand and Achilles tendon.

INTERACTIONS

Drug
Antacids, sucralfate: May decrease absorption and effects of ofloxacin.
Caffeine: May increase the effects of caffeine.
Procainamide: May increase risk of life-threatening arrhythmias.
Theophylline: May increase theophylline blood concentration and risk of toxicity.
Herbal
None known.
Food
None known.

DIAGNOSTIC TEST EFFECTS

None known.

SIDE EFFECTS

Frequent (7%-10%)
Nausea, headache, insomnia.
Occasional (3%-5%)
Abdominal pain, diarrhea, vomiting, dry mouth, flatulence, dizziness, fatigue, drowsiness, rash, pruritus, fever.
Rare (< 1%)
Constipation, paraesthesia.

SERIOUS REACTIONS

• Antibiotic-associated colitis and other superinfections may occur from altered bacterial balance.
• Hypersensitivity reactions, including photosensitivity (as evidenced by rash, pruritus, blisters, edema, and burning skin), have occurred in patients receiving fluoroquinolones.

• Arthropathy (swelling, pain, and clubbing of fingers and toes, degeneration of stress-bearing portion of a joint) may occur if the systemic drug is given to Children (rare).
• Tendonitis or tendon rupture.

PRECAUTIONS & CONSIDERATIONS

Caution is warranted in patients with central nervous system (CNS) disorders, renal impairment, or seizures and those taking caffeine or theophylline. Caution should also be used regarding syphilis because ofloxacin may mask or delay symptoms of syphilis; serologic test for syphilis should be done at diagnosis and 3 mo after treatment. Ofloxacin is distributed in breast milk. If possible, pregnant or breastfeeding women should avoid taking the drug because of the risk of arthropathy in the fetus or infant. The safety and efficacy of ofloxacin have not been established in children (children younger than 6 mo for otic form). Age-related renal impairment may require a dosage adjustment for oral and parenteral forms in elderly patients. No age-related precautions for the otic form have been noted in elderly patients. Avoid exposure to sunlight and ultraviolet light and wear sunscreen and protective clothing if photosensitivity develops.

Caution is warranted with systemic use in children under age 18 yr because of the possible development of arthropathy. Care is important in high sun exposure situations as a result of increased photosensitivity.

Dizziness, drowsiness, headache, and insomnia may occur while taking ofloxacin. Avoid tasks requiring mental alertness or motor skills until response to ofloxacin is established.

Signs and symptoms of infection, mental status, WBC count, skin for rash, pattern of daily bowel activity and stool consistency should be monitored. Be alert for signs of superinfection, such as anal or genital pruritus, fever, stomatitis, and vaginitis, which should be reported immediately to the health care provider.

Caution is warranted in individuals who are physically active, exercise, and are generally mobile; ruptures of the tendons in the hand, shoulder, and Achilles tendon have been reported with fluoroquinolone use; such injury may require surgical repair and extended disability. Patients experiencing pain or inflammation in a tendon should be advised to rest and refrain from exercise until the situation can be medically evaluated.

Storage
Store at room temperature.

Administration
Do not take ofloxacin with food. The preferred dosing time is 1 h before or 2 h after a meal. Take with 8 oz of water and provide additional liquids between meals. Consume citrus fruits and cranberry juice to acidify urine. Take antacids containing aluminum or magnesium or products containing iron or zinc within 2 h before or after taking ofloxacin.

For ophthalmic use, tilt the head back and place the solution in the conjunctival sac. Close the eye; then press gently on the lacrimal sac for 1 min. Do not use ophthalmic solutions for injection. Unless the infection is very superficial, expect to also administer systemic drug therapy.

For otic use, lie down with the head turned so that the affected ear is upright. Warm solution in hands for 1-2 min. Instill drops toward the canal wall, not directly on the eardrum. Pull the auricle down and back in children and up and back in adults. Maintain position for 5 min per ear treated to ensure penetration into ear.

Olanzapine
oh-lan′za-peen
(Zyprexa, Zyprexa Intramuscular, Zyprexa Zydis)
Do not confuse olanzapine with olsalazine, or Zyprexa with Zyrtec or Zyvox.

CATEGORY AND SCHEDULE
Pregnancy Risk Category: C

Classification: Antipsychotics, Atypical

MECHANISM OF ACTION
A dibenzepin derivative that antagonizes α_1-adrenergic, dopamine, histamine, muscarinic, and serotonin receptors. Produces anticholinergic, histaminic, and central nervous system (CNS) depressant effects. *Therapeutic Effect:* Diminishes manifestations of psychotic symptoms.

PHARMACOKINETICS
Well absorbed after PO administration. Protein binding: 93%. Extensively distributed throughout the body. Undergoes extensive first-pass metabolism in the liver. Excreted primarily in urine and, to a lesser extent, in feces. Not removed by dialysis. *Half-life:* 21-54 h.

AVAILABILITY
Tablets (Zyprexa): 2.5 mg, 5 mg, 7.5 mg, 10 mg, 15 mg, 20 mg).
Tablets (Orally Disintegrating

[Zyprexa Zydis]): 5 mg, 10 mg, 15 mg, 20 mg.
Injection (Zyprexa Intramuscular): 10 mg. Powder for solution.

INDICATIONS AND DOSAGES
▸ **Schizophrenia**
PO
Adults. Initially, 5-10 mg once daily. Target dose: 10 mg/day within several days. If further adjustments are indicated, may increase by 5-10 mg/day at 7-day intervals. Range: 10-20 mg/day.
Children. Initially, 2.5 mg/day. Titrate as necessary up to 20 mg/day.
▸ **Bipolar mania**
PO
Adults. Initially, 10-15 mg/day (monotherapy) or 10 mg/day (with lithium or valproate). May increase by 5 mg/day at intervals of at least 24 h. Maximum: 20 mg/day.
Children. Initially, 2.5 mg/day. Titrate as necessary up to 20 mg/day.
▸ **Dosage for elderly or debilitated patients and those predisposed to hypotensive reactions**
PO
The initial dosage for these patients is 5 mg/day, then titrate with caution according to indication.
▸ **Control of agitation in schizophrenic or bipolar patients**
IM
Adults, Elderly. 2.5-10 mg. May repeat 2 h after first dose and 4 h after 2nd dose. Maximum: 30 mg/day. Use lower doses (5-7.5 mg) if at risk for hypotension or if debilitated.

OFF-LABEL USES
Use for the above indications orally in children 6 yr and older, behavioral disturbance secondary to dementia.

CONTRAINDICATIONS
Hypersensitivity.

INTERACTIONS
Drug
Alcohol, other CNS depressants, diazepam: May increase CNS depressant effects.
Anticholinergic agents: May increase anticholinergic effects.
Antihypertensives: May increase the hypotensive effects of these drugs.
Carbamazepine: Increases olanzapine clearance.
Ciprofloxacin, fluvoxamine: May increase the olanzapine blood concentration.
Dopamine agonists, levodopa: May antagonize the effects of these drugs.
Imipramine, theophylline: May inhibit the metabolism of these drugs.
Herbal
None known.
Food
None known.

DIAGNOSTIC TEST EFFECTS
May significantly increase serum GGT, prolactin, AST (SGOT), and ALT (SGPT) levels, cholesterol or triglycerides, blood sugar.

SIDE EFFECTS
Frequent
Somnolence (26%), agitation (23%), insomnia (20%), headache (17%), nervousness (16%), hostility (15%), dizziness (11%), rhinitis (10%), weightgain.
Occasional
Anxiety, constipation (9%); nonaggressive atypical behavior (8%); dry mouth (7%); weight gain (6%); orthostatic hypotension, fever, arthralgia, restlessness, cough, pharyngitis, visual changes (dim vision) (5%).
Rare
Tachycardia; back, chest, abdominal, or extremity pain; tremor.

O

SERIOUS REACTIONS

• Rare reactions include seizures and neuroleptic malignant syndrome, a potentially fatal syndrome characterized by hyperpyrexia, muscle rigidity, irregular pulse or BP, tachycardia, diaphoresis, and cardiac arrhythmias.

• Extrapyramidal symptoms and dysphagia may also occur.

• Overdose (300 mg) produces drowsiness and slurred speech.

• Development of hyperglycemia/diabetes.

• QT prolongation (rare).

PRECAUTIONS & CONSIDERATIONS

Caution is warranted with a hypersensitivity to clozapine, hepatic impairment, cerebrovascular disease, cardiovascular disease (such as conduction abnormalities, heart failure, or history of myocardial infarction [MI] or ischemia), history of seizures or conditions that lower the seizure threshold (such as Alzheimer disease), and conditions predisposing to hypotension (such as dehydration, hypovolemia, and use of antihypertensives). Extreme caution should be used with elderly patients who are at risk for aspiration pneumonia, those who are concurrently taking hepatotoxic drugs, and those who should avoid anticholinergics (such as persons with benign prostatic hyperplasia). It is unknown whether olanzapine crosses the placenta or is distributed in breast milk. The safety and efficacy of olanzapine have not been established in children. No age-related precautions have been noted in elderly patients, although there may be an increased risk of mortality in patients with dementia-associated psychosis.

Drowsiness may occur but generally subsides with continued therapy. Tasks requiring mental alertness or motor skills should be avoided. Dehydration, particularly during exercise; exposure to extreme heat; and concurrent use of medications that cause dry mouth or other drying effects should also be avoided. A healthy diet and exercise program should be maintained to prevent weight gain. Notify the physician of extrapyramidal symptoms. BP and therapeutic response should be assessed. Rapid postural changes should be avoided due to possible development of orthostatic hypotension.

Symptoms including sore tongue, problems eating or swallowing, fever, or infection need to be reported immediately.

Storage

Store at room temperature. Keep orally disentegrating tablets in blister until time of use. Unopened injection should be protected from light; do not freeze.

Once constituted, drug is stable for 1 h at room temperature.

Administration

Caution should be used with each dosage increase. Take olanzapine without regard to food. Take as ordered and do not abruptly discontinue the drug or increase the dosage. Orally dissolving tablets may be dissolved on tongue without water.

Zyprexa IM is for IM use only. Dissolve vial contents with 2.1 mL of sterile water for injection (resulting solution is 5 mg/mL). Inject slowly, deep into muscle mass. Incompatible with diazepam, lorazepam, and haloperidol.

Olmesartan Medoxomil

ohl-me-sar′-tan med-ox-o-myl
(Benicar, Benicar HCT [in combination])

CATEGORY AND SCHEDULE

Pregnancy Risk Category: C (D if used in second or third trimester)

Classification: Angiotensin II (AT1) receptor antagonists

MECHANISM OF ACTION

An angiotensin II receptor, type AT_1, antagonist that blocks the vasoconstrictor and aldosterone-secreting effects of angiotensin II, inhibiting the binding of angiotensin II to the AT_1 receptors. *Therapeutic Effect*: Causes vasodilation, decreases peripheral resistance, and decreases BP.

PHARMACOKINETICS

Rapidly and completely absorbed after PO administration. Metabolized in the liver. Recovered primarily in feces and, to a lesser extent, in urine. Not removed by hemodialysis. *Half-life:* 13 h.

AVAILABILITY

Tablets: 5 mg, 20 mg, 40 mg.

INDICATIONS AND DOSAGES

▸ **Hypertension**
PO
Adults, Elderly, Patients with mildly impaired hepatic or renal function. 20 mg once a day in patients who are not volume depleted. After 2 wks of therapy, if further reduction in BP is needed, may increase dosage to 40 mg/day.

CONTRAINDICATIONS

Bilateral renal artery stenosis, hypersensitivity.

INTERACTIONS

Drug
No significant drug interactions have been reported; however, increased hypotensive effects are always possible when used with other antihypertensives or sedatives.
Herbal
None known.
Food
None known.

DIAGNOSTIC TEST EFFECTS

May increase blood hemoglobin and hematocrit levels.

SIDE EFFECTS

Occasional (3%)
Dizziness.
Rare (< 2%)
Headache, diarrhea, upper respiratory tract infection.

SERIOUS REACTIONS

• Overdosage may manifest as hypotension and tachycardia. Bradycardia occurs less often.

PRECAUTIONS & CONSIDERATIONS

Caution is warranted in patients with hepatic and renal impairment and renal arterial stenosis. It is unknown whether olmesartan is distributed in breast milk. It may cause fetal or neonatal morbidity or mortality. Therefore, caution is warranted in lactation; discontinue use in pregnancy; assess patient for pregnancy before prescribing. Safety and efficacy of olmesartan have not been established in children. No age-related precautions have been noted in elderly patients.

Dizziness may occur. Tasks that require mental alertness or motor skills should be avoided. Apical pulse and BP should be assessed immediately before each olmesartan

O

dose and regularly throughout therapy. Be alert to fluctuations in apical pulse and BP. If an excessive reduction in BP occurs, place the patient in the supine position with feet slightly elevated and notify the physician. Diagnostic tests, such as hemoglobin and hematocrit levels and liver function tests, should be assessed. Maintain adequate hydration; exercising outside during hot weather should be avoided to decrease the risk of dehydration and hypotension. Caution is warranted when sedation or general anesthesia is required due to risk of hypotensive episode.

Administration
Take olmesartan without regard to meals.

Olopatadine
oh-loe-pa-ta´-deen
(Patanase, Patanol, Pataday)

CATEGORY AND SCHEDULE
Pregnancy Risk Category: C

Classification: Antihistamine; mast cell stabilizer

MECHANISM OF ACTION
An antihistamine that inhibits histamine release from the mast cell. *Therapeutic Effect:* Inhibits symptoms associated with allergic conjunctivitis/allergic rhinitis.

PHARMACOKINETICS
The time to peak concentration is < 2 h and duration of action is 8 h. Minimal absorption after topical administration. Metabolized to inactive metabolites. Primarily excreted in urine. *Half-life:* 3 h.

AVAILABILITY
Nasal spray Solution: 0.6%.
Ophthalmic Solution: 0.1%, 0.2%.

INDICATIONS AND DOSAGES
▶ **Allergic conjunctivitis**
OPHTHALMIC
Adults, Elderly, Children 3 yr and older. 0.1% Solution: 1-2 drops in affected eye(s) twice daily q6-8h; 0.2% solution: 1 drop in affected eye(s) once daily.
▶ **Seasonal allergic rhinitis**
INTRANASAL
Adults, Elderly, Children 12 yr and older. 2 sprays per nostril once daily.

CONTRAINDICATIONS
Hypersensitivity to olopatadine hydrochloride or any other component of the formulation.

INTERACTIONS
Drug
Anticholinergics: Enhanced anticholinergic effects.
CNS depressants: Enhanced somnolence.
Herbal
None known.
Food
None known.

SIDE EFFECTS
Occasional
Ophthalmic Use: Headache, weakness, cold syndrome, taste perversion, burning, stinging, dry eyes, foreign body sensation, hyperemia, keratitis, eyelid edema, itching, pharyngitis, rhinitis, sinusitis.
Nasal spray: bitter taste, nasal ulceration, epistaxis, pharyngolaryngeal pain, postnasal drip, cough, throat irritation, somnolence, dry mouth.

SERIOUS REACTIONS
• None reported.

PRECAUTIONS & CONSIDERATIONS
Do not use olopatadine while wearing contacts. To avoid contamination, to not touch the dropper tip to the eye area.

Storage

Store at room temperature.

Administration

Do not use ophthalmic olopatadine while wearing contacts. To avoid contamination, to not touch the dropper tip to the eye area.

Prime nasal spray before initial use and when not used for more than 7 days.

Olsalazine Sodium
ohl-sal'ah-zeen soo-dee-um
(Dipentum)
Do not confuse olsalazine with olanzapine.

CATEGORY AND SCHEDULE
Pregnancy Risk Category: C

Classification:
Anti-inflammatory, salicylate derivatives, 5-aminosalicylates

MECHANISM OF ACTION
A salicylic acid derivative that is converted to mesalamine in the colon by bacterial action. Blocks prostaglandin production in bowel mucosa. *Therapeutic Effect:* Reduces colonic inflammation in inflammatory bowel disease.

PHARMACOKINETICS
PO: Partially absorbed; peak attained in 1.5 h. Excreted in urine as 5-aminosalicylic acid and metabolites; crosses placenta. *Half-life:* 5-10 h.

AVAILABILITY
Capsules: 250 mg.

INDICATIONS AND DOSAGES
▸ **Maintenance of controlled ulcerative colitis**
PO
Adults, Elderly. 1 g/day in 2 divided doses, preferably q12h.

OFF-LABEL USES
Treatment of Crohn's disease.

CONTRAINDICATIONS
History of hypersensitivity to 5-aminosalicylates or other salicylates.

Caution

Lacation, impaired hepatic function, severe allergy, bronchial asthma, renal disease.

INTERACTIONS
Drug

Antacids: Do not administer olsalazine sodium with antacids.
Azithoprine, mercaptopurine: May increase side effects of these anineoplastics.

Herbal

None known.

Food

None known.

DIAGNOSTIC TEST EFFECTS
May increase AST (SGOT) and ALT (SGPT) levels.

SIDE EFFECTS
Frequent (5%-10%)
Headache, diarrhea (17%), abdominal pain or cramps, nausea.

O

Occasional (1%-5%)
Depression, fatigue, dyspepsia,
upper respiratory tract infection,
decreased appetite, rash, itching,
arthralgia.
Rare (1%)
Dizziness, vomiting, stomatitis.

SERIOUS REACTIONS
• Sensitivity may occur in
susceptible patients, manifested by
cramping, headache, diarrhea, fever,
rash, hives, itching, and wheezing.
Discontinue drug immediately.
• Excessive diarrhea associated with
extreme fatigue is noted rarely.
• Hepatotoxicity (rare).

PRECAUTIONS & CONSIDERATIONS
Caution is warranted with
preexisting renal disease. Serum
alkaline phosphatase, AST, and ALT
levels should be obtained before
therapy. Adequate fluid intake
should be maintained. Daily bowel
activity and stool consistency and
skin for rash should be assessed.
Notify physician if persistent or
increasing cramping, diarrhea, fever,
pruritus, or rash occurs; olsalazine
should be discontinued. Avoid
adiminstration of any drug that
could aggravate inflammatory colon
disease; medical consultation is
necessary for appropriate antibiotic
selection.
Administration
Take olsalazine with food in evenly
divided doses.

Omalizumab
oh-mah-liz'uw-mab
(Xolair)

CATEGORY AND SCHEDULE
Pregnancy Risk Category: B

Classification: Anti-IgE
Monoclonal antibodies

MECHANISM OF ACTION
A monoclonal antibody that
selectively binds to human
immunoglobulin E (IgE), preventing
it from binding to the surface of mast
cells and basophiles. *Therapeutic
Effect*: Prevents or reduces the
number of asthmatic attacks because
of allergens.

PHARMACOKINETICS
Absorbed slowly after SC
administration, with peak
concentration in 7-8 days. Excreted
in the liver, reticuloendothelial
system, and endothelial cells.
Half-life: 26 days.

AVAILABILITY
Powder for Injection: 202.5 mg,
provides 150 mg/1.2 mL after
reconstitution.

INDICATIONS AND DOSAGES
▸ **Moderate to severe persistent
asthma in patients who are reactive
to a perennial allergen and whose
asthma symptoms have been
inadequately controlled with inhaled
corticosteroids**
SC
*Adults, Elderly, Children 12 yr
and older.* 150-375 mg every 2 or
4 wks; dose and dosing frequency
are individualized based on weight
and pretreatment immunoglobulin E
(IgE) level (as shown below).

4-wks Dosing Table

Pretreatment Serum IgE Levels (units/mL)	Weight 30-60 kg	Weight 61-70 kg	Weight 71-90 kg	Weight 91-150 kg
30-100 mg	150 mg	150 mg	150 mg	300 mg
101-200 mg	300 mg	300 mg	300 mg	See next table
201-300 mg	300 mg	See next table	See next table	See next table

2-wks Dosing Table

Pretreatment Serum IgE Levels (units/mL)	Weight 30-60 kg	Weight 61-70 kg	Weight 71-90 kg	Weight 91-150 kg
101-200	See preceding table	See preceding table	See preceding table	225 mg
201-300	See preceding table	225 mg	225 mg	300 mg
301-400	225 mg	225 mg	300 mg	Do not dose
401-500	300 mg	300 mg	375 mg	Do not dose
501-600	300 mg	375 mg	Do not dose	Do not dose
601-700	375 mg	Do not dose	Do not dose	Do not dose

OFF-LABEL USES
Treatment of asthma resulting from food allergies.

CONTRAINDICATIONS
Hypersensitivity.

INTERACTIONS
Drug
None known.
Herbal
None known.
Food
None known.

DIAGNOSTIC TEST EFFECTS
May increase serum IgE levels.

SIDE EFFECTS
Frequent (11%-45%)
Injection site ecchymosis, redness, warmth, stinging, and urticaria; viral infections; sinusitis; headache; pharyngitis.

Occasional (3%-8%)
Arthralgia, leg pain, fatigue, dizziness.
Rare (2%)
Arm pain, earache, dermatitis, pruritus.

SERIOUS REACTIONS
• Anaphylaxis occurs within 2 h of the first dose or subsequent doses in 0.1% of patients.
• Malignant neoplasms occur in 0.5% of patients.

PRECAUTIONS & CONSIDERATIONS
Omalizumab is not intended to reverse acute bronchospasm or status asthmaticus. Because IgE is present in breast milk, omalizumab is also believed to be present in breast milk. Use omalizumab only if clearly needed. The safety and efficacy of omalizumab have not been established in children younger than

O

12 yr. No age-related precautions have been noted in elderly patients. Drink plenty of fluids to decrease the thickness of lung secretions.

Serum total IgE levels should be obtained before beginning omalizumab therapy because the drug dosage is based on these pretreatment levels. Pulse rate and quality as well as respiratory depth, rate, rhythm, and type should be monitored. Fingernails and lips should also be assessed for a blue or dusky color in light-skinned patients and a gray color in dark-skinned patients, which may be signs of hypoxemia. Rapidly acting sympathomimetic inhalants should be available for emergency use.

Storage

Store omalizumab in the refrigerator. The reconstituted solution is stable for 8 h if refrigerated or 4 h if stored at room temperature. Protect from direct sunlight.

Administration

! Expect to base omalizumab dosage on serum IgE levels obtained before beginning treatment. Do not use serum IgE levels obtained during treatment to determine omalizumab dosage because IgE levels remain elevated for up to 1 yr after the drug has been discontinued.

Use only clear or slightly opalescent solution; the solution is slightly viscous. Use only sterile water for injection to prepare for SC administration. Draw 1.4 mL sterile water for injection into a 3-mL syringe with a 1-inch, 18-gauge needle, and inject contents into the vial of powder. Swirl the vial for approximately 1 min; do not shake it. Then swirl the vial again for 5-10 s every 5 min until no gel-like particles appear in the solution. The drug takes 15-20 min to dissolve. Do not use the solution if the contents fail to dissolve completely in 40 min. Invert the vial for 15 s to allow the solution to drain toward the stopper. Using a new 3-mL syringe with a 1-in., 18-gauge needle, withdraw the required 1.2-mL dose and replace the 18-gauge needle with a 25-gauge needle for SC administration. SC administration may take 5-10 s because of omalizumab's viscosity.

Omeprazole

om-eh-pray′zole
(Losec [CAN], Maxor [AUS], Prilosec, Prilosec OTC, Probitor [AUS])

Do not confuse Prilosec with prilocaine, Prinivil, or Prozac or Prevacid or omeprazole with olmesartan.

CATEGORY AND SCHEDULE

Pregnancy Risk Category: C

Classification: Antisecretory proton pump inhibitors

MECHANISM OF ACTION

A benzimidazole that is converted to active metabolites that irreversibly bind to and inhibit hydrogen-potassium adenosine triphosphatase, an enzyme on the surface of gastric parietal cells. Inhibits hydrogen ion transport into gastric lumen. *Therapeutic Effect:* Increases gastric pH, reduces gastric acid production.

PHARMACOKINETICS

Route	Onset	Peak	Duration
PO	1 h	2 h	72 h

Rapidly absorbed from the GI tract. Protein binding: 99%. Primarily distributed into gastric parietal cells. Metabolized extensively in the liver. Primarily excreted in urine. Unknown whether removed by hemodialysis. *Half-life:* 0.5-1 h (increased in patients with hepatic impairment).

AVAILABILITY
Capsules (Delayed-Release [Prilosec]): 10 mg, 20 mg, 40 mg.
Tablets (OTC): 20 mg.
Delayed-Release Granules for Oral Suspension: 2.5-mg, 10-mg packets.

INDICATIONS AND DOSAGES
▸ **Erosive esophagitis, poorly responsive gastroesophageal reflux disease (GERD), active duodenal ulcer, prevention and treatment of NSAID-induced ulcers**
PO
Adults, Elderly. 20 mg/day.
▸ **To maintain healing of erosive esophagitis**
PO
Adults, Elderly. 20 mg/day.
▸ **Pathologic hypersecretory conditions**
PO
Adults, Elderly. Initially, 60 mg/day up to 120 mg 3 times a day.
▸ **Duodenal ulcer caused by** *Helicobacter pylori*
PO
Adults, Elderly. 20 mg twice a day for 10 days, with antibiotics.
▸ **Active benign gastric ulcer**
PO
Adults, Elderly. 40 mg/day for 4-8 wks.
▸ **Dyspepsia (OTC use)**
Adults. 20 mg once daily for no more than 14 days. Contact physician if heartburn continues regarding long-term treatment.
▸ **Usual pediatric dosage**
Children older than 2 yr weighing ≥ 20 kg. 20 mg/day.
Children older than 2 yr weighing < 20 kg. 10 mg/day (usually 1 mg/kg/day).

OFF-LABEL USES
Prevention of NSAID-induced ulcers.

CONTRAINDICATIONS
Hypersensitivity to the drugs or related drugs, including interstitial nephritis.

INTERACTIONS
Drug
Diazepam, oral anticoagulants (warfarin), phenytoin: May increase the blood concentration of diazepam, oral anticoagulants, and phenytoin.
Ketoconazole: Decreases ketoconazole absorption.
Protease inhibitors: Reduce absorption of many.
Tacrolimus: May increase serum levels.
Herbal
None known.
Food
None known.

DIAGNOSTIC TEST EFFECTS
May increase serum alkaline phosphatase, AST (SGOT), and ALT (SGPT) levels.

SIDE EFFECTS
Frequent (7%)
Headache.
Occasional (2%-3%)
Diarrhea, abdominal pain, nausea.
Rare (2%)
Dizziness, asthenia or loss of strength, vomiting, constipation, upper respiratory tract infection, back pain, rash, cough.

SERIOUS REACTIONS
• Anaphylaxis/angioedema.
• Interstitial nephritis.

O

PRECAUTIONS & CONSIDERATIONS

It is unknown whether omeprazole crosses the placenta or is distributed in breast milk; caution warranted in lactation and pregnancy. Safety and efficacy of omeprazole have not been established in children under 1 yr. No age-related precautions have been noted in elderly patients. Consider dose reduction in chronic use in chronic hepatic disease or Asian patients.

Notify the physician if headache, diarrhea, discomfort, or nausea occurs during omeprazole therapy. Serum chemistry laboratory values, particularly serum alkaline phosphatase, AST, and ALT levels should be obtained to assess liver function. Loose or soft stool may be noted early in the therapy protocol. Do not use Prilosec OTC for more than 2 wks without medical consultation.

Administration

Take omeprazole before meals. Do not crush capsules; swallow capsules whole. If patient has difficulty swallowing, capsule may be opened and contents sprinkled on a tablespoon of cool applesauce. Swallow without chewing and follow with a sip of water. The oral suspension is prepared as follows: Mix 2.5- or 10- mg packet into 5 or 15 mL of water, respectively. Stir and allow to thicken 2-3 min. Stir and drink. Can also be given via nasogastric tube.

Ondansetron Hydrochloride
on-dan-seh′tron high-droh-klor-ide
(Zofran, Zofran ODT)
Do not confuse Zofran with Zantac or Zosyn.

CATEGORY AND SCHEDULE
Pregnancy Risk Category: B

Classification: Antiemetics, selective 5-HT3 serotonin receptor antagonists

MECHANISM OF ACTION
An antiemetic that blocks serotonin, both peripherally on vagal nerve terminals and centrally in the chemoreceptor trigger zone. *Therapeutic Effect:* Prevents nausea and vomiting.

PHARMACOKINETICS
Readily absorbed from the GI tract. Protein binding: 70%-76%. Metabolized in the liver. Primarily excreted in urine. Unknown whether removed by hemodialysis. All tablets are bioequivalently interchangeable. *Half-life:* 4 h.

AVAILABILITY
Oral Solution (Zofran): 4 mg/5 mL.
Tablets (Zofran): 4 mg, 8 mg, 24 mg.
Tablets (Orally Disintegrating [Zofran ODT]): 4 mg, 8 mg.
Injection (Zofran): 2 mg/mL.
Injection (Premix): 32 mg/50 mL.

INDICATIONS AND DOSAGES
▸ **Prevention of chemotherapy-induced nausea and vomiting**
PO
Adults, Elderly, Children older than 11 yr. 24 mg as a single dose 30 min before starting chemotherapy,

or 8 mg 30 min before chemotherapy and again 8 h after first dose; then q12h for 1-2 days.

Children 4-11 yr. 4 mg 30 min before chemotherapy and again 4 and 8 h after chemotherapy, then q8h for 1-2 days.

IV INFUSION

Adults, Elderly, Children 4-18 yr. 32 mg as a single dose, or 0.15 mg/kg/dose 30 min before chemotherapy, then 4 and 8 h after chemotherapy.

▸ **Prevention of radiation-induced nausea and vomiting**

PO

Adults, Elderly. 8 mg 1-2 h before radiation, followed by 8 mg 3 times a day, or if radiation is intermittent, 8-mg single dose 1-2 h before radiation.

▸ **Prevention of postoperative nausea and vomiting**

IV, IM

Adults, Elderly. 4 mg undiluted over 2-5 min.

Children weighing < 40 kg. 0.1 mg/kg.

Children weighing ≥ 40 kg. 4 mg.

PO

Adults, Elderly. 16 mg given as 2 8-mg tablets 1 h before anesthesia.

OFF-LABEL USES

Treatment of postoperative nausea and vomiting.

CONTRAINDICATIONS

Hypersensitivity to ondansetron or other selective 5-HT3 receptor antagonists.

Caution

Pregnancy only if the benefit greater than risk, children younger than 4 yr.

INTERACTIONS

Drug

Phenytoin, Carbamazepine, Rifampicin: May decrease levels of ondansetron.

Tramadol: May increase patient controlled administration of tramadol.

Herbal and Food

None known.

DIAGNOSTIC TEST EFFECTS

May transiently increase serum bilirubin, AST (SGOT), and ALT (SGPT) levels.

🅘 IV INCOMPATIBILITIES

Acyclovir (Zovirax), allopurinol (Aloprim), aminophylline, amphotericin B (Fungizone), amphotericin B complex (Abelcet, AmBisome, Amphotec), ampicillin (Polycillin), ampicillin and sulbactam (Unasyn), cefepime (Maxipime), cefoperazone (Cefobid), ertapenem, 5-fluorouracil, furosemide, insulin (regular), lansoprazole, lorazepam (Ativan), meropenem (Merrem IV), methylprednisolone (Solu-Medrol), micafungin pantoprazole.

🅘 IV COMPATIBILITIES

Carboplatin (Paraplatin), cisplatin (Platinol), cyclophosphamide (Cytoxan), cytarabine (Cytosar), dacarbazine (DTIC-Dome), daunorubicin (Cerubidine), dexamethasone (Decadron), diphenhydramine (Benadryl), docetaxel (Taxotere), dopamine (Intropin), etoposide (VePesid), gemcitabine (Gemzar), heparin, hydromorphone (Dilaudid), ifosfamide (Ifex), magnesium, mannitol, mesna (Mesnex), methotrexate, metoclopramide (Reglan), mitomycin (Mutamycin), mitoxantrone (Novantrone), morphine, paclitaxel (Taxol), potassium chloride, teniposide (Vumon), topotecan (Hycamtin), vinblastine (Velban), vincristine (Oncovin), vinorelbine (Navelbine).

SIDE EFFECTS

Frequent (5%-13%)

Anxiety, dizziness, somnolence,

headache, fatigue, constipation, diarrhea, hypoxia, urine retention.
Occasional (2%-4%)
Abdominal pain, xerostomia, fever, feeling of cold, redness and pain at injection site, paresthesia, asthenia.
Rare (1%)
Hypersensitivity reaction (including rash and pruritus), blurred vision.

SERIOUS REACTIONS
• Overdose may produce a combination of central nervous system (CNS) stimulant and depressant effects.

PRECAUTIONS & CONSIDERATIONS
It is unknown whether ondansetron crosses the placenta or is distributed in breast milk. The safety and efficacy of ondansetron have not been established in children. No age-related precautions have been noted in elderly patients. Alcohol, barbiturates, and tasks that require mental alertness or motor skills should be avoided.

Dizziness or drowsiness may occur. Pattern of daily bowel activity and stool consistency, hydration status, bilirubin, AST (SGOT), and ALT (SGPT) levels should be monitored. Onset of sudden blindness, which usually resolves in 2-3 h, should be immediately reported as it may indicate overdosage.
Storage
Store vials at room temperature. The solution is stable for 48 h after dilution.
Administration
! Give all oral doses 30 min before chemotherapy and repeat at 8-h intervals, as prescribed.

Take ondansetron without regard to food. Orally disentegrating tablets may be dissolved on tongue without water.

For IV use, ondansetron may be given undiluted as an IV push over 2-5 min for doses up to 4 mg only. For IV infusion, dilute with 50 mL D5W or 0.9% NaCl before administration, and infuse over 15 min. May also give IM if dose is 4 mg or less.

Oprelvekin (Interleukin-11 [IL-11])
oh-prel′ve-kin in-teer-loo-kin
(Neumega)
Do not confuse Neumega with Neupogen. Do not confuse with interleukin-2.

CATEGORY AND SCHEDULE
Pregnancy Risk Category: C

Classification: Hematopoietic agents; platelet growth factor, interleukins.

MECHANISM OF ACTION
A hematopoietic recombinant version of human interleukin-11 (IL-11) that stimulates production of blood platelets, essential to the blood-clotting process. *Therapeutic Effect*: Increases platelet production.

PHARMACOKINETICS
Peak 3.2 h following single subcutaneous dose. Rapidly excreted by the kidneys. *Half-life:* 6.9 h.

AVAILABILITY
Injection: 5 mg.

INDICATIONS AND DOSAGES
▸ **Prevention of thrombocytopenia as a result of chemotherapy**
SC
Adults. 50 mcg/kg once a day, beginning 6-24 h after completion

of chemotherapy, and usually for 10-21 days.

▸ **Dosage in renal impairment**
If CrCl < 30 mL/min, reduce to 25 mcg/kg once daily.

CONTRAINDICATIONS
Hypersensitivity.

INTERACTIONS
Drug
Platelet inhibitors, aspirin: Caution is warranted with NSAIDs and aspirin, which can affect platelet function.
Thiazide loop diuretics: Increase risk of hypokalemia.
Herbal
None known.
Food
None known.

DIAGNOSTIC TEST EFFECTS
May decrease hemoglobin and hematocrit, usually within 3-5 days of initiation of therapy; reverses about 1 wk after therapy discontinued.

SIDE EFFECTS
Frequent
Nausea or vomiting (77%), fluid retention (59%), neutropenic fever (48%), diarrhea (43%), rhinitis (42%), headache (41%), dizziness (38%), fever (36%), insomnia (33%), cough (29%), rash or pharyngitis (25%), tachycardia (20%), vasodilation (19%).

SERIOUS REACTIONS
• Transient atrial fibrillation or flutter occurs in 10% of patients and may be caused by increased plasma volume; oprelvekin is not directly arrhythmogenic. Arrhythmias usually are brief and spontaneously convert to normal sinus rhythm.
• Papilledema, especially in children.
• Serious acute hypersensitivity.
• Congestive heart failure, dyspnea, pulmonary edema.

PRECAUTIONS & CONSIDERATIONS
Caution is warranted in patients with or susceptible to developing congestive heart failure (CHF) and in those with a history of atrial arrhythmia or heart failure. An electric razor and soft toothbrush should be used to prevent bleeding until platelet count is within normal range. Although drug has been used in children, a safe and effective dose is not established; the effective dose often exceeds the maximum tolerated dose of 50 mcg/kg/day.

Notify the physician of palpitations or dyspnea. Fluid and electrolyte status should be closely monitored, particularly if the patient is receiving diuretic therapy. Fluid retention should be assessed as evidenced by dyspnea on exertion and peripheral edema; fluid retention generally occurs during the first week of therapy and continues for the duration of treatment. An ECG should be obtained to assess for an underlying arrhythmia. Platelet count should also be periodically assessed for therapeutic response. CBC should be obtained before chemotherapy and at regular intervals thereafter; discontinue oprelvekin more than 2 days before starting next round of chemotherapy.
Storage
Store in refrigerator. Once reconstituted, use within 3 h.
Administration
! Begin oprelvekin administration 6-24 h following completion of chemotherapy dose.

For SC use, add 1 mL sterile water for injection to provide concentration of 5 mg/mL oprelvekin. Inject along inside surface of vial, and swirl contents gently to avoid excessive agitation. Discard unused portion. Give single injection in the abdomen, thigh, hip, or upper arm. Continue drug dosing until postnadir platelet count is > 50,000 cells/mcL. Expect drug to be discontinued at least 2 days before next planned chemotherapy cycle.

Orlistat
ohr'lih-stat
(Xenical, Alli [OTC])
Do not confuse Xenical with Xeloda.

CATEGORY AND SCHEDULE
Pregnancy Risk Category: B
OTC (Alli)

Classification: Gastrointestinals, lipase inhibitors

MECHANISM OF ACTION
A gastric and pancreatic lipase inhibitor that inhibits absorption of dietary fats by inactivating gastric and pancreatic enzymes. *Therapeutic Effect*: Resulting caloric deficit may positively affect weight control.

PHARMACOKINETICS
Minimal absorption after administration. Protein binding: 99%. Primarily eliminated unchanged in feces. Unknown if removed by hemodialysis. *Half-life:* 1-2 h.

AVAILABILITY
Capsules: 120 mg (Rx).
Capsules: 60 mg (OTC).

INDICATIONS AND DOSAGES
▸ **Weight reduction in patients with body mass indexes of 27 kg/m² or over**
PO
Adults, Elderly, Children aged 12 yr and older. 120 mg 3 × a day (Xenical); 60 mg 3 ×/day (Alli).

CONTRAINDICATIONS
Cholestasis, chronic malabsorption syndrome, hypersensitivity.

INTERACTIONS
Drug
Cyclosporine: Reduces cyclosporine absorption; do not co-administer. If necessary, give cyclosporine 2 h before or after orlistat.
Fat-soluble vitamins: Orlistat reduces absortion; take multivitamin supplement to ensure adequate nutrition. Take 2 h before or after orlistat.
Levothyroxine: May decrease absorption of thyroid hormone. Administer at least 4 h apart.
Herbal and Food
None known.

DIAGNOSTIC TEST EFFECTS
Decreases: blood glucose, total cholesterol, and serum LDL levels. Decreases absorption and levels of vitamins A and E.

SIDE EFFECTS
Frequent (20%-30%)
Headache, abdominal discomfort, flatulence, fecal urgency, fatty or oily stool.
Occasional (5%-14%)
Back pain, menstrual irregularity, nausea, fatigue, diarrhea, dizziness.
Rare (< 4%)
Anxiety, rash, myalgia, dry skin, vomiting.

SERIOUS REACTIONS
• None known.

PRECAUTIONS & CONSIDERATIONS
It is unknown whether orlistat is excreted in breast milk. Orlistat use is not recommended during pregnancy or in breastfeeding women. Safety and efficacy of

orlistat have not been established in children. No age-related precautions have been noted in elderly patients.

Unpleasant side effects, such as flatulence and urgency, may occur but should diminish with time. Laboratory studies, such as blood glucose levels and lipid profile, should be obtained before and during therapy. Changes in coagulation parameters as well as height and weight should also be monitored. Monitor patients who are severely obese for diabetes or cardiovascular disease before beginning therapy.

Administration

! Orlistat's side effects tend to be mild and transient in nature, gradually diminishing during treatment as long as patient adheres to low-fat diet.

A nutritionally balanced, reduced-calorie diet should be maintained. Carbohydrates, fats, and protein should be distributed over three main meals. Give orlistat with each main meal or up to 1 h after such meals.

Orphenadrine

or-fen′a-dreen
(Norflex, Orphenace [CAN], Rhoxal-orphenadrine [CAN])

CATEGORY AND SCHEDULE
Pregnancy Risk Category: C

Classification: Skeletal muscle relaxants

MECHANISM OF ACTION
A skeletal muscle relaxant that is structurally related to diphenhydramine and may be thought to affect skeletal muscle indirectly by central atropine-like effects. *Therapeutic Effect*: Relieves musculoskeletal pain.

PHARMACOKINETICS
Well absorbed after PO and IM absorption. Protein binding: low. Metabolized in liver. Primarily excreted in urine and feces. *Half-life:* 14 h.

AVAILABILITY
Injection: 30 mg/mL (Norflex).
Tablets (Extended-Release): 100 mg (Norflex).

INDICATIONS AND DOSAGES
▸ **Musculoskeletal pain**
IM/IV
Adults, Elderly. 60 mg 2 times/day. Switch to oral form for maintenance.
PO
Adults, Elderly. 100 mg 2 times/day.

OFF-LABEL USES
Drug-induced extrapyramidal reactions.

CONTRAINDICATIONS
Angle-closure glaucoma, myasthenia gravis, pyloric or duodenal obstruction, stenosing peptic ulcer, prostatic hypertrophy, obstruction of the bladder neck, achalasia, cardiospasm (megaesophagus), hypersensitivity to orphenadrine or any component of the formulation.

INTERACTIONS
Drug
Alcohol, central nervous system (CNS) depressants, propoxyphene: May increase CNS sedative effects.
Anticholinergics: May increase anticholinergic effects.
Propoxyphene: Reports of confusion, tremors anxiety.

Herbal
St. John's wort, kava kava, gotu kola: May increase CNS depression.
Food
None known.

DIAGNOSTIC TEST EFFECTS
None known.

ⓘ IV INCOMPATIBILITIES
None known.

ⓘ IV COMPATIBILITIES
None known.

SIDE EFFECTS
Frequent
Drowsiness, dizziness, muscular weakness, hypotension, dry mouth, nose, throat, and lips, urinary retention, thickening of bronchial secretions.
Elderly, Frequent
Sedation, dizziness, hypotension.
Occasional
Flushing, visual or hearing disturbances, paresthesia, diaphoresis, chill.

SERIOUS REACTIONS
• Hypersensitivity reaction, such as eczema, pruritus, rash, cardiac disturbances, and photosensitivity, may occur.
• Overdosage may vary from CNS depression, including sedation, apnea, hypotension, cardiovascular collapse, or death to severe paradoxical reaction, such as hallucinations, tremor, and seizures.

PRECAUTIONS & CONSIDERATIONS
Caution is warranted with tachycardia or urinary retention. It is unknown whether orphenadrine crosses the placenta or is distributed in breast milk; therefore, caution in lactation and pregnancy is warranted. Safety and efficacy of orphenadrine

have not been established in children. No age-related precautions have been noted in elderly patients.

Drowsiness and dizziness may occur but usually diminish with continued therapy. Avoid alcohol and tasks that require mental alertness or motor skills.

If bloody or tarry stools, continued weakness, diarrhea, fatigue, itching, nausea, or skin rash occurs, notify the physician.
Storage
Store oral and injection formulations at room temperature. Solution for injection normally appears clear, colorless; discard if cloudy or precipitate is present.
Administration
Do not crush extended-release product. Take two tablets per day, one in the morning and one in the evening. Give without regard to food.

For IV, may administer undiluted. Give slowly over 5 min, with patient in the supine position. Keep patient supine for at least 10 min. IM is injected deeply into a large muscle, such as the deltoid.

Oseltamivir
ah-suhl-tahm'ah-veer
(Tamiflu)

CATEGORY AND SCHEDULE
Pregnancy Risk Category: C

Classification: Antivirals

MECHANISM OF ACTION
A selective inhibitor of influenza virus neuraminidase, an enzyme essential for viral replication. Acts against both influenza A and

B viruses. *Therapeutic Effect*:
Suppresses the spread of infection
within the respiratory system and
reduces the duration of clinical
symptoms.

PHARMACOKINETICS

Readily absorbed. Protein binding:
3%. Extensively converted to active
drug in the liver. Primarily excreted
in urine. *Half-life*: 6-10 h.

AVAILABILITY

Capsules: 30 mg, 45 mg, 75 mg.
Oral Suspension: 12 mg/mL.

INDICATIONS AND DOSAGES

▶ **Influenza A or B infection**
PO
Adults, Elderly. 75 mg 2 times a day
for 5 days
Children weighing >40 kg. 75 mg
twice a day for 5 days.
Children weighing 24-40 kg. 60 mg
twice a day for 5 days.
Children weighing 15-23 kg. 45 mg
twice a day for 5 days.
Children weighing < 15 kg. 30 mg
twice a day for 5 days. Not indicated
in infants < 1 yr of age.
▶ **Prevention of influenza**
PO
Adults, Elderly. 75 mg once a day for
10 days-6 weeks.
▶ **Dosage in renal impairment**
PO
CrCL 30 mL/min or less.
Adult, Elderly. Dosage is decreased
to 75 mg once a day for 5 days for
active treatment. For prophylaxis,
decrease to 75 mg every other day
or 30 mg once daily.
Children. Reduce usual dose
by 50%.

CONTRAINDICATIONS

Hypersensitivity to oseltamivir or
any of its components, use in infants
and neonates.

INTERACTIONS

Drug
Intranasal influenza vaccine. Do not
give at same time; oseltamivir may
interfere with response to vaccine.
Herbal and Food
None known.

DIAGNOSTIC TEST EFFECTS

None known.

SIDE EFFECTS

Frequent (5%)
Nausea, vomiting, diarrhea.
Occasional (1%-4%)
Abdominal pain, bronchitis,
dizziness, headache, cough,
insomnia, fatigue, vertigo.

SERIOUS REACTIONS

• Colitis, pneumonia, and pyrexia
occur rarely.

PRECAUTIONS & CONSIDERATIONS

Caution is warranted in patients
with renal function impairment. Be
aware that it is unknown whether
oseltamivir is excreted in breast
milk; therefore, caution in lactation
is warranted. Oseltamivir is most
suitable for treating influenza Type
A. Be aware that the safety and
efficacy of this drug have not been
established in children younger
than 1 yr. No age-related
precautions have been noted in
elderly patients. Be aware that
oseltamivir is not a substitute for
a flu shot. Blood glucose should
be monitored. Oseltamivir is on
the Center for Disease Control and
Prevention (CDC) list of approved
medications for use in pandemic
H5N1 flu.
Storage
Store capsules at room temperature.
After reconstitution, store
suspension in refrigerator for
up to 10 days. Do not freeze.

Administration

Give oseltamivir without regard to food. The drug should be started as soon as possible within the first 24 h of the first appearance of flu symptoms. The entire duration of therapy should be followed. Shake oral suspension well before each use.

Oxacillin
ox-a-sill′in

CATEGORY AND SCHEDULE
Pregnancy Risk Category: B

Classification: Broad-spectrum anti-infective; penicillinase-resistant penicillin.

MECHANISM OF ACTION
A penicillin that binds to bacterial membranes. *Therapeutic Effect:* Bactericidal.

PHARMACOKINETICS
PO/IM: Peak 30-60 min; duration 4-6 h. IV: Peak 5 min; duration 4-6 h. Metabolized in the liver, excreted in bile, urine and breast milk; crosses the placenta. *Half-life:* 30-60 min.

AVAILABILITY
Powder for Injection: 1-g vials, 2-g vials.

INDICATIONS AND DOSAGES
▸**Upper respiratory tract, skin and skin-structure infections**
IV, IM
Adults, Elderly, Children weighing 40 kg or more. 250-500 mg q4-6h. Maximum: 12 g/day.
Children weighing < 40 kg.
50 mg/kg/day in divided doses q6h.
▸**Lower respiratory tract and other serious infections**

IV, IM
Adults, Elderly, Children weighing ≥ 40 kg. 1 g q4-6h. Maximum: 12 g/day.
Children and Infants weighing < 40 kg. 100 mg/kg/day in divided doses q4-6 h. Neonates require extended dosage intervals and lower total daily dosage (e.g., 25-75 mg/kg/day).

CONTRAINDICATIONS
Hypersensitivity to any penicillin.

INTERACTIONS
Drug
Aminoglycosides: Infusions must be separated by 1 h.
Erythromycin, lincosamides, tetracyclines: Possible decrease in antimicrobial effectiveness.
Methotrexate: Possible increase in methotrexate toxicity.
Oral contraceptives: May decrease effectiveness of these medications.
Probenecid: May increase oxacillin blood concentration and risk of toxicity.
Herbal and Food
None known.

DIAGNOSTIC TEST EFFECTS
May increase AST (SGOT) levels. May cause a positive Coombs' test.

⚧ IV INCOMPATIBILITIES
Amphotericin B, calcium chloride, calcium gluconate, diazepam, dobutamine, haloperidol, inamrinone, phenytoin, tobramycin.

SIDE EFFECTS
Frequent
Mild hypersensitivity reaction (fever, rash, pruritus), GI effects (nausea, vomiting, diarrhea).
Occasional
Phlebitis, thrombophlebitis (more common in elderly), hepatotoxicity (with high IV dosage).

SERIOUS REACTIONS

• Antibiotic-associated colitis and other superinfections may result from altered bacterial balance.
• A mild to severe hypersensitivity reaction may occur in those allergic to penicillins.

PRECAUTIONS & CONSIDERATIONS

Caution is warranted in with patients impaired renal function or a history of allergies, especially to cephalosporins. History of allergies, especially to cephalosporins or penicillins, should be determined before giving the drug. Withhold and promptly notify the physician if rash or diarrhea occurs. Severe diarrhea with abdominal pain, blood or mucus in stool, and fever may indicate antibiotic-associated colitis. Signs and symptoms of superinfection, including anal or genital pruritus, black hairy tongue, diarrhea, increased fever, sore throat, ulceration or changes of oral mucosa, and vomiting should be monitored. Intake and output, renal function tests, urinalysis, and the injection sites should be assessed.

For patients using oral contraceptives, there is a potential risk for decreased effectiveness; the patient should be advised to comply with the oral dosing schedule of contraceptives while taking this medication, as well as use an additional nonhormonal birth control method throughout the duration of treatment.

Storage
Store vials at room temperature. Once reconstituted, the solution remains stable for 3 days at room temperature or 7 days refrigerated. When further diluted with D5W or 0.9% NaCl, the solution is stable for 24 h.

Administration
For IV use add 5 mL to each 250-mg vial (concentration 50 mg/mL) or add 10 mL sterile water for injection to each 1-g vial to provide a concentration of 100 mg/mL. For piggyback administration, further dilute with 50-100 mL D5W or 0.9% NaCl. Administer IV piggyback over 30 min-1h. Slower infusion time and IV concentrations of 20 mg/mL or less may help limit phlebitis. If needed, the drug may be given IV push slowly over 10 min after vial reconstitution.

For IM use, reconstitute each 1.5-g vial with 3.2 mL or each 3-g vial with 6.4 mL of sterile water for injection to provide a concentration of 250 mg ampicillin/125 mg sulbactam per milliliter. Administer the injection deep into a large muscle mass within 1 h of preparation.

Oxaliplatin
ahks-al-eh-plah´-tin
(Eloxatin)

CATEGORY AND SCHEDULE
Pregnancy Risk Category: D

Classification: Antineoplastic; platinum coordination complex

MECHANISM OF ACTION
A platinum-containing complex that cross-links with DNA strands, preventing cell division. Cell cycle-phase nonspecific. *Therapeutic Effect:* Inhibits DNA replication.

PHARMACOKINETICS
Rapidly distributed. Protein binding: 90%. Undergoes rapid, extensive nonenzymatic biotransformation. Excreted in urine. *Half-life:* 70 h.

AVAILABILITY
Injection Solution: 5 mg/mL.

INDICATIONS AND DOSAGES

▸ **Metastatic colon or rectal cancer in patients whose disease has recurred or progressed during or within 6 mo of completing first-line therapy with bolus 5-fluorouracil (5-FU), leucovorin, and irinotecan**
IV

Adults. Day 1: Oxaliplatin 85 mg/m^2 in 250-500 mL D5W and leucovorin 200 mg/m^2, both given simultaneously over more than 2 h in separate bags using a Y-line, followed by 5-FU 400 mg/m^2 IV bolus given over 2-4 min, followed by 5-FU 600 mg/m^2 in 500 mL D5W as a 22-h continuous IV infusion. Day 2: Leucovorin 200 mg/m^2 IV infusion given over more than 2 h, followed by 5-FU 400 mg/m^2 IV bolus given over 2-4 min, followed by 5-FU 600 mg/m^2 in 500 mL D5W as a 22-h continuous IV infusion.

CONTRAINDICATIONS

History of allergy to platinum compounds.

DRUG INTERACTIONS

Drug
None reported.
Herbal
None known.
Food
None known.

ⓘ IV INCOMPATIBILITIES

Alkaline medications or solutions (e.g., 5-fluorouracil), aluminum needles or IV sets, sodium chloride solution or chloride-containing solutions, diazepam.

SIDE EFFECTS

Frequent
Peripheral or sensory neuropathy (usually occurs in hands, feet, perioral area, and throat but may present as jaw spasm, abnormal tongue sensation, eye pain, chest pressure, or difficulty walking, swallowing, or writing), nausea, fatigue, diarrhea, vomiting, constipation, abdominal pain, fever, anorexia.
Occasional
Stomatitis, earache, insomnia, cough, difficulty breathing, backache, edema.
Rare
Dyspepsia, dizziness, rhinitis, flushing, alopecia.

SERIOUS REACTIONS

• Peripheral or sensory neuropathy can occur, sometimes precipitated or exacerbated by drinking or holding a glass of cold liquid during the IV infusion.
• Pulmonary fibrosis, characterized by a nonproductive cough, dyspnea, crackles, and radiologic pulmonary infiltrates, may require drug discontinuation.
• Hypersensitivity reaction (rash, urticaria, pruritus) occurs rarely.
• Hepatotoxicity.
• Extravasation necrosis.

PRECAUTIONS & CONSIDERATIONS

Use with caution in patients with renal function impairment. Dose adjustments may be necessary in patients with renal impairment, neurosensory toxicity, gastrointestinal toxicity, neutropenia, or thrombocytopenia. Premedication with antiemetics is recommended. Avoid mucositis prophylaxis with ice chips during oxaliplatin infusion. Elderly may be more sensitive to adverse effects. Safety and efficacy not established in children. Avoid use in pregnancy or breast-feeding.
Storage
Store at room temperature in original carton. After dilution, can be kept up

to 6 h at room temperature or up to 24 h under refrigeration.

Administration

Must be diluted in D5W. Administer over 2 to 6 h. Flush infusion line with D5W before administration of any concomitant medications.

Oxandrolone

ox-an'droe-lone

(Lonavar [AUS], Oxandrin)

Do not confuse with testolactone or nandrolone, or oxymethalone

CATEGORY AND SCHEDULE

Pregnancy Risk Category: X
Controlled Substance: Schedule III

Classification: Androgenic anabolic steroid

MECHANISM OF ACTION

A synthetic testosterone derivative that promotes growth and development of male sex organs, maintains secondary sex characteristics in androgen-deficient males. *Therapeutic Effect*: Androgenic and anabolic actions.

PHARMACOKINETICS

Well absorbed from the GI tract. Protein binding: 94%-97%. Metabolized in liver. Primarily excreted in urine. Unknown whether removed by hemodialysis. *Half-life:* 5-13 h.

AVAILABILITY

Tablets: 2.5 mg, 10 mg (Oxandrin).

INDICATIONS AND DOSAGES
▸ **Cachexia**

Adults, Elderly. 2.5-20 mg in divided doses 2-4 times/day usually for 2-4 wks. Course of therapy is based on individual response. Repeat intermittently as needed.

Children. Total daily dose is less than or equal to 0.1 mg/kg. Repeat intermittently as needed.

OFF-LABEL USES

AIDS wasting syndrome, growth failure, Turner syndrome.

CONTRAINDICATIONS

Nephrosis, carcinoma of breast or prostate hypercalcemia, pregnancy, hypersensitivity to oxandrolone or any component of the formulation, nephrosis.

Caution

Diabetes meellitus, cardiovascular disease, myocardial infarction (MI), increased risk of benign prostatic hypertrophy, prostatic carcinoma, virilization (women), increased PT.

INTERACTIONS

Drug

Adrenocorticotropic hormone (ACTH), adrenal steroids: May increase the risk of edema and acne.

Adrenal steroids: May increase the effects of the adrenal steroids.

Insulin, oral hypoglycemic agents: May increase the effects of hypoglycemic agents.

Oral anticoagulants: May increase the effects of oral anticoagulants. Monitor INR.

Herbal

Chaparral: May increase liver enzymes.

Comfrey: May increase liver enzymes.

Eucalyptus: May increase risk of hepatoxicity.

Germander: May increase liver enzymes.

Jin bu huan: May increase liver enzymes.

Kava kava: May increase liver enzymes.

O

Pennyroyal: May increase liver enzymes.
Skullcap: May increase the risk of liver damage.
Velerian: May increase risk of hepatotoxicity.
Food
None known.

DIAGNOSTIC TEST EFFECTS

May decrease levels of thyroxine-binding globulin, resulting in decreased total T_4 serum levels and increased resin uptake of T_3 and T_4. May increase PBI and radioactive iodine uptake.

SIDE EFFECTS

Frequent
Gynecomastia, acne, amenorrhea, other menstrual irregularities. Females: Hirsutism, deepening of voice, clitoral enlargement that may not be reversible when drug is discontinued.
Occasional
Edema, nausea, insomnia, oligospermia, priapism, male pattern of baldness, bladder irritability, hypercalcemia in immobilized patients or those with breast cancer, hypercholesterolemia.
Rare
Polycythemia with high dosage.

SERIOUS REACTIONS

• Peliosis hepatitis of the liver, spleen replaced with blood-filled cysts, hepatic neoplasms, and hepatocellular carcinoma have been associated with prolonged high-dosage, anaphylactic reactions.
• Children: compromised adult stature.
• Cholestatic jaundice.
• Priapism.

PRECAUTIONS & CONSIDERATIONS
Caution is warranted in patients with diabetes, epilepsy, and liver, cardiac, and renal disease. Oxandrolone use is contraindicated during lactation and is excreted in breast milk. Oxandrolone may accelerate bone maturation more rapidly than linear growth in children, and the effect may continue for 6 mo after the drug has been stopped. Its use in elderly patients may increase the risk of hyperplasia or stimulate growth of occult prostate carcinoma. Salt intake should be reduced.

Acne, nausea, pedal edema, or vomiting may occur. Women should report deepening of voice, hoarseness, and menstrual irregularities. Men should report difficulty urinating, frequent erections, and gynecomastia. Weight should be obtained each day. Weekly weight gains of more than 5 lb should be reported. Signs of anemia should be reported to health care provider. Avoid unnecessary activities that could result in unnecessary injury and bleeding.
Storage
Store oxandrolone at room temperature away from moisture, heat, and direct light.
Administration
Take oxandrolone with or without food. Take with a full glass of water. Duration of therapy will depend on the response of the patient.

Oxaprozin

ox-a-pro'zin
(Daypro)
Do not confuse oxaprozin with oxazepam.

CATEGORY AND SCHEDULE

Pregnancy Risk Category: C (D if used in third trimester or near delivery)

Classification: Nonsteroidal anti-inflammatory drugs

MECHANISM OF ACTION

An NSAID that produces analgesic and anti-inflammatory effects by inhibiting prostaglandin synthesis. *Therapeutic Effect*: Reduces the inflammatory response and intensity of pain.

PHARMACOKINETICS

Well absorbed from the GI tract. Protein binding: 99%. Widely distributed. Metabolized in the liver. Primarily excreted in urine; partially eliminated in feces. Not removed by hemodialysis. *Half-life:* 42-50 h.

AVAILABILITY

Tablets: 600 mg.

INDICATIONS AND DOSAGES

▸ **Osteoarthritis**
PO
Adults, Adults. 1200 mg once a day (600 mg in patients with low body weight or mild disease). Maximum: 1800 mg/day.
▸ **Rheumatoid arthritis**
PO
Adults, Elderly. 1200 mg once a day. Range: 600-1800 mg/day.
▸ **Juvenile rheumatoid arthritis (6 yr and older)**
Children weighing > 54 kg.
1200 mg/day.

Children weighing 32-54 kg.
900 mg/day.
Children weighing 22-31 kg.
600 mg/day.
▸ **Dosage in renal impairment**
For adults and elderly patients with renal impairment, the recommended initial dose is 600 mg/day; may be increased up to 1200 mg/day.

CONTRAINDICATIONS

Active peptic ulcer disease, chronic inflammation of GI tract, GI bleeding or ulceration, history of hypersensitivity to aspirin or NSAIDs.
Caution
Lactation, children, bleeding disorders, GI disorders, cardiac disorders, hypersensitivity to other antiinflammatory agents, diabetes.

INTERACTIONS

Drug
Antihypertensives, diuretics: May decrease the effects of these drugs.
Aspirin, other salicylates, alcohol, corticosteroids: May increase the risk of GI side effects such as bleeding.
Bone marrow depressants: May increase the risk of hematologic reactions.
Cyclosporine: May increase risk of decreased renal function.
Diuretics, β-adrenergic blockers, ACE inhibitors: May decrease antihypertensive effects.
First-time users of SSRIs also taking NSAIDs: May have a higher risk of GI effects.
Heparin, oral anticoagulants, thrombolytics: May increase the effects of these drugs.
Lithium: May increase the blood concentration and risk of toxicity of lithium.
Methotrexate: May increase the risk of methotrexate toxicity.
Probenecid: May increase the oxaprozin blood concentration.

O

Herbal
Feverfew: May decrease the effects of feverfew.
Ginkgo biloba: May increase the risk of bleeding.
Food
None known.

DIAGNOSTIC TEST EFFECTS
May increase BUN, serum creatinine, AST (SGOT), and ALT (SGPT) levels.

SIDE EFFECTS
Occasional (3%-9%)
Nausea, diarrhea, constipation, dyspepsia, edema.
Rare (< 3%)
Vomiting, abdominal cramps or pain, flatulence, anorexia, confusion, tinnitus, insomnia, somnolence.

SERIOUS REACTIONS
• Hypertension, acute renal failure, respiratory depression, GI bleeding, and coma occur rarely.

PRECAUTIONS & CONSIDERATIONS
Caution is warranted in patients with a history of GI tract disease, hepatic or renal impairment, and a predisposition to fluid retention. It is unknown whether oxaprozin is excreted in breast milk; therefore, caution is warranted in lactation. Oxaprozin should not be used during the third trimester of pregnancy because it may cause adverse effects in the fetus, such as premature closure of the ductus arteriosus. The safety and efficacy of oxaprozin have not been established in children. In elderly patients, GI bleeding or ulceration is more likely to cause serious complications, and age-related renal impairment may increase the risk of hepatotoxicity or renal toxicity; a decreased dosage is recommended. Avoid alcohol and aspirin during therapy because these substances

increase the risk of GI bleeding. Tasks that require mental alertness or motor skills should also be avoided.

Notify the physician if bleeding, ecchymosis, edema, confusion or weight gain occurs. BUN, serum alkaline phosphatase, bilirubin, creatinine, AST (SGOT), and ALT (SGPT) levels to assess hepatic and renal function should be assessed during therapy. Therapeutic response, such as decreased pain, stiffness, swelling, and tenderness, improved grip strength, and increased joint mobility, should be evaluated. Signs of blood dyscrasias including infection, poor circulation, bleeding, and poor healing should be reported to the health care provider immediately.
Administration
Take oxaprozin with food, milk, or antacids if GI distress occurs.

Oxazepam
ox-a′ze-pam
(Alepam [AUS], Apo-Oxazepam [CAN], Murelax [AUS], Serax, Serepax [AUS])
Do not confuse oxazepam with oxaprozin, or Serax with Eurax or Xerac.

CATEGORY AND SCHEDULE
Pregnancy Risk Category: D
Controlled Substance: Schedule IV

Classification: Anxiolytics, benzodiazepines

MECHANISM OF ACTION
A benzodiazepine that potentiates the effects of γ-aminobutyric acid and other inhibitory neurotransmitters by binding to specific receptors in the central nervous system. *Therapeutic*

Effect: Produces anxiolytic effect and skeletal muscle relaxation.

PHARMACOKINETICS

Well absorbed from the GI tract. Protein binding: 97%. Metabolized in the liver. Primarily excreted in urine. Not removed by hemodialysis. *Half-life:* 5-20 h.

AVAILABILITY

Capsules: 10 mg, 15 mg, 30 mg.
Tablets: 15 mg.

INDICATIONS AND DOSAGES

▶ **Mild to moderate anxiety**
PO
Adults. 10-15 mg 3-4 times a day.
▶ **Severe anxiety**
PO
Adults. 15-30 mg 3-4 times a day.
▶ **Alcohol withdrawal**
PO
Adults. 15-30 mg 3-4 times a day.
Elderly. Initially, 10 mg 3 times a day. May gradually increase up to 15 mg 3-4 times daily.

CONTRAINDICATIONS

Hypersensitivity, psychoses.
Caution
Elderly, debilitated, hepatic disease, renal diseaes, lactation, pregnancy.

INTERACTIONS

Drug
Alcohol, other CNS depressants, anticonvulsant medications: May potentiate CNS depression.
Herbal
Kava kava, valerian: May increase CNS depression.
Food
None known.

DIAGNOSTIC TEST EFFECTS

May elevate serum alkaline phosphatase, bilirubin, LDH, AST (SGOT), and ALT (SGPT) levels.

May produce abnormal renal function test results. Therapeutic serum drug level is 0.2-1.4 mcg/mL; toxic serum drug level has not been established.

SIDE EFFECTS

Frequent
Mild, transient somnolence at beginning of therapy.
Occasional
Dizziness, headache.
Rare
Paradoxical CNS reactions, such as hyperactivity or nervousness in children and excitement or restlessness in the elderly or debilitated (generally noted during the first 2 wks of therapy).

SERIOUS REACTIONS

• Abrupt or too-rapid withdrawal may result in pronounced restlessness, irritability, insomnia, hand tremor, abdominal or muscle cramps, diaphoresis, vomiting, and seizures.
• Overdose results in somnolence, confusion, diminished reflexes, and coma.

PRECAUTIONS & CONSIDERATIONS

Caution is warranted in patients with a history of drug dependence. Women on long-term therapy should use effective contraception during therapy and notify the physician if she becomes or may be pregnant. Alcohol and other CNS depressants should be avoided while taking oxazepam. While has been used in children > 6 years of age, absolute dosage has not been established.

Drowsiness and dizziness may occur. Tasks requiring mental alertness or motor skills should be avoided. CBC, blood chemistry, and hepatic and renal function should be monitored, especially during long-term therapy because of possible cardiovascular effects.

Psychological and physical dependence may occur with chronic administration. Elderly patients should be evaluated for adjustments in dosage. Abrupt withdrawal may result in pronounced irritability, restlessness, hand tremors, abdominal or muscle cramps, diaphoresis, vomiting, seizures.

Administration

! Plan to use the smallest effective dose in elderly or debilitated patients and in those with hepatic disease or a low serum albumin level. Do not abruptly discontinue after long-term use. The therapeutic serum level for oxazepam is 0.2-1.4 mcg/mL; the toxic serum level is not established.

Oxcarbazepine
oks-kar-bays′uh-peen
(Trileptal)
Do not confuse with carbamazepine

CATEGORY AND SCHEDULE
Pregnancy Risk Category: C

Classification: Anticonvulsants

MECHANISM OF ACTION
An anticonvulsant that blocks sodium channels, resulting in stabilization of hyperexcited neural membranes, inhibition of repetitive neuronal firing, and diminishing synaptic impulses. *Therapeutic Effect*: Prevents seizures.

PHARMACOKINETICS
Completely absorbed from GI tract and extensively metabolized in the liver to active metabolite. Protein binding: 40%. Primarily excreted in urine. *Half-life:* 2 h; metabolite, 6-10 h.

AVAILABILITY
Oral Suspension: 300 mg/5 mL.
Tablets: 150 mg, 300 mg, 600 mg.

INDICATIONS AND DOSAGES
▶ **Adjunctive treatment of seizures**
PO
Adults, Elderly. Initially, 600 mg/day in 2 divided doses. May increase by up to 600 mg/day at weekly intervals. Maximum: 2400 mg/day.
Children aged 4-16 yr. 8-10 mg/kg. Maximum: 600 mg/day. Maintenance (based on weight): 1800 mg/day for children weighing >39 kg; 1200 mg/day for children weighing 29.1-39 kg; and 900 mg/day for children weighing 20-29 kg.
▶ **Conversion to monotherapy**
PO
Adults, Elderly. 600 mg/day in 2 divided doses (while decreasing concomitant anticonvulsant over 3-6 wks). May increase by 600 mg/day at weekly intervals up to 2400 mg/day.
Children aged 4 years and older. Initially, 8-10 mg/kg/day in 2 divided doses with simultaneous initial reduction of dose of concomitant antiepileptic.
▶ **Initiation of monotherapy**
PO
Adults, Elderly. 600 mg/day in 2 divided doses. May increase by 300 mg/day every 3 days up to 1200 mg/day.
Children aged 4 years and older. Initially, 8-10 mg/kg/day in 2 divided doses. Increase at 3 day intervals by 5 mg/kg/day to achieve maintenance dose by weight;
(70 kg): 1500-2100 mg/day;
(60-69 kg): 1200-2100 mg/day;
(50-59 kg): 1200-1800 mg/day;

(41-49 kg): 1200-1500 mg/day;
(35-40 kg): 900-1500 mg/day;
(25-34 kg): 900-1200 mg/day;
(20-24 kg): 600-900 mg/day.
▸ **Dosage in renal impairment**
For patients with creatinine clearance
< 30 mL/min, give 50% of normal
starting dose, then titrate slowly to
desired dose.

OFF-LABEL USES
Atypical panic disorder.

CONTRAINDICATIONS
Hypersensitivity to this drug or to
carbamazepine.

INTERACTIONS
Drug
**All central nervous system
(CNS) depressants, alcohol:** May
increase CNS depressive
effects.
Calcium channel blockers:
Oxcarbazepine may lower blood
levels.
**Carbamazepine, phenobarbital,
phenytoin, valproic acid,
verapamil:** May decrease the
blood concentration and effects of
oxcarbazepine.
CYP450 3A4/5 enzyme inducers:
May decrease plasma levels.
Oral contraceptives: May decrease
the effectiveness of birth control.
Phenobarbital, phenytoin: May
increase the blood concentration and
risk of toxicity of these drugs.
Herbal
None known.
Food
None known.

DIAGNOSTIC TEST EFFECTS
May increase GGT level and other
hepatic function test results. May
increase or decrease blood glucose
level. May decrease serum calcium,
potassium, and sodium levels.

SIDE EFFECTS
Frequent (13%-22%)
Dizziness, nausea, headache.
Occasional (5%-7%)
Vomiting, diarrhea, ataxia,
nervousness, heartburn, indigestion,
epigastric pain, constipation.
Rare (4%)
Tremor, rash, back pain, epistaxis,
sinusitis, diplopia.

SERIOUS REACTIONS
• Clinically significant hyponatremia
may occur.
• Serious hypersensitivity or rashes,
including Stevens-Johnson syndrome
and TENS.
• Aplastic anemia, agranulocytosis
(rare).

PRECAUTIONS & CONSIDERATIONS
Caution is warranted in patients
with renal impairment and a
hypersensitivity to carbamazepine.
Oxcarbazepine crosses the placenta
and is distributed in breast milk.
Oxcarbazepine is related to
carbamazepine, considered to
be teratogenic. No age-related
precautions have been noted in
children older than 4 yr. In elderly
patients, age-related renal impairment
may require dosage adjustment.
    Drowsiness may occur, so alcohol
and tasks requiring mental alertness
or motor skills should be avoided.
Notify the physician if dizziness,
headache, nausea, and rash occur.
Seizure disorder, including the onset,
duration, frequency, intensity, and
type of seizures, should be assessed
before and during treatment. Serum
sodium levels should be monitored;
signs and symptoms of hyponatremia
include confusion, headache,
lethargy, malaise, and nausea.
Administration
! Plan to give all doses in a twice-
daily regimen.

O

Take oxcarbazepine without regard to food.

Shake oral suspension well before each use.

Oxiconazole
ox-i-con′a-zole
(Oxistat, Oxizole [CAN])
Do not confuse with Nitrostat.

CATEGORY AND SCHEDULE
Pregnancy Risk Category: B

Classification: Antifungals, topical, dermatologics

MECHANISM OF ACTION
An antifungal agent that inhibits ergosterol synthesis. *Therapeutic Effect*: Destroys cytoplasmic membrane integrity of fungi. Fungicidal.

PHARMACOKINETICS
Low systemic absorption. Absorbed and distributed in each layer of the dermis. Excreted in the urine.

AVAILABILITY
Cream: 1% (Oxistat).
Lotion: 1% (Oxistat).

INDICATIONS AND DOSAGES
▸**Tinea pedis**
TOPICAL
Adults, Elderly, Children aged 12 yr and older. Apply 1-2 times daily for 1 mo or until signs and symptoms significantly improve.
▸**Tinea cruris, tinea corporis**
TOPICAL
Adults, Elderly, Children aged 12 yr and older. Apply 1-2 times daily for 2 wks or until signs and symptoms significantly improve.

CONTRAINDICATIONS
Not for ophthalmic use, hypersensitivity to oxiconazole or any other azole fungals.

INTERACTIONS
Drug
None known.
Herbal
None known.
Food
None known.

DIAGNOSTIC TEST EFFECTS
None known.

SIDE EFFECTS
Occasional
Itching, local irritation, stinging, dryness.

SERIOUS REACTIONS
• Hypersensitivity reactions characterized by rash, swelling, pruritus, maceration, and a sensation of warmth may occur.

PRECAUTIONS & CONSIDERATIONS
Caution should be used in patients with known hypersensitivity to other antifungal agents. It is unknown ehether oxiconazole is distributed in breast milk; caution is warranted during lactation. Safety and efficacy of oxiconazole have not been established in children younger than 12 yr. No age-related precautions have been noted in elderly patients.

Signs and symptoms of a local reaction include blistering, burning, irritation, itching, oozing, redness, and swelling. Oxiconazole should be discontinued and the physician should be notified immediately. Hypersensitivity manifests as rash, swelling, pruritus, maceration, and sense of warmth and should be reported.

Administration
Oxiconazole is for external use only. Shake lotion well before using. Apply and rub gently into the affected and surrounding area. Avoid contact with eyes, mouth, nose, or other mucous membranes. Topical therapy may be used for 2-4 wks. Area should not be covered with an occlusive dressing. Keep area clean and dry and wear light clothing to promote ventilation.

Oxybutynin
ox-i-byoo′ti-nin
(Ditropan, Ditropan XL, Oxytrol)
Do not confuse oxybutynin with Oxycontin, or Ditropan with diazepam.

CATEGORY AND SCHEDULE
Pregnancy Risk Category: B

Classification: Antispasmodic (papaverine-like)

MECHANISM OF ACTION
An anticholinergic that exerts antispasmodic (papaverine-like) and antimuscarinic (atropine-like) action on the detrusor smooth muscle of the bladder. *Therapeutic Effect:* Increases bladder capacity and delays desire to void.

PHARMACOKINETICS

Route	Onset	Peak	Duration
PO	0.5-1 h	3-6 h	6-10 h

Rapidly absorbed from the GI tract. Metabolized in the liver. Primarily excreted in urine. Unknown if removed by hemodialysis.
Half-life: 1-2.3 h.

AVAILABILITY
Syrup (Ditropan): 5 mg/5 mL.
Tablets (Ditropan): 5 mg.
Tablets (Extended-Release [Ditropan XL]): 5 mg, 10 mg, 15 mg.
Transdermal (Oxytrol): 3.9 mg.

INDICATIONS AND DOSAGES
▸ **Neurogenic bladder**
PO
Adults. 5 mg 2-3 times a day up to 5 mg 4 times a day.
Elderly. 2.5-5 mg twice a day. May increase by 2.5 mg/day every 1-2 days.
Children 5 yr and older. 5 mg twice a day up to 5 mg 4 times a day.
Children aged 1-4 yr. 0.2 mg/kg/dose 2-4 times a day.
PO (EXTENDED RELEASE)
Adults. 5-10 mg/day up to 30 mg/day.
TRANSDERMAL
Adults. 3.9 mg applied twice a week. Apply every 3-4 days.

CONTRAINDICATIONS
GI or genitourinary obstruction, glaucoma, myasthenia gravis, toxic megacolon, ulcerative colitis. Lactation, suspected glaucoma, children under age 12 yr, hiatal hernia, esophageal reflux, coronary heart disease, congestive heart failure (CHF), hypertension.

INTERACTIONS
Drug
Anticholinergics (such as antihistamines): May increase the anticholinergic effects of oxybutynin.
Alcohol, central nervous system (CNS) depressants: May increase CNS depressant effects.
Herbal
None known.
Food
None known.

O

DIAGNOSTIC TEST EFFECTS

None known.

SIDE EFFECTS

Frequent

Constipation, dry mouth, somnolence, decreased perspiration.

Occasional

Decreased lacrimation or salivation, impotence, urinary hesitancy and retention, suppressed lactation, blurred vision, mydriasis, nausea or vomiting, insomnia.

SERIOUS REACTIONS

• Overdose produces CNS excitation (including nervousness, restlessness, hallucinations, and irritability), hypotension or hypertension, confusion, tachycardia, facial flushing, and respiratory depression.

PRECAUTIONS & CONSIDERATIONS

Caution is warranted in patients with cardiovascular disease, glaucoma, suspected glaucoma, hypertension, hyperthyroidism, hepatic or renal impairment, neuropathy, benign prostatic hyperplasia, and reflux esophagitis. It is unknown whether oxybutynin crosses the placenta or is distributed in breast milk; therefore, caution in lactation is warranted. No age-related precautions have been noted in children older than 5 yr. Elderly patients may be more sensitive to the drug's anticholinergic effects, such as dry mouth and urine retention. Avoid alcohol and tasks that require mental alertness and motor skills until response to the drug is established.

Drowsiness and dizziness may occur. Intake and output, pattern of daily bowel activity and stool consistency, and symptomatic relief should be assessed. Overdose manifests as CNS excitation (restlessness, nervousness, hallucinations, irritability), hypotension or hypertension, confusion, tachycardia, facial flushing, and respiratory depression; these symptoms need to be reported to the health care provider immediately. The physician should be informed of xerostomic effects such as sore tongue, problems eating or swallowing, so that medication change can be evaluated.

Administration

Take oxybutynin without regard to food. Extended-release tablets should not be crushed or chewed. Transdermal patch is applied to clear, dry skin of abdomen, hip, or buttock. Do not cut patch. Rotate application sites with each use.

Oxycodone

ox-ee-koe′done

(Endone [AUS], OxyContin, Oxydose, OxyFast, OxyIR, Oxynorm [AUS], Roxicodone, Roxicodone Intensol)

Do not confuse oxycodone with hydrocodone or oxybutynin.

CATEGORY AND SCHEDULE

Pregnancy Risk Category: B (D if used for prolonged periods or at high dosages at term)

Controlled Substance: Schedule II

Classification: Synthetic opioid analgesic.

MECHANISM OF ACTION

An opioid analgesic that binds with opioid receptors in the central nervous system (CNS). *Therapeutic Effect*: Alters the perception of and emotional response to pain.

PHARMACOKINETICS

Route	Onset	Peak	Duration
PO, Immediate-release	NA	NA	4-5 h
PO, Controlled-release	NA	NA	12 h

Moderately absorbed from the GI tract. Protein binding: 38%-45%. Widely distributed. Metabolized in the liver. Excreted in urine. Unknown whether removed by hemodialysis. *Half-life:* 2-3 h (3.2 h controlled-release).

AVAILABILITY

Capsules (Immediate-Release [OxyIR]): 5 mg.
Oral Concentrate (Oxydose, OxyFast, Roxicodone Intensol): 20 mg/mL.
Oral Solution (Roxicodone): 5 mg/5 mL.
Tablets (Roxicodone): 5 mg, 15 mg, 30 mg.
Tablets (Extended-Release [OxyContin]): 10 mg, 20 mg, 40 mg, 80 mg, 160 mg.

INDICATIONS AND DOSAGES
Analgesia
PO (CONTROLLED-RELEASE)
Adults, Elderly. Initially, 10 mg q12h. May increase every 1-2 days by 25%-50%. Usual: 40 mg/day (100 mg/day for cancer pain).
PO (IMMEDIATE-RELEASE)
Adults, Elderly. Initially, 5 mg q6h as needed. May increase up to 30 mg q4h. Usual: 10-30 mg q4h as needed.
Children. 0.05-0.15 mg/kg/dose q4-6h.

CONTRAINDICATIONS
Hypersensitivity, narcotic addiction, Severe respiratory depression in unmonitored setting, paralytic ileus.

INTERACTIONS
Drug
Alcohol, other CNS depressant, other narcotics, sedative-hypnotics, skeletal muscle relaxants, phenothiazines, benzodiazepines: May increase CNS or respiratory depression and hypotension.
Anticholinergics (e.g., antihistamines): May increase anticholinergic effects.
Potent CYPZD6 inhibitors: May increase oxycodone exposure.
Herbal
None known.
Food
None known.

DIAGNOSTIC TEST EFFECTS
May increase serum amylase and lipase levels.

SIDE EFFECTS
Frequent
Somnolence, dizziness, hypotension (including orthostatic hypotension), anorexia.
Occasional
Confusion, diaphoresis, facial flushing, urine retention, constipation, dry mouth, nausea, vomiting, headache.
Rare
Allergic reaction, depression, paradoxical CNS hyperactivity or nervousness in children, paradoxical excitement and restlessness in elderly or debilitated patients.

SERIOUS REACTIONS
• Overdose results in respiratory depression, skeletal muscle flaccidity, cold or clammy skin, cyanosis, and extreme somnolence progressing to seizures, stupor, and coma.
• Hepatotoxicity may occur with overdose of the acetaminophen

component of fixed-combination products.

• The patient who uses oxycodone repeatedly may develop a tolerance to the drug's analgesic effect and physical dependence.

PRECAUTIONS & CONSIDERATIONS

Extreme caution should be used in patients with acute alcoholism, anoxia, CNS depression, hypercapnia, respiratory depression or dysfunction, seizures, shock, or untreated myxedema. Caution is also warranted with acute abdominal conditions, Addison disease, chronic obstructive pulmonary disease (COPD), hypothyroidism, hepatic impairment, increased intracranial pressure, prostatic hypertrophy, and urethral stricture. Oxycodone readily crosses the placenta and is distributed in breast milk. Regular use of opioids during pregnancy may produce withdrawal symptoms in the neonate, including irritability, diarrhea, excessive crying, fever, hyperactive reflexes, irritability, seizures, sneezing, tremors, vomiting, and yawning. The neonate may develop respiratory depression if the mother receives oxycodone during labor. Children are more prone to experience paradoxical excitement. Children younger than 2 yr and elderly patients are more susceptible to the drug's respiratory depressant effects. Age-related renal impairment may increase the risk of urine retention in elderly patients.

Dizziness and drowsiness may occur, so change positions slowly and avoid alcohol, CNS depressants, and tasks that require mental alertness or motor skills until response to the drug is established. BP, respiratory rate, mental status, pattern of daily bowel activity, and clinical improvement should be monitored. The drug should be withheld and the physician should be notified if the respiratory rate is 12 breaths/min or less in an adult or 20 breaths/min or less in a child.

Overdose manifests as respiratory depression, skeletal muscle flaccidity, cold or clammy skin, cyanosis, and extreme somnolence progressing to seizures and stupor and need to be reported immediately. Hepatotoxicity may result from overdose of the acetaminophen component of fixed-combination products. Some predisposed patients may develop a tolerance to the drug's analgesic effect and physical dependence. Abrupt discontinuation of the drug may result in withdrawal effects.

Storage

Store products at room temperature.

Administration

! Be aware that oxycodone's side effects are dependent on the dosage. Know that ambulatory patients and patients not in severe pain are more likely to experience dizziness, hypotension, nausea, and vomiting than those in the supine position or those in severe pain.

! Swallow controlled-release tablets (OxyContin) whole because crushing, breaking, or chewing them may lead to the rapid release and absorption of a potentially fatal dose. Be aware that OxyContin has a potential for abuse and accidental overdose may result in death.

Take oral oxycodone without regard to food. Crush immediate-release tablets as needed.

Concentrated oral solution: Use care in measuring dose—highly concentrated. May add to 30 mL of liquid or semi-solid food just before administration.

Oxymetazoline
ox-ee-met-az'oh-leen
(Afrin, Afrin 12-Hour, Afrin
Children's Strength Nose
Drops, Ocuclear, Sinex 12-Hour
Long-Acting)

CATEGORY AND SCHEDULE
Pregnancy Risk Category: C
OTC

Classification: Imidazoline
derivative, decongestant

MECHANISM OF ACTION
A direct-acting sympathomimetic
amine that acts on α-adrenergic
receptors in arterioles of the nasal
mucosa to produce constriction.
Therapeutic Effect: Causes vasoconstriction resulting in decreased blood
flow and decreased nasal congestion.

PHARMACOKINETICS
Onset of action is about 10 min, and
duration of action is 7 h or longer.
Absorption occurs from the nasal
mucosa and can produce systemic
effects, primarily following overdose
or excessive use. Excreted mostly
in the urine as well as the feces.
Half-life: 5-8 h.

AVAILABILITY
Eyedrops: 0.025% (Ocuclear).
Nasal Drops: 0.025% (Afrin
Children's Strength Nose Drops),
0.05% (Afrin).
Nasal Spray: 0.05% (Afrin, Afrin
12-Hour, Sinex 12-Hour Long-Acting).

INDICATIONS AND DOSAGES
▸ **Rhinitis**
INTRANASAL
*Adults, Elderly, Children older
than 6 yr.* 2-3 drops/sprays (0.05%
nasal solution) in each nostril q12hr.

Children aged 2-5 yr. 2-4 drops/
sprays (0.025% nasal solution) in
each nostril q12hr for up to 3 days.
▸ **Conjunctival hyperemia**
OPHTHALMIC
*Adults, Elderly, Children older than
6 yr.* 1-2 drops (0.025% ophthalmic
solution) q6hr for 3-4 days.

OFF-LABEL USES
Otitis media surgical procedures.

CONTRAINDICATIONS
Narrow-angle glaucoma or
hypersensitivity to oxymetazoline or
other adrenergic agents, MAOI use.

INTERACTIONS
Drug
MAOIs: Systemic absorption
of oxymetazoline may cause
hypertensive crisis.
**Maprotiline, tricyclic
antidepressants:** May increase the
effects of oxymetazoline.
Herbal
None known.
Food
None known.

DIAGNOSTIC TEST EFFECTS
None known.

SIDE EFFECTS
Occasional
Burning, stinging, drying nasal
mucosa, sneezing, rebound
congestion, insomnia, nervousness.

SERIOUS REACTIONS
• Large doses may produce
tachycardia, hypertension,
arrhythmias, palpitations, light-
headedness, nausea, and vomiting.

PRECAUTIONS & CONSIDERATIONS
Caution is warranted in patients
with cerebral arteriosclerosis,
coronary artery disease, diabetes,

O

heart disease, hypertension, hypertensive cardiovascular disease, concurrent monoamine oxidase inhibitors or tricyclic antidepressants, prostatic enlargement, or hyperthyroidism. It is unknown whether oxymetazoline crosses the placenta and is distributed in breast milk; therefore, caution is warranted in lactation and pregnancy. Safety and efficacy of oxymetazoline have not been established in children younger than 2 yr of age using oxymetazoline intranasally and younger than 6 yr of age using the drug ophthamologically. No age-related precautions have been noted in elderly patients. Excessive or prolonged use of oxymetazoline intranasally should be monitored for rebound nasal congestion or rhinitis medicamentosa or cardiovascular effects. Care using decongestant medications is always warranted in hypertension, even if only applied intranasally. Medical consultation should occur before using this or similar decongestant medications.

Be aware that if oxymetazoline is systemically absorbed it may cause fast, irregular, and pounding heartbeat, headache, insomnia, lightheadedness, nausea, nervousness, and trembling.

Administration

Be aware that oxymetazoline should be used up to 3 days.

Blow nose gently before using the nasal drops. Tilt head back while standing or sitting and squeeze drop in nostril. Keep head tilted back for few minutes. Rinse the dropper with hot water and dry with a clean tissue.

Blow nose gently before using the nasal spray. Stand upright, and spray the medicine once into the nostril, sniffing while squeezing the bottle quickly and firmly. Wait 3-5 min to allow the drug to work, and then blow nose again. Rinse tip of nasal spray with hot water and dry with a clean tissue.

Wash hands before administering oxymetazoline eyedrops. With the middle finger, put pressure to the inside corner of the eye. Tilt the head back and with the index finger of the same hand, and pull the lower eyelid away from the eye to form a pouch. Drop the medicine into the pouch and gently close the eyes. Tell the patient not to blink. Keep the eyes closed for 1-2 min to allow the medicine to be absorbed.

Oxymetholone
ox-ee-meth'oh-lone
(Anadrol, Anapolon [CAN])
Do not confuse with oxycodone or oxandrolone.

CATEGORY AND SCHEDULE
Pregnancy Risk Category: X
Controlled Substance: Schedule III

Classification: Androgenic anabolic steroid.

MECHANISM OF ACTION
An androgenic-anabolic steroid that is a synthetic derivative of testosterone synthesized to accentuate anabolic as opposed to androgenic effects. *Therapeutic Effect:* Improves nitrogen balance in conditions of unfavorable protein metabolism with adequate caloric and protein intake, stimulates erythropoiesis, suppress gonadotropic functions of pituitary and may exert a direct effect upon the testes.

PHARMACOKINETICS

The pharmacokinetics of oxymetholone has been studied. Metabolized in the liver via reduction and oxidation. Unchanged oxymetholone and its metabolites are excreted in urine. *Half-life:* Unknown.

AVAILABILITY

Tablets: 50 mg (Anadrol).

INDICATIONS AND DOSAGES

▸ **Anemia, chronic renal failure, acquired aplastic anemia, chemotherapy-induced myelosuppression, fanconi's anmia, red cell aplasia**
PO
Adults, Elderly, Children.
1-5 mg/kg/day. Response is not immediate, and a minimum of 3-6 mo should be given.

CONTRAINDICATIONS

Cardiac impairment, pregnancy, prostatic or breast cancer in males, metastatic breast cancer in women with active hypercalcemia, nephrosis or nephritic phase nephritis, severe liver disease, hypersensitivity to oxymetholone or any of its components.
Caution
Diabetes mellitus, cardiovascular disease, myocardial infarction (MI), increased risk of benign prostatic hypertrophy, prostatic carcinoma, virilization (women), increased PT.

INTERACTIONS

Drug
ACTH, adrenal steroids: May increase effects of adrenal steroids.
Hepatotoxic medications: May increase liver toxicity.
Insulin, oral hypoglycemics: May increase the effects of hypoglycemic agents.

Oral anticoagulants: May increase effects of oral anticoagulants.
Herbal
Chaparral, comfrey, germander, Jin bu huan: May increase liver enzymes.
Eucalyptus, valerian: May increase risk of heptotoxicity.
Kava kava, pennyroyal, skullcap: May increase risk of liver damage.
Food
None known.

DIAGNOSTIC TEST EFFECTS

May increase blood hemoglobin and hematocrit, LDL concentrations, serum alkaline phosphatase, bilirubin, calcium, potassium, SGOT (AST) levels, and sodium levels. May decrease HDL concentrations.

SIDE EFFECTS

Frequent
Gynecomastia, acne, amenorrhea, menstrual irregularities.
Females: Hirsutism, deepening of voice, clitoral enlargement that may not be reversible when drug is discontinued.
Occasional
Edema, nausea, insomnia, oligospermia, priapism, male pattern of baldness, bladder irritability, hypercalcemia in immobilized patients or those with breast cancer, hypercholesterolemia.
Rare
Liver damage, hypersensitivity.

SERIOUS REACTIONS

• Cholestatic jaundice, hepatic necrosis, and death occur rarely but have been reported in association with long-term androgenic-anabolic steroid use.
• Priapism.

PRECAUTIONS & CONSIDERATIONS

Caution is warranted in patients with diabetes, liver or renal impairment, congestive heart failure, hypertension, coronary artery disease, previous myocardial infarction, lipid-lipoprotein abnormalities, benign prostatic hyperplasia, suppression of clotting factors II, V, VII, and X, and an increase in prothrombin time. Oxymetholone use is contraindicated during lactation and is excreted in breast milk. Safety and efficacy of oxymethalone have not been established in children and elderly patients. Adequate calories and protein should be consumed.

Acne, nausea, pedal edema, or vomiting may occur. Women should report deepening of voice, hoarseness, and menstrual irregularities. Men should report difficulty urinating, frequent erections, and gynecomastia. Weight should be obtained each day. Weekly weight gains of more than 5 lb should be reported.

Administration

Dose should be individualized. Response is not often immediate and a minimum trial of 3-6 mo should be given.

Oxymorphone Hydrochloride

ox-ee-mor'fone high-droh-klor-ide
(Numorphan, Opana, Opana ER)

CATEGORY AND SCHEDULE

Pregnancy Risk Category B, D if used for prolonged periods or at high dosages at term
Controlled Substance: Schedule II

Classification: Opioid analgesics

MECHANISM OF ACTION

An opioid agonist, similar to morphine, that binds at opiate receptor sites in the central nervous system (CNS). *Therapeutic Effec*t: Reduces intensity of pain stimuli incoming from sensory nerve endings, altering pain perception and emotional response to pain; suppresses cough reflex.

PHARMACOKINETICS

Route	Onset (min)	Peak (min)	Duration (h)
SC	5-10	30-90	4-6
IM	5-10	30-60	3-6
IV	5-10	15-30	3-6

Well absorbed from the GI tract after IM administration. Widely distributed. Metabolized in liver via glucuronidation. Excreted in urine. *Half-life:* 1-2 h.

AVAILABILITY

Numorphan
Injection: 1 mg/mL, 1.5 mg/mL
Rectal Suppository: 5 mg.
OPANA
Tablet: 5mg, 10 mg
Injection: 1 mg/mL
OPANA ER
Tablets: 5 mg, 10 mg, 20 mg, 40 mg.

INDICATIONS AND DOSAGES

▸ **Analgesic, anxiety, preanesthesia**
IV
Adults, Elderly, Children 12 yr and older. Initially 0.5 mg.
SC/IM
Adults, Elderly, Children 12 yr and older. 1-1.5 mg IM or SC q4-6h as needed
▸ **Acute or chronic moderate to severe pain**
PO

Adults, Elderly, Children 12 yr and older. 10-20 mg q4-6h (Opana) *or* 5 mg q12h, increasing by 5-10 mg q12h. every 3-7 days (Opana ER). NOTE: Opana ER is not for as-needed use and should be given only to patients needing continuous, around-the-clock pain relief.

▸ **Obstetric analgesic**
IM
Adults, Elderly, Children 12 yr and older. 0.5-1 mg IM during labor.

OFF-LABEL USES
Cancer pain, intractable pain in narcotic-tolerant patients.

CONTRAINDICATIONS
Paralytic ileus, acute asthma attack, pulmonary edema secondary to chemical respiratory irritant, severe respiratory depression, upper airway obstruction, hypersensitivity.

INTERACTIONS
Drug
Anticholinergics: May increase urinary retention and severe constipation.
Alcohol, CNS depressants, tricyclic antidepressants: May increase CNS or respiratory depression, hypotension, profound sedation or coma.
Cimetidine: May increase activity of oxymorphone.
MAOIs: May produce severe, fatal reaction; plan to reduce dose to one quarter usual dose.
Mixed antagonist/agonist opioid analgesics (buprenorphine, butorphanol, nalbuphine, pentazocine): May reduce oxymorphone effects and precipitate withdrawal.
Phenothiazines: May decrease effect of oxymorphone.
Propafol: May increase risk of bradycardia.

Herbal
Ginseng: May decrease opioid analgesic effectiveness.
Gotu kola, kava kava, valerian: May increase CNS or respiratory depression.
St. John's wort: May increase sedation.
Food
Alcohol: Alcohol administration with Opana ER can cause immediate release of high doses and potential fatal overdose.

DIAGNOSTIC TEST EFFECTS
May increase serum amylase levels and plasma lipase concentrations.

Ⓓ IV INCOMPATIBILITIES
No data available.

🖟 IV COMPATIBILITIES
Glycopyrrolate (Robinul), hydroxyzine (Vistaril), ranitidine (Zantac)

SIDE EFFECTS
Frequent
Drowsiness, dizziness, hypotension, decreased appetite, tolerance, or dependence.
Occasional
Confusion, diaphoresis, facial flushing, urinary retention, constipation, dry mouth, nausea, vomiting, headache, pain at injection site, abdominal cramps.
Rare
Allergic reaction, depression.

SERIOUS REACTIONS
• Hypotension, paralytic ileus, respiratory depression, and toxic megacolon rarely occur.
• Overdosage results in respiratory depression, skeletal muscle flaccidity, cold or clammy skin, cyanosis, extreme somnolence progressing to seizures, stupor, and coma.

• Tolerance to analgesic effect and physical dependence may occur with repeated use.
• Prolonged duration of action and cumulative effect may occur in patients with impaired liver or renal function.

PRECAUTIONS & CONSIDERATIONS

Caution is warranted with acute alcoholism, anoxia, CNS depression, hypercapnia, respiratory depression or dysfunction, seizures, shock, untreated myxedema, acute abdominal conditions, Addison disease, chronic obstructive pulmonary disease (COPD), hypothyroidism, impaired liver function, increased intracranial pressure, and urethral stricture. Oxymorphone readily crosses the placenta, and it is unknown whether oxymorphone is distributed in breast milk. Its use may prolong labor if administered in the latent phase of the first stage of labor or before cervical dilation of 4-5 cm has occurred. Respiratory depression may occur in a neonate if the mother receives opiates during labor. Regular use of opiates during pregnancy may produce withdrawal symptoms in the neonate, including diarrhea, excessive crying, fever, hyperactive reflexes, irritability, seizures, sneezing, tremors, vomiting, and yawning. Safety and efficacy of oxymorphone have not been established in children younger than 12 yr. Elderly patients may be more susceptible to respiratory depression, and the drug may cause paradoxical excitement. Age-related prostatic hypertrophy or obstruction and renal impairment may increase the risk of urinary retention, and dosage adjustment is recommended in elderly patients. Alcohol and tasks that require mental alertness and motor skills should be avoided during therapy. Drug dependence and tolerance may occur with prolonged use at high dosages.

Excessive sedation or drowsiness, slow or shallow breathing, low BP, slow heart rate, and severe constipation should be reported to health care providers immediately.

Dizziness, hypotension, nausea, and vomiting may be experienced more frequently than those in supine position or having severe pain.

Storage
Store injection formulation at room temperature and protect from light. Discard unused medication according to procedures for Schedule II controlled substances.

Administration
Oxymorphone's side effects depend on the dosage amount and route of administration but occur infrequently with oral antitussives. A high concentration injection should be used only in patients currently receiving high doses of another opiate agonist for severe, chronic pain caused by cancer or tolerance to opiate agonists. Slight yellow discoloration of parenteral form does not indicate a loss of potency. May give undiluted as IV push.

Unwrap rectal suppository before inserting. Moisten suppository with cold water before inserting well up into rectum.

Opana ER: Do not crush, break, cut or chew; swallow whole. Do not consume with alcohol.

Oxytocin

ox-ee-toe'sin
(Pitocin, Syntocinon INJ [AUS])
**Do not confuse Pitocin with
Pitressin.**

CATEGORY AND SCHEDULE
Pregnancy Risk Category: X

Classification: Exogenous
hormone

MECHANISM OF ACTION
An oxytocic that affects uterine
myofibril activity and stimulates
mammary smooth muscle.
Therapeutic Effect: Contracts
uterine smooth muscle. Enhances
lactation.

PHARMACOKINETICS

Route	Onset	Peak	Duration
IV	Immediate	NA	1 h
IM	3-5 min	NA	2-3 h

Onset of activity almost immediate
with IV administration; 3-5 min
with IM administration. Protein
binding: 30%. Distributed in
extracellular fluid. Metabolized
in the liver and kidney. Primarily
excreted in urine. *Half-life:*
1-6 min.

AVAILABILITY
Injection: 10 units/mL.

INDICATIONS AND DOSAGES
▸ **Induction or stimulation of labor**
IV
Adults. 0.5-1 milliunit/min. May
gradually increase in increments of
1-2 milliunit/min. Rates of
9-10 milliunit/min are rarely
required.

▸ **Abortion, adjunct**
IV
Adults. 10-20 milliunit/min.
Maximum: 30 units in any 12-h period.
▸ **Control of postpartum bleeding**
IV INFUSION
Adults. 10-40 units in 1 L IV fluid at a
rate sufficient to control uterine atony.
IM
Adults. 10 units (total dose) after
delivery.

CONTRAINDICATIONS
Adequate uterine activity that fails to
progress, cephalopelvic disproportion,
fetal distress without imminent
delivery, grand multiparity, hyperactive
or hypertonic uterus, obstetric
emergencies that favor surgical
intervention, prematurity, unengaged
fetal head, unfavorable fetal position or
presentation, when vaginal delivery is
contraindicated, such as active genital
herpes infection, placenta previa, or
cord presentation, invasive cervical
carcinoma, elective induction of labor.

INTERACTIONS
Drug
**Caudal block anesthetics,
vasopressors:** May increase pressor
effects.
Cyclopropane anesthetics: May
cause maternal hypotension,
bradycardia, abnormal AV rhythm.
Other oxytocics: May cause cervical
lacerations, uterine hypertonus, or
uterine rupture.
Herbal
None known.
Food
None known.

DIAGNOSTIC TEST EFFECTS
None known.

ⓘ IV INCOMPATIBILITIES
Amphotericin B, diazepam,
phenytoin, remifentanil.

O

IV COMPATIBILITIES

Heparin, insulin, multivitamins, potassium chloride, sodium bicarbonate, sodium bisulfite.

SIDE EFFECTS

Occasional
Tachycardia, premature ventricular contractions, hypotension, nausea, vomiting.

SERIOUS REACTIONS

• Hypertonicity may occur with tearing of the uterus, increased bleeding, abruptio placentae, and cervical and vaginal lacerations.
• In the fetus, bradycardia, CNS or brain damage, trauma due to rapid propulsion, low Apgar score at 5 min, and retinal hemorrhage occur rarely.
• Prolonged IV infusion of oxytocin with excessive fluid volume has caused severe water intoxication with seizures, coma, and death.

PRECAUTIONS & CONSIDERATIONS

Induction of labor should be for medical, not elective, reasons. Oxytocin should be used as indicated and is not known to cause fetal abnormalities. Oxytocin is present in small amounts in breast milk. Oxytocin is not recommended for use in pregnant women because it may precipitate contractions and abortions. Oxytocin is contraindicated in elective induction of labor. Oxytocin is not used in children or elderly patients.

BP, pulse, respiration rates, intake and output, uterine contractions, including duration, frequency and strength, and fetal heart rate should be monitored every 15 min. If uterine contractions last longer than 1 min, occur more frequently than every 2 min, or stop, notify the physician. Be alert to potential water intoxication and for unexpected or increased blood loss.

Storage
Store at room temperature.
Administration
Dilute 10-40 units (1-4 mL) in 1000 mL of 0.9% NaCl, lactated Ringer's solution, or D5W to provide a concentration of 10-40 mUnits/mL solution. Give by IV infusion and use an infusion device to control prescribed rate of flow.

Paclitaxel

Pak-leh-tax′-ell
(Abraxane, Anzatax [AUS], Onxol,
Taxol)
**Do not confuse paclitaxel with
Paxil or Taxol with Taxotere.**

CATEGORY AND SCHEDULE

Pregnancy Risk Category: D

Classification: Antineoplastic

MECHANISM OF ACTION

An antineoplastic agent in the taxoid
family that disrupts the microtubular
cell network, which is essential for
cellular function. Blocks cells in the
late G2 phase and M phase of the
cell. *Therapeutic Effect:* Inhibits
cellular mitosis and replication.

PHARMACOKINETICS

Does not readily cross the blood-
brain barrier. Protein binding:
89%-98%. Metabolized in the liver
to active metabolites; eliminated
by the bile. Not removed by
hemodialysis. *Half-life:* 1.3-8.6 h.

AVAILABILITY

Injection. 6 mg/mL.
*Injection, Protein-Bound
(Abraxane).* 100 mg.

INDICATIONS AND DOSAGES

▸ **Ovarian cancer**
IV
Adults. 135-175 mg/m²/dose over
3-24 h q3wk.
▸ **Breast carcinoma**
IV (ONXOL, TAXOL)
Adults, Elderly. 175 mg/m²/dose over
3 h q3wk or 135 mg/m² over 24 h.
IV (ABRAXANE)
Adults, Elderly. 260 mg/m² over
30 min q3wk.

▸ **Non–small cell lung carcinoma**
IV
Adults, Elderly. 135 mg/m² over 24 h,
followed by cisplatin 75 mg/m² q3wk.
▸ **Kaposi sarcoma**
IV
Adults, Elderly. 135 mg/m²/dose over
3 h q3wk or 100 mg/m²/dose over 3
h q2wk.
▸ **Dosage in hepatic impairment**
No specific recommendations are
available; dosage adjustment may
be needed based on liver enzymes,
bilirubin levels, disease being treated,
and product selected for use.

CONTRAINDICATIONS

History of hypersensitivity to
paclitaxel or other drugs formulated
in polyoxyethylated castor oil
(Cremophor EL); patients with
solid tumors who have baseline
neutrophils counts < 1500 cells/
mm³ or patients with AIDS-related
Kaposi sarcoma who have baseline
neutrophils counts < 1000 cells/mm³.

INTERACTIONS

Drugs
**Strong CYP2C8 and CYP3A4
isoenzyme inhibitors (diazepam,
ketoconazole, midazolam):** Possible
increase in action.
Herbal
St. John's wort: May decrease
paclitaxel levels.
Food
None known.

Ⓘ IV INCOMPATIBILITIES

Polyvinylchloride (PVC) infusion sets.

SIDE EFFECTS

Expected
Diarrhea, alopecia, nausea, vomiting,
neutropenia.
Frequent
Myalgia or arthralgia, peripheral
neuropathy.

Occasional
Mucositis, hypotension during infusion, pain or redness at injection site, thrombocytopenia.
Rare
Bradycardia, severe hypotension, angioedema, generalized uticaria.

SERIOUS REACTIONS
Severe hypersensitivity reactions, severe cardiac conduction abnormalities, severe peripheral neuropathy.

PRECAUTIONS & CONSIDERATIONS
Administer only under supervision of experienced cancer chemotherapy physician. Caution should be exercised in patients with bone marrow depression, AV block, hepatic impairment, recent myocardial infarction, angina pectoris, history of congestive heart failure, or currently using drug with effect on cardiac conduction system. Neutropenic nadir occurs at approximately day 11 of paclitaxel therapy. Elderly may have higher incidence of severe neuropathy, severe myelosuppression, or cardiovascular events. Avoid use in pregnant or breast-feeding patients. Safety and efficacy not established in children.
Storage
Store at room temperature in original package. Paclitaxel solutions for infusion stable at room temperature for up to 27 h. Paclitaxel protein-bound (Abraxane) solutions prepared for infusion are stable at room temperature up to 8 h.
Administration
Premedicate with dexamethasone, diphenhydramine, and an H_2 antagonist. Infuse through in-line filter. Protein-bound paclitaxel (Abraxane) is not interchangeable with conventional paclitaxel.

Palifermin
pal-ih-fur′min
(Kepivance)

CATEGORY AND SCHEDULE
Pregnancy Risk Category: C

Classification: Keratinocyte growth factor

MECHANISM OF ACTION
An antineoplastic adjunct that binds to the keratinocyte growth factor receptor, present on epithelial cells of the buccal mucosa and tongue, resulting in the proliferation, differentiation, and migration of epithelial cells. *Therapeutic Effect:* Reduces incidence and duration of severe oral mucositis.

PHARMACOKINETICS
Linear pharmacokinetics and extravascular distribution. Total body clearance is twofold to fourfold higher in cancer patients than in healthy volunteers. *Half-life:* 3.3-5.7 h.

AVAILABILITY
Injection: 6.25-mg vials.

INDICATIONS AND DOSAGES
▸ **Mucositis (premyelotoxic therapy)**
IV
Adults, Elderly. 60 mcg/kg/day for 3 consecutive days, with the 3rd dose 24-48 h before chemotherapy.
▸ **Mucositis (postmyelotoxic therapy)**
IV
Adults, Elderly. The last three 60-mcg/kg/day doses should be administered after myelotoxic therapy; the first of these doses should be administered after, but on the same day of, hematopoietic stem cell infusion and at least 4 days after the most recent administration of palfermin.

CONTRAINDICATIONS

Patients allergic to *Escherichia coli*—derived proteins or any component of the product.

INTERACTIONS

Drug
Heparin: Palfermin binds to heparin.
Myelotoxic chemotherapy:
Administration of palifermin during or within 24 h before or after myelotoxic chemotherapy results in increased severity and duration of oral mucositis.
Herbal
None known.
Food
None known.

DIAGNOSTIC TEST EFFECTS

May elevate serum lipase and serum amylase levels.

⊘ IV INCOMPATIBILITIES

Heparin. No other data available.

SIDE EFFECTS

Frequent (28%-62%)
Rash, fever, pruritus, erythema, edema, pain at injection site.
Occasional (10%-17%)
Mouth and tongue thickness or discoloration, altered taste, dysesthesia (hyperesthesia, hypoesthesia, paresthesia), arthralgia.

SERIOUS REACTIONS

• Transient hypertension occurs occasionally.

PRECAUTIONS & CONSIDERATIONS

Use palifermin cautiously in women who are pregnant or breastfeeding. Excretion in breast milk is unknown. Safety and efficacy in children have not been established.
Storage
If not used immediately, the reconstituted solution may be stored in the refrigerator for 24 h. Protect it from light. The reconstituted solution may be warmed to room temperature for up to 1 h before administration. Discard the solution if it is left at room temperature for longer than 1 h or if it becomes discolored or contains particles.
Administration
Reconstitute palifermin using aseptic technique. Slowly inject 1.2 mL of sterile water for injection to yield a final concentration of 5 mg/mL. Swirl gently to dissolve. Do not shake or agitate the solution. Dissolution takes < 3 min. Administer by IV bolus injection. If heparin is being used to maintain an IV line, use 0.9% NaCl to rinse the IV line before and after palifermin administration.

Palonosetron

pal-oh-noe′seh-tron
(Aloxi) [US; not available in Canada]

CATEGORY AND SCHEDULE

Pregnancy Risk Category: B

P

Classification: 5-HT$_3$ receptor antagonist: Antiemetic/antivertigo, serotonin receptor antagonists

MECHANISM OF ACTION

A 5-HT$_3$ receptor antagonist that acts centrally in the chemoreceptor trigger zone and peripherally at the vagal nerve terminals. *Therapeutic Effect:* Prevents nausea and vomiting associated with chemotherapy.

PHARMACOKINETICS

Protein binding: 62%. Eliminated in urine. *Half-life:* 40 h.

AVAILABILITY

Injection: 0.25 mg.

INDICATIONS AND DOSAGES
▶ **Chemotherapy-induced nausea and vomiting associated with moderately and highly emetogenic cancer chemotherapy**
IV
Adults, Elderly. 0.25 mg as a single dose 30 min before starting chemotherapy.

CONTRAINDICATIONS
Hypersensitivity to palonosetron or any inactive ingredient of the product.

INTERACTIONS
Drug
None known.
Herbal
None known.
Food
None known.

DIAGNOSTIC TEST EFFECTS
None are well documented but may transiently increase serum bilirubin, AST (SGOT), and ALT (SGPT) levels.

Ⓟ IV INCOMPATIBILITIES
Do not mix palonosetron with any other drugs.

SIDE EFFECTS
Occasional (5%-9%)
Headache, constipation.
Rare (< 1%)
Diarrhea, dizziness, fatigue, abdominal pain, insomnia, anxiety, hyperkalemia, weakness.

SERIOUS REACTIONS
• Overdose may produce a combination of central nervous system (CNS) stimulant and depressant effects: Nonsustained tachycardia, bradycardia, hypotension.

PRECAUTIONS & CONSIDERATIONS
Caution is warranted in patients with history of cardiovascular disease. It is unknown whether palonosetron is excreted in breast milk. The safety and efficacy of palonosetron have not been established in children. No age-related precautions have been noted for elderly patients.

Hypersensitivity may occur in patients who have exhibited hypersensitivity to other selective 5-HT$_3$ receptor antagonists.

Administer with caution in patients who have or may develop prolongation of cardiac conduction intervals, particularly QTc.

Alcohol, barbiturates, and tasks that require mental alertness or motor skills should be avoided.

Dizziness or drowsiness may occur. Pattern of daily bowel activity and stool consistency and hydration status should be monitored. Intolerable headache, persistent or intolerable constipation or diarrhea could be indicative of a serious reaction and should be reported immediately.
Storage
Store vials at room temperature. The solution normally appears clear and colorless. Discard it if it appears cloudy or contains precipitate.
Administration
Give the drug undiluted as an IV push over 30 s. Flush the IV line with 0.9% NaCl before and after administration.

Pamidronate Disodium
pam-id'drow-nate
(Aredia)
Do not confuse with Adriamycin.

CATEGORY AND SCHEDULE
Pregnancy Risk Category: D

Drug Class: Bone resorption inhibitor, electrolyte modifier

Classification: Bisphosphonates

MECHANISM OF ACTION
A bisphosphate that binds to bone and inhibits osteoclast-mediated calcium resorption. *Therapeutic Effect:* Lowers serum calcium concentrations.

USES
Treatment of moderate to severe Paget disease, mild to moderate hypercalcemia associated with malignancy with or without bone metastases, osteolytic bone metastases in bone cancer, and multiple myeloma patients.

PHARMACOKINETICS

Route	Onset	Peak	Duration
IV	24-48 h	5-7 days	NA

After IV administration, rapidly absorbed by bone. Slowly excreted unchanged in urine. Unknown whether removed by hemodialysis. *Half-life:* bone, 300 days; unmetabolized, 2.5 h.

AVAILABILITY
Powder for Injection: 30 mg, 90 mg.
Injection Solution: 3 mg/mL, 6 mg/mL, 9 mg/mL.

INDICATIONS AND DOSAGES
▸ **Hypercalcemia**
IV INFUSION
Adults, Elderly. Moderate hypercalcemia (corrected serum calcium level 12-13.5 mg/dL): 60-90 mg over 2-24 h. Severe hypercalcemia (corrected serum calcium level >13.5 mg/dL): 90 mg over 2-24 h.
▸ **Paget disease**
IV INFUSION
Adults, Elderly. 30 mg/day over 4 h for 3 days.
▸ **Osteolytic bone lesion**
IV INFUSION
Adults, Elderly. 90 mg over 4 h once a month.

OFF-LABEL USES
Postmenopausal osteoporosis; hyperparathyroidism; prevention of glucocorticoid-induced osteoporosis; reduction of bone pain in patients with prostatic carcinoma; immobilization-related hypercalcemia.

CONTRAINDICATIONS
Hypersensitivity to other bisphosphonates, such as etidronate, tiludronate, risedronate, and alendronate.

INTERACTIONS
Drug
Calcium-containing medications, vitamin D, and antacids: Possible antagonism of pamidronate in treatment of hypercalcemia.
Herbal and Food
None known.

DIAGNOSTIC TEST EFFECTS
May decrease serum phosphate, magnesium, calcium, and potassium levels.

ⓦ IV INCOMPATIBILITIES
Calcium-containing IV fluids, including lactated Ringer's solutions.

P

SIDE EFFECTS

Frequent (> 10%)
Temperature elevation (at least 1° C)
24-48 h after administration; redness,
swelling, induration, pain at catheter
site in patients receiving 90 mg;
anorexia, nausea, fatigue.
Occasional (1%-10%)
Constipation, rhinitis.

SERIOUS REACTIONS

• Hypophosphatemia, hypokalemia,
hypomagnesemia, and hypocalcemia
occur more frequently with higher
dosages.
• Anemia, hypertension, tachycardia,
atrial fibrillation, and somnolence
occur more frequently with 90-mg
doses.
• GI hemorrhage occurs rarely.
• Deterioration in renal function that
may lead to renal failure.
• Osteonecrosis of the jaw.

PRECAUTIONS & CONSIDERATIONS

Hypersensitivity to other
bisphosphonates: etidronate,
tiledronate, risedronate, alendronate,
and zoledronic acid. Dental
implants are contraindicated for
patients taking this drug. Caution
is warranted with cardiac failure
and renal impairment. Because no
adequate and well-controlled studies
have been conducted in pregnant
women, it is unknown whether
pamidronate causes fetal harm or
is excreted in breast milk. Safety
and efficacy of pamidronate have
not been established in children.
Elderly patients may become
overhydrated and require careful
monitoring of fluid and electrolytes.
Dilute the drug in a smaller volume
for elderly patients. Avoid drugs
containing calcium and vitamin D,
such as antacids, because they
might antagonize the effects of
pamidronate.

Hematocrit, hemoglobin, BUN,
creatinine levels, and serum
electrolyte levels, including serum
calcium levels, should be established.
Pattern of daily bowel activity
and stool consistency, BP, pulse,
and temperature should also be
monitored.

Storage
Store parenteral form at room
temperature. The reconstituted vial
is stable for 24 h when refrigerated;
the IV solution is stable for 24 h after
dilution.

Administration
Reconstitute each 30-mg vial with
10 mL sterile water for injection to
provide concentration of 3 mg/mL.
Allow the drug to dissolve before
withdrawing. Further dilute with
1000 mL sterile 0.45% or 0.9%
NaCl or D5W. Administer as IV
infusion over 2-24 h for treatment of
hypercalcemia and over 4 h for other
indications. Adequate hydration
is essential during pamidronate
administration. Avoid overhydration
in those with the potential for heart
failure. Be alert for potential GI
hemorrhage in those receiving a
90-mg dose.

Pancrelipase
pan-kre-li'pase
(Ku-Zyme, Pancreatin)(Cotazym-S
[AUS], Cotazym-S Forte [AUS], Creon,
Pancrease [CAN], Pancrease MT,
Ultrase, Viokase)

CATEGORY AND SCHEDULE
Pregnancy Risk Category: B
(Pancrease MT)
Pregnancy Risk Category: C
(Creon, Kuzyme, Kuzyme HP,
Kutrase, Lipram, Pancrelipase,
Panokase, Plaretase, ultrase,
Ultrase MT, Viokase)

Drug Class: Digestant

Classification: Enzymes,
gastrointestinal, gastrointestinals

MECHANISM OF ACTION
Digestive enzymes that replace
endogenous pancreatic enzymes.
Therapeutic Effect: Assist in
digestion of protein, starch, and fats.

AVAILABILITY
Capsules (Delayed Release): Creon
5 [US, CAN], Creon 10 [US, CAN],
Creon 20 [US, CAN].
Capsules: Kutrase, Kuzyme,
Kuzyme HP, Lipram 4500, Lipram
PN-10, Lipram PN-16, Lipram
PN-20, Pancrease MT [CAN]
Pancrease MT-4, Pancrease MT-10,
Pancrease MT-20, Pancrecarb MS-4,
Pancrecarb MS-8, Ultrase, Ultrase
MT-12, Ultrase MT-18, Ultrase
MT-20
Tablets: Pancrelipase, Panokase,
Plaretase 8000, Viokase 8, Viokase 16.
Powder: Viokase.

PHARMACOKINETICS
Not studied.

INDICATIONS AND DOSAGES
▶ **Pancreatic enzyme replacement
or supplement when enzymes are
absent or deficient, such as with
chronic pancreatitis, cystic fibrosis,
or ductal obstruction from cancer of
the pancreas or common bile duct;
to reduce malabsorption; treatment
of steatorrhea associated with
bowel resection or postgastrectomy
syndrome**
Dosages are adjusted based on
severity of the exocrine pancreatic
enzyme deficiency, and dosage varies
with the brand and formulation. Take
with meals or snacks.
PO
Adults, Elderly. KuZyme,
Pancrecarb, Ultrase, Ultrase MT:
Start with 1-2 capsules with each
meal or snack.
   Kutrase: Take 1 capsule with each
meal or snack.
   Ku-Zyme HP: Take 1-3 capsules
with each meal or snack; with severe
deficiencies, increase the dose to 8
capsules with meals or increase the
frequency to hourly intervals if nausea,
diarrhea, or vomiting does not occur.
   Pancrease, Lipram: Take 4000-
20,000 lipase units with each meal
or snack.
   Creon 5: Start with 2-4 capsules
with each meal or snack.
   Creon 10: Start with 1-2 capsules
with each meal or snack.
   Creon 20: Start with 1 capsule
with each meal or snack.
   Panokase, Plaretase, Viokase
(tablets): Adults with cystic fibrosis
or chronic pancreatitis patients: Dose
ranges from 8000 to 32,000 lipase
units (1-4 tablets [Plaretase, Panokase,
Viokase 8] or 1-2 tablets [Viokase
16]) with each meal or snack. Adults
with pancreatectomy or obstruction
of pancreatic ducts: Dose 1-2 tablets
(Plaretase, Panokase or Viokase 8) or
1 tablet (Viokase 16) every 2 h.

P

Viokase *Powder:* Adults with cystic fibrosis: Dose up to 7 g (¼ tsp) with each meal.

Children. Pancrease MT-4: Children 4 yr or older: Start with 400 lipase units/kg/meal. Maximum: 2500 lipase units/kg/meal. Children younger than 4 yr: Start with 1000 lipase units/kg with each meal. Maximum: 2500 lipase units/kg with each meal: Infants up to 12 mo: 2000-4000 lipase units/120 mL of formula or breast milk.

Pancrease, Lipram: Children 7-12 yr: take 4000-12,000 lipase units with each meal or snack. Children 1-6 yr: take 4000-8000 lipase units with each meal or snack. Children 6 mo to < 1 yr: Take 2000 lipase units with each meal.

Creon 5: Children 6 yr or older: Start with 2-4 capsules with each meal or snack. Children younger than 6 yr: Start with 1-2 capsules with each meal or snack; select exact dose based on clinical experience with age group. Children with cystic fibrosis: Usual dose is 1500-3000 lipase units/kg with each meal. Maximum: 6000 lipase units/kg/meal.

Creon 10: Children 6 yr or older: Start with 1-2 capsules with each meal or snack. Children younger than 6 yr: Start with 1 capsule per meal or snack. Children with cystic fibrosis: Usual dose is 1500-3000 lipase units/kg with each meal. Maximum: 6000 lipase units/kg/meal.

Creon 20: Children 6 yr or older: Select exact dose based on clinical experience with this age group. Children with cystic fibrosis: Usual starting dose is 1500-3000 lipase units/kg with each meal. Maximum: 6000 lipase units/kg/meal.

CONTRAINDICATIONS

Acute pancreatitis, exacerbation of chronic pancreatitis, hypersensitivity to pork protein or enzymes.

INTERACTIONS
Drug
Antacids: May decrease the effects of pancreatin and pancrelipase.
Iron supplements: May decrease the absorption of iron supplements.
Herbal
None known.
Food
None known.

DIAGNOSTIC TEST EFFECTS
None well documented; may increase serum uric acid level.

SIDE EFFECTS
Rare
Allergic reaction, mouth irritation, shortness of breath, wheezing.
GI
Colonic strictures, diarrhea, abdominal pain, intestinal obstruction, vomiting, intestinal stenosis, constipation, flatulence, nausea, bloating and cramping.
Dermatologic
Perianal irritation.

SERIOUS REACTIONS
• Excessive dosage may produce nausea, vomiting, bloating, constipation, cramping, and diarrhea.
• Hyperuricosuria and hyperuricemia have occurred with extremely high dosages.

PRECAUTIONS & CONSIDERATIONS
Products are not bioequivalent; drugs should not be changed or substituted without the advice of a medical practitioner. Pancreatin and pancrelipase should be used cautiously because inhalation of the powder form may precipitate an asthma attack. It is unknown whether pancreatin or pancrelipase crosses the placenta or is distributed in breast milk. Information is not available on pancreatin or pancrelipase

P

use in children. No age-related precautions have been noted in elderly patients. Tell the physician if the patient is allergic to pork because hypersensitivity to pancreatin and pancrelipase may exist. Colonic strictures are reported primarily in cystic fibrosis patients, often at dosages above the recommended range.

Administration

Take pancreatin or pancrelipase before or with meals or snacks. Do not crush enteric-coated form. Do not chew capsules or tablets to minimize irritation to the mouth, lips, and tongue. If patient is unable to swallow capsules, open capsules and spread contents over applesauce, mashed fruit, or rice cereal. Spilling Viokase powder on the hands may irritate skin. Inhaling powder may irritate mucous membranes and produce bronchospasm.

Panitumumab

Pan-ih-tu-mue′-mab
(Vectibix)

CATEGORY AND SCHEDULE

Pregnancy Risk Category: C.

Classification: Antineoplastic agent

MECHANISM OF ACTION

An antineoplastic agent that binds specifically to epidermal growth factor receptor (EGFR) on normal and tumor cells and competitively inhibits the binding of ligands for EGFR. Blocks phosphorylation and activation of intracellular tyrosine kinases, resulting in inhibition of cell survival, growth, proliferation and transformation. *Therapeutic Effect:* Inhibits growth and survival of selected human tumor cell lines expressing EGFR.

PHARMACOKINETICS

Pharmacokinetic parameters other than *half-life* have not been established. Half-life: 4-11 days.

AVAILABILITY

Injection Solution: 20 mg/mL.

INDICATIONS AND DOSAGES

▸ **EGFR-positive metastatic colorectal cancer**

IV

Adults. 6 mg/kg administered over 60 min every 14 days. Doses >1000 mg should be administered over 90 min.

▸ **Dosing adjustments**

INFUSION REACTIONS

Infusion reactions, mild to moderate (grade 1 or 2): Reduce the infusion rate by 50% for the duration of infusion.

Infusion reactions, severe (grade 3 or 4): Immediately and permanently discontinue.

▸ **Dermatologic toxicity**

Dermatologic toxicity (grade 3 or 4): Withhold panitumumab if skin toxicity does not improve to grade 2 or lower within 1 mo; permanently discontinue.

Dermatologic toxicity (grade 2 or lower) and the patient is symptomatically improved after withholding no more than 2 doses of panitumumab. Treatment may be resumed at 50% the original dose. If toxicities recur, permanently discontinue drug. If toxicities do not recur, subsequent doses may be increased in increments of 25% of the original dose until the recommended dose of 6 mg/kg is obtained.

P

INTERACTIONS

Drug

Aspirin, NSAIDs: Increased GI irritation, nausea, vomiting.
Irinotecan: Increased frequency and severity of diarrhea.
Chemotherapy: Increased toxicity with combination chemotherapy.

Food and Herbal

None reported.

SIDE EFFECTS

Frequent

Dermatologic toxicity, erythema, acneiform rash, pruritus, hypomagnesemia, fatigue, exfoliation, abdominal pain, paronychia, nausea, rash, diarrhea, constipation, fissures, vomiting, cough, acne, peripheral edema, dry skin.

Occasional

Nail disorder, stomatitis, mucositis, eyelash growth, conjunctivitis, ocular hyperemia, lacrimation increased.

Rare

Infusion reactions, eye/eyelid irritation.

SERIOUS REACTIONS

Dermatologic toxicities, severe infusion-related reactions, pulmonary fibrosis.

PRECAUTIONS & CONSIDERATIONS

EGFR testing necessary to identify patients eligible for therapy. Use caution in patients with any hypersensitivities to panitumumab or its components. Sunlight may exacerbate skin reactions. Increased toxicity has been observed in patients receiving panitumumab in combination with chemotherapy. Safety and efficacy in children have not been established. Avoid use in pregnancy; use contraception during and for 6 mo after the last dose. Avoid breastfeeding during and for 2 mo after the last dose.

Storage

Store vials in original cartons in refrigerator. Protect from sunlight. Use diluted solution within 6 h of preparation if stored at room temperature or within 24 h if stored in the refrigerator.

Administration

Dilute solution with NS. Infuse over 60 min; doses over 1000 mg should be infused over 90 min. Administer with IV infusion pump using a low-protein binding 0.2- or 0.22-micrometer in-line filter. Flush line with NS before and after administration.

Pantoprazole

pan-toe-pra′zole
(Protonix, Pantoloc, Somac [AUS])
Do not confuse Protonix with Lotronex.

CATEGORY AND SCHEDULE

Pregnancy Risk Category: B

Classification: Gastrointestinals, proton pump inhibitors

MECHANISM OF ACTION

A benzimidazole that is converted to active metabolites that irreversibly bind to and inhibit hydrogen-potassium adenosine triphosphate, an enzyme on the surface of gastric parietal cells. Inhibits hydrogen ion transport into gastric lumen. *Therapeutic Effect:* Increases gastric pH and reduces gastric acid production.

PHARMACOKINETICS

Route	Onset	Peak	Duration
PO	NA	NA	24 h

Rapidly absorbed from the GI tract. Protein binding: 98%. Primarily

distributed into gastric parietal cells. Metabolized extensively in the liver. Excreted primarily in urine. Not removed by hemodialysis.
Half-life: 1 h.

AVAILABILITY

Tablets (Delayed-Release): 20 mg, 40 mg.
Powder for Injection: 40 mg.

INDICATIONS AND DOSAGES
▸ **Erosive esophagitis**
PO
Adults, Elderly. 40 mg/day for up to 8 wks. If not healed after 8 wks, may continue an additional 8 wks.
IV
Adults, Elderly. 40 mg/day for 7-10 days.
▸ **Hypersecretory conditions: Zollinger-Ellison syndrome**
PO
Adults, Elderly. Initially, 40 mg twice a day. May increase to 240 mg/day.
IV
Adults, Elderly. 80 mg twice a day. May increase to 80 mg q8h.

CONTRAINDICATIONS
Contraindicated in patients with known hypersensitivity to any component of the formulation.

INTERACTIONS
Drug
Atazanavir: Pantoprazole substantially decreases therapeutic effect.
Warfarin: Possible increases in INR and prothrombin time.
Ketoconazole, ampicillin esters, iron salts: Pantoprazole may interfere with drug absorption.
Herbal
None known.
Food
None known.

DIAGNOSTIC TEST EFFECTS
May increase serum creatinine, cholesterol, and uric acid levels.

⊘ IV INCOMPATIBILITIES
Do not mix with other medications. Flush IV with D5W, 0.9% NaCl, or lactated Ringer's solution before and after administration.

SIDE EFFECTS
Rare (< 2%)
Diarrhea, headache, dizziness, pruritus, rash.

SERIOUS REACTIONS
• Anaphylaxis (rare), other serious hypersensitivity reactions.

PRECAUTIONS & CONSIDERATIONS
Caution is warranted in patients with a chronic or current hepatic disease. It is unknown whether pantoprazole crosses the placenta or is distributed in breast milk. Safety and efficacy of pantoprazole have not been established in children. No age-related precautions have been noted in elderly patients. Serum chemistry laboratory values, including serum creatinine and cholesterol levels, should be obtained before therapy.
Storage
Refrigerate vials and protect from light; do not freeze reconstituted vials. Once diluted, the drug is stable for 2 h at room temperature.
Administration
Take oral pantoprazole without regard to meals. Do not crush or split tablet; swallow tablet whole.
    For IV use, mix 40-mg vial with 10 mL 0.9% NaCl injection. Infuse over 2 min or 15 min.
    Do not administer by IV push or any other parenteral routes other than IV infusion.

P

Paregoric
par-e-gor'ik
Do not confuse with opium tincture.

CATEGORY AND SCHEDULE
Pregnancy Risk Category: B, D if used for prolonged periods, high dosages at term
Controlled Substance: It is now Schedule II (since it is derived from schedule II opium tincture)

Classification: Opioid analgesic

MECHANISM OF ACTION
An opioid agonist that contains many narcotic alkaloids including morphine. It inhibits gastric motility because of its morphine content. *Therapeutic Effect:* Decreases digestive secretions and increases in GI muscle tone. Inhibits propulsive contractions of circular and longitudinal GI muscles.

PHARMACOKINETICS
Variably absorbed from the GI tract. Protein binding: low. Rapidly metabolized in liver following oral administration. Excreted primarily in urine primarily as morphine glucuronide conjugates and unchanged drug—morphine, codeine, papaverine, etc. Unknown whether removed by hemodialysis. *Half-life:* 2-3 h.

AVAILABILITY
Liquid Anhydrous Morphine Equivalent per Milliliter to Paregoric: Liquid 2 mg anhydrous morphine/5 mL.

INDICATIONS AND DOSAGES
▸ **Antidiarrheal**
PO

Adults, Elderly. As paregoric. 5-10 mL 1-4 times/day.
Children. 0.25-0.5 mL/kg/dose 1-4 times/day.

OFF-LABEL USES
Narcotic withdrawal symptoms in neonates.

CONTRAINDICATIONS
Children: Diarrhea caused by poisoning until the toxic material is removed; Diarrhea caused by infectious agent; hypersensitivity to morphine sulfate or any component of the formulation; pregnancy (prolonged use or high dosages near term); liver disease; addiction-prone individuals.

INTERACTIONS
Drug
Alcohol, central nervous system (CNS) depressants: May increase CNS or respiratory depression, and hypotension.
Cimetidine: Monitor for increased respiratory and CNS depression, apnea, confusion, and muscle twitching.
MAOIs, tricyclic antidepressants: May produce severe reactions.
Herbal
None known.
Food
None known.

DIAGNOSTIC TEST EFFECTS
None known.

SIDE EFFECTS
Frequent
Constipation, drowsiness, nausea, vomiting.
Occasional
Paradoxical excitement, confusion, pounding heartbeat, facial flushing, decreased urination, blurred vision, dizziness, dry mouth, headache,

hypotension, decreased appetite, redness, burning, respiratory depression.

Rare

Hallucinations, depression, stomach pain, insomnia.

SERIOUS REACTIONS

• Overdosage results in nausea, vomiting, miosis, cold or clammy skin, confusion, convulsions, decreased BP, restlessness, pinpoint pupils, bradycardia, CNS or respiratory depression, decreased level of consciousness (LOC), and severe weakness, skeletal muscle flaccidity, noncardiogenic pulmonary edema, hypoglycemia, circulatory collapse, cardiac arrest, death.

• Tolerance to analgesic effect and physical dependence may occur with repeated use.

PRECAUTIONS & CONSIDERATIONS

Cautious use in debilitated individuals, patients with increased intracranial pressure, cerebral arteriosclerosis, hepatic cirrhosis or liver insufficiency, GI hemorrhage, myxedema, emphysema, and bronchial asthma.

Extreme caution is warranted in patients with acute alcoholism; CNS or respiratory depression; hepatic, renal, or respiratory dysfunction; severe prostatic hyperplasia; history of narcotic abuse; and seizures. Paregoric crosses the placenta and is distributed in breast milk. Be aware that respiratory depression may occur in the neonate if the mother received opiates during labor. Regular use of opiates during pregnancy may produce withdrawal symptoms in the neonate, such as diarrhea, excessive crying, fever, hyperactive reflexes, irritability, seizures, sneezing, tremors, vomiting, and yawning. Children may experience paradoxical excitement.

Safety and efficacy in children have not been established. Be aware that children younger than 3 mo and elderly patients are more susceptible to the respiratory depressant effects of paregoric. Paregoric use in elderly patients may mask dehydration and electrolyte depletion.

Drowsiness and dizziness may occur during treatment. Avoid tasks that require mental alertness or motor skills until response to the drug is established. Change positions slowly to avoid orthostatic hypotension.

Storage

Store away from heat and direct light.

Administration

! Be aware that paregoric, or camphorated tincture of opium, is not the same as opium tincture. Paregoric has just 0.4 mg/mL of morphine, whereas opium tincture contains 10 mg/mL—a 25-fold difference.

Use a dosing syringe, dosing cup, or dosing spoon to ensure proper dosing. Can be given with or without regard to food.

P

Paricalcitol
pare-i-cal′sih-tal
(Zemplar)

CATEGORY AND SCHEDULE
Pregnancy Risk Category: C

Classification: Vitamins/minerals

MECHANISM OF ACTION

A fat-soluble vitamin that is essential for absorption, utilization of calcium phosphate, and normal calcification

of bone. *Therapeutic Effect:*
Stimulates calcium and phosphate
absorption from the small intestine,
promotes the secretion of calcium
from bone to blood, promotes renal
tubule phosphate resorption, acts on
bone cells to stimulate skeletal growth
and on parathyroid gland to suppress
hormone synthesis and secretion.

PHARMACOKINETICS

Protein binding: more than 99%.
Metabolized in the liver by multiple
hepatic enzymes, including
CYP3A4. Eliminated primarily in
feces; minimal excretion in urine.
Not removed by hemodialysis. *Half-life:* 13-17 h.

AVAILABILITY

Injection: 5 mcg/mL (Zemplar).

USES

Hyperparathyrodism associated
with chronic kidney disease stage
3, 4, and 5.

INDICATIONS AND DOSAGES

▸ **Hyperparathyrodism**
IV (STAGE 5)
Adults, Elderly, Children.
0.04-0.1 mcg/kg (2.8-7.0 mcg) given
as a bolus dose no more frequently
than every other day during dialysis;
dose as high as 0.24 mcg/kg
(16.8 mcg) has been administered
safely. Usually start with 0.04 mcg/kg
3 times/wk as a bolus, increased by
0.04 mcg/kg every 2 wks.
*Dose adjustment based on serum
PTH levels:*
Serum PTH level decreased by
< 30%, is same or increasing:
Increase dose by 2-4 mg/dose.
Serum PTH level decreased > 30%
or < 60% or are 1.5-3 times upper
limit of normal. Maintain dose.
Serum PTH level decreased > 60%:
Decrease dose.

PO
*Dose adjustment (stages 3 and 4)
based on baseline serum intact
(IPTH) PTH levels:*
iPTH ≤ 500 pg/mL. Initially with
PTH, > 500 pg/mL. 1 mcg daily or
2 mcg 3 times/wk.
Initially, 2 mcg daily or 4 mcg
3 times/wk.
Serum iPTH level decreased by < 30%:
Increase dose by 1 mcg daily or 2 mcg
3 times/wk.
Serum iPTH level decreased by > 30%
and < 60%: Maintain dose
Serum iPTH level decrease by > 60%
or iPTH < 60 pg/mL: Decrease dose
by 1 mcg daily or 2 mcg 3times/wk.

CONTRAINDICATIONS

Hypercalcemia, malabsorption
syndrome, vitamin D toxicity,
hypersensitivity to other vitamin D
products or analogues.

INTERACTIONS

Drug
**Aluminum-containing antacid
(long-term use):** May increase
aluminum concentration and
aluminum bone toxicity.
**Calcium-containing preparations,
thiazide diuretics:** May increase the
risk of hypercalcemia.
**Cholestyramine and other
fat-absorbing impairing drugs:**
May decrease absorption.
Digoxin: May increase the risk of
digitalis toxicity.
Magnesium-containing antacids:
May increase magnesium
concentration.
Strong CYP3A4 inhibitors:
Atazanavir, clarithromycin,
indinavir, itraconazole, ketoconazole,
nefazodone, nelfinavir, ritonavir,
saquinavir, telithromycin,
variconazole: increases risk of toxicity.
Herbal
None known.

Food
None known.

DIAGNOSTIC TEST EFFECTS
May decrease serum alkaline phosphatase.

SIDE EFFECTS
Occasional
Edema, nausea, vomiting, headache, dizziness.
Rare
Palpitations.

SERIOUS REACTIONS
• Early signs of overdosage are manifested as headache, somnolence, hypercalcemia, anorexia, nausea, vomiting, dry mouth, constipation, muscle and bone pain, and metallic taste sensation, weakness.
• Later signs of overdosage are evidenced by hypercalcemia, hypercalciuria, hyperphosphatemia, oversuppression of PTH, polyuria, polydipsia, anorexia, weight loss, nocturia, photophobia, rhinorrhea, pruritus, disorientation, hallucinations, hyperthermia, hypertension, and cardiac arrhythmias.
• Hypercalcemia occurs rarely.

PRECAUTIONS & CONSIDERATIONS
Caution is necessary in concomitant use of digoxin. It is unknown whether paricalcitol crosses the placenta or is distributed in breast milk. Safety and efficacy have not been established in children younger than 5 yr. No age-related precautions have been noted in elderly patients. Consume foods rich in vitamin D, including eggs, leafy vegetables, margarine, meats, milk, vegetable oils, and vegetable shortening.

Serum alkaline phosphatase, BUN, serum calcium, serum creatinine, serum magnesium, serum phosphate,

and urinary calcium levels should be monitored monthly once therapeutic dosage is established for 3 mo, then every 3 mo thereafter. The therapeutic serum calcium level is 9-10 mg/dL.
Storage
Store at room temperature.
Administration
Give injection form as an IV bolus dose no more frequently than every other day, given at any time during dialysis. Capsules may be administered without regard to food. Discard any unused portion.

Paromomycin
par-oh-moe-mye′sin
(Humatin)
Do not confuse with Humira.

CATEGORY AND SCHEDULE
Pregnancy Risk Category: C

Classification: Amebicide: antibiotics, aminoglycosides, antiprotozoals

P

MECHANISM OF ACTION
An antibacterial agent that acts directly on amoebas and against normal and pathogenic organisms in the GI tract. Interferes with bacterial protein synthesis by binding to 30S ribosomal subunits. *Therapeutic Effect*: Produces amoebicidal effects.

PHARMACOKINETICS
Poorly absorbed from the GI tract; most of the dose is eliminated unchanged in feces.

AVAILABILITY
Capsules: 250 mg (Humantin).

INDICATIONS AND DOSAGES
▶ **Intestinal amebiasis**
PO
Adults, Elderly, Children.
25-35 mg/kg/day q8h for 9-10 days.
▶ **Hepatic coma**
PO
Adults, Elderly. 4 g/day q6-12h for
5-10 days.

OFF-LABEL USES
Cryptosporidiosis, giardiasis,
leishmaniasis, microsporidiosis,
mycobacterial infections, tapeworm
infestation, trichomoniasis, typhoid
carriers.

CONTRAINDICATIONS
Intestinal obstruction, ileus,
renal failure, hypersensitivity
to paromomycin or any of its
components.

INTERACTIONS
Drug
Digoxin: May decrease digoxin
serum concentrations and efficacy.
Herbal
None known.
Food
Xylose, sucrose, fats: May cause
decreased absorption of xylose,
sucrose, and fats.

DIAGNOSTIC TEST EFFECTS
May increase LDH concentrations,
SGOT (AST) and SGPT (ALT) levels.

SIDE EFFECTS
Occasional
Diarrhea, abdominal cramps, nausea,
vomiting, heartburn.
Rare
Rash, pruritus, vertigo.

SERIOUS REACTIONS
• Nephrotoxicity (rare), ototoxicity
(rare). Overdosage may result in
nausea, vomiting, and diarrhea.

PRECAUTIONS & CONSIDERATIONS
Caution should be used in patients
with proven ulcerative bowel disease.
Be aware that paromomycin is
contraindicated in renal failure.
Liver and renal function tests should
be performed before administering
paromomycin. It is unknown whether
paromomycin crosses the placenta
and is distributed in breast milk.
No precautions have been noted
in children or elderly patients.
Impaired hearing should be reported
immediately.
   Sore throat, oral burning
sensations, fever or fatigue,
any or all can be indicative of
superinfection and should be
reported immediately.
Administration
Give with meals. Take full course of
therapy and do not skip doses.

Paroxetine Hydrocholoride
par-ox′e-teen
(Paxeva, Paxil, Paxil CR)
**Do not confuse paroxetine with
pyridoxine or Paxil with Doxil
or Taxol.**

CATEGORY AND SCHEDULE
Pregnancy Risk Category: C

Classification: Antidepressants,
serotonin specific reuptake
inhibitors

MECHANISM OF ACTION
An antidepressant, anxiolytic,
and antiobsessional agent that

selectively blocks uptake of the neurotransmitter serotonin at neuronal presynaptic membranes, thereby increasing its availability at postsynaptic receptor sites. *Therapeutic Effect:* Relieves depression, reduces obsessive-compulsive behavior, decreases anxiety.

PHARMACOKINETICS

Well absorbed from the GI tract. Protein binding: 95%. Widely distributed. Metabolized in the liver. Excreted in urine. Not removed by hemodialysis. *Half-life:* 15-20 h.

AVAILABILITY

Oral Suspension (Paxil):
10 mg/5 mL.
Tablets (Paxil, Pexeva): 10 mg, 20 mg, 30 mg, 40 mg.
Tablets (Controlled-Release [Paxil CR]): 12.5 mg, 25 mg, 37.5 mg.

INDICATIONS AND DOSAGES
▸ **Major depressive disorder**
PO
Adults. Initially, 20 mg/day. May increase by 10 mg/day at intervals of more than 1 wk. Maximum: 50 mg/day.
PO (CONTROLLED-RELEASE)
Adults. Initially, 25 mg/day. May increase by 12.5 mg/day at intervals of more than 1 wk. Maximum: 62.5 mg/day.
▸ **Generalized anxiety disorder**
PO
Adults. Initially, 20 mg/day. May increase by 10 mg/day at intervals of more than 1 wk. Range: 20-50 mg/day.
▸ **Obsessive compulsive disorder**
PO
Adults. Initially, 20 mg/day. May increase by 10 mg/day at intervals of more than 1 wk. Range: 20-60 mg/day.

▸ **Panic disorder**
PO
Adults. Initially, 10-20 mg/day. May increase by 10 mg/day at intervals of more than 1 wk. Range: 10-60 mg/day.
PO (CONTROLLED-RELEASE)
Adults. Initially 12.5 mg/day. May increase by 12.5 mg/day at intervals of more than 1 wk. Maximum: 75 mg/day.
▸ **Social anxiety disorder**
PO
Adults. Initially 20 mg/day. May increase by 10 mg/day at intervals of > 1 wk. Range: 20-60 mg/day.
PO (CONTROLLED-RELEASE)
Adults. Initially, 12.5 mg/day. May increase by 12.5 mg/day at intervals of more than 1 wk. Maximum: 37.5 mg/day.
▸ **Posttraumatic stress disorder**
PO
Adults. Initially, 20 mg/day. May increase by 10 mg/day at intervals of more than 1 wk. Range: 20-60 mg/day.
▸ **Premenstrual dysphoric disorder**
PO
Adults. (Paxil CR) Initially, 12.5 mg/day. May increase by 12.5 mg at weekly intervals to a maximum of 37.5 mg/day.

CONTRAINDICATIONS

Use within 14 days of MAOIs.
Caution
Lactation, elderly patients, oral anticoagulants, renal or hepatic impairment, children with higher risk of suicide ideation, other serotonergic drugs.

INTERACTIONS

Drug
Cimetidine: May increase paroxetine blood concentration.
Diazepam: Increased half-life of diazepam in the presence of paroxetine.

P

MAOIs: May cause serotonin syndrome, marked by excitement, diaphoresis, rigidity, hyperthermia, autonomic hyperactivity, coma, and neuroleptic malignant syndrome.

Macrolide antibiotics: Possible inhibition of paroxetine metabolism.

NSAIDs in first-time users: Little available data but may increase GI side effects and risk of GI bleed.

Phenytoin: May decrease paroxetine blood concentration.

Pimozide and thiroidazine: May result in prolonged QT intervals.

Protein highly bound drugs (e.g., aspirin): Possible increased side effects.

Other antidepressants and alcohol: Possible increased side effects.

Risperidone: May increase risperidone blood concentration and cause extrapyramidal symptoms.

Herbal

St. John's wort: May increase paroxetine's pharmacologic effects and risk of toxicity.

Tryptophan: May cause headache, nausea, sweating and dizziness similar to serotonin syndrome.

Food

None known.

DIAGNOSTIC TEST EFFECTS

May increase serum hepatic enzyme levels. May decrease blood hemoglobin level, hematocrit, and WBC count.

SIDE EFFECTS

Frequent

Nausea (26%); somnolence (23%); headache, dry mouth (18%); asthenia (15%); constipation (15%); dizziness, insomnia (13%); diarrhea (12%); diaphoresis (11%); tremor (8%).

Occasional

Decreased appetite, respiratory disturbance (such as increased cough) (6%); anxiety, nervousness (5%); flatulence, paresthesia, yawning (4%); decreased libido, sexual dysfunction, abdominal discomfort (3%).

Rare

Palpitations, vomiting, blurred vision, altered taste, confusion.

SERIOUS REACTIONS

• Abnormal bleeding, hyponatremia, seizures, hypomania, suicidal thoughts have been reported.

PRECAUTIONS & CONSIDERATIONS

Caution is warranted in patients with suicidal tendency, cardiac disease, a history of seizures, impaired platelet aggregation, mania, hepatic and renal impairment, in volume-depleted patients, and in those using diuretics. Paroxetine use may impair reproductive function; it is distributed in breast milk. The safety and efficacy of this drug have not been established in children. In elderly patients, age-related renal impairment may require dosage adjustment. Be aware that St. John's wort should be avoided while taking paroxetine.

Alcohol and tasks that require mental alertness or motor skills should be avoided. CBC and liver and renal function tests should be performed before and periodically during therapy, especially with long-term use.

Administration

! Make sure at least 14 days elapse between the use of MAOIs and paroxetine. Expect to reduce paroxetine dosage in elderly patients and patients with severe hepatic or renal impairment. Keep in mind that dosage changes should occur at intervals of 1 wk or longer.

Take paroxetine as a single morning dose. Give it with food or milk if GI distress occurs. Scored tablets may be crushed or broken.

Pegaspargase
peg-as′par-jase
(Oncaspar)

CATEGORY AND SCHEDULE
Pregnancy Risk Category: C

Classification: Antineoplastics, modified enzymes

MECHANISM OF ACTION
An enzyme that breaks down extracellular supplies of the amino acid asparagine, which is necessary for the survival of leukemic cells. Binding to polyethylene glycol decreases the antigenicity of pegaspargase, making it less likely to cause a hypersensitivity reaction. Cell cycle–phase specific for G1 phase of cell division. *Therapeutic Effect:* Interferes with DNA, RNA, and protein synthesis in leukemic cells.

AVAILABILITY
Injection: 750 international units/mL.

INDICATIONS AND DOSAGES
▸ **Acute lymphocytic leukemia in combination with other chemotherapeutic agents**
IV, IM
Adults, Elderly, Children with a body surface area ≥0.6 m². 2500 international units/m² every 14 days. Children with a body surface area <0.6 m². 82.5 international units/kg every 14 days.

⊘ IV INCOMPATIBILITIES
Do not mix with other drugs at Y-site. Compatible only with dextrose 5% and 0.9% NaCl.

CONTRAINDICATIONS
Previous anaphylactic reaction or significant hemorrhagic event or thrombosis associated with L-asparaginase or pegaspargase therapy, pancreatitis (current or previous).

INTERACTIONS
Drug
Drug interactions are not well documented.
Antigout medications: May decrease the effects of these drugs.
Live-virus vaccine: May potentiate virus replication, increase vaccine side effects, and decrease the patient's antibody response to the vaccine.
Methotrexate: May block the effects of methotrexate.
Steroids, vincristine: May increase hyperglycemia, risk of neuropathy, and disturbances of erythropoiesis.
Herbal
None known.
Food
None known.

DIAGNOSTIC TEST EFFECTS
May increase BUN, blood ammonia, and blood glucose levels; serum alkaline phosphatase, bilirubin, uric acid, AST (SGOT), and ALT (SGPT) levels; PT; and aPTT. May decrease blood clotting factors (including plasma fibrinogen, antithrombin, and plasminogen) as well as serum albumin, calcium, and cholesterol levels.

SIDE EFFECTS
Frequent
Allergic reaction (including rash, urticaria, arthralgia, facial edema,

P

hypotension, and respiratory distress).

Occasional

Central nervous system (CNS) effects (including confusion, drowsiness, depression, nervousness, and fatigue), stomatitis, hypoalbuminemia, uric acid nephropathy (manifested as edema of the feet or lower legs), hyperglycemia.

Rare

Hyperthermia (fever or chills), CNS thrombosis.

SERIOUS REACTIONS

• The patient may have a hypersensitivity reaction, including anaphylaxis, during therapy.

• Pancreatitis, as evidenced by severe abdominal pain with nausea and vomiting, is a common reaction.

• Hepatotoxicity, as evidenced by jaundice and abnormal hepatic enzyme test results, may occur, especially in patients with pre-existing hepatic impairment.

• An increased risk of hematologic toxicity and coagulation disorders occurs occasionally.

• Seizures occur rarely.

PRECAUTIONS & CONSIDERATIONS

Caution is warranted in those concurrently taking aspirin, NSAIDs, and anticoagulants. Vaccinations and coming in contact with crowds and people with known infections should be avoided.

Any hypersensitivity reactions with L-asparginase therapy previously warrants careful consideration as to whether this drug should be used. Nausea may occur but will decrease during therapy. Notify the physician if fever, signs of local infection, or unusual bleeding from any site occurs. Antihistamines, epinephrine, and corticosteroids should be kept readily available before and during pegaspargase administration to ensure an adequate airway and treat any allergic reaction.

Adequate hydration should be maintained to protect against renal impairment. CBC, bone marrow tests, fibrinogen level, PT, aPTT, liver, pancreatic and renal function test results should be monitored before beginning therapy and whenever a week or longer has elapsed between drug doses.

Storage

Refrigerate—do not freeze—vials. Discard the solution if it is cloudy or contains a precipitate. Also discard it if it has been stored at room temperature for longer than 48 h or if the vial has been previously frozen because freezing destroys the drug's potency.

Administration

! Handle pegaspargase with care because the drug is a contact irritant. Wear gloves, avoid inhaling vapors, and avoid contact with skin or mucous membranes. In case of contact, wash with a copious amount of water for at least 15 min. Avoid excessive agitation of the vial (do not shake). The IM administration route is preferred because it poses less risk of coagulopathy, hepatotoxicity, and GI or renal disorders than the IV route. Use one dose per vial; do not re-enter the vial. Discard any unused portion.

Administer no more than 2 mL at any one IM site. Use multiple injection sites if more than 2 mL is being administered.

For IV, add dose to 100 mL 0.9% NaCl or D5W and administer the drug through IV infusion that is already running. Infuse over 1-2 h.

P

Pegfilgrastim

pehg-phil-gras′tim
(Neulasta)
Do not confuse Neulasta with Neumega.

CATEGORY AND SCHEDULE
Pregnancy Risk Category: C

Classification: Hematopoietic agents

MECHANISM OF ACTION
A colony-stimulating factor that regulates the production of neutrophils within bone marrow. Also a glycoprotein that primarily affects neutrophil progenitor proliferation, differentiation, and selected end-cell functional activation. *Therapeutic Effect:* Increases phagocytic ability and antibody-dependent destruction; decreases incidence of infection.

PHARMACOKINETICS
Readily absorbed after subcutaneous administration. *Half-life:* 15-80 h.

AVAILABILITY
Solution for Injection:
6 mg/0.6 mL prefilled syringe equivalent to 10 mg/mL.

USES
Nonmyeloid malignancies receiving myelosuppressive anticancer drugs, febrile neutropenia.

INDICATIONS AND DOSAGES
▸ **Myelosuppression**
SC
Adults, Elderly. > 45 kg. Give as a single 6-mg injection once per chemotherapy cycle.

CONTRAINDICATIONS
Hypersensitivity to *Escherichia coli*–derived proteins, pegfilgrastim, filgrastim, or any other components of the product. Do not use for peripheral blood progenitor cell mobilization.

INTERACTIONS
Drug
G-CSF, other exogenous growth factors: May result in development of antibodies causing immune-mediated neutropenia.
Lithium: May potentiate the release of neutrophils.
Herbal
None known.
Food
None known.

DIAGNOSTIC TEST EFFECTS
May increase LDH concentrations, leukocyte alkaline phosphatase scores, and serum alkaline phosphatase and uric acid levels.

SIDE EFFECTS
Frequent (15%-72%)
Bone pain, nausea, fatigue, alopecia, diarrhea, vomiting, constipation, anorexia, abdominal pain, arthralgia, generalized weakness, peripheral edema, dizziness, stomatitis, mucositis, neutropenic fever.

SERIOUS REACTIONS
• Allergic reactions, such as anaphylaxis, rash, and urticaria, occur rarely.
• Cytopenia resulting from an antibody response to growth factors occurs rarely.
• Splenomegaly occurs rarely; assess for left upper abdominal or shoulder pain.
• Adult respiratory distress syndrome (ARDS) may occur in patients with sepsis.

P

PRECAUTIONS & CONSIDERATIONS

Caution is warranted with concurrent use of medications with myeloid properties and in those with sickle cell disease. It is unknown whether pegfilgrastim crosses the placenta or is distributed in breast milk. Safety and efficacy of pegfilgrastim have not been established in children. The 6-g prefilled syringe should not be used in infants, children, and adolescents weighing < 45 kg. No age-related precautions have been noted in elderly patients.

CBC, hematocrit value and platelet count should be obtained before initiation of pegfilgrastim therapy and routinely thereafter. Pattern of daily bowel activity and stool consistency should be assessed. Be aware of signs of peripheral edema, particularly behind the medial malleolus, which is usually the first area to show peripheral edema, and for evidence of mucositis (such as red mucous membranes, white patches, and extreme mouth soreness) and stomatitis.

Storage
Store in refrigerator at 36°-46° F in the carton until use but may warm to room temperature up to 48 h before use. Discard if left at room temperature for longer than 48 h. Protect from light. Avoid freezing, but if accidentally frozen, may allow to thaw in refrigerator before administration. Discard if freezing takes place a second time. Discard if discoloration or precipitate is present.

Administration
! Do not administer from 14 days before to 24 h after cytotoxic chemotherapy, as prescribed. Do not use pegfilgrastim in infants, children, or adolescents weighing < 45 kg.

Do not shake prefilled syringe as this may disrupt the drug. If syringe is shaken, discard; do not use.

Pegfilgrastim should be injected subcutaneously. Compliance with pegfilgrastim regimen is important.

Peginterferon Alfa-2a
peg-inn-ter-fear′on
(Pegasys)

CATEGORY AND SCHEDULE
Pregnancy Risk Category: C

Classification: Biologic response modulators, interferons

MECHANISM OF ACTION
An immunomodulator that binds to specific membrane receptors on the cell surface, inhibiting viral replication in virus-infected cells, suppressing cell proliferation, and producing reversible decreases in leukocyte and platelet counts. *Therapeutic Effect:* Inhibits hepatitis C virus.

PHARMACOKINETICS
Readily absorbed after SC administration, with peak serum levels attained at 72-96 h. Excreted by the kidneys. *Half-life:* 80 h.

AVAILABILITY
Injection: 180 mcg/mL.

INDICATIONS AND DOSAGES
▸ Hepatitis C
SC (AS MONOTHERAPY)
Adults 18 yr and older, Elderly.
180 mcg (1 mL) injected in abdomen or thigh once weekly for 48 wks.

SC (IN COMBINATION WITH RIBAVIRIN)

180 mcg (1 mL) once weekly plus ribavirin (800-1200 mg/day in 2 divided doses) for 24-48 wks.

▶ **Dosage in renal impairment**

For patients who require hemodialysis, dosage is 135 mcg injected in the abdomen or thigh once weekly for 48 wks.

▶ **Dosage in hepatic impairment**

For patients with progressive ALT (SGPT) increases above baseline values, dosage is 135 mcg injected in the abdomen or thigh once weekly for 48 wks.

For patients with an absolute neutrophil count <750 cells/mm^3, reduce dose to 135 mcg (0.75 mL). For those with an absolute neutrophil count <500 cells/mm^3, discontinue treatment until the count returns to 1000 cells/mm^3. For those with a platelet count <50,000 cells/mm^3, reduce dose to 90 mcg.

OFF-LABEL USE

Antiviral agent.

CONTRAINDICATIONS

Hypersensitivity to *E. coli,* protein, autoimmune hepatitis, decompensated hepatic disease, infants, neonates, benzyl alcohol hypersensitivity.

INTERACTIONS

Drug

Bone marrow depressants: May increase myelosuppression.

Theophylline: May increase the serum level of theophylline.

Herbal

None known.

Food

None known.

DIAGNOSTIC TEST EFFECTS

May increase ALT (SGPT) level. May decrease the absolute neutrophil, platelet, and WBC counts. May cause a slight decrease in blood hemoglobin level and hematocrit.

SIDE EFFECTS

Frequent

Headache.

Occasional

Alopecia, nausea, insomnia, anorexia, dizziness, diarrhea, abdominal pain, flulike symptoms, psychiatric reactions (depression, irritability, anxiety), injection site reaction, impaired concentration, diaphoresis, dry mouth, nausea, vomiting.

SERIOUS REACTIONS

• Serious, acute hypersensitivity reactions, such as urticaria, angioedema, bronchoconstriction, and anaphylaxis, may occur. Other rare reactions include pancreatitis, colitis, hyperthyroidism or hypothyroidism, endocrine disorders (e.g., diabetes mellitus), benzyl alcohol hypersensitivity ophthalmologic disorders, and pulmonary disorders.

PRECAUTIONS & CONSIDERATIONS

Caution is warranted in patients with autoimmune, hepatitis, decompensated hepatic disease, infants and neonates and preexisting cardiac disease. May aggravate hypothroidism and hyperthyroidism, diabetes, or hyperglycemia. Peginterferon alfa-2a may cause spontaneous abortion. It is unknown whether peginterferon alfa-2a is distributed in breast milk. The safety and efficacy of peginterferon alfa-2a have not been established in children younger than 18 yr. Cardiac, central nervous system (CNS), and systemic effects may be more severe in elderly patients, particularly in those with renal impairment. Avoid performing tasks requiring mental alertness or motor skills until response to the drug has been established.

Caution is recommended in patients having compromised CNS function, myelosuppression, history of neuropsychiatric disorders, and renal impairment characterized by a creatinine clearance < 50 mL/min.

Flulike symptoms may occur but usually diminish with continued therapy. Notify the physician of depression or suicidal thoughts. CBC, ECG, urinalysis, BUN level, and serum alkaline phosphatase, creatinine, AST (SGOT), and ALT (SGPT) levels should be obtained before and routinely during therapy. Chest radiographs should be assessed for pulmonary infiltrates.

Storage
Refrigerate vials.

Administration
! For moderate to severe adverse reactions, expect to decrease the dose to 135 mcg (0.75 mL) or 90 mcg (0.5 mL), as prescribed.

Vials are for single use only; discard unused portions. Inject the drug subcutaneously in the abdomen or thigh. The drug's therapeutic effect should appear in 1-3 mo.

Peginterferon Alfa-2b

peg-in-ter-feer′on
(PEG-Intron)

CATEGORY AND SCHEDULE
Pregnancy Risk Category: C

Classification: Biologic response modifier, interferons

MECHANISM OF ACTION
An immunomodulator that inhibits viral replication in virus-infected cells, suppresses cell proliferation, increases phagocytic action of macrophages, and augments specific cytotoxicity of lymphocytes for target cells. *Therapeutic Effect:* Inhibits hepatitis C virus.

USES
Treatment of adults with chronic hepatitis C with compensated liver disease who have not been previously treated with interferon-alfa. Peg-interferon alfa 2b can be used with ribivarin.

AVAILABILITY
Injection Powder for Reconstitution: 50 mcg, 80 mcg, 120 mcg, 150 mcg.

INDICATIONS AND DOSAGES
▶ **Chronic hepatitis C, monotherapy**
SC
Adults 18 yr and older, Elderly. Administer appropriate dosage (see chart below) once weekly for 1 yr on the same day each wk.

Vial (mcg/mL)	Weight (kg)	Strength	
		mcg*	mL*
100	37-45	40	0.4
160	46-56	50	0.5
240	57-72	64	0.4
300	73-88	80	0.5
	89-106	96	0.4
	107-136	120	0.5
	137-160	150	0.5

*Of peginterferon alpha-2b to administer.

▶ **Chronic hepatitis C**
SC
Combination therapy with ribavirin (dose varies). Initially, 1.5 mcg/kg/wk.

OFF-LABEL USE
Antiviral agent.

CONTRAINDICATIONS
Autoimmune hepatitis, cardiac disease, decompensated hepatic disease, history of psychiatric disorders.

INTERACTIONS
Drug
Acetaminophen: Risk of hepatotoxicity in severe liver disease.
Bone marrow depressants: May increase myelosuppression.
Herbal
None known.
Food
None known.

DIAGNOSTIC TEST EFFECTS
May increase blood glucose and ALT (SGPT) levels. May decrease blood neutrophil and platelet counts.

SIDE EFFECTS
Frequent
Flulike symptoms; inflammation, bruising, pruritus, and irritation at injection site.
Occasional
Psychiatric reactions (depression, anxiety, emotional lability, irritability), insomnia, alopecia, diarrhea.
Rare
Rash, diaphoresis, dry skin, dizziness, flushing, vomiting, dyspepsia.

SERIOUS REACTIONS
• Serious, acute hypersensitivity reactions (such as urticaria, angioedema, bronchoconstriction, and anaphylaxis), pulmonary disorders, endocrine disorders (e.g., diabetes mellitus), hypothyroidism, hyperthyroidism, and pancreatitis occur rarely.

• Ulcerative colitis may occur within 12 wks of starting treatment.

PRECAUTIONS & CONSIDERATIONS
Caution is warranted in patients with preexisting cardiac disease; may aggravate hypothyroidism, hyperthyroidism, hyperglycemia, hypoglycemia, diabetes, ophthalmologic disorders; use cautiously in lactating women and children, in those with compromised CNS function, myelosuppression, renal impairment (creatinine clearance <50 mL/min), and in elderly patients. Closely monitor patients as severe life-threatening neuropsychiatric, autoimmune, ischemic, or infectious disorders may cause or aggravate these conditions while using peginterferon alfa-2b. Peginterferon alfa-2b may cause spontaneous abortion. It is unknown whether peginterferon alfa-2b is distributed in breast milk. The safety and efficacy of peginterferon alfa-2b have not been established in children younger than 18 yr. Cardiac, CNS, and systemic effects may be more severe in elderly patients, particularly in patients with renal impairment.

Flulike symptoms may occur but usually diminish with continued therapy. Notify the physician of bloody diarrhea, fever, persistent abdominal pain, depression, signs of infection, or unusual bruising or bleeding. CBC, ECG, urinalysis, BUN level, and serum alkaline phosphatase, creatinine, AST (SGOT), and ALT (SGPT) levels should be obtained before and routinely during therapy. Chest radiographs should be assessed for pulmonary infiltrates.
Storage
Store vials at room temperature. Use it immediately or after reconstitution

P

or, if necessary, refrigerate it for up to 24 h.

Administration

! If severe adverse reactions occur, modify the dosage or temporarily discontinue the drug, as prescribed. Dosage is based on weight. Remember that the drug's side effects are dose related.

Reconstitute the drug by adding 0.7 mL sterile water for injection (the supplied diluent) to the vial. Administer as SC injection.

Pegvisomant
peg-vis'oh-mant
(Somavert)
Do not confuse Somavert with somatrem or somatropin.

CATEGORY AND SCHEDULE
Pregnancy Risk Category: B

Classification: Acromegaly agent, growth hormone analog

MECHANISM OF ACTION
A protein that selectively binds to growth hormone (GH) receptors on cell surfaces, blocking the binding of endogenous growth hormones and interfering with growth hormone signal transduction. *Therapeutic Effect:* Decreases serum concentrations of insulin-like growth factor 1 (IGF-1) and other GH-responsive serum proteins.

PHARMACOKINETICS
Not distributed extensively into tissues after SC administration. Less than 1% excreted in urine. *Half-life:* 6 days.

AVAILABILITY
Powder for Injection: 10-mg, 15-mg, 20-mg vials.

INDICATIONS AND DOSAGES
▶ **Acromegaly**
SC
Adults, Elderly. Initially, 40 mg as a loading dose, then 10 mg daily. After 4-6 wks, adjust dosage in 5-mg increments based on serum IGF-1 concentrations.

CONTRAINDICATIONS
Latex allergy (stopper on vial contains latex), intravenous administration.

INTERACTIONS
Drug
Insulin, oral antidiabetics:
May enhance the effects of these drugs, possibly resulting in hypoglycemia. Dosage should be decreased when initiating pegvisomant therapy.
Opioids: Decreased serum pegvisomant levels.
Herbal
None known.
Food
None known.

DIAGNOSTIC TEST EFFECTS
Interferes with measurement of serum growth hormone concentration. May markedly increase AST (SGOT), ALT (SGPT), and serum transaminase levels. Decreases effect of insulin on carbohydrate metabolism.

SIDE EFFECTS
Frequent
Infection (cold symptoms, upper respiratory tract infection, blister, ear infection).
Occasional
Back pain, dizziness, injection site reaction, peripheral edema, sinusitis, nausea.

Rare
Diarrhea, paresthesia.

SERIOUS REACTIONS

• Pegvisomant use may markedly elevate liver function test results, including serum transaminase levels.

• Substantial weight gain occurs rarely.

PRECAUTIONS & CONSIDERATIONS

Caution is warranted in patients with diabetes mellitus and in elderly patients. It is unknown whether pegvisomant is excreted in breast milk. The safety and efficacy of pegvisomant have not been established in children. In elderly patients, treatment should begin at the low end of the dosage range.

Notify the physician of yellowing of the skin or sclera of eyes or any other adverse effects. Serum alkaline phosphatase, bilirubin, AST (SGOT), and ALT (SGPT) levels should be monitored. Serum IGF-1 concentrations should be obtained 4-6 wks after therapy begins and periodically thereafter. The drug dosage should be adjusted based on these results, not on growth hormone assays. Progressive tumor growth with periodic imaging scans of the sella turcica should be monitored with tumors that secrete growth hormone. Diabetics should be assessed for hypoglycemia.

Storage
Store unreconstituted vials in the refrigerator. Administer the drug within 6 h of reconstitution.

Administration
The solution normally appears clear after reconstitution. Discard the solution if it appears cloudy or contains particles. Withdraw 1 mL sterile water for injection and inject it into the vial of pegvisomant, aiming the stream against the glass wall. Hold the vial between the palms of both hands and roll it gently to dissolve the powder; do not shake. Administer only one dose from each vial subcutaneously.

Pemetrexed
pem-eh-trex'ed
(Alimta)

CATEGORY AND SCHEDULE
Pregnancy Risk Category: D

Classification: Antineoplastics, antimetabolites

MECHANISM OF ACTION

An antimetabolite that disrupts folate-dependent enzymes essential for cell replication. *Therapeutic Effect:* Inhibits the growth of mesothelioma cell lines.

PHARMACOKINETICS

Protein binding: 81%. Drug is not metabolized; excreted in urine. *Half-life:* 3.5 h.

AVAILABILITY

Powder for Injection: 500 mg.

INDICATIONS AND DOSAGES

! Pretreatment with corticosteroid (e.g., dexamethasone), the day before, day of, and 1 day after infusion, as prescribed, to reduce the incidence and severity of cutaneous reactions. Folic acid and vitamin B_{12} supplementation (IM) 7 days before the first dose of pemetrexed, during therapy, and for 21 days after the last dose will reduce treatment-related hematologic and GI toxicity. IM administered B_{12} should be administered again every 3 cycles and can be administered the same day as pemetrexed.

▸ **Malignant pleural mesothelioma, unresectable**

IV

Adults, Elderly. 500 mg/m² infused over 10 min on day 1 of each 21-day cycle when used in combination with cisplatin 75 mg/m². Reductions in dosages are indicated as follows:

For absolute neutrophil count (ANC) <500 mm³, nadir platelets equal to 50,000/mm³, grade 3 or grade 4 toxicities, diarrhea requiring hospitalization: Reduce IV dose to 75% of previous dose.

For nadir platelets <50,000/mm³ regardless of nadir ANC or grades 3 or 4 mucositis: Reduce IV dose to 50% of previous dose.

For grades 3 or 4 neurotoxicities or any hematologic or nonhematologic grades 3 or 4 toxicity after 2 dose reductions: Discontinue drug.

CONTRAINDICATIONS

Mannitol hypersensitivity.

INTERACTIONS

Drug

Calcium (including lactated Ringer's injection and Ringer's injection): Incompatible.

Cisplatin: Concomitant therapy may augment any adverse reactions.

Nephrotoxic agents, probenecid: May delay pemetrexed clearance.

NSAIDs (short-acting, particularly ibuprofen, and long-acting, e.g., piroxicam): Increase the risk of myelosuppression and GI and renal toxicity.

Herbal

None known.

Food

None known.

DIAGNOSTIC TEST EFFECTS

May decrease platelet, RBC, and WBC counts.

ⓘ IV INCOMPATIBILITIES

Use only 0.9% NaCl to reconstitute; flush the line before and after the infusion. Do not add any other medications to the IV line.

SIDE EFFECTS

Frequent

Fatigue, nausea, vomiting, constipation, anorexia, stomatitis, pharyngitis, diarrhea, neutropenia, leukopenia, anemia, thrombocytopenia, chest pains, rash, desquamation, mood alteration or depression, dypsnea.

Occasional

Allergic reaction, hypersensitivity, dehydration, creatinine elevation, fever, infection without neutropenia, infection with grade 3 or 4 neutropenia, hypertension, thrombosis, embolism.

Rare

Febrile neutropenia, renal failure, esophagitis, odynophagia, dysphagia.

SERIOUS REACTIONS

• Myelosuppression, manifested as neutropenia, thrombocytopenia, or anemia, may occur.

PRECAUTIONS & CONSIDERATIONS

CBC with differential platelet count should be assessed before starting therapy and again on days 8 and 15 of each cycle and before starting a new cycle. New cycles should not be started with ANC <1500 mm³, platelet count ≤ 100,000 mm³ and creatinine clearance rate of at least 45 mL/min. Do not administer in patients with CrCl <45 mL/min.

Caution is warranted with liver and renal impairment as well as concurrent therapy with aspirin or other NSAIDs. Short-acting NSAIDs (e.g., ibuprofen) should be discontinued 2 days before, the day of, and for 2 days after pemetrexed administration; long-acting NSAIDs (e.g., piroxicam) should be discontinued 5 days before, the day of, and for 2 days after pemetrexed administration. Pemetrexed may be harmful to a fetus, and it is unknown whether pemetrexed is distributed in breast milk. Do not breastfeed once treatment has been initiated. Safety and efficacy of pemetrexed in children younger than 18 yr of age have not been established. Be aware that elderly patients may have higher incidence of fatigue, leukopenia, neutropenia, and thrombocytopenia.

Fastidious oral hygiene should be maintained. Do not have immunizations without physician's approval (drug lowers body's resistance). Crowds and those with infection should be avoided. Contraceptive measures should be used during therapy. Report fever, sore throat, signs of local infection, easy bruising, and unusual bleeding from any site immediately.

Storage

Store undiluted vial at room temperature. Reconstituted solution is stable for up to 24 h at room temperature or if refrigerated. Discard any reconstituted material after 24 h.

Administration

Be aware that pretreatment with dexamethasone (or equivalent) will reduce the risk and incidence and severity of cutaneous reaction; treatment with folic acid and vitamin B$_{12}$ beginning 1 wk before treatment and for 21 days after the last pemetrexed dose will reduce risk of side effects.

Dilute 500-mg vial with 20 mL 0.9% NaCl to provide a concentration of 25 mg/mL. Gently swirl each vial until powder is completely dissolved. Solution appears clear and ranges in color from colorless to yellow or green-yellow. Further dilute prescribed amount of reconstituted solution to 100 mL with preservative-free sodium chloride (0.9% NaCl) injection and administer as IV infusion over 10 min.

Do not use if particular matter or cloudiness is evident. Do not save any unused portions for future use.

Pemirolast Potassium

peh-meer´-oh-last poe-tass´-ee-um (Alamast)

P

CATEGORY AND SCHEDULE

Pregnancy Risk Category: C

Classification: Ophthalmic

MECHANISM OF ACTION

An antiallergic agent that prevents the activation and release of mediators of inflammation (e.g., mast cells). *Therapeutic Effect:* Reduces symptoms of allergic conjunctivitis.

PHARMACOKINETICS

Detected in plasma. Excreted in urine. *Half-life:* 4.5 h.

AVAILABILITY

Ophthalmic Solution: 0.1%

INDICATIONS AND DOSAGES
▶ **Allergic conjunctivitis**
OPHTHALMIC
Adults, Elderly, Children 3 yr and older. 1-2 drops in affected eye(s) 4 times/day.

CONTRAINDICATIONS
Hypersensitivity to any component of the formulation.

INTERACTIONS
None reported.

SIDE EFFECTS
Ophthalmic: Transient ocular stinging, burning, itching, dry eye, foreign-body sensation, tearing. Other: Headache, rhinitis, cold and flu symptoms, sinusitis, sneezing/nasal congestion.

SERIOUS REACTIONS
None reported.

PRECAUTIONS & CONSIDERATIONS
Safety and efficacy not established in children less than 3 yr of age. Caution if breastfeeding.
Storage
Store at room temperature.
Administration
Do not wear contact lens if eyes are red. If eyes are not red, remove contact lens before administration and wait 10 min before reinserting.

Pemoline
pem'oh-leen
(Cylert, PemADD, PemADD CT)
Discontinued in the United States

CATEGORY AND SCHEDULE
Pregnancy Risk Category: B
Controlled Substance: Schedule IV

Classification: Oxazolidine central nervous system (CNS) stimulant.

MECHANISM OF ACTION
A CNS stimulant that blocks the reuptake mechanism present in dopaminergic neurons in the cerebral cortex and subcortical structures with minimal sympathomimetic efffects. Exact mechanism and site of action are unknown. *Therapeutic Effect:* Reduces motor restlessness and fatigue, increases alertness, elevates mood.

PHARMACOKINETICS
Rapidly absorbed from the GI tract; 50% bound to plasma proteins. Peak serum levels attained 2-4 h after ingestion. Metabolized in the liver and 50% excreted unchanged through the kidneys.

AVAILABILITY
Tablets (Cylert, PemADD): 18.75 mg, 37.5 mg, 75 mg.
Tablets (Chewable [PemADD CT]): 37.5 mg.

INDICATIONS AND DOSAGES
▶ **Attention Deficit Hyperactivity Disorder (ADHD)**
PO
Children 6 yr and older. Initially, 37.5 mg/day as a single dose in morning. May increase by 18.75 mg at weekly intervals until therapeutic

response is achieved. Range:
56.25-75 mg/day. Maximum:
112.5 mg/day.

CONTRAINDICATIONS

Family history of Tourette syndrome,
hepatic impairment, motor tics,
phonic tics, known hypersensitivity
or idiosyncrasy to the drug, renal
disease, breast-feeding, drug abuse,
children younger than 6 yr.

INTERACTIONS

Drug
Antiepileptic agents: May decrease
seizure threshold.
Other CNS stimulants: May
increase CNS stimulation.
Herbal
None known.
Food
**Caffeine-containing products and
food:** May increase irritability.

DIAGNOSTIC TEST EFFECTS

May increase serum LDH, AST
(SGOT), and ALT (SGPT) levels.
Monitor weight gain and height
periodically during long-term use
of drug.

SIDE EFFECTS

Frequent
Anorexia, insomnia.
Occasional
Nausea, abdominal discomfort,
diarrhea, headache, dizziness,
somnolence, growth suppression.
Rare
Elevated acid phosphatase
in association with prostate
enlargement.

SERIOUS REACTIONS

Black Box Warning
Because of its association with
life-threatening hepatic failure,
pemoline should not ordinarily
be considered as first-line drug

therapy for ADHD. Because
pemoline provides an observable
symptomatic benefit, patients who
fail to show substantial clinical
benefit within 3 wks of completing
dose titration should be withdrawn
from therapy.
• Visual disturbances, rash, and
dyskinetic movements of the tongue,
lips, face, and extremities have
occurred.
• Large doses of pemoline may
produce extreme nervousness and
tachycardia.
• Hepatic effects, such as hepatitis
and jaundice, appear to be reversible
when the drug is discontinued.
• Prolonged administration
to children with ADHD may
temporarily delay growth.

PRECAUTIONS & CONSIDERATIONS

Caution is warranted in patients
with hypertension, psychosis,
renal impairment, seizures, and
a history of drug abuse. Hepatic
function tests should be performed
before and periodically during
therapy. Height and weight
should be measured before and
during pemoline therapy. Notify
the physician if dark urine, GI
complaints, loss of appetite, or
yellow skin occurs. Tasks that
require mental alertness or motor
skills, alcohol, and caffeine
should be avoided. Use caution in
pregnancy; it is not known whether
the drug is excreted in breast milk.
Safety and efficacy in children
under 6 yr are not established.
Long-term effects in children are
not established. Dose selection in
elderly patients should be cautious,
starting at the low end of the
dosing range, to avoid the greater
frequency of decreased hepatic,
renal, or cardiac function. Pemoline
should not be used by patients until

P

there is a complete discussion of the risks and benefits of therapy and written informed consent has been obtained.

Administration

Do not abruptly discontinue the drug.

Penbutolol

pen-beaut-oh-lol
(Levatol)
Do not confuse with pindolol

CATEGORY AND SCHEDULE

Pregnancy Risk Category: C (D if used in the second or third trimester)

Classification: Non-specific β-adrenergic blocking agent

MECHANISM OF ACTION

An antihypertensive that possesses nonselective β-blocking. Has moderate intrinsic sympathomimetic activity. *Therapeutic Effect:* Decreases heart rate, cardiac contractility, and BP; increases airway resistance, promoting bronchospasm, and decreases myocardial ischemia severity.

PHARMACOKINETICS

Rapidly and completely (100%) absorbed from the GI tract. Protein binding: 80%-98%. Metabolized in liver. 90% excreted in urine. *Half-life:* 17-26 h.

AVAILABILITY

Tablets: 20 mg (Levatol).

INDICATIONS AND DOSAGES

▸ Hypertension

PO
Adults, Elderly. Initially, 20 mg/day as a single dose. May increase to 40-80 mg/day.

CONTRAINDICATIONS

Bronchial asthma or related bronchospastic conditions, chronic obstructive pulmonary disease (COPD), congestive heart failure (CHF) unless secondary to tachyarrhythmia or untreated hypertension treatable with β-blockers, overt cardiac failure cardiogenic shock, pulmonary edema, second- or third-degree atrioventricular (AV) block, severe bradycardia, hypersensitivity to penbutolol or any component of the formulation.

INTERACTIONS

Drug

Calcium blockers: Increase risk of conduction disturbances.
Clonidine: May potentiate BP effects, especially upon withdrawal.
Cimetidine: May increase penbutolol concentrations.
Digoxin: Increases concentrations of this drug.
Diuretics, other hypotensives: May increase hypotensive effect.
Ergot derivatives: May cause peripheral ischemia.
Fentanyl: May cause severe hypotension.
Hydrocarbon inhalation anesthetics: May increase hypotension, myocardial depression.
Indomethacin, NSAIDs: May decrease antihypertensive effect.
Insulin, oral hypoglycemics: May mask symptoms of hypoglycemia and prolong hypoglycemic effect of these drugs.

Lidocaine: May prolong the elimination of lidocaine leading to toxicity.

Theophylline: May reduce elimination of theophylline; may reduce effects of both drugs by pharmacologic antagonism.

Verapamil: May increase risk of hypotension and bradycardia.

Sympathomimetics, xanthines: May mutually inhibit effects.

Herbal

Dong quai: May decrease BP.

St. John's wort, yohimbine: May decrease effectiveness of penbutolol.

Food

None known.

DIAGNOSTIC TEST EFFECTS

May increase ANA titer, SGOT (AST), SGPT (ALT), alkaline phosphatase, LDH, bilirubin, BUN, creatinine, potassium, uric acid, lipoproteins, triglycerides.

SIDE EFFECTS

Frequent

Decreased sexual ability, drowsiness, unusual tiredness or weakness, dizziness, fatigue, headache, insomnia, alteration of blood sugar levels, cough, bronchospasm.

Occasional

Diarrhea, bradycardia, depression, cold hands or feet, constipation, anxiety, nasal congestion, nausea, vomiting.

Rare

Altered taste; dry eyes; itching; numbness of fingers, toes, scalp; bradycardia; edema; AV block; worsening angina; adrenal insufficiency.

SERIOUS REACTIONS

• Abrupt withdrawal may result in sweating, palpitations, headache, and tremors.

• May cause insulin-induced hypoglycemia in patients with previously controlled diabetes.

PRECAUTIONS & CONSIDERATIONS

Caution is warranted in patients with inadequate cardiac function, impaired renal or hepatic function, diabetes mellitus, COPD, myasthenia gravis, peripheral vascular disease, hypotension, and hyperthyroidism. It is unknown whether penbutolol crosses the placenta or is distributed in breast milk. Safety and efficacy of penbutolol have not been established in children. In elderly patients, the incidence of dizziness may be increased.

Dizziness and drowsiness may be experienced during treatment. Avoid alcohol and tasks that require mental alertness or motor skills. In addition, avoid nasal decongestants and over-the-counter (OTC) cold preparations, especially those containing stimulants, without physician approval. Medication should not be taken when pulse is irregular or <60 beats/min without advice of health care provider.

Abrupt withdrawal should be avoided, especially in hyperthyroidism, which could cause reactions similar to thyroid storm; rebound effects may produce angina or myocardial infarction (MI).

Storage

Store at room temperature.

Administration

Take with food, which slows the rate of absorption and reduces the risk of orthostatic hypotension. To assess the tolerance of the drug, assess a standing systolic BP 1 h after giving penbutolol. The full antihypertensive effect of penbutolol should take 1-2 wks. Do not abruptly discontinue penbutolol but withdraw over a period of 1-2 wks.

P

Penciclovir Triphosphatepen-sye′kloe-veer

(Denavir, Vectavir [SOUTH AFRICA, COSTA RICA, DOMINICAN REPUBLIC, EL SALVADOR, GERMANY, GUATEMALA, HONDURAS, ISRAEL, NICARAGUA, PANAMA])

Do not confuse with acyclovir.

CATEGORY AND SCHEDULE
Pregnancy Risk Category: B

Classification: Antivirals

MECHANISM OF ACTION
Penciclovir triphosphate selectively inhibits herpes simplex virus (HSV) polymerase competitively with deoxyguanosine triphosphate. Consequently, herpes viral DNA synthesis and, therefore, replication are selectively inhibited. *Therapeutic Effect:* An antiviral compound that has inhibitory activity against HSV-1 and HSV-2.

PHARMACOKINETICS
Measurable penciclovir concentrations were not detected in plasma or urine. The systemic absorption of penciclovir following topical administration has not been evaluated.

AVAILABILITY
Cream: 10 mg/g.

INDICATIONS AND DOSAGES
▸ **Herpes labialis (cold sores)**
TOPICAL
Adolescents, Adults. Penciclovir should be applied every 2 h during waking h for a period of 4 days. Treatment should be started as early as possible (i.e., during the prodrome or when lesions appear).

OFF-LABEL USES
Varicella-zoster virus.

CONTRAINDICATIONS
Hypersensitivity to penciclovir or any of its components or any related compound.

INTERACTIONS
Drug
OTC creams or ointments: May delay healing or increase risk of spreading the infection.
Herbal
None known.
Food
None known.

DIAGNOSTIC TEST EFFECTS
None known.

SIDE EFFECTS
Frequent
Headache.
Occasional
Change in sense of taste; decreased sensitivity of skin, particularly to touch; redness of the skin, skin rash (maculopapular, erythematous), local edema; skin discoloration; pruritis; hypoesthesia; parasthesias; parosmia; urticaria; oral or pharyngeal edema.
Rare
Mild pain, burning, or stinging.

PRECAUTIONS & CONSIDERATIONS
Hypersensitivity to penciclovir or any of its components. Acyclovir-resistant herpes viruses, patients younger than 12 yr, use in mucous membranes.

It is unknown whether penciclovir crosses the placenta or is distributed into breast milk. Safety and efficacy have not been established in children. No age-related precautions have been noted in elderly patients. Headache may occur while taking penciclovir. Do not apply near eyes, ears, or mucous membranes. Local irritation should be reported to the health care provider.

Storage

Store at room temperature.

Administration

Penciclovir is for external use only. Apply every 2 h during waking h for 4 days. Continue medication for the full time of treatment.

Penicillamine

pen-i-sil-a-meen
(Cuprimine, Depen)
Do not confuse with penicillin.

CATEGORY AND SCHEDULE

Pregnancy Risk Category: D

Classification: Chelators, cysteine-depleting agents, disease-modifying antirheumatic drugs (DMARD)

MECHANISM OF ACTION

A heavy metal antagonist that chelates copper, iron, mercury, lead to form complexes, promoting excretion of copper. Combines with cysteine-forming complex, thus reducing concentration of cysteine to below levels for formation of cysteine stones. Exact mechanism for rheumatoid arthritis is unknown. May decrease cell-mediated immune response. May inhibit collagen formation. *Therapeutic Effect:* Promotes excretion of copper, prevents renal calculi, dissolves existing stones, acts as anti-inflammatory drug

PHARMACOKINETICS

Moderately absorbed from the GI tract. Protein binding: 80% to albumin. Metabolized in small amounts in the liver. Excreted unchanged in urine. *Half-life:* 1.7-3.2 h.

AVAILABILITY

Capsules: 125 mg, 250 mg (Cuprimine).
Tablets, Titratable: 250 mg (Depen).

INDICATIONS AND DOSAGES

▸ **Wilson disease**

PO

Adults, Elderly. Initially, 250 mg 4 times/day (some patients may begin at 250 mg/day; gradually increase). Dosages of 750-1500 mg/day that produce initial 24-h cupriuresis >2 mg should be continued for 3 mo. Maintenance: Based on serum-free copper concentration (<10 mcg/dL indicative of adequate maintenance). Maximum: 2 g/day.

▸ **Cystinuria**

PO

Adults, Elderly. Initially, 250 mg/day. Gradually increase dose. Maintenance: 2 g/day. Range: 1-4 g/day.
Children. 30 mg/kg/day in 4 divided doses or larger portion given at bedtime.

▸ **Rheumatoid arthritis**

PO

Adults, Elderly.
Initially, 125-250 mg/day. May increase by 125-250 mg/day at intervals of 1-3 mo. Maintenance: 500-750 mg/day. After 2-3 mo with no improvement or toxicity, may increase by 250 mg/day at intervals of 2-3 mo until remission or toxicity. Maximum: 1 g up to 1.5 g/day.

OFF-LABEL USES

Treatment of rheumatoid vasculitis, heavy metal toxicity.

P

CONTRAINDICATIONS

History of penicillamine-related aplastic anemia or agranulocytosis, rheumatoid arthritis patients with history or evidence of renal insufficiency, pregnancy (unless treating Wilson disease or certain cases of cystinuria), breastfeeding.

INTERACTIONS

Drug

Aluminum salts, sucralfate: May decrease absorption of penicillamine.

Bone marrow depressants, gold compounds, immunosuppressants: May increase risk of hematologic and renal adverse effects.

Iron supplements, antacids: May decrease absorption of penicillamine.

Herbal

None known.

Food

May decrease absorption of penicillamine.

DIAGNOSTIC TEST EFFECTS

None known.

IV INCOMPATIBILITIES

None known.

IV COMPATIBILITIES

None known.

SIDE EFFECTS

Frequent

Rash (pruritic, erythematous, maculopapular, morbilliform, pemphigus), reduced or altered sense of taste (hypogeusia), GI disturbances (anorexia, epigastric pain, nausea, vomiting, diarrhea), oral ulcers, glossitis, polymyositis.

Occasional

Proteinuria, hematuria, hot flashes, drug fever.

Rare

Alopecia, tinnitus, pemphigoid rash (water blisters), thrombocytopenia, leukopenia, eosinophilia, thrombocytosis, renal failure.

SERIOUS REACTIONS

• Aplastic anemia, agranulocytosis, thrombocytopenia, Goodpasture syndrome, proteinuria, hematuria, leukopenia, myasthenia gravis, obliterative bronchiolitis, erythematous-like syndrome, evening hypoglycemia, skin friability at sites of pressure or trauma producing extravasation or white papules at venipuncture, surgical sites reported.

• Iron deficiency (particularly children, menstruating women) may develop.

PRECAUTIONS & CONSIDERATIONS

Caution should be used in elderly patients who may have age-related decreased renal function. Caution should also be used with penicillin allergy and impaired renal and hepatic function. Be aware that penicillamine crosses the placenta and is distributed in breast milk and breastfeeding is contraindicated. Use only when the drug's benefits outweigh the possible hazard to the fetus. No age-related precautions have been noted in children. Baseline WBC, differential, hemoglobin, and platelet count should be performed before therapy begins, every 2 wks thereafter for first 6 mo, then monthly during therapy. Liver function tests (GGT, SGOT, SGPT, LDH) and radiography for renal stones should also be ordered. If WBC < 3500, neutrophils < 2000/mm^3, monocytes > 500/mm^3, or platelet counts < 100,000, or if a progressive fall in either platelet count or WBC in three successive determinations are noted, inform the physician (drug withdrawal is necessary).

If missed menstrual periods or other indications of pregnancy, fever, sore throat, chills, bruising, bleeding, difficulty breathing on exertion, unexplained cough or wheezing occurs, notify the physician promptly.

Storage
Store in tight, well-closed containers.

Administration
Take 1 h before or 2 h after meals or at least 1 h from any other drug, food, or milk. May mix contents of capsule with fruit juice or chilled fruit if the patient cannot swallow capsules.

A 2-h interval is necessary between iron and penicillamine therapy.

In the event of upcoming surgery, dosage should be reduced to 250 mg/day.

Be aware that for Wilson disease, base dosage on urinary copper excretion, serum-free copper concentration that produces or maintains negative copper balance.

Be alert for the presence of cystinuria; give in 4 equal doses; if not feasible, give larger dose at bedtime. Dose based on urinary cysteine excretion. Maintain high fluid intake.

Penicillin
pen-i-sil′in

Amoxicillin, ampicillin, bacampicillin, carbenicillin, cloxacillin, dicloxacillin, flucloxacillin, methicillin, mezlocillin, nafcillin, oxacillin, penicillin G benzathine, penicillin G potassium, penicillin V potassium, piperacillin, pivampicillin, pivmecillinam, ticarcillin; Penicillin and β-lactamase inhibitors; amoxicillin/clavulanate potassium, ampicillin/ sulbactam sodium, piperacillin sodium/tazobactam sodium, ticarcillin disodium/ clavulanate potassium.

CATEGORY AND SCHEDULE
Pregnancy Risk Category: B

Classification: Penicillin, natural, antibiotic

MECHANISM OF ACTION
Penicillins: Bind to bacterial cell wall, inhibiting bacterial cell wall synthesis. *Therapeutic Effect:* Inhibits bacterial cell wall synthesis.

β-Lactamase inhibitors: Inhibit the action of bacterial β-lactamase. *Therapeutic Effect:* Protects the penicillin from enzymatic degradation.

PHARMACOKINETICS
Penicillins are generally well absorbed from the GI tract after oral administration. Widely distributed to most tissues and body fluids. Protein binding: 20%. Partially metabolized in liver. Excreted primarily in urine. *Half-life:* Varies (half-life increased in reduced renal function).

P

AVAILABILITY

Penicillins are available in tablets, chewable tablets, capsules, powder for oral suspension, powder for injection, prefilled syringes for injection, premixed dextrose solutions for injection, and solutions for infusion.

INDICATIONS AND DOSAGES

Penicillins may be used to treat a large number of infections, including pneumonia and other respiratory diseases, urinary tract infections, septicemia, meningitis, intra-abdominal infections, gonorrhea, syphilis, and bone and joint infections.

Doses vary depending on the drug used. In general, penicillins should be taken on an empty stomach. Patients with impaired renal function may require dose adjustment.

OFF-LABEL USES

Some penicillins, such as amoxicillin, have been used in the treatment of Lyme disease and typhoid fever.

CONTRAINDICATIONS

Hypersensitivity to any penicillin, β-lactam, or cephalosporin antibiotics; infectious mononucleosis.

INTERACTIONS

Drug
Penicillin, Penicillin G Potassium, Aqueous (Pfizerpen), Penicillin V Potassium/Penicillin V
Allopurinol: May increase incidence of rash.
Oral contraceptives: May decrease effectiveness of oral contraceptives.
Probenecid, Aspirin: May increase penicillin blood concentration and risk for penicillin toxicity.

Tetracyclines, erythromycin, lincosamides: Possible decreased antimicrobial effect.
Herbal
None known.
Food
None known.

DIAGNOSTIC TEST EFFECTS

May increase BUN, LDH, serum bilirubin, serum creatinine, SGOT (AST), and SGPT (ALT) levels. May cause positive Coombs' test.

SIDE EFFECTS

Frequent
GI disturbances (mild diarrhea, nausea, or vomiting), headache, oral or vaginal candidiasis.
Occasional
Generalized rash, urticaria.

SERIOUS REACTIONS

• Altered bacterial balance may result in potentially fatal superinfections and antibiotic-associated colitis as evidenced by abdominal cramps, watery or severe diarrhea, and fever.
• Severe hypersensitivity reactions, including anaphylaxis and acute interstitial nephritis, occur rarely.

PRECAUTIONS & CONSIDERATIONS

Caution is warranted in patients with antibiotic-associated colitis or a history of allergies, especially to cephalosporins β-lactamases. Be aware that penicillins cross the placenta and are distributed in breast milk in low concentrations Penicillin administration may lead to allergic sensitization, candidiasis, diarrhea, and skin rash in infants. Many penicillins are used in children and are generally well tolerated. Be aware that immature renal function in neonates and young infants may delay renal excretion of penicillins.

In elderly patients, age-related renal impairment may require dosage adjustment.

Notify the physician of signs and symptoms of superinfection, including anal or genital pruritus, black hairy tongue, diarrhea, increased fever, sore throat, ulceration or changes of oral mucosa, and vomiting.

Storage

Store capsules or tablets at room temperature.

In general, after reconstitution, oral solutions are stable for 14 days whether at room temperature or refrigerated.

Store solutions for injection according to manufacturer's instructions.

Administration

Take oral formulations without regard to meals. If GI upset occurs, take with food. Chew or crush chewable tablets thoroughly before swallowing. Take full length of treatment and space doses evenly around the clock.

For IM use, reconstitution and stability vary with each penicillin for injection. Reconstitute and store based on manufacturer's instructions. Give injection deeply into a large muscle mass.

For IV use, reconstitution, rate of infusion, and stability vary with each penicillin for injection. Reconstitute, administer, and store based on manufacturer's instructions.

Penicillin G Benzathine

pen-i-sill'in G ben'za-theen
(Bicillin LA, Permapen)
Do not confuse with penicillin G potassium, penicillin G procaine.

CATEGORY AND SCHEDULE

Pregnancy Risk Category: B

Classification: Antibiotics, benzathine salt of natural penicillin G

MECHANISM OF ACTION

A penicillin that inhibits bacterial cell wall synthesis by binding to one or more of the penicillin-binding proteins of bacteria. *Therapeutic Effect:* Bactericidal.

PHARMACOKINETICS

IM
Very slow absorption; hydrolyzed to penicillin G. Duration 21-28 days. *Half-life:* 30-60 min; excreted in urine, breast milk; crosses placenta.

AVAILABILITY

Injection (Prefilled Syringe [Bicillin LA, Permapen]): 600,000 units/mL.

INDICATIONS AND DOSAGES

Treatment of respiratory infections, scarlet fever, erysipelas, otitis media, pneumonia, skin and soft tissue infections, bejel, pinta, yaws; effective for some gram-positive cocci (*Staphylococcus, S. pyogenes, S. viridans, S. faecalis, S. bovis, S. pneumoniae*), gram-negative cocci (*Neisseria gonorrhoeae*), gram-positive bacilli (*Bacillus anthracis, Clostridium perfringens, C. tetani, C. diptheriae, Listeria monocytogenes*), gram-negative

P

bacilli (*Escherichia coli, Proteus mirabilis, Salmonella, Shigella* spp., *Enterobacter* spp., *S. moniliformis*), spirochetes (*Treponema palladium, Actinomyces* spp).

▸ **Group A streptococcal infections**
IM
Adults, Children > 27 kg. Elderly.
1.2 million units as a single dose.
Children ≤ 27 kg. 600,000 units as a single dose.

▸ **Prevention of rheumatic fever**
IM
Adults, Elderly. 1.2 million units every 3-4 wks or 600,000 units twice monthly.
*Children.*25,000-50,000 units/kg every 3-4 wks.

▸ **Early syphilis**
IM
Adults, Elderly. 2.4 million units divided and administered in two separate injection sites.

▸ **Congenital syphilis**
IM
Children. 50,000 units/kg as single injection after a 10-day course of aqueous penicillin G.

▸ **Syphilis of more than 1-yr duration**
IM
Adults, Elderly. 2.4 million units divided and administered in two separate injection sites weekly for 3 wks.
Children. 50,000 units/kg weekly for 3 wks.

CONTRAINDICATIONS
Hypersensitivity to any penicillin.
Caution
Hypersensitivity to any cephalosporin.

INTERACTIONS
Drug
Erythromycin, lincomycins, tetracyclines: Possible decreased antimicrobial effect.
Methotrexate: Suspected increased risk of toxicity.

Probenecid, aspirin: Increases serum concentration of penicillin.
Oral contraceptives:
Advise patient of a low risk for decreased contraception action, to maintain compliance with oral contraceptive use while taking antibiotics like penicillin, and to consider using additional nonhormonal based contraceptions for the duration of therapy.
Herbal
None known.
Food
None known.

DIAGNOSTIC TEST EFFECTS
May cause a positive Coombs' test.

SERIOUS REACTIONS
• Hypersensitivity reactions, ranging from chills, fever, and rash to anaphylaxis, may occur.

SIDE EFFECTS
Occasional
Lethargy, fever, dizziness, rash, pain at injection site.
Rare
Seizures, interstitial nephritis.

PRECAUTIONS & CONSIDERATIONS
Caution is warranted with a hypersensitivity to cephalosporins, impaired cardiac or renal function, or seizure disorders. History of allergies, especially to cephalosporins or penicillins, should be determined before giving the drug. Signs and symptoms of superinfection, including anal or genital pruritus, black hairy tongue, diarrhea, increased fever, sore throat, ulceration or changes of oral mucosa, and vomiting should be monitored. CBC, renal function test results, and urinalysis should be assessed.

Storage
Store prefilled syringes in the refrigerator. Do not freeze them.
Administration
Administer the drug undiluted by deep IM injection.
! Do not administer penicillin G benzathine IV, intra-arterially, or subcutaneously because doing so may cause heart attack, severe neurovascular damage, thrombosis, and death.

Penicillin G Potassium
pen-i-sill'in G
(Megacillin [CAN], Novepen-G [CAN], Pfizerpen)
Do not confuse with penicillin G benzathine, penicillin G procaine.

CATEGORY AND SCHEDULE
Pregnancy Risk Category: B

Classification: Antibiotics, penicillins

MECHANISM OF ACTION
A penicillin that inhibits bacterial cell wall synthesis by binding to one or more of the penicillin-binding proteins of bacteria. *Therapeutic Effect:* Bactericidal.

PHARMACOKINETICS
Completely absorbed from IM injection sites. Peak blood levels reached rapidly after IV infusion. Bound primarily to albumin. Widely distributed but has limited penetration into cerebrospinal fluid. 60% excreted within 5 h by kidney. *Half-life:* varies.

AVAILABILITY
Injection IM: 5 million units.

Premixed Dextrose Solution:
1 million units, 2 million units, 3 million units.

INDICATIONS AND DOSAGES
▸ **Sepsis, meningitis, pericarditis, endocarditis, pneumonia due to susceptible gram-positive organisms (not *Staphylococcus aureus*) and some gram-negative organisms**
IV, IM
Adults, Elderly. 2-24 million units/day in divided doses q4-6h.
Children. 100,000-400,000 units/kg/day in divided doses q4-6h.
▸ **Dosage in renal impairment**
Dosage interval is modified based on creatinine clearance.

Creatinine Clearance (mL/min)	Dosage Interval
10-50	Usual dose q8-12h
< 10	Usual dose q12-18h

CONTRAINDICATIONS
Hypersensitivity to any penicillin.

INTERACTIONS
Drug
Erythromycin, lincosamides, tetracyclines: May antagonize effects of penicillin.
Oral contraceptives: Advise patient of a potential low risk for decreased contraceptive action, to maintain compliance with oral contraceptive while using antibiotics, and to consider using additional nonhormonal contraception for the duration of therapy.
Probenecid, aspirin: Increased or prolonged plasma levels of penicillin.
Herbal
None known.

P

Food
Food, milk: Decreases penicillin absorption.

DIAGNOSTIC TEST EFFECTS
May cause a positive Coombs' test.

⦸ IV INCOMPATIBILITIES
Include aminophylline, amphotericin B, dextran, diazepam, dobutamine, erythromycin, fat (lipid) emulsion, haloperidol, inamrinone, pentobarbital, phenytoin, protamine, quinidine.

🛡 IV COMPATIBILITIES
Include amiodarone, aztreonam, calcium gluconate, cimetidine, clindamycin, digoxin, dopamine, famotidine, furosemide, magnesium sulfate, metoclopramide, morphine, nitroglycerin, oxytocin.

SIDE EFFECTS
Occasional
Lethargy, fever, dizziness, rash, electrolyte imbalance, diarrhea, thrombophlebitis.
Rare
Seizures, interstitial nephritis.

SERIOUS REACTIONS
• Hypersensitivity reactions ranging from rash, fever, and chills to anaphylaxis occur.

PRECAUTIONS & CONSIDERATIONS
Caution is warranted in patients with a hypersensitivity to cephalosporins, impaired hepatic or renal function, a history of antibiotic-associated colitis, or seizure disorders. CBC, electrolyte levels, renal function test results, and urinalysis results should be monitored. Hypersensitivity to penicillin or cephalosporin should be established before beginning therapy. Any indications of

superinfection, such as sore throat, oral burning sensation, fever, or fatigue, should be reported.
Storage
The reconstituted solution is stable for 7 days if refrigerated and 24 hr at room temperature.
Administration
For IV use, follow the manufacturer's guidelines for dilution. After reconstitution, further dilute with 50-100 mL D5W or 0.9% NaCl to yield a final concentration of 100,000-500,000 units/mL (50,000 units/mL for infants and neonates). Infuse the solution over 1-2 hr for adults, 15-30 min for infants and children.

Penicillin V Potassium
pen-i-sill'in V
(Abbocillin VK [AUS], Apo-Pen-VK [CAN], Cilicaine VK [AUS], L.P.V. [AUS], Novo-Pen-VK [CAN], Veetids, V-Cillin-K)

CATEGORY AND SCHEDULE
Pregnancy Risk Category: B

Classification: Antibiotics, semisynthetic penicillins

MECHANISM OF ACTION
A penicillin that inhibits cell wall synthesis by binding to bacterial cell membranes. *Therapeutic Effect:* Bactericidal.

PHARMACOKINETICS
Moderately absorbed from the GI tract. Protein binding: 80%. Widely distributed. Metabolized in the liver. Primarily excreted in urine. *Half-life:* 1 h (increased in impaired renal function).

AVAILABILITY
Tablets: 250 mg, 500 mg.
Powder for Oral Solution:
125 mg/5 mL, 250 mg/5 mL.

INDICATIONS AND DOSAGES
Effective for treatment of gram-positive cocci (*Staphylococcus aureus, S. viridans, S. faecalis, S. bovis, S. pneumoiae*), gram-negative cocci *(Neisseria gnorrhoeae, N. meningitis)*, gram-positive bacilli (*Bacillus anthracis, Clostridium perfrignens, C. tetani, C. dipththeriae*), gram-negative bacilli (*S. moniliformis*), spirochetes (*Treponema palladium*), *Actinomyces, Peptococcus,* and *Peptostreptococcus* spp.
▸ **Mild to moderate respiratory tract or skin or skin-structure infections, otitis media, necrotizing ulcerative gingivitis**
PO
Adults, Elderly, Children 12 yr and older. 125-500 mg q6-8h.
Children younger than 12 yr.
25-50 mg/kg/day in divided doses q6-8h. Maximum: 3 g/day.
▸ **Primary prevention of rheumatic fever**
PO
Adults, Elderly. 125-250 q6-8h for 10 days.
Children. 250 mg 2-3 times/day for 10 days.

CONTRAINDICATIONS
Hypersensitivity to any penicillin.

INTERACTIONS
Drug
Oral contraceptives: Advise patient of potential low risk for decreased contraceptive action, to maintain compliance with oral contraceptive use while taking antibiotics and to consider using additional nonhormonal contraception during therapy.

Probenecid, aspirin: May increase penicillin blood concentration and risk of toxicity.
Tetracyclines, lincomycins, and erythromycin: Decreased antimicrobial effectiveness.
Herbal and Food
None known.

DIAGNOSTIC TEST EFFECTS
May cause a positive Coombs' test.

SIDE EFFECTS
Frequent
Mild hypersensitivity reaction (chills, fever, rash), nausea, vomiting, diarrhea.
Rare
Bleeding, allergic reaction.

SERIOUS REACTIONS
• Severe hypersensitivity reactions, including anaphylaxis, may occur.
• Nephrotoxicity, antibiotic-associated colitis, and other superinfections may result from high dosages or prolonged therapy.

PRECAUTIONS & CONSIDERATIONS
Caution is warranted in patients with renal impairment, a history of seizures, or a history of allergies, particularly to cephalosporins. Penicillin V readily crosses the placenta, appears in cord blood and amniotic fluid, and is distributed in breast milk in low concentrations. Penicillin V may lead to allergic sensitization, candidiasis, diarrhea, and skin rash in infants. Use caution when giving to neonates and young infants because their immature renal function may delay renal excretion of the drug. Age-related renal impairment may require dosage adjustment in elderly patients.
    History of allergies, especially to cephalosporins or penicillins, should be determined before giving the drug.

Withhold and promptly notify the physician if rash or diarrhea occurs. Severe diarrhea with abdominal pain, blood or mucus in stool, and fever may indicate antibiotic-associated colitis. Signs of bleeding, including ecchymosis, overt bleeding, and swelling, should be assessed. Signs and symptoms of superinfection, including anal or genital pruritus, black hairy tongue, diarrhea, increased fever, sore throat, ulceration or changes of oral mucosa, and vomiting, should also be monitored. Intake and output, renal function tests, hemoglobin levels, and urinalysis should be obtained and reviewed. Possible superinfection evidenced by sore throat, oral burning sensation, fatigue, or fever should be reported immediately to the health care provider.

Storage
Store tablets at room temperature. After reconstitution, the oral solution is stable for 14 days if refrigerated.

Administration
Take the drug without regard to food. Space drug doses evenly around the clock.

Pentamidine Isethionate

pen-tam′i-deen ice-ethy-eye-oh-nate
(NebuPent, Pentacarinat [CAN], Pentam-300)

CATEGORY AND SCHEDULE
Pregnancy Risk Category: C

Classification: Antiprotozoals

MECHANISM OF ACTION
An anti-infective that interferes with nuclear metabolism and incorporation of nucleotides, inhibiting DNA, RNA, phospholipid, and protein synthesis. *Therapeutic Effect:* Produces antibacterial and antiprotozoal effects.

PHARMACOKINETICS
Well absorbed after IM administration; minimally absorbed after inhalation. Widely distributed. Primarily excreted in urine. Minimally removed by hemodialysis. *Half-life:* 6.4 h (IV), 9.1-13.2 h (IV/IM) (increased in impaired renal function).

AVAILABILITY
Injection (Pentam-300): 300 mg.
Powder for Nebulization (Nebupent): 300 mg.

INDICATIONS AND DOSAGES
▸ **Treatment of *Pneumocystis carinii* infections in immunocompromised patients (injection); prevention in high-risk HIV-infected patients (inhalant)**
▸ **P. carinii pneumonia (PCP)**
IV, IM
Adults, Elderly, Children. 4 mg/kg/ day once a day for 14-21 days.
▸ **Prevention of PCP**
INHALATION
Adults, Elderly. 300 mg q4wk.
Children 5 yr and older. 300 mg q4 wk.

OFF-LABEL USES
Treatment of African trypanosomiasis, cutaneous or visceral leishmaniasis.

CONTRAINDICATIONS
Concurrent use with didanosine.

INTERACTIONS
Drug
Blood dyscrasia–producing medications, bone marrow

depressants: May increase the abnormal hematologic effects of pentamidine.

Didanosine: May increase the risk of pancreatitis.

Foscarnet: May increase the risk of hypocalcemia, hypomagnesemia, and nephrotoxicity of pentamidine.

Nephrotoxic medications: May increase the risk of nephrotoxicity.

Herbal
None known.

Food
None known.

DIAGNOSTIC TEST EFFECTS

May increase BUN and serum alkaline phosphatase, bilirubin, creatinine, AST (SGOT), and ALT (SGPT) levels. May decrease serum calcium and magnesium levels. May alter blood glucose levels.

Ⓓ IV INCOMPATIBILITIES

Do not mix with other medications.

SIDE EFFECTS

Frequent
Injection (> 10%): Abscess, pain at injection site.
Inhalation (> 5%): Fatigue, metallic taste, shortness of breath, decreased appetite, dizziness, rash, cough, nausea, vomiting, chills.

Occasional
Injection (1%-10%): Nausea, decreased appetite, hypotension, fever, rash, altered taste, confusion.
Inhalation (1%-5%): Diarrhea, headache, anemia, muscle pain.

Rare
Injection (< 1%): Neuralgia, thrombocytopenia, phlebitis, dizziness.

SERIOUS REACTIONS

• Rare reactions include life-threatening or fatal hypotension, cardiac arrhythmias, hypoglycemia, leukopenia, nephrotoxicity or renal failure, anaphylactic shock, Stevens-Johnson syndrome, and toxic epidural necrolysis are reported with IM and IV routes; monitor BP continuously throughout the infusion, and every 30 min for 2 h thereafter and every 4 h after that until BP stabilizes..

• Hyperglycemia and insulin-dependent diabetes mellitus (often permanent) may occur even months after therapy has stopped.

PRECAUTIONS & CONSIDERATIONS

Caution is warranted in patients with diabetes mellitus, hypertension, hypotension, or renal or hepatic impairment. It is unknown whether pentamidine crosses the placenta or is distributed in breast milk. No age-related precautions have been noted in children, although safety and efficacy of the inhalation formulation are not established. No information is available regarding pentamidine use in elderly patients. Avoid alcohol.

Report any lightheadedness, palpitations, shakiness or sweating, shortness of breath, cough, or fever. Drowsiness, decreased appetite, and increased thirst and urination may develop in the months following therapy, which may be indicative of drug-induced hyperglycemia. Adequate hydration should be maintained.

IV and IM sites should be evaluated for abscess development. Skin should be examined for rash. Hematology, liver, and renal function tests should be performed. Be alert for respiratory difficulty when administering pentamidine by inhalation.

Storage
Store vials at room temperature. After reconstitution, the IV solution

P

is stable at room temperature for 48 h. Store the aerosol at room temperature for 48 h.

Administration

! Make sure the person is in the supine position during administration and has frequent BP checks until stable because of the risk of a life-threatening hypotensive reaction. Have resuscitative equipment readily available.

For intermittent IV infusion (piggyback), reconstitute each vial with 3-5 mL D5W or sterile water for injection. Withdraw the desired dose and further dilute with 50-250 mL D5W. Infuse the drug over 60 min. Discard any unused portion. Do not give the drug by IV injection or rapid IV infusion because this increases the risk of severe hypotension.

For IM use, reconstitute each 300-mg vial with 3 mL sterile water for injection to provide a concentration of 100 mg/mL.

For aerosol (nebulizer) use, reconstitute each 300-mg vial with 6 mL sterile water for injection. Avoid using 0.9% NaCl because it may cause a precipitate to form. Do not mix pentamidine with other medications in the nebulizer reservoir.

Pentazocine Hydrochloride

pen-tah-zoe-seen high-droh-klor-ide (Talwin)

Combination Products:
With naloxone, a narcotic antagonist (oral) (Talwin NX); with aspirin (oral) (Talwin Compound); with acetaminophen (oral) (Talacen)

CATEGORY AND SCHEDULE

With naloxone, a narcotic antagonist (oral) (Talwin NX); with aspirin (oral) (Talwin Compound); with acetaminophen (oral) (Talacen)

Classification: Analgesics, narcotic mixed agonist-antagonist

MECHANISM OF ACTION

Narcotic antagonist and agonist that induces analgesia by stimulating the κ- and σ-receptors within the central nervous system (CNS). *Therapeutic Effect:* Alters processes affecting pain perception, emotional response to pain.

PHARMACOKINETICS

Well absorbed after administration. Widely distributed, including the cerebrospinal fluid (CSF). Metabolized in liver via oxidative and glucuronide conjugation pathways, extensive first-pass effect. Excreted in small amounts in the bile and feces as unchanged drug. *Half-life:* 2-3 h, prolonged with hepatic impairment.

AVAILABILITY

Tablets: 12.5 mg and 325 mg aspirin (Talwin Compound), 25 mg and 650 mg acetaminophen (Talacen), 50 mg pentazocine and 0.5 mg

naloxone (Talwin NX), 50 mg (Talwin).
Injection: 30 mg (Talwin).

INDICATIONS AND DOSAGES

Treatment of moderate to severe pain alone or in combination with aspirin or acetaminophen.

▸ **Pain, analgesia, moderate to severe**

PO
Adults, elderly, children 12 yr and older. 50 mg q3-4h. May increase to 100 mg q3-4h, if needed. Maximum: 600 mg/day.

IM/IV
Adults. 30 mg q3-4h. Do not exceed 30 mg IV or 60 mg IM per dose. Maximum: 360 mg/day.

IM

▸ **Obstetric labor**

IM
Adults. 30 mg as a single dose.
IV
Adults. 20 mg when contractions are regular. May repeat 2-3 times q2-3h.

CONTRAINDICATIONS

Hypersensitivity to pentazocine or any component of the formulation, elderly.

INTERACTIONS

Drug
Alcohol, central nervous system (CNS) depressants: May increase CNS or respiratory depression and hypotension.
Anticholinergics: Increased effect.
Fluoxetine: May cause hypertension, diaphoresis, ataxia, flushing, nausea, dizziness, and anxiety.
MAOIs: May produce severe, fatal reaction.
Opioid analgesics: May increase withdrawal symptoms or cause additive effects.
Sibutramine: May increase risk of serotonin syndrome.

Herbal
None known.
Food
None known.

DIAGNOSTIC TEST EFFECTS

May increase amylase and lipase.

SIDE EFFECTS

Frequent
Drowsiness, euphoria, nausea, vomiting.
Occasional
Allergic reaction, histamine reaction (decreased BP, increased sweating, flushing, wheezing), decreased urination, altered vision, constipation, dizziness, dry mouth, headache, hypotension, pain/burning at injection site.

SERIOUS REACTIONS

• Overdosage results in severe respiratory depression, skeletal muscle flaccidity, cyanosis, extreme somnolence progressing to convulsions, stupor, and coma.
• Abrupt withdrawal after prolonged use may produce symptoms of narcotic withdrawal (abdominal cramps, rhinorrhea, lacrimation, nausea, vomiting, restlessness, anxiety, increased temperature, piloerection).

P

PRECAUTIONS & CONSIDERATIONS

Caution is warranted in patients with head injury or increased intracranial pressure, respiratory disease, or respiratory depression before biliary tract surgery (produces spasm of spinchter of Oddi), acute myocardial infarction, severe heart disease, opioid dependence or abuse, addictive personality, impaired hepatic and renal function, acute abdominal conditions, Addison disease, prostatic hypertrophy, and patients taking other narcotics.

It is unknown whether pentazocine crosses the placenta or is distributed in breast milk. Safety and efficacy have not been established in children 12 yr or older. Age-related renal or liver impairment may require decreased dosage. Not recommended for use in the elderly, because of potential for increase CNS adverse reactions.

Pentazocine may cause withdrawal in patients currently dependent on narcotics. It may cause drowsiness and impaired judgment or coordination, so driving and tasks requiring alertness and coordination should be avoided. Alcohol should be avoided. Psychological and physical dependence may occur with chronic administration.

Storage
Store parenteral form at room temperature.

Administration
Rotate injection site for IM use. SC route not recommended because of potential for severe local reactions. Avoid intra-arterial injection. Do not mix with barbiturates in solution or syringe.

May take oral pentazocine with food if GI upset occurs.

Pentobarbital
pen-toe-bar'bi-tal
(Nembutal, Phenobarbitone [AUS])
Do not confuse with phenobarbital.

CATEGORY AND SCHEDULE
Pregnancy Risk Category: D
Controlled Substance: Schedule II (capsules, injection), Schedule III (suppositories)

Classification: Anticonvulsants,, preanesthetics, sedative/hypnotic, barbiturates

MECHANISM OF ACTION
A barbiturate that binds at the γ-amino butyric acid (GABA) receptor complex, enhancing GABA activity. *Therapeutic Effect:* Depresses central nervous system (CNS) activity and reticular activating system.

PHARMACOKINETICS
Well absorbed after PO, parenteral administration. Protein binding: 35%-55%. Rapidly, widely distributed. Metabolized in liver. Primarily excreted in urine. Removed by hemodialysis. *Half-life:* 15-48 h.

AVAILABILITY
Capsules: 50 mg, 100 mg.
Injection: 50 mg/mL.
Suppositories: 30 mg, 120 mg, 200 mg.

INDICATIONS AND DOSAGES
▸ **Treatment of insomnia, sedation, preoperative medication, increased intracranial pressure (ICP) or dental anesthetic**
▸ **Preanesthetic**
PO
Adults, Elderly. 100 mg.
Children. 2-6 mg/kg. Maximum: 100 mg/dose.
IM
Adults, Elderly. 150-200 mg.
Children. 2-6 mg/kg. Maximum: 100 mg/dose.
RECTAL
Children aged 12-14 yr. 60 or 120 mg.
Children aged 5-12 yr. 60 mg.
Children aged 1-4 yr. 30-60 mg.
Children aged 2-12 mo. 30 mg.
▸ **Hypnotic**
PO
Adults, Elderly. 100 mg at bedtime.
IM
Adults, Elderly. 150-200 mg at bedtime.
Children. 2-6 mg/kg. Maximum: 100 mg/dose at bedtime.

IV
Adults, Elderly. 100 mg initially then, after 1 min, may give additional small doses at 1-min intervals, up to 500 mg total.
RECTAL
Adults, Elderly. 120-200 mg at bedtime.
Children aged 12-14 yr. 60 or 120 mg at bedtime.
Children aged 5-12 yr. 60 mg at bedtime.
Children aged 1-4 yr. 30-60 mg at bedtime.
Children aged 2-12 mo to 1 yr. 30 mg at bedtime.
▸ **Anticonvulsant**
IV
Adults, Elderly. 10-15 mg/kg loading dose given slowly over 1-2 h. Maintenance infusion: 0.5 mg/kg/h.
Children. 10-15 mg/kg loading dose given slowly over 1-2 h. Maintenance infusion: 0.5 mg/kg/h.

OFF-LABEL USES

Intracranial hypertension, psychiatric interviews, sedative withdrawal, drug abuse withdrawal.

CONTRAINDICATIONS

Porphyria, hypersensitivity to barbiturates.

INTERACTIONS

Drug
Alcohol, CNS depressants: May increase the depressive effects of pentobarbital.
Alprenolol, metoprolol: May decrease effectiveness.
Antihistamines, cold remedies (OTC): May have additive effect with any other CNS depressant ingredients.
Barbituates, chloral hydrate, opioid analgesics: May increase the risk of respiratory depression.
Carbamazepine: May increase metabolism.

Dicumarol: May decrease the anticoagulant effectiveness.
Doxycycline: May decrease half-life.
Glucocorticoids and corticosteroids: May increase metabolism and decrease therapeutic effects.
Halogenated hydrocarbon anesthetics: May cause hepatotoxicity.
Procarbazine: May increase the risk of CNS depression.
Quetiapine: May decrease serum quetiapine concentrations.
Theophylline: May decrease theophylline effectiveness.
Tricyclic antidepressants and MAOIs: May increase metabolism and decrease effectiveness.
Herbal
Catnip oil: May increase risk of CNS depression.
Eucalyptol: May decrease effectiveness of barbiturates.
Kava kava, valerian: May increase CNS depression.
St. John's wort: May decrease CNS depressive effect of barbiturates.
Food
None known.

DIAGNOSTIC TEST EFFECTS

None known.

ⓘ IV INCOMPATIBILITIES

In general, do not mix or infuse with other drugs. Amikacin (Amikin), aminophylline, atracurium (Tacrium), benzquinamide, butorphanol, cefazolin (Ancef), chlorpheniramine, clindamycin (Cleocin), codeine, cyclizine, diphenhydramine (Benadryl), droperidol (Inapsine), fenoldopam (Corlopam), fentanyl, glycopyrrolate (Robinul), hyaluronidase (Wydase), hydrocortisone (Solu-Cortef),hydromorphone (Dilaudid), insulin, kanamycin

(Kantrex), levorphanol (Levo-Dromoran),lidocaine, meperidine (Demerol), metaraminol (Aramin), methadone, methyldopa (Aldomet), metocurine (Metubine), midazolam (Versed), nalbuphine (Nubain), neostigmine (Prostigmin), opium alkaloids, oxytetracycline, pancuronium (Pavulon), penicillin G (Pfizerpen), pentazocine (Talwin), perphenazine (Trilafon), prochlorperazine (Compazine), promazine (Sparine), propofol (Diprivan), ranitidine (Zantac), scopolamine, sodium bicarbonate, sodium iodide, streptomycin, thiamine, thiopental (Pentothal), triflupromazine (Stelazine), tripelennamine (PBZ), vancomycin (Vancocin), verapamil.

SIDE EFFECTS

Occasional
Agitation, confusion, dizziness, somnolence.
Rare
Confusion, paradoxical CNS hyperactivity or nervousness in children, excitement or restlessness in elderly

SERIOUS REACTIONS

• Agranulocytosis, megaloblastic anemia, apnea, hypoventilation, bradycardia, hypotension, syncope, hepatic damage, and Stevens-Johnson syndrome occur rarely.
• Abrupt withdrawal after prolonged therapy may produce effects ranging from markedly increased dreaming, nightmares or insomnia, tremor, sweating and vomiting, to hallucinations, delirium, seizures, and status epilepticus.
• Skin eruptions appear as hypersensitivity reactions.
• Overdosage produces cold or clammy skin, hypothermia, severe CNS depression, cyanosis, and rapid pulse.

PRECAUTIONS & CONSIDERATIONS

Caution is warranted in patients with liver or renal impairment, in elderly patients, or in patients with debilitated, suicidal tendencies, or a history of drug or alcohol abuse. Pentobarbital readily crosses the placenta and is distributed in breast milk. Withdrawal symptoms may appear in neonates born to women receiving barbiturates during the last trimester of pregnancy. Its use may cause paradoxical excitement in children. Elderly patients taking pentobarbital may exhibit confusion, excitement, and mental depression. Alcohol consumption and caffeine should be avoided while taking pentobarbital. Tasks that require mental alertness or motor skills should be avoided because pentobarbital may cause dizziness and drowsiness. Drug should not be given if respirations drop to 10/min or less or pupils become dilated.

Storage
Store vials at room temperature.
　Refrigerate suppositories.

Administration
Be aware that dosage must be individualized based on patient's age, weight, and condition.
　Give oral pentobarbital on an empty stomach.
　Do not inject more than 5 mL in any one IM injection site because it produces tissue irritation. Inject IM dorsogluteally or into lateral aspect of thigh.
　May give IV injection undiluted or may dilute with 0.45% NaCl or 0.9% NaCl to final concentration of 4-10 mg/mL.
　Expect to hydrate adequately before and immediately after infusion to decrease the risk of adverse renal effects. Parenteral routes should be pursued only when oral administration is impossible or

impractical. Beware that inadvertent intra-arterial injection may result in arterial spasm with severe pain and tissue necrosis. Also know that extravasation in SC tissue may produce redness, tenderness, and tissue necrosis. If either occurs, treat with 0.5% procaine solution injected into affected area and apply moist heat.

Unwrap rectal suppository before insertion. Moisten suppository with cold water before inserting well up into rectum.

Pentosan Polysulfate
pen-toe-san poll-ee-sull-fate
(Elmiron)
Do not confuse with pentostatin.

CATEGORY AND SCHEDULE
Pregnancy Risk Category: B

Classification: Anticoagulant

MECHANISM OF ACTION
A negatively charged synthetic sulfated polysaccharide with heparin-like properties that appears to adhere to bladder wall mucosal membrane; it may act as a buffering agent to control cell permeability, preventing irritating solutes in the urine. Has anticoagulant/fibrinolytic effects. *Therapeutic Effect:* Relieves bladder pain.

PHARMACOKINETICS
Poorly and erratically absorbed from the GI tract. Distributed in uroepithelium of the genitourinary tract, with lesser amount found in the liver, spleen, lung, skin, periosteum, and bone marrow. Metabolized in the liver and kidney (secondary). Eliminated in the urine. *Half-life:* 4.8 h.

AVAILABILITY
Capsules: 100 mg (Elmiron).

INDICATIONS AND DOSAGES
Relief of interstitial cystitis symptoms.
▶ **Interstitial cystitis**
PO
Adults, Elderly. 100 mg 3 times/day.

OFF-LABEL USES
Urolithiasis

CONTRAINDICATIONS
Hypersensitivity to pentosan polysulfate sodium or structurally related compounds.

INTERACTIONS
Drug
Anticoagulants, high-dose aspirin: May increase risk of bleeding.
NSAIDs: May increase risk of bleeding and GI effects.
Herbal
Alfalfa, coenzyme Q, green tea: May decrease anticoagulant effectiveness.
Arnica, bilberry, black currant, bromelain, cat's claw, chamomile, clove oil, curcumin, dong quai, primrose oil, fenugreek, garlic, ginger, kava kava, licorice, red clover, skullcap, tan-shen, vitamin A: May increase risk of bleeding.
Chondroitin, ginseng: May increase INR serum values and increase anticoagulant effects.
Food
Avocado: May decrease anticoagulant effectiveness.
Rhubarb: May increase risk of bleeding.

P

DIAGNOSTIC TEST EFFECTS

May increase transaminase (ALT), alkaline phosphatase (SGOT), PTT, PT. May decrease WBC count, thrombocytes.

SIDE EFFECTS

Frequent

Alopecia areata (a single area on the scalp), diarrhea, nausea, headache, rash, abdominal pain, dyspepsia.

Occasional

Dizziness, depression, increased liver function tests.

SERIOUS REACTIONS

• Ecchymosis, epistaxis, gum hemorrhage have been reported (drug produces weak anticoagulant effect).

• Overdose may produce liver function abnormalities.

PRECAUTIONS & CONSIDERATIONS

Caution is warranted with GI ulcerations, polyps, diverticula, history of heparin-induced thrombocytopenia, hepatic or splenic function impairment, concurrent anticoagulant, thrombolytic or antiplatelet therapy, and recent intracranial, intraspinal, or ophthalmologic surgery. It is unknown whether pentosan polysulfate sodium is distributed in breast milk. Safety and efficacy of pentosan polysulfate sodium have not been established in children younger than 16 yr. No age-related precautions have been noted in elderly patients.

The physician should be notified if any bleeding from gums or nose, bloody or black bowel movements, coughing up blood, bloody vomit or vomit that looks like coffee grounds, or severe stomach pain or diarrhea that does not stop occurs.

Administration

Take with water at least 1 h before or 2 h after meals.

Pentostatin

Pen-toe-stat-in

(Nipent)

Do not confuse with pravastatin.

CATEGORY AND SCHEDULE

Pregnancy Risk Category: D

Classification: Antineoplastic, enzyme inhibitor

MECHANISM OF ACTION

An antimetabolite that inhibits the enzyme adenosine deaminase (ADA) (increases intracellular levels of adenine deoxynucleotide). Greatest activity in T cells of lymphoid system. Inhibits ADA and RNA synthesis. Produces DNA damage. *Therapeutic Effect:* Leads to tumor cell death.

PHARMACOKINETICS

After IV administration, rapidly distributed to body tissues (poorly distributed to cerebrospinal fluid). Protein binding: 4%. Excreted primarily in urine unchanged or as active metabolite. *Half-life:* 5.7 h (2.6-10 h).

AVAILABILITY

Powder for Injection. 10 mg (Nipent), 2 mg/mL once reconstituted.

INDICATIONS AND DOSAGES

Treatment of α-interferon-refractory hairy cell leukemia.

▸ **Hairy cell leukemia**

IV
Adults, Elderly. 4 mg/m² q2wk
until complete response is attained
(without any major toxicity).
Discontinue if no response in 6 mo;
partial response in 12 mo.
▶ **Dosage in renal cell impairment**
Only when benefits justify risks, give
2-3 mg/m² in patients with creatinine
clearance of < 60 mL/min.

UNLABELED USES
Palliative therapy of chronic
lymphocytic leukemia,
prolymphocytic leukemia, cutaneous
T-cell lymphoma.

CONTRAINDICATIONS
Pentostatin hypersensitivity.

INTERACTIONS
Drug
Allopurinol: May increase
pentostatin toxicity.
**Carmustine, cyclophosphamide,
etoposide:** Acute pulmonary edema,
hypotension, and death when
coadministered.
Fludarabine: Coadministration can
cause severe pulmonary toxicity.
Vidarabine: May increase toxic
effect of vidarabine.
Herbal
None known.
Food
None known.

DIAGNOSTIC TEST EFFECTS
May elevate creatinine (3%-10%),
hypercalcemia, hyponatremia (< 3%).
Monitor CBC with differential and
platelet count and renal function
before each dose.

SIDE EFFECTS
Frequent
Nausea, vomiting, fever, fatigue,
rash, pain, cough, upper respiratory
tract infection, anorexia, diarrhea.

Occasional
Headache, pharyngitis, sinusitis,
myalgia, chills, peripheral
edema, anorexia, blurred vision,
conjunctivitis, skin discoloration,
sweating, anxiety, depression,
dizziness, confusion.

SERIOUS REACTIONS
• Bone marrow depression is
manifested as hematologic toxicity
(principally leukopenia, anemia,
thrombocytopenia). Doses higher
than recommended (20-50 mg/m² in
divided doses for more than 5 days)
may produce severe renal, hepatic,
pulmonary, or central nervous system
(CNS) toxicity.

PRECAUTIONS &CONSIDERATIONS
Do not exceed recommended doses
as nephrotoxicity, hepatoxicity,
pulmonary and CNS toxicities
have occurred at doses higher
than recommended. Any of the
following symptoms should be
reported immediately: rash, hives,
difficulty breathing, fever, chills;
these symptoms can be indicators
of possible infection: bleeding or
unusual bruising, mouth sores, dark
urine, yellowing of skin or eyes, pain,
redness, swelling at injection site;
persistent nausea, vomiting, diarrhea,
appetite loss or worsening general
body weakness. Maintain adequate
hydration during therapy to avoid
developing hyperuricemia and urate
precipitation. Rashes, occasionally
severe, are common and may
worsen with continued treatment;
development of such rashes need to
be reported immediately because
discontinuation of the drug therapy
may be warranted.

Care is warranted with handling,
administration, and disposal of
the drug. Appropriate protective
equipment should be worn when

P

preparing and administering the dose. Avoid exposure by inhalation or direct skin, mucous membrane or eye contact. Spills should be treated with 5% sodium hypochlorite solution prior to disposal. If accidental skin or mucous membrane contact occurs, wash immediately with soap and water; if ocular contact occurs, immediately institute copious plain-water irrigation.

Storage
Refrigerate unopened vials; use reconstituted solution or reconstituted solution further diluted within 8 h of reconstitution.

Administration
Administer only by bolus IV infusion; do not use intradermally, subcutaneously, intramuscularly, intra-arterially, or orally.

Reconstitute powder for injection with 5 mL sterile water for injection. Mix thoroughly to obtain complete dissolution to a 2 mg/mL concentration of pentostatin. Do not administer if particulate matter, cloudiness, or discoloration is noted. May administer reconstituted solution as a bolus injection or may further dilute reconstituted solution with 25-50 mL of dextrose 5% in water or sodium chloride 0.9% injection for IV infusion over 20-30 min.

Pentoxifylline
pen-tox-if'ih-lin
(Albert [CAN], Apo-Pentoxifylline SR [CAN], Pentoxifylline [CAN], Pentoxyl, Trental)
Do not confuse Trental with Tegretol, Trandate.

CATEGORY AND SCHEDULE
Pregnancy Risk Category: C

Classification: Hemorrheologic agents, xanthine derivatives

MECHANISM OF ACTION
A blood viscosity-reducing agent that alters the flexibility of RBCs; inhibits production of tumor necrosis factor, neutrophil activation, and platelet aggregation. *Therapeutic Effect:* Reduces blood viscosity and improves blood flow.

PHARMACOKINETICS
Well absorbed after oral administration. Undergoes first-pass metabolism in the liver. Excreted primarily in urine. Unknown whether removed by hemodialysis.
Half-life: 24-48 min; metabolite, 60-90 min.

AVAILABILITY
Tablets (Controlled-Release [Pentoxil, Trental]): 400 mg.

INDICATIONS AND DOSAGES
▸ **Intermittent claudication related to chronic occlusive arterial disease of the limbs.**
PO
Adults, Elderly. 400 mg 3 times a day. Decrease to 400 mg twice a day if GI or CNS adverse effects occur. Continue for at least 8 wks.

CONTRAINDICATIONS

History of intolerance to xanthine derivatives, such as caffeine, theophylline, or theobromine; recent cerebral or retinal hemorrhage.

INTERACTIONS

Drug
Antihypertensives: May increase the effects of antihypertensives.
Aspirin, NSAIDs: May increase anticoagulant effects and risk of bleeding.
Herbal
None known.
Food
None known.

DIAGNOSTIC TEST EFFECTS

None known.

SIDE EFFECTS

Occasional (2%-5%)
Dizziness, nausea, altered taste, dyspepsia, marked by heartburn, epigastric pain, and indigestion.
Rare (< 2%)
Rash, pruritus, anorexia, constipation, dry mouth, blurred vision, edema, nasal congestion, anxiety.

SERIOUS REACTIONS

• Angina and chest pain occur rarely and may be accompanied by palpitations, tachycardia, and arrhythmias.
• Signs and symptoms of overdose, such as flushing, hypotension, nervousness, agitation, hand tremor, fever, and somnolence, appear 4-5 h after ingestion and last for 12 h.

PRECAUTIONS & CONSIDERATIONS

Caution is warranted in patients with chronic occlusive arterial disease, insulin-treated diabetes, hepatic or renal impairment, peptic ulcer disease, and recent surgery. It is unknown whether pentoxifylline crosses the placenta and is distributed in breast milk. Safety and efficacy of pentoxifylline have not been established in children. In elderly patients, age-related renal impairment may require cautious use. Caffeine should be limited and smoking should be avoided; smoking causes vasoconstriction and occlusion of peripheral blood vessels.

Dizziness may occur. Avoid tasks requiring mental alertness or motor skills until response to the drug has been established. Notify the physician of hand tremor. Notify the physician of red or dark urine, muscular pain or weakness, abdominal or back pain, gingival bleeding, black or red stool, coffee-ground vomitus, or blood-tinged mucus from cough. BP, heart rate and rhythm, pulse rate, serum creatinine (SCr), and AST (SGOT) levels should be monitored. Relief of signs and symptoms of intermittent claudication should be monitored; symptoms generally occur while walking or exercising or with weight bearing in the absence of walking or exercising. Patient's ability to tolerate stress should be considered as stress responses may compromise cardiovascular functions.

Administration
Do not crush or break film-coated tablets. Take with meals to avoid GI upset. Therapeutic effect is generally noted in 2-4 wks.

Pergolide Mesylate
per'go-lide mez-il-ate
(Permax)
**Do not confuse Permax with
Pentrax or Pernox.**
Discontinued in the United States

CATEGORY AND SCHEDULE
Pregnancy Risk Category: B

Classification: Antiparkinson
agents, dermatologics, ergot
alkaloids and derivatives

MECHANISM OF ACTION
A centrally active dopamine agonist
that directly stimulates dopamine
receptors. *Therapeutic Effect:*
Decreases signs and symptoms of
Parkinson disease.

PHARMACOKINETICS
Well absorbed from the GI tract. Protein
binding: 90%. Undergoes extensive
first-pass metabolism in the liver.
Primarily excreted in urine. Unknown
whether removed by hemodialysis.

AVAILABILITY
Tablets: 0.05 mg, 0.25 mg, 1 mg.

INDICATIONS AND DOSAGES
▶ **Adjunctive treatment of Parkinson
disease, parkinsonism**
PO
Adults, Elderly. Initially,
0.05 mg/day for 2 days. May increase
by 0.1-0.15 mg/day every 3 days
over the next 12 days; afterward
may increase by 0.25 mg/day
every 3 days. Range: 2-3 mg/day
in 3 divided doses. Maximum:
5 mg/day.

CONTRAINDICATIONS
Hypersensitivity to pergolide or other
ergot derivatives.

INTERACTIONS
Drug
**Haloperidol, phenothiazines,
droperidol, thiothixenes,
metoclopramide:** May decrease the
effectiveness of pergolide.
**Hypotension-producing
medications:** May increase the
hypotensive effect.
Herbal
None known.
Food
None known.

DIAGNOSTIC TEST EFFECTS
May increase the serum growth
hormone level.

SIDE EFFECTS
Frequent (10%-24%)
Nausea, dizziness, hallucinations,
constipation, rhinitis, dystonia,
confusion, somnolence.
Occasional (3%-9%)
Orthostatic hypotension, insomnia,
dry mouth, peripheral edema, anxiety,
diarrhea, dyspepsia, abdominal pain,
headache, abnormal vision, anorexia,
tremor, depression, rash.
Rare (< 2%)
Urinary frequency, vivid dreams,
neck pain, hypotension, vomiting.

SERIOUS REACTIONS
• Symptoms of overdose may
vary from central nervous system
(CNS) depression, characterized
by sedation, apnea, cardiovascular
collapse, and death, to severe
paradoxic reactions, such as
hallucinations, tremor, and seizures.

PRECAUTIONS & CONSIDERATIONS
Caution is warranted with
preexisting pleuritis, pulmonary
fibrosis, pericarditis, pericardial
effusion, and cardiac valvulopathy
have been reported in patients taking
pergolide. Cardiac arrhythmias,

confusion, and hallucinations. It is unknown whether pergolide crosses the placenta or is distributed in breast milk. Pergolide may interfere with lactation. The safety and efficacy of this drug have not been established in children. No age-related precautions have been noted in elderly patients.

Dizziness, drowsiness, and dry mouth may occur. Alcohol and tasks that require mental alertness or motor skills should be avoided. Notify the physician if agitation, headache, lethargy, or confusion occurs. A baseline ECG should be performed in those with a history of cardiac disease. BP and pulse rate should be monitored to detect hypotension and irregularities that could indicate an arrhythmia. Also, ABG and serum electrolyte levels should be monitored. Relief of parkinsonian symptoms, such as improvement of masklike facial expression, muscular rigidity, shuffling gait, and resting tremors of the hands and head, should be assessed.

Administration

! Pergolide is usually given in 3 divided doses daily.

Crush scored tablets as needed. Take pergolide without regard to food.

Perindopril
per-in′doh-pril
(Aceon)

CATEGORY AND SCHEDULE
Pregnancy Risk Category: C (D if used in second or third trimester)

Classification:
Angiotensin-converting enzyme (ACE) inhibitors

MECHANISM OF ACTION
An ACE inhibitor that suppresses the renin-angiotensin-aldosterone system and prevents conversion of angiotensin I to angiotensin II, a potent vasoconstrictor; may also inhibit angiotensin II at local vascular and renal sites. *Therapeutic Effect:* Reduces peripheral arterial resistance and BP.

AVAILABILITY
Tablets: 2 mg, 4 mg, 8 mg.

INDICATIONS AND DOSAGES
▶ **Hypertension: Treatment of essential hypertension as monotherapy or in combination with other hypertensive medications.**
PO
Adults, Elderly. 2-8 mg/day as single dose or in 2 divided doses. Maximum: 16 mg/day.

OFF-LABEL USES
Management of heart failure.

CONTRAINDICATIONS
History of angioedema from previous treatment with ACE inhibitors.

INTERACTIONS
Drug
Alcohol, antihypertensives, diuretics: May increase the effects of perindopril.
Lithium: May increase lithium blood concentration and risk of lithium toxicity.
NSAIDs, aspirin: May decrease hypotensive effects.
Other hypotensive agents: May increase hypotensive effects.
Potassium-sparing diuretics, potassium supplements: May cause hyperkalemia.
Salicylates: Suspected reduction in antihypertensive and vasodilator effects; monitor BP if used concurrently.
Herbal
None known.

P

Food
None known.

DIAGNOSTIC TEST EFFECTS

May increase BUN, serum alkaline phosphatase, serum bilirubin, serum creatinine, serum potassium, AST (SGOT), and ALT (SGPT) levels. May decrease serum sodium levels. May cause positive antinuclear antibody titer.

SIDE EFFECTS

Occasional (1%-5%)
Cough, back pain, sinusitis, upper extremity pain, dyspepsia, fever, palpitations, hypotension, dizziness, fatigue, syncope.

SERIOUS REACTIONS

• Excessive hypotension (first-dose syncope) may occur in patients with congestive heart failure (CHF) and in those who are severely salt or volume depleted.
• Angioedema (swelling of face and lips) and hyperkalemia occur rarely.
• Agranulocytosis and neutropenia may be noted in those with collagen vascular disease, including scleroderma and systemic lupus erythematosus, and impaired renal function.
• Nephrotic syndrome may be noted in those with history of renal disease.

PRECAUTIONS & CONSIDERATIONS

Caution is warranted with patients having a history of angioedema from previous treatment with ACE inhibitors, renal insufficiency, hypertension with CHF, renal artery stenosis, autoimmune disease, collagen vascular disease, pregnancy category C (first trimester), pregnancy category D (second and third trimesters), lactation. Perindopril crosses the placenta; it is unknown whether it is distributed in breast milk. Perindopril has caused fetal or neonatal morbidity or mortality. Safety and efficacy of perindopril have not been established in children. In elderly patients, age-related renal impairment may require cautious use of perindopril.

Dizziness may occur. Be alert to fluctuations in BP. If an excessive reduction in BP occurs, place the person in the supine position with legs elevated. CBC and blood chemistry should be obtained before beginning perindopril therapy, then every 2 wks for the next 3 mo, and periodically thereafter in patients with autoimmune disease, or renal impairment, and in those who are taking drugs that affect immune response or leukocyte count. BUN, serum creatinine, serum potassium, AST (SGOT), and ALT (SGPT) levels should also be monitored.

Administration
Take perindopril 1 h before meals. Do not skip doses or voluntarily discontinue the drug to avoid severe rebound hypertension.

Permethrin

per-meth′ren
(A200 Lice, Acticin, Elimite, Kwellada-P [CAN], Nix, RID Spray)

CATEGORY AND SCHEDULE

Pregnancy Risk Category: B

Classification: Anti-infectives, topical, dermatologics, scabicides/pediculicides

MECHANISM OF ACTION

An antiparasitic agent that inhibits sodium influx through nerve cell membrane channels. *Therapeutic Effect:* Results in delayed repolarization, paralysis, and death of parasites.

PHARMACOKINETICS

Less than 2% absorption after topical application. Detected in residual amounts on hair for ≥10 days following treatment. Metabolized by liver to inactive metabolites. Excreted in urine.

AVAILABILITY

Cream: 5% (Acticin).
Liquid, Topical: 1% (Nix).
Shampoo: 0.33% (A200 Lice).
Solution: 0.25% (Nix), 0.5% (A200 Lice, RID).

INDICATIONS AND DOSAGES
▸ **Head lice**
SHAMPOO
Adults, Elderly, Children 2 mo and older. Shampoo hair, towel dry, apply to scalp, leave on for 10 min and rinse. Remove nits with nit comb. Repeat application if live lice are present 7 days after initial treatment.
▸ **Scabies**
TOPICAL
Adults, Elderly, Children 2 mo and older. Apply from head to feet, leave on for 8-14 h. Wash with soap and water. Repeat application if living mites are present 14 days after initial treatment.

OFF-LABEL USES

Demodicidosis, insect bite prophylaxis, leishmaniasis prophylaxis, malaria prophylaxis.

CONTRAINDICATIONS

Infants younger than 2 mo, hypersensitivity to pyrethroid, pyrethrin, chrysanthemums or any component of the formulation.

INTERACTIONS
Drug
None known.

Herbal
None known.
Food
None known.

DIAGNOSTIC TEST EFFECTS
None known.

SIDE EFFECTS
Occasional
Burning, pruritus, stinging, erythema, rash, swelling.

SERIOUS REACTIONS
• Shortness of breath and difficulty breathing have been reported.

PRECAUTIONS & CONSIDERATIONS
Caution should be used during pregnancy and in patients with asthma, pruritus, edema, and erythema. It is unknown whether permethrin is distributed in breast milk. No age-related precautions have been noted for suspension or topical use in children over 2 mo of age. Permethrin is not recommended for use in children 2 mo or younger. No age-related precautions have been noted in elderly patients.
Administration
Because scabies and lice are contagious, use caution to avoid spreading or infecting oneself. Use gloves when applying.

Shampoo hair, towel dry, apply rinse to scalp, leave on for 10 min then rinse. Remove nits with nit comb. Repeat application if live lice are present 7 days after initial treatment. If live lice are detected 14 days after the initial application of permethrin, retreatment is indicated. Also, in epidemic settings, a second application is recommended 2 wks after the first.

When using the topical formulation, apply and rub gently into the affected and surrounding

P

area. Apply from head to feet and leave on for 8-14 h. Wash with soap and water. Repeat application if living mites are present 14 days after initial treatment.

Perphenazine
per-fen-ah-zeen
(Trilafon)
Do not confuse with promazine.

CATEGORY AND SCHEDULE
Pregnancy Risk Category: C

Classification:
Antiemetic/antivertigo, phenothiazine antipsychotic

MECHANISM OF ACTION
An antipsychotic agent and antiemetic that blocks postsynaptic dopamine receptor sites in the brain. *Therapeutic Effect:* Suppresses behavioral response in psychosis and relieves nausea and vomiting.

AVAILABILITY
Oral Concentrate: 15 mg/5 mL.
Tablets: 2 mg, 4 mg, 8 mg, 16 mg.

INDICATIONS AND DOSAGES
▸ **Treatment of psychotic disorders, schizophrenia**
▸ **Severe schizophrenia**
PO
Adults. 4-16 mg 2-4 times/day. Maximum: 64 mg/day.
Elderly. Initially, 2-4 mg/day. May increase at intervals of 4-7 days by 2-4 mg/day up to 32 mg/day.
▸ **Severe nausea and vomiting**
PO
Adults. 8-16 mg/day in divided doses up to 24 mg/day.

CONTRAINDICATIONS
Coma, myelosuppression, severe cardiovascular disease, phenothiazine or sulfite hypersensitivity, severe central nervous system (CNS) depression, subcortical brain damage.

INTERACTIONS
Drug
Alcohol, other CNS depressants, barbiturate anesthetics, opioid analgesics: May increase hypotensive effects and CNS and respiratory depression.
Anticholinergics: May increase anticholinergic effects.
Antihypertensives: May increase the risk of hypotension.
Antithyroid agents: May increase the risk of agranulocytosis.
Epinephrine: May cause hypotension, tachycardia.
Haloperidol, droperidol, phenothiazines and related drugs, metoclopramide: May increase the severity and frequency of extrapyramidal symptoms.
Levodopa: May decrease the effects of this drug.
Lithium: May decrease perphenazine absorption and produce adverse neurologic effects.
MAOIs, tricyclic antidepressants: May increase anticholinergic and sedative effects.
Tetracyclines, fluoroquinolones, thiazide diuretics: Additive photosensitization.
Herbal
None known.
Food
Apple juice, caffeine- or tannic-containing beverages (such as tea): Do not mix oral concentrate with these beverages.

DIAGNOSTIC TEST EFFECTS
May produce false-positive pregnancy and phenylketonuria test

results. May produce ECG changes, including prolonged QT and QTc intervals and T-wave depression or inversion.

SIDE EFFECTS

Occasional

Marked photosensitivity, somnolence, dry mouth, blurred vision, lethargy, constipation or diarrhea, nasal congestion, peripheral edema, urine retention.

Rare

Ocular changes, altered skin pigmentation, hypotension, dizziness, syncope.

SERIOUS REACTIONS

• Extrapyramidal symptoms appear to be dose-related and are divided into 3 categories: akathisia (characterized by inability to sit still, tapping of feet), parkinsonian symptoms (including masklike face, tremors, shuffling gait, hypersalivation), and acute dystonias (such as torticollis, opisthotonos, and oculogyric crisis).

• Tardive dyskinesia occurs rarely.

• Abrupt withdrawal after long-term therapy may precipitate nausea, vomiting, gastritis, dizziness, and tremors.

PRECAUTIONS & CONSIDERATIONS

Caution is warranted in patients with impaired respiratory, hepatic, renal, or cardiac function; alcohol withdrawal; history of seizures; urinary retention; glaucoma; prostatic hypertrophy; or hypocalcemia (increases susceptibility to dystonias). Be aware that perphenazine crosses the placenta and is distributed in breast milk. Be aware that children may develop extrapyramidal symptoms (EPS) or neuromuscular symptoms, especially dystonias. Elderly patients are more prone to anticholinergic effects, such as dry mouth, EPS, orthostatic hypotension, and sedation symptoms.

Urine may darken. Drowsiness may occur. Alcohol and tasks that require mental alertness or motor skills should be avoided. Exposure to artificial light and sunlight should also be avoided during therapy. EPS, tardive dyskinesia, and potentially fatal, rare neuroleptic malignant syndrome, such as altered mental status, fever, irregular pulse or BP, and muscle rigidity should be monitored. Hydration status should also be assessed.

Notify health care provider if significant xerostomic side effects occur (sore tongue, problems eating or swallowing, difficulty wearing prosthesis) for possible medication change.

Administration

Skin should not come in contact with solutions (contact dermatitis). Therapeutic effect may take up to 6 wks to appear. Do not abruptly discontinue perphenazine.

P

Phenazopyridine hydrochloride

fen-az′o-peer′i-deen
high-droh-klor-ide
(Azo-Gesic, Azo-Standard,
Phenazo [CAN], Prodium,
Pyridium, Uristat)
**Do not confuse phenazopyridine
with pyridoxine or Prodium
with Perdiem.**

CATEGORY AND SCHEDULE
Pregnancy Risk Category: B

Classification: Urinary tract
analgesic, non-narcotic

MECHANISM OF ACTION
An interstitial cystitis agent that
exerts topical analgesic effect on
urinary tract mucosa. *Therapeutic
Effect:* Relieves urinary pain,
burning, urgency, and frequency.

PHARMACOKINETICS
Well absorbed from the GI tract.
Partially metabolized in the liver.
Primarily excreted in urine.

AVAILABILITY
*Tablets (Azo-Gesic, Azo-Standard,
Prodium, Uristat):* 100 mg, 200 mg.
Tablets (Pyridium): 95 mg.

INDICATIONS AND DOSAGES
▶ **Treatment of urinary tract irritation
from infection**
▶ **Urinary analgesic**
PO
Adults. 200 mg 3 times a day.
Use for 2 days when used with an
antibacterial agent.
Children 6 yr and older. 12 mg/kg/
day in 3 divided doses for 2 days.
Use for 2 days when used with an
antibacterial agent.

▶ **Dosage in renal impairment**
Dosage interval is modified based on
creatinine clearance.

Creatinine Clearance (mL/min)	Dosage Interval
50-80	Usual dose q8-16h
< 50	Avoid use

CONTRAINDICATIONS
Hepatic or renal insufficiency, G6PD
deficiency.

INTERACTIONS
Drug
None known.
Herbal
None known.
Food
None known.

DIAGNOSTIC TEST EFFECTS
May interfere with urinalysis tests
based on color reactions, such as
urinary glucose, ketones, protein,
and 17-ketosteroids.

SIDE EFFECTS
Occasional
Headache, GI disturbance, rash,
pruritus.

SERIOUS REACTIONS
• Overdose may lead to hemolytic
anemia, nephrotoxicity, or
hepatotoxicity. Patients with renal
impairment or severe hypersensitivity
to the drug may also develop these
reactions.
• A massive, acute overdose may
result in methemoglobinemia.

PRECAUTIONS & CONSIDERATIONS
Caution is warranted in patients with
hepatic or renal insufficiency or renal
disease.
   Notify the physician, and expect
to discontinue the drug if skin or

sclera turns yellow because this signifies impaired renal excretion. It is unknown whether phenazopyridine crosses the placenta or is distributed in breast milk. No age-related precautions have been noted in children older than 6 yr. Age-related renal impairment may increase the risk of toxicity in elderly patients.

Urine may turn a reddish orange color and may permanently stain clothing. Irreversible staining of soft contact lenses has been reported. Therapeutic response, including relief of urinary frequency, pain, and burning, should be assessed.

Administration

Take phenazopyridine with food. Expect to discontinue the drug after 2 days as there is no evidence that it is effective after this period.

Phendimetrazine

fen-dye-me′tra-zeen

(Adipost, Bontril PDM, Bontril Slow-Release, Melfiat, Obezine, Phendiet, Phendiet-105, Plegine, Prelu-2)

CATEGORY AND SCHEDULE

Pregnancy Risk Category: C

Classification: Anorexiants, amphetamine-like central nervous system (CNS) stimulant

MECHANISM OF ACTION

A phenylalkylamine sympathomimetic agent with activity similar to amphetamines that stimulates the central nervous system CNS and elevates BP most likely mediated via norepinephrine and dopamine metabolism. Causes stimulation of the hypothalamus. *Therapeutic Effect:* Decreases appetite.

PHARMACOKINETICS

The pharmacokinetics of phendimetrazine tartrate has not been well established. Metabolized to active metabolite, phendimetrazine. Excreted in urine. *Half-life:* 2-4 h.

AVAILABILITY

Tablets: 35 mg (Bontril PDM, Obezine, Phendiet, Plegine).
Capsules (Extended-Release): 105 mg (Adipost, Bontril Slow-Release, Melfiat, Phendiet-105, Prelu-2).

INDICATIONS AND DOSAGES

Treatment of exogenous obesity.
▸ **Obesity**
PO
Adults, Elderly. 105 mg/day in the morning or before the morning meal (sustained-release); 35 mg 2-3 times/day (immediate-release). Maximum: 70 mg 3 times/day.

CONTRAINDICATIONS

Advanced arteriosclerosis, agitated states, glaucoma, history of drug abuse, history of hypersensitivity to sympathomimetic amines, hyperthyroidism, moderate to severe hypertension, symptomatic cardiovascular disease, use within 14 days of discontinuation MAOI, hypersensitivity to phendimetrazine or sympathomimetics.
Caution
Drug abuse, anxiety, lactation.

INTERACTIONS

Drug
Caffeine, caffeine-containing products: May increase risk of insomnia or dry mouth.
Guanethidine: May decrease hypotensive effect of guanethidine.
Hydrocarbon inhalants, general anesthetics: May increase risk of dysrhythmias.

P

MAOIs or within 14 days of MAOIs: May increase risk of hypertensive crisis.
Sibutramine: May increase risk of hypertension and tachycardia.
Tricyclic antidepressants, phenothiazines, ascorbic acid: May increase cardiovascular effects.
Herbal and Food
None known.

DIAGNOSTIC TEST EFFECTS
None known.

SIDE EFFECTS
Occasional
Constipation, nausea, diarrhea, dry mouth, dysuria, libido changes, flushing, hypertension, insomnia, nervousness, headache, dizziness, irritability, agitation, restlessness, palpitations, increased heart rate, sweating, tremor, urticaria.

SERIOUS REACTIONS
• Multivalvular heart disease, primary pulmonary hypertension, and arrhythmias occur rarely.
• Overdose may produce flushing, arrhythmias, and psychosis.
• Abrupt withdrawal following prolonged administration of high doses may produce extreme fatigue and depression.

PRECAUTIONS & CONSIDERATIONS
Caution is warranted in patients with diabetes mellitus or mild hypertension. Caution should be used with pregnancy. It is unknown whether phendimetrazine is excreted in breast milk. Be aware that safety and efficacy of this drug have not been established in children. No age-related precautions have been noted in elderly patients. Tasks that require mental alertness or motor skills should be avoided. Palpitations, dizziness, dry mouth, and pronounced nervousness should be reported.

Care should be used in patients with advanced arteriosclerosis, agitated states, glaucoma, history of drug abuse, hypersensitivity to sympathomimetic amines, hyperthroidsm, moderate to severe hypertension, symptomatic cardiovascular disease, hypersensitivity to phendimetrazine. Psychological and physical dependence may occur with chronic administration.
Administration
Take extended-release capsule in the morning, 60 min before the morning meal. Do not chew, crush, or open the capsules. Take immediate-release tablets 1 h before meals.

Phenelzine Sulfate
fen'el-zeen sull-fate
(Nardil)

CATEGORY AND SCHEDULE
Pregnancy Risk Category: C

Classification: Antidepressant, monoamine oxidase inhibitors (MAOIs)

MECHANISM OF ACTION
An MAOI that inhibits the activity of the enzyme monoamine oxidase at central nervous system (CNS) storage sites, leading to increased levels of the neurotransmitters epinephrine, norepinephrine, serotonin, and dopamine at neuronal receptor sites. *Therapeutic Effect:* Relieves depression.

AVAILABILITY
Tablets: 15 mg.

INDICATIONS AND DOSAGES
▸ **Treatment of depression when uncontrolled by other means**
PO
Adults. 15 mg 3 times a day. May increase to 60-90 mg/day.
Elderly. Initially, 7.5 mg/day. May increase by 7.5-15 mg/day q3-4wk up to 60 mg/day in divided doses.

OFF-LABEL USES
Treatment of panic disorder, vascular or tension headaches.

CONTRAINDICATIONS
Includes, but not limited to, cardiovascular or cerebrovascular disease, hepatic or renal impairment, pheochromocytoma.

INTERACTIONS
Drug
Alcohol, other CNS depressants: May increase CNS depression and sedative effects.
Amphetamine, ephedrine, indirect acting sympathomimetics: Increased pressor effects.
Buspirone: May increase BP.
Caffeine-containing medications: May increase the risk of cardiac arrhythmias and hypertension.
Carbamazepine, cyclobenzaprine, maprotiline, other MAOIs: May precipitate hypertensive crisis, convulsions, hyperpyretic crisis.
Dopamine, tryptophan: May cause sudden, severe hypertension.
Fluoxetine, trazodone, tricyclic antidepressants: May cause serotonin syndrome.
Insulin, oral antidiabetics: May increase the effects of these drugs.
Meperidine, other opioid analgesics: May produce diaphoresis, immediate excitation, rigidity, and severe hypertension or hypotension, sometimes leading to severe respiratory distress,

vascular collapse, seizures, coma, and death.
Methylphenidate: May increase the CNS stimulant effects of methylphenidate.
Herbal
None known.
Food
Caffeine, chocolate, tyramine-containing foods (such as aged cheese): May cause sudden, severe hypertension.

DIAGNOSTIC TEST EFFECTS
None known.

SIDE EFFECTS
Frequent
Orthostatic hypotension, restlessness, GI upset, insomnia, dizziness, headache, lethargy, asthenia, dry mouth, peripheral edema.
Occasional
Flushing, diaphoresis, rash, urinary frequency, increased appetite, transient impotence.
Rare
Visual disturbances.

SERIOUS REACTIONS
• Hypertensive crisis occurs rarely and is marked by severe hypertension, occipital headache radiating frontally, neck stiffness or soreness, nausea, vomiting, diaphoresis, fever or chilliness, clammy skin, dilated pupils, palpitations, tachycardia or bradycardia, and constricting chest pain.
• Intracranial bleeding occurs rarely in cases of severe hypertension.

PRECAUTIONS & CONSIDERATIONS
Caution is warranted in patients with cardiac arrhythmias, frequent or severe headaches, hypertension, suicidal tendencies, and within several hours of ingestion of a

P

contraindicated substance, such as tyramine-containing foods. Foods that require bacteria or molds for their preparation or preservation (such as yogurt and aged cheese), foods containing tyramine (including avocados, bananas, broad beans, figs, papayas, raisins, sour cream, soy sauce, beer, wine, yeast extracts, meat tenderizers, and smoked or pickled meats), and excessive amounts of caffeine-containing foods or beverages (such as chocolate, coffee, and tea) should be avoided during therapy.

Phenelzine sulfate is not recommended for use in children.

Alcohol and tasks that require mental alertness or motor skills should be avoided. Notify the physician if headache or neck soreness or stiffness occurs. If hypertensive crisis occurs, phentolamine 5-10 mg IV should be administered. Liver function tests should be performed before and periodically during therapy, especially with long-term use.
Storage
Store phenelzine tablets at room temperature. Do not freeze.
Administration
Take the drug with food or milk to alleviate GI symptoms. Crush them and give with food or fluids. Depression may start to lift during the first week of therapy but phenelzine's full therapeutic effect may require 2-6 wks of therapy.

Phenobarbital
fee-noe-bar′bi-tal
(Luminal, Phenobarbitone [AUS])
Do not confuse Phenobarbital with pentobarbital or Luminal with Tuinal.

CATEGORY AND SCHEDULE
Pregnancy Risk Category: D
Controlled Substance: Schedule IV

Classification: Barbiturate anticonvulsant, preanesthetics, sedatives/ hypnotics

MECHANISM OF ACTION
A barbiturate that enhances the activity of γ-aminobutyric acid (GABA) by binding to the GABA receptor complex. *Therapeutic Effect:* Depresses central nervous system (CNS) activity.

PHARMACOKINETICS

Route	Onset	Peak	Duration
PO	20-60 min	NA	6-10 h
IV	5 min	30 min	4-10 h

Well absorbed after PO or parenteral administration. Protein binding: 35%-50%. Rapidly and widely distributed. Metabolized in the liver. Excreted primarily in urine. Removed by hemodialysis. *Half-life:* 53-118 h.

AVAILABILITY
Elixir: 20 mg/5 mL.
Tablets: 30 mg, 100 mg.
Injection: 60 mg/mL, 130 mg/mL.

INDICATIONS AND DOSAGES
▸ **Status epilepticus**

IV
Adults, Elderly, Children, Neonates.
Loading dose of 15-20 mg/kg as a
single dose or in divided doses.
▸ **Seizure control**
PO, IV
*Adults, Elderly, Children 12 yr and
older.* 1-3 mg/kg/day.
Children aged 6-12 yr. 3-6 mg/kg/day.
Children aged 1-5 yr. 6-8 mg/kg/day.
Children younger than 1 yr.
5-6 mg/kg/day.
Neonates. 3-4 mg/kg/day.
▸ **Sedation**
PO, IM
Adults, Elderly. 30-120 mg/day in
2-3 divided doses.
Children. 2 mg/kg 3 times a day.
▸ **Hypnotic**
PO, IV, IM, SC
Adults, Elderly. 100-320 mg at
bedtime.
Children. 3-5 mg/kg at bedtime.

OFF-LABEL USES

Prevention and treatment of
hyperbilirubinemia, chronic
cholestasis.

CONTRAINDICATIONS

Porphyria, preexisting CNS
depression, severe pain, severe
respiratory disease.
Caution
Anemia.

INTERACTIONS

Drug
**Alcohol, other CNS depressants,
saquinavir:** May increase the effects
of phenobarbital.
Barbiturates: May induce liver
microsomal enzymes altering
metabolism of other drugs.
Carbamazepine: May increase the
metabolism of carbamazepine.
**Digoxin, glucocorticoids,
metronidazole, oral
anticoagulants, quinidine, tricyclic**

antidepressants: May decrease the
effects of these drugs.
Valproic acid: Increases the blood
concentration and risk of toxicity of
phenobarbital.
Herbal
None known.
Food
None known.

DIAGNOSTIC TEST EFFECTS

May decrease serum bilirubin level.
Therapeutic serum level is
10-40 mcg/mL; toxic serum level is
> 50 mcg/mL.

🚫 IV INCOMPATIBILITIES

Amphotericin B complex (Abelcet,
AmBisome, Amphotec), fentanyl
(Sublimaze), fosphenytoin (cerebyx),
hydrocortisone (Solu-Cortef),
hydromorphone (Dilaudid), insulin,
morphine.

SIDE EFFECTS

Occasional (1%-3%)
Somnolence.
Rare (< 1%)
Confusion; paradoxical CNS
reactions, such as hyperactivity
or nervousness in children and
excitement or restlessness in elderly
patients (generally noted during first
2 wks of therapy, particularly in the
presence of uncontrolled pain).

SERIOUS REACTIONS

• Abrupt withdrawal after prolonged
therapy may produce increased
dreaming, nightmares, insomnia,
tremor, diaphoresis, vomiting,
hallucinations, delirium, seizures,
and status epilepticus.
• Skin eruptions may be a sign of a
hypersensitivity reaction.
• Blood dyscrasias, hepatic disease,
and hypocalcemia occur rarely.
• Overdose produces cold or clammy
skin, hypothermia, severe CNS

P

depression, cyanosis, tachycardia, and Cheyne-Stokes respirations.
• Toxicity may result in severe renal impairment.

PRECAUTIONS & CONSIDERATIONS

Caution is warranted in patients with hepatic and renal impairment. Phenobarbital readily crosses the placenta and is distributed in breast milk. Phenobarbital use lowers serum bilirubin concentrations in neonates, produces respiratory depression in neonates during labor, and may increase the risk of maternal bleeding and neonatal hemorrhage during delivery. Neonates born to women who use barbiturates during the last trimester of pregnancy may experience withdrawal symptoms. Phenobarbital use may cause paradoxical excitement in children. Elderly patients taking phenobarbital may exhibit confusion, excitement, and mental depression.

Drowsiness and dizziness may occur, so alcohol and tasks requiring mental alertness or motor skills should be avoided. Notify the physician if headache, nausea, and rash occur. BP, heart rate, respiratory rate, CNS status, renal and hepatic function, and seizure activity should be monitored.

Storage
Store vials at room temperature.

Administration
PO
Take oral phenobarbital without regard to food. Crush tablets as needed. The elixir may be mixed with fruit juice, milk, or water.
! Expect to administer the maintenance dose 12 h after the loading dose. Therapeutic serum drug level is 10-40 mcg/mL; the toxic serum drug level is > 50 mcg/mL.

IV, IM
Phenobarbital may be given undiluted or may be diluted with NaCl, D5W, or lactated Ringer's solution. Expect to hydrate the patient adequately before and immediately after infusion to decrease the risk of adverse renal effects. Do not exceed an injection rate of 30 mg/min for children and 60 mg/min for adults. Injecting too rapidly may produce marked respiratory depression and severe hypotension. Be aware that inadvertent intra-arterial injection may result in arterial spasm with severe pain and tissue necrosis and that extravasation in subcutaneous tissue may produce redness, tenderness, and tissue necrosis. If either occurs, inject 0.5% procaine solution into the affected area and apply moist heat, as ordered.

For IM use, do not inject more than 5 mL in any one injection site because doing so may cause tissue irritation. Inject the drug deep intramuscularly.

Phenoxybenzamine
fen-ox-ee-ben′za-meen
(Dibenzyline)

CATEGORY AND SCHEDULE
Pregnancy Risk Category: C

Classification: Antiadrenergics, antihypertensive α-blocking agent

MECHANISM OF ACTION
An antihypertensive that produces long-lasting noncompetitive α-adrenergic blockade of

postganglionic synapses in exocrine glands and smooth muscles. Relaxes urethra and increases opening of the bladder. *Therapeutic Effect:* Controls hypertension.

PHARMACOKINETICS
Well absorbed from the GI tract. Distributed into fatty tissue. Metabolized in liver. Eliminated in urine and feces. Not removed by hemodialysis. *Half-life:* 24 h.

AVAILABILITY
Tablets: 10 mg (Dibenzyline).

INDICATIONS AND DOSAGES
▸ **Treatment of hypertension caused by pheocromocytoma**
PO
Adults. Initially, 10 mg twice daily. May increase dose every other day to 20-40 mg 2-3 times/day

OFF-LABEL USES
Bladder instability, complex regional pain syndrome (CRPS), contraception, prostatic obstruction, Raynaud disease.

CONTRAINDICATIONS
Any condition compromised by hypotension, hypersensitivity to phenoxybenzamine, or any component of the formulation.

INTERACTIONS
Drug
α-**Adrenergic agonists:**
May decrease the effects of phenoxybenzamine
β-**blockers (used concurrently):**
May increase risk of toxicity (hypotension, tachycardia).
CNS depressants: May increase risk of CNS depression.
Ephedrine and OTC cold medicines containing ephedrine:
May counteract hypotensive effects.

Hypotensive-producing medications: May increase the effects of phenoxybenzamine.
Herbal
Licorice, Ma huang, yohimbine:
May decrease the effects of phenoxybenzamine.
Food
None known.

DIAGNOSTIC TEST EFFECTS
None known.

SIDE EFFECTS
Frequent
Headache, lethargy, confusion, fatigue.
Occasional
Nausea, postural hypotension, syncope, dry mouth.
Rare
Palpitations, diarrhea, constipation, inhibition of ejaculation, weakness, altered vision, dizziness.

SERIOUS REACTIONS
• Overdosage produces severe hypotension, irritability, lethargy, tachycardia, dizziness, and shock.

P

PRECAUTIONS & CONSIDERATIONS
Caution is warranted in patients with congestive heart failure, coronary artery disease, and renal function impairment. It is unknown whether phenoxybenzamine crosses the placenta or is distributed into breast milk. Safety and efficacy have not been established in children. Elderly patients may be more sensitive to hypotensive effects and may be at risk of developing phenoxybenzamine-induced hypothermia.

Miosis, nasal congestion, dizziness, lightheadedness, and fast heartbeat may occur. Caution when driving and change positions slowly. Alcohol should be avoided.

Administration
Dosage increments should not be made more frequently than every 4 days. If GI irritation occurs, take with meals or milk.

Phentermine
(Adipex-P, Fastin, Ionamin, Oby-Cap, Phentercot, Pro-Fast HS, Pro-Fast SA, Pro-Fast SR, T-Diet, Teramine, Zantryl)

CATEGORY AND SCHEDULE
Pregnancy Risk Category: B
Controlled Substance: Schedule IV

Classification: Anorexiants, Sympathomimetics

MECHANISM OF ACTION
A sympathomimetic amine structurally similar to dextroamphetamine and most likely mediated via norephinephrine and dopamine metabolism. Causes stimulation of the hypothalamus. *Therapeutic Effect:* Decreased appetite.

PHARMACOKINETICS
Well absorbed from the GI tract; resin absorbed slower. Excreted unchanged in urine. *Half-life:* 20 h.

AVAILABILITY
Capsules (as Hydrochloride): 15 mg, 18.75 mg, 30 mg (Fastin), 37.5 mg (Adipex-P).
Capsules (as Resin Complex): 15 mg (Ionamin), 30 mg (Ionamin).
Tablets (as Hydrochloride): 8 mg, 37.5 mg (Adipex-P).

INDICATIONS AND DOSAGES
Treatment of exogenous obesity.
▸ **Obesity**
PO
Adults, Children older than 16 yr.
Adipex-P: 37.5 mg as a single daily dose or in divided doses. Ionamin: 15-37.5 mg/day before breakfast or 1-2 h. after breakfast. Fastin: 30 mg/day taken in the morning

CONTRAINDICATIONS
Advanced arteriosclerosis, agitated states, cardiovascular disease, anorexia nervosa, concurrent use or within 14 days of discontinuation of MAOI therapy, glaucoma, history of drug abuse, hypertension (moderate-to-severe), hyperthyroidism, hypersensitivity to phentermine or sympathomimetic amines.

INTERACTIONS
Drug
Caffeine and caffeine-containing products: Increased risk of insomnia.
Fenfluramine: May increase risk of pulmonary hypertension and valvular heart disease.
Hydrocarbon inhalants, general anesthetics: Increased risk of dysrhythmia.
MAOIs: May increase risk of hypertensive crisis (headache, hyperpyrexia, hypertension).
Sibutramine: May increase risk of hypertension and tachycardia.
Tricyclic antidepressants, ascorbic acid, phenothiazines: Decreased effect of phentermine.
Herbal
None known.
Food
None known.

DIAGNOSTIC TEST EFFECTS

May interfere and give false positive amphetamine EMIT assay result.

SIDE EFFECTS

Occasional

Restlessness, insomnia, tremor, palpitations, tachycardia, elevation in BP, headache, dizziness, dry mouth, unpleasant taste, diarrhea or constipation, changes in libido.

SERIOUS REACTIONS

• Primary pulmonary hypertension (PPH), psychotic episodes, and valvular heart disease rarely occur.
• Anorectic agents have been associated with regurgitant multivalvular heart disease involving mitral, aortic, or tricuspid valves.
• Prolonged use may cause physical or psychological dependence.

PRECAUTIONS & CONSIDERATIONS

Caution is warranted in patients with cardiovascular disease, psychosis, diabetes, insomnia, porphyria, mild hypertension, Tourette syndrome, seizure disorders, and history of substance abuse. It is unknown whether phentermine is excreted in breast milk. Be aware that the safety and efficacy of this drug have not been established in children younger than 16 yr. Age-related liver or renal impairment may require decreased dosage in elderly patients. Phentermine may be habit forming, and it should not be abruptly discontinued.

Fast, pounding, or irregular heartbeat; chest pain; severe headache; trouble breathing; skin rash; blurred vision; confusion; or unexplained sore throat should be reported immediately.

Caution is warranted in patients having a history of drug abuse or addictive personality as prolonged use can cause physical or psychological dependence. Patients on chronic drug therapy may rarely have symptoms of blood dyscrasias, which include infection, bleeding, and poor healing.

Administration

Do not take phentermine in the afternoon or evening because it can cause insomnia. May take before breakfast or 1-2 h after breakfast.

Phentolamine
fen-tole′a-meen
(Regitine)

CATEGORY AND SCHEDULE

Pregnancy Risk Category: C

Classification: Antiadrenergics, α-blocking antihypertensives.

MECHANISM OF ACTION

An α-adrenergic blocking agent that produces peripheral vasodilation and cardiac stimulation. *Therapeutic Effect:* Decreases BP.

PHARMACOKINETICS

Poorly absorbed from the GI tract. Protein binding: 72%. Metabolized in liver. Eliminated in urine and feces. Not removed by hemodialysis. *Half-life:* 19 min.

AVAILABILITY

Injection: 5 mg/mL (Regitine).

INDICATIONS AND DOSAGES

▸ **Acute treatment of hypertension, pheochromocytoma, prevention or treatment of dermal necrosis following extravasation of norepinephrine or dopamine**

P

▸ **Extravasation—norepinephrine**
SC
Adults, Elderly. Infiltrate area with
a small amount (1 mL) of solution
(made by diluting 5-10 mg in 10 mL
of NS) within 12 h of extravasation.
Do not exceed 0.1-0.2 mg/kg or 10 mg
total. If dose is effective, normal skin
color should return to the blanched
area within 1 h.
Children. Infiltrate area with a
small amount (1 mL) of solution
(made by diluting 5-10 mg in
10 mL of NS) within 12 h of
extravasation. Do not exceed
0.1-0.2 mg/kg or 5 mg total.
▸ **Diagnosis of pheochromocytoma**
IM/IV
Adults, Elderly. 5 mg as a single
dose.
Children. 0.05-0.1 mg/kg/dose.
Maximum single dose: 5 mg.
▸ **Surgery for pheochromocytoma:
Hypertension**
IM/IV
Adults, Elderly. 5 mg given 1-2 h
before procedure and repeated as
needed every 2-4 h.
Children. 0.05-0.1 mg/kg/dose
given 1-2 h before procedure.
Repeat as needed every 2-4 h
until hypertension is controlled.
Maximum single dose: 5 mg.
▸ **Hypertensive crisis**
IV
Adults, Elderly. 5-15 mg as a single
dose.

OFF-LABEL USES

Treatment of pralidoxime-induced
hypertension, erectile dysfunction
(with papaverine for intracavernous
injection), extravasation-dopamine,
epinephrine, hyperhidrosis.

CONTRAINDICATIONS

Renal impairment, coronary or
cerebral arteriosclerosis, concurrent
use with phosphodiesterase-5

(PDE-5) inhibitors including
sildenafil (>25 mg), tadalafil, or
vardenafil, hypersensitivity to
phentolamine or related compounds.

INTERACTIONS
Drug
Alcohol: May increase the risk of
disulfiram-type reactions.
β-Blockers: May exaggerate
hypotensive effects.
Epinephrine, ephedrine: May
decrease the effects of phentolamine;
may cause tachycardia.
Sildenafil, tadalafil, vardenafil:
May increase BP-lowering effects.
Herbal
None known.
Food
None known.

DIAGNOSTIC TEST EFFECTS
May increase liver function tests.

IV COMPATIBILITIES
Amiodarone (Cordarone),
dobutamine (Dobutrex),
norepinephrine (Levophed),
papaverine (Papacon), verapamil.

SIDE EFFECTS
Occasional
Hypotension, tachycardia,
arrhythmia, flushing, orthostatic
hypotension, weakness, dizziness,
nausea, vomiting, diarrhea, nasal
congestion, pulmonary hypertension.

SERIOUS REACTIONS
• Symptoms of overdosage include
tachycardia, shock, vomiting, and
dizziness.
• Mixed agents, such as epinephrine,
may cause more hypotension.

PRECAUTIONS & CONSIDERATIONS
Caution is warranted in patients
with arrhythmias, cerebral vascular
spasm or occlusion, hypotension,

and tachycardia. Be aware that it is unknown whether phentolamine crosses the placenta or is distributed into breast milk. No age-related precautions have been noted in children or elderly patients.

Nasal congestion, increased heartbeat, palpitations, dizziness, headache, and hypotension are common side effects of phentolamine. BP should be monitored during its use. Symptoms including tachycardia, shock, vomiting and dizziness may indicate overdosage and should be reported immediately.

Storage

Store at room temperature.

Administration

Phentolamine mesylate for injection is reconstituted for parenteral use by adding 1 mL of sterile water for injection to the vial, producing a solution containing 5 mg of phentolamine mesylate per milliliter. Discard any unused portion.

Persons undergoing diagnostic testing for pheochromocytoma should be maintained in the supine position during phentolamine administration.

Phenylephrine (Systemic)

(AD-Nephrin, AK-Dilate, Mydrfrin, Neo-Synephrine, Prefrin [US], IsoptoFrin, Neo-Synephrine Ophthalmic Viscous 10% [AUS], Af-Taf [ISRAEL]; AK-Dilate; Albalon Relief [NEW ZEALAND]; Despec-SF; Drosin [INDIA]; Efrin-10 [ISRAEL]; Efrisel [INDONESIA]; Isopto Frin [BELGIUM, CZECH REPUBLIC, ECUADOR, MALAYSIA]; Metaoxedrin [DEN, NOR, SWE]; Minims Phenylephrine HCL 10% [SOUTH AFRICA]; Minims Phenylephrine Hydrochloride [ENG]; Mydfrin; Nefrin-Ofteno [COSTA RICA, DOMINICAN REPUBLIC, EL SALVADOR, GUATEMALA, HONDURAS, NICARAGUA, PANAMA]; Neofrin; Neosynephrine [BELGIUM, SWE]; Neosynephrine 10% Chibret [FRA]; Neosynephrine Faure 10% [FRA]; Neo-Synephrine Ophthalmic; Neosynephrin-POS [KOR]; Ocu-Phrin; Oftan-Metaoksedrin [FIN]; Optistin [ITL]; Phenoptic; Phenylephrine [NETHERLANDS]; Prefrin [AUSTRIA, ECUADOR, GREECE, HONG KONG, INDONESIA, NEW ZEALAND, SOUTH AFRICA, THAILAND]; Pupiletto Forte [INDIA]; Rectasol; Vistafrin [SPA]; Vistosan [GER]). **Do not confuse with pseudo-ephedrine, epinephrine.**

CATEGORY AND SCHEDULE

Pregnancy Risk Category: C

Classification: Decongestant, sympathomimetic

MECHANISM OF ACTION

Phenylephrine is a powerful postsynaptic α-receptor stimulant that acts on the α-adrenergic receptors of vascular smooth muscle, with little effect on the β-receptors of the heart, lacking chronotropic and inotropic actions on the heart. Causes vasoconstriction of arterioles of nasal mucosa or conjunctiva, activates dilator muscles of the pupil to cause contraction, and produces systemic arterial vasoconstriction. *Therapeutic Effect:* Vasoconstriction, decreases heart rate, increases stroke output, increases blood pressure, decreases mucosal blood flow and relieves congestion, and increases systolic BP.

PHARMACOKINETICS

Phenylephrine is irregularly absorbed from and readily metabolized in the GI tract. After IV administration, a pressor effect occurs almost immediately and persists for 15-20 min. After IM administration, a pressor effect occurs within 10-15 min and persists for 50 min to 1 h. After oral inhalation of phenylephrine in combination with isoproterenol, pulmonary effects occur within a few minutes and persist for about 3 h. Minimal absorption occurs after intranasal and intraocular administration. The pharmacologic effects of phenylephrine are terminated at least partially by the uptake of the drug into the tissues. Phenylephrine is metabolized in the liver and intestine by the enzyme monoamine oxidase (MAO). The metabolites and their route and rate of excretion have not been identified. *Half-life:* up to 2.5 h, variable.

Route	Onset	Peak	Duration
IV	Immediate	NA	15-20 min
IM	10-15 min	NA	0.5-2 h
SC	10-15 min	NA	1 h

AVAILABILITY

Solution (Ophthalmic): 2.5%, 10%.
Solution (Nasal): 0.125%, 0.16%, 0.25%, 0.5%.

Solution (Injection): 10 mg/mL.
Solution (Oral): 5 mg/mL.
Suppository (Rectal): 0.25%.

INDICATIONS AND DOSAGES

Treatment of nasal congestion (temporary relief), mild to moderate hypotension, paroxysmal supraventricular tachycardia (PSVT), hypotensive prophylaxis during spinal anesthesia, vasoconstriction during anesthesia

▸ **Paroxysmal supraventricular tachycardia (PSVT)**
Adults. The initial dose, given by rapid IV injection, should not exceed 0.5 mg. Subsequent doses may be increased in increments of 0.1-0.2 mg. Maximum single dose is 1 mg IV.
Children. 5-10 mcg/kg IV over 20-30 s.

▸ **Mild to moderate hypotension**
SC/IM
Adults. 2-5 mg IM or SC (range 1-10 mg), repeated no more than every 10-15 min. Maximum initial IM or SC dose is 5 mg.
Children. 0.1 mg/kg IM or SC every 1-2 h as needed. Maximum dose is 5 mg.
IV
Adults. 0.2 mg IV (range 0.1-0.5 mg), given no more frequently than every 10-15 min. Maximum initial IV dose is 0.5 mg.

▸ **Severe hypotension or shock**
IM, SC
Adults, Elderly. 2-5 mg/dose q1-2 h.
Children. 0.1 mg/kg/dose q1-2 h.
IV BOLUS
Adults, Elderly. 0.1-0.5 mg/dose q10-15 min as needed.
Children. 5-20 mcg/kg/dose q10-15 min.
IV INFUSION
Adults. Initially, 100-180 mcg/min IV infusion, with dose titration to the desired MAP and SVR.

A maintenance infusion rate of 40-60 mcg/min IV is usually adequate after BP stabilizes.
Children. 5-20 mcg/kg IV bolus, followed by an initial IV infusion of 0.1-0.5 mcg/kg/min, titrated to desired effect. Titrate to achieve desired effect.

▸ **Hypotensive emergencies during spinal anesthesia**
IV
Adults. Initially, 0.2 mg IV. Subsequent doses should not exceed the previous dose by more than 0.1-0.2 mg. Maximum of 0.5 mg per dose.

▸ **Hypotension during spinal anesthesia in children**
IM/SC
Children. A dose of 0.044-0.088 mg/kg IM or SC is recommended by the manufacturer.

▸ **Hypotension prophylaxis during spinal anesthesia**
IM/SC
Adults. 2-3 mg SC or IM, 3 or 4 min before anesthesia. A dose of 2 mg SC or IM is usually adequate with low spinal anesthesia; 3 mg IM or SC may be necessary with high spinal anesthesia.

▸ **Vasoconstriction in regional anesthesia**
IV
Adults. The manufacturer states that the optimum concentration of phenylephrine HCl is 0.05 mg/mL (1:20,000). Solutions may be prepared for regional anesthesia by adding 1 mg of phenylephrine HCl to each 20 mL of local anesthesia solution. Some pressor response can be expected when at least 2 mg is injected.

▸ **Prolongation of spinal anesthesia**
IV
Adults. The addition of 2-5 mg to the anesthetic solution increases the duration of motor block by as much as 50% without an increase in the incidence of complications such as nausea, vomiting, or BP disturbances.

▸ **Nasal decongestion**
NASAL SPRAY, NASAL SOLUTION
Adults, Elderly, Children 12 yr and older. 2-3 drops or 1-2 sprays of 0.25%-0.5% solution into each nostril q4h as needed. Do not use more than 3 consecutive days.
Children aged 6-11 yr. 2-3 drops or 1-2 sprays of 0.25% solution into each nostril q4h as needed. Do not use more than 3 consecutive days.
Children younger than 6 yr. 2-3 drops of 0.125% solution (dilute 0.5% solution with 0.9% NaCl to achieve 0.125%) in each nostril. Repeat q4h as needed. Do not use for more than 3 consecutive days.

CONTRAINDICATIONS

Phenylephrine HCl injection should not be used with patients with severe hypertension, ventricular tachycardia or fibrillation, acute myocardial infarction (MI), atrial flutter or fibrillation, cardiac arrhythmias, cardiac disease, cardiomyopathy, closed-angle glaucoma, coronary artery disease, women who are in labor, during obstetric delivery, or in patients who have a known hypersensitivity to phenylephrine, sulfitres, or to any one of its components.

INTERACTIONS

Drug
β-Adrenergic blockers: Risk of bradycardia with systemic absorption.
Halothane: Vasopressors may cause serious cardiac arrhythmias during halothane anesthesia and therefore should be used only with great caution or not at all.
MAO Inhibitors: The pressor effect of sympathomimetic pressor amines and adrenergic agents is markedly

potentiated in patients receiving MAO inhibitors.

Nitrous oxide/oxygen gas inhalation: May complicate nasal administration.

Oxytocics: The pressure effect of sympathomimetic pressor amines is potentiated.

Tricyclic antidepressants: Increased risk of dysrhythmias and hypertension.

Herbal
None known.

Food
None known.

DIAGNOSTIC TEST EFFECTS
None known.

SIDE EFFECTS

Frequent
Nasal: Rebound nasal congestion due to overuse, especially when used for more than 3 days.

Occasional
Mild central nervous system (CNS) stimulation (restlessness, nervousness, tremors, headache, insomnia), headache, reflex bradycardia, excitability, restlessness, and rarely arrhythmias.
Nasal: stinging, burning, drying of nasal mucosa.
Ophthalmic: Transient burning or stinging, brow ache, blurred vision.

SERIOUS REACTIONS
• Overdose may induce ventricular extrasystoles and short paroxysms of ventricular tachycardia, a sensation of fullness in the head, and tingling of the extremities. If an excessive elevation of BP occurs, it can be immediately relieved by an α-adrenergic blocking agent (e.g., phentolamine).

PRECAUTIONS & CONSIDERATIONS
Caution is warranted in patients with metabolic acidosis, acute pancreatitis, heart disease, pheochromocytoma, severe hypertension, thrombosis, ventricular tachycardia, hypercapnia, phenylketonuria, hypoxia, atrial fibrillation, narrow-angle glaucoma, pulmonary hypertension, hypovolemia, mechanical obstruction such as severe valvular aortic stenosis, myocardial infarction, arterial embolism, atherosclerosis, Buerger disease, cold injury such as frostbite, diabetic endarteritis, Raynaud syndrome, and sensitivity to other sympathomimetics. It is unknown whether phenylephrine (systemic) crosses the placenta or is distributed into breast milk. Phenylephrine (systemic) should be used cautiously in children and elderly patients. Particular caution is warranted in children under 6 yr of age with diabetes, cardiovascular disease, hypertension, hyperthyroidism, increased intraocular pressure, prostatic hypertrophy, glaucoma, ischemic heart disease.

Storage
Store at room temperature.

Administration
To prepare a solution of phenylephrine for direct IV injection, 10 mg (1 mL) of phenylephrine hydrochloride injection should be diluted with 9 mL of sterile water for injection to provide a solution containing 1 mg of phenylephrine per milliliter.
Infuse over 20-30 s.

Phenylephrine (Topical)

(Af-Taf [ISRAEL]; AK-Dilate; Albalon Relief [NEW ZEALAND]; Despec-SF; Drosin [INDIA]; Efrin-10 [ISRAEL]; Efrisel [INDONESIA]; Isopto Frin [BELGIUM, CZECH REPUBLIC, ECUADOR, MALAYSIA]; Metaoxedrin [AEN, NOR, SWE]; Minims Phenylephrine HCL 10% [SOUTH AFRICA]; Minims Phenylephrine Hydrochloride [ENG]; Mydfrin; Nefrin-Ofteno [COSTA RICA, DOMINICAN REPUBLIC, EL SALVADOR, GUATEMALA, HONDURAS, NICARAGUA, PANAMA]; Neofrin; Neosynephrine [BELGIUM, SWE]; Neosynephrine 10% Chibret [FRA]; Neosynephrine Faure 10% [FRA]; Neo-Synephrine Ophthalmic Viscous 10% [AUS]; Neo-Synephrine Ophthalmic; Neosynephrin-POS [KOR]; Ocu-Phrin; Oftan-Metaoksedrin [FIN]; Optistin [ITL]; Phenoptic; Phenylephrine [NETHERLANDS]; Prefrin [AUSTRIA, ECUADOR, GREECE, HONG KONG, INDONESIA, NEW ZEALAND, SOUTH AFRICA, THAILAND]; Pupiletto Forte [INDIA]; Rectasol; Vistafrin [SPA]; Vistosan [GER]). **Do not confuse with pseudo-ephedrine, epinephrine.**

CATEGORY AND SCHEDULE

Pregnancy Risk Category: C

Classification: Substituted phenylethylamine, decongestant, mydriatic

MECHANISM OF ACTION

Phenylephrine HCl is an α-receptor sympathetic agonist used in local ocular disorders because of its vasoconstrictor and mydriatic action.

It exhibits rapid and moderately prolonged action, and it produces little rebound vasodilatation. Systemic side effects are uncommon. *Therapeutic Effect:* Vasoconstriction and pupil dilation.

PHARMACOKINETICS

Some absorption occurs systemically. The duration of action of intranasal administration ranges from 30 min to 4 h. The duration of the mydriatic effect is roughly 3 h after administration of the 2.5% solution but may be as long as 7 h after the 10% solution.

AVAILABILITY

Solution (Ophthalmic): 2.5%, 10%.
Solution (Nasal): 0.125%, 0.16%, 0.25%, 0.5%.
Solution (Injection): 10 mg/mL.
Solution (Oral): 5 mg/mL.
Suppository (Rectal): 0.25%.

INDICATIONS AND DOSAGES

Treatment of mydriasis, uveitis, conjunctival congestion, cycloplegia, nasal congestion
▶ **Mydriasis induction (ophthalmic)**
TOPICAL
Adults, Adolescents, Elderly. Instill 1 or 2 drops of a 2.5% or 10% solution in eye before procedure. May be repeated in 10-60 min if needed. In general, the 2.5% solution is preferred in elderly patients to avoid cardiac reactions.
Children. Instill 1 or 2 drops of a 2.5% solution in the eye before procedure. May be repeated in 10-60 min if needed.
Infants younger than 1 yr. 1 drop of 2.5% solution 15-30 min before procedure.
▶ **Uveitis (posterior synechia)**
TOPICAL
Adults, Elderly. Instill 1 drop of 10% solution in eye 3 or more times daily with atropine sulfate. In general, the

P

2.5% solution is preferred in elderly patients to avoid adverse cardiac reactions.

▸ **Conjunctival congestion**
TOPICAL
Adults, Elderly. 1-2 drops of a 0.12%-0.25% solution applied to the conjunctiva every 3-4 h as needed. In general, the 2.5% solution is preferred in elderly patients to avoid cardiac reactions.

▸ **Postoperative malignant glaucoma**
TOPICAL
Adults, Elderly. Instill 1 drop of a 10% solution with 1 drop of a 1%-4% solution 3 or more times per day. In general, the 2.5% solution is preferred in elderly to avoid cardiac reactions.

▸ **Vasoconstriction and pupil dilatation**
TOPICAL
Adults. A drop of a suitable topical anesthetic may be applied, followed in a few minutes by 1 drop on the upper limbus.
TOPICAL
Adults. When a short-acting mydriatic is needed for wide dilatation of the pupil before intraocular surgery, phenylephrine HCl 2.5% (or the 10%) may be applied topically from 30 to 60 min before the operation.

▸ **Cycloplegia**
TOPICAL
Adults. One drop of the preferred cycloplegic is placed in each eye, followed in 5 min by one drop of phenylephrine HCl 2.5%.
Children. For a "one application method," phenylephrine HCl 2.5% may be combined with one of the preferred rapid acting cycloplegics to produce adequate cycloplegia.

▸ **Ophthalmoscopic examination**
TOPICAL
Adults. One drop of phenylephrine HCl 2.5% is placed in each eye.

▸ **Blanching test**
TOPICAL
Adults. One or two drops of phenylephrine HCl 2.5% should be applied to the injected eye.

▸ **Glaucoma**
TOPICAL
Adults. In certain patients with glaucoma, temporary reduction of intraocular tension may be attained by producing vasoconstriction of the intraocular vessels; this may be accompanied by placing 1 drop of the 10% solution on the upper surface of the cornea. This treatment may be repeated as often as necessary.

▸ **Nasal congestion**
INTRANASAL
Adults, Children 12 and older. Use 2 or 3 drops or sprays of a 0.25%-0.5% solution in the nose every 4 h as needed
Children aged 6-12 yr. Use 2 or 3 drops or sprays of a 0.25% solution in the nose every 4 h as needed.
Children 2-6 yr. Use 2 or 3 drops of a 0.125%-0.16% solution in the nose every 4 h as needed.

CONTRAINDICATIONS

Ophthalmic solutions (both strengths) of phenylephrine HCl are contraindicated in patients with anatomically narrow angles or narrow-angle glaucoma, some low-birth-weight infants and some elderly adults with severe arteriosclerotic cardiovascular or cerebrovascular disease, use during intraocular operative procedures when the corneal epithelial barrier has been disturbed and in persons with a known sensitivity to phenylephrine, sulfites, or any of its components, including preservatives. The 10% solution is contraindicated in infants and in patients with aneurysms.

INTERACTIONS
Drug
Adrenergic drugs: May increase adrenergic effects.

β-Adrenergic blockers: Risk of bradycardia with systemic absorption; may potentiate the cardiovascular depressant effects of potent inhalation anesthetics.

Halothane: Vasopressors may cause serious cardiac arrhythmias during halothane anesthesia and therefore should be used only with great caution or not at all.

MAO Inhibitors: The pressor effect of sympathomimetic pressor amines and adrenergic agents is markedly potentiated in patients receiving MAO inhibitors.

Nitrous oxide/oxygen gas inhalation: May complicate nasal administration.

Oxytocics: The pressure effect of sympathomimetic pressor amines is potentiated.

Tricyclic antidepressants: Increased risk of dysrhythmias and hypertension. May increase the pressor response of adrenergic agents.

Herbal
None known.

Food
None known.

DIAGNOSTIC TEST EFFECTS
None known.

SIDE EFFECTS
Frequent
Burning or stinging of eyes, headache or brow ache, sensitivity to light, watering of the eyes, increase in runny or stuffy nose, burning, stinging, dryness of inside the nose.
Occasional
Rare
Irritation, dizziness, fast or irregular or pounding heartbeat, increased sweating, increase in BP, paleness, trembling, headache, nervousness, trouble sleeping.

SERIOUS REACTIONS
• There have been reports associating the use of phenylephrine HCl 10% ophthalmic solutions with the development of serious cardiovascular reactions, including ventricular arrhythmias and myocardial infarctions. These episodes, some ending fatally, have usually occurred in elderly patients with preexisting cardiovascular diseases.

PRECAUTIONS & CONSIDERATIONS
Caution is necessary with advanced arteriosclerotic changes, cardiac disease, diabetes mellitus, angle-closure glaucoma, hypertension, idiopathic orthostatic hypotension, and sensitivity to sulfites. It is unknown whether phenylephrine (topical) crosses the placenta or is distributed into breast milk. Children may be more sensitive to the effects of phenylephrine. The 10% strength is not recommended in infants. Repeated use may increase the chance of adverse effects, such as miosis and reduced mydriatic effects in elderly patients.

Burning or stinging of the eyes, headache, brow ache, sensitivity of eyes to light, and watering of eyes may occur.

Intranasal applications is not recommended for chronic or long-term use to avoid developing congestion rebound. Particular caution is warranted in children under 6 yr of age with diabetes, cardiovascular disease, hypertension, hyperthyroidism, increased intraocular pressure, prostatic hypertrophy, glaucoma, ischemic heart disease.

P

Storage
Store at room temperature.
Prolonged exposure to strong
light may cause oxidation and
discoloration. Do not use if solution
is brown or precipitate is present.
Administration
Apply digital pressure to the
lacrimal sac during and for 2 or
3 min following instillation. The
recommended dose should not be
exceeded.

Phenylephrine Hydrochloride

fen-ill-ef′rin

(AK-Dilate, AD-Nephrin, Isopto
Frin [AUS], Mydfrin, Neo-Synephrine, Prefrin)

CATEGORY AND SCHEDULE

Pregnancy Risk Category: C
OTC (nasal solution, nasal spray,
ophthalmic solution)

Classification: Adrenergic
agonists, decongestants,
ophthalmics

MECHANISM OF ACTION

A sympathomimetic, α-receptor
stimulant that acts on the α-adrenergic
receptors of vascular smooth muscle.
Causes vasoconstriction of arterioles
of nasal mucosa or conjunctiva,
activates dilator muscle of the pupil to
cause contraction, produces systemic
arterial vasoconstriction. *Therapeutic
Effect:* Decreases mucosal blood flow
and relieves congestion and increases
systolic BP.

PHARMACOKINETICS

Route	Onset	Peak	Duration
IV	Immediate	NA	15-20 min
IM	10-15 min	NA	0.5-2 h
SC	10-15 min	NA	1 h

Minimal absorption after intranasal
and ophthalmic administration.
Metabolized in the liver and GI tract.
Primarily excreted in urine. *Half-life:*
2.5 h.

AVAILABILITY

Injection: 1% (10 mg/mL).
*Nasal Solution Drops
(Neosynephrine):* 0.5%, 1%.
Nasal Spray (Neosynephrine):
0.25%, 0.5%, 1%.
Ophthalmic Solution (Ak-Nephrin):
0.12%.
Ophthalmic Solution (AK-Dilate):
2.5%, 10%.
*Ophthalmic Solution (Mydfrin,
Neosynephrine):* 2.5%.

INDICATIONS AND DOSAGES
▶ **Nasal decongestant**
NASAL SPRAY, NASAL
SOLUTION
*Adults, Elderly, Children 12 yr and
older.* 2-3 drops or 1-2 sprays of
0.25%-0.5% solution into each nostril.
Children aged 6-11 yr. 2-3 drops or
1-2 sprays of 0.25% solution into
each nostril.
Children younger than 6 yr.
2-3 drops of 0.125% solution (dilute
0.5% solution with 0.9% NaCl to
achieve 0.125%) in each nostril.
Repeat q4h as needed. Do not use for
more than 3 days.
▶ **Conjunctival congestion, itching,
and minor irritation; whitening of
sclera**
OPHTHALMIC
*Adults, Elderly, Children 12 yr and
older.* 1-2 drops of 0.12% solution
q3-4h.

▸ **Hypotension, shock**
IM, SC
Adults, Elderly. 2-5 mg/dose q1-2h.
Children. 0.1 mg/kg/dose q1-2h.
IV BOLUS
Adults, Elderly. 0.1-0.5 mg/dose
q10-15min as needed.
Children. 5-20 mcg/kg/dose q10-15min.
IV INFUSION
Adults, Elderly. 100-180 mcg/min.
Children. 0.1-0.5 mcg/kg/min.
Titrate to desired effect.

CONTRAINDICATIONS

Acute pancreatitis, heart disease,
hepatitis, narrow-angle glaucoma,
pheochromocytoma, severe
hypertension, thrombosis, ventricular
tachycardia.

INTERACTIONS

Drug
β-Blockers: May have mutually
inhibitory effects.
Digoxin: May increase risk of
arrhythmias.
Ergonovine, oxytocin: May increase
vasoconstriction.
MAOIs: May increase vasopressor
effects.
**Maprotiline, tricyclic
antidepressants:** May increase
cardiovascular effects.
Methyldopa: May decrease effects
of methyldopa.
Herbal
None known.
Food
None known.

DIAGNOSTIC TEST EFFECTS

None known.

Ⓟ IV INCOMPATIBILITIES

Thiopentothal (Pentothal).

Ⓟ IV COMPATIBILITIES

Amiodarone (Cordarone),
dobutamine (Dobutrex), lidocaine,

potassium chloride, propofol
(Diprivan).

SIDE EFFECTS

Frequent
Nasal: Rebound nasal congestion
due to overuse, especially when used
longer than 3 days.
Occasional
Mild central nervous system
(CNS) stimulation (restlessness,
nervousness, tremors, headache,
insomnia, particularly in those
hypersensitive to sympathomimetics,
such as elderly patients).
Nasal: Stinging, burning, drying of
nasal mucosa.
Ophthalmic: Transient burning or
stinging, brow ache, blurred vision.

SERIOUS REACTIONS

• Large doses may produce
tachycardia and palpitations
(particularly in those with cardiac
disease), light-headedness, nausea,
and vomiting.
• Overdose in those older than 60 yr
may result in hallucinations, CNS
depression, and seizures.
• Prolonged nasal use may produce
chronic swelling of nasal mucosa and
rhinitis.

PRECAUTIONS & CONSIDERATIONS

Caution is warranted in patients
with bradycardia, heart block,
hyperthyroidism, and severe
arteriosclerosis. If phenylephrine 10%
ophthalmic is instilled into denuded or
damaged corneal epithelium, corneal
clouding may result. Phenylephrine
crosses the placenta and is distributed
in breast milk. Children may exhibit
increased absorption and toxicity with
nasal preparation. No age-related
precautions have been noted with
systemic use in children. Elderly
patients are more likely to experience
adverse effects.

P

The drug should be immediately discontinued if dizziness, feeling of irregular heartbeat, insomnia, tremor, or weakness occurs. BP and heart rate should be monitored before and during therapy.

Storage

Store vials at room temperature.

Administration

For nasal administration, blow nose before giving the medication. Tilt head back and instill the drops in one nostril, as prescribed. Remain in the same position; wait 5 min before applying drops in other nostril. Administer nasal spray into each nostril with the head erect. Sniff briskly while squeezing container; then wait 3-5 min before blowing nose gently. Rinse tip of spray bottle. Do not use for longer than 5 days because of the risk of rebound nasal congestion.

For ophthalmic use, tilt head backward and look up. With a gloved finger, gently pull the lower eyelid down to form a pouch; instill medication into the pouch. Do not touch tip of applicator to eyelids or any surface. When lower eyelid is released, keep eye open without blinking for at least 30 s. Apply gentle finger pressure to lacrimal sac, which is located at the bridge of the nose at the inside corner of the eye, for 1-2 min. Remove excess solution around eye with tissue. Wash hands immediately to remove medication on hands. Notify the physician if swelling of eyelids or itching occurs.

For IV push, dilute 1 mL of 10 mg/mL solution with 9 mL sterile water for injection to provide a concentration of 1 mg/mL. Give over 20-30 s. For IV infusion, dilute 10-mg vial with 500 mL D5W or 0.9% NaCl to provide a concentration of 2 mcg/mL. Maximum concentration: 500 mg/250 mL. Titrate as prescribed.

Phenytoin

fen′-i-toyn

Dilantin Infatab, Dilantin-125, Phenytoin sodium, Dilantin, Dilantin Kapseals

Do not confuse phenytoin with mephenytoin, or Dilantin with Dilaudid.

CATEGORY AND SCHEDULE

Pregnancy Risk Category: D

Classification: Anticonvulsants, hydantoins

MECHANISM OF ACTION

A hydantoin anticonvulsant that stabilizes neuronal membranes in the motor cortex by decreasing sodium and calcium ion influx into the neurons. Also acts as an antiarrhythmic agent by decreasing abnormal ventricular automaticity and shortening the refractory period, QT interval, and action potential duration. *Therapeutic Effect:* Limits the spread of seizure activity. Restores normal cardiac rhythm.

PHARMACOKINETICS

Slowly and variably absorbed after PO administration; slowly but completely absorbed after IM administration. Protein binding: 90%-95% (adults), 84% (neonates). Widely distributed; Crosses the placenta into breast milk. Metabolized in the liver. Excreted primarily in urine. Not removed by hemodialysis. *Half-life:* 22 h (oral), 14 h (infatabs).

AVAILABILITY

Capsules (Prompt-Release): 100 mg (92 mg phenytoin).

Capsules (Extended-Release [Dilantin]): 30 mg (27.6 mg phenytoin).
Capsules (Extended-Release [Phenytek]): 200 mg, 300 mg.
Oral Suspension (Dilantin): 125 mg/5 mL.
Tablets (Chewable [Dilantin]): 50 mg.
Injection: 50 mg/mL.

INDICATIONS AND DOSAGES
▸ **Used in the treatment of status epilepticus of the grand mal type, prevention and treatment of seizures occurring during neurosurgery. Control of arrhythmias is common (off-label)**
▸ **Status epilepticus**
IV
Adults, Elderly, Children. 15-20 mg/kg by slow IV, followed by a maintenance dose of 100 mg every 6-8 h, PO or IV. Maintenance dose: 300 mg/day in 2-3 divided doses for adults and elderly; 6-7 mg/kg/day for children 10-16 yr; 7-8 mg/kg/day for children 7-9 yr; 7.5-9 mg/kg/day for children 4-6 yr; 8-10 mg/kg/day for children 6 mo to 3 yr. IV rate should not exceed 1-3 mg/kg/min.
Neonates. Loading dose: 15-20 mg/kg. Maintenance dose: 5-8 mg/kg/day.
▸ **Seizure control**
PO
Adults, Elderly. 100 mg or 125 mg suspension 3 times/day initially, followed by 300-400 mg/day, not to exceed 600 mg/day. Can administer 1 g loading dose in 3 divided doses (400 mg, 300 mg, 300 mg) given at 2-h intervals. Once control is established, extended release 300 mg/day may be administered once daily.
Children 16 yr or younger. PO 5 mg/kg/day in 2-3 divided doses initially. Once control is established, follow with 4-8 mg/kg/day, not to exceed 300 mg/day.

▸ **Neurosurgery prophylaxis**
Adults. 10-20 mg/kg IV load. Maintenance: 4-6 mg/kg/day in 2 doses during surgery and postoperatively.

OFF-LABEL USES
Control of arrhythmias (particularly glycoside-induced arrhythmias), control of convulsions in severe preeclampsia, Adjunctive treatment of tricyclic antidepressant toxicity; treatment of muscle hyperirritability, digoxin-induced arrhythmias, and trigeminal neuralgia (tic douloureux), recessive dystrophic epidermolysis bullosa and junctional epidermolysis bullosa.

CONTRAINDICATIONS
Hypersensitivity to hydantoins, seizures due to hypoglycemia.
IV: Adam-Stokes syndrome, second- and third-degree AV block, sinoatrial block, sinus bradycardia.

INTERACTIONS
Drug
There are many drug interactions.
Acetaminophen: May increase hepatotoxicity potential with chronic use.
Alcohol, other central nervous system (CNS) depressants: May increase CNS depression.
Amiodarone, anticoagulants, cimetidine, disulfiram, estrogens, felbamate, fluconzaole, isoniazid, oxyphenbutazone, phenylbutazone, phenacemide, sulfonamides, trimethoprim: May increase phenytoin blood concentration, effects, and risk of toxicity.
Antacids: May decrease phenytoin absorption.
Carbamazepine, sucralfaate, antineoplastic agents, rifampin, rifabutin: May decrease serum levels of phenytoin.

P

Corticosteroids, coumarin anticoagulants, doxycycline, estrogens, levodopa, felodipine, methadone, loop diuretics, oral contraceptives, quinidine, rifampin, rifabutin: May impair the effects of these agents.

CNS depressants, alcohol: May increase depressant effects.

Cyclosporine: May reduce serum levels.

Disopyramide: May cause decreased bioavailability and serum concentrations; may enhance anticholinergic effect.

Fluconazole, ketoconazole, miconazole: May increase phenytoin blood concentration.

Folic acid: May cause folic acid deficiency.

Glucocorticoids: May decrease the effects of glucocorticoids.

Lidocaine, propranolol: May increase cardiac depressant effects.

Metyrapone: May cause a subnormal response to metyrapone.

Mexiletine: May decrease cardiac effects and serum concentration.

Nondepolarizing muscle relaxants: May cause decreased effect or shorter duration of activity.

Phenobarbital, sodium valproate, valproic acid: May alter phenytoin levels, may increase phenobarbital levels and decrease valproic acid levels.

Primidone: May increase serum levels leading to toxicity.

Sympathomimetics (e.g., dopamine): May cause profound hypotension and cardiac arrest.

Theophylline: May decrease effects of both theophylline and phenytoin.

Valproic acid: May decrease the metabolism and increase the blood concentration of phenytoin.

Xanthine: May increase the metabolism of these drugs.

Herbal
None known.

Food
Enteral nutrition therapy: May reduce serum concentrations of phenytoin.

DIAGNOSTIC TEST EFFECTS
May increase blood glucose level and serum GGT and alkaline phosphatase levels. Therapeutic serum level is 10-20 mcg/mL; toxic serum level is > 25 mcg/mL.

ⓘ IV INCOMPATIBILITIES
Do not mix with any other medications.

SIDE EFFECTS
Frequent
Drowsiness, lethargy, confusion, slurred speech, irritability, gingival hyperplasia, hypersensitivity reaction (including fever, rash, and lymphadenopathy), constipation, dizziness, nausea, vomiting, pink-colored urine.

Occasional
Headache, hirsutism, coarsening of facial features, insomnia, muscle twitching.

Rare
Dermatologic manifestations with fever: Scarlatiniform or morbiliform rashes.

SERIOUS REACTIONS
• Abrupt withdrawal may precipitate status epilepticus.
• Local irritation, inflammation, tenderness, necrosis and sloughing with or without extravasation at site of injection or IV infusion.
• Because of variances in bioavailability, brand interchange is not recommended and should be avoided.
• Blood dyscrasias, lymphadenopathy, and osteomalacia

(caused by impaired vitamin D metabolism) may occur.

• Toxic phenytoin blood concentration (25 mcg/mL or more) may produce ataxia, nystagmus, or diplopia. As the level increases, extreme lethargy may lead to coma.

• There is no known antidote.

• Drug should not be given to anyone having a known sensitivity to phenytoin or any of its components.

PRECAUTIONS & CONSIDERATIONS

! Extreme caution should be used in patients with congestive heart failure (CHF), myocardial damage, myocardial infarction (MI), and respiratory depression. Caution is also warranted with hyperglycemia, hypotension, hepatic and renal impairment, and severe myocardial insufficiency, alcohol abuse, hypotension, acute intermittent porphyria. Phenytoin crosses the placenta and is distributed in small amounts in breast milk. Fetal hydantoin syndrome, marked by craniofacial abnormalities, digital or nail hypoplasia, and prenatal growth deficiency, have been reported. Pregnant women may experience more frequent seizures because of altered drug absorption and metabolism. Phenytoin use may increase the risk of neonatal hemorrhage and maternal bleeding during delivery. Children are more susceptible to coarsening of facial hair, hirsutism, and gingival hyperplasia. Lower dosages are recommended for elderly patients, although no age-related precautions have been noted for this age group.

The lethal dose is not known but is estimated to be 2-5 g. Toxicity is evidenced by nystagmus, ataxia and dysarthria, tremor, hyperflexia, slurred speech, nausea and vomiting. Coma and hypertension may occur.

Death is due to respiratory and circulatory depression.

Skin rash, nystagmus, ataxia, drowsiness, severe nausea or vomiting, gingival hyperplasia, or jaundice should be reported. Blood sugar levels may be affected by phenytoin, and changes in levels beyond normal should be reported.

Drowsiness, dizziness, and lethargy may occur, so alcohol and tasks that require mental alertness or motor skills should be avoided. Notify the physician if fever, swollen glands, sore throat, a skin reaction, or signs of hematologic toxicity (such as a bleeding tendency, bruising, fatigue, or fever) occur. History of the seizure disorder, including the duration, frequency, and intensity of seizures, should be assessed. CBC and blood chemistry tests should be performed to assess hepatic function before and periodically during phenytoin therapy. Repeat the CBC 2 wks after beginning phenytoin therapy and 2 wks after the phenytoin maintenance dose is established. CBC should be performed every month for 1 yr after the maintenance dose is established and every 3 mo thereafter. Therapeutic serum drug level is 10-20 mcg/mL; the toxic serum drug level is > 25 mcg/mL.

Discontinuation of the drug abruptly should be avoided as this could precipitate seizures or status epilepticus. Dosages should be reduced or other anticonvulsant medication should be introduced gradually. Do not use phenytoin to treat seizures because of hypoglycemia or other metabolic disorders as this may cause petit mal or absence seizures to occur.

Storage

If refrigerated or frozen, the solution may form a precipitate that dissolves at room temperature; clear or slightly yellow solution is usable.

P

Administration
Take oral phenytoin with food if
GI distress occurs. Do not chew,
open, or break capsules or take any
discolored capsules. Tablets may be
chewed. Shake the oral suspension
well before using.

If administering with tube
feedings, delay feeding 1-2 hr before
and after administration of phenytoin.
! Give phenytoin by IV push directly
into a large vein through a large gauge
needle or IV catheter. Remember that
the maintenance dose is usually given
12 h after the loading dose.

A slight yellow discoloration of the
solution will not affect its potency.
Phenytoin may be given undiluted
or may be diluted with 0.9% NaCl.
Do not exceed an injection rate
of 50 mg/min for adults to avoid
cardiovascular collapse and severe
hypotension. For elderly patients,
administer 50 mg over 2-3 min. For
neonates, do not exceed 1-3 mg/kg/min.
To minimize pain from chemical
irritation of the vein, flush the catheter
with sterile saline solution after each
bolus dose of phenytoin.

Phosphates, Potassium
Poe-tass-eeum fos-fates
(Fleet Enema, Fleet Phospho
Soda, K-Phos ME, K-Phos
Neutral, Neutra-Phos,
Uro-KP-Neutral[CAN])

CATEGORY AND SCHEDULE
Pregnancy Risk Category: C

Classification: Urinary acidifier,
antiurolithic

MECHANISM OF ACTION
Electrolytes that participate in bone
deposition, calcium metabolism, and
utilization of B complex vitamins
and act as a buffer in maintaining
acid-base balance. Also exert an
osmotic effect in the small intestine,
producing distention and promoting
peristalsis. *Therapeutic Effect:*
Correct hypophosphatemia, acidify
urine in urinary tract infections,
help to prevent calcium deposits in
urinary tract (unapproved use), and
promote evacuation of the bowel.

PHARMACOKINETICS
Poorly absorbed after PO
administration. PO form excreted in
feces; IV form excreted in urine.

AVAILABILITY
Oral Solution (Fleet Phospha-Soda):
4 mmol phosphate per mL.
*Powder (Neutra-Phos, Neutra-Phos
K):* 250 mg (8 mmol) phosphate.
Tablets (K-Phos ME): 125 mg
(4 mmol) phosphate.
*Tablets (K-Phos Neutral, Uro-KP-
Neutral):* 250 mg (8 mmol) phosphate.
Enema (Fleet Enema): 2.25 oz, 4.5 oz.
Injection (potassium phosphate):
3 mmol phosphate and 4.4 mEq
potassium per mL.
Injection (sodium phosphate): 3 mmol
phosphate and 4 mEq sodium per mL.

INDICATIONS AND DOSAGES
▸ **Hypophosphatemia**
PO (NEUTRA-PHOS, NEUTRA-
PHOS K, K-PHOS ME, K-PHOS-
NEUTRAL, URO-KP-NEUTRAL)
Adults, Elderly. 800 mg.
Children > 10 yr of age. 1200 mg
Children 1-10 yr of age. 800 mg
Children 6-12 mo of age. 360 mg
Children up to 6 mo of age. 240 mg
IV
Adults, Elderly. 0.5 mmol/kg IV over
4-6 h.
Children. 0.25 mmol/kg over 4-6 h.
▸ **Laxative or to increase GI
peristaltic action**

PO (NEUTRA-PHOS, NEUTRA-PHOS K, URO-KP-NEUTRAL)
Adults, Elderly, Children 4 yr and older. 1-2 capsules/packets 4 times a day.
Children younger than 4 yr.
1 capsule/packet 4 times a day.
RECTAL
Adults, Elderly, Children 12 yr and older. 4.5-oz enema as single dose. May repeat.
Children younger than 12 yr. 2.25-oz enema as single dose. May repeat.
▸ **Urine acidification**
PO
Adults, Elderly. 8 mmol 4 times a day (250 mg).

OFF-LABEL USES
Prevention of calcium renal calculi.

CONTRAINDICATIONS
Abdominal pain or fecal impaction (from rectal dosage form), CHF, hyperkalemia, hypernatremia, hyperphosphatemia, hypocalcemia, hypomagnesemia, phosphate renal calculi, severe renal impairment

INTERACTIONS
Drug
Amiloride, ACE inhibitors, NSAIDs, potassium-containing medications, potassium-sparing diuretics, salt substitutes containing potassium phosphate: May increase potassium blood concentration.
Antacids: May decrease the absorption of phosphates.
Calcium-containing medications: May increase the risk of calcium deposition in soft tissues and decrease phosphate absorption.
Digoxin: May increase the risk of heart block caused by hyperkalemia when given with potassium phosphates.
Glucocorticoids: May cause edema when given with sodium phosphate.

Iron and iron-containing products: May inhibit absorption if taken within 2 h of phosphate dose.
Phosphate-containing medications: May increase the risk of hyperphosphatemia.
Sodium-containing medications: May increase the risk of edema when given with sodium phosphate.
Triamterine and other potassium-sparing diuretics: Concurrent use may increase the risk of hyperkalemia developing.
Herbal
None known.
Food
None known.

DIAGNOSTIC TEST EFFECTS
None known.

🖥 IV COMPATIBILITIES
Diltiazem (Cardizem), enalapril (Vasotec), famotidine (Pepcid), magnesium sulfate, metoclopramide (Reglan).

SIDE EFFECTS
Frequent
Mild laxative effect (in first few days of therapy), decrease in frequency and amount of urination.
Occasional
Diarrhea, nausea, abdominal pain, vomiting, slow or irregular heart beat.
Rare
Headache; dizziness; confusion; heaviness of lower extremities; fatigue; muscle cramps; paraesthesia; peripheral edema; arrhythmias; weight gain; thirst.

SERIOUS REACTIONS
• Hyperphosphatemia may produce extra-skeletal calcification.

PRECAUTIONS & CONSIDERATIONS
Caution is warranted in patients with adrenal insufficiency, cirrhosis,

P

renal impairment, and concurrent use of potassium-sparing drugs. It is unknown whether phosphates cross the placenta or are distributed in breast milk. No age-related precautions have been noted in children or elderly patients.

Notify the physician of abdominal pain. Baseline phosphate levels and urinary pH should be obtained. Serum alkaline phosphatase, bilirubin, calcium, phosphorus, potassium, sodium, AST (SGOT), and ALT (SGPT) levels should be monitored throughout therapy. Pattern of daily bowel activity and stool consistency should also be assessed.

Injectible form contains aluminum, which may reach toxic levels with prolonged use; care is warranted in neonates.

Storage

Store vials at room temperature.

Administration

For oral use, dissolve tablets in water. Give phosphates after meals or with food to decrease GI upset. Maintain high fluid intake to prevent renal calculi.

For IV use, dilute the drug before using. Generally, infuse over 4-6 h.

Phosphorated Carbohydrate Solution

(Emetrol)

CATEGORY AND SCHEDULE

Pregnancy Risk Category: NR
OTC

Classification: Hyperosmolar carbohydrate with phosphoric acid, antiemetic

MECHANISM OF ACTION

An antiemetic whose mechanism of action has not been determined. Phosphorated carbohydrate solution consists of fructose, dextrose, and phosphoric acid, and it may directly act on the wall of the GI tract and reduce smooth muscle contraction and delays gastric emptying time through high osmotic pressure exerted by the solution of simple sugars. *Therapeutic Effect:* Relieves nausea and vomiting.

PHARMACOKINETICS

Fructose is slowly absorbed from the GI tract. Metabolized in liver by phosphorylation and partly converted to liver glycogen and glucose. Excreted in urine.

Dextrose is rapidly absorbed from GI tract. Distributed and stored throughout tissues. Metabolized in liver to carbon dioxide and water.

AVAILABILITY

Solution: 1.87 g fructose/1.87 g dextrose/21.5 mg phosphoric acid/ 5 mL (Emetrol).

INDICATIONS AND DOSAGES

▸ **Antiemetic**

PO

Adults, Elderly. 15-30 mL initially. May repeat dose every 15 min until distress subsides. Maximum: 5 doses in a 1-h period.

Children 2 yr and older. 5-10 mL initially. May repeat dose every 15 min until distress subsides. Maximum: 5 doses in a 1-h period.

Children under 2 yr. Do not use.

CONTRAINDICATIONS

Symptoms of appendicitis or inflamed bowel, hereditary fructose intolerance, hypersensitivity to any component of the formulation.

INTERACTIONS
Drug
None known.
Herbal
None known.
Food
None known.

DIAGNOSTIC TEST EFFECTS
May increase blood glucose concentrations.

SIDE EFFECTS
Frequent
Diarrhea, abdominal pain.

SERIOUS REACTIONS
• Fructose intolerance includes symptoms of fainting, swelling of face, arms and legs, unusual bleeding, vomiting, weight loss, and yellow eyes and skin.

PRECAUTIONS & CONSIDERATIONS
Caution is warranted with diabetes mellitus because the condition may be aggravated because of the solution's high carbohydrate content as well as with children and elderly because of the risk of fluid and electrolyte loss as a result of vomiting. It is unknown whether phosphorated carbohydrate solution crosses the placenta or is distributed in breast milk. Safety and efficacy of phosphorated carbohydrate solution have not been established in children younger than 2 yr of age. Be aware of the risk of fluid and electrolyte loss in elderly patients.
Administration
Take 1 or 2 tbsp until nausea stops. May repeat dose after 15 min if distress does not subside. Do not dilute phosphorated carbohydrate solution. Do not drink any other fluids immediately before or after taking this drug. Do not exceed more than 5 doses in 1-h period.

Physostigmine
fi-zoe-stig′meen
(Antilirium)
Do not confuse physostigmine with Prostigmin or pyridostigmine.

CATEGORY AND SCHEDULE
Pregnancy Risk Category: C

Classification: Cholinergic parasympathomimetic

MECHANISM OF ACTION
A cholinergic that inhibits destruction of acetylcholine by enzyme acetylcholinesterase, thus enhancing impulse transmission across the myoneural junction.
Therapeutic Effect: Improves skeletal muscle tone, stimulates salivary and sweat gland secretions.

AVAILABILITY
Injection: 1 mg/mL.

INDICATIONS AND DOSAGES
▶ **To reverse central nervous system (CNS) effects of anticholinergic drugs and tricyclic antidepressants**
IV, IM
Adults, Elderly. Initially, 0.5-2 mg. If no response, repeat 10-30 min until response or adverse cholinergic effects occur. If initial response occurs, may give additional doses of 1-2 mg q30-60min as life-threatening signs, such as arrhythmias, seizures, and deep coma, recur.
Children. 0.01-0.03 mg/kg. May give additional doses q5-10min until response or adverse cholinergic effects occur or total dose of 2 mg is given.

OFF-LABEL USES
Treatment of hereditary ataxia.

P

CONTRAINDICATIONS

Active uveal inflammation, angle-closure glaucoma before iridectomy, asthma, cardiovascular disease, concurrent use of ganglionic-blocking agents, diabetes, gangrene, glaucoma associated with iridocyclitis, hypersensitivity to cholinesterase inhibitors or their components, mechanical obstruction of intestinal or urogenital tract, vagotonic state.

INTERACTIONS

Drug
Broad-spectrum antibiotics, salicylates: May decrease action.
Cholinesterase agents, including bethanechol and carbachol: May increase the effects of these drugs.
Oral anticoagulants: May cause antagonistic activity.
Succinylcholine: May prolong the action of succinylcholine.
Herbal
None known.
Food
None known.

DIAGNOSTIC TEST EFFECTS

None known.

SIDE EFFECTS

Expected
Miosis, increased GI and skeletal muscle tone, bradycardia.
Occasional
Marked drop in BP (hypertensive patients).
Rare
Allergic reaction.

SERIOUS REACTIONS

• Parenteral overdose produces a cholinergic crisis manifested as abdominal discomfort or cramps, nausea, vomiting, diarrhea, flushing, facial warmth, excessive salivation, diaphoresis, urinary urgency, and blurred vision. If overdose occurs, stop all anticholinergic drugs and immediately administer 0.6-1.2 mg atropine sulfate IM or IV for adults or 0.01 mg/kg for infants and children younger than 12 yr.

PRECAUTIONS & CONSIDERATIONS

Caution is warranted in patients with bradycardia, bronchial asthma, epilepsy, GI disturbances, hypotension, parkinsonism, peptic ulcer disease, and disorders that may be adversely affected by drug's vagotonic effects and in those who have recently had an myocardial infarction. Avoid driving at night and activities requiring visual acuity in dim light during physostigmine therapy.

Adverse effects usually subside after the first few days of therapy. Vital signs should be assessed immediately before and every 15-30 min after physostigmine administration. Cholinergic reactions, such as abdominal pain, dyspnea, hypotension, arrhythmias, muscle weakness, and diaphoresis, after drug administration should be assessed.
Administration
For adults, administer at a rate not exceeding 1 mg/min. For children, administer at a rate not exceeding 0.5 mg/min.

Phytonadione
(vitamin K₁)
fye-toe-na-dye´-own
(Aqua Mephyton, Mephyton)

Category and Schedule:
Pregnancy Risk Category: C

Drug Class: Vitamin K₁,
fat-soluble vitamin

MECHANISM OF ACTION
Needed for adequate blood clotting
(factors II, VII, IX, X).

USES
Treatment of vitamin K
malabsorption,
hypoprothrombinemia, prevention of
hypoprothrombinemia caused by oral
anticoagulants.

PHARMACOKINETICS
PO/Injection: Readily absorbed
from duodenum and requires bile
salts, rapid hepatic metabolism,
onset of action 6-12 h, normal PT in
12-24 h, crosses placenta, renal and
biliary excretion; because of severe
side effects, restrict IV route when
other administration routes are not
available.

INDICATIONS AND DOSAGES
▸ **Hypoprothrombinemia caused by
vitamin K malabsorption**
PO/IM
Adults. 2-25 mg; may repeat or
increase to 50 mg.
Children, Infants. 2.5-5 mg as a
single dose.
▸ **Prevention of hemorrhagic disease
of the newborn**
SC/IM
Neonates. 0.5-1 mg after birth;
repeat in 6-8 h if required.

▸ **Hypoprothrombinemia caused by
oral anticoagulants**
PO/SC/IM
Adults. 2.5-10 mg; may repeat
12-48 h after PO dose or 6-8 h
after subcutaneous/IM dose, based
on PT.

SIDE EFFECTS/ADVERSE REACTIONS
Occasional
Taste alterations, headache, cardiac
irregularities (tachycardia), nausea,
vomiting, hemoglobinuria, rash,
urticaria, flushing, erythema,
sweating, bronchospasms, dyspnea,
cramplike pain.
Rare
Hyperbilirubinemia.

CONTRAINDICATIONS
Hypersensitivity, severe hepatic
disease, last few weeks of pregnancy.

DRUG INTERACTIONS
**Broad-spectrum antibiotics,
salicylates (high doses):** Decreased
action.
Oral anticoagulants: Antagonist to
oral anticoagulants.

SERIOUS REACTIONS
• Severe hypersensitivity reactions.

PRECAUTIONS & CONSIDERATIONS
General
Determine why the patient is taking
this drug. Medical consultation should
be made before dental treatment.
 Patients on chronic drug therapy
may rarely have symptoms of
blood dyscrasias, which can
include infection, bleeding, and
poor healing.
Administration
Protect tablets from light. Oral
administration is preferred. Avoid
IM administration in patients with
coagulopathy. SC administration

results in erratic and delayed absorption. Dilute IV with normal saline or preservative-free D5W. Protect from light. Infuse at a rate not to exceed 1 mg/min.

Pilocarpine Hydrochloride
pye-loe-kar'peen high-dro-clor-ide
(IsoptoCarpin, Ocusert, Pilo-20, Ocusert Pilo-40, Pilopt Eyedrops, P.V. Carpine Liquifilm Ophthalmic Solution[AUS], Salagen)

CATEGORY AND SCHEDULE
Pregnancy Risk Category: C

Classification: Cholinergic agonist

MECHANISM OF ACTION
A cholinergic that increases exocrine gland secretions by stimulating cholinergic receptors. *Therapeutic Effect:* Improves symptoms of dry mouth in patients with salivary gland hypofunction.

PHARMACOKINETICS

Route	Onset	Peak	Duration
PO	20 min	1 h	3-5 h

Absorption decreased if taken with a high-fat meal. Inactivation of pilocarpine thought to occur at neuronal synapses and probably in plasma. Excreted in urine. *Half-life:* 4-12 h.

AVAILABILITY
Tablets: 5 mg.

INDICATIONS AND DOSAGES
▶ **Dry mouth associated with radiation treatment for head and neck cancer**
PO
Adults, Elderly. 5 mg three times a day. Range: 15-30 mg/day. Maximum: 2 tablets/dose.
▶ **Dry mouth associated with Sjögren syndrome**
PO
Adults, Elderly. 5 mg four times a day. Range: 10-30 mg/day.
▶ **Dosage in hepatic impairment**
Adults, Elderly. Dosage decreased to 5 mg twice a day for adults and elderly with hepatic impairment.

CONTRAINDICATIONS
Conditions in which miosis is undesirable, such as acute iritis and angle-closure glaucoma; uncontrolled asthma.
Caution
Bronchial asthma, hypertension.

INTERACTIONS
Drug
Anticholinergics: May antagonize the effects of anticholinergics.
β-Blockers: May produce conduction disturbances.
Herbal
None known.
Food
High-fat meals: May decrease the absorption rate of pilocarpine.

DIAGNOSTIC TEST EFFECTS
None known.

SIDE EFFECTS
Frequent (29%)
Diaphoresis.
Occasional (5%-11%)
Headache, dizziness, urinary frequency, flushing, dyspepsia, nausea, asthenia, lacrimation, visual disturbances.

Rare (< 4%)
Diarrhea, abdominal pain, peripheral edema, chills.

SERIOUS REACTIONS
• Patients with diaphoresis who do not drink enough fluids may develop dehydration.

PRECAUTIONS & CONSIDERATIONS
Caution is warranted with hepatic impairment, pulmonary disease, and significant cardiovascular disease. Pilocarpine use may impair reproductive function. The safety and efficacy of pilocarpine have not been established in children. Elderly patients have an increased incidence of diarrhea, dizziness, and urinary frequency. Adequate hydration should be maintained. Avoid tasks that require mental alertness or motor skills until response to the drug has been established.

Visual changes may occur, especially at night. Caution when driving at night or when performing hazardous activities in reduced lighting due to visual blurring. Pattern of daily bowel activity and stool consistency and urinary frequency should be assessed.
Administration
Take pilocarpine without regard to food.

Pimecrolimus
pim-eh-crow-leh-mus
(Elidel)

CATEGORY AND SCHEDULE
Pregnancy Risk Category: C

Classification: Dermatologics, immunosuppressives, topical anti-inflammatory

MECHANISM OF ACTION
An immunomodulator that inhibits release of cytokine, an enzyme that produces an inflammatory reaction. *Therapeutic Effect:* Produces anti-inflammatory activity.

PHARMACOKINETICS
Minimal systemic absorption with topical application. Metabolized in liver. Excreted in feces.

AVAILABILITY
Cream: 1% (Elidel).

INDICATIONS AND DOSAGES
▸ **Atopic dermatitis (eczema)**
TOPICAL
Adults, Elderly, Children 2-17 yr. Apply to affected area twice daily for up to 3 wks (up to 6 wks in adolescents, children 2-17 yr). Rub in gently and completely.

OFF-LABEL USES
Allergic contact dermatitis, irritant contact dermatitis, psoriasis.

CONTRAINDICATIONS
Hypersensitivity to pimecrolimus or any component of the formulation, Netherton syndrome (potential for increased systemic absorption), application to active cutaneous viral infections.

INTERACTIONS
Drug
None known.
Herbal
None known.
Food
None known.

DIAGNOSTIC TEST EFFECTS
None known.

P

SIDE EFFECTS

Rare

Transient application-site sensation of burning or feeling of heat.

SERIOUS REACTIONS

• Lymphadenopathy and phototoxicity occur rarely.

PRECAUTIONS & CONSIDERATIONS

Caution should be used in immunocompromised patients and in those who are at an increased risk of varicella zoster virus infection, herpes simplex virus infection, or eczema herpeticum. Be aware that clinical infection at treatment sites should be cleared before commencing treatment. Consider discontinuing therapy if lymphadenopathy or in the presence of acute infectious or if mononucleosis develops. It is unknown whether pimecrolimus is distributed in breast milk. Safety and efficacy of pimecrolimus have not been established in children younger than 2 yr of age. No age-related precautions have been noted in elderly patients.

Do not use for active cutaneous viral infections, infected dermatitis, natural or artifical light exposures.

Pimecrolimus may cause a mild to moderate feeling of warmth or a sensation of burning at the site of application. Artificial sunlight or tanning beds should be avoided.

Administration

Gently cleanse area before application. Use occlusive dressings only as ordered. Apply sparingly and rub into area thoroughly. Do not use topical pimecrolimus on broken skin or in areas of infection, and do not apply to the face, inguinal areas, or wet skin.

Pimozide

pi'moe-zide

(Orap)

CATEGORY AND SCHEDULE

Pregnancy Risk Category: C

Classification: Antipsychotics, antidyskinetic

MECHANISM OF ACTION

A diphenylbutylpiperidine that blocks dopamine at postsynaptic receptor sites in the brain. *Therapeutic Effect:* Suppresses behavioral response in psychosis.

PHARMACOKINETICS

PO: Onset erratic, peak 6-8 h. *Half-life:* 50-55 h. Metabolized in the liver, excreted in the urine, feces.

AVAILABILITY

Tablets: 1 mg, 2 mg (Orap).

INDICATIONS AND DOSAGES

▶ **Tourette disorder**

PO

Adults, Elderly. 1-2 mg/day in a single dose or divided doses 3 times/day. Maximum: 10 mg/day. *Children older than 12 yr.* Initially, 0.05 mg/kg/day. Maximum: 10 mg/day.

OFF-LABEL USE

Psychotic disorders.

CONTRAINDICATIONS

Aggressive schizophrenics when sedation is required, concurrent administration of pemoline, methylphenidate or amphetamines, concurrent administration with dofetilide, sotalol, quinidine, other Class IA and III anti-arrhythmics, mesoridazine, thioridazine, chlorpromazine, droperidol, sparfloxacin, gatifloxacin, moxifloxacin, halofantrine, mefloquine, pentamidine, arsenic trioxide, levomethadyl acetate, dolasetron mesylate, probucol, tacrolimus, ziprasidone, sertraline, macrolide antibiotics, drugs that cause QT prolongation, and less potent inhibitors of CYP3A, congenital or drug-induced long QT syndrome, doses > 10 mg daily, history of cardiac arrhythmias, Parkinson disease, patients with known hypokalemia or hypomagnesemia, severe central nervous system (CNS) depression, simple tics or tics not associated with Tourette syndrome, hypersensitivity to pimozide or any of its components.

INTERACTIONS
Drug
Alcohol, CNS depressants: May increase CNS and respiratory depression.
Aprepitant: May increase pimozide plasma concentrations.
Class IA and II antiarrhythmics: May increase risk for QT prolongation and cardiotoxicity.
Drugs that prolong QT interval: May increase risk for QT prolongation and cardiotoxicity.
Belladonna alkaloids: May increase anticholinergic effects.
Lithium: May increase extrapyramidal symptoms.
Phenylalanine: May increase incidence of tardive dyskinesia.
Sertraline: May increase plasma pimozide levels.
Tramadol: May increase risk of seizures.
Vitex: May decrease effectiveness of dopamine antagonists.
Herbal
Betel nut: May increase extrapyramidal side effects of pimozide.

Kava kava: May increase dopamine antagonist effects.
Food
Grapefruit juice: May inhibit metabolism of pimozide.

DIAGNOSTIC TEST EFFECTS
None known.

SIDE EFFECTS
Occasional
Akathisia, dystonic extrapyramidal effects, parkinsonian extrapyramidal effects, tardive dyskinesia, blurred vision, ocular changes, constipation, decreased sweating, dry mouth, nasal congestion, dizziness, drowsiness, orthostatic hypotension, urinary retention, somnolence.
Rare
Rash, cholestatic jaundice, priapism.

SERIOUS REACTIONS
• Serious reactions such as blood dyscrasias, agranulocytosis, leukocytopenia, thrombocytopenia, cholestatic jaundice, neuroleptic malignant syndrome (NMS), constipation or paralytic ileus, priapism, QT prolongation and torsades de pointes, seizure, systemic lupus erythematosus-like syndrome, and temperature-regulation dysfunction (heatstroke or hypothermia) occur rarely.
• Abrupt withdrawal following long-term therapy may precipitate nausea, vomiting, gastritis, dizziness, and tremors.

PRECAUTIONS & CONSIDERATIONS
Caution is necessary with history of neuroleptic malignant syndrome, tardive dyskinesia, and impaired liver or kidney function. Caution is warranted with concomitant administration with inhibitors of cytochrome P450 1A2 and 3A4 enzymes as well as CNS

P

depressants and fluoxetine. Safety and effectiveness have not been established in children under the age of 12 yr. Elderly and debilitated patients may require a lower initial dose. Avoid grapefruit juice and alcohol consumption.

Akathisia, dystonic extrapyramidal effects, parkinsonian extrapyramidal effects, tardive dyskinesia, tardive dystonia, urinary retention, blurred vision, ocular changes, epithelial keratopathy, pigmentary retinopathy, constipation, decreased sweating, dry mouth, nasal congestion, dizziness, drowsiness, hypotension, and orthostatic hypotension may occur. Signs of tardive dyskinesia or akathias should be immediately reported.

Administration
The suppression of tics by pimozide requires a slow and gradual introduction of the drug. The dose should be carefully adjusted to a point where the suppression of tics and the relief afforded is balanced against the unpleasant side effects.

Pindolol
pin′doe-loll
(Apo-Pindol [CAN], Visken)

CATEGORY AND SCHEDULE
Pregnancy Risk Category: B (D if used in second or third trimester)

Classification: Nonselective β-adrenergic antagonist

MECHANISM OF ACTION
A nonselective β-blocker that blocks β_1- and β_2-adrenergic receptors. *Therapeutic Effect:* Slows heart rate, decreases cardiac output, decreases BP, and exhibits antiarrhythmic activity. Decreases myocardial ischemia severity by decreasing oxygen requirements.

PHARMACOKINETICS
Completely absorbed from GI tract. Metabolized in liver. Primarily excreted in urine. *Half-life:* 3-4 h (half-life increased with impaired renal function, elderly).

AVAILABILITY
Capsules: 5 mg, 10 mg (Visken).

INDICATIONS AND DOSAGES
▸ **Mild to moderate hypertension**
PO
Adults. Initially, 5 mg 2 times/day. Gradually increase dose by 10 mg/day at intervals of 2-4 wks. Maintenance: 10-30 mg/day in 2-3 divided doses. Maximum: 60 mg/day.
Elderly. Usual elderly dosage: Initially, 5 mg/day. May increase by 5 mg q3-4 wk.

OFF-LABEL USES
Treatment of chronic angina pectoris, hypertrophic cardiomyopathy, tremors, and mitral valve prolapse syndrome. Increases antidepressant effect with fluoxetine and other SSRIs.

CONTRAINDICATIONS
Bronchial asthma, chronic obstructive pulmonary disease (COPD), uncontrolled cardiac failure, sinus bradycardia, heart block greater than first degree, cardiogenic shock, congestive heart failure (CHF), unless secondary to tachyarrhythmias.

INTERACTIONS
Drug
Anticholinergics, hydrocarbon inhalation anesthetics, fentanyl

derivatives: May increase risk of hypotension.
Diuretics, other hypotensives: May increase hypotensive effect of pindolol.
Epinephrine, ephedrine: May cause hypertension or bradycardia.
Fluoxetine and other SSRI antidepressants: May increase antidepressant effect.
Indomethacin: May decrease antihypertensive effects.
Insulin and oral hypoglycemics: May mask symptoms of hypoglycemia and/or prolong hypoglycemic effect.
Lidocaine: May slow metabolism of drug.
Sympathomimetics, phenothiazines, xanthines: May mutually inhibit effects of pindolol.
Theophylline: May decrease bronchodilation effects.
Herbal
None known.
Food
None known.

DIAGNOSTIC TEST EFFECTS
May increase ANA titer, SGOT (AST), SGPT (ALT), alkaline phosphatase, LDH, bilirubin, BUN, creatinine, potassium, uric acid, lipoproteins, and triglycerides.

SIDE EFFECTS
Frequent
Decreased sexual ability, drowsiness, trouble sleeping, unusual tiredness or weakness.
Occasional
Bradycardia, depression, cold hands or feet, diarrhea, constipation, anxiety, nasal congestion, nausea, vomiting.
Rare
Altered taste, dry eyes, itching, numbness of fingers, toes, and scalp

SERIOUS REACTIONS
• Overdosage may produce profound bradycardia and hypotension.
• Abrupt withdrawal may result in sweating, palpitations, headache, and tremulousness.
• May precipitate CHF or myocardial infarction (MI) in patients with heart disease; thyroid storm in those with thyrotoxicosis; or peripheral ischemia in those with existing peripheral vascular disease.
• Hypoglycemia may occur in previously controlled diabetics.
• Signs of thrombocytopenia, such as unusual bleeding or bruising, occur rarely.

PRECAUTIONS & CONSIDERATIONS
Caution is warranted with bronchospastic disease, diabetes, hyperthyroidism, impaired renal or liver function, inadequate cardiac function, or peripheral vascular disease. Pindolol readily crosses the placenta and is distributed in breast milk. During delivery, pindolol may produce apnea, bradycardia, hypoglycemia, and hypothermia as well as low-birth-weight infants. Safety and efficacy have not been established in children. Caution should be used in elderly patients who may have age-related peripheral vascular disease. Nasal decongestants or over-the-counter (OTC) cold preparations (stimulants) should be avoided without physician approval. Excess salt and alcohol consumption should be limited.
Excessive fatigue, headache, prolonged dizziness, shortness of breath, or weight gain should be reported.
Administration
May be given with or without regard to meals. Tablets may be crushed. Do not abruptly discontinue the drug.

Pioglitazone
pye-oh-gli′ta-zone
(Actos)

CATEGORY AND SCHEDULE
Pregnancy Risk Category: C

Classification: Antidiabetic
agents, thiazolidinedione

MECHANISM OF ACTION
An antidiabetic that improves
target-cell response to insulin
without increasing pancreatic
insulin secretion. Decreases hepatic
glucose output and increases insulin-
dependent glucose utilization in
skeletal muscle. *Therapeutic Effect:*
Lowers blood glucose concentration.

PHARMACOKINETICS
Rapidly absorbed. Highly protein
bound (99%), primarily to albumin.
Metabolized in the liver. Excreted in
urine. Unknown whether removed by
hemodialysis. *Half-life:* 16-24 h.

AVAILABILITY
Tablets: 15 mg, 30 mg, 45 mg.

INDICATIONS AND DOSAGES
▸ **Diabetes mellitus, combination
therapy with sulfonylureas**
PO
Adults, Elderly. With insulin:
Initially, 15-30 mg once a day.
Initially continue current insulin
dosage; then decrease insulin dosage
by 10%-25% if hypoglycemia occurs
or plasma glucose level decreases to
< 100 mg/dL. Maximum: 45 mg/day.
As monotherapy: Monotherapy
is not to be used if patient is well
controlled with diet and exercise
alone. Initially, 15-30 mg/day.
May increase dosage in increments

until 45 mg/day is reached.
With sulfonylureas: Initially,
15-30 mg/day. Decrease sulfonylurea
dosage if hypoglycemia occurs. With
metformin: Initially, 15-30 mg/day.

CONTRAINDICATIONS
Active hepatic disease; diabetic
ketoacidosis; increased serum
transaminase levels, including ALT
(SGPT) > 2.5 times normal serum
level; type 1 diabetes mellitus; known
NYHA class III or IV heart failure.

INTERACTIONS
Drug
Gemfibrozil: May increase the effect
and toxicity of pioglitazone.
Ketoconazole: May significantly
inhibit metabolism of pioglitazone.
Oral contraceptives: May alter the
effects of oral contraceptives.
Rifampin: May decrease the
effectiveness of pioglitazone.
Food
None known.
Herbal
None known.

DIAGNOSTIC TEST EFFECTS
May increase creatine kinase (CK)
level. May decrease hemoglobin
levels by 2%-4% and serum
alkaline phosphatase, bilirubin, and
transaminase ALT (SGOT) levels to
2.5 times normal serum levels.
Fewer than 1% of patients experience
ALT values 3 times the normal level.

SIDE EFFECTS
Frequent (9%-13%)
Headache, upper respiratory tract
infection.
Occasional (5%-6%)
Sinusitis, myalgia, pharyngitis,
aggravated diabetes mellitus.

SERIOUS REACTIONS
• None known.

PRECAUTIONS & CONSIDERATIONS

Black Box Warning regarding congestive heart failure (CHF): May cause or exacerbate heart failure in some patients. Patients should be monitored for signs and symptoms of heart failure, including excessive, rapid weight gain, dypsnea, or edema. Pioglitazone should not be used in patients with symptomatic heart failure or New York Heart Association (NYHA) Class III or IV heart failure.

Caution is warranted with edema, and hepatic impairment. It is unknown whether pioglitazone crosses the placenta or is distributed in breast milk. Pioglitazone use is not recommended in pregnant or breastfeeding women. Safety and efficacy of pioglitazone have not been established in children. No age-related precautions have been noted in elderly patients. Avoid alcohol.

Food intake, blood glucose, and hemoglobin levels should be monitored before and during therapy. Hepatic enzyme levels should also be obtained before beginning pioglitazone therapy and periodically thereafter. Notify the physician of abdominal or chest pain, dark urine or light stool, hypoglycemic reactions, fever, nausea, palpitations, rash, vomiting, or yellowing of the eyes or skin. Be aware of signs and symptoms of hypoglycemia (anxiety, cool wet skin, diplopia, dizziness, headache, hunger, numbness in mouth, tachycardia, tremors), or hyperglycemia (deep rapid breathing, dim vision, fatigue, nausea, polydipsia, polyphagia, polyuria, vomiting); carry candy, sugar packets, or other sugar supplements for immediate response to hypoglycemia. Consult the physician when glucose demands are altered (such as with fever, heavy physical activity, infection, stress, trauma). Exercise, good personal hygiene (including foot care), not smoking, and weight control are essential parts of therapy.

Administration
Take pioglitazone without regard to meals.

Piperacillin; Piperacillin/ Tazobactam
(Tazocin [CAN], Zosyn)
Do not confuse Zosyn with Zofran or Zyvox.

CATEGORY AND SCHEDULE
Pregnancy Risk Category: B

MECHANISM OF ACTION
Piperacillin inhibits cell wall synthesis by binding to bacterial cell membranes. Tazobactam inactivates bacterial β-lactamase. *Therapeutic Effect:* Piperacillin is bactericidal in susceptible organisms. Tazobactam protects piperacillin from enzymatic degradation, extends its spectrum of activity, and prevents bacterial overgrowth.

PHARMACOKINETICS
Protein binding: 16%-30%. Widely distributed. Primarily excreted unchanged in urine. Removed by hemodialysis. *Half-life:* 0.7-1.2 h (increased in hepatic cirrhosis and impaired renal function).

AVAILABILITY
! Piperacillin/tozobactam is a combination product in a ratio of piperacillin to tazobactam.

Powder for Injection: 2.25 g, 3.375 g, 4.5 g.
Premix Ready To Use: 2.25 g, 3.375 g, 4.5 g.

INDICATIONS AND DOSAGES
▸ **Severe infections**
IV
Adults, Elderly, Children 12 yr and older. 4 g/0.5 g q6-8h or 3 g/0.375 g q6h.
▸ **Moderate infections**
IV
Adults, Elderly, Children 40 kg. 2 g/0.225g q6-8h or 3.375 q6h.
▸ **Dosage in renal impairment**
Dosage and frequency are modified based on creatinine clearance.

Creatinine Clearance (mL/min)	Dosage
20-40	3.375 q6h for nosocomial pneumonia, 2.25 IV q6h for all other indications.
< 20	2.25 g q8h for all indications except nosocomial pneumonia (2.25 g q6h)

▸ **Dosage in hemodialysis patients**
IV
Adults, Elderly. 2.25 g q8h with additional dose of 0.75 g after each dialysis session.

CONTRAINDICATIONS
Hypersensitivity to any penicillin.

INTERACTIONS
Drug
Hepatotoxic medications: May increase the risk of hepatotoxicity.
Probenecid: May increase piperacillin blood concentration and risk of toxicity.
Herbal
None known.
Food
None known.

DIAGNOSTIC TEST EFFECTS
May increase serum sodium, alkaline phosphatase, bilirubin, LDH, AST (SGOT), and ALT (SGPT) levels. May decrease serum potassium level. May cause a positive Coombs' test.

💊 IV INCOMPATIBILITIES
Amiodarone amphotericin B (Fungizone), amiodarone, amphotericin B complex (Abelcet, AmBisome, Amphotec), chlorpromazine (Thorazine), ciprofloxacin, dacarbazine (DTIC), daunorubicin (Cerubidine), dobutamine (Dobutrex), doxorubicin (Adriamycin), doxorubicin liposomal (Doxil), droperidol (Inapsine), drotrecogin alfa, famotidine (Pepcid), haloperidol (Haldol), hydroxyzine (Vistaril), idarubicin (Idamycin), minocycline (Minocin), nalbuphine (Nubain), prochlorperazine (Compazine), promethazine (Phenergan), vancomycin (Vancocin).

💊 IV COMPATIBILITIES
Aminophylline, bumetanide (Bumex), calcium gluconate, diphenhydramine (Benadryl), dopamine (Intropin), enalapril (Vasotec), furosemide (Lasix), granisetron (Kytril), heparin, hydrocortisone (Solu-Cortef), hydromorphone (Dilaudid), lorazepam (Ativan), magnesium sulfate, methylprednisolone (Solu-Medrol), metoclopramide (Reglan), morphine, ondansetron (Zofran), potassium chloride.

SIDE EFFECTS
Frequent
Diarrhea, headache, constipation, nausea, insomnia, rash.
Occasional
Vomiting, dyspepsia, pruritus, fever, agitation, candidiasis, dizziness, abdominal pain, edema, anxiety, dyspnea, rhinitis.

SERIOUS REACTIONS

• Antibiotic-associated colitis and other superinfections may result from altered bacterial balance.

• Seizures and other neurologic reactions are more likely to occur in patients with renal impairment and in those who have received an overdose.

• Severe hypersensitivity reactions, including anaphylaxis, occur rarely.

PRECAUTIONS & CONSIDERATIONS

Caution is warranted in patients with a history of allergies, especially to penicillin and cephalosporins, a preexisting seizure disorder, or renal impairment. Piperacillin readily crosses the placenta, appears in cord blood and amniotic fluid, and is distributed in breast milk in low concentrations. Piperacillin may lead to allergic sensitization, candidiasis, diarrhea, and skin rash in infants. The safety and efficacy of piperacillin have not been established in children younger than 12 yr. Age-related renal impairment may require dosage adjustment in elderly patients.

History of allergies, especially to cephalosporins or penicillins, should be determined before giving the drug. Withhold and promptly notify the physician if rash or diarrhea occurs. Severe diarrhea with abdominal pain, blood or mucus in stool, and fever may indicate antibiotic-associated colitis. Signs and symptoms of superinfection, including anal or genital pruritus, black hairy tongue, diarrhea, increased fever, sore throat, ulceration or changes of oral mucosa, and vomiting should be monitored. Electrolytes (especially potassium), intake and output, renal function tests, urinalysis, and the injection sites should be assessed.

Storage
The reconstituted vial is stable for 24 h at room temperature and 48 h if refrigerated.

Administration
For each gram of zosyn, reconstitute with 5 mL D5W or 0.9% NaCl. Shake vigorously to dissolve. Further dilute with at least 50-100 mL D5W, 0.9% NaCl, dextrose 5% in 0.9% NaCl, or lactated Ringer's solution. After further dilution, the solution is stable for 24 h at room temperature and 7 days if refrigerated. Infuse the drug over 30 min.

Pirbuterol
peer-beut-er-all
(Maxair, Maxair Autohaler)

CATEGORY AND SCHEDULE
Pregnancy Risk Category: C

Classification: Adrenergic agonists, bronchodilators

P

MECHANISM OF ACTION
A sympathomimetic, adrenergic agonist, that stimulates β_2-adrenergic receptors in the lungs, resulting in relaxation of bronchial smooth muscle. *Therapeutic Effect:* Relieves bronchospasm, reduces airway resistance.

PHARMACOKINETICS
Absorbed from bronchi following inhalation. Metabolized in liver. Primarily excreted in urine. Unknown if removed by hemodialysis. *Half-life:* 2-3 h.

AVAILABILITY
Oral Inhalation: 0.2 mg/actuation (Autohaler).

INDICATIONS AND DOSAGES
▸ **Prevention of bronchospasm**
INHALATION
Adults, Elderly, Children 12 yr and older. 2 inhalations q4-6h. Maximum: 12 inhalations daily.
▸ **Treatment of bronchospasm**
INHALATION
Adults, Elderly, Children 12 yr and older. 2 inhalations q4-6h. Maximum: 12 inhalations daily.

CONTRAINDICATIONS
History of hypersensitivity to pirbuterol, albuterol, or any of its components, children.

INTERACTIONS
Drug
Aspirin or sulfite preservatives: Can exacerbate asthma.
β-Adrenergic blocking agents: Antagonizes effects of pirbuterol.
MAOIs, tricyclic antidepressants: May potentiate cardiovascular effects.
Herbal
None known.
Food
None known.

DIAGNOSTIC TEST EFFECTS
May decrease serum potassium levels.

SIDE EFFECTS
Occasional (1%-7%)
Nervousness, tremor, headache, palpitations, nausea, dizziness, tachycardia, cough.

SERIOUS REACTIONS
• Excessive sympathomimetic stimulation may produce palpitations, extrasystoles, tachycardia, chest pain, slight increases in BP followed by a substantial decrease, chills, sweating, and blanching of skin.
• Too frequent or excessive use may lead to loss of bronchodilating effectiveness and severe, paradoxical bronchoconstriction.

PRECAUTIONS & CONSIDERATIONS
Caution is necessary in patients with a history of hypersensitivity to pirbuterol, albuterol, or any of its components; cardiovascular disease; diabetes mellitus; hypertension; or hyperthyroidism. Pirbuterol appears to cross the placenta, but it is unknown whether it is distributed in breast milk. Safety and efficacy have not been established in children younger than 12 yr. Elderly patients may be more likely to develop tremors or tachycardia because of the age-related increased sympathetic sensitivity. Increase fluid intake to decrease the viscosity of pulmonary secretions. Excessive use of caffeine derivatives, such as chocolate, cocoa, coffee, cola, and tea, should be avoided.
Administration
Shake container for inhalation well and exhale completely through the mouth. Place the mouthpiece into the mouth and close the lips while holding the inhaler upright. Inhale deeply through the mouth while fully depressing the top of the canister and hold breath as long as possible before exhaling slowly. Wait 2 min before inhaling second dose to allow for deeper bronchial penetration. Rinse mouth with water immediately after inhalation to prevent mouth and throat dryness.

Piroxicam
peer-ox′i-kam
(Apo-Piroxicam [CAN], Candyl-D [AUS], Feldene, Fexicam [CAN], Mobilis [AUS], Novopirocam [CAN], Pirohexal-D [AUS], Rosig [AUS], Rosig-D [AUS])
Do not confuse Feldene with Seldane.

CATEGORY AND SCHEDULE
Pregnancy Risk Category: C (D if used in third trimester or near delivery)

Classification: Analgesics, non-narcotic, nonsteroidal anti-inflammatory

MECHANISM OF ACTION
An NSAID that produces analgesic, antipyretic and anti-inflammatory effects by inhibiting the cyclo-oxygenase pathway in prostaglandin synthesis. *Therapeutic Effect:* Reduces inflammatory response and intensity of pain.

PHARMACOKINETICS
PO: Peak 2 h. *Half-life:* 3-3.5 h; 99% protein binding; metabolized in the liver; metabolites excreted in urine and breast milk.

AVAILABILITY
Capsules: 10 mg, 20 mg.

INDICATIONS AND DOSAGES
▶ **Acute or chronic rheumatoid arthritis and osteoarthritis**
PO
Adults, Elderly. Initially, 10-20 mg/day as a single dose or in divided doses. Some patients may require up to 30-40 mg/day.

OFF-LABEL USES
Treatment of acute gouty arthritis, ankylosing spondylitis, dysmenorrheal.

CONTRAINDICATIONS
Active peptic ulcer disease, chronic inflammation of the GI tract, GI bleeding or ulceration, history of hypersensitivity to aspirin or NSAIDs, myocardial infarction, coronartery artery bypass graft surgery.

INTERACTIONS
Drug
Acetaminophen: Possible nephrotoxicity with prolonged use and high doses.
Antihypertensives, diuretics, α-adrenergic blockers, ACE inhibitors: May decrease the antihypertensive effects of these drugs.
Aspirin, other salicylates, alcohol, corticosteroids: May increase the risk of GI side effects such as bleeding and decrease anti-inflammatory effects.
Bone marrow depressants: May increase the risk of hematologic reactions.
Cyclosporine: Possible risk of decreased renal function if used concurrently.
Heparin, oral anticoagulants, oral antihyperglycemic agents, thrombolytics: May increase the effects of these drugs.
Lithium: May increase the blood concentration and risk of toxicity of lithium.
Methotrexate: May increase the risk of methotrexate toxicity.
Probenecid: May increase the piroxicam blood concentration.
Herbal
Feverfew: May decrease the effects of feverfew.

P

Ginkgo biloba: May increase the risk of bleeding.
St. John's wort: May increase the risk of phototoxicity.
Food
None known.

DIAGNOSTIC TEST EFFECTS
May increase AST (SGOT) and ALT (SGPT) levels. May decrease serum uric acid levels.

SIDE EFFECTS
Frequent (4%-9%)
Dyspepsia, nausea, dizziness.
Occasional (1%-3%)
Diarrhea, constipation, abdominal cramps or pain, flatulence, stomatitis.
Rare (< 1%)
Hypertension, urticaria, dysuria, ecchymosis, blurred vision, insomnia, phototoxicity.

SERIOUS REACTIONS
• Rare reactions with long-term use include peptic ulcer disease, GI bleeding, gastritis, severe hepatic reaction (cholestasis, jaundice), nephrotoxicity (dysuria, hematuria, proteinuria, nephrotic syndrome), hematologic sensitivity (anemia, leukopenia, eosinophilia, thrombocytopenia), and a severe hypersensitivity reaction (fever, chills, bronchospasm).
Caution
Breast-feeding, children, bleeding disorders, GI disorders, cardiac disorders, hypersensitivity to other antiinflammatories, hypertension.

PRECAUTIONS & CONSIDERATIONS
First-time users of SSRIs also taking NSAIDs may have an increased risk of GI side effects; until more data are available, it may be advisable to avoid using NSAIDs in these patients (*Br J Clin Pharmacol* 2003; 55:591-595). Caution is warranted with GI disease, hypertension, impaired cardiac or hepatic function, and concurrent anticoagulant use. Notify the physician of pregnancy. Avoid alcohol and aspirin during therapy because these substances increase the risk of GI bleeding. Tasks that require mental alertness or motor skills should also be avoided.

CBC, hepatic and renal function test results, and pattern of daily bowel activity and stool consistency should be assessed before and during therapy. Therapeutic response, such as decreased pain, stiffness, swelling, and tenderness, improved grip strength, and increased joint mobility, should be evaluated.
Administration
Do not crush or break capsules. Take piroxicam with food, milk, or antacids if GI distress occurs.

Podofilox
po-doe-fil′ox
(Condyline [CAN], Condyline Paint [AUS], Condylox)

CATEGORY AND SCHEDULE
Pregnancy Risk Category: C

Classification: Antimitotic agent, dermatologic

MECHANISM OF ACTION
An active component of podophyllin resin that binds to tubulin to prevent formation of microtubules, resulting in mitotic arrest. Many biological effects, such as it damages endothelium of small blood vessels, attenuates nucleoside transport,

suppresses immune responses, inhibits macrophage metabolism, induces interleukin-1 and interleukin-2, decreases lymphocytes response to mitogens and enhances macrophage growth. *Therapeutic Effect:* Removes genital warts.

PHARMACOKINETICS

Time to peak occurs in 1-2 h. Some degree of absorption. *Half-life:* 1-4.5 h.

AVAILABILITY

Gel: 0.5% (Condylox).
Solution: 0.5% (Condylox).

INDICATIONS AND DOSAGES
▶ **Anogenital warts**
TOPICAL
Adults. Apply 0.5% gel twice daily for 3 days, then withhold for 4 days. Repeat cycle up to 4 times.
▶ **Genital warts (condylomata acuminate)**
TOPICAL
Adults. Apply 0.5% solution or gel q12hr in the morning and evening for 3 days, then withhold for 4 days. Repeat cycle up to 4 times.

OFF-LABEL USES

Systemic: Treatment of fungal pneumonia, prostate cancer, septicemia, general warts (nonbleeding) on the outside of skin.

CONTRAINDICATIONS

Bleeding warts, moles, birthmarks, or unusual warts with hair, diabetes, poor blood circulation, pregnancy, ocular exposure, steroid use, hypersensitivity to podofilox or any component of its formulation.

INTERACTIONS
Drug
None known.

Herbal
None known.
Food
None known.

DIAGNOSTIC TEST EFFECTS
None known.

SIDE EFFECTS
Occasional
Erosion, inflammation, itching, pain, burning.
Rare
Nausea, vomiting.

SERIOUS REACTIONS
• Nausea and vomiting occur rarely and usually after cumulative doses.

PRECAUTIONS & CONSIDERATIONS
Caution is necessary with mucous membrane warts, bleeding warts, moles, birthmarks or warts with hair; in patients with poor circulation or diabetes or pregnancy. It is unknown whether podofilox is distributed in breast milk. Safety and efficacy of podofilox have not been established in children or elderly. Nausea, vomiting, blood in urine, or dizziness should be reported immediately.

Tactful conversation related to STD may be appropriate.
Administration
Apply on warts with supplied cotton-tip applicator. Allow to dry completely before putting legs together. Use no more than 10 cm^2/day and no more than 0.5 g/day of topical gel. Use no more than 10 cm^2/day and no more than 0.5 mL/day of topical solution.

P

Podophyllum resin
po-dof-fil-um rez-in
(Podocon-25, Pododerm)

CATEGORY AND SCHEDULE
Pregnancy Risk Category: X

Classification: Dermatologics, cytotoxic, topical

MECHANISM OF ACTION
A cytotoxic agent that directly affects epithelial cell metabolism by arresting mitosis through binding to a protein subunit of spindle microtubules. *Therapeutic Effect:* Removes soft genital warts.

PHARMACOKINETICS
Topical podophyllum is systemically absorbed. Absorption may be increased if applied to bleeding, friable, or recently biopsied warts.

AVAILABILITY
Liquid: 25% (Podocon-25, Pododerm).

INDICATIONS AND DOSAGES
▸ **Genital warts (condylomata acuminate)**
TOPICAL
Adults, Elderly, Children. Apply 10%-25% solution in compound benzoin tincture to dry surface. Use 1 drop at a time allowing drying between drops until area is covered. Total volume should be limited to < 0.5 mL per treatment session.

OFF-LABEL USES
Epitheliomatosis, laryngeal papilloma.

CONTRAINDICATIONS
Diabetes mellitus, concomitant steroid therapy, circulation disorders, bleeding warts, moles, birthmarks or unusual warts with hair growing from them, pregnancy, hypersensitivity to podophyllum resin preparations.

INTERACTIONS
Drug
None known.
Herbal
None known.
Food
None known.

DIAGNOSTIC TEST EFFECTS
May increase BUN, serum alkaline phosphatase, serum creatinine, SGOT (AST), and SGPT (ALT) levels.

SIDE EFFECTS
Occasional (1%-10%)
Pruritus, nausea, vomiting, abdominal pain, diarrhea.

SERIOUS REACTIONS
• Paresthesia, polyneuritis, paralytic ileus, pyrexia, leukopenia, thrombocytopenia, coma, and death have been reported with podophyllum resin use.
Caution
Hypersensitivity to podophyllum resin preparations.

PRECAUTIONS & CONSIDERATIONS
Caution is warranted in patients with diabetes mellitus, concomitant steroid therapy, circulation disorders, bleeding warts, moles, birthmarks or unusual warts with hair, pregnancy. Caution should be used on skin that appears irritated as well as area surrounding the eyes. Contact should be avoided with the eyes because podophyllum resin can cause corneal damage. Podophyllum resin use should be avoided during pregnancy. It is unknown whether podophyllum is distributed in breast milk. No

age-related precautions have been noted in children or elderly patients.

Painful urination, dizziness, lightheadedness, increased heart rate, constipation, or tingling in hands or feet should be reported.

Tasteful discussion about STD may be appropriate.

Administration

Podophyllum resin is to be applied only by a physician. It may not be dispensed to the patient. Apply with gloved hands. Apply only to intact lesion (no bleeding). Large areas or numerous warts should not be treated at once. Use concentration of 5%-10% for very large lesions (>10-20 cm) to minimize the risk of toxicity.

Thoroughly cleanse affected area before use. The first application of podophyllum resin is recommended to be left on contact for only a short time (30-40 min) to determine sensitivity. Use supplied applicator to apply podophyllum resin sparingly to lesion. Avoid contact with healthy tissue. Allow to dry thoroughly. After treatment time has elapsed, remove dried podophyllum resin thoroughly with alcohol or soap and water.

Poly-L-Lactic Acid

CATEGORY AND SCHEDULE

Pregnancy Risk Category: Not established

Classification: Physical adjunct, lipoatrophy agent

MECHANISM OF ACTION

A lipoatrophy agent containing microparticles of a synthetic polymer

that is used as an injectable implant.
Therapeutic Effect: Restores facial fat.

PHARMACOKINETICS

Biodegradable, biocompatible synthetic polymer.

AVAILABILITY

Powder for Injection (Freeze-Dried).

INDICATIONS AND DOSAGES

▸ **Facial lipoatrophy**
SC

Adults, Elderly. For severe facial fat loss, one vial is usually injected into multiple points of each cheek during each injection session. Volume of drug for each injection and number of injection sessions depend on severity of condition. Typically, 3-6 injection sessions, separated by intervals of at least 2 wks, are required.

CONTRAINDICATIONS

None known.

INTERACTIONS

Drug
None known.
Herbal
None known.
Food
None known.

DIAGNOSTIC TEST EFFECTS

None known.

SIDE EFFECTS

Frequent
Ecchymosis.
Occasional
Discomfort, edema.
Rare
Erythema.

SERIOUS REACTIONS

• Subcutaneous papules at injection sites and hematoma occur occasionally.

PRECAUTIONS & CONSIDERATIONS

Be aware of the tendency of keloid formation. It is unknown whether poly-L-lactic acid is excreted in breast milk. Safety and efficacy of poly-L-lactic acid have not been established in children younger than 18 yr. Age-related liver impairment may require decreased dosage in elderly patients.

Redness, swelling or bruising that typically resolves in hours to 1 wk. Avoid excessive sunlight or UV lamp exposure until initial swelling and redness has resolved.

Storage
Reconstituted product is stable for up to 72 h at room temperature.

Administration and Handling
For IV infusion, reconstitute by drawing 3-5 mL sterile water for injection. Using an 18-gauge sterile needle, slowly add all sterile water for injection into the vial. Let vial stand for at least 2 h. Do not shake during this period. After 2 h, agitate vial until a uniform translucent suspension is obtained. Withdraw amount of the suspension (usually 1 mL) into a syringe using a new 18-gauge needle and replace with a 26-gauge needle before injecting the product into the deep dermis or subcutaneous layer.

Polycarbophil
polly-car'bow-fill
(Fibercon, Replens [CAN])

CATEGORY AND SCHEDULE
Pregnancy Risk Category: C

Classification: OTC

MECHANISM OF ACTION

A bulk-forming laxative and antidiarrheal. As a laxative, retains water in the intestine and opposes dehydrating forces of the bowel. *Therapeutic Effect:* Promotes well-formed stools. As an antidiarrheal, absorbs fecal-free water, restores normal moisture level, and provides bulk. *Therapeutic Effect:* Forms gel and produces formed stool.

PHARMACOKINETICS

Route	Onset	Peak	Duration
PO	12-72 h	NA	NA

Acts in small and large intestines.

AVAILABILITY

Tablets: 500 mg, 625 mg.
Tablets (Chewable): 500 mg.

INDICATIONS AND DOSAGES
▸ **Constipation, diarrhea**
PO
Adults, Elderly, Children 12 yr and older. 1 g 1-4 times a day, or as needed. Maximum: 4 g/24 h.
Children aged 6-11 yr. 500 mg 1-4 times a day or as needed. Maximum: 2 g/24 h.
Children younger than 6 yr. Consult product labeling.

CONTRAINDICATIONS

Abdominal pain, dysphagia, nausea, partial bowel obstruction, symptoms of appendicitis, vomiting, hypercalcemia, hypercalciuria, esophageal stricture.

INTERACTIONS
Drug
Digoxin, oral anticoagulants, salicylates, tetracyclines: May

decrease the effects of digoxin, salicylates, and tetracyclines.
Potassium-sparing diuretics, potassium supplements: May interfere with the effects of potassium-sparing diuretics and potassium supplements.
Herbal
None known.
Food
None known.

DIAGNOSTIC TEST EFFECTS
May increase blood glucose level. May decrease serum potassium levels.

SIDE EFFECTS
Rare
Some degree of abdominal discomfort, nausea, mild cramps, griping, syncope or near syncope.

SERIOUS REACTIONS
• Esophageal or bowel obstruction may occur if administered with < 250 mL or 1 full glass of liquid.

PRECAUTIONS & CONSIDERATIONS
This drug may be used safely in pregnancy. Polycarbophil use is not recommended in children younger than 6 yr of age. No age-related precautions have been noted in elderly patients.
Pattern of daily bowel activity and stool consistency and serum electrolyte levels should be monitored. Adequate fluid intake should be maintained.
Administration
! For severe diarrhea, give every half hour up to maximum daily dosage; for constipation, give with 8 oz liquid, as prescribed.
Drink 6-8 glasses of water a day to aid in stool softening. To promote defecation, increase fluid intake, exercise, and eat a high-fiber diet.

Polyethylene Glycol-Electrolyte Solution
pol-ee-eth′-ill-een
(CoLyte, GoLYTELY, Klean-Prep [CAN], MiraLax[OTC], NuLytely, Peglyte [CAN], Pro-Lax [CAN], TriLyte)

CATEGORY AND SCHEDULE
Pregnancy Risk Category: C

Classification: Bowel evacuants, laxatives

MECHANISM OF ACTION
A laxative that has an osmotic effect. *Therapeutic Effect:* Induces diarrhea and cleanses bowel without depleting electrolytes.

PHARMACOKINETICS

Route	Onset	Peak	Duration
PO	1-2 h	NA	NA (bowel cleansing)
PO	2-4 days	NA	NA (constipation)

AVAILABILITY
Powder for Oral Solution.
Oral Solution.

INDICATIONS AND DOSAGES
▸ **Bowel cleansing**
PO
Adults, Elderly. Before GI examination: 240 mL (8 oz) q10min until 4 L consumed or rectal effluent clear. Nasogastric tube: 20-30 mL/min until 4 L given.
Children. 25 mL/kg/h until rectal effluent clear.
▸ **Constipation**
PO (MIRALAX)
Adults. 17 g or 1 heaping tbsp a day dissolved into water or juice.

P

CONTRAINDICATIONS

Bowel perforation, gastric retention, GI obstruction, megacolon, toxic colitis, toxic ileus.

INTERACTIONS

Drug
Oral medications: May decrease the absorption of oral medications if given within 1 h because they may be flushed from GI tract.
Herbal
None known.
Food
None known.

DIAGNOSTIC TEST EFFECTS

None known.

SIDE EFFECTS

Frequent (50%)
Some degree of abdominal fullness, nausea, bloating.
Occasional (1%-10%)
Abdominal cramping, vomiting, anal irritation.
Rare (< 1%)
Urticaria, rhinorrhea, dermatitis.

SERIOUS REACTIONS

• None known.

PRECAUTIONS & CONSIDERATIONS

Caution is warranted in patients with ulcerative colitis. It is unknown whether polyethylene crosses the placenta or is distributed in breast milk. No age-related precautions have been noted in children or elderly patients.

Notify the physician if severe abdominal pain or bloating occurs. Blood glucose, BUN, serum electrolyte levels, urine osmolality, and pattern of daily bowel activity and stool consistency should be monitored.
Storage
Refrigerate reconstituted solutions; use within 48 h.

Administration
May use tap water to prepare solution. Shake vigorously for several minutes to ensure complete dissolution of powder. Take nothing by mouth 3 h or more before ingestion of solution. Give only clear liquids after administration. May give via nasogastric tube. Rapid drinking preferred. Chilled solution is more palatable.

Polymyxin B
polly-mix-in
(Aerosporin)

CATEGORY AND SCHEDULE
Pregnancy Risk Category: B

Classification: Antibiotics, polymyxins

MECHANISM OF ACTION

An antibiotic that al*ters cell membrane permeability in susceptible microorganisms.* *Therapeutic Effect:* Bactericidal activity.

PHARMACOKINETICS

Negligible absorption. Protein binding: low. Excreted in urine. Poor removal in hemodialysis. *Half-life:* 6 h.

AVAILABILITY

Powder: 500,000 units (Aerosporin).

INDICATIONS AND DOSAGES

▸ **Mild to moderate infections**
IV
Adults, Elderly, Children 2 yr and older. 15,000-25,000 units/kg/day in divided doses q12hr.
Infants. 15,000-40,000 units/kg/day in divided doses q12h.

IM
Adults, Elderly, Children 2 yr and older. 25,000-30,000 units/kg/day in divided doses q4-6h.
Infants. 25,000-40,000 units/kg/day in divided doses q4-6h.
▸ **Usual irrigation dosage**
CONTINUOUS BLADDER IRRIGATION
Adults, Children > 2 yr of age. 200,000-400,000 units/day as a continuous bladder irrigation.
▸ **Usual ophthalmic dosage**
OPHTHALMIC
Adults, Elderly, Children. 1-3 drops containing 10,000-20,000 units/mL/hr until a favorable response occurs. Maximum: 25,000 units/kg/day or 2 million units/day.

⊘ IV INCOMPATIBILITIES

Cefoxitin, diazepam, cefoperazone, furosemide, heparin, hydrocortisone, regular insulin, oxacillin, pantoprazole, penicillin-class antibiotics.

CONTRAINDICATIONS

Hypersensitivity to polymyxin B or any component of the formulation, neuromuscular disease.

INTERACTIONS

Drug
Aminoglycosides, other nephrotoxic drugs: May increase nephrotoxicity.
Muscle relaxants: May cause nephrotoxic reaction, especially in patients with renal impairment.
Neuromuscular blocking agents or anesthetics: May produce muscle paralysis and prolonged or increased skeletal muscle relaxation.
Herbal
None known.
Food
None known.

SIDE EFFECTS

Frequent
Severe pain, irritation at IM injection sites, phlebitis, thrombophlebitis with IV administration.
Occasional
Fever, urticaria.

SERIOUS REACTIONS

• Nephrotoxicity, especially with concurrent/sequential use of other nephrotoxic drugs, renal impairment, concurrent/sequential use of muscle relaxants.
• Superinfection, especially with fungi, may occur.
Caution
Hypokalemia, renal disease, hepatic disease, gout, chronic obstructive pulmonary disease (COPD), lupus erythematosus, diabetes mellitus.

PRECAUTIONS & CONSIDERATIONS

Caution should be used with impaired renal function. Safety and efficacy of polymyxin B have not been established in pregnant women or children younger than 2 yr. No age-related precautions have been noted in elderly patients.
Renal function should be carefully monitored. Serum concentrations >5 mcg/mL are toxic in adults. Neurotoxic reactions may be manifested by drowsiness, irritability, blurred vision, weakness, ataxia, and numbness of the extremities.
Storage
Store at room temperature before reconstitution and protect from light. After reconstitution, store under refrigeration. Discard any unused solution after 72 h.
Administration
For IV use, dissolve 500,000 units in 300-500 mL D5W for continuous IV infusion. Administer every 12 h.

P

For IM injection, dissolve 500,000 units in 2 mL water for injection, 0.9% NaCl, or 1% procaine solution. IM injection is not routinely recommended because of severe pain at the injection sites.

For intrathecal administration, dissolve 500,000 units in 10 mL physiologic solution. Administer once daily for 3-4 days, then every other day for at least 2 wks after cerebrospinal fluid (CSF) cultures are negative.

For ophthalmic use, 500,000 units in 20-50 mL sterile water for injection or 0.9% NaCl. Instill drops and close the eye gently for 1-2 min and roll eyeball to increase contact area of drug to eye. Remove excess solution around the eye with a tissue.

Polymyxin B sulfate; trimethoprim sulfate

pol-ee-mix´-in bee sul´-fate; trye-meth´-oh-prim sul´-fate
(Polytrim)

CATEGORY AND SCHEDULE
Pregnancy Risk Category: C

Classification: Anti-infective (ophthalmic)

MECHANISM OF ACTION
Polymyxin B damages bacterial cytoplasmic membrane, which causes leakage of intracellular components. Trimethoprim is a folate antagonist that blocks bacterial biosynthesis of nucleic acids and proteins by interfering with metabolism of folinic acid. *Therapeutic Effect:* Prevents inflammatory process. Interferes with bacterial protein synthesis. Produces antibacterial activity.

PHARMACOKINETICS
Absorption through intact skin and mucous membranes is insignificant.

AVAILABILITY
Ophthalmic Drops, Solution: 10,000 units/mL.

INDICATIONS AND DOSAGES
▸ **Treatment of surface ocular bacterial conjunctivitis and blepharoconjunctivitis**
OPHTHALMIC
Adults, Elderly, Children. Instill 1 drop in affected eye(s) every 3 h for 7–10 days. Maximum: 6 doses/day.

CONTRAINDICATIONS
Polymixin or trimethoprim hypersensitivity.

INTERACTIONS
Drug
None reported.
Herbal
None known.
Food
None known.

SIDE EFFECTS
Occasional
Local irritation, redness, burning, stinging, itching.

SERIOUS REACTIONS
• Prolonged use may result in overgrowth of nonsusceptible organisms, including superinfection.
• Hypersensitivity reactions consisting of lid edema, itching, increased redness, tearing, and/or circumocular rash have been reported.
• Photosensitivity has been reported in patients taking oral trimethoprim.

PRECAUTIONS & CONSIDERATIONS
Hypersensitivity to polymyxin B, trimethoprim sulfate, or any component of the formulation.

Administration
Wash hands before and after use.
Tilt head back and pull lower eyelid
down to form a pouch. Squeeze the
prescribed number of drops into pouch
and gently close eyes for 1-2 min.

Poractant Alfa
poor-ak'tant
(Curosurf)

CATEGORY AND SCHEDULE
Pregnancy Risk Category: This
drug is not indicated for use in
pregnant women.

Classification: Surfactants, lung

MECHANISM OF ACTION
A pulmonary surfactant that reduces
alveolar surface tension during
ventilation and stabilizes the alveoli
against collapse that may occur at
resting transpulmonary pressures.
Therapeutic Effect: Improves lung
compliance and respiratory gas
exchange.

PHARMACOKINETICS
Biophysical effects occur directly
on the alveolar surface where the
drug is administered. No human
pharmacokinetic studies on
absorption, biotransformation or
excretion are available.

AVAILABILITY
Intratracheal Suspension: 1.5 mL
(120 mg), 3 mL (240 mg).

INDICATIONS AND DOSAGES
▶ **Respiratory distress syndrome
(RDS)**
INTRATRACHEAL
Infants. Initially, 2.5 mL/kg of birth
weight. May give up to 2 subsequent

doses of 1.25 mL/kg of birth weight
at 12-h intervals. Maximum: 5 mL/kg
(total dose).

OFF-LABEL USES
Adult RDS from viral pneumonia or
near-drowning, *Pneumocystis carinii*
pneumonia in HIV-infected patients,
prevention of RDS.

CONTRAINDICATIONS
Porcine protein hypersensitivity.

INTERACTIONS
Drug
None known.
Herbal
None known.
Food
None known.

DIAGNOSTIC TEST EFFECTS
None known.

SIDE EFFECTS
Frequent
Transient bradycardia, oxygen
(O_2) desaturation, increased carbon
dioxide (CO_2) retention.
Occasional
Endotracheal tube reflux.
Rare
Apnea, endotracheal tube blockage,
hypotension or hypertension, pallor,
vasoconstriction.

SERIOUS REACTIONS
• None known.

PRECAUTIONS & CONSIDERATIONS
Caution should be used with persons at
risk for circulatory overload. This drug
is for use only in neonates. No age-
related precautions have been noted.
　The infant's oxygenation and
ventilation should be monitored using
arterial or transcutaneous measurement
of systemic oxygen (O_2) and carbon
dioxide (CO_2). Heart rate and breath

P

sounds should also be assessed. Visitors should be limited during treatment. Handwashing and other infection control measures should be enforced to minimize the risk of nosocomial infections.

It is important to understand that although this drug may control or eliminate problems associated with neonatal RDS, it will not prevent the morbidity and mortality normally associated with premature birth.

Storage

Refrigerate vials. Unopened, unused vials may be returned to the refrigerator only once after having been warmed to room temperature.

Administration

Warm the vial by letting it stand at room temperature for 20 min or warming it in your hand for 8 min. Turn the vial upside down and gently swirl it, if needed, to obtain a uniform suspension. Do not shake the vial.

Withdraw the entire contents of the vial into a 3- or 5-mL plastic syringe through a large-gauge needle (20 gauge or larger). Attach the syringe to a catheter that is inserted into the infant's endotracheal tube, and instill the solution through the catheter. Monitor the infant for bradycardia and decreased SaO$_2$ during administration. Stop the procedure if the infant experiences these effects, and take appropriate measures before reinstituting therapy.

Posaconazole
poe-sah-kone´-ah-zole
(Noxafil)

CATEGORY AND SCHEDULE
Pregnancy Risk Category: C

Classification: Antifungal

MECHANISM OF ACTION
A tirazole antifungal that blocks the synthesis of ergosterol, a key component of fungal cell membrane, through the inhibition of the enzyme lanosterol 14α-demethylase and accumulation of methylated sterol precursors. *Therapeutic Effect:* Inhibits fungal cell membrane formation.

PHARMACOKINETICS
Food increases absorption. Protein binding: > 98%. Not significantly metabolized; undergoes glucuronidation into metabolites. Primarily eliminated in feces (71%, 66% unchanged); partial excretion in urine (13%, < 0.2% unchanged). *Half-life:* 35 h.

AVAILABILITY
Oral Suspension: 40 mg/mL.

INDICATIONS AND DOSAGES
▸ **Prophylaxis of invasive *Aspergillus* and *Candida* fungal infections in patients who are severely immunocompromised**
PO
Adults, Children 13 yr and older. 200 mg (5 mL) three times/day.
▸ **Oropharyngeal candidiasis**
PO
Adults. 100 mg (2.5 mL) twice a day on the first day, then 100 mg (2.5 mL) once a day for 13 days.
▸ **Oropharyngeal candidiasis, refractory to itraconazole and/or fluconazole**
PO
Adults, Children 13 yr and older. 400 mg (10 mL) twice a day.

CONTRAINDICATIONS
Hypersensitivity to azole antifungals, posaconazole or its components; avoid co-administration with ergot alkaloids, sirolimus, or

QTc-prolonging CYP3A4 substrates (pimozide, quinidine).

DRUG INTERACTIONS

Calcium channel blockers: May increase the levels and effects of calcium channel blockers.

Cimetidine: May decrease the levels and effects of posaconazole; avoid concurrent use.

Cyclosporine: May increase the levels and effects of cyclosporine.

CYP3A4 substrates: May increase the levels and effects of CYP3A4 substrates.

Ergot alkaloids: May increase the levels and effects of ergot alkaloids.

HMG-CoA reductase inhibitors: May increase the levels and effects of HMG-CoA reductase inhibitors.

Midazolam: May increase the levels and effects of midazolam.

Phenytoin: May increase the levels and effects of phenytoin; avoid concurrent use.

QT-prolonging agents: Increased risk of arrhythmia (torsade de pointes).

Rifabutin: May increase the levels and effects of rifabutin; avoid concurrent use.

Sirolimus: May increase the levels and effects of sirolimus.

Tacrolimus: May increase the levels and effects of tacrolimus.

Vinca alkaloids: May increase the levels and effects of vinca alkaloids.

Herbal:
None known.

Food
Grapefruit juice: May decrease posaconzole levels; avoid.

SIDE EFFECTS/ADVERSE REACTIONS:

Frequent
Diarrhea.
Occasional
Nausea, neutropenia, headache, vomiting, abdominal pain, flatulence, QTc prolongation, rash, hypokalemia, anemia, fever, bilirubin increased, ALT increased, AST increased, GGT increased, dizziness, weakness, anorexia, fatigue, insomnia, mucositis, thrombocytopenia, alkaline phosphatase increased, serum creatinine increased, myalgia, pruritus, dyspepsia, xerostoma.
Rare
Hypertension, blurred vision, tremor, hepatocellular damage, taste perversion, constipation, somnolence.

Serious Reactions
• Hepatic dysfunction may occur.
• Arrhythmia (torsade de pointes) has been reported.

PRECAUTIONS & CONSIDERATIONS
Caution in patients with severe renal impairment, hepatic impairment, arrhythmia risk, electrolyte abnormalities, severe diarrhea or vomiting. Safety and efficacy not established in children less than 13 yr of age. No unique precaution in the elderly. Teratogenic in animal studies; use in pregnancy only if benefit to mother justifies risk to fetus. Do not breastfeed.
Storage
Store at room temperature.
Administration.
Shake well before use. Dose with a full meal or liquid nutritional supplement. Use dosing spoon provided with product. Rinse spoon with water after each use.

P

Potassium Iodide
Poe-tass-ee-um i-o-died
(Pima, SSKI, Thyro-Block [CAN])

CATEGORY AND SCHEDULE
Pregnancy Risk Category: D
OTC (tablets)

Classification: Antithyroid
agents, hormones/hormone
modifiers

MECHANISM OF ACTION
An agent that reduces viscosity of
mucus by increasing respiratory
tract secretions. Inhibits secretion
of thyroid hormone, fosters colloid
accumulation in thyroid follicles.
Therapeutic Effect: Blocks thyroid
radioiodine uptake.

PHARMACOKINETICS
Oral onset 24-48 h, peak 10-15 days,
duration 6 wks. Primarily excreted in
the urine.

AVAILABILITY
Solution: 1 mg/mL (SSKI),
100 mg/mL (Lugol's solution).
Syrup: 325/5 mL (Pima).
Tablets: 130 mg (Iosat).

INDICATIONS AND DOSAGES
▸ **Expectorant**
PO
*Adults, Elderly, Children 3 yr and
older.* 325-650 mg q8h (Pima);
300-600 mg 3-4 times/day (SSKI).
Children younger than 3 yr.
162 mg q8h.
▸ **Preoperative thyroidectomy**
PO
Adults, Elderly, Children. 0.1-0.3 mL
(3-5 drops of Lugol's solution) q8h
or 50-250 mg (1-5 drops of SSKI)
q8h. Administer 10 days before
surgery.

▸ **Radiation protectant to radioactive
isotopes of iodine**
PO
Adults, Elderly. 195 mg/day (Pima) for
10 days. Start 24 h before exposure.
Children more than 1 yr. 130 mg/day
for 10 days. Start 24 h before exposure.
Children < 1 yr. 65 mg/day for
10 days. Start 24 h before exposure.
▸ **Reduce risk of thyroid cancer
following nuclear accident**
PO
*Adults, Elderly, Children weighing
>68 kg.* 130 mg/day
Children aged 3-18 yr. 65 mg/day.
Children aged 1 mo to 3 yr.
32 mg/day.
Children 1 mo and younger. 16 mg/day.
▸ **Sporotrichosis**
PO
Adults, Elderly. Initally, 5 drops
(SSKI) q8h and increase to 40-50
drops q8h as tolerated for 3-6 mo.
▸ **Thyrotoxic crisis**
PO
Adults, Elderly. 300-500 mg (6-19
drops SSKI) q8h or 1 mL (Lugol's
solution) q8h.

CONTRAINDICATIONS
Hypersensitivity to potassium,
iodine compounds, or any of its
components, pulmonary edema,
hyperkalemia, impaired renal
function, hyperthyroidism, iodine-
induced goiter, pregnancy.

INTERACTIONS
Drug
ACE inhibitors: May increase
risk of hyperkalemia, cardiac
arrhythmias, or cardiac arrest.
Diuretics, potassium-sparing:
May increase risk of hyperkalemia,
cardiac arrhythmias, or cardiac arrest.
Lithium: May increase the
hypothyroid effects.
**Potassium (and potassium-
containing products):** May increase

risk of hyperkalemia, cardiac arrhythmias, or cardiac arrest.
Herbal
None known.
Food
None known.

DIAGNOSTIC TEST EFFECTS
May alter thyroid function tests.

SIDE EFFECTS
Occasional
Irregular heart beat, confusion, drowsiness, fever, rash, diarrhea, GI bleeding, metallic taste, nausea, stomach pain, vomiting, numbness, tingling, weakness.
Rare
Goiter, salivary gland swelling and tenderness, thyroid adenoma, swelling of the throat and neck, myxedema, lymph node swelling.

SERIOUS REACTIONS
• Hypersensitivity symptoms include angioedema, muscle weakness, paralysis, peaked T-waves, flattened P-waves, prolongation of QRS complex, ventricular arrhythmias.

PRECAUTIONS & CONSIDERATIONS
Caution is warranted with congestive heart failure (CHF), hypertension, and pulmonary edema. Be aware citrate use may increase the risk of urolithiasis.

CBC (particularly blood hematocrit and hemoglobin level), serum acid-base balance, and serum creatinine should be monitored. ECG and urinary pH should be assessed in those with cardiac disease.

Any indications of swelling in the throat or neck or salivary glands should be reported immediately.
Administration
Take after meals with food or milk to minimize GI side effects. Mix SSKI dose in water, juice, milk, or broth.

Potassium Salts: Potassium Acetate/ Potassium Bicarbonate-Citrate/ Potassium Chloride/ Potassium Gluconate

Poe-tah-see-um ass-eh-tay-te
(Potassium bicarbonate-citrate: K-Lyte, Klor-Con EF, Effer K, K-Lyte DS)
(Potassium chloride: Apo-K [CAN], Kaochlor, K-Dur, K-Lor, K-Lor-Con M 15, Kaon-Cl, KSR [AUS], KSR-600 [AUS], Micro-K, Slow-K [AUS], Span-K [AUS])
(Potassium gluconate: Kaon)
Do not confuse K-Dur with Cardura.

CATEGORY AND SCHEDULE
Pregnancy Risk Category: C
(A for potassium chloride)

Classification: Potassium electrolytes, minerals

MECHANISM OF ACTION
An electrolyte that is necessary for multiple cellular metabolic processes. Primary action is intracellular. *Therapeutic Effect:* Is necessary for nerve impulse conduction and contraction of cardiac, skeletal, and smooth muscle; maintains normal renal function and acid-base balance.

PHARMACOKINETICS
Well absorbed from the GI tract. Enters cells by active transport from extracellular fluid. Primarily excreted in urine.

AVAILABILITY
Potassium Acetate
Injection: 2 mEq/mL.

**Potassium Bicarbonate and
Potassium Citrate**
*Tablet for Solution (Klor-Con EF,
Effer-K, K-Lyte):* 25 mEq.
Tablet for Solution (K-Lyte DS):
50 mEq.
Potassium Chloride
*Capsules (Controlled-Release
[Micro-K]):* 8 mEq, 10 mEq.
Liquid (Kaochlor): 20 mEq/15 mL.
Liquid (Kaon-Cl): 40 mEq/15 mL.
Powder for Oral Solution (K-Lor):
20 mEq.
Injection: 2 mEq/mL.
*Tablets (Extended-Release [Klor-Con,
Micro-K]):* 8 mEq, 10 mEq.
*Tablets (Extended-Release [Kaon-Cl,
K-Tab]):* 10 mEq.
Tablets (Extended-Release [K-Dur]):
10 mEq, 20 mEq.
Potassium Gluconate
Elixir (Kaon): 20 mEq/15 mL.

INDICATIONS AND DOSAGES
▸ **Prevention of hypokalemia (in
patients on diuretic therapy)**
PO
Adults, Elderly. 20-40 mEq/day in
1-2 divided doses.
Children. 1-2 mEq/kg/day in
1-2 divided doses.
▸ **Treatment of hypokalemia**
PO
Adults, Elderly. 40-100 mEq/day
given in 2-4 doses; further doses
based on laboratory values.
Children. 2-5 mEq/day; further doses
based on laboratory values.
IV
Adults, Elderly. Usual dose is not
more than 3 mEq/h. Maximum:
400 mEq/day.
Children. 2-5 mEq/kg/day usual rate
0.3-0.5 mEq 11g/hr. Max rate
1 mEq/kg/hr.

CONTRAINDICATIONS
Concurrent use of potassium-sparing
diuretics, digitalis toxicity, heat cramps,

hyperkalemia, postoperative oliguria,
severe burns, severe renal impairment,
shock with dehydration or hemolytic
reaction, untreated Addison disease.

INTERACTIONS
Drug
**ACE inhibitors, β-adrenergic
blockers, cyclosporine, heparin,
NSAIDs, potassium-containing
medications, potassium-sparing
diuretics, salt substitutes:**
May increase potassium blood
concentration.
Anticholinergics, NSAIDs: May
increase the risk of GI lesions or side
effects.
Corticosteroids: May decrease
potassium requirement.
**Iodine and iodine-containing
products:** Do not use.
Herbal
None known.
Food
Iodine-containing shellfish:
Contraindicated.

DIAGNOSTIC TEST EFFECTS
None known.

⊘ IV INCOMPATIBILITIES
Amphotericin B complex
(Abelcet, AmBisome, Amphotec),
methylprednisolone (Solu-Medrol),
phenytoin (Dilantin).

⬛ IV COMPATIBILITIES
Aminophylline, amiodarone
(Cordarone), atropine, aztreonam
(Azactam), calcium gluconate,
cefepime (Maxipime), ciprofloxacin
(Cipro), clindamycin (Cleocin),
dexamethasone (Decadron), digoxin
(Lanoxin), diltiazem (Cardizem),
diphenhydramine (Benadryl),
dobutamine (Dobutrex), dopamine
(Intropin), enalapril (Vasotec),
famotidine (Pepcid), fluconazole
(Diflucan), furosemide (Lasix),

granisetron (Kytril), heparin, hydrocortisone (Solu-Cortef), insulin, lidocaine, lorazepam (Ativan), magnesium sulfate, methylprednisolone (Solu-Medrol), metoclopramide (Reglan), midazolam (Versed), milrinone (Primacor), morphine, norepinephrine (Levophed), ondansetron (Zofran), oxytocin (Pitocin), piperacillin and tazobactam (Zosyn), procainamide (Pronestyl), propofol (Diprivan), propranolol (Inderal).

SIDE EFFECTS
Frequent
Skin rash.
Occasional
Nausea, vomiting, diarrhea, flatulence, abdominal discomfort with distention, phlebitis with IV administration (particularly when potassium concentration of > 40 mEq/L is infused).
Rare
Rash

SERIOUS REACTIONS
• Hyperkalemia (more common in elderly patients and those with impaired renal function) may be manifested as paresthesia, feeling of heaviness in the lower extremities, cold skin, grayish pallor, hypotension, confusion, irritability, flaccid paralysis, and cardiac arrhythmias.

PRECAUTIONS & CONSIDERATIONS
Caution is warranted with cardiac disease and concurrent use of potassium-sparing diuretics, digitalis toxicity, systemic acidosis, renal impairment, and tartrazine sensitivity (most common in those with aspirin hypersensitivity). It is unknown whether potassium crosses the placenta or is distributed in breast milk. No age-related precautions have been noted in children. Elderly patients may be at

increased risk for hyperkalemia because of an impaired ability to excrete potassium. Consuming potassium-rich foods, including apricots, avocados, bananas, beans, beef, broccoli, brussel sprouts, cantaloupe, chicken, dates, fish, ham, lentils, milk, molasses, potatoes, prunes, raisins, spinach, turkey, watermelon, veal, and yams, is encouraged.

Notify the physician of a feeling of heaviness in the lower extremities and paraesthesia. Serum potassium levels should be obtained before and throughout therapy. Intake and output, pattern of daily bowel activity, and stool consistency should also be monitored. Be alert for signs and symptoms of hyperkalemia, including cold skin, feeling of heaviness in lower extremities, paraesthesia, and skin pallor.

Hypersensitivity to seafood, iodine or iodine-containing products should be noted and if present, should not use this drug.
Storage
Store vials at room temperature.
Administration
! Potassium dosage must be individualized.

Give oral potassium with or after meals and with a full glass of water to decrease GI upset. Mix effervescent tablets, liquids, and powder with juice or water, and let them dissolve before administering. Swallow the tablets whole, and do not chew or crush them.

Dilute the drug to a concentration of no more than 40 mEq/L, and mix it well before IV infusion. Do not add potassium to a hanging IV line. Usual infusion rate is 10 mEq/h. Rate should not exceed 1mEq/min for adults. Maximum and recommended rates of infusion differ according to the institution and patient care setting (e.g., ICU vs. medical floor). Check the IV site closely during the infusion

P

for evidence of phlebitis (hardness of vein; heat, pain, and red streaking of skin over vein) and extravasation (cool skin, little or no blood return, pain, and swelling).

Pralidoxime
pra-li-doks-eem
(Protopam Chloride)

CATEGORY AND SCHEDULE
Pregnancy Risk Category: C

Classification: Antidotes

MECHANISM OF ACTION
Reactivates cholinesterase activity by 2-formyl-1-methylpyridinium ion. *Therapeutic Effect:* Restores cholinesterase activity following organophosphate anticholinesterase poisoning.

PHARMACOKINETICS
Onset of activity is 1 h and duration of action is short, which may require readministration. Not protein bound. Excreted in urine. *Half-life:* 1.2-2.6 h.

AVAILABILITY
Injection, Powder for Reconstitution: 1 g (Protopam Chloride).

INDICATIONS AND DOSAGES
▸ **Anticholinesterase overdosage**
IV
Adults, Elderly. 1-2 g initially, followed by increments of 250 mg q5min until response is observed.
▸ **Organophosphate poisoning**
IV
Adults, Elderly. 1-2 g initially in 100 mL 0.9% NaCl infused over 15-30 min or 5% solution in sterile water for injection over not <5 min. Repeat 1-2 g in 1 h if muscle weakness persists.
Children. 25-50 mg/kg/dose. Repeat in 1-2 h if muscle weakness has not been relieved, then at 8-12 h intervals if cholinergic signs recur.

CONTRAINDICATIONS
Use of aminophylline, morphine, theophylline, and succinylcholine; hypersensitivity to pralidoxime or any of its components.

INTERACTIONS
Drug
Aminophylline, caffeine, theophylline: May exacerbate effects of organophosphate poisoning.
Atropine: May decrease effects of pralidoxime.
Barbiturates: May increase effect of pralidoxime.
Reserpine, phenothiazines: May exacerbate effects of organophosphate poisoning.
Succinylcholine: May prolong respiratory paralysis.
Thiamine: May delay excretion of pralidoxime due to competition at renal excretory site.
Herbal
None known.
Food
None known.

DIAGNOSTIC TEST EFFECTS
May increase SGOT (AST) and creatine kinase levels.

SIDE EFFECTS
Occasional
Blurred vision, dizziness, headache, laryngospasm, hyperventilation, nausea, tachycardia, hypertension, pain at injection site.
Rare
Rash, muscle rigidity, decreased renal function.

SERIOUS REACTIONS

• Excessive doses may cause blurred vision, nausea, tachycardia and dizziness.

PRECAUTIONS & CONSIDERATIONS

Caution is warranted with myasthenia gravis and renal impairment as well as in elderly patients. It is unknown whether pralidoxime crosses the placenta and is distributed in breast milk. Safety and efficacy of pralidoxime have not been established in children. Age-related renal impairment may require dosage adjustment in elderly patients. Avoid consuming an excessive amount of caffeine derivatives such as chocolate, cocoa, coffee, cola, or tea.

Resolution of clinical symptoms (muscle weakness, respiratory difficulty, muscarinic effects such as salivation, lacrimation, urination, and defecation) should be assessed.

Storage

Store vials for injection at room temperature.

Administration

Initiation of therapy must not be delayed until results of tests are available. Dilute 1 g with 20 mL of sterile water for injection. Solution may be further diluted and administered as 1-2 g in 100 mL 0.9% NaCl. Slow IV infusion prevents tachycardia, laryngospasm, and muscle rigidity. Do not use if solution appears discolored or contains a precipitate.

Pramipexole

pram-eh-pex′ol

(Mirapex)

Do not confuse Mirapex with Mifeprex or MiraLax.

CATEGORY AND SCHEDULE

Pregnancy Risk Category: C

Classification: Antiparkinson agents, dopaminergics

MECHANISM OF ACTION

An antiparkinson agent that stimulates dopamine receptors in the striatum. *Therapeutic Effect:* Relieves signs and symptoms of Parkinson's disease.

PHARMACOKINETICS

Rapidly and extensively absorbed after PO administration. Protein binding: 15%. Widely distributed. Steady-state concentrations achieved within 2 days. Primarily eliminated in urine. Not removed by hemodialysis. *Half-life:* 8 h (12 h in patients older than 65 yr).

AVAILABILITY

Tablets: 0.125 mg, 0.25 mg, 0.5 mg, 1 mg, 1.5 mg.

INDICATIONS AND DOSAGES

▶ **Parkinson's disease**

PO

Adults, Elderly. Initially, 0.375 mg/day in 3 divided doses. Do not increase dosage more frequently than every 5-7 days. Maintenance: 1.5-4.5 mg/day in 3 equally divided doses.

▶ **Dosage in renal impairment**

Dosage and frequency are modified based on creatinine clearance.

Creatinine Clearance (mL/min)	Initial Dose (mg/day)	Maximum Dose
> 60	0.125	1.5 mg 3×/day
35-59	0.125	1.5 mg 2×/day
15-34	0.125	1.5 mg 1×/day

CONTRAINDICATIONS
History of hypersensitivity to pramipexole.

INTERACTIONS
Drug
Carbidopa and levodopa, levodopa: May increase plasma level of levodopa.
Cimetidine: Increases pramipexole plasma concentration and half-life.
Cimetidine, diltiazem, quinidine, quinine, ranitidine, triamterene, verapamil: May decrease pramipexole clearance.
Central nervous system (CNS) depressants: May increase CNS depressive effects.
Phenothiazines, butyrophenones, thioxanthenes, metoclopramide: May decrease effectiveness.
Herbal
None known.
Food
All foods: Delay peak drug plasma levels by 1 h but do not affect drug absorption.

DIAGNOSTIC TEST EFFECTS
None known.

SIDE EFFECTS
Frequent
Early Parkinson's disease (10%-28%): Nausea, asthenia, dizziness, somnolence, insomnia, constipation. Advanced Parkinson's disease (17%-53%): Orthostatic hypotension, extrapyramidal reactions, insomnia, dizziness, hallucinations.
Occasional
Early Parkinson's disease (2%-5%): Edema, malaise, confusion, amnesia, akathisia, anorexia, dysphagia, peripheral edema, vision changes, impotence.
Advanced Parkinson's disease (7%-10%): Asthenia, somnolence, confusion, constipation, abnormal gait, dry mouth.
Rare
Advanced Parkinson's disease (2%-6%): General edema, malaise, chest pain, amnesia, tremor, urinary frequency or incontinence, dyspnea, rhinitis, vision changes.

SERIOUS REACTIONS
• None known.

PRECAUTIONS & CONSIDERATIONS
Caution is warranted in patients with hallucinations, syncope, renal impairment, history of orthostatic hypotension, and in those using central nervous system (CNS) depressants concurrently. It is unknown whether pramipexole is distributed in breast milk. The safety and efficacy of pramipexole have not been established in children. Elderly patients are at increased risk for hallucinations.

Dizziness, drowsiness, lightheadedness, and constipation may occur. Alcohol and tasks that require mental alertness or motor skills should be avoided. Change positions slowly to prevent orthostatic hypotension. Baseline vital signs and renal function should be assessed at baseline. Relief of symptoms, such as improvement of masklike facial expression, muscular rigidity, shuffling gait, and resting tremors of the hands and head should be assessed during treatment.

Administration
Take pramipexole without regard to food. Take with food if nausea is a problem. Do not abruptly discontinue pramipexole.

Pramoxine
pra-mox'een
(Analpram-HC, Anusol, Enzone, Epifoam, Pramosome, Pramox HC [CAN], Prasone [TAIWAN], Prax, Proctofoam [US, ENG, GERMANY], Proctocream, Rectocort, Tronolane, Zone-A)
Do not confuse with pralidoxime, Apisol, Aquasol, Tronothane.

CATEGORY AND SCHEDULE
Pregnancy Risk Category: C

Classification: Morpholine derivative, anesthetic, topical

MECHANISM OF ACTION
A surface or local anesthetic that is not chemically related to the "caine" types of local anesthetics. Decreases the neuronal membranes' permeability to sodium ions, blocking both the initiation and conduction of nerve impulses, therefore inhibiting depolarization of the neuron.
Therapeutic Effect: Temporarily relieves pain and itching associated with anogenital pruritus or irritation.

PHARMACOKINETICS
Onset of action occurs within a few minutes of application. Peak effect is reached in 3-5 min. Duration is several days.

AVAILABILITY
Foam: 1% (Proctofoam NS).
Cream: 1% (Tranolane).
Gel: 1% (Itch-X).
Lotion: 1% (Prax).
Ointment: 1% (Anusol).
Solution: 1% (Itch-X).
Suppository: 1% (Tronolane).

INDICATIONS AND DOSAGES
▸ **Anogenital pruritus or irritation, dermatosis, minor burns, hemorrhoids**
TOPICAL
Adults, Elderly. Apply to affected area 3 or 4 times daily.

CONTRAINDICATIONS
Hypersensitivity to any component of the product.

INTERACTIONS
Drug
None known.
Herbal
None known.
Food
None known.

DIAGNOSTIC TEST EFFECTS
None known.

SIDE EFFECTS
Occasional
Angioedema, contact dermatitis, burning, itching, irritation, stinging.
Rare
Dryness, folliculitis, hypopigmentation, perianal dermatitis, maceration of the skin, secondary infection, skin atrophy, striae, miliaria.

SERIOUS REACTIONS
• None known.

PRECAUTIONS & CONSIDERATIONS
Caution is warranted with children and elderly patients. It is unknown whether pramoxine crosses the placenta and is distributed in the breast milk.

P

Redness, irritation, swelling, burning, stinging, pain, and dryness may occur. If bleeding at affected area, hoarseness, hives, rash, severe itching, difficulty breathing or swallowing, or swelling of the face, throat, lips, eyes, hands, feet, or ankles occurs, notify physician immediately.

Storage

Store at room temperature.

Administration

To use pramoxine cream, gel, spray, or lotion, wash hands first. Clean the affected area with mild soap and warm water. Rinse thoroughly. Pat affected area dry with a clean, soft cloth or tissue. Apply small amount of pramoxine to affected area. Wash hands thoroughly.

To use pramoxine pledgets, wash hands first. Clean affected rectal area with mild soap and warm water. Rinse thoroughly. Gently dry by patting or blotting with a clean, soft cloth or tissue. Open sealed pouch and remove pledget. Apply medication from pledget to affected rectal area by patting. If needed, fold pledget and leave in place for up to 15 min. Remove pledget, and throw away. Wash hands thoroughly.

To use pramoxine hemorrhoidal foam, wash hands first. Clean affected area with mild soap and warm water. Rinse thoroughly. Gently dry by patting or blotting with a clean, soft cloth or tissue. Shake the foam container. Squirt a small amount of foam onto a clean tissue and apply to affected rectal area. Wash hands thoroughly.

Pravastatin
prav-i-sta′tin
(Pravachol)
Do not confuse pravastatin with Prevacid, or Pravachol with propranolol.

CATEGORY AND SCHEDULE
Pregnancy Risk Category: X

Classification: Antihyperlip-idemics, HMG CoA reductase inhibitors

MECHANISM OF ACTION
An HMG-CoA reductase inhibitor that interferes with cholesterol biosynthesis by preventing the conversion of HMG-CoA reductase to mevalonate, a precursor to cholesterol. *Therapeutic Effect:* Lowers serum low density lipoprotein (LDL) and very low density lipoprotein (VLDL) cholesterol and plasma triglyceride levels; increases serum high density lipoprotein (HDL) concentration.

PHARMACOKINETICS
Poorly absorbed from the GI tract. Protein binding: 50%. Metabolized in the liver (minimal active metabolites). Primarily excreted in feces via the biliary system. Not removed by hemodialysis. *Half-life:* 2.7 h.

AVAILABILITY
Tablets: 10 mg, 20 mg, 40 mg, 80 mg.

INDICATIONS AND DOSAGES
▶ **Hyperlipidemia, primary and secondary prevention of cardiovascular events in patient with elevated cholesterol levels**

PO
Adults, Elderly. Initially, 40 mg/day.
Titrate to desired response. Range:
10-80 mg/day.
Children 14-18 yr. 40 mg/day.
Children 8-13 yr. 20 mg/day.
▶ **Dosage in hepatic and renal impairment**
For adults, give 10 mg/day initially.
Titrate to desired response.

CONTRAINDICATIONS

Pregnancy, active hepatic disease or unexplained, persistent elevations of liver function test results.

INTERACTIONS

Drug
Cyclosporine, erythromycin, clarithromycin, azithromycin, itraconazole: Increases the risk of acute renal failure and rhabdomyolysis or myopathy.
Herbal
None known.
Food
None known. Alcohol should be avoided during therapy.

DIAGNOSTIC TEST EFFECTS

May increase serum CK and transaminase concentrations.

SIDE EFFECTS

Pravastatin is generally well tolerated. Side effects are usually mild and transient.
Occasional (4%-7%)
Nausea, vomiting, diarrhea, constipation, abdominal pain, headache, rhinitis, rash, pruritus.
Rare (2%-3%)
Heartburn, myalgia, dizziness, cough, fatigue, flulike symptoms.

SERIOUS REACTIONS

• Malignancy and cataracts may occur.
• Hypersensitivity occurs rarely.

PRECAUTIONS & CONSIDERATIONS

Caution is warranted in patients with a history of acute hepatic disease or unexplained persistent elevations of liver function test results. Additional caution is warranted in patients with past liver disease, severe acute infection, tauma, severe metabolic or seizure disorders, severe electrolyte, endocrine, and metabolic disorders and in any patient who consumes a substantial amount of alcohol. Withholding or discontinuing pravastatin may be necessary when the person is at risk for renal failure secondary to rhabdomyolysis. Pravastatin is contraindicated in pregnancy (category X) and may cause fetal harm. It is unknown whether pravastatin is distributed in breast milk; because there is risk of serious adverse reactions in breastfeeding infants, pravastatin is contraindicated during lactation. Safety and efficacy of pravastatin have not been established in children. No age-related precautions have been noted in elderly patients.

Dizziness and headache may occur. Tasks that require mental alertness or motor skills should be avoided until response to the drug is established. Notify the physician of muscle weakness, myalgia, severe gastric upset, or rash. Pattern of daily bowel activity and stool consistency should be assessed. Serum lipid cholesterol and triglyceride levels and hepatic function should be checked at baseline and periodically during treatment.

Administration
! Before the patient begins pravastatin therapy, he or she should be on a standard cholesterol-lowering diet for a minimum of 3-6 mo. The patient should continue the diet throughout pravastatin therapy.

Take pravastatin without regard to meals and administer in the evening.

Praziquantel
pray-zih-kwon-tel
(Biltricide)

CATEGORY AND SCHEDULE
Pregnancy Risk Category: B

Classification: Antihelmintics

MECHANISM OF ACTION
An antihelmintic that increases cell permeability in susceptible helminths resulting in loss of intracellular calcium, massive contractions, and paralysis of their musculature, followed by attachment of phagocytes to the parasites. *Therapeutic Effect:* Vermicidal. Dislodges the dead and dying worms.

PHARMACOKINETICS
Well absorbed from GI tract. Protein binding: 80%. Widely distributed, including cerebrospinal fluid (CSF). Metabolized in liver. Primarily excreted in urine. Not removed by hemodialysis. *Half-life:* 4-5 h.

AVAILABILITY
Tablets: 600 mg (Biltricide).

INDICATIONS AND DOSAGES
▸ **Schistosomiasis**
PO
Adults, Elderly, Children > 4 yr of age. 3 doses of 20 mg/kg as 1-day treatment. Do not give doses <4 h or >6 h apart.
▸ **Clonorchiasis/opisthorchiasis**
PO
Adults, Elderly, Children > 4 yr of age. 3 doses of 25 mg/kg as 1-day treatment.

CONTRAINDICATIONS
Ocular cysticercosis, hypersensitivity to praziquantel or any component of the formulation.

INTERACTIONS
Drug
Albendazole: May increase risk of albendazole adverse effects.
Carbamazepine, phenytoin, fosphenytoin: May decrease praziquantel effectiveness.
Cimetidine: May increase praziquantel concentrations.
Herbal
None known.
Food
None known.

DIAGNOSTIC TEST EFFECTS
None known.

SIDE EFFECTS
Frequent
Headache, dizziness, malaise, abdominal pain.
Occasional
Anorexia, vomiting, diarrhea, severe cramping abdominal pain may occur within 1 h of administration with fever, sweating, bloody stools.
Rare
Dizziness, urticaria.

SERIOUS REACTIONS
• Overdose should be treated with fast-acting laxative.

PRECAUTIONS & CONSIDERATIONS
Caution should be used in patients with severe liver impairment and cardiac irregularities. It is unknown whether praziquantel is distributed in breast milk. Safety and efficacy have not been established in children. No age-related precautions have been noted in elderly patients. Indications of giddiness or uticaria may indicate a hypersensitivity reaction and should be reported.
Storage
Store at room temperature.

Administration
Doses should not be spaced not <4 h and not >6 h apart. Tablets are scored and may be broken for dosage adjustment. If iron supplements are ordered, continue as directed which may be up to 6 mo post therapy.

Prazosin Hydrochloride
pra′zoe-sin high-droh-klor-eye-d
(Minipress, Prasig [AUS], Pratisol [AUS], Pressin [AUS])

CATEGORY AND SCHEDULE
Pregnancy Risk Category: C

Classification: α-adrenergic antagonist

MECHANISM OF ACTION
An antidote, antihypertensive, and vasodilator that selectively blocks α_1-adrenergic receptors, decreasing peripheral vascular resistance. *Therapeutic Effect:* Produces vasodilation of veins and arterioles, decreases total peripheral resistance, and relaxes smooth muscle in bladder neck and prostate.

PHARMACOKINETICS
PO: Onset 2 h, peak 1-3 h, duration 6-12 h. *Half-life:* 2-4 h; metabolized in liver, excreted in bile, feces (> 90%), in urine (< 10%).

AVAILABILITY
Capsules: 1 mg, 2 mg, 5 mg.

INDICATIONS AND DOSAGES
▶ **Mild to moderate hypertension**
PO
Adults, Elderly. Initially, 1 mg 2-3 times a day. Maintenance: 6-15 mg/day in divided doses. Maximum: 20 mg/day.
Children. 5 mcg/kg/dose q6h. Gradually increase up to 25 mcg/kg/dose.

OFF-LABEL USES
Treatment of urinary retention in benign prostatic hypertrophy, congestive heart failure (CHF), ergot alkaloid toxicity, pheochromocytoma, Raynaud phenomenon.

CONTRAINDICATIONS
Hypersensitivity to prazosin.

INTERACTIONS
Drug
Estrogen, NSAIDs, indomethacin, and other sympathomimetics: May decrease the effects of prazosin.
Hypotension-producing medications, such as antihypertensives, epinephrine and diuretics: May increase the effects of prazosin.
Herbal
Licorice: Causes sodium and water retention and potassium loss.
Food
None known.

DIAGNOSTIC TEST EFFECTS
None known.

SIDE EFFECTS
Frequent (7%-10%)
Dizziness, somnolence, headache, asthenia (loss of strength, energy).
Occasional (4%-5%)
Palpitations, nausea, dry mouth, nervousness.
Rare (< 1%)
Angina, urinary urgency.

SERIOUS REACTIONS
• First-dose syncope (hypotension with sudden loss of consciousness)

P

may occur 30-90 min following initial dose of more than 2 mg, a too rapid increase in dosage, or addition of another antihypertensive agent to therapy. First-dose syncope may be preceded by tachycardia (pulse rate of 120-160 beats/min).

PRECAUTIONS & CONSIDERATIONS

Caution is warranted in patients with chronic renal failure. Caution should be used when driving or operating machinery. Tasks that require mental alertness or motor skills should be avoided until response to the drug is established.

Dizziness, lightheadedness, and fainting may occur. Rise slowly from a lying to a sitting position, and permit legs to dangle momentarily before standing to avoid the hypotensive effect. Notify the physician if dizziness or palpitations become bothersome. BP and pulse should be obtained immediately before each dose, and every 15-30 min thereafter until BP is stabilized. Be alert for fluctuations in BP. Pattern of daily bowel activity and stool consistency should also be assessed.

Assess patient's tolerance to stress, which could compromise cardiovascular function.

Administration

Take prazosin without regard to food. Take the first dose at bedtime to minimize the risk of fainting from first-dose syncope.

Prednisolone

pred-niss'oh-lone
(AK-Pred, AK-Tate [CAN], Inflamase Forte, Inflamase Mild, Minims-Prednisolone [CAN], Novo-Prednisolone [CAN], Orapred, Pediapred, Pred Forte, Pred Mild, Prelone, Solone [AUS])
Do not confuse prednisolone with prednisone or Primidone.

CATEGORY AND SCHEDULE

Pregnancy Risk Category: C (D if used in first trimester)

Classification: Glucocorticoid, immediate acting

MECHANISM OF ACTION

An adrenocortical steroid that inhibits accumulation of inflammatory cells at inflammation sites, phagocytosis, lysosomal enzyme release and synthesis, and release of mediators of inflammation. *Therapeutic Effect:* Prevents or suppresses cell-mediated immune reactions. Decreases or prevents tissue response to inflammatory process.

PHARMACOKINETICS

PO: Peak 1-2 h, duration 2 days.

AVAILABILITY

Oral Solution (Pediapred): 6.7 mg/5 mL.
Oral Solution (Orapred): 20 mg/5 mL.
Tablets: 5 mg.
Orally-Disintegrating Tablets (Orapred OTD): 10 mg, 15 mg, 30 mg.
Syrup (Prelone): 5 mg/5 mL.
Ophthalmic Solution (Inflamase Mild): 0.125%.
Ophthalmic Solution (AK-Pred, Inflamase Forte): 1%.

Ophthalmic Suspension (Pred Mild):
0.12%.
*Ophthalmic Suspension (Pred Forte):*1%.

INDICATIONS AND DOSAGES

▸ **Substitution therapy for deficiency states: acute or chronic adrenal insufficiency, congenital adrenal hyperplasia, and adrenal insufficiency secondary to pituitary insufficiency; nonendocrine disorders: arthritis; rheumatic carditis; allergic, collagen, intestinal tract, liver, ocular, renal, skin diseases; bronchial asthma; cerebral edema; malignancies**
PO
Adults, Elderly. 5-60 mg/day in divided doses.
Children. 0.1-2 mg/kg/day in 3-4 divided doses.
▸ **Treatment of conjuctivitis and corneal injury**
OPHTHALMIC
Adults, Elderly. 1-2 drops every hour during day and q2h during night. After response, decrease dosage to 1 drop q4h, then 1 drop 3-4 times a day.

CONTRAINDICATIONS

Acute superficial herpes simplex keratitis, systemic fungal infections, varicella, Cushing's syndrome.

INTERACTIONS

Drug
Acetaminophen (chronic use or high dose, alone or in combination products): May increase risk of hepatotoxicity.
Alcohol, salicylates, NSAIDs: May increase side effects.
Amphotericin: May increase hypokalemia.
Barbiturates, rifampin, rifabutin: May result in decreased glucocorticoid activity.

Digoxin: May increase the risk of digoxin toxicity caused by hypokalemia
Diuretics, insulin, oral hypoglycemics, potassium supplements: May decrease the effects of these drugs.
Hepatic enzyme inducers: May decrease the effects of prednisolone.
Ketoconazole, macrolide antibiotics (erythromycin, clarithromycin, azithromycin): May result in increased glucocorticoid activity.
Live virus vaccines: May decrease the patient's antibody response to vaccine, increase vaccine side effects, and potentiate virus replication.
Herbal
None known.
Food
None known.

DIAGNOSTIC TEST EFFECTS

May increase blood glucose and serum lipid, amylase, and sodium levels. May decrease serum calcium, potassium, and thyroxine levels.

SIDE EFFECTS

Frequent
Insomnia, heartburn, nervousness, abdominal distention, increased sweating, acne, mood swings, increased appetite, facial flushing, delayed wound healing, increased susceptibility to infection, diarrhea or constipation.
Occasional
Headache, edema, change in skin color, frequent urination.
Rare
Tachycardia, allergic reaction (such as rash and hives), psychological changes, hallucinations, depression. Ophthalmic: stinging or burning, posterior subcapsular cataracts.

P

SERIOUS REACTIONS

• Long-term therapy may cause hypocalcemia, hypokalemia, muscle wasting (especially in the arms and legs), osteoporosis, spontaneous fractures, amenorrhea, cataracts, glaucoma, peptic ulcer disease, and congestive heart failure (CHF).

• Abruptly withdrawing the drug after long-term therapy may cause anorexia, nausea, fever, headache, severe or sudden joint pain, rebound inflammation, fatigue, weakness, lethargy, dizziness, and orthostatic hypotension.

• Suddenly discontinuing prednisolone may be fatal.

• Oral medication doses should be taken with a light meal or milk.

PRECAUTIONS & CONSIDERATIONS

Caution is warranted in patients with cirrhosis, CHF, diabetes mellitus, hypertension, hypothyroidism, myasthenia gravis, ocular herpes simplex, osteoporosis, peptic ulcer disease, thromboembolic disorders, and ulcerative colitis. Monitor the growth and development of children receiving long-term steroid therapy. Avoid alcohol and limit caffeine intake during therapy.

Use contraindicated in acute superficial herpes simplex keratitis, systemic fungal infections, and varicella.

May cause changes in blood glucose levels; levels should be monitored closely during therapy.

Mood swings, ranging from euphoria to depression, may occur. Notify the physician of fever, muscle aches, sore throat, and sudden weight gain or swelling. The mouth should be assessed daily for signs and symptoms of candidal infection, such as white patches and painful mucous membranes and tongue. Blood glucose level, intake and output, BP, serum electrolyte levels, pattern of daily bowel activity, height, and weight should be monitored before and during therapy. Be alert to signs and symptoms of infection caused by reduced immune response, including fever, sore throat, and vague symptoms, as normal infection symptoms may be masked.

Administration

Shake ophthalmic preparation well before using. Instill drops into conjunctival sac, as prescribed. Avoid touching the applicator tip to the conjunctiva to avoid contamination. Do not abruptly discontinue the drug without physician approval.

Prednisone

pred′ni-sone

(Aristocort, Aristospan, Kenalog, Apo-Prednisone [CAN], Deltasone, Panafcort [AUS], Prednisone Intensol, Sone [AUS], Sterapred, Sterapred DS, Winpred [CAN])

Do not confuse prednisone with prednisolone or Primidone.

CATEGORY AND SCHEDULE

Pregnancy Risk Category: C, D if used in first trimester

Classification: Glucocorticoid, immediate acting

MECHANISM OF ACTION

An adrenocortical steroid that inhibits accumulation of inflammatory cells at inflammation sites, phagocytosis, lysosomal enzyme release and synthesis, and release of mediators of inflammation. *Therapeutic Effect:* Prevents or suppresses cell-mediated immune reactions. Decreases or prevents tissue response to inflammatory process.

PHARMACOKINETICS

Well absorbed from the GI tract. Protein binding: 70%-90%. Widely distributed. Metabolized in the liver and converted to prednisolone. Metabolized in the liver and converted to predinsolone. Excreted primarily in urine. Not removed by hemodialysis.
Half-life: 3.4-3.8 h.

AVAILABILITY

Oral Concentrate (Prednisone Intensol): 5 mg/mL.
Oral Solution: 5 mg/5 mL.
Tablets (Deltasone): 2.5 mg, 5 mg, 10 mg, 20 mg, 50 mg.
Tablets (Sterapred): 5 mg, 10 mg.
Tablets (Generic): 1 mg, 2 mg, 5 mg, 10 mg, 20 mg, 40 mg.
Injection (Kenalog): 10 mg/mL, 40 mg/mL.
Injection (Aristocort): 2.5 mg/mL, 40 mg/mL
Injection (Aristospan): 5 mg/mL, 20 mg/mL

INDICATIONS AND DOSAGES

▶ **Substitution therapy in deficiency states: acute or chronic adrenal insufficiency, congenital adrenal hyperplasia, and adrenal insufficiency secondary to pituitary insufficiency; nonendocrine disorders: arthritis; rheumatic carditis; allergic, collagen, intestinal tract, liver, ocular, renal, skin diseases; bronchial asthma; cerebral edema; malignancies**
PO
Adults, Elderly. 5-60 mg/day in divided doses.
Children. 0.05-2 mg/kg/day in 1-4 divided doses.
▶ **Immunosuppression or anti-inflammation**
PO
Adults, Elderly. 5-60 mg/day divided into 1-4 doses.

CONTRAINDICATIONS

Acute superficial herpes simplex keratitis, systemic fungal infections, varicella.

INTERACTIONS

Drug
Acetaminophen (chronic long-term or high-dose, alone or in combination products): May increase risk of hepatotoxicity.
Alcohol, salicylates, NSAIDs: May cause increased side effects.
Amphotericin: May increase hypokalemia.
Barbiturates, rifampin, rifabutin: May decrease glucocorticoid activity.
Digoxin: May increase the risk of digoxin toxicity caused by hypokalemia
Diuretics, insulin, oral hypoglycemics, potassium supplements: May decrease the effects of these drugs.
Hepatic enzyme inducers: May decrease the effects of prednisone.
Ketoconazole, macrolide antibiotics (erythromycin, clarithromycin, azithromycin): May increase glucocorticoid activity.
Live virus vaccines: May decrease the patient's antibody response to vaccine, increase vaccine side effects, and potentiate virus replication.
Herbal
None known.
Food
None known.

DIAGNOSTIC TEST EFFECTS

May increase blood glucose and serum lipid, amylase, and sodium levels. May decrease serum calcium, potassium, and thyroxine levels.

SIDE EFFECTS

Frequent
Insomnia, heartburn, nervousness, abdominal distention, increased

P

sweating, acne, mood swings, increased appetite, facial flushing, delayed wound healing, increased susceptibility to infection, diarrhea or constipation; pain at injection site.

Occasional
Headache, edema, change in skin color, frequent urination.

Rare
Tachycardia, allergic reaction (including rash and hives), psychological changes, hallucinations, depression.

SERIOUS REACTIONS

• Long-term therapy may cause muscle wasting in the arms and legs, osteoporosis, spontaneous fractures, amenorrhea, cataracts, glaucoma, peptic ulcer disease, and CHF.
• Abruptly withdrawing the drug following long-term therapy may cause anorexia, nausea, fever, headache, sudden or severe joint pain, rebound inflammation, fatigue, weakness, lethargy, dizziness, and orthostatic hypotension.
• Suddenly discontinuing prednisone may be fatal.
• Oral medication doses should be taken with a light meal or milk.

PRECAUTIONS & CONSIDERATIONS

Prednisone therapy is contraindicated in cases of acute superficial herpes simplex keratitis, systemic fungal infections, varicella. Caution is warranted in patients with CHF, cirrhosis, diabetes mellitus, glaucoma, hypertension, hyperthyroidism, myasthenia gravis, ocular herpes simplex, osteoporosis, renal disease, and esophagitis. Prednisone crosses the placenta and is distributed in breast milk. Prolonged prednisone use in the first trimester of pregnancy causes cleft palate in the neonate. Prolonged treatment or high dosages may decrease the cortisol secretion and short-term growth rate in children. Elderly patients may be more susceptible to developing hypertension or osteoporosis. Never give prednisone with live virus vaccines, such as smallpox vaccine; avoid exposure to chickenpox or measles. A dentist or other physician should be informed of prednisone therapy if taken within the past 12 mo. May cause changes in blood glucose levels and levels should be monitored closely during therapy.

Conversion to prednisolone may be impaired in liver disease.

Mood swings, ranging from euphoria to depression, may occur. Notify the physician of fever, muscle aches, sore throat, and sudden weight gain or swelling. Initially, tuberculosis skin test, radiographs, and ECG should be checked. Blood glucose level, intake and output, BP, serum electrolyte levels, height, and weight should be monitored before and during therapy. Be alert to signs and symptoms of infection caused by reduced immune response, including fever, sore throat, and vague symptoms. The mouth should be assessed daily for signs and symptoms of candidal infection, such as white patches and painful mucous membranes and tongue.

Administration
Take prednisone without regard to meals; give with food if GI upset occurs. Take single doses before 9:00 AM; give multiple doses at evenly spaced intervals. Do not abruptly discontinue prednisone without physician approval.

Primaquine
prim-a-kween
(Primacin [AUS])
Do not confuse with primidone.

CATEGORY AND SCHEDULE
Pregnancy Risk Category: C

Classification: Antiprotozoals

MECHANISM OF ACTION
An antimalarial and antirheumatic that eliminates tissue exoerythrocytic forms of *Plasmodium falciparum*. Disrupts mitochondria and binds to DNA. *Therapeutic Effect:* Inhibits parasite growth.

PHARMACOKINETICS
Well absorbed. Metabolized in the liver to the active metabolite, carboxyprimaquine. Excreted in the urine in small amounts as unchanged drug. *Half-life:* 4-6 h.

AVAILABILITY
Tablets: 26.3 mg (Primaquine phosphate).

INDICATIONS AND DOSAGES
▸ **Treatment of malaria (caused by *Plasmodium vivax*)**
PO
Adults, Elderly. 15-mg base daily for 14 days.
Children. 0.5-0.6 mg base/kg/day once daily for 14 days.
▸ **Malaria prophylaxis (off label use)**
Adults, Elderly. 30-mg base daily. Begin 1 day before departure and continue for 7 days after leaving malarious area.

OFF-LABEL USES
With clindamycin in treatment of *Pneumocystis carinii* in AIDS.

CONTRAINDICATIONS
Concomitant medications that cause bone marrow suppression, rheumatoid arthritis, lupus erythematosus, glucose-6-phosphate dehydrogenase (G-6-PD) deficiency, pregnancy, hypersensitivity to primaquine or any of its components.

INTERACTIONS
Drug
Aurothioglucose: May increase risk of blood dyscrasias.
Levomethadyl: May increase risk of cardiotoxicity (QT prolongation, torsade de pointes, cardiac arrest).
Herbal
None known.
Food
None known.

DIAGNOSTIC TEST EFFECTS
None known.

SIDE EFFECTS
Frequent
Abdominal pain, nausea, vomiting.
Rare
Leukopenia, hemolytic anemia, methemoglobinemia.

SERIOUS REACTIONS
• Leukopenia, hemolytic anemia, methemoglobinemia occur rarely.
• Overdosage include symptoms of abdominal cramps, vomiting, burning epigastric distress, central nervous system and cardiovascular disturbances, cyanosis, methemoglobinemia, moderate leukocytosis or leukopenia, and anemia.
• Acute hemolysis occurs, but patients recover completely if the dosage is discontinued.

PRECAUTIONS & CONSIDERATIONS
Caution is warranted with erythrocytic G6PD deficiency or

nicotinamide adenine dinucleotide (NADH) methemoglobin reductase deficiency, a family personal history of favism, and a previous idiosyncrasy to primaquine phosphate (as manifested by hemolytic anemia, methemoglobinemia, or leukopenia). Primaquine crosses the placenta, but it is unknown whether it is distributed in breast milk. Children are especially susceptible to primaquine's fatal effects.

Signs suggestive of hemolytic anemia such as darkening of urine, marked fall of hemoglobin or erythrocytic count, should be reported and primaquine should be discontinued promptly.

Administration

26.3 mg primaquine = 15 mg base. The dose of 1 tablet (15 mg base) daily for 14 days should not be exceeded. Take dose with food.

Primidone

pri'mi-done

(Apo-Primidone [CAN], Mysoline)

Do not confuse primidone with prednisone.

CATEGORY AND SCHEDULE

Pregnancy Risk Category: D

Classification: Anticonvulsant, barbiturate derivative

MECHANISM OF ACTION

A barbiturate that decreases motor activity from electrical and chemical stimulation and stabilizes the seizure threshold against hyperexcitability. *Therapeutic Effect:* Reduces seizure activity.

PHARMACOKINETICS

PO: Peak 4 h. *Half-life:* 3-24 h. Excreted through kidneys, breast milk. Metabolized in the liver.

AVAILABILITY

Tablets: 50 mg, 250 mg.

INDICATIONS AND DOSAGES

▸ **Seizure control (general tonic-clonic (grand mal), complex partial psychomotor seizures)**

PO

Adults, Elderly, Children 8 yr and older. 125-250 mg/day at bedtime. May increase by 125-250 mg/day every 3-7 days. Maximum: 2 g/day. *Children younger than 8 yr.* Initially, 50-125 mg/day at bedtime. May increase by 50-125 mg/day every 3-7 days. Usual dose: 10-25 mg/kg/day in divided doses. *Neonates.* 12-20 mg/kg/day in divided doses.

OFF-LABEL USES

Treatment of essential tremor.

CONTRAINDICATIONS

History of bronchopneumonia, porphyria, barbiturate hypersensitivity.

INTERACTIONS

Drug

Acetaminophen, corticosteroids, doxycycline, fenoprofen: May decrease effects of these drugs.

Alcohol, other central nervous system (CNS) depressants: May increase the effects of primidone.

Carbamazepine: May increase the metabolism of carbamazepine causing lower blood concentration.

Digoxin, glucocorticoids, metronidazole, oral anticoagulants, quinidine, tricyclic

antidepressants: May decrease the effects of these drugs.
Halothane, halogenated hydrocarbon inhalation anesthetics, haloperidol, phenothiazines: May cause increased metabolism and hepatotoxicity.
Valproic acid: Increases the blood concentration and risk of toxicity of primidone.
Herbal
None known.
Food
None known.

DIAGNOSTIC TEST EFFECTS

May decrease serum bilirubin level. Therapeutic serum level is 4-12 mcg/mL; toxic serum level is > 12 mcg/mL.

SIDE EFFECTS

Frequent
Ataxia, dizziness.
Occasional
Anorexia, drowsiness, mental changes, nausea, vomiting, paradoxical excitement.
Rare
Rash.

SERIOUS REACTIONS

• Abrupt withdrawal after prolonged therapy may produce effects ranging from increased dreaming, nightmares, insomnia, tremor, diaphoresis, and vomiting to hallucinations, delirium, seizures, and status epilepticus.
• Skin eruptions may be a sign of a hypersensitivity reaction.
• Blood dyscrasias, hepatic disease, and hypocalcemia occur rarely.
• Overdose produces cold or clammy skin, hypothermia, and severe CNS depression, followed by high fever and coma.

PRECAUTIONS & CONSIDERATIONS

Caution is warranted in patients with hepatic and renal impairment. Dizziness may occur, so change positions slowly—from recumbent to sitting position before standing. Alcohol and tasks requiring mental alertness or motor skills should be avoided. CBC, neurologic status (including duration, frequency, and severity of seizures) and serum concentrations of primidone should be assessed before and during treatment.

Signs of overdose including cold or clammy skin, hypothermia, CNS depression with high fever or coma should be reported immediately.
Administration
Administer primidone at the same time each day. Do not abruptly discontinue primidone after long-term use because this may precipitate seizures. Strict maintenance of drug therapy is essential for seizure control. Be aware that the therapeutic serum drug level is 4-12 mcg/mL; the toxic serum drug level is > 12 mcg/mL.

P

Probenecid
proe-ben′e-sid
(Benuryl [CAN], Pro-cid [AUS])
Do not confuse probenecid with procainamide.

CATEGORY AND SCHEDULE
Pregnancy Risk Category: C

Classification: Antigout agents, uricosurics

MECHANISM OF ACTION
A uricosuric that competitively inhibits reabsorption of uric acid at the proximal convoluted tubule.

Also inhibits renal tubular secretion of weak organic acids, such as penicillins. *Therapeutic Effect:* Promotes uric acid excretion, reduces serum uric acid level, and increases plasma levels of penicillins and cephalosporins.

AVAILABILITY
Tablets: 500 mg.

INDICATIONS AND DOSAGES
▶ **Gout**
PO
Adults, Elderly. Initially, 250 mg twice a day for 1 wk; then 500 mg twice a day. May increase by 500 mg q4wk. Maximum: 2 g/day. Maintenance: Dosage that maintains normal uric acid level.
▶ **As an adjunct to penicillin or cephalosporin therapy to prolong antibiotic plasma levels**
PO
Adults, Elderly. 2 g/day in divided doses.
Children weighing >50 kg. Receive adult dosage.
Children aged 2-14 yr. Initially, 25 mg/kg. Maintenance: 40 mg/kg/day in 4 divided doses.
▶ **Gonorrhea**
PO
Adults, Elderly. 1 g 30 min before penicillin, ampicillin, amoxicillin, or cefoxitin.

CONTRAINDICATIONS
Blood dyscrasias, children younger than 2 yr, concurrent high-dose aspirin therapy, severe renal impairment, uric acid calculi.

INTERACTIONS
Drug
Alcohol, salicylates: May increase serum urate level, decrease uricosuric activity.

Antineoplastics: May increase the risk of uric acid nephropathy.
Benzodiazepines: May result in increased sedative effects.
Cephalosporins, penicillins, methotrexate, nitrofurantoin, NSAIDs, penicillins, zidovudine: May increase blood concentrations of these drugs.
Dapsone, indomethacin, other NSAIDs, acyclovir: May result in increased toxicity.
Heparin: May increase and prolong the effects of heparin.
Ketorolac: Contraindicated.
Salicylates: May decrease uricosuric effect.
Herbal
None known.
Food
None known.

DIAGNOSTIC TEST EFFECTS
May inhibit renal excretion of serum PSP (phenolsulfonphthalein), 17-ketosteroids, and BSP (sulfobromophthalein).

SIDE EFFECTS
Frequent (6%-10%)
Headache, anorexia, nausea, vomiting.
Occasional (1%-5%)
Lower back or side pain, rash, hives, itching, dizziness, flushed face, frequent urge to urinate, gingivitis.

SERIOUS REACTIONS
• Severe hypersensitivity reactions, including anaphylaxis, occur rarely and usually within a few hours after administration following previous use. If severe hypersensitivity reactions develop, discontinue the drug immediately and contact the physician.
• Pruritic maculopapular rash, possibly accompanied by malaise, fever, chills, arthralgia, nausea,

vomiting, leukopenia, and aplastic anemias, should be considered a toxic reaction.

PRECAUTIONS & CONSIDERATIONS

Caution is warranted in patients with hematuria, peptic ulcer disease, and renal colic. Avoid alcohol and large doses of aspirin or other salicylates. Limit intake of high purine foods, such as fish and organ meats.

High fluid intake (3000 mL/day) should be encouraged; intake and output should be monitored; output should be at least 2000 mL/day. CBC, serum uric acid level, and urine for cloudiness, odor, and unusual color should also be monitored. Signs and symptoms of a therapeutic response, including improved joint range of motion and reduced joint tenderness, redness, and swelling, should be evaluated.

Do not use with ketorolac therapy (Toradol).

Storage

Store at room temperature.

Administration

! Do not start giving probenecid until acute gouty attack has subsided; continue drug if acute attack occurs during therapy. Probenecid should not be used in those with renal impairment.

Give probenecid orally with or immediately after meals or milk. Drink at least 6-8 eight-oz. glasses of fluid each day to prevent renal calculi. It may take more than 1 wk for the full therapeutic effect of the drug to be evident.

Procainamide Hydrochloride

proe-kane′a-mide high-droh-clor-ide
(Pronestyl)

Do not confuse Pronestyl with Pregnyl, procainamide with procaine.

CATEGORY AND SCHEDULE

Pregnancy Risk Category: C

Classification: Antiarrhythmics, Group IA

MECHANISM OF ACTION

Increases the effective refractory period of atria, bundle of His-Purkinje system and ventricles of the heart. *Therapeutic Effect:* Reduces conduction velocity in the atria and resolves ventricular arrhythmia.

PHARMACOKINETICS

Irreversible protein binding (< 20%); *Half-life:* 4 h (prolonged in renal impairment). IM, IV: Rapidly absorbed, peak 15-60 min. PO: Less readily absorbed, peak 90-120 min.

AVAILABILITY

Tablets, Capsules: 250 mg, 375 mg, 500 mg.
IM, IV: 100 mg/10 mL, 500 mg/2 mL.

INDICATIONS AND DOSAGES

▸ **Treat ventricular arrhythmias**
PO
Adults, Elderly, Children. By weight.

Weight (lb)	Dosage
88-100	250 mg q3h or 500 mg q6h
132-154	375 mg q3h or 750 mg q6h
176-198	500 mg q3h or 1 g q6h
>220	625 mg q3h or 1.25 mg q6h

P

IV
Adults.15-17 mg/kg at a rate or 20-30 mg/min load. Or 100 mg IV q5min by slow IV push until arrhythmia resolves, up to 1000 mg.
Children. 3-6 mg/kg over 5 min. Do not exceed 100 mg as a single dose. May repeat q5-10min to a maximum dose of 15 mg/kg.

ⓘ IV INCOMPATIBILITIES
Include ceftizoxime, diazepam, hydralazine, lansoprazole, milrinone, phanytoin, dextrose 5%.

OFF-LABEL USES
None noted.

CONTRAINDICATIONS
Complete heart block due to possible asystole, idiosyncratic hypersensitivity to procainamide, lupus erythromatosus, torsade de pointes.

INTERACTIONS
Drug
Alcohol, other CNS depressants: May decrease effectiveness.
Astemizole, cisapride, dofetilide, phenothiazines, type 5 photodiesterase inhibitors (e.g., sildenafil, vardenafil), terfenadine, ziprasidone: May cause potent vasodilation, increased irregular heartbeat, and increased side effects.
Digoxin, glucocorticoids, metronidazole, oral anticoagulants, quinidine, disopyramide, tricyclic antidepressants: May decrease the effects of these drugs.
Macrolide antibiotics (erythromycin, clarithromycin, azithromycin), cimetidine, ketolide antibiotics (telithromycin), H_2-agonists: May increase side effects and risk of irregular heartbeat.

Succinylcholine and neuromuscular blockers: May increase risk of side effects.
Herbal
None known.
Food
None known.

DIAGNOSTIC TEST EFFECTS
May decrease serum bilirubin level. Therapeutic serum level is up to 10 mcg/mL; toxic serum level is > 12 mcg/mL. May cause positive antinuclear antibody (ANA) test. Elevated liver enzymes, alkaline phosphatase (ALT, SGOT) and bilirubin.

SIDE EFFECTS
Frequent
Ataxia, dizziness.
Occasional
Dizziness, giddiness, weakness, mental depression, psychosis with hallucinations.
Rare
Neutropenia, thrombocytopenia, hemolytic anemia.

SERIOUS REACTIONS
• Neutropenia, thrombocytopenia, and hemolytic anemia may develop over time; usually reverses upon discontinuation of drug therapy.
• Skin eruptions may be a sign of a hypersensitivity reaction.
• Blood dyscrasias, hepatic disease, and hypocalcemia occur rarely.

PRECAUTIONS & CONSIDERATIONS
Caution is warranted in patients with bundle-branch block, congestive heart failure (CHF), liver and renal impairment, marked AV-conduction disturbances, severe digoxin toxicity, and supraventricular tachyarrhythmias. Be aware that procainamide crosses the placenta and that procainamide is distributed

in breast milk and is absorbed by nursing infants. No age-related precautions have been noted in children. Elderly patients are more susceptible to the drug's hypotensive effect. In elderly patients, age-related renal impairment may require dosage adjustment. Be aware that cardiotoxic effects occur most commonly with IV administration, observed as conduction changes (50% widening of QRS complex, frequent ventricular premature contractions, ventricular tachycardia, complete atrioventricular [AV] block); prolonged PR and QT intervals, flattened T waves occur less frequently. Nasal decongestants or over-the-counter (OTC) cold preparations, especially those containing stimulants, should be avoided without consulting the physician for approval. Alcohol and salt consumption should be restricted while taking procainamide.

GI upset, headache, dizziness, and joint pain may occur. Notify the physician if fever, joint pain or stiffness, and signs of upper respiratory infection occur. ECG for cardiac changes, particularly widening of QRS and prolongation of PR and QT intervals, should be monitored. Pulse, pattern of daily bowel activity and stool consistency, skin for hypertensive reaction, intake and output, serum electrolyte levels, including chloride, potassium, and sodium, and BP should be assessed during therapy.

Oral dosing results in dizziness, blurred vision. Care in driving, operating machinery, and engaging in exercises requiring mental acuity or alertness should be avoided until the patient knows how he/she reacts to the drug.

Storage
When diluted with D5W, solution is stable for up to 24 h at room temperature or for 7 days if refrigerated. Solutions darker than light amber in color should be discarded.

Administration
❗ Know that procainamide dosage and the interval of administration are individualized based on age, clinical response, renal function, and underlying myocardial disease. Also be aware that extended-release tablets are used for maintenance therapy.

Do not crush or break tablets or capsules; swallow whole.

❗ May give procainamide by IM injection, IV push, or IV infusion. Therapeutic serum level is 4-8 mcg/mL, and a toxic serum level is >10 mcg/mL.

Solution normally appears clear, colorless to light yellow. Discard if solution darkens or appears discolored or if precipitate forms. For IV push, dilute with 5-10 mL D5W. For initial loading IV infusion, add 1 g to 50 mL D5W to provide a concentration of 20 mg/mL. For IV infusion, add 1 g to 250-500 mL D5W to provide concentration of 2-4 mg/mL. Know that the maximum concentration is 4 g/250 mL. For IV push, with patient in the supine position, administer at a rate not exceeding 25-50 mg/min. For initial loading infusion, infuse 1 mL/min for up to 25-30 min. For IV infusion, infuse at 1-3 mL/min. Check BP every 5-10 min during infusion. If a fall in BP exceeds 15 mm Hg, discontinue drug and contact physician. Monitor ECG for cardiac changes, particularly widening of QRS and prolongation of PR and QT intervals. Notify physician of any significant interval changes. Continuously monitor BP and ECG during IV administration. Continuously adjust the rate of infusion to eliminate arrhythmias.

Procaine
proe'kane
(Novocain, Mericaine)

CATEGORY AND SCHEDULE
Pregnancy Risk Category: C

Classification: Anesthetics, local

MECHANISM OF ACTION
Procaine causes a reversible blockade of nerve conduction by decreasing nerve membrane permeability to sodium. *Therapeutic Effect:* Local anesthesia.

PHARMACOKINETICS
Highly plasma protein-bound and distributed to all body tissues. Excreted in the urine (80%).
Half-life: 40 ± 9 s in adults, 84 ± 30 s in neonates.

AVAILABILITY
Solution: 0.25%, 0.5%, 10% (Novocaine).

INDICATIONS AND DOSAGES
▸ **Spinal anesthesia**
INTRATHECAL
Adults. 0.5-1 mL of a 10% solution (50-100 mg) mixed with an equal volume of diluent injected into the third or fourth lumber interspace (perineum and lower extremities). 2 mL of a 10% solution (200 mg) mixed with 1 mL of diluent injected into the second, third, or fourth interspace.
▸ **Infiltration anesthesia, dental anesthesia, control of severe pain (postherpatic neuralgia, cancer pain, or burns)**
TOPICAL
Adults. A single dose of 350-600 mg using a 0.25% or 0.5% solution. Use 0.9% sodium chloride for dilution.

Children. 15 mg/kg of a 0.5% solution is the maximum recommended dose.
▸ **Peripheral or sympathetic nerve block (regional anesthesia)**
TOPICAL
Adults. Up to 200 mL of a 0.5% solution (1 g), 100 mL of a 1% solution (1 g), or 50 mL of a 2% solution (1 g). The 2% solution should only be used when a small volume of anesthetic is required.

OFF-LABEL USES
Severe pain.

CONTRAINDICATIONS
Hypersensitivity to ester local anesthetics, sulfites, PABA, patients on anticoagulant therapy, and in patients with coagulopathy, infection, thrombocytopenia. Should not be given intrarterially, intrathecally or intravenously.

INTERACTIONS
Drug
Antihypertensives, nitrates: May experience additive hypotensive effects.
Central nervous system (CNS) depressants: May cause additive suppression, especially in children and when larger doses are used.
Cholinesterase inhibitors, succincholine: Procaine may antagonize the effect of these medications.
Local anesthetics: May cause a toxic additive effect.
MAOIs: Increased risk of hypotension.
Medications that cause QT prolongation: May cause additive cardiotoxic effects, especially on rapid intravascular injection.
Sulfonamides: Suspected interference with antimicrobial activity.

Herbal
None known.
Food
None known.

DIAGNOSTIC TEST EFFECTS
None known.

SIDE EFFECTS
Frequent
Numbness or tingling of the face
or mouth, pain at the injection
site, dizziness, drowsiness,
lightheadedness, nausea, vomiting,
back pain, headache
Rare
Anxiety, restlessness, difficulty
breathing, shortness of breath,
seizures (convulsions), skin rash,
itching (hives), slow irregular
heartbeat (palpitations), swelling
of the face or mouth, tremors, QT
prolongation, PR prolongation,
atrial fibrillation, sinus bradycardia,
hypotension, angina, cardiovascular
collapse, fecal or urinary
incontinence, loss of perineal
sensation and sexual function,
persistent motor, sensory, or
autonomic (sphincter control) deficit.

SERIOUS REACTIONS
• Procaine-induced CNS toxicity
usually presents with symptoms
of stimulation, such as anxiety,
apprehension, restlessness,
nervousness, disorientation,
confusion, dizziness, blurred vision,
tremor, nausea/vomiting, shivering,
or seizures. Subsequently, depressive
symptoms can occur, including
drowsiness, unconsciousness, and
respiratory arrest.
• If higher concentrations are
introduced into the bloodstream,
depression of cardiac excitability and
contractility may cause AV block,
ventricular arrhythmias, or cardiac
arrest. CNS toxicity, including

dizziness, tongue numbness, visual
impairment and disturbances, and
muscular twitching appear to occur
before cardiotoxic effects.
Caution
! Procaine should be used with
caution in patients who have asthma
because there is an increased
risk of anaphylactoid reactions,
including bronchospasm and status
asthmaticus.
Alert
! Local anesthetics can cause
varying degrees of maternal, fetal,
and neonatal toxicities during labor
and obstetric delivery. Fetal heart
rate should be monitored as well as
the presence of symptoms indicating
fetal bradycardia, fetal acidosis,
and maternal hypotension. Epidural
procaine may cause decreased
uterine contractility or maternal
expulsion efforts and alter the forces
of parturition.
Alert
! Unintentional fetal intracranial
injection of procaine occurring
during pudenal or paracervical block
has been shown to lead to neonatal
depression at birth and can lead to
seizures within 6 h as a result of high
serum concentrations.

PRECAUTIONS & CONSIDERATIONS
Caution is warranted in
patients with cardiac disease,
hyperthyroidism, or other endocrine
disease. It is unknown whether
procaine crosses the placenta or is
distributed in the breast milk. No
age-related precautions have been
noted in elderly patients. A burning
sensation may occur at the site of
injection.
Administration
Dosage varies based on procedure,
desired depth and duration
of anesthesia, desired muscle
relaxation, vascularity of tissues,

physical condition, and age of patient. Before instillation of anesthetic agent, withdraw plunger to ensure needle is not in artery or vein. Resuscitative equipment should be available when local anesthetic is administered.

Procarbazine Hydrochloride

pro-kar′ba-zeen high-dro-klor-ide
(Matulane, Natulan [CAN])
Do not confuse procarbazine with dacarbazine.

CATEGORY AND SCHEDULE
Pregnancy Risk Category: D

Classification: Antineoplastics, miscellaneous

MECHANISM OF ACTION
A methylhydrazine derivative that inhibits DNA, RNA, and protein synthesis. May also directly damage DNA. Cell cycle-phase specific for S phase of cell division. *Therapeutic Effect:* Causes cell death.

PHARMACOKINETICS
PO: Peak levels 1 h; concentrates in liver, kidney, skin; metabolized in liver, excreted in urine.

AVAILABILITY
Capsules: 50 mg.

INDICATIONS AND DOSAGES
▸ **Advanced Hodgkin disease**
PO
Adults, Elderly. Initially, 2-4 mg/kg/ day as a single dose or in divided doses for 1 wk, then 4-6 mg/kg/day. Maintenance: 1-2 mg/kg/day.

Children. 50-100 mg/m^2/day for 10-14 days of a 28-day cycle. Continue until maximum response occurs, leukocyte count falls below 4000/mm^3, or platelet count falls below 100,000/mm^3. Maintenance: 50 mg/m^2/day.

OFF-LABEL USES
Treatment of lung carcinoma, malignant melanoma, multiple myeloma, non-Hodgkin lymphoma, polycythemia vera, primary brain tumors.

CONTRAINDICATIONS
Myelosuppression, breast-feeding, MAOI therapy.

INTERACTIONS
Drug
Alcohol: May cause a disulfiram-like reaction.
Antihistamines, barbiturates, narcotics: May increase CNS depressive effects.
Anticholinergics, antihistamines: May increase the anticholinergic effects of these drugs.
Bone marrow depressants: May increase myelosuppression.
Buspirone, caffeine-containing medications: May increase BP.
Carbamazepine, cyclobenzaprine, MAOIs, maprotiline: May cause hyperpyretic crisis, seizures, or death.
CNS depressants: May increase CNS depression.
Indirect-acting sympathomimetics: May cause hypertension.
Insulin, oral antidiabetics: May increase the effects of these drugs.
Meperidine and other opioids, tyramine-containing foods: May produce coma, seizures, immediate excitation, rigidity, severe hypertension or hypotension, severe respiratory distress, diaphoresis, and vascular collapse.

Tricyclic antidepressants, antihistamines: May increase anticholinergic effects; may cause seizures and hyperpyretic crisis.
Herbal
None known.
Food
Caffeine-containing beverages: May increase BP.

DIAGNOSTIC TEST EFFECTS
None known.

SIDE EFFECTS
Frequent
Severe nausea, vomiting, respiratory disorders (cough, effusion), myalgia, arthralgia, drowsiness, nervousness, insomnia, nightmares, diaphoresis, hallucinations, seizures.
Occasional
Hoarseness, tachycardia, nystagmus, retinal hemorrhage, photophobia, photosensitivity, urinary frequency, nocturia, hypotension, diarrhea, stomatitis, paraesthesia, unsteadiness, confusion, decreased reflexes, foot drop.
Rare
Hypersensitivity reaction (dermatitis, pruritus, rash, urticaria), hyperpigmentation, alopecia.

SERIOUS REACTIONS
• Procarbazine's major toxic effects are myelosuppression manifested as hematologic toxicity (mainly leukopenia, thrombocytopenia, and anemia) and hepatotoxicity manifested as jaundice and ascites.
• Urinary tract infections may occur secondary to leukopenia.

PRECAUTIONS & CONSIDERATIONS
Caution is warranted in patients with hepatic and renal impairment. Alcohol should be avoided because it may cause nausea and vomiting, sedation, severe headache, and visual disturbances.

Caution is warranted if general anesthesia or sedation is required because of the increased risk for hypotensive episode.

Notify the physician if bleeding, easy bruising, fever, or sore throat occurs. WBC count with differential, platelet count, and reticulocyte count, bone marrow test results, urinalysis results, BUN level, blood hematocrit and hemoglobin levels, serum alkaline phosphatase, AST (SGOT), and ALT (SGPT) levels should be monitored before and periodically during procarbazine therapy. Procarbazine should be discontinued if stomatitis, diarrhea, paraesthesia, neuropathy, confusion, or a hypersensitivity reaction occurs, WBC count falls to <4000/mm^3, or if the platelet count falls to <100,000/mm^3.
Administration
Administer procarbazine with food or fluids if the patient has severe GI side effects or difficulty swallowing.

P

Prochlorperazine
proe-klor-per'a-zeen
(Compazine, Stemetil [CAN], Stemzine [AUS])
Do not confuse prochlorperazine with chlorpromazine or Compazine with Copaxone.

CATEGORY AND SCHEDULE
Pregnancy Risk Category: C

Classification: Antiemetics/antivertigo, antipsychotics, phenothiazines

MECHANISM OF ACTION

A phenothiazine that acts centrally to inhibit or block dopamine receptors in the chemoreceptor trigger zone and peripherally to block the vagus nerve in the GI tract. *Therapeutic Effect:* Relieves nausea and vomiting and improves psychotic conditions.

PHARMACOKINETICS

Route	Onset* (min)	Peak	Duration (h)
Tablets, oral solution	30-40	NA	3-4
Capsules (extended release)	30-40	NA	10-12
Rectal	60	NA	3-4

*As an antiemetic.

Variably absorbed after PO administration. Widely distributed. Metabolized in the liver and GI mucosa. Excreted primarily in urine. Unknown whether removed by hemodialysis. *Half-life:* 23 h.

AVAILABILITY

Capsules (Extended-Release): 10 mg, 15 mg.
Oral Solution: 5 mg/5 mL.
Tablets: 5 mg, 10 mg.
Suppositories: 2.5 mg, 5 mg, 25 mg. Injection (Compazine): 5 mg/mL.

INDICATIONS AND DOSAGES

▸ **Nausea and vomiting**
PO
Adults, Elderly. 5-10 mg 3-4 times a day.
Children weighing 18-39 kg. 2.5 mg 3 times/day or 5 mg 2 times/day.
Children weighing 14-17 kg. 2.5 mg 2-3 times/day.
Children weighing 9-13 kg. 2.5 mg 1-2 times/day.

PO (EXTENDED-RELEASE)
Adults, Elderly. 10-15 mg twice daily.
IV
Adults, Elderly. 5-10 mg. May repeat q3-4h.
Children. 0.132 mg/kg/dose q6-8 h.
Adults, Elderly. 5-10 mg q3-4h.
Children. 0.132 mg/kg/dose q6-8h.
RECTAL
Adults, Elderly. 25 mg twice a day.
Children weighing 18-39 kg. 2.5 mg 3 times/day or 5 mg 2 times/day.
Children weighing 14-17 kg. 2.5 mg 2-3 times/day.
Children weighing 9-13 kg. 2.5 mg 1-2 times/day.
▸ **Psychosis**
PO
Adults, Elderly. 5-10 mg 3-4 times a day. Maximum: 150 mg/day.
Children. 2.5 mg 2-3 times a day. Maximum: 25 mg for children aged 6-12 yr; 20 mg for children aged 2-5 yr.
IM
Adults, Elderly. 10-20 mg q1-4h.
Children. 0.132 mg/kg/dose.

CONTRAINDICATIONS

Angle-closure glaucoma, central nervous system (CNS) depression, coma, myelosuppression, severe cardiac or hepatic impairment, severe hypotension or hypertension, agranulocytosis, phenothiazine hypersensitivity, dementia.
Caution
Children younger than 2 yr, elderly.

INTERACTIONS

Drug
Alcohol, other CNS depressants, barbiturate anesthetics, opioid analgesics: May increase CNS and respiratory depression and the hypotensive effects of prochlorperazine.
Anticholinergics: May increase anticholinergic effects.

Antihypertensives: May increase hypotension.
Antithyroid agents: May increase the risk of agranulocytosis.
Epinephrine: Possible risk of hypotension, tachycardia.
Levodopa: May decrease the effects of levodopa.
Lithium: May decrease the absorption of prochlorperazine and produce adverse neurologic effects.
MAOIs, tricyclic antidepressants: May increase the anticholinergic and sedative effects of prochlorperazine.
Phenothiazines and related drugs (haloperidol, droperidol), metoclopramide: May increase extrapyramidal symptoms.
Tetracyclines: Possible additive photosensitization.
Herbal
None known.
Food
None known.

DIAGNOSTIC TEST EFFECTS
None known.

ⓘ IV INCOMPATIBILITIES
Manufacturer recommends that drug not be mixed with other agents in the syringe. For IV infusion, the drug is incompatible with many drugs; refer to specialty references to check compatibilities.

SIDE EFFECTS
Frequent
Somnolence, hypotension, dizziness, fainting (commonly occurring after first dose, occasionally after subsequent doses, and rarely with oral form).
Occasional
Dry mouth, blurred vision, lethargy, constipation, diarrhea, myalgia, nasal congestion, peripheral edema, urine retention.

SERIOUS REACTIONS
• Extrapyramidal symptoms appear to be dose-related and are divided into three categories: akathisia (marked by inability to sit still, tapping of feet), parkinsonian symptoms (including masklike face, tremors, shuffling gait, hypersalivation), and acute dystonias (such as torticollis, opisthotonos, and oculogyric crisis). A dystonic reaction may also produce diaphoresis or pallor.
• Tardive dyskinesia, manifested as tongue protrusion, puffing of the cheeks, and puckering of the mouth, is a rare reaction that may be irreversible.
• Abrupt withdrawal after long-term therapy may precipitate nausea, vomiting, gastritis, dizziness, and tremors.
• Blood dyscrasias, particularly agranulocytosis and mild leukopenia, may occur.
• Prochlorperazine use may lower the seizure threshold.

PRECAUTIONS & CONSIDERATIONS
Caution is warranted in patients with Parkinson disease or seizures and in children younger than 2 yr.

Prochlorperazine crosses the placenta and is distributed in breast milk. The safety and efficacy of this drug have not been established in children younger than 2 yr or weighing < 9 kg. A decreased prochlorperazine dosage is recommended for elderly patients, who are more susceptible to the drug's sedative, anticholinergic, extrapyramidal, and hypotensive effects. Alcohol, barbiturates, and tasks that require mental alertness or motor skills should be avoided and limit caffeine consumption. Orthostatic hypotension may occur; avoid rapid postural changes.

BP, CBC for blood dyscrasias, and hydration status should

be monitored. Be alert for extrapyramidal symptoms such as rapid tongue movement.

Signs of tardive dyskinesia or akathisia need to be immediately reported to the health care provider.
Storage
Store prochlorperazine at room temperature and protect from light. Solution should be clear or slightly yellow.
Administration
Take oral prochlorperazine without regard to food. Avoid skin contact with prochlorperazine oral solution because it may cause contact dermatitis.

For IV use, keep the person recumbent—head low and legs raised—for 30-60 min after drug administration to minimize the drug's hypotensive effect. May give by IV push slowly over 5-10 min. May give by IV infusion over 30 min. IM injection should be made deeply into the dorsogluteal muscle.

For rectal use, moisten the suppository with cold water before inserting it well into the rectum.

Procyclidine
proe-sye-kli-deen
(Kemadrin)

CATEGORY AND SCHEDULE
Pregnancy Risk Category: C

Classification: Anticholinergics, antidyskinetic

MECHANISM OF ACTION
An anticholinergic agent that exerts an atropine-like action and produces an antispasmodic effect on smooth muscle, is a potent mydriatic, and inhibits salivation. *Therapeutic Effect:* Relieves symptoms of Parkinson disease and drug-induced extrapyramidal symptoms.

PHARMACOKINETICS
Well absorbed from the GI tract. Protein binding: extensive. Metabolized in liver—undergoes extensive first-pass effect. Primarily excreted in urine. Unknown whether removed by hemodialysis. *Half-life:* 7.7-16.1 h.

AVAILABILITY
Tablets: 5 mg (Kemadrin).

INDICATIONS AND DOSAGES
▸ **Drug-induced extrapyramidal reactions**
PO
Adults, Elderly. Initially, 2.5 mg 3 times/day. May increase by 2.5 mg/day as needed. Maintenance: 10-20 mg/day in divided doses 3 times/day.
▸ **Parkinson disease**
PO
Adults, Elderly. Initially, 2.5 mg 3 times/day after meals. Maintenance: 2.5-5 mg/day in divided doses 3 times/day after meals.
▸ **Hepatic function impairment**
PO
Adults, Elderly. 2.5-5 mg/day in divided doses twice a day after meals.

CONTRAINDICATIONS
Angle-closure glaucoma, elderly, breast-feeding, tachycardia, prostatic hypertrophy, children, kidney or liver disease, drug abuse, hypotension, myasthenia gravis, megacolin, hypertension, psychiatric patients.

INTERACTIONS
Drug
Alcohol, central nervous system (CNS) depressants: May increase sedation.

Amantadine, narcotic analgesics (meperidine), phenothiazines, tricyclic antidepressants, quinidine, antihistamines: May increase anticholinergic effects.
Bicarbonate-containing products: Delay taking for 1 h after procyclidine dosage.
Levodopa: May increase gastric degradation of levodopa and decrease the amount of levodopa absorbed by gastric emptying.
Paroxetine: May increase anticholinergic effects.
Herbal
Betel nut: May decrease anticholinergic effect of procyclidine.
Food
None known.

DIAGNOSTIC TEST EFFECTS

None known.

SIDE EFFECTS

Frequent
Blurred vision, mydriasis, disorientation, lightheadedness, nausea, vomiting, dry mouth, nose, throat, and lips.

SERIOUS REACTIONS

• Overdosage may vary from severe anticholinergic effects, such as unsteadiness; severe drowsiness; severe dryness of mouth, nose, or throat; tachycardia, shortness of breath; and skin flushing.
• Also produces severe paradoxical reaction, marked by hallucinations, tremor, seizures, and toxic psychosis.

PRECAUTIONS & CONSIDERATIONS

Caution is necessary with hypotension, mental disorders, prostatic hypertrophy, tachycardia, and urinary retention. It is unknown whether procyclidine is distributed in breast milk. Procyclidine is not indicated for pediatric use. Elderly patients

may exhibit increased sensitivity to procyclidine's anticholinergic effects. Tasks that require mental alertness or motor skills should be avoided. Alcoholic beverages should be avoided during procyclidine therapy.

Dizziness, drowsiness, and dry mouth are expected responses to the drug. These symptoms tend to diminish or disappear with continued therapy. Orthostatic hypotension may occur; avoid rapid postural changes.
Administration
Take procyclidine after meals to minimize GI upset.

Progesterone
proe-jess'ter-one
(Crinone, Prochieve, Prometrium)

CATEGORY AND SCHEDULE
Pregnancy Risk Category: D

Classification: Contraceptives, hormones/hormone modifiers, progestins

P

MECHANISM OF ACTION
A natural steroid hormone that promotes mammary gland development and relaxes uterine smooth muscle. *Therapeutic Effect:* Decreases abnormal uterine bleeding; transforms endometrium from proliferative to secretory in an estrogen-primed endometrium.

PHARMACOKINETICS
IM, rectal, vaginal: Duration 24 h; excreted in urine, feces; metabolized in liver.

AVAILABILITY
Capsules (Prometrium): 100 mg, 200 mg.
Injection: 50 mg/mL.

Vaginal Gel (Crinone, Prochieve):
4% (45 mg), 8% (90 mg).
Suppository (Progesterone): 10 mg,
25 mg.

INDICATIONS AND DOSAGES
▶ **Amenorrhea**
PO
Adults. 400 mg daily in evening for
10 days.
IM
Adults. 5-10 mg for 6-8 days.
Withdrawal bleeding expected in
48-72 h if ovarian activity produced
proliferative endometrium.
VAGINAL
Adults. Apply 45 mg (4% gel) every
other day for 6 or fewer doses.
▶ **Abnormal uterine bleeding**
IM
Adults. 5-10 mg for 6 days. When
estrogen given concomitantly, begin
progesterone after 2 wks of estrogen
therapy; discontinue when menstrual
flow begins.
▶ **Prevention of endometrial
hyperplasia**
PO
Adults. 200 mg in evening for 12 days
per 28-day cycle in combination with
daily conjugated estrogen.
▶ **Infertility**
VAGINAL
Adults. 90 mg (8% gel) once a day
(2 twice a day in women with partial
or complete ovarian failure).

OFF-LABEL USES
Treatment of corpus luteum
dysfunction, premenstrual syndrome,
preterm delivery prophylaxis.

CONTRAINDICATIONS
Breast cancer; history of active
cerebral apoplexy; thromboembolic
disorders or thrombophlebitis;
missed abortion; severe hepatic
dysfunction; undiagnosed vaginal
bleeding; use as a pregnancy test.

INTERACTIONS
Drug
Bromocriptine: May interfere with
the effects of bromocriptine.
Herbal
None known.
Food
None known.

DIAGNOSTIC TEST EFFECTS
May increase serum LDL and serum
alkaline phosphatase levels. May
decrease glucose tolerance and HDL
concentrations. May cause abnormal
serum thyroid, metapyrone, hepatic,
and endocrine function test results.

SIDE EFFECTS
Frequent
Breakthrough bleeding or spotting
at beginning of therapy, amenorrhea,
change in menstrual flow, breast
tenderness.
Gel: drowsiness.
Occasional
Edema, weight gain or loss, rash,
pruritus, photosensitivity, skin
pigmentation.
Rare
Pain or swelling at injection site,
acne, depression, alopecia, hirsutism.

SERIOUS REACTIONS
• Thrombophlebitis, cerebrovascular
disorders, retinal thrombosis, and
pulmonary embolism occur rarely.
Caution
Some formulations include peanut or
sesame oil; possible hypersensitivity
possible. Cervical and vaginal
cancer, Uterine cancer, IV
administration, ectopic pregnancy.

PRECAUTIONS & CONSIDERATIONS
Caution is warranted in patients
with conditions aggravated by fluid
retention, diabetes mellitus, and
history of depression. Progesterone
use should be avoided during

pregnancy. Progesterone is distributed in breast milk. Safety and efficacy of progesterone have not been established in children. No age-related precautions have been noted in elderly patients. Women using progesterone vaginal gel form should avoid performing tasks that require mental alertness or motor skills until response to the drug has been established. Use sunscreen and wear protective clothing until tolerance to sunlight and ultraviolet light has been determined. Avoid smoking because of the increased risk of blood clot formation and myocardial infarction (MI). Some patients experience drowsiness; do not drive or perform other tasks requiring mental alertness.

Notify the physician of chest pain, migraine headache, peripheral paresthesia, sudden decrease in vision, sudden shortness of breath, pain, redness, swelling, warmth in the calf, abnormal vaginal bleeding, or other symptoms. BP and weight should be monitored.

Patient should be assessed for allergy to peanuts and sesame seed as some formulations (Prometrium) include these oils and should be avoided in hypersensitive individuals.
Storage
Store progesterone at room temperature.
Administration
Take the daily dose of oral progesterone in the evening to minimize the effects of dizziness and drowsiness. If the dose is taken in the morning, take it 2 h after breakfast.

Shake vial well before withdrawing dose. Administer deep IM injection only in the upper arm or outer quadrant of gluteal muscle. Rarely, a residual lump, change in skin color, or sterile abscess occurs at the injection site. Rotate injection sites.

Promethazine Hydrochloride
proe-meth′a-zeen high-droh-clor-ide
(Insomn-Eze [AUS], Phenadoz, Phenergan)
Do not confuse promethazine with promazine.

CATEGORY AND SCHEDULE
Pregnancy Risk Category: C

Classification: Antiemetics/ antivertigo, antihistamines, H1 receptor antagonist, phenothiazines

MECHANISM OF ACTION
A phenothiazine that acts as an antihistamine, antiemetic, and sedative-hypnotic. As an antihistamine, inhibits histamine at histamine receptor sites. As an antiemetic, diminishes vestibular stimulation, depresses labyrinthine function, and acts on the chemoreceptor trigger zone. As a sedative-hypnotic, produces central nervous system (CNS) depression by decreasing stimulation to the brain stem reticular formation. *Therapeutic Effect:* Prevents allergic responses mediated by histamine, such as rhinitis, urticaria, and pruritus. Prevents and relieves nausea and vomiting.

PHARMACOKINETICS

Route	Onset (min)	Peak	Duration (h)
PO	20	NA	2-8
IV	3-5	NA	2-8
IM	20	NA	2-8
Rectal	20	NA	2-8

P

Well absorbed from the GI tract after IM administration. Widely distributed. Metabolized in the liver. Excreted primarily in urine. Not removed by hemodialysis. *Half-life:* 16-19 h.

AVAILABILITY

Syrup (Phenergan): 6.25 mg/mL.
Tablets (Phenergan): 12.5 mg, 25 mg, 50 mg.
Injection (Phenergan): 25 mg/mL, 50 mg/mL.
Suppositories (Phenergan): 12.5 mg, 25 mg, 50 mg.
Suppositories (Phenadoz): 25 mg.

INDICATIONS AND DOSAGES
▶ **Allergic symptoms**
PO
Adults, Elderly. 12.5 mg 3 times a day and at bedtime.
Children. 6.25-12.5 mg 3 times/day as needed.
IV, IM
Adults, Elderly. 25 mg. May repeat in 2 h.
▶ **Motion sickness**
PO
Adults, Elderly. 25 mg 30-60 min before departure; may repeat q12h as needed.
Children. 12.5-25 mg twice daily as needed, with first dose given 30-60 min before departure.
▶ **Prevention of nausea and vomiting**
PO, IV, IM, RECTAL
Adults, Elderly. 12.5-25 mg q4-6h as needed.
Children. 0.5 mg/lb every 4-6h as needed.
▶ **Preoperative and postoperative sedation; adjunct to analgesics**
IV, IM
Adults, Elderly. 25-50 mg as a single dose.
Children. 12.5-25 mg as a single dose.
▶ **Sedative**
PO, IV, IM, RECTAL

Adults, Elderly. 25-50 mg at bedtime.
Children. 0.5 mg/lb at bedtime. Maximum: 25 mg/dose.

CONTRAINDICATIONS

Angle-closure glaucoma, GI or genitourinary obstruction, severe CNS depression or coma
Caution
Increaseed intraocular pressure, renal disease, cardiac disease, hypertension, bronchial asthma, seizure disorder, stenosed peptic ulcers, hyperthroidism, benign prostatic hypertrophy, bladder neck obstruction, jaundice, bone marrow suppression.

INTERACTIONS
Drug
Alcohol, other CNS depressants: May increase CNS depressant effects.
Anticholinergics: May increase anticholinergic effects.
General anesthetics: May cause hypotensive effects.
MAOIs: May intensify and prolong the anticholinergic and CNS depressant effects of promethazine.
Herbal
None known.
Food
None known.

DIAGNOSTIC TEST EFFECTS

May suppress wheal and flare reactions to antigen skin testing unless the drug is discontinued 4 days before testing.

ⓦ IV INCOMPATIBILITIES

Allopurinol (Aloprim), amphotericin B complex (Abelcet, AmBisome, Amphotec), heparin, ketorolac (Toradol), nalbuphine (Nubain), piperacillin and tazobactam (Zosyn).

⚗ IV COMPATIBILITIES

Atropine, diphenhydramine (Benadryl), glycopyrrolate (Robinul), hydromorphone (Dilaudid), hydroxyzine (Vistaril), meperidine (Demerol), midazolam (Versed), morphine, nalbuphine (Nubain), prochlorperazine (Compazine).

SIDE EFFECTS

Expected
Somnolence, disorientation; in elderly, hypotension, confusion, syncope.
Frequent
Dry mouth, nose, or throat; urine retention; thickening of bronchial secretions.
Occasional
Epigastric distress, flushing, visual disturbances, hearing disturbances, wheezing, paresthesia, diaphoresis, chills.
Rare
Dizziness, urticaria, photosensitivity, nightmares.

SERIOUS REACTIONS

• Children may experience paradoxical reactions, such as excitation, nervousness, tremor, hyperactive reflexes, and seizures.
• Infants and young children have experienced CNS depression manifested as respiratory depression, sleep apnea, and sudden infant death syndrome.
• Long-term therapy may produce extrapyramidal symptoms, such as dystonia (abnormal movements), pronounced motor restlessness (most frequently in children), and parkinsonian (most frequently in elderly patients).
• Blood dyscrasias, particularly agranulocytosis, occur rarely.

PRECAUTIONS & CONSIDERATIONS

Caution is warranted in patients with asthma, history of seizures, cardiovascular disease, hepatic impairment, peptic ulcer disease, sleep apnea, and possible Reye syndrome. Promethazine readily crosses the placenta and may produce extrapyramidal symptoms and jaundice in neonates if taken during pregnancy. It is unknown whether the drug is excreted in breast milk. Children are more likely to experience paradoxical reactions, such as increased excitement, nervousness, and tremor. Promethazine is not recommended for children younger than 2 yr. Elderly patients are more sensitive to the drug's anticholinergic effects, such as dry mouth, confusion, dizziness, hypotension, syncope, and sedation. Avoid CNS depressants, drinking alcoholic beverages, and tasks that require alertness or motor skills until response to the drug is established.

Drowsiness and dry mouth may occur. Pulse rate, electrolytes, BP, and therapeutic response should be monitored.

Assess vital signs 30 min after dosing if used as a sedative.
Storage
Store vials at room temperature. Refrigerate rectal suppositories.
Administration
Take promethazine without regard to food. Crush scored tablets as needed.

For IV use, promethazine may be given undiluted or diluted with 0.9% NaCl; final dilution should not exceed 25 mg/mL. Inject the drug at a rate of 25 mg/min through the tubing of an infusing IV solution, as prescribed. Injecting the drug too rapidly may cause a transient drop in BP, resulting in orthostatic hypotension and reflex tachycardia. ! Avoid giving subcutaneously because significant tissue necrosis may occur. Inject the drug carefully because inadvertent intra-arterial

P

injection may produce severe arteriospasm, possibly resulting in gangrene.

For IM use, inject deep into a large muscle mass.

For rectal use, unwrap and moisten the suppository with cold water before inserting it well into the rectum.

Propafenone Hydrochloride
proe-pa-fen′one high-droh-clor-ide
(Rythmol, Rythmol SR)

CATEGORY AND SCHEDULE
Pregnancy Risk Category: C

Classification: Antiarrhythmics, class IC

MECHANISM OF ACTION
An antiarrhythmic that decreases the fast sodium current in Purkinje or myocardial cells. Decreases excitability and automaticity; prolongs conduction velocity and the refractory period. *Therapeutic Effect:* Suppresses arrhythmias.

PHARMACOKINETICS
Peak 3-5 h. *Half-life:* 2-10 h. Metabolized in liver; excreted in urine (metabolite).

AVAILABILITY
Tablets (Rythmol): 150 mg, 225 mg, 300 mg.
Capsules (Extended-Release [Rythmol SR]): 225 mg, 325 mg, 425 mg.

INDICATIONS AND DOSAGES
▸ **Documented life-threatening ventricular arrhythmias, such as sustained ventricular tachycardia**

PO, PROMPT-RELEASE
Adults, Elderly. Initially, 150 mg q8h; may increase at 3- to 4-day intervals to 225 mg q8h, then to 300 mg q8h. Maximum: 900 mg/day.
PO, EXTENDED-RELEASE
Adults, Elderly. Initially, 225 mg q12h. May increase at 5-day intervals. Maximum: 425 mg q12h.

OFF-LABEL USES
Treatment of supraventricular arrhythmias. Wolff-Parkinson-White syndrome.

CONTRAINDICATIONS
Bradycardia; bronchospastic disorders; cardiogenic shock; electrolyte imbalance; sinoatrial, AV, and intraventricular impulse generation or conduction disorders, such as sick sinus syndrome or AV block, without the presence of a pacemaker; uncontrolled congestive heart failure (CHF).
Caution
CHF, hypokalemia, hyperkalemia, recent myocardial infarction (MI), nonallergic bronchospasm, breast-feeding, children, hepatic or renal disease.

INTERACTIONS
Drug
No specific interactions are reported; however, any drug that could affect the cardiac action of propafenone (other local anesthetics, vasoconstrictors, anticholinergics) should be used in the lowest effective dose.
Herbal
None known.
Food
None known.

DIAGNOSTIC TEST EFFECTS
May cause ECG changes, such as QRS widening and PR interval prolongation, and positive ANA titers.

SIDE EFFECTS
Frequent (7%-13%)
Dizziness, nausea, vomiting, altered taste, constipation.
Occasional (3%-6%)
Headache, dyspnea, blurred vision, dyspepsia (heartburn, indigestion, epigastric pain).
Rare (< 2%)
Rash, weakness, dry mouth, diarrhea, edema, hot flashes.

SERIOUS REACTIONS
• Propafenone may produce or worsen existing arrhythmias.
• Overdose may produce hypotension, somnolence, bradycardia, and atrioventricular conduction disturbances.

PRECAUTIONS & CONSIDERATIONS
Caution is warranted with CHF, conduction disturbances, impaired hepatic or renal function, and recent MI.

Altered taste sensation may occur while taking propafenone. Notify the physician if blurred vision, GI upset, dizziness, or headache occurs. Tasks that require mental alertness or motor skills should be avoided until response to the drug has been established. Electrolyte imbalances should be corrected before beginning propafenone therapy. Pulse rate for quality and irregularity, pattern of daily bowel activity and stool consistency, serum electrolyte levels, and hepatic enzymes should be assessed. Patient should be assessed for stress responses that can have adverse cardiovascular effects.
Administration
Take without regard to meals. Do not skip doses. Therapeutic serum level is 0.06-1 mcg/mL.

Propantheline
proe-pan-the-leen
(Pro-Banthine, Propanthl [CAN])

CATEGORY AND SCHEDULE
Pregnancy Risk Category: C

Classification: Anticholinergics

MECHANISM OF ACTION
A quaternary ammonium compound that has anticholinergic properties and that inhibits action of acetylcholine at postganglionic parasympathetic sites. *Therapeutic Effect:* Reduces gastric secretions and urinary frequency, urgency and urge incontinence.

PHARMACOKINETICS
Onset occurs within 90 min but < 50% is absorbed from the GI tract. Extensive hepatic metabolism. Excreted in the urine and feces. *Half-life:* 2.9 h.

AVAILABILITY
Tablets: 7.5 mg, 15 mg (Pro-Banthine).

INDICATIONS AND DOSAGES
▶ **Peptic ulcer**
PO
Adults, Elderly. 15 mg 3 times/day 30 min before meals and 30 mg at bedtime.
Children. 1-2 mg/kg/day in 3-4 divided doses.

CONTRAINDICATIONS
GI or genitourinary (GU) obstruction, myasthenia gravis, narrow-angle glaucoma, autonomic neuropathy, toxic megacolon, severe ulcerative colitis, unstable cardiovascular adjustment in acute hemorrhage, hypersensitivity to propantheline or other anticholinergics.

INTERACTIONS
Drug
Digoxin: May increase serum digoxin levels by increasing absorption due to decreased gastrointestinal motility.
Herbal
None known.
Food
None known.

SIDE EFFECTS
Frequent
Dry mouth, decreased sweating, constipation.
Occasional
Blurred vision, intolerance to light, urinary hesitancy, drowsiness, agitation, excitement.
Rare
Confusion, increased intraocular pressure, orthostatic hypotension, tachycardia.

SERIOUS REACTIONS
• Overdosage may produce temporary paralysis of ciliary muscle, pupillary dilation, tachycardia, palpitations, hot, dry, or flushed skin, absence of bowel sounds, hyperthermia, increased respiratory rate, ECG abnormalities, nausea, vomiting, rash over face or upper trunk, central nervous system stimulation, and psychosis, marked by agitation, restlessness, rambling speech, visual hallucinations, paranoid behavior, and delusions, followed by depression.
Caution
Hyperthyroidism, coronary artery disease, dysrhythmias, CHF, ulcerative colitis, hypertension, hiatal hernia, hepatic disease, renal disease, pregnancy category C, urinary retention, benign prostatic hypertrophy.
Hypersensitivity to propantheline or other anticholinergics.

PRECAUTIONS & CONSIDERATIONS
Caution is warranted with chronic obstructive pulmonary disease (COPD), CHF, coronary artery disease, esophageal reflux or hiatal hernia associated with reflux esophagitis, gastric ulcer, hyperthyroidism, hypertension, liver or renal disease, tachyarrhythmias, autonomic neuropathy, diarrhea, known or suspected GI infections, and mild to moderate ulcerative colitis. It is unknown whether propantheline crosses the placenta or is distributed in breast milk. Infants and young children are more susceptible to the drug's toxic effects. Propantheline use in elderly patients may cause agitation, confusion, drowsiness, or excitement. Hot baths and saunas should be avoided.

Tasks that require mental alertness or motor skills should be avoided.

Dry mouth may be experienced during therapy. Good oral hygiene should be practiced. Physicians should be alerted to any significant xerostomic side effects such as increased caries, sore tongue, problems eating or swallowing, difficulty wearing prosthesis, as a medication change may need to be considered.
Administration
Give propantheline 30 min before meals and at bedtime.

Propofol
pro-poe-fall
(Diprivan Recofol[AUS])

CATEGORY AND SCHEDULE
Pregnancy Risk Category: B

Classification: Anesthetics, general

MECHANISM OF ACTION

A rapidly acting general anesthetic that inhibits sympathetic vasoconstrictor nerve activity and decreases vascular resistance. *Therapeutic Effect:* Produces hypnosis rapidly.

PHARMACOKINETICS

Route	Onset	Peak	Duration
IV	40 s	N/A	3-10 min

Rapidly and extensively distributed. Protein binding: 97%-99%. Metabolized in the liver. Excreted primarily in urine. Unknown whether removed by hemodialysis. *Half-life:* 3-12 h.

AVAILABILITY

Injection: 10 mg/mL.

INDICATIONS AND DOSAGES
▸ **Intensive care unit sedation**
IV

Adults, Elderly. Initially, 0.3 mg/kg/h. May increase by 0.3-0.6 mg/kg/h q5-10 min until desired effect is obtained. Maintenance: 0.3-3 mg/kg/h.
▸ **Anesthesia**
IV

Adults, American Society of Anesthesiologists (ASA) I and II patients. 2-2.5 mg/kg (about 40 mg q10sec until onset of anesthesia). Maintenance: 0.1-0.2 mg/kg/min. *Elderly, Debilitated, Hypovolemic, ASA III or IV patients.* 1-1.5 mg/kg (about 20 mg q10sec until onset of anesthesia). Maintenance: 0.05-0.1 mg/kg/min. *Children aged 3 yr and older, ASA I or II patients.* 2.5-3.5 mg/kg (lower dosage for ASA III or IV patients). *Children aged 2 mo to 16 yr.* Maintenance dose: 0.125-0.3 mg/kg/min.

CONTRAINDICATIONS

Impaired cerebral circulation, increased intracranial pressure (ICP).
Caution
Elderly, debilitated, respiratory depression, severe respiratory disorders, cardiac dysrhythmias, pregnancy Category B, labor and delivery, lactation, children younger than 3 yr, epilepsy, egg hypersensitivity, soy lecithin hypersensitivity.

INTERACTIONS
Drug
Alcohol, narcotics, sedative-hypnotics, antipsychotics, skeletal muscle relaxants, inhalational anesthetics, other CNS depressants: May increase hypotensive and CNS and respiratory depressant effects of propofol.
Herbal
None known.
Food
None known.

DIAGNOSTIC TEST EFFECTS
None known.

Ⓓ IV INCOMPATIBILITIES
Amikacin (Amikin), amphotericin B complex (Abelcet, AmBisome, Amphotec), bretylium (Bretylol), calcium chloride, ciprofloxacin (Cipro), diazepam (Valium), digoxin (Lanoxin), doxorubicin (Adriamycin), gentamicin (Garamycin), methylprednisolone (Solu-Medrol), minocycline (Minocin), phenytoin (Dilantin), tobramycin (Nebcin), verapamil (Isoptin).

Ⓔ IV COMPATIBILITIES
Acyclovir (Zovirax), bumetanide (Bumex), calcium gluconate, ceftazidime (Fortaz), dobutamine (Dobutrex), dopamine (Intropin), enalapril (Vasotec), fentanyl, heparin,

P

insulin, labetalol (Normodyne, Trandate), lidocaine, lorazepam (Ativan), magnesium, milrinone (Primacor), nitroglycerin, norepinephrine (Levophed), potassium chloride, vancomycin (Vancocin).

SIDE EFFECTS
Frequent
Involuntary muscle movements, apnea (common during induction; lasts longer than 60 s), hypotension, nausea, vomiting, IV site burning or stinging or phlebitis.
Occasional
Twitching, bucking, jerking, thrashing, headache, dizziness, bradycardia, hypertension, fever, abdominal cramps, paresthesia, coldness, cough, hiccups, facial flushing, greenish-colored urine.
Rare
Rash, dry mouth, agitation, confusion, myalgia, thrombophlebitis.

SERIOUS REACTIONS
• A continuous infusion or repeated intermittent infusions of propofol may result in extreme somnolence, respiratory depression, and circulatory depression.
• Too-rapid IV administration may produce severe hypotension, respiratory depression, and involuntary muscle movements.
• The patient may experience an acute allergic reaction, characterized by abdominal pain, anxiety, restlessness, dyspnea, erythema, hypotension, pruritus, rhinitis, and urticaria.

PRECAUTIONS & CONSIDERATIONS
Caution is warranted in patients with circulatory, hepatic, lipid metabolism, renal, or respiratory disorder, history of epilepsy and in debilitated patients. Propofol crosses the placenta and is not recommended

for obstetric use. Propofol is distributed in breast milk and is not recommended for breast-feeding women. The safety and efficacy of propofol have not been established in children. However, the Food and Drug Administration has approved the drug for use in children older than 3 yr. Lower propofol dosages are recommended for elderly patients.

Drug should only be administered by qualified personnel trained in anesthesia; resuscitative equipment should be available. Changes in PVC, PAC, ST segment may be evidenced; frequent monitoring of ECG is recommended. Physician should be notified if patient's respirations are <10/min for possible CNS changes or respiratory dysfunction.

Be aware that urine may turn green. Vital signs should be obtained before propofol administration. ABG levels, BP, heart and respiratory rates, oxygen saturation, depth of sedation, and lipid and triglyceride levels should be monitored if propofol is given for longer than 24 h.

Overdosage is treated by discontinuing the drug, using artificial ventilation, vasopressor agents or anticholinergics.
Storage
Store propofol at room temperature. Do not use propofol if the emulsion separates.
Administration
! Don't give propofol through the same IV line as blood or plasma.

Shake well before using. Propofol may be given undiluted, or it may be diluted only with D5W to a concentration of no < 2 mg/mL (4 mL D5W to 1 mL propofol yields 2 mg/mL). Discard any unused portions of the drug. Too-rapid IV administration of propofol may produce irregular muscle movements, respiratory depression, and severe hypotension. Observe for signs of inadvertent intra-arterial injection, such as delayed onset of drug action, pain or discolored skin near the injection site, or blue or white discoloration of the hand if a hand or arm IV site is used.

Propoxyphene Hydrochloride/ Propoxyphene Napsylate

Pro-pox-y-feen high-droh-clo-ride/ nap-sigh-late
(Darvon, Doloxene [AUS])
(Darvon-N [CAN])
Do not confuse with Diovan.

CATEGORY AND SCHEDULE
Pregnancy Risk Category: C (D if used for prolonged periods)

Classification: Sythetic opioid narcotic analgesic

MECHANISM OF ACTION
An opioid agonist that binds with opioid receptors in the central nervous system (CNS). *Therapeutic Effect:* Alters the perception of and emotional response to pain.

PHARMACOKINETICS

Route	Onset	Peak	Duration
PO	15-60 min	N/A	4-6 h

Well absorbed from the GI tract. Protein binding: High. Widely distributed. Metabolized in the liver. Primarily excreted in urine. Not removed by hemodialysis. *Half-life:* 6-12 h; metabolite: 30-36 h.

AVAILABILITY
Capsules (Hydrochloride): 65 mg.
Tablets (Napsylate): 100 mg.

INDICATIONS AND DOSAGES
▸ **Mild to moderate pain**
PO (PROPOXYPHENE HYDROCHLORIDE)
Adults, Elderly. 65 mg q3-4h as needed. Maximum: 390 mg/day.
PO (PROPOXYPHENE NAPSYLATE)
Adults, Elderly. 100 mg q4h as needed. Maximum: 600 mg/day.

CONTRAINDICATIONS
Alcoholism, substance abuse, suicidal ideation.

INTERACTIONS
Drug
Acetaminophen, acetaminophen-containing products: May increase risk of hepatotoxicity.
Alcohol, other CNS depressants, narcotics, sedative-hypnotics, skeletal muscle relaxants: May increase CNS or respiratory depression and risk of hypotension.
Anticholinergics, antihypertensives: May cause increased effects of these drugs.
Buprenorphine: May decrease the effects of propoxyphene.
Carbamazepine: May increase the blood concentration and risk of toxicity of carbamazepine.
MAOIs: May produce a severe, sometimes fatal reaction. Use is contraindicated.
Herbal
None known.
Food
None known.

DIAGNOSTIC TEST EFFECTS
May increase serum alkaline phosphatase, lipase, amylase, bilirubin, LDH, AST (SGOT), and

P

ALT (SGPT) levels. Therapeutic serum drug level is 100-400 ng/mL; toxic serum drug level is > 500 ng/mL.

SIDE EFFECTS
Frequent
Dizziness, somnolence, dry mouth, euphoria, hypotension (including orthostatic hypotension), nausea, vomiting, fatigue.
Occasional
Allergic reaction (including decreased BP), diaphoresis, flushing, and wheezing), trembling, urine retention, vision changes, constipation, headache.
Rare
Confusion, increased BP, depression, abdominal cramps, anorexia.

SERIOUS REACTIONS
• Overdose results in respiratory depression, skeletal muscle flaccidity, cold or clammy skin, cyanosis, and extreme somnolence progressing to seizures, stupor, and coma.
• Hepatotoxicity may occur with overdose of the acetaminophen component of fixed-combination products.
• The patient who uses propoxyphene repeatedly may develop a tolerance to the drug's analgesic effect and physical dependence.
Caution
Addictive personality, lactation, increased intracranial pressure, myocardial infarction (acute), severe heart disease, respiratory depression, hepatic disease, renal disease, children younger than 18 yr, alcoholism.

PRECAUTIONS & CONSIDERATIONS
Caution is warranted in patients with hepatic or renal impairment and in those who are narcotic dependent. Propoxyphene crosses the placenta and a minimal amount of the drug is distributed in breast milk. Be aware that regular use of opioids during pregnancy may produce withdrawal symptoms in the neonate, including diarrhea, excessive crying, fever, hyperactive reflexes, irritability, seizures, sneezing, tremors, vomiting, and yawning. The neonate may develop respiratory depression if the mother receives propoxyphene during labor. The pediatric dosage of this drug has not been established. Avoid use in elderly patients, if possible. They may be more susceptible to propoxyphene's CNS effects and constipation. Psychological and physical dependence may occur with chronic use.

Dizziness and drowsiness may occur, so change positions slowly and avoid alcohol, CNS depressants, and tasks that require mental alertness or motor skills until response to the drug is established. Vital signs, pattern of daily bowel activity, and clinical improvement should be monitored. The drug should be held and the physician should be notified if the respiratory rate is 12 breaths/min or less in an adult or 20 breaths/min or less in a child.
Storage
Store at room temperature.
Administration
! Be aware that propoxyphene's side effects are dependent on the dosage. Know that ambulatory patients and patients not in severe pain are more likely to experience dizziness, hypotension, nausea, and vomiting than patients in the supine position and those in severe pain. Expect to reduce the initial dosage with Addison disease, hypothyroidism, and renal insufficiency, for the debilitated or elderly, and for those concurrently

taking CNS depressants. Be aware that the therapeutic serum level of propoxyphene is 100-400 ng/mL, and the toxic serum level is over 500 ng/mL.

Take oral propoxyphene without regard to food. Empty capsules and mix with food as needed. Do not crush or break film-coated tablets.

Administration with nonopioid analgesics (aspirin, NSAIDs, acetaminophen) permits better quality pain relief but may increase risk of GI side effects; hepatotoxicity with long-term or high-dose use.

Propranolol Hydrochloride

proe-pran′oh-lole high-droh-clo-ride (Apo-Propranolol [CAN], Deralin [AUS], Inderal, Inderal LA, InnoPran XL, Nu-Propranolol [CAN], Propranolol Intensol)
Do not confuse Inderal with Adderall or Isordil or Indocin or propranolol with Pravachol.

CATEGORY AND SCHEDULE
Pregnancy Risk Category: C (D if used in second or third trimester)

Classification: Nonselective β-adrenergic antagonist, class II

MECHANISM OF ACTION
An antihypertensive, antianginal, antiarrhythmic, and antimigraine agent that blocks β_1- and β_2-adrenergic receptors. Decreases oxygen requirements. Slows AV conduction and increases refractory period in AV node. Large doses increase airway resistance. *Therapeutic Effect:* Slows sinus heart rate; decreases cardiac output, BP, and myocardial ischemia severity. Exhibits antiarrhythmic activity.

PHARMACOKINETICS

Route	Onset	Peak	Duration
PO	1-2 h	N/A	6 h

Well absorbed from the GI tract. Protein binding: 93%. Widely distributed. Metabolized in the liver. Primarily excreted in urine. Not removed by hemodialysis. *Half-life:* 3-5 h.

AVAILABILITY
Tablets (Inderal): 10 mg, 20 mg, 40 mg, 60 mg, 80 mg.
Tablets (Propranolol): 10 mg, 20 mg, 40 mg, 60 mg, 80 mg, 120 mg, 160 mg.
Capsules (Extended-Release [Inderal LA]): 60 mg, 80 mg, 120 mg, 160 mg.
Capsules (Extended-Release [InnoPran XL]): 80 mg, 120 mg.
Oral Solution (Inderal): 4 mg/mL.
Oral Concentrate (Propranolol Intensol): 80 mg/mL.
Injection (Inderal): 1 mg/mL.

INDICATIONS AND DOSAGES
▶ **Hypertension**
PO
Adults, Elderly. Initially, 40 mg twice a day. May increase dose q3-7 days. Range: Up to 480 mg/day in divided doses. Maximum: 640 mg/day.
Children. Initially, 0.5-1 mg/kg/day in 4 divided doses. Usual dose: 1-5 mg/kg/day. Maximum: 8 mg/kg/day.
▶ **Angina**
PO
Adults, Elderly. 160-320 mg/day in divided doses. (long-acting): Initially, 80 mg/day. Maximum: 320 mg/day.

P

▸ **Arrhythmias**

IV

Adults, Elderly. Usual dose is 1-3 mg IV. Second dose can be give after 2-3 min if needed. Subsequent doses can be given every 4-6 h if needed.

PO

Adults, Elderly. Initially, 10-30 mg q6-8h. May gradually increase dose. Range: 80-320 mg/day.

▸ **Life-threatening arrhythmias**

IV

Adults, Elderly. Usual dose is 1-3 mg IV. Second dose can be give after 2-3 min if needed. Subsequent doses can be given every 4-6 h if needed.

▸ **Hypertrophic subaortic stenosis**

PO

Adults, Elderly. Usual dose is 1-3 mg IV. Second dose can be give after 2-3 min if needed. Subsequent dose can be given every 4-6 h if needed.

▸ **Adjunct to α-blocking agents to treat pheochromocytoma**

PO

Adults, Elderly. 60 mg/day in divided doses with α-blocker for 3 days before surgery. Maintenance (inoperable tumor): 30 mg/day with α-blocker.

▸ **Migraine headache**

PO

Adults, Elderly. 80 mg/day in divided doses. Or 80 mg once daily as extended-release capsule. Increase up to 160-240 mg/day in divided doses.

Children weighing > 35 kg. 20-40 mg 3 times/day.

Children weighing ≤ 35 kg. 10-20 mg 3 times/day.

▸ **Reduction of cardiovascular mortality and reinfarction in patients with previous myocardial infarction (MI)**

PO

Adults, Elderly. 180-240 mg/day in divided doses.

▸ **Essential tremor**

PO

Adults, Elderly. Initially, 40 mg twice a day increased up to 120-320 mg/day in 2-3 divided doses.

OFF-LABEL USES

Treatment adjunct for anxiety, mitral valve prolapse syndrome, thyrotoxicosis, acute myocardial infarction, esophageal varices, hemangioma, portal hypertension, scleroderma, renal crisis, unstable aneurysm, variceal bleeding prophylaxis.

CONTRAINDICATIONS

Asthma, bradycardia, cardiogenic shock, chronic obstructive pulmonary disease (COPD), heart block, Raynaud syndrome, uncompensated congestive heart failure (CHF).

INTERACTIONS

Drug

Didanosine: Possible decreased hypotensive effects.

Diphenhydramine: Suspected plasma level increases.

Diuretics, other antihypertensives: May increase hypotensive effect.

Epinephrine, ephedrine, OTC and Rx combination cold products, other sympathomimetics: Possible hypertensive effects or bradycardia.

Halogen, hydrocarbon inhalation anesthetics: May increase hypotensive effects and risk of myocardial depression.

Indomethacin, NSAIDs: May decrease hypotensive effect.

Insulin, oral hypoglycemics: May mask symptoms of hypoglycemia and prolong the hypoglycemic effect of insulin and oral hypoglycemics.

IV phenytoin: May increase cardiac depressant effect.

Lidocaine: Possible slower metabolism of lidocaine.

NSAIDs: May decrease antihypertensive effect.

Sympathomimetics, xanthines:
May mutually inhibit effects.
Herbal
None known.
Food
None known.

DIAGNOSTIC TEST EFFECTS

May increase serum antinuclear antibody titer and BUN, serum LDH, serum lipoprotein, serum alkaline phosphatase, serum bilirubin, serum creatinine, serum potassium, serum uric acid, AST (SGOT), ALT (SGPT), and serum triglyceride levels.

IV INCOMPATIBILITIES

Amphotericin B complex (Abelcet, AmBisome, Amphotec).

IV COMPATIBILITIES

Alteplase (Activase), heparin, milrinone (Primacor), potassium chloride, propofol (Diprivan).

SIDE EFFECTS

Frequent
Diminished sexual ability, drowsiness, difficulty sleeping, unusual fatigue or weakness.
Occasional
Bradycardia, depression, sensation of coldness in extremities, diarrhea, constipation, anxiety, nasal congestion, nausea, vomiting.
Rare
Altered taste, dry eyes, pruritus, paresthesia.

SERIOUS REACTIONS

• Overdose may produce profound bradycardia and hypotension.
• Abrupt withdrawal may result in sweating, palpitations, headache, and tremors.
• Propranolol administration may precipitate CHF and myocardial infarction (MI) in patients with cardiac disease; thyroid storm in those with thyrotoxicosis; and peripheral ischemia in those with existing peripheral vascular disease.
• Hypoglycemia may occur in patients with previously controlled diabetes.
Caution
Diabetes mellitus, renal disease, breast-feeding, hyperthroidism, COPD, hepatic disease, children, myasthenia gravis, peripheral vascular disease, hypotension.

PRECAUTIONS & CONSIDERATIONS

Caution should be used in those who are also receiving calcium channel blockers, especially when giving propranolol IV. Caution is also warranted with diabetes and hepatic and renal impairment. Propranolol crosses the placenta and is distributed in breast milk. Propranolol use should be avoided in pregnant women after the first trimester because it may result in low-birth-weight infants. The drug may also produce apnea, bradycardia, hypoglycemia, hypothermia during childbirth. No age-related precautions have been noted in children. In elderly patients, age-related peripheral vascular disease may increase susceptibility to decreased peripheral circulation. Be aware that salt and alcohol intake should be restricted. Nasal decongestants or OTC cold preparations (stimulants) should not be used without physician approval. Tasks that require mental alertness or motor skills should be avoided.

Notify the physician of behavioral changes, fatigue, rash, dizziness, excessively slow pulse rate (<60 beats/min), or peripheral numbness. BP for hypotension, respiratory status for shortness of breath, pattern of daily bowel activity and stool

P

consistency, ECG for arrhythmias, and pulse for quality, rate and rhythm should be monitored during treatment. If pulse rate is 60 beats/min or lower or systolic BP is < 90 mm Hg, withhold the medication and contact the physician. In those receiving propranolol for treatment of angina, the onset, type (sharp, dull, squeezing), radiation, location, intensity, and duration of anginal pain and its precipitating factors, including exertion and emotional stress should be recorded. Signs and symptoms of CHF, such as decreased urine output, distended neck veins, dyspnea (particularly on exertion or lying down), night cough, peripheral edema, and weight gain should also be assessed.

Abrupt withdrawal is contraindicated because it can result in palpitations, headache, tremors and sweating. Blood glucose levels should be monitored regularly after initiating therapy in patients with diabetes mellitus because propranolol can cause hyperglycemic effects. Rapid postural changes should be avoided because orthostatic hypotensive effects may occur.

Storage
Store at room temperature.

Administration
For oral use, crush scored tablets if necessary. Take at same time each day. Do not abruptly discontinue the drug. Compliance with the therapy regimen is essential to control anginal pain, arrhythmias, and hypertension.

For IV use, give undiluted for IV push. For IV infusion, may dilute each 1 mg in 10 mL D5W. Do not exceed 1 mg/min injection rate. For IV infusion, give 1 mg over 10-15 min.

Propylthiouracil
proe-pill-thye-oh-yoor'a-sill
(Propylthiouracil, Propyl-Thyracil [CAN])

CATEGORY AND SCHEDULE
Pregnancy Risk Category: D

Classification: Thyroid hormone antagonist

MECHANISM OF ACTION
A thiourea derivative that blocks oxidation of iodine in the thyroid gland and blocks synthesis of thyroxine and tri-iodothyronine. *Therapeutic Effect:* Inhibits synthesis of thyroid hormone.

PHARMACOKINETICS
Onset 30-40 min., duration 2-4 h. *Half-life:* 1-2 h; excreted in urine, bile and breast milk; crosses placental barrier.

AVAILABILITY
Tablets: 50 mg.

INDICATIONS AND DOSAGES
▸ **Hyperthyroidism**
PO
Adults, Elderly. Initially: 300-450 mg/day in divided doses q8h. Maintenance: 100-150 mg/day in divided doses q8-12h.
Children. Initially: 5-7 mg/kg/day in divided doses q8h. Maintenance: 33%-66% of initial dose in divided doses q8-12h.
Neonates. 5-10 mg/kg/day in divided doses q8h.

CONTRAINDICATIONS
Infection, bone marrow depression, hepatic disease.

Caution
Infection, bone marrow depression, hepatic disease.

INTERACTIONS
Drug
Amiodarone, iodinated glycerol, iodine, potassium iodide: May decrease response of propylthiouracil.
Anticholinergics, sympathomimetics: May increase side effects in uncontrolled patients.
Central nervous ystem (CNS) depressants: May be more responsive to depressant effects in uncontrolled hypothyroidism.
Digoxin: May increase digoxin blood concentration as patient becomes euthyroid.
I^{131}: May decrease thyroid uptake of I^{131}.
Oral anticoagulants: May decrease the effects of oral anticoagulants.
Vasoconstrictors: May increase risk in patients with uncontrolled hypothroidism.
Herbal
None known.
Food
None known.

DIAGNOSTIC TEST EFFECTS
May increase LDH, serum alkaline phosphatase, bilirubin, AST (SGOT), and ALT (SGPT) levels and prothrombin time.

SIDE EFFECTS
Frequent
Urticaria, rash, pruritus, nausea, skin pigmentation, hair loss, headache, paraesthesia.
Occasional
Somnolence, lymphadenopathy, vertigo.
Rare
Drug fever, lupus-like syndrome.

SERIOUS REACTIONS
• Agranulocytosis as long as 4 mo after therapy, pancytopenia, and fatal hepatitis have occurred.

PRECAUTIONS & CONSIDERATIONS
Caution is warranted with concurrent use of other agranulocytosis-inducing drugs and in persons older than 40 yr. Propylthiouracil crosses the placenta and should be avoided during pregnancy. Breast-feeding should be avoided. Use cautiously in children because of the risk of hepatic dysfunction. Restrict the consumption of iodine products and seafood.
Notify the physician of somnolence, jaundice, nausea, vomiting, illness, unusual bleeding or bruising, rash, itching, swollen lymph glands, or a pulse rate < 60 beats/min. Weight, pulse, prothrombin time, LDH, serum alkaline phosphatase, bilirubin, AST, and ALT levels should be monitored. Prolonged therapy may cause blood dyscrasias, evidenced by bleeding, infection, and poor healing.
Administration
Space doses evenly around the clock.

Protamine Sulfate
proe′ta-meen sull-fate
(Protamine [CAN], Protamine sulfate)
Do not confuse protamine with ProAmatine, Protopam, or Protropin.

CATEGORY AND SCHEDULE
Pregnancy Risk Category: C

Classification: Heparin antagonist

MECHANISM OF ACTION
A protein that complexes with heparin to form a stable salt.
Therapeutic Effect: Reduces anticoagulant activity of heparin.

P

PHARMACOKINETICS
IV: Onset 5 min; duration 2 h.

AVAILABILITY
Injection: 10 mg/mL.

INDICATIONS AND DOSAGES
▸ **Heparin overdose (antidote and treatment), hemorrhage**
IV
Adults, Elderly. 1 mg protamine sulfate neutralizes 90-115 units of heparin. Heparin disappears rapidly from circulation, reducing the dosage demand for protamine as time elapses.

OFF-LABEL USES
Treatment of enoxaparin toxicity.

CONTRAINDICATIONS
None known.

INTERACTIONS
Drug
Oral anticoagulants, including aspirin and NSAIDs: May increase anticoagulant effects, possible hemorrhage and should be avoided.
Herbal
None known.
Food
None known.

DIAGNOSTIC TEST EFFECTS
None known. Assessment of PPT, PT or INR, CBC, should be performed periodically to assess effectiveness.

SIDE EFFECTS
Frequent
Decreased BP, dyspnea.
Occasional
Hypersensitivity reaction (urticaria, angioedema); nausea and vomiting, which generally occur in those sensitive to fish and seafood, vasectomized men, infertile men, those on isophane (NPH) insulin,

or those previously on protamine therapy.
Rare
Back pain.

SERIOUS REACTIONS
• Too rapid IV administration may produce acute hypotension, bradycardia, pulmonary hypertension, dyspnea, transient flushing, and feeling of warmth.
• Heparin rebound may occur several hours after heparin has been neutralized (usually 8-9 h after protamine administration). Heparin rebound occurs most often after arterial or cardiac surgery.

PRECAUTIONS & CONSIDERATIONS
This drug is intended for use only in acute care situations in hospitals and emergency rooms. Caution is warranted with a history of allergy to fish and seafood, in those previously on protamine therapy because of a propensity to hypersensitivity reaction, and in infertile or vasectomized men and those on isophane (NPH) or insulin therapy. An electric razor or soft toothbrush should be used to prevent bleeding until coagulation studies normalize.

Notify the physician of black or red stool, coffee-ground vomitus, dark or red urine, or red-speckled mucus from cough. Activated clotting time, aPTT, BP, cardiac function, and other coagulation tests should be monitored.
Storage
Store vials at room temperature.
Administration
May give undiluted over 10 min. Do not exceed 5 mg/min or 50 mg in any 10-min period. Make sure the patient is supine while protamine is being administered to prevent injury from a hypotensive episode or other complication.

Protriptyline
proe-trip′-ti-leen
(Vivactil, Triptil [CAN])

CATEGORY AND SCHEDULE
Pregnancy Risk Category: C

Classification: Antidepressants, tricyclic

MECHANISM OF ACTION
A tricyclic antidepressant that increases synaptic concentration of norepinephrine and serotonin by inhibiting their reuptake by presynaptic membranes. *Therapeutic Effect:* Produces antidepressant effect.

PHARMACOKINETICS
Well absorbed from the GI tract. Protein binding: 92%. Widely distributed. Extensively metabolized in liver. Excreted in urine. Not removed by hemodialysis. *Half-life:* 54-92 h.

AVAILABILITY
Tablets: 5 mg, 10 mg (Vivactil).

INDICATIONS AND DOSAGES
▶ **Depression**
PO
Adults. 15-40 mg/day divided into 3-4 doses/day. Maximum: 60 mg/day.
Elderly. 5 mg 3 times/day. May increase gradually. Maximum: 30 mg/day.

OFF-LABEL USES
Narcolepsy, sleep apnea, sleep hypoxemia, obstructive apnea, chronic obstructive pulmonary disease.

CONTRAINDICATIONS
Acute recovery period after myocardial infarction, coadministration with cisapride, use of MAOIs within 14 days, hypersensitivity to protriptyline or any component of the formulation, QT prolongation.
Caution
Suicidal patients, severe depression, increased intraocular pressure, narrow-angle glaucoma, urinary retention, cardiac disease, hepatic disease, hyperthyroidism, electroshock therapy, elective surgery, MAOIs.

INTERACTIONS
Drug
Alcohol, barbiturates, benzodiazepines and other central nervous system (CNS) depressants: May increase CNS and respiratory depression and the hypotensive effects of protriptyline.
Antithyroid agents: May increase risk of agranulocytosis.
Cimetidine: May increase protriptyline blood concentration and risk of toxicity.
Clonidine, guanadrel, guanethidine: May decrease the effects of clonidine and guanadrel.
Direct-acting sympathomimetics, epinephrine, levonordefrin: Possible increased cardiac sympathomimetic effects.
MAOIs: May increase the risk of hyperpyrexia, hypertensive crisis, and seizures.
Phenothiazines, muscarinic blockers, antihistamines: May increase the anticholinergic and sedative effects of protriptyline.
Phenytoin: May decrease protriptyline blood concentration.
Herbal
St. John's wort: May have additive effects.
Food
None known.

DIAGNOSTIC TEST EFFECTS
None known.

P

SIDE EFFECTS
Frequent
Drowsiness, weight gain, fatigue, dry mouth, blurred vision, constipation, delayed micturition, postural hypotension, diaphoresis, disturbed concentration, increased appetite, urinary retention.
Occasional
GI disturbances, such as nausea, diarrhea, GI distress, metallic taste sensation.
Rare
Paradoxical reaction, marked by agitation, restlessness, nightmares, insomnia, extrapyramidal symptoms, particularly fine hand tremor.

SERIOUS REACTIONS
• High dosage may produce confusion, seizures, severe drowsiness, arrhythmias, fever, hallucinations, agitation, shortness of breath, vomiting, and unusual tiredness or weakness.
• Abrupt withdrawal from prolonged therapy may produce severe headache, malaise, nausea, vomiting, and vivid dreams.

PRECAUTIONS & CONSIDERATIONS
Caution is warranted in patients with increased intraocular pressure, overactive or agitated patients, seizure disorder, bipolar disorder, suicidal ideation, cardiovascular disease, hyperthyroidism, urinary retention, and concurrent use of guanethidine or other peripherally acting antihypertensives. Be aware that protriptyline crosses the placenta and is minimally distributed in breast milk. Safety and efficacy have not been established in children. Expect to use lower dosages in elderly patients. Higher dosages are not tolerated well and increase the risk of toxicity in elderly patients.

Caution is warranted within 14 days of MAOI therapy, after acute myocardial infarction, and with coadministration with cisapride. Significant xerostomic side effects such as sore tongue or problems eating or swallowing should be reported as medication change may be needed.

Protriptyline serum levels should be monitored. The therapeutic serum level for protriptyline is 70-250 ng/mL, and the toxic serum level for protriptyline is >500 ng/mL.

Anticholinergic, sedative effects, and postural hypotension usually develop during early therapy. Avoid unnecessary exposure to sunlight.
Storage
Store at room temperature.
Administration
May be taken with food to decrease GI distress. Dose increases should occur during the morning dose.

Pseudoephedrine
soo-doe-e-fed′rin
(Balminil Decongestant [CAN], BioContac Cold 12 Hour Relief Non Drowsy [CAN], Decofed, Dimetapp 12 Hour Non Drowsy Extentabs, Dimetapp Decongestant, Dimetapp sinus liquid caps [AUS], Genaphed, PMS-Pseudoephedrine [CAN], Robidrine [CAN], Sudafed, Sudafed 12hr [AUS], Sudafed 12 Hour, Sudafed 24 Hour)

CATEGORY AND SCHEDULE
Pregnancy Risk Category: C
Restricted OTC (dosages ≤120 mg/12 h) due to Methamphet-amine Drug Act (2007).

Classification: Direct acting α-adrenergic and β-adrenergic sympathomimetic

MECHANISM OF ACTION
A sympathomimetic that directly stimulates α-adrenergic and β-adrenergic receptors. *Therapeutic Effect:* Produces vasoconstriction of respiratory tract mucosa; shrinks nasal mucous membranes; reduces edema, and nasal congestion.

PHARMACOKINETICS

Route	Onset	Peak	Duration (h)
PO	15-30 min	NA	4-6 (tablets, syrup)
PO	NA	NA	8-12 (extended-release)

Well absorbed from the GI tract. Partially metabolized in the liver. Primarily excreted in urine. Not removed by hemodialysis. *Half-life:* 9-16 h (children, 3.1 h).

AVAILABILITY
Gelcaps (Dimetapp Decongestant): 30 mg.
Liquigels (Advil Cold & Sinus, Aleve Cold & Sinus): 30 mg
Liquid (Sudafed): 15 mg/5 mL.
Oral Drops (Dimetapp Infant Drops): 7.5 mg/0.8 mL.
Syrup (Biofed, Decofed): 30 mg/5 mL.
Tablets (Genaphed, Sudafed): 30 mg.
Tablets (Chewable [Sudafed]): 15 mg.
Tablets (Extended-Release [Dimetapp 12 Hour Non Drowsy Extentabs, Sudafed 12 Hour]): 120 mg.
Tablets (Extended-Release [Sudafed 24 Hour]): 240 mg.

INDICATIONS AND DOSAGES
▶ **Decongestant**
PO
Adults, Children 12 yr and older. 60 mg q4-6h. Maximum: 240 mg/day.
Children aged 6-11 yr. 30 mg q4-6h. Maximum: 120 mg/day.
Children 2-5 yr. 15 mg q4-6h. Maximum: 60 mg/day.
Children younger than 2 yr. Safety and effective use has not been established.
Elderly. 30-60 mg q6h as needed.
PO (EXTENDED-RELEASE)
Adults, Children 12 yr and older. 120 mg q12h.

CONTRAINDICATIONS
Breastfeeding women, coronary artery disease, severe hypertension, use within 14 days of MAOIs.
Caution
Cardiac disorders, hyperthyroidism, diabetes mellitus, benign prostatic hypertrophy.

INTERACTIONS
Drug
Antihypertensive, β-blockers, diuretics: May decrease the effects of these drugs.
Hydrocarbon inhalation anesthetics: May cause dysrhythmias.
MAOIs: May increase cardiac stimulant and vasopressor effects.
Sympathomimetics: Possible increased CNS, cardiovascular effects.
Herbal
None known.
Food
None known.

DIAGNOSTIC TEST EFFECTS
None known.

SIDE EFFECTS
Occasional (5%-10%)
Nervousness, restlessness, insomnia, tremor, headache.
Rare (1%-4%)
Diaphoresis, weakness.

SERIOUS REACTIONS
• Large doses may produce tachycardia, palpitations (particularly in patients with cardiac disease), light-headedness, nausea, and vomiting.
• Overdose in patients older than 60 yr may result in hallucinations, CNS depression, and seizures.

PRECAUTIONS & CONSIDERATIONS
Caution is warranted with diabetes, heart disease, hyperthyroidism, benign prostatic hyperplasia, and in elderly patients. Pseudoephedrine crosses the placenta and is distributed in breast milk. The safety and efficacy of pseudoephedrine have not been established in children younger than 2 yr. Age-related benign prostatic hyperplasia may require a dosage adjustment in elderly patients.

BP should be monitored for increases. Tell the physician if taking antihypertensives, β-blockers, diuretics, or MAOIs before administering pseudoephedrine.
Administration
Do not crush extended-release tablets; swallow them whole. Discontinue therapy and notify the physician if dizziness, insomnia, irregular or rapid heartbeat, tremors, or other side effects occur.

Psyllium
sill'ee-yum
(Fiberall, Hydrocil, Konsyl, Metamucil, Novo-Mucilax [CAN], Perdiem)

CATEGORY AND SCHEDULE
Pregnancy Risk Category: B
OTC

Classification: Psyllium colloid, laxative

MECHANISM OF ACTION
A bulk-forming laxative that dissolves and swells in water providing increased bulk and moisture content in stool. *Therapeutic Effect:* Promotes peristalsis and bowel motility.

PHARMACOKINETICS

Route	Onset	Peak	Duration
PO	12-24 h	2-3 days	NA

Acts in small and large intestines.

AVAILABILITY
Powder (Fiberall, Hydrocil, Konsyl, Metamucil).
Wafer(Metamucil): 3.4 g/dose.
Capsules(Metamucil): 0.52 g.
Granules (Perdiem): 4 g/5 mL.

INDICATIONS AND DOSAGES
▸ **Constipation, irritable bowel syndrome**
PO
! 3.4 µg powder equals 1 rounded tsp, 1 packet or 1 wafer.
Adults, Elderly. 2-5 capsules/dose 1-3 times a day. 1-2 tsp granules 1-2 times a day. 1 rounded tsp or 1 tbsp of powder 1-3 times a day. 2 wafers 1-3 times a day.
Children 6-11 yr. One half-1 tsp powder in water 1-3 times a day.

CONTRAINDICATIONS
Fecal impaction, GI obstruction, appendicitis, dysphagia.

INTERACTIONS
Drug
Digoxin, oral anticoagulants, salicylates: May decrease the effects of digoxin, oral anticoagulants, and salicylates by decreasing absorption.
Potassium-sparing diuretics, potassium supplements: May interfere with the effects of potassium- sparing diuretics and potassium supplements.

Herbal
None known.
Food
None known.

DIAGNOSTIC TEST EFFECTS
May increase blood glucose level.
May decrease serum potassium
level.

SIDE EFFECTS
Rare
Some degree of abdominal
discomfort, nausea, mild abdominal
cramps, griping, faintness.

SERIOUS REACTIONS
• Esophageal or bowel obstruction
may occur if administered < 250 mL
of liquid.

PRECAUTIONS & CONSIDERATIONS
Caution is warranted with
esophageal strictures, intestinal
adhesions, stenosis, and ulcers.
This drug may be used safely in
pregnancy. Safety and efficacy of
psyllium have not been established
in children younger than 6 yr of age.
No age-related precautions have been
noted in elderly patients.
    Pattern of daily bowel activity
and stool consistency and serum
electrolyte levels should be
monitored. Adequate fluid intake
should be maintained.
Administration
Administer at least 2 h before or after
other medication administration.
Drink 6-8 glasses of water a day
to aid in stool softening. Drugs
should not be swallowed in dry
form but should be mixed with at
least 1 full glass (8 oz) of liquid
and then followed by 8 oz of liquid;
inadequate amount of fluid may
cause GI obstruction. To promote
defecation, increase fluid intake,
exercise, and eat a high-fiber diet.

Pyrantel Pamoate
pi-ran-tel pam-oh-ate
(Antiminth, Combantrin [CAN],
Pin-Rid, Pin-X, Reese's Pinworm
Caplets, Reese's Pinworm
Medicine)

CATEGORY AND SCHEDULE
Pregnancy Risk Category: C
OTC (capsules, liquid, suspension)

Classification: Pyrimidine
derivative, antihelmintic

MECHANISM OF ACTION
A depolarizing neuromuscular
blocking agent that causes the
release of acetylcholine and
inhibits cholinesterase. *Therapeutic
Effect:* Results in a spastic paralysis
of the worm and consequent
expulsion from the host's intestinal
tract.

PHARMACOKINETICS
Poorly absorbed through GI tract.
Time to peak occurs in 1-3 h.
Partially metabolized in liver.
Primarily excreted in feces; minimal
elimination in urine.

AVAILABILITY
Caplets: 180 mg (Reese's Pinworm
Caplets).
Capsules: 180 mg (Pin-Rid).
Liquid: 50 mg/mL (Reese's Pinworm
Medicine).
Suspension, Oal: 50 mg/mL
(Antiminth, Pin-X).

INDICATIONS AND DOSAGES
▸ **Enterobiasis vermicularis
(pinworm)**
PO
*Adults, Elderly, Children older than
2 yr.* 11 mg base/kg once. Repeat in
2 wks. Maximum: 1 g/day.

P

CONTRAINDICATIONS
Hypersensitivity to pyrantel or any of its components.

INTERACTIONS
Drug
Piperazine: May decrease effects of pyrantel.
Herbal
None known.
Food
None known.

DIAGNOSTIC TEST EFFECTS
None known.

SIDE EFFECTS
Occasional
Nausea, vomiting, headache, dizziness, drowsiness, GI distress, weakness.

SERIOUS REACTIONS
• Overdosage includes symptoms of anorexia, nausea, abdominal cramps, vomiting, diarrhea, and ataxia.

PRECAUTIONS & CONSIDERATIONS
Caution is necessary in pregnancy and in patients with liver disease. Pyrantel should not be used concurrently with piperazines. It is unknown whether pyrantel is distributed in breast milk. No age-related precautions have been noted in children or elderly. The entire family should be treated for pinworms. Wash bedding and clothes in hot soapy water to avoid being reinfected. Tactful discussion regarding proper toileting techniques should be discussed to avoid transmission of infection or reinfection.
Storage
Refrigerate suspension.
Administration
2.9 g pamoate salt = 1 g base. May be taken with or without food. Shake suspension well before using.

Pyrazinamide
pye-ra-zin'a-mide
(Pyrazinamide, Tebrazid [CAN], Zinamide [AUS])

CATEGORY AND SCHEDULE
Pregnancy Risk Category: C

Classification: Antitubercular agent

MECHANISM OF ACTION
An antitubercular whose exact mechanism of action is unknown. *Therapeutic Effect:* Either bacteriostatic or bactericidal, depending on the drug's concentration at the infection site and the susceptibility of infecting bacteria.

PHARMACOKINETICS
PO: Peak 2 h. *Half-life:* 9-10 h. Metabolized in liver, excreted in urine (metabolites and unchanged drug).

AVAILABILITY
Tablets: 500 mg.

INDICATIONS AND DOSAGES
▸ **Tuberculosis (in combination with other antituberculars)**
PO
Adults. 15-30 mg/kg/daily.
Maximum: 3 g/day.
Children. 15-30 mg/kg/day.
Maximum: 3 g/day.

CONTRAINDICATIONS
Severe hepatic dysfunction.

INTERACTIONS
Drug
Allopurinol, colchicine, probenecid, sulfinpyrazone: May decrease the effects of these drugs.

Herbal
None known.
Food
None known.

DIAGNOSTIC TEST EFFECTS
May increase AST (SGOT), ALT (SGPT), and serum uric acid concentrations.

SIDE EFFECTS
Frequent
Arthralgia, myalgia (usually mild and self-limiting).
Rare
Hypersensitivity reaction (rash, pruritus, urticaria), photosensitivity, gouty arthritis.

SERIOUS REACTIONS
• Hepatotoxicity, gouty arthritis, thrombocytopenia, and anemia occur rarely.
Caution
Use in children under 13 yr.

PRECAUTIONS & CONSIDERATIONS
Caution is warranted in patients with diabetes mellitus, a history of gout, and renal impairment. Caution should be used with possible cross-sensitivity to ethionamide, isoniazid, and niacin. Be aware that the safety and efficacy of pyrazinamide have not been established in Children.Liver function test results should be monitored. Side effects such as anorexia, fever, jaundice, liver tenderness, malaise, nausea, and vomiting may occur. If any liver reactions occur, stop the drug and notify the physician promptly. Serum uric acid levels should be monitored and signs and symptoms of gout, such as hot, painful, swollen joints, especially the ankle, big toe, or knee, should be assessed. Blood glucose levels should be evaluated, especially in persons with diabetes mellitus, because pyrazinamide administration may make diabetic management difficult. Skin should be assessed for rash or eruptions.

It is important to test for noninfectious status by ensuring that compliance with anti-TB for 3 wks or longer has occurred; that culture has confirmed TB susceptiblity to antiinfectives; patient has 3 consecuetive negative sputum smears; and patient is not coughing.
Administration
Take pyrazinamide with food to reduce GI upset.

Pyridostigmine bromide
peer-id-oh-stig′meen brom-ide
(Mestinon, Mestinon SR [CAN], Mestinon Timespan)
Do not confuse pyridostigmine with physostigmine or Mesitonin with Mesantoin or Metatensin.

CATEGORY AND SCHEDULE
Pregnancy Risk Category: C

Classification: Cholinergic

MECHANISM OF ACTION
A cholinergic that prevents destruction of acetylcholine by inhibiting the enzyme acetylcholinesterase, thus enhancing impulse transmission across the myoneural junction.
Therapeutic Effect: Produces miosis; increases tone of intestinal, skeletal muscle tone; stimulates salivary and sweat gland secretions.

PHARMACOKINETICS
PO: Onset 20-30 min, duration 3-6 h.
IV/IM/SC: Onset 2-15 min, duration 2.5-4 h.
Metabolized in liver, excreted in urine.

AVAILABILITY
Syrup (Mestinon): 60 mg/5 mL.
Tablets (Mestinon): 60 mg.
Tablets (Extended-Release [Mestinon Timespan]): 180 mg.
Injection (Mestinon): 5 mg/mL.

INDICATIONS AND DOSAGES
▸ **Myasthenia gravis**
PO
Adults, Elderly. Initially, 60 mg
3 times a day. Dosage increased at
48-h intervals. Maintenance: 60 mg
to 1.5 g a day.
PO (EXTENDED-RELEASE)
Adults, Elderly. 180-540 mg once
or twice a day with at least a 6-h
interval between doses.
IV, IM
Adults, Elderly. 2 mg q2-3h.
Children, Neonates.
0.05-0.15 mg/kg/dose. Maximum
single dose: 10 mg.
▸ **Reversal of nondepolarizing
neuromuscular blockade**
IV
Adults, Elderly. 0.1-0.25 mg/kg with,
or shortly after, 0.6-1.2 mg atropine
sulfate or an equipotent dose of
glycopyrrolate.
Children. 0.25 mg/kg.

CONTRAINDICATIONS
Mechanical GI or urinary tract
obstruction, cholmesterase inhibitor
toxicity.
Caution
Seizure disorders, bronchial asthma,
coronary occlusion, hyperthyroidism,
dysrhythmias, peptic ulcer,
megacolon, poor GI motility, elderly,
breast-feeding.

INTERACTIONS
Drug
**Anticholinergics, atropine,
scopolamine, methocarbamol:**
Prevent or reverse the effects of
pyridostigmine.

Cholinesterase inhibitors: May
increase the risk of toxicity.
Ester local anesthetics: May reduce
metabolic rate.
Neuromuscular blockers:
Antagonizes the effects of these
drugs.
Procainamide, quinidine:
May antagonize the action of
pyridostigmine.
Herbal
None known.
Food
None known.

DIAGNOSTIC TEST EFFECTS
None known.

ⓘ IV INCOMPATIBILITIES
Do not mix pyridostigmine with any
other medications.

💉 IV COMPATIBILITIES
None known.

SIDE EFFECTS
Frequent
Miosis, increased GI and skeletal
muscle tone, bradycardia,
constriction of bronchi and ureters,
diaphoresis, increased salivation.
Occasional
Headache, rash, temporary decrease
in diastolic BP with mild reflex
tachycardia, short periods of atrial
fibrillation (in hyperthyroid patients),
marked drop in BP (in hypertensive
patients).

SERIOUS REACTIONS
• Overdose may produce a
cholinergic crisis, manifested as
increasingly severe muscle weakness
that appears first in muscles
involving chewing and swallowing
and is followed by muscle weakness
of the shoulder girdle and upper
extremities, respiratory muscle
paralysis, and pelvis girdle and

leg muscle paralysis. If overdose occurs, stop all cholinergic drugs and immediately administer 1-4 mg atropine sulfate IV for adults or 0.01 mg/kg for infants and children younger than 12 yr.

PRECAUTIONS & CONSIDERATIONS

Caution is warranted in patients with bradycardia, bronchial asthma, cardiac arrhythmias, epilepsy, hyperthyroidism, peptic ulcer disease, recent coronary occlusion, and vagotonia. Keep a log of energy level and muscle strength to help guide drug dosing.

Notify the physician of diarrhea, difficulty breathing, profuse salivation or sweating, irregular heartbeat, muscle weakness, severe abdominal pain, or nausea and vomiting. Therapeutic response to the drug, such as decreased fatigue, improved chewing and swallowing, and increased muscle strength, should be monitored. Respirations should be closely assessed.

Caution is warranted with postural changes because of possible orthostatic hypotensive effects.

Administration

! Drug dosage and frequency of administration are dependent on the daily clinical response, including exacerbations, physical and emotional stress, and remissions.

Crush tablets as needed. Take larger doses at times of increased fatigue, for example 30-45 min before meals. May break extended-release tablets but do not chew or crush them.

For IV and IM use, give large doses concurrently with 0.6-1.2 mg atropine sulfate IV, as prescribed, to minimize side effects.

Pyridoxine Hydrochloride (Vitamin B₆)

peer-i-dox′een high-droh-clo-ride

(Aminoxin, Beesix, Doxine, Nestrex, Pryi, Pyroxin [AUS], Rodex, Vitabee 6)

Do not confuse pyridoxine with paroxetine, pralidoxime, or Pyridium.

CATEGORY AND SCHEDULE

Pregnancy Risk Category: A

OTC (tablets, capsules), Rx (injectible)

Classification: Vitamin B₆, water-soluble

MECHANISM OF ACTION

Acts as a coenzyme for various metabolic functions, including metabolism of proteins, carbohydrates, and fats. Aids in the breakdown of glycogen and in the synthesis of γ-aminobutyric acid in the central nervous system (CNS). *Therapeutic Effect:* Prevents pyridoxine deficiency. Increases the excretion of certain drugs, such as isoniazid, that are pyridoxine antagonists.

PHARMACOKINETICS

Readily absorbed primarily in jejunum. Stored in the liver, muscle, and brain. Metabolized in the liver. Primarily excreted in urine. Removed by hemodialysis. *Half-life:* 15-20 days.

AVAILABILITY

Capsules: 250 mg.
Tablets: 20 mg, 25 mg, 50 mg, 100 mg, 250 mg, 500 mg.
Injection: 100 mg/mL.

INDICATIONS AND DOSAGES
▶ **Pyridoxine deficiency**
PO
Adults, Elderly. Initially,
2.5-10 mg/day; then 2-5 mg/day
when clinical signs are corrected.
Children. Initially, 5-25 mg/day for
3 wks, then 1.5-2.5 mg/day.
▶ **Pyridoxine dependent seizures**
PO, IV, IM
Infants. Initially,10-100 mg/day.
Maintenance: PO: 50-100 mg/day.
▶ **Drug-induced neuritis**
PO (TREATMENT)
Adults, Elderly. 100-200 mg/day in
divided doses
Children. 10-50 mg/day.
PO (PROPHYLAXIS)
Adults, Elderly. 25-100 mg/day.
Children. 1-2 mg/kg/day.

CONTRAINDICATIONS
Hypersensitivity to pyroxidine or
any of its components, Parkinson
disease.

INTERACTIONS
Drug
Immunosuppressants,
isoniazid, penicillamine:
May antagonize pyridoxine,
causing anemia or peripheral
neuritis.
Levodopa: Reverses the effects of
levodopa.
Herbal
None known.
Food
None known.

DIAGNOSTIC TEST EFFECTS
None known.

ⓘ IV INCOMPATIBILITIES
Do not mix pyridoxine with any
other medications.

▣ IV COMPATIBILITIES
None known.

SIDE EFFECTS
Occasional
Stinging at IM injection site.
Rare
Headache, nausea, somnolence;
sensory neuropathy (paraesthesia,
unstable gait, clumsiness of hands)
with high doses.

SERIOUS REACTIONS
• Long-term megadoses (2-6 g
over >2 mo) may produce sensory
neuropathy (reduced deep tendon
reflexes, profound impairment of
sense of position in distal limbs,
gradual sensory ataxia). Toxic
symptoms subside when drug is
discontinued.
• Seizures have occurred after IV
megadoses.

PRECAUTIONS & CONSIDERATIONS
Pyridoxine crosses the placenta
and is excreted in breast milk. High
doses of pyridoxine in pregnancy
may produce seizures in neonates.
No age-related precautions have been
noted in children or elderly patients.
Foods rich in pyridoxine, including
avocados, bananas, bran, carrots,
eggs, organ meats, tuna, shrimp,
hazelnuts, legumes, soybeans,
sunflower seeds, and wheat germ, are
encouraged.
   Improvement of deficiency
symptoms, including CNS
abnormalities (anxiety, depression,
insomnia, motor difficulty,
paraesthesia and tremors) and skin
lesions (glossitis, seborrhea-like
lesions around eyes, mouth, nose),
should be monitored.
Storage
Store vials for parenteral use at
room temperature. Use the solution
immediately if reconstituted with
sterile water for injection and
within 7 days if reconstituted with
bacteriostatic water for injection.

Administration
Scored tablets may be crushed.
! Give pyridoxine orally unless malabsorption, nausea, or vomiting occurs. Avoid IV use in cardiac patients.

Take extended-release capsules and tablets whole without crushing or breaking them. Have the patient avoid chewing the capsule or tablet.

For IV use, pyridoxine may be given undiluted or may be added to IV solutions and given as an infusion.

IM injections may cause discomfort.

Pyrimethamine
pye-ri-meth′a-meen
(Daraprim, Malocide [France])
Do not confuse with Dantrium, Daranide.

CATEGORY AND SCHEDULE
Pregnancy Risk Category: C

Classification: Antiprotozoals, antimalarial

MECHANISM OF ACTION
An antiprotozoal with blood and some tissue schizonticidal activity against malaria parasites of humans. Highly selective activity against plasmodia and *Toxoplasma gondii.* *Therapeutic Effect:* Inhibition of tetrahydrofolic acid synthesis.

PHARMACOKINETICS
Well absorbed, peak levels occurring between 2 and 6 h following administration. Protein binding: 87%. Eliminated slowly. *Half-life:* approximately 96 h.

AVAILABILITY
Tablets: 25 mg (Daraprim).

INDICATIONS AND DOSAGES
▸ **Toxoplasmosis**
PO
Adults. Initially, 50-75 mg daily, with 1-4 g daily of a sulfonamide of the sulfapyrimidine type (e.g., sulfadoxine). Continue for 1-3 wks, depending on response of patient and tolerance to therapy then reduce dose to one-half that previously given for each drug and continue for additional 4-5 wks.
Children. 1 mg/kg/day divided into 2 equal daily doses; after 2-4 days reduce to one half and continue for approximately 1 mo. The usual pediatric sulfonamide dosage is used in conjunction with pyrimethamine.
▸ **Acute malaria**
PO
Adults (in combination with sulfonamide). 25 mg daily for 2 days with a sulfonamide
Adults (without concomitant sulfonamide). 50 mg for 2 days
Children aged 4-10 yr. 25 mg daily for 2 days.
▸ **Chemoprophylaxis of malaria**
PO
Adults and pediatric patients older than 10 yr. 25 mg once weekly.
Children aged 4-10 yr. 12.5 mg once weekly.
Infants and children under 4 yr. 6.25 mg once weekly.

OFF-LABEL USES
Prophylaxis for first episode and recurrence of *Pneumocystis carinii* pneumonia and *Toxoplasma gondii* in HIV-infected patients, isosporiasis.

CONTRAINDICATIONS
Hypersensitivity to pyrimethamine, megaloblastic anemia due to folate deficiency, monotherapy for treatment of acute malaria, breast-feeding, IM injection.

INTERACTIONS
Drug
Antifolic drugs: Pyrimethamine may be used with sulfonamides, quinine, and other antimalarials, and with other antibiotics. However, the concomitant use of other antifolic drugs, such as sulfonamides or trimethoprim-sulfamethoxazole combinations, while the patient is receiving pyrimethamine, may increase the risk of bone marrow suppression. If signs of folate deficiency develop, pyrimethamine should be discontinued. Folinic acid (leucovorin) should be administered until normal hematopoiesis is restored.
Benzodiazepines: Mild hepatotoxicity has been reported in some patients when lorazepam and pyrimethamine were administered concomitantly.
Herbal
None known.
Food
None known.

DIAGNOSTIC TEST EFFECTS
None known.

SIDE EFFECTS
Frequent
Anorexia, vomiting.
Occasional
Hypersensitivity reactions, Stevens-Johnson syndrome, toxic epidermal necrolysis, erythema multiforme, anaphylaxis, hyperphenylalaninemia, megaloblastic anemia, leukopenia, thrombocytopenia, pancytopenia, atrophic glossitis, hematuria, and disorders of cardiac rhythm.
Rare
Pulmonary eosinophilia.

SERIOUS REACTIONS
• Megaloblastic anemia, leukopenia, thrombocytopenia, pancytopenia, atrophic glossitis, hematuria, and disorders of cardiac rhythm. Hematologic effects may be severe and require leucovorin rescue or prophylaxis, depending on the indication for use.
• Pulmonary eosinphilia (rare).

PRECAUTIONS & CONSIDERATIONS
Caution is warranted in patients with megaloblastic anemia resulting from folate deficiency, seizures or epilepsy, kidney disease, and liver disease. It is unknown whether pyrimethamine crosses the placenta. It passes through the breast milk and may be harmful to the infant. No age-related precautions have been noted in elderly patients.
Storage
Store at room temperature away from heat and moisture.
Administration
Take with food to decrease stomach upset. Take each dose with a full glass of water.

Quazepam
kwaz'ze-pam
(Doral)

CATEGORY AND SCHEDULE
Pregnancy Risk Category: X
Controlled Substance: Schedule IV

Classification: Benzodiazepines,
sedatives/hypnotics

MECHANISM OF ACTION
BZ-1 receptor-selective
benzodiazepine with sedative
properties. *Therapeutic Effect:*
Produces sedative effect from its
central nervous system (CNS)
depressant action.

PHARMACOKINETICS
Rapidly absorbed from GI tract.
Protein binding: 95%. Extensively
metabolized in liver. Excreted in
urine and feces. Unknown whether
removed by hemodialysis.
Half-life: 39-73 h.

AVAILABILITY
Tablets: 7.5 mg, 15 mg (Doral).

INDICATIONS AND DOSAGES
▶ **Insomnia**
PO
Adults. Initially, 15 mg at bedtime.
Adjust from 7.5 mg to 15 mg at
bedtime, depending on initial
response. Optimal effective dose is
thought to be 15 mg.
Elderly, debilitated, liver disease.
Initially, 7.5-15 mg at bedtime.
Adjust dose depending on initial
response.

CONTRAINDICATIONS
Pregnancy, sleep apnea,
hypersensitivity to quazepam or any
component of the formulation.

INTERACTIONS
Drug
**Alcohol, CNS depressants,
antihistamines, psychotropic
medications:** Potentiates effects of
quazepam.
Azole antifungals: May
inhibit liver metabolism and
increase quazepam blood serum
concentrations.
Theophylline: May decrease
quazepam effectiveness.
Herbal
**Dong quai, kava, magnolia,
passionflower, skullcap, tan-shen,
valerian:** May increase CNS-
depressant effect of quazepam.
Food
Caffeine: May decrease sedative and
anxiolytic effects of quazepam.

DIAGNOSTIC TEST EFFECTS
None known.

SIDE EFFECTS
Frequent
Muscular incoordination (ataxia),
light-headedness, transient mild
drowsiness, slurred speech (particularly
in elderly or debilitated patients).
Occasional
Confusion, depression, blurred
vision, constipation, diarrhea, dry
mouth, headache, nausea.
Rare
Behavioral problems such as anger,
impaired memory, paradoxical
reactions such as insomnia,
nervousness, or irritability.

SERIOUS REACTIONS
• Abrupt or too-rapid withdrawal may
result in pronounced restlessness,
irritability, insomnia, hand tremors,
abdominal and muscle cramps,
sweating, vomiting, and seizures.
• Overdosage results in somnolence,
confusion, diminished reflexes, and
coma.

• Blood dyscrasias have been reported rarely.

PRECAUTIONS & CONSIDERATIONS

Caution should be used in patients with impaired renal or liver function, and smaller initial doses should be used. Quazepam crosses the placenta and is distributed in breast milk. Chronic ingestion of quazepam during pregnancy may produce withdrawal symptoms in women and CNS depression in neonates; therefore, the benefit of taking in patients who desire to become pregnant should be weighed against the risk to the fetus and neonate. Safety and efficacy of quazepam have not been established in children. In elderly patients, use small initial doses and gradually increase them to avoid excessive sedation or ataxia as evidenced by muscular incoordination.

Drowsiness and dizziness are expected side effects. Avoid tasks that require mental alertness or motor skills. Concomitant use with alcohol should also be avoided.

Administration

May be taken on an empty stomach. Take quazepam at bedtime. Tablets may be crushed. Do not abruptly stop quazepam.

Quetiapine

kwe-tye'a-peen
(Seroquel) and quetiapine extended-release tablets (Seroquel XR)
Do not confuse with Serzone.

CATEGORY AND SCHEDULE

Pregnancy Risk Category: C

Classification: Antipsychotics, atypical

MECHANISM OF ACTION

A dibenzepin derivative that antagonizes dopamine, serotonin, histamine, and α_1-adrenergic receptors. *Therapeutic Effect:* Diminishes manifestations of psychotic disorders. Produces moderate sedation, few extrapyramidal effects, and no anticholinergic effects.

PHARMACOKINETICS

Well absorbed after PO administration. Protein binding: 83%. Widely distributed in tissues; central nervous system (CNS) concentration exceeds plasma concentration. Undergoes extensive first-pass metabolism in the liver. Primarily excreted in urine. *Half-life:* 6 h.

AVAILABILITY

Tablets: 25 mg, 50 mg, 100 mg, 200 mg, 300 mg, 400 mg.
Extended-Release Tablets: 200 mg, 300 mg, 400 mg.

INDICATIONS AND DOSAGES

▸ **Management of manifestations of psychotic disorders, bipolar disorder (depressed and manic phases), and schizophrenia**
PO
Adults, Elderly: Initially, 25 mg twice a day, then 25-50 mg 2-3 times a day on the second and third days, up to 300-400 mg/day in divided doses 2-3 times a day by the fourth day. Further adjustments of 25-50 mg twice a day may be made at intervals of 2 days or longer. For patients with schizophrenia, if extended-release tablets are used, 300-mg tablets once daily increasing by up to 300 mg/day. Maintenance: *Immediate-Release Tablets:* 300-800 mg/day administered in 2-3 divided doses (adults);

Extended-Release Tablets:
400-800 mg/day administered as one daily dose; 50-200 mg/day (elderly).

▶ **Dosage in hepatic impairment, elderly or debilitated patients, and those predisposed to hypotensive reactions**

These patients should receive a lower initial dose and lower dosage increases.

CONTRAINDICATIONS

Hypersensitivity to quetiapine.

INTERACTIONS

Drug
Alcohol, other central nervous system (CNS) depressants: May increase CNS depression.
Antihypertensives: May increase the hypotensive effects of these drugs.
Hepatic enzyme inducers (such as carbamazepine, cimetidine, phenytoin): May increase quetiapine clearance.
Herbal
None known.
Food
High-fat meals: Increase the effects of quetiapine.

DIAGNOSTIC TEST EFFECTS

May decrease serum total and free thyroxine (T_4) serum levels. May increase serum cholesterol, triglyceride, AST (SGOT), and ALT (SGPT) levels. May produce a false-positive pregnancy test result.

SIDE EFFECTS

Frequent (10%-19%)
Headache, somnolence, dizziness.
Occasional (3%-9%)
Constipation, orthostatic hypotension, tachycardia, dry mouth, dyspepsia, rash, asthenia, abdominal pain, rhinitis.

Rare (2%)
Back pain, fever, weight gain.

SERIOUS REACTIONS

• Overdosage may produce heart block, hypotension, hypokalemia, and tachycardia.

PRECAUTIONS & CONSIDERATIONS

There is a black box warning against use in elderly patients with dementia-related psychosis because of the increased risk of death when treated with atypical antipsychotics vs. placebo. Caution is warranted with Alzheimer disease, cardiovascular disease (such as congestive heart failure or history of myocardial infarction), cerebrovascular disease, seizures, hepatic impairment, dehydration, hypothyroidism, hypovolemia, a history of breast cancer, and a history of drug abuse or dependence. It is unknown whether quetiapine is distributed in breast milk. However, this drug is not recommended for breastfeeding women. The safety and efficacy of quetiapine have not been established in children. For elderly patients, lower initial and target dosages may be necessary.

Drowsiness and dizziness may occur but generally subside with continued therapy. Tasks requiring mental alertness or motor skills should be avoided. Dehydration, particularly during exercise, exposure to extreme heat, and concurrent use of medications that cause dry mouth or other drying effects, should also be avoided. BP, pulse rate, weight, pattern of daily bowel activity, and stool consistency should be assessed.
Administration
Take quetiapine without food or with a light meal. With immediate-release quetiapine, dosage

Q

adjustments should occur at 2-day intervals. With extended-release quetiapine, dosage adjustments may occur daily. When restarting therapy for persons who have been off quetiapine for longer than 1 wk, follow the initial titration schedule, as prescribed. When restarting therapy for persons who have been off quetiapine for < 1 wk, titration is not required and the maintenance dose can be reinstituted. Do not abruptly discontinue or increase the dosage.

Quinapril
kwin′a-pril
(Accupril, Asig [AUS])
Do not confuse Accupril with Accolate or Accutane.

CATEGORY AND SCHEDULE
Pregnancy Risk Category: C (D if used in second or third trimester)

Classification: Angiotensin-converting enzyme inhibitors

Q

MECHANISM OF ACTION
An ACE inhibitor that suppresses the renin-angiotensin-aldosterone system and prevents the conversion of angiotensin I to angiotensin II, a potent vasoconstrictor; may also inhibit angiotensin II at local vascular and renal sites. *Therapeutic Effect:* Reduces peripheral arterial resistance, BP, and pulmonary capillary wedge pressure; improves cardiac output.

PHARMACOKINETICS

Route	Onset	Peak	Duration
PO	1 h	NA	24 h

Readily absorbed from the GI tract. Protein binding: 97%. Metabolized in the liver, GI tract, and extravascular tissue to active metabolite. Excreted primarily in urine. Minimal removal by hemodialysis. *Half-life:* 1-2 h; metabolite, 3 h (increased in those with impaired renal function).

AVAILABILITY
Tablets: 5 mg, 10 mg, 20 mg, 40 mg.

INDICATIONS AND DOSAGES
▸ **Hypertension (monotherapy)**
PO
Adults. Initially, 10-20 mg/day. May adjust dosage at intervals of at least 2 wks or longer. Maintenance: 20-80 mg/day as single dose or 2 divided doses. Maximum: 80 mg/day.
Elderly. Initially, 10 mg/day. May increase by 2.5-5 mg q1-2wk.
▸ **Hypertension (combination therapy)**
PO
Adults. Initially, 5 mg/day titrated to patient's needs.
Elderly. Initially, 5 mg/day.
May increase by 2.5-5 mg q1-2wk.
▸ **Adjunct to manage heart failure**
PO
Adults, Elderly. Initially, 5 mg twice a day. Range: 20-40 mg/day divided into 2 doses.
▸ **Dosage in renal impairment**
Dosage is titrated to the patient's needs after the following initial doses:

Creatinine Clearance (mL/min)	Initial Dose (mg)
> 60	10
30-60	5
10-29	2.5

OFF-LABEL USES

Treatment of hypertension and renal crisis in scleroderma, diabetic nephropathy, valvular regurgitation.

CONTRAINDICATIONS

Bilateral renal artery stenosis; angioedema related to this or another ACE inhibitor.

INTERACTIONS

Drug

Alcohol, antihypertensives, diuretics: May increase the effects of quinapril.

Lithium: May increase lithium blood concentration and risk of lithium toxicity.

NSAIDs: May decrease the effects of quinapril.

Potassium-sparing diuretics, potassium supplements: May cause hyperkalemia.

Tetracycline, quinolones, and magnesium: May reduce the absorption of the co-administered medications due to magnesium content in quinapril tablets.

Herbal

Garlic: May increase antihypertensive effect.

Ginseng, yohimbe: May worsen hypertension.

Food

None known.

DIAGNOSTIC TEST EFFECTS

May increase BUN, serum alkaline phosphatase, serum bilirubin, serum creatinine, serum potassium, AST (SGOT), and ALT (SGPT) levels. May decrease serum sodium levels. May cause positive antinuclear antibody titer.

SIDE EFFECTS

Frequent (5%-7%)

Headache, dizziness.

Occasional (3%-4%)

Fatigue, vomiting, nausea, hypotension, chest pain, cough, syncope.

Rare (< 2%)

Diarrhea, cough, dyspnea, rash, palpitations, impotence, insomnia, drowsiness, malaise.

SERIOUS REACTIONS

• Excessive hypotension (first-dose syncope) may occur in patients with congestive heart failure (CHF) and in those who are severely salt or volume depleted.

• Angioedema and hyperkalemia occur rarely.

• Agranulocytosis and neutropenia may be noted in those with collagen vascular disease, including scleroderma and systemic lupus erythematosus, and impaired renal function.

• Nephrotic syndrome may be noted in those with history of renal disease.

PRECAUTIONS & CONSIDERATIONS

Caution is warranted with CHF, collagen vascular disease, hyperkalemia, hypovolemia, renal impairment, and renal stenosis. Quinapril crosses the placenta, and it is unknown whether it is distributed in breast milk. Quinapril may cause fetal or neonatal morbidity or mortality, so it should be avoided in women of childbearing age. Safety and efficacy of quinapril have not been established in children. Elderly patients may be more sensitive to the hypotensive effect of quinapril.

Dizziness and headache may occur. Tasks that require mental alertness or motor skills should be avoided. Be alert to fluctuations in BP. If an excessive reduction in BP occurs, place the patient in the supine position with legs elevated.

Q

CBC and blood chemistry should be obtained before beginning quinapril therapy, then every 2 wks for the next 3 mo, and periodically thereafter in patients with autoimmune disease, or renal impairment, and in those who are taking drugs that affect immune response or leukocyte count. BUN, serum creatinine, serum potassium levels, and WBC count should also be monitored.

Administration

If possible, expect to discontinue diuretics 2-3 days before beginning quinapril therapy and then restart the diuretic if goal BP reduction is not obtained.

Take quinapril without regard to food. Crush tablets as desired.

Quinidine

(Apo-Quin-G [CAN], Apo-Quinidine [CAN], Biquinate [AUS], BioQuin Durules [CAN], Kinidin Durules [AUS], Myoquin [AUS], Quinaglute Dura-Tabs, Quinate [CAN], Quinbisu [AUS], Quinidex Extentabs, Quinoctal [AUS], Quinsul [AUS]).
Do not confuse quinidine with clonidine or quinine.

CATEGORY AND SCHEDULE
Pregnancy Risk Category: C

Classification: Antiarrhythmics, class IA, antiprotozoals

MECHANISM OF ACTION

An antiarrhythmic that decreases sodium influx during depolarization, decreases potassium efflux during repolarization, and reduces calcium transport across the myocardial cell membrane. Decreases myocardial excitability, conduction velocity, and contractility. *Therapeutic Effect:* Suppresses arrhythmias.

AVAILABILITY
Injection: 80 mg/mL.
Tablets: 200 mg, 300 mg.
Tablets (Extended-Release [Quinidex Extentabs]): 300 mg.
Tablets (Extended-Release [Quinaglute Dura-Tabs]): 324 mg.

INDICATIONS AND DOSAGES
▶ **Maintenance of normal sinus rhythm after conversion of atrial fibrillation or flutter; prevention of premature atrial, AV, and ventricular contractions; paroxysmal atrial tachycardia; paroxysmal AV junctional rhythm; atrial fibrillation; atrial flutter; paroxysmal ventricular tachycardia not associated with complete heart block**
PO
Adults, Elderly. 200-600 mg q6-8h (long-acting): 324-972 mg q8-12h.
Children. 30 mg/kg/day in divided doses q6h.
IV
Adults, Elderly. 5-10 mg/kg.

OFF-LABEL USES
Treatment of malaria (IV only).

CONTRAINDICATIONS
Complete AV block, intraventricular conduction defects (widening of QRS complex). Known quinidine allergy or a history of thrombocytopenia or thrombocytic purpura during quinidine therapy.

INTERACTIONS
Drug
Antimyasthenics: May decrease effects of these drugs on skeletal muscle.
Digoxin: May increase digoxin serum concentration.

Other antiarrhythmics, pimozide:
May increase cardiac effects.
Neuromuscular blockers, oral anticoagulants: May increase effects of these drugs.
Urinary alkalizers such as antacids: May decrease quinidine renal excretion.
Herbal
None known.
Food
None known.

DIAGNOSTIC TEST EFFECTS

Therapeutic serum level is 2-5 mcg/mL; toxic serum level is > 5 mcg/mL.

ⓦ IV INCOMPATIBILITIES

Furosemide (Lasix), heparin.

ⓦ IV COMPATIBILITIES

Milrinone (Primacor).

SIDE EFFECTS

Frequent
Abdominal pain and cramps, nausea, diarrhea, vomiting (can be immediate, intense).
Occasional
Mild cinchonism (ringing in ears, blurred vision, hearing loss) or severe cinchonism (headache, vertigo, diaphoresis, light-headedness, photophobia, confusion, delirium).
Rare
Hypotension (particularly with IV administration), hypersensitivity reaction (fever, anaphylaxis, photosensitivity reaction).

SERIOUS REACTIONS

• Cardiotoxic effects occur most commonly with IV administration, particularly at high concentrations, and are observed as conduction changes (50% widening of QRS complex, prolonged QT interval, flattened T waves, and disappearance of P wave), ventricular tachycardia or flutter, frequent premature ventricular contractions (PVCs), or complete AV block.
• Quinidine-induced syncope may occur with the usual dosage.
• Severe hypotension may result from high dosages.
• Patients with atrial flutter and fibrillation may experience a paradoxical, extremely rapid ventricular rate that may be prevented by prior digitalization.
• Hepatotoxicity with jaundice due to drug hypersensitivity may occur.

PRECAUTIONS & CONSIDERATIONS

Caution is warranted in patients with digoxin toxicity, incomplete AV block, hepatic and renal impairment, myasthenia gravis, myocardial depression, and sick sinus syndrome. Direct sunlight and artificial light should be avoided.

BP and pulse rate should be checked for 1 full minute before giving quinidine unless the person is on a continuous cardiac monitor. Notify the physician if fever, ringing in the ears, or visual disturbances occur. CBC; BUN; serum alkaline phosphatase, bilirubin, creatinine, AST (SGOT), and ALT (SGPT) levels; intake and output; pattern of bowel activity and stool consistency; and serum potassium should be monitored in those receiving long-term therapy. ECG for cardiac changes, particularly prolongation of PR or QT interval and widening of the QRS complex, should also be assessed; notify the physician of significant ECG changes.
Storage
Solution is stable for 24 h at room temperature when diluted with D5W.
Administration
! Quinidine's therapeutic serum level is 2-5 mcg/mL, and the toxic level is > 5 mcg/mL.

Q

Do not crush or chew sustained-release tablets. Take quinidine with food to reduce GI upset.

! Continuously monitor BP and ECG during IV administration; adjust the rate of the infusion as appropriate and as ordered to minimize arrhythmias and hypotension.

Use only clear, colorless solution. For IV infusion, dilute 800 mg with 50 mL D5W to provide concentration of 16 mg/mL. Give at rate of 1 mL (16 mg)/min because a rapid rate may markedly decrease arterial pressure. Administer with patient in supine position.

Quinine
kwye′nine
(Qualaquin)
Do not confuse with quinidine.

CATEGORY AND SCHEDULE
Pregnancy Risk Category: X

Classification: Antiprotozoals

Q

MECHANISM OF ACTION
A cinchona alkaloid that relaxes skeletal muscle by increasing the refractory period, decreasing excitability of motor endplates (curare-like), and affecting distribution of calcium with muscle fiber. Antimalaria: Depresses oxygen uptake and carbohydrate metabolism, elevates pH in intracellular organelles of parasites. *Therapeutic Effect:* Relaxes skeletal muscle; produces parasite death.

PHARMACOKINETICS
Rapidly absorbed mainly from upper small intestine. Protein binding: 70%-95%. Metabolized in liver. Excreted in feces, saliva, and urine. *Half-life:* 8-14 h (adults), 6-12 h (children).

AVAILABILITY
Capsules: 324 mg (Qualaquin).

INDICATIONS AND DOSAGES
▸ **Treatment of malaria**
PO
Adults, Elderly, Children ≥ 16 yr.
648 mg PO q8hr for 7 days.
▸ **Dosage in renal impairment**
In patients with severe chronic renal failure, the following modified dosage is recommended: Give one dose of 648 mg; then 12 h after, begin maintenance dose of 324 mg q12h.

CONTRAINDICATIONS
Known hypersensitivity to quinine or to mefloquine or quinidine because of cross-sensitivity, such reactions include thrombocytopenia, thrombotic thrombocytopenic purpura or hemolytic uremic syndrome; prolonged QT intervals, G6PD deficiency; myasthenia gravis, blackwater fever, optic neuritis.

INTERACTIONS
Drug
Alkalinizing agents, cimetidine, ranitidine: May increase quinine serum concentrations.
Digoxin: May increase blood concentration of digoxin.
Mefloquine: May increase risk of seizures and ECG abnormalities.
Phenobarbital, phenytoin, rifampin: May decrease quinine serum concentrations.
Warfarin: May increase anticoagulant effect.
Herbal
St. John's wort: May decrease quinine levels.

Food
None known.

DIAGNOSTIC TEST EFFECTS
May interfere with 17-OH steroid determinations. May result in positive Coombs' test.

SIDE EFFECTS
Frequent
Nausea, headache, tinnitus, slight visual disturbances (mild cinchonism).
Occasional
Extreme flushing of skin with intense generalized pruritus is most typical hypersensitivity reaction; also rash, wheezing, dyspnea, angioedema. Prolonged therapy: cardiac conduction disturbances, decreased hearing.

SERIOUS REACTIONS
• Overdosage (severe cinchonism) may result in cardiovascular effects, severe headache, intestinal cramps with vomiting and diarrhea, apprehension, confusion, seizures, blindness, and respiratory depression.
• Hypoprothrombinemia, thrombocytopenic purpura, hemoglobinuria, asthma, agranulocytosis, hypoglycemia, deafness, and optic atrophy occur rarely.

PRECAUTIONS & CONSIDERATIONS
Caution is warranted in patients with cardiovascular disease, myasthenia gravis, and asthma. Be aware that quinine is contraindicated in pregnant women. Quinine readily crosses the placenta and is distributed in breast milk. Be aware that quinine may cause congenital malformations such as deafness, limb abnormalities, visceral defects, visual changes, and stillbirths. Nonhormonal contraception should be used. No age-related precautions have been noted in children. In elderly patients, age-related renal impairment may require dosage adjustment.

Fasting blood sugar should be checked. Watch for signs of hypoglycemia such as cold sweating, tremors, tachycardia, hunger, and anxiety. Visual or hearing difficulties, shortness of breath, rash, itching, and nausea should be reported. Aluminum-containing antacids should be avoided because of drug absorption problems.

Storage
Store at room temperature.

Administration
Take quinine with food. Do not crush tablets or capsules to avoid bitter taste.

Q

Rabeprazole
rah-bep'rah-zole
(Aciphex, Novo-Rabeprazole
EC [CAN], Pariet [CAN], Ran-
Rabeprazole [CAN])
**Do not confuse Aciphex with
Accupril or Aricept.**

CATEGORY AND SCHEDULE
Pregnancy Risk Category: B

Classification: Gastrointestinals,
proton-pump inhibitors

MECHANISM OF ACTION
A proton-pump inhibitor that
converts to active metabolites that
irreversibly bind to and inhibit
hydrogen-potassium adenosine
triphosphate, an enzyme on the
surface of gastric parietal cells.
Actively secretes hydrogen ions
for potassium ions, resulting in an
accumulation of hydrogen ions in
gastric lumen. *Therapeutic Effect:*
Increases gastric pH, reducing gastric
acid production.

PHARMACOKINETICS
Rapidly absorbed from the GI tract
after passing through the stomach
relatively intact. Protein binding:
96%. Metabolized extensively in the
liver to inactive metabolites. Excreted
primarily in urine. Unknown whether
removed by hemodialysis. *Half-life:*
1-2 h is dose-dependent (increased
with hepatic impairment).

AVAILABILITY
Tablets (Delayed-Release): 20 mg.
Pariet [CAN]: 10 mg, 20 mg.

INDICATIONS AND DOSAGES
▸ **Erosive/ulcerative or symptomatic
gastroesophageal reflux disease
(GERD)**

PO
Adults, Elderly. 20 mg/day for
4-8 wks. Maintenance: 20 mg/day.
Children. 20 mg/day for up to 8 wks.
▸ **Erosive/ulcerative GERD:
[CAN labeling]**
PO
Adults, Elderly. 20 mg/day for
4 wks. May repeat an additional
4 wks but warrants further
evaluation. Maintenance: 10 mg/day
(maximum, 20 mg/day).
▸ **Symptomatic GERD: [CAN labeling]**
PO
Adults, Elderly. 10 mg/day for 4 wks
(Maximum, 20 mg/day). If symptom
control is not achieved after 4 wks,
additional evaluation is warranted.
▸ **Duodenal ulcer**
PO
Adults, Elderly. 20 mg/day before
morning meal for 4 wks. Some
patients may require an additional
4 wks of therapy.
▸ **Gastric ulcers: [CAN labeling]**
PO
Adults, Elderly. 20 mg/day for up to
6 wks. Some patients may require
additional therapy.
▸ **Pathologic hypersecretory
conditions, including
Zollinger-Ellison syndrome**
PO
Adults, Elderly. Initially, 60 mg
once a day. May increase to 100 mg
once a day or 60 mg twice a day.
Continue as long as necessary, even
up to 1 yr.
▸ ***Helicobacter pylori* infection**
PO
Adults, Elderly. 20 mg twice a
day for 7 days administered with
amoxicillin 1000 mg twice daily for
7 days and clarithromycin 500 mg
twice daily for 7 days.

CONTRAINDICATIONS
Hypersensitivity to rabeprazole or
any other proton-pump inhibitor.

INTERACTIONS
Drug
Atazanavir: Avoid co-administration due to decreased concentrations of atazanavir.
Digoxin: May increase the plasma concentration of digoxin.
Ethanol: Avoid because of increased GI irritation.
Iron salts: May interfere with absorption of iron salts.
Ketoconazole, itraconazole: May decrease the blood concentration of ketoconazole and itraconazole.
Warfarin: May incease availability of warfarin. Monitor PT/INR closely.
Herbal
St. John's wort: May decrease the levels of rabeprazole.
Food
High-fat meal: May delay absorption.

DIAGNOSTIC TEST EFFECTS
May increase serum alkaline phosphatase, AST (SGOT), and ALT (SGPT) levels.

SIDE EFFECTS
Rare (< 2%)
Headache, nausea, dizziness, rash, diarrhea, malaise.

SERIOUS REACTIONS
• Hyperglycemia, hypokalemia, hyponatremia, and hyperlipemia occur rarely.

PRECAUTIONS & CONSIDERATIONS
Caution is warranted in patients with severely impaired hepatic function. It is unknown whether rabeprazole crosses the placenta or is distributed in breast milk. Safety and efficacy of rabeprazole have been established in children 12 yr and older. No age-related precautions have been noted in elderly patients.

Notify the physician if diarrhea, GI discomfort, headache, nausea, or skin rash occurs. Laboratory values, especially serum chemistries and liver function test results, should be assessed before therapy.
Administration
Take rabeprazole before meals. Do not crush, chew, or split tablet; swallow it whole.

Raloxifene
ra-lox′i-feen
(Evista)
Do not confuse raloxifene with propoxyphene or Avinza.

CATEGORY AND SCHEDULE
Pregnancy Risk Category: X

Classification: Estrogen-receptor modulators, selective, hormones/hormone modifiers

MECHANISM OF ACTION
A selective estrogen receptor modulator that affects some receptors like estrogen. *Therapeutic Effect:* Like estrogen, prevents bone loss and improves lipid profiles.

PHARMACOKINETICS
Rapidly absorbed after PO administration. Highly bound to plasma proteins (95%) and albumin. Undergoes extensive first-pass metabolism in liver. Excreted mainly in feces and, to a lesser extent, in urine. Unknown whether removed by hemodialysis. *Half-life:* 28-33 h.

AVAILABILITY
Tablets: 60 mg.

R

INDICATIONS AND DOSAGES
▸ **Prevention or treatment of osteoporosis**
PO
Adults, Elderly. 60 mg a day.
▸ **For invasive breast cancer prophylaxis in postmenopausal women with osteoporosis or in postmenopausal women who are at high risk for developing the disease**
PO
Adults, Elderly. 60 mg a day.

CONTRAINDICATIONS
Active or history of venous thromboembolic events, such as deep vein thrombosis, pulmonary embolism, and retinal vein thrombosis; women who are at risk for stroke; women who are or may become pregnant or are breastfeeding.

INTERACTIONS
Drug
Cholestyramine: Reduces raloxifene absorption.
Drugs highly protein-bound (i.e., diazepam, diaoxide, lidocaine): Use with caution because raloxifene may affect protein binding of other drugs.
Hormone replacement therapy, systemic estrogen: Do not use raloxifene concurrently with these drugs.
Levothyroxine: May decrease levothyroxine's absorption.
Warfarin: May decrease PT and the effects of warfarin.
Herbal
Ethanol: Avoid because of the potential to increase risk of osteoporosis.
Food
None known.

DIAGNOSTIC TEST EFFECTS
Lowers serum total cholesterol and LDL levels but does not affect HDL or triglyceride levels. Slightly decreases platelet count and serum inorganic phosphate, albumin, calcium, and protein levels.

SIDE EFFECTS
Frequent (10%-25%)
Hot flashes, flulike symptoms, arthralgia, sinusitis.
Occasional (5%-9%)
Weight gain, nausea, myalgia, pharyngitis, cough, dyspepsia, leg cramps, rash, depression.
Rare (3%-4%)
Vaginitis, urinary tract infection, peripheral edema, flatulence, vomiting, fever, migraine, diaphoresis.

SERIOUS REACTIONS
• Pneumonia, chest pain, vaginal bleeding, and breast pain occur rarely.

PRECAUTIONS & CONSIDERATIONS
Caution is warranted in patients with cardiovascular disease, hepatic or renal impairment, and a history of cervical or uterine cancer. It is unknown whether raloxifene is distributed in breast milk; however, this drug is not recommended for breastfeeding women. Raloxifene is not used in children. No age-related precautions have been noted in elderly patients. Avoid alcohol consumption and cigarette smoking during raloxifene therapy. Also avoid prolonged immobility during travel because limited movement increases the risk of venous thromboembolic events. Exercise is encouraged.

Bone mineral density, platelet count, serum levels of inorganic phosphate, calcium, total and LDL cholesterol, and protein should be monitored.

Administration

Take raloxifene without regard to food at any time of day. Discontinue the drug 72 h before and during prolonged immobilization, such as postoperative recovery and prolonged bed rest. Resume therapy, as prescribed, only after the patient is fully ambulatory. Take supplemental calcium and vitamin D if daily dietary intake is inadequate.

Ramipril
ram'i-pril
(Altace, Apo-Ramipril [CAN], CO Ramipril [CAN], Novo-Ramipril [CAN], ratio-Ramipril [CAN], Sandoz-Ramipril [CAN])
Do not confuse Altace with Alteplase or Artane.

CATEGORY AND SCHEDULE
Pregnancy Risk Category: C (D if used in second or third trimester)

Classification: Angiotensin-converting enzyme (ACE) inhibitors

MECHANISM OF ACTION

An ACE inhibitor that suppresses the renin-angiotensin-aldosterone system. Decreases plasma angiotensin II, increases plasma renin activity, and decreases aldosterone secretion. *Therapeutic Effect:* Reduces peripheral arterial resistance and BP.

PHARMACOKINETICS

Route	Onset	Peak	Duration
PO	1-2 h	3-6 h	24 h

Well absorbed from the GI tract. Protein binding: 73%. Metabolized in the liver to active metabolite. Primarily excreted in urine (60%). Not removed by hemodialysis. *Half-life:* 2-17 h.

AVAILABILITY

Capsules: 1.25 mg, 2.5 mg, 5 mg, 10 mg.

INDICATIONS AND DOSAGES
▸ **Hypertension (monotherapy)**
PO
Adults, Elderly. Initially, 2.5 mg/day. Maintenance: 2.5-20 mg/day as single dose or in 2 divided doses.
▸ **Hypertension (in combination with other antihypertensives)**
PO
Adults, Elderly. Initially, 1.25-5 mg/day titrated to recovery's needs.
▸ **Congestive heart failure (CHF) post myocardial infarction (MI)**
PO
Adults, Elderly. Initially, 1.25-2.5 mg twice a day. Maximum: 5 mg twice a day; doses should be increased about 3 wks apart.
▸ **Risk reduction for MI, stroke, and death form cardiovascular causes**
PO
Adults, Elderly. Initially, 2.5 mg twice a day. If hypotensive, decrease to 1.25 mg twice a day, and after 1 wk at starting dose, dose can be titrated to 5 mg twice a day.
▸ **Dosage in renal impairment**
Creatinine clearance ≤ 40 mL/min. 25% of normal dose.
Renal failure and hypertension. Initially, 1.25 mg/day titrated upward to a maximum daily dose of 5 mg.
Renal failure and CHF. Initially, 1.25 mg/day, titrated up to 2.5 mg twice a day.

OFF-LABEL USES

Treatment of hypertension and renal crisis in scleroderma.

R

CONTRAINDICATIONS

Prior hypersensitivity (i.e., angioedema); bilateral renal artery stenosis; pregnancy second and third trimesters.

INTERACTIONS

Drug

Alcohol, antihypertensives, diuretics: May increase the effects of ramipril.

Angiotensin II receptor blockers, potassium-sparing diuretics, potassium supplements: May cause hyperkalemia.

Lithium: May increase lithium blood concentration and risk of lithium toxicity.

NSAIDs: May decrease the effects of ramipril and decrease renal function.

Herbal

Dong quai: May increase estrogenic activity.

Garlic: May increase antihypertensive effect.

Ephedra, ginseng, yohimbe: May worsen hypertension.

Food

None known.

DIAGNOSTIC TEST EFFECTS

May increase BUN, serum alkaline phosphatase, serum bilirubin, serum creatinine, serum potassium, AST (SGOT), and ALT (SGPT) levels. May decrease serum sodium levels. May cause positive antinuclear antibody titer.

SIDE EFFECTS

Frequent (5%-12%)
Cough, headache.
Occasional (2%-4%)
Dizziness, fatigue, nausea, asthenia (loss of strength).
Rare (< 2%)
Palpitations, insomnia, nervousness, malaise, abdominal pain, myalgia.

SERIOUS REACTIONS

• Excessive hypotension (first-dose syncope) may occur in patients with CHF and and in those who are severely salt or volume depleted.

• Angioedema and hyperkalemia occur rarely.

• Agranulocytosis and neutropenia may be noted in those with collagen vascular disease, including scleroderma and systemic lupus erythematosus, and impaired renal function.

• Nephrotic syndrome may be noted in those with history of renal disease.

PRECAUTIONS & CONSIDERATIONS

Caution is warranted in patients with CHF, collagen vascular disease, hyperkalemia, hypovolemia, renal impairment, and renal stenosis. Ramipril crosses the placenta, is distributed in breast milk, and may cause fetal or neonatal morbidity or mortality. Safety and efficacy of ramipril have not been established in children. Elderly patients may be more sensitive to the hypotensive effect of ramipril.

Dizziness and lightheadedness may occur. Tasks that require mental alertness or motor skills should be avoided. Notify the physician if chest pain, cough, or palpitations occur. Be alert to fluctuations in BP. If an excessive reduction in BP occurs, place the patient in the supine position with legs elevated. CBC and blood chemistry, including BUN and serum creatinine should be obtained before beginning ramipril therapy, then every 2 wks for the next 3 mo, and periodically thereafter in patients with autoimmune disease or renal impairment and in those who are taking drugs that affect immune response or leukocyte count. BUN, serum creatinine, serum potassium levels, and WBC count should also be monitored. Crackles and wheezing should be assessed in persons with CHF.

Administration

! Expect to reduce the dosage of diuretics 2-3 days before beginning ramipril therapy.

Take ramipril without regard to food. Swallow the capsules whole, and do not chew or break them. Mix with apple juice, applesauce, or water as needed.

Ranitidine

ra-ni′ti-deen
(Apo-Ranitidine [CAN], Ausran [AUS], Novo-Ranidine [CAN], Rani-2 [AUS], Ranihexal [AUS], Zantac, Zantac-75, Zantac EFFERdose)
Do not confuse Zantac with Xanax, Zarontin, Ziac, Zofran, or Zyrtec.

CATEGORY AND SCHEDULE

Pregnancy Risk Category: B
OTC (Tablets, 75 mg)

Classification: Antihistamines, H_2, gastrointestinals

MECHANISM OF ACTION

An antiulcer agent that inhibits histamine action at H_2 receptors of gastric parietal cells. *Therapeutic Effect:* Inhibits gastric acid secretion when fasting, at night, or when stimulated by food, caffeine, or insulin. Reduces volume and hydrogen ion concentration of gastric acid.

PHARMACOKINETICS

Rapidly absorbed from the GI tract. Protein binding: 15%. Widely distributed. Metabolized in the liver. Excreted primarily in urine. Not removed by hemodialysis. *Half-life:* 2.5 h; (increased with impaired renal function).

AVAILABILITY

Tablets (Effervescent [Zantac EFFERdose]): 25 mg.
Capsules: 150 mg, 300 mg.
Granules (Zantac EFFERdose): 150 mg.
Syrup (Zantac): 15 mg/mL.
Tablets (Zantac 75): 75 mg (OTC).
Tablets (Zantac): 150 mg, 300 mg.
Infusion, Premixed: 50 mL (Zantac 50 mg).
Injection (Zantac): 25 mg/mL.

INDICATIONS AND DOSAGES

▸ **Duodenal ulcers, gastric ulcers, gastroesophageal reflux disease (GERD)**
PO
Adults, Elderly. 150 mg twice a day or 300 mg after evening meal or at bedtime. Maintenance: 150 mg at bedtime.
Children aged 1 mo to 16 yr. 2-4 mg/kg/day in divided doses twice a day. Maximum: 300 mg/day. Maintenance for children: 150 mg/day.
▸ **Erosive esophagitis**
PO
Adults, Elderly. 150 mg 4 times a day. Maintenance: 150 mg 2 times/day or 300 mg at bedtime.
Children. 5-10 mg/kg/day in 2 divided doses.
▸ **Hypersecretory conditions**
PO
Adults, Elderly. 150 mg twice a day. May increase up to 6 g/day.
▸ **Usual parenteral dosage**
IV, IM
Adults, Elderly. 50 mg/dose q6-8h. Maximum: 400 mg/day.

R

Children. 2-4 mg/kg/day in divided doses q6-8h. Maximum: 200 mg/day.

▸ **_Helicobacter pylori_ eradication**
PO
Adults, Elderly. 150 mg twice daily in combination with antibiotics.

▸ **Prevention of heartburn**
PO
Adults, Elderly. 75 mg-150 mg before meals which cause heartburn. Max 150 mg/day. Do not use more the 14 days.
Children older than 2 yr. 75 mg before meals which cause heartburn. Max 150 mg/day. Do not use more the 14 days.

▸ **Usual neonatal dosage**
PO
Neonates. 2 mg/kg/day in divided doses q12h-24 hr.
IV
Neonates. Initially, 1.5 mg/kg/dose; then 1.5-2 mg/kg/day in divided doses q12h-24 hr.

▸ **Dosage in renal impairment**
For patients with creatinine clearance < 50 mL/min, give 150 mg PO q24h or 50 mg IV or IM q18-24h.

OFF-LABEL USES
Prevention of aspiration pneumonia.

CONTRAINDICATIONS
Hypersensitivity or history of acute porphyria.

INTERACTIONS
Drug
Antacids: May decrease the absorption of ranitidine.
Atazanavir, cyanocobalamin: Ranitidine may decrease absorption of these medications.
Cefuroxime, cefpodoxime: Rantidine may decrease the absorption so separate administration by 2 h.

Cyclosporin: Increased effect/toxicity of cyclosporin.
Ketoconazole: May decrease the absorption of ketoconazole.
Ethanol: Avoid since may worsen gastric irritation.
Warfarin: Variable effects on warfarin requires monitoring of PT/INR.
Herbal
None known.
Food
None known.

DIAGNOSTIC TEST EFFECTS
Interferes with skin tests using allergen extracts. May increase hepatic function enzyme, γ-glutamyl transpeptidase, and serum creatinine levels.

ⓦ IV INCOMPATIBILITIES
Amphotericin B complex (Abelcet, AmBisome, Amphotec).

ⓦ IV COMPATIBILITIES
Diltiazem (Cardizem), dobutamine (Dobutrex), dopamine (Intropin), heparin, hydromorphone (Dilaudid), insulin, lidocaine, lorazepam (Ativan), morphine, norepinephrine (Levophed), potassium chloride, propofol (Diprivan).

SIDE EFFECTS
Occasional (2%)
Diarrhea.
Rare (1%)
Constipation, headache (may be severe).

SERIOUS REACTIONS
• Reversible hepatitis and blood dyscrasias occur rarely.

PRECAUTIONS & CONSIDERATIONS
Caution is warranted in patients with impaired hepatic or renal function and in elderly patients.

Ranitidine does cross the placenta and is distributed in breast milk; use with caution. No age-related precautions have been noted in children. Elderly patients are more likely to experience confusion, especially those with hepatic or renal impairment. Smoking should be avoided. Also avoid alcohol, aspirin, and coffee, all of which may cause GI distress, during ranitidine therapy.

Notify the physician if headache occurs. Blood chemistry laboratory test results, including BUN, serum alkaline phosphatase, bilirubin, creatinine, AST (SGOT), and ALT (SGPT) levels to assess hepatic and renal function, should be obtained before and during therapy.

Storage

IV infusion (piggyback) is stable for 48 h at room temperature. Discard if discolored or precipitate forms.

Administration

Take oral ranitidine without regard to meals; however it is best given after meals or at bedtime. Do not administer within 1 h of magnesium- or aluminum-containing antacids because they decrease ranitidine absorption by 33%. Give 2 h after ketoconazole, cefuroxime, or cefpodoxime administration.

Effervescent dose should be dissolved in at least 5 mL (1 tsp of water) and administered once completely dissolved. Effervescent dose should not be chewed, swallowed whole, or dissolved on the tongue.

IV solutions normally appear clear and are colorless to yellow; slight darkening does not affect potency. For IV push, dilute each 50 mg with 20 mL 0.9% NaCl or D5W. For intermittent IV infusion (piggyback), dilute each 50 mg with 50 mL 0.9% NaCl or D5W. For IV infusion, dilute with 250-1000 mL 0.9% NaCl or D5W. Administer IV push over minimum of 5 min to prevent arrhythmias and hypotension. Infuse IV piggyback over 15-20 min. Infuse IV infusion over 24 h.

For IM use, ranitidine may be given undiluted. Give deep IM into large muscle mass, such as the gluteus maximus.

Repaglinide
re-pag′lih-nide
(GlucoNorm [CAN], Prandin)

CATEGORY AND SCHEDULE
Pregnancy Risk Category: C

Classification: Antidiabetic agents, meglitinides

MECHANISM OF ACTION
An antihyperglycemic that stimulates release of insulin from β-cells of the pancreas by depolarizing β-cells, leading to an opening of calcium channels. Resulting calcium influx induces insulin secretion. *Therapeutic Effect:* Lowers blood glucose concentration.

PHARMACOKINETICS
Rapidly, completely absorbed from the GI tract. Protein binding: > 98%. Metabolized in the liver to inactive metabolites. Excreted primarily in feces with a small amount in urine. Unknown whether removed by hemodialysis. *Half-life:* 1 h.

AVAILABILITY
Tablets: 0.5 mg, 1 mg, 2 mg.

INDICATIONS AND DOSAGES
▶ **Diabetes mellitus**
PO
Adults, Elderly. 0.5-4 mg with
each meal, up to 4 times/day.
Maximum: 16 mg/day. *Note:*
The starting dose for patients not
previously treated or with A1c
< 8% is 0.5 mg taken with meals.
For patients previously treated or
with A1c ≥ 8.0%, the initial dose
is 1-2 mg taken with each meal.

CONTRAINDICATIONS
Diabetic ketoacidosis, type 1
diabetes mellitus.

INTERACTIONS
Drug
**Azole antifungals, atazanavir,
β-blockers, chloramphenicol,
gemfibrozil, macrolide
antibiotics, MAOIs, NSAIDs,
probenecid, protease
inhibitors, ritonavir, salicylates,
sulfonamides, trimethoprim,
warfarin:** May increase the effects
of repaglinide.
**Carbamazepine, phenobarbital,
phenytoin, rifampin, nevirapine,
rifamycins:** May decrease the
effects of repaglinide.
Herbal
Gymenma, garlic: May cause
hypoglycemia.
St. John's wort: May decrease
repaglinide levels.

DIAGNOSTIC TEST EFFECTS
None known.

SIDE EFFECTS
Frequent (6%-16%)
Upper respiratory tract infection,
headache, rhinitis, bronchitis, back
pain.
Occasional (3%-5%)
Diarrhea, dyspepsia, sinusitis, nausea,
arthralgia, urinary tract infection.

Rare (2%)
Constipation, vomiting, paresthesia,
allergy.

SERIOUS REACTIONS
• Hypoglycemia occurs in 16% to
31% of patients.
• Chest pain occurs rarely.

PRECAUTIONS & CONSIDERATIONS
Caution is warranted in patients
with hepatic or moderate to
severe renal impairment. It is
unknown whether repaglinide is
distributed in breast milk. Safety
and efficacy of repaglinide have
not been established in children.
No age-related precautions
have been noted in the elderly,
but hypoglycemia may be more
difficult to recognize in this patient
population.
   Food intake and blood glucose
should be monitored before
and during therapy. Be aware
of the signs and symptoms of
hypoglycemia (anxiety, cool
wet skin, diplopia, dizziness,
headache, hunger, numbness in
mouth, tachycardia, tremors)
or hyperglycemia (deep rapid
breathing, dim vision, fatigue,
nausea, polydipsia, polyphagia,
polyuria, vomiting); carry candy,
sugar packets, or other sugar
supplements for immediate response
to hypoglycemia. Consult the
physician when glucose demands
are altered (such as with fever,
heavy physical activity, infection,
stress, trauma). Exercise, good
personal hygiene (including foot
care), not smoking, and weight
control are essential parts of
therapy.
Administration
Ideally, take repaglinide within
15 min of a meal 2- 4 times/day;
however, it may be taken

immediately or as long as 30 min before a meal. Allow at least 1 wk to elapse to assess response to the drug before new dosage adjustment is made.

Reserpine
reh-zer′peen
Do not confuse with Risperdal, risperidone.

CATEGORY AND SCHEDULE
Pregnancy Risk Category: C

Classification: Antiadrenergics, peripheral

MECHANISM OF ACTION
An antihypertensive that depletes stores of catecholamines and 5-hydroxytryptamine in many organs, including the brain and adrenal medulla. Depression of sympathetic nerve function results in a decreased heart rate and a lowering of arterial BP. Depletion of catecholamines and 5-hydroxytryptamine from the brain is thought to be the mechanism of the sedative and tranquilizing properties. *Therapeutic Effects:* Decrease BP and heart rate; sedation.

PHARMACOKINETICS
Characterized by slow onset of action and sustained effects. Both cardiovascular and central nervous system (CNS) effects may persist for a period following withdrawal of the drug. Mean maximum plasma levels were attained after a median of 3.5 h. Bioavailability was approximately 50% of that of a corresponding intravenous dose. Protein binding: 96%. *Half life:* 33 h.

AVAILABILITY
Tablets: 0.25 mg, 0.1 mg (reserpine).

INDICATIONS AND DOSAGES
▸ **Hypertension**
PO
Adults. Usual initial dosage 0.5 mg daily for 1 or 2 wks. For maintenance, reduce to 0.1-0.25 mg daily.
Children. Reserpine is not recommended for use in children.
▸ **Psychiatric disorders**
PO
Adults. Initial dosage, 0.5 mg daily; may range from 0.1 to 1 mg. Adjust dosage upward (in increments of 0.1-0.25 mg) or downward according to response. Max dose 5 mg/day.

OFF-LABEL USES
Cerebral vasospasm, migraines, Raynaud syndrome, reflex sympathetic dystrophy, refractory depression, tardive dyskinesia, thyrotoxic crisis.

CONTRAINDICATIONS
Hypersensitivity, mental depression or history of mental depression (especially with suicidal tendencies), active peptic ulcer, ulcerative colitis, patients receiving electroconvulsive therapy.

INTERACTIONS
Drug
β-Blockers: Reserpine may increase effect.
CNS depressants/ethanol: Reserpine may increase effects.
Levodopa, quinidine, procainamide, digitalis glycosides: Reserpine may increase effects/ toxicity.

R

MAO inhibitors: May cause hypertensive reactions.
Tricyclic antidepressants: May increase antihypertensive effects.
Herbal
Dong quai: Has estrogenic activity.
Ephedra/yohimbe: May worsen hypertension.
Valerian, St John's wort, kava kava, gotu kola: May increase CNS depression.
Garlic: May have increased antihypertensive effects.
Food
Ethanol: May increase CNS depression.

DIAGNOSTIC TEST EFFECTS
None known.

SIDE EFFECTS
Occasional
Burning in the stomach, nausea, vomiting, diarrhea, dry mouth, nosebleed, stuffy nose, dizziness, headache, nervousness, nightmares, drowsiness, muscle aches, weight gain, redness of the eyes.
Rare
Difficulty breathing, swelling, gynecomastia, decreased libido.

SERIOUS REACTIONS
• Irregular heart beat.
• Heart problems.
• Feeling faint.

PRECAUTIONS & CONSIDERATIONS
Caution is warranted in patients with kidney disease, gallstones, ulcers, ulcerative colitis, history of depression, electric shock therapy, and allergy to tartrazine. The physician should be aware of other medications being taken especially quinidine, digoxin, and tricyclic antidepressants such as imipramine, amitriptyline, doxepin, and nortriptyline. Be aware that reserpine is excreted in the breast milk. Elderly patients may be more susceptible to the hypotensive effects of reserpine. A low-salt diet should be followed. Change positions slowly to avoid orthostatic hypotension.

Dizziness, loss of appetite, diarrhea, upset stomach, vomiting, headache, dry mouth, and decreased sexual ability may occur. Notify physician immediately if depression, nightmares, fainting, slow heartbeat, chest pain, or swollen ankles, and feet occur.
Storage
Store at room temperature.
Administration
Take with food or milk to avoid GI irritation. Take at the same time each day.

Respiratory Syncytial Immune Globulin
res′purr-ah-tore-ee sin-sish′ee-al ih-mewn′ glah′byew-lin
(RespiGam)

CATEGORY AND SCHEDULE
Pregnancy Risk Category: C

Classification: Immune globulins

MECHANISM OF ACTION
An immune serum with a high concentration of neutralizing and protective antibodies specific for respiratory syncytial virus (RSV).
Therapeutic Effect: Provides protection against RSV infection and decreases the severity of existing infection.

AVAILABILITY
Injection: 2500 mcg RSV immune globulin.

INDICATIONS AND DOSAGES
▸ **Prevention of RSV in children with bronchopulmonary dysplasia and history of premature birth**
IV
Children younger than 24 mo.
750 mg/kg (15 mL/kg). Give prior to the beginning of RSV season and continue monthly throughout the season. RSV season typically begins in November and continues through April. Administer at a rate of 1.5 mL/kg/hr for the first 15 min. If tolerated, increase the rate to 3 mL/kg/hr for 15 min, then to a maximum rate of 6 mL/kg/hr until infusion is complete. Do not exceed maximum infusion rate.

Ⓓ IV INCOMPATIBILITIES
Manufacturer states do not mix or infuse with any other medications.

CONTRAINDICATIONS
IgA deficiency.

INTERACTIONS
Drug
Live-virus vaccines: May decrease immune response to live virus vaccines.
Herbal
None known.
Food
None known.

DIAGNOSTIC TEST EFFECTS
None known.

SIDE EFFECTS
Occasional (2%-6%)
Fever, vomiting, wheezing.

Rare (< 1%)
Diarrhea, rash, tachycardia, hypertension, hypoxia, injection-site inflammation.

SERIOUS REACTIONS
• Hypersensitivity reactions, characterized by dizziness, flushing, anxiety, palpitations, pruritus, myalgia, and arthralgia, occur rarely.

PRECAUTIONS & CONSIDERATIONS
Caution is warranted in patients with pulmonary disease. ABG, blood chemistry, serum osmolality electrolyte, and total protein levels should be monitored. Cardiopulmonary status and vital signs should be assessed before giving the drug, before each dosage or rate increase, every 30 min during the infusion, and 30 min after the infusion is completed. Child's body weight should be recorded. Baseline pulmonary assessment, including breath sounds, the presence of intercostal retractions, and respiratory rate, should be performed.
Storage
Refrigerate vials. Do not freeze.
Administration
Do not shake the vials. Start the infusion within 6 h and complete it within 12 h of opening the vial.

Reteplase
reh′te-place
(Rapilysin [AUS], Retavase)
Do not confuse reteplase or Retavase with Restasis.

CATEGORY AND SCHEDULE
Pregnancy Risk Category: C

Classification: Thrombolytics

R

MECHANISM OF ACTION
A tissue plasminogen activator that activates the fibrinolytic system by directly cleaving plasminogen to generate plasmin, an enzyme that degrades the fibrin of the thrombus. *Therapeutic Effect:* Exerts thrombolytic action.

PHARMACOKINETICS
Rapidly cleared from plasma. Eliminated primarily in the feces and urine. *Half-life:* 13-16 min.

AVAILABILITY
Powder for Injection: 10.4 units (18.1 mg).

INDICATIONS AND DOSAGES
▸ **Acute myocardial infarction (MI), congestive heart failure (CHF)**
IV BOLUS
Adults, Elderly. 10 units over 2 min; repeat in 30 min.

CONTRAINDICATIONS
Active internal bleeding, AV malformation or aneurysm, bleeding diathesis, history of cerebrovascular accident, intracranial neoplasm, recent intracranial or intraspinal surgery, or trauma, severe uncontrolled hypertension.

INTERACTIONS
Drug
Aminocaproic acid: May decrease the effectiveness of reteplase.
Clopidogrel, heparin, low-molecular-weight heparin, nonsteroidal anti-inflammatory agents (NSAIDs), platelet aggregation antagonists (such as abciximab, aspirin, dipyridamole), ticlopidine, warfarin: Increase the risk of bleeding.
Herbal
Ginkgo biloba: May increase the risk of bleeding.

Food
None known.

DIAGNOSTIC TEST EFFECTS
May decrease fibrinogen and serum plasminogen levels.

Ⓦ IV INCOMPATIBILITIES
Do not mix with other medications.

SIDE EFFECTS
Frequent
Bleeding at superficial sites, such as venous injection sites, catheter insertion sites, venous cutdowns, arterial punctures, and sites of recent surgical procedures, gingival bleeding.

SERIOUS REACTIONS
• Bleeding at internal sites may occur, including intracranial, retroperitoneal, GI, genitourinary, and respiratory sites.
• Lysis or coronary thrombi may produce atrial or ventricular arrhythmias and stroke.

PRECAUTIONS & CONSIDERATIONS
Caution is warranted in patients with acute pericarditis, bacterial endocarditis, cerebrovascular disease, diabetic retinopathy; severe hepatic or renal impairment; hypertension, major surgery, including coronary artery bypass graft, obstetric delivery, organ biopsy, mitral stenosis with atrial fibrillation, occluded AV cannula at an infected site, ophthalmic hemorrhage, recent GI or GU bleeding, septic thrombophlebitis, concurrent use of oral anticoagulants, and in the elderly (> 75 yr old). It is unknown whether reteplase is distributed in breast milk. Safety and efficacy of reteplase have not been established in children. Elderly patients are

more susceptible to bleeding. Use reteplase cautiously in this population. An electric razor and a soft toothbrush should be used to reduce the risk of bleeding.

Notify the physician of black or red stool, coffee-ground vomitus, dark or red urine, red-speckled mucus from cough, chest pain, headache, palpitations, or shortness of breath. Continuous cardiac monitoring should be performed. BP and pulse and respiration rates should be checked every 15 min until stable; then check hourly. Serum creatine kinase (CK), and CK-MB concentrations, 12-lead ECG, electrolyte levels, hematocrit, platelet count, aTT, aPTT, PT, and fibrinogen level should be evaluated before therapy starts.

Storage

Use within 4 h of reconstitution. Discard any unused portion.

Administration

Reconstitute only with sterile water for injection immediately before use. Reconstituted solution contains 1 unit/mL. Do not shake the vial. Slight foaming may occur; let stand for a few minutes to allow bubbles to dissipate. Give through a dedicated IV line. Give as a 10-unit plus 10-unit double bolus, with each IV bolus administered over 2 min. Give the second bolus 30 min after the first bolus injection. Do not add other medications to the bolus injection solution. Do not give second IV bolus if serious bleeding occurs after first bolus.

Rho (D) Immune Globulin
(HyperRHO S/D Full Dose, HyperRHO S/D Mini Dose MICRhogam, RhoGAM, Rhophylac,WinRho SDF)

CATEGORY AND SCHEDULE
Pregnancy Risk Category: C

Classification: Immune globulins

MECHANISM OF ACTION
$Rh_o(D)$ immune globulin contains anti-$Rh_o(D)$ antibody to the RBC antigen $Rh_o(D)$. $Rh_o(D)$ immune globulin suppresses the active antibody response and formation of anti-$Rh_o(D)$ in $Rh_o(D)$-negative women exposed to Rh_o-positive blood from a pregnancy with an $Rh_o(D)$-positive fetus or transfusion with $Rh_o(D)$-positive blood. The anti-$Rh_o(D)$ antibody in $Rh_o(D)$ immune globulin may bind to $Rh_o(D)$ antigen in maternal circulation, preventing stimulation of the primary immune response to $Rh_o(D)$ and subsequent active productiuon of anti-$Rh_o(D)$. Injection of $Rh_o(D)$ immune globulin into an Rh-positive patient with idiopathic thrombocytopenic purpura (ITP) may result in the formation of anti-$Rh_o(D)$-coated RBC complexes; as the RBCs are cleared by the spleen, they saturate the capacity of the spleen to clear antibody-coated cells, sparing antibody-coated platelets. *Therapeutic Effect:* Prevents antibody response and hemolytic disease of the newborn in women who have previously conceived an $Rh_o(D)$-positive fetus. Prevents

R

Rh$_o$(D) sensitization in patients who have received Rh$_o$(D)-positive blood. Decreases bleeding in patients with ITP.

AVAILABILITY

Injection, Powder for Reconstitution for IM or IV use (WinRho SDF): 120 mcg, 300 mcg, 500 mcg, 1000 mcg, 3000 mcg.
Injection solution, IM only (HyperRHO S/D Full Dose): 300 mcg.
Injection solution, IM only (HyperRHO S/D Mini Dose): 50 mcg.
Injection solution, IM only (RhoGAM): 300 mcg.
Injection solution, IM only (MICRORhoGAM): 50 mcg.
Injection solution, IM or IV use (Rhophylac): 300 mcg/2 mL.

INDICATIONS AND DOSAGES
▸ **ITP**
IV (WINRHO SDF, RHINOPHYLAC)
Adults, Elderly, Children. Initially, 50 mcg/kg as single dose (Rhinophylac) (WinRho SDF reduce to 25-40 mcg/kg if Hgb is < 10 g/dL). Maintenance: 25-60 mcg/kg based on platelet count and hemoglobin level.
▸ **Suppression of the active antibody response and formation of anti-Rh$_o$(D) in Rh$_o$(D)-negative women exposed to Rh$_o$ positive blood from a pregnancy with an Rh$_o$(D)-positive fetus**
IM (HYPERRHO S/D FULL DOSE, RHOGAM) OR IM, IV (RHOPHYLAC, WINRHO)
Adults. 300 mcg (HyperRHO S/D Full Dose, RhoGAM, Rhophylac) or 120 mcg (WinRho), preferably within 72 h of delivery but may be given up to 28 days following delivery.

IV, IM (RHOPHLAC, WINRHO SDF)
Adults. 300 mcg at 28-wks gestation. After delivery: 120 mcg, preferably within 72 h.
▸ **Suppression of active antibody response and formation of anti-Rh$_o$(D) in Rh$_o$(D)-negative women exposed to Rh$_o$-positive blood from a miscarriage with an Rh$_o$(D)-positive fetus**
IM (HYPERRHO S/D FULL DOSE, RHOGAM)
Adults. 300 mcg as soon as possible.
▸ **Suppression of the active antibody response and formation of anti-Rh$_o$(D) in Rh$_o$(D)-negative women exposed to Rh$_o$-positive blood from an abortion, miscarriage, or termination of an ectopic pregnancy with an Rh$_o$(D)-positive fetus**
IM (RHOGAM)
Adults. 300 mcg if > 13-wks gestation, 50 mcg if < 13-wks gestation.
IV, IM (WINRHO SDF)
Adults. 120 mcg after 34-wks gestation; administer immediately or within 72 h.
▸ **Transfusion incompatibility**
IV (WINRHO SDF)
Children, Adults. 3000 units (600 mcg) q8h until total dose given; exposure to Rh$_o$(D)-positive whole blood 9 mcg/mL blood; exposure to Rh$_o$(D)-positive red blood cells (RBCs) 18 mcg/mL blood.
IM (WINRHO SDF)
Children, Adults. 6000 units (1200 mcg) q12h until total dose given; exposure to Rh$_o$(D)-positive whole blood 12 mcg/mL blood; exposure to Rh$_o$(D)-positive red blood cells 24 mcg/mL blood.
IM (HYPERRHO S/D FULL DOSE, RHOGAM)
Adults. Multiply the volume of Rh-positive whole blood administered by the hematocrit of

the donor unit to equal the volume of RBCs transfused. Divide the volume of RBCs by 15 mL = 300 mcg doses to administer. Round up fractions to the higher whole 300-mcg dose.
IM, IV (RHOPHYLAC)
Adults. 20 mcg/2 mL transfused blood to 20 mcg/2 mL erythrocyte concentrate.

CONTRAINDICATIONS

Hypersensitivity to any component, IgA deficiency, mothers whose Rh group or immune status is uncertain, prior sensitization to $Rh_o(D)$, $Rh_o(D)$-positive mother or pregnant woman, transfusion of $Rh_o(D)$-positive blood in previous 3 mo.

INTERACTIONS

Drug
Live-virus vaccines: May interfere with the patient's immune response to the vaccine.
Herbal
None known.
Food
None known.

DIAGNOSTIC TEST EFFECTS
None known.

SIDE EFFECTS

Hypotension, pallor, vasodilation (IV formulation), fever, headache, chills, dizziness, somnolence, lethargy, rash, pruritus, abdominal pain, diarrhea, discomfort and swelling at injection site, back pain, myalgia, arthralgia, asthenia.

SERIOUS REACTIONS

• None known.

PRECAUTIONS & CONSIDERATIONS

Caution is warranted in patients with bleeding disorders, particularly thrombocytopenia, and blood hemoglobin (Hgb) < 8 g/dL. Notify the physician of chills, dizziness, fever, headache, or rash. CBC (especially Hgb and platelet count), BUN and serum creatinine levels, reticulocyte count, and urinalysis results should be monitored. Do not give live vaccines within 3 mo after $Rh_o(D)$.

Storage
Refrigerate vials. Do not freeze. Once reconstituted, the solution is stable for 12 h at room temperature.

Administration
For IV use, reconstitute the 120-mcg and 300-mcg vials with 2.5 mL 0.9% NaCl (the 1000-mcg vials with 8.5 mL 0.9% NaCl). Gently swirl—do not shake—the vial. Infuse the solution over 3-5 min.

For IM use, reconstitute the 120-mcg and 300-mcg vials with 2.5 mL 0.9% NaCl (the 1000-mg vials with 8.5 mL 0.9% NaCl). Inject the IM solution into the deltoid muscle of the upper arm or the anterolateral aspect of the upper thigh.

Ribavirin

rye-ba-vye′rin
(Copegus, Rebetol, RibaPak, Ribasphere, Virazole)
Do not confuse ribavirin with riboflavin.

CATEGORY AND SCHEDULE
Pregnancy Risk Category: X

Classification: Antivirals

MECHANISM OF ACTION

A synthetic nucleoside that inhibits replication of RNA and DNA viruses, inhibits influenza virus RNA polymerase activity, and interferes with expression of messenger RNA. *Therapeutic Effect:* Inhibits viral protein synthesis and replication of viral RNA and DNA.

PHARMACOKINETICS

Readily absorbed from the respiratory tract or GI tract. Protein binding: None. Widely distributed into erythrocytes. Metabolized in the liver and intracellularly. Excreted in urine and feces. Unknown whether removed by hemodialysis. *Half-life:* Inhalation 6.5-11 h (children), oral capsules 44-298 h, oral tablets 120-170 h.

AVAILABILITY

Capsules (Rebetol, Ribasphere): 200 mg.
Tablets (Cepegus): 200 mg.
Tablet (dose pack) (RibaPak): 400 mg, 600 mg and RibaPak 400/600: 400 mg, 600 mg.
Powder for Reconstitution (Aerosol [Virazole]): 6 g.
Oral Solution (Rebetol): 40 mg/mL.

INDICATIONS AND DOSAGES
▸ **Chronic hepatitis C**
PO (CAPSULE OR ORAL SOLUTION IN COMBINATION WITH INTERFERON ALFA-2B)
Adults, Elderly weighing ≤ 75 kg. 400 mg in morning, 600 mg in evening, > 75 kg 600 mg in morning, 600 mg in evening.
Children weighing ≥ 61 kg or more. Use adult dosage. Weight 51-61 kg: 400 mg twice/day; 37-50 kg: 200 mg in morning, 400 mg in evening; 24-36 kg: 200 mg twice/day.
PO (CAPSULES IN COMBINATION WITH PEGINTERFERON ALFA-2B)
Adults, Elderly. 400 mg/day twice/day.

PO (TABLETS IN COMBINATION WITH PEGINTERFERON ALFA-2B)
Adults, Elderly. Monoinfection, genotype 1,4: < 75 kg: 1000 mg/day in 2 divided doses, ≥ 75 kg 1200 mg/day in 2 divided doses. Monoinfection, genotype 2, 3: 800 mg/day in 2 divided doses. Coinfection: 800 mg/day in 2 divided doses. (800-1200 mg/day in 2 divided doses).
▸ **Severe lower respiratory tract infection caused by respiratory syncytial virus (RSV)**
INHALATION
Children, Infants. Use with Viratek small-particle aerosol generator at a concentration of 20 mg/mL (6 g reconstituted with 300 mL sterile water) over 12-18 h/day for 3-7 days.

OFF-LABEL USES

Treatment of influenza A or B and west Nile virus.

CONTRAINDICATIONS

Pregnancy, women of childbearing age who will not use contraception reliably.

INTERACTIONS
Drug
Didanosine: May increase the risk of pancreatitis and peripheral neuropathy and decrease the effects of didanosine.
Interferons, alpha: May increase the risk of hemolytic anemia.
Live influenza vaccine: May diminish the effects of the vaccine.
Nucleoside analogues (including adefovir, didanosine, emtricitabine, entecavir, lamivudine, stavudine, zalcitabine, zidovudine): May increase the risk of lactic acidosis.
Stavudine: May decrease effect of stavudine.

Herbal
None known.
Food
None known.

DIAGNOSTIC TEST EFFECTS
None known.

SIDE EFFECTS
Frequent (> 10%)
Dizziness, headache, fatigue, fever, insomnia, irritability, depression, emotional lability, impaired concentration, alopecia, rash, pruritus, nausea, anorexia, dyspepsia, vomiting, decreased hemoglobin, hemolysis, arthralgia, musculoskeletal pain, dyspnea, sinusitis, flulike symptoms.
Occasional (10%-1%)
Nervousness, altered taste, weakness.

SERIOUS REACTIONS
• Cardiac arrest, apnea, ventilator dependence, bacterial pneumonia, pneumonia, and pneumothorax occur rarely.
• Anemia may occur if ribavirin therapy exceeds 7 days.

PRECAUTIONS & CONSIDERATIONS
Use inhaled ribavirin cautiously with asthma, chronic obstructive pulmonary disease (COPD), and those requiring mechanical ventilation. Caution should be used with oral ribavirin in the elderly and with cardiac or pulmonary disease and a history of psychiatric disorders.

Report any difficulty breathing or itching, redness, or swelling of the eyes. Respiratory tract secretions should be obtained for diagnostic testing before giving the first dose of ribavirin or at least during the first 24 h of therapy. Complete blood count (CBC) with differential should be obtained. Pretreat and test women of childbearing age monthly for pregnancy. Hematology reports should be assessed for anemia from reticulocytosis when therapy exceeds 7 days. For ventilator-assisted patients, watch for "rainout" in tubing and empty frequently.

Storage
Solution normally appears clear and colorless and is stable for 24 h at room temperature. Discard solution for nebulization after 24 h. Discard solution if discolored or cloudy. Oral solution may be stored at room temperature or refrigerated.

Administration
! Ribavirin may be given via nasal or oral inhalation. Add 50-100 mL sterile water for injection or inhalation to 6-g vial. Transfer to a flask, serving as reservoir for aerosol generator. Further dilute to final volume of 300 mL, giving a solution concentration of 20 mg/mL. Use only aerosol generator available from the drug manufacturer. Do not give at the same time with other drug solutions for nebulization. Discard reservoir solution when fluid levels are low and at least every 24 h. Be aware that there is controversy over the safety of administering ribavirin to ventilator-dependent patients; only experienced personnel should administer the drug.

Capsules should not be opened, crushed, chewed or broken. Capsules or solution may be taken without regard to food. Tablets should be given with food.

R

Rifabutin
rif'a-byoo-ten
(Mycobutin)
Do not confuse rifabutin with rifampin.

CATEGORY AND SCHEDULE
Pregnancy Risk Category: B

Classification:
Antimycobacterials

MECHANISM OF ACTION
An antitubercular agent that inhibits DNA-dependent RNA polymerase, an enzyme in susceptible strains of *Escherichia coli* and *Bacillus subtilis*. Rifabutin has a broad spectrum of antimicrobial activity, including activity against mycobacteria such as *Mycobacterium avium* complex (MAC). *Therapeutic Effect:* Prevents MAC disease.

PHARMACOKINETICS
Readily absorbed from the GI tract (high-fat meals delay absorption). Protein binding: 85%. Widely distributed. Crosses the blood-brain barrier. Extensive intracellular tissue uptake. Metabolized in the liver to active and inactive metabolites. Excreted in urine; eliminated in feces. Unknown if removed by hemodialysis. *Half-life:* 16-69 h.

AVAILABILITY
Capsules: 150 mg.

INDICATIONS AND DOSAGES
▸ **Prevention of MAC disease (first episode) in HIV-infected patients with < 50 CD4+ cells/mm³**
PO
Adults, Elderly. 300 mg as a single dose or in 2 divided doses if GI upset occurs.

Children ≥ 6 yr of age: 300 mg as a single dose.
▸ **Prevention of recurrent MAC disease**
PO
Adults, Elderly. 300 mg/day (in combination with azithromycin).
▸ **Dosage in renal impairment**
Dosage is modified based on creatinine clearance. If creatinine clearance is < 30 mL/min, reduce dosage by 50%.

CONTRAINDICATIONS
Active tuberculosis; hypersensitivity to other rifamycins, including rifampin.

INTERACTIONS
Drug
Clopidogrel: May increase therapeutic effect of clopidogrel.
CYP3A4 inducers (carbamazepines, phenobarbital, phenytoin): May decrease effects of rifabutin.
Isoniazid: May increase the risk of hepatotoxicity.
Oral contraceptives: May decrease contraceptive effectiveness.
Zidovudine: May decrease blood concentration of zidovudine but does not affect the drug's inhibition of HIV. Note: Rifabutin may decrease the effects of numerous drugs, including CYP3A4 substrates.
Herbal
None known.
Food
High-fat meals: May decrease the rate of absorption.

DIAGNOSTIC TEST EFFECTS
May increase serum alkaline phosphatase, AST (SGOT), and ALT (SGPT) levels.

SIDE EFFECTS
Frequent (30%)
Red-orange or red-brown discoloration of urine, feces,

saliva, skin, sputum, sweat, or tears.
Occasional (3%-11%)
Rash, nausea, abdominal pain, diarrhea, dyspepsia, belching, headache, altered taste, uveitis, corneal deposits.
Rare (< 2%)
Anorexia, flatulence, fever, myalgia, vomiting, insomnia.

SERIOUS REACTIONS
• Hepatitis and thrombocytopenia occur rarely. Anemia and neutropenia may also occur.

PRECAUTIONS & CONSIDERATIONS
Caution should be used with liver or renal impairment. The safety of this drug for use in children is not established. Be aware that it is unknown whether rifabutin crosses the placenta or is excreted in breast milk. No age-related precautions have been noted in children or in elderly patients. Avoid crowds and those with known infection.

Feces, perspiration, saliva, skin, sputum, tears, and urine may be discolored red-brown or red-orange during drug therapy. Soft contact lenses may be permanently discolored. Rifabutin may decrease the effectiveness of oral contraceptives. Alternative methods of contraception should be used. Expect to perform a biopsy of suspicious nodes, if present. Also, expect to obtain blood or sputum cultures and a chest x-ray to rule out active tuberculosis. If ordered, obtain baseline complete blood count (CBC) and liver function test results.
Administration
Should take on an empty stomach. Take with food if GI irritation occurs. May mix with applesauce

if unable to swallow capsules whole.

Rifampin
rye'fam-pin
(Rifadin, Rimactane, Rimycin [AUS], Rofact [CAN])
Do not confuse rifampin with rifabutin, Rifamate, rifapentine, or Ritalin.

CATEGORY AND SCHEDULE
Pregnancy Risk Category: C

Classification:
Antimycobacterials

MECHANISM OF ACTION
An antitubercular agent that interferes with bacterial RNA synthesis by binding to DNA-dependent RNA polymerase, thus preventing its attachment to DNA and blocking RNA transcription. *Therapeutic Effect:* Bactericidal in susceptible microorganisms.

PHARMACOKINETICS
Well absorbed from the GI tract (food delays absorption). Protein binding: 80%. Widely distributed. Metabolized in the liver to active metabolite. Eliminated primarily by the biliary system. Not removed by hemodialysis. *Half-life:* 3-4 h (increased in hepatic impairment).

AVAILABILITY
Capsules (Rifadin): 150 mg, 300 mg.
Capsules (Rimactane): 300 mg.
Injection, Powder for Reconstitution (Rifadin): 600 mg.

R

INDICATIONS AND DOSAGES
▶ **Tuberculosis**
PO, IV
Adults, Elderly. 10 mg/kg/day in divided doses q12-24h. Maximum: 600 mg/day.
Children. 10-20 mg/kg/day in divided doses q12-24h.
▶ **Prevention of meningococcal infections**
PO, IV
Adults, Elderly. 600 mg q12h for 2 days.
Children 1 mo and older. 20 mg/kg/day in divided doses q12-24h. Maximum: 600 mg/dose.
Infants younger than 1 mo. 10 mg/kg/day in divided doses q12h for 2 days.
▶ **Staphylococcal infections**
PO, IV
Adults, Elderly. 600 mg once a day.
Children. 15 mg/kg/day in divided doses q12h.
▶ ***Staphylococcus aureus* infections (in combination with other anti-infectives)**
PO
Adults, Elderly. 300-600 mg twice a day.
▶ **Prevention of *Haemophilus influenzae* infection**
PO
Adults, Elderly. 600 mg/day for 4 days.
Children 1 mo and older. 20 mg/kg/ day in divided doses q12h for 5-10 days.
Children younger than 1 mo. 10 mg/kg/day in divided doses q12h for 2 days.

OFF-LABEL USES
Prophylaxis of *H. influenzae* type b infection; treatment of atypical mycobacterial infection.

CONTRAINDICATIONS
Concomitant therapy with amprenavir, saquinavir/ritonovir, hypersensitivity to rifampin or any other rifamycins.

INTERACTIONS
Drug
Alcohol, hepatotoxic medications: May increase the risk of hepatotoxicity.
Aminophylline, theophylline: May increase clearance of these drugs.
Amiodarone, chloramphenicol, digoxin, disopyramide, fluconazole, methadone, mexiletine, oral anticoagulants, oral antidiabetics, phenytoin, quinidine, tocainide, verapamil: May decrease the effects of these drugs.
Clopidogrel: May increase the therapeutic effects.
Isoniazid, pyrazaminde or amprenavir, saquinavir/ ritonavir: May increase the risk of hepatotoxicity.
Macrolide antibiotics: May increase levels/toxicity of rifampin.
Oral contraceptives: May decrease oral contraceptive effectiveness.
NOTE: Rifampin may decrease the effects of numerous drugs, including CYP1A2, 2A6, 2B6, 2C8, 2C9, 2C19, 3A4 substrates.
Herbal
St. John's wort: May decrease rifampin levels.
Food
All foods: Food may decrease rifampin concentrations.

DIAGNOSTIC TEST EFFECTS
May increase serum alkaline phosphatase, bilirubin, uric acid, AST (SGOT), and ALT (SGPT) levels.

🌀 IV INCOMPATIBILITIES

Diltiazem (Cardizem), amiodarone, minocycline, tramadol.

SIDE EFFECTS

Expected
Red-orange or red-brown discoloration of urine, feces, saliva, skin, sputum, sweat, or tears.
Occasional (2%-5%)
Hypersensitivity reaction (such as flushing, pruritus, or rash).
Rare (1%-2%)
Diarrhea, dyspepsia, nausea, candida as evidenced by sore mouth or tongue.

SERIOUS REACTIONS

• Rare reactions include hepatotoxicity (risk is increased when rifampin is taken with isoniazid), hepatitis, blood dyscrasias, Stevens-Johnson syndrome, and antibiotic-associated colitis.

PRECAUTIONS & CONSIDERATIONS

Caution is warranted with active alcoholism, a history of alcohol abuse, or liver dysfunction. Be aware that rifampin crosses the placenta and is distributed in breast milk. No age-related precautions have been noted in children or in elderly patients. Avoid alcohol and any other medications, including antacids, without consulting with the physician. The reliability of oral contraceptives may be affected by rifampin, so alternative methods of contraception should be used.

Feces, sputum, sweat, tears, or urine may become red-orange or red-brown, and soft contact lenses may be permanently stained. Notify the physician of any new symptoms or if fatigue, fever, flu, nausea, unusual bleeding or bruising, vomiting, weakness, or yellow eyes and skin occurs. CBC results should be evaluated for blood dyscrasias and bleeding, bruising, infection manifested as a fever or sore throat, and unusual tiredness and weakness should be assessed.

Storage
Reconstituted vial is stable for 24 h. Once the reconstituted vial is further diluted, it is stable for 4 h in D5W or 24 h in 0.9% NaCl.

Administration
Preferably give oral rifampin 1 h before or 2 h after meals with 8 oz of water. Rifampin may be given with food to decrease GI upset, but this will delay the drug's absorption. For those unable to swallow capsules, rifampin's contents may be mixed with applesauce or jelly. Give rifampin at least 1 h before administering antacids, especially antacids containing aluminum.

! Administer rifampin by IV infusion only. Avoid IM and SC administration. Reconstitute 600-mg vial with 10 mL sterile water for injection to provide a concentration of 60 mg/mL. Withdraw the desired dose and further dilute with 500 mL D5W. Evaluate periodically for extravasation as evidenced by local inflammation and irritation. Infuse over 3 h (may dilute with 100 mL D5W and infuse over 30 min).

R

Rifapentine
rif-a-pen'teen
(Priftin)
Do not confuse with Rifampin.

CATEGORY AND SCHEDULE
Pregnancy Risk Category: C

Classification:
Antimycobacterials

MECHANISM OF ACTION
An antitubercular agent that
inhibits bacterial RNA synthesis by
binding to DNA-dependent RNA
polymerase in *Mycobacterium
tuberculosis.* This action prevents
the enzyme from attaching to
DNA, thereby blocking RNA
transcription. *Therapeutic Effect:*
Bactericidal.

AVAILABILITY
Tablets: 150 mg.

INDICATIONS AND DOSAGES
▸ **Tuberculosis (in combination with
at least one other antituberculosis
agent)**
PO
Adults, Elderly. Intensive phase:
600 mg twice weekly for 2 mo
(interval between doses not
< 3 days). Continuation phase:
600 mg weekly for 4 mo.

CONTRAINDICATIONS
Hypersensitivity to rifapentine,
rifampin, rifabutin.

INTERACTIONS
Drug
**Amiodarone, chloramphenicol,
digoxin, disopyramide, fluconazole,
methadone, mexiletine, oral
anticoagulants, oral antidiabetics,
phenytoin, quinidine, tocainide,**
verapamil: May decrease the effects
of these drugs.
Clopidogrel: May increase the
therapeutic effects.
Isoniazid: May increase the risk of
hepatoxocity.
NOTE: Rifapentine may decrease the
effects of numerous drugs, including
CYP2C8, 2C9, and 3A4 substrates.
Herbal
None known.
Food
All foods: Increases maximum
serum concentrations.

DIAGNOSTIC TEST EFFECTS
May increase serum AST
(SGOT), ALT (SGPT), and
bilirubin levels.

SIDE EFFECTS
Rare (< 4%)
Red-orange or red-brown
discoloration of urine, feces, saliva,
skin, sputum, sweat, or tears;
arthralgia, pain, nausea, vomiting,
headache, dyspepsia, hypertension,
dizziness, diarrhea.

SERIOUS REACTIONS
• Hyperuricemia, neutropenia,
proteinuria, hematuria, and hepatitis
occur rarely.

PRECAUTIONS & CONSIDERATIONS
Caution is warranted in alcoholic
patients and in those with liver
function impairment. Feces, sputum,
sweat, tears, and urine may become
red-orange or red-brown, and soft
contact lenses may be permanently
stained. The reliability of oral
contraceptives may be affected by
rifapentine, so alternative methods of
contraception should be used. Initial
complete blood count (CBC) and
liver function test results should be
evaluated. Evaluate for diarrhea, GI
upset, nausea, or vomiting as well as

R

pattern of daily bowel activity and stool consistency.
Administration
! Be aware that rifapentine is used only in combination with another antituberculosis agent.

Rifaximin
rye-faks′eh-men
(Xifaxan)

CATEGORY AND SCHEDULE
Pregnancy Risk Category: C

Classification: Antibiotics, miscellaneous

MECHANISM OF ACTION
An anti-infective that inhibits bacterial RNA synthesis by binding to a subunit of bacterial DNA-dependent RNA polymerase. *Therapeutic Effect:* Bactericidal.

PHARMACOKINETICS
< 0.4% absorbed after PO administration. Widely distributed in the GI tract. *Half-life:* 6 h. Excreted primary in feces as unchanged drug.

AVAILABILITY
Tablets: 200 mg.

INDICATIONS AND DOSAGES
▸ **Traveler's diarrhea**
PO
Adults, Elderly, Children 12 yr and older. 200 mg 3 times a day for 3 days.

OFF-LABEL USES
Treatment of hepatic encephalopathy.

CONTRAINDICATIONS
Hypersensitivity to rifaximin or other rifamycin antibiotics or diarrhea with fever or blood in the stool.

INTERACTIONS
Drug
None known.
Herbal
None known.
Food
None known.

DIAGNOSTIC TEST EFFECTS
None known.

SIDE EFFECTS
Occasional (5%-11%)
Flatulence, headache, abdominal discomfort, rectal tenesmus, defecation urgency, nausea.
Rare (2%-4%)
Constipation, fever, vomiting.

SERIOUS REACTIONS
• Hypersensitivity reactions, including dermatitis, angioneurotic edema, pruritus, rash, and urticaria, may occur.
• Superinfection occurs rarely.

PRECAUTIONS & CONSIDERATIONS
Caution should be used with diarrhea complicated by fever and/or blood in the stool, or diarrhea due to pathogens other than Escherichia coli (rifaximin is not considered effective) as well as with diarrhea believed to be caused by Campylobacter jejuni, Shigella spp., or Salmonella spp. It is unknown if rifaximin is distributed in breast milk. Safety and efficacy of rifaximin have not been established in children younger than 12 yr. In elderly patients with normal renal function, no age-related precautions are noted.

If diarrhea worsens or within 48 h, if blood in the stool occurs, or if fever develops, notify the physician.
Storage
Store tablets at room temperature.
Administration
Take with or without food. Do not break or crush film-coated tablets.

Riluzole
rye′loo-zole
(Rilutek)

CATEGORY AND SCHEDULE
Pregnancy Risk Category: C

Classification: Neuroprotectives, glutamate inhibitor

MECHANISM OF ACTION
An amyotrophic lateral sclerosis (ALS) agent that inhibits presynaptic glutamate release in the central nervous system (CNS) and interferes postsynaptically with the effects of excitatory amino acids. *Therapeutic Effect:* Extends survival of ALS patients.

PHARMACOKINETICS
Well absorbed from the GI tract (high-fat meal decreases absorption). Protein binding: 96%. Metabolized extensively in the liver to major and minor metabolites. Primarily eliminated in the urine as metabolites. *Half-life:* 12 h.

AVAILABILITY
Tablets: 50 mg.

INDICATIONS AND DOSAGES
▸ **ALS**
PO
Adults, Elderly. 50 mg q12h.

CONTRAINDICATIONS
None significant.

INTERACTIONS
Drug
Amiodarone, amitriptyline, fluvoxamine, ketoconazole, quinolones, theophylline: May increase the effects and risk of toxicity of riluzole.
Carbamazepine, omeprazole, phenobarbital, rifampin: May decrease the effects of riluzole.
Herbal
None known.
Ethanol
Alcohol: May increase CNS depression.
Food
Caffeine: May increase the effects and risk of toxicity of riluzole.
High-fat meals: May decrease the absorption and effects of riluzole.

DIAGNOSTIC TEST EFFECTS
May increase liver function test results.

SIDE EFFECTS
Frequent (> 10%)
Nausea, asthenia, reduced respiratory function.
Occasional (1%-10%)
Edema, tachycardia, headache, dizziness, somnolence, depression, vertigo, tremor, pruritus, alopecia, abdominal pain, diarrhea, anorexia, dyspepsia, vomiting, stomatitis, increased cough.

SERIOUS REACTIONS
• Hepatic insufficiency and potential for hepatic failure.

PRECAUTIONS & CONSIDERATIONS
Caution is warranted in patients with renal or hepatic impairment. Alcohol should be avoided as well as tasks requiring mental alertness

or motor skills until response to the medication has been established.

Notify the physician of fever. Blood chemistry tests to evaluate hepatic function should be obtained before and during therapy. The drug should be discontinued if the ALT level exceeds 10 times the upper normal limit.

Administration
Take riluzole at least 1 h before or 2 h after a meal at the same time each day.

Rimantadine
ri-man'ti-deen
(Flumadine)
Do not confuse rimantadine with ranitidine or Flumadine with flunisolide or flutamide.

CATEGORY AND SCHEDULE
Pregnancy Risk Category: C

Classification: Antivirals

MECHANISM OF ACTION
An antiviral that appears to exert an inhibitory effect early in the viral replication cycle. May inhibit uncoating of the virus. *Therapeutic Effect:* Prevents replication of influenza A virus.

AVAILABILITY
Syrup: 50 mg/5 mL.
Tablets: 100 mg.

INDICATIONS AND DOSAGES
▶ **Treatment of influenza A virus infection**
PO
Adults, Elderly. 100 mg twice a day for 7 days.
Elderly nursing home patients, patients with severe hepatic or renal impairment. 100 mg once a day for 7 days.
▶ **Prevention of influenza A virus**
PO
Adults, Elderly, Children 10 yr and older. 100 mg twice a day for at least 10 days after known exposure (usually for 6-8 wks).
Children younger than 10 yr. 5 mg/kg once a day. Maximum: 150 mg.
Elderly nursing home patients, patients with severe hepatic or renal impairment. 100 mg once a day.

CONTRAINDICATIONS
Hypersensitivity to amantadine or rimantadine.

INTERACTIONS
Drug
Acetaminophen, aspirin: May decrease rimantadine blood concentration.
Anticholinergics, central nervous system (CNS) stimulants: May increase side effects of rimantadine.
Cimetidine: May increase rimantadine blood concentration.
Live influenza vaccine: May decrease the efficacy of the vaccine.
Herbal
None known.
Food
None known.

DIAGNOSTIC TEST EFFECTS
None known.

SIDE EFFECTS
Occasional (2%-3%)
Insomnia, nausea, nervousness, impaired concentration, dizziness.
Rare (< 2%)
Vomiting, anorexia, dry mouth, abdominal pain, asthenia, fatigue.

SERIOUS REACTIONS
• None known.

R

PRECAUTIONS & CONSIDERATIONS

Caution is warranted in patients with a history of recurrent eczematoid dermatitis, liver disease, renal impairment, seizures, uncontrolled psychosis, and concomitant use of CNS stimulants. Avoid taking acetaminophen, aspirin, or compounds containing these drugs. Avoid contact with those who are at high risk for developing influenza A (rimantadine-resistant virus may be shed during therapy).

Dry mouth may occur while taking rimantadine. Do not drive or perform tasks that require mental alertness if decreased concentration or dizziness occurs. Nervousness, sleep pattern, insomnia, and dizziness should be assessed.

Administer the live influenza vaccine at least 48 h after rimantadine and do not give rimantadine within 2 wks of live vaccine.

Note: In June 2006 the Centers for Disease Control and Prevention (CDC) recommended that rimatadine not be used for treatment or prophylaxis of influenza A due to resistance.

Administration
Give rimantadine without regard to food.

Risedronate
rye-se-droe′nate
(Actonel)

CATEGORY AND SCHEDULE
Pregnancy Risk Category: C

Classification: Bisphosphonates

MECHANISM OF ACTION
A bisphosphonate that binds to bone hydroxyapatite and inhibits osteoclasts. *Therapeutic Effect:* Reduces bone turnover (the number of sites at which bone is remodeled) and bone resorption.

AVAILABILITY
Tablets: 5 mg, 30 mg, 35 mg, 75 mg.

INDICATIONS AND DOSAGES
▸ **Paget disease**
PO
Adults, Elderly. 30 mg/day. Retreatment may occur after 2-mo post-treatment observation period.
▸ **Prevention and treatment of postmenopausal osteoporosis**
PO
Adults, Elderly. 5 mg/day or 35 mg once weekly or 75 mg/day on 2 consecutive days/mo.
▸ **Glucocorticoid-induced osteoporosis**
PO
Adults, Elderly. 5 mg/day.
▸ **Treatment of male osteoporosis.**
PO
Adults, Elderly. 35 mg once weekly.

CONTRAINDICATIONS
Hypersensitivity to other bisphosphonates, including etidronate, ibandronate, tiludronate, risedronate, and alendronate; hypocalcemia; inability to stand or sit upright for at least 30 min; renal impairment when serum creatinine clearance is < 30 mL/min.

INTERACTIONS
Drug
Antacids containing aluminum, calcium, magnesium; oral calcium, iron, and magnesium salts; vitamin D: May decrease the absorption of risedronate.

NSAIDs: May enhance GI toxic effects.
Phosphate supplements: May enhance hypocalcemic effects.
Herbal
None known.
Food
Food: Reduces absorption.

DIAGNOSTIC TEST EFFECTS
May interfere with diagnostic imaging, technetium-99m-diphosphonate in bone scans.

SIDE EFFECTS
Frequent (30%)
Arthralgia.
Occasional (8%-12%)
Rash, flu-like symptoms, peripheral edema.
Rare (3%-5%)
Bone pain, sinusitis, asthenia, dry eye, tinnitus.

SERIOUS REACTIONS
• Overdose causes hypocalcemia, hypophosphatemia, and significant GI disturbances.
• Osteonecrosis of the jaw.

PRECAUTIONS & CONSIDERATIONS
Caution is warranted in patients with cardiac failure or renal impairment. Because there are no adequate and well-controlled studies in pregnant women, it is unknown whether risedronate causes fetal harm or is excreted in breast milk. Safety and efficacy of risedronate have not been established in children. Elderly patients may become overhydrated and require careful monitoring of fluid and electrolytes. Dilute the drug in a smaller volume for elderly patients. Consider beginning weight-bearing exercises and modifying behavioral factors, such as avoiding alcohol consumption and cigarette smoking.

Hypocalcemia and vitamin D deficiency, if present, should be corrected before beginning risedronate therapy. BUN, creatinine levels, and serum electrolyte levels, including serum calcium and creatinine levels, should be established before and monitored during therapy.

Because of concern about osteonecrosis, preventative dental care, including exams, should be done before beginning therapy, and invasive dental procedures should be avoided while on therapy.

Administration
Take the drug with a full glass (6-8 oz) of plain water first thing in the morning and at least 30 min before first beverage, food, or medication of the day. Taking risedronate with other beverages, including coffee, mineral water, and orange juice, significantly reduces the absorption of the drug. Avoid lying down or bending over for at least 30 min after taking risedronate to potentiate delivery to the stomach and reduce the risk of esophageal irritation. Do not crush or chew the tablet.

Risperidone
ris-per′i-done
(Risperdal, Risperdal Consta, Risperdal M-Tabs)
Do not confuse risperidone with reserpine.

CATEGORY AND SCHEDULE
Pregnancy Risk Category: C

Classification: Antipsychotics, atypical

MECHANISM OF ACTION
A benzisoxazole derivative that may antagonize dopamine and serotonin receptors. *Therapeutic Effect:* Suppresses psychotic behavior.

PHARMACOKINETICS
Oral form is well absorbed from the GI tract; unaffected by food. Protein binding: 90%. Extensively metabolized in the liver to active metabolite. Excreted primarily in urine. *Half-life,* Oral: 3-20 h; metabolite: 21-30 h (increased in elderly); *Injection:* 3-6 days. Excreted primarily in urine and feces.

AVAILABILITY
Oral Solution (Risperdal): 1 mg/mL.
Tablets (Risperdal): 0.25 mg, 0.5 mg, 1 mg, 2 mg, 3 mg, 4 mg.
Tablets (Orally Disintegrating [Risperdal M-Tabs]): 0.5 mg, 1 mg, 2 mg, 3 mg, 4 mg.
Injection (Risperdal Consta): 12.5 mg, 25 mg, 37.5 mg, 50 mg.

INDICATIONS AND DOSAGES
▸ **Schizophrenia**
PO
Adolescents aged 13-17 yr. Initially, 0.5 mg once a day, adjusted in increments of 0.5-1 mg/day. Range: 1-6 mg/day, but doses > 3 mg/day do not yield additional benefits.
Adults. Initially, 1 mg twice a day. May increase dosage slowly, 1-2 mg/day on a weekly basis. Range 4-16 mg/day. Maintenance: 4 mg/day. Range: 2-8 mg/day.
Elderly. Initially, 0.25-2 mg/day in 2 divided doses. May increase dosage slowly. Range: 2-6 mg/day.
IM
Adults, Elderly. 25 mg q2wk. Maximum: 50 mg q2wk.

▸ **Mania, bipolar**
PO
Children and adolescents aged 10-17 yr. Initially 0.5 mg/day, May increase at 24-h intervals of 0.5-1 mg/day. Range: 0.5-6 mg, but doses > 2.5 mg/day do not yield additional benefits.
Adults, Elderly. Initially, 2-3 mg as a single daily dose. May increase at 24-h intervals of 1 mg/day. Range: 1-6 mg/day. No maintenance dosing beyond 3 wks recommended.

▸ **Autism**
PO
Children 5 yr and older and adolescents. < 15 kg, use with caution; < 20 kg, 0.25 mg/day. After 4 days, may increase to 0.5 mg/day. Maintain dose for at least 14 days, then increase dose by 0.25 mg/day q2wk. Clinical response peaks at 1 mg/day; > 20 kg, 0.5 mg/day. After 4 days, may increase to 1 mg/day. Maintain dose for at least 14 days, then increase dose by 0.5 mg/day q2wk. Clinical response peaks at 2.5 mg/day.

▸ **Dosage in renal impairment**
Initial dosage for adults and elderly patients is 0.25-0.5 mg twice a day. Dosage is titrated slowly to desired effect.

OFF-LABEL USES
Behavioral symptoms associated with dementia, pervasive developmental disorder, Tourette disorder.

CONTRAINDICATIONS
Dementia-related psychosis in the elderly (Black Box).

INTERACTIONS
Drug
Alcohol, other CNS depressants: May increase CNS depression.
Carbamazepine: May decrease the risperidone blood concentration.
Clozapine: May increase the risperidone blood concentration.

CYP2D6 inhibitors: May increase the levels/effects of risperidone.
Dopamine agonists, levodopa: May decrease the effects of these drugs.
Paroxetine: May increase the risperidone blood concentration and the risk of extrapyramidal symptoms.
Valproic acid: May increase the adverse effects/toxicity of risperidone.
Verapamil, SSRIs, and lithium: May increase the levels/effects of risperidone.
Herbal
Kava kava, gotu kola, St. John's wort, valerian: May increase central nervous system (CNS) depression.
Food
Food: None known.
Ethanol: Avoid; may increase CNS depression.

DIAGNOSTIC TEST EFFECTS

May increase serum prolactin, creatinine, alkaline phosphatase, uric acid, AST (SGOT), ALT (SGPT), and triglyceride levels. May decrease blood glucose and serum potassium, protein, and sodium levels. May cause ECG changes.

SIDE EFFECTS

Frequent (13%-26%)
Agitation, anxiety, insomnia, headache, constipation.
Occasional (4%-10%)
Dyspepsia, rhinitis, somnolence, dizziness, nausea, vomiting, rash, abdominal pain, dry skin, tachycardia.
Rare (3%-2%)
Visual disturbances, fever, back pain, pharyngitis, cough, arthralgia, angina, aggressive behavior, orthostatic hypotension, breast swelling.

SERIOUS REACTIONS

• Rare reactions include tardive dyskinesia (characterized by tongue protrusion, puffing of the cheeks, and chewing or puckering of the mouth) and neuroleptic malignant syndrome (marked by hyperpyrexia, muscle rigidity, change in mental status, irregular pulse or BP, tachycardia, diaphoresis, cardiac arrhythmias, rhabdomyolysis, and acute renal failure).
Warnings
Patients with dementia-related psychosis who are treated with an atypical antipsychotic are at an increased risk of death compared with those taking placebo.

PRECAUTIONS & CONSIDERATIONS

Caution is warranted in patients with cardiac disease, breast cancer, hepatic or renal impairment, seizure disorders, recent MI, those at risk for aspiration pneumonia, suicidal tendencies, and dementia (may increase risk of cerebrovascular accident [CVA]). Be aware that risperidone may increase the risk of hyperglycemia. It is unknown whether risperidone crosses the placenta or is excreted in breast milk. Breastfeeding is not recommended for patients taking this drug. The safety and efficacy of this drug have not been established in children. Elderly patients are more susceptible to orthostatic hypotension and may require a dosage adjustment because of age-related renal or hepatic impairment.

Drowsiness and dizziness may occur but generally subsides with continued therapy. Tasks requiring mental alertness or motor skills should be avoided. Notify the physician if altered gait, difficulty breathing, palpitations, pain or

R

swelling in breasts, severe dizziness or fainting, trembling fingers, unusual movements, rash, fever, or visual changes occur. BP, heart rate, liver function test results, ECG, and weight should be assessed.

Storage
The drug may be given up to 6 h after reconstitution, but immediate administration is recommended. If 2 min pass before the injection, reconstitute the solution by shaking the upright vial vigorously back and forth for as long as it takes to resuspend the microspheres. Store the drug below 77° F (25° C) once it is in suspension.

Administration
Take risperidone without regard to food. Mix the oral solution with water, orange juice, coffee, or low-fat milk, but not with cola or tea.

For M-Tabs, once removed from blister pack, place immediately on tongue. Do not split or chew tablet because it will dissolve within seconds and may be swallowed with or without liquid.

For IM administration, use only the diluent and needle supplied in the dose pack. All the components in the dose pack will be required for administration. Do not substitute any components. Prepare the suspension according to the manufacturer's directions. Inject the drug intramuscularly into the upper outer quadrant of the gluteus maximus. Do not administer the drug by the IV route.

Ritonavir
ri-tone′a-veer
(Norvir, Norvisec [CAN])
Do not confuse ritonavir with Retrovir or Norvir with Norvasc.

CATEGORY AND SCHEDULE
Pregnancy Risk Category: B

Classification: Antivirals, protease inhibitors

Mechanism of Action
Inhibits HIV-1 and HIV-2 proteases, rendering these enzymes incapable of processing the polypeptide precursors; this results in the production of noninfectious, immature HIV particles. *Therapeutic Effect:* Impedes HIV replication, slowing the progression of HIV infection.

PHARMACOKINETICS
Well absorbed after PO administration (absorption increased with food). Protein binding: 98%-99%. Extensively metabolized in the liver to active metabolite. Eliminated primarily in feces. Unknown whether removed by hemodialysis. *Half-life:* 3-5 h.

AVAILABILITY
Oral Solution: 80 mg/mL.
Soft Gelatin Capsules: 100 mg.

INDICATIONS AND DOSAGES
▸ **HIV infection**
PO
Children > 1 mo. Initiate 250 mg/m^2 twice a day, titrating upward every 2-3 days by 50 mg/m^2 to a maximum of 600 mg twice a day.
Adults, Children 12 yr and older. 600 mg twice a day. If nausea

occurs at this dosage, give 300 mg twice a day for 1 day, 400 mg twice a day for 2 days, 500 mg twice a day for 1 day, then 600 mg twice a day thereafter.
Children younger than 12 yr.
Initially, 250 mg/m^2 twice a day. Increase by 50 mg/m^2 up to 400 mg/m^2. Maximum: 600 mg twice a day.

CONTRAINDICATIONS
Concurrent use of amiodarone, astemizole, bepridil, bupropion, cisapride, clozapine, encainide, flecainide, meperidine, piroxicam, propafenone, propoxyphene, quinidine, rifabutin, terfenadine, or voriconazole (increased risk of serious or life-threatening drug interactions, such as arrhythmias, hematologic abnormalities, and seizures); concurrent use of alprazolam, clorazepate, diazepam, estazolam, flurazepam, midazolam, triazolam, or zolpidem (may produce extreme sedation and respiratory depression).

INTERACTIONS
Drug
Desipramine, fluoxetine, other antidepressants: May increase the blood concentration of these drugs.
Disulfiram, drugs causing disulfiram-like reaction (such as metronidazole): May produce a disulfiram-like reaction.
Enzyme inducers (including carbamazepine, dexamethasone, nevirapine, phenobarbital, phenytoin, rifabutin, rifampin): May increase the metabolism and decrease the efficacy of ritonavir.
Oral contraceptives, theophylline: May decrease the effectiveness of these drugs.
NOTE: Interactions are numerous.

Herbal
St. John's wort: May decrease the blood concentration and effect of ritonavir.
Food
Food: Enhances absorption.

DIAGNOSTIC TEST EFFECTS
May alter serum CK, GGT, triglyceride, uric acid, AST (SGOT), and ALT (SGPT) levels as well as creatinine clearance.

SIDE EFFECTS
Frequent
GI disturbances (abdominal pain, anorexia, diarrhea, nausea, vomiting), circumoral and peripheral paresthesias, altered taste, headache, dizziness, fatigue, asthenia.
Occasional
Allergic reaction, flu-like symptoms, hypotension.
Rare
Diabetes mellitus, hyperglycemia.

SERIOUS REACTIONS
• None known.

PRECAUTIONS & CONSIDERATIONS
Caution should be used in patients with impaired hepatic function. Be aware that breastfeeding is not recommended in this population because of the possibility of HIV transmission. No age-related precautions have been noted in children older than 2 yr. There are no known effects of this drug's use in elderly patients.

When beginning combination therapy with ritonavir and nucleosides, it may promote GI tolerance by first beginning ritonavir alone and then by adding nucleosides before completing 2 wks of ritonavir monotherapy. Check baseline laboratory test results, if ordered, especially

R

liver function tests and serum triglycerides, before beginning ritonavir therapy and at periodic intervals during therapy. Monitor for signs and symptoms of GI disturbances or neurologic abnormalities, particularly paresthesias.

When used as "booster" in combination with other protease inhibitors, be sure to consult specific dosage recommendations of both agents.

Storage

Store capsules or solution in the refrigerator. Protect the drug from light. Refrigerate the oral solution unless it is used within 30 days and stored below 77° F.

Administration

Administer with food. May improve the taste of the oral solution by mixing it with Advera, chocolate milk, or Ensure within 1 h of dosing. Continue therapy for the full length of treatment, and evenly space drug doses around the clock. Separate administration from buffered didanosine or antacids by 2.5 h.

R

Rituximab

rye-tucks′ih-mab
(monoclonal antibody, antineoplastic)
(Mabthera [AUS], Rituxan)
Do not confuse Rituxan with Remicade or rituximab with infliximab.

CATEGORY AND SCHEDULE

Pregnancy Risk Category: C

Classification: Antineoplastics, monoclonal antibodies

MECHANISM OF ACTION

Binds to CD20, the antigen found on the surface of B lymphocytes and B-cell non-Hodgkin lymphomas. *Therapeutic Effect:* Produces cytotoxicity, reducing tumor size.

PHARMACOKINETICS

Rapidly depletes B cells. Distribution: 4.3 L. *Half-life* proportional to dose: 3.2 days after first infusion and 8.6 days after fourth infusion. Excretion: uncertain.

AVAILABILITY

Injection: 10 mg/mL.

INDICATIONS AND DOSAGES

▸ **Non-Hodgkin lymphoma: different treatment protocols depending on type**
IV
Adults. 375 mg/m^2 once weekly for 4 wks. May administer a second 4-wk course.
▸ **Rheumatoid arthritis**
IV
Adults. 1000 mg on days 1 and 15 in combination with methotrexate.

CONTRAINDICATIONS

Hypersensitivity to murine proteins.

INTERACTIONS

Drug
Antihypertensives: May intensify hypotensive effects.
Live vaccines: Decrease effect of rituximab.
Monoclonal antibiodies: May increase the risk of allergic reactions to rituximab.
Herbal
Hypoglycemic herbs (alfalfa, bilberry, bitter melon, burdock, celery, daminana, fenugreek, garcinia, garlic, ginger, ginseng, symnema, marshmallow, and stinging nettle: May enhance hypoglycemic effects of rituximab.

Food
None known.

DIAGNOSTIC TEST EFFECTS
None known.

⍟ IV INCOMPATIBILITIES
Do not mix rituximab with any other medications.

SIDE EFFECTS
In general, patients receiving treatment for RA may see fewer side effects.
Frequent
Fever (49%), chills (32%), asthenia (16%), headache (14%), angioedema (13%), hypotension (10%), nausea (18%), rash or pruritus (10%).
Occasional (< 10%)
Myalgia, dizziness, abdominal pain, throat irritation, vomiting, neutropenia, rhinitis, bronchospasm, urticaria.

SERIOUS REACTIONS
• A hypersensitivity reaction marked by hypotension, bronchospasm, and angioedema may occur.
• Arrhythmias may occur, particularly in those with a history of preexisting cardiac conditions.
Warning
Progressive multifocal leukoencephalopathy (PML) due to JC virus has been reported with use. Tumor lysis syndrome leading to acute renal failure requiring dialysis may occur 12-24 h following the first dose. Severe, sometimes fatal mucocutaneous reactions have been reported.

PRECAUTIONS & CONSIDERATIONS
Caution is warranted in patients with a history of cardiac disease. Be aware that rituximab may cause fetal B-cell depletion. Women with childbearing potential should use contraceptive methods during treatment and for up to 12 mo afterward. It is unknown whether rituximab is distributed in breast milk. The safety and efficacy of rituximab have not been established in children. No age-related precautions have been noted in elderly patients.

Infusion-related reactions, including chills, fever, hypotension, and rigors, which usually occur 30 min to 2 h after beginning the first rituximab infusion, should be monitored; slowing the infusion resolves these symptoms. CBC should be obtained before and regularly during therapy.
Storage
Refrigerate unopened vials. The diluted solution is stable for up to 24 h if refrigerated and at room temperature for an additional 24 hr.
Administration
❗ Expect to pretreat the patient with acetaminophen and diphenhydramine before each infusion to help prevent infusion-related reactions. With rheumatoid arthritis, pretreat with a corticosteroid before each rituximab dose. Do not give rituximab by IV push or bolus.

Withdraw the needed amount into an infusion bag, and dilute it with 0.9% NaCl or D5W to a final concentration of 1-4 mg/mL. For the initial infusion, infuse the drug at 50 mg/h. The infusion rate may be increased, as necessary, in increments of 50 mg/h every 30 min to a maximum rate of 400 mg/h. For subsequent infusions, the drug may be administered initially at 100 mg/h and increased in increments of 100 mg/h every 30 min to a maximum rate of 400 mg/h.

R

Rizatriptan
rize-a-trip′tan
(Maxalt, Maxalt-MLT)

CATEGORY AND SCHEDULE
Pregnancy Risk Category: C

Classification: Serotonin
receptor agonists

MECHANISM OF ACTION
A serotonin receptor agonist
that binds selectively to
vascular receptors, producing a
vasoconstrictive effect on cranial
blood vessels. *Therapeutic Effect:*
Relieves migraine headache.

PHARMACOKINETICS
Well absorbed after PO
administration. Protein binding:
14%. Crosses the blood-brain barrier.
Metabolized by the liver to inactive
metabolite. Eliminated primarily in
urine and, to a lesser extent, in feces.
Half-life: 2-3 h.

AVAILABILITY
Tablets (Maxalt): 5 mg, 10 mg.
*Oral Disintegrating Tablets
(Maxalt-MLT):* 5 mg, 10 mg.

INDICATIONS AND DOSAGES
▸ **Acute migraine attack**
PO (TABLETS OR ODT)
Adults older than 18 yr, Elderly. 5-10
mg. If headache improves, but then
returns, dose may be repeated after
2 h. Maximum: 30 mg/24 h.

CONTRAINDICATIONS
Basilar or hemiplegic migraine,
coronary artery disease, ischemic
heart disease (including angina
pectoris, history of myocardial
infarction [MI], silent ischemia, and
Prinzmetal's angina), uncontrolled

hypertension, use within 24 h of
ergotamine-containing preparations
or another serotonin receptor
agonist; use within 14 days of
MAOIs.

INTERACTIONS
Drug
**Dextromethorphan, fluoxetine,
fluvoxamine, paroxetine,
sertraline, tramadol:** May produce
hyperreflexia, incoordination, and
weakness.
**Selective 5-HT1 antagonist,
ergotamine-containing
medications:** May produce a
vasospastic reaction.
MAOIs, propranolol: May
dramatically increase plasma
concentration of rizatriptan.
Herbal
None known.
Food
All foods: Delays peak drug
concentration by 1 h.

DIAGNOSTIC TEST EFFECTS
None known.

SIDE EFFECTS
Frequent (7%-9%)
Dizziness, somnolence, paresthesia,
fatigue.
Occasional (3%-6%)
Nausea, chest pressure, dry mouth.
Rare (2%)
Headache; neck, throat, or jaw
pressure; photosensitivity.

SERIOUS REACTIONS
• Cardiac reactions (such as
ischemia, coronary artery
vasospasm, and MI) and noncardiac
vasospasm-related reactions
(including hemorrhage and
cerebrovascular accident) occur
rarely, particularly in patients with
hypertension, diabetes, or a strong
family history of coronary artery

disease; obese patients; smokers; males older than 40 yr; and postmenopausal women.

PRECAUTIONS & CONSIDERATIONS

Caution is warranted in patients with mild to moderate hepatic or renal impairment and cardiovascular risk factors. It is unknown whether rizatriptan is excreted in breast milk. The safety and efficacy of rizatriptan have not been established in children. Rizatriptan is not recommended for elderly patients. Smoking, exposure to sunlight and ultraviolet rays, and tasks that require mental alertness or motor skills should be avoided.

Dizziness may occur. Notify the physician immediately if anxiety, chest pain, palpitations, or tightness in the throat occurs. BUN level and serum alkaline phosphatase, bilirubin, creatinine AST (SGOT), and ALT (SGPT) levels should be obtained before treatment to assess renal and hepatic function. ECG should also be obtained at baseline. Migraines and associated symptoms, including nausea and vomiting, photophobia, and phonophobia (sound sensitivity), should be assessed before and during treatment.

Administration

Do not crush, chew, or split tablets. Preferably take without food. The orally disintegrating tablets come packaged in individual aluminum blister packs. Do not remove the orally disintegrating tablet from the blister pack until just before taking it. Open packet with dry hands, and place tablet on the tongue to dissolve. Then swallow it. Do not administer the orally disintegrating tablets with water.

Ropinirole
ro-pin'i-role
(Requip)

CATEGORY AND SCHEDULE
Pregnancy Risk Category: C

Classification: Antiparkinson agents, dopaminergics

MECHANISM OF ACTION
An antiparkinson agent that stimulates dopamine receptors in the striatum. *Therapeutic Effect:* Relieves signs and symptoms of Parkinson disease.

PHARMACOKINETICS
Rapidly absorbed after PO administration. Protein binding: 40%. Extensively distributed throughout the body. Extensively metabolized. Steady-state concentrations achieved within 2 days. Eliminated in urine. Unknown whether removed by hemodialysis. *Half-life:* 6 h.

AVAILABILITY
Tablets: 0.25 mg, 0.5 mg, 1 mg, 2 mg, 3 mg, 4 mg, 5 mg.

INDICATIONS AND DOSAGES
▸ **Parkinson disease**
PO (IMMEDIATE-RELEASE TABLETS)
Adults, Elderly. Initially, 0.25 mg 3 times a day. May increase dosage every 7 days.
PO (EXTENDED-RELEASE)
Adults, Elderly. Initially, 2 mg once daily for 1-2 wks, followed by increases of 2 mg/day at 1 wk or longer intervals as appropriate. Maximum: 24 mg/day.
▸ **Restless legs syndrome**
PO
Adults, Elderly. Initially, 0.25 mg daily 1-3 h before bedtime. May

R

increase dosage after 2 days to
0.5 mg daily then 1 mg daily after
7 days. May titrate dose 0.5 mg/wk
every 7 days. Maximum: 4 mg/day.

CONTRAINDICATIONS
Hypersensitivity to ropinirole.

INTERACTIONS
Drug
**Antipsychotics, butyrophenones,
carbamazepine, cigarette smoking,
phenobarbital, metoclopramide,
phenothiazines, rifampin,
thioxanthenes:** Decrease the
effectiveness of ropinirole.
**Central nervous system (CNS)
depressants:** May increase CNS
depressant effects.
**Cimetidine, diltiazem, enoxacin,
erythromycin, fluvoxamine,
mexiletine, norfloxacin, tacrine:**
Alter ropinirole blood
concentration.
Estrogens: Reduce the clearance of
ropinirole.
Levodopa: Increases the blood
concentration of levodopa.
Quinolones: Increase ropinirole
blood concentration.
Herbal
**Kava kava, gotu kola, valerian,
St. John's wort:** May increase CNS
depression.
Ethanol
Food
All foods: Delay peak plasma
levels by 1 h but do not affect drug
absorption.
Ethanol: May increase CNS
depression.

DIAGNOSTIC TEST EFFECTS
May increase serum alkaline
phosphatase level.

SIDE EFFECTS
Frequent (40%-60%)
Nausea, dizziness, somnolence.

Occasional (4%-12%)
Syncope, vomiting, fatigue, viral
infection, dyspepsia, diaphoresis,
asthenia, orthostatic hypotension,
abdominal discomfort, pharyngitis,
abnormal vision, dry mouth,
hypertension, hallucinations,
confusion.
Rare (< 4%)
Anorexia, peripheral edema, memory
loss, rhinitis, sinusitis, palpitations,
impotence.

SERIOUS REACTIONS
• None known.

PRECAUTIONS & CONSIDERATIONS
Caution is warranted in patients with
hallucinations (especially elderly),
syncope, history of orthostatic
hypotension, and those who take
CNS depressants concurrently.
Because ropinirole is distributed in
breast milk, it may cause drug-related
effects in the breastfeeding infant.
The safety and efficacy of ropinirole
have not been established in children.
No age-related precautions have been
noted in elderly patients, but they are
more likely than other age groups to
experience hallucinations.
    Dizziness, drowsiness, and
orthostatic hypotension are common
initial responses to the drug. Alcohol
and tasks that require mental
alertness or motor skills should be
avoided. Change positions slowly
to prevent orthostatic hypotension.
Baseline vital signs and serum
alkaline phosphatase levels should
be assessed at baseline. Relief of
symptoms, such as improvement of
masklike facial expression, muscular
rigidity, shuffling gait, and resting
tremors of the hands and head should
be assessed during treatment.
Administration
For Parkinson disease, expect
the dosage schedule to increase

gradually, as follows: wk 1, 0.25 mg 3 times a day to total daily dose of 0.75 mg; wk 2, 0.5 mg 3 times a day to total daily dose of 1.5 mg; wk 3, 0.75 mg 3 times a day to total daily dose of 2.25 mg; wk 4, 1 mg 3 times a day to total daily dose of 3 mg, as prescribed. After wk 4, dosage may be increased every week, if needed, by 1.5-3 mg/day to a total dose of 24 mg/day.

For Parkinson disease, plan to discontinue the drug gradually at 7-day intervals, as follows: first decrease the frequency from 3 times a day to twice a day for 4 days; for the remaining 3 days, decrease the frequency to once a day before complete withdrawal, as prescribed. For restless legs syndrome, doses up to 4 mg/day may be discontinued without tapering.

Rosiglitazone
roz-ih-gli'ta-zone
(Avandia)
Do not confuse with Avalide, Avinza, or Prandin.

CATEGORY AND SCHEDULE
Pregnancy Risk Category: C

Classification: Antidiabetic agents, thiazolidinediones

MECHANISM OF ACTION
An antidiabetic that improves target-cell response to insulin without increasing pancreatic insulin secretion. Decreases hepatic glucose output and increases insulin-dependent glucose utilization in skeletal muscle. *Therapeutic Effect:* Lowers blood glucose concentration.

PHARMACOKINETICS
Rapidly absorbed. Protein binding: 99.8%. Metabolized in the liver. Excreted primarily in urine, with a lesser amount in feces. Not removed by hemodialysis. *Half-life:* 3-4 h.

AVAILABILITY
Tablets: 2 mg, 4 mg, 8 mg.

INDICATIONS AND DOSAGES
▸ **Diabetes mellitus, combination therapy**
PO
Adults, Elderly. Initially, 4 mg as a single daily dose or in divided doses twice a day. May increase to 8 mg/day after 12 wks of therapy if fasting glucose level is not adequately controlled.
▸ **Diabetes mellitus, monotherapy**
Adults, Elderly. Initially, 4 mg as single daily dose or in divided doses twice a day. May increase to 8 mg/ day after 12 wks of therapy.

CONTRAINDICATIONS
Hypersensitivity to rosiglitazone, active hepatic disease, diabetic ketoacidosis, increased serum transaminase levels, including ALT (SGPT) > 2.5 times the normal serum level, type 1 diabetes mellitus, New York Heart Association (NYHA) class III/IV heart failure before initiation.

INTERACTIONS
Drug
Amiodarone, paclitaxel, pioglitazone, repaglinide: May have increased levels.
Atazanavir, gemfibrozil, ritonavir, trimethoprim: Levels and effects of rosiglitazone may be increased.
Bile acide sequestrants, carbamazepine, corticosteroids, lutenizing hormone-releasing

R

hormone, phenobarbital, phenytoin, rifampin, rifapentine: Levels and effects of rosiglitazone may be decreased.

Insulin, pregabalin: May exacerbate fluid retention.

Herbal

Hypoglycemic herbs (alfalfa, bilberry, bitter melon, burdock, celery, daminana, fenugreek, garcinia, garlic, ginger, ginseng, symnema, marshmallow, and stinging nettle: May enhance hypoglycemic effects.

Food

All foods: Delay peak concentrations but not significantly.

Ethanol: Avoid; may cause hypoglycemia.

DIAGNOSTIC TEST EFFECTS

May decrease hematocrit and hemoglobin and serum alkaline phosphatase, bilirubin, and AST (SGOT) levels. < 1% of patients experience ALT values that are 3 times the normal level.

SIDE EFFECTS

Frequent (9%)
Upper respiratory tract infection.
Occasional (2%-4%)
Headache, edema, back pain, fatigue, sinusitis, diarrhea.

SERIOUS REACTIONS

• None known.
WARNING
Because thiazolidinediones, including rosiglitazone, may exacerbate congestive heart failure, closely monitor patients for signs/symptoms of congestive heart failure (CHF).

PRECAUTIONS & CONSIDERATIONS

Caution is warranted with CHF, edema, and hepatic impairment. It is unknown whether rosiglitazone crosses the placenta or is distributed in breast milk. Rosiglitazone use is not recommended in pregnant or breastfeeding women. Safety and efficacy of rosiglitazone have not been established in children. No age-related precautions have been noted in elderly patients.

Food intake, blood glucose, and hemoglobin should be monitored before and during therapy. Hepatic enzyme levels should also be obtained before beginning rosiglitazone therapy and periodically thereafter. Notify the physician of abdominal or chest pain, dark urine or light stool, hypoglycemic reactions, fever, nausea, palpitations, rash, vomiting, or yellowing of the eyes or skin. Be aware of signs and symptoms of hypoglycemia (anxiety, cool wet skin, diplopia, dizziness, headache, hunger, numbness in mouth, tachycardia, tremors) or hyperglycemia (deep rapid breathing, dim vision, fatigue, nausea, polydipsia, polyphagia, polyuria, vomiting); carry candy, sugar packets, or other sugar supplements for immediate response to hypoglycemia. Consult the physician when glucose demands are altered (such as with fever, heavy physical activity, infection, stress, trauma). Exercise, good personal hygiene (including foot care), not smoking, and weight control are essential parts of therapy.

Administration

Take rosiglitazone without regard to meals.

Rosuvastatin
ross-uh-vah-stah'tin
(Crestor)

CATEGORY AND SCHEDULE
Pregnancy Risk Category: X

Classification: Antihyperlipidemics, HMG CoA reductase inhibitors

MECHANISM OF ACTION
An antihyperlipidemic that interferes with cholesterol biosynthesis by inhibiting the conversion of the enzyme HMG-CoA to mevalonate, a precursor to cholesterol. *Therapeutic Effect:* Decreases LDL cholesterol, VLDL, and plasma triglyceride levels, increases HDL concentration.

PHARMACOKINETICS
Protein binding: 88%. Minimal hepatic metabolism. Primarily eliminated in the feces. *Half-life:* 19 h (increased in patients with severe renal dysfunction).

AVAILABILITY
Tablets: 5 mg, 10 mg, 20 mg, 40 mg.

INDICATIONS AND DOSAGES
▸ **Hyperlipidemia, dyslipidemia**
PO
Adults, Elderly. 5-40 mg/day. Usual starting dosage is 10 mg/day, with adjustments based on lipid levels at intervals of 2-4 wks until desired level is achieved. Doses may be increased by 5-10 mg once daily. Maximum: 40 mg/day.
▸ **Renal impairment (creatinine clearance < 30 mL/min)**
PO
Adults, Elderly. 5 mg/day; do not exceed 10 mg/day.

▸ **Concurrent lopinavir; ritonavir use**
PO
Adults, Elderly. 10 mg/day.
▸ **Concurrent cyclosporine use**
PO
Adults, Elderly. 5 mg/day.
▸ **Concurrent lipid-lowering therapy**
PO
Adults, Elderly. 10 mg/day.

CONTRAINDICATIONS
Active hepatic disease, breastfeeding, pregnancy, unexplained, persistent elevations of serum transaminase levels.

INTERACTIONS
Drug
Cyclosporine, gemfibrozil, niacin, or lopinavir/ritonavir: Increase the risk of myopathy with cyclosporine, gemfibrozil, and niacin.
Erythromycin: Reduces the plasma concentration of erythromycin.
Ethinylestradiol, norgestrel: Increase the plasma concentrations of ethinylestradiol and norgestrel.
Warfarin: Enhances anticoagulant effect.
Herbal
None known.
Food
Ethanol: Avoid; may increase hepatic effects.

DIAGNOSTIC TEST EFFECTS
May increase serum creatinine kinase and transaminase concentrations. May produce hematuria and proteinuria.

SIDE EFFECTS
Rosuvastatin is generally well tolerated. Side effects are usually mild and transient.
Occasional (3%-9%)
Pharyngitis, headache, diarrhea, dyspepsia, including heartburn and epigastric distress, nausea.

R

Rare (< 3%)
Myalgia, asthenia or unusual fatigue and weakness, back pain.

SERIOUS REACTIONS
• Lens opacities may occur.
• Hypersensitivity reaction and hepatitis occur rarely.

PRECAUTIONS & CONSIDERATIONS
Caution is warranted in patients with a history of hepatic disease, hypotension, severe acute infection; severe electrolyte, endocrine, metabolic imbalances or disorders; trauma; and uncontrolled seizures. Caution should also be used in those who consume a substantial amount of alcohol and those who have had recent major surgery. Rosuvastatin use is contraindicated in pregnancy because the suppression of cholesterol biosynthesis may cause fetal toxicity. Rosuvastatin is contraindicated during lactation because it carries the risk of serious adverse reactions in breastfeeding infants. Safety and efficacy of rosuvastatin have not been established in children. No age-related precautions have been noted in elderly patients.

Notify the physician of headache, sore throat, muscle weakness and aches, severe gastric upset, or rash. Pattern of daily bowel activity and stool consistency should be assessed. Serum lipid cholesterol and triglyceride levels and hepatic function should be checked at baseline and periodically during treatment. At initiation of rosuvastatin therapy, a standard cholesterol-lowering diet should be practiced and continued throughout rosuvastatin therapy.

Administration
Take rosuvastatin without regard to meals and administer in the evening.

Salicylic Acid
Salicylic Acid
sal-i-sill′ik
(Compound W, Compound
W One Step Wart Remover,
DHS Sal, Dr. Scholl's, Callus
Remover, Dr. Scholl's Clear
Away, DuoFilm, DuoPlant,
Freezone, Fung-O, Gordofilm,
Hydrisalic, Ionil, Ionil Plus,
Keralyt, LupiCare, Dandruff,
LupiCare II Psoriasis, LupiCare
Psoriasis, Mediplast, MG217
Sal-Acid, Mosco Corn and
Callus Remover, NeoCeuticals
Acne Spot Treatment,
Neutrogena Acne Wash,
Neutrogena Body Clear,
Neutrogena Clear Pore,
Neutrogena Clear Pore Shine
Control, Neutrogena Healthy
Scalp, Neutrogena Maximum
Strength T/Sal, Neutrogena On
The Spot Acne Patch, Occlusal
[CAN], Occlusal-HP, Oxy
Balance, Oxy Balance Deep
Pore, Palmer's Skin Success
Acne Cleanser, Pedisilk, Propa
pH, SalAc, Sal-Acid, Salactic,
Sal-Plant, Stri-dex, Stri-dex
Body Focus, Stri-dex Facewipes
To Go, Stri-dex Maximum
Strength, Sunspot Cream [AUS],
Tinamed, Tiseb, Trans-Ver-Sal,
Wart-Off Maximum Strength,
Zapzyt Acne Wash, Zapzyt Pore
Treatment, Salac)

CATEGORY AND SCHEDULE
Pregnancy Risk Category: C
OTC (cream, gel, foam, liquid,
ointment, pads, patch, plaster,
soap, shampoo, solution)

Classification: Antipsoriatics,
dermatologics, keratolytics,
salicylates

MECHANISM OF ACTION
A keratolytic agent that produces
desquamation of hyperkeratotic
epithelium by dissolution of
intercellular cement and causes
the cornified tissue to swell,
soften, macerate, and desquamate.
Therapeutic Effect: Decreases acne,
psoriasis, and wart removal.

PHARMACOKINETICS
Absorption differs between
formulations. Protein binding:
50%-80%. Bound to serum
albumin. Metabolized to salicylate
glucoronides and salicyluric acid.
Excreted in urine.

AVAILABILITY
Cream: 2% (Neutrogena Acne
Wash), 2.5% (LupiCare Dandruff,
LupiCare Psoriasis, LupiCare II).
Gel: 0.5% (Neutrogena Clean Pore
Shine Control), 2% (NeuCeuticals
Acne Spot Treatment, Neutrogena
Clean Pore, Oxy Balance,
Stri-dex Body Focus, Zapzyt Acne
Wash, Zapzyt Pore Treatment),
6% (Hydrisalic, Keralyt), 17%
(Compound W, DuoPlant, Sal-Plant).
Foam: 2% (Neutrogena Acne Wash,
Salac).
Liquid: 2% (NeoCeuticals Acne
Spot Treatment, Neutrogena Acne
Wash, Neutrogena Body Clear,
Propa pH, SalAc), 17% (Compound
W, DuoFilm, Freezone, Fung-O,
Gordofilm, Mosco Corn and Callus
Remover, Occlusal-HP, Pedisilk,
Salactic, Tinamed, Wart-Off).
Ointment: 3% (MG217 Sal-Acid).
Pads: 0.5% (Oxy Balance, Oxy
Balance Deep Pore, Stri-dex,
Stri-dex Facewipes To Go), 2%
(Neutrogena Acne Wash, Stri-dex
Maximum Strength).
Patch: 2% (Neutrogena On The Spot
Acne Patch), 15% (Trans-Ver-Sal),
40% (Compound W, Dr. Scholl's

Callus Remover, Dr. Scholl's Clear Away, DuoFilm).
Plaster: 40% (Mediplast, Sal-Acid, Tinamed).
Shampoo: 1.8% (Neutrogena Healthy Scalp), 2% (Ionil, Ionil Plus, LupiCare Dandruff, LupiCare Psoriasis, Tiseb), 3% (Neutrogena Maximum Strength T/Sal).
Soap: 2%.
Solution: 17% (Compound W).

INDICATIONS AND DOSAGES
▸ **Acne**
TOPICAL
Adults, Elderly, Children. Apply cream, foam, gel, liquid, pads, patch, or soap 1-3 times/day.
▸ **Callus, corn, wart removal**
TOPICAL
Adults, Elderly, Children. Apply gel, liquid, plaster, or patch to wart 1-2 times/day.
▸ **Dandruff, psoriasis, seborrheic dermatitis**
TOPICAL
Adults, Elderly, Children. Apply cream, ointment, or shampoo 3-4 times/day.

OFF-LABEL USES
Tinea pedis.

CONTRAINDICATIONS
Children younger than 2 yr, diabetes, impaired circulation, hypersensitivity to salicylic acid or any of its components.

INTERACTIONS
Drug
Ammonium sulfate: May increase plasma salicylate levels.
Corticosteroids: May decrease plasma salicylate levels.
Heparin: May decrease platelet adhesiveness and interfere with hemostasis in heparin-treated patients.

Methotrexate: May increase risk of methotrexate toxicity.
Pyranzinamide: May inhibit pyrazinamide-induced hyperuricemia.
Tolbutamide: May increase risk of hypoglycemia.
Uricosuric agents: May decrease the effects of probenecid, sulfinpyrazone, and phenylbutazone.
Varicella virus vaccine: May increase risk of developing Reye syndrome.
Herbal
Tamarind: May increase risk of salicylate toxicity.
Food
None known.

DIAGNOSTIC TEST EFFECTS
May interfere with thyroid function tests (decreasing protein-bound iodine and increase T_3 uptake). May give false-negative results with glucose oxidase test and fluorometric test. May give false-positive results with Clinitest with high-dose salicylate therapy and $FeCl_3$ in Gerhardt reaction. May give false reduced values with 17-OH corticosteroid tests and vanilmandelic acid test. May increase or decrease uric acid levels. May decrease prothrombin levels and slightly increase prothrombin time.

SIDE EFFECTS
Occasional
Burning, erythema, irritation, pruritus, stinging.
Rare
Dizziness, nausea, vomiting, diarrhea, hypoglycemia.

SERIOUS REACTIONS
• Symptoms of salicylate toxicity include lethargy, hyperpnea, diarrhea, and psychic disturbances.

PRECAUTIONS & CONSIDERATIONS

Salicylic acid should not be applied to areas that are irritated, infected, or reddened; birthmarks; genital or facial warts; or mucous membranes. It is unknown whether salicylic acid crosses the placenta or is distributed in breast milk. Salicylic acid is not recommended for use in children younger than 2 yr. No age-related precautions have been noted in elderly patients. Use of abrasive soaps and cleansers, alcohol-containing preparations, other topical acne preparations, cosmetic soaps that dry skin, and medicated cosmetics should be avoided.

Administration

Use 2% cream, pads, foam, or liquid cleansers for acne by cleansing the skin 1-2 times/day. Massage gently into skin, work into lather, and rinse thoroughly. Pads should be wet with water before using and disposed of after use. Do not flush pads.

Use gel (0.5% or 2%) for acne by applying a small amount to clean, dry skin on the face in the morning or evening. If peeling or drying occurs, use every other day. Some products may be used up to 3-4 times/day.

Use pads (0.5% or 2%) for acne to cover clean, dry skin with thin layer 1-3 times/day. Do not leave pad on skin.

Use patches (2%) for acne by washing face, and allow skin to dry for at least 5 min. Apply patch directly over pimple being treated at bedtime. Remove in the morning.

When using shower/bath gels or soap (2%), use once daily in shower or bath. Massage over skin prone to acne. Rinse well.

Use gel or liquid (17%) for callus, corns, or warts by cleaning and drying the area. Apply to each wart and allow to dry. Repeat 1-2 times/day for up to 12 wks as needed.

Apply gel (6%) to callus, corns, or warts once daily. Use at night and rinse off in the morning.

Apply plaster or patch (40%) for callus, corns, or warts by cleaning and drying skin. Apply directly over affected area. Leave on for 48 h. Repeat procedure for up to 12 wks as needed.

Use patch (15%) for callus, corns, or warts by applying directly over affected area at bedtime. Leave in place overnight and remove in the morning. Repeat daily for up to 12 wks as needed. May trim patch to fit area.

Use cream (2.5%) for dandruff, psoriasis, or seborrheic dermatitis by cleaning and drying skin. Apply to affected area 3-4 times/day. Apply to clean, dry skin. Some products may remain overnight.

Apply ointment (3%) for dandruff, psoriasis, or seborrheic dermatitis to scales or plaques on skin up to 4 times/day. Do not apply to scalp or face.

Massage shampoo (1.8%-3%) for dandruff, psoriasis, or seborrheic dermatitis into wet hair. Leave in place for several minutes and rinse thoroughly. Some products may be used 2-3 times/wk.

S

Salmeterol

sal-me'te-rol
(Serevent Diskus, Serevent Inhaler
and Disks [AUS])
**Do not confuse Serevent with
Serentil.**

CATEGORY AND SCHEDULE
Pregnancy Risk Category: C

Classification: Adrenergic
agonists, bronchodilators

MECHANISM OF ACTION
An adrenergic agonist that
stimulates β_2-adrenergic receptors
in the lungs, resulting in relaxation
of bronchial smooth muscle.
Therapeutic Effect: Relieves
bronchospasm and reduces airway
resistance.

PHARMACOKINETICS

Route	Onset	Peak	Duration
Inhalation	30-48 min	2-4 h	12 h

Low systemic absorption; acts
primarily in the lungs. Protein
binding: 96%. Metabolized by
hydroxylation. Primarily eliminated
in feces. *Half-life:* 5.5 h.

AVAILABILITY
*Powder for Oral Inhalation (Serevent
Diskus):* 50 mcg.

INDICATIONS AND DOSAGES
▸ **Prevention and maintenance
treatment of asthma**
INHALATION (DISKUS)
*Adults, Elderly, Children 4 yr and
older.* 1 inhalation (50 mcg)
q12h.
▸ **Prevention of exercise-induced
bronchospasm**

INHALATION (DISKUS)
*Adults, Elderly, Children 4 yr and
older.* 1 inhalation (50 mcg) at least
30 min before exercise.
▸ **Chronic obstructive pulmonary
disease (COPD)**
INHALATION
Adults, Elderly. 1 inhalation q12h.

CONTRAINDICATIONS
History of hypersensitivity to
sympathomimetics.

INTERACTIONS
Drug
β-Blockers: May decrease the effects
of β-blockers.
Nonselective β-blockers: May
decrease the effects of salmeterol.
Sympathomimetics: May
increase the adverse effects of
salmeterol.
Herbal
None known.
Food
None known.

DIAGNOSTIC TEST EFFECTS
May decrease serum potassium
level.

SIDE EFFECTS
Frequent (28%)
Headache.
Occasional (3%-7%)
Cough, tremor, dizziness, vertigo,
throat dryness or irritation,
pharyngitis.
Rare (3%)
Palpitations, tachycardia, tremors,
nausea, heartburn, GI distress,
diarrhea.

SERIOUS REACTIONS
• At high doses, salmeterol may
prolong the QT interval, which may
precipitate ventricular arrhythmias.
• Hypokalemia and hyperglycemia
may occur.

SERIOUS REACTIONS

• Long-acting β_2-agonists may increase the risk of asthma-related deaths.

PRECAUTIONS & CONSIDERATIONS

Caution is warranted in patients with cardiovascular disorders (such as coronary insufficiency, arrhythmias, and hypertension), seizure disorders, and thyrotoxicosis. Salmeterol is not for acute asthma symptoms and may cause paradoxical bronchospasm. It is unknown whether salmeterol is excreted in breast milk. No age-related precautions have been noted in children older than 4 yr. Elderly patients may require a lower dosage because of increased sensitivity to sympathomimetics and increased susceptibility to tachycardia and tremors. Avoid excessive use of caffeinated products, such as chocolate, cocoa, cola, coffee, and tea.

Notify the physician of chest pain or dizziness. Pulse rate and quality, respiratory rate, depth, rhythm and type, BP, and serum potassium levels should be monitored. Evidence of cyanosis, a blue or a dusky color in light-skinned patients or a gray color in dark-skinned patients, should also be assessed. NOTE: This drug is not for the relief of acute attacks.

Storage

Keep the drug canister at room temperature because cold decreases the drug's effects.

Administration

Instruct the patient to open and prepare mouthpiece of Diskus device and slide device lever to activate the first dose (see package instructions). Do not advance the lever more than once at any one time as this will release further doses that will be wasted. Holding the Diskus mouthpiece level to, but away from, the mouth, exhale.

Then, put the mouthpiece to the lips and breathe in the dose deeply and slowly. Remove the Diskus from the mouth, hold breath for at least 10 sec, and then exhale slowly. Instruct patient to close the Diskus, which will also reset the dose lever for the next scheduled dose. After administration, instruct patient to rinse mouth with water to minimize dry mouth. The Diskus device and mouthpiece should be kept dry; do not wash.

To prevent exercise-induced bronchospasm, administer the dose at least 30-60 min before exercising.

Saquinavir

sa-kwin'a-veer
(Invirase)
Do not confuse saquinavir with Sinequan.

CATEGORY AND SCHEDULE

Pregnancy Risk Category: B

Classification: Antivirals, protease inhibitors

MECHANISM OF ACTION

Inhibits HIV protease, rendering the enzyme incapable of processing the polyprotein precursors needed to generate functional proteins in HIV-infected cells. *Therapeutic Effect:* Intereferes with HIV replication, slowing the progression of HIV infection.

PHARMACOKINETICS

Poorly absorbed after PO administration (absorption increased with high-calorie and high-fat meals). Protein binding: 98%. Metabolized in the liver to inactive metabolite. Eliminated primarily in feces. Unknown

S

whether removed by hemodialysis.
Half-life: 13 h.

AVAILABILITY

Capsules: 200 mg.
Tablet: 500 mg.

INDICATIONS AND DOSAGES
▸ **HIV infection in combination with other antiretrovirals**
PO
Adults, Elderly. 1000 mg twice a day within 2 h after a full meal. Should be given only in combination with ritonavir 100 mg twice a day.
▸ **Dosage adjustments when given in combination therapy**
Lopinavir/ritonavir. 1000 mg 2 times a day.
Concurrent use with ergot medications, lovastatin, midazolam, simvastatin, or triazolam. Clinically significant increases in plasma concentration of these medications when given with saquinavir.

INTERACTIONS
Drug
Calcium channel blockers, clindamycin, dapsone, quinidine, triazolam: May increase the plasma concentrations of these drugs.
Carbamazepine, dexamethasone, phenobarbital, phenytoin, rifampin: May reduce saquinavir plasma concentration.
Ketoconazole: Increases saquinavir plasma concentration.
Herbal
Garlic, St. John's wort: May decrease the plasma concentration and effect of saquinavir.
Food
High-fat meal: Maximally increases saquinavir's bioavailability.
Grapefruit juice: May increase saquinavir plasma concentration.

DIAGNOSTIC TEST EFFECTS
May alter serum CK levels, elevate liver function test results, and lower blood glucose levels.

SIDE EFFECTS
Occasional
Diarrhea, abdominal discomfort and pain, nausea, photosensitivity, stomatitis.
Rare
Confusion, ataxia, asthenia, headache, rash.

SERIOUS REACTIONS
• Ketoacidosis occurs rarely.

PRECAUTIONS & CONSIDERATIONS
Caution is warranted in patients with diabetes mellitus or liver impairment. Breastfeeding is not recommended in this population because of the possibility of HIV transmission. Be aware that the safety and efficacy of saquinavir have not been established in children. There is no information on the effects of this drug's use in elderly patients, so it should be used with caution. Avoid exposure to artificial light sources and sunlight and grapefruit products. Saquinavir is not a cure for HIV infection, nor does it reduce the risk of transmission to others; illnesses associated with advanced HIV infection may occur.

Check the baseline laboratory and diagnostic test results, especially liver function test results, if ordered, before beginning saquinavir therapy and at periodic intervals during therapy. Closely monitor for signs and symptoms of GI discomfort.

Assess the patient's pattern of daily bowel activity and stool consistency. Inspect the mouth for signs of mucosal ulceration. Notify

S

the physician if nausea, numbness, persistent abdominal pain, tingling, or vomiting occurs.

Administration
Give within 2 h after a full meal. Keep in mind that if saquinavir is taken on an empty stomach, the drug might not produce antiviral activity. When used with ritonavir, saquinavir should be administered at the same time. Continue therapy for the full length of treatment and evenly space drug doses around the clock.

Sargramostim (Granulocyte Macrophage Colony-Stimulating Factor, GM-CSF)
sar-gram′oh-stim
(Leukine)
Do not confuse Leukine with Leukeran.

CATEGORY AND SCHEDULE
Pregnancy Risk Category: C

Classification: Hematopoietic agents, recombinant DNA origin

MECHANISM OF ACTION
A colony-stimulating factor that stimulates proliferation and differentiation of hematopoietic cells to activate mature granulocytes and macrophages. *Therapeutic Effect:* Assists bone marrow in making new WBCs and increases their chemotactic, antifungal, and antiparasitic activity. Increases cytoneoplastic cells and activates neutrophils to inhibit tumor cell growth.

PHARMACOKINETICS

Effect	Onset	Peak	Duration
Increase WBCs	7-14 days	NA	1 wk

Detected in serum within 15 min after SC administration. *Half-life:* IV, 1 h; SC, 2.7 h.

AVAILABILITY
Injection Solution: 500 mcg/mL: Discontinued.
Injection Powder for Reconstitution: 250 mcg: Available as limited access from manufacturer.

INDICATIONS AND DOSAGES
▸ **Myeloid recovery following bone marrow transplant (BMT)**
IV INFUSION
Adults, Elderly. Usual parenteral dosage: 250 mcg/m^2/day (as 2-h infusion) beginning 2-4 h after autologous bone marrow infusion and not < 24 h after the last dose of chemotherapy or radiation treatment. Discontinue if blast cells appear or underlying disease progresses.
▸ **Bone marrow transplant failure, engraftment delay**
IV INFUSION
Adults, Elderly. 250 mcg/m^2/day for 14 days. Infuse over 2 h. May repeat after 7 days off therapy if engraftment has not occurred with 500 mcg/m^2/day for 14 days.
▸ **Stem cell transplant**
IV, SC
Adults. 250 mcg/m^2/day.
▸ **Mobilization of peripheral blood progenitor cells (PBPCs)**
IV, SC
Adults. 250 mcg/m^2/day IV over 24 h or SC daily continued through the period of PBPCs, according to protocol.

S

▸ Postperipheral blood progenitor cell transplantation
IV, SC
Adults. 250 mcg/m^2/day IV over 24 h or SC daily, continuing until ANC > 1500 cells/mm^3 for 3 consecutive days.
▸ Neutrophil recovery following chemotherapy in acute myelogenic leukemia (AML)
IV
Adults. 250 mcg/m^2/day IV over 4 h starting 4 days after completion of induction chemotherapy, continuing until ANC > 1500 cells/mm^3 for 3 consecutive days. Maximum: 42 days.

OFF-LABEL USES

Treatment of AIDS-related neutropenia; chronic, severe neutropenia; drug-induced neutropenia; myelodysplastic syndrome.

CONTRAINDICATIONS

24 h before or after chemotherapy or radiotherapy; excessive leukemic myeloid blasts in bone marrow or peripheral blood (> 10%); known hypersensitivity to GM-CSF, yeast-derived products, or components of drug.

INTERACTIONS

Drug
Lithium, steroids: May increase the effects of sargramostim.
Herbal
None known.
Food
None known.

DIAGNOSTIC TEST EFFECTS

May increase serum bilirubin, creatinine, and hepatic enzyme levels. May decrease serum albumin level.

IV INCOMPATIBILITIES

Amphotericin B complex (Abelcet, AmBisome, Amphotec), hydromorphone (Dilaudid), lorazepam (Ativan), morphine.

IV COMPATIBILITIES

Calcium gluconate, dopamine (Intropin), heparin, magnesium, potassium chloride.

SIDE EFFECTS

Frequent
GI disturbances, including nausea, diarrhea, vomiting, stomatitis, anorexia, and abdominal pain; arthralgia or myalgia; headache; malaise; rash; pruritus.
Occasional
Peripheral edema, weight gain, dyspnea, asthenia, fever, leukocytosis, capillary leak syndrome (such as fluid retention, irritation at local injection site, and peripheral edema).
Rare
Rapid or irregular heartbeat, thrombophlebitis.

SERIOUS REACTIONS

• Pleural or pericardial effusion occurs rarely after infusion.

PRECAUTIONS & CONSIDERATIONS

Caution is warranted with congestive heart failure (CHF), hypoxia, impaired hepatic or renal function, preexisting cardiac disease, preexisting fluid retention, and pulmonary infiltrates. It is unknown whether sargramostim crosses the placenta or is distributed in breast milk. Safety and efficacy of this drug have not been established in children. No age-related precautions have been noted in elderly patients. Avoid situations that might place risk for contracting an infectious disease such as influenza.

Notify the physician of chest pain, chills, fever, palpitations, or dyspnea. Follow-up blood tests should be maintained to evaluate the effectiveness of drug therapy. CBC, pulmonary, liver, and kidney function test results, platelet count, vital signs, and weight should be monitored.

Storage
Refrigerate powder, reconstituted solution, and diluted solution for injection. Do not shake. Do not use past expiration date. Reconstituted solution is normally clear and colorless. Use reconstituted solution within 6 h; discard unused portion. Use one dose/vial; do not reenter vial.

Administration
For IV use, to reconstitute, add 1 mL preservative-free sterile water for injection to 250-mcg vial. Direct sterile water for injection to side of vial, and gently swirl contents to avoid foaming. Do not shake or vigorously agitate. After reconstitution, further dilute with 0.9% NaCl. If final concentration is < 10 mcg/mL, add 1 mg albumin per mL 0.9% NaCl to provide a final albumin concentration of 0.1%.
! Albumin is added before sargramostim to prevent drug adsorption to components of drug delivery system. Give each single dose over 2, 4, or 24 h, as directed by physician. Consider administration with analgesics and antipyretics. When given subcutaneously, rotate injection sites.

Scopolamine
skoe-pol'a-meen
(Isopto Hyoscine, Trans-Derm Scop, Scopace, Transderm-V [CAN])

CATEGORY AND SCHEDULE
Pregnancy Risk Category: C

Classification: Anticholinergics, antiemetics/antivertigo, cycloplegics, gastrointestinals, mydriatics, ophthalmics, preanesthetics, sedatives/hypnotics.

MECHANISM OF ACTION
An anticholinergic that reduces excitability of labyrinthine receptors, depressing conduction in the vestibular cerebellar pathway. *Therapeutic Effect:* Prevents motion-induced nausea and vomiting.

AVAILABILITY
Tablet: 0.4 mg.
Transdermal System: 1.5 mg.

INDICATIONS AND DOSAGES
▸ **Postoperative nausea or vomiting**
TRANSDERMAL
Adults, Elderly. 1 system no sooner than 1 h before surgery and removed 24 h after surgery.
▸ **Motion sickness**
Adults, Elderly. 1 system at least 4 h (ideally 12 h) before exposure, reapplying every 3 days as needed.

CONTRAINDICATIONS
Angle-closure glaucoma, GI or genitourinary obstruction, myasthenia gravis, paralytic ileus, tachycardia, thyrotoxicosis.

S

INTERACTIONS
Drug
Antihistamines, tricyclic antidepressants: May increase the anticholinergic effects of scopolamine.
Central nervous system (CNS) depressants: May increase CNS depression.
Pramlintide: May enhance GI effects of scopolamine.
Herbal
None known.
Food
Ethanol: May increase CNS depression.

DIAGNOSTIC TEST EFFECTS
May interfere with gastric secretion test.

SIDE EFFECTS
Frequent (> 15%)
Dry mouth, somnolence, blurred vision.
Rare (1%-5%)
Dizziness, restlessness, hallucinations, confusion, difficulty urinating, rash.

SERIOUS REACTIONS
• None known.

PRECAUTIONS & CONSIDERATIONS
Caution is warranted in patients with cardiac disease, renal or hepatic impairment, psychoses, and seizures. Tasks that require mental alertness or motor skills should be avoided.

BUN level, blood chemistry test results, and serum alkaline phosphatase, bilirubin, creatinine, AST (SGOT) and ALT (SGPT) levels to assess hepatic and renal function should be monitored.
Administration
Wash hands. Apply transdermal patch to the hairless area behind one ear. Replace the patch after 72 h or if it becomes dislodged. Wash hands after applying the patch. Use only one patch at a time and do not cut it.

Secobarbital
see-koe-bar'bi-tal
(Seconal)

CATEGORY AND SCHEDULE
Pregnancy Risk Category: D
Controlled Substance: Schedule II

Classification: Barbiturates, preanesthetics, sedatives/hypnotics

MECHANISM OF ACTION
A barbiturate that depresses the central nervous system (CNS) activity by binding to barbiturate site at the GABA-receptor complex enhancing GABA activity and depressing reticular activity system. *Therapeutic Effect:* Produces hypnotic effect as a result of central nervous system (CNS) depression.

PHARMACOKINETICS
Well absorbed from the GI tract. Protein binding: 52%-57%. Crosses blood-brain barrier. Widely distributed. Metabolized in liver by microsomal enzyme system to inactive and active metabolites. Excreted primarily in urine. Not removed by hemodialysis. *Half-life:* 15-40 h.

AVAILABILITY
Capsules: 50 mg (Seconal sodium).

INDICATIONS AND DOSAGES
▸ **Insomnia**
PO
Adults. 100 mg at bedtime, range 100-200 mg.

▸ **Preoperative sedation**
PO
Adults. 100-300 mg 1-2 h before procedure.
Children. 2-6 mg/kg 1-2 h before procedure. Maximum: 100 mg/dose.

OFF-LABEL USES

Chemotherapy-induced nausea and vomiting.

CONTRAINDICATIONS

History of manifest or latent porphyria, marked liver dysfunction, marked respiratory disease in which dyspnea or obstruction is evident, and hypersensitivity to secobarbital or barbiturates.

INTERACTIONS

Drug
Alcohol, CNS depressants: May increase the CNS depressant effects.
Anticoagulants: May decrease anticoagulant activity.
Corticosteroids: May increase metabolism of corticosteroids.
Doxycycline: May shorten the half-life of doxycycline.
Griseofulvin: May decrease levels of griseofulvin by interfering with its metabolism.
Estradiol, estrone, progesterone, other steroidal hormones: May decrease the effect of these hormones by increasing their metabolism.
MAOIs: May prolong the effects of secobarbital by inhibiting its metabolism.
Phenytoin, sodium valproate, valproic acid: May decreases the metabolism and increase the concentration and risk of toxicity with secobarbital.
Herbal
St. John's wort, kava kava, gotu kola, valerian: May increase CNS depressant effects.

Food
None known.

DIAGNOSTIC TEST EFFECTS

None known.

SIDE EFFECTS

Frequent
Somnolence.
Occasional
Agitation, confusion, hyperkinesia, ataxia, CNS depression, nightmares, nervousness, psychiatric disturbance, hallucinations, insomnia, anxiety, dizziness, abnormality in thinking, hypoventilation, apnea, bradycardia, hypotension, syncope, nausea, vomiting, constipation, headache.
Rare
Hypersensitivity reactions, fever, liver damage, megaloblastic anemia.

SERIOUS REACTIONS

• Agranulocytosis, megaloblastic anemia, apnea, hypoventilation, bradycardia, hypotension, syncope, hepatic damage, and Stevens-Johnson syndrome rarely occur.
• Tolerance and physical dependence may occur with repeated use.

PRECAUTIONS & CONSIDERATIONS
Secobarbital crosses the placenta and is distributed in breast milk. Its use may cause paradoxical excitement in children. Elderly patients taking secobarbital may exhibit confusion, excitement, and mental depression. Alcohol consumption and caffeine intake should be limited while taking secobarbital. Avoid tasks that require mental alertness or motor skills because this drug may cause dizziness and drowsiness.
Administration
Give secobarbital without regard to meals.

S

Selegiline
seh-leg′ill-ene
(Apo-Selegiline [CAN], Eldepryl,
Emsam, Novo-Selegiline [CAN],
Selgene [AUS], Zelapar)
**Do not confuse selegiline with
Stelazine, or Eldepryl with
enalapril.**

CATEGORY AND SCHEDULE
Pregnancy Risk Category: C

Classification: Antiparkinson
agents, dopaminergics

MECHANISM OF ACTION
An antiparkinson agent that
irreversibly inhibits the activity of
monoamine oxidase type B, the
enzyme that breaks down dopamine,
thereby increasing dopaminergic
action. *Therapeutic Effect:* Relieves
signs and symptoms of Parkinson
disease.

PHARMACOKINETICS
Rapidly absorbed from the GI tract.
Crosses the blood-brain barrier.
Metabolized in the liver to the active
metabolites. Excreted primarily in
urine. *Half-life:* 17 h (amphetamine),
20 h (methamphetamine).

AVAILABILITY
Capsules: 5 mg.
Tablets: 5 mg.
*Tablets, Oral Disintegrating
(Zelapar):* 1.25 mg.
Transdermal System (Emsam): 6 mg,
9 mg, 12 mg.

INDICATIONS AND DOSAGES
▸ **Adjunctive treatment for
parkinsonism**
PO
Adults. 10 mg/day in divided doses,
such as 5 mg at breakfast and lunch,
given concomitantly with each dose
of carbidopa and levodopa.
Elderly. Initially, 5 mg in the
morning. May increase up to
10 mg/day.
ORAL DISINTEGRATING
TABLETS
Adults. Initially 1.25 mg daily for
6 wks. May increase to 2.5 mg
daily.
▸ **Depression**
TRANSDERMAL
Adults. Initially 6 mg/24 h applied
once a day. May increase by 3 mg/day
every 2 wks. Maximum of
12 mg/24 h.
Elderly. 6 mg/ 24 h.

CONTRAINDICATIONS
Hypersensitivity to selegiline. Oral
disintegrating *Tablets:* concomitant
use of dextromaethorphan,
methadone, propoxyphene,
tramadol, other MAOIs. Numerous
contraindications with transdermal
selegiline.

INTERACTIONS
Drug
Fluoxetine: May cause serotonin
syndrome.
Meperidine: May cause a
diaphoresis, excitation, hypertension
or hypotension, coma, and even
death.
Herbal
None known.
Food
Tyramine-rich foods: May
produce a severe hypertensive
reaction.

DIAGNOSTIC TEST EFFECTS
None known.

SIDE EFFECTS
Frequent (4%-10%)
Nausea, dizziness, lightheadedness,
syncope, abdominal discomfort.

Occasional (2%-3%)
Confusion, hallucinations, dry mouth, vivid dreams, dyskinesia.
Rare (1%)
Headache, myalgia, anxiety, diarrhea, insomnia.

SERIOUS REACTIONS
• Symptoms of overdose may vary from CNS depression, characterized by sedation, apnea, cardiovascular collapse, and death, to severe paradoxical reactions, such as hallucinations, tremor, and seizures.
• Other serious effects may include involuntary movements, impaired motor coordination, loss of balance, blepharospasm, facial grimaces, feeling of heaviness in the lower extremities, depression, nightmares, delusions, overstimulation, sleep disturbance, and anger.
Warning
Transdermal: Selegeline is not approved for use in children. Antidepressants increase the risk of suicidal thinking and behavior in children, adolescents, and young adults (aged 18-24 yr) with major depressive disorder and other psychiatric disorders. Selegeline is not approved for treating bipolar depression.

PRECAUTIONS & CONSIDERATIONS
Caution is warranted in patients with cardiac arrhythmias, dementia, history of peptic ulcer disease, profound tremor, psychosis, and tardive dyskinesia. It is unknown whether selegiline crosses the placenta or is distributed in breast milk. The safety and efficacy of selegiline have not been established in children. No age-related precautions have been noted in elderly patients. Be aware that tyramine-rich foods, such as wine and aged cheese, should be avoided to prevent a hypertensive reaction.

Dizziness, drowsiness, light-headedness, and dry mouth are common side effects of the drug but will diminish or disappear with continued treatment. Alcohol and tasks that require mental alertness or motor skills should be avoided. Change positions slowly to prevent orthostatic hypotension. Notify the physician if agitation, headache, lethargy, or confusion occurs. Baseline vital signs should be assessed. Relief of symptoms, such as improvement of masklike facial expression, muscular rigidity, shuffling gait, and resting tremors of the hands and head should be assessed during treatment.
Administration
! Expect to take selegiline with carbidopa and levodopa therapy. Keep in mind that therapy should begin with the lowest dosage, then increase gradually over 3-4 wks. With oral disintegrating tablets, administer in the morning before breakfast allowing tablet to dissolve. Food or drink should be avoided 5 min before and after administration. Transdermal patches should be applied to clean, dry, hairless area of skin on upper torso, thigh, or arm at the same time every day. Application area should not be exposed to heat. Application sites should be rotated. Hands should be washed before and after patch application.

S

Senna

sen′na

(Ex-lax, Senexon, Senna-Glen, Sennatural, Senokot, X-Prep)

CATEGORY AND SCHEDULE
Pregnancy Risk Category: C
OTC

Classification: Anthraquinone derivative, laxative, stimulant

MECHANISM OF ACTION

A GI stimulant that has a direct effect on intestinal smooth musculature by stimulating the intramural nerve plexi. *Therapeutic Effect:* Increases peristalsis and promotes laxative effect.

PHARMACOKINETICS

Route	Onset	Peak	Duration
PO	6-12 h	NA	NA
Rectal	0.5-2 h	NA	NA

Minimal absorption after oral administration. Hydrolyzed to active form by enzymes of colonic flora. Absorbed drug metabolized in the liver. Eliminated in feces via biliary system.

AVAILABILITY

Granules (Senokot): 15 mg/tsp.
Liquid (X-Prep): 8.8 mg/5 mL.
Syrup (Senokot): 8.8 mg/5 mL.
Tablets (Sennatural, Senokot, Senexon, Senna-Gen): 8.6 mg, 15 mg.
Tablets (Ex-Lax).

INDICATIONS AND DOSAGES
▸ **Constipation**
PO (TABLETS)
Adults, Elderly. 2 tablets at bedtime. Maximum: 4 tablets twice a day.
Children >27 kg. 1 tablet at bedtime.

Maximum: 2 tablets twice a day. twice a day.
SYRUP
Adults, Elderly. 10-15 mL at bedtime. Maximum: 15 mL twice a day.
Children aged 5-15 yr. 5-10 mL at bedtime. Maximum: 10 mL twice a day.
Children aged 1-5 yr. 2.5-5 mL at bedtime. Maximum: 1 tsp twice a day.
Infants 1-12 mo > 27 kg.
1.25-2.5 mL at bedtime. Maximum: 2.5 mL twice daily.
PO (GRANULES)
Adults, Elderly. 1 tsp at bedtime. Maximum: 2 tsp twice a day.
Children weighing > 27 kg.
Half (½) teaspoon at bedtime up to 1 tsp twice/day.
▸ **Bowel evacuation**
PO
Adults, Elderly. 1-2 tablets or 1-2 tsp 12-14 hr before examination. 75 mL between 2:00 and 4:00 PM on day before procedure.

CONTRAINDICATIONS

Abdominal pain, appendicitis, intestinal obstruction, nausea, vomiting.

INTERACTIONS

Drug
Oral medications: May decrease transit time of concurrently administered oral medications, decreasing absorption of senna.
Herbal
None known.
Food
None known.

DIAGNOSTIC TEST EFFECTS

May increase blood glucose level. May decrease serum potassium level.

SIDE EFFECTS

Frequent
Pink-red, red-violet, red-brown, or yellow-brown discoloration of urine.

Occasional
Some degree of abdominal discomfort, nausea, mild cramps, griping, faintness.

SERIOUS REACTIONS
• Long-term use may result in laxative dependence, chronic constipation, and loss of normal bowel function.
• Prolonged use or overdose may result in electrolyte and metabolic disturbances (such as hypokalemia, hypocalcemia, and metabolic acidosis or alkalosis), vomiting, muscle weakness, persistent diarrhea, malabsorption, and weight loss.

PRECAUTIONS & CONSIDERATIONS
Senna should be used cautiously for extended periods (> 1 wk). It is unknown whether senna is distributed in breast milk. Safety and efficacy of senna have not been established in children younger than 6 yr. No age-related precautions have been noted in elderly patients, but this population should be monitored for signs and symptoms of dehydration and electrolyte loss.

Urine may turn pink-red, red-violet, red-brown, or yellow-brown. Pattern of daily bowel activity and stool consistency and serum electrolyte levels should be monitored. Adequate fluid intake should be maintained.

Administration
Take senna on an empty stomach for faster results. Drink at least 6-8 glasses of water a day to aid in stool softening. Avoid giving within 1 h of other oral medications because drug absorption is decreased. To promote defecation, increase fluid intake, exercise, and eat a high-fiber diet. Oral senna generally produces a laxative effect in 6-12 h, but it can take 24 h.

Sertaconazole
sir-tah-con'ah-zole
(Ertaczo)

CATEGORY AND SCHEDULE
Pregnancy Risk Category: C

Classification: Antifungals, topical, dermatologics

MECHANISM OF ACTION
An imidazole derivative that inhibits synthesis of ergosterol, a vital component of fungal cell formation. *Therapeutic Effect:* Damages the fungal cell membrane, altering its function.

AVAILABILITY
Cream: 2%.

INDICATIONS AND DOSAGES
▸ **Tinea pedis**
TOPICAL
Adults, Elderly, Children 12 yr and older. Apply to affected area twice a day for 4 wks.

CONTRAINDICATIONS
None known.

INTERACTIONS
Drug
None known.
Herbal
None known.
Food
None known.

DIAGNOSTIC TEST EFFECTS
None known.

SIDE EFFECTS
Rare (2%)
Burning, tenderness, erythema, dryness, pruritus, hyperpigmentation, and contact dermatitis at application site.

S

SERIOUS REACTIONS
• None known.

PRECAUTIONS & CONSIDERATIONS
It is unknown whether sertaconazole is excreted in breast milk. No age-related precautions have been noted in patients younger than 12 yr or in elderly patients. Skin should be assessed for dermatitis, dryness, erythema, hyperpigmentation, burning sensation, or pruritus.
Administration
Rub gently into affected, surrounding areas. Avoid contact with eyes, nose, and mouth. Keep the affected area clean and dry. Continue sertaconazole treatment for the full length of therapy.

Sertraline
sir′trall-een
(Apo-Sertraline [CAN], Novo-Sertraline [CAN], PMS-Sertraline [CAN], Zoloft)
Do not confuse sertraline with Serentil.

CATEGORY AND SCHEDULE
Pregnancy Risk Category: C

Classification: Antidepressants, serotonin specific reuptake inhibitors

MECHANISM OF ACTION
An antidepressant, anxiolytic, and obsessive-compulsive disorder agent that blocks the reuptake of the neurotransmitter serotonin at central nervous system (CNS) neuronal presynaptic membranes, increasing its availability at postsynaptic receptor sites. *Therapeutic Effect:* Relieves depression, reduces obsessive-compulsive behavior, decreases anxiety.

PHARMACOKINETICS
Incompletely and slowly absorbed from the GI tract; food increases absorption. Protein binding: 98%. Widely distributed. Undergoes extensive first-pass metabolism in the liver to active compound. Excreted in urine and feces. Not removed by hemodialysis. *Half-life:* 26 h.

AVAILABILITY
Oral Concentrate: 20 mg/mL.
Tablets: 25 mg, 50 mg, 100 mg.

INDICATIONS AND DOSAGES
▸ **Depression, obsessive-compulsive disorder (OCD)**
PO
Adults, Children aged 13-17 yr. Initially, 50 mg/day with morning or evening meal. May increase by 50 mg/day at 7-day intervals. *Elderly, Children 6-12 yr.* Initially, 25 mg/day. May increase by 25-50 mg/day at 7-day intervals. Maximum: 200 mg/day.
▸ **Panic disorder, posttraumatic stress disorder, social anxiety disorder**
PO
Adults, Elderly. Initially, 25 mg/day. May increase by 50 mg/day at 7-day intervals. Range: 50-200 mg/day. Maximum: 200 mg/day.
▸ **Premenstrual dysphoric disorder**
PO
Adults. Initially, 50 mg/day either every day or during the luteal phase of menstrual cycle. May increase up to 150 mg/day in 50-mg increments/menstrual cycle.

CONTRAINDICATIONS
Use within 14 days of MAOIs, concurrent use of pimozide or disulfiram.

INTERACTIONS
Drug
Highly protein-bound medications (such as digoxin and warfarin): May increase the blood concentration and risk of toxicity of these drugs.

MAOIs, amphetamines, busipirone, meperidine, nefazodone, sumatriptan, ritonavir, tramadol, venlafaxine: May cause neuroleptic malignant syndrome, hypertensive crisis, hyperpyrexia, seizures, and serotonin syndrome (marked by diaphoresis, diarrhea, fever, mental changes, restlessness, and shivering).

Thioridazine, mesoridazine: May increase risk of serious ventricular arrhythmias.
Herbal
Gotu kola, kava kava, St. John's wort, valerian: May increase CNS depression.
Food
Ethanol: May increase CNS depression.

DIAGNOSTIC TEST EFFECTS
May increase serum total cholesterol, triglyceride, AST (SGOT), and ALT (SGPT) levels. May decrease serum uric acid level.

SIDE EFFECTS
Frequent (12%-26%)
Headache, nausea, diarrhea, insomnia, somnolence, dizziness, fatigue, rash, dry mouth.
Occasional (4%-6%)
Anxiety, nervousness, agitation, tremor, dyspepsia, diaphoresis, vomiting, constipation, abnormal ejaculation, visual disturbances, altered taste.
Rare (< 3%)
Flatulence, urinary frequency, paraesthesia, hot flashes, chills.

SERIOUS REACTIONS
• None known.

WARNINGS
Sertraline is not approved for use in children with major depressive disorder but is approved for the treatment of OCD in children aged 6 yr and older. Antidepressants increase the risk of suicidal thinking and behavior in children, adolescents, and young adults (18-24 yr) with major depressive disorder and other psychiatric disorders. Sertraline is not approved for treating bipolar depression.

PRECAUTIONS & CONSIDERATIONS
Caution is warranted in patients with cardiac disease, hepatic impairment, seizure disorders, those who have had a recent myocardial infarction (MI), and in those with suicidal tendency. It is unknown whether sertraline crosses the placenta or is distributed in breast milk. Notify the physician if pregnancy occurs. No age-related precautions have been noted in children older than 6 yr. Lower initial sertraline dosages are recommended for elderly patients, although no age-related precautions have been noted in this age group.

Dizziness may occur, so alcohol and tasks that require mental alertness or motor skills should be avoided. Notify the physician if fatigue, headache, sexual dysfunction, or tremor occurs. CBC and liver and renal function tests should be performed before and periodically during therapy, especially with long-term use.
Administration
! Make sure at least 14 days elapse between the use of MAOIs and sertraline.

Take sertraline with food or milk if GI distress occurs. Oral solution must be diluted immediately before use with 4 oz of *only* water, orange juice, ginger ale, lemon/lime soda,

S

or lemonade. Once diluted the oral solution must be taken immediately.

Sevelamer
seh-vel'a-mer
(Renagel)
Do not confuse Renagel with Reglan or Regonol.

CATEGORY AND SCHEDULE
Pregnancy Risk Category: C

Classification: Metabolics

MECHANISM OF ACTION
An antihyperphosphatemia agent that binds with dietary phosphorus in the GI tract, thus allowing phosphorus to be eliminated through the normal digestive process and decreasing the serum phosphorus level. *Therapeutic Effect:* Decreases incidence of hypercalcemic episodes in patients receiving calcium acetate treatment. Decreases serum phosphate in patients with end-stage renal disease without the risk of increasing serum calcium levels.

PHARMACOKINETICS
Not absorbed systemically. Unknown whether removed by hemodialysis. Excreted in feces.

AVAILABILITY
Tablets: 400 mg, 800 mg.

INDICATIONS AND DOSAGES
▸ **Hyperphosphatemia**
PO
Adults, Elderly. 800-1600 mg with each meal, depending on severity of hyperphosphatemia. Maintenance dose is based on goal of lowering serum phosphate to < 5.5 mg/dL.

CONTRAINDICATIONS
Hypersensitivity to any ingredients, bowel obstruction, hypophosphatemia.

INTERACTIONS
Drug
Ciprofloxacin, antiarrhythmics, antiseizure medications: Binding may result in decreased absorption.
Herbal and Food
None known.

DIAGNOSTIC TEST EFFECTS
None known.

SIDE EFFECTS
Frequent (11%-20%)
Infection, pain, hypotension, diarrhea, dyspepsia, nausea, vomiting.
Occasional (1%-10%)
Headache, constipation, hypertension, thrombosis, increased cough.

SERIOUS REACTIONS
• None known.

PRECAUTIONS & CONSIDERATIONS
Caution is warranted in patients with dysphagia, severe GI tract motility disorders, swallowing disorders, and in those who have undergone major GI tract surgery. Sevelamer is not distributed in breast milk. The safety and efficacy of sevelamer have not been established in children. No age-related precautions have been noted in elderly patients.

Serum bicarbonate, chloride, calcium, and phosphorus levels should be monitored. Notify the physician of diarrhea, signs of hypotension (such as lightheadedness), nausea or vomiting, or a persistent headache.
Administration
Take sevelamer with food. Do not break, crush, or chew capsules apart because the contents expand in water. Take other medications at least 1 h before or 3 h after sevelamer.

Sibutramine
sih-byoo'tra-meen
(Meridia)

CATEGORY AND SCHEDULE
Pregnancy Risk Category: C
Controlled Substance: Schedule IV

Classification: Anorexiants, stimulants, central nervous system (CNS)

MECHANISM OF ACTION
A CNS stimulant inhibits reuptake of serotonin (enhancing satiety) and norepinephrine (raises the metabolic rate) centrally. *Therapeutic Effect:* Induces and maintains weight loss.

PHARMACOKINETICS
Rapidly absorbed from the GI tract. Protein binding: 95%-97%. Metabolized in liver, undergoes first-pass metabolism. Primarily excreted in urine, minimal elimination in feces. *Half-life:* 1.1 h.

AVAILABILITY
Capsules: 5 mg, 10 mg, 15 mg (Meridia).

INDICATIONS AND DOSAGES
▸ **Weight loss**
PO
Adults aged 16 yr and older. Initially, 10 mg/day after 9 wks. May increase up to 15 mg/day.

CONTRAINDICATIONS
Anorexia nervosa, concomitant MAOI use or within 2 wks, concomitant use of centrally acting appetite suppressants, hypersensitivity to sibutramine or any component of the formulation.

INTERACTIONS
Drug
CNS-acting appetite suppressants: May increase risk of hypertension and tachycardia.
Dextromethorphan, dihydroergotamine, ergotamine, fentanyl, lithium, meperidine, MAOIs, pentazocine, SSRIs, serotonin agonists, tramadol, tryptophan, venlafaxine: May increase the risk of serotonin syndrome.
Herbal
SAMe, St. John's wort: May decrease sibutramine levels.
Yohimbine: May increase risk of adverse cardiovascular effects.
Food
None known.

DIAGNOSTIC TEST EFFECTS
None known.

SIDE EFFECTS
Frequent
Headache, dry mouth, anorexia, constipation, insomnia, rhinitis, pharyngitis.
Occasional
Back pain, flu syndrome, dizziness, nausea, asthenia (loss of strength, energy), arthralgia, nervousness, dyspepsia, sinusitis, abdominal pain, anxiety, dysmenorrhea.
Rare
Depression, rash, cough, sweating, tachycardia, migraine, increased BP, paresthesia, altered taste.

SERIOUS REACTIONS
• Seizures, thrombocytopenia, and deaths have been reported.
• Serotonin syndrome can occur with concomitant use of drugs that increase serotonin.
• Large doses may produce extreme nervousness and tachycardia.

S

PRECAUTIONS & CONSIDERATIONS

Caution is warranted in patients with arrhythmias, congestive heart failure, coronary artery disease, gallstones, hypertension (uncontrolled or poorly controlled), narrow-angle glaucoma, seizures, severe liver or renal impairment, and stroke. It is unknown whether sibutramine crosses the placenta or is distributed in breast milk. Safety and efficacy have not been established in children younger than 16 yr. Be aware that sibutramine is not recommended for elderly patients. Avoid alcohol. Do not take any OTC medications without consulting with the physician.

Storage
Store at room temperature.

Administration
Take with or without food usually in the morning. Administer sibutramine with a low-calorie diet.

Sibutramine is intended for obese persons with an initial body mass index ≥ 30 kg/m^2 or ≥ 27 kg/m^2 in the presence of other risk factors, such as hypertension, diabetes, dyslipidemia. Sibutramine may be habit forming. Do not abruptly discontinue the medication.

Sildenafil

sill-den'a-fill
(Revatio, Viagra)
Do not confuse Viagra with Vaniqa.

CATEGORY AND SCHEDULE

Pregnancy Risk Category: B

Classification:
phosphodiesterase-5 enzyme inhibitors

MECHANISM OF ACTION

An agent that inhibits phosphodiesterase type 5, the enzyme responsible for degrading cyclic guanosine monophosphate (cGMP) in the corpus cavernosum of the penis or the smooth muscle of pulmonary vasculature, resulting in smooth muscle relaxation and increased blood flow. *Therapeutic Effect:* Facilitates an erection in ED. In PAH, results in vasodilation in pulmonary vasculature.

AVAILABILITY

Tablets (Viagra): 25 mg, 50 mg, 100 mg.
Tablets (Revatio): 20 mg.

INDICATIONS AND DOSAGES

▸ **Erectile dysfunction**
PO
Adults. 50 mg (30 min-4 h before sexual activity). Range: 25-100 mg. Maximum dosing frequency is once daily.
Elderly (> 65 yr). Consider starting dose of 25 mg.

▸ **Pulmonary arterial hypertension (PAH)**
PO
Adults, Elderly. 20 mg 3 times daily, administered 4-6 h apart.

OFF-LABEL USES

Treatment of diabetic gastroparesis, sexual dysfunction associated with the use of selective serotonin reuptake inhibitors (SSRIs).

CONTRAINDICATIONS

Concurrent use of sodium nitroprusside or nitrates in any form.

INTERACTIONS

Drug
α-Blockers, nitrates: Potentiates the hypotensive effects of nitrates.

Azole antifungals, cimetidine, erythromycin, itraconazole, ketoconazole, protease inhibitors, other CYP3A4 substrates: May increase the effects of sildenafil.
Herbal
St. John's wort: May decrease sildenafil levels.
Food
Grapefruit juice: May increase sildenafil levels.
High-fat meals: Delay drug's maximum effectiveness by 1 h.

DIAGNOSTIC TEST EFFECTS
None known.

SIDE EFFECTS
Frequent
Headache (16%), flushing (10%).
Occasional (3%-7%)
Dyspepsia, nasal congestion, UTI, abnormal vision, diarrhea.
Rare (2%)
Dizziness, rash.

SERIOUS REACTIONS
• Prolonged erections (lasting over 4 h) and priapism (painful erections lasting > 6 h) occur rarely.

PRECAUTIONS & CONSIDERATIONS
Caution is warranted with an anatomic deformity of the penis, cardiac, hepatic or renal impairment, and conditions that increase the risk of priapism, including leukemia, multiple myeloma, and sickle cell anemia. Be aware that sildenafil is not effective without sexual stimulation. Avoid using nitrate drugs concurrently with sildenafil. Seek treatment immediately if an erection lasts longer than 4 h.

Avoid use of itraconazole, ketoconazole, and ritonavir with sildenafil.

Administration
Sildenafil is usually taken 1 h before sexual activity, but it may be taken anywhere from 4 h to 30 min beforehand. When sildenafil (Revatio) is used for PAH, administer doses at least 4-6 h apart. High-fat meals may affect the drug's absorption rate and effectiveness.

Silver Nitrate

CATEGORY AND SCHEDULE
Pregnancy Risk Category: C

Classification: Anti-infectives, ophthalmics

MECHANISM OF ACTION
Free silver ions precipitate bacterial proteins by combining with chloride in tissue-forming silver chloride; coagulates cellular protein to form an eschar or scab. The germicidal action is credited to precipitation of bacterial proteins by free silver ions. *Therapeutic Effect:* Inhibits growth of both gram-positive and gram-negative bacteria.

PHARMACOKINETICS
Minimal GI tract and cutaneous absorption. Minimal excretion in urine.

AVAILABILITY
Applicator sticks: 75% silver nitrate and 25% potassium nitrate.
Ophthalmic Solution: 1%.
Topical Solution: 10%, 25%, 50%.

INDICATIONS AND DOSAGES
▶ **Exuberant granulations**
APPLICATOR STICKS
Adults, Elderly, Children. Apply to mucous membranes and other moist

S

skin surfaces only on area to be treated 2-3 times/wk for 2-3 wks.
TOPICAL, SOLUTION
Adults, Elderly, Children. Apply a cotton applicator dipped in solution on the affected area 2-3 times/wk for 2-3 wks.

▸ **Gonococcal ophthalmia neonatorum**
OPHTHALMIC
Children. Instill 2 drops in each eye immediately after delivery.

CONTRAINDICATIONS
Broken skin, cuts, or wounds, hypersensitivity to silver nitrate or any of its components.

INTERACTIONS
Drug
None known.
Herbal
None known.
Food
None known.

DIAGNOSTIC TEST EFFECTS
None known.

SIDE EFFECTS
Occasional
Ophthalmic: Chemical conjunctivitis. Topical: Burning, irritation, staining of the skin.
Rare
Hyponatremia, methemoglobinemia.

SERIOUS REACTIONS
• Symptoms of overdose include blackening of skin and mucous membranes, pain and burning of the mouth, salivation, vomiting, diarrhea, shock, convulsions, coma, and death.
• Methemoglobinemia is caused by absorbed silver nitrate but occurs rarely.
• Cauterization of the cornea and blindness occur rarely.

PRECAUTIONS & CONSIDERATIONS
Topical preparations should be used cautiously and should not be applied to abraded areas or near the eyes. It is unknown whether silver nitrate crosses the placenta and is distributed in breast milk. No age-related precautions have been noted in children or elderly patients.

Prolonged use may cause skin discoloration. Repeated applications of silver nitrate ophthalmic solution can cause cauterization of the cornea and blindness.
Storage
Store silver nitrate in a dry place and in a tight, light-resistant container. Exposure to light causes silver to oxidize and turn brown.
Administration
Apply topical preparation by rubbing gently into the affected and surrounding area.

Instill ophthalmic drops of solution in each lower conjunctival sac. Gently massage the closed eyelids to help spread the solution to all areas of the conjunctiva. Gently wipe away excess solution from the eyelids and surrounding skin with sterile cotton.

Silver Sulfadiazine
sul-fa-dye′a-zeen
(Flamazine [CAN], SSD, SSD AF, Silvadene)

CATEGORY AND SCHEDULE
Pregnancy Risk Category: B; near-term pregnancy: Category D

Classification: Anti-infectives, topical, dermatologics

MECHANISM OF ACTION

An anti-infective that acts on cell wall and cell membrane. Releases silver slowly in concentrations selectively toxic to bacteria. *Therapeutic Effect:* Produces bactericidal effect.

PHARMACOKINETICS

Variably absorbed. Significant systemic absorption may occur if applied to extensive burns. Absorbed medication excreted unchanged in urine. *Half-life:* 10 h (half-life increased with impaired renal function).

AVAILABILITY

Cream: 1% (Silvadene, SSD, SSD AF).

INDICATIONS AND DOSAGES
▸ **Burns**
TOPICAL
Adults, Elderly Children. Apply topically to a thickness of approximately 1.66 mu (⅟₁₆ inch) 2 times daily.

OFF-LABEL USES

Treatment of minor bacterial skin infection, dermal ulcer.

CONTRAINDICATIONS

Hypersensitivity to silver sulfadiazine or any component of the formulation.

INTERACTIONS
Drug
Collagenase, papain, sutilains: May be inactivated.
Herbal and Food
None known.

DIAGNOSTIC TEST EFFECTS

None known.

SIDE EFFECTS

Side effects characteristic of all sulfonamides may occur when systemically absorbed such as with extensive burn areas, anorexia, nausea, vomiting, headache, diarrhea, dizziness, photosensitivity, joint pain.
Frequent
Burning feeling at treatment site.
Occasional
Brown-gray skin discoloration, rash, itching.
Rare
Increased sensitivity or skin to sunlight.

SERIOUS REACTIONS

• If significant systemic absorption occurs, serious reactions such as hemolytic anemia, hypoglycemia, diuresis, peripheral neuropathy, Stevens-Johnson syndrome, agranulocytosis, disseminated lupus erythematosus, anaphylaxis, hepatitis, and toxic nephrosis may occur.
• Fungal superinfections may occur.
• Interstitial nephritis occurs rarely.

PRECAUTIONS & CONSIDERATIONS

Caution is warranted in patients with impaired renal or hepatic function, G6PD deficiency, premature neonates, and infants younger than 2 mo. Be aware that silver sulfadiazine is not recommended during pregnancy unless burn area is > 20% of body surface. Be aware that it is unknown whether silver sulfadiazine is distributed in breast milk. There is a risk of kernicterus in neonates. No age-related precautions have been noted in children or elderly patients.

Skin should be assessed for burns, surrounding areas for pain, burning, itching, and rash. Antihistamines may provide relief. Silver sulfadiazine therapy should continue unless reactions are severe.
Storage
Store at room temperature. Cream will occasionally darken either in the jar or after application to the skin.

S

This color change results from a light catalyzed reaction, which is a common characteristic of all silver salts. The antimicrobial activity of the product is not substantially diminished because the color change reaction involves such a small amount of the active drug.

Administration

Apply topical preparation to cleansed and debrided burns using sterile glove. Keep burn areas covered with silver sulfadiazine cream at all times. Reapply to areas where removed by activity. Dressings may be ordered on individual basis.

Simethicone
si-meth'i-kone
(Alka-Seltzer Gas Relief, Gas-X, Genasym, Infant Mylicon, Mylanta Gas, Ovol [CAN], Phazyme)

CATEGORY AND SCHEDULE
Pregnancy Risk Category: C
OTC

Classification: Siloxane polymer, antiflatulent

MECHANISM OF ACTION
An antiflatulent that changes surface tension of gas bubbles, allowing easier elimination of gas. *Therapeutic Effect:* Drug dispersal, prevents formation of gas pockets in the GI tract.

PHARMACOKINETICS
Does not appear to be absorbed from GI tract. Excreted unchanged in feces.

AVAILABILITY
Oral Drops (Infants Mylicon): 40 mg/0.6 mL.
Softgel (Alka-Seltzer Gas Relief, Gas-Z, Mylanta Gas): 125 mg.
Softgel (Phazyme): 180 mg.
Tablets (Chewable [Gas-X, Mylanta Gas]): 80 mg, 125 mg.

INDICATIONS AND DOSAGES
▸ **Antiflatulent**
PO
Adults, Elderly, Children 12 yr and older. 125 mg after meals and at bedtime. Maximum: 500 mg/day.
Children aged 2-11 yr. 40 mg 4 times a day.
Children younger than 2 yr. 20 mg 4 times a day.

OFF-LABEL USES
Adjunct to bowel radiography and gastroscopy.

CONTRAINDICATIONS
None known.

INTERACTIONS
Drug
None known.
Herbal
None known.
Food
None known.

DIAGNOSTIC TEST EFFECTS
None known.

SIDE EFFECTS
None known.

SERIOUS REACTIONS
• None known.

PRECAUTIONS & CONSIDERATIONS
It is unknown whether simethicone crosses the placenta or is distributed in breast milk. Simethicone may be used safely in children and elderly patients. Before simethicone administration, the abdomen should be assessed for signs of tenderness,

rigidity, and the presence of bowel sounds. Avoid carbonated beverages during simethicone therapy.

Administration

Take simethicone after meals and at bedtime, as needed. Chew tablets thoroughly before swallowing. Shake suspension well before using.

Simvastatin

sim'va-sta-tin

(Apo-Simvastatin [CAN], Lipex [AUS], Zocor)

Do not confuse Zocor with Cozaar.

CATEGORY AND SCHEDULE

Pregnancy Risk Category: X

Classification:

Antihyperlipidemics, HMG CoA reductase inhibitors

MECHANISM OF ACTION

An HMG-CoA reductase inhibitor that interferes with cholesterol biosynthesis by inhibiting the conversion of the enzyme HMG-CoA to mevalonate. *Therapeutic Effect:* Decreases serum LDL, cholesterol, VLDL, and plasma triglyceride levels; slightly increases serum HDL concentration.

Well absorbed from the GI tract. Protein binding: 95%. Undergoes extensive first-pass metabolism. Hydrolyzed to active metabolite. Eliminated primarily in feces. Unknown whether removed by hemodialysis.

AVAILABILITY

Tablets: 5 mg, 10 mg, 20 mg, 40 mg, 80 mg.

INDICATIONS AND DOSAGES

▸ **To decrease elevated total and LDL cholesterol in hypercholesterolemia (types IIa and IIb), lower triglyceride levels, and increase HDL levels; to reduce the risk of death and prevent myocardial infarction (MI) in patients with heart disease and elevated cholesterol level; to reduce risk of revascularization procedures; to decrease risk of stroke or transient ischemic attack; to prevent cardiovascular events**

PO

Children aged 10-17 yr. 10 mg/day in evening. Range: 10-40 mg/day. Maximum 40 mg/day.

Adults. Initially, 10-40 mg/day in evening. Dosage adjusted at 4-wks intervals. Range: 5-80 mg/day. Maximum: 80 mg/day.

Elderly. Initially, 10 mg/day in evening. May increase by 5-10 mg/day q4wk. Range: 5-80 mg/day. Maximum: 80 mg/day.

CONTRAINDICATIONS

Active hepatic disease or unexplained, persistent elevations of liver function test results, pregnancy.

INTERACTIONS

Drug

Amiodarone, verapamil: May increase simvastatin levels, limit dose to 20 mg/day.

Cyclosporin, danazol, gemfibrozil: May increase simvastatin levels, limit dose to 10 mg/day.

Cyclosporine, erythromycin, gemfibrozil, immunosuppressants, niacin: Increases the risk of acute renal failure and rhabdomyolysis.

Erythromycin, itraconazole, ketoconazole: May increase simvastatin blood concentration and cause muscle inflammation, myalgia, or weakness.

S

Warfarin: May increase warfarin's anticoagulant effects.
Herbal
St. John's wort: May increase simvastatin levels.
Food
None known.

DIAGNOSTIC TEST EFFECTS

May increase serum CK and serum transaminase concentrations.

SIDE EFFECTS

Simvastatin is generally well tolerated. Side effects are usually mild and transient.
Occasional (2%-3%)
Headache, abdominal pain or cramps, constipation, upper respiratory tract infection.
Rare (< 2%)
Diarrhea, flatulence, asthenia (loss of strength and energy), nausea, or vomiting.

SERIOUS REACTIONS

• Lens opacities may occur.
• Hypersensitivity reaction and hepatitis occur rarely.

PRECAUTIONS & CONSIDERATIONS

Caution is warranted in patients with history of hepatic disease; severe electrolyte, endocrine, or metabolic disorders; and who consume substantial amounts of alcohol. Withholding or discontinuing simvastatin may be necessary when the person is at risk for renal failure secondary to rhabdomyolysis. Simvastatin use is contraindicated in pregnancy because suppression of cholesterol biosynthesis may cause fetal toxicity. Simvastatin is contraindicated in lactation because there is a risk of serious adverse reactions in breastfeeding infants. Safety and efficacy of simvastatin

have not been established in children. No age-related precautions have been noted in elderly patients.

Notify the physician of headache or muscle weakness and aches. Pattern of daily bowel activity and stool consistency should be assessed. Serum lipid cholesterol and triglyceride levels and hepatic function should be checked at baseline and periodically during treatment. Before beginning therapy, a standard cholesterol-lowering diet for a minimum of 3-6 mo should be practiced and then continued throughout simvastatin therapy.
Administration
Take simvastatin without regard to meals and administer in the evening.

Sirolimus
sir-oh-leem′us
(Rapamune)

CATEGORY AND SCHEDULE
Pregnancy Risk Category: C

Classification:
Immunosuppressives

MECHANISM OF ACTION

An immunosuppressant that inhibits T-lymphocyte proliferation induced by stimulation of cell-surface receptors, mitogens, alloantigens, and lymphokines. Prevents activation of the enzyme target of rapamycin, a key regulatory kinase in cell-cycle progression. *Therapeutic Effect:* Inhibits proliferation of T and B cells, essential components of the immune response; prevents organ transplant rejection.

AVAILABILITY
Oral Solution: 1 mg/mL.
Tablets: 1 mg, 2 mg.

INDICATIONS AND DOSAGES
▶ **Prevention of organ transplant rejection**
PO
Adults. Loading dose: 6 mg. Maintenance: 2 mg/day.
Children 13 yr and older weighing < 40 kg. Loading dose: 3 mg/m². Maintenance: 1 mg/m²/day.
NOTE: Dosing is by body weight and depends on whether patient is low-moderate risk or high risk.

CONTRAINDICATIONS
Hypersensitivity to sirolimus, malignancy.

INTERACTIONS
Drug
Cyclosporine, diltiazem, ketoconazole, protease inhibitors, quinidine, verapamil: May increase the blood concentration and risk of toxicity of sirolimus.
Carbamazepine, phenobarbital, phenytoin, rifampin: May decrease the blood concentration and effects of sirolimus.
Herbal
None known.
Food
Grapefruit, grapefruit juice: May decrease the metabolism of sirolimus.

DIAGNOSTIC TEST EFFECTS
May decrease blood hemoglobin level, hematocrit, and platelet count. May increase serum cholesterol, creatinine, and triglyceride levels.

SIDE EFFECTS
Occasional
Hypercholesterolemia, hyperlipidemia, hypertension, rash; with high doses (5 mg/day): anemia, arthralgia, diarrhea, hypokalemia, and thrombocytopenia.

SERIOUS REACTIONS
• None known.
Warnings
Sirolimus is not recommended for de novo use in liver or lung transplant patients. Sirolimus increases the risk of infection and may be associated with the development of lymphoma.

PRECAUTIONS & CONSIDERATIONS
Caution is warranted in patients with chickenpox, herpes zoster, hepatic impairment, and infection. Avoid consuming grapefruit or grapefruit juice during therapy. Also, avoid coming in contact with people with colds or other infections. Liver function tests, CBCs, and sirolimus levels should be monitored.
Storage
Store vials at room temperature. Use it immediately or after reconstitution or, if necessary, refrigerate it for up to 24 h.
Administration
Take the drug at the same time each day. Notify the physician if a dose is missed.

S

Sodium Bicarbonate

CATEGORY AND SCHEDULE
Pregnancy Risk Category: C
OTC

Classification: Alkalinizing agents, electrolyte replacements

MECHANISM OF ACTION

An alkalinizing agent that dissociates to provide bicarbonate ion. *Therapeutic Effect:* Neutralizes hydrogen ion concentration, raises blood and urinary pH.

PHARMACOKINETICS

Route	Onset	Peak	Duration
PO	15 min	NA	1-3 h
IV	Immediate	NA	8-10 min

After administration, sodium bicarbonate dissociates to sodium and bicarbonate ions. With increased hydrogen ion concentrations, bicarbonate ions combine with hydrogen ions to form carbonic acid, which then dissociates to CO_2, which is excreted by the lungs.

AVAILABILITY

Tablets: 325 mg, 650 mg.
Injection: 0.5 mEq/mL (4.2%), 0.6 mEq/mL (5%), 0.9 mEq/mL (7.5%), 1 mEq/mL (8.4%).

INDICATIONS AND DOSAGES

▸ **Cardiac arrest**
IV
Adults, Elderly. Initially, 1 mEq/kg (as 7.5%-8.4% solution). May repeat with 0.5 mEq/kg q10min during continued cardiopulmonary arrest. Use in the postresuscitation phase is based on arterial blood pH, partial pressure of carbon dioxide in arterial blood ($Paco_2$), and base deficit calculation.
Children, Infants. Initially, 1 mEq/kg.
▸ **Metabolic acidosis (not severe)**
IV
Adults, Elderly, Children. 2-5 mEq/kg over 4-8 h. May repeat based on laboratory values.
▸ **Metabolic acidosis (associated with chronic renal failure)**
PO
Adults, Elderly. Initially, 20-36 mEq/day in divided doses.

▸ **Renal tubular acidosis (distal)**
PO
Adults, Elderly. 0.5-2 mEq/kg/day in 4-5 divided doses.
Children. 2-3 mEq/kg/day in 4-5 divided doses.
▸ **Renal tubular acidosis (proximal)**
PO
Adults, Elderly, Children. 5-10 mEq/ kg/day in 4-5 divided doses.
▸ **Urine alkalinization**
PO
Adults, Elderly. Initially, 4 g, then 1-2 g q4h. Maximum: 16 g/day.
Children. 84-840 mg/kg/day in 4-6 divided doses.
▸ **Antacid**
PO
Adults, Elderly. 300 mg-2 g 1-4 times a day.
▸ **Hyperkalemia**
IV
Adults, Elderly. 44.6-50 mEq over 5 min.

CONTRAINDICATIONS

Excessive chloride loss due to diarrhea, vomiting, or GI suctioning; hypocalcemia; metabolic or respiratory alkalosis.

INTERACTIONS

Drug
Calcium-containing products: May result in milk-alkali syndrome.
Corticosteroids: May cause edema and hypertension.
Lithium, salicylates: May increase the excretion of these drugs.
Methenamine: May decrease the effects of methenamine.
Herbal
None known.
Food
Milk, other dairy products: May result in milk-alkali syndrome.

DIAGNOSTIC TEST EFFECTS

May increase serum and urinary pH.

ⓘ IV INCOMPATIBILITIES
Ascorbic acid, diltiazem (Cardizem), dobutamine (Dobutrex), dopamine (Intropin), hydromorphone (Dilaudid), magnesium sulfate, midazolam (Versed), morphine, norepinephrine (Levophed).

ⓘ IV COMPATIBILITIES
Aminophylline, furosemide (Lasix), heparin, insulin, mannitol, milrinone (Primacor), phenylephrine (Neo-Synephrine), potassium chloride propofol (Diprivan).

SIDE EFFECTS
Frequent
Abdominal distention, flatulence, belching.

SERIOUS REACTIONS
• Excessive or chronic use may produce metabolic alkalosis (characterized by irritability, twitching, paresthesias, cyanosis, slow or shallow respirations, headache, thirst, and nausea).
• Fluid overload results in headache, weakness, blurred vision, behavioral changes, incoordination, muscle twitching, elevated BP, bradycardia, tachypnea, wheezing, coughing, and distended neck veins.
• Extravasation may occur at the IV site, resulting in tissue necrosis and ulceration.

PRECAUTIONS & CONSIDERATIONS
Caution is warranted with congestive heart failure (CHF), renal insufficiency, edema, and concurrent corticosteroid therapy. Sodium bicarbonate use may produce hypernatremia and increased deep tendon reflexes in the neonate or fetus whose mother is administered chronically high doses. Sodium bicarbonate may be distributed in breast milk. No age-related precautions have been noted in children; however sodium bicarbonate should not be used as an antacid in children younger than 6 yr. In elderly patients, age-related renal impairment may require cautious use. Check with the physician before taking any OTC drugs because they may contain sodium.

Serum calcium, phosphate and uric acid levels, blood and urinary pH, $Paco_2$ and CO_2, plasma bicarbonate, and serum electrolyte levels should be monitored. Pattern of daily bowel activity and stool consistency and clinical improvement of metabolic acidosis, including relief from disorientation, hyperventilation, and weakness, should also be assessed.

Storage
Store vials at room temperature.

Administration
! Sodium bicarbonate may be given by IV push, IV infusion, or orally. Dosage is individualized based on age, weight, clinical conditions, and laboratory values and on the severity of acidosis. Metabolic alkalosis may result if the bicarbonate deficit is fully corrected during the first 24 h.

Take oral sodium bicarbonate 1-3 h after meals. Do not take other oral drugs within 2 h of sodium bicarbonate administration.
! With acidosis, administer sodium bicarbonate when the plasma bicarbonate level is < 15 mEq/L. Use a 0.5 mEq/mL concentration for direct IV administration to neonates and infants.

Sodium bicarbonate may be given undiluted. For IV push, give up to 1 mEq/kg over 1-3 min for cardiac arrest. Do not exceed an infusion rate of 1 mEq/kg/h. For children younger than 2 yr,

S

premature infants, and neonates, administer by slow infusion, up to 8 mEq/min.

Sodium Chloride
(Muro 128, Nasal Mist, Nasal Moist, Ocean, SalineX, SeaMist, Slo-Salt)

CATEGORY AND SCHEDULE
Pregnancy Risk Category: C
OTC (Tablets, nasal solution, ophthalmic solution, ophthalmic ointment)

Classification: Electrolyte replacements, vitamins/minerals

MECHANISM OF ACTION
Sodium is a major cation of extracellular fluid that controls water distribution, fluid and electrolyte balance, and osmotic pressure of body fluids; it also maintains acid-base balance.

PHARMACOKINETICS
Well absorbed from the GI tract. Widely distributed. Excreted primarily in urine.

AVAILABILITY
Tablets: 1 g.
Injection (Concentrate): 23.4% (4 mEq/mL).
Injection: 0.45%, 0.9%, 3%.
Irrigation: 0.45%, 0.9%.
Nasal Gel (Nasal Moist): 0.65%.
Nasal Solution (OTC [SalineX]): 0.4%.
Nasal Solution (OTC [Nasal Moist, SeaMist]): 0.65%.
Ophthalmic Solution (OTC [Muro 128]): 5%.
Ophthalmic Ointment (OTC [Muro 128]): 5%.

INDICATIONS AND DOSAGES
▶ **Prevention and treatment of sodium and chloride deficiencies; source of hydration**
IV
Adults, Elderly. 1-2 L/day 0.9% or 0.45%. Assess serum electrolyte levels before giving additional fluid.
▶ **Prevention of heat prostration and muscle cramps from excessive perspiration**
PO
Adults, Elderly. 1-2 g 3 times a day.
▶ **Relief of dry and inflamed nasal membranes**
INTRANASAL
Adults, Elderly. Use as needed.
▶ **Diagnostic aid in ophthalmoscopic exam, treatment of corneal edema**
OPHTHALMIC SOLUTION
Adults, Elderly. Apply 1-2 drops q3-4h.
OPHTHALMIC OINTMENT
Adults, Elderly. Apply once a day or as directed.

CONTRAINDICATIONS
Fluid retention, hypernatremia.

INTERACTIONS
Drug
Hypertonic saline solution, oxytocics: May cause uterine hypertonus, ruptures, or lacerations.
Herbal
None known.
Food
None known.

DIAGNOSTIC TEST EFFECTS
None known.

SIDE EFFECTS
Frequent
Facial flushing.

Occasional
Fever; irritation, phlebitis, or extravasation at injection site. Ophthalmic: Temporary burning or irritation.

SERIOUS REACTIONS
• Too rapid administration may produce peripheral edema, congestive heart failure (CHF), and pulmonary edema.
• Excessive dosage may cause hypokalemia, hypervolemia, and hypernatremia.

PRECAUTIONS & CONSIDERATIONS
Caution is warranted with cirrhosis, CHF, hypertension, and renal impairment. Do not administer sodium and chloride preserved with benzyl alcohol to neonates. No age-related precautions have been noted in children or elderly patients.

Notify the physician of acute redness of eyes, floating spots, severe eye pain or pain on exposure to light, a rapid change in vision (side and straight ahead), or headache after ophthalmic administration. Fluid balance, weight, acid-base balance, BP, and serum electrolyte levels should be monitored. Be alert for signs and symptoms of hypernatremia (edema, hypertension, and weight gain) and hyponatremia (dry mucous membranes, muscle cramps, nausea, and vomiting).
Storage
Store vials at room temperature.
Administration
! Dosage is based on acid-base status, age, weight, clinical condition, and fluid and electrolyte status.

Do not crush or break enteric-coated or slow-release tablets. Take tablets with a full glass of water.

For IV use, administer hypertonic solutions (3% or 5%) through a large vein at a rate not exceeding 1 mEq/kg/h. Avoid infiltration. Dilute vials containing 2.5-4 mEq/mL (concentrated NaCl) with D5W or $D_{10}W$ before administration.

For nasal use, inhale slowly just before releasing the drug into nose. Then release air gently through the mouth. Continue this technique for 20-30 s.

For ophthalmic use, place a finger on the lower eyelid, and pull it out until a pocket is formed between the eye and lower lid. Hold the dropper above the pocket and instill the prescribed number of drops (or apply a thin strip of ointment) in the pocket. Close the eyes gently so that the drug is not squeezed out of the sac. After administering the solution, apply gentle finger pressure to the lacrimal sac for 1-2 min to reduce systemic absorption. Release the lower lid, and keep solution in the affected eye open without blinking for at least 30 s; close the affected eye with ointment and roll the eyeball to distribute the drug.

Sodium Ferric Gluconate Complex
sew-dee'um fair'ick glue'koe-nate calm'plex
(Ferrlecit)

S

CATEGORY AND SCHEDULE
Pregnancy Risk Category: B

Classification: Hematinics, vitamins and minerals

MECHANISM OF ACTION
A trace element that repletes total iron content in body. Replaces iron found in hemoglobin, myoglobin,

and specific enzymes; allows oxygen transport via hemoglobin. *Therapeutic Effect:* Prevents and corrects iron deficiency.

AVAILABILITY

Ampules: 12.5 mg/mL elemental iron.

INDICATIONS AND DOSAGES

▸ **Iron deficiency anemia**
IV INFUSION
Adults, Elderly. 125 mg in 100 mL 0.9% NaCl infused over 1 h. May administer undiluted, at a rate ≤ 12.5 mg/min. Minimum cumulative dose 1 g elemental iron given over 8 sessions at sequential dialysis treatments. May be given during dialysis session.
Children younger than 6 yr. 1.5 mg/kg elemental iron diluted in 0.9% NaCl infused over 1 h. Maximum 125 mg/dose given over 8 sessions at sequential dialysis treatments. May be given during dialysis session.

CONTRAINDICATIONS

All anemias not associated with iron deficiency.

INTERACTIONS

Drug
None known.
Herbal
None known.
Food
None known.

DIAGNOSTIC TEST EFFECTS

None known.

ⓘ IV INCOMPATIBILITIES

Do not mix with other medications.

SIDE EFFECTS

Frequent (> 3%)
Flushing, hypotension, hypersensitivity reaction.

Occasional (1%-3%)
Injection-site reaction, headache, abdominal pain, chills, flulike syndrome, dizziness, leg cramps, dyspnea, nausea, vomiting, diarrhea, myalgia, pruritus, edema.

SERIOUS REACTIONS

• A potentially fatal hypersensitivity reaction occurs rarely, characterized by cardiovascular collapse, cardiac arrest, dyspnea, bronchospasm, angioedema, and urticaria.
• Rapid administration may cause hypotension associated with flushing, lightheadedness, fatigue, weakness, or severe pain in the chest, back, or groin.

PRECAUTIONS & CONSIDERATIONS

Caution is warranted in patients with asthma, iron overload, hepatic impairment, rheumatoid arthritis, and significant allergies. It is unknown whether sodium ferric gluconate complex is distributed in breast milk. No age-related precautions have been noted in elderly patients. However, lower initial dosages of sodium ferric gluconate complex are recommended in elderly patients.

Stools may become black during iron therapy, but this effect is harmless unless accompanied by abdominal cramping or pain and red streaking and sticky consistency of stool. Notify the physician of abdominal cramping or pain or red streaking or sticky consistency of stool. Laboratory test results, especially CBC, serum iron concentrations, and vital signs, should be monitored. Test results may not be meaningful for 3 wks after beginning sodium ferric gluconate complex therapy. Patients with rheumatoid arthritis or iron deficiency anemia should be assessed for acute exacerbation of joint pain and swelling.

Storage
Store at room temperature.
Administration
! May give undiluted as slow IV injection or IV infusion without test dose.
   Use immediately after dilution. The standard recommended dose is 125 mg (10 mL) diluted with 100 mL 0.9% NaCl. Infused over 1 h. Do not give concurrently with oral iron because excessive iron intake may produce excessive iron storage (hemosiderosis). The drug may be administered during dialysis treatments.

Sodium Oxybate
sew-dee'um ox'ee-bate
(Xyrem)

CATEGORY AND SCHEDULE
Pregnancy Risk Category: B
Controlled Substance: Schedule III

Classification: Depressants, central nervous system (CNS)

MECHANISM OF ACTION
A naturally occurring inhibitory neurotransmitter that binds to γ-aminobutyric acid (GABA)-B receptors and sodium oxybate specific receptors with its highest concentrations in the basal ganglia, which meditates sleep cycles, temperature regulation, cerebral glucose metabolism and blood flow, memory, and emotion control. *Therapeutic Effect:* Reduces the number of sleep episodes.

PHARMACOKINETICS
Rapidly and incompletely absorbed. Absorption is delayed and decreased by a high fat meal. Protein

binding: < 1%. Widely distributed, including cerebrospinal fluid (CSF). Metabolized in liver. Excretion is < 5% in the urine and negligible in feces. Unknown whether removed by hemodialysis. *Half-life:* 20-53 min.

AVAILABILITY
Oral Solution: 500 mg/mL (Xyrem).

INDICATIONS AND DOSAGES
▸ **Cataplexy of narcolepsy**
PO
Adults aged 16 yr or older, Elderly.
4.5 g/day in 2 equal doses of 2.25 g, the first taken at bedtime while in bed and the second 2.5-4 h later. Maximum: 9 g/day in 2-wks increments of 1.5 g/day. Maximum dose: 9 g/day.

CONTRAINDICATIONS
Metabolic/respiratory alkalosis, current treatment with sedative hypnotics, succinic semialdehyde dehydrogenase deficient, history of substance abuse including active alcoholism, hypersensitivity to sodium oxybate or any component of the formulation.

INTERACTIONS
Drug
Alcohol, barbiturates, benzodiazepines, centrally acting muscle relaxants, opioid analgesics: May increase CNS and respiratory depressant effects.
Methamphetamine: May increase risk of unconsciousness and seizure-like tremor.
Herbal
None known.
Food
None known.

DIAGNOSTIC TEST EFFECTS
May increase sodium and glucose level.

S

SIDE EFFECTS
Frequent
Mild bradycardia.
Occasional
Headache, vertigo, dizziness, restless legs, abdominal pain, muscle weakness.
Rare
Dream-like state of confusion.

SERIOUS REACTIONS
• Agitation, excitation, increased BP, and insomnia may occur on abrupt discontinuation of sodium oxybate.

PRECAUTIONS & CONSIDERATIONS
Caution is warranted in patients with a history of depression, hypertension, pregnancy, concurrent ingestion of alcohol, other CNS depressants and liver impairment. It is unknown whether sodium oxybate is excreted in breast milk. Use caution if giving sodium oxybate to pregnant women. Safety and efficacy of this drug have not been established in children. Age-related liver or renal impairment may require decreased dosage in elderly patients. High-fat meals should be avoided because they will delay absorption of the drug.

Dizziness and lightheadedness may occur. Avoid alcohol and tasks that require mental alertness or motor skills. Notify physician of signs of metabolic alkalosis or irritability, twitching, numbness or tingling of extremities, cyanosis, slow or shallow respiration, headache, thirst, nausea.
Storage
Store at room temperature.
Administration
Be aware that sodium oxybate is available only through restricted distribution. Take sodium oxybate without regard to meals. Mix this medicine with 2 oz (¼ cup) of water before using. Mix both doses of medicine before going to bed, and store the second dose close to the bed. Take the second dose 2 ½ to 4 h of taking the first dose. Set an alarm clock to wake up to take the second dose on time.

Sodium Polystyrene Sulfonate
pol-ee-stye′reen
(Kayexalate, Kionex, PMS-Sodium Polystyrene Sulfonate [CAN], SPS)

CATEGORY AND SCHEDULE
Pregnancy Risk Category: C

Classification: Resins

MECHANISM OF ACTION
An ion exchange resin that releases sodium ions in exchange primarily for potassium ions. *Therapeutic Effect:* Moves potassium from the blood into the intestine so it can be expelled from the body.

AVAILABILITY
Suspension (SPS): 15 g/60 mL.
Powder for Suspension (Kayexalate, Kionex): 15g/60 mL.

INDICATIONS AND DOSAGES
▸ **Hyperkalemia**
PO
Adults, Elderly. 60 mL (15 g) 1-4 times a day.
Children. 1 g/kg/dose q6h.
RECTAL
Adults, Elderly. 30-50 g as needed q 1-2 h initially, as needed to correct hyperkalemia, then q6h.
Children. 1 g/kg q2-6h.

CONTRAINDICATIONS

Hypokalemia, hypocalcemia, intestinal obstruction, or perforation.

INTERACTIONS

Drug
Cation-donating antacids, laxatives (such as magnesium hydroxide): May decrease effect of sodium polystyrene sulfonate and cause systemic alkalosis in patients with renal impairment.
Herbal
None known.
Food
None known.

DIAGNOSTIC TEST EFFECTS

May decrease serum calcium and magnesium levels.

SIDE EFFECTS

Frequent
High dosage: Anorexia, nausea, vomiting, constipation.
High dosage in elderly: Fecal impaction characterized by severe stomach pain with nausea or vomiting.
Occasional
Diarrhea, sodium retention marked by decreased urination, peripheral edema, and increased weight.

SERIOUS REACTIONS

• Potassium deficiency may occur. Early signs of hypokalemia include confusion, delayed thought processes, extreme weakness, irritability, and ECG changes (including prolonged QT interval; widening, flattening, or inversion of T wave; and prominent U waves).
• Hypocalcemia, manifested by abdominal or muscle cramps, occurs occasionally.
• Arrhythmias and severe muscle weakness may be noted.

PRECAUTIONS & CONSIDERATIONS

Caution is warranted in patients with edema, hypertension, and severe CHF. It is unknown whether sodium polystyrene sulfonate crosses the placenta or is distributed in breast milk. No age-related precautions have been noted in children. Elderly patients may be at increased risk for fecal impaction. Foods rich in potassium should be consumed.

Because sodium polystyrene sulfonate does not rapidly correct severe hyperkalemia (it may take hours to days), consider other measures, such as dialysis, IV glucose and insulin, IV calcium, and IV sodium bicarbonate to correct severe hyperkalemia in a medical emergency. Serum potassium levels, calcium and magnesium, and pattern of daily bowel activity and stool consistency should be assessed. Clinical condition and ECG is valuable when determining when treatment should be discontinued.
Administration
Give oral sodium polystyrene sulfonate with 20-100 mL of water to aid in potassium removal, facilitate passage of resin through the intestinal tract, and prevent constipation. Do not mix this drug with foods or liquids containing potassium. Drink the entire amount of the resin for best results. Chilling oral suspension will help improve the taste.

For rectal use, after initial cleansing enema, insert large rubber tube well into sigmoid colon and tape in place. Introduce suspension with 100 mL sorbitol by gravity. Flush with 50-100 mL fluid and clamp. Retain for several hours, if possible. Irrigate colon with a non–sodium-containing solution to remove resin.

S

Solifenacin
sohl-e-fen'ah-sin
(VESIcare)
Do not confuse VESIcare with Viscol.

CATEGORY AND SCHEDULE
Pregnancy Risk Category: C

Classification: Anticholinergics, relaxants, urinary tract

MECHANISM OF ACTION
A urinary antispasmodic that acts as a direct antagonist at muscarinic acetylcholine receptors in cholinergically innervated organs. Reduces tonus (elastic tension) of smooth muscle in the bladder and slows parasympathetic contractions. *Therapeutic Effect:* Decreases urinary bladder contractions, increases residual urine volume, and decreases detrusor muscle pressure.

AVAILABILITY
Tablets: 5 mg, 10 mg.

INDICATIONS AND DOSAGES
▸ **Overactive bladder**
PO
Adults, Elderly. 5 mg/day; if tolerated, may increase to 10 mg/day.
▸ **Dosage in renal or hepatic impairment**
For patients with severe renal impairment, moderate hepatic impairment, or concomitant use of CYP3A4 inhibitors, maximum dosage is 5 mg/day.

CONTRAINDICATIONS
Breastfeeding, GI obstruction, uncontrolled angle-closure glaucoma, urine retention, patients at risk for torsades de pointes.

INTERACTIONS
Drug
Aminoglutethimide, carbamazepine, nafcillin, nevirapine, phenobarbital, phenytoin: May decrease the effects and serum level of solifenacin.
Azole antifungals, ciprofloxacin, clarithromycin, diclofenac, doxycycline, erythromycin, imatinib, isoniazid, nefazodone, nicardipine, propofol, protease inhibitors, quinidine, verapamil: May increase the effects and serum level of solifenacin.
Ketoconazole: May increase the serum level of solifenacin.
Herbal
St John's wort: May decrease the effects and serum level of solifenacin.
Food
Grapefruit, grapefruit juice: May increase the effects and serum level of solifenacin.

DIAGNOSTIC TEST EFFECTS
None known.

SIDE EFFECTS
Frequent (5%-11%)
Dry mouth, constipation, blurred vision.
Occasional (3%-5%)
Urinary tract infection, dyspepsia, nausea.
Rare (1%-2%)
Dizziness, dry eyes, fatigue, depression, edema, hypertension, upper abdominal pain, vomiting, urinary retention.

SERIOUS REACTIONS
• Angioneurotic edema and GI obstruction occur rarely.
• Overdose can result in severe central anticholinergic effects.

PRECAUTIONS & CONSIDERATIONS
Caution is warranted with bladder outflow obstruction, congenital or acquired prolonged QT interval,

controlled angle-closure glaucoma, decreased GI motility, GI obstructive disorders, hepatic or renal impairment, and in pregnant women.
Administration
Take solifenacin without regard to food but with liquid; swallow tablets whole.

Somatrem
soe'-ma-trem
(Protropin)
Do not confuse with Proloprim, Protamine, Protopam, or somatropin.

CATEGORY AND SCHEDULE
Pregnancy Risk Category: C

Classification: Hormones/hormone modifiers, recombinant DNA origin

MECHANISM OF ACTION
A polypeptide hormone that increases the number and size of muscle cells; increases red blood cell (RBC) mass. Affects carbohydrate metabolism by antagonizing action of insulin, increasing the mobilization of fats, and increasing cellular protein synthesis. *Therapeutic Effect:* Stimulates linear growth.

AVAILABILITY
Powder for Injection: 5 mg, 10 mg.

INDICATIONS AND DOSAGES
▸ **Long-term treatment of children who have growth failure due to endogenous growth hormone deficiency**
IM/SC
Children. Initially, 0.025-0.05 mg/kg 3 times/wk or every other day; may be increased to 0.1 mg/kg 3 times/wk. Up to 0.1 mg/kg (0.26 international units/kg) 3 times/wk.

CONTRAINDICATIONS
None known.

INTERACTIONS
Drug
Corticosteroids: May inhibit growth response.
Herbal
None known.
Food
None known.

DIAGNOSTIC TEST EFFECTS
May increase serum parathyroid hormone levels, serum alkaline phosphatase, and inorganic phosphorus levels.

SIDE EFFECTS
Frequent (30%)
Persistent antibodies to growth hormone, but these generally do not cause failure to respond to somatrem.
Occasional
Headache, muscle pain, weakness, mild hyperglycemia, allergic reaction, including rash and itching, pain and swelling at injection site, pain in hip or knee.

PRECAUTIONS & CONSIDERATIONS
Caution is warranted in patients with diabetes mellitus, malignancy, and untreated hypothyroidism. Blood glucose levels, bone age, growth rate, parathyroid, phosphorus, renal function, serum calcium, and thyroid function studies should be monitored.
Administration
May be administered as IM or SC injection.

S

Sorbitol
sor′bi-tole

CATEGORY AND SCHEDULE
Pregnancy Risk Category: C

Classification: Irrigants, genitourinary

MECHANISM OF ACTION
A polyalcoholic sugar with osmotic cathartic actions. Specific mechanism unknown. *Therapeutic Effect:* Catharsis, urinary irrigation.

PHARMACOKINETICS
Onset of action within 15-60 min. Poorly absorbed by both oral and rectal route. Metabolized in liver to primary metabolite, fructose.

AVAILABILITY
Solution, Genitourinary Irrigation: 3%.
Solution, Oral: 70%.

INDICATIONS AND DOSAGES
▶ **Hyperosmotic laxative**
PO
Adults, Elderly, Children 12 yr and older. 30-150 mL as a 70% solution.
Children aged 2-11 yr. 2 mL/kg as a 70% solution.
RECTAL
Adults, Elderly, Children 12 yr and older. 120 mL as a 25%-30% solution.
Children aged 2-11 yr. 30-60 mL as a 25%-30% solution.
▶ **Transurethral surgical procedure**
TOPICAL
Adults, Elderly. 3%-3.3% as transurethral surgical procedure irrigation.

CONTRAINDICATIONS
Anuria.

INTERACTIONS
Drug
None known.
Herbal
None known.
Food
None known.

DIAGNOSTIC TEST EFFECTS
None known.

SIDE EFFECTS
Acidosis, electrolyte loss, marked diuresis, urinary retention, edema, dryness of mouth and thirst, dehydration, pulmonary congestion, hypotension, tachycardia, angina-like pains, blurred vision, convulsions, nausea, vomiting, diarrhea, rhinitis, chills, vertigo, backache, urticaria.

PRECAUTIONS & CONSIDERATIONS
Caution is warranted in patients with cardiopulmonary dysfunction, diabetes mellitus, fructose intolerance, hyponatremia, and renal dysfunction. Be aware that it is unknown whether sorbitol crosses the placenta or is distributed in breast milk. No age-related precautions have been noted in children or elderly patients.
Storage
Store at room temperature. Protect from freezing and heat.
Administration
Do not use unless solution is clear.

Do not use oral formulation for more than 1 wk, and do not take with additional laxatives or stool softeners. Prolonged use can result in dependence.

Sotalol
soe'ta-lole

(Apo-Sotalol [CAN], Betapace, Betapace AF, Cardol [AUS], Novo-Sotalol [CAN], PMS-Sotalol [CAN], Solavert [AUS], Sorine, Sotab [AUS], Sotacor [AUS], Sotahexal [AUS])

Do not confuse sotalol with Stadol.

CATEGORY AND SCHEDULE
Pregnancy Risk Category: B (D if used in second or third trimester)

Classification: Antiadrenergics, β-blocking, antiarrhythmics, class III

MECHANISM OF ACTION
A β-adrenergic blocking agent that prolongs action potential, effective refractory period, and QT interval. Decreases heart rate and AV node conduction; increases AV node refractoriness. *Therapeutic Effect:* Produces antiarrhythmic activity.

PHARMACOKINETICS
Well absorbed from the GI tract. Protein binding: None. Widely distributed. Excreted primarily unchanged in urine. Removed by hemodialysis. *Half-life:* 12 h (increased in elderly patients and in patients with impaired renal function).

AVAILABILITY
Tablets (Betapace): 80 mg, 120 mg, 160 mg, 240 mg.
Tablets (Betapace AF): 80 mg, 120 mg, 160 mg.
Tablets (Sorine): 80 mg, 120 mg, 160 mg, 240 mg.

INDICATIONS AND DOSAGES
▸ **Documented, life-threatening arrhythmias**
PO
Adults, Elderly. Initially, 80 mg twice a day. May increase gradually at 2- to 3-day intervals. Range: 240-320 mg/day in 2 divided doses.
▸ **Dosage in renal impairment**
Dosage interval is modified based on creatinine clearance.

Creatinine Clearance (mL/min)	Dosage Interval
30-59	24 h
10-29	36-48 h
< 10	Individualized

OFF-LABEL USES
Maintenance of normal heart rhythm in chronic or recurring atrial fibrillation or flutter; treatment of anxiety, chronic angina pectoris, hypertension, hypertrophic cardiomyopathy, myocardial infarction, mitral valve prolapse syndrome, pheochromocytoma, thyrotoxicosis, tremors.

CONTRAINDICATIONS
Bronchial asthma, cardiogenic shock, hypokalemia, prolonged QT syndrome (unless functioning pacemaker is present), second- and third-degree heart block, sinus bradycardia, uncontrolled cardiac failure.

INTERACTIONS
Drug
Antiarrhythmics, phenothiazine, tricyclic antidepressants: May prolong QT interval.
Calcium channel blockers: May increase effect on AV conduction and BP.
Clonidine: May potentiate rebound hypertension after clonidine is discontinued.

S

Digoxin: May increase risk of proarrhythmias.
Insulin, oral hypoglycemics: May mask signs of hypoglycemia and prolong the effects of insulin and oral hypoglycemics.
Sympathomimetics: May inhibit the effects of sympathomimetics.
Herbal
Ephedra: May worsen arrhythmias.
Food
None known.

DIAGNOSTIC TEST EFFECTS

May increase blood glucose, serum alkaline phosphatase, serum LDH, serum lipoprotein, AST (SGOT), ALT (SGPT), and serum triglyceride levels.

SIDE EFFECTS

Frequent
Diminished sexual function, drowsiness, insomnia, unusual fatigue or weakness.
Occasional
Depression, cold hands or feet, diarrhea, constipation, anxiety, nasal congestion, nausea, vomiting.
Rare
Altered taste, dry eyes, itching, numbness of fingers, toes, or scalp.

SERIOUS REACTIONS

• Bradycardia, congestive heart failure (CHF), hypotension, bronchospasm, hypoglycemia, prolonged QT interval, torsade de pointes, ventricular tachycardia, and premature ventricular complexes may occur.

PRECAUTIONS & CONSIDERATIONS

Caution is warranted with cardiomegaly, CHF, diabetes mellitus, excessive QT-interval prolongation, history of ventricular tachycardia, hypokalemia, hypomagnesemia, severe and prolonged diarrhea, sick sinus syndrome, ventricular fibrillation, and those at risk for developing thyrotoxicosis. Sotalol crosses the placenta and is excreted in breast milk. The safety and efficacy of sotalol have not been established in children. In elderly patients, age-related peripheral vascular disease may increase susceptibility to decreased peripheral circulation. Tasks that require mental alertness or motor skills should be avoided.

Monitor BP for hypotension and pulse for bradycardia during treatment. If pulse rate is 60 beats/min or lower or systolic BP is < 90 mm Hg, withhold the medication and contact the physician. Continuous cardiac monitoring should be performed when beginning sotalol therapy. If the pulse rate is 60 beats/min or less, consult the physician before beginning sotalol therapy. Arrhythmias should also be assessed. Signs and symptoms of CHF, such as decreased urine output, distended neck veins, dyspnea (particularly on exertion or lying down), night cough, peripheral edema, and weight gain should also be assessed.
Administration
! Some people may require 480-640 mg/day. Sotalol has a long half-life and administering the drug more than twice a day is usually not necessary. Avoid abrupt withdrawal.

Take sotalol without regard to food. Do not abruptly discontinue the drug.

Spectinomycin
spek-ti-noe-mye'sin
(Trobicin)
**Do not confuse with
streptomycin or tobramycin.**

CATEGORY AND SCHEDULE
Pregnancy Risk Category: B

Classification: Antibiotics,
miscellaneous

MECHANISM OF ACTION
An anti-infective that inhibits
protein synthesis of bacterial cells.
Therapeutic Effect: Produces
bacterial cell death.

PHARMACOKINETICS
Rapid, complete absorption after
IM administration. Protein binding:
Unknown. Widely distributed.
Excreted unchanged in urine.
Partially removed by hemodialysis.
Half-life: 1.7 h.

AVAILABILITY
Powder for Reconstitution: 2 g
(Trobicin).

INDICATIONS AND DOSAGES
▶ **Treatment of acute gonococcal
urethritis, proctitis in men, acute
gonococcal cervicitis, and proctitis
in women**
IM
*Children weighing ≥ 45 kg, Adults,
Elderly.* 2 g once. In areas where
antibiotic resistance is known to
be prevalent, 4 g (10 mL) divided
between 2 injection sites is preferred.
Children < 45 kg. 40 mg/kg/dose.

OFF-LABEL USES
Treatment of disseminated
gonorrhea.

CONTRAINDICATIONS
Hypersensitivity to spectinomycin or
any component of the formulation.

INTERACTIONS
Drug
None known.
Herbal
None known.
Food
None known.

DIAGNOSTIC TEST EFFECTS
None known.

SIDE EFFECTS
Frequent
Pain at IM injection site.
Occasional
Dizziness, insomnia.
Rare
Decreased urine output.

SERIOUS REACTIONS
• Hypersensitivity reaction
characterized as chills, fever, nausea,
vomiting, urticaria, and anaphylaxis.

PRECAUTIONS & CONSIDERATIONS
Caution should be used in patients
with history of allergies. Be
aware that it is unknown whether
spectinomycin crosses the placenta
or is distributed in breast milk.
Safety and efficacy have not been
established in children. No age-
related precautions have been noted
in elderly patients.
Storage
Store at room temperature. After
reconstitution, use within 24 h.
Administration
Shake vial vigorously immediately
after adding diluent and before
withdrawing dose. Inject deep IM
into upper outer quandrant of gluteal
muscle.

S

Spironolactone

speer-on-oh-lak'tone
(Aldactone, Novospiroton [CAN],
Spiractin [AUS])
Do not confuse with Aldactazide.

CATEGORY AND SCHEDULE

Pregnancy Risk Category: C
(D if used in pregnancy-induced
hypertension)

Classification: Diuretics,
potassium sparing

MECHANISM OF ACTION

A potassium-sparing diuretic that
interferes with sodium reabsorption
by competitively inhibiting the action
of aldosterone in the distal tubule, thus
promoting sodium and water excretion
and increasing potassium retention.
Therapeutic Effect: Produces diuresis;
lowers BP; diagnostic aid for primary
aldosteronism.

PHARMACOKINETICS

Route	Onset	Peak	Duration
PO	24-48 h	48-72 h	48-72 h

Well absorbed from the GI tract
(absorption increased with food). Protein binding: 91%-98%. Metabolized
in the liver to active metabolite.
Excreted primarily in urine. Unknown
whether removed by hemodialysis.
Half-life: 1.3-2 h (metabolite, 10-35 h).

AVAILABILITY

Tablets: 25 mg, 50 mg, 100 mg.

INDICATIONS AND DOSAGES

▸ **Edema or the treatment of Ascites
due to Cirrhosis**
PO
Adults, Elderly. 25-200 mg/day as a
single dose or in 2 divided doses.

Children (unlabeled use).
1.5-3.3 mg/kg/day once daily or in
2-4 divided doses.
Neonates (unlabeled use).
1-3 mg/kg/day in 1-2 divided
doses once daily or in 2-4 divided
doses.
▸ **CHF, severe with ACEI and loop
diuretic**
Adults. 12.5-25 mg/day. Maximum:
50 mg/day.
▸ **Hypertension**
PO
Adults, Elderly. 50-100 mg/day in
1-2 doses/day. After 2 wks, may be
titrated to 200 mg/day in 2-4 divided
doses.
Children. 1.5-3.3 mg/kg/day in
divided doses.
▸ **Hypokalemia**
PO
Adults, Elderly. 25-100 mg/day as
a single dose or in 2 divided
doses.
▸ **Hirsutism (unlabeled use)**
PO
Adults, Elderly. 50-200 mg/day as
a single dose or in 2 divided doses.
▸ **Primary aldosteronism**
PO
Adults, Elderly. 100-400 mg/day as
a single dose or in 2 divided doses.
▸ **Dosage in renal impairment**
Dosage interval is modified based on
creatinine clearance.

Creatinine Clearance (mL/min)	Dosage Interval
10-50	Usual dose q24h
< 10	Avoid use

OFF-LABEL USES

Treatment of female hirsutism,
polycystic ovary disease, indications
in children.

CONTRAINDICATIONS

Acute renal insufficiency, anuria,
BUN and serum creatinine levels

more than twice normal values, hyperkalemia.

INTERACTIONS
Drug
ACE inhibitors (such as captopril), potassium-containing medications, potassium supplements: May increase the risk of hyperkalemia.
Anticoagulants, heparin: May decrease the effects of these drugs.
Digoxin: May increase the half-life of digoxin.
Lithium: May decrease the clearance and increase the risk of toxicity of lithium.
NSAIDs: May decrease the antihypertensive effect of spironolactone.
Herbal
Natural licorice: May increase mineralocorticoid effects of spironolactone.
Food
None known.

DIAGNOSTIC TEST EFFECTS
May increase urinary calcium excretion; BUN and blood glucose levels; serum creatinine, magnesium, potassium, and uric acid levels. May decrease serum sodium level.

SIDE EFFECTS
Frequent
Hyperkalemia (in patients with renal insufficiency and those taking potassium supplements), dehydration, hyponatremia, lethargy.
Occasional
Nausea, vomiting, anorexia, abdominal cramps, diarrhea, headache, ataxia, somnolence, confusion, fever.
Male: Gynecomastia, impotence, decreased libido.
Female: Menstrual irregularities (including amenorrhea and postmenopausal bleeding), breast tenderness.

Rare
Rash, urticaria, hirsutism.

SERIOUS REACTIONS
• Severe hyperkalemia may produce arrhythmias, bradycardia, and ECG changes (tented T waves, widening QRS complex and ST segment depression). These may proceed to cardiac standstill or ventricular fibrillation.
• Cirrhosis patients are at risk for hepatic decompensation if dehydration or hyponatremia occurs.
• Patients with primary aldosteronism may experience rapid weight loss and severe fatigue during high-dose therapy.

PRECAUTIONS & CONSIDERATIONS
Caution is warranted in patients with hyponatremia, hepatic or renal impairment, dehydration, and concurrent use of potassium supplements. An active metabolite of spironolactone is excreted in breast milk. Breastfeeding is not recommended for patients taking this drug. No age-related precautions have been noted in children. Elderly patients may be more susceptible to hyperkalemia. In addition, age-related renal impairment may require cautious use in this age group. Avoid foods high in potassium, such as apricots, bananas, legumes, meat, orange juice, raisins, whole grains, including cereals, and white and sweet potatoes. Also, avoid performing tasks that require mental alertness or motor skills until response to the drug has been established.

An increase in the frequency and volume of urination may occur. Notify the physician of an irregular heartbeat, diarrhea, muscle twitching, cold and clammy skin, confusion, drowsiness, dry mouth, or excessive thirst. BP, vital signs, electrolytes, and

S

intake and output should be monitored before and during treatment. Be especially alert for evidence of hyperkalemia, such as arrhythmias, colic, diarrhea, and muscle twitching, followed by paralysis and weakness. Also be aware signs of hyponatremia may result in cold and clammy skin, confusion, and thirst.

Storage
Store tablets at room temperature.

Administration
Take spironolactone with food to enhance its absorption. Crush scored tablets as needed. The drug's therapeutic effect takes several days to begin and can last for several days once the drug is discontinued (unless taking a potassium-losing drug concomitantly).

Stanozolol
stan-oh′zoe-lole
(Winstrol)
Discontinued in the United States.

CATEGORY AND SCHEDULE
Pregnancy Risk Category: X

Classification: Anabolic steroids, hormones and hormone modifiers

MECHANISM OF ACTION
A synthetic testosterone derivative that increases circulating levels of C1 INH and C4 through an increase in general protein anabolism and, more specifically, through an increase in the synthesis of messenger RNA.
Therapeutic Effect: Decreases swelling of the face, extremities, genitalia, bowel wall, and upper respiratory tract.

PHARMACOKINETICS
Metabolized in liver. Primarily excreted in urine. Unknown whether removed by hemodialysis.

AVAILABILITY
Tablets: 2 mg (Winstrol).

INDICATIONS AND DOSAGES
▶ **Hereditary angioedema prophylaxis**
PO
Adults. Initially, 2 mg 2 times/day. Decrease at intervals of 1-3 mo. Maintenance: 2 mg/day.

OFF-LABEL USES
Antithrombin III deficiency, arterial occlusions, hemophilia A, lichen sclerosus et atrophicus, liposclerosis, necrobiosis lipoidica, osteoporosis, protein C deficiency, rheumatoid arthritis, thrombosis, urticaria.

CONTRAINDICATIONS
Cardiac impairment, hypercalcemia, pregnancy, prostatic or breast cancer in men, severe liver or renal disease, hypersensitivity to stanozolol or its components.

INTERACTIONS
Drug
ACTH: May increase the risk of edema and acne.
Bupropion: May lower seizure threshold. Insulin, oral hypoglycemics: May increase hypoglycemic effects of insulin and oral hypoglycemics.
Oral anticoagulants: May increase the effects of oral anticoagulants.
Herbal
Chaparral, comfrey, germander, jin bu huan, kava kava, pennyroyal: May increase liver enzymes.
Eucalyptus, valerian: May increase risk of hepatotoxicity.
Skullcap: May increase the risk of liver damage.

Food
None known.

DIAGNOSTIC TEST EFFECTS
May increase blood hemoglobin and hematocrit, LDL concentrations, serum alkaline phosphatase, bilirubin, calcium, potassium, SGOT (AST) levels, and sodium levels. May decrease HDL concentrations.

SIDE EFFECTS
Frequent
Gynecomastia, acne. Females: Amenorrhea or other menstrual irregularities, hirsutism, deepening of voice, clitoral enlargement that may not be reversible when drug is discontinued.
Occasional
Edema, nausea, insomnia, oligospermia, male pattern of baldness, bladder irritability, hypercalcemia in immobilized patients or those with breast cancer, hypercholesterolemia.

SERIOUS REACTIONS
• Peliosis hepatitis or liver, spleen replaced with blood-filled cysts, hepatic neoplasms, and hepatocellular carcinoma have been associated with prolonged high-dosage.

PRECAUTIONS & CONSIDERATIONS
Caution is warranted in patients with diabetes, epilepsy, and liver or renal impairment. Stanozolol use is contraindicated during lactation. Stanozolol is not recommended for children. Its use in elderly patients may increase the risk of hyperplasia or stimulate growth of occult prostate carcinoma.

Acne, nausea, pedal edema, or vomiting may occur. Women should report deepening of voice, hoarseness, and menstrual irregularities. Men should report difficulty urinating, frequent erections, and gynecomastia. Weight should be obtained each day. Weekly weight gains of more than 5 lb should be reported.
Administration
Take with or without regard to food. Decrease dose to 2 mg/day after 1-3 mo. Some people may be maintained on 2 mg every other day.

Stavudine (d4T)
stav′yoo-deen
(Zerit)

CATEGORY AND SCHEDULE
Pregnancy Risk Category: C

Classification: Antivirals, nucleoside reverse transcriptase inhibitors

MECHANISM OF ACTION
Inhibits HIV reverse transcriptase by terminating the viral DNA chain. Also inhibits RNA- and DNA-dependent DNA polymerase, an enzyme necessary for HIV replication. *Therapeutic Effect:* Impedes HIV replication, slowing the progression of HIV infection.

PHARMACOKINETICS
Rapidly and completely absorbed after PO administration. Undergoes minimal metabolism. Excreted in urine. *Half-life:* 1.2-1.6 h (increased in renal impairment).

AVAILABILITY
Capsules: 15 mg, 20 mg, 30 mg, 40 mg.
Oral Solution: 1 mg/mL.

INDICATIONS AND DOSAGES
▸ **HIV infection (in combination with other antiretrovirals)**
PO
Adults, Children weighing ≥60 kg.
40 mg twice a day.
Adults weighing < 60 kg. 30 mg twice a day.
Children weighing ≥ 30-60 kg. 30 mg twice a day.
Children weighing < 30 kg. 1 mg/kg twice a day.
Newborns (< 14 days old). 0.5 mg/kg every 12 h.
▸ **HIV infection in patients with a recent history and complete resolution of peripheral neuropathy or elevated liver function test results (50% of recommended dose)**
Adults weighing ≥60 kg. 20 mg twice a day.
Adults weighing < 60 kg. 15 mg twice a day.
▸ **Dosage in renal impairment**
Dosage and frequency are modified based on creatinine clearance and patient weight.

Creatinine Clearance (mL/min)	Weight ≥60 kg	Weight < 60 kg
> 50	40 mg q12h	30 mg q12h
26-50	20 mg q12h	15 mg q12h
10-25	20 mg q24h	15 mg q24h Note: Administer after hemodialysis dose on day of dialysis

CONTRAINDICATIONS
None known.

INTERACTIONS
Drug
Didanosine, ethambutol, isoniazid, lithium, phenytoin, zalcitabine: May increase the risk of peripheral neuropathy development.
Didanosine, hydroxyurea: May increase the risk of hepatotoxicity.
Doxorubicin, zidovudine: May have antagonistic antiviral effect.
Herbal
None known.
Food
None known.

DIAGNOSTIC TEST EFFECTS
Commonly increases AST (SGOT) and ALT (SGPT) levels. May decrease neutrophil count.

SIDE EFFECTS
Frequent
Headache (55%), diarrhea (50%), chills and fever (38%), nausea and vomiting, myalgia (35%), rash (33%), asthenia (28%), insomnia, abdominal pain (26%), anxiety (22%), arthralgia (18%), back pain (20%), diaphoresis (19%), malaise (17%), depression (14%).
Occasional
Anorexia, weight loss, nervousness, dizziness, conjunctivitis, dyspepsia, dyspnea.
Rare
Constipation, vasodilation, confusion, migraine, urticaria, abnormal vision.

SERIOUS REACTIONS
• Peripheral neuropathy (numbness, tingling, or pain in the hands and feet) occurs in 15%-21% of patients.
• Ulcerative stomatitis (erythema or ulcers of oral mucosa, glossitis, gingivitis), pneumonia, and benign skin neoplasms occur occasionally.
• Pancreatitis and lactic acidosis occur rarely.

PRECAUTIONS & CONSIDERATIONS
Caution is warranted in patients with a history of peripheral neuropathy or liver or renal impairment. Breastfeeding is not recommended

in this population because of the possibility of HIV transmission. No age-related precautions have been noted in children. There is no information on the effects of this drug's use in elderly patients. Avoid taking any medications, including over-the-counter (OTC) drugs, without first notifying the physician. Stavudine is not a cure for HIV infection, nor does it reduce risk of transmission to others, and illnesses, including opportunistic infections, may develop.

Check baseline laboratory test results, if ordered, especially liver function test results, before beginning stavudine therapy and at periodic intervals during therapy. Monitor for signs and symptoms of peripheral neuropathy, which is characterized by numbness, pain, or tingling in the feet or hands. Be aware that peripheral neuropathy symptoms resolve promptly if stavudine therapy is discontinued. Also, know that symptoms may worsen temporarily after the drug is withdrawn. If symptoms resolve completely, expect to resume drug therapy at a reduced dosage. Assess for dizziness, headache, muscle or joint aches, myalgia, weight loss, conjunctivitis, nausea, and vomiting. Monitor for evidence of a rash and signs of chills or a fever. Determine sleep pattern and pattern of daily bowel activity and stool consistency.

Administration
Take without regard to meals. If oral solution is used, it should be shaken vigorously before use. Continue stavudine therapy for the full length of treatment and evenly space doses around the clock.

Streptokinase
strep-toe-kye′nase
(Streptase)

CATEGORY AND SCHEDULE
Pregnancy Risk Category: C

Classification: Thrombolytics

MECHANISM OF ACTION
An enzyme that activates the fibrinolytic system by converting plasminogen to plasmin, an enzyme that degrades fibrin clots. Acts indirectly by forming a complex with plasminogen, which converts plasminogen to plasmin. Action occurs within the thrombus, on its surface, and in circulating blood. *Therapeutic Effect:* Destroys thrombi.

PHARMACOKINETICS
Rapidly cleared from plasma by antibodies and the reticuloendothelial system. Route of elimination unknown. Duration of action continues for several hours after the drug has been discontinued. *Half-life:* 23 min.

AVAILABILITY
Powder for Injection: 250,000 International Units, 750,000 International Units, 1.5 million International Units.

INDICATIONS AND DOSAGES
▸ **Acute evolving transmural myocardial infarction (MI; given as soon as possible after symptoms occur)**
IV INFUSION
Adults, Elderly (1.5 million International Units diluted to 45 mL). 1.5 million International Units infused over 60 min.
INTRACORONARY INFUSION
Adults, Elderly (250,000 International Units diluted to 125 mL). Initially,

S

20,000-International Unit (10-mL) bolus; then, 2000 International Units/min for 60 min. Total dose: 140,000 International Units.
▸ **Pulmonary embolism, deep vein thrombosis (DVT), arterial thrombosis and embolism (given within 7 days of onset)**
IV INFUSION
Adults, Elderly (1.5 million International Units diluted to 90 mL). Initially, 250,000 International Units infused over 30 min; then 100,000 International Units/h for 24-72 h for arterial thrombosis or embolism and pulmonary embolism, 72 h for DVT.
INTRA-ATERIAL INFUSION
Adults, Elderly (1.5 million International Units diluted to 45 mL). Initially, 250,000 International Units infused over 30 min; then 100,000 International Units/h for maintenance.

CONTRAINDICATIONS
Carcinoma of the brain, cerebrovascular accident, internal bleeding, intracranial surgery, recent streptococcal infection, severe hypertension.

INTERACTIONS
Drug
Anticoagulants, heparin: May increase the risk of hemorrhage.
Platelet aggregation inhibitors such as aspirin: May increase the risk of bleeding.
Herbal and Food
None known.

DIAGNOSTIC TEST EFFECTS
Decreases serum plasminogen and fibrinogen level during infusion, decreasing clotting time and confirming presence of lysis.

Ⓓ IV INCOMPATIBILITIES
Do not mix with other medications.

SIDE EFFECTS
Frequent
Fever, superficial bleeding at puncture sites, decreased BP.
Occasional
Allergic reaction, including rash and wheezing; ecchymosis.

SERIOUS REACTIONS
• Severe internal hemorrhage may occur.
• Lysis of coronary thrombi may produce life-threatening arrhythmias.

PRECAUTIONS & CONSIDERATIONS
Caution is warranted in patients with GI bleeding or recent trauma and in those who have had major surgery within past 10 days. Streptokinase should be used during pregnancy only when the benefit to the mother outweighs the risk to the fetus. It is unknown whether streptokinase crosses the placenta or is distributed in breast milk. Safety and efficacy of streptokinase have not been established in children. Elderly patients may have an increased risk of intracranial hemorrhage. Streptokinase should be used cautiously in this population. Women may experience an increase in menstrual flow. An electric razor and a soft toothbrush should be used to reduce the risk of bleeding.

Notify the physician of bruises, back or abdominal pain, black or red stool, coffee-ground vomitus, dark or red urine, red-speckled mucus from cough, chest pain, headache, palpitations, or shortness of breath. Stool should be monitored for occult blood. BP and pulse and respiration rates should be checked every 15 min until stable; then check hourly. Hematocrit and hemoglobin, platelet count, aPTT, PT, and fibrinogen level should be evaluated before and during therapy.

Storage
Store unopened vials at room temperature. Refrigerate reconstituted solution, and use within 24 h.
Administration
! Streptokinase must be administered within 12 h of clot formation. The greatest benefit in mortality reduction was seen when administered within 4 h. It has little effect on older, organized clots. Do not use within 5 days-6 mo of previous streptokinase treatment if administered for streptococcal infection, such as acute glomerulonephritis secondary to streptococcal infection, pharyngitis, and rheumatic fever.

Reconstitute vial with 5 mL D5W or 0.9% NaCl (preferred). Add diluent slowly to side of vial; roll and tilt to avoid foaming. Do not shake vial. May dilute further with 50-500 mL of D5W or 0.9% NaCl in 45-mL increments. For peripheral IV administration for coronary artery thrombi, give 1.5 million International Units over 60 min. For direct intracoronary administration of coronary artery thrombi, give bolus dose over 25-30 s using coronary catheter. Follow with 2000-4000 International Units/min for 60 min. For treatment of DVT, pulmonary arterial embolism, or arterial thrombi, give single dose over 30 min. Follow with maintenance dose of 100,000 or more International Units every hour for 24-72 h (72 h for DVT). Monitor BP during infusion. Hypotension, which may be severe, occurs in 1%-10% of patients. If necessary, decrease the infusion rate, as prescribed. Discontinue the infusion immediately, and notify the physician if uncontrolled hemorrhage occurs. Slowing the rate of infusion instead of discontinuing it may produce worsening hemorrhage. Do not use dextran to control hemorrhage.

Streptomycin
strep-toe-mye′sin

CATEGORY AND SCHEDULE
Pregnancy Risk Category: D

Classification: Antibiotics, aminoglycosides, antimycobacterials

MECHANISM OF ACTION
An aminoglycoside that binds directly to the 30S ribosomal subunits causing a faulty peptide sequence to form in the protein chain. *Therapeutic effect:* Inhibits bacterial protein synthesis.

AVAILABILITY
Injection: 1 g.

INDICATIONS AND DOSAGES
▸ **Tuberculosis**
IM
Adults. 15 mg/kg/day. Maximum: 1 g/day.
Elderly. 10 mg/kg/day. Maximum: 750 mg/day.
Children. 20-40 mg/kg/day. Maximum: 1 g/day.
NOTE: May also give as directly observed therapy 2-3 times/wk.
Other indications for adults:
Brucellosis, endocarditis, *Mycobacterium avium* complex, plague, tularemia, given every 12 h; duration depends on indication.
▸ **Dosage in renal impairment**

Creatinine Clearance (mL/min)	Dosage Interval
10-50	q24-72h
< 10	q72-96h

CONTRAINDICATIONS
Pregnancy.

S

INTERACTIONS
Drug
Amphotericin, loop diuretics:
May increase the nephrotoxicity of streptomycin.
Neuromuscular blockers: May increase the effects of streptomycin.
Herbal and Food
None known.

DIAGNOSTIC TEST EFFECTS
None known.

SIDE EFFECTS
Occasional
Hypotension, drowsiness, headache, drug fever, paresthesia, rash, nausea, vomiting, anemia, arthralgia, weakness, tremor.

SERIOUS REACTIONS
• Nephrotoxicity (as evidenced by increased BUN and serum creatinine levels and decreased creatinine clearance) may be reversible if the drug is stopped at the first sign of nephrotoxic symptoms.
• Irreversible ototoxicity (manifested as tinnitus, dizziness, ringing or roaring in the ears, and impaired hearing) and neurotoxicity (as evidenced by headache, dizziness, lethargy, tremor, and visual disturbances) occur occasionally. Symptoms of ototoxicity, nephrotoxicity, and neuromuscular toxicity may occur.

PRECAUTIONS & CONSIDERATIONS
Caution is warranted in patients with tinnitus, vertigo, neuromuscular disorders, and renal impairment. Before giving streptomycin, determine whether hypersensitive to aminoglycosides, pregnant, or being treated for other medical conditions such as myasthenia gravis or parkinsonism. Hearing, renal function, and serum concentrations

of streptomycin should be monitored. If symptoms of hearing loss, dizziness, or fullness or roaring in the ears occur, notify the physician.
Administration
For IM use, inject streptomycin deep into a large muscle mass. Be aware that for patients who are unable to tolerate IM injections, streptomycin may be given as an IV infusion over 30-60 min. (Dilute desired dose in at least 100 mL NS).

Succimer
sux′sim-mer
(Chemet)

CATEGORY AND SCHEDULE
Pregnancy Risk Category: C

Classification: Antidotes, chelators

MECHANISM OF ACTION
An analogue of dimercaprol that forms water-soluble chelates with heavy metals, which are excreted renally. *Therapeutic Effect:* Treats lead intoxication in children.

PHARMACOKINETICS
Rapidly absorbed from the GI tract. Extensively metabolized. Excreted in feces (39%), urine (9%-25%), and lungs (1%). Removed by hemodialysis. *Half-life:* 2 h-2 days.

AVAILABILITY
Capsules: 100 mg (Chemet).

INDICATIONS AND DOSAGES
▸ **Lead poisoning, in pediatric patients with blood lead levels about 45 mcg/L**

PO
Children 12 mo and older. 10 mg/kg
q8h for 5 days, then 10 mg/kg q12h
for 14 days.

OFF-LABEL USES
Lead poisoning in adults, arsenic
intoxication, mercury intoxication.

CONTRAINDICATIONS
Hypersensitivity to succimer or any
component of its formulation.

INTERACTIONS
Drug
None known.
Herbal
None known.
Food
None known.

DIAGNOSTIC TEST EFFECTS
May decrease serum creatine
phophokinase and serum uric acid
measurements. May cause false-
positive results for urinary ketones
using nitroprusside reagents such as
Ketostix.

SIDE EFFECTS
Occasional
Anorexia, diarrhea, nausea,
vomiting, rash, odor to breath and
urine, increased liver function tests.
Rare
Neutropenia.

SERIOUS REACTIONS
• Elevated blood lead levels and
symptoms of intoxication may occur
after succimer therapy because of
redistribution of lead from bone to
soft tissues and blood.
• Elevated liver function tests have
been reported.

PRECAUTIONS & CONSIDERATIONS
It is unknown whether succimer is
distributed in breast milk. Safety

and efficacy of succimer complex
have not been established in children
younger than 12 mo. No age-related
precautions have noted in elderly
patients. Plasma lead levels should
be monitored and kept < 15 mcg/dL.

Sulfurous odor to breath and urine
may occur but will subside when
succimer is discontinued.
Administration
Keep in mind that succimer is not
a substitute for effective abatement
of lead exposure. Capsules may be
opened and contents sprinkled onto
soft food. Make sure all food is
eaten. Capsule contents may also be
placed on a spoon and followed by a
fruit drink.

Sucralfate
soo-kral′fate
(Apo-Sucralate [CAN], Carafate,
Novo-Sucralate [CAN], Ulcyte
[AUS])
**Do not confuse Carafate with
Cafergot.**

CATEGORY AND SCHEDULE
Pregnancy Risk Category: B

Classification: Cytoprotectives,
gastrointestinals

S

MECHANISM OF ACTION
An antiulcer agent that forms
an ulcer-adherent complex with
proteinaceous exudate, such as
albumin, at the ulcer site. Also
forms a viscous, adhesive barrier on
the surface of intact mucosa of the
stomach or duodenum. *Therapeutic
Effect:* Protects damaged mucosa
from further destruction by
absorbing gastric acid, pepsin, and
bile salts.

PHARMACOKINETICS

Minimally absorbed from the GI tract. Eliminated in feces, with small amount excreted in urine. Not removed by hemodialysis.

AVAILABILITY

Oral Suspension: 500 mg/5 mL.
Tablets: 1 g.

INDICATIONS AND DOSAGES

▸ **Active duodenal ulcers**
PO
Adults, Elderly. 1 g 4 times a day (before meals and at bedtime) for up to 8 wks.
▸ **Maintenance therapy after healing of acute duodenal ulcers**
PO
Adults, Elderly. 1 g twice a day.

OFF-LABEL USES

Prevention and treatment of stress-related mucosal damage, especially in acutely or critically ill patients; treatment of gastric ulcer and rheumatoid arthritis; relief of GI symptoms associated with NSAIDs; treatment of gastroesophageal reflux disease.

CONTRAINDICATIONS

None known.

INTERACTIONS

Drug
Antacids: May interfere with binding of sucralfate.
Digoxin, phenytoin, quinolones, such as ciprofloxacin, theophylline: May decrease the absorption of these drugs.
Herbal
None known.
Food
None known.

DIAGNOSTIC TEST EFFECTS

None known.

SIDE EFFECTS

Frequent (2%)
Constipation.
Occasional (< 2%)
Dry mouth, backache, diarrhea, dizziness, somnolence, nausea, indigestion, rash, hives, itching, abdominal discomfort.

SERIOUS REACTIONS

• None known.

PRECAUTIONS & CONSIDERATIONS

It is unknown whether sucralfate crosses the placenta or is distributed in breast milk. Safety and efficacy of sucralfate have not been established in children. No age-related precautions have been noted in elderly patients.

Dry mouth may occur, so take sips of tepid water or suck on sour hard candy to relieve it. Before sucralfate administration, the abdomen should be assessed for signs of tenderness, rigidity, and the presence of bowel sounds. Pattern of daily bowel activity and stool consistency should be monitored throughout therapy.
Administration
! 1 g equals 10 mL suspension.

Shake suspension well before each use.

Take 1 h before meals on an empty stomach and at bedtime. Tablets may be crushed or dissolved in water. Do not take antacids within 30 min of sucralfate. Do not take digoxin, phenytoin, quinolones, or theophylline within 2-3 h of sucralfate.

Sulfabenzamide/ Sulfacetamide/ Sulfathiazole

sul-fa-ben′za-mide/sul-fa-see′ta-mide/sul-fa-thye′a-zole
(V.V.S.)

CATEGORY AND SCHEDULE
Pregnancy Risk Category: C

Classification: Anti-infectives, topical, antibiotics, sulfonamides, dermatologics

MECHANISM OF ACTION
Interferes with synthesis of folic acid that bacteria require for growth by inhibition of para-aminobenzoic acid metabolism. *Therapeutic Effect:* Prevents further bacterial growth.

PHARMACOKINETICS
Absorption from vagina is variable and unreliable. Primarily metabolized by acetylation. Excreted in urine. *Half-life:* unknown.

AVAILABILITY
Vaginal Cream: 3.7% sulfabenzamide, 2.86% sulfacetamide, 3.42% sulfathiazole (V.V.S.).

INDICATIONS AND DOSAGES
▶ **Treatment of *Haemophilus vaginalis* vaginitis**
VAGINAL
Adults, Elderly. Insert one applicatorful into vagina twice daily for 4-6 days. Dosage may then be decreased to ¼-½ of an applicatorful twice daily.

CONTRAINDICATIONS
Renal dysfunction, pregnancy (or near term), hypersensitivity to sulfabenzamide, sulfacetamide, sulfathiazole or any component of preparation.

INTERACTIONS
Drug
None known.
Herbal
None known.
Food
None known.

DIAGNOSTIC TEST EFFECTS
None known.

SIDE EFFECTS
Occasional
Local irritation.
Rare
Pruritus urticaria, allergic reactions.

SERIOUS REACTIONS
• Superinfection and Stevens-Johnson syndrome occur rarely.

PRECAUTIONS & CONSIDERATIONS
Be aware that sulfabenzamide, sulfacetamide, sulfathiazole has been associated with Stevens-Johnson syndrome, and therapy should be discontinued if local irritation occurs. It is unknown whether sulfabenzamide, sulfacetamide, or sulfathiazole crosses the placenta or is distributed in breast milk. Do not use sulfabenzamide, sulfacetamide, or sulfathiazole in patients during the third trimester of pregnancy. Safety and efficacy of sulfabenzamide, sulfacetamide, and sulfathiazole have not been established in children. No age-related precautions have been noted in elderly patients.
Administration
Cream is for intravaginal use only. Complete full course of therapy.

S

Sulfacetamide

sul-fa-see'ta-mide
(AK-Sulf, Bleph-10, Isopto
Cetamide, Diosulf [CAN],
Ophthacet, Sodium Sulamyd,
Sulfair)

CATEGORY AND SCHEDULE

Pregnancy Risk Category: C

Classification: Anti-infectives,
ophthalmics, antibiotics,
sulfonamides

MECHANISM OF ACTION

Interferes with synthesis of folic
acid that bacteria require for growth.
Therapeutic Effect: Prevents further
bacterial growth. Bacteriostatic.

PHARMACOKINETICS

Small amounts may be absorbed into
the cornea. Excreted rapidly in urine.
Half-life: 7-13 h.

AVAILABILITY

Lotion: 10% (Carmol, Klaron,
Ovace).
Ophthalmic Ointment: 10%
(AK-Sulf).
Ophthalmic Solution: 10%
(Bleph-10, Ocusulf, Sulf-10).

INDICATIONS AND DOSAGES

▸ **Treatment of corneal ulcers,
conjunctivitis, and other superficial
infections of the eye, prophylaxis
after injuries to the eye/removal
of foreign bodies, adjunctive
therapy for trachoma and inclusion
conjunctivitis**
OPHTHALMIC
Adults, Elderly. Ointment: Apply
small amount in lower conjunctival
sac 1-4 times/day and at bedtime.

Solution: 1-3 drops to lower
conjunctival sac q2-3h.
▸ **Seborrheic dermatitis, seborrheic
sicca (dandruff), secondary bacterial
skin infections**
TOPICAL
Adults, Elderly. Apply 1-4 times/day.

OFF-LABEL USES

Treatment of bacterial blepharitis,
blepharoconjunctivitis, bacterial
keratitis, keratoconjunctivitis.

CONTRAINDICATIONS

Hypersensitivity to sulfonamides or
any component of preparation (some
products contain sulfite), use in
combination with silver-containing
products.

INTERACTIONS

Drug
Silver-containing preparations:
These products are incompatible
together.
Herbal
None known.
Food
None known.

DIAGNOSTIC TEST EFFECTS

None known.

SIDE EFFECTS

Frequent
Transient ophthalmic burning,
stinging.
Occasional
Headache.
Rare
Hypersensitivity (erythema, rash,
itching, swelling, photosensitivity).

SERIOUS REACTIONS

• Superinfection, drug-induced
lupus erythematosus, Stevens-
Johnson syndrome occur
rarely; nephrotoxicity with high
dermatologic concentrations.

PRECAUTIONS & CONSIDERATIONS

Caution should be used with extremely dry eye. It is unknown if whether sulfacetamide crosses the placenta or is distributed in breast milk. Do not use sulfacetamide during the third trimester of pregnancy. Safety and efficacy of sulfacetamide have not been established in children. No age-related precautions have been noted in elderly patients. Be aware that sulfacetamide application of lotion to large infected, denuded, or debrided areas should be avoided.

Eyedrops may burn upon instillation. Eye ointment will cause blurred vision.

Sulfacetamide may cause sensitivity to light. Sunglasses should be worn and avoid bright light.

Storage

Store at room temperature and protect from light. Discolored solution should not be used. Discard Sulfacet-R lotion after 4 mo.

Administration

For ophthalmic use, tilt the head back. Place solution in conjunctival sac. Close eyes, and then press gently on the lacrimal sac for 1 min. Wait at least 10 min before using another eye preparation.

For topical treatment, cleanse area before application to ensure direct contact with affected area. Apply at bedtime and allow to remain overnight.

Sulfasalazine

sul-fa-sal′a-zeen
(Alti-Sulfasalazine [CAN],
Azulfidine, Azulfidine EN-tabs,
Pyralin EN [AUS], Salazopyrin
[CAN], Salazopyrin EN [AUS],
Salazopyrin EN-Tabs [CAN])
Do not confuse Azulfidine with azathioprine, sulfasalazine with sulfadiazine, or sulfisoxazole.

CATEGORY AND SCHEDULE

Pregnancy Risk Category: B (D if given near term)

Classification:

Disease-modifying antirheumatic drugs, gastrointestinals, 5-aminosalicylates

MECHANISM OF ACTION

A sulfonamide that inhibits prostaglandin synthesis, acting locally in the colon. *Therapeutic Effect:* Decreases inflammatory response, interferes with GI secretion.

PHARMACOKINETICS

Poorly absorbed from the GI tract. Cleaved in colon by intestinal bacteria, forming sulfapyridine and mesalamine (5-ASA). Absorbed in colon. Widely distributed. Metabolized in the liver. Primarily excreted in urine. *Half-life:* sulfapyridine, 6-14 h; 5-ASA, 0.6-1.4 h.

AVAILABILITY

Tablets (Azulfidine): 500 mg.
Tablets (Delayed-Release [Azulfidine EN-Tabs]): 500 mg.

INDICATIONS AND DOSAGES
▸ **Ulcerative colitis**
PO
Adults, Elderly. 1 g 3-4 times a day in divided doses q6-8h.

S

Maintenance: 2 g/day in divided doses q6-12h. Maximum: 4 g/day.
Children. 40-60 mg/kg/day in divided doses q4-6h. Maintenance: 30 mg/kg/day in divided doses q6h. Maximum: 2 g/day.

▸ **Rheumatoid arthritis**
PO
Adults, Elderly. Initially, 0.5-1 g/day for 1 wk. Increase by 0.5 g/wk, up to 2 g/day.

▸ **Juvenile rheumatoid arthritis**
PO
Children > 6 yr. Initially, 10 mg/kg/day. May increase by 10 mg/kg/day at weekly intervals. Range: 30-50 mg/kg/day. Maximum: 2 g/day.

OFF-LABEL USES
Treatment of ankylosing spondylitis.

CONTRAINDICATIONS
Intestinal or urinary obstruction; porphyria; hypersensitivity to sulfasalazine, its metabolites, other 5-aminosalicylates, sulfonamides, or salicylates.

INTERACTIONS
Drug
Anticonvulsants, methotrexate, oral anticoagulants, oral antidiabetics: May increase the effects of these drugs.
Hemolytics: May increase the toxicity of sulfasalazine.
Hepatotoxic medications: May increase the risk of hepatotoxicity.
Thioguanince or 6-marcaptopurine: 5-Aminosalicylates may increase sensitivity to myelosuppressive effects.
Herbal
None known.
Food
None known.

DIAGNOSTIC TEST EFFECTS
None known.

SIDE EFFECTS
Frequent (33%)
Anorexia, nausea, vomiting, headache, oligospermia (generally reversed by withdrawal of drug).
Occasional (3%)
Hypersensitivity reaction (rash, urticaria, pruritus, fever, anemia).
Rare (< 1%)
Tinnitus, hypoglycemia, diuresis, photosensitivity.

SERIOUS REACTIONS
• Anaphylaxis, Stevens-Johnson syndrome, hematologic toxicity (leukopenia, agranulocytosis), hepatotoxicity, and nephrotoxicity occur rarely.

PRECAUTIONS & CONSIDERATIONS
Caution is warranted with bronchial asthma, G6PD deficiency, impaired hepatic or renal function, or severe allergies. Sulfasalazine may produce infertility and oligospermia in men. Sulfasalazine readily crosses the placenta and is excreted in breast milk. Lactating patients should not breastfeed premature infants or those with hyperbilirubinemia or G6PD deficiency. If given near term, sulfasalazine may produce hemolytic anemia, jaundice, and kernicterus in the newborn. No age-related precautions have been noted in children older than 2 yr or elderly patients. Avoid the sun and ultraviolet light; photosensitivity may last for months after the last dose of sulfasalazine.

Adequate hydration should be maintained (minimum output 1500 mL/24 h) and to prevent nephrotoxicity. Skin should be examined for rash; withhold the drug at the first sign of a rash. Pattern of daily bowel activity and stool consistency should be monitored; drug dosage may need to be increased if diarrhea continues or recurs. Report hematologic effects such as bleeding, ecchymosis, fever, jaundice, pallor, purpura, pharyngitis, and weakness.

Administration

Space drug doses evenly at intervals not to exceed 8 h. Administer sulfasalazine after meals, if possible, to prolong intestinal passage. Swallow delayed-release tablets whole without chewing or crushing them. Take the drug with 8 oz of water.

Sulfinpyrazone

sul-fin-pyr′a-zone

(Anturane, Apo-Sulfinpyrazone [CAN], Nu-Sufinpyrazone [CAN])

Do not confuse with Accutane.

CATEGORY AND SCHEDULE

Pregnancy Risk Category: C/D (near term)

Classification: Uricosurics

MECHANISM OF ACTION

A uricosuric that increases urinary excretion of uric acid, thereby decreasing blood urate levels. *Therapeutic Effect:* Promotes uric acid excretion and reduces serum uric acid levels.

PHARMACOKINETICS

Rapidly and completely absorbed from the GI tract. Widely distributed. Metabolized in liver to two active metabolites, *p*-hydroxy-sulfinpyrazone and a sulfide analogue. Excreted primarily in urine. Not removed by hemodialysis. *Half-life:* 2.7-6 h.

AVAILABILITY

Tablets: 100 mg (Anturane).

INDICATIONS AND DOSAGES

▸ **Gout**

PO

Adults, Elderly. 100-200 mg 2 times/day. Maximum: 800 mg/day.

OFF-LABEL USES

Mitral valve replacement, myocardial infarction.

CONTRAINDICATIONS

Active peptic ulcer, blood dyscrasias, GI inflammation, pregnancy (near term), hypersensitivity to sulfinpyrazone, phenylbutazone, other pyrazoles, or any of its components.

INTERACTIONS

Drug

Acetaminophen: May increase risk of heptotoxicity and decrease effect of sulfinpyrazone.

Aspirin: May decrease uricosuric effect.

Oral anticoagulants: May increase anticoagulant effect.

Oral hypoglycemics: May increase hypoglycemic effect.

Salicylates, niacin: May decrease uricosuric activity.

Theophylline, verapamil: May decrease effects and levels of theophylline and verapamil.

Herbal

Arnica, astragalus, bilberry, black currant, cat's claw, chaparral, chondroitin, clove oil, evening primrose, feverfew, ginger, Ginkgo biloba, hawthorn, kava kava, skullcap, tan-shen: May increase risk of bleeding.

Dong quai, St. John's wort: May increase risk of photosensitization.

Food

Rhubarb: May increase risk of bleeding.

S

DIAGNOSTIC TEST EFFECTS
May alter serum uric acid levels.

SIDE EFFECTS
Frequent
Nausea, vomiting, stomach pain.
Occasional
Flushed face, headache, dizziness, frequent urge to urinate, rash.
Rare
Increased bleeding time, hepatic necrosis, nephrotic syndrome, uric acid stones.

SERIOUS REACTIONS
• Hematologic toxicity, including anemia, leukopenia, agranulocytosis, thrombocytopenia, and aplastic anemia, occur rarely.
• Overdose causes a drowsiness, dizziness, anorexia, abdominal pain, hemolytic anemia, acidosis, jaundice, fever, and agranulocytosis.

PRECAUTIONS & CONSIDERATIONS
Caution is necessary in patients with urolithiasis. It is unknown whether sulfinpyrazone crosses the placenta or is distributed in breast milk. Safety and efficacy of sulfinpyrazone have not been established in children older than 18 yr. Age-related renal impairment may increase risk of toxicity in elderly patients. Avoid citrate containing products as well as use of aspirin or aspirin-containing products.
Administration
Do not use in the presence of renal impairment. Give sulfinpyrazone with meals or milk to decrease GI irritation. Drink at least 8-10 glasses (8 oz) of water each day to prevent renal stone development.

Sulfisoxazole
sul-fi-sox′a-zole
Gantrisin, Novo-Soxazole [CAN], Sulfizole [CAN], Truxazole)
Do not confuse with sulfadiazine, sulfamethoxazole, sulfasalazine, or Gastrosed.

CATEGORY AND SCHEDULE
Pregnancy risk category: B/D (near term)

Classification: Antibiotics, sulfonamides

MECHANISM OF ACTION
An antibacterial sulphonamide that inhibits bacterial synthesis of dihydrofolic acid by preventing condensation of pteridine with aminobenzoic acid through competitive inhibition of the enzyme dihydropteroate synthetase. *Therapeutic Effect:* Bacteriostatic.

PHARMACOKINETICS
Rapidly and completely absorbed. Small intestine is major site of absorption, but some absorption occurs in the stomach. Exists in the blood as unbound, protein-bound and conjugated forms. Sulfisoxazole is metabolized primarily by acetylation and oxidation in the liver. The free form is considered the therapeutically active form. Protein binding: 85%-88%. *Half-life:* 4-7 h.

AVAILABILITY
Tablet: 500 mg. Suspension: 500 mg/5 mL (Gantrisin).

INDICATIONS AND DOSAGES
▸ **Acute, recurrent or chronic urinary tract infections, meningococcal meningitis, acute otitis media due to** *Haemophilus influenzae*

PO
Infants older than 2 mo, Children.
75 mg/kg or 2 g/m^2 initially, followed
by 150 mg/kg daily or 4 g/m^2 daily
for maintenance divided q4-6h.
Maximum dose: 6 g daily.
Adults. 2-4 g initially, then 4-8 g daily
divided q4-6h. Maximum:12 g/day.

CONTRAINDICATIONS

Patients with a known
hypersensitivity to sulfonamides,
children younger than 2 mo (except
in the treatment of congenital
toxoplasmosis as adjunctive therapy
with pyrimethamine), pregnant
women at term, and mothers nursing
infants younger than 2 mo.

INTERACTIONS

Drug
Methotrexate: May increase free
methotrexate concentrations.
Sulfonylureas: May increase
hypoglycemic effect of sulfonylureas.
Thiopental: May increase effect of
thiopental.
Warfarin: May prolong prothrombin
time.
Herbal
Dong quai, St. John's wort: May
cause photosensitization.
Food
Folate: May decrease folate
absorption.

DIAGNOSTIC TEST EFFECTS

May cause false-positive for protein
in urine and urine glucose with
Clinitest.

SIDE EFFECTS

Anaphylaxis, erythema multiforme
(Stevens-Johnson syndrome),
toxic epidermal necrolysis,
exfoliative dermatitis, angioedema,
arteritis and vasculitis, allergic
myocarditis, serum sickness, rash,
urticaria, pruritus, photosensitivity,
conjunctival and scleral injection,
generalized allergic reactions,
generalized skin eruptions,
tachycardia, palpitations, syncope,
cyanosis, goiter, diuresis,
hypoglycemia, arthralgia, myalgia,
headache, dizziness, peripheral
neuritis, paresthesia, convulsions,
tinnitus, vertigo, ataxia, intracranial
hypertension, cough, shortness of
breath, pulmonary infiltrates.

SERIOUS REACTIONS

• Fatalities associated with the
administration of sulfonamides,
including Stevens-Johnson
syndrome, toxic epidermal
necrolysis, fulminant hepatic
necrosis, agranulocytosis, aplastic
anemia, and other blood dyscrasias
occur rarely.
• Clinical signs such as rash, sore
throat, fever, arthralgia, pallor,
purpura, or jaundice may be early
indications of serious reactions.

PRECAUTIONS & CONSIDERATIONS

Caution is necessary with G6PD
deficiency and liver or kidney
disease. Avoid prolonged exposure
to sunlight. Sunscreen and protective
clothing should be worn if sunlight
is not avoidable. Be aware that it
is unknown whether sulfisoxazole
crosses the placenta. Sulfisoxazole
enters the breast milk. No age-
related precautions have been noted
in children or elderly patients.
Alcohol should be avoided. If rash,
hives, itching, shortness of breath,
wheezing, cough, or swelling of face,
lips, tongue, and throat occurs, notify
physician.
Administration
Take with or without food and with a
full glass of water. Take with food if
GI upset occurs. Administer around
the clock to promote less variation in
peak and trough levels.

S

Sulindac
sul-in'dak
(Aclin [AUS], Apo-Sulin [CAN],
Clinoril, Novo Sundac [CAN])
**Do not confuse Clinoril with
Clozaril.**

CATEGORY AND SCHEDULE
Pregnancy Risk Category: C
(D if used in third trimester or
near delivery)

Classification: Analgesics,
non-narcotic, nonsteroidal
anti-inflammatory drugs (NSAID)

MECHANISM OF ACTION
An NSAID that produces analgesic
and anti-inflammatory effects by
inhibiting prostaglandin synthesis.
Therapeutic Effect: Reduces
inflammatory response and intensity
of pain.

PHARMACOKINETICS

Route	Onset	Peak	Duration
PO (antirheu-matic)	7 days	2-3 wks	NA

Well absorbed from the GI tract.
Metabolized in liver to active
metabolite. Primarily excreted in
urine. Not removed by hemodialysis.
Half-life: 7.8 h; metabolite: 16.4 h.

AVAILABILITY
Tablets: 150 mg, 200 mg.

INDICATIONS AND DOSAGES
▸ **Rheumatoid arthritis, osteoarthritis,
ankylosing spondylitis**
PO
Adults, Elderly. Initially, 150 mg
twice a day; may increase up to
maximum 400 mg/day.

▸ **Acute shoulder pain, gouty
arthritis, bursitis, tendinitis**
PO
Adults, Elderly. 200 mg twice a day.
Usually 7-14 days.

CONTRAINDICATIONS
Active peptic ulcer disease,
chronic inflammation of GI tract,
GI bleeding or ulceration, history
of hypersensitivity to aspirin or
NSAIDs.

INTERACTIONS
Drug
Antacids: May decrease the sulindac
blood concentration.
Antihypertensives, diuretics:
May decrease the effects of these
drugs.
Aspirin, other salicylates:
May increase the risk of GI
side effects such as
bleeding.
Bone marrow depressants: May
increase the risk of hematologic
reactions.
**Heparin, oral anticoagulants,
thrombolytics:** May increase the
effects of these drugs.
Lithium: May increase the blood
concentration and risk of toxicity of
lithium.
Methotrexate: May increase the risk
of methotrexate toxicity.
Probenecid: May increase the
sulindac blood concentration.
Herbal
Feverfew: May decrease the effects
of feverfew.
Ginkgo biloba: May increase the
risk of bleeding.
Food
None known.

DIAGNOSTIC TEST EFFECTS
May increase liver function
test results and serum alkaline
phosphatase level.

SIDE EFFECTS
Frequent (4%-9%)
Diarrhea or constipation, indigestion, nausea, maculopapular rash, dermatitis, dizziness, headache.
Occasional (1%-3%)
Anorexia, abdominal cramps, flatulence.

SERIOUS REACTIONS
• Rare reactions with long-term use include peptic ulcer disease, GI bleeding, gastritis, nephrotoxicity (glomerular nephritis, interstitial nephritis, nephrotic syndrome), severe hepatic reactions (cholestasis, jaundice), and severe hypersensitivity reactions (fever, chills, and joint pain).
WARNINGS
Use in perioperative pain for CABG surgery is contraindicated. NSAIDs may increase risk of GI irritation, inflammation, ulceration, bleeding, and perforation.

PRECAUTIONS & CONSIDERATIONS
Caution is warranted in patients with a history of GI tract disease, hepatic or renal impairment, a predisposition to fluid retention, and concurrent use of anticoagulant therapy. It is unknown whether sulindac is excreted in breast milk. Sulindac should not be used during the third trimester of pregnancy because it might cause adverse effects in the fetus, such as premature closure of the ductus arteriosus. The safety and efficacy of naproxen have not been established in children. In elderly patients, GI bleeding or ulceration is more likely to cause serious complications, and age-related renal impairment may increase the risk of hepatotoxicity and renal toxicity; a reduced drug dosage is recommended. Avoid alcohol and aspirin during therapy because these substances increase the risk of GI bleeding. Tasks that require mental alertness or motor skills should also be avoided.

CBC, especially platelet count, skin for rash, and liver and renal function test results should be assessed before and periodically during therapy. Therapeutic response, such as decreased pain, stiffness, swelling, and tenderness, improved grip strength, and increased joint mobility, should be evaluated.
Administration
Take sulindac orally with food, milk, or antacids if GI distress occurs. Sulindac's therapeutic antiarthritic effect will occur 1-3 wks after therapy begins.

Sumatriptan
soo-ma-trip′tan
(Imigran [AUS], Imitrex, Suvalan [AUS])
Do not confuse sumatriptan with somatropin.

CATEGORY AND SCHEDULE
Pregnancy Risk Category: C

Classification: Serotonin receptor agonists

S

MECHANISM OF ACTION
A serotonin receptor agonist that binds selectively to vascular receptors, producing a vasoconstrictive effect on cranial blood vessels. *Therapeutic Effect:* Relieves migraine headache.

PHARMACOKINETICS

Route	Onset (min)	Peak (h)	Duration (h)
Nasal	15	NA	24-48
PO	30	2	24-48
SC	10	1	24-48

Rapidly absorbed after SC administration. Absorption after PO administration is incomplete, with significant amounts undergoing hepatic metabolism, resulting in low bioavailability (about 14%). Protein binding: 10%-21%. Widely distributed. Undergoes first-pass metabolism in the liver. Excreted in urine. *Half-life:* 2 h.

AVAILABILITY

Tablets: 25 mg, 50 mg, 100 mg.
Injection: 6 mg/0.5 mL.
Nasal Spray: 5 mg, 20 mg.

INDICATIONS AND DOSAGES
▸ **Acute migraine attack**
PO
Adults, Elderly. 25-100 mg. Dose may be repeated after at least 2 h. Maximum: 100 mg/single dose; 200 mg/24 h.
SC
Adults, Elderly. 6 mg. Maximum: Two 6-mg injections/24 h (separated by at least 1 h).
INTRANASAL
Adults, Elderly. 5 or 10 mg (1 or 2 sprays) into 1 nostril as a single dose or 20 mg into 1 nostril as a single dose. Maximum: 40 mg/24 h.

CONTRAINDICATIONS
Cerebrovascular accident, ischemic heart disease (including angina pectoris, history of myocardial infarction (MI), silent ischemia, and Prinzmetal's angina), severe hepatic impairment, transient ischemic attack, uncontrolled hypertension, use within 14 days of MAOIs, use within 24 h of ergotamine preparations.

INTERACTIONS
Drug
Ergotamine-containing medications: May produce vasospastic reaction.

MAOIs: May increase sumatriptan blood concentration and half-life.
Serotonin agonists, SSRI, or SNRI antidepressants: May increase risk of serotonin syndrome.
Herbal
St. John's wort: May increase serotonergic effects.
Food
None known.

DIAGNOSTIC TEST EFFECTS
None known.

SIDE EFFECTS
Frequent
Oral (5%-10%): Tingling, nasal discomfort.
SC (> 10%): Injection site reactions, tingling, warm or hot sensation, dizziness, vertigo.
Nasal (> 10%): Bad or unusual taste, nausea, vomiting.
Occasional
Oral (1%-5%): Flushing, asthenia, visual disturbances.
Subcutaneous (2%-10%): Burning sensation, numbness, chest discomfort, drowsiness, asthenia.
Nasal (1%-5%): Nasopharyngeal discomfort, dizziness.
Rare
Oral (< 1%): Agitation, eye irritation, dysuria.
Subcutaneous (< 2%): Anxiety, fatigue, diaphoresis, muscle cramps, myalgia.
Nasal (< 1%): Burning sensation.

SERIOUS REACTIONS
• Excessive dosage may produce tremor, red extremities, reduced respirations, cyanosis, seizures, and paralysis.
• Serious arrhythmias occur rarely, especially in patients with hypertension, diabetes, or a strong family history of coronary artery disease; obese patients; and smokers.

PRECAUTIONS & CONSIDERATIONS

Caution is warranted in patients with epilepsy, a hypersensitivity to sumatriptan, and hepatic or renal impairment. It is unknown whether sumatriptan is distributed in breast milk. The safety and efficacy of sumatriptan have not been established in children. No age-related precautions have been noted in elderly patients.

Dizziness may occur. Notify the physician immediately if palpitations, a rash, wheezing, pain or tightness in the chest or throat, or facial edema occurs. ECG should be obtained at baseline. Migraines and associated symptoms, including nausea and vomiting, photophobia, and phonophobia (sound sensitivity), should be assessed before and during treatment.

Administration

Swallow oral tablets whole with a full glass of water.

Expect to administer first SC dosage in physician's office if patient has identifiable cardiovascular risk factors. Never give intravenously because this drug may precipitate coronary vasospasm.

Patients using autoinjector should be thoroughly instructed in autoinjection technique.

For SC use, follow the manufacturer's instructions for using the autoinjection device. Inject the drug into an area with adequate SC tissue because the needle will penetrate the skin and adipose tissue as deeply as 6 mm. Do not administer more than two SC injections during any 24-h period and allow at least 1 h between injections. After injecting the medication, discard the syringe.

For nasal use, each unit contains only one spray, so do not test the spray before use. Blow the nose gently to clear nasal passages. With the head upright, close one of the nostrils with an index finger and breathe gently through the mouth. Insert the nozzle about 1/2 in. into the open nostril. Close mouth, then breathe through the nose while depressing the blue plunger and releasing the spray. Remove the nozzle from the nose, and gently breathe in through the nose and out through the mouth for 10-20 s. Do not breathe in deeply.

S

Tacrine
Tacrine
tack'rin
(Cognex)

CATEGORY AND SCHEDULE
Pregnancy Risk Category: C

Classification: Cholinesterase inhibitors

MECHANISM OF ACTION
A cholinesterase inhibitor that inhibits the enzyme acetylcholinesterase, thus increasing the concentration of acetylcholine at cholinergic synap ses and enhancing cholinergic function in the central nervous system (CNS). *Therapeutic Effect:* Slows the progression of Alzheimer disease.

PHARMACOKINETICS
Rapid oral absorption. Protein binding: 55%. Extensively metabolized in the liver. *Half-Life:* 24-36 h.

AVAILABILITY
Capsules: 10 mg, 20 mg, 30 mg, 40 mg.

INDICATIONS AND DOSAGES
▶ **Alzheimer disease**
PO
Adults, Elderly. Initially, 10 mg 4 times a day for 4 wks, followed by 20 mg 4 times a day for 4 wks, 30 mg 4 times a day for 4 wks, then 40 mg 4 times a day if needed.
▶ **Dosage in hepatic impairment**
For patients with transaminase levels > 3-5 times normal, decrease the dose by 40 mg/day and resume the normal dose when transaminase levels returns to normal. For patients with transaminase levels > 5 times normal, stop treatment and resume it when transaminare levels returns to normal.

CONTRAINDICATIONS
Active, severe hepatic disease; active and untreated duodenal or gastric ulcers; breastfeeding women; concurrent use of other cholinesterase inhibitors; hypersensitivity to cholinergics; mechanical obstruction of intestine or urinary tract; pregnancy; women with childbearing potential.

INTERACTIONS
Drug
Anticholinergics: May decrease the effects of tacrine or anticholinergics.
Azole antifungals, cimetidine, fluvoxamine, quinalone antibiotics: May increase the tacrine blood concentration.
β-Blockers: May produce additive bradycardia.
Carbamazepine, cigarette smoking, phenobarbital, rifampin: May decrease the effects of tacrine.
NSAIDs: May increase the adverse effects of NSAIDs.
Theophylline: May increase the theophylline blood concentration.
Herbal
None known.
Food
Food: May decrease absorption.

DIAGNOSTIC TEST EFFECTS
Increases AST (SGOT) and ALT (SGPT) levels. Alters blood hemoglobin, hematocrit, and serum electrolyte levels.

SIDE EFFECTS
Frequent (11%-28%)
Headache, nausea, vomiting, diarrhea, dizziness.
Occasional (4%-9%)
Fatigue, chest pain, dyspepsia, anorexia, abdominal pain, flatulence,

constipation, confusion, agitation, rash, depression, ataxia, insomnia, rhinitis, myalgia.
Rare (< 3%)
Weight loss, anxiety, cough, facial flushing, urinary frequency, back pain, tremor.

SERIOUS REACTIONS
• Overdose can cause cholinergic crisis, marked by increased salivation, lacrimation, bradycardia, respiratory depression, hypotension, and increased muscle weakness. Treatment usually consists of supportive measures and an anticholinergic such as atropine.

PRECAUTIONS & CONSIDERATIONS
Caution is warranted in patients with alcohol abuse, asthma, bradycardia, cardiac arrhythmias, chronic obstructive pulmonary disease (COPD), peptic ulcer disease, hyperthyroidism, hepatic dysfunction, and a history of seizures. Be aware that tacrine is not a cure for Alzheimer disease but may slow the progression of its symptoms. Smoking should be avoided because it reduces the drug's blood level. Liver function tests should be monitored every other week beginning 4 wks after the initiation of treatment and continuing for at least the first 16 wks, then once every 3 mo. ECG and rhythm strips should be periodically monitored. Patients with jaundice confirmed by elevated total bilirubin should not be rechallenged with tacrine.
Administration
! If tacrine therapy is stopped for longer than 14 days, reinstitute therapy as prescribed.

Take tacrine at regular intervals, 1 h before or 2 h after meals on an empty stomach. Take with food if GI upset occurs. Do not abruptly discontinue or adjust the dosage of tacrine.

Tacrolimus
tak-roe-leem'us
(Prograf, Protopic)
Do not confuse Protopic with Protonix, Protopam, Protopin.

CATEGORY AND SCHEDULE
Pregnancy Risk Category: C

Classification: Dermatologics, immunosuppressives

MECHANISM OF ACTION
An immunologic agent that inhibits T-lymphocyte activation by binding to intracellular proteins, forming a complex, and inhibiting phosphatase activity. *Therapeutic Effect:* Suppresses the immunologically mediated inflammatory response; prevents organ transplant rejection.

Pharmacokinetics
Variably absorbed after PO administration (food reduces absorption). Protein binding: 75%-97%. Extensively metabolized in the liver. Excreted in urine. Not removed by hemodialysis. *Half-life:* 11.7 h.

AVAILABILITY
Capsules (Prograf): 0.5 mg, 1 mg, 5 mg.
Injection (Prograf): 5 mg/mL.
Ointment (Protopic): 0.03%, 0.1%.

INDICATIONS AND DOSAGES
▸ **Prevention of liver transplant rejection**
PO
Adults, Elderly. 0.1-0.15 mg/kg/day in 2 divided doses 12 h apart.

Children. 0.15-0.2 mg/kg/day in
2 divided doses 12 h apart.
IV
Adults, Elderly, Children.
0.03-0.05 mg/kg/day as a continuous
infusion.
▸ **Prevention of kidney transplant
rejection**
PO
Adults, Elderly. 0.2 mg/kg/day in
2 divided doses 12 h apart.
IV
Adults, Elderly. 0.03-0.05 mg/kg/day
as continuous infusion.
▸ **Atopic dermatitis**
TOPICAL
Adults, Elderly, Children 2 yr and older.
Apply 0.03% ointment to affected area
twice a day; 0.1% ointment may be
used in adolescents >15 yr, adults, and
elderly patients. Continue until 1 wk
after symptoms have cleared.

OFF-LABEL USES
Prevention of organ rejection in
patients receiving allogeneic bone
marrow, heart, pancreas, pancreatic
island cell, or small-bowel
transplant; treatment of autoimmune
disease; severe recalcitrant
psoriasis.

CONTRAINDICATIONS
Concurrent use with cyclosporine
(increases the risk of nephrotoxicity),
hypersensitivity to HCO-60
polyoxyl 60 hydrogenated castor
oil (used in solution for injection),
hypersensitivity to tacrolimus.

INTERACTIONS
Drug
**Aminoglycosides, amphotericin B,
cisplatin:** Increase the risk of renal
dysfunction.
Antacids: Decrease the absorption
of tacrolimus.
**Antifungals, bromocriptine,
calcium channel blockers,**
cimetidine, clarithromycin,
cyclosporine, danazol, diltiazem,
erythromycin, methylprednisolone,
metoclopramide, voriconazole:
Increase tacrolimus blood
concentration.
**Carbamazepine, phenobarbital,
phenytoin, rifamycin:** Decrease
tacrolimus blood concentration.
Cyclosporine: Increases the risk of
nephrotoxicity.
Live-virus vaccines: May potentiate
virus replication, increase vaccine
side effects, and decrease the
patient's antibody response to the
vaccine.
Other immunosuppressants: May
increase the risk of infection or
lymphomas.
Herbal
St. John's wort, echinacea: May
decrease the effects of tacrolimus.
Food
Grapefruit, grapefruit juice: May
alter the effects of the drug.
High-fat food: May decrease the
absorption.

DIAGNOSTIC TEST EFFECTS
May increase blood glucose, BUN,
and serum creatinine levels, as well
as WBC count. May decrease serum
magnesium level and RBC and
thrombocyte counts. May alter serum
potassium level.

ⓘ IV INCOMPATIBILITIES
Do not mix tacrolimus with other
medications if possible.

⚑ IV COMPATIBILITIES
Calcium gluconate, dexamethasone
(Decadron), diphenhydramine
(Benadryl), dobutamine (Dobutrex),
dopamine (Intropin), furosemide
(Lasix), heparin, hydromorphone
(Dilaudid), insulin, leucovorin,
lorazepam (Ativan), morphine,
nitroglycerin, potassium chloride.

SIDE EFFECTS

Frequent (> 30%)
Headache, tremor, insomnia, paresthesia, diarrhea, nausea, constipation, vomiting, abdominal pain, hypertension.
Occasional (10%-29%)
Rash, pruritus, anorexia, asthenia, peripheral edema, photosensitivity.

SERIOUS REACTIONS

• Nephrotoxicity (characterized by increased serum creatinine level and decreased urine output), neurotoxicity (including tremor, headache, and mental status changes), and pleural effusion are common adverse reactions.
• Thrombocytopenia, leukocytosis, anemia, atelectasis, sepsis, and infection occur occasionally.
Warnings
Increased suspectibility to infection and the possible development of lymphoma may occur after administration of tacrolimus. Because topical calcineurin inhibitors have been associated with rare cases of malignancy, they should be used only for short-term and intermittent treatment to control symptoms. The use of Protopic is not recommended in children younger than 2 yr.

PRECAUTIONS & CONSIDERATIONS

Caution is warranted in patients with immunosuppression and hepatic or renal impairment. Tacrolimus crosses the placenta and is distributed in breast milk. Women taking this drug should not breastfeed. Hyperkalemia and renal dysfunction have been noted in neonates. Children may require a higher dosage because of decreased bioavailability and increased clearance of the drug. Post-transplant lymphoproliferative disorder is more common in children, especially children younger than 3 yr. Age-related renal impairment may require a dosage adjustment in elderly patients. Avoid crowds and people with infection. Also avoid exposure to sunlight and artificial light because these may cause a photosensitivity reaction.

Notify the physician of change in mental status, chest pain, dizziness, headache, decreased urination, rash, respiratory infection, or unusual bleeding or bruising. CBC should be monitored weekly during the first month of therapy, twice monthly during the second and third months of treatment, then monthly for the rest of the first year. Liver function test results and serum creatinine and potassium levels should also be assessed.
Storage
Store the diluted solution in a glass or polyethylene containers and discard after 24 h. Do not store it in a polyvinyl chloride container because the container may absorb the drug or affect its stability.
Administration
! If unable to take capsules, initiate therapy with IV infusion. Give oral dose 8-12 h after discontinuing IV infusion. Titrate dosage based on clinical assessments of rejection and tolerance. With hepatic or renal impairment, give the lowest IV and oral doses, as prescribed. Plan to delay administration for 48 h or longer with postoperative oliguria.

Take oral tacrolimus on an empty stomach at the same time each day. If GI intolerance occurs, be consistent with taking oral tacrolimus with regard to timing and type of meal. Notify the physician if a dose is missed. Do not give this drug with grapefruit or grapefruit juice or within 2 h of antacids.

T

Keep oxygen and an aqueous solution of epinephrine 1:1000 available at the bedside before beginning the IV infusion. Dilute the drug with 250-1000 mL 0.9% NaCl or D5W, depending on the desired dose, to provide a concentration of 4-20 mcg/mL. Administer tacrolimus as a continuous IV infusion. Monitor continuously for the first 30 min of the infusion and at frequent intervals thereafter. Stop the infusion immediately at the first sign of a hypersensitivity reaction.

Tacrolimus ointment is for external use only. Rub the ointment gently and completely into clean, dry skin. Do not cover the treated area with an occlusive dressing.

Tadalafil
(Cialis)

CATEGORY AND SCHEDULE
Pregnancy Risk Category: B

Classification:
Phosphodiesterase-5 enzyme inhibitors

MECHANISM OF ACTION
An erectile dysfunction agent that inhibits phosphodiesterase type 5, the enzyme responsible for degrading cyclic guanosine monophosphate in the corpus cavernosum of the penis, resulting in smooth muscle relaxation and increased blood flow. *Therapeutic Effect:* Facilitates an erection.

PHARMACOKINETICS

Route	Onset	Peak	Duration
PO	16 min	2 h	36 h

Rapidly absorbed after PO administration. Drug has no effect on penile blood flow without sexual stimulation. Metabolized in liver to inactive metabolites. *Half-life:* 17.5 h. Excreted in feces and urine.

AVAILABILITY
Tablets: 2.5 mg, 5 mg, 10 mg, 20 mg.

INDICATIONS AND DOSAGES
▸ **Erectile dysfunction**
PO
Adults, Elderly. 10 mg 30 min before sexual activity. Dose may be increased to 20 mg or decreased to 5 mg, based on patient tolerance. Daily treatment as 2.5 mg once daily is also an option. Dose may be increased to 5 mg based on patient tolerance. Maximum dosing frequency is once daily.
▸ **Dosage in renal impairment**
For patients with a creatinine clearance of 31-50 mL/min, the starting dose is 5 mg before sexual activity once a day and the maximum dose is 10 mg no more frequently than once q48h.
For patients with a creatinine clearance of ≤ 30 mL/min, the starting dose is 5 mg before sexual activity given no more than q72h.
▸ **Dosage in mild or moderate hepatic impairment**
Patients with Child-Pugh class A or B hepatic impairment should take no more than 10 mg once a day.

CONTRAINDICATIONS
Concurrent use of sodium nitroprusside or nitrates in any form, severe hepatic impairment.

INTERACTIONS
Drug
α-Adrenergic blockers, nitrates: Potentiate the hypotensive effects of these drugs.

Strong CY3A4 inhibitors (apenavir, atazanavir, azole antifungals, clarithromycin, delavirdine, fosamprenavir, indinavir, isoniazid, nefazodone, nelfinavir, ritonavir, troleandomycin): May increase tadalafil blood concentration.
Alcohol: Increases the risk of orthostatic hypotension.
Doxazosin: May produce additive hypotensive effects.
Herbal
None known.
Food
None known.

DIAGNOSTIC TEST EFFECTS
None known.

SIDE EFFECTS
Occasional
Headache, dyspepsia, back pain, myalgia, nasal congestion, flushing.

SERIOUS REACTIONS
• Prolonged erections (lasting over 4 h) and priapism (painful erections lasting over 6 h) occur rarely.

PRECAUTIONS & CONSIDERATIONS
Caution is warranted in patients with an anatomic deformity of the penis; cardiac, hepatic, or renal impairment; and conditions that increase the risk of priapism, including leukemia, multiple myeloma, and sickle cell anemia. No age-related precautions have been noted in elderly patients. This drug is not indicated for use in women and children. Be aware that tadalafil is not effective without sexual stimulation. Avoid using nitrate drugs concurrently with tadalafil. If α-adrenergic blockers are used concurrently with tadalafil, initiate therapy at the lowest possible dose. If strong CYP3A4 inhibitors are used, do not exceed 10 mg

tadalafil every 72 h on as-needed basis or tadalafil 2.5 mg daily. Seek treatment immediately if an erection lasts longer than 4 h.
Administration
Take tadalafil without regard to food. Do crush or break film-coated tablets. When used as needed, take at least 30 min before sexual activity. When taken on a daily basis, tadalafil should be taken at the same time every day without regard to sexual activity.

Talc Powder, Sterile
(Sclerosal)

CATEGORY AND SCHEDULE
Pregnancy Risk Category: B

Classification: Sclerosing agents

MECHANISM OF ACTION
A sclerosing agent that induces inflammatory reaction. *Therapeutic Effect:* Obliterates the pleural space and prevents reaccumulation of pleural fluid.

PHARMACOKINETICS
Systemic absorption after intrapleural administration has not been studied.

AVAILABILITY
Aerosol Spray, Intrapleural: 4 g (Sclerosol).

INDICATIONS AND DOSAGES
▸ **Pleural effusions**
AEROSOL
Adults. 8 g as single treatment.

CONTRAINDICATIONS
Sensitivity to talc powder or any component of the formulation.

T

INTERACTIONS
Drug
None known.
Herbal
None known.
Food
None known.

DIAGNOSTIC TEST EFFECTS
None known.

SIDE EFFECTS
Rare
Pain.

SERIOUS REACTIONS
• Atrial arrhythmias, hypotension, cardiac arrest, chest pain, tachycardia, hypovolemia, asystolic arrest, myocardial infarction, and respiratory complications have been reported.

PRECAUTIONS & CONSIDERATIONS
Be aware that pulmonary complications can occur with talc use. It is unknown whether talc crosses the placenta or is distributed in breast milk. Safety and efficacy have not been established in children. No age-related precautions have been noted in elderly patients.
Storage
Store aerosol at room temperature. Protect from direct sunlight.
Administration
Shake canister well, remove protective cap, and securely attach the actuator button with the selected delivery tube (either 15 or 25 cm long) to the valve stem. The total dose should be administered in several short bursts, given with the delivery tube pointing in different directions. Delivery depends on the extent and duration of manual compression of the actuator button. The canister should be kept in an upright position during administration. The spray valve delivers talc at a rate of approximately 0.4 g/s, but the medication is not delivered as a metered dose.

Tamoxifen
ta-mox'i-fen
(Apo-Tamox [CAN], Genox [AUS], Istubol, Nolvadex, Nolvadex-D [CAN], Novo-Tamoxifen [CAN], Tamofen [CAN], Tamosin [AUS])

CATEGORY AND SCHEDULE
Pregnancy Risk Category: D

Classification: Antineoplastics, antiestrogens, estrogen receptor modulators, selective hormones/hormone modifiers

MECHANISM OF ACTION
A nonsteroidal antiestrogen that competes with estradiol for estrogen-receptor binding sites in the breasts, uterus, and vagina. *Therapeutic Effect:* Inhibits DNA synthesis and estrogen response.

PHARMACOKINETICS
Well absorbed from the GI tract. Protein binding: 99%. Metabolized in the liver. Eliminated primarily in feces by the biliary system. *Half-life:* 5-7 days.

AVAILABILITY
Tablets: 10 mg, 20 mg.

INDICATIONS AND DOSAGES
▸ **Adjunctive treatment of breast cancer**
PO
Adults, Elderly. 20-40 mg/day in divided doses twice daily.

▸ **Metastatic breast cancer (males and females)**
PO
Adults, Elderly. 20-40 mg/day in divided doses twice daily.
▸ **Prevention of breast cancer in high-risk women**
PO
Adults, Elderly. 20 mg/day.
▸ **Ductal carcinoma in situ (DCIS)**
PO
Adults, Elderly. 20 mg/day for 5 yr.

OFF-LABEL USES
Induction of ovulation.

CONTRAINDICATIONS
Hypersensitivity to tamoxifen, pregnancy, concurrent warfarin therapy, history of deep vein thrombosis or pulmonary embolism.

INTERACTIONS
Drug
Anastrozole: May decrease the effects of anastrozole.
Carbamazepine, phenobarbital, phenytoin, rifampin, estrogens: May decrease the effects of tamoxifen.
Warfarin: May inhance the anticoagulant effects of warfarin.
NOTE: Because of extensive metabolism, many other drugs may be affected by tamoxifen.
Herbal
Black cohosh, dong quai: May increase effects in estrogen-dependent tumors.
St. John's wort: May decrease effects of tamoxifen.
Food
None known.

DIAGNOSTIC TEST EFFECTS
May increase serum cholesterol, calcium, and triglyceride levels.

SIDE EFFECTS
Frequent
Women (> 10%): Hot flashes, nausea, vomiting.
Occasional
Women (≤ 1%): Changes in menstruation, genital itching, vaginal discharge, endometrial hyperplasia or polyps.
Men: Impotence, decreased libido.
Men and women: Headache, nausea, vomiting, rash, bone pain, confusion, weakness, somnolence.

SERIOUS REACTIONS
• Retinopathy, corneal opacity, and decreased visual acuity have been noted in patients receiving extremely high dosages (240-320 mg/day) for longer than 17 mo.

PRECAUTIONS & CONSIDERATIONS
Caution is warranted in patients with leukopenia and thrombocytopenia. Tamoxifen use should be avoided during pregnancy, especially during the first trimester, because it can cause fetal harm. Nonhormonal contraception should be used during treatment. It is unknown whether tamoxifen is distributed in breast milk; however, breastfeeding is not recommended. Tamoxifen use is safe and effective in girls aged 2-10 yr with McCune-Albright syndrome and precocious puberty. No age-related precautions have been noted in elderly patients.

Initially, an increase in bone and tumor pain may occur, which indicates a good tumor response to tamoxifen. Notify the physician if nausea and vomiting, leg cramps, weakness, weight gain, or vaginal bleeding, itching, or discharge develops. Intake and output, weight, CBC, and serum calcium levels should be monitored before and periodically during tamoxifen therapy. An estrogen receptor assay test should be performed before beginning treatment. Signs and symptoms for hypercalcemia, including constipation, deep bone or flank pain, excessive thirst, hypotonicity of muscles, increased urine output, nausea and vomiting, and renal calculi, should be assessed.

Storage
Store at room temperature.

Administration
Take oral tamoxifen without regard to food.

Tamsulosin
tam-sool′o-sin
(Flomax)
Do not confuse Flomax with Fosamax or Volmax.

CATEGORY AND SCHEDULE
Pregnancy Risk Category: B (Not indicated for use in women.)

Classification: Antiadrenergics, α-blocking

MECHANISM OF ACTION
An α$_1$ antagonist that targets receptors around the bladder neck and prostate capsule. *Therapeutic Effect:* Relaxes smooth muscle and improves urinary flow and symptoms of prostatic hyperplasia.

PHARMACOKINETICS
Well absorbed and widely distributed. Protein binding: 94%-99%. Metabolized in the liver. Excreted primarily in urine. Unknown whether it is removed by hemodialysis. *Half-life:* 9-13 h.

AVAILABILITY
Capsules: 0.4 mg.

INDICATIONS AND DOSAGES
▸ **Benign prostatic hyperplasia**
PO
Adults. 0.4 mg once a day, approximately 30 min after same meal each day. May increase dosage to 0.8 mg if inadequate response in 2-4 wks.

CONTRAINDICATIONS
History of sensitivity to tamsulosin.

INTERACTIONS
Drug
α-Adrenergic blocking agents (such as doxazosin, prazosin, terazosin): May increase the α-blockade effects of both drugs.
β-Blockers, calcium channel blockers, phosphodiasterase-5 inhibitors: May increase the potential for hypotension.
Warfarin: May alter the effects of warfarin.
Herbal
Herbs with hypotensive properties (black cohosh, coleus, golden seal, hawthorn, mistletoe, periwinkle, quinine): May increase the potential for hypotension.
Saw palmetto: Unknown whether it will interact but it is recommended to avoid use.
St. John's wort: May decrease tamulosin's effects.
Food
None known.

DIAGNOSTIC TEST EFFECTS
None known.

SIDE EFFECTS
Frequent (7%-9%)
Dizziness, somnolence.
Occasional (3%-5%)
Headache, anxiety, insomnia, orthostatic hypotension.
Rare (< 2%)
Nasal congestion, pharyngitis, rhinitis, nausea, vertigo, impotence.

SERIOUS REACTIONS

• First-dose syncope (hypotension with sudden loss of consciousness) may occur within 30-90 min after administration of initial dose and may be preceded by tachycardia (pulse rate of 120-160 beats/min).

PRECAUTIONS & CONSIDERATIONS

Caution is warranted in patients with renal impairment. Tamsulosin is not indicated for use in women or children. No age-related precautions have been noted in elderly patients. Tell the physician if using other α-adrenergic blocking agents or warfarin.

Dizziness and lightheadedness may occur. Tasks that require mental alertness or motor skills should be avoided until response to the drug is established. Caution should be used when getting up from a sitting or lying position. BP and renal function should be monitored.

Administration

Take at the same time each day, 30 min after the same meal. Do not crush or open capsule.

Tazarotene

ta-zare'oh-teen
(Tazorac, Avage)

CATEGORY AND SCHEDULE

Pregnancy Risk Category: X

Classification: Dermatologics, retinoids

MECHANISM OF ACTION

Modulates differentiation and proliferation of epithelial tissue, binds, selectively to retinoic acid receptors. *Therapeutic Effect:* Restores normal differentiation of the epidermis and reduction in epidermal inflammation.

PHARMACOKINETICS

Minimal systemic absorption occurs through the skin. Binding to plasma proteins is > 99%. Metabolism is in the skin and liver. Elimination occurs through the fecal and renal pathways. *Half-life:* 18 h.

AVAILABILITY

Gel: 0.05%, 0.1% (Tazorac).
Cream: 0.05% (Tazorac), 0.1% (Avage, Tazorac).

INDICATIONS AND DOSAGES

▶ **Psoriasis**
TOPICAL
Adults, adolescents, children older than 12 yr. Thin film applied once daily in the evening; only cover the lesions, and area should be dry before application

▶ **Acne vulgaris**
TOPICAL
Adults, adolescents, children older than 12 yr. Thin film applied to affected areas once daily in the evening after the face is gently cleansed and dried.

▶ **Fine facial wrinkles, facial mottled hyperpigmentation (liver spots), hypopigmentation associated with photoaging**
TOPICAL
Adults, children older than 17 yr. Thin film applied to affected areas once daily in the evening, after face is gently cleansed and dried.

CONTRAINDICATIONS

Should not be used in pregnant women, patients with hypersensitivity to tazarotene, benzyl alcohol, any one of its components, or other retinoid or vitamin A derivatives.

T

INTERACTIONS
Drug
Ethanol, benzoyl peroxide, resorcinol, salicylic acid, sulfur:
Increases the drying effect.
Quinolones, phenothiazines, sulfonamides, sulfonylureas, tetracyclines, thiazide diuretics:
Increase the risk of photosensitivity.
Herbal
None known.
Food
None known.

DIAGNOSTIC TEST EFFECTS
None known.

SIDE EFFECTS
Frequent
Desquamation, burning or stinging, dry skin, itching, erythema, worsening of psoriasis, irritation, skin pain, pruritis, xerosis, photosensitivity.
Occasional
Irritation, skin pain, fissuring, localized edema, skin discoloration, rash, desquamation, contact dermatitis, skin inflammation, bleeding, dry skin, hypertriglyceridema, peripheral edema, acne vulgaris, cheilitis.

PRECAUTIONS & CONSIDERATIONS
Caution is warranted in patients with other skin conditions such as eczema, sunburn, and undiagnosed skin lesions. Tazarotene is contraindicated during pregnancy. It is unknown whether it enters the breast milk. Safety and efficacy have not been established in children or elderly patients.

Burning or stinging after application, dryness, itching, peeling, or redness of the skin may occur during tazarotene therapy. Avoid direct exposure to sunlight.

Storage
Store at room temperature away from heat and direct light.
Administration
Tazarotene is for external use only. Apply only on face, once daily at bedtime, or as directed by physician. Remove any makeup, gently wash face with a mild cleanser, and pat skin dry. Wait at least 20 min to make sure face is dry before applying a small, pea-sized amount (about ¼-in. wide) of medication. Apply in a thin layer over wrinkles and discolored spots avoiding eye and mouth areas. Wash hands after using the medication. In the morning, apply a moisturizing sunscreen with SPF 15 or greater.

Telithromycin
tell-ith'roe-my-sin
(Ketek)

CATEGORY AND SCHEDULE
Pregnancy Risk Category: C

Classification: Antibiotics, ketolides

MECHANISM OF ACTION
A ketolide that blocks protein synthesis by binding to ribosomal receptor sites on the bacterial cell wall. *Therapeutic Effect:* Bactericidal.

PHARMACOKINETICS
Protein binding: 60%-70%. More of drug is concentrated in WBCs than in plasma, and drug is eliminated more slowly from WBCs than from plasma. Partially metabolized by the liver. Minimally excreted in feces and urine. *Half-life:* 10 h.

AVAILABILITY
Tablets: 400 mg.

INDICATIONS AND DOSAGES
▶ **Community-acquired pneumonia**
PO
Adults, Elderly. 800 mg once a day
for 7-10 days.

CONTRAINDICATIONS
Hypersensitivity to macrolide
antibiotics, concurrent use of
cisapride or pimozide, myasthenia
gravis, congenital QT prolongation.

INTERACTIONS
Drug
Antiarrhythmics: May result in
additive effects even resulting in
serious arrhythmias.
**Atorvastatin, digoxin, lovastatin,
metoprolol, pimozide, simvastatin,
theophylline:** May increase the
blood concentration and toxicity of
these drugs.
**Carbamazepine, phenobarbital,
phenytoin, rifampin:** May
decrease the blood concentration of
telithromycin.
Cisapride: Increases blood
concentration of cisapride, resulting
in significantly increased QT interval.
Itraconazole, ketoconazole: May
increase the blood concentration of
telithromycin.
Sotolol: Decreases the blood
concentration of sotalol.
Herbal
None known.
Food
None known.

DIAGNOSTIC TEST EFFECTS
May increase platelet count and AST
(SGOT) and ALT (SGPT) levels.

SIDE EFFECTS
Occasional (4%-11%)
Diarrhea, nausea, headache, dizziness.

Rare (2%-3%)
Vomiting, loose stools, altered
taste, dry mouth, flatulence, visual
disturbances.

SERIOUS REACTIONS
• Hepatic dysfunction, severe
hypersensitivity reaction, and atrial
arrhythmias occur rarely.
• Myastenia gravis with life-
threatening and fatal respiratory
depression occurs rarely.
• Antibiotic-associated colitis and
other superinfections may result from
altered bacterial balance.

PRECAUTIONS & CONSIDERATIONS
Caution is warranted in patients
with uncorrected hypokalemia,
hypomagnesemia, bradycardia,
concomitant use of class IA or
III antiarrhythmics, QTc interval
prolongation, and history of
hepatitis or jaundice associated with
telithromycin use. It is unknown
whether telithromycin is distributed
in breast milk. Safety and efficacy
of telithromycin have not been
established in children. In elderly
patients with normal renal function,
no age-related precautions have been
noted.
   Be aware that there is a potential
for visual disturbances. Nausea,
vomiting, diarrhea, headache, and
dizziness are other possible side
effects.
Storage
Store at room temperature.
Administration
May administer without regard to
meals. Do not break or crush
film-coated tablets.

T

Telmisartan
tel-meh-sar′tan
(Micardis, Pritor [AUS])

CATEGORY AND SCHEDULE
Pregnancy Risk Category: C (D if
used in second or third trimester)

Classification: Angiotensin II
receptor antagonists

MECHANISM OF ACTION
An angiotensin II receptor, type
AT_1, antagonist that blocks
vasoconstrictor and aldosterone-
secreting effects of angiotensin II,
inhibiting the binding of angiotensin
II to the AT_1 receptors. *Therapeutic
Effect:* Causes vasodilation,
decreases peripheral resistance, and
decreases BP.

PHARMACOKINETICS
Rapidly and completely absorbed
after PO administration. Protein
binding: > 99.5%. Undergoes
metabolism in the liver to inactive
metabolite. Excreted in feces.
Unknown whether removed by
hemodialysis. *Half-life:* 24 h.

AVAILABILITY
Tablets: 20 mg, 40 mg, 80 mg.

INDICATIONS AND DOSAGES
▶ **Hypertension**
PO
Adults, Elderly. 40 mg once a day.
Range: 20-80 mg/day.

OFF-LABEL USES
Treatment of congestive heart failure
(CHF).

CONTRAINDICATIONS
Hypersentivity to telmisartan.

INTERACTIONS
Drug
Digoxin: Increases digoxin plasma
concentration.
**Potassium supplements,
potassium-sparing diuretics,
ACE inhibitors, eplerenone:** May
increase risk of hyperkalemia.
Warfarin: Slightly decreases
warfarin plasma concentration.
Herbal
Dong quai, garlic: May increase
antihypertensive effect.
Ephedra, ginseng, yohimbe: May
decrease antihypertensive effect.
Food
None known.

DIAGNOSTIC TEST EFFECTS
May increase serum creatinine and
potassium levels. May decrease
blood hemoglobin and hematocrit
levels.

SIDE EFFECTS
Occasional (3%-7%)
Upper respiratory tract infection,
sinusitis, back or leg pain, diarrhea.
Rare (1%)
Dizziness, headache, fatigue,
nausea, heartburn, myalgia, cough,
peripheral edema.

SERIOUS REACTIONS
• Overdosage may manifest as
hypotension and tachycardia.
Bradycardia occurs less often.

PRECAUTIONS & CONSIDERATIONS
Caution is warranted in patients with
hepatic and renal impairment, renal
artery stenosis (bilateral or unilateral),
and volume depletion. It is unknown
whether telmisartan is excreted in
breast milk; it may cause fetal harm.
Safety and efficacy of telmisartan
have not been established in children.
No age-related precautions have been
noted in elderly patients.

Dizziness may occur. Tasks that require mental alertness or motor skills should be avoided. Notify the physician if fever or sore throat occurs. Apical pulse and BP should be assessed immediately before each olmesartan dose and regularly throughout therapy. Be alert to fluctuations in apical pulse and BP. If an excessive reduction in BP occurs, place the person in the supine position with feet slightly elevated and notify the physician. Pulse rate and BUN, serum creatinine, and serum electrolyte levels should be assessed. Maintain adequate hydration; exercising outside during hot weather should be avoided in order to decrease the risk of dehydration and hypotension.

Administration

! May be given concurrently with other antihypertensives. If BP is not controlled by telmisartan alone, a diuretic may be added.

Take telmisartan without regard to meals.

Temazepam
te-maz′e-pam
(Apo-Temazepam [CAN], Novo-Temazepam [CAN], PMS-Temazepam [CAN], Restoril)
Do not confuse Restoril with Vistaril or Zestril.

CATEGORY AND SCHEDULE
Pregnancy Risk Category: X
Controlled Substance: Schedule IV

Classification: Benzodiazepines, sedatives/hypnotics

MECHANISM OF ACTION
A benzodiazepine that enhances the action of the inhibitory neurotransmitter gamma-aminobutyric acid, resulting in central nervous system (CNS) depression. *Therapeutic Effect:* Induces sleep.

PHARMACOKINETICS
Well absorbed from the GI tract. Protein binding: 96%. Widely distributed. Crosses the blood-brain barrier. Metabolized in the liver. Primarily excreted in urine. Not removed by hemodialysis. *Half-life:* 4-18 h.

AVAILABILITY
Capsules: 7.5 mg, 15 mg, 30 mg.

INDICATIONS AND DOSAGES
▸ **Insomnia**
PO
Adults, Children 18 yr and older. 15-30 mg at bedtime.
Elderly, Debilitated. 7.5-15 mg at bedtime.

CONTRAINDICATIONS
Angle-closure glaucoma; CNS depression; pregnancy or breastfeeding; severe, uncontrolled pain; sleep apnea.

INTERACTIONS
Drug
Alcohol, other CNS depressants: May increase CNS depression.
Herbal
Kava kava, valerian: May increase CNS depression.
Food
None known.

DIAGNOSTIC TEST EFFECTS
None known.

SIDE EFFECTS
Frequent
Somnolence, sedation, rebound
insomnia (may occur for 1-2 nights
after drug is discontinued), dizziness,
confusion, euphoria.
Occasional
Asthenia, anorexia, diarrhea.
Rare
Paradoxical CNS excitement or
restlessness (particularly in elderly
or debilitated patients).

SERIOUS REACTIONS
• Abrupt or too-rapid withdrawal
may result in pronounced
restlessness, irritability, insomnia,
hand tremor, abdominal or muscle
cramps, vomiting, diaphoresis, and
seizures.
• Overdose results in somnolence,
confusion, diminished reflexes,
respiratory depression, and coma.

PRECAUTIONS & CONSIDERATIONS
Caution is warranted in patients with
mental impairment and the potential
for drug dependence. Temazepam
is pregnancy risk category X and
crosses the placenta and may be
distributed in breast milk. Long-term
use of temazepam during pregnancy
may produce withdrawal symptoms
and CNS depression in neonates.
Temazepam use is not recommended
for children younger than 18 yr. To
avoid ataxia or excessive sedation in
elderly patients, plan to administer
small doses initially and to increase
dosage gradually.

Avoid alcohol, CNS depressants,
and tasks that require mental
alertness and motor skills. BP,
pulse rate, respiratory rate, rhythm,
and depth should be assessed
before administering temazepam.
Cardiovascular, mental, and
respiratory status should be
monitored throughout therapy.

Administration
If desired, open temazepam capsules
and mix the contents with food. Take
temazepam 30 min before bedtime.

Temozolomide
tem-oh-zohl'oh-mide
(Temodal [AUS], Temodar)

CATEGORY AND SCHEDULE
Pregnancy Risk Category: D

Classification: Antineoplastics,
alkylating agents

MECHANISM OF ACTION
An imidazotetrazine derivative that
acts as a prodrug and is converted to
a highly active cytotoxic metabolite.
Its cytotoxic effect is associated with
methylation of DNA. *Therapeutic
Effect:* Inhibits DNA replication,
causing cell death.

PHARMACOKINETICS
Rapidly and completely absorbed
after PO administration. Protein
binding: 15%. Peak plasma
concentration occurs in 1 h.
Penetrates the blood-brain barrier.
Eliminated primarily in urine and, to
a much lesser extent, in feces.
Half-life: 1.6-1.8 h.

AVAILABILITY
Capsules: 5 mg, 20 mg, 100 mg,
250 mg.

INDICATIONS AND DOSAGES
▶ **Anaplastic astrocytoma**
PO
Adults, Elderly. Initially,
150 mg/m^2/day on days 1-5 of a
28-day treatment cycle. Subsequent
doses based on platelet count
and absolute neutrophil count

(>1500/mm³ANC) during previous cycle. ANC > 1500 and platelet >100,000/mm³. Maintenance: 200 mg/m²/day for 5 days q4wk. Continue until disease progression. Minimum: 100 mg/m²/day for 5 days for subsequent cycle. Dosage adjustments are based on ANC and platelets.

CONTRAINDICATIONS
Hypersensitivity to dacarbazine, pregnancy.

INTERACTIONS
Drug
Live-virus vaccines: May potentiate virus replication, increase vaccine side effects, and decrease the patient's antibody response to the vaccine.
Valproic acid: Decreases the clearance of temozolomide.
Herbal
None known.
Food
All foods: Decrease the rate of drug absorption.

DIAGNOSTIC TEST EFFECTS
May decrease blood hemoglobin levels and neutrophil, platelet, and WBC counts.

SIDE EFFECTS
Frequent (33%-53%)
Nausea, vomiting, headache, fatigue, constipation.
Occasional (10%-16%)
Diarrhea, asthenia, fever, dizziness, peripheral edema, incoordination, insomnia.
Rare (5%-7%)
Paraesthesia, drowsiness, anorexia, urinary incontinence, anxiety, pharyngitis, cough.

SERIOUS REACTIONS
• Elderly patients and women are at increased risk for developing severe myelosuppression, characterized by neutropenia and thrombocytopenia and usually occurring within the first few cycles. Neutrophil and platelet counts reach their nadirs approximately 26-28 days after administration and recover within 14 days of the nadir.

PRECAUTIONS & CONSIDERATIONS
Caution is warranted in patients with severe hepatic or renal impairment. Temozolomide use should be avoided during pregnancy because the drug may cause fetal harm. Although it is unknown whether temozolomide is excreted in breast milk, women taking this drug should avoid breastfeeding. The safety and efficacy of temozolomide have not been established in children. Elderly patients (i.e., older than 70 yr) have a higher risk of developing grade 4 neutropenia and grade 4 thrombocytopenia. Vaccinations and coming in contact with crowds and people with known infections should be avoided.

Notify the physician if the patient experiences easy bruising, fever, signs of local infection, sore throat, or unusual bleeding from any site. Before administration, ANC must be > 1500/mm³ and the platelet count must be > 100,000/mm³. To control nausea and vomiting, antiemetics should be administered. A CBC on day 22 (21 days after the first dose) or within 48 h of that day and then weekly until the ANC is > 1500/mm³ and the platelet count is > 100,000/mm³ should be ordered.
Administration
! Because temozolomide is cytotoxic, avoid touching the contents of an open capsule during preparation and administration.

Administer temozolomide on an empty stomach because food

reduces the rate and extent of drug absorption and increases the risk of nausea and vomiting. For best results, take temozolomide at bedtime. Swallow the capsule whole with a glass of water. If the patient cannot swallow, open the capsule and mix the contents with applesauce or apple juice.

as soon as possible after onset of symptoms.

Weight (kg)	(mg)	(mL)
≥ 90	50	10
80-< 89	45	9
70-< 79	40	8
60-< 69	35	7
< 60	30	6

Tenecteplase
ten′neck-te-place
(Metalyse [AUS], TNKase)
Do not confuse TNKase with t-PA.

CATEGORY AND SCHEDULE
Pregnancy Risk Category: C

Classification: Thrombolytics

MECHANISM OF ACTION
A tissue plasminogen activator produced by recombinant DNA that binds to fibrin and converts plasminogen to plasmin. Initiates fibrinolysis by degrading fibrin clots, fibrinogen, and other plasma proteins. *Therapeutic Effect:* Exerts thrombolytic action.

PHARMACOKINETICS
Extensively distributed to tissues. Completely eliminated by hepatic metabolism. *Half-life:* 20-24 min.

AVAILABILITY
Powder for Injection: 50 mg.

INDICATIONS AND DOSAGES
▸ **Acute myocardial infarction (MI)**
IV
Adults. Dosage is based on patient's weight. Treatment should be initiated

CONTRAINDICATIONS
Active internal bleeding, aneurysm, AV malformation, bleeding diathesis, history of cerebrovascular accident, intracranial or intraspinal surgery or trauma within past 2 mo, intracranial neoplasm, coagulopathy, severe uncontrolled hypertension.

INTERACTIONS
Drug
Aminocaproic acid: May decrease effectiveness of tenecteplase.
Anticoagulants (such as heparin, warfarin), aspirin, dipyridamole, glycoprotein IIb/IIIa inhibitors: Increase the risk of bleeding.
Herbal
Ginkgo biloba: May increase the risk of bleeding.
Food
None known.

DIAGNOSTIC TEST EFFECTS
Decreases plasminogen and fibrinogen levels during infusion, decreasing clotting time and confirming presence of lysis. Decreases hematocrit and hemoglobin.

⊘ IV INCOMPATIBILITIES
Do not mix with other medications.

SIDE EFFECTS
Frequent
Bleeding (major, 4.7%; minor, 21.8%).

SERIOUS REACTIONS
• Bleeding at internal sites may occur, including intracranial, retroperitoneal, GI, genitourinary, and respiratory sites.
• Lysis or coronary thrombi may produce atrial or ventricular arrhythmias and stroke.

PRECAUTIONS & CONSIDERATIONS
Caution is warranted in patients with severe hepatic impairment and in those who have previously received tenecteplase. It is unknown whether tenecteplase is distributed in breast milk. Safety and efficacy of tenecteplase have not been established in children. Elderly patients may have an increased risk of intracranial hemorrhage, major bleeding, and stroke. Tenecteplase should be used cautiously in this population. An electric razor and a soft toothbrush should be used to reduce the risk of bleeding.

Patients should also receive aspirin and heparin as soon as possible with tenecteplase.

Notify the physician of bruises, back or abdominal pain, black or red stool, coffee-ground vomitus, dark or red urine, red-speckled mucus from cough, chest pain, headache, palpitations, or shortness of breath. Continuous cardiac monitoring for arrhythmias, BP, and pulse and respiration rates every 15 min should be performed until the patient is stable, then hourly. Cardiac enzyme concentrations, 12-lead ECG, electrolyte levels, aPTT, hematocrit, hemoglobin, fibrinogen level, platelet count, and thrombin time should be evaluated before and during therapy.
Storage
Store at room temperature. If possible, use immediately after reconstitution but may refrigerate for up to 8 h. Discard after 8 h.

Administration
! Give as a single IV bolus over 5 s. Precipitate may occur when given in an IV line containing dextrose. Flush line with saline before and after administration.

Tenecteplase is normally a colorless to pale yellow solution. Do not use if solution is discolored or contains particulates. Add 10 mL sterile water for injection without preservative to vial to provide concentration of 5 mg/mL. Gently swirl until dissolved. Do not shake. If foaming occurs, allow vial to sit undisturbed for several minutes.

Teniposide
ten-i-poe′side
(Vumon)
Do not confuse teniposide with etoposide.

CATEGORY AND SCHEDULE
Pregnancy Risk Category: D

Classification: Antineoplastics, epipodophyllotoxins

MECHANISM OF ACTION
An epipodophyllotoxin that induces single- and double-strand breaks in DNA, inhibiting or altering DNA synthesis. Acts in the late S and early G_2 phases of cell cycle. *Therapeutic Effect:* Prevents cells from entering mitosis.

AVAILABILITY
Injection: 50 mg (10 mg/mL).

Ⓥ IV INCOMPATIBILITIES
Amphotericin B, Phenytoin.

INDICATIONS AND DOSAGES
▸ **Induction therapy in patients with refractory childhood**

acute lymphoblastic leukemia (in combination with other antineoplastic agents)
IV
Children. 165 mg/m^2 IV twice weekly for 8-9 doses or 250 mg/m^2 IV once weekly for 4-8 wk.

CONTRAINDICATIONS

Absolute neutrophil count < 500/mm^3; hypersensitivity to Cremophor EL (polyoxyethylated castor oil), etoposide, or teniposide; platelet count < 50,000/mm^3.

INTERACTIONS

Drug
Bone marrow depressants: May increase myelosuppression.
Live-virus vaccines: May potentiate virus replication, increase vaccine side effects, and decrease the patient's antibody response to the vaccine.
Methotrexate: May increase intracellular accumulation of this drug.
Vincristine: May increase the severity of peripheral neuropathy.
Herbal
None known.
Food
None known.

DIAGNOSTIC TEST EFFECTS

None significant.

SIDE EFFECTS

Frequent (> 30%)
Mucositis, nausea, vomiting, diarrhea, anemia.
Occasional (3%-5%)
Alopecia, rash.
Rare (< 3%)
Hepatic dysfunction, fever, renal dysfunction, peripheral neurotoxicity.

SERIOUS REACTIONS

• Myelosuppression manifested as hematologic toxicity (principally leukopenia, neutropenia, and thrombocytopenia) may be severe and may increase the risk of infection or bleeding.
• Hypersensitivity reaction may include anaphylaxis (marked by chills, fever, tachycardia, bronchospasm, dyspnea, and facial flushing).

PRECAUTIONS & CONSIDERATIONS

Caution is warranted with brain tumors, hepatic dysfunction, Down syndrome, and neuroblastoma (increases the risk of anaphylaxis). Women of childbearing age should be cautioned to avoid pregnancy during teniposide therapy. Contraceptive methods should be practiced. Vaccinations and coming in contact with crowds and people with known infections should be avoided.

Notify the physician if fever, signs of local infection, or unusual bleeding from any site occurs.

Appropriate medication and equipment should be readily available before giving the first dose in case life-threatening anaphylaxis occurs. Hematologic test results should be assessed before and frequently during teniposide therapy.
Storage
Refrigerate unopened ampules and protect them from light. Reconstituted solutions are stable for 24 h at room temperature. They should not be refrigerated.
Administration
! Wear gloves when preparing the solution. If the solution comes in contact with your skin, wash immediately and thoroughly with soap and water.

Dilute with 0.9% NaCl or D5W to provide a concentration of 0.1-1 mg/mL. Prepare and administer the drug in glass containers or polyolefin plastic bags. Do not use polyvinyl chloride containers. Use the 1-mg/mL solution within 4 h of preparation to reduce the risk of precipitation. Discard the solution if precipitation occurs. Infuse teniposide over at least 30-60 min. Avoid rapid IV injection.

Tenofovir
ten-oh'foh-veer
(Viread)

CATEGORY AND SCHEDULE
Pregnancy Risk Category: B

Classification: Antivirals, nucleotide reverse transcriptase inhibitors

MECHANISM OF ACTION
A nucleotide analogue that inhibits HIV reverse transcriptase by being incorporated into viral DNA, resulting in DNA chain termination. *Therapeutic Effect:* Slows HIV replication and reduces HIV RNA levels (viral load).

AVAILABILITY
Tablets: 300 mg.

INDICATIONS AND DOSAGES
▶ **HIV infection (in combination with other antiretrovirals)**
PO
Adults, Elderly, Children 18 yr and older. 300 mg once a day.

CONTRAINDICATIONS
Hypersensitivity to tenofovir, concurrent use of tenofovir-containing combinations.

INTERACTIONS
Drug
Acyclovir, cidofovir, ganciclovir, valacyclovir, valganciclovir: May increase the blood concentrations of tenofovir.
Didanosine: May increase didanosine blood concentration.
Indinavir, lamivudine, lopinavir, ritonavir: May decrease the blood concentrations of these drugs.
Herbal
None known.
Food
High-fat food: Increases tenofovir bioavailability.

DIAGNOSTIC TEST EFFECTS
May elevate liver function test results. May alter serum CK, GGT, uric acid, AST (SGOT), ALT (SGPT), and triglyceride levels as well as creatinine clearance.

SIDE EFFECTS
Frequent
Pain, GI disturbances (diarrhea, flatulence, nausea, vomiting), weakness.
Occasional
Headache, depression, insomnia, fever, dizziness, myalgia, sweating.

SERIOUS REACTIONS
• Lactic acidosis and hepatomegaly with steatosis occur rarely but may be severe.

T

PRECAUTIONS & CONSIDERATIONS
Caution should be used with impaired liver or renal function. Check baseline laboratory test results, if ordered, especially liver function test results and serum triglyceride levels before beginning tenofovir therapy and at periodic intervals during therapy. Tenofovir is not a cure for HIV infection, nor does it reduce risk of transmission

to others; illnesses associated with advanced HIV infection.

Monitor CD4 cell count, complete blood count (CBC), hemoglobin levels, HIV RNA plasma levels, liver function test results, and reticulocyte count. Assess pattern of daily bowel activity and stool consistency. Notify the physician if nausea, persistent abdominal pain, or vomiting occurs.

Administration

Give with food to increase absorption. Continue drug therapy for the full length of treatment.

Terazosin
ter-a′zoe-sin
(Apo-Terazosin [CAN],
Novo-Terazosin [CAN])

CATEGORY AND SCHEDULE
Pregnancy Risk Category: C

Classification: Antiadrenergics, α-blocking, peripheral

MECHANISM OF ACTION
An antihypertensive and benign prostatic hyperplasia agent that blocks α-adrenergic receptors. Produces vasodilation, decreases peripheral resistance, and targets receptors around bladder neck and prostate. *Therapeutic Effect:* In hypertension, decreases BP. In benign prostatic hyperplasia, relaxes smooth muscle and improves urine flow.

PHARMACOKINETICS

Route	Onset	Peak	Duration
PO	15 min	1-2 h	12-24 h

Rapidly, completely absorbed from the GI tract. Protein binding: 90%-94%. Metabolized in the liver to active metabolite. Eliminated primarily in feces via the biliary system; excreted in urine. Not removed by hemodialysis.
Half-life: 9.2-12 h.

AVAILABILITY
Capsules: 1 mg, 2 mg, 5 mg, 10 mg.

INDICATIONS AND DOSAGES
▸ **Mild to moderate hypertension**
PO
Adults, Elderly. Initially, 1 mg at bedtime. Slowly increase dosage to desired levels. Range: 1-5 mg/day as single or 2 divided doses. Maximum: 20 mg.
▸ **Benign prostatic hyperplasia**
PO
Adults, Elderly. Initially, 1 mg at bedtime. May increase up to 10 mg/day. Maximum: 20 mg/day.

CONTRAINDICATIONS
Hypersensitivity to terazosin or other α_1-blockers. Concurrent use with phosphodiesterase-5 inhibitors.

INTERACTIONS
Drug
Estrogen, NSAIDs, other sympathomimetics: May decrease the effects of terazosin.
Hypotension-producing medications, such as antihypertensives and diuretics: May increase the effects of terazosin.
Tadalafil, vardenafil: May increase the hypotensive effects. Use is contraindicated.
Herbal
Dong quai, ginseng, garlic, yohimbe: May decrease the effects of terazosin.

Saw palmetto: May interfere with effects of terazosin.
Food
None known.

DIAGNOSTIC TEST EFFECTS
May decrease blood hemoglobin and hematocrit levels, serum albumin level, total serum protein level, and WBC count.

SIDE EFFECTS
Frequent (5%-9%)
Dizziness, headache, unusual tiredness.
Rare (< 2%)
Peripheral edema, orthostatic hypotension, myalgia, arthralgia, blurred vision, nausea, vomiting, nasal congestion, somnolence.

SERIOUS REACTIONS
• First-dose syncope (hypotension with sudden loss of consciousness) may occur 30-90 min after initial dose of 2 mg or more, a too-rapid increase in dosage, or addition of another antihypertensive agent to therapy. First-dose syncope may be preceded by tachycardia (pulse rate of 120-160 beats/min).

PRECAUTIONS & CONSIDERATIONS
Caution is warranted in patients with confirmed or suspected coronary artery disease. It is unknown whether terazosin crosses the placenta or is distributed in breast milk. The safety and efficacy of terazosin have not been established in children. No age-related precautions have been noted in elderly patients, but this age group may be more sensitive to the drug's hypotensive effects. Caution should be used when driving or operating machinery. Tasks that require mental alertness or motor skills should be avoided until response to the drug is established.

Nasal congestion, dizziness, lightheadedness, and fainting may occur. Rise slowly from a lying to a sitting position, and permit legs to dangle momentarily before standing to avoid the hypotensive effect. BP and pulse should be obtained immediately before each dose, and every 15-30 min thereafter until BP is stabilized. Be alert for fluctuations in BP. Genitourinary symptoms and peripheral edema should also be assessed.
Administration
! If terazosin is discontinued for several days, expect to restart therapy with a 1-mg dose at bedtime.
Take terazosin without regard to food. Administer first dose at bedtime to minimize the risk of fainting at the first dose.

Terbinafine
ter-been'a-feen
(Apo-Terbinafine [CAN], Lamisil, Lamisil AT, Novo-Terbinafine [CAN])
Do not confuse terbinafine with terbutaline or Lamisil with Lamictal.

CATEGORY AND SCHEDULE
Pregnancy Risk Category: B

Classification: Antifungals, topical, dermatologics

MECHANISM OF ACTION
A fungicidal antifungal that inhibits the enzyme squalene epoxidase, thereby interfering with fungal biosynthesis. *Therapeutic Effect:* Results in death of fungal cells.

AVAILABILITY
Tablets (Lamisil): 250 mg.
Cream (Lamisil AT): 1%.
Granules (Lamisil): 125 mg/packet,
187.5 mg/packet
*Topical Solution (Lamisil, Lamisil
AT):* 1%.

INDICATIONS AND DOSAGES
▸ **Tinea pedis**
TOPICAL
*Adults, Elderly, Children 12 yr
and older.* Apply twice a day until
signs and symptoms significantly
improve.
▸ **Tinea cruris, tinea corporis**
TOPICAL
*Adults, Elderly, Children 12 yr
and older.* Apply twice a day until
signs and symptoms significantly
improve.
▸ **Onychomycosis**
PO
*Adults, Elderly, Children 12 yr
and older.* 250 mg/day for 6 wks
(fingernails) or 12 wks (toenails).
▸ **Tinea versicolor**
TOPICAL SOLUTION
Adults, Elderly. Apply to the affected
area twice a day at least 7 days and
no longer than 4 wks.

CONTRAINDICATIONS
Oral: Children younger than
12 yr, preexisting hepatic or renal
impairment (creatinine clearance
of ≤ 50 mL/min).

INTERACTIONS
Drug
**Alcohol, other hepatotoxic
medications:** May increase the risk
of hepatotoxicity.
**Hepatic enzyme inducers,
including rifampin:** May increase
terbinafine clearance.
**Hepatic enzyme inhibitors,
including cimetidine:** May decrease
terbinafine clearance.

Herbal
None known.
Food
None known.

DIAGNOSTIC TEST EFFECTS
May increase SGOT (AST) and
SGPT (ALT) levels.

SIDE EFFECTS
Frequent (13%)
Oral: Headache.
Occasional (3%-6%)
Oral: Diarrhea, rash, dyspepsia,
pruritus, taste disturbance, nausea.
Rare
Oral: Abdominal pain, flatulence,
urticaria, visual disturbance.
Topical: Irritation, burning, pruritus,
dryness.

SERIOUS REACTIONS
• Hepatobiliary dysfunction
(including cholestatic hepatitis),
serious skin reactions, and severe
neutropenia occur rarely.
• Ocular lens and retinal changes
have been noted.

PRECAUTIONS & CONSIDERATIONS
As appropriate, monitor liver
function when receiving treatment
for longer than 6 wks.
❗ Topical therapy may be used for
a minimum of 1 wk and is not to
exceed 4 wks. Discontinue the
medication and notify the physician
if a local reaction occurs. Signs
and symptoms of a local reaction
include blistering, burning, irritation,
itching, oozing, redness, and
swelling. Separate personal items
that come in contact with affected
areas.
Administration
Rub the topical form well into the
affected and surrounding area.
Keep affected areas clean and dry
and wear light clothing to promote

ventilation. Avoid contact with eyes, mouth, nose, or other mucous membranes. The treated area should not be covered with an occlusive dressing.

When taking terbinafine tablets, take without regard to food. Granules may be sprinkled on a spoonful of nonacidic food that should be swallowed without chewing.

Terbutaline
ter-byoo′te-leen
(Bricanyl [CAN])
Do not confuse terbutaline with tolbutamide or terbinafine, or Brethine with Brethaire.

CATEGORY AND SCHEDULE
Pregnancy Risk Category: B

Classification: Adrenergic agonists, bronchodilators

MECHANISM OF ACTION
An adrenergic agonist that stimulates β_2-adrenergic receptors, resulting in relaxation of uterine and bronchial smooth muscle. *Therapeutic Effect:* Relieves bronchospasm and reduces airway resistance. Also inhibits uterine contractions.

AVAILABILITY
Tablets: 2.5 mg, 5 mg.
Injection: 1 mg/mL.

INDICATIONS AND DOSAGES
▶ **Bronchospasm**
PO
Adults, Elderly, Children 15 yr and older. Initially, 2.5 mg 3-4 times a day. Maintenance: 2.5-5 mg 3 times a day q6h while awake. Maximum: 15 mg/day.
Children aged 12-14 yr. 2.5 mg 3 times a day. Maximum: 7.5 mg/day.
Children 6-11 yr. Initially, 0.05 mg/kg/dose q8h. May increase up to 0.15 mg/kg/dose. Maximum: 5 mg/day.
SC
Adults, Children 12 yr and older. Initially, 0.25 mg. Repeat in 15-30 min if substantial improvement does not occur. Maximum: 0.5 mg/4 h.
Children younger than 12 yr. 0.005-0.01 mg/kg/dose to a maximum of 0.25 mg q15-20 min for 3 doses.

CONTRAINDICATIONS
History of hypersensitivity to sympathomimetics.

INTERACTIONS
Drug
β-Blockers: May decrease the effects of β-blockers.
Digoxin, sympathomimetics: May increase the risk of arrhythmias.
MAOIs: May increase the risk of hypertensive crisis.
Tricyclic antidepressants: May increase cardiovascular effects.
Herbal
Ephedra, yohimbe: May increase central nervous system (CNS) stimulation.
Food
None known.

DIAGNOSTIC TEST EFFECTS
May decrease serum potassium level.

SIDE EFFECTS
Frequent (18%-23%)
Tremor, anxiety.
Occasional (10%-11%)
Somnolence, headache, nausea, heartburn, dizziness.

T

Rare (1%-3%)
Flushing, asthenia, mouth and throat dryness or irritation (with inhalation therapy).

SERIOUS REACTIONS
• Too-frequent or excessive use may lead to decreased drug effectiveness and severe, paradoxical bronchoconstriction.
• Excessive sympathomimetic stimulation may cause palpitations, extrasystoles, tachycardia, chest pain, a slight increase in BP followed by a substantial decrease, chills, diaphoresis, and blanching of skin.

PRECAUTIONS & CONSIDERATIONS
Caution is warranted in patients with cardiovascular disorders, hypertension, diabetes mellitus, a history of seizures, and hyperthyroidism. Avoid excessive use of caffeinated products, such as chocolate, cocoa, cola, coffee, and tea.

Anxiety, nervousness, and shakiness may occur. Notify the physician of chest pain, difficulty breathing, dizziness, flushing, headache, muscle tremors, or palpitations. Pulse rate and quality, respiratory rate, depth, rhythm, and type, BP, ABG levels, and serum potassium levels should be monitored. Fingernails and lips should be assessed for a blue or dusky color in light-skinned patients and a gray color in dark-skinned patients, which are signs of hypoxemia.

Administration
Take terbutaline with food if the patient experiences GI upset. Crush tablets as needed.

The drug may be injected subcutaneously into the lateral deltoid region. Do not use solution if it appears discolored.

Terconazole
ter-kon'a-zole
(Terazol [CAN], Terazol 3, Terazol 7, Zazole)

CATEGORY AND SCHEDULE
Pregnancy Risk Category: C

Classification: Antifungals, topical, dermatologics

MECHANISM OF ACTION
An antifungal that disrupts fungal cell membrane permeability. *Therapeutic Effect:* Produces antifungal activity.

PHARMACOKINETICS
Extent of systemic absorption varies 5%-8% in women who have had a hysterectomy versus 12%-16% in women with a uterus.

AVAILABILITY
Suppository: 80 mg (Terazol 3).
Cream: 0.4 % (Terazol 7, Zazole), 0.8% (Terazol 3, Zazole).

INDICATIONS AND DOSAGES
▶ **Vulvovaginal candidiasis**
INTRAVAGINAL
Adults, Elderly. 1 suppository vaginally at bedtime for 3 days.
Adults, Elderly. One applicatorful at bedtime for 7 days (0.4% cream) or for 3 days (0.8% cream).

CONTRAINDICATIONS
Hypersensitivity to terconazole or any component of the formulation.

INTERACTIONS
Drug
None known.

Herbal
None known.
Food
None known.

DIAGNOSTIC TEST EFFECTS
None known.

SIDE EFFECTS
Frequent
Headache, vulvovaginal burning.
Occasional
Dysmenorrhea, pain in female
genitalia, abdominal pain, fever,
itching.
Rare
Chills.

SERIOUS REACTIONS
• Flulike syndrome has been
reported.

PRECAUTIONS & CONSIDERATIONS
Caution should be used in the
first trimester of pregnancy. It is
unknown whether terconazole
crosses the placenta or is distributed
in breast milk. Safety and efficacy
of terconazole have not been
established in children. No age-
related precautions have been noted
in elderly patients.
Storage
Store at room temperature.
Administration
Insert suppository or administer
cream at bedtime. Complete full
course of therapy. Contact physician
if burning or irritation occurs.

Teriparatide
ter-i-par′a-tide
(Forteo)

CATEGORY AND SCHEDULE
Pregnancy Risk Category: C

Classification: Hormones/
hormone modifiers, parathyroid
hormone analogue

MECHANISM OF ACTION
A synthetic polypeptide hormone
that acts on bone to mobilize
calcium; also acts on kidney to
reduce calcium clearance, increase
phosphate excretion. *Therapeutic
Effect:* Promotes an increased rate
of release of calcium from bone
into blood, stimulates new bone
formation.

AVAILABILITY
Injection: 3-mL prefilled pen
containing 750 mcg teriparatide
(Forteo).

INDICATIONS AND DOSAGES
▸ **Osteoporosis**
SC
Adults, Elderly. 20 mcg once daily
into the thigh or abdominal wall.

CONTRAINDICATIONS
Serum calcium above normal
level, those at increased risk for
osteosarcoma (Paget disease,
unexplained elevations of alkaline
phosphatase, open epiphyses, prior
radiation therapy that includes the
skeleton), hypercalcemic disorder
(e.g., hyperparathyroidism),
hypersensitivity to teriparatide
or any of the components of the
formulation.

INTERACTIONS
Drug
Digoxin: May increase serum digoxin concentration.
Herbal
None known.
Food
None known.

DIAGNOSTIC TEST EFFECTS
May increase serum calcium.

Ⓓ IV INCOMPATIBILITIES
Do not mix with other medications.

SIDE EFFECTS
Occasional
Leg cramps, nausea, dizziness, headache, orthostatic hypotension, increased heart rate.

SERIOUS REACTIONS
• None known.
WARNINGS
In animal studies, teriparatide has been associated with an increase in osteosarcoma.

PRECAUTIONS & CONSIDERATIONS
Caution is warranted in patients with bone metastases, cardiovascular disease, history of skeletal malignancies, metabolic bone diseases other than osteoporosis, and concurrent therapy with digoxin. Be aware that teriparatide use for more than 2 yr is not recommended. Teriparatide should be used in women who have passed menopause and cannot become pregnant or breastfeed. Teriparatide is not indicated for Children. Teriparatide may cause fast heartbeat, dizziness, lightheadedness, and fainting. Avoid alcohol and tasks that require mental alertness and change positions slowly. Signs of toxicity are rash, nausea, dizziness, and leg cramps.

Storage
Refrigerate and minimize the time out of the refrigerator. Do not freeze. Discard if frozen or if solid particles appear or if the solution is cloudy or colored.
Administration
Administer SC injection into the thigh or abdominal wall. Administration sites should be rotated. For the first administration, patients should sit or lie down to minimize hypotension.

Testosterone
tess-toss′ter-one
(Andriol [CAN], Androderm, AndroGel, Andropository [CAN], Delatestryl, Depotest [CAN], Depo-Testosterone, Everone [CAN], Striant, Testim, Testoderm, Testoprel, Virilon IM [CAN])
Do not confuse testosterone with testolactone.

CATEGORY AND SCHEDULE
Pregnancy Risk Category: X

Classification: Androgens, hormones/hormone modifiers
Restrictions: C-III

MECHANISM OF ACTION
A primary endogenous androgen that promotes growth and development of male sex organs and maintains secondary sex characteristics in androgen-deficient males. *Therapeutic Effect:* Helps relieve androgen deficiency.

PHARMACOKINETICS
Well absorbed after IM administration. Protein binding: 98%. Undergoes first-pass

metabolism in the liver. Excreted primarily in urine. Unknown whether removed by hemodialysis. *Half-life:* 10-100 min.

AVAILABILITY

Cypionate Injection (Depo-Testosterone): 100 mg/mL, 200 mg/mL.
Ethanate Injection (Delatestryl): 200 mg/mL.
Kit (Prescription Compounding) (First Testosterone): 100 mg/mL mixed to cream or gel
Subcutaneous Pellets (Testopel): 75 mg.
Topical Gel (AndroGel): 25 mg/2.5 g, 50 mg/5 g.
Topical Gel (Testim): 50 mg/5 g.
Transdermal Patch (Androderm): 2.5 mg/day, 5 mg/day.
Transdermal Patch (Testoderm): 4 mg/day, 6 mg/day.
Buccal (Striant): 30 mg.

INDICATIONS AND DOSAGES
▶ **Male hypogonadism**
IM
Adults. 50-400 mg q2-4wk.
Adolescents. Initially 40-50 mg/m²/ dose monthly until growth rate falls to prepubertal levels. 100 mg/m²/dose until growth ceases. Maintanence virilizing dose: 100 mg/m²/dose twice a month.
SC (PELLETS)
Adults, Adolescents. 150-450 mg q3-6mo.
TRANSDERMAL (PATCH [TESTODERM])
Adults, Elderly. Start therapy with 6 mg/day patch. Apply patch to scrotal area.
TRANSDERMAL (PATCH [TESTODERM TTS])
Adults, Elderly. Apply TTS patch (5 mg/day) to arm, back, or upper buttocks.

TRANDERMAL (PATCH [ANDRODERM])
Adults, Elderly. Start therapy with 5 mg/day patch applied at night. Apply patch to abdomen, back, thighs, or upper arms.
TRANSDERMAL (GEL [ANDROGEL])
Adults, Elderly. Initial dose of 5 mg of 1% gel delivers 50 mg testosterone and is applied once daily to the abdomen, shoulders, or upper arms. May increase to 7.5 g, then to 10 g, if necessary.
TRANSDERMAL (GEL [TESTIM])
Adults, Elderly. Initial dose of 5 g delivers 50 mg testosterone and is applied once a day to the shoulders or upper arms. May increase to 10 g.
BUCCAL SYSTEM (STRIANT)
Adults, Elderly. 30 mg q12h.
▶ **Delayed puberty**
IM
Adults. 50-200 mg q2-4wk.
Adolescents. 40-50 mg/m²/dose every month for 6 mo.
SC (PELLETS)
Adults, Adolescents. 150-450 mg q3-6mo.
▶ **Breast carcinoma**
IM (AQUEOUS)
Adults. 50-100 mg 3 times a week.
IM (CYPIONATE OR ETHANATE)
Adults. 200-400 mg q2-4wk.
IM (PROPIONATE)
Adults. 50-100 mg 3 times a week.

CONTRAINDICATIONS
Cardiac impairment, hypercalcemia, pregnancy, prostate or breast cancer in males, severe hepatic or renal disease.

INTERACTIONS
Drug
Hepatotoxic medications: May increase the risk of hepatotoxicity.
Oral anticoagulants: May increase the effects of oral anticoagulants.

Herbal
None known.
Food
None known.

DIAGNOSTIC TEST EFFECTS

May increase blood hemoglobin level and hematocrit, as well as serum LDL, alkaline phosphatase, bilirubin, calcium, potassium, sodium, and AST (SGOT) levels. May decrease serum HDL level.

SIDE EFFECTS

Frequent
Gynecomastia, acne.
Females: Hirsutism, amenorrhea or other menstrual irregularities, deepening of voice, clitoral enlargement that may not be reversible when drug is discontinued.
Occasional
Edema, nausea, insomnia, oligospermia, priapism, male-pattern baldness, bladder irritability, hypercalcemia (in immobilized patients or those with breast cancer), hypercholesterolemia, inflammation and pain at IM injection site.
Transdermal: Pruritus, erythema, skin irritation.
Rare
Polycythemia (with high dosage), hypersensitivity.

SERIOUS REACTIONS

• Peliosis hepatitis (presence of blood-filled cysts in parenchyma of liver), hepatic neoplasms, and hepatocellular carcinoma have been associated with prolonged high-dose therapy.
• Anaphylactic reactions occur rarely.

PRECAUTIONS & CONSIDERATIONS

Caution is warranted in patients with diabetes and hepatic or renal impairment. Testosterone use is contraindicated during breastfeeding. Use testosterone with caution in children because its safety and efficacy have not been established. Testosterone use in elderly patients may increase the risk of hyperplasia or stimulate growth of occult prostate carcinoma. Avoid taking any other medications, including OTC drugs, without first consulting the physician. Consume a diet high in calories and protein; food may be better tolerated if small, frequent meals are eaten.

Notify the physician of weight gain of ≥5 lb/wk, acne, nausea, vomiting, or foot swelling. Females should report deepening of voice, hoarseness, or menstrual irregularities; males should report difficulty urinating, frequent erections, or gynecomastia. Blood hemoglobin and hematocrit, BP, intake and output, weight, serum cholesterol, electrolyte levels, and liver function tests should be monitored. Hand or wrist radiographs should be obtained when using the drug in prepubertal children.

Storage
IM formulations should be kept refrigerated. Other formulations may be kept at room temperature.

Administration
Do not give testosterone IV. For IM use, inject testosterone deep into the gluteal muscle. Warming and shaking redissolves crystals that may form in long-acting preparations. A wet needle may cause the solution to become cloudy; this does not affect potency.

Apply Testoderm to clean, dry scrotal skin that has been dry-shaved for optimal skin contact. Apply Testoderm TTS to the arm, back, or upper buttocks. Apply Androderm to clean, dry skin on the back, abdomen, upper arms, or thighs. Do not apply it to the scrotum, bony prominences, such as the shoulder; or oily, damaged, or irritated skin. Do not apply Androderm to the same site for 7 days.

Apply the transdermal gel to clean, dry, intact skin of shoulder or upper arm, preferably in the morning. Androgel may also be applied to the abdomen. Open the packet, squeeze the entire contents into the palm of the hand, and apply at once to the affected site. Allow the gel to dry. Do not apply the gel to the genital areas.

Apply Striant to the gum area above the incisor tooth, alternating sides of the mouth with each application. Striant is not affected by consumption of alcohol or food, gum chewing, or tooth brushing. Remove Striant product before placing the new one.

Tetracaine

tet′ra-cane
(Ametop [CAN], Pontocaine, Pontocaine Niphanoid)
Do not confuse with procaine, lidocaine.

CATEGORY AND SCHEDULE
Pregnancy Risk Category: C

Classification: Anesthetics, local, spinal

MECHANISM OF ACTION
Tetracaine causes a reversible blockade of nerve conduction by decreasing nerve membrane permeability to sodium. *Therapeutic Effect:* Local anesthetic.

PHARMACOKINETICS
Systemic absorption of tetracaine is variable. Metabolized by plasma pseudocholinesterasis. Excreted in the urine.

AVAILABILITY
Solution for Injection:
1% (Pontocaine).
Powder for Reconstitution: 20 mg (Pontocaine Niphanoid).
Solution, Ophthalmic: 0.5%.
Solution, Topical: 2%.

INDICATIONS AND DOSAGES
▸ **Anesthetize lower abdomen**
SPINAL
Adults. 3-4 mL (9-12 mg) of a 0.3% solution
▸ **Anesthetize perineum**
SPINAL
Adults. 1-2 mL (3-6 mg) of a 0.3% solution.
▸ **Anesthetize upper abdomen**
SPINAL
Adults. 5 mL (15 mg) of a 0.3% solution.
▸ **Obstetric anesthesia, low spinal (saddle block) anesthesia**
SPINAL
Adults. 1-2 mL (2-4 mg) of a 0.2% solution.
▸ **Anesthesia of the perineum**
INTRATHECAL
Adults. 0.5 mL (5 mg) as a 1% solution, diluted with equal amount of cerebrospinal fluid (CSF) or 10% dextrose injection.
▸ **Anesthesia of the perineum and lower extremeties**
INTRATHECAL
Adults. 1 mL (10 mg) as a 1% solution, diluted with equal amount of CSF or 10% dextrose injection.
▸ **Anesthesia up to the costal margin**
INTRATHECAL
Adults. 1.5-2 mL (15-20 mg) as a 1% solution, diluted with equal amount of CSF.

T

▸ **Topical anesthesia**
TOPICAL
Adults. Apply to the affected areas as needed. Maximum dosage is 28 g per 24 h.
Children. Apply to the affected areas as needed. Maximum dosage is 7 g in a 24-h period.
▸ **Topical anesthesia of nose and throat, abolish laryngeal and esophageal reflexes before diagnostic procedure**
TOPICAL
Adults. Direct application of a 0.25% or 0.5% topical solution or by oral inhalation of a nebulized 0.5% solution. Total dose should not exceed 20 mg.
▸ **Mild pain, burning or pruritis associated with herpes labialis (cold sores or fever blisters)**
TOPICAL
Adults and children 2 yr and older. Apply to the affected area no more than 3-4 times a day.
▸ **Ophthalmic anesthesia**
TOPICAL
Adults. 1-2 drops of a 0.5% solution.

CONTRAINDICATIONS

Hypersensitivity, to ester local anesthetics, sulfites, PABA, infection or inflammation at the injection site, bacteremia, platelet abnormalities, thrombocytopenia, increased bleeding time, uncontrolled coagulopathy, or anticoagulant therapy, sulfonamide therapy.

INTERACTIONS
Drug
Anihypertensives, nitrates, vasodilators: Additive hypotensive effects.
Cholinesterase inhibitors: Local anesthetics can antagonize the effects of these medications.
Class IA and III antiarrhythmics, macrolide and ketolide antibiotics, quinolone antibiotics, alfuzosin, arsenic trioxide, astemizole, beta agonists, amoxapine, bepridil, cisapride, chloroquine, clozapine, cyclobenzaprine, dolasetron, droperidol, flecainide, halofantrine, haloperidol, halogenated anesthetics, levomethadyl, maprotiline, methadone, octreotide, palonosetron, pentamidine, chlorpromazine, fluphenazine, mesoridazine, pimozide, probucol, propafenone, risperidone, sertindole, tacrolimus, terfenadine, vardenafil, ziprasidone: May increase the risk of cardiotoxicity, including QT prolongation.
Local anesthetics: The toxic effects are additive.
Neuromuscular blockers: Local anesthetics prolong and enhance the effects of these medications.
MAOIs: Increased risk of hypotension.
Opiate agonists: May lead to increased depression of the central nervous system (CNS).
Herbal
None known.
Food
None known.

DIAGNOSTIC TEST EFFECTS
None known.

🖗 IV COMPATIBILITIES
Physiologic saline solution, dextrose solution, CSF.

SIDE EFFECTS
Frequent
Burning, stinging, or tenderness, skin rash, itching, redness, or inflammation, numbness or tingling of the face or mouth, pain at the injection site, sensitivity to light, swelling of the eye or eyelid, watering or the eyes, acute ocular

pain and ocular irritation (burning, stinging, or redness).

Occasional

Paresthesias, weakness and paralysis of lower extremity, hypotension, high or total spinal block, urinary retention or incontinence, fecal incontinence, headache, back pain, septic meningitis, meningismus, arachnoiditis, shivering cranial nerve palsies due to traction on nerves from loss of CSF, and loss of perineal sensation and sexual function.

Rare

Anxiety, restlessness, difficulty breathing, shortness of breath, dizziness, drowsiness, lightheadedness, nausea, vomiting, seizures (convulsions), slow, irregular heartbeat (palpitations), swelling of the face or mouth, skin rash, itching (hives), tremors, visual impairment.

SERIOUS REACTIONS

• Tetracaine-induced CNS toxicity usually presents with symptoms of a CNS stimulation, such as anxiety, apprehension, restlessness, nervousness, disorientation, confusion, dizziness, tinnitus, blurred vision, tremor, or seizures. Subsequently, depressive symptoms may occur, including drowsiness, respiratory arrest, or coma.

• Depression or cardiac excitability and contractility may cause AV block, ventricular arrhythmias, or cardiac arrest. Symptoms of local anesthetic CNS toxicity, such as dizziness, tongue numbness, visual impairment or disturbances, and muscular twitching appear to occur before cardiotoxic effects. Cardiotoxic effects include angina, QT prolongation, PR prolongation, atrial fibrillation, sinus bradycardia, hypotension, palpitations, and cardiovascular collapse. Maternal

seizures and cardiovascular collapse may occur following paracervical block in early pregnancy as a result of rapid systemic absorption.

• Tetracaine is more likely than any other topical anesthetic to cause contact reactions, including skin rash (unspecified), mucous membrane irritation, erythema, pruritis, urticaria, burning, stinging, edema, or tenderness.

• During labor and obstetric delivery, local anesthetics can cause varying degrees of maternal, fetal, and neonatal toxicities. Fetal heart rate should be monitored continuously because fetal bradycardia may occur in patients receiving tetracaine anesthesia and may be associated with fetal acidosis. Maternal hypotension can result from regional anesthesia; patient position can alleviate this problem. Spinal tetracaine may cause decreased uterine contractility or maternal expulsion efforts and alter the forces of parturition.

PRECAUTIONS & CONSIDERATIONS

Caution is warranted with heart or liver disease, myasthenia gravis, and history of drug allergies. Be aware that it is unknown whether tetracaine crosses the placenta or is distributed in the breast milk. No age-related precautions have been noted in children or elderly patients.

Administration

To apply eye drops, wash hands first. To avoid contamination, do not touch the dropper tip or let it touch the eye or any other surface. Tilt head back, gaze upward, and pull down the lower eyelid to make a pouch. Place dropper directly over eye, and administer the prescribed number of drops. Look downward and gently close eye for 1-2 min. Place one finger at the corner of the eye near

T

the nose and apply gentle pressure. This will prevent the medication from draining away from the eye. Try not to blink initially and do not rub the eye. Do not rinse the dropper. Replace cap after use. If using another kind of eye drop, wait at least 5 min before applying other medications. Administer eye drops before eye ointments to allow the eye drops to enter the eye. The usual dosage is 1 or 2 drops in the affected eye before the procedure.

After applying to the eye, do not rub or wipe the eye until the anesthetic has worn off and feeling in the eye returns. Doing so may cause injury or damage to the eye. The effects of tetracaine last for about 20 min. However, if more than one dose is applied, the effects may last longer. If tetracaine is in contact with fingers, it may cause a rash with dryness and cracking of the skin. If the patient touches the eye after this medicine has been applied, the hands must be washed as soon as possible.

Administration as spinal anesthesia will have specific considerations.

Tetracycline

tet-ra-sye′kleen

(Apo-Tetra [CAN], Latycin [AUS], Mysteclin [AUS], Novotetra [CAN], Nu-Tetra [CAN], Sumycin, Tetrex [AUS])

CATEGORY AND SCHEDULE

Pregnancy Risk Category: D

Classification: Anti-infectives, ophthalmic, topical, antibiotics, tetracyclines, dermatologics

MECHANISM OF ACTION

A tetracycline antibiotic that inhibits bacterial protein synthesis by binding to ribosomes. *Therapeutic Effect:* Bacteriostatic.

PHARMACOKINETICS

Readily absorbed from the GI tract. Protein binding: 30%-60%. Widely distributed. Excreted in urine; eliminated in feces through biliary system. Not removed by hemodialysis. *Half-life:* 6-11 h (increased in impaired renal function).

AVAILABILITY

Capsules: 250 mg, 500 mg.
Oral Suspension: 125 mg/5 mL.
Tablets: 250 mg, 500 mg.

INDICATIONS AND DOSAGES

▸ **Inflammatory acne vulgaris, Lyme disease, mycoplasmal disease, *Legionella* infections, Rocky Mountain spotted fever, chlamydial infections in patients with gonorrhea**
PO
Adults, Elderly. 250-500 mg q6-12h. Duration of therapy and exact dose is based on indication.
Children 8 yr and older.
25-50 mg/kg/day in 4 divided doses. Maximum: 3 g/day.
▸ **Helicobacter pylori infections**
PO
Adults, Elderly. 500 mg 2-4 times a day (in combination with another antibiotic and acid suppressant therapy).
▸ **Dosage in renal impairment**
Dosage interval is modified based on creatinine clearance.

Creatinine Clearance (mL/min)	Dosage Interval
50-80	Usual dose q8-12h
10-50	Usual dose q12-24h
< 10	Usual dose q24h

CONTRAINDICATIONS

Children 8 yr and younger, hypersensitivity to tetracyclines or sulfites.

INTERACTIONS

Drug
Aluminum-, calcium-, or magnesium-containing antacids, iron, zinc, sodium bicarbonate, sucralfate, didanosine, quinapril: May decrease tetracycline absorption.
Retinoic acid derivatives: May enhance retinoic acid's adverse effects.
Carbamazepine, phenobarbital, phenytoin, rifamycin: May decrease tetracycline blood concentration.
Cholestyramine, colestipol: May decrease tetracycline absorption.
Oral contraceptives: May decrease the effects of oral contraceptives.
Warfarin: May increase warfarin's anticoagulant effects.
Herbal
Dong quai, St. John's wort: May increase the risk of photosensitivity.
Food
Dairy products: Inhibit tetracycline absorption.

DIAGNOSTIC TEST EFFECTS

May increase BUN and serum alkaline phosphatase, amylase, bilirubin, AST (SGOT), and ALT (SGPT) levels.

SIDE EFFECTS

Frequent
Dizziness, lightheadedness, diarrhea, nausea, vomiting, abdominal cramps, possibly severe photosensitivity.
Occasional
Pigmentation of skin or mucous membranes, rectal or genital pruritus, stomatitis.

SERIOUS REACTIONS

• Superinfection (especially fungal), anaphylaxis, and benign intracranial hypertension may occur.
• Bulging fontanelles occur rarely in infants.

PRECAUTIONS & CONSIDERATIONS

Caution is warranted with those who cannot avoid the sun or ultraviolet exposure because such exposure can produce a severe photosensitivity reaction. Tetracycline readily crosses the placenta and is distributed in breast milk. Women in the last half of pregnancy should avoid using tetracycline because it may inhibit skeletal growth of the fetus. Tetracycline use is not recommended for children 8 yr and younger because it may cause permanent discoloration of teeth or enamel hypoplasia and may inhibit skeletal growth. No age-related precautions have been noted in elderly patients.

History of allergies, especially to tetracyclines or sulfites, should be determined before drug therapy. Pattern of daily bowel activity, stool consistency, food intake and tolerance, and skin for rash should be assessed. Be alert for signs and symptoms of superinfection, such as anal or genital pruritus, diarrhea, and ulceration or changes of the oral mucosa or tongue. BP and level of consciousness should be monitored because of the potential for increased intracranial pressure.
Administration
! Space drug doses evenly around the clock. Take capsules and tablets with a full glass of water 1 h before or 2 h after a meal. Doses should be separated from antacids; administer 1-2 h before or 4 h after.

Tetrahydrozoline Hydrochloride

tet-ra-hi-droz'o-leen
(Visine, Tyzine, Tyzine Pediatric)

CATEGORY AND SCHEDULE

Pregnancy Risk Category: C

Classification: Decongestants, nasal, ophthalmics

MECHANISM OF ACTION

A vasoconstrictor that stimulates α-adrenergic receptors in sympathetic nervous system. Constricts arterioles. *Therapeutic Effect:* Reduces redness, irritation, and congestion.

PHARMACOKINETICS

May be systemically absorbed. Metabolic, elimination rates unknown.

AVAILABILITY

Nasal Solution: 0.05% (Tyzine Pediatric), 0.1% (Tyzine).
Ophthalmic Solution: 0.05% (Visine, Murine Tear Plus, Opti-Clear, etc.).

INDICATIONS AND DOSAGES

▸ **Relief of itching, minor irritation and to control hyperemia with superficial corneal vascularity**
OPHTHALMIC
Adults, Elderly, Children. 1-2 drops 2-4 times/day.
▸ **Relief of nasal congestion of rhinitis, the common cold, sinusitis, hay fever, or other allergies; reduces swelling and improves visualization for surgery or diagnostic procedures; opens obstructed eustachian ostia with ear inflammation**
INTRANASAL
Adults, Elderly, Children older than 6 yr. 2-4 drops (0.1% solution) or 3-4 sprays (0.1% solution) to each nostril q4-6h (no sooner than q3h).
Children aged 2-6 yr. 2-3 drops (0.05% solution) to each nostril q4-6hr (no sooner than q3h).

CONTRAINDICATIONS

Children < 2 yr of age, the 0.1% nasal solution is contraindicated in children < 6 yr of age, angle-closure glaucoma or other serious eye diseases, hypersensitivity to tetrahydrozyline or any component of the formulation.

INTERACTIONS

Drug
Maprotiline, tricyclic antidepressants: May increase pressor effects.
MAOIs: May cause severe hypertensive reaction.
Herbal
Ma huang: May increase CNS stimulation.
Food
None known.

DIAGNOSTIC TEST EFFECTS

None known.

SIDE EFFECTS

Occasional
Intranasal: Transient burning, stinging, sneezing, dryness of mucosa.
Ophthalmic: Irritation, blurred vision, mydriasis.
Systemic sympathomimetic effects may occur with either route: headache, hypertension, weakness, sweating, palpitations, tremors. Prolonged use may result in rebound congestion.

SERIOUS REACTIONS

• Overdosage may result in CNS depression with drowsiness, decreased body temperature, bradycardia, hypotension, coma, and apnea.

Caution is warranted with cardiac disease, hyperthyroidism, hypertension, diabetes mellitus, cerebral arteriosclerosis, bronchial asthma, and concurrent use of MAOIs. Be aware that safety in pregnancy and lactation has not been established. Safety and efficacy have not been established in children younger than 2 yr. No age-related precautions have been noted in elderly patients.

Storage
Store at room temperature.

Administration
For ophthalmic use, first tilt head backward and look up. Place finger on lower eyelid and pull out until a pocket is formed between eye and lower lid. Hold dropper above pocket and place correct number of drops into pocket. Close eye gently. Apply gentle finger pressure to lacrimal sac (bridge of the nose, inside corner of the eye) for 1-2 min. Remove excess solution around eye with tissue. Discontinue and consult physician immediately if ocular pain or visual changes occur or if condition worsens or continues for > 72 h.

For intranasal use, drops or spray should be administered while in lateral, head-low position or reclining with head tilted back as far as possible. Maintain same position for 5 min. Then add drops/spray to other nostril. Dropper containers should be used by only one person. Tips of dispensers or droppers should be rinsed well with hot water after use. Discontinue and consult physician if rebound congestion occurs.

Thalidomide
thal-e-doe-mide
(Thalomid)

CATEGORY AND SCHEDULE
Pregnancy Risk Category: X

Classification:
Immunomodulators, tumor necrosis factor modulators

MECHANISM OF ACTION
An immunomodulator whose exact mechanism is unknown. Has sedative, anti-inflammatory, and immunosuppressive activity, which may be due to selective inhibition of the production of tumor necrosis factor-α. *Therapeutic Effect:* Improves muscle wasting in HIV patients; reduces local and systemic effects of leprosy.

AVAILABILITY
Capsules: 50 mg, 100 mg, 200 mg.

INDICATIONS AND DOSAGES
▶ **AIDS-related muscle wasting (unlabeled)**
PO
Adults. 100-200 mg a day.
▶ **Leprosy**
PO
Adults, Elderly. Initially, 100-300 mg/day as single bedtime dose, at least 1 h after the evening meal. Continue until active reaction subsides, then reduce dose q2-4 wk in 50-mg increments.
▶ **Multiple myeloma**
PO
Adults. 200 mg a day (as a single bedtime dose, at least 1 h after the evening meal in combination with dextromethorphan on specified days as determined by regimen).

T

OFF-LABEL USES

Behçet syndrome, discoid lupus erythematosus, treatment of Crohn disease, recurrent aphthous ulcers in HIV patients, wasting syndrome associated with HIV or cancer.

CONTRAINDICATIONS

Pregnancy, neutropenia, peripheral neuropathy; sensitivity to thalidomide.

INTERACTIONS

Drug
Alcohol, other CNS depressants: May increase sedative effects.
Medications associated with peripheral neuropathy (such as isoniazid, lithium, metronidazole, phenytoin): May increase peripheral neuropathy.
Medications that decrease effectiveness of hormonal contraceptives (such as carbamazepine, protease inhibitors, rifampin): May decrease the effectiveness of the contraceptive; patient must use two other methods of contraception.
Herbal
Cat's claw, echinacea: May intensify thalidomide's immunosuppressant effects.
Food
None known.

DIAGNOSTIC TEST EFFECTS

None known.

SIDE EFFECTS

Frequent
Somnolence, dizziness, mood changes, constipation, dry mouth, peripheral neuropathy.
Occasional
Increased appetite, weight gain, headache, loss of libido, edema of face and limbs, nausea, alopecia, dry skin, rash, hypothyroidism.

SERIOUS REACTIONS

• Neutropenia, peripheral neuropathy, and thromboembolism occur rarely.
WARNINGS
As a known tetratogen, contraception must be used 4 wks before, during, and 4 wks following discontinuation of thalidomide. Because thromboembolic events have been reported with thalidomide, especially in patients at risk for thromboembolic events, patients should be monitored closely, and prophylactic anticoagulation may be considered. Risk may be greater with concomitant dexamethasone use.

PRECAUTIONS & CONSIDERATIONS

Caution is warranted with history of seizures. Thalidomide is contraindicated in pregnant women. Women of childbearing age should perform a pregnancy test within 24 h before beginning thalidomide therapy and then every 2-4 wks. Avoid consuming alcohol or using other drugs that cause drowsiness during thalidomide therapy. Also avoid tasks that require mental alertness or motor skills until response to the drug has been established.

Notify the physician if symptoms of peripheral neuropathy occur. HIV viral load, nerve conduction studies, and WBC count should be monitored.
Administration
Administer thalidomide with water at least 1 h after the evening meal and, if possible, at bedtime because of the risk of developing somnolence.

Theophylline
thee-off'i-lin
(Aerobin [GERMANY]; Aerodyne
Retard [AUSTRIA]; Afonilum
Forte [GERMANY]; Afonilum Mite
[GERMANY]; Afonilum Retard
[GERMANY]; Almarion [THAILAND];
Armophylline [France];
Asmasalon [PHILIPPINES]; Asperal-T
[Belgium]; Austyn [KOREA];
Bronchoretard [GERMANY];
Bronsolvan [Indonesia]; Cronasma
[GERMANY]; Deo-Q Syrup [KOREA];
Ditenaten [GERMANY]; Elixofilina
[MEXICO, PERU]; Elixophyllin;
Euphylong [ISRAEL, HONG KONG];
Euphylong Retardkaps [GERMANY];
Euphylong SR [PHILIPPINES];
Godafilin [SPAIN]; Lasma [ISRAEL,
ENGLAND]; Nefoben [ARGENTINA];
Neobiphyllin [CHINA]; Neulin
SA [SOUTH AFRICA]; Neulin-SR
[TAIWAN]; Nuelin [PUERTO RICO,
COSTA RICA, DENMARK, DOMINICAN
REPUBLIC, EL SALVADOR, FINLAND,
HONDURAS, MALAYSIA, NORWAY,
PANAMA, PHILIPPINES]; Nuelin SA
[SOUTH AFRICA, ISRAEL, COSTA RICA,
DOMINICAN REPUBLIC, EL SALVADOR,
GUATEMALA, HONDURAS, PANAMA];
Nuelin SR [ISRAEL, AUSTRALIA,
HONG KONG, MALAYSIA, THAILAND];
Pharphylline [NETHERLANDS];
Phylobid [SOUTH AFRICA, INDIA];
Protheo [CHINA]; Pulmidur
[AUSTRIA, GERMANY]; Slo-Bid
Gyrocaps; Quibron-T; Quibron
T SR [US, CANADA, INDONESIA];
Slo-Theo [HONG KONG]; Solosin
[GERMANY]; Somofillina [ITALY];
Teobid [COLOMBIA]; Teoclear
[KOREA]; Teoclear LA [ARGENTINA];
Teofilina Retard [COLOMBIA];
Teolixir [SPAIN]; Teolong [MEXICO];
Teosona [ARGENTINA]; Theo-2
[BELGIUM]; Theo-24; Theo-Bros
[GREECE]; Theochron; Theo-Dur;
Theolair; Theolair SR; Theolair S
[PERU]; Theolan [KOREA, TAIWAN];
Theolin [SINGAPORE]; Theolin SR
[SINGAPORE]; Theolong [JAPAN];
Theomax [SPAIN]; Theon
[SWITZERLAND]; Theo PA [INDIA];
Theoplus [BULGARIA, SINGAPORE,
SPAIN]; Theoplus Retard [AUSTRIA,
GREECE]; Theospirex Retard
[AUSTRIA, SWITZERLAND]; Theostat
LP [FRANCE]; Theotard [ISRAEL];
Theo-Time; Theotrim [ISRAEL];
Theovent LA [HONG KONG]; Theo
von CT [GERMANY]; Tiodilax
[ARGENTINA]; T-Phyl; Truxophyllin;
Tyrex [PERU]; Unicontin-400
Continus [INDIA]; Uni-Dur; Unifyl
Retard [SWITZERLAND]; Uniphyl;
Uniphyl CR [KOREA]; Uniphyllin
[TAIWAN]; UniphyllinContinus
[SOUTH AFRICA]; Xanthium
[SINGAPORE]; Xantivent
[SWITZERLAND])

CATEGORY AND SCHEDULE
Pregnancy risk category: C

Classification: Bronchodilators,
xanthine derivatives

MECHANISM OF ACTION
An antiasthmatic medication
with two distinct actions in the
airways of patients with reversible
obstruction: smooth muscle
relaxation and suppression of the
response of airways to stimuli.
Mechanisms of action are not
known with certainty. Theophylline
is known to increase the force
of contraction of diaphragmatic
muscles by enhancing calcium
uptake through adenosine-mediated
channels. *Therapeutic Effect:*
Causes bronchodilation and
decreased airway reactivity.

PHARMACOKINETICS

The pharmacokinetics of theophylline vary widely among similar patients and cannot be predicted by age, sex, body weight, or other demographic characteristics. Rapidly and completely absorbed after oral administration in solution or immediate-release solid oral dosage form. Distributed freely into fat-free tissues. Extensively metabolized in liver. *Half-life:* 4-8 h.

AVAILABILITY

Capsule, Extended Release: 100 mg (Slo-Bid Gyrocaps); 125 mg; 200 mg (Slo-Bid Gyrocaps); 300 mg (Slo-Bid Gyrocaps).
Elixir: 80 mg/15 mL (Elixophyllin).
Solution, IV: 40 mg/100 mL, 80 mg/100 mL, 160 mg/100 mL, 200 mg/100 mL, 200 mg/50 mL, 320 mg/100 mL, 400 mg/100 mL.
Solution, Oral: 80 mg/15 mL (Truxophyllin).
Tablets: 100 mg.
Tablet, Extended Release: 100 mg (Theo-Dur, Theochron, Theo-Time); 200 mg (Theo-Dur, Theochron, Theo-Time); 300 mg (Theo-Dur, Theochron, Theo-Time); 400 mg (Uni-Dur); 450 mg (Theochron).

INDICATIONS AND DOSAGES
▸ **Chronic asthma/lung diseases**
PO
Adults, Adolescents, Children.
Acute symptoms: 5 mg/kg using immediate-release product.
▸ **Maintenance therapy**
Adults, Children weighing > 45 kg.
10 mg/kg/day (maximum: 300 mg/day) divided q6-8h. After 3 days, increase to 400 mg/day divided q6-8h. After 3 more days, increase to 600 mg/day. Maximum: 800 mg.
IV
5 mg/kg load over 20 min, maintenance 0.25 mg/kg/h (CHF,

elderly), 0.4 mg/kg/h (nonsmokers), 0.7 mg/kg/h (young adult smokers).
Slow titration: Initial dose 16 mg/kg/day or 400 mg daily, whichever is less, doses divided every 6-8 h.
Dosage adjustment after serum theophylline measurement: Serum level 5-10 mcg/mL if symptoms not controlled, increase dose by 25% and recheck in 3 days. Serum level 10-20 mcg/mL, maintain dosage if tolerated, recheck level every 6-12 mo. Serum level 20-25 mcg/mL, decrease dose by 25%, recheck level in 3 days. Serum level 25-30 mcg/mL, skip next dose, decrease dose by 25%, recheck level in 3 days. Serum level > 30 mcg/mL, skip next 2 doses, decrease dose by 50%, recheck level in 3 days.
Children 9-16 yr. 5 mg/kg as a loading dose, maintenance 3 mg/kg every 6 h; IV 5 mg/kg load over 20 min, maintenance 0.7 mg/kg/h.
Children 1-9 yr. 5 mg/kg as a loading dose, maintenance 4 mg/kg every 6 h; IV 5 mg/kg load over 20 min, maintenance 0.8 mg/kg/h.
Infants. $[(0.2 \times$ age in week$) + 5] \times 24$ = 24-h dose in mg; divide into every 8-h dosing (6 wks to 6 mo), every 6-h dosing (6-12 mo); IV 5 mg/kg load over 20 min, maintenance dose in mg/kg/h $[(0.0008 \times$ age in week$) + 0.21]$

OFF-LABEL USES
Apnea, bradycardia of prematurity.

CONTRAINDICATIONS
Hypersensitivity to theophylline or any component of the formulation, active peptic ulcer disease, underlying seizure disorders unless receiving appropriate anticonvulsant medication.

INTERACTIONS
Drug
Adenosine, diazepam, flurazepam, lorazepam, midazolam: May

T

decrease therapeutic effect at adenosine receptors.
Alcohol, allopurinol, cimetidine, ciprofloxacin, clarithromycin, disulfiram, erythromycin, enoxacin, estrogen, fluvoxamine, interferon alpha-A, methotrexate, mexiletine, pentoxifylline, propafenone, propranolol, thiabendazole, ticlopidine, troleandomycin, verapamil: May decrease theophylline clearance.
Aminoglutethimide, carbamazepine, isoproterenol, moricizinel, phenobarbital, phenytoin, rifampin, sulfinpyrazone: May increase theophylline clearance.
Ephedrine: May cause synergistic CNS effects.
Halothane: May cause ventricular arrhythmia.
Ketamine: May decrease seizure threshold.
Lithium: May increase lithium clearance.
Herbal
Capsicum: May increase absorption and effect.
St. John's wort: May increase metabolism of theophylline.
Food
High-fat content meals: May decrease theophylline absorption.
Caffeine, dietary protein, and carbohydrates: May increase the activity and side effects caused by theophylline. Large amounts should be avoided. Low-carbohydrate, high-protein diets, charbroiled beef, and large amounts of cruciferous vegetables (broccoli, Brussels sprouts, cabbage, and cauliflower) can reduce theophylline activity.
Charbroiled foods: May increase elimination of theophylline.

DIAGNOSTIC TEST EFFECTS
None known.

SIDE EFFECTS
Anxiety, dizziness, headache, insomnia, lightheadedness, muscle twitching, restlessness, seizures, dysrhythmias, fluid retention with tachycardia, hypotension, palpitations, pounding heartbeat, sinus tachycardia, anorexia, bitter taste, diarrhea, dyspepsia, gastroesophageal reflux, nausea, vomiting, urinary frequency, increased respiratory rate, flushing, urticaria.

SERIOUS REACTIONS
• Severe toxicity from theophylline overdose is a relatively rare event.

PRECAUTIONS & CONSIDERATIONS
Caution is warranted in patients with peptic ulcer, hyperthyroidism, seizure disorders, hypertension, and cardiac arrhythmias (excluding bradyarrhythmias). Be aware that dose adjustments must be made for smokers. Be aware that theophylline crosses the placenta and is distributed in breast milk. A dose reduction should be used when starting theophylline in elderly patients. Avoid excessive amounts of caffeine as well as extremes in dietary protein and carbohydrates. Charbroiled foods may increase elimination and reduce the half-life.

Nervousness, restlessness, and increased heart rate may occur during theophylline therapy. Signs and symptoms of theophylline toxicity are persistent; repetitive vomiting and serum theophylline level should be drawn and dose should be withheld.
Administration
Take this medication with a full glass of water on an empty stomach, at least 1 h before or 2 h after a meal. Do not chew or crush the extended-release tablets; swallow them whole. Extended-release capsules may be swallowed whole or opened and the contents mixed with soft food and swallowed without chewing.

Thiabendazole
thye-a-ben′da-zole
(Mintezol)

CATEGORY AND SCHEDULE
Pregnancy Risk Category: C

Classification: Antihelmintics

MECHANISM OF ACTION
An antihelmintic agent that inhibits helminth-specific mitochondrial fumarate reductase. *Therapeutic Effect:* Suppresses parasite production.

PHARMACOKINETICS
Rapidly and well absorbed from the GI tract. Rapidly metabolized in liver. Excreted primarily in urine; partially eliminated in feces. Removed *Half-life:* 1.2 h.

AVAILABILITY
Suspension: 500 mg/5 mL (Mintezol).
Tablets: 500 mg (Mintezol).

INDICATIONS AND DOSAGES
▸ **Cutaneous larva migrans**
Adults, Children weighing ≥ 68 kg. 1.5 g twice daily for 2-5 days. Maximum: 3 g.
Children weighing 57-67 kg. 1.25 g twice daily for 2-5 days.
Children weighing 46-56 kg. 1 g twice daily for 2-5 days.
Children weighing 35-45 kg. 750 mg twice daily for 2-5 days or 25 mg/kg twice daily for 2-5 days.
Children weighing 23-34 kg. 500 mg twice daily for 2-5 days.
Children weighing 13.6-22 kg. 250 mg twice daily for 2-5 days.
▸ **Intestinal roundworms and strongyloidiasis**
Adults, Children weighing ≥ 68 kg. 1.5 g twice daily for 2 days. Maximum: 3 g.

Children weighing 57-67 kg. 1.25 g twice daily for 2 days.
Children weighing 46-56 kg. 1 g twice daily for 2 days.
Children weighing 35-45 kg. 750 mg twice daily for 2 days or 25 mg/kg twice daily for 2 days.
Children weighing 23-34 kg. 500 mg twice daily for 2 days.
Children weighing 13.6-22 kg. 250 mg twice daily for 2 days.
▸ **Trichinosis**
Adults, Children weighing ≥ 68 kg. 1.5 g twice daily for 2-4 days.
Children weighing 57-67 kg. 1.25 g twice daily for 2-4 days.
Children weighing 46-56 kg. 1 g twice daily for 2-4 days.
Children weighing 35-45 kg. 750 mg twice daily for 2-4 days or 25 mg/kg twice daily for 2-4 days.
Children weighing 23-34 kg. 500 mg twice daily for 2-4 days.
Children weighing 13.6-22 kg. 250 mg twice daily for 2-4 days. Maximum: 3 g.
▸ **Visceral larva migrans**
Adults, Children weighing ≥ 68 kg. 1.5 g twice daily for 7 days. Maximum: 3 g.
Children weighing 57-67 kg. 1.25 g twice daily for 7 days.
Children weighing 46-56 kg. 1 g twice daily for 7 days.
Children weighing 35-45 kg. 750 mg twice daily for 7 days or 25 mg/kg twice daily for 7 days.
Children weighing 23-34 kg. 500 mg twice daily for 7 days.
Children weighing 13.6-22 kg. 250 mg twice daily for 7 days.

OFF-LABEL USES
Angiostrongyliasis, capillaria infestations, dracunculus infestations, pediculosis capitis, tinea infections.

CONTRAINDICATIONS

Prophylactic treatment of pinworm infestation, hypersensitivity to thiabendazole or its components.

INTERACTIONS

Drug
Theophylline, other xanthines:
May increase levels of theophylline or other xanthines.
Herbal and Food
None known.

DIAGNOSTIC TEST EFFECTS

None known.

SIDE EFFECTS

Occasional
Dizziness, drowsiness, nausea, vomiting, diarrhea.
Rare
Erythema multiform, liver damage.

SERIOUS REACTIONS

• Overdose includes symptoms of altered mental status and visual problems.
• Erythema multiform, liver damage, and Stevens-Johnsons syndrome occur rarely.

PRECAUTIONS & CONSIDERATIONS

Caution is necessary in patients with malnutrition or anemia, mixed helminthic infections, liver or renal dysfunction. Thiabendazole is not for prophylactic use, and it is not suitable for treatment of mixed infections with ascaris. It is unknown whether thiabendazole crosses the placenta and is distributed in breast milk. No age-related precautions have been noted in children or elderly patients.

Urine may be red-brown or dark during drug therapy. Thiabendazole may also cause drowsiness. Tasks requiring mental alertness or motor skills should be avoided.

Chew tablets before swallowing.
Take with meals or milk to minimize GI irritation.

Thiamine (vitamin B₁)

thy′a-min
(Beta-Sol [AUS], Betaxin [CAN], Thiamilate)

CATEGORY AND SCHEDULE

Pregnancy Risk Category: A (C if used in doses above recommended daily allowance)
OTC (tablets)

Classification: Vitamins/minerals

MECHANISM OF ACTION

A water-soluble vitamin that combines with adenosine triphosphate in the liver, kidneys, and leukocytes to form thiamine diphosphate, a coenzyme that is necessary for carbohydrate metabolism. *Therapeutic Effect:* Prevents and reverses thiamine deficiency.

PHARMACOKINETICS

Readily absorbed from the GI tract, primarily in duodenum, after IM administration. Widely distributed. Metabolized in the liver. Primarily excreted in urine.

AVAILABILITY

Tablets: 50 mg, 100 mg, 250 mg, 500 mg.
Injection: 100 mg/mL.

INDICATIONS AND DOSAGES

▸ **Dietary supplement**
PO
Adults, Elderly. 1-2 mg/day.
Children. 0.5-1 mg/day.
Infants. 0.2-0.3 mg/day.

▸ **Thiamine deficiency**
PO
Adults, Elderly. 5-30 mg/day, as a single dose or in 3 divided doses, for 1 mo.
Children. 10-50 mg/day in 3 divided doses for 1 mo.

▸ **Thiamine deficiency in patients who are critically ill or have malabsorption syndrome**
IV, IM
Adults, Elderly. 5-30 mg, 3 times a day for 1 mo.
Children. 10-25 mg/day for 1 mo.

▸ **Treatment of Wernicke/Korsakoff syndrome**
IV
Adults, Elderly. Initially, 100 mg, followed by 50-100 mg/day until normal dietary intake of thiamine is established.

CONTRAINDICATIONS
None known.

INTERACTIONS
Drug
None known.
Herbal
None known.
Food
None known.

DIAGNOSTIC TEST EFFECTS
None known.

⍟ IV COMPATIBILITIES
Famotidine (Pepcid), multivitamins.

SIDE EFFECTS
Frequent
Pain, induration, and tenderness at IM injection site.

SERIOUS REACTIONS
• IV administration may result in a rare, severe hypersensitivity reaction marked by a feeling of warmth, pruritus, urticaria, weakness, diaphoresis, nausea, restlessness, tightness in throat, angioedema, cyanosis, pulmonary edema, GI tract bleeding, and cardiovascular collapse.

PRECAUTIONS & CONSIDERATIONS
Caution is warranted with Wernicke encephalopathy. Thiamine crosses the placenta; it is unknown whether it is excreted in breast milk. No age-related precautions have been noted in children or elderly patients. Consuming foods rich in thiamine, including legumes, nuts, organ meats, pork, rice bran, seeds, wheat germ, whole grain and enriched cereals, and yeast, is encouraged.

Urine may appear bright yellow during therapy. Before and during treatment, signs and symptoms of thiamine deficiency, including peripheral neuropathy, ataxia, hyporeflexia, muscle weakness, nystagmus, ophthalmoplegia, confusion, peripheral edema, bounding arterial pulse, and tachycardia, should be assessed.

Administration
! IM and IV administration routes are used only in acutely ill patients and in those who are unresponsive to the PO route, such as those with malabsorption syndrome. The IM route is preferred over the IV route. The solution may be given by IV push or may be added to most IV solutions and given as an IV infusion.

IM injection may cause discomfort. Discomfort may be reduced by applying cool compresses.

Thioridazine
thye-or-rid′a-zeen
(Aldazine [AUS], Apo-Thioridazine
[CAN], Mellaril, Melleril [AUS],
Thioridazine Intensol)
**Do not confuse thioridazine with
thiothixene or Thorazine, or
Mellaril with Mebaral.**

CATEGORY AND SCHEDULE
Pregnancy Risk Category: C

Classification: Antipsychotics,
phenothiazines

MECHANISM OF ACTION
A phenothiazine that blocks
dopamine at postsynaptic
receptor sites. Possesses strong
anticholinergic and sedative effects.
Therapeutic Effect: Suppresses
behavioral response in psychosis;
reduces locomotor activity and
aggressiveness.

AVAILABILITY
*Oral Solution (Concentrate
[Thioridazine Intensol]):* 30 mg/mL.
Tablets (Melleril): 10 mg, 15 mg,
25 mg, 50 mg, 100 mg, 150 mg,
200 mg.

INDICATIONS AND DOSAGES
▶ **Psychosis**
PO
*Adults, Elderly, Children 12 yr and
older.* Initially, 10-50 mg 3 times
a day; dosage increased gradually
q4-7 days. Maximum: 300 mg/day.
Children aged 2-11 yr. Initially,
0.5 mg/kg/day in 2-3 divided doses.
Maximum: 3 mg/kg/day.

OFF-LABEL USES
Treatment of behavioral problems
in children, dementia, depressive
neurosis.

CONTRAINDICATIONS
Angle-closure glaucoma, blood
dyscrasias, cardiac arrhythmias,
cardiac or hepatic impairment,
concurrent use of drugs that prolong
QT interval, severe central nervous
system (CNS) depression.

INTERACTIONS
Drug
Alcohol, other CNS depressants:
May increase respiratory depression
and the hypotensive effects of
thioridazine.
Antithyroid agents: May increase
the risk of agranulocytosis.
**Extrapyramidal symptom–
producing medications:** May increase
the risk of extrapyramidal symptoms.
Hypotension-producing agents:
May increase hypotension.
Levodopa: May decrease the effects
of levodopa.
Lithium: May decrease the
absorption of thioridazine and
produce adverse neurologic effects.
MAOIs, tricyclic antidepressants:
May increase the anticholinergic and
sedative effects of thioridazine.
Herbal
None known.
Food
None known.

DIAGNOSTIC TEST EFFECTS
May cause ECG changes.

SIDE EFFECTS
Occasional
Drowsiness during early therapy,
dry mouth, blurred vision, lethargy,
constipation or diarrhea, nasal
congestion, peripheral edema, urine
retention.
Rare
Ocular changes, altered skin
pigmentation (in those taking
high doses for prolonged periods),
photosensitivity, darkening of urine.

T

SERIOUS REACTIONS
• Prolonged QT interval may produce torsades de pointes, a form of ventricular tachycardia, and sudden death.

PRECAUTIONS & CONSIDERATIONS
Caution is warranted in patients with benign prostatic hypertrophy, decreased GI motility, seizures, urinary retention, and visual problems. Urine may darken and drowsiness and dizziness may occur but generally subsides with continued therapy. Alcohol, tasks requiring mental alertness or motor skills, and exposure to artificial light and sunlight should be avoided. BP, CBC, ECG, serum potassium level, and liver function test results, including serum alkaline phosphatase, bilirubin, AST (SGOT), and ALT (SGPT) levels, should be monitored. Extrapyramidal symptoms should be assessed.
Administration
Avoid skin contact with the oral solution because it can cause contact dermatitis. Full therapeutic effect may take up to 6 wks to appear. Do not abruptly discontinue the drug after long-term use.

Thiothixene
thye-oh-thix′een
(Navane)
Do not confuse thiothixene with thioridazine.

CATEGORY AND SCHEDULE
Pregnancy Risk Category: C

Classification: Antipsychotics

MECHANISM OF ACTION
An antipsychotic that blocks postsynaptic dopamine receptor sites in brain. Has α-adrenergic blocking effects and depresses the release of hypothalamic and hypophyseal hormones. *Therapeutic Effect:* Suppresses psychotic behavior.

PHARMACOKINETICS
Well absorbed from the GI tract after IM administration. Widely distributed. Metabolized in the liver. Excreted primarily in urine. Unknown whether removed by hemodialysis. *Half-life:* 34 h.

AVAILABILITY
Capsules: 1 mg, 2 mg, 5 mg, 10 mg, 20 mg.
Oral Concentrate: 5 mg/mL.
Injection: 5 mg of thiothixene and 59.6 mg of mannitol per mL when reconstituted with 2.2 mL of sterile water for injection.

INDICATIONS AND DOSAGES
▸ **Psychosis**
PO
Adults, Elderly, Children older than 12 yr. Initially, 2 mg 3 times a day or 5 mg twice daily. Maximum: 60 mg/day.
IM
Adults, Elderly. Initially, 4 mg 2-4 times a day. Maximum: 30 mg/day.

CONTRAINDICATIONS
Blood dyscrasias, circulatory collapse, central nervous system (CNS) depression, coma, history of seizures.

INTERACTIONS
Drug
Alcohol, other CNS depressants: May increase CNS and respiratory depression and the hypotensive effects of thiothixene.
Extrapyramidal symptom–producing medications: May increase the risk of extrapyramidal symptoms.

Levodopa: May inhibit the effects of levodopa.
Quinidine: May increase cardiac effects.
Herbal
Kava kava, St. John's wort, valerian: May increase CNS depression.
Food
None known.

DIAGNOSTIC TEST EFFECTS

May decrease serum uric acid level.

SIDE EFFECTS

Expected
Hypotension, dizziness, syncope (occur frequently after first injection, occasionally after subsequent injections, and rarely with oral form).
Frequent
Transient drowsiness, dry mouth, constipation, blurred vision, nasal congestion.
Occasional
Diarrhea, peripheral edema, urine retention, nausea.
Rare
Ocular changes, altered skin pigmentation (in those taking high doses for prolonged periods), photosensitivity.

SERIOUS REACTIONS

• The most common extrapyramidal reaction is akathisia, characterized by motor restlessness and anxiety. Akinesia, marked by rigidity, tremor, increased salivation, masklike facial expression, and reduced voluntary movements, occurs less frequently. Dystonias, including torticollis, opisthotonos, and oculogyric crisis, occur rarely.
• Tardive dyskinesia, characterized by tongue protrusion, puffing of the cheeks, and chewing or puckering of the mouth, occurs rarely but may be irreversible. Elderly women have a greater risk of developing this reaction.

• Grand mal seizures may occur in epileptic patients, especially those receiving the drug by IM administration.
• Neuroleptic malignant syndrome occurs rarely.

PRECAUTIONS & CONSIDERATIONS

Caution is warranted in patients with alcohol withdrawal, dementia-related psychosis in the elderly, severe cardiovascular disorders, glaucoma, benign prostatic hyperplasia, and exposure to extreme heat. Thiothixene crosses the placenta and is distributed in breast milk. Children are more prone to develop extrapyramidal and neuromuscular symptoms, especially dystonias. Elderly patients are more prone to anticholinergic effects (such as dry mouth), extrapyramidal symptoms, orthostatic hypotension, and increased sedation.

Drowsiness and dizziness may occur but generally subside with continued therapy. Alcohol, tasks requiring mental alertness or motor skills, and exposure to artificial light and sunlight should be avoided. Notify the physician if fluid retention, fever, or visual disturbances occur. Pattern of daily bowel activity and stool consistency, BP, and signs of extrapyramidal reactions should be assessed.
Administration
Take thiothixene without regard to food. Avoid skin contact with the oral solution because it can cause contact dermatitis. The drug's full therapeutic effect may take up to 6 wks to appear.

For IM use, reconstitute drug with 2.2 mL of sterile water.

T

Thyroid
thye′roid
(Armour Thyroid, Nature-Thyroid
NT, Westhyroid)

CATEGORY AND SCHEDULE
Pregnancy Risk Category: A

Classification: Hormones/
hormone modifiers, thyroid agents

MECHANISM OF ACTION
A natural hormone derived from
animal sources, usually beef or pork,
that is involved in normal metabolism,
growth, and development, especially
the central nervous system (CNS)
of infants. Possesses catabolic and
anabolic effects. Provides both
levothyroxine and liothyronine
hormones. *Therapeutic Effect:*
Increases basal metabolic rate,
enhances gluconeogenesis, stimulates
protein synthesis.

PHARMACOKINETICS
Partially absorbed from the GI
tract. Protein binding: 99%. Widely
distributed. Metabolized in liver
to active, liothyronine (T_3), and
inactive, reverse triiodothyronine
(rT_3), metabolites. Eliminated by
biliary excretion. *Half-life:* 2-7 days.

AVAILABILITY
Capsules: 15 mg, 30 mg, 60 mg,
90 mg, 120 mg, 180 mg, 240 mg.
Tablets: 30 mg, 32.5 mg, 60 mg,
65 mg, 120 mg, 130 mg, 180 mg,
15 mg, 30 mg, 60 mg, 90 mg,
120 mg, 180 mg, 240 mg, 300 mg
(Armour Thyroid). 32.4 mg,
64.8 mg, 129.6 mg, 194.4 mg
(Nature-Thyroid NT, Westhyroid).

INDICATIONS AND DOSAGES
▸ **Hypothyroidism**

PO
Adults, Elderly. Initially, 15-30 mg.
May increase by 15 mg increments
q2-4wk. Maintenance: 60-130 mg/day.
Use 15 mg in patients with
cardiovascular disease or myxedema.
Children 12 yr and older. 90 mg/day.
Children 6-12 yr. 60-90 mg/day.
Children older than 1-5 yr.
45-60 mg/day.
Children older than 6-12 mo.
30-45 mg/day.
Children 3 mo. and younger.
15-30 mg/day.

CONTRAINDICATIONS
Uncontrolled adrenal cortical
insufficiency, untreated thyrotoxicosis,
treatment of obesity, uncontrolled
angina, uncontrolled hypertension,
uncontrolled myocardial infarction,
and hypersensitivity to any
component of the formulations.

INTERACTIONS
Drug
Cholestyramine, colestipol: May
decrease absorption of thyroid
hormones.
Estrogens, oral contraceptives: May
decrease effects of thyroid hormones.
Insulin, oral hypoglycemics: May
decrease effects of insulin and oral
hypoglycemics.
Oral anticoagulants: May increase
hypoprothrombinemic effects of oral
anticoagulants
Tricyclic antidepressants: May
increase risk of toxicity of both drugs.
Herbal
Bugleweed: May decrease effects of
thyroid hormones.
Food
None known.

SIDE EFFECTS
Rare
Dry skin, GI intolerance, skin rash,
hives, severe headache.

T

SERIOUS REACTIONS
• Excessive dosage produces signs and symptoms of hyperthyroidism, including weight loss, palpitations, increased appetite, tremors, nervousness, tachycardia, hypertension, headache, insomnia, and menstrual irregularities.
• Cardiac arrhythmias occur rarely.

PRECAUTIONS & CONSIDERATIONS
Caution is warranted in patients with angina pectoris, hypertension, or other cardiovascular disease as well as adrenal insufficiency, cardiovascular disease, coronary artery disease, diabetes insipidus, and diabetes mellitus. Thyroid hormone does not cross the placenta and is minimally excreted in breast milk. No age-related precautions have been noted in children. Be aware that thyroid hormone should be used cautiously in neonates in interpreting thyroid function tests. Elderly patients may be more sensitive to thyroid effects. Individualized dosages are recommended for this population. Signs of nervousness or tremors should be reported.
Administration
The following are equivalent doses between the thyroid preparations: thyroid 60 mg, thyroglobulin 65 mg, Thyroid Strong 43 mg, levothyroxine 0.1 mg, liothyronine 25 mcg, and liotrix 50-60 mcg of levothyroxine and 12.5-15 mcg of liothyronine.

Begin therapy with small doses and increase the dosage gradually, as prescribed. Take at the same time each day to maintain hormone levels. Take on an empty stomach.

Tiagabine
ti-ah-ga'bean
(Gabitril)

CATEGORY AND SCHEDULE
Pregnancy Risk Category: C

Classification: Anticonvulsants

MECHANISM OF ACTION
An anticonvulsant that enhances the activity of gamma-aminobutyric acid, the major inhibitory neurotransmitter in the central nervous system (CNS). *Therapeutic Effect:* Inhibits seizures.

AVAILABILITY
Tablets: 2 mg, 4 mg, 12 mg, 16 mg.

INDICATIONS AND DOSAGES
▶ **Adjunctive treatment of partial seizures**
PO
Adults, Elderly. Initially, 4 mg once a day. May increase by 4-8 mg/day at weekly intervals. Maximum: 56 mg/day.
Children aged 12-18 yr. Initially, 4 mg once a day. May increase by 4 mg at week 2 and by 4-8 mg at weekly intervals thereafter. Maximum: 32 mg/day.

CONTRAINDICATIONS
None known.

INTERACTIONS
Drug
Carbamazepine, phenobarbital, phenytoin: May increase tiagabine clearance.
Valproic acid: May alter the effects of valproic acid.
Herbal
None known.
Food
None known.

DIAGNOSTIC TEST EFFECTS
None known.

SIDE EFFECTS
Frequent (20%-34%)
Dizziness, asthenia, somnolence, nervousness, confusion, headache, infection, tremor.
Occasional
Nausea, diarrhea, abdominal pain, impaired concentration.

SERIOUS REACTIONS
• Overdose is characterized by agitation, confusion, hostility, and weakness. Full recovery occurs within 24 h.

PRECAUTIONS & CONSIDERATIONS
Caution is warranted in patients with hepatic impairment and in those who take other CNS depressants concurrently. Dizziness may occur, so change positions slowly—from recumbent to sitting position before standing—and alcohol and tasks requiring mental alertness or motor skills should be avoided. History of the seizure disorder, including the duration, frequency, and intensity of seizures, should be reviewed before and during therapy. CBCs and blood chemistry tests to assess hepatic and renal function should be performed before and during treatment.
Administration
Tiagabine should be taken with food.

Ticarcillin
tie-car-sill′in
(Ticar)

CATEGORY AND SCHEDULE
Pregnancy Risk Category: B

Classification: Antibiotics, penicillins

MECHANISM OF ACTION
Binds to bacterial cell wall, inhibiting bacterial cell wall synthesis. *Therapeutic Effect:* Causes cell lysis, death. Bactericidal.

PHARMACOKINETICS
Well absorbed. Widely distributed. Protein binding: 45%-60%. Minimal metabolism in liver. Primarily excreted unchanged in urine. Moderately dialyzable. *Half-life:* 1.2 h (half-life is increased in those with impaired renal function).

AVAILABILITY
Powder for Reconstitution: 1g, 3 g, 20 g (Ticar).

INDICATIONS AND DOSAGES
▸ **Septicemia; skin and skin-structure, bone, joint, and lower respiratory tract infections; and endometriosis**
IV/IM
Adults, Elderly, Children weighing > 40 kg. 200-300 mg/kg/day IV or IM q4-6h or 3 g q4h or 4 g q6h. Maximum: 18 g/day.
Children and infants weighing < 40 kg. 200-300 mg/kg/day IV q4-6h. Maximum: 18 g/day.
Neonates weighing > 2000 g. 75 mg/kg IV or IM q8h < 7 days old; 100 mg/kg IV or IM q8h > 7 old.
Neonates weighing < 2000 g. 75 mg/kg IV or IM q12h < 7 days old; 75 mg/kg q8h > 7 days old.
▸ **Urinary tract infection (UTI), complicated**
IV
Adults, Elderly, Children weighing > 40 kg. 150-200 mg/kg/day divided q4-6h.
Children weighing < 40 kg. 150-200 mg/kg/day in divided doses q6-8h.
▸ **UTI, uncomplicated**
IV/IM

Adults, Elderly, Children weighing > 40 kg. 1 g q6h IV or IM.
Children weighing < 40 kg. 50-100 mg/kg/day IV or IM in divided doses q6-8h.

▸ **Dosage in renal impairment**

Adults: Creatinine Clearance (mL/min)	Dosage Interval
30-60	2 g q4h
10-30	2 g q8h
< 10 with hepatic impairment 2 g IV q24h	2 g q12h or 1 g IM q6h

CONTRAINDICATIONS
Hypersensitivity to any penicillin.

INTERACTIONS
Drug
Anticoagulants, heparin, NSAIDs, thrombolytics: May increase the risk of hemorrhage with high dosages of ticarcillin.
Probenecid: May increase ticarcillin blood concentration and risk of toxicity.
Herbal and Food
None known.

DIAGNOSTIC TEST EFFECTS
May cause positive Coombs' test. May increase bleeding time, serum alkaline phosphatase, serum bilirubin, serum creatinine, serum LDH, SGOT (AST), and SGPT (ALT) levels. May decrease serum potassium, sodium, and uric acid levels.

Ⓓ IV INCOMPATIBILITIES
Amphotericin B complex (Abelcet, AmBisome, Amphotec), caspofungin, calcium chloride, ciprofloxacin, dobutamine, vancomycin (Vancocin).

Ⓥ IV COMPATIBILITIES
Diltiazem (Cardizem), heparin, insulin, morphine, propofol (Diprivan).

SIDE EFFECTS
Frequent
Phlebitis, thrombophlebitis with IV dose, rash, urticaria, pruritus, smell or taste disturbances.
Occasional
Nausea, diarrhea, vomiting.
Rare
Headache, fatigue, hallucinations, bleeding, or bruising.

SERIOUS REACTIONS
• Overdosage may produce seizures and neurologic reactions.
• Superinfections, including potentially fatal antibiotic-associated colitis, may result from bacterial imbalance.
• Severe hypersensitivity reactions, including anaphylaxis, occur rarely.

PRECAUTIONS & CONSIDERATIONS
Caution is warranted in patients with a history of allergies, especially to cephalosporins, penicillius, and renal impairment. Be aware that ticarcillin readily crosses the placenta, appears in amniotic fluid and cord blood, and is distributed in breast milk in low concentrations. Ticarcillin use in infants may lead to allergic sensitization, candidiasis, diarrhea, and skin rash.

Be aware that the safety and efficacy of this drug have not been established in children younger than 3 mo. Age-related renal impairment may require dosage adjustment in elderly patients.

Notify the physician if severe diarrhea, a rash or itching, or any other unusual sign or symptom occurs.
Storage
After reconstitution for IM injection, ticarcillin solution retains potency for 12 h at room temperature or 24 h if refrigerated. After reconstitution for IV administration, solutions in

T

concentrations of 10-50 mg/mL retain most of their potency for 48-72 h at room temperature or 14 days if refrigerated or 30 days when frozen.

Administration
Ticarcillin is generally given intravenously.

For direct IV use of ticarcillin, add at least 4 mL of D5W, 0.9% NaCl, or lactated Ringer's injection to each 1 g vial. Each gram of ticarcillin may be further diluted if desired. The resulting solution should be administered as slowly as possible to avoid vein irritation.

For intermittent infusions of ticarcillin, administer over 30 min to 2 h in adults. For neonates, administer over a 10- to 20-min period. Because of the potential for hypersensitivity reactions such as anaphylaxis, start initial dose at a few drops per minute, increase slowly to ordered rate; monitor the patient the first 10-15 min, then check the patient every 10 min.

For IM injection of ticarcillin, add 2 mL of sterile water for injection, 1% lidocaine hydrochloride injection (without epinephrine), or sodium chloride injection to each 1 g vial to provide a concentration of 1 g/2.6 mL.

Ticarcillin Disodium/Clavulanate Potassium
tyekar-sill'in klav'yoo-la-nate
(Timentin)

CATEGORY AND SCHEDULE
Pregnancy Risk Category: B

Classification: Antibiotics, penicillins

MECHANISM OF ACTION
Ticarcillin binds to bacterial cell walls, inhibiting cell wall synthesis. Clavulanate inhibits the action of bacterial β-lactamase. *Therapeutic Effect:* Ticarcillin is bactericidal in susceptible organisms. Clavulanate protects ticarcillin from enzymatic degradation.

PHARMACOKINETICS
Widely distributed. Protein binding: ticarcillin 45%-60%, clavulanate 9%-30%. Minimally metabolized in the liver. Primarily excreted unchanged in urine. Removed by hemodialysis. *Half-life:* 1-1.2 h (increased in impaired renal function).

AVAILABILITY
Powder for Injection: 3.1 g.
Premixed Solution for Infusion: 3.1 g/100 mL.

INDICATIONS AND DOSAGES
▸ **Skin and skin structure, bone, joint, and lower respiratory tract infections; septicemia; endometriosis; urinary tract infection**
IV
Adults, Elderly ≥ 60 kg. 3.1 g (3 g ticarcillin) q4-6h. Maximum: 18-24 g/day.
Adults, Elderly < 60 kg. 200-300 mg/kg/day divided q4-6h.
Children 3 mo and older. Mild to moderate infections, 200 mg/kg/day (based on ticarcillin content) divided q6h; severe infections, 300 mg/kg/day (based on ticarcillin content) divided q4-6h. Maximum 18-24 g/day.
▸ **Dosage in renal impairment**
Dosage interval is modified based on creatinine clearance.
Adult CrCl 30-60 mL/min: loading dose of 3.1 g, then 2 g q4h.
Adult CrCl 10-30 mL/min: loading dose of 3.1 g, then 2 g IV q8h.

Adult CrCl < 10 mL/min: loading dose of 3.1 g, then 2 g IV q12h. *Adult* CrCl < 10 mL/min with hepatic impairment: 3.1 g IV, then 2 g IV q24h.

CONTRAINDICATIONS
Hypersensitivity to any penicillin.

INTERACTIONS
Drug
Anticoagulants, heparin, NSAIDs, thrombolytics: May increase the risk of hemorrhage with high dosages of ticarcillin.
Probenecid: May increase ticarcillin blood concentration and risk of toxicity.
Herbal and Food
None known.

DIAGNOSTIC TEST EFFECTS
May increase bleeding time and serum alkaline phosphatase, bilirubin, creatinine, sLDH, AST (SGOT), and ALT (SGPT) levels. May decrease serum potassium, sodium, and uric acid levels. May cause a positive Coombs' test.

Ⓓ IV INCOMPATIBILITIES
Amphotericin B complex (Abelcet, AmBisome, Amphotec), azithromycin, caspofungin, cefamandole, erythromycin, ganciclovir, quinupristin-dalfopristin, vancomycin (Vancocin).

Ⓓ IV COMPATIBILITIES
Diltiazem (Cardizem), heparin, insulin, morphine, propofol (Diprivan).

SIDE EFFECTS
Frequent
Phlebitis or thrombophlebitis (with IV dose), rash, urticaria, pruritus, altered smell or taste.
Occasional
Nausea, diarrhea, vomiting.

Rare
Headache, fatigue, hallucinations, bleeding, or ecchymosis.

SERIOUS REACTIONS
• Overdosage may produce seizures and other neurologic reactions.
• Antibiotic-associated colitis and other superinfections may result from bacterial imbalance.
• Severe hypersensitivity reactions, including anaphylaxis, occur rarely.

PRECAUTIONS & CONSIDERATIONS
Caution is warranted in patients with renal impairment or a history of allergies, especially to penicillins and cephalosporins. Ticarcillin readily crosses the placenta, appears in cord blood and amniotic fluid, and is distributed in breast milk in low concentrations. Ticarcillin may lead to allergic sensitization, candidiasis, diarrhea, and skin rash in infants. The safety and efficacy of ticarcillin have not been established in children younger than 3 mo. Age-related renal impairment may require dosage adjustment in elderly patients.

History of allergies, especially to cephalosporins or penicillins, should be determined before giving the drug. Withhold and promptly notify the physician if rash or diarrhea occurs. Severe diarrhea with abdominal pain, blood or mucus in stool, and fever may indicate antibiotic-associated colitis. Signs and symptoms of superinfection, including anal or genital pruritus, black hairy tongue, diarrhea, increased fever, sore throat, ulceration or changes of oral mucosa, and vomiting should be monitored. Food tolerance, intake and output, renal function tests, urinalysis, and the injection sites should be assessed.
Storage
The solution normally appears colorless to pale yellow; a darker

color indicates a loss of potency. The reconstituted IV infusion (piggyback) is stable for 6 h at room temperature and 3 days if refrigerated. Discard the solution if a precipitate forms.
Administration
This drug is available in ready-to-use containers. For IV infusion (piggyback), reconstitute each 3.1-g vial with 13 mL sterile water for injection or 0.9% NaCl to provide a concentration of 200 mg ticarcillin and 6.7 mg clavulanic acid per milliliter. Shake the vial to assist reconstitution. Further dilute with D5W or 0.9% NaCl to a concentration between 10 and 100 mg/mL. Infuse the drug over 30 min. Because of the potential for hypersensitivity reactions such as anaphylaxis, start the initial dose at a few drops per minute, and then increase it slowly to the ordered rate. Stay with the patient for the first 10-15 min during the initial dose; then check every 10 min during the infusion for signs and symptoms of hypersensitivity or anaphylaxis.

Ticlopidine
tye-klo′pa-deen
(Apo-Ticlopidine [CAN], Ticlid, Tilodene [AUS])

CATEGORY AND SCHEDULE
Pregnancy Risk Category: B

Classification: Platelet inhibitors

MECHANISM OF ACTION
An aggregation inhibitor that inhibits the release of adenosine diphosphate from activated platelets, which prevents fibrinogen from binding to glycoprotein IIb/IIIa receptors on the surface of activated platelets.

Therapeutic Effect: Inhibits platelet aggregation and thrombus formation.

AVAILABILITY
Tablets: 250 mg.

INDICATIONS AND DOSAGES
▶ **Prevention of stroke**
PO
Adults, Elderly. 250 mg twice a day.

OFF-LABEL USES
Treatment of intermittent claudication, sickle cell disease, subarachnoid hemorrhage.

CONTRAINDICATIONS
Active pathologic bleeding, such as bleeding peptic ulcer and intracranial bleeding, hematopoietic disorders, including neutropenia and thrombocytopenia; presence of hemostatic disorder; severe hepatic impairment.

INTERACTIONS
Drug
Aspirin, heparin, oral anticoagulants, thrombolytics: May increase the risk of bleeding with these drugs.
Herbal
None known.
Food
None known.

DIAGNOSTIC TEST EFFECTS
May increase serum cholesterol, serum alkaline phosphatase, bilirubin, triglyceride, AST (SGOT), and ALT (SGPT) levels. May prolong bleeding time. May decrease neutrophil and platelet counts.

SIDE EFFECTS
Frequent (5%-13%)
Diarrhea, nausea, dyspepsia, including heartburn, indigestion, GI discomfort, and bloating.

Rare (1%-2%)
Vomiting, flatulence, pruritus,
dizziness.

SERIOUS REACTIONS
• Neutropenia occurs in
approximately 2% of patients.
• Thrombotic thrombocytopenia
purpura, agranulocytosis, hepatitis,
cholestatic jaundice, and tinnitus
occur rarely.

Caution is warranted in patients
with an increased risk of bleeding
and severe hepatic or renal disease.
Safety and efficacy of ticlopidine in
children have not been established.
No age-related precautions have been
noted in elderly patients.
    Laboratory studies, particularly
hepatic enzyme tests and CBC,
should be obtained. Pattern of daily
bowel activity and stool consistency,
BP for hypotension, and skin for
rash, should be monitored.
Administration
Take ticlopidine with food or just
after meals to increase bioavailability
and decrease GI discomfort.
Ticlopidine should be discontinued
10-14 days before surgery if
antiplatelet effect is not desired.

Tiludronate
ti-loo'dro-nate
(Skelid)

CATEGORY AND SCHEDULE
Pregnancy Risk Category: C

Classification: Bisphosphonates

MECHANISM OF ACTION
A calcium regulator that inhibits
functioning osteoclasts through
disruption of cytoskeletal
ring structure and inhibition
of osteoclastic proton pump.
Therapeutic Effect: Inhibits bone
resorption.

AVAILABILITY
Tablets: 200 mg.

INDICATIONS AND DOSAGES
▸ **Paget disease**
PO
Adults, Elderly. 400 mg once a day
for 3 mo.

CONTRAINDICATIONS
GI disease, such as dysphagia and
gastric ulcer, impaired renal function,
biphosphonate hypersensitivity, renal
failure (CrCl < 30 mL/min).

INTERACTIONS
Drug
**Antacids containing aluminum or
magnesium, calcium, salicylates:**
May interfere with the absorption of
tiludronate.
Herbal
None known.
Food
All foods: Administration with food
interferes with bioavailability.

DIAGNOSTIC TEST EFFECTS
None known.

SIDE EFFECTS
Frequent (6%-9%)
Nausea, diarrhea, generalized body
pain, back pain, headache.
Occasional
Rash, dyspepsia, vomiting, rhinitis,
sinusitis, dizziness.
! See serious reactions under
Alendronate.

Caution is warranted in patients with
hyperparathyroidism, hypocalcemia,
and vitamin D deficiency. Because

there are no adequate and well-controlled studies in pregnant women, it is unknown whether tiludronate causes fetal harm or is excreted in breast milk. Safety and efficacy of tiludronate have not been established in children. No age-related precautions have been noted in elderly patients.

Serum calcium, serum alkaline phosphatase, osteocalcin, and urinary hydroxyproline levels should be adjusted to assess the effectiveness of tiludronate.

! See precautions and considerations for Alendronate for further instruction.

Administration

Take tiludronate at least 2 h before or after beverages, food, other medications, calcium or other mineral supplements, and vitamin D. Take with 6-8 oz of plain water (not mineral water).

Timolol

tim′oh-lole

(Apo-Timol [CAN], Apo-Timop [CAN], Betimol, Blocadren, Gen-Timolol [CAN], Istadol, Optimol [AUS], PMS-Timolol [CAN], Tenopt [AUS], Timoptic, Timoptic OccuDose, Timoptic XE, Timoptol [AUS], Timoptol XE [AUS])

Do not confuse timolol with atenolol, or Timoptic with Viroptic.

CATEGORY AND SCHEDULE

Pregnancy Risk Category: C (D if used in second or third trimester)

Classification: Antiadrenergics, β-blocking, ophthalmics

MECHANISM OF ACTION

An antihypertensive, antimigraine, and antiglaucoma agent that blocks β_1- and β_2-adrenergic receptors. *Therapeutic Effect:* Reduces intraocular pressure (IOP) by reducing aqueous humor production, lowers BP, slows the heart rate, and decreases myocardial contractility.

PHARMACOKINETICS

Route	Onset	Peak	Duration
PO	15-45 min	0.5-2.5 h	4 h
Ophthalmic	30 min	1-2 h	12-24 h

Well absorbed from the GI tract. Protein binding: 10%. Minimal absorption after ophthalmic administration. Metabolized in the liver. Excreted primarily in urine. Not removed by hemodialysis. *Half-life:* 4 h. Systemic absorption may occur with ophthalmic administration.

AVAILABILITY

Tablets (Blocadren): 5 mg, 10 mg, 20 mg.
Ophthalmic Gel (Timoptic-XE): 0.25%, 0.5%.
Ophthalmic Solution (Betimol, Timoptic, Timoptic OccuDose): 0.25%, 0.5%.

INDICATIONS AND DOSAGES

▸ **Mild to moderate hypertension**
PO
Adults, Elderly. Initially, 10 mg twice a day, alone or in combination with other therapy. Gradually increase at intervals of not < 1 wk. Usual dose is 10-20 mg twice daily. Maximum: 60 mg.

▸ **Reduction of cardiovascular mortality in definite or suspected acute myocardial infarction (MI)**
PO
Adults, Elderly. 10 mg twice a day, beginning 1-4 wks after MI.

▸ **Migraine prevention**
PO
Adults, Elderly. Initially, 10 mg twice a day. Range: 10-30 mg/day.
▸ **Reduction of IOP in open-angle glaucoma, aphakic glaucoma, ocular hypertension, and secondary glaucoma**
OPHTHALMIC
Adults, Elderly, Children. 1 drop of 0.25% solution in affected eye(s) twice a day. May be increased to 1 drop of 0.5% solution in affected eye(s) twice a day. When IOP is controlled, dosage may be reduced to 1 drop once a day. If patient is switched to timolol from another antiglaucoma agent, administer concurrently for 1 day. Discontinue other agent on following day.

OFF-LABEL USES

Systemic: Treatment of anxiety, cardiac arrhythmias, chronic angina pectoris, hypertrophic cardio-myopathy, migraine, pheochromo-cytoma, thyrotoxicosis, tremors. Ophthalmic: To decrease IOP in acute or chronic angle-closure glaucoma, treatment of angle-closure glaucoma during and after iridectomy, malignant glaucoma, secondary glaucoma.

CONTRAINDICATIONS

Bronchial asthma, cardiogenic shock, congestive heart failure (CHF) unless secondary to tachyarrhythmias, chronic obstructive pulmonary disease (COPD), patients receiving MAOI therapy, second- or third-degree heart block, sinus bradycardia, abrupt discontinuation of therapy.

INTERACTIONS

Drug
Diuretics, other antihypertensives: May increase hypotensive effect.

Insulin, oral hypoglycemics: May mask symptoms of hypoglycemia and prolong hypoglycemic effects of these drugs.
NSAIDs: May decrease antihypertensive effect.
Sympathomimetics, xanthines: May mutually inhibit effects.
Herbal
None known.
Food
None known.

DIAGNOSTIC TEST EFFECTS

May increase antinuclear antibody titer and BUN, serum LDH, serum lipoprotein, serum alkaline phosphatase, serum bilirubin, serum creatinine, serum potassium, serum uric acid, AST (SGOT), ALT (SGPT), and serum triglyceride levels.

SIDE EFFECTS

Frequent
Diminished sexual function, drowsiness, difficulty sleeping, unusual tiredness or weakness. Ophthalmic: Eye irritation, visual disturbances.
Occasional
Depression, cold hands or feet, diarrhea, constipation, anxiety, nasal congestion, nausea, vomiting, bradycardia, bronchospasm.
Rare
Altered taste, dry eyes, itching, numbness of fingers, toes, or scalp.

SERIOUS REACTIONS

• Overdose may produce profound bradycardia, hypotension, and bronchospasm.
• Abrupt withdrawal may result in diaphoresis, palpitations, headache, and tremors.
• Timolol administration may precipitate CHF and MI in patients with cardiac disease; thyroid storm in those with thyrotoxicosis; and

T

peripheral ischemia in those with existing peripheral vascular disease.

• Hypoglycemia may occur in patients with previously controlled diabetes.

• Ophthalmic overdose may produce bradycardia, hypotension, bronchospasm, and acute cardiac failure.

PRECAUTIONS & CONSIDERATIONS

Caution is warranted with hyperthyroidism, impaired hepatic or renal function, and inadequate cardiac function. Precautions apply to both oral and ophthalmic administration because of the possible systemic absorption of ophthalmic timolol. Timolol is distributed in breast milk and is not for use in breastfeeding women because of the potential for serious adverse effects in the breast-fed infant. Timolol use should be avoided in pregnant women after the first trimester because it may result in low-birth-weight infants. The drug may also produce apnea, bradycardia, hypoglycemia, or hypothermia during childbirth. The safety and efficacy of timolol have not been established in children. In elderly patients, age-related peripheral vascular disease increases susceptibility to decreased peripheral circulation. Be aware that salt and alcohol intake should be restricted. Nasal decongestants or OTC cold preparations (stimulants) should not be used without physician approval. Tasks that require mental alertness or motor skills should be avoided.

Notify the physician of excessive fatigue, prolonged dizziness or headache, or shortness of breath. Pattern of daily bowel activity and stool consistency, ECG for arrhythmias (particularly premature ventricular contractions), BP, heart rate, IOP (with ophthalmic preparation), and liver and renal function test results should be monitored during treatment. If pulse rate is 60 beats/min or lower or systolic BP is < 90 mm Hg, withhold the medication and contact the physician.

Administration

Take timolol without regard to meals. Tablets may be crushed. Do not abruptly discontinue timolol. Compliance is essential to control angina, arrhythmias, glaucoma, and hypertension.

! When administering ophthalmic gel, invert container and shake once before each use.

For ophthalmic administration, place a finger on the lower eyelid and pull it out until pocket is formed between the eye and lower lid. Hold the dropper above the pocket and place the prescribed number of drops or amount of prescribed gel into pocket. Close eyes gently so that medication will not be squeezed out of the sac. Apply gentle digital pressure to the lacrimal sac at the inner canthus for 1 min after installation to lessen the risk of systemic absorption.

Tinidazole
ty-ni′da-zole
(Tindamax)

CATEGORY AND SCHEDULE
Pregnancy Risk Category: C

Classification: Antiprotozoals

MECHANISM OF ACTION
A nitroimidazole derivative that is converted to the active metabolite by reduction of cell extracts of *Trichomonas.* The active metabolite causes DNA damage in pathogens. *Therapeutic Effect:* Produces antiprotozoal effect.

PHARMACOKINETICS
Rapidly and completely absorbed.
Protein binding: 12%. Distributed in
all body tissues and fluids; crosses
blood-brain barrier. Significantly
metabolized. Excreted primarily in
urine; partially eliminated in feces.
Half-life: 12-14 h.

AVAILABILITY
Tablets: 250 mg, 500 mg.

INDICATIONS AND DOSAGES
▶ **Intestinal amebiasis**
PO
Adults, Elderly. 2 g/day for 3 days.
Children 3 yr and older.
50 mg/kg/day (up to 2 g) for 3 days.
▶ **Amebic hepatic abscess**
PO
Adults, Elderly. 2 g/day for 3-5 days.
Children 3 yr and older. 50 mg/kg/day
(up to 2 g) for 3-5 days.
▶ **Giardiasis**
PO
Adults, Elderly. 2 g as a single dose.
Children 3 yr and older. 50 mg/kg
(up to 2 g) as a single dose.
▶ **Trichomoniasis**
PO
Adults, Elderly. 2 g as a single
dose.

CONTRAINDICATIONS
First trimester of pregnancy,
hypersensitivity to nitroimidazole
derivatives.

INTERACTIONS
Drug
Alcohol: May cause a disulfiram-
type reaction.
Cholestyramine, oxytetracycline:
May decrease the effectiveness of
tinidazole; separate dosage times.
**Cimetidine, fosphenytoin,
ketoconazole, phenobarbital,
rifampin:** Decreases the metabolism
of tinidazole.

**Cyclosporine, fluorouracil, lithium,
phenytoin (IV), tacrolimus:** May
increase blood levels of these drugs.
Disulfiram: May increase the risk
of psychotic reactions (separate dose
by 2 wks).
Oral anticoagulants: Increase the
risk of bleeding.
Herbal
None known.
Food
None known.

DIAGNOSTIC TEST EFFECTS
May increase serum LDH, triglyceride,
AST (SGOT), and ALT (SGPT) levels.

SIDE EFFECTS
Occasional (2%-4%)
Metallic or bitter taste, nausea,
weakness, fatigue, or malaise.
Rare (< 2%)
Epigastric distress, anorexia,
vomiting, headache, dizziness, red-
brown or darkened urine.

SERIOUS REACTIONS
• Peripheral neuropathy,
characterized by paresthesia, is
usually reversible if tinidazole
treatment is stopped as soon as
neurologic symptoms appear.
• Superinfection, hypersensitivity
reaction, and seizures occur rarely.

PRECAUTIONS & CONSIDERATIONS
Caution is warranted in patients with
blood dyscrasia, candidiasis (may
present more prominent symptoms
during tinidazole therapy), central
nervous system disease (risk of
seizure or peripheral neuropathy),
liver impairment, and concurrent
treatment with related agents such as
metronidazole. Tinidazole crosses the
placenta and is distributed in breast
milk. Safety and efficacy of tinidazole
have not established in children
younger than 3 yr. No age-related

precautions have been noted in elderly patients. Avoid alcohol while taking tinidazole and for at least 3 days after discontinuing the medication.

Storage

Store at room temperature.

Administration

Score tablets may be crushed. Take with meals or snack to minimize GI irritation. Do not miss a dose; complete the full length of treatment.

Tinzaparin
tin-za-pair′in
(Innohep)

CATEGORY AND SCHEDULE
Pregnancy Risk Category: B

Classification: Anticoagulants, low-molecular-weight heparin (LMWH)

MECHANISM OF ACTION
A low-molecular-weight heparin that inhibits factor Xa. Causes less inactivation of thrombin, inhibition of platelets, and bleeding than standard heparin. Does not significantly influence bleeding time, PT, aPTT. *Therapeutic Effect:* Produces anticoagulation.

PHARMACOKINETICS
Well absorbed after SC administration. Eliminated primarily in urine. *Half-life:* 3-4 h.

AVAILABILITY
Injection: 20,000 anti-Xa international units/mL.

INDICATIONS AND DOSAGES
▸ **Deep vein thrombosis**
SC
Adults, Elderly. 175 anti-Xa international units/kg once a day.

Continue for at least 6 days and until patient is sufficiently anticoagulated with warfarin (International Normalizing Ratio [INR] of 2 or more for 2 consecutive days).

CONTRAINDICATIONS
Elderly with renal insufficiency; active major bleeding; concurrent heparin therapy, hypersensitivity to heparin, sulfite, benzyl alcohol, or pork products; thrombocytopenia associated with positive in vitro test for antiplatelet antibody.

INTERACTIONS
Drug
Anticoagulants, platelet inhibitors: May increase the risk of bleeding.
Herbal
Ginkgo biloba: May increase the risk of bleeding.
Food
None known.

DIAGNOSTIC TEST EFFECTS
Increases (reversible) LDH, serum alkaline phosphatase, AST (SGOT), and ALT (SGPT) levels.

SIDE EFFECTS
Frequent (16%)
Injection site reaction, such as inflammation, oozing, nodules, and skin necrosis.
Rare (< 2%)
Nausea, asthenia, constipation, epistaxis.

SERIOUS REACTIONS
• Overdose may lead to bleeding complications ranging from local ecchymoses to major hemorrhage. Antidote: Dose of protamine sulfate (1% solution) should be equal to dose of tinzaparin injected. 1 mg protamine sulfate neutralizes 100 anti-Xa International Units (IU) of tinzaparin. A second dose of 0.5 mg protamine

per 100 anti-Xa IU of tinzaparin may be given if aPTT tested 2-4 h after the initial infusion remains prolonged.

PRECAUTIONS & CONSIDERATIONS

Caution is warranted in patients with conditions associated with increased risk of hemorrhage, history of recent GI ulceration and hemorrhage, history of heparin-induced thrombocytopenia, impaired renal function, uncontrolled arterial hypertension, and in elderly patients. Patients should be monitored closely for bleeding if tinzaparin is administered during or immediately after lumbar puncture, spinal anesthesia, or epidural anesthesia. Tinzaparin should be used with caution in pregnant women, particularly during the last trimester and immediately postpartum because it increases the risk of maternal hemorrhage. It is unknown whether tinzaparin is excreted in breast milk. Safety and efficacy of tinzaparin have not been established in children. Elderly patients may be more susceptible to bleeding.

Notify the physician of chest pain, injection site reaction, such as inflammation, nodules, oozing, numbness, pain, swelling or tingling of joints, unusual bleeding, or bruising. PT, INR, and CBC, including platelet count, should be monitored before and during therapy. Be aware of signs of bleeding, including bleeding at injection or surgical sites or from gums, blood in stool, bruising, hematuria, and petechiae.

Storage
Store at room temperature.
Administration
! Do not mix with other injections or infusions. Do not give intramuscularly. Administer tinzaparin by subcutaneous route only.

The parenteral form normally appears clear and colorless to pale yellow. Lie down before administering by deep SC injection.

Tioconazole
tyo-con′a-zole
(Gynecure [CAN], Monistat-1, Trosyd [CAN], Vagistat)

CATEGORY AND SCHEDULE
Pregnancy Risk Category: C

Classification: Antifungals, topical, dermatologics

MECHANISM OF ACTION
An imidazole derivative that inhibits synthesis of ergosterol (vital component of fungal cell formation). *Therapeutic Effect:* Damaging fungal cell membrane. Fungistatic.

PHARMOCOKINETICS
Negligible absorption from vaginal application.

AVAILABILITY
Vaginal Ointment: 6.5% (Monistat-1, Vagistat).

INDICATIONS AND DOSAGES
▶ **Vulvovaginal candidiasis**
INTRAVAGINAL
Adults, Elderly. 1 applicatorful just before bedtime as a single dose.

CONTRAINDICATIONS
Hypersensitivity to tioconazole or other imidazole antifungal agents.

INTERACTIONS
Drug
None known.
Herbal
None known.
Food
None known.

T

DIAGNOSTIC TEST EFFECTS
None known.

SIDE EFFECTS
Frequent (25%)
Headache.
Occasional (1%-6%)
Burning, itching.
Rare (< 1%)
Irritation, vaginal pain, dysuria, dryness of vaginal secretions, vulvar edema/swelling.

SERIOUS REACTIONS
• None reported.

PRECAUTIONS & CONSIDERATIONS
Caution is warranted in patients with diabetes and HIV or AIDS infection. It is unknown whether tioconazole is distributed in breast milk. Safety and efficacy have not been established in children. No age-related precautions have been noted in elderly patients. Separate personal items that come in contact with affected areas.
Storage
Store at room temperature.
Administration
Insert applicatorful high into vagina just before bedtime. Contact physician if itching or burning continues. Be aware that tioconazole base may interact with latex or rubber. Condoms or diaphragms should not be used within 72 h of administration.

Tiopronin
tye-o-pro′nin
Thiola

CATEGORY AND SCHEDULE
Pregnancy Risk Category: C

Classification: Cystine depleting agents

MECHANISM OF ACTION
A sulfhydryl compound with similar properties to those of penicillamine and glutathione that undergoes thiol-disulfide exchange with cysteine to form tiopronin-cysteine, a mixed disulfide. This disulfide is water soluble, unlike cysteine, and does not crystallize in the kidneys. May break disulfide bonds present in bronchial secretions and break the mucus complexes. *Therapeutic Effect:* Decreases cysteine excretion.

PHARMACOKINETICS
Moderately absorbed from the GI tract. Excreted primarily in urine. Following oral administration, up to 48% of dose appears in urine during the first 4 h and up to 78% by 72 h. *Half-life:* 53 h.

AVAILABILITY
Tablets: 100 mg (Thiola).

INDICATIONS AND DOSAGES
▶ **Crystinuria**
PO
Adults, Elderly. Initially, 800 mg in 3 divided doses. Adjust and maintain crystine concentration below its solubility limit (usually < 250 mg/L). *Children 9 yr and older.* 15 mg/kg/day in 3 divided doses. Adjust and maintain crystine concentration below its solubility limit (usually < 250 mg/L).

OFF-LABEL USES
Cataracts, epilepsy, hepatitis, rheumatoid arthritis.

CONTRAINDICATIONS
History of agranulocytosis, aplastic anemia, or thrombocytopenia while on tiopronin, pregnancy and lactation, hypersensitivity to tiopronin or its components.

INTERACTIONS
Drug
None known.
Herbal
None known.
Food
Sodium: May increase cystine in urine.

DIAGNOSTIC TEST EFFECTS
None known.

ⓘ IV INCOMPATIBILITIES
None known.

ⓘ IV COMPATIBILITIES
None known.

SIDE EFFECTS
Frequent
Pain, swelling, tenderness of skin,
rash, hives, itching, oral ulcers.
Occasional
GI upset, taste or smell impairment,
bloody or cloudy urine, chills,
difficulty in breathing, high blood
pressure, hoarseness, joint pain,
swelling of feet or lower legs,
tenderness of glands.
Rare
Chest pain; cough; difficulty in
chewing, talking, swallowing,
double vision, a general feeling
of discomfort; illness; weakness;
muscle weakness; spitting up blood;
swelling of lymph glands.

SERIOUS REACTIONS
• Hematologic abnormalities,
including myelosuppression,
unusual bleeding, drug fever,
renal complications, and lupus
erythematous-like reaction
including fever, arthralgia, and
lymphadenopathy rarely occur.

PRECAUTIONS & CONSIDERATIONS
Caution is warranted with a history
of penicillamine exposure; serious
adverse reactions are more likely

to occur. It is unknown whether
tiopronin crosses the placenta or is
distributed in breast milk. Safety and
efficacy of tiopronin have not been
established in children younger than
9 yr old. No age-related precautions
have been noted in elderly patients.
Drastic dietary changes, especially
in sodium, should be avoided. Fluid
intake should be increased to maintain
urine pH at a normal range of 6.5-7.
Administration
Take tiopronin on an empty stomach.

Tiotropium
ty-oh′tro-pee-um
(Spiriva)

CATEGORY AND SCHEDULE
Pregnancy Risk Category: C

Classification: Anticholinergics,
bronchodilators

MECHANISM OF ACTION
An anticholinergic that binds to
recombinant human muscarinic receptors at the smooth muscle, resulting
in long-acting bronchial smooth-
muscle relaxation. *Therapeutic Effect:*
Relieves bronchospasm.

PHARMACOKINETICS

Route	Onset	Peak	Duration
Inhalation	NA	NA	24-36 h

Binds extensively to tissue. Protein
binding: 72%. Metabolized by
oxidation. Excreted in urine.
Half-life: 5-6 days

AVAILABILITY
Powder for Inhalation: 18 mcg/
capsule (in blister packs containing
6 capsules with inhaler).

T

INDICATIONS AND DOSAGES
▸ **Chronic obstructive pulmonary disease (COPD)**
INHALATION
Adults, Elderly. 18 mcg (1 capsule)/day via HandiHaler inhalation device.

CONTRAINDICATIONS
History of hypersensitivity to atropine or its derivatives, including ipratropium.

INTERACTIONS
Drug
Ipratropium: Concurrent administration with this drug is not recommended.
Herbal
None known.
Food
None known.

DIAGNOSTIC TEST EFFECTS
None known.

SIDE EFFECTS
Frequent (6%-16%)
Dry mouth, sinusitis, pharyngitis, dyspepsia, urinary tract infection, rhinitis
Occasional (4%-5%)
Abdominal pain, peripheral edema, constipation, epistaxis, vomiting, myalgia, rash, oral candidiasis.

SERIOUS REACTIONS
• Angina pectoris, depression, and flulike symptoms occur rarely.

PRECAUTIONS & CONSIDERATIONS
Caution is warranted with angle-closure glaucoma, benign prostatic hyperplasia, and bladder neck obstruction. It is unknown whether tiotropium is distributed in breast milk. The safety and efficacy of tiotropium have not been established in children. Elderly patients are more likely to experience constipation, dry mouth, and urinary tract infection. Drink plenty of fluids to decrease the thickness of lung secretions. Avoid excessive use of caffeinated products, such as chocolate, cocoa, cola, coffee, and tea.

Pulse rate and quality, respiratory rate, depth, rhythm and type, ABG levels, and clinical improvement should be monitored. Fingernails and lips should be assessed for cyanosis, including a blue or dusky color in light-skinned patients and a gray color in dark-skinned patients, which are signs of hypoxemia.
Storage
Store tiotropium capsules at room temperature. Protect them from extreme temperatures and moisture. Do not store capsules in the HandiHaler device.
Administration
For inhalation, open the HandiHaler dustcap by pulling it up; then open the mouthpiece. Place the capsule in the center chamber and firmly close the mouthpiece until you hear a click, leaving the dustcap open. Use only 1 capsule for inhalation at a time. Holding the HandiHaler device with the mouthpiece up, press the piercing button completely once and then release it. Exhale completely before inhaling slowly and deeply, at a rate sufficient to hear the capsule vibrate. Hold breath for as long as is comfortable and then exhale slowly. Repeat this process a second time to ensure the full dose is received. Rinse mouth with water immediately after inhalation to prevent mouth and throat dryness and oral candidiasis.

Tirofiban
tye-roe-fye′ban
(Aggrastat)
Do not confuse Aggrastat with Aggrenox.

CATEGORY AND SCHEDULE
Pregnancy Risk Category: B

Classification: Platelet inhibitors

MECHANISM OF ACTION
An antiplatelet and antithrombotic agent that binds to platelet receptor glycoprotein IIb/IIIa, preventing binding of fibrinogen. *Therapeutic Effect:* Inhibits platelet aggregation and thrombus formation.

PHARMACOKINETICS
Poorly bound to plasma proteins; unbound fraction in plasma: 35%. Limited metabolism. Eliminated primarily in the urine (65%) and, to a lesser amount, in the feces. Removed by hemodialysis. *Half-life:* 2 h. Clearance is significantly decreased in severe renal impairment (creatinine clearance < 30 mL/min).

AVAILABILITY
Injection Premix: 12.5 mg/250 mL, 25 mg/500 mL (50 mcg/mL).
Vial: 250 mcg/mL.

INDICATIONS AND DOSAGES
▸ **Inhibition of platelet aggregation**
IV
Adults, Elderly. Initially, 0.4 mcg/kg/min for 30 min; then continue at 0.1 mcg/kg/min through procedure and for 12-24 h after procedure. In clinical trials, tirofiban was administered with heparin for 48-108 h.
▸ **Severe renal insufficiency (creatinine clearance < 30 mL/min)**
Adults, Elderly. Half the usual rate of infusion.

CONTRAINDICATIONS
Active internal bleeding or a history of bleeding diathesis within previous 30 days, arteriovenous malformation or aneurysm, coagulopathy, hemophilia, stroke, trauma, history of intracranial hemorrhage, history of thrombocytopenia after prior exposure to tirofiban, intracranial neoplasm, major surgical procedure within previous 30 days, severe hypertension, stroke.

INTERACTIONS
Drug
Drugs that affect hemostasis (such as aspirin, heparin, NSAIDs, and warfarin): May increase the risk of bleeding.
Herbal and Food
None known.

DIAGNOSTIC TEST EFFECTS
Decreases hematocrit, hemoglobin, and platelet count.

Ⓓ IV INCOMPATIBILITIES
Do not mix with other medications.

SIDE EFFECTS
Occasional (3%-6%)
Pelvis pain, bradycardia, dizziness, leg pain.
Rare (1%-2%)
Edema and swelling, vasovagal reaction, diaphoresis, nausea, fever, headache.

SERIOUS REACTIONS
• Signs and symptoms of overdose include generally minor mucocutaneous bleeding and bleeding at the femoral artery access site.
• Thrombocytopenia occurs rarely.

PRECAUTIONS & CONSIDERATIONS

Caution is warranted in patients with hemorrhagic retinopathy, platelet counts < 150,000/mm^3, renal impairment, and those who are also receiving drugs affecting hemostasis, such as warfarin. It is unknown whether tirofiban is distributed in breast milk. Safety and efficacy of tirofiban have not been established in children. There is an increased risk of bleeding in elderly patients. Use tirofiban with caution in this population. Be aware that it may take longer to stop bleeding during tirofiban therapy.

Notify the physician of any unusual bleeding or before a surgery or new drugs are prescribed. aPTT should be monitored 6 h after the beginning of the heparin infusion. Heparin dosage should be adjusted to maintain aPTT at approximately twice control. Nasogastric tube and urinary catheter should be avoided, if possible.

Storage

Store at room temperature and protect from light. Use only clear solution. Discard unused solution 24 h after start of infusion.

Administration

! Heparin and tirofiban can be administered through the same IV line.

For injection for solution (250 mcg/mL), withdraw and discard 100 mL from a 500-mL bag of 0.9% NaCl or D5W and replace this volume with 100 mL of tirofiban drawn from two 50-mL vials, or withdraw and discard 50 mL from a 250-mL bag and replace with 50 mL of tirofiban drawn from one 50-mL vial to achieve a final concentration of 50 mcg/mL. Mix injection for solution (250 mcg/mL) well before administration. For injection (50 mcg/mL), premix in 500-mL

IntraVia container, and tear off the dust cover to open the IntraVia container. Check the IntraVia container for leaks by squeezing the inner bag firmly; if a leak is found or if the solution is not clear, discard the solution. Do not add other drugs or remove injection (50 mcg/mL); premix solution directly from the bag with a syringe. Do not use plastic containers in series connections because doing so may result in air embolism caused by drawing air from the first container that holds no solution. For loading dose, give 0.4 mcg/kg/min for 30 min. For maintenance infusion, give 0.1 mcg/kg/min.

Tizanidine
tye-zan'i-deen
(Zanaflex)

CATEGORY AND SCHEDULE
Pregnancy Risk Category: C

Classification: Adrenergic agonists, musculoskeletal agents, relaxants, skeletal muscle

MECHANISM OF ACTION
A skeletal muscle relaxant that increases presynaptic inhibition of spinal motor neurons mediated by α_2-adrenergic agonists, reducing facilitation to postsynaptic motor neurons. *Therapeutic Effect:* Reduces muscle spasticity.

Pharmacokinetics

Route	Onset	Peak	Duration
PO	NA	1-2 h	3-6 h

Metabolized in the liver. *Half-life:* 4-8 h.

AVAILABILITY
Tablets: 2 mg, 4 mg.

INDICATIONS AND DOSAGES
▸ **Muscle spasticity**
PO
Adults, Elderly. Initially 2-4 mg, gradually increased in 2- to 4-mg increments and repeated q6-8h. Maximum: 3 doses/day or 36 mg/24 h.

OFF-LABEL USES
Spasticity associated with multiple sclerosis or spinal cord injury.

CONTRAINDICATIONS
None known.

INTERACTIONS
Drug
Alcohol, other central nervous system (CNS) depressants: May increase CNS depressant effects.
Antihypertensives: May increase tizanidine's hypotensive potential.
Oral contraceptives: May reduce tizanidine clearance.
Phenytoin: May increase serum levels and risk of toxicity of phenytoin.
Herbal
None known.
Food
None known.

DIAGNOSTIC TEST EFFECTS
May increase serum alkaline phosphatase, AST (SGOT), and ALT (SGPT) levels.

SIDE EFFECTS
Frequent (41%-49%)
Dry mouth, somnolence, asthenia.
Occasional (4%-16%)
Dizziness, urinary tract infection, constipation.
Rare (3%)
Nervousness, amblyopia, pharyngitis, rhinitis, vomiting, urinary frequency.

SERIOUS REACTIONS
• Hypotension (a reduction in either diastolic or systolic BP) may be associated with bradycardia, orthostatic hypotension, and rarely syncope. The risk of hypotension increases as dosage increases; BP may decrease within 1 h after administration.

PRECAUTIONS & CONSIDERATIONS
Caution is warranted in patients with hypotension and cardiac, hepatic, or renal disease. The safety and efficacy of tizanidine have not been established in children. In elderly patients, age-related renal impairment may warrant cautious use.
   Low BP, impaired coordination, and sedation may occur. Avoid alcohol, CNS depressants, and tasks that require mental alertness or motor skills. Change positions slowly to prevent dizziness. Baseline serum alkaline phosphatase and total bilirubin levels should be obtained. Therapeutic response, such as decreased stiffness, tenderness, and intensity of skeletal muscle pain and improved mobility, should be assessed.
Administration
Do not abruptly discontinue the medication.

Tobramycin Sulfate
toe-bra-mye′sin
(AK-Tob, Apo-Tobramycin [CAN], Nebcin, PMS-Tobramycin, TOBI, Tobrex)

CATEGORY AND SCHEDULE
Pregnancy Risk Category: C (B, ophthalmic form)

Classification: Antibiotics, aminoglycosides

MECHANISM OF ACTION

An aminoglycoside antibiotic that irreversibly binds to protein on bacterial ribosomes. *Therapeutic Effect:* Interferes with protein synthesis of susceptible microorganisms.

PHARMACOKINETICS

Rapid, complete absorption after IM administration. Protein binding: 30%. Widely distributed (does not cross the blood-brain barrier; low concentrations in cerebrospinal fluid. Excreted unchanged in urine. Removed by hemodialysis. *Half-life:* 2-4 h (increased in impaired renal function and neonates; decreased in cystic fibrosis and febrile or burn patients).

AVAILABILITY

Injection Solution (Nebcin): 10 mg/mL, 40 mg/mL.
Injection Powder for Reconstitution (Nebcin): 1.2 g.
Ophthalmic Ointment (Tobrex): 0.3%.
Ophthalmic Solution (AKTob, Tobrex): 0.3%.
Nebulization Solution (TOBI): 60 mg/mL.

INDICATIONS AND DOSAGES
▶ **Skin and skin structure, bone, joint, respiratory tract, postoperative, intra-abdominal, and burn wound infections; complicated urinary tract infection; septicemia; meningitis**
IV, IM
Adults, Elderly. 3-6 mg/kg/day in 2-3 divided doses or 5-7 mg/kg once a day.
▶ **Superficial eye infections, including blepharitis, conjunctivitis, keratitis, and corneal ulcers**
OPHTHALMIC OINTMENT
Adults, Elderly. Usual dosage; apply a thin strip to conjunctiva q8-12h (q3-4h for severe infections).

OPHTHALMIC SOLUTION
Adults, Elderly. Usual dosage, 1-2 drops in affected eye q4h (2 drops/hr for severe infections).
▶ **Bronchopulmonary infections in patients with cystic fibrosis**
INHALATION SOLUTION (ToBi)
Adults, Children ≥ 6 yr. Usual dosage, 300 mg (1 ampule) twice a day for 28 days, then off for 28 days.
▶ **Dosage in renal impairment**
Dosage and frequency are modified based on the degree of renal impairment and the serum drug concentration.

CONTRAINDICATIONS

Hypersensitivity to tobramycin, other aminoglycosides (cross-sensitivity), and their components.

INTERACTIONS
Drug
Nephrotoxic medications, other aminoglycosides, ototoxic medications: May increase the risk of nephrotoxicity and ototoxicity.
Neuromuscular blockers: May increase neuromuscular blockade.
Herbal and Food
None known.

DIAGNOSTIC TEST EFFECTS

May increase serum bilirubin, BUN, serum creatinine, serum LDH, SGOT (AST), and SGPT (ALT) levels. May decrease serum calcium, magnesium, potassium, and sodium concentrations. Traditional therapeutic peak serum level is 5-8 mcg/mL; peaks up to 20 mcg/mL may be required for some infections. Therapeutic trough serum level is < 1-2 mcg/mL. Toxic peak serum level is > 20 mcg/mL; toxic trough serum level is > 2 mcg/mL.

🐾 IV INCOMPATIBILITIES

Amphotericin B complex (Abelcet, AmBisome, Amphotec), heparin, hetastarch (Hespan), indomethacin (Indocin), propofol (Diprivan), sargramostim (Leukine, Prokine).

🐾 IV COMPATIBILITIES

Amiodarone (Cordarone), calcium gluconate, diltiazem (Cardizem), hydromorphone (Dilaudid), magnesium sulfate, midazolam (Versed), morphine, theophylline.

SIDE EFFECTS

Occasional
IM: Pain, induration.
IV: Phlebitis, thrombophlebitis.
Topical: Hypersensitivity reaction (fever, pruritus, rash, urticaria).
Ophthalmic: Tearing, itching, redness, eyelid swelling.
Rare
Hypotension, nausea, vomiting.

SERIOUS REACTIONS

• Nephrotoxicity (as evidenced by increased BUN and serum creatinine levels and decreased creatinine clearance) may be reversible if the drug is stopped at the first sign of nephrotoxic symptoms.
• Irreversible ototoxicity (manifested as tinnitus, dizziness, ringing or roaring in ears, and hearing loss) and neurotoxicity (manifested as headache, dizziness, lethargy, tremor, and visual disturbances) occur occasionally. The risk of these reactions increases with higher dosages or prolonged therapy and when the solution is applied directly to the mucosa.
• Superinfections, particularly fungal infections, may result from bacterial imbalance with any administration route.
• Anaphylaxis may occur.

PRECAUTIONS & CONSIDERATIONS

Caution is warranted in patients with concomitant use of neuromuscular blockers and in those with impaired renal function or auditory or vestibular impairment. Tobramycin readily crosses the placenta and is distributed in breast milk. Tobramycin may cause fetal nephrotoxicity. The ophthalmic form should not be used in breastfeeding mothers and only when specifically indicated in pregnant women. Immature renal function in neonates and premature infants may increase the risk of toxicity. Age-related renal impairment may require a dosage adjustment in elderly patients.

Determine the patient's history of allergies, especially to aminoglycosides, sulfites, and parabens (for topical and ophthalmic routes), before giving the drug. Intake and output and urinalysis results, as appropriate, should be monitored. To maintain adequate hydration, encourage the patient to drink fluids. Monitor urinalysis results for casts, RBCs, WBCs, and decreased specific gravity. Be alert for ototoxic and neurotoxic side effects. If giving ophthalmic tobramycin, monitor the patient's eye for burning, itching, redness, eyelid swelling and tearing. If giving topical tobramycin, monitor for itching and redness. Be alert for signs and symptoms of superinfection, particularly changes in the oral mucosa, diarrhea, and genital or anal pruritus. Monitor peak and trough serum drug levels.
Storage
Store ophthalmic preparation and solution vials for injection at room temperature. Solutions may be discolored by light or air, but

T

discoloration does not affect drug potency.

Administration

! Space parenteral doses evenly around the clock. Be aware that dosages are based on ideal body weight. Expect to monitor peak and trough serum drug levels. The therapeutic peak serum level is 5-20 mcg/mL, and the therapeutic trough level is 1-2 mcg/mL; the toxic peak serum level is > 20 mcg/mL, and the toxic trough level is > 2 mcg/mL.

For IV use, dilute with 50-100 mL of D5W or 0.9% NaCl. The amount of diluent for infant and children dosages depends on individual needs. Infuse over 20-60 min.

For IM use, to minimize injection site discomfort, administer the IM injection slowly and deep into the gluteus maximus rather than the lateral aspect of the thigh.

For ophthalmic use, place a gloved finger on the lower eyelid, and pull it out until a pocket is formed between the eye and lower lid. Hold the dropper above the pocket and place the correct number of drops (or ¼-½ inch of ointment) into the pocket. Close the eye gently. After administering ophthalmic solution, apply digital pressure to the lacrimal sac for 1-2 min to minimize drainage into the nose and throat, thereby reducing the risk of systemic effects. After applying ophthalmic ointment, close the eye for 1-2 min. Roll the eyeball to increase the drug's contact with the eye. Use a tissue to remove excess solution or ointment around the eye.

Tolazamide

tole-az′a-mide
(Tolinase)
Do not confuse with tolbutamide, tocainide, or tolazine.

CATEGORY AND SCHEDULE

Pregnancy Risk Category: D

Classification: Antidiabetic agents, sulfonylureas, first generation

MECHANISM OF ACTION

A first-generation sulfonylurea that promotes release of insulin from β-cells of the pancreas. *Therapeutic Effect:* Lowers blood glucose concentration.

PHARMACOKINETICS

Well absorbed from the GI tract. Extensively metabolized in liver to five metabolites, three which are active. Primarily excreted in urine. Unknown whether removed by hemodialysis. *Half-life:* 7 h.

AVAILABILITY

Tablets: 100 mg, 250 mg, 500 mg; 100 mg, 250 mg (Tolinase).

INDICATIONS AND DOSAGES
▶ **Diabetes mellitus**
PO
Adults, Elderly. Initially, 100-250 mg once a day, with breakfast or first main meal.
Maintenance: 100-1000 mg once a day.
May increase by increments of 100-250 mg weekly, based on blood glucose response. Maximum: 1000 mg/day. Doses more than 500 mg/day should be given in 2 divided doses with meals.

OFF-LABEL USES
None known.

CONTRAINDICATIONS
Diabetic complications, such as ketosis, acidosis, and diabetic coma, sole therapy for type 1 diabetes mellitus, hypersensitivity to sulfonylurea or tolazamide or its components.

INTERACTIONS
Drug

β-Blockers: May increase hypoglycemic effect and mask signs of hypoglycemia.

Cimetidine, fluoroquinolones, fluconazole, MAOIs, quinidine, ranitidine, large doses of salicylates: May increase effects of tolazamide.

Corticosteroids, lithium, thiazide diuretics: May decrease effects of tolazamide.

Oral anticoagulants: May increase effects of oral anticoagulants.

Herbal

Bitter melon, fenugreek, ginseng, glucomannan, glucosamine, gymnema extracts, licorice, psyllium, St. John's wort: May increase risk of hypoglycemia.

Food

None known.

DIAGNOSTIC TEST EFFECTS
May increase BUN, LDH concentrations, serum alkaline phosphatase, creatinine, and SGOT (AST) levels.

ⓘ IV INCOMPATIBILITIES
None known.

ⓘ IV COMPATIBILITIES
None known.

SIDE EFFECTS
Frequent

Altered taste sensation, dizziness, drowsiness, weight gain, constipation, diarrhea, heartburn, nausea, vomiting, stomach fullness, headache.

Occasional

Increased sensitivity of skin to sunlight, peeling of skin, itching, rash.

SERIOUS REACTIONS
• Severe hypoglycemia may occur due to overdosage and insufficient food intake, especially with increased glucose demands.
• GI hemorrhage, cholestatic hepatic jaundice, leukopenia, thrombocytopenia, pancytopenia, agranulocytosis and aplastic or hemolytic anemia occurs rarely.

PRECAUTIONS & CONSIDERATIONS
Caution is necessary in patients with hypoglycemia or loss of glycemic control as a result of secondary failure. Replace with insulin if necessary if stress from fever, infection, trauma, or surgery has occurred. Tolazamide use is not recommended during pregnancy. It is unknown whether tolazamide is distributed in breast milk. Safety and efficacy of tolazamide have not been established in children. Be aware that hypoglycemia may be difficult to recognize in elderly patients.

Signs and symptoms of hypoglycemia, such as anxiety, cool wet skin, diplopia, dizziness, headache, hunger, numbness in mouth, tachycardia, and tremors, or hyperglycemia, including deep, rapid breathing, dim vision, fatigue, nausea, polydipsia, polyphagia, polyuria, and vomiting, may occur during treatment. Candy, sugar packets, or other sugar supplements should be carried for immediate response to hypoglycemia. Sunscreen and protective eyewear should be worn to prevent the effects of light sensitivity.

Administration

Take tolazamide with breakfast or first main meal. Divide into 2 doses if taking more than 500 mg/day.

Tolbutamide
tole-byoo′ta-mide
(Apo-Tolbutamide [CAN], Orinase, Orinase Diagnostic, Rastinon [AUS], Tol-Tab)
Do not confuse with tolazamide, tocainide, or tolazine.

CATEGORY AND SCHEDULE
Pregnancy Risk Category: C

Classification: Antidiabetic agents, sulfonylureas, first generation

MECHANISM OF ACTION
A first-generation sulfonylurea that promotes the release of insulin from beta cells of pancreas. *Therapeutic Effect:* Lowers blood glucose concentration.

PHARMACOKINETICS

Route	Onset	Peak	Duration
PO	1 h	5-8 h	12-24 h
IV	NA	30-45 min	90-181 min

Well absorbed from the GI tract. Protein binding: 80%-99%. Extensively metabolized in liver to 2 inactive metabolites, primarily via oxidation. Excreted in urine. Removed by hemodialysis. *Half-life:* 4.5-6.5 h.

AVAILABILITY
Tablets: 500 mg (Orinase, Tol-Tab). *Injection, Powder for Reconstitution:* 1 g (Orinase Diagnostic).

INDICATIONS AND DOSAGES
▸ **Diabetes mellitus**
PO
Adults. Initially, 1 g daily, with breakfast or first main meal, or in divided doses. Maintenance: 0.25-3 g once a day.

▸ **Endocrine tumor diagnosis**
IV
Adults. 1 g infused over 2-3 min.

CONTRAINDICATIONS
Diabetic ketoacidosis with or without coma, sole therapy for type 1 diabetes mellitus, use in children, hypersensitivity to tolbutamide or any component of its formulation.

INTERACTIONS
Drug
β-Blockers: May increase the hypoglycemic effect and mask signs of hypoglycemia.
Cimetidine, fluoroquinolones, fluconazole, MAOIs, quinidine, ranitidine, large doses of salicylates: May increase the effects of tolbutamide.
Corticosteroids, lithium, thiazide diuretics: May decrease the effects of tolbutamide.
Fosphenytoin, phenytoin: May increase the risk of phenytoin toxicity.
Oral anticoagulants: May increase the effects of oral anticoagulants.
Rifampin: May decrease effectiveness of tolbutamide.
Sertraline: May decrease the clearance of tolbutamide.
Herbal
Bitter melon, fenugreek, ginseng, glucomannan, glucosamine, gymnema extracts, licorice, psyllium, St. John's wort: May increase the risk of hypoglycemia.
Food
None known.

DIAGNOSTIC TEST EFFECTS
May increase BUN, LDH concentrations, serum alkaline phosphatase, creatinine, and SGOT (AST) levels.

SIDE EFFECTS
Frequent
Increased sensitivity of skin to
sunlight, peeling of skin, itching, rash,
dizziness, drowsiness, weight gain,
constipation, diarrhea, heartburn,
nausea, headache, pain at injection site.
Occasional
Altered taste sensation, constipation,
vomiting, stomach fullness.

SERIOUS REACTIONS
• Severe hypoglycemia may occur
because of overdosage or insufficient
food intake, especially those with
increased glucose demands.
• Cardiovascular mortality has been
reported higher in patients treated
with tolbutamide.
• GI hemorrhage, cholestatic
hepatic jaundice, leukopenia,
thrombocytopenia, pancytopenia,
agranulocytosis and aplastic or
hemolytic anemia occur rarely.

PRECAUTIONS & CONSIDERATIONS
Caution is warranted in patients with
adrenal or pituitary insufficiency,
hypoglycemic reactions, loss of
glycemic control due to secondary
failure, and impaired liver function.
Replacement with insulin may
be necessary during stress from
infection, fever, trauma, or surgery.
It is unknown whether tolbutamide
is distributed in breast milk. Safety
and efficacy of this drug have
not been established in children.
Hypoglycemia may be difficult
to recognize in elderly patients.
Age-related renal impairment may
increase sensitivity to glucose-
lowering in elderly patients.

Signs and symptoms of
hypoglycemia, such as anxiety,
cool wet skin, diplopia, dizziness,
headache, hunger, numbness in
mouth, tachycardia, and tremors, or
hyperglycemia, including deep, rapid

breathing, dim vision, fatigue, nausea,
polydipsia, polyphagia, polyuria, and
vomiting may occur during treatment.
Candy, sugar packets, or other sugar
supplements should be carried for
immediate response to hypoglycemia.
Sunscreen and protective eyewear
should be worn to prevent the effects
of light sensitivity.
Administration
Take oral tolbutamide with breakfast
or first main meal or in divided
doses.

Give IV tolbutamide 1 g over
2-3 min. Reconstitute tolbutamide
with 20 mL of diluent provided in an
ampule in tolbutamide package.

Tolcapone
toll′ka-pone
(Tasmar)

CATEGORY AND SCHEDULE
Pregnancy Risk Category: C

Classification: Antiparkinson
agents, dopaminergics

MECHANISM OF ACTION
An antiparkinson agent that
inhibits the enzyme catechol-
O-methyltransferase (COMT),
potentiating dopamine activity and
increasing the duration of action
of levodopa. *Therapeutic Effect:*
Relieves signs and symptoms of
Parkinson disease.

PHARMACOKINETICS
Rapidly absorbed after PO
administration. Protein binding:
99%. Metabolized in the liver.
Eliminated primarily in urine (60%)
and, to a lesser extent, in feces
(40%). Unknown whether removed
by hemodialysis. *Half-life:* 2-3 h.

AVAILABILITY
Tablets: 100 mg, 200 mg.

INDICATIONS AND DOSAGES
▸ **Adjunctive treatment of Parkinson disease**
PO
Adults, Elderly. Initially, 100 mg 3 times a day concomitantly with each dose of carbidopa and levodopa. May increase dose to 200 mg three times/day if benefit outweighs risk of hepatotoxicity. Maximum: 600 mg/day.

CONTRAINDICATIONS
Hepatic disease. Use with nonselective MAO inhibitors.

INTERACTIONS
Drug
Levodopa: Increases the duration of action of this drug.
Herbal
None known.
Food
All foods: Decrease tolcapone bioavailability by 10%-20% if given within 1 h before or 2 h after drug administration.

DIAGNOSTIC TEST EFFECTS
May increase AST (SGOT) and ALT (SGPT) levels.

SIDE EFFECTS
! Frequency of side effects increases with dosage. The following effects are based on a 200-mg dose.
Frequent (16%-35%)
Nausea, insomnia, somnolence, anorexia, diarrhea, muscle cramps, orthostatic hypotension, excessive dreaming.
Occasional (4%-11%)
Headache, vomiting, confusion, hallucinations, constipation, diaphoresis, bright yellow urine, dry eyes, abdominal pain, dizziness, flatulence.

Rare (2%-3%)
Dyspepsia, neck pain, hypotension, fatigue, chest discomfort.

SERIOUS REACTIONS
• Upper respiratory tract infection and urinary tract infection occur in 5%-7% of patients.
• Too-rapid withdrawal from therapy may produce withdrawal-emergent hyperpyrexia, characterized by fever, muscular rigidity, and altered level of consciousness.
• Dyskinesia and dystonia occur frequently.
• Hepatocellular injury.

PRECAUTIONS & CONSIDERATIONS
Caution is warranted in patients with baseline hypotension, renal impairment, a history of hallucinations, and orthostatic hypotension. Because of a risk of acute fulminant liver failure, tolcapone should be reserved for patients not responding to other therapies. Notify the physician if a female patient is planning to become pregnant. It is unknown whether tolcapone is distributed in breast milk. Tolcapone is not used in children. Elderly patients are at increased risk for hallucinations. Typically, hallucinations in elderly patients occur within the first 2 wks of therapy.

Dizziness, drowsiness, and nausea may occur initially but will diminish or disappear with continued treatment. Alcohol and tasks that require mental alertness or motor skills should be avoided. Change positions slowly to prevent orthostatic hypotension. Also, urine may turn bright yellow. Notify the physician if dark urine, falls, fatigue, itching, loss of appetite, persistent nausea, yellowing of the skin and sclera of the eyes, or abnormal contractions of the head, neck, or trunk occur. Baseline vital signs should be assessed. AST (SGOT) and ALT (SGPT) levels should be monitored before increasing dose and then q2-4 wks for next 6 mo. Relief of symptoms, such as improvement of masklike facial expression, muscular rigidity, shuffling gait, and resting tremors of the hands and head, should also be assessed during treatment.

Administration
! Always administer tolcapone with carbidopa and levodopa. Expect to discontinue tolcapone if ALT and AST levels exceed the upper limits of normal or signs and symptoms of hepatic failure develop.

Take tolcapone without regard to food.

Tolmetin
tole′met-in
(Novo-Tolmetin [CAN], Tolectin, Tolectin DS)

CATEGORY AND SCHEDULE
Pregnancy Risk Category: C, D if used in third trimester or near delivery

Classification: Analgesics, non-narcotic, nonsteroidal anti-inflammatory drugs

MECHANISM OF ACTION
A nonsteroidal anti-inflammatory (NSAID) that produces analgesic and anti-inflammatory effect by inhibiting prostaglandin synthesis. *Therapeutic Effect:* Reduces inflammatory response and intensity of pain stimulus reaching sensory nerve endings.

PHARMACOKINETICS
Rapidly absorbed from the GI tract. Metabolized in liver. Excreted in urine. Minimally removed by hemodialysis. *Half-life:* 5 h.

AVAILABILITY
Tablets: 200 mg, 600 mg (Tolectin).
Capsules: 400 mg (Tolectin DS).

INDICATIONS AND DOSAGES
▶ **Rheumatoid arthritis, osteoarthritis**
PO
Adults, Elderly. Initially, 400 mg 3 times/day (including 1 dose upon arising, 1 dose at bedtime). Adjust dose at intervals of 1-2 wks. Maintenance: 600-1800 mg/day in 3-4 divided doses.
▶ **Juvenile rheumatoid arthritis**
PO
Children more than 2 yr. Initially, 20 mg/kg/day in 3-4 divided doses. Maintenance: 15-30 mg/kg/day in 3-4 divided doses.

OFF-LABEL USES
Treatment of ankylosing spondylitis, psoriatic arthritis.

CONTRAINDICATIONS
MI, hypersensitivity to aspirin or other NSAIDs, coronary artery bypass graft surgery. Use within 14 days of CABG.

INTERACTIONS
Drug
Antacids: May decrease concentrations of tolmetin.
Antihypertensives, diuretics: May decrease the effects of antihypertensives and diuretics.
Aspirin, salicylates: May increase the risk of GI bleeding and side effects.
Bone marrow depressants: May increase the risk of hematologic reactions.

Heparin, oral anticoagulants, thrombolytics: May increase the effects of heparin, oral anticoagulants and thrombolytics.

Lithium: May increase the blood concentration and risk of toxicity of lithium.

Methotrexate: May increase the risk of toxicity of methotrexate.

Probenecid: May increase tolmetin blood concentration.

Herbal

Ginkgo biloba: May increase the risk of bleeding.

Feverfew: May decrease the effects of feverfew.

Food

None known.

DIAGNOSTIC TEST EFFECTS

May increase BUN, potassium, liver function tests. May decrease hemoglobin, hematocrit. May prolong bleeding time.

SIDE EFFECTS

Occasional

Nausea, vomiting, diarrhea, abdominal cramping, dyspepsia (heartburn, indigestion, epigastric pain), flatulence, dizziness, headache, weight decrease or increase.

Rare

Constipation, anorexia, rash, pruritus.

SERIOUS REACTIONS

• Peptic ulcer, GI bleeding, gastritis, and severe hepatic reaction (cholestasis, jaundice) occur rarely.

• Nephrotoxicity (dysuria, hematuria, proteinuria, nephrotic syndrome) and severe hypersensitivity reaction (fever, chills, bronchospasm) occur rarely.

PRECAUTIONS & CONSIDERATIONS

Caution is warranted in patients with impaired renal function, impaired cardiac function, coagulation disorders, and history of upper GI disease. Tolmetin should not be administered to patients with MI or in the setting of coronary artery bypass graft surgery. Tolmetin crosses the placenta. It is unknown whether the drug is distributed in breast milk. Tolmetin use should be avoided during the last trimester of pregnancy as the drug may adversely affect the fetal cardiovascular system causing premature closure of ductus arteriosus. Safety and efficacy of tolmetin have not been established in children younger than 2 yr. GI bleeding or ulceration is more likely to cause serious adverse effects in elderly patients. Age-related renal impairment may increase the risk of liver or renal toxicity, and a reduced dosage is recommended in elderly patients. Avoid alcohol and aspirin during tolmetin therapy as these substances increase the risk of GI bleeding.

Storage

Store at room temperature.

Administration

Take with food, milk, or antacids if GI distress occurs. Therapeutic effect is noted in 1-3 wks.

Tolnaftate

tole-naf´tate

(Absorbine Jr. Antifungal, Aftate Antifungal, Fungi-Guard, Pitrex [CAN], Tinactin Antifungal, Tunactin Antifungal Jock Itch, Tinaderm, Ting)

CATEGORY AND SCHEDULE

Pregnancy Risk Category: B

OTC (aerosol liquid, aerosol powder, cream, gel, powder, solution)

Classification: Carbamothioic acid derivative, antifungal

MECHANISM OF ACTION

An antifungal that distorts hyphae and stunts mycelial growth in susceptible fungi. *Therapeutic Effect:* Results in fungal cell death.

AVAILABILITY

Aerosol, Liquid, Topical: 1 % (Aftate, Tinactin Antifungal, Ting).
Aerosol, Powder, Topical: 1% (Aftate, Tinactin Antifungal, Tinactin Antifungal Jock Itch, Ting).
Cream: 1% (Fungi-Guard, Tinactin Antifungal, Tinactin Antifungal Jock Itch).
Gel: 1% (Absorbine Jr. Antifungal).
Powder: 1% (Tinactin Antifungal).
Solution, Topical: 1% (Absorbine Jr. Antifungal, Tinaderm).

INDICATIONS AND DOSAGES
▸ **Tinea pedis, tinea cruris, tinea corporis**
TOPICAL
Adults, Elderly, Children 2 yr and older.
Spray aerosol or apply 1-3 drops of solution or a small amount of cream, gel, or powder 2 times daily for 2-4 wks.

CONTRAINDICATIONS

Nail and scalp infections, hypersensitivity to tolnaftate or any component of its formulation.

INTERACTIONS

Drug
None known.
Herbal
None known.
Food
None known.

DIAGNOSTIC TEST EFFECTS

None known.

SIDE EFFECTS

Rare
Irritation, burning, pruritus, contact dermatitis.

SERIOUS REACTIONS

• None known.

PRECAUTIONS & CONSIDERATIONS

It is unknown whether tolnaftate is excreted in breast milk. No age-related precautions have been noted in children. Age-related renal impairment may require dosage adjustment in elderly patients. Affected areas should be kept clean and dry. Light clothing should be worn to promote ventilation as well as ventilated shoes. Shoes and socks should be changed at least once a day.
Administration
Apply and rub gently into the affected and surrounding area. Wash hands before and after applying tolnaftate to the skin. Topical therapy may be used for up to 4 wks for tinea pedis or tinea corporis and up to 2 wks for tinea cruris.

Tolterodine
tol-tare′oh-deen
(Detrol, Detrol LA)

CATEGORY AND SCHEDULE
Pregnancy Risk Category: C

Classification: Anticholinergics, relaxants, urinary tract

T

MECHANISM OF ACTION

An antispasmodic that exhibits potent antimuscarinic activity by interceding via cholinergic muscarinic receptors, thereby inhibiting urinary bladder contraction. *Therapeutic Effect:* Decreases urinary frequency, urgency.

PHARMACOKINETICS
Rapidly and well absorbed after PO administration. Protein binding: 96%. Extensively metabolized in the liver to active metabolite. Excreted primarily in urine. Unknown whether removed by hemodialysis. *Half-life:* 1.9-3.7 h.

AVAILABILITY
Tablets (Detrol): 1 mg, 2 mg.
Capsules (Extended-Release [Detrol LA]): 2 mg, 4 mg.

INDICATIONS AND DOSAGES
▸ **Overactive bladder**
PO (EXTENDED RELEASE)
Adults, Elderly. 4 mg once a day.
PO (IMMEDIATE-RELEASE)
Adults, Elderly. 1-2 mg twice a day.
▸ **Dosage in severe renal or hepatic impairment**
PO
Adults, Elderly. 1 mg twice a day.
PO (EXTENDED-RELEASE)
Adults, Elderly. 2 mg once a day.

CONTRAINDICATIONS
Uncontrolled angle-closure glaucoma, urinary retention.

INTERACTIONS
Drug
Clarithromycin, erythromycin, itraconazole, ketoconazole, miconazole: May increase tolterodine blood concentration.
Fluoxetine: May inhibit tolterodine metabolism.
Herbal and Food
None known.

DIAGNOSTIC TEST EFFECTS
None known.

SIDE EFFECTS
Frequent (40%)
Dry mouth.

Occasional (4%-11%)
Headache, dizziness, fatigue, constipation, dyspepsia (heartburn, indigestion, epigastric discomfort), upper respiratory tract infection, urinary track infection, dry eyes, abnormal vision (accommodation problems), nausea, diarrhea.
Rare (3%)
Somnolence, chest or back pain, arthralgia, rash, weight gain, dry skin.

SERIOUS REACTIONS
• Overdose can result in severe anticholinergic effects, including abdominal cramps, facial warmth, excessive salivation or lacrimation, diaphoresis, pallor, urinary urgency, blurred vision, and prolonged QT interval.

PRECAUTIONS & CONSIDERATIONS
Caution is warranted in patients with renal impairment, clinically significant bladder outflow obstruction (increases risk of urine retention), GI obstructive disorders such as pyloric stenosis (increases risk of gastric retention), and treated angle-closure glaucoma. It is unknown whether tolterodine is distributed in breast milk. However, breastfeeding is not recommended. The safety and efficacy of this drug have not been established in children. No age-related precautions have been noted in elderly patients.

Blurred vision, GI upset, constipation, and dry eyes and mouth may occur. Notify the physician of a change in vision. Incontinence and residual urine in the bladder should be determined.
Administration
Take tolterodine without regard to food.

T

Topiramate
toe-peer′a-mate
(Topamax)
Do not confuse with Toprol XL.

CATEGORY AND SCHEDULE
Pregnancy Risk Category: C

Classification: Anticonvulsants

MECHANISM OF ACTION
An anticonvulsant that blocks repetitive, sustained firing of neurons by enhancing the ability of γ-aminobutyric acid to induce an influx of chloride ions into the neurons; may also block sodium channels. *Therapeutic Effect:* Decreases seizure activity.

PHARMACOKINETICS
Rapidly absorbed after PO administration. Protein binding: 13%-17%. Not extensively metabolized. Excreted primarily unchanged in urine. Removed by hemodialysis. *Half-life:* 21 h.

AVAILABILITY
Capsules (Sprinkle): 15 mg, 25 mg.
Tablets: 25 mg, 50 mg, 100 mg, 200 mg.

INDICATIONS AND DOSAGES
▸ **Initial monotherapy**
Adults, Children > 10 yr. Initiate therapy at 50 mg/day in 2 divided doses. Increase by 50 mg/day (in divided doses) weekly to a recommended maintenance dose of 400 mg/day in 2 divided doses.
▸ **Adjunctive treatment of partial seizures, Lennox-Gastaut syndrome, generalized tonic-clonic seizures**
PO
Adults, Elderly, Children older than 16 yr. Initially, 25-50 mg for 1 wk.
May increase by 25-50 mg/day at weekly intervals. Maintenance dose is individualized. Usual range: 200-400 mg/day in 2 divided doses, dependent on seizure type. Maximum: 1600 mg/day.
Children 2-16 yr. Initially, 1-3 mg/kg/day (maximum: 25 mg); initial dose given nightly. May increase by 1-3 mg/kg/day at weekly intervals. Maintenance: 5-9 mg/kg/day in 2 divided doses.
▸ **Migraine prevention**
PO
Adults, Elderly. 25 mg/day for 1 wk, followed by titration of 25 mg/wk to a target of 100 mg/day in 2 divided doses.
▸ **Dosage in renal impairment**
For adults, expect to reduce drug dosage by 50% if CrCl < 70 mL/min. A supplemental dose may be required if on hemodialysis.

OFF-LABEL USES
Treatment of alcohol dependence.

CONTRAINDICATIONS
Hypersensitivity to topiramate or other carbonic anhydrase inhibitors.

INTERACTIONS
Drug
Alcohol, other central nervous system (CNS) depressants: May increase CNS depression.
Carbamazepine, phenytoin, valproic acid: May decrease topiramate blood concentration.
Carbonic anhydrase inhibitors: May increase the risk of renal calculi.
Oral contraceptives: May decrease the effectiveness of oral contraceptives.
Herbal and Food
None known.

DIAGNOSTIC TEST EFFECTS
None known.

T

SIDE EFFECTS

Frequent (10%-30%)
Somnolence, dizziness, ataxia, nervousness, nystagmus, diplopia, paresthesia, nausea, tremor.
Occasional (3%-9%)
Confusion, breast pain, dysmenorrhea, dyspepsia, depression, asthenia, pharyngitis, weight loss, anorexia, rash, musculoskeletal pain, abdominal pain, difficulty with coordination, sinusitis, agitation, flulike symptoms.
Rare (2%-3%)
Mood disturbances, such as irritability and depression; dry mouth; aggressive behavior, kidney stones.

SERIOUS REACTIONS

• Psychomotor slowing, impaired concentration, language problems (such as word-finding difficulties), and memory disturbances occur occasionally. These reactions are generally mild to moderate but may be severe enough to require discontinuation of drug therapy.
• Serious and potentially fatal exfoliative dermatologic reactions.
• Metabolic acidosis (rare) secondary to bicarbonate loss; action may also lead to kidney stones.

PRECAUTIONS & CONSIDERATIONS

Caution is warranted in patients with impaired hepatic and renal function, a predisposition to renal calculi, and hypersensitivity to topiramate. It is unknown whether topiramate is distributed in breast milk. Be aware that topiramate decreases oral contraceptive effectiveness, and an alternative means of contraception should be used during therapy. No age-related precautions have been noted in children older than 2 yr. In elderly patients, age-related renal impairment may require dosage adjustment.

Drowsiness and dizziness may occur, so alcohol and tasks requiring mental alertness or motor skills should be avoided. Notify the physician of blurred vision or other visual changes. Seizure disorder, including the onset, duration, frequency, intensity, and type of seizures, should be assessed before and during treatment. Renal function, including BUN and serum creatinine levels, should also be monitored. Adequate hydration should be maintained to decrease the risk of kidney stones.
Administration
Do not break tablets because they have a bitter taste. Take topiramate without regard to food. Capsules may be swallowed whole or contents sprinkled on a teaspoonful of soft food and swallowed immediately. They should not be chewed. Do not abruptly discontinue topiramate because this may precipitate seizures. Strict maintenance of drug therapy is essential for seizure control.

Topotecan
toe-poe-tee′kan
(Hycamtin)

CATEGORY AND SCHEDULE
Pregnancy Risk Category: D

Classification: Antineoplastics, topoisomerase inhibitors

MECHANISM OF ACTION

A DNA topoisomerase inhibitor that interacts with topoisomerase I, an enzyme that allows DNA replication by producing reversible single-strand breaks in DNA that relieve torsional strain. Topotecan prevents religation of the DNA strand, resulting in damage to double-strand

DNA and cell death. *Therapeutic Effect:* Destroys cancer cells.

PHARMACOKINETICS
Hydrolyzed to active form after IV administration. Protein binding: 35%. Excreted in urine. *Half-life:* 2-3 h (increased in impaired renal function).

AVAILABILITY
Powder for Injection: 4 mg (single-dose vial).

INDICATIONS AND DOSAGES
▸ **Ovarian carcinoma, small-cell lung cancer**
IV
Adults, Elderly. 1.5 mg/m^2/day over 30 min for 5 consecutive days, beginning on day 1 of a 21-day course. Minimum of four courses is recommended. If severe neutropenia (neutrophil count < 1500/mm^2) or if platelet count < 25,000 mm^3 occurs during treatment, reduce dose for subsequent courses by 0.25 mg/m^2, or administer filgrastim (G-CSF) no sooner than 24 h after the last dose of topotecan.
▸ **Dosage in renal impairment**
No dosage adjustment is necessary in patients with mild renal impairment (creatinine clearance of 40-60 mL/min). For moderate renal impairment (creatinine clearance of 20-39 mL/min), give 0.75 mg/m^2.

OFF-LABEL USES
Treatment of solid tumors including osteosarcoma, neuroblastoma, pediatric leukemia, rhabdomyosarcoma.

CONTRAINDICATIONS
Baseline neutrophil count < 1500 cells/mm^3, breastfeeding, pregnancy, severe myelosuppression.

INTERACTIONS
Drug
Cisplatin: May increase the severity of myelosuppression.
Live-virus vaccines: May potentiate virus replication, increase vaccine side effects, and decrease the patient's antibody response to the vaccine.
Other bone marrow depressants: May increase the risk of myelosuppression.
Herbal and Food
None known.

DIAGNOSTIC TEST EFFECTS
May increase serum bilirubin, AST (SGOT), and ALT (SGPT) levels. May decrease RBC, leukocyte, neutrophil, and platelet counts.

🔟 IV INCOMPATIBILITIES
Dexamethasone (Decadron), 5-fluorouracil, mitomycin (Mutamycin).

🔟 IV COMPATIBILITIES
Carboplatin (Paraplatin), cisplatin (Platinol AQ), cyclophosphamide (Cytoxan), doxorubicin (Adriamycin), etoposide (VePesid), gemcitabine (Gemzar), granisetron (Kytril), ondansetron (Zofran), paclitaxel (Taxol), vincristine (Oncovin).

SIDE EFFECTS
Frequent
Nausea (77%), vomiting (58%), diarrhea and total alopecia (42%), headache (21%), dyspnea (21%).
Occasional
Paraesthesia (9%), constipation and abdominal pain (3%)
Rare
Anorexia, malaise, arthralgia, asthenia, myalgia.

SERIOUS REACTIONS
• Severe neutropenia (neutrophil count < 500 cells/mm^3) occurs in

60% of patients, usually during the first course of therapy. The neutrophil nadir usually occurs at a median of 11 days after starting therapy.

• Thrombocytopenia (platelet count < 25,000/mm³) occurs in 26% of patients, and severe anemia (RBC count < 8 g/dL) occurs in 40% of patients. The platelet and RBC nadirs usually occur at a median of 15 days after starting the first course of therapy.

PRECAUTIONS & CONSIDERATIONS

Caution is warranted with hepatic and renal impairment and mild myelosuppression.

Because of the risk of fetal harm, pregnant women should not take topotecan, especially in the first trimester. It is unknown whether topotecan is distributed in breast milk; however, breastfeeding is not recommended. The safety and efficacy of topotecan have not been established in children. In elderly patients, age-related renal impairment may require dosage adjustment. Vaccinations and coming in contact with crowds and people with known infections should be avoided.

CBC, especially blood hemoglobin levels, and platelet count, should be assessed before each topotecan dose. Myelosuppression may precipitate life-threatening anemia, hemorrhage, and infection. If platelet count drops, minimize trauma (for example, by avoiding IM or rectal drug administration and by gently repositioning the person). Premedicate with antiemetics, if ordered, on the day of treatment, starting at least 30 min before topotecan administration. Electrolyte levels, hydration status, and intake and output should also be monitored because diarrhea and vomiting are common side effects of topotecan.

Storage

Store vials at room temperature in original cartons. Reconstituted vials diluted for infusion are stable at room temperature in ambient lighting for up to 24 h.

Administration

! As prescribed, do not give topotecan if baseline neutrophil count is < 1500 cells/mm³ and platelet count is < 100,000/mm³.

Reconstitute each 4-mg vial with 4 mL sterile water for injection. Further dilute with 50-100 mL 0.9% NaCl or D5W. Administer the drug by IV infusion over 30 min. Be aware that extravasation is associated with only mild local reactions, such as ecchymosis and erythema.

Toremifene
(Fareston)

CATEGORY AND SCHEDULE
Pregnancy Risk Category: D

Classification: Antineoplastics, antiestrogens, estrogen receptor modulators, selective, hormones/hormone modifiers.

MECHANISM OF ACTION
A nonsteroidal antiestrogen and antineoplastic agent that binds to estrogen receptors on tumors, producing a complex that decreases DNA synthesis and inhibits estrogen effects. *Therapeutic Effect:* Blocks growth-stimulating effects of estrogen in breast cancer.

PHARMACOKINETICS
Well absorbed after PO administration. Metabolized in the

liver. Eliminated in feces. *Half-life:* Approximately 5 days.

AVAILABILITY
Tablets: 60 mg.

INDICATIONS AND DOSAGES
▸ **Breast cancer**
PO
Adults. 60 mg/day until disease progression is observed.

OFF-LABEL USES
Treatment of desmoid tumors, endometrial carcinoma.

CONTRAINDICATIONS
History of thromboembolic disease.

INTERACTIONS
Drug
Carbamazepine, phenobarbital, phenytoin: May decrease toremifene blood concentration.
Warfarin: May increase PT.
Herbal
None known.
Food
None known.

DIAGNOSTIC TEST EFFECTS
May increase serum alkaline phosphatase, bilirubin, calcium, and AST (SGOT) levels.

SIDE EFFECTS
Frequent
Hot flashes (35%); diaphoresis (20%); nausea (14%); vaginal discharge (13%); dizziness, dry eyes (9%).
Occasional (2%-5%)
Edema, vomiting, vaginal bleeding.
Rare
Fatigue, depression, lethargy, anorexia.

SERIOUS REACTIONS
• Ocular toxicity (cataracts, glaucoma, decreased visual acuity) and hypercalcemia may occur.

PRECAUTIONS & CONSIDERATIONS
Caution is warranted in patients with preexisting endometrial hyperplasia, leukopenia, and thrombocytopenia. Toremifene use should be avoided during pregnancy because this drug may cause fetal harm. Nonhormonal methods of contraception should be used during treatment. It is unknown whether toremifene is distributed in breast milk; however, breastfeeding is not recommended. Toremifene is not prescribed for children; the safety and efficacy of this drug in children have not been established. No age-related precautions have been noted in elderly patients.

Initial flare-up of symptoms, including bone pain and hot flashes, may occur but will subside with continued therapy. Notify the physician if nausea and vomiting, leg cramps, shortness of breath, weakness, weight gain, or vaginal bleeding, discharge, or itching occurs. Estrogen receptor assay test should be performed before starting therapy. CBC and serum calcium levels should be monitored before and periodically during toremifene therapy. Be aware of signs and symptoms of hypercalcemia, including constipation, deep bone or flank pain, excessive thirst, hypotonicity of muscles, increased urine output, nausea and vomiting, and renal calculi.
Administration
Take oral toremifene without regard to food.

Torsemide

tor´se-mide
(Demadex)
Do not confuse torsemide with furosemide.

CATEGORY AND SCHEDULE

Pregnancy Risk Category: B

Classification: Diuretics, loop

MECHANISM OF ACTION

A loop diuretic that enhances the excretion of sodium, chloride, potassium, and water at the ascending limb of the loop of Henle; also reduces plasma and extracellular fluid volume. *Therapeutic Effect:* Produces diuresis; lowers BP.

PHARMACOKINETICS

Route	Onset	Peak	Duration
PO	1 h	1-2 h	6-8 h
IV	10 min	1 h	6-8 h

Rapidly and well absorbed from the GI tract. Protein binding: 97%-99%. Metabolized in the liver. Primarily excreted in urine. Not removed by hemodialysis. *Half-life:* 3.3 h.

AVAILABILITY

Tablets: 5 mg, 10 mg, 20 mg, 100 mg.
Injection: 10 mg/mL.

INDICATIONS AND DOSAGES
▸ **Hypertension**
PO
Adults, Elderly. Initially, 5 mg/day. May increase to 10 mg/day if no response in 4-6 wks. If no response, additional antihypertensive added.

▸ **Edema associated with congestive heart failure (CHF)**
PO, IV
Adults, Elderly. Initially, 10-20 mg/day. May increase by approximately doubling dose until desired therapeutic effect is attained. Doses > 200 mg have not been adequately studied.
▸ **Edema associated with chronic renal failure**
PO, IV
Adults, Elderly. Initially, 20 mg/day. May increase by approximately doubling dose until desired therapeutic effect is attained. Doses > 200 mg have not been adequately studied.
▸ **Hepatic cirrhosis**
PO, IV
Adults, Elderly. Initially, 5 mg/day given with aldosterone antagonist or potassium-sparing diuretic. May increase by approximately doubling dose until desired therapeutic effect is attained. Doses > 40 mg have not been adequately studied.

CONTRAINDICATIONS

Anuria, hepatic coma, severe electrolyte depletion.

INTERACTIONS
Drug
Amphotericin B, nephrotoxic medications, ototoxic medications: May increase the risk of nephrotoxicity and ototoxicity.
Anticoagulants, heparin, thrombolytics: May decrease the effects of these drugs.
Digoxin: May increase the risk of digoxin toxicity associated with torsemide-induced hypokalemia.
Lithium: May increase the risk of lithium toxicity.
NSAIDs, probenecid: May decrease the diuretic effect of torsemide.

Other antihypertensives: May increase the risk of hypotension.
Other hypokalemia-causing medications: May increase the risk of hypokalemia.
Herbal and Food
None known.

DIAGNOSTIC TEST EFFECTS

May increase BUN, serum creatinine, and serum uric acid levels. May decrease serum calcium, chloride, magnesium, potassium, and sodium levels.

⊘ IV INCOMPATIBILITIES

Do not mix torsemide with any other medications except for milrinone (Primacor).

⊌ IV COMPATIBILITIES

Milrinone (Primacor).

SIDE EFFECTS

Frequent (10%-40%)
Headache, dizziness, rhinitis.
Occasional (1%-3%)
Asthenia, insomnia, nervousness, diarrhea, constipation, nausea, dyspepsia, edema, ECG changes, pharyngitis, cough, arthralgia, myalgia.
Rare (< 1%)
Syncope, hypotension, arrhythmias.

SERIOUS REACTIONS

• Ototoxicity may occur with high doses or a too-rapid IV administration.
• Overdose produces acute, profound water loss; volume and electrolyte depletion; dehydration; decreased blood volume; and circulatory collapse.

PRECAUTIONS & CONSIDERATIONS

Caution is warranted in patients with ascites, hepatic cirrhosis, renal impairment, systemic lupus erythematosus, history of ventricular arrhythmias, hypersensitivity to sulfonamides, with cardiac patients and elderly patients. It is unknown whether torsemide is excreted in breast milk. The safety and efficacy of this drug have not been established in children. No age-related precautions have been noted in elderly patients. Consuming foods high in potassium, such as apricots, bananas, legumes, meat, orange juice, raisins, whole grains, including cereals, and white and sweet potatoes, is encouraged. Avoid taking other medications, including OTC drugs, without first consulting the physician.

An increase in the frequency and volume of urination may occur. Notify the physician of cramps, dizziness, an irregular heartbeat, muscle weakness, nausea, or hearing abnormalities. BP, vital signs, electrolytes, intake and output, and weight should be monitored before and during treatment. Be aware of signs of electrolyte disturbances such as hypokalemia or hyponatremia. Hypokalemia may cause arrhythmias, altered mental status, muscle cramps, asthenia, and tremor. Less potassium is lost with torsemide than with furosemide.
Storage
Store torsemide at room temperature.
Administration
Take torsemide with food to avoid GI upset, preferably with breakfast to prevent nocturia.
! Flush IV line with 0.9% NaCl before and after torsemide administration.

Torsemide may be given undiluted as IV push over 2 min. For continuous IV infusion, dilute with 0.9% or 0.45% NaCl or D5W and infuse over 24 h. Administer

T

IV push slowly because too-rapid administration may cause ototoxicity.

Tositumomab and Iodine 131 I-Tositumomab
toe-sit-two′mo-mab
(Bexxar)

CATEGORY AND SCHEDULE
Pregnancy Risk Category: X

Classification: Antineoplastics, monoclonal antibodies, radiopharmaceuticals

MECHANISM OF ACTION
A monoclonal antibody composed of an antibody conjoined with a radiolabeled antitumor antibody. The antibody portion binds specifically to the CD20 antigen, which is found on pre-B and B lymphocytes and on more than 90% of B-cell non-Hodgkin lymphomas resulting in formation of a complex. *Therapeutic Effect:* Induces cytotoxicity associated with ionizing radiation from the radioisotope. Depletes circulating CD20-positive cells.

PHARMACOKINETICS
Elimination of iodine 131 (^{131}I) occurs by decay and excretion in urine. *Half-life:* 8 days. Patients with high tumor burden, splenomegaly, or bone marrow involvement have a faster clearance, shorter half-life, and larger volume of distribution.

AVAILABILITY
Kit (dosimetric): (Bexxar) tositumomab 225 mg/16.1 mL (2 vials), tositumomab 35 mg/2.5 mL (1 vial), and ^{131}I tositumomab 0.1 mg/mL (1 vial).
Kit (therapeutic): (Bexxar) tositumomab 225 mg/16.1 mL (2 vials), tositumomab 35 mg/2.5 mL (1 vial), and ^{131}I tositumomab 1.1 mg/mL (1 or 2 vials).

INDICATIONS AND DOSAGES
▸ **Non-Hodgkin lymphoma**
IV
Adults, Elderly. Dosage contains 4 components. Day 0: tositumomab 450 mg/50 NaCl over 60 min. Then ^{131}I tositumomab 35 mg in 30 mL NaCl over 20 min. Day 7: tositumomab 450 mg/50 NaCl over 60 min. Then ^{131}I tositumomab to deliver 65-75 cGy total body irradiation and tositumomab 35 mg over 20 min.

CONTRAINDICATIONS
Hypersensitivity to murine proteins or iodine.

INTERACTIONS
Drug
Anticoagulants, medications that interfere with platelet function: Increase the risk of bleeding and hemorrhage.
Herbal
None known.
Food
None known.

DIAGNOSTIC TEST EFFECTS
May decrease blood hematocrit and hemoglobin levels, platelet and WBC counts, and thyroid-stimulating hormone level.

SIDE EFFECTS
Frequent (18%-46%)
Asthenia, fever, nausea, cough, chills.
Occasional (10%-17%)
Rash, headache, abdominal pain, vomiting, anorexia, myalgia,

T

diarrhea, pharyngitis, arthralgia, rhinitis, pruritus.

Rare (5%-9%)
Peripheral edema, diaphoresis, constipation, dyspepsia, back pain, hypotension, vasodilation, dizziness, somnolence.

SERIOUS REACTIONS

• Infusion toxicity, characterized by fever, rigors, diaphoresis, hypotension, dyspnea, and nausea, may occur during or within 48 h of the infusion.
• Severe, prolonged myelosuppression, characterized by neutropenia, anemia, and thrombocytopenia, occurs in 71% of patients.
• Sepsis occurs in 45% of patients.
• Hemorrhage occurs in 12% of patients.
• Myelodysplastic syndrome occurs in 8% of patients.

PRECAUTIONS & CONSIDERATIONS

Caution is warranted with active systemic infection, immunosuppression, and impaired renal function. The use of the ^{131}I-tositumomab component is contraindicated during pregnancy and causes severe, possibly irreversible hypothyroidism in neonates. Because ^{131}I is excreted in breast milk, breastfeeding is not recommended. The safety and efficacy of this drug have not been established in children. Elderly patients (i.e., older than 65 yr) have exhibited a lower overall response rate to the drug. They have also had a lower incidence, but longer duration, of severe hematologic toxicity. Immunizations during therapy and contact with those who have recently received a live-virus vaccine should be avoided.

Notify the physician if bruising, fever, signs of local infection, sore throat, or unusual bleeding from any site occurs. CBC should be obtained before beginning therapy and at least weekly after administration for at least 10 wks. Laboratory values should be monitored for evidence of severe and prolonged anemia, neutropenia, and thrombocytopenia. Know that time to nadir is 4-7 wks and the duration of cytopenias (predominantly grade 3 and 4 thrombocytopenia and grade 3 and 4 neutropenia) is approximately 30 days. Signs and symptoms for hematologic toxicity (including excessive fatigue and weakness, chills, fever, ecchymosis, and unusual bleeding from any site) and hypothyroidism (including fatigue, sensitivity to cold, unexplained weight gain, and constipation) should be assessed.

Storage
Refrigerate tositumomab vials before dilution. Protect from strong light. After dilution, tositumomab solution is stable for 24 h if refrigerated and 8 h at room temperature. Discard any unused portion left in the vial. Do not shake.

Administration
! Pretreat by administering diphenhydramine 50 mg and acetaminophen 650-1000 mg 1 h before administering tositumomab, followed by acetaminophen 650-1000 mg every 4 h for 2 doses, then every 4 h as needed. Full recovery from hematologic toxicities is not a requirement for giving the second dose. Be aware that the regimen consists of 4 components given in 2 separate steps: the dosimetric step, followed 7-14 days later by the therapeutic step. During the infusion, use IV tubing with an in-line 0.22-μm filter, and use the same tubing for both the dosimetric and therapeutic steps because changing

T

the filter results in drug loss. Plan to reduce the infusion rate by 50% for mild to moderate infusion toxicity and to interrupt the infusion for severe infusion toxicity. Expect to resume therapy at 50% of the infusion rate when toxic reactions have resolved.

! Administer a thyroid protective agent such as potassium iodide, as prescribed, beginning 24 h before administration of the ^{131}I-tositumomab dosimetric step and continuing for 2 wks after administration of the therapeutic step. Remember that reconstitution amounts and rates of administration are the same for both the dosimetric and therapeutic steps.

Use strict aseptic technique in preparing the drug to protect the patient from infection. Follow radiation safety protocols. Reconstitute 450 mg tositumomab in 50 mL 0.9% NaCl. Reconstitute 450 mg tositumomab in 50 mL 0.9% NaCl. Infuse tositumomab over 60 min. Keep ^{131}I-tositumomab frozen until thawing it before drug administration. Thawed ^{131}I-tositumomab doses are stable for 8 h if refrigerated. Discard any unused portion. Reconstitute ^{131}I-tositumomab in 30 mL 0.9% NaCl. Infuse ^{131}I-tositumomab over 20 min.

Tramadol
tray′mah-doal
(Tramal [AUS], Tramal SR [AUS], Ultram, Zydol [AUS])
Do not confuse tramadol with Toradol, or Ultram with Ultane.

CATEGORY AND SCHEDULE
Pregnancy Risk Category: C

Classification: Analgesics, narcotic-like

MECHANISM OF ACTION
An analgesic that binds to μ-opioid receptors and inhibits reuptake of norepinephrine and serotonin. Reduces the intensity of pain stimuli reaching sensory nerve endings. *Therapeutic Effect:* Alters the perception of and emotional response to pain.

PHARMACOKINETICS

Route	Onset	Peak	Duration
PO	< 1 h	2-3 h	4-6 h

Rapidly and almost completely absorbed after PO administration. Protein binding: 20%. Extensively metabolized in the liver to active metabolite (reduced in patients with advanced cirrhosis). Primarily excreted in urine. Minimally removed by hemodialysis. *Half-life:* 6-7 h.

AVAILABILITY
Tablets: 50 mg.

INDICATIONS AND DOSAGES
▸ **Moderate to moderately severe pain**
PO (IMMEDIATE RELEASE)
Adults, Elderly. 50-100 mg q4-6h. Maximum: 400 mg/day for patients

younger than 75 yr; 300 mg/day for patients older than 75 yr.

▸ **Dosage in renal impairment**
For patients with creatinine clearance of < 30 mL/min, increase dosing interval to q12h. Do not use extended-release tablets. Maximum: 200 mg/day.

▸ **Dosage in hepatic impairment**
Dosage is decreased to 50 mg q12h. Do not use extended-release tablets.

CONTRAINDICATIONS
Opiate agonist hypersensitivity, acute alcohol intoxication; concurrent use of centrally acting analgesics, hypnotics, opioids, or psychotropic drugs.

INTERACTIONS
Drug
Alcohol, other central nervous system (CNS) depressants: May increase CNS or respiratory depression and hypotension.
Carbamazepine: Decreases tramadol blood concentration.
MAOIs: Increase tramadol blood concentration.
Herbal and Food
None known.

DIAGNOSTIC TEST EFFECTS
May increase serum creatinine, AST (SGOT), and ALT (SGPT) hepatic levels. May decrease blood hemoglobin level. May cause proteinuria.

SIDE EFFECTS
Frequent (5%-15%)
Dizziness or vertigo, nausea, constipation, headache, somnolence.
Occasional (5%-10%)
Vomiting, pruritus, CNS stimulation (such as nervousness, anxiety, agitation, tremor, euphoria, mood swings, and hallucinations), asthenia, diaphoresis, dyspepsia, dry mouth, diarrhea.

Rare (< 5%)
Malaise, vasodilation, anorexia, flatulence, rash, blurred vision, urine retention or urinary frequency, menopausal symptoms.

SERIOUS REACTIONS
• Overdose results in respiratory depression and seizures.
• Tramadol may have a prolonged duration of action and cumulative effect in patients with hepatic or renal impairment.

PRECAUTIONS & CONSIDERATIONS
Extreme caution should be used with acute abdominal conditions, hepatic or renal impairment, increased intracranial pressure, opioid dependence, and a sensitivity to opioids. Tramadol crosses the placenta and is distributed in breast milk. The safety and efficacy of tramadol have not been established in children. Age-related renal impairment may require a dosage adjustment in elderly patients. Alcohol and OTC drugs, such as analgesics and sedatives, should be avoided.

Blurred vision, dizziness, and drowsiness may occur, so tasks requiring mental alertness or motor skills should be avoided. Notify the physician of any chest pain, difficulty breathing, excessive sedation, muscle weakness, palpitations, seizures, severe constipation, or tremors. Liver and renal function studies should be obtained before therapy. BP, pulse rate, pattern of daily bowel activity and stool consistency, bladder for urine retention, and therapeutic response should be monitored during tramadol use.

Administration
! Be aware that dialysis patients can receive their regular dose on the day of dialysis.

Take tramadol without regard to food.

Trandolapril
tran-doe′la-pril
(Gopten [AUS], Mavik, Odrik [AUS])
Do not confuse with tramadol.

CATEGORY AND SCHEDULE
Pregnancy Risk Category: C (D if used in second or third trimester)

Classification: Angiotensin-converting enzyme inhibitors

MECHANISM OF ACTION
An ACE inhibitor that suppresses the renin-angiotensin-aldosterone system and prevents the conversion of angiotensin I to angiotensin II, a potent vasoconstrictor; may also inhibit angiotensin II at local vascular and renal sites. Decreases plasma angiotensin II, increases plasma renin activity, and decreases aldosterone secretion. *Therapeutic Effect:* Reduces peripheral arterial resistance and pulmonary capillary wedge pressure; improves cardiac output and exercise tolerance.

PHARMACOKINETICS
Slowly absorbed from the GI tract. Protein binding: 80%. Metabolized in the liver and GI mucosa to active metabolite. Primarily excreted in urine. Removed by hemodialysis. *Half-life:* 24 h.

AVAILABILITY
Tablets: 1 mg, 2 mg, 4 mg.

INDICATIONS AND DOSAGES
▶ **Hypertension (without diuretic)**
PO
Adults, Elderly. Initially, 1 mg once a day in nonblack patients, 2 mg once a day in black patients. Adjust dosage at least at 7-day intervals. Maintenance: 2-4 mg/day. Maximum: 8 mg/day.
▶ **Congestive heart failure (CHF)**
PO
Adults, Elderly. Initially, 0.5-1 mg, titrated to target dose of 4 mg/day.

CONTRAINDICATIONS
History of angioedema from previous treatment with ACE inhibitors.

INTERACTIONS
Drug
Alcohol, antihypertensives, diuretics: May increase the effects of trandolapril.
Lithium: May increase lithium blood concentration and risk of lithium toxicity.
NSAIDs: May decrease the effects of trandolapril.
Potassium-sparing diuretics, potassium supplements: May cause hyperkalemia.
Herbal
None known.
Food
None known.

DIAGNOSTIC TEST EFFECTS
May increase BUN, serum alkaline phosphatase, serum bilirubin, serum creatinine, serum potassium, AST (SGOT), and ALT (SGPT) levels. May decrease serum sodium levels. May cause positive antinuclear antibody titer.

SIDE EFFECTS
Frequent (23%-35%)
Dizziness, cough.
Occasional (3%-11%)
Hypotension, dyspepsia (heartburn, epigastric pain, indigestion),

syncope, asthenia (loss of strength), tinnitus.

Rare (< 1%)
Palpitations, insomnia, drowsiness, nausea, vomiting, constipation, flushed skin.

SERIOUS REACTIONS
• Excessive hypotension (first-dose syncope) may occur in patients with CHF and in those who are severely salt or volume depleted.
• Angioedema and hyperkalemia occur rarely.
• Agranulocytosis and neutropenia may be noted in those with collagen vascular disease, including scleroderma and systemic lupus erythematosus, and impaired renal function.
• Nephrotic syndrome may be noted in those with history of renal disease.

PRECAUTIONS & CONSIDERATIONS
Caution is warranted in patients with CHF, collagen vascular disease, hyperkalemia, hypovolemia, renal impairment, and renal stenosis. Trandolapril crosses the placenta, is distributed in breast milk, and may cause fetal or neonatal morbidity or mortality. Safety and efficacy of trandolapril have not been established in children. No age-related precautions have been noted in elderly patients.

Dizziness and light-headedness may occur. Tasks that require mental alertness or motor skills should be avoided. Notify the physician of chest pain, cough, diarrhea, difficulty swallowing, fever, palpitations, sore throat, swelling of the face, or vomiting. Be alert to fluctuations in BP. If an excessive reduction in BP occurs, place the person in the supine position with legs elevated. CBC and blood chemistry should be obtained before beginning trandolapril

therapy, then every 2 wks for the next 3 mo, and periodically thereafter in patients with autoimmune disease or renal impairment and in those who are taking drugs that affect immune response or leukocyte count. Crackles and wheezing should be assessed in persons with CHF. BUN, serum creatinine, and serum potassium levels, WBC count, urinalysis, intake and output, and pattern of daily bowel activity and stool consistency should also be monitored.

Administration
Take trandolapril without regard to food. Crush tablets as necessary.

Tranylcypromine
tran-ill-sip'roe-meen
(Parnate)

CATEGORY AND SCHEDULE
Pregnancy Risk Category: C

Classification: Antidepressants, monoamine oxidase inhibitors

MECHANISM OF ACTION
An MAOI that inhibits the activity of the enzyme monoamine oxidase at central nervous system (CNS) storage sites, leading to increased levels of the neurotransmitters epinephrine, norepinephrine, serotonin, and dopamine at neuronal receptor sites. *Therapeutic Effect:* Relieves depression.

AVAILABILITY
Tablets: 10 mg.

INDICATIONS AND DOSAGES
▸ **Depression refractory to or intolerant of other therapy**

PO
Adults, Elderly. Initially, 10 mg twice a day. May increase by 10 mg/day at 1- to 3-wk intervals up to 60 mg/day in divided doses.

CONTRAINDICATIONS
Ethanol intoxication, CHF, children younger than 16 yr, pheochromocytoma, severe hepatic or renal impairment, uncontrolled hypertension, concurrent MAOI therapy.

INTERACTIONS
Drug
Alcohol, other CNS depressants: May increase CNS depressant effects.
Buspirone: May increase BP.
Caffeine-containing medications: May increase the risk of cardiac arrhythmias and hypertension.
Carbamazepine, cyclobenzaprine, maprotiline, other MAOIs: May precipitate hypertensive crisis.
Dopamine, tryptophan: May cause sudden, severe hypertension.
Fluoxetine, trazodone, tricyclic antidepressants: May cause serotonin syndrome and neuroleptic malignant syndrome.
Insulin, oral antidiabetics: May increase the effects of these drugs.
Meperidine, other opioid analgesics: May produce diaphoresis, immediate excitation, rigidity, and severe hypertension or hypotension, sometimes leading to severe respiratory distress, vascular collapse, seizures, coma, and death.
SSRI: May cause serotonin syndrome.
Herbal
None known.
Food
Caffeine, chocolate, tyramine-containing foods (such as aged cheese): May cause sudden, severe hypertension.

DIAGNOSTIC TEST EFFECTS
None known.

SIDE EFFECTS
Frequent
Orthostatic hypotension, restlessness, GI upset, insomnia, dizziness, lethargy, weakness, dry mouth, peripheral edema.
Occasional
Flushing, diaphoresis, rash, urinary frequency, increased appetite, transient impotence.
Rare
Visual disturbances.

SERIOUS REACTIONS
• Hypertensive crisis occurs rarely and is marked by severe hypertension, occipital headache radiating frontally, neck stiffness or soreness, nausea, vomiting, diaphoresis, fever or chills, clammy skin, dilated pupils, palpitations, tachycardia or bradycardia, and constricting chest pain.

PRECAUTIONS & CONSIDERATIONS
Caution is warranted in patients with cardiac arrhythmias, frequent or severe headaches, hypertension, suicidal tendencies, and within several hours of ingestion of contraindicated substance, such as tyramine-containing food. Foods that require bacteria or molds for their preparation or preservation (such as yogurt and aged cheese), foods containing tyramine (such as avocados, bananas, broad beans, meat tenderizers, liver, smoked or pickled meats and fish, papayas, figs, raisins, sour cream, soy sauce, beer, wine, and yeast extracts), and excessive amounts of caffeine-containing foods or beverages (including chocolate, coffee, and tea) should be avoided.

Dizziness may occur, so change positions slowly, and alcohol and tasks that require mental alertness or motor skills should be avoided. Notify the physician if headache or neck soreness or stiffness occurs. If hypertensive crisis occurs, phentolamine 5-10 mg IV should be administered. BP, temperature, and weight should be assessed.

Administration

! Make sure at least 14 days elapse between the use of tranylcypromine and a selective serotonin reuptake inhibitor (5 wk for fluoxetine).

Take the second daily dose no later than 4:00 PM to avoid insomnia. Depression may start to lift during the first week of therapy and the drug's full therapeutic benefit will occur within 3 wks.

Trastuzumab

tras-too′-ze-mab
(Herceptin)

CATEGORY AND SCHEDULE

Pregnancy Risk Category: B

Classification: Antineoplastics, monoclonal antibodies

MECHANISM OF ACTION

Binds to the HER-2 protein, which is overexpressed in 25%-30% of primary breast cancers, thereby inhibiting proliferation of tumor cells. *Therapeutic Effect:* Inhibits the growth of tumor cells and mediates antibody-dependent cellular cytotoxicity.

PHARMACOKINETICS

Half-life: 5.8 days (range: 1-32 days).

AVAILABILITY

Injection, Powder for Reconstitution: 440 mg.

INDICATIONS AND DOSAGES

▶ **Breast cancer**

IV

Adults, Elderly. Initially, 4 mg/kg as an infusion of 90-min on wk 1 then 2 mg/kg weekly as at least a 30-min infusion.

CONTRAINDICATIONS

Preexisting cardiac disease.

INTERACTIONS

Drug

Cyclophosphamide, doxorubicin, epirubicin: May increase the risk of cardiac dysfunction.

Herbal

None known.

Food

None known.

DIAGNOSTIC TEST EFFECTS

None known.

⊘ IV INCOMPATIBILITIES

Do not mix trastuzumab with any other medications or with D5W.

SIDE EFFECTS

Frequent (> 20%)

Pain, asthenia, fever, chills, headache, abdominal pain, back pain, infection, nausea, diarrhea, vomiting, cough, dyspnea.

Occasional (5%-15%)

Tachycardia, CHF, flulike symptoms, anorexia, edema, bone pain, arthralgia, insomnia, dizziness, paresthesia, depression, rhinitis, pharyngitis, sinusitis.

Rare (< 5%)

Allergic reaction, anemia, leukopenia, neuropathy, herpes simplex.

SERIOUS REACTIONS

• Cardiomyopathy, ventricular dysfunction, and CHF occur rarely.
• Pancytopenia may occur.

T

PRECAUTIONS & CONSIDERATIONS

Caution should be used in those who have previously received cardiotoxic drug therapy or radiation therapy to the chest wall and in those with a known hypersensitivity to the drug. It is unknown whether trastuzumab is distributed in breast milk. The safety and efficacy of trastuzumab have not been established in children. Age-related cardiac dysfunction may require cautious use in elderly patients. Vaccinations and coming in contact with crowds, people with known infections, and anyone who has recently received an oral polio vaccine should be avoided.

Notify the physician of nausea and vomiting, abdominal pain, back pain, chills, and fever. Left ventricular function and baseline ECG and multigated acquisition (MUGA) scan should be obtained before starting therapy. CBC should be monitored before and periodically during therapy. Signs and symptoms of deteriorating cardiac function should also be assessed.

Storage
Refrigerate unopened vials. After reconstitution of the vial with bacteriostatic water for injection, the solution is stable for 28 days if refrigerated. After reconstitution of the vial with sterile water for injection without a preservative, use the solution immediately; discard unused portions.

Administration
! Do not give trastuzumab by IV push or IV bolus. Do not use dextrose solutions for reconstitution.

Reconstitute the vial with 20 mL bacteriostatic water for injection (with benzyl alcohol) to yield a concentration of 21 mg/mL. If the patient is hypersensitive to benzyl alcohol, use sterile water for injection. Add the calculated dose from the vial to an IV solution of 250 mL 0.9% NaCl (do not use D5W). Gently mix contents in bag. The reconstituted IV solution normally appears colorless to pale yellow. IV solution reconstituted in 0.9% NaCl is stable for up to 24 h if refrigerated. Give loading dose (4 mg/kg) over 90 min. If tolerated, give maintenance infusion (2 mg/kg) over 30 min.

Trazodone
tray′zoe-done
(Apo-Trazodone [CAN], Desyrel, Novo-Trazodone [CAN], PMS-Trazodone [CAN])
Do not confuse Desyrel with Delsym or Zestril.

CATEGORY AND SCHEDULE
Pregnancy Risk Category: C

Classification: Antidepressants, miscellaneous

MECHANISM OF ACTION
An antidepressant that blocks the reuptake of serotonin at neuronal presynaptic membranes, increasing its availability at postsynaptic receptor sites. *Therapeutic Effect:* Relieves depression.

PHARMACOKINETICS
Well absorbed from the GI tract. Protein binding: 85%-95%. Metabolized in the liver. Excreted primarily in urine. Unknown whether removed by hemodialysis. *Half-life:* 5-9 h.

AVAILABILITY
Tablets: 50 mg, 100 mg, 150 mg, 300 mg.

INDICATIONS AND DOSAGES
▶ **Depression**
PO
Adults. Initially, 150 mg/day in equally divided doses. Increase by 50 mg/day at 3- to 4-day intervals until therapeutic response is achieved. Maximum: 600 mg/day.
Elderly. Initially, 25-50 mg at bedtime. May increase by 25-50 mg every 3-7 days. Range: 75-150 mg/day.
Children 6-18 yr. Initially, 1.5-2 mg/kg/day in divided doses. May increase gradually to 6 mg/kg/day in 3 divided doses.

OFF-LABEL USES
Treatment of neurogenic pain.

CONTRAINDICATIONS
None known.

INTERACTIONS
Drug
Alcohol, CNS depression-producing medications: May increase CNS depression.
Antihypertensives: May increase the effects of antihypertensives.
Digoxin, phenytoin: May increase the blood concentration of these drugs.
Indinavir, ketoconazole, ritonavir: May increase the blood concentration and toxicity of trazodone.
Herbal
St. John's wort: May increase the adverse effects of trazodone.
Food
None known.

DIAGNOSTIC TEST EFFECTS
May decrease serum WBC and neutrophil counts.

SIDE EFFECTS
Frequent (3%-9%)
Somnolence, dry mouth, light-headedness, dizziness, headache, blurred vision, nausea, vomiting.
Occasional (1%-3%)
Nervousness, fatigue, constipation, generalized aches and pains, mild hypotension.
Rare
Photosensitivity reaction.

SERIOUS REACTIONS
• Priapism, diminished or improved libido, retrograde ejaculation, and impotence occur rarely.
• Trazodone appears to be less cardiotoxic than other antidepressants, although arrhythmias may occur in patients with preexisting cardiac disease.

PRECAUTIONS & CONSIDERATIONS
Caution is warranted with arrhythmias and cardiac disease. Trazodone crosses the placenta and is minimally distributed in breast milk. The use of trazodone in children is not FDA approved. Should not be used in patients with a history of suicidal ideation. Lower dosages are recommended for elderly patients, who are more likely to experience hypotensive or sedative effects.

Anticholinergic and sedative effects may occur, so avoid alcohol and tasks that require mental alertness or motor skills. Tolerance usually develops to these side effects. Notify the physician if a painful, prolonged penile erection occurs. CBC, neutrophil and WBC counts, and liver and renal function tests should be assessed during therapy. ECG should also be obtained to assess for arrhythmias.
Administration
Take trazodone shortly after a meal or snack to reduce the risk of dizziness or lightheadedness. Crush tablets, as needed.

T

Treprostinil
treh-prost'in-ill
(Remodulin)

CATEGORY AND SCHEDULE
Pregnancy Risk Category: B

Classification: Platelet inhibitors, prostaglandins, vasodilators

MECHANISM OF ACTION
An antiplatelet that directly dilates pulmonary and systemic arterial vascular beds, inhibiting platelet aggregation. *Therapeutic Effect:* Reduces symptoms of pulmonary arterial hypertension associated with exercise.

PHARMACOKINETICS
Rapidly, completely absorbed after subcutaneous infusion; 91% bound to plasma protein. Metabolized by the liver. Excreted mainly in the urine with a lesser amount eliminated in the feces. *Half-life:* 2-4 h.

AVAILABILITY
Injection: 1 mg/mL, 2.5 mg/mL, 5 mg/mL, 10 mg/mL.

INDICATIONS AND DOSAGES
▸ **Pulmonary arterial hypertension**
CONTINUOUS SC OR IV INFUSION
Adults, Elderly. Initially, 1.25 ng/kg/min. Reduce infusion rate to 0.625 ng/kg/min if initial dose cannot be tolerated. Increase infusion rate in increments of no more than 1.25 ng/kg/min weekly for the first 4 wks and then no more than 2.5 ng/kg/min per week for the duration of infusion.
▸ **Hepatic impairment (mild to moderate)**
Adults, Elderly. Decrease the initial dose to 0.625 ng/kg/min based on ideal body weight and increase cautiously.

CONTRAINDICATIONS
Hypersensitivity to treprostinil.

INTERACTIONS
Drug
Anticoagulants, aspirin, heparin, thrombolytics: May increase the risk of bleeding.
Drugs that alter BP, including antihypertensive agents, diuretics, vasodilators: Reduced BP caused by treprostinil may be exacerbated by these drugs.
Herbal
None known.
Food
None known.

DIAGNOSTIC TEST EFFECTS
None known.

SIDE EFFECTS
Frequent
Infusion site pain, erythema, induration, rash.
Occasional
Headache, diarrhea, jaw pain, vasodilation, nausea.
Rare
Dizziness, hypotension, pruritus, edema.

SERIOUS REACTIONS
• Abrupt withdrawal or sudden large reductions in dosage may result in worsening of pulmonary arterial hypertension symptoms.

PRECAUTIONS & CONSIDERATIONS
Caution is warranted in patients with liver or renal impairment and in elderly patients. It is unknown whether treprostinil is distributed in breast milk. Safety and efficacy of treprostinil have not been established in children.

T

In elderly patients, age-related decreased cardiac, hepatic, and renal function as well as concurrent disease or other drug therapy may require dosage adjustment. Consider dosage selection carefully in elderly patients because of the increased incidence of diminished organ function. Notify the physician of signs of increased pulmonary artery pressure, such as dyspnea, cough, or chest pain.

Storage

Store at room temperature and administer without further dilution. Do not use a single vial for longer than 30 days after initial use.

Administration

Give as a continuous SC infusion via SC catheter, using an infusion pump designed for SC drug delivery. Calculate the infusion rate using the following formula: Infusion rate (mL/h) = Dose (ng/kg/min) multiplied by Weight (kg) multiplied by (0.00006/treprostinil dosage strength concentration [mg/mL]). To avoid potential interruptions in drug delivery, provide the patient with immediate access to a backup infusion pump and spare subcutaneous infusion sets. Abrupt withdrawal or sudden large reductions in dosage may result in worsening of pulmonary arterial hypertension symptoms.

Tretinoin
tret'i-noyn
(Altinac, Avita, Renova, Retin-A, Retin-A Micro, Vesanoid)

CATEGORY AND SCHEDULE
Pregnancy Risk Category: D (oral), C (topical)

Classification: Antineoplastics, retinoids, dermatologics, keratolytics

MECHANISM OF ACTION
A retinoid that decreases cohesiveness of follicular epithelial cells. Increases turnover of follicular epithelial cells. Bacterial skincounts are not altered. Transdermal: Exerts its effects on growth and differentiation of epithelial cells. Antineoplastic: Induces maturation, decreases proliferation of acute promyelocytic leukemia (APL) cells. *Therapeutic Effect:* Causes expulsion of blackheads; alleviates fine wrinkles, hyperpigmentation; causes repopulation of bone marrow and blood by normal hematopoietic cells.

PHARMACOKINETICS
Topical: Minimally absorbed. Oral: Well absorbed following oral administration. Protein binding: 95%. Metabolized in liver. Primarily excreted in urine, minimal excretion in feces. *Half-life:* 0.5-2 h.

AVAILABILITY
Capsules: 10 mg (Vesanoid).
Cream: 0.025% (Altinac, Avita, Retin-A), 0.02% (Renova), 0.05% (Altinac, Renova, Retin-A), 0.1 % (Altinac, Retin-A).
Gel: 0.01% (Retin-A), 0.025% (Avita, Retin-A), 0.04% (Retin-A

T

Micro), 0.1% (Retin-A Micro).
Topical Liquid: 0.05% (Retin-A).

INDICATIONS AND DOSAGES
▸ **Acne**
TOPICAL
Adults. Apply once daily at bedtime.
▸ **Acute promyelocytic leukemia**
PO
Adults, Children > 1 yr. 45 mg/m²/
day given as two evenly divided
doses until complete remission is
documented. Discontinue therapy
30 days after complete remission or
after 90 days of treatment, whichever
comes first.

OFF-LABEL USES
Treatment of disorders of
keratinization, including photo-aged
skin, liver spots.

CONTRAINDICATIONS
Sensitivity to parabens (used as
preservative in gelatin capsule).

INTERACTIONS
Drug
TOPICAL
**Keratolytic agents (e.g., sulfur,
benzoyl peroxide, salicylic acid),
medicated soaps, shampoos,
astringents, spice or lime cologne,
permanent wave solutions, hair
depilatories:** May increase skin
irritation.
**Photosensitive medication
(thiazides, tetracyclines,
fluoroquinolones, phenothiazines,
sulfonamides):** May augment
phototoxicity.
PO
Ketoconazole: May increase
tretinoin concentration.
Herbal
Vitamin A: May increase risk of
vitamin A toxicity.
Food
None known.

DIAGNOSTIC TEST EFFECTS
PO
Leukocytosis occurs commonly
(40%). May elevate liver function
tests, cholesterol, triglycerides.

SIDE EFFECTS
Expected
TOPICAL
Temporary change in pigmentation,
photosensitivity, local
inflammatory reactions (peeling,
dry skin, stinging, erythema,
pruritus) are to be expected and are
reversible with discontinuation of
tretinoin.
Frequent
PO
Headache, fever, dry skin/oral
mucosa, bone pain, nausea,
vomiting, rash.
Occasional
PO
Mucositis, earache or feeling
of fullness in ears, flushing,
pruritus, increased sweating, visual
disturbances, hypo/hypertension,
dizziness, anxiety, insomnia,
alopecia, skin changes.
Rare
PO
Change in visual acuity, temporary
hearing loss.

SERIOUS REACTIONS
PO
• Retinoic acid syndrome (fever,
dyspnea, weight gain, abnormal
chest auscultatory findings, episodic
hypotension) occurs commonly as
does leukocytosis.
• Syndrome generally occurs
during first month of therapy
(sometimes occurs following first
dose).
• Pseudo tumor cerebri may
be noted, especially in children
(headache, nausea, vomiting, visual
disturbances).

• Possible tumorigenic potential when combined with ultraviolet radiation.

TOPICAL

• Possible tumorigenic potential when combined with ultraviolet radiation.

PRECAUTIONS & CONSIDERATIONS

Caution should be used in patients with elevated cholesterol and/or triglycerides and considerable sun exposure in their occupation or hypersensitivity to sun. Be aware that tretinoin should be avoided in pregnant women. Be aware that it is unknown whether tretinoin is distributed in breast milk; exercise caution in nursing mother. Tretinoin may have a teratogenic and embryotoxic effect.

All women of childbearing potential should be warned of risk to fetus if pregnancy occurs. Two reliable forms of contraceptives should be used concurrently during therapy and for 1 mo after discontinuation of therapy, even in infertile, premenopausal women. A pregnancy test should be obtained within 1 wk before institution of therapy. Liver function tests and cholesterol and triglyceride levels should be monitored before and during therapy.

Avoid exposure to sunlight or sunbeds; sunscreens and protective clothing should also be protected from wind, cold. If skin is already sunburned, do not use until fully recovered. Keep tretinoin away from eyes, mouth, angles of nose, and mucous membranes. Do not use medicated, drying, or abrasive soaps; wash face no more than 2-3 times daily with bland soap. Avoid use of preparations containing alcohol, menthol, spice, or lime such as shaving lotions, astringents, and perfume. Mild redness, peeling are expected; decrease frequency or discontinue medication if excessive reaction occurs. Nonmedicated cosmetics may be used; however, cosmetics must be removed before tretinoin application.

Storage

Store at room temperature.

Administration

Take oral tretinoin with food. Do not crush or break capsule.

For topical administration, thoroughly cleanse area before applying tretinoin. Lightly cover only the affected area. Liquid may be applied with fingertip, gauze, or cotton, taking care to avoid running onto unaffected skin. Keep medication away from eyes, mouth, angles of nose, mucous membranes. Wash hands immediately after application. Improvement noted during first 24 wks of therapy. Therapeutic results noted in 2-3 wks; optimal results in 6 wks.

Triamterene

try-am′ter-een
(Dyrenium)
Do not confuse triamterene with trimipramine.

CATEGORY AND SCHEDULE

Pregnancy Risk Category: C (D if used in pregnancy-induced hypertension)

Classification: Diuretics, potassium sparing

T

MECHANISM OF ACTION

A potassium-sparing diuretic that inhibits sodium, potassium, ATPase. Interferes with sodium and potassium exchange in distal tubule, cortical collecting tubule, and collecting duct. Increases sodium and decreases potassium excretion. Also increases magnesium, decreases calcium loss. *Therapeutic Effect:* Produces diuresis and lowers BP.

PHARMACOKINETICS

Route	Onset	Peak	Duration
PO	2-4 h	NA	7-9 h

Incompletely absorbed from the GI tract. Widely distributed. Metabolized in the liver. Primarily eliminated in feces via biliary route. *Half-life:* 1.5-2.5 h (increased in renal impairment).

AVAILABILITY

Capsules: 50 mg, 100 mg.

INDICATIONS AND DOSAGES
▶ **Edema, hypertension**
PO
Adults, Elderly. 25-100 mg/day as a single dose or in 2 divided doses. Maximum: 300 mg/day.
Children. 2-4 mg/kg/day as a single dose or in 2 divided doses. Maximum: 6 mg/kg/day or 300 mg/day.

OFF-LABEL USES

Treatment adjunct for hypertension, prevention and treatment of hypokalemia.

CONTRAINDICATIONS

Diabetic neuropathy, drug-induced or preexisting hyperkalemia, progressive or severe renal disease, anuria, severe hepatic disease.

INTERACTIONS
Drug
ACE inhibitors (such as captopril), potassium-containing medications, potassium supplements: May increase the risk of hyperkalemia.
Anticoagulants, heparin: May decrease the effects of these drugs.
Lithium: May decrease the clearance and increase the risk of toxicity of lithium.
NSAIDs: May decrease the antihypertensive effect of triamterene.
Herbal
None known.
Food
None known.

DIAGNOSTIC TEST EFFECTS

May increase urinary calcium excretion; BUN and blood glucose levels; and serum calcium, creatinine, potassium, magnesium, and uric acid levels. May decrease serum sodium levels.

SIDE EFFECTS
Occasional
Fatigue, nausea, diarrhea, abdominal pain, leg cramps, headache.
Rare
Anorexia, asthenia, rash, dizziness.

SERIOUS REACTIONS

• Triamterene use may result in hyponatremia (somnolence, dry mouth, increased thirst, lack of energy) or severe hyperkalemia (irritability, anxiety, heaviness of legs, paresthesia, hypotension, bradycardia, ECG changes [tented T waves, widening QRS complex, ST segment depression]).
• Agranulocytosis, nephrolithiasis, and thrombocytopenia occur rarely.

PRECAUTIONS & CONSIDERATIONS
Caution is warranted in patients with diabetes mellitus, history of renal

calculi, hepatic or renal impairment, and concurrent use of potassium-sparing diuretics or potassium supplements. Triamterene crosses the placenta and is distributed in breast milk. Breastfeeding is not recommended for patients taking this drug. The safety and efficacy of this drug have not been established in children. Elderly patients may be at increased risk for developing hyperkalemia. Avoid consuming salt substitutes and foods high in potassium.

An increase in the frequency and volume of urination may occur. Notify the physician of dry mouth, fever, headache, nausea and vomiting, persistent or severe weakness, sore throat, or unusual bleeding or bruising blood pressure (BP), vital signs, electrolytes, intake and output, and weight should be monitored before and during treatment. Be aware of signs of electrolyte disturbances such as hypokalemia or hyponatremia. Hypokalemia may cause arrhythmias, altered mental status, muscle cramps, asthenia, and tremor.

Administration

Take triamterene with food if GI disturbances occur. Do not crush or break capsules. Therapeutic effect takes several days to begin and can last for several days after the drug is discontinued.

Triazolam
trye-ay′zoe-lam
(Apo-Triazo [CAN], Halcion)
Do not confuse Halcion with Haldol or Healon.

CATEGORY AND SCHEDULE
Pregnancy Risk Category: X
Controlled Substance Schedule: IV

Classification: Benzodiazepines, sedatives/hypnotics

MECHANISM OF ACTION
A benzodiazepine that enhances the action of the inhibitory neurotransmitter γ-aminobutyric acid, resulting in central nervous system (CNS) depression.
Therapeutic Effect: Induces sleep.

AVAILABILITY
Tablets: 0.125 mg, 0.25 mg.

INDICATIONS AND DOSAGES
▸ **Insomnia**
PO
Adults, Children older than 18 yr.
Typically, 0.25 mg at bedtime, 0.125 mg may be sufficient for some patients. Maximum: 0.5 mg.
Elderly. 0.125-0.25 mg at bedtime. Maximum: 0.25 mg.

CONTRAINDICATIONS
Angle-closure glaucoma; CNS depression; pregnancy or breastfeeding; severe, uncontrolled pain; sleep apnea, ethanol intoxication. Triazolam is contraindicated with ketoconazole, itraconazole, nefazodone, and other medications that potentially impair CYP3A4 metabolism.

T

INTERACTIONS

Drug

Alcohol, other CNS depressants:
May increase CNS depression.

Herbal

Kava kava, valerian: May increase
CNS depression.

Food

Grapefruit, grapefruit juice: May
alter the absorption of triazolam.

DIAGNOSTIC TEST EFFECTS

None known.

SIDE EFFECTS

Frequent

Somnolence, sedation, dry mouth,
headache, dizziness, nervousness,
light-headedness, incoordination,
nausea, rebound insomnia (may
occur for 1-2 nights after drug is
discontinued).

Occasional

Euphoria, tachycardia, abdominal
cramps, visual disturbances.

Rare

Paradoxical CNS excitement or
restlessness (particularly in elderly
or debilitated patients).

SERIOUS REACTIONS

• Abrupt or too-rapid withdrawal may
result in pronounced restlessness,
irritability, insomnia, hand tremors,
abdominal or muscle cramps,
vomiting, diaphoresis, and seizures.
• Overdose results in somnolence,
confusion, diminished reflexes,
respiratory depression, and coma.

PRECAUTIONS & CONSIDERATIONS

Caution is warranted in persons
with a potential for drug abuse.
Pregnancy should be determined
before therapy begins. Drowsiness
may occur. Avoid alcohol, CNS
depressants, and tasks that require
mental alertness or motor skills.
Smoking should also be avoided

because it can reduce the drug's
effectiveness. Cardiovascular,
mental, and respiratory status
and hepatic function should be
monitored throughout therapy.

Administration

Take triazolam without regard to
food. Crush tablets as needed. Do not
administer the drug with grapefruit
juice.

Trientine

trye-en′teen
(Syprine)

CATEGORY AND SCHEDULE

Pregnancy Risk Category: C

Classification: Antidotes,
chelators

MECHANISM OF ACTION

An oral chelating agent that forms
complexes by binding metal ions,
particularly copper. *Therapeutic
Effect:* Binds to copper and induces
cupruresis.

PHARMACOKINETICS

None reported.

AVAILABILITY

Capsules: 250 mg (Syprine).

INDICATIONS AND DOSAGES

▸ **Wilson disease**

PO

Adults, Elderly. 750-1250 mg/day in
2-4 divided doses. Maximum: 2 g/day.
Children 12 yr and older.
500-750 mg/day in 2-4 divided
doses. Maximum: 1500 mg/day.

CONTRAINDICATIONS

Hypersensitivity to trientine or its
components.

INTERACTIONS
Drug
Iron preparations: May decrease absorption of both drugs.
Herbal and Food
None known.

DIAGNOSTIC TEST EFFECTS
None known.

SIDE EFFECTS
Occasional
Contact dermatitis, dystonia, muscular spasm, myasthenia gravis.

SERIOUS REACTIONS
• Iron deficiency anemia and systemic lupus erythematosus rarely occur.

PRECAUTIONS & CONSIDERATIONS
Caution is necessary with cystinuria, rheumatoid arthritis, and biliary cirrhosis.

It is unknown whether trientine is distributed in breast milk. Safety and efficacy of trientine have not been established in children younger than 12 yr. No age-related precautions have been noted in elderly patients. Serum-free copper level and copper analysis should be obtained every 6-12 mo. Adequate fluid intake should be maintained.
Storage
Store trientine bottles in the refrigerator.
Administration
Be aware that trientine is second-line therapy for people intolerant of penicillamine. Do not open or chew capsules. Take 1 h before or 2 h after meals and at least 1 h apart from milk or other drugs. Long-term maintenance dose should be determined at intervals of 6-12 mo.

Trifluridine
trye-flure′i-deen
(Viroptic)
Do not confuse with Zostrix.

CATEGORY AND SCHEDULE
Pregnancy Risk Category: C

Classification: Antivirals, ophthalmics

MECHANISM OF ACTION
An antiviral agent that incorporates into DNA causing increased rate of mutation and errors in protein formation. *Therapeutic Effect:* Prevents viral replication.

PHARMACOKINETICS
Intraocular solution is undetectable in serum. *Half-life:* 12 min.

AVAILABILITY
Ophthalmic Solution: 1% (Viroptic).

INDICATIONS AND DOSAGES
▸ **Herpes simplex virus ocular infections**
OPHTHALMIC
Adults, Elderly, Children older than 6 yr. 1 drop into affected eye q2h while awake. Maximum: 9 drops/day. Continue until corneal ulcer has completely reepithelialized; then, 1 drop q4h while awake (minimum: 5 drops/day) for an additional 7 days.

CONTRAINDICATIONS
Hypersensitivity to trifluridine or any component of the formulation.

INTERACTIONS
Drug
None known.
Herbal
None known.

T

Food
None known.

DIAGNOSTIC TEST EFFECTS
None known.

SIDE EFFECTS
Frequent
Transient stinging or burning with instillation.
Occasional
Edema of eyelid.
Rare
Hypersensitivity reaction.

SERIOUS REACTIONS
• Ocular toxicity may occur if used longer than 21 days.

PRECAUTIONS & CONSIDERATIONS
Be aware that trifluridine use should not exceed 21 days because of the potential for ocular toxicity. It may cause transient irritation of the conjunctiva and cornea. Be aware that trifluridine is not recommended during pregnancy or lactation because of its mutagenic effects in vitro. Safety and efficacy have not been established in children younger than 6 yr. No age-related precautions have been noted in elderly patients.

If no improvement occurs after 7 days or complete healing after 14, contact the physician. Report any itching, swelling, redness, or increased irritation.
Storage
Refrigerate trifluridine; avoid freezing.
Administration
For ophthalmic use, do not touch applicator tip to any surface. Place finger on lower eyelid and pull out until pocket is formed between eye and lower lid. Hold dropper above pocket and place prescribed number of drops in pocket. Close eyes gently so medication will not be squeezed out of sac. Apply gentle finger pressure to the lacrimal sac at inner canthus for 1 min following installation (lessens risk of systemic absorption). If more than 1 ophthalmic drug is being used, separate administration by at least 5-10 min.

Trihexyphenidyl
trye-hex-ee-fen'i-dill
(Artane, Apo-Trihex [CAN])

CATEGORY AND SCHEDULE
Pregnancy Risk Category: C

Classification: Anticholinergics, antiparkinson agents

MECHANISM OF ACTION
An anticholinergic agent that blocks central cholinergic receptors (aids in balancing cholinergic and dopaminergic activity). *Therapeutic Effect:* Decreases salivation, relaxes smooth muscle.

PHARMACOKINETICS
Well absorbed from GI tract. Primarily excreted in urine. *Half-life:* 3.3-4.1 h.

AVAILABILITY
Elixer: 2 mg/5 mL (Artane).
Tablets: 2 mg, 5 mg (Artane).

INDICATIONS AND DOSAGES
▸ **Parkinsonism**
PO
Adults, Elderly. Initially, 1 mg on first day. May increase by 2 mg/day at intervals of 3-5 days up to 6-10 mg/day (12-15 mg/day in patients with postencephalitic parkinsonism).
▸ **Drug-induced extrapyramidal symptoms**

PO
Adults, Elderly. Initially, 1 mg/day.
Range: 5-15 mg/day.

CONTRAINDICATIONS

Angle-closure glaucoma, GI
obstruction, paralytic ileus, intestinal
atony, severe ulcerative colitis,
prostatic hypertrophy, myasthenia
gravis, megacolon, hypersensitivity
to trihexyphenidyl or any component
of the formulation.

INTERACTIONS

Drug
**Alcohol, central nervous system
(CNS) depressants:** May increase
sedative effect.
**Amantadine, anticholinergics,
MAOIs:** May increase
anticholinergic effects.
Antacids, antidiarrheals: May
decrease absorption and effects of
trihexyphenidyl.
Herbal
None known.
Food
None known.

DIAGNOSTIC TEST EFFECTS

None known.

SIDE EFFECTS

Elderly (older than 60 yr) tend
to develop mental confusion,
disorientation, agitation, psychotic-
like symptoms.
Frequent
Drowsiness, dry mouth.
Occasional
Blurred vision, urinary retention,
constipation, dizziness, headache,
muscle cramps.
Rare
Seizures, depression, rash.

SERIOUS REACTIONS

• Hypersensitivity reaction
(eczema, pruritus, rash, cardiac
disturbances, photosensitivity) may
occur.
• Overdosage may vary from
CNS depression (sedation, apnea,
cardiovascular collapse, death)
to severe paradoxical reaction
(hallucinations, tremor, seizures).

PRECAUTIONS & CONSIDERATIONS

Caution is warranted in
patients with treated open-angle
glaucoma, autonomic neuropathy,
pulmonary disease, esophageal
reflux, hiatal hernia, heart
disease, hyperthyroidism, and
hypertension. It is unknown
whether trihexyphenidyl crosses the
placenta or is distributed in breast
milk. Safety and efficacy have
not been established in children.
Elderly patients are more sensitive
to the effects of trihexyphenidyl
as well as anxiety, confusion, and
nervousness.

Dry mouth, drowsiness, and
dizziness are expected side effects of
this drug. Avoid alcohol and do not
drive, use machinery, or engage in
other activities that require mental
acuity if dizziness or blurred vision
occurs.
Storage
Store at room temperature.
Administration
Be aware not to use sustained-release
capsules for initial therapy. Once
stabilized, may switch, on mg-for-
mg basis, giving in 2 daily doses
and with food. High doses may be
divided into 4 doses, at mealtimes,
and at bedtime.

T

Trimethobenzamide
trye-meth-oh-ben′za-mide
(Tigan)

CATEGORY AND SCHEDULE
Pregnancy Risk Category: C

Classification: Anticholinergics,
antiemetics/antivertigo

MECHANISM OF ACTION
An anticholinergic that acts at the
chemoreceptor trigger zone in the
medulla oblongata. *Therapeutic
Effect:* Relieves nausea and
vomiting.

PHARMACOKINETICS

Route	Onset	Peak	Duration
PO	10-40 min	NA	3-4 h
IM	15-30 min	NA	2-3 h

Partially absorbed from the GI tract.
Distributed primarily to the liver.
Metabolic fate unknown. Excreted in
urine. *Half-life:* 7-9 h.

AVAILABILITY
Capsules: 100 mg, 300 mg.
Injection: 100 mg/mL.

INDICATIONS AND DOSAGES
▶ Nausea and vomiting
PO
Adults, Elderly. 300 mg 3-4 times
a day.
Children weighing 30-100 lb.
100-200 mg 3-4 times a day.
IM
Adults, Elderly. 200 mg 3-4 times
a day.
Rectal
Adults, Elderly. 200 mg 3-4 times
a day.

Children weighing 30-100 lb.
100-200 mg 3-4 times a day.
Children weighing < 30 lb. 100 mg
3-4 times a day.

CONTRAINDICATIONS
Hypersensitivity to benzocaine
or similar local anesthetics;
agranulocytosis; use of parenteral
form in children.

INTERACTIONS
Drug
CNS depressants: May increase
CNS depression.
Herbal
None known.
Food
None known.

DIAGNOSTIC TEST EFFECTS
None known.

SIDE EFFECTS
Frequent
Somnolence.
Occasional
Blurred vision, diarrhea, dizziness,
headache, muscle cramps.
Rare
Rash, seizures, depression,
opisthotonos, parkinsonian
syndrome, Reye's syndrome
(marked by vomiting, seizures).

SERIOUS REACTIONS
• A hypersensitivity reaction,
manifested as extrapyramidal
symptoms such as muscle rigidity
and allergic skin reactions, occurs
rarely.
• Children may experience
paradoxical reactions, marked by
restlessness, insomnia, euphoria,
nervousness, and tremor.
• Overdose may produce CNS
depression (manifested as sedation,
apnea, cardiovascular collapse,
and death) or severe paradoxical

reactions (such as hallucinations, tremor, and seizures).

PRECAUTIONS & CONSIDERATIONS

Caution is warranted with dehydration, electrolyte imbalances, high fever, and the debilitated or elderly. It is unknown whether trimethobenzamide crosses the placenta or is distributed in breast milk. No age-related precautions have been noted in elderly patients. Do not administer the parenteral form to children. Tasks that require mental alertness or motor skills should be avoided until response to the drug has been established.

Drowsiness may occur. Notify the physician of headache, visual disturbances, restlessness, or involuntary muscle movements. BP, intake and output, vomitus, and skin for hydration status should be assessed.

Administration

! Elderly patients (older than 60 yr) are at increased risk for developing agitation, disorientation, confusion, and psychotic-like symptoms. Do not administer trimethobenzamide by the IV route because it produces severe hypotension.

Take oral trimethobenzamide without regard to food. Don't crush, open, or break the capsules.

For IM use, inject the drug deep into a large muscle mass, usually the upper outer gluteus maximus.

Trimethoprim
trye-meth'oh-prim
(Apo-Tremethoprim [CAN], Primsol, Proloprim)

CATEGORY AND SCHEDULE
Pregnancy Risk Category: C

Classification: Antibiotics, folate antagonists

MECHANISM OF ACTION
A folate antagonist that blocks bacterial biosynthesis of nucleic acids and proteins by interfering with the metabolism of folinic acid. *Therapeutic Effect:* Bacteriostatic.

PHARMACOKINETICS
Rapidly and completely absorbed from the GI tract. Protein binding: 42%-46%. Widely distributed, including to the cerebrospinal fluid (CSF). Metabolized in the liver. Primarily excreted in urine. Moderately removed by hemodialysis. *Half-life:* 8-10 h (increased in impaired renal function and newborns; decreased in children).

AVAILABILITY
Oral Solution (Primsol): 50 mg/5 mL.
Tablets (Proloprim): 100 mg, 200 mg.

INDICATIONS AND DOSAGES
▸ **Acute, uncomplicated urinary tract infection**
PO
Adults, Elderly, Children 12 yr and older. 100 mg q12hr or 200 mg once a day for 10-14 days.
Children younger than 12 yr. 4-6 mg/kg/day in 2 divided doses for 10 days.

▸**Dosage in renal impairment**
Dosage and frequency are modified based on creatinine clearance.

Creatinine Clearance (mL/min)	Dosage Interval
> 30	No change
15-29	Reduce dose by 50%

OFF-LABEL USES
Prevention of bacterial urinary track infection, treatment of pneumonia caused by *Pneumocystis carinii*.

CONTRAINDICATIONS
Infants younger than 2 mo, megaloblastic anemia caused by folic acid deficiency.

INTERACTIONS
Drug
Folate antagonists (including methotrexate): May increase the risk of megaloblastic anemia.
Herbal
None known.
Food
None known.

DIAGNOSTIC TEST EFFECTS
May increase BUN and serum bilirubin, creatinine, AST (SGOT), and ALT (SGPT) levels.

SIDE EFFECTS
Occasional
Nausea, vomiting, diarrhea, decreased appetite, abdominal cramps, headache.
Rare
Hypersensitivity reaction (pruritus, rash), methemoglobinemia (bluish fingernails, lips, or skin; fever; pale skin; sore throat; unusual tiredness), photosensitivity.

SERIOUS REACTIONS
• Stevens-Johnson syndrome, erythema multiforme, exfoliative dermatitis, and anaphylaxis occur rarely.
• Hematologic toxicity (thrombocytopenia, neutropenia, leukopenia, megaloblastic anemia) is more likely to occur in elderly, debilitated, or alcoholic patients; in patients with impaired renal function; and in those receiving prolonged high dosage.

PRECAUTIONS & CONSIDERATIONS
Caution is warranted in patients with impaired hepatic or renal function or folic acid deficiency. Trimethoprim readily crosses the placenta and is distributed in breast milk. No age-related precautions have been noted in elderly patients, but they may have an increased incidence of thrombocytopenia. Avoid sun and ultraviolet light.

Report bleeding, bruising, skin discoloration, fever, pallor, rash, sore throat, and tiredness. Hematology and renal function tests should be assessed before and during therapy.

Administration
Space doses evenly around the clock to maintain a constant drug level in urine. Take trimethoprim without regard to food (or with food if stomach upset occurs). Space drug doses evenly around the clock and complete the full course of trimethoprim therapy, which usually lasts 10-14 days.

Trimipramine

trye-mih-prah-meen
(Apo-Trimip [CAN],
Novo-Tripramine [CAN],
Nu-Tripramine [CAN],
Rhotrimine [CAN], Surmontil)
**Do not confuse with
desipramine.**

CATEGORY AND SCHEDULE
Pregnancy Risk Category: D

Classification: Antidepressants,
tricyclic

MECHANISM OF ACTION
A tricyclic antibulimic,
anticataplectic, antidepressant,
antinarcoleptic, antineuralgic,
antineuritic, and antipanic
agent that blocks the reuptake
of neurotransmitters, such as
norepinephrine and serotonin, at
presynaptic membranes, increasing
their concentration at postsynaptic
receptor sites. May demonstrate
less autonomic toxicity than other
tricyclic antidepressants. *Therapeutic
Effect:* Results in antidepressant
effect. Anticholinergic effect controls
nocturnal enuresis.

PHARMACOKINETICS
Rapidly, completely absorbed after
PO administration and not affected
by food. Protein binding: 95%.
Metabolized in liver (significant first-
pass effect). Primarily excreted in
urine. Not removed by hemodialysis.
Half-life: 16-40 h.

AVAILABILITY
Capsules: 25 mg, 50 mg, 100 mg
(Surmontil).

INDICATIONS AND DOSAGES
▸ **Depression**

PO
Adults. 50-150 mg/day at
bedtime. Maximum: 200 mg/day
for outpatients, 300 mg/day for
inpatients.
Elderly. Initially, 25 mg/day at
bedtime. May increase by 25 mg
q3-7 days. Maximum: 100 mg/day.

CONTRAINDICATIONS
Acute recovery period after
myocardial infarction (MI), cardiac
conduction defects, within 14 days
of MAOI ingestion, hypersensitivity
to trimipramine or any component of
the formulation.

INTERACTIONS
Drug
**Alcohol, central nervous system
(CNS) depressants:** May increase
CNS and respiratory depression
and the hypotensive effects of
trimipramine.
Anticoagulants: May increase risk
of bleeding.
**Antipsychotics (amisulpride,
haloperidol, risperidone,
sertindole, quetiapine, sultopride,
zotepine):** May increase the cardiac
effects (QT prolongation, torsades
de pointes, cardiac arrest).
Antithyroid agents: May increase
the risk of agranulocytosis.
Amprenavir, atazanavir: May
increase serum concentrations and
risk of toxicity of trimipramine.
Atomoxetine: May increase plasma
concentrations of atomoxetine.
Barbiturates: May decrease
trimipramine serum concentrations
and possible additive adverse effects.
Baclofen: May increase the risk of
memory loss and/or muscle tone.
Cimetidine: May increase
trimipramine blood concentration
and risk of toxicity.
**Class 1, 1A, and III
antiarrhythmic agents; cisapride;**

T

cotrimoxazole; fluconazole; gatifloxacin; gemifloxacin; grepafloxacin; sparfloxacin; telithromycin; halofantrine; halothane; sympathomimetics; vasopressin; zolmitriptan: May increase the cardiac effects.
Clonidine, guanadrel: May decrease the effects of clonidine and guanadrel.
Duloxetine, fluoxetine, paroxetine, sertraline: May increase serum concentrations and risk of toxicity.
Estrogens: May increase the antidepressant effectiveness and risk of tricyclic toxicity.
MAOIs: May increase the risk of hyperpyrexia, hypertensive crisis, and seizures.
Phenothiazines: May increase anticholinergic and sedative effects of trimipramine.
Phenytoin: May decrease trimipramine blood concentration.
Quinidine: May increase the risk of trimipramine toxicity.
Herbal
Ginkgo biloba: May decrease seizure threshold.
St. John's wort: May have additive effect.

DIAGNOSTIC TEST EFFECTS
May alter blood glucose levels and ECG readings.

SIDE EFFECTS
Frequent
Drowsiness, fatigue, dry mouth, blurred vision, constipation, delayed micturition, postural hypotension, diaphoresis, disturbed concentration, increased appetite, urinary retention, photosensitivity.
Occasional
GI disturbances, such as nausea, and a metallic taste sensation.
Rare
Paradoxical reaction, marked by

agitation, restlessness, nightmares, insomnia, extrapyramidal symptoms, particularly fine hand tremors.

SERIOUS REACTIONS
• High dosage may produce cardiovascular effects, such as severe postural hypotension, dizziness, tachycardia, palpitations, arrhythmias, and seizures. High dosage may also result in altered temperature regulation, including hyperpyrexia or hypothermia.
• Abrupt withdrawal from prolonged therapy may produce headache, malaise, nausea, vomiting, and vivid dreams.

PRECAUTIONS & CONSIDERATIONS
Caution is warranted in patients with cardiac disease, diabetes mellitus, glaucoma, hiatal hernia, history of seizures, history or urinary obstruction or retention, hyperthyroidism, increased intraocular pressure (IOP) decreased GI motility, liver disease, prostatic hypertrophy, renal disease, and schizophrenia. It is unknown whether trimipramine crosses the placenta or is distributed in breast milk. Be aware that trimipramine is not recommended in children younger than 18 yr. Dose reduction may be required in elderly patients.
   Tolerance usually develops to anticholinergic effects, postural hypotension, and sedative effects during therapy. Avoid tasks that require mental alertness or motor skills until response to trimipramine is established.
Administration
Take with food or milk if GI distress occurs.

Trioxsalen
trye-ox′a-len
(Trisoralen)
Discontinued in the United States

CATEGORY AND SCHEDULE
Pregnancy Risk Category: C

Classification: Photosensitizers,
psoralens

MECHANISM OF ACTION
A member of the family of
psoralens that induces the process of
melanogenesis by a mechanism that
is not known. *Therapeutic Effect:*
Enhances pigmentation.

PHARMACOKINETICS
Rapidly absorbed from the GI tract.
Half-life: 2 h. (Skin sensitivity to
light remains for 8-12 h.)

AVAILABILITY
Tablets: 5 mg (Trisoralen).

INDICATIONS AND DOSAGES
▸ **Pigmentation**
PO
*Adults, Elderly, Children 12 yr and
older.* 10 mg/day 2 h before exposure
to UVA light or sun exposure.
▸ **Vitiligo**
PO
*Adults, Elderly, Children 12 yr
and older.* 10 mg/day 2-4 h before
exposure to UVA light.

OFF-LABEL USES
Polymorphous light eruption,
psoriasis, sunlight sensitivity.

CONTRAINDICATIONS
Concomitant disease states
associated with photosensitivity
(acute lupus erythematosus,
porphyria, leukoderma of infectious
origin), concomitant use of
preparations with any internal or
external photosensitizing capacity,
children younger than 12 yr,
hypersensitivity to trioxsalen or any
component of the formulation

INTERACTIONS
Drug
None known.
Herbal
None known.
Food
Furocoumarin foods: May increase
risk of severe burns.

SIDE EFFECTS
Occasional
Gastric discomfort, photosensitivity,
pruritus.

SERIOUS REACTIONS
• Overdose or overexposure may
result in serious blistering and
burning.

PRECAUTIONS & CONSIDERATIONS
Caution is warranted in patients
with alibinism, hydroa, leukoderma
of infectious origin, lupus
erythematosus, polymorphic light
eruptions, porphyria, xeroderma
pigmentosum, aphakia, severe
cardiovascular disease, cataracts,
and skin cancer. It is unknown
whether trioxsalen crosses the
placenta or is distributed in breast
milk. Safety and efficacy have
not been determined in children
younger than 12 yr. No age-related
precautions have been noted in
elderly patients. Furocoumarin-
containing foods, such as carrots,
celery, limes, figs, mustard, parsley,
and parsnips, which contain natural
psoralens, should be avoided
because they can increase the risk
of severe burns and blistering.
Direct and indirect sunlight should

T

be avoided for 8 h after therapy. If sunlight cannot be avoided, protective clothing or sunscreens should be worn.

If burning, blistering, or intractable pruritus occurs, trioxsalen should be discontinued.

Administration
Therapy with trioxsalen should not exceed 14 days nor should the dosage be increased. Take with food or milk to reduce gastric discomfort.

Triptorelin Pamoate
trip'toe-rel-in
(Trelstar Depot, Trelstar LA)

CATEGORY AND SCHEDULE
Pregnancy Risk Category: X

Classification: Antineoplastics, hormones/hormone modifiers, gonadotropin-releasing hormone analogues.

MECHANISM OF ACTION
A gonadotropin-releasing hormone (GnRH) analogue and antineoplastic agent that inhibits gonadotropin hormone secretion through a negative feedback mechanism. Circulating levels of luteinizing hormone, follicle-stimulating hormone, testosterone, and estradiol rise initially, then subside with continued therapy. *Therapeutic Effect:* Suppresses growth of abnormal prostate tissue.

AVAILABILITY
Powder for Injection (Trelstar Depot): 3.75 mg.
Powder for Injection (Trelstar LA): 11.25 mg.

INDICATIONS AND DOSAGES
▸ **Prostate cancer**
IM
Adults, Elderly. 3.75 mg once q28 days (Trelstar Depot). 11.25 mg q84 days (Trelstar LA).

CONTRAINDICATIONS
Hypersensitivity to luteinizing hormone-releasing hormone (LHRH) or LHRH agonists, pregnancy.

INTERACTIONS
Drug
Hyperprolactinemic drugs: Reduce the number of pituitary gonadotropin-releasing hormone (GnRH) receptors.
Herbal
None known.
Food
None known.

DIAGNOSTIC TEST EFFECTS
May alter serum pituitary-gonadal function test results. May cause transient increase in serum testosterone levels, usually during first week of treatment.

SIDE EFFECTS
Frequent (> 5%)
Hot flashes, skeletal pain, headache, impotence.
Occasional (2%-5%)
Insomnia, vomiting, leg pain, fatigue.
Rare (< 2%)
Dizziness, emotional lability, diarrhea, urinary retention, urinary tract infection, anemia, pruritus.

SERIOUS REACTIONS
• Bladder outlet obstruction, skeletal pain, hematuria, and spinal cord compression (with weakness or paralysis of the lower extremities) may occur.

PRECAUTIONS & CONSIDERATIONS

Women who are or might be pregnant should not use this drug. Pregnancy should be determined before beginning triptorelin therapy. It is unknown whether triptorelin is excreted in breast milk. The safety and efficacy of triptorelin have not been established in children. No age-related precautions have been noted in elderly patients.

Blood in urine, increased skeletal pain, and urine retention may occur initially, but these symptoms usually subside within 1 wk. Notify the physician if difficulty breathing, infection at the injection site, numbness of the arms or legs, breast pain or swelling, persistent nausea or vomiting, or rapid heartbeat develop. Prostatic acid phosphatase (PAP), prostate-specific antigen (PSA), and serum testosterone levels should be obtained periodically during therapy. Serum testosterone and PAP levels should increase during the first week of therapy. The testosterone level should then decrease to baseline level or less within 2 wks, and the PAP level should decrease within 4 wks.

A worsening of signs and symptoms of prostatic cancer, especially during the first week of therapy, because of a transient increase in testosterone level should be carefully assessed.

Administration

Administer under the supervision of a physician. Do not miss monthly injections.

Trospium
trose′pee-um
(Sanctura)

CATEGORY AND SCHEDULE
Pregnancy Risk Category: C

Classification: Anticholinergics, relaxants, urinary tract

MECHANISM OF ACTION
An anticholinergic that antagonizes the effect of acetylcholine on muscarinic receptors, producing parasympatholytic action. *Therapeutic Effect:* Reduces smooth muscle tone in the bladder.

PHARMACOKINETICS
Minimally absorbed after PO administration. Protein binding: 50%-85%. Distributed in plasma. Excreted mainly in feces and, to a lesser extent, in urine. *Half life:* 20 h.

AVAILABILITY
Tablets: 20 mg.

INDICATIONS AND DOSAGES
▸ **Overactive bladder**
PO
Adults. 20 mg 2 times/day.
Elderly (75 yr and older). Initially, 20 mg 2 times/day. Titrate dosage down to 20 mg once a day, based on tolerance.
▸ **Dosage in renal impairment**
For patients with creatinine clearance < 30 mL/min, dosage reduced to 20 mg once a day at bedtime.

CONTRAINDICATIONS
Decreased GI motility, gastric retention, toxic megacolon, uncontrolled angle-closure glaucoma, urinary retention.

INTERACTIONS

Drug

Other anticholinergic agents:
Increases the severity and frequency of side effects and may alter the absorption of other drugs because of anticholinergic effects on GI motility.

Digoxin, metformin, morphine, pancuronium, procainamide, tenofovir, vancomycin:
May increase trospium blood concentration.

Herbal
None known.

Food
High-fat meal: May reduce trospium absorption.

DIAGNOSTIC TEST EFFECTS

None known.

SIDE EFFECTS

Frequent (20%)
Dry mouth.

Occasional (≤ 4%)
Constipation, headache.

Rare (< 2%)
Fatigue, upper abdominal pain, dyspepsia, flatulence, dry eyes, urine retention.

SERIOUS REACTIONS

• Overdose may result in severe anticholinergic effects, such as abdominal pain, nausea and vomiting, confusion, depression, diaphoresis, facial flushing, hypertension, hypotension, respiratory depression, irritability, lacrimation, nervousness, and restlessness.

• Supraventricular tachycardia and hallucinations occur rarely.

PRECAUTIONS & CONSIDERATIONS

Caution is warranted with renal or hepatic impairment, intestinal atony, obstructive GI disorders, significant bladder obstruction, ulcerative colitis, myasthenia gravis, and angle-closure glaucoma. It is unknown whether trospium crosses the placenta or is distributed in breast milk. The safety and efficacy of trospium have not been established in Children. Elderly patients (age 75 and older) have a higher incidence of constipation, dry mouth, dyspepsia, urine retention, and urinary track infection.

Notify the physician of increased salivation or sweating, an irregular heartbeat, nausea and vomiting, or severe abdominal pain. Intake and output, pattern of daily bowel activity and stool consistency, and symptomatic relief should be assessed.

Storage
Store trospium at room temperature.

Administration
Don't break or crush the tablets. Take the drug at least 1 h before meals or on an empty stomach. Do not take trospium with high-fat meals because it may reduce absorption.

Undecylenic Acid
un-de-sye-len'ik
(Blis-To-Sol Powder, Caldesene Powder, Cruex Aerosol, Cruex Cream, Cruex Powder, Desenex Powder, Desenex Soap, Elon Dual Defense Anti-Fungal Formula Solution, Fungoid AF Solution, Godochom Solution)

CATEGORY AND SCHEDULE
Pregnancy Risk Category: NR
OTC

Classification: Antifungals, topical, dermatologics

MECHANISM OF ACTION
An antifungal that inihibits the growth and reproduction of fungal cells. *Therapeutic Effect:* Fungistatic.

AVAILABILITY
Aerosol Powder: 19% (Cruex Aerosol).
Cream: 8% (Phicon F), 20% (Cruex Cream).
Solution, Topical: 25% (Elon Dual Defense Anti-Fungal Formula, Fungoid AF, Gordochom Solution).
Powder: 10% (Caldesene Powder, Cruex Powder), 12% (Blis-To-Sol Powder), 25% (Desenex Powder).
Soap: (Desenex).

INDICATIONS AND DOSAGES
▸ **Tinea pedis, tinea corporis**
Topical
Adults, Children 2 yr and older. Apply twice daily to affected area for 4 wks.

CONTRAINDICATIONS
Hypersensitivity to undecylenic acid or any component of its formulation.

INTERACTIONS
Drug
None known.
Herbal
None known.
Food
None known.

DIAGNOSTIC TEST EFFECTS
None known.

SIDE EFFECTS
Occasional
Skin irritation, rash.

SERIOUS REACTIONS
• Hypersensitivity reactions characterized by rash, facial swelling, pruritus, and a sensation of warmth occur.

PRECAUTIONS & CONSIDERATIONS
Products are for external use only. Caution should be used when administering to children younger than 2 yr and in those with diabetes mellitus. No precautions have been noted in pregnant women. Safety and efficacy of undecylenic acid have not been established in children younger than 2 yr. No age-related precautions have been noted for elderly patients. These products have not been proven safe and effective in the treatment of the scalp or nails. Skin should be kept clean and dry. Light clothing should be worn to promote ventilation. Affected area should not be covered with occlusive dressing. The physician should be notified if skin irritation occurs or if there is no improvement after 4 wks of use.
Administration
Topical therapy should not be used on scalp or nails. Apply and rub gently into the affected and surrounding area.

Ursodiol
your-soo´dee-ol
(Actigall, DOM-Ursodiol C [CAN],
PHL-Ursodiol C [CAN],
PMS-Ursodiol C [CAN],
Urso,Urso [CAN])

CATEGORY AND SCHEDULE
Pregnancy Risk Category: B

Classification: Gallstone
dissolution agent

MECHANISM OF ACTION
A gallstone-solubilizing agent that
suppresses the hepatic synthesis and
secretion of cholesterol; inhibits the
intestinal absorption of cholesterol.
Therapeutic Effect: Changes the
bile of patients with gallstones from
precipitating (capable of forming
crystals) to cholesterol solubilizing
(capable of being dissolved).

AVAILABILITY
Capsules: 300 mg.
Tablets: 250 mg.

PHARMACOKINETICS
With the capsules, ~90% is
absorbed in the small bowel, with
sites of action in the liver, bile, and
gut lumen. Tablets are absorbed
and undergo hepatic extraction;
also distributed in bile and small
intestine. Steady-state concentrations
are reached in ~ 3 wks. Most active
ingredients in tablets and capsules
are metabolized in the colon and
excreted as metabolites in the feces.

INDICATIONS AND DOSAGES
▸ **Dissolution of radiolucent,
noncalcified gallstones
when cholecystectomy is not
recommended**

PO
Adults, Elderly. 8-10 mg/kg/day in
2-3 divided doses. Treatment may
require months. Obtain ultrasound
image of gallbladder at 6-mo
intervals for first year. If gallstones
have dissolved, continue therapy and
repeat ultrasound within 1-3 mo.
▸ **Primary biliary cirrhosis**
PO
Adults, Elderly. 13-15 mg/kg/day in
2-4 divided doses with food.
▸ **Prevention of gallstones**
PO
Adults, Elderly. 300 mg twice a day.

OFF-LABEL USES
Treatment of alcoholic cirrhosis,
biliary atresia, biliary cirrhosis,
cystic fibrosis, cholestatic jaundice
syndrome, chronic hepatitis,
congenital dilation of lobar
intrahepatic duct, gallstone formation,
sclerosing cholangitis, prophylaxis of
liver transplant rejection.

INTERACTIONS
Drug
**Aluminum-based antacids,
cholestyramine:** May decrease the
absorption and effects of ursodiol.
Estrogens, oral contraceptives:
May decrease the effects of ursodiol.
Herbal
None known.
Food
None known.

DIAGNOSTIC TEST EFFECTS
May alter liver function test results.

SIDE EFFECTS
All were similar to placebo.
Frequent
Abdominal pain, diarrhea, dyspepsia,
flatulence, nausea.
Common
Cholecystitis, constipation,
gastrointestinal disorder, vomiting.

SERIOUS REACTIONS
• None significant.

PRECAUTIONS & CONSIDERATIONS

Allergy to bile acids, calcified cholesterol stones, chronic hepatic disease, compelling reason for cholestectomy, radiolucent bile pigment stones, radiopaque stones.
❗ Patients with ascites, hepatic encephalopathy, variceal bleeding, or in need of liver transplant should be treated for those specific causes; lactation, children.

Blood serum chemistry values, including BUN, serum alkaline phosphatase, bilirubin, creatinine, AST (SGOT), and ALT (SGPT) levels, should be obtained before the start of ursodiol therapy, 1 and 3 mo after therapy begins, and every 6 mo thereafter to assess hepatic function.

Administration

Take with meals or a snack because the drug dissolves more readily in the presence of bile acid and pancreatic juice. Avoid taking antacids within hours of taking ursodiol. Therapy with ursodiol is usually for several months.

U

Valacyclovir
val-a-sye′kloe-veer
(Valtrex)
Do not confuse valacyclovir with valganciclovir.

CATEGORY AND SCHEDULE
Pregnancy Risk Category: B

Classification: Antivirals

MECHANISM OF ACTION
A virustatic antiviral that is converted to acyclovir triphosphate, becoming part of the viral DNA chain. *Therapeutic Effect:* Interferes with DNA synthesis and replication of herpes simplex virus and varicella zoster virus.

PHARMACOKINETICS
Rapidly absorbed after PO administration. Protein binding: 13%-18%. Rapidly converted by hydrolysis to the active compound acyclovir. Widely distributed to tissues and body fluids (including cerebrospinal fluid [CSF]). Eliminated primarily in urine. Removed by hemodialysis. *Half-life:* 2.5-3.3 h (increased in impaired renal function).

AVAILABILITY
Caplets: 500 mg, 1000 mg.

INDICATIONS AND DOSAGES
▸ **Herpes zoster (shingles)**
PO
Adults, Elderly. 1 g 3 times a day for 7 days.
▸ **Herpes labialis (cold sores)**
PO
Adults, Elderly. 2 g twice a day for 2 doses starting at the first sign of symptom of lesions.

▸ **Initial episode of genital herpes**
PO
Adults, Elderly. 1 g twice a day for 10 days.
▸ **Recurrent episodes of genital herpes**
PO
Adults, Elderly. 500 mg twice a day for 3 days.
▸ **Prevention of genital herpes**
PO
Adults, Elderly. 500-1000 mg/day.
▸ **Dosage in renal impairment**
Dosage and frequency are modified based on creatinine clearance.

Creatinine Clearance (mL/min)	Herpes Zoster	Genital Herpes (recurrence)
30-49	1 g q12h	500 mg q12h
10-29	1 g q24h	500 mg q24h
< 10	500 mg q24h	500 mg q24h

OFF-LABEL USES
To reduce the risk of heterosexual transmission of genital herpes.

CONTRAINDICATIONS
Hypersensitivity to or intolerance of acyclovir, valacyclovir, or their components.

INTERACTIONS
Drug
Cimetidine, probenecid:
May increase acyclovir blood concentration.
Herbal
None known.
Food
None known.

DIAGNOSTIC TEST EFFECTS
None known.

SIDE EFFECTS
Frequent
Herpes zoster (10%-17%): Nausea, headache.
Genital herpes (17%): Headache.
Occasional
Herpes zoster (3%-7%): Vomiting, diarrhea, constipation (50 yr or older), asthenia, dizziness (50 yr or older).
Genital herpes (3%-8%): Nausea, diarrhea, dizziness.
Rare
Herpes zoster (1%-3%): Abdominal pain, anorexia.
Genital herpes (1%-3%): Asthenia, abdominal pain.

SERIOUS REACTIONS
• Thrombotic thrombocytopenic purpura/hemolytic uremic syndrome.

PRECAUTIONS & CONSIDERATIONS
Caution is warranted in patients with advanced HIV infection, bone marrow or renal transplantation, concurrent use of nephrotoxic agents, dehydration, fluid or electrolyte imbalance, neurologic abnormalities, and renal or liver impairment. Be aware that valacyclovir may cross the placenta and be distributed in breast milk. The safety and efficacy of this drug have not been established in children. In elderly patients, age-related renal impairment may require dosage adjustment. Do not touch lesions with fingers to avoid spreading infection to new sites. Avoid sexual intercourse during the duration of lesions to prevent infecting partner.

Tissue cultures should be obtained from those with herpes simplex and herpes zoster before giving the first dose of valacyclovir. Therapy may proceed before test results are known. Complete blood count (CBC), liver or renal function tests,

fluid intake, and urinalysis should be monitored. Maintain adequate fluids. Fingernails should be kept short and hands clean. Pap smears should be done at least annually because of increased risk of cervical cancer in women with genital herpes.
Administration
! Be aware that therapy should be initiated at the first sign of shingles and that valacyclovir is most effective within 48 h of the onset of zoster rash.

Give oral valacyclovir without regard to meals. Do not crush or break tablets. Continue therapy for the full length of treatment, and evenly space doses around the clock.

Valganciclovir
val-gan-sye'kloh-veer
(Valcyte)
Do not confuse valganciclovir with valacyclovir.

CATEGORY AND SCHEDULE
Pregnancy Risk Category: C

Classification: Antivirals

MECHANISM OF ACTION
A synthetic nucleoside that competes with viral DNA esterases and is incorporated directly into growing viral DNA chains. *Therapeutic Effect:* Interferes with DNA synthesis and viral replication.

PHARMACOKINETICS
Well absorbed and rapidly converted to ganciclovir by intestinal and hepatic enzymes. Widely distributed. Slowly metabolized intracellularly. Excreted primarily unchanged in

V

urine. Removed by hemodialysis.
Half-life: 18 h (increased in impaired renal function).

AVAILABILITY
Tablets: 450 mg.

INDICATIONS AND DOSAGES
▶ **Cytomegalovirus (CMV) retinitis in patients with normal renal function**
PO
Adults. Initially, 900 mg (two 450-mg tablets) twice a day for 21 days. Maintenance: 900 mg once a day.
▶ **Prevention of CMV after transplant**
PO
Adults, Elderly. 900 mg once a day beginning within 10 days of transplant and continuing until 100 days post-transplant.
▶ **Dosage in renal impairment**
Dosage and frequency are modified based on creatinine clearance.

Creatinine Clearance (mL/min)	Induction Dosage (mg)	Maintenance Dosage
40-59	450 twice/day	450 mg min once/day
25-39	450 once/day	450 mg once/day
10-24	450 q2 days	450 mg twice/week

CONTRAINDICATIONS
Hypersensitivity to acyclovir or ganciclovir.

INTERACTIONS
Drug
Amphotericin B, cyclosporine: May increase the risk of nephrotoxicity.
Bone marrow depressants: May increase bone marrow depression.
Imipenem and cilastatin: May increase the risk of seizures.

Mycophenolate: May increase serum concentration of valganciclovir.
Probenecid: Decreases renal clearance of valganciclovir.
Tenofovir: May decrease excretion of tenofovir.
Zidovudine (AZT): May increase the risk of hematologic toxicity.
Herbal
None known.
Food
All foods: Maximize drug bioavailability.

DIAGNOSTIC TEST EFFECTS
May decrease blood hematocrit and hemoglobin levels, serum creatinine level, platelet count, and WBC count.

SIDE EFFECTS
Frequent (9%-41%)
Diarrhea, neutropenia, headache, fever, insomnia, nausea, vomiting, abdominal pain, anemia.
Occasional (3%-8%)
Thrombocytopenia, paresthesia.
Rare (1%-3%)
Herpes zoster: Abdominal pain, anorexia.
Genital herpes: Asthenia, abdominal pain.

SERIOUS REACTIONS
• Hematologic toxicity, including severe neutropenia (most common), anemia, and thrombocytopenia may occur.
• Retinal detachment occurs rarely.
• An overdose may result in renal toxicity.
• Valganciclovir may decrease sperm production and fertility.

PRECAUTIONS & CONSIDERATIONS
Extreme caution should be used in children because of long-term carcinogenicity and risk of reproductive toxicity. Caution

should also be used in patients with a history of cytopenic reactions to other drugs, preexisting cytopenias, and renal impairment and in elderly patients, who are at a greater risk of renal impairment. Valganciclovir should not be used during pregnancy and effective contraception should be used during therapy because of the mutagenic and teratogenic potential of valganciclovir. Women taking valganciclovir should avoid breastfeeding. Breastfeeding may be resumed no sooner than 72 h after the last dose of valganciclovir. Be aware that the safety and efficacy of this drug have not been established in children younger than 12 yr. In elderly patients, age-related renal impairment may require dosage adjustment.

Blood chemistry, hematologic baselines, and serum creatinine levels should be evaluated. Intake and output should be monitored, and ensure that the patient maintains adequate hydration (minimum 1500 mL/24 h). Ophthalmologic examinations should be obtained every 4-6 wks during treatment. Valganciclovir may temporarily or permanently inhibit sperm production in men; valganciclovir may temporarily or permanently suppress fertility in women.

Administration
Do not break or crush tablets (potentially carcinogenic and teratogenic). Avoid contact with skin. Wash skin with soap and water if contact occurs. Give valganciclovir with food. Cannot be substituted for ganciclovir on a one-to-one basis.

Valproic Acid/ Valproate Sodium/ Divalproex Sodium

val-pro′ick
Valproic acid
(Depakene, Stavzor)
Valproate sodium
(Depakene Syrup)
Divalproex sodium (Depacon, Depakote, Depakote ER, Depakote Sprinkle)

CATEGORY AND SCHEDULE

Pregnancy Risk Category: D

Classification: Anticonvulsants

MECHANISM OF ACTION

An anticonvulsant, antimanic, and antimigraine agent that directly increases concentration of the inhibitory neurotransmitter γ-aminobutyric acid. *Therapeutic Effect:* Reduces seizure activity.

PHARMACOKINETICS

Well absorbed from the GI tract. Protein binding: 80%-90%. Metabolized in the liver. Excreted primarily in urine. Not removed by hemodialysis. *Half-life:* 6-16 h (may be increased in patients with hepatic impairment, elderly patients, and children younger than 18 mo).

AVAILABILITY

Capsules (Depakene): 250 mg.
Capsules (Delayed-Release [Stavzor]): 125 mg, 250 mg, 500 mg.
Syrup (Depakene): 250 mg/5 mL.
Tablets (Delayed-Release [Depakote]): 125 mg, 250 mg, 500 mg.
Tablets (Extended-Release [Depakote ER]): 500 mg.
Capsules Sprinkles (Depakote Sprinkle): 125 mg.
Injection (Depacon): 100 mg/mL.

V

INDICATIONS AND DOSAGES
▶ **Seizures**
PO
Adults, Elderly, Children 10 yr and older. Initially, 10-15 mg/kg/day in 2-3 divided doses. May increase by 5-10 mg/kg/day at weekly intervals up to 30-60 mg/kg/day. Usual adult dosage: 1000-2500 mg/day.
IV
Adults, Elderly, Children. Same as oral dose but given q6h.
▶ **Manic episodes**
PO
Adults, Elderly. Initially, 750 mg/day in divided doses twice daily. Maximum: 60 mg/kg/day.
▶ **Prevention of migraine headaches**
PO (EXTENDED-RELEASE TABLETS)
Adults, Elderly. Initially, 500 mg/day for 7 days. May increase up to 1000 mg/day.
PO (DELAYED-RELEASE TABLETS, DELAYED-RELEASE CAPSULES)
Adults, Elderly. Initially, 250 mg twice a day. May increase up to 1000 mg/day.

OFF-LABEL USES
Treatment of myoclonic, simple partial, and tonic-clonic seizures.

CONTRAINDICATIONS
Active hepatic disease or significant hepatic function impairment; hypersensitivity to the drug; known urea cycle disorders.

INTERACTIONS
Drug
Alcohol, other central nervous system (CNS) depressants: May increase CNS-depressant effects.
Amitriptyline, primidone: May increase the blood concentration of these drugs.

Anticoagulants, heparin, platelet aggregation inhibitors, thrombolytics: May increase the risk of bleeding.
Carbamazepine: May decrease valproic acid blood concentration.
Hepatotoxic medications: May increase the risk of hepatotoxicity.
Phenytoin: May increase the risk of phenytoin toxicity and decrease the effects of valproic acid.
Topiramate: Increased risk of hyperammonemia.
Herbal
None known.
Food
None known.

DIAGNOSTIC TEST EFFECTS
May increase serum LDH, bilirubin, AST (SGOT), and ALT (SGPT) levels. Therapeutic serum level is 50-100 mcg/mL; toxic serum level is > 100 mcg/mL. May cause false-positive urine ketone test.

🕭 IV INCOMPATIBILITIES
Do not mix valproic acid with any other medications.

SIDE EFFECTS
Frequent
Epilepsy: Abdominal pain, irregular menses, diarrhea, transient alopecia, indigestion, nausea, vomiting, tremors, weight gain or loss.
Mania (19%-22%): Nausea, somnolence.
Occasional
Epilepsy: Constipation, dizziness, drowsiness, headache, skin rash, unusual excitement, restlessness.
Mania (6%-12%): Asthenia, abdominal pain, dyspepsia (heartburn, indigestion, epigastric distress), rash.
Rare
Epilepsy: Mood changes, diplopia, nystagmus, spots before eyes, unusual bleeding or ecchymosis.

SERIOUS REACTIONS

• Hepatotoxicity may occur, particularly in the first 6 mo of valproic acid therapy. It may be preceded by loss of seizure control, malaise, weakness, lethargy, anorexia, and vomiting rather than by abnormal serum liver function test results.
• Blood dyscrasias may occur.
• Life-threatening pancreatitis.
• Hyperammonemia and encephalopathy.
• Multiorgan hypersensitivity reaction.

PRECAUTIONS & CONSIDERATIONS

Caution is warranted in patients with bleeding abnormalities and a history of hepatic disease. Valproic acid crosses the placenta and is distributed in breast milk. Children younger than 2 yr are at increased risk for hepatotoxicity. Lower dosages are recommended for elderly patients, although no age-related precautions have been noted for this age group. Congenital malformations have been associated with valproate exposure during pregnancy; administer to women of childbearing potential only if essential for seizure management.

Drowsiness and dizziness may occur, so alcohol and tasks requiring mental alertness or motor skills should be avoided. Notify the physician of abdominal pain, altered mental status, bleeding, easy bruising, lethargy, loss of appetite, nausea, vomiting, weakness, or yellowing of skin. Seizure disorder, including the onset, duration, frequency, intensity, and type of seizures, should be assessed before and during treatment. CBC and serum alkaline phosphatase, ammonia, bilirubin, AST (SGOT), and ALT (SGPT) levels should also

be monitored. CBC and platelet count should be obtained before beginning valproic acid therapy, 2 wks later, and again 2 wks after the maintenance dose has been established.

Storage

Store vials at room temperature. Diluted solutions are stable for 24 h; discard unused portion.

Administration

! Regular-release and delayed-release formulations are given in 2-4 divided doses daily; extended-release formulations are given once a day.

Take oral valproic acid without regard to food. Do not take it with carbonated drinks. Capsule contents may be sprinkled on applesauce and given immediately; however, do not break, chew, or crush the sprinkle beads. Give delayed-release or extended-release tablets and capsules whole. Do not abruptly discontinue valproic acid after long-term use, because this may precipitate seizure. Strict maintenance of drug therapy is essential for seizure control.

For IV use, dilute each single dose with at least 50 mL D5W, 0.9% NaCl, or lactated Ringer's solution. Infuse over 5-10 min. The recommended infusion rate is 20 mg/min. Faster infusion rates of up to 15 mg/kg over 5-10 min (1.5-3 mg/kg/min) have been used; however, the incidence of adverse events may be higher. Be aware that the therapeutic serum drug level is 50-100 mcg/mL and the toxic serum level is > 100 mcg/mL.

V

Valrubicin
val-rue´bih-sin
(VaHaxan [CAN], Valstar)
Do not confuse valrubicin with valsartan.

CATEGORY AND SCHEDULE
Pregnancy Risk Category: C

Classification: Antineoplastic

MECHANISM OF ACTION
An anthracycline that inhibits incorporation of nucleosides into nucleic acids after penetrating cells. *Therapeutic Effect:* Causes chromosomal damage, arresting cells in the G_2 phase of cell division, and interferes with DNA synthesis.

PHARMACOKINETICS
Concentrated in bladder wall; minimal absorption into circulation. Excreted in urine.

AVAILABILITY
Concentrate Solution: 40 mg/mL for intravesical instillation.

INDICATIONS AND DOSAGES
▶ Bladder cancer
INTRAVESICAL
Adults, Elderly. 800 mg once weekly for 6 wks.

CONTRAINDICATIONS
Perforated bladder; sensitivity to valrubicin, anthracyclines, or polyoxyl castor oil; severe irritated bladder; small bladder capacity; urinary tract infection.

INTERACTIONS
Drug
None known.
Herbal
None known.

Food
None known.

DIAGNOSTIC TEST EFFECTS
None known.

⊘ IV INCOMPATIBILITIES
Do not mix with other drugs.

SIDE EFFECTS
Frequent
Local intravesical reaction: Local bladder symptoms, urinary frequency or urgency, dysuria, hematuria, bladder pain, cystitis, bladder spasms.
Systemic: Abdominal pain, nausea, urinary tract infection.
Occasional
Local intravesical reaction: Nocturia, local burning, urethral pain, pelvic pain, gross hematuria.
Systemic: Diarrhea, vomiting, urine retention, microscopic hematuria, asthenia, headache, malaise, back pain, chest pain, dizziness, rash, anemia, fever, vasodilation.
Rare
Systemic: Flatus, peripheral edema, hyperglycemia, pneumonia, myalgia.

SERIOUS REACTIONS
Serious systemic toxicity if bladder wall is perforated.

PRECAUTIONS & CONSIDERATIONS
Evaluate bladder status before administration; delay administration in patients with perforated bladder or compromised mucosal integrity. All patients of reproductive age should be advised to use an effective contraceptive method during the treatment period. Monitor for disease recurrence or progression by using cystoscopy, biopsy, and urine cytology every 3 mo.

Storage

Unopened vials should be stored under refrigeration in the carton; diluted solution is stable for 12 h at temperatures up to 25° C (77° F).

Administration

Use of gloves during dose preparation and administration is recommended; avoid skin contact. Prepare and store instillation solution in glass, polypropylene, or polyolefin containers. Non-DEHP-containing administration sets are recommended for administration. For each instillation, contents of four 200 mg/5 mL vials should be allowed to warm to room temperature. 20 mL should be withdrawn from the four vials and diluted with 55 mL NaCl 0.9% injection, providing 75 mL diluted valrubicin solution. The diluted soultion should be instilled in the bladder slowly via gravity flow over several minutes. Drug should be retained in the bladder for 2 h before voiding. At the end of 2 h, all patients should void. Instillation solution is red; advise patients that red-tinged urine is typical for the first 24 h after administration.

Valsartan
val-sar'tan
(Diovan)
Do not confuse Valsartan with Valstan.

CATEGORY AND SCHEDULE
Pregnancy Risk Category: C (D if used in second or third trimester)

Classification: Angiotensin II receptor antagonists

MECHANISM OF ACTION

An angiotensin II receptor, type AT_1, antagonist that blocks vasoconstrictor and aldosterone-secreting effects of angiotensin II, inhibiting the binding of angiotensin II to the AT_1 receptors. *Therapeutic Effect:* Causes vasodilation, decreases peripheral resistance, and decreases BP.

PHARMACOKINETICS

Poorly absorbed after PO administration. Food decreases peak plasma concentration. Protein binding: 95%. Metabolized in the liver. Recovered primarily in feces and, to a lesser extent, in urine. Unknown whether removed by hemodialysis. *Half-life:* 6 h.

AVAILABILITY

Tablets: 40 mg, 80 mg, 160 mg, 320 mg.

INDICATIONS AND DOSAGES
▶ **Hypertension**
PO
Adults, Elderly. Initially, 80-160 mg/day in patients who are not volume depleted, up to a maximum of 320 mg/day.
▶ **Congestive heart failure (CHF)**
PO
Adults, Elderly. Initially, 40 mg twice a day. May increase up to 160 mg twice a day. Maximum: 320 mg/day.
▶ **Post-myocardial infarction (MI)**
PO
Adults, Elderly. May be initiated as early as 12 h after an MI. Initially 20 mg twice daily. Titrate to target dose of 160 mg twice daily, as tolerated.

CONTRAINDICATIONS

Bilateral renal artery stenosis, biliary cirrhosis or obstruction,

V

hypoaldosteronism, severe hepatic impairment.

INTERACTIONS
Drug
Diuretics: Produces additive hypotensive effects.
Lithium: Elevated lithium concentrations and risk of toxic effects.
Potassium-sparing diuretics, potassium supplements: Increased serum potassium.
Herbal
None known.
Food
Decreases peak plasma concentration of valsartan.

DIAGNOSTIC TEST EFFECTS
May increase AST (SGOT), ALT (SGPT), and serum bilirubin, creatinine, and potassium levels. May decrease blood hemoglobin and hematocrit levels.

SIDE EFFECTS
Rare (1%-2%)
Insomnia, fatigue, heartburn, abdominal pain, dizziness, headache, diarrhea, nausea, vomiting, arthralgia, edema.

SERIOUS REACTIONS
• Overdosage may manifest as hypotension and tachycardia. Bradycardia occurs less often.
• Viral infection and upper respiratory tract infection (cough, pharyngitis, sinusitis, rhinitis) occur rarely.

PRECAUTIONS & CONSIDERATIONS
Caution is warranted in patients with coronary artery disease, mild to moderate hepatic impairment, renal impairment, and unilateral renal artery stenosis and in those receiving potassium-sparing diuretics or potassium supplements. For those with severe CHF, signs and symptoms of impaired renal function, which may develop during valsartan therapy, should be monitored. It is unknown whether valsartan is distributed in breast milk; it may cause fetal harm. Women should avoid valsartan during the second and third trimester of pregnancy. Safety and efficacy of valsartan have not been established in children. No age-related precautions have been noted in elderly patients.

Dizziness may occur. Tasks that require mental alertness or motor skills should be avoided. Notify the physician if fever or sore throat occurs. Apical pulse and BP should be assessed immediately before each olmesartan dose and regularly throughout therapy. Be alert to fluctuations in apical pulse and BP. If an excessive reduction in BP occurs, place the person in the supine position with feet slightly elevated and notify the physician. Serum electrolyte levels, liver and renal function tests, urinalysis, and pulse rate should be assessed. Maintain adequate hydration; exercising outside during hot weather should be avoided to decrease the risk of dehydration and hypotension.

Administration
! Valsartan may be given concurrently with other antihypertensives. If BP is not controlled by valsartan alone, expect to administer a diuretic, as prescribed.

Take valsartan without regard to meals.

Vancomycin
van-koe-mye′sin
(Vancocin, Vancocin CP [AUS],
Vancocin HCL Pulvules [AUS])

CATEGORY AND SCHEDULE
Pregnancy Risk Category: B

Classification: Antibiotics,
glycopeptides

MECHANISM OF ACTION
A tricyclic glycopeptide antibiotic
that binds to bacterial cell
walls, altering cell membrane
permeability and inhibiting RNA
synthesis. *Therapeutic Effect:*
Bactericidal.

PHARMACOKINETICS
PO: Poorly absorbed from the GI
tract. Primarily eliminated in feces.
Parenteral: Widely distributed.
Protein binding: 55%. Primarily
excreted unchanged in urine. Not
removed by hemodialysis. *Half-life:*
4-11 h (increased in impaired renal
function).

AVAILABILITY
Capsules: 125 mg, 250 mg.
*Powder for Oral Suspension
(Vancocin):* 1 g (provides 250 mg/
5 mL after mixing).
Powder for Injection: 500 mg, 1 g,
5 g, 10 g.
Infusion (Premix): 500 mg/100 mL,
1 g/200 mL.

INDICATIONS AND DOSAGES
▸ **Treatment of bone, respiratory
tract, skin, and soft-tissue infections,
endocarditis, peritonitis, and
septicemia; prevention of bacterial
endocarditis in those at risk (if
penicillin is contraindicated) when
undergoing biliary, dental, GI,
genitourinary, or respiratory surgery
or invasive procedures**
IV
Adults, Elderly. 15 mg/kg or
1 g q12h.
Children older than 1 mo.
40 mg/kg/day in divided doses
q6-8h.
Neonates. Initially, 10-15 mg/kg
q8-12h.
▸ **Staphylococcal enterocolitis,
antibiotic-associated
pseudomembranous colitis caused
by *Clostridium difficile***
PO
Adults, Elderly. 125-500 mg
q6h for 7-10 days.
Children. 40 mg/kg/day in
3-4 divided doses for 7-14 days.
Maximum: 2 g/day.
▸ **Dosage in renal impairment**
After a loading dose, subsequent
dosages and frequency are
modified based on creatinine
clearance, the severity of
the infection, and the serum
concentration of the drug.

OFF-LABEL USES
Treatment of brain abscess,
perioperative infections,
staphylococcal or streptococcal
meningitis.

CONTRAINDICATIONS
Hypersensitivity.

INTERACTIONS
Drug
**Aminoglycosides, amphotericin B,
aspirin, bumetanide, carmustine,
cisplatin, cyclosporine, ethacrynic
acid, furosemide, streptozocin:**
May increase the risk of ototoxicity
and nephrotoxicity of parenteral
vancomycin.
Cholestyramine, colestipol:
May decrease the effects of oral
vancomycin.

V

Herbal
None known.
Food
None known.

DIAGNOSTIC TEST EFFECTS
May increase BUN level. Therapeutic peak serum level is 20-40 mcg/mL; therapeutic trough serum level is 5-15 mcg/mL. Toxic peak serum level is > 40 mcg/mL; toxic trough serum level is > 15 mcg/mL.

ⓘ IV INCOMPATIBILITIES
Albumin, amphotericin B complex (Abelcet, AmBisome, Amphotec), aztreonam (Azactam), cefazolin (Ancef), cefepime (Maxipime), cefotaxime (Claforan), cefotetan (Cefotan), cefoxitin (Mefoxin), ceftazidime (Fortaz), ceftriaxone (Rocephin), cefuroxime (Zinacef), foscarnet (Foscavir), heparin, idarubicin (Idamycin), nafcillin (Nafcil), piperacillin and tazobactam (Zosyn), propofol (Diprivan), ticarcillin and clavulanate (Timentin).

ⓘ IV COMPATIBILITIES
Amiodarone (Cordarone), calcium gluconate, diltiazem (Cardizem), hydromorphone (Dilaudid), insulin, lorazepam (Ativan), magnesium sulfate, midazolam (Versed), morphine, potassium chloride.

SIDE EFFECTS
Frequent
PO: Bitter or unpleasant taste, nausea, vomiting, mouth irritation (with oral solution).
Rare
Parenteral: Phlebitis, thrombophlebitis, or pain at peripheral IV site; dizziness; vertigo; tinnitus; chills; fever; rash; necrosis with extravasation.
PO: Rash.

SERIOUS REACTIONS
• Nephrotoxicity and ototoxicity may occur.
• "Red man" syndrome (redness on face, neck, arms, and back; chills; fever; tachycardia; nausea or vomiting; pruritus; rash; unpleasant taste) may result from too-rapid injection.
• Neutropenia

PRECAUTIONS & CONSIDERATIONS
Caution is warranted in patients with preexisting hearing impairment or renal dysfunction and in those taking other ototoxic or nephrotoxic medications concurrently. Vancomycin crosses the placenta; it is unknown whether it is distributed in breast milk. Close monitoring of serum drug levels is recommended in premature neonates and young infants. Age-related renal impairment may increase the risk of ototoxicity and nephrotoxicity in elderly patients. Dosage adjustment is recommended.

Notify the physician if rash, tinnitus, or signs and symptoms of nephrotoxicity occur. Laboratory tests are an important part of therapy. Know that the vancomycin therapeutic peak serum level is 20-40 mcg/mL and the trough level is 5-15 mcg/mL. The toxic peak serum level is > 40 mcg/mL, and the trough level is > 15 mcg/mL. Assess skin for rash, intake and output, renal function, balance and hearing acuity; assess IV site during vancomycin therapy.
Storage
The refrigerated oral solution is stable for 2 wks. After reconstitution, the IV solution may be refrigerated and should be used within 14 days.

Administration

Be aware that oral vancomycin is not given for systemic infections because it is poorly absorbed from the GI tract; however, some patients with colitis may absorb the drug effectively. Reconstitute powder for oral solution as appropriate and administer it orally or by nasogastric tube. Do not use powder for oral solution for IV administration.

! Give vancomycin by intermittent IV infusion (piggyback) or continuous IV infusion. Do not give by IV push, because this may result in exaggerated hypotension. For intermittent IV infusion (piggyback), reconstitute each 500-mg or 1-g vial with 10 mL or 20 mL, respectively, of sterile water for injection to provide a concentration of 50 mg/mL. Further dilute to a final concentration of no more than 5 mg/mL. Discard the solution if a precipitate forms. Administer the solution over 60 min or longer. Monitor the patient's BP closely during the infusion. ADD-Vantage vials should not be used in neonates, infants, and children requiring less than a 500-mg dose.

Vardenafil

(Levitra)
Do not confuse Levitra with Lexiva.

CATEGORY AND SCHEDULE

Pregnancy Risk Category: B

Classification: Impotence agents, phosphodiesterase inhibitors

MECHANISM OF ACTION

An erectile dysfunction agent that inhibits phosphodiesterase type 5, the enzyme responsible for degrading cyclic guanosine monophosphate in the corpus cavernosum of the penis, resulting in smooth muscle relaxation and increased blood flow. *Therapeutic Effect:* Facilitates an erection.

PHARMACOKINETICS

Rapidly absorbed after PO administration. Extensive tissue distribution. Protein binding: 95%. Metabolized in the liver. Excreted primarily in feces; a lesser amount eliminated in urine. Drug has no effect on penile blood flow without sexual stimulation. *Half-life:* 4-5 h.

AVAILABILITY

Tablets: 2.5 mg, 5 mg, 10 mg, 20 mg.

INDICATIONS AND DOSAGES

▸ **Erectile dysfunction**
PO
Adults. 10 mg approximately 1 h before sexual activity. Dose may be increased to 20 mg or decreased to 5 mg, based on patient tolerance. Maximum dosing frequency is once daily.
Elderly (older than 65 yr). 5 mg.
▸ **Dosage in moderate hepatic impairment**
PO
For patients with Child-Pugh class B hepatic impairment, dosage is 5 mg 60 min before sexual activity.
▸ **Dosage with concurrent ritonavir**
PO
Adults. 2.5 mg in a 72-h period.
▸ **Dosage with concurrent ketoconazole or itraconazole (at 400 mg/day), indinavir, atazanavir, saquinavir, clarithromycin, ketoconazole, or itraconazole (400 mg/day)**

V

PO
Adults. 2.5 mg in a 24-h period.
▸ **Dosage with concurrent
ketoconazole or itraconazole
(at 200 mg/day) or erythromycin**
PO
Adults. 5 mg in a 24-h period.
▸ **Stable α-adrenergic blocker therapy**
PO
Adults. 5-mg initial dose.

OFF-LABEL USES
Raynaud phenomenon.

CONTRAINDICATIONS
Concurrent use of sodium
nitroprusside, or nitrates in any form.

INTERACTIONS
Drug
α-Adrenergic blockers, nitrates:
Potentiates the hypotensive effects of
these drugs. Use of vardenafil with
nitrates is contraindicated.
**Erythromycin, indinavir,
itraconazole, ketoconazole,
ritonavir:** May increase vardenafil
blood concentration.
Herbal
None known.
Food
High-fat meals: Delay drug's
maximum effectiveness.

DIAGNOSTIC TEST EFFECTS
None known.

SIDE EFFECTS
Occasional
Headache, flushing, rhinitis,
indigestion.
Rare (< 2%)
Dizziness, changes in color vision,
blurred vision.

SERIOUS REACTIONS
• Prolonged erections (lasting over
4 h) and priapism (painful erections
lasting > 6 h) occur rarely.

• Hypotension.
• Vision loss.

PRECAUTIONS & CONSIDERATIONS
Caution is warranted in patients
with an anatomic deformity of
the penis; cardiac, hepatic, or
renal impairment; and conditions
that increase the risk of priapism,
including leukemia, multiple
myeloma, and sickle cell anemia.
No age-related precautions have
been noted in elderly patients, but
their initial dose should be 5 mg.
Be aware that vardenafil is not
effective without sexual stimulation.
Avoid using nitrate drugs and
α-adrenergic blockers concurrently
with vardenafil. Seek treatment
immediately if an erection lasts
longer than 4 h.
Administration
Take vardenafil approximately
1 h before sexual activity. Do not
crush or break film-coated tablets.
High-fat meals delay the drug's
maximum effectiveness.

Varenicline
var-e-ni-kleen
(Chantix)

CATEGORY AND SCHEDULE
Pregnancy Risk Category: C

Classification: Smoking
deterrent

MECHANISM OF ACTION
Selectively binds $\alpha_4\beta_2$ neuronal
nicotinic acetylcholine receptors;
possesses agonist activity at lower
level than nicotine while blocking
nicotine binding to receptors, thus
blocking ability of nicotine to
stimulate central nervous mesolimbic
dopamine system.

PHARMACOKINETICS

Extensively absorbed, peak concentration within 3-4 h of oral administration. Minimal metabolism; 92% excreted unchanged in the urine. *Half-life:* 24 h (increased in renal impairment).

AVAILABILITY

Tablets: 0.5 mg, 1 mg.

INDICATIONS AND DOSAGES
▸ **Smoking cessation aid**
PO
Adults, Elderly. Days 1-3: 0.5 mg once daily; days 4-7: 0.5 mg twice daily; day 8–end of treatment: 1 mg twice daily. Administer for 12 wks; additional 12 wks may increase likelihood of long-term abstinence.
▸ **Dosage in renal impairment**
Severe renal impairment. Titrate from 0.5 mg once daily to maximum dose of 0.5 mg twice daily.
End-stage renal disease. Maximum dose 0.5 mg once daily.

CONTRAINDICATIONS

None.

INTERACTIONS
Drug
None known.
Herbal
None known.
Food
None known.

DIAGNOSTIC TEST EFFECTS

Abnormal liver function test results reported.

SIDE EFFECTS
Frequent (> 10%)
Nausea, insomnia, abnormal dreams.
Occasional (5%-10%)
Constipation, flatulence, vomiting.

SERIOUS REACTIONS

Depressed mood, suicidal ideation, suicidal behavior.

PRECAUTIONS & CONSIDERATIONS

All patients should be monitored for neuropsychiatric symptoms, such as changes in behavior, agitation, depressed mood, suicidal ideation, and suicidal behavior, and worsening of preexisting psychiatric illness; varenicline therapy should be discontinued in the presence of such symptoms. Varenicline has not been studied in pregnant women. May be excreted in human milk; use in nursing mothers is not recommended.
Administration
Start varenicline 1 wk before date set to stop smoking. Take after eating with a full glass of water.

Vasopressin
vay-soe-press′in
(Pitressin, Pressyn [CAN])
Do not confuse Pitressin with Pitocin.

CATEGORY AND SCHEDULE
Pregnancy Risk Category: B

Classification: Antidiuretics, hormones/hormone modifiers

MECHANISM OF ACTION

A posterior pituitary hormone that increases reabsorption of water by the renal tubules. Increases water permeability at the distal tubule and collecting duct. Directly stimulates smooth muscle in the GI tract. *Therapeutic Effect:* Causes peristalsis and vasoconstriction.

PHARMACOKINETICS

Route	Onset	Peak	Duration
IV	NA	NA	0.5-1 h
IM	1-2 h	NA	2-8 h SC

Distributed throughout extracellular fluid. Metabolized in the liver and kidney. Excreted in urine. *Half-life:* 10-20 min.

AVAILABILITY

Injection: 20 units/mL.

INDICATIONS AND DOSAGES
▸ **Cardiac arrest**
IV
Adults, Elderly. 40 units as a one-time bolus.
▸ **Diabetes insipidus**
IV INFUSION
Adults, Children. 0.5 milliunits/kg/h. May double dose q30min. Maximum: 10 milliunits/kg/h.
IM, SC
Adults, Elderly. 5-10 units 2-4 times a day. Range: 5-60 units/day.
Children. 2.5-10 units, 2-4 times a day.
▸ **Abdominal distention, intestinal paresis**
IM
Adults, Elderly. Initially, 5 units. Subsequent doses, 10 units q3-4h.
▸ **GI hemorrhage**
IV INFUSION
Adults, Elderly. Initially, 0.2-0.4 unit/min may titrate to maximum of 0.8 unit/min.
Children. 0.002-0.005 unit/kg/min. Titrate as needed. Maximum: 0.01 unit/kg/min.
▸ **Vasodilatory shock**
IV
Adults, Elderly. Initially, 0.01-0.04 units/min. Titrate to desired effect.

OFF-LABEL USES
Adjunct in treatment of acute, massive hemorrhage.

CONTRAINDICATIONS
Hypersensitivity.

INTERACTIONS
Drug
Alcohol, demeclocycline, lithium, norepinephrine: May decrease the effects of vasopressin.
Carbamazepine, chlorpropamide, clofibrate: May increase the effects of vasopressin.
Herbal
None known.
Food
None known.

DIAGNOSTIC TEST EFFECTS
None known.

ⓘ IV INCOMPATIBILITIES
Amphotericin B complex (Abelcet, AmBisome, Amphotec), diazepam (Valium), etomidate (Amidate), furosemide (Lasix), thiopentothal.

ⓘ IV COMPATIBILITIES
Dobutamine (Dobutrex), dopamine (Intropin), heparin, lorazepam (Ativan), midazolam (Versed), milrinone (Primacor), verapamil (Calan, Isoptin).

SIDE EFFECTS
Frequent
Pain at injection site (with vasopressin tannate).
Occasional
Abdominal cramps, nausea, vomiting, diarrhea, dizziness, diaphoresis, pale skin, circumoral pallor, tremors, headache, eructation, flatulence.
Rare
Chest pain; confusion; allergic reaction, including rash or hives,

pruritus, wheezing or difficulty
breathing, facial and peripheral
edema; sterile abscess (with
vasopressin tannate).

SERIOUS REACTIONS
• Anaphylaxis, MI, and water
intoxication have occurred.
• Elderly patients and very young
patients are at higher risk for water
intoxication.

PRECAUTIONS & CONSIDERATIONS
Caution is warranted in patients
with arteriosclerosis, asthma,
cardiac disease, goiter with cardiac
complications, migraine, nephritis,
renal disease, seizures, and vascular
disease. Vasopressin should be
used cautiously in breastfeeding
women. Vasopressin should be used
cautiously in children and in elderly
patients because of the risk of water
intoxication and hyponatremia in
these age groups.
Notify the physician of chest
pain, headache, shortness of breath,
or other symptoms. BP, serum
electrolyte levels, pulse rate, urine
specific gravity, intake and output,
and weight should be monitored
before and during therapy. Be alert
for early signs of water intoxication,
such as somnolence, headache, and
listlessness.
Storage
Store at room temperature.
Administration
! May administer intranasally on
cotton pledgets or by nasal spray;
individualize dosage.
For IV use, dilute with D5W or
0.9% NaCl to concentration of
0.1-1 unit/mL. Give as IV infusion.
For IM or SC, give with 1-2 glasses
of water to reduce side effects.

Venlafaxine
ven-la-fax´een
(Effexor, Effexor XR)

CATEGORY AND SCHEDULE
Pregnancy Risk Category: C

Classification: Antidepressants,
serotonin and norepinephrine
reuptake inhibitors

MECHANISM OF ACTION
A phenethylamine derivative that
potentiates central nervous system
(CNS) neurotransmitter activity by
inhibiting the reuptake of serotonin,
norepinephrine, and, to a lesser
degree, dopamine. *Therapeutic
Effect:* Relieves depression.

PHARMACOKINETICS
Well absorbed from the GI tract.
Protein binding: 25%-30%.
Metabolized in the liver to active
metabolite. Excreted primarily in
urine. Not removed by hemodialysis.
Half-life: 3-7 h; metabolite, 9-13 h
(increased in hepatic or renal
impairment).

AVAILABILITY
*Capsules (Extended-Release [Effexor
XR]):* 37.5 mg, 75 mg, 150 mg.
Tablets (Effexor): 25 mg, 37.5 mg,
50 mg, 75 mg, 100 mg.

INDICATIONS AND DOSAGES
▸ **Depression**
PO
Adults, Elderly. Initially, 75 mg/day
in 2-3 divided doses with food. May
increase by 75 mg/day at intervals
of 4 days or longer. Maximum:
375 mg/day in 3 divided doses.
PO (EXTENDED-RELEASE)
Adults, Elderly. 75 mg/day as a
single dose with food. May increase

by 75 mg/day at intervals of 4 days or longer. Maximum: 225 mg/day.

▸ **Anxiety disorder, panic disorder**
PO (EXTENDED-RELEASE)
Adults. 37.5-225 mg/day. Dosage may be increased by 75 mg/day at intervals ≥ 4 days.

▸ **Dosage in renal and hepatic impairment**
Expect to decrease venlafaxine dosage by 50% in patients with moderate hepatic impairment, 25% in patients with mild to moderate renal impairment, and 50% in patients on dialysis (withhold dose until completion of dialysis).

OFF-LABEL USES

Prevention of relapses of depression; treatment of attention-deficit hyperactivity disorder, autism, chronic fatigue syndrome, obsessive-compulsive disorder, hot flashes.

CONTRAINDICATIONS

Hypersensitivity; use within 14 days of MAOIs.

INTERACTIONS

Drug
MAOIs, serotonergic agents, linezolid, SSRIs, triptans: May cause neuroleptic malignant syndrome, autonomic instability (including rapid fluctuations of vital signs), extreme agitation, hyperthermia, mental status changes, myoclonus, rigidity, and coma.
Herbal
St. John's wort: May increase the sedative-hypnotic effect of venlafaxine; increased risk of serotonin syndrome.
Food
None known.

DIAGNOSTIC TEST EFFECTS

May increase BUN level and serum alkaline phosphatase, bilirubin, cholesterol, uric acid, AST (SGOT), and ALT (SGPT) levels. May decrease serum phosphate and sodium levels. May alter blood glucose and serum potassium levels.

SIDE EFFECTS

Frequent (> 20%)
Nausea, somnolence, headache, dry mouth.
Occasional (10%-20%)
Dizziness, insomnia, constipation, diaphoresis, nervousness, asthenia, ejaculatory disturbance, anorexia.
Rare (< 10%)
Anxiety, blurred vision, diarrhea, vomiting, tremor, abnormal dreams, impotence, weight loss.

SERIOUS REACTIONS

• A sustained increase in diastolic BP of 10-15 mm Hg occurs occasionally.
• Serotonin syndrome.

PRECAUTIONS & CONSIDERATIONS

Caution is warranted in patients with suicidal tendencies and those with abnormal platelet function, congestive heart failure, volume depletion, hyperthyroidism, mania, angle-closure glaucoma, hepatic and renal impairment, and seizure disorder. Notify the physician if pregnant or planning to become pregnant. Complications have been observed in neonates exposed to venlafaxine in the third trimester; consider tapering in the third trimester. It is unknown whether venlafaxine is excreted in breast milk. The safety and efficacy of venlafaxine have not been established in children. No age-related precautions have been noted in elderly patients.

Drowsiness, dizziness, and light-headedness may occur, so avoid alcohol and tasks that require mental alertness or motor skills. Monitor for clinical worsening, suicidality, and unusual changes in behavior. BP, pulse rate, and weight should be assessed during therapy.

Administration

! When discontinuing venlafaxine, plan to taper the dosage slowly over 2 wks. Allow at least 14 days to elapse before switching from an MAOI to venlafaxine and at least 7 days to elapse before switching from venlafaxine to an MAOI.

Take venlafaxine with food or milk if the patient experiences GI distress. Crush scored tablets if needed. Do not break, open, or crush extended-release capsules.

Verapamil

ver-ap′a-mill
(Anpec [AUS], Apo-Verap [CAN], Calan, Calan SR, Chronovera [CAN], Cordilox SR [AUS], Covera-HS, Isoptin SR, Novo-Veramil [CAN], Novo-Veramil SR [CAN], Veracaps SR [AUS], Verahexal [AUS], Verelan, Verelan PM)
Do not confuse Isoptin with Intropin, or Verelan with Virilon, Vivarin, or Voltaren.

CATEGORY AND SCHEDULE
Pregnancy Risk Category: C

Classification: Antiarrhythmics, class IV, calcium channel blockers

MECHANISM OF ACTION
A calcium channel blocker and antianginal, antiarrhythmic, and antihypertensive agent that inhibits calcium ion entry across cardiac and vascular smooth-muscle cell membranes. This action causes the dilation of coronary arteries, peripheral arteries, and arterioles. *Therapeutic Effect:* Decreases heart rate and myocardial contractility and slows SA and AV conduction. Decreases total peripheral vascular resistance by vasodilation.

PHARMACOKINETICS

Route	Onset	Peak	Duration
PO	30 min	1-2 h	6-8 h
PO (extended-release)	30 min	NA	NA
IV	1-2 min	3-5 min	0-60 min

Well absorbed from the GI tract. Protein binding: 90% (60% in neonates). Undergoes first-pass metabolism in the liver to active metabolite. Primarily excreted in urine. Not removed by hemodialysis. *Half-life:* 2-8 h.

AVAILABILITY
Capsules (Extended-Release [Verelan PM]): 100 mg, 200 mg, 300 mg.
Capsules (Extended-Release [Verelan]): 120 mg, 180 mg, 240 mg, 360 mg.
Tablets (Calan): 40 mg, 80 mg, 120 mg.
Tablets (Sustained-Release [Calan SR, Isoptin SR]): 120 mg, 180 mg, 240 mg.
Injection: 2.5 mg/mL.

INDICATIONS AND DOSAGES
▶ **Supraventricular tachyarrhythmias, temporary control of rapid ventricular rate with atrial fibrillation or flutter**
IV
Adults, Elderly. Initially, 5-10 mg; repeat in 30 min with 10-mg dose. *Children 1-15 yr.* 0.1 mg/kg (up to 5 mg maximum single dose). May repeat in 30 min up to a maximum

second dose of 10 mg. Not recommended in children younger than 1 yr.

▸ **Arrhythmias, including prevention of recurrent paroxysmal supraventricular tachycardia and control of ventricular resting rate in chronic atrial fibrillation or flutter**
PO
Adults, Elderly. 240-480 mg/day in 3-4 divided doses.

▸ **Vasospastic angina (Prinzmetal's variant), unstable (crescendo or preinfarction) angina, chronic stable (effort-associated) angina**
PO
Adults. Initially, 80-120 mg 3 times a day. For elderly patients and those with hepatic dysfunction, 40 mg 3 times a day. Titrate to optimal dose. Maintenance: 240-480 mg/day in 3-4 divided doses.
PO (COVERA-HS)
Adults, Elderly. 180-480 mg/day at bedtime.

▸ **Hypertension**
PO
Adults, Elderly. Initially, 40-80 mg 3 times a day. Maintenance: 480 mg or less a day.
PO (COVERA-HS)
Adults, Elderly. 180-480 mg/day at bedtime.
PO (EXTENDED-RELEASE)
Adults, Elderly. 120-240 mg/day. May give 480 mg or less a day in 2 divided doses.
PO (VERELAN PM)
Adults, Elderly. Initially, 200 mg/day at bedtime. Dosage may be increased by 100 mg/day up to 400 mg/day.

OFF-LABEL USES
Treatment of hypertrophic cardiomyopathy, vascular headaches.

CONTRAINDICATIONS
Atrial fibrillation or flutter and an accessory bypass tract, cardiogenic shock, heart block, sinus bradycardia, ventricular tachycardia; hypersensitivity.

INTERACTIONS
Drug
Amiodarone: Monitor closely for cardiotoxicity with bradycardia and decreased cardiac output.
β-Blockers: May have additive effect.
Carbamazepine, quinidine, theophylline: May increase verapamil blood concentration and risk of toxicity.
Digoxin: May increase digoxin blood concentration.
Disopyramide: May increase negative inotropic effect.
Procainamide, quinidine: May increase risk of QT-interval prolongation.
Statins (atorvastatin, lovastatin, simvastatin): Statin levels may be increased.
Herbal
None known.
Food
Grapefruit, grapefruit juice: May increase verapamil blood concentration.

DIAGNOSTIC TEST EFFECTS
ECG waveform may show increased PR interval.

ⓘ IV INCOMPATIBILITIES
Amphotericin B complex (Abelcet, AmBisome, Amphotec), nafcillin (Nafcil), propofol (Diprivan), sodium bicarbonate.

ⓘ IV COMPATIBILITIES
Amiodarone (Cordarone), calcium chloride, calcium gluconate, dexamethasone (Decadron), digoxin (Lanoxin), dobutamine (Dobutrex), dopamine (Intropin), heparin, hydromorphone (Dilaudid),

lidocaine, magnesium sulfate, metoclopramide (Reglan), milrinone (Primacor), morphine, multivitamins, nitroglycerin, norepinephrine (Levophed), potassium chloride, potassium phosphate, procainamide (Pronestyl), propranolol (Inderal).

SIDE EFFECTS
Frequent (7%)
Constipation.
Occasional (2%-4%)
Dizziness, light-headedness, headache, asthenia (loss of strength, energy), nausea, peripheral edema, hypotension.
Rare (< 1%)
Bradycardia, dermatitis or rash.

SERIOUS REACTIONS
• Rapid ventricular rate in atrial flutter or fibrillation, marked hypotension, extreme bradycardia, congestive heart failure (CHF), asystole, and second- and third-degree AV block occur rarely.

PRECAUTIONS & CONSIDERATIONS
Caution is warranted in patients with CHF, hepatic or renal impairment, and sick sinus syndrome and in those concurrently receiving β-blockers or digoxin. Verapamil crosses the placenta and is distributed in breast milk. Breastfeeding is not recommended for patients taking this drug. No age-related precautions have been noted in children. In elderly patients, age-related renal impairment may require cautious use. Grapefruit juice, which may increase verapamil blood concentration, should be avoided. Alcohol and tasks that require alertness and motor skills should also be avoided.

Be aware that ECG should be monitored for changes, particularly PR-interval prolongation. Notify the physician of significant PR interval or other ECG changes. BP, pulse, and stool consistency and frequency should be assessed. The onset, type (sharp, dull, or squeezing), radiation, location, intensity, and duration of anginal pain and its precipitating factors, such as exertion and emotional stress, should be recorded. Be aware that concurrent administration of sublingual nitroglycerin therapy may be used for relief of anginal pain.

Storage
Store at room temperature.

Administration
Take tablets that are not sustained-release with or without food. Sustained-release form should be given on an empty stomach. Swallow extended-release or sustained-released preparations whole and without chewing or crushing. If needed, open sustained-release capsules and sprinkle contents on applesauce. Swallow the applesauce immediately, without chewing. Do not abruptly discontinue verapamil. Compliance is essential to control anginal pain.

For IV use, give undiluted, if desired. Administer IV push over more than 2 min for adults and children and over > 3 min for elderly patients. Continuous ECG monitoring during IV injection is required for children and recommended for adults.

Monitor ECG for asystole, extreme bradycardia, heart block, PR-interval prolongation, and rapid ventricular rates. Notify the physician of significant ECG changes. Monitor BP every 5-10 min

V

or as ordered. Keep the patient in a recumbent position for at least 1 h after IV administration.

Verteporfin
ver-te-por'-fin
(Visudyne)

CATEGORY AND SCHEDULE
Pregnancy Risk Category: C

Classification: Phototherapy

MECHANISM OF ACTION
Light-activated agent. Produces oxygen-free radicals resulting in local damage to neovascular endothelium and vessel occlusion.

PHARMACOKINETICS
Limited metabolism by liver and plasma esterases. Fecal elimination; < 0.01% of dose recovered in urine. *Half-life:* 5-6 h.

AVAILABILITY
Lyophilized cake for injection 15 mg.

INDICATIONS AND DOSAGES
Predominantly classic subfoveal choroidal neovascularization resulting from age-related macular degeneration, pathologic myopia, or presumed ocular histoplasmosis.
IV
Adults. 6 mg/m^2 followed by activation with light from a nonthermal diode laser. May be repeated every 3 mo.

CONTRAINDICATIONS
Porphyria; known hypersensitivity to any product ingredients.

INTERACTIONS
Drug
None known.
Herbal
None known.
Food
None known.

DIAGNOSTIC TEST EFFECTS
None known.

⊘ IV INCOMPATIBILITIES
May precipitate in saline solutions. Do not mix with other medications.

SIDE EFFECTS
Frequent (10%-30%)
Injection site reactions, visual disturbances.
Occasional (1%-10%)
Severe vision reduction, cataracts, conjunctivitis, fever, back pain during infusion, photosensitivity reactions, atrial fibrillation, hypertension, eczema, constipation, nausea, arthralgia, hypesthesia, sleep disorder, vertigo, cough.
Rare (< 1%)
Retinal detachment, retinal or choroidal vessel nonperfusion, chest pain, musculoskeletal pain, hypersensitivity reactions, syncope, vasovagal reactions.

SERIOUS REACTIONS
• Severe chest pain, vasovagal reactions, hypersenstivity reactions.

PRECAUTIONS & CONSIDERATIONS
Avoid exposure of skin and eyes to direct sunlight or bright indoor light for 5 days after administration. Do not re-treat patients experiencing severe loss of vision within 1 wk after treatment unless vision completely recovers to pretreatment levels. Take precautions to avoid extravasation; if extravasation occurs, protect area from direct light until

V

swelling and discoloration have faded. Use with caution in patients with moderate to severe hepatic impairment.

Storage
Store verteporfin at room temperature. Reconstituted solution must be protected from light and used within 4 h.

Administration
Each vial is reconstituted with 7 mL sterile water to produce 7.5 mL dark green solution containing verteporfin 2 mg/mL. Dilute required quantity with 5% dextrose for a total infusion volume of 30 mL. Administered over 10 min at a rate of 3 mL/min with an in-line filter. Following IV dose, initiate 689-nm wavelength laser light delivery to the patient 15 min after the start of the 10-min infusion.

Vinblastine Sulfate

vin-blass′teen sul′fate
(Oncovin [AUS], Velban, Velbe [AUS])
Do not confuse vinblastine with vincristine or vinorelbine.

CATEGORY AND SCHEDULE
Pregnancy Risk Category: D

Classification: Antineoplastic

MECHANISM OF ACTION
A vinca alkaloid that binds to microtubular protein of mitotic spindle, causing metaphase arrest. *Therapeutic Effect:* Inhibits cell division.

PHARMACOKINETICS
Does not cross the blood-brain barrier. Protein binding: 75%.

Metabolized in the liver to active metabolite. Primarily eliminated in feces by biliary system. *Half-life:* 24.8 h.

AVAILABILITY
Powder for Injection: 10 mg.
Injection: 1 mg/mL.

INDICATIONS AND DOSAGES
▸ **Remission induction in advanced testicular carcinoma, advanced mycosis fungoides, breast carcinoma, choriocarcinoma, disseminated Hodgkin disease, non-Hodgkin lymphoma, Kaposi sarcoma (KS), or Letterer-Siwe disease**
IV
Adults, Elderly. Initially, 3.7 mg/m^2 as a single dose. Increase dose by about 1.8 mg/m^2 at weekly intervals until desired therapeutic response is attained, WBC count falls below 3000/mm^3, or maximum weekly dose of 18.5 mg/m^2 is reached.
Children. Initially, 2.5 mg/m^2 as a single dose. Increase dose by about 1.25 mg/m^2 at weekly intervals until desired therapeutic response is attained, WBC count falls below 3000/mm^3, or maximum weekly dose of 7.5-12.5 mg/m^2 is reached.
▸ **Maintenance dose for treatment of advanced testicular carcinoma, advanced mycosis fungoides, breast carcinoma, choriocarcinoma, disseminated Hodgkin disease, non-Hodgkin's lymphoma, KS, or Letterer-Siwe disease**
IV
Adults, Elderly, Children. Administer one increment less than dose required to produce WBC count of 3000/mm^3. Each subsequent dose given when WBC count returns to 4000/mm^3 and at least 7 days have elapsed since previous dose.

V

▸ **Dose in hepatic impairment**
IV
Reduce dose by 50% if total bilirubin is 1.5-3 mg/dL. Reduce dose by 75% if total bilirubin > 3 mg/dL.

CONTRAINDICATIONS
Bacterial infection, severe leukopenia, significant granulocytopenia (unless it stems from disease being treated); intrathecal administration.

INTERACTIONS
Drug
Strong inhibitors of CYP3A4 isoenzymes (erythromycin, clarithromycin, fluconazole, itraconazole, ketoconazole, metronidazole): Increase concentrations of vinblastine.
Herbal
None known.
Food
None known.

DIAGNOSTIC TEST EFFECTS
Decreases WBC.

ⓦ IV INCOMPATIBILITIES
Do not mix with other medications.

SIDE EFFECTS
Frequent
Nausea, vomiting, alopecia.
Occasional
Constipation or diarrhea, rectal bleeding, headache, paraesthesia (occur 4-6 h after administration and persist for 2-10 h); malaise; asthenia; dizziness; pain at tumor site; jaw or face pain; depression; dry mouth.
Rare
Dermatitis, stomatitis, phototoxicity, hyperuricemia.

SERIOUS REACTIONS
• Hematologic toxicity is manifested as leukopenia and, less commonly, anemia. The WBC count reaches its nadir 4-10 days after initial therapy and recovers within 7-14 days (21 days with high vinblastine dosages).
• Thrombocytopenia is usually mild and transient, with recovery occurring in a few days.
• Hepatic insufficiency may increase the risk of toxic drug effects.
• Acute shortness of breath or bronchospasm may occur, particularly when vinblastine is administered concurrently with mitomycin.

PRECAUTIONS & CONSIDERATIONS
Leukopenia is common; may be more severe in older patients with cachexia or ulcerated skin surfaces. Toxicity may be greater in patients with hepatic impairment.
 For IV use only. Must be dispensed with overwrap with the statement, "Do not remove covering until the moment of injection. Fatal if given intrathecally. For IV use only." Syringes should be labeled, "Fatal if given intrathecally. For IV use only."
Storage
Refrigerate unopened vials. Refrigerate reconstituted solution for up to 28 days.
Administration
Reconstitute power for injection with 10 mL NS injection (with or without preservative) to a concentration of 1 mg/mL. Inject into tubing of a running IV infusion or directly into a vein over 1 min. Do not dilute in large volumes or infuse over prolonged period to reduce risk of vein irritation and extravasation.

V

Vincristine Sulfate

vin-cris´teen sul´fate
(Oncovin, Vincasar PFS)
**Do not confuse vincristine with
vinblastine, or Oncovin with
Ancobon.**

CATEGORY AND SCHEDULE

Pregnancy Risk Category: D

Classification: Antineoplastic

MECHANISM OF ACTION

A vinca alkaloid that binds to
microtubular protein of mitotic spindle,
causing metaphase arrest. *Therapeutic
Effect:* Inhibits cell division.

PHARMACOKINETICS

Does not cross the blood-brain barrier.
Protein binding: 75%. Metabolized in
the liver. Primarily eliminated in feces
by biliary system. *Half-life:* 10-37 h.

AVAILABILITY

Injection: 1 mg/mL.

INDICATIONS AND DOSAGES

▸ **Acute leukemia, advanced
non-Hodgkin lymphoma,
disseminated Hodgkin disease,
neuroblastoma, rhabdomyosarcoma,
Wilms tumor**
IV
Adults, Elderly. 0.4-1.4 mg/m^2 once
a week.
Children. 1-2 mg/m^2 once a week
during induction phase.
*Children weighing < 10 kg or
with a body surface area < 1 m^2.*
0.05 mg/kg once a week during
induction phase. Maximum: 2 mg.
▸ **Dosage in hepatic impairment**
Reduce dosage by 50% if total
bilirubin concentration is 1.5-3 mg/dL.
Reduce dosage by 75% if total
bilirubin concentration > 3 mg/dL.

CONTRAINDICATIONS

Patients receiving radiation therapy
through ports that include the liver;
patients with demyelinating form
of Charcot-Marie-Tooth syndrome;
intrathecal administration.

INTERACTIONS

Drug
**Strong inhibitors of CYP3A4
isoenzymes (erythromycin,
clarithromycin, fluconazole,
intraconazole, metronidazole):**
Increase concentrations of
vincristine.
Mitomycin: Increased risk of
pulmonary reactions.
Herbal
None known.
Food
None known.

DIAGNOSTIC TEST EFFECTS

Decreased WBC and platelets.

⊘ IV INCOMPATIBILITIES

Do not mix with other medications.

SIDE EFFECTS

Expected
Peripheral neuropathy (occurs in
nearly every patient; first clinical
sign is depression of Achilles tendon
reflex).
Frequent
Peripheral paraesthesia, alopecia,
constipation or obstipation (upper
colon impaction with empty rectum),
abdominal cramps, headache, jaw
pain, hoarseness, diplopia, ptosis
or drooping of eyelid, urinary tract
disturbances.
Occasional
Nausea, vomiting, diarrhea,
abdominal distention, stomatitis,
fever.
Rare
Mild leukopenia, mild anemia,
thrombocytopenia.

V

SERIOUS REACTIONS
• Acute shortness of breath and bronchospasm may occur, especially when vincristine is administered concurrently with mitomycin.
• Prolonged or high-dose therapy may produce foot or wrist drop, difficulty walking, slapping gait, ataxia, and muscle wasting.
• Acute uric acid nephropathy may occur.

For IV administration only. Intrathecal administration is fatal. Perform complete blood count before each dose.
Storage
Store unopened vials under refrigeration. Diluted solution stable for 7 days under refrigeration or 2 days at room temperature. In ambulatory pumps, solution is stable for 7-10 days at room temperature.
Administration
May be diluted with normal saline or D5W. Inject into tubing of a running IV infusion or directly into a vein. May be injected in about 1 min. Carefully position IV to avoid extravasation.

Vinorelbine
vin-oh-rel′bean
(Navelbine)
Do not confuse vinorelbine with vinblastine.

CATEGORY AND SCHEDULE
Pregnancy Risk Category: D

Classification: Antineoplastic

MECHANISM OF ACTION
A semisynthetic vinca alkaloid that interferes with mitotic microtubule assembly. *Therapeutic Effect:* Prevents cell division.

PHARMACOKINETICS
Widely distributed after IV administration. Protein binding: 80%-90%. Metabolized in the liver. Primarily eliminated in feces by biliary system. *Half-life:* 28-43 h.

AVAILABILITY
Injection: 10 mg/mL.

INDICATIONS AND DOSAGES
▸ **Unresectable, advanced non–small-cell lung cancer (as monotherapy or in combination with cisplatin)**
IV
Adults, Elderly. 30 mg/m^2 administered weekly over 6-10 min.
▸ **Dosage adjustment guidelines**
Dosage adjustments should be based on granulocyte count obtained on the day of treatment, as follows:

Granulocyte Count (cells/mm^3) on Day of Treatment	% of Starting Dose
> 1500	100%
1000-1499	50%
< 1000	Do not administer

Additional dosage adjustments are required for patients experiencing fever or sepsis during granulocytopenia or patients who had two consecutive doses withheld because of granulocytopenia:

Granulocyte Count (cells/mm^3) on Day of Treatment	% of Starting Dose
> 1500	75%
1000-1499	37.5%
< 1000	Do not administer

Dosage adjustments based on total bilirubin:

Total Bilirubin (mg/dL)	% of Starting Dose
≤ 2	100%
2.1-3	50%
> 3	25%

▶ **Combination therapy (with cisplatin)**
IV INJECTION
Adults, Elderly: 25 mg/m^2 every week or 30 mg/m^2 on days 1 and 29, then q6wk.

CONTRAINDICATIONS

Pretreatment granulocyte counts < 1000 cells/mm^3. Intrathecal administration.

INTERACTIONS

Drug
Cisplatin: Increased risk of granulocytopenia.
Mitomycin: Increased risk of pulmonary toxicity.
Paclitaxel: Increased risk of neurotoxicity.
Herbal
None known.
Food
None known.

DIAGNOSTIC TEST EFFECTS

Decreased WBC. Increased AST, bilirubin.

Ⓘ IV INCOMPATIBILITIES

Do not mix with other medications.

SIDE EFFECTS

Frequent
Asthenia; mild or moderate nausea; constipation; erythema, pain, or vein discoloration at injection site; fatigue; peripheral neuropathy manifested as paresthesia and hyperesthesia; diarrhea; alopecia.
Occasional
Phlebitis, dyspnea, loss of deep tendon reflexes.

Rare
Chest pain, jaw pain, myalgia, arthralgia, rash.

SERIOUS REACTIONS

• Bone marrow depression is manifested mainly as granulocytopenia, which may be severe. Other hematologic toxicities, including neutropenia, thrombocytopenia, leukopenia, and anemia, increase the risk of infection and bleeding.
• Acute shortness of breath and severe bronchospasm occur infrequently, particularly in patients with preexisting pulmonary dysfunction and in those receiving mitomycin concurrently. Fatal interstitial pulmonary changes and acute respiratory distress syndrome have occurred.
• Severe, sometimes fatal, constipation, paralytic ileus, intestinal obstruction, necrosis, or perforation.

PRECAUTIONS & CONSIDERATIONS

Granulocyte count before treatment should be at least 1000 cells/mm^3. Obtain complete blood count with differentials on the day of treatment. Caution if bone marrow reserve is compromised by previous radiation therapy or chemotherapy. Use with caution in hepatic impairment. Discontinue therapy if grade 2 or greater neurotoxicity occurs.

For IV administration only. Syringes should be labeled as follows: "Warning—for IV use only. Fatal if given intrathecally."
Storage
Store unopened vials in cartons under refrigeration. Unopened vials are stable at temperatures up to 25° C (77° F) for up to 72 h. Diluted solution may be used for up to 24 h under normal room light when stored in polypropylene syringes

V

or polyvinyl chloride bags under refrigeration or at room temperature.
Administration
Dilute injection solution in the syringe or IV bag. Doses in a syringe should be diluted to 1.5-3 mg/mL with D5W or normal Saline (NS). Doses diluted in an IV bag should be diluted to 0.5-2 mg/mL with D5W, normal Saline (NS), 0.45% NaCl injection, 5% dextrose with 0.45% NaCl injection, Ringer's injection, or lactated Ringer's injection. Diluted solution should be administered over 6-10 min into the side port of a free-flowing IV closest to the IV bag, followed by flushing with at least 75-125 mL of a recommended dilution solution. Carefully position IV needle to minimize extravasation risk.

Vitamin A
vight'ah-myn A
(Aquasol A, Palmitate A)
Do not confuse Aquasol A with Anusol.

CATEGORY AND SCHEDULE
Pregnancy Risk Category: A (X if used in doses above recommended daily allowance)

Classification: Vitamin/mineral; fat-soluble vitamin

MECHANISM OF ACTION
A fat-soluble vitamin that may act as a cofactor in biochemical reactions. *Therapeutic Effect:* Essential for normal function of retina, visual adaptation to darkness, bone growth, testicular and ovarian function, and embryonic development; preserves integrity of epithelial cells.

PHARMACOKINETICS
Rapidly absorbed from the GI tract if bile salts, pancreatic lipase, protein, and dietary fat are present. Transported in blood to the liver, where it is metabolized; stored in parenchymal hepatic cells, then transported in plasma as retinol, as needed. Excreted primarily in bile and, to a lesser extent, in urine.

AVAILABILITY
Capsules: 10,000 units, 15,000 units, 25,000 units.
Injection (Aquasol A): 50,000 units/mL.
Tablets (Palmitate A): 5000 units, 15,000 units.

INDICATIONS AND DOSAGES
▸ **Severe vitamin A deficiency**
PO
Adults, Elderly, Children 8 yr and older. 100,000 units/day for 3 days, then 50,000 units/day for 14 days, then 10,000-20,000 units/day for 2 mo.
Children 1-8 yr. 10,000 units/kg/day for 5 days, then 5000-10,000 units/day for 2 mo.
Children younger than 1 yr. 10,000 units/day for 5 days, then 7500-15,000 units for 10 days.
IM
Adults, Elderly, Children 8 yr and older. 100,000 units/day for 3 days; then 50,000 units/day for 14 days, followed by 10,000-20,000 units/day PO for 2 mo.
Children aged 1-8 yr. 17,500-35,000 units/day for 10 days.
Children younger than 1 yr. 7500-15,000 units/day.
▸ **Malabsorption syndrome**
PO
Adults, Elderly, Children 8 yr and older. 10,000-50,000 units/day.
▸ **Dietary supplement**
Females ≥ 14 yr. 2333 International Units/day.

V

Males ≥ 14 yr. 3000 International Units/day.
Pregnant Adolescent Females aged 14-18 yr. 2500 International Units/day.
Pregnant Adult Female. 2566 International Units/day.
Lactating Adolescent Females aged 14-18 yr. 4000 International Units/day during first 6 mo of breast-feeding.
Lactating Adult Female. 4333 Internationl Units during first 6 mo of breast-feeding.
Children aged 9-13 yr. 2000 International Units/day.
Children aged 4-8 yr. 1333 International Units/day.
Children aged 1-3 yr. 1000 International Units/day.
Infants (term) aged 7-12 mo. 1666 International Units/day, based on dietary intake of breast milk, formula, or other food sources.
Infants (term) aged birth-6 mo. 1333 International Units/day, based on dietary intake of human breast milk.

CONTRAINDICATIONS

Hypervitaminosis A; oral use in malabsorption syndrome; hypersensitivity, IV administration.

INTERACTIONS

Drug
Cholestyramine, colestipol, mineral oil: May decrease the absorption of vitamin A.
Isotretinoin: May increase the risk of toxicity.
Mineral oil: May decrease oral vitamin A absorption.
Herbal and Food
None known.

DIAGNOSTIC TEST EFFECTS

May increase BUN and serum cholesterol, calcium, and triglyceride levels. May decrease blood erythrocyte and leukocyte counts.

SIDE EFFECTS

Occasional (1%-10%)
Fever, headache, irritability, lethargy, malaise, vertigo, drying or cracking of the skin, hypercalcemia, weight loss, visual changes, hypervitaminosis A.

SERIOUS REACTIONS

• Chronic overdosage produces malaise, nausea, vomiting, drying or cracking of skin or lips, inflammation of tongue or gums, irritability, alopecia, and night sweats.
• Bulging fontanelles have occurred in infants.

PRECAUTIONS & CONSIDERATIONS

Caution is warranted in patients with renal impairment. Vitamin A crosses the placenta and is distributed in breast milk. Use caution when administering high doses of vitamin A to children and elderly patients. Consuming foods rich in vitamin A, including cod, halibut, tuna, and shark, is encouraged; naturally occurring vitamin A is found only in animal sources. Avoid taking cholestyramine (Questran), colestipol, and mineral oil during vitamin A therapy.

Before and during treatment, assess for signs and symptoms of vitamin A deficiency, including night blindness, dry and brittle nails, alopecia, and drying of corneas. Be alert for symptoms of overdose when receiving prolonged administration of > 25,000 units/day. The therapeutic serum vitamin A level is 80-300 units/mL.
Administration
! IM administration is used only in acutely ill patients or patients unresponsive to the oral route, such as those with malabsorption syndrome.

Do not administer intravenously.

Do not crush, open, or break capsules. Take vitamin A without regard to food.

V

For adults, an IM injection dose of 1 mL (50,000 units) may be given in the deltoid muscle; a dose > 1 mL should be given in a large muscle mass, such as the gluteus maximus muscle. The anterolateral thigh is the preferred site for infants younger than 7 mo.

Vitamin D (Cholecalciferol, Vitamin D₃; Ergocalciferol, Vitamin D₂)

vight'ah-myn D
(Calciferol, Drisdol, Ostoforet [CAN])

CATEGORY AND SCHEDULE

Pregnancy Risk Category: A (D if used in doses above recommended daily allowance)

Classification: Vitamin; fat-soluble vitamin

MECHANISM OF ACTION

A fat-soluble vitamin that stimulates calcium and phosphate absorption from small intestine, promotes secretion of calcium from bone to blood, and promotes resorption of phosphate in renal tubules; also acts on bone cells to stimulate skeletal growth and on parathyroid gland to suppress hormone synthesis and secretion. *Therapeutic Effect:* Essential for absorption and utilization of calcium and phosphate and normal bone calcification. Reduces parathyroid hormone level. Improves phosphorus and calcium homeostasis in chronic renal failure.

PHARMACOKINETICS

Readily absorbed from small intestine; vitamin D₃ may be absorbed more rapidly and more completely than vitamin D₂. Concentrated primarily in liver and fat deposits. Activated in the liver and kidneys. Eliminated by biliary system; excreted in urine. *Half-life:* 14 h for cholecalciferol; 19-48 h for ergocalciferol.

AVAILABILITY

Capsules (Ergocalciferol, Drisdol): 50,000 units (1.25 mg).
Injection (Calciferol): 500,000 units/mL (12.5 mg).
Oral Liquid Drops (Calciferol, Drisdol): 8000 units/mL.
Tablets (Cholecalciferol, Vitamin D₃): 400 units, 1000 units.
Capsules (Cholecalciferol, Vitamin D₃): 10,000 units.

INDICATIONS AND DOSAGES

! Oral dosing is preferred. Administer the drug IM only in patients with GI, hepatic, or biliary disease associated with malabsorption of vitamin D.
▸ **Dietary supplement**
PO
Adults, Elderly. 10 mcg (400 units)/day.
Children. 5 mcg.
Neonates. 5 mcg (400-800 units)/day.
▸ **Renal failure**
PO
Adults, Elderly. 0.5 mg/day.
Children. 0.1-1 mg/day.
▸ **Hypoparathyroidism**
PO
Adults, Elderly. 1250-5000 mcg/day (with calcium supplements).
Children. 1250-5000 mcg/day (with calcium supplements).
▸ **Nutritional rickets, osteomalacia**
PO
Adults, Elderly, Children. 25-125 mcg/day for 8-12 wks.
Adults, Elderly (with malabsorption syndrome). 250-7500 mcg/day.

Children (with malabsorption syndrome). 250-625 mcg/day.
▸ **Vitamin D–dependent rickets**
PO
Adults, Elderly. 250 mcg to 1.5 mg/day.
Children. 75-125 mcg/day. Maximum: 1500 mcg/day.
▸ **Vitamin D–resistant rickets**
PO
Adults, Elderly. 250-1500 mcg/day (with phosphate supplements).
Children. Initially 1000-2000 mcg/day (with phosphate supplements). May increase in 250- to 600-mcg increments q3-4mo.

CONTRAINDICATIONS

Hypercalcemia, malabsorption syndrome, vitamin D toxicity.

INTERACTIONS

Drug
Aluminum-containing antacids (long-term use): May increase aluminum blood concentration and risk of aluminum bone toxicity.
Calcium-containing preparations, thiazide diuretics: May increase the risk of hypercalcemia.
Magnesium-containing antacids: May increase magnesium blood concentration.
Mineral oil: Excessive use of mineral oil decreases vitamin D absorption.
Herbal
None known.
Food
None known.

DIAGNOSTIC TEST EFFECTS

May increase serum cholesterol, calcium, magnesium, and phosphate levels. May decrease serum alkaline phosphatase level.

SIDE EFFECTS

None known.

SERIOUS REACTIONS

• Early signs and symptoms of overdose are weakness, headache, somnolence, nausea, vomiting, dry mouth, constipation, muscle and bone pain, and metallic taste.
• Later signs and symptoms of overdose include polyuria, polydipsia, anorexia, weight loss, nocturia, photophobia, rhinorrhea, pruritus, disorientation, hallucinations, hyperthermia, hypertension, and cardiac arrhythmias.

PRECAUTIONS & CONSIDERATIONS

Caution is warranted in patients with coronary artery disease, renal calculi, and renal impairment. It is unknown whether vitamin D crosses the placenta or is distributed in breast milk. Children may be more sensitive to the effects of vitamin D. No age-related precautions have been noted in elderly patients. Avoid taking mineral oil. Those receiving chronic renal dialysis should not take magnesium-containing antacids during vitamin D therapy. Consuming foods rich in vitamin D, including milk, eggs, leafy vegetables, margarine, meats, and vegetable oils and shortening, is encouraged.

BUN, serum alkaline phosphatase, calcium, creatinine, magnesium, and phosphate levels, and urinary calcium levels should be monitored.
Administration
! Be aware that 1 mcg of vitamin D = 40 International Units.

Begin vitamin D therapy at the lowest possible dosage. Take vitamin D without regard to food. Swallow the capsules whole and avoid crushing, chewing, or opening them.

V

Vitamin E
vight′ah-myn E
(Aqua Gem-E, Aquasol E,
E-Gems, Key-E, Key-E Kaps)
**Do not confuse Aquasol E with
Anusol.**

CATEGORY AND SCHEDULE
Pregnancy Risk Category: A (C if
used in doses above recommended
daily allowance)
OTC

Classification: Vitamins/
minerals; fat-soluble vitamin

MECHANISM OF ACTION
An antioxidant that prevents
oxidation of vitamins A and C,
protects fatty acids from attack by
free radicals, and protects RBCs
from hemolysis by oxidizing agents.
Therapeutic Effect: Prevents and
treats vitamin E deficiency.

PHARMACOKINETICS
Variably absorbed from the GI tract
(requires bile salts, dietary fat,
and normal pancreatic function).
Concentrated primarily in adipose
tissue. Metabolized in the liver.
Eliminated primarily by the biliary
system.

AVAILABILITY
Capsules (E-Gems): 100 units,
600 units, 800 units, 1000 units,
1200 units.
*Capsules (Vitamin E, Aqua Gem-E,
Key-E Kaps):* 100 units, 200 units,
400 units, 1000 units.
Tablets (Vitamin E, Key-E): 100 units,
200 units, 400 units, 500 units,
800 units.
Oral Drops: 15 units/0.3 mL.

Oral Liquid: 15 units/30 mL,
200 units/30 mL, 798 units/30 mL.

INDICATIONS AND DOSAGES
▸ **Vitamin E deficiency**
PO
Adults, Elderly. 60-75 units/day.
Children. 1 unit/kg/day.
1.5 Units = 1 mg α-tocopherol
equivalents.

OFF-LABEL USES
To decrease the severity of tardive
dyskinesia.

CONTRAINDICATIONS
None known.

INTERACTIONS
Drug
**Cholestyramine, colestipol,
mineral oil:** May decrease the
absorption of vitamin E.
Iron (large doses): May increase
vitamin E requirements.
Oral anticoagulants: Increased
anticoagulant effects with vitamin E
doses exceeding 400 units/day.
Herbal
None known.
Food
None known.

DIAGNOSTIC TEST EFFECTS
None known.

SIDE EFFECTS
None known.

SERIOUS REACTIONS
• Chronic overdose may produce
fatigue, weakness, nausea, headache,
blurred vision, flatulence, and
diarrhea.

PRECAUTIONS & CONSIDERATIONS
Vitamin E use may impair the
hematologic response with iron
deficiency anemia. It is unknown

whether vitamin E crosses the placenta or is distributed in breast milk. No age-related precautions have been noted with normal dosages in children or in elderly patients. Consuming foods high in vitamin E, including eggs, meats, milk, leafy vegetables, margarine, and vegetable oils and shortening, is encouraged.

Notify the physician of signs and symptoms of toxicity including blurred vision, diarrhea, nausea, dizziness, flu-like symptoms, or headache.

Administration

Do not crush, open, or break capsules or tablets. Take vitamin E without regard to food.

Voriconazole

vohr-ee-con′ah-zole
(Vfend)

CATEGORY AND SCHEDULE

Pregnancy Risk Category: D

Classification: Antifungals

MECHANISM OF ACTION

A triazole derivative that inhibits the synthesis of ergosterol, a vital component of fungal cell wall formation. *Therapeutic Effect:* Damages fungal cell wall membrane.

PHARMACOKINETICS

Rapidly and completely absorbed after PO administration. Widely distributed. Protein binding: 98%. Metabolized in the liver. Primarily excreted as a metabolite in urine. *Half-life:* 6 h.

AVAILABILITY

Tablets: 50 mg, 200 mg.
Injection Powder for Reconstitution: 200 mg.
Powder for Oral Suspension: 200 mg/5 mL.

INDICATIONS AND DOSAGES

▸ **Invasive aspergillosis, other serious fungal infections caused by *Scedosporium apiospermum* and *Fusarium* spp**

PO

Adults, Elderly weighing ≥ 40 kg. Initially, 400 mg q12h for 2 doses on day 1. Maintenance: 200 mg q12h.

Adults, Elderly weighing < 40 kg. Initially, 200 mg q12h for 2 doses on day 1. Maintenance: 100 mg q12h (may increase to 150 mg q12h).

▸ **Usual parenteral dosage**

IV

Adults, Elderly, Children. Initially, 6 mg/kg/dose q12h for 2 doses, then 4 mg/kg/dose q12h (may decrease to 3 mg/kg/dose if patient is unable to tolerate 4 mg/kg/dose). Candidemia in nonneutropenic patients; deep tissue *Candida* infections.

PO

Adults, Elderly weighing ≥ 40 kg. After initial IV loading dose, 200 mg q12h.

Adults, Elderly weighing < 40 kg. After initial IV loading dose, 100 mg q12h.

IV

Adults. Elderly. Initially, 6 mg/kg/dose q12h for 2 doses, then 3-4 mg/kg/dose q12h.

▸ **Esophageal candidiasis**

PO

Adults, Elderly weighing ≥ 40 kg. 200 mg q12h for minimum of 14 days, then at least 7 days following resolution of symptoms.

V

*Adults, Elderly weighing
< 40 kg.* 100 mg q12h for
minimum 14 days, then at least
7 days following resolution of
symptoms.

CONTRAINDICATIONS

Concurrent administration with
CYP3A4 substrates, such as
carbamazepine; ergot alkaloids;
pimozide or quinidine (may cause
prolonged QT interval or torsade
de pointes); rifabutin; rifampin;
sirolimus.

INTERACTIONS

Drug
**Cyclosporine, omeprazole,
phenytoin, rifabutin, sirolimus,
tacrilimus, warfarin:** May increase
plasma concentrations of these
drugs.
Phenytoin, rifabutin, rifampin:
May decrease voriconazole plasma
concentration.
Herbal
None known.
Food
Absorption reduced with high-fat
meal.

DIAGNOSTIC TEST EFFECTS

May increase serum alkaline
phosphatase and SGPT (ALT)
levels.

ⓘ IV INCOMPATIBILITIES

Do not mix voriconazole with any
other medications.

SIDE EFFECTS

Frequent (5%-20%)
Abnormal vision, fever, nausea, rash,
vomiting.
Occasional (2%-5%)
Headache, chills, hallucinations,
photophobia, tachycardia,
hypertension.

SERIOUS REACTIONS

• Hepatotoxicity occurs rarely.

PRECAUTIONS & CONSIDERATIONS

Caution should be used in patients
with hypersensitivity to other
antifungal agents, impaired renal
or liver function, or proarrhythmic
conditions. Correct hypocalemia,
hypokalemia, and hypomagnesemia
before initiating voriconazole.
Be aware that voriconazole may
cause fetal harm. Use effective
contraception during voriconazole
treatment. Be aware that the safety
and efficacy of voriconazole have
not been established in children
younger than 12 yr. No age-related
precautions have been noted in
elderly patients.

Expect to monitor liver and renal
function test results. Evaluate and
monitor visual function, including
color perception, visual acuity, and
visual field, for drug therapy lasting
longer than 28 days. Avoid driving
at night because voriconazole
may cause visual changes, such
as blurred vision or photophobia.
Avoid performing hazardous tasks if
changes in vision occur. Avoid direct
sunlight.
Storage
Store powder for injection at room
temperature. Use reconstituted
solution immediately. Do not use
reconstituted solution after 24 h
when refrigerated.

Powder for oral suspension
should be stored in refrigerator until
reconstituted. Reconstituted oral
suspension stable for 14 days at room
temperature.
Administration
Give oral voriconazole 1 h before or
1 h after a meal.

Reconstitute 200-mg vial with
19 mL sterile water for injection to
provide a concentration of 10 mg/mL.

Further dilute with 0.9% NaCl or D5W to provide a concentration not < 0.5 mg/mL or > 5 mg/mL. Infuse over 1-2 h at a concentration of 5 mg/mL or less.

Vorinostat
vor-in-o-stat
(Zolinza)

CATEGORY AND SCHEDULE
Pregnancy Risk Category: D

Classification: Antineoplastic

MECHANISM OF ACTION
Inhibits histone deacetylase enzymes HDAC1, HDAC2, HDAC3, and HDAC6, which catalyze removal of acetyl groups from the lysine residues of proteins. Inhibition of histone deacylase enzymes results in accumulation of acetyl groups on the histone lysine residues, resulting in open chromatin structure and transcriptional activation, which results in cell cycle arrest and/or apoptosis.

PHARMACOKINETICS
Vorinostat is extensively metabolized. *Half-life:* 2 h.

AVAILABILITY
Capsules: 100 mg.

INDICATIONS AND DOSAGES
▶ Cutaneous T-cell lymphoma
PO
Adults, Elderly. 400 mg once daily; if not tolerated, may reduce to 300 mg once daily or 300 mg once daily 5 days/wk.

CONTRAINDICATIONS
None known.

INTERACTIONS
Drug
Valproic acid (other HDAC inhibitors): Severe thrombocytopenia and GI bleeding.
Warfarin: Prolonged PT.
Herbal
None known.
Food
Administration with food resulted in a small (33%) increase in the extent of absorption and a delay in the time to peak concentration.

DIAGNOSTIC TEST EFFECTS
Increased serum glucose, serum creatinine.

SIDE EFFECTS
Frequent (> 20%)
Fatigue, anorexia, diarrhea, dysgeusia, nausea, thrombocytopenia, weight loss.
Occasional (10%-20%)
Dizziness, headache, alopecia, pruritus, constipation, decreased appetite, dry mouth, vomiting, anemia, muscle spasms, cough, upper respiratory tract infection, increased serum creatinine, chills, peripheral edema, pyrexia.

SERIOUS REACTIONS
Pulmonary embolism, deep vein thrombosis, squamous cell carcinoma, thrombocytopenia, anemia, QT prolongation.

V

PRECAUTIONS & CONSIDERATIONS
Monitor for signs and symptoms of thromboembolic disease; monitor glucose, electrolytes, blood cell counts, serum creatinine. ECG is required at baseline and periodically

during treatment. Antiemetics, antidiarrheals, and fluid and electrolyte replacement may be necessary in patients with severe GI side effects. Patients should be instructed to drink at least 2 L of fluid per day to prevent dehydration. Use with caution in patients with renal or hepatic impairment.

Storage

Store at room temperature.

Administration

Take with food. Do not open or crush capsules; avoid contact with powder.

Warfarin Sodium
war'far-in soe'dee-um
(Apo-Warfarin [CAN], Coumadin,
Gen-Warfarin [CAN], Jantoven,
Marevan [AUS], Novo-Warfarin [CAN],
Taro-Warfarin [CAN])
**Do not confuse Coumadin with
Kemadrin.**

CATEGORY AND SCHEDULE
Pregnancy Risk Category: D

Classification: Oral anticoagulant

MECHANISM OF ACTION
A coumarin derivative that interferes
with hepatic synthesis of vitamin
K–dependent clotting factors,
resulting in depletion of coagulation
factors II, VII, IX, and X. *Therapeutic
Effect:* Prevents further extension
of formed existing clot; prevents
new clot formation or secondary
thromboembolic complications.

PHARMACOKINETICS

Route	Onset	Peak	Duration
PO	1.5-3 days	5-7 days	2-5 days

Well absorbed from the GI tract.
Metabolized in the liver. Excreted
primarily in urine. Not removed by
hemodialysis. *Half-life:* 1-2.5 days,
but highly variable among individuals.

AVAILABILITY
Tablets (Coumadin, Jantoven): 1 mg,
2 mg, 2.5 mg, 3 mg, 4 mg, 5 mg,
6 mg, 7.5 mg, 10 mg.
Injection (Coumadin): 5-mg vial.

INDICATIONS AND DOSAGES
▸ **Anticoagulant**
PO
Adults, Elderly. Initially, 5-15 mg/day
for 2-5 days; then adjust based on
International Normalized Ratio
(INR). Maintenance: 2-10 mg/day.
Children. Initially, 0.1-0.2 mg/kg
(maximum 10 mg). Maintenance:
0.05-0.34 mg/kg/day.
▸ **Usual Elderly Dosage
(Maintenance)**
PO, IV
Elderly. 2-5 mg/day.

OFF-LABEL USES
Antiphospholipid antibody
syndrome; impaired left
ventricular function; percutaneous
transluminal coronary angioplasty;
prevention of recurrent cerebral
embolism; MI; prophylaxis of
coronary arteriosclerosis; treatment
adjunct in transient ischemic
attacks.

CONTRAINDICATIONS
Known hypersensitivity to warfarin
or to any other components of
this product. Anticoagulation is
contraindicated in any circumstance
in which the risk of hemorrhage
is greater than the potential
benefit of anticoagulation such as
(1) pregnancy; (2) hemorrhagic
tendencies or blood dyscrasias;
(3) recent or contemplated
surgery of the eye, CNS, or major
trauma; (4) bleeding tendencies
associated with active ulceration
or overt bleeding of the GI, GU,
or respiratory tracts; cerebral
aneurysms, dissecting aorta; or
pericarditis or pericardial effusions,
and bacterial endocarditis;
(5) threatened abortion, eclampsia
and preeclampsia; (6) Inadequate
laboratory facilities to monitor
the patient; (7) unsupervised
patients with senility, alcoholism,
or psychosis or other lack of
patient cooperation; (8) spinal
puncture and other diagnostic
or therapeutic procedures with

potential for uncontrollable bleeding; (9) miscellaneous, including major regional or lumbar block anesthesia, malignant hypertension.

! Alcoholism, elderly, any disease state where an increased risk of bleeding would be detrimental.

Caution

! Known or suspected deficiency in protein C–mediated anticoagulant response.

INTERACTIONS
Drug
Alcohol: Acute alcohol use (binge drinking) may enhance warfarin's anticoagulant effect (increased PT/INR). Chronic alcohol use may decrease warfarin's anticoagulant effect through increased metabolism (decreased PT/INR).
Barbiturates, carbamazepine, cholestyramine, estrogens, griseofulvin, primidone, rifampin, vitamin K: Decreased action.
Acetaminophen, celecoxib, rofecoxib: Possible increase in anticoagulant effects; monitor INR levels.
Acetaminophen, amiodarone, chloral hydrate, cimetidine, ciprofloxacin, clarithromycin, diflunisal, erythromycin, fluconazole, fluoroquinolones, gemfibrozil, HMG CoA reductase inhibitors, indomethacin, itraconazole, ketoconazole, levofloxacin, metronidazole, NSAIDs, oral hypoglycemics, orlistat, phenytoin, propoxyphene, proton pump inhibitors, salicylates, SSRIs, sulfamethoxazole/ trimethoprim, sulfonamides, systemic corticosteroids, tetracyclines, thyroid products, vitamins A and E: Increased action.

NSAIDs: If NSAIDs must be used, monitor patient (avoid aspirin).
Herbal
Herbal products with some anticoagulant activity (cranberry, dong quai, evening primrose oil, feverfew, garlic, ginger, ginkgo, glucosamine, green tea, omega-3-acids, SAM-e): May increase the risk of bleeding.
Herbal products with decreased anticoagulant effect (American ginseng, coenzyme Q_{10}, St. John's wort): May decrease the effectiveness of warfarin.
Many herbal products: *Can interfere with warfarin, so caution should be used.*
Food
Foods with a high vitamin K content: Decreased effect (decreased PT/INR).
Cranberry juice and vitamin E: Increased effect (increased PT/INR).

DIAGNOSTIC TEST EFFECTS
None known.

SIDE EFFECTS
Occasional
GI distress, such as nausea, anorexia, abdominal cramps, diarrhea.
Rare
Hypersensitivity reaction, including dermatitis and urticaria, especially in those sensitive to aspirin.

SERIOUS REACTIONS
• Bleeding complications ranging from local ecchymoses to major hemorrhage may occur. Drug should be discontinued immediately and vitamin K or phytonadione administered. Mild hemorrhage: Vitamin K 1-10 mg PO, SC, or IV. Severe hemorrhage: Vitamin K 1-10 mg IV and repeated q4h as necessary.

W

• Hepatotoxicity, blood dyscrasias, necrosis, vasculitis, and local thrombosis occur rarely.

PRECAUTIONS & CONSIDERATIONS

Caution is warranted in patients at risk for hemorrhage and in those with active tuberculosis, diabetes, gangrene, heparin-induced thrombocytopenia, or necrosis. Warfarin use is contraindicated in pregnancy because it causes fetal and neonatal hemorrhage and intrauterine death. Warfarin crosses the placenta and is distributed in breast milk. Children are more susceptible to the effects of warfarin. In elderly patients, because there is an increased risk of hemorrhage, a lower dose of warfarin is recommended. Other medications, including OTC drugs, should be avoided. An electric razor and soft toothbrush should be used to prevent bleeding during therapy. Avoid alcohol, drastic dietary changes, and salicylates.

Notify the physician before having dental work or surgery. Notify the physician of abdominal or back pain; gingival bleeding; black stool; bleeding; brown, dark, or red urine; coffee ground vomitus; or red-speckled mucus from cough. INR should be determined before administration and daily after therapy begins until INR stabilizes. Once INR is stabilized, INR determinations should be followed every 4 to 6 wks. Pulse, hematocrit, platelet count, AST (SGOT) and ALT (SGPT) levels, and stool and urine cultures for occult blood, regardless of administration route, should be monitored periodically.

Storage

Store at room temperature and protect from light. Do not refrigerate. Use reconstituted solution within 4 h; discard unused portion.

Administration

Remember that warfarin dosage is highly individualized based on PT and INR.

Split scored tablets as needed. Give oral warfarin without regard to food, but if GI upset occurs, give with food. Take warfarin exactly as prescribed at the same time each day. Do not take or discontinue other medications without physician approval. Do not change from one brand of warfarin to another.

For IV use, to reconstitute, add 2.7 mL sterile water for injection to 5-mg vial to produce a solution of 2 mg of warfarin per milliliter. Administer as a slow bolus injection over 1-2 min, but do not administer intramuscularly.

W

Xylometazoline

Xylometazoline
zye-loe-met-az′oh-leen
(4-Way Decongestant Moisturizing
Relief, Otrivin with M-D Pump
[CAN], Otrivin with Moisturizers
Measured-Dose Pump [CAN],
Otrivin Nasal Drops, Otrivin Nasal
Spray, Otrivin Nasal Spray with
Eucalyptol [CAN], Otrivin Nasal
Spray with Moisturizers [CAN],
Otrivin Pediatric Nasal Drops,
Otrivin Pediatric Nasal Spray,
Otrivin with Measured-Dose
Pump [CAN])

CATEGORY AND SCHEDULE
Pregnancy Risk Category: C

Classification: Decongestant,
imidazoline derivative

MECHANISM OF ACTION
A sympathomimetic that directly
acts on α-adrenergic receptors
in arterioles of the nasal mucosa
to produce vasoconstriction
resulting in decreased blood flow.
Therapeutic Effect: Decreased
nasal congestion.

PHARMACOKINETICS
Onset of action occurs within
5-10 min for a duration of action
of 5-6 h. Well absorbed through
the nasal mucosa. May also be
systemically absorbed from both
nasal mucosa and GI tract.
Half-life: Unknown.

AVAILABILITY
Nasal Drops: 0.05% (Otrivin
Pediatric Nasal Drops), 0.1%
(Otrivin Nasal Drops).
Nasal Spray: 0.1% (Otrivin Nasal
Spray).

INDICATIONS AND DOSAGES
▸ **Rhinitis**
INTRANASAL
*Adults, Elderly, Children 12 yr
 and older.* 2-3 drops (0.1%) in each
nostril q8-10h or 1-3 sprays (0.1%)
in each nostril q8-10h. Maximum:
3 doses/day for no longer than 72 hr.
▸ **Relief of nasal pressure and
congestion from a cold**
INTRANASAL
Children aged 2-12 yr. 2 or 3 drops
(0.05%) or 1 spray in each nostril
q8-10h. Maximum: 3 doses/day for
no longer than 72 hr.

CONTRAINDICATIONS
Narrow-angle glaucoma, rhinitis
sicca, children younger than 6 yr;
hypersensitivity to xylometazoline
or other adrenergic agents.

INTERACTIONS
Drug
MAOIs: May increase the risk of
hypertensive crisis.
**Maprotiline, tricyclic
antidepressants:** May increase
effects of xylometazoline.
Herbal
None known.
Food
None known.

DIAGNOSTIC TEST EFFECTS
None known.

SIDE EFFECTS
OCCASIONAL
Nasal: Burning, stinging, drying
nasal mucosa, sneezing, rebound
congestion.

SERIOUS REACTIONS
• Large doses may produce
tachycardia, palpitations, light-
headedness, nausea, vomiting.
• Overdosage in patients older than
60 yr may produce hallucinations,

central nervous system (CNS) depression, and seizures.

Caution is warranted in patients with cardiovascular disease, diabetes mellitus, hypertension, pheochromocytoma, prostatic enlargement, and thyroid disease. It is unknown whether xylometazoline crosses the placenta or is distributed in breast milk. Safety and efficacy of xylometazoline have not been established in children younger than 2 yr. Children younger than 12 yr should not use the 0.1% nasal solution. Age-related prostatic hypertrophy may require dosage adjustment in elderly patients.

Fast, irregular, and pounding heartbeat; headache; insomnia; light-headedness; nausea; nervousness; and trembling can occur if xylometazoline is systemically absorbed. If used too frequently, rebound effects (increased nasal congestion) can occur. Xylometazoline should not be used longer than 72 h. Use of the same product container by more than 1 person may spread infection.

Administration

For adults, instill 2-3 drops or 1-3 sprays in each nostril every 8-10 h. For children, instill 2-3 drops or 1 spray in each nostril q8-10h. Do not exceed 3 doses each day. Do not use for longer than 3 days because of the risk of rebound congestion.

X

Yohimbine
Yohimbine
yoe-him′been
(Aphrodyne, Yocon, Yohimbe)

CATEGORY AND SCHEDULE
Pregnancy Risk Category: NA
Do not use during pregnancy.

Classification: Antiadrenergics, α-blocking, impotence agents

MECHANISM OF ACTION
An herb that produces genital blood vessel dilation, improves nerve impulse transmission to genital area. Increases penile blood flow, central sympathetic excitation impulses to genital tissues. *Therapeutic Effect:* Improves sexual vigor, affects impotence.

PHARMACOKINETICS
Rapidly absorbed. Extensive metabolism in liver and kidneys. Minimal excretion in urine as unchanged drug. *Half-life:* < 30 min.

AVAILABILITY
Tablets: 5.4 mg (Aphrodyne, Yocon).

INDICATIONS AND DOSAGES
NOTE: There are no FDA-approved indications.
▶ Impotence
PO
Adults, Elderly. 5.4 mg 3 times/day.

OFF-LABEL USES
Treatment of SSRI-induced sexual dysfunction, weight loss; sympathicolytic and mydriatic, aphrodisiac.

CONTRAINDICATIONS
Renal disease, hypersensitivity to yohimbine or any component of the formulation.

INTERACTIONS
Drug
Antidiabetics, antihypertensives: May interfere with the effects of these drugs.
Clonidine: May antagonize the effects of clonidine.
MAOIs, linezolid, sympathomimetics, tricyclic antidepressants: Has additive effects with these drugs.
Use with MAOIs is not recommended due to additive effect of yohimbine on MAO.
Herbal
Ephedra: May increase the risk of hypertensive crises.
Ginkgo biloba, St. John's wort: May have additive therapeutic and adverse effects.
Food
Caffeine-containing products (such as coffee, tea, and chocolate), tyramine-containing foods (such as aged cheese and Chianti wine): May increase the risk of hypertensive crises.

DIAGNOSTIC TEST EFFECTS
None known.

SIDE EFFECTS
Excitement, tremors, insomnia, anxiety, hypertension, tachycardia, dizziness, headache, irritability, salivation, dilated pupils, nausea, vomiting, hypersensitivity reaction.

SERIOUS REACTIONS
• Paralysis, severe hypotension, irregular heartbeats, and cardiac failure may occur.
• Overdose can be fatal.

PRECAUTIONS & CONSIDERATIONS
Caution is warranted in patients with anxiety, diabetes mellitus, hypertension, posttraumatic stress disorder, and schizophrenia.

Yohimbine is generally not used in females. Its use is contraindicated in breastfeeding and pregnant women. Safety and efficacy of yohimbine have not been established in children. Age-related liver and renal impairment may require discontinuation of yohimbine in elderly patients.

Over-the-counter drugs should be avoided without first consulting with the physician.

Administration

Reduce dose if side effects occur. May reduce to ½ tablet 3 times a day followed by gradual increases to 1 tablet 3 times a day.

Zafirlukast
za-feer'loo-kast
(Accolate)
**Do not confuse Accolate with
Accupril or Aclovate.**

CATEGORY AND SCHEDULE
Pregnancy Risk Category: B

Classification: Selective
leukotriene receptor antagonist

MECHANISM OF ACTION
Antiasthmatic that binds to
leukotriene receptors, inhibiting
bronchoconstriction caused by
sulfur dioxide, cold air, and
specific antigens, such as grass, cat
dander, and ragweed. *Therapeutic
Effect:* Reduces airway edema and
smooth muscle constriction; alters
cellular activity associated with the
inflammatory process.

PHARMACOKINETICS
Rapidly absorbed after PO
administration (food reduces
absorption). Protein binding:
99%. Extensively metabolized
in the liver. Primarily excreted in
feces. Unknown if removed by
hemodialysis. *Half-life:* 10 h.

AVAILABILITY
Tablets: 10 mg, 20 mg.

INDICATIONS AND DOSAGES
▸ **Bronchial asthma**
PO
*Adults, Elderly, Children 12 yr and
older.* 20 mg twice a day.
Children aged 5-11 yr. 10 mg twice
a day.

INTERACTIONS
Drug
Aspirin: Increased plasma levels.
**Erythromycin, terfenadine,
theophylline:** Reduced plasma
levels.
**Drugs metabolized by CYP2C9
and CYP3A4 isoenzymes
(carbamazepine, erythromycin,
fluoxetine, glimepiride, glipizide,
nateglinide, phenobarbital,
rifampin, rifapentine, phenytoin):**
Inhibits CYP2C9 and CYP3A4
isoenzymes.
Warfarin: Increased PT with
concurrent use of warfarin.
Herbal
None known.
Food
None known.

DIAGNOSTIC TEST EFFECTS
May increase ALT (SGPT) level.

SIDE EFFECTS
Frequent
Headache.
Occasional
Nausea, diarrhea, dizziness, fever,
infection, myalgia, pain, vomiting,
weakness, increased ALT.
Rare
Agranulocytosis, bleeding,
eosinophilia, hepatic failure,
hepatitis, vasculitis with clinical
features of Churg-Strauss syndrome.

SERIOUS REACTIONS
• Concurrent administration of
inhaled corticosteroids increases
the risk of upper respiratory tract
infections.

PRECAUTIONS & CONSIDERATIONS
Caution is warranted in patients
with impaired hepatic function,
whether from prior use of
zafirlukast or not. Caution is also
warranted if hypersensitivity has
been experienced with zafirlukast.
Zafirlukast is pregnancy category B
and is distributed in breast milk. It is

not recommended for breastfeeding women. The safety and efficacy of this drug have not been established in children younger than 5 yr. Although no specific age-related precautions have been noted in elderly patients, they may be more at risk for infection. Be aware that zafirlukast is not intended to treat acute asthma episodes. Drink plenty of fluids to decrease the thickness of lung secretions.

Liver function, pulse rate and quality, as well as respiratory depth, rate, rhythm, and type should be monitored. Fingernails and lips should be assessed for cyanosis, manifested as a blue or dusky color in light-skinned patients and a gray color in dark-skinned patients. Notify the physician of any abdominal pain, nausea, flulike symptoms, jaundice, or worsening of asthma.

Administration

Take zafirlukast 1 h before or 2 h after meals. Do not crush or break tablets. Take zafirlukast as prescribed, even during symptom-free periods. Do not alter the dosage or abruptly discontinue other asthma medications.

Zaleplon
zal´eh-plon
(Sonata, Stamoc [CAN])

CATEGORY AND SCHEDULE
Pregnancy Risk Category: C
Controlled Substance Schedule IV

Classification: Hypnotic, nonbenzodiazepine

MECHANISM OF ACTION
A nonbenzodiazepine that enhances the action of the inhibitory neurotransmitter γ-aminobutyric acid. *Therapeutic Effect:* Induces sleep.

AVAILABILITY
Capsules: 5 mg, 10 mg.

PHARMACOKINETICS
PO: Rapid absorption, but heavy, high-fat meals delay absorption; peak plasma levels in 1 h; wide tissue distribution; rapid hepatic metabolism (CYP3A4 minor pathway); excretion in urine.

INDICATIONS AND DOSAGES
▸ **Insomnia**
PO
Adults. 10 mg at bedtime. Range: 5-20 mg. Has been studied up to 5 wks in trials.
Elderly. 5 mg at bedtime with a recommended maximum of 10 mg.

INTERACTIONS
Drug
All CNS-depressant drugs (anticonvulsants, antipsychotics, barbiturates, benzodiazepines, opioid agonists) and alcohol: Central nervous system (CNS) depression.
Cimetidine: Increased concentration of zaleplon.
Flumazenil and rifamycin derivatives: Decreased effects of zaleplon.
Herbal
None known.
Food
Heavy, high-fat meals: Onset of sleep may be delayed by approximately 2 h.

SIDE EFFECTS
Expected
Somnolence, sedation, mild rebound insomnia (on first night after drug is discontinued).

Z

Frequent
Nausea, headache, myalgia, dizziness, weakness.
Occasional
Amnesia, abdominal pain, asthenia, dysmenorrhea, dyspepsia, eye pain, paresthesia, somnolence.
Rare
Anaphylaxis, angioedema, bundle-branch block, cerebral ischemia, intestinal obstruction, tremors, amnesia, hyperacusis (acute sense of hearing), fever, glaucoma, abnormal liver function tests, pericardial effusion, pulmonary embolus, ventricular tachycardia, ventricular extrasystoles.

SERIOUS REACTIONS
• Zaleplon may produce altered concentration, behavior changes, and impaired memory.
• Taking the drug while up and about may result in adverse CNS effects, such as hallucinations, impaired coordination, dizziness, and light-headedness.
• Overdosage results in somnolence, confusion, diminished reflexes, and coma.

PRECAUTIONS & CONSIDERATIONS
Use is contraindicated in patients with hypersensitivity to zaleplon. Caution is warranted in patients with mild to moderate hepatic impairment, signs or symptoms of depression, and a hypersensitivity to aspirin (it may cause an allergic-type reaction). Use is not recommended in pregnancy or breastfeeding because it enters the breast milk. Drowsiness may occur. Avoid alcohol, CNS depressants, and tasks that require mental alertness or motor skills. Zaleplon should be administered with caution in elderly or smaller patients or those with compromised respiratory,

hepatic, or renal function. Safety and efficacy in children have not been established. Disturbed sleep may occur for 1 or 2 nights after discontinuing the drug.
Administration
Avoid taking this drug with or immediately after a high-fat meal to avoid delayed absorption. Can be taken at bedtime or if the patient is in bed and cannot fall asleep.

Zanamivir
za-na´mi-veer
(Relenza)

CATEGORY AND SCHEDULE
Pregnancy Risk Category: B

Classification: Antiviral, neuraminidase inhibitor

MECHANISM OF ACTION
An antiviral that appears to inhibit the influenza virus enzyme neuraminidase, which is essential for viral replication. *Therapeutic Effect:* Prevents viral release from infected cells.

AVAILABILITY
Powder for Inhalation: 5 mg/blister.

PHARMACOKINETICS
Inhalation: 4%-17% of inhaled dose is absorbed, peak serum levels 1-2 h, low plasma protein binding (< 10%), excreted unchanged in urine.

INDICATIONS AND DOSAGES
▸ **Influenza virus**
INHALATION
Adults, Elderly, Children aged 7 yr and older. 2 inhalations (one 5-mg blister per inhalation for a total dose of 10 mg) twice a day (about 12 h apart) for 5 days.

▸ **Prevention of influenza virus**
INHALATION
*Adults, Elderly, Children aged 5 yr
and older.* 2 inhalations once a day
for 28 days.

INTERACTIONS
Drug
Decreased effect of zanamivir: Use
of zanamivir is not recommended
48 h before and up to 2 wks after the
administration of the live, attenuated
influenza vaccine (FluMist).
Herbal
None known.
Food
None known.

DIAGNOSTIC TEST EFFECTS
May increase serum creatine kinase
level and liver function test results.

SIDE EFFECTS
Frequent
More with prophylaxis: Headache,
throat or tonsil discomfort and pain,
nasal signs and symptoms, cough,
viral infections.
Occasional
Diarrhea, sinusitis, nausea, bronchitis,
cough, dizziness, headache, vomiting,
infection, sinusitis.
More with prophylaxis: Fever or
chills, cough, fatigue, malaise,
anorexia or an increased or
decreased appetite, muscle pain,
musculoskeletal pain.
**RARE AND SERIOUS
REACTIONS**
Allergic or allergic-like reaction,
arrhythmia, bronchospasm if a
history of chronic obstructive
pulmonary disease (COPD) or
asthma, central nervous system
(CNS) effects (confusion, delusions,
altered consciousness, delirium,
delusions, hallucinations),
hemorrhage, serious cutaneous rash,
seizure.

PRECAUTIONS & CONSIDERATIONS
Use with caution in patients with a
history of hypersensitivity. Caution
should be used in patients with
asthma or COPD; these patients
should still be given the influenza
vaccine. Be aware that persons
requiring an inhaled bronchodilator
at the same time as zanamivir
should receive the bronchodilator
before zanamivir. Dizziness may
occur. Avoid contact with those
who are at high risk for influenza.
Use in pregnancy has not been well
established. Use with caution in
breastfeeding patients. Safety has
not been established for prophylaxis
in children younger than 5 yr and in
treatment of patients younger than
7 yr. One concern about children is
their ability to use the Diskhaler.
Administration
Using the Diskhaler device provided,
exhale completely; then put the white
mouthpiece to the lips and breathe in
the dose deeply and slowly. Remove
mouthpiece from mouth, hold
breathe for at least 10 seconds, and
exhale slowly. Continue treatment
for the full 5-day course, and evenly
space doses around the clock (~12 h
apart). For prophylactic therapy,
patients should use therapy once
daily for 28 days. Patients should
be made aware that they should
immediately report any signs or
symptoms of bronchospasm or
respiratory depression.

Z

Ziconotide
zi-koe´no-tide
(Prialt)

CATEGORY AND SCHEDULE
Pregnancy Risk Category: C

Classification: Analgesic, nonopioid, calcium channel blocker

MECHANISM OF ACTION
A synthetic peptide that selectively binds to N-type voltage-sensitive calcium channels located on afferent nerves in the spinal cord. This binding is thought to block N-type calcium channels. *Therapeutic Effect:* Blocks excitatory neurotransmitter release, reducing sensitivity to painful stimuli.

AVAILABILITY
Injection Solution: 25 mcg/mL (20 mL), 100 mcg/mL (1-mL, 2-mL, 5-mL) vials.

PHARMACOKINETICS
Elimination half-life: 4.6 h after intrathecal administration. 50% bound to plasma proteins; metabolized in multiple organs. Excreted in urine as proteolytic degradation products.

INDICATIONS AND DOSAGES
▸ **Pain control**
INTRATHECAL
Adults, Elderly. Initially, 2.4 mcg/day (0.1 mcg/h). May titrate to maximum of 19.2 mcg/day (0.8 mcg/h).

INTERACTIONS
Drug
All CNS depressants: Enhanced central nervous system (CNS) depression.

Alcohol: May increase CNS effects.
Herbal
None known.
Food
None known.

DIAGNOSTIC TEST EFFECTS
May increase CPK levels; monitor every other week for the first month, then monthly.

SIDE EFFECTS
Frequent
Dizziness, nausea, somnolence, weakness, diarrhea, confusion, ataxia, headache, vomiting, gait disturbance, memory impairment, hypertonia, aphasia, hallucination, increased creatine kinase levels, blurred vision.
Occasional
Abnormal thinking, amnesia, anorexia, dysarthia, visual disturbances, anxiety, urinary retention, speech disorder, aphasia, nystagmus, paresthesia, rigors, tremor, muscle spasm, limb pain, fever, nervousness, vertigo, taste perversion, sinusitis, diaphoresis, myoclonus, and psychosis occur rarely.
Rare
Acute renal failure, atrial fibrillation, cerebrovascular accident, meningitis, respiratory distress, seizure, sepsis, suicide attempt or ideation.

PRECAUTIONS & CONSIDERATIONS
Ziconotide should be used with caution in patients with a history of psychosis, presence of infection at the injection site, uncontrolled bleeding, IV administration, or spinal canal obstruction that impairs cerebrospinal fluid (CSF) circulation. The same dose used in other adults can be used in elderly patients but should be used cautiously because these patients are at increased risk of developing confusion.

Z

Administration
For intrathecal use, administer ziconotide only with a Medtronic SynchroMed EL or SynchroMed II Infusion System or the Simms Deltec CADD Micro External Microinfusion Device and Catheter. Refer to the manufacturer's manuals for instructions for initial filling and refilling of the reservoir.

Zidovudine
zyde-oh´vue-deen
(Apo-Zidovudine [CAN], AZT, Novo-AZT [CAN], Retrovir)
Do not confuse Retrovir with ritonavir.

CATEGORY AND SCHEDULE
Pregnancy Risk Category: C

Classification: Antiviral thymidine analogue

MECHANISM OF ACTION
A nucleoside reverse transcriptase inhibitor that interferes with viral RNA-dependent DNA polymerase, an enzyme necessary for viral HIV replication. *Therapeutic Effect:* Interferes with HIV replication, slowing the progression of HIV infection.

PHARMACOKINETICS
Rapidly and completely absorbed from the GI tract. Protein binding: 25%-38%. Undergoes first-pass metabolism in the liver. Crosses the blood-brain barrier and is widely distributed, including to cerebrospinal fluid. Excreted primarily in urine. Minimal removal by hemodialysis. *Half-life:* 0.8-1.2 h (increased in impaired renal function).

AVAILABILITY
Injection: 10 mg/mL.
Capsule: 100 mg.
Tablet: 300 mg.
Oral Solution: 50 mg/5 mL.

INDICATIONS AND DOSAGES
▶ **HIV infection**
PO
Adults, Elderly, Children older than 12 yr. 200 mg q8h or 300 mg q12h.
Children 12 yr and younger. 160 mg/m^2/dose q8h. Range: 90-180 mg/m^2/dose q6-8h.
Neonates. 2 mg/kg/dose q6h.
IV
Adults, Elderly, Children older than 12 yr. 1-2 mg/kg/dose q4h.
Children 12 yr and younger. 120 mg/m^2/dose q6h.
Neonates. 1.5 mg/kg/dose q6h.
▶ **Renal failure**
Dosage adjustments recommended for all patients maintained on hemodialysis or peritoneal dialysis, or those with CrCl < 15 mL/min (see manufacturer's literature).

INTERACTIONS
Drug
Acetaminophen, clarithromycin: Decreased blood levels.
Fluconazole: Increased serum levels.

🍷 IV INCOMPATIBILITIES
Lansoprazole.

SIDE EFFECTS
Expected
Nausea, headache.
Frequent
Abdominal pain, asthenia, rash, fever, acne.
Occasional
Diarrhea, anorexia, malaise, myalgia, somnolence.

Z

Rare
Dizziness, paresthesia, vomiting, insomnia, dyspnea, altered taste.

SERIOUS REACTIONS

• Serious reactions include anemia, which occurs most commonly after 4-6 wks of therapy, and granulocytopenia; both effects are more likely to occur in patients who have a low hemoglobin level or granulocyte count before beginning therapy.
• Neurotoxicity (as evidenced by ataxia, fatigue, lethargy, nystagmus, and seizures) may occur.

PRECAUTIONS & CONSIDERATIONS

Life-threatening allergic reactions to zidovudine or its components.
Caution
Granulocyte count < 1000/mm³ or hemoglobin < 9.5 g/dL, lactation, children, severe renal disease, severe hepatic dysfunction, risk of severe neutropenia and anemia.

Zileuton
zye-lew´ton
(Zyflo)
Do not confuse Zyflo with Zyban.

CATEGORY AND SCHEDULE
Pregnancy Risk Category: C

Classification: Leukotriene pathway inhibitor

MECHANISM OF ACTION

A leukotriene inhibitor that inhibits the enzyme responsible for producing inflammatory response. Prevents formation of leukotrienes (leukotrienes induce bronchoconstriction response, enhance vascular permeability, stimulate mucus secretion).
Therapeutic Effect: Prevents airway edema, smooth-muscle contraction, and the inflammatory process, relieving signs and symptoms of bronchial asthma.

PHARMACOKINETICS

Rapidly absorbed from GI tract. Protein binding: 93%. Metabolized in liver. Excreted primarily in urine. Unknown whether removed by hemodialysis. *Half-life:* 2.1-2.5 h.

INDICATIONS AND DOSAGES
▸ **Bronchial asthma**
PO (IMMEDIATE RELEASE)
Adults, Elderly, Children 12 yr and older. 1200 mg twice daily.

CONTRAINDICATIONS

Active liver disease or with transaminase elevations ≥ 3 times ULN, not effective for status asthmaticus, known hypersensitivity to zileuton.

INTERACTIONS
Drug
Dental drugs that are strong inhibitors of CYP1A2 isoenzymes: Use caution when prescribing dental drugs that are strong inhibitors of CYP1A2 isoenzymes.
Theophylline, propranolol: Increased plasma levels of these drugs. Reduce theophylline or aminophylline by 50% when zileuton is started.
Warfarin: Significant increase in PT when taking warfarin.

SIDE EFFECTS
Frequent
Headache.
Occasional
Dyspepsia, nausea, abdominal pain, asthenia (loss of strength), myalgia.

Rare
Conjunctivitis, constipation, dizziness, flatulence, insomnia.

SERIOUS REACTIONS
• Liver dysfunction occurs rarely and may be manifested as right upper-quadrant pain, nausea, fatigue, lethargy, pruritus, jaundice, or flulike symptoms.

PRECAUTIONS & CONSIDERATIONS
Active liver disease, impaired liver function, hypersensitivity to zileuton or any component of the formulation.
Caution
Not for acute bronchospasm; status asthmaticus; theophylline, warfarin, propranolol; hepatic impairment; lactation; children younger than 12 yr; monitor ALT (SGPT) levels.

Zinc Oxide/Zinc Sulfate
zinkox´eyed/zink sul´fate
(zinc oxide: Balmex, Desitin; zinc sulfate: Orazinc, Zincaps [AUS])

CATEGORY AND SCHEDULE
Pregnancy Risk Category: C

Classification: Mineral

MECHANISM OF ACTION
A mineral that acts as a cofactor for enzymes that are important for protein and carbohydrate metabolism. *Therapeutic Effect:* Zinc oxide acts as a mild astringent and skin protectant. Zinc sulfate helps maintain normal growth and tissue repair, as well as skin hydration.

INDICATIONS AND DOSAGES
▶ **Mild skin irritations and abrasions (such as chapped skin, diaper rash)**
TOPICAL (ZINC OXIDE)
Adults, Elderly, Children. Apply as needed.
▶ **Treatment and prevention of zinc deficiency, wound healing**
PO (ZINC SULFATE)
Adults, Elderly. 220 mg 3 times a day.

INTERACTIONS
Drug
Decreased absorption: Tetracyclines, fluoroquinolones.

SIDE EFFECTS
None known.

SERIOUS REACTIONS
• None known.

Ziprasidone
zye-pray´za-done
(Geodon)

CATEGORY AND SCHEDULE
Pregnancy Risk Category: C

Classification: Antipsychotic, atypical

MECHANISM OF ACTION
A piperazine derivative that antagonizes α-adrenergic, dopamine, histamine, and serotonin receptors; also inhibits reuptake of serotonin and norepinephrine. *Therapeutic Effect:* Diminishes symptoms of schizophrenia and depression.

PHARMACOKINETICS
Well absorbed after PO administration. Food increases bioavailability. Protein binding: 99%.

Z

Extensively metabolized in the liver. Not removed by hemodialysis.
Half-life: 7 h.

INDICATIONS AND DOSAGES
▶ **Schizophrenia**
PO
Adults, Elderly. Initially, 20 mg twice a day with food. Titrate at intervals of no < 2 days. Maximum: 80 mg twice a day.
IM
Adults, Elderly. 10 mg q2h or 20 mg q4h. Maximum: 40 mg/day.
▶ **Bipolar mania**
PO
Adults, Elderly. 40 mg 2 times a day.

CONTRAINDICATIONS
Known hypersensitivity to ziprasidone, cardiac conduction defects, or a known history of QT prolongation (e.g., AV block, congenital long QT syndrome); uncompensated heart failure or recent acute myocardial infarction, significant untreated electrolyte imbalance, do not give IM injection intravenously.

INTERACTIONS
Drug
Carbamazepine: Reduced plasma levels.
Central nervous system (CNS) depressants: Increased risk of CNS depressant effects; use caution.
Drugs that lower blood pressure: Increased risk of hypotension.
Drugs that prolong the QT interval: Avoid use of these drugs.
Ketoconazole and other strong inhibitors of CYP3A4 isoenzymes: Increased plasma levels.
Phenothiazines and related drugs (haloperidol, droperidol), metoclopramide: Increased extrapyramidal effects.

SIDE EFFECTS
Frequent
Headache, somnolence, dizziness.
Occasional
Rash, orthostatic hypotension, weight gain, restlessness, constipation, dyspepsia, hyperglycemia, onset of diabetes mellitus.

SERIOUS REACTIONS
• Prolongation of QT interval may produce torsade de pointes, a form of ventricular tachycardia. Patients with bradycardia, hypokalemia, or hypomagnesemia are at increased risk.

PRECAUTIONS & CONSIDERATIONS
Conditions that prolong the QT interval, such as congenital long QT syndrome.
Caution
May antagonize levodopa, dopamine agonists. QT prolongation and risk of sudden death; bradycardia; hypokalemia; hypomagnesemia; electrolyte depletion caused by diarrhea, diuretics, or vomiting; neuromalignant syndrome; tardive dyskinesia; seizures; suicide; lactation; pediatric use, dementia-related psychosis in the elderly.

Zoledronic Acid
zole-eh-drone´ick ass´id
(Zometa)

CATEGORY AND SCHEDULE
Pregnancy Risk Category: C

Classification: Osteoporosis therapy adjunct, bisphosphonate

MECHANISM OF ACTION
A bisphosphonate that inhibits the resorption of mineralized bone and cartilage; inhibits

increased osteoclastic activity and skeletal calcium release induced by stimulatory factors produced by tumors. *Therapeutic Effect:* Increases urinary calcium and phosphorus excretion; decreases serum calcium and phosphorus levels.

PHARMACOKINETICS
IV INFUSION
Shows triphasic half-life; plasma protein binding 22%; little to no metabolism; excreted mainly in urine; a high percentage of the dose remains bound to bone.

AVAILABILITY
Zometa Injection: 4 mg/5 mL for further dilution.
Reclast Infusion: 5 mg/100 mL solution for infusion.

INDICATIONS AND DOSAGES
▸ **Hypercalcemia**
IV INFUSION (ZOMETA)
Adults, Elderly. 4 mg IV infusion given over not < 15 min.
Retreatment may be considered, but at least 7 days should elapse to allow for full response to initial dose.
▸ **Multiple myeloma**
IV INFUSION (ZOMETA)
Adults, Elderly. 4 mg IV infusion over a minimum of 15 min.
▸ **Dose adjustment for Zometa for renal impairment**
CrCl 50-60 ml/min: Reduce dose to 3.5 mg.
CrCl 40-49 ml/min: Reduce dose to 3.3 mg.
CrCl 30-39 ml/min: Reduce dose to 3 mg.
CrCl < 30 ml/min: Do not use.
▸ **Osteoporosis, Paget's Disease**
IV INFUSION (RECLAST)
Adults. 5 mg IV once yearly.
▸ **Dose adjustment for once-yearly Reclast for renal impairment**

CrCl 35 ml/min or over: No dosage adjustment needed.
CrCl < 35 ml/min: Not recommended due to lack of clinical data. Zoledronic acid is usually contraindicated when SCr > 4.5 mg/dL.

CONTRAINDICATIONS
Hypersensitivity to the drug or other bisphosphonates, hypocalemia, pregnancy, severe renal impairmet.

INTERACTIONS
Drug
None reported.

SIDE EFFECTS
Frequent
Fever, nausea, vomiting, constipation.
Occasional
Hypotension, anxiety, insomnia, flu-like symptoms (fever, chills, bone pain, myalgia, and arthralgia).
Rare
Conjunctivitis.

SERIOUS REACTIONS
• Renal toxicity may occur if IV infusion is administered in < 15 min.

PRECAUTIONS & CONSIDERATIONS
Hypersensitivity to other bisphosphonates, including alendronate, etidronate, pamidronate, risedronate, and tiludronate. Dental implants are contraindicated for patients taking this drug.
Caution
Data for use in children are not available; monitor hypercalcemic parameters, ensure good hydration; renal impairment; bronchospasm in aspirin-sensitive asthmatic patients; hypocalcemia; hypoparathyroidism; lactation.

Z

Zolmitriptan
zohl-mih-trip´tan
(Zomig, Zomig Rapimelt [CAN], Zomig-ZMT)

CATEGORY AND SCHEDULE
Pregnancy Risk Category: C

Classification: Serotonin agonist

MECHANISM OF ACTION
A serotonin receptor agonist that binds selectively to vascular receptors, producing a vasoconstrictive effect on cranial blood vessels. *Therapeutic Effect:* Relieves migraine headache.

PHARMACOKINETICS
Rapidly but incompletely absorbed after PO administration. Protein binding: 15%. Undergoes first-pass metabolism in the liver to active metabolite. Eliminated primarily in urine (60%) and, to a lesser extent, in feces (30%). *Half-life:* 3 h.

CONTRAINDICATIONS
! Known ischemic heart disease (angina, coronary vasospasm, MI) or other significant CV disease (e.g., uncontrolled HTN). Do not use within 24 hr of use of other 5-HT1 agonists or an ergot-type drug. Not for use in hemiplegic or basilar migraine. Use within 2 wk of MAOI therapy. Hypersensitivity to zolmitriptan.

INDICATIONS AND DOSAGES
▸ **Acute migraine attack**
PO
Adults, Elderly, Children older than 18 yr. Initially, 2.5 mg or less. If headache returns, may repeat dose in 2 h. Maximum: 10 mg/24 h.
INTRANASAL
Adults, Elderly. 5 mg. May repeat in 2 h. Maximum: 10 mg/24 h.

INTERACTIONS
Drug
Selective serotonin reuptake inhibitors, ergot-containing drugs (avoid use within 24 h of taking this drug): Potential serotonin crises.
Cimetidine: Decreased plasma levels.

SIDE EFFECTS
Frequent
Oral: Dizziness; tingling; neck, throat, or jaw pressure; somnolence.
Nasal: Altered taste, paraesthesia.
Occasional
Oral: Warm or hot sensation, asthenia, chest pressure.
Nasal: Nausea, somnolence, nasal discomfort, dizziness, asthenia, dry mouth.
Rare
Diaphoresis, myalgia, paresthesia.

SERIOUS REACTIONS
Cardiac reactions (including ischemia, coronary artery vasospasm, and myocardial infarction [MI]) and noncardiac vasospasm-related reactions (such as hemorrhage and cerebrovascular accident) occur rarely, particularly in patients with hypertension, diabetes, or a strong family history of coronary artery disease; obese patients; smokers; men older than 40 yr; and postmenopausal women.

PRECAUTIONS & CONSIDERATIONS
Arrhythmias associated with conduction disorders, basilar or hemiplegic migraine, coronary artery disease, ischemic heart disease (including angina pectoris, history of MI, silent ischemia, and Prinzmetal's angina), uncontrolled hypertension, use within 24 h of ergotamine-containing preparations or another serotonin receptor

agonist, use within 14 days of MAOIs, Wolff-Parkinson-White syndrome.

Caution
Renal or hepatic impairment may cause coronary vasospasm; caution should be used in lactating patients, elderly patients, and children.

Zolpidem Tartrate
zole-pi′dem tar′trate
(Ambien, Stilnox [AUS])
Do not confuse Ambien with Amen.

CATEGORY AND SCHEDULE
Pregnancy Risk Category: B
Controlled Substance:
Schedule IV

Classification: Nonbarbiturate, nonbenzodiazepine sedative-hypnotic

MECHANISM OF ACTION
A nonbenzodiazepine that enhances the action of the inhibitory neurotransmitter γ-aminobutyric acid. *Therapeutic Effect:* Induces sleep and improves sleep quality.

PHARMACOKINETICS

Route	Onset	Peak	Duration
PO	30 min	NA	6-8 h

Rapidly absorbed from the GI tract. Protein binding: 92%. Metabolized in the liver; excreted in urine. Not removed by hemodialysis.
Half-life: 1.4-4.5 h (increased in hepatic impairment).

AVAILABILITY
Tablets: 5 mg, 10 mg.

Controlled-Release Tablets: 6.25 mg, 12.5 mg (Ambien CR).

INDICATIONS AND DOSAGES
▸ **Insomnia**
PO
Adults. 10 mg at bedtime.
Elderly, Debilitated. 5 mg at bedtime.

INTERACTIONS
Drug
Alcohol, all CNS depressants, fluconazole, ketoconazole, itraconazole: Increased central nervous system (CNS) depression.

SIDE EFFECTS
Occasional
Headache.
Rare
Dizziness, nausea, diarrhea, muscle pain.

Serious Reactions
• Overdosage may produce severe ataxia, bradycardia, altered vision (such as diplopia), severe drowsiness, nausea and vomiting, difficulty breathing, and unconsciousness.
• Abrupt withdrawal of the drug after long-term use may produce asthenia, facial flushing, diaphoresis, vomiting, and tremor.
• Drug tolerance or dependence may occur with prolonged, high-dose therapy.

PRECAUTIONS & CONSIDERATIONS
Hypersensitivity.
Caution
May cause abnormal thinking and complex behavior; use with caution in elderly, depression, hepatic disease, COPD, and sleep apnea.

Z

Zonisamide
zoh-nis´ah-mide
(Zonegran)

CATEGORY AND SCHEDULE
Pregnancy Risk Category: C

Classification: Anticonvulsant
(sulfonamide derivative)

MECHANISM OF ACTION
A succinimide that may stabilize
neuronal membranes and suppress
neuronal hypersynchronization
by blocking sodium and calcium
channels. *Therapeutic Effect:*
Reduces seizure activity.

PHARMACOKINETICS
Well absorbed after PO
administration. Extensively bound
to RBCs. Protein binding: 40%.
Primarily excreted in urine. *Half-life:*
63 h (plasma), 105 h (RBCs).

INDICATIONS AND DOSAGES
▸ **Partial seizures**
PO
*Adults, Elderly, Children older
than 16 yr.* Initially, 100 mg/day for
2 wks. May increase by 100 mg/day
at intervals of 2 wks or longer.
Range: 100-600 mg/day.

INTERACTIONS
Drug
It has been proposed that drugs that
either induce or inhibit CYP3A4
enzymes might alter zonisamide
serum levels.
Carbamazepine: Increases renal
clearance.

SIDE EFFECTS
Frequent
Somnolence, dizziness, anorexia,
headache, agitation, irritability,
nausea.
Occasional
Fatigue, ataxia, confusion,
depression, impaired memory or
concentration, insomnia, abdominal
pain, diplopia, diarrhea, speech
difficulty.
Rare
Paresthesia, nystagmus, anxiety, rash,
dyspepsia, weight loss.

SERIOUS REACTIONS
• Overdose is characterized by
bradycardia, hypotension, respiratory
depression, and coma.
• Leukopenia, anemia, and
thrombocytopenia occur rarely.

PRECAUTIONS & CONSIDERATIONS
Allergy to sulfonamides.
    Discontinue if skin rash
occurs; pediatric patients at risk
for oligohidrosis, hyperthermia;
seizures with abrupt withdrawal;
use contraception in women of
childbearing age; hepatic or renal
dysfunction; lactation; kidney stones.
Administration
May be taken without regard to
food.
    Swallow capsules whole.

Z

APPENDIX A

General Anesthetics

Uses

MECHANISMS OF ACTION

IV anesthetic agents are used to induce general anesthesia. The general anesthetic state consists of unconsciousness, amnesia, analgesia, immobility, and attenuation of autonomic responses to noxious stimuli.

IV anesthetic agents act on the γ-aminobutyric acid (GABA) receptor complex to produce central nervous system (CNS) depression. GABA is the primary inhibitory neurotransmitter in the CNS. Ketamine produces dissociation between the thalamus and the limbic system.

Volatile inhalation agents produce all the components of the anesthetic state but are administered through the lungs via an anesthesia machine. Agents for use include desflurane, enflurane, halothane, isoflurane, and sevoflurane. They are used in practice to maintain general anesthesia.

The specific actions of volatile inhalation agents are not all fully understood but may disrupt neuronal transmission throughout the CNS. These agents may either block excitatory transmission or enhance inhibitory transmission through axons or synapses.

General Anesthetics

Name	Availability	Uses	Dosage Range	Side Effects
Etomidate (Amidate)	I: 2 mg/mL	IV induction	0.2-0.6 mg/kg	Myoclonus, pain on injection, nausea, vomiting, respiratory depression
Ketamine (Ketalar)	I: 10 mg/mL, 50 mg/mL, 100 mg/mL	Analgesia, sedation, IV induction	1-4.5 mg/kg	Delirium, euphoria, nausea, vomiting
Methohexital (Brevital)	Powder for injection: 500 mg	IV induction, sedation	50-120 mg	Cardiovascular depression, myoclonus, nausea, vomiting, respiratory depression
Midazolam (Versed)	I: 1 mg/mL, 5 mg/mL	Anxiolytic, amnesic, sedation	1-5 mg titrated slowly	Respiratory depression
Propofol (Diprivan)	I: 10 mg/mL	Sedation IV induction maintenance	0.5 mg/kg, 2-2.5 mg/kg, 100-200 mcg/kg/min	Cardiovascular depression, delirium, euphoria, pain on injection, respiratory depression
Thiopental (Pentothal)	Powder for injection: 2.5% (25 mg/mL)	IV induction	Titrate vs. pt response. Average: 50-75 mg	Cardiovascular depression, nausea, vomiting, respiratory depression

I, Injection; *pt,* patient.
From *Mosby's 2006 drug consult for nurses,* St. Louis, 2006, Mosby.

APPENDIX B
English-to-Spanish Drug Phrases Translator

English
Spanish
Pronunciation

TAKING THE MEDICATION HISTORY

Are you allergic to any medications? (If yes:)
¿Es alérgico a algún medicamento? (sì:)
(Ehs ah-lehr-hee-koh ah ahl-goon meh-dee-kah-mehn-toh) (see:)

Which medications are you allergic to?
¿A cuál medicamento es alérgico?
(ah koo-ahl meh-dee-kah-mehn-toh ehs ah-lehr-hee-koh)

What happens when you develop an allergic reaction?
¿Qué le pasa cuando desarrolla una reacción alérgica?
(Keh leh pah-sah koo-ahn-doh deh-sah-roh-yah oo-nah reh-ahk-see-ohn
    ah-lehr-hee-kah)

What did you do to relieve or stop the allergic reaction?
¿Qué hizo para aliviar o detener la reacción alérgica?
(Keh ee-soh pah-rah ah-lee-bee-ahr oh deh-teh-nehr lah reh-ahk-see-ohn
    ah-lehr-hee-kah)

Do you take any over-the-counter, prescription, or herbal medications? (If yes:)
¿Toma medicamentos sin receta, con receta, o naturistas (hierbas
    medicinales)? (sì:)
(Toh-mah meh-dee-kah-mehn-tohs seen reh-seh-tah, kohn reh-seh-tah,
    oh nah-too-rees-tahs [ee-ehr-bahs meh-dee-see-nah-lehs]) (see:)

Why do you take each medication?
¿Porqué toma cada medicamento?
(Pohr-keh toh-mah kah-dah meh-dee-kah-mehn-toh)

What is the dosage for each medication?
¿Cuál es la dosis de cada medicamento?
(Koo-ahl ehs lah doh-sees deh kah-dah meh-dee-kah-mehn-toh)

How often do you take each medication?
¿Con qué frequencia toma cada medicamento?
(Kohn keh freh-koo-ehn-see-ah toh-mah kah-dah meh-dee-kah-mehn-toh)

Once a day?
¿Una vez por dìa; diariamente?
(Oo-nah behs pohr dee-ah; dee-ah-ree-ah-mehn-teh)

Twice a day?
¿Dos veces por dìa?
(dohs beh-sehs pohr dee-ah)

Three times a day?
¿Tres veces por dìa?
(Trehs beh-sehs pohr dee-ah)

Four times a day?
¿Cuatro veces por dìa?
(Koo-ah-troh beh-sehs pohr-dee-ah)

Every other day?
¿Cada tercer dìa?
(Kah-dah tehr-sehr dee-ah)

Once a week?
¿Una vez por semana?
(Oo-nah behs pohr seh-mah-nah)

How does each medication make you feel?
¿Como le hace sentir cada medicamento?
(Koh-moh leh ah-seh sehn-teer kah-dah meh-dee-kah-mehn-toh)

Does the medication make you feel better?
¿Le hace sentir mejor el medicamento?
(Heh ah-seh sehn-teer meh-hohr ehl meh-dee-kah-mehn-toh)

Does the medication make you feel the same or unchanged?
¿Le hace sentir igual o sin cambio el medicamento?
(Leh ah-seh sehn-teer ee-goo-ahl oh seen kam-bee-oh ehl meh-dee-kah-mehn-toh)

Does the medication make you feel worse? (If yes:)
¿Se siente peor con el medicamento? (si:)
(Seh see-ehn teh peh-ohr kohn ehl meh-dee-kah-mehn-toh) (see:)

What do you do to make yourself feel better?
¿Qué hace para sentirse mejor?
(Keh ah-seh pah-rah sehn-teer-seh meh-hohr)

PREPARING FOR TREATMENT TO MEDICATION THERAPY
Medication Purpose

This medication will help relieve:
Este medicamento le ayudará a alivir:
(Ehs-teh meh-dee-kah-mehn-toh leh ah-yoo-dah-rah ah ah-lee-bee-ahr)

—abdominal gas
gases intestinales
(gah-sehs een-tehs-tee-nah- lehs)

—abdominal pain
dolor intestinal; dolor en el abdomen
(doh-lohr een-tehs-tee-nahl; doh-lohr eh ehl ahb-doh-mehn)

—chest congestion
congestión del pecho
(kohn-hehs-tee-ohn dehl peh-choh)

—chest pain
dolor del pecho
(doh-lohr dehl peh-choh)

—constipation
constipación; estreñimiento
(Kohns-tee-pah-see-ohn; ehs-treh-nyee-mee-ehn-toh)

—cough
tos
(tohs)

—headache
dolor de cabeza
(doh-lohr-deh kah-beh-sah)

—muscle aches and pains
achaques musculares y dolores
(ah-chah-kehs moos-koo-lah-rehs ee doh-loh-rehs)

—pain
dolor
(doh-lohr)

This medication will prevent:
Este medicamento prevendrá:
(Ehs-teh meh-dee-kah-mehn-toh preh-behn-drah)

—blood clots
coágulos de sangre
(koh-ah-goo-lohs deh sahn-greh)

—constipation
constipación; estreñimiento
(Kohns-tee-pah-see-ohn; ehs-treh-nyee-mee-ehn-toh)

—contraception
contracepción; embarazo
(kohn-trah-sehp-see-ohn; ehm-bah-rah-soh)

—diarrhea
diarrea
(dee-ah-reh-ah)

—infection
infección
(een-fehk-see-ohn)

—seizures
convulciónes; ataque epiléptico
(kohn-bool-see-ohn-ehs; ah-tah-keh eh-pee-lehp-tee-koh)

—shortness of breath
respiración corta; falta de aliento
(rehs-pee-rah-see-ohn kohr-tah; fahl-tah deh ah-lee-ehn-toh)

—wheezing
el resollar; la respiración ruidosa
(ehl reh-soh-yahr; lah rehs-pee-rah-see-ohn roo-ee-doh- sibilante sah,
    see-bee-lahn-teh)

This medication will increase your:
Este medicamento aumentará su:
(Ehs-teh meh-dee-kah-mehn-toh ah-oo-mehn-tah-rah soo:)

—ability to fight infections
habilidad a combatir infecciones
(ah-bee-lee-dahd ah kohm-bah-teer een-fehk-see-oh-nehs)

—appetite
apetito
(ah-peh-tee-toh)

—blood iron levels
nivel de hierro en la sangre
(nee-behl deh ee-eh-roh ehn lah sahn-greh)

—blood sugar
azúcar en la sangre
(ah-soo-kahr ehn lah sahn-greh)

—heart rate
pulso; latido
(pool-soh; lah-tee-doh)

—red blood cell count
cuenta de células rojas
(koo-ehn-tah deh seh-loo-lahs roh-hahs)

—thyroid hormone levels
niveles de hormona tiroide
(nee-beh-lehs deh ohr-moh-nah tee-roh-ee-deh)

—urine volume
volumen de orina
(boh-loo-mehn deh oh-ree-nah)

This medication will decrease your:
Este medicamento reducirá su:
(Ehs-teh meh-dee-kah-mehn-toh reh-doo-see-rah soo:)

—anxiety
ansiedad
(ahn-see-eh-dahd)

—blood cholesterol level
nivel de colesterol en la sangre
(nee-behl deh koh-lehs-the-rohl ehn lah sahn-greh)

—blood lipid level
nivel de lipido en la sangre
(nee-behl deh lee-pee-doh ehn lah sahn-greh)

—blood pressure
presión arterial de sangre
(preh-see-ohn ahr teh-ree-ahl; deh sahn-greh)

—blood sugar level
nivel de azúcar en la sangre
(nee-behl deh ah-soo-kahr ehn lah sahn-greh)

—heart rate
pulso; latido
(pool-soh; lah-tee-doh)

—stomach acid
ácido en el estómago
(ah-see-doh ehn ehl ehs-toh-mah-goh)

—thyroid hormone levels
niveles de hormona tiroide
(nee-beh-lehs deh ohr-moh-nah tee-roh-ee-deh)

—weight
peso
(peh-soh)

This medication will treat:
Este medicamento sirve para:
(Ehs-teh meh-dee-kah-mehn-toh seer-beh pah-rah)

—cancer of your _____
cancer de su _____
(kahn-sehr deh soo)

depression
—depression
(deh-preh-see-ohn)

—HIV infection
infección de VIH
(een-fehk-see-ohn deh beh ee ah-cheh)

—inflammation
inflamación
(een-flah-mah-see-ohn)

—swelling
hinchazón
(een-chah-sohn)

—the infection in your _____
la infección en su _____
(lah een-fehk-see-ohn ehn soo)

—your abnormal heart rhythm
su ritmo anormal de corazón
(soo reet-moh ah-nohr-mahl deh koh-rah-sohn)

—your allergy to _____
su alergia a _____(soo eh-lehr-hee-ah ah)

—your rash
su erupción; sarpullido
(soo eh-roop-see-ohn; sahr-poo-yee-doh)

ADMINISTERING MEDICATION

Swallow this medication with water or juice.
Tragüe este medicamento con agua o jugo
(Trah-geh ehs-teh meh dee-kah-mehn-toh kohn ah-goo-ah oh hoo-goh)

If you cannot swallow the medication whole, I can crush it and put it in food.
Si no puede tragar el medicamento entero puedo aplastarlo (triturarlo) y ponerlo en el
    alimento.
(See noh poo-eh-deh trah-gahr ehl meh-dee-kah-mehn-toh ehn-teh-roh poo-eh-doh ah-
    plahs-tahr-loh [tree-too-rahr-loh] ee poh-nehr-loh ehn ehl ah lee-mehn-toh)

I need to mix this medication with water or juice before you drink it.
Necesito mezclar este medicamento en agua o jugo antes de que lo tome.
(Neh-seh-see-toh mehs-klahr ehs-teh meh-dee-kah-mehn-toh ehn ah-goo-ah oh hoo-goh
    ahn-tehs deh keh loh toh-meh)

Do not chew this medication. Swallow it whole.
No mastique este medicamento. Tragüelo entero.
(Noh mahs-tee-keh ehs-teh meh-dee-kah-mehn-toh. Trah-geh-loh ehn-teh-roh)

Gargle with this medication and then swallow it.
Haga gargaras con este medicamento y luego tragüelo.
(Ah-gah gahr-gah-rahs koh ehs-teh meh-dee-kah-mehn-toh ee loo-eh-goh
    trah-geh-loh)

Place this medication under your tongue and let it dissolve.
Ponga este medicamento bajo la lengua y deje que se disuelva
(Pohn-gah ehs-teh meh-dee-kah-mehn-toh bah-hoh lah lehn-goo-ah ee deh-heh keh seh
    dee-soo-ehl-bah)

I would like to give this injection in your:
Quiero aplicar esta injección en su:
(Kee-eh-roh ah-plee-kahr ehs-tah een-yehk-see-ohn ehn soo:)

—abdomen
abdomen
(ahb-doh-mehn)

—arm
brazo
(brah-soh)

—buttocks
nalga
(nahl-gah)

—hip
cadera
(kah-deh-rah)

—thigh
muslo
(moos-loh)

I will give you this medication through your intravenous line.
Le daré este medicamento por el tubo de suero intravenoso.
(Leh dah-reh ehs-teh meh-dee-kah-mehn-toh pohr ehl too-boh deh soo-eh-roh
   een-trah-beh-noh-soh)

Let me know if you feel burning or pain at the intravenous site.
Digame si siente ardor o dolor en el sitio del suero intravenoso.
(Dee-gah-meh see see-ehn-teh ahr-dohr oh doh-lohr ehn ehl see-tee-oh dehl soo-eh-roh
   een-trah-beh-noh-soh)

I need to insert this suppository into your rectum (or vagina).
Necesito meter este supositorio en el recto (o vagina).
(Neh-seh-see-toh meh-tehr ehs-teh soo-poh-see-toh-ree-oh ehn ehl rehk-toh
   [oh bah-hee-nah])

I need to put this medication into each ear; left ear; right ear.
Necesito poner este medicamento en cada oreja; oreja izquierda; oreja derecha.
(Neh-seh-see-toh poh-nehr ehs-teh meh-dee-kah-mehn-toh ehn kah-dah oh-reh-hah;
   oh-reh-hah ees-kee-ehr-dah; -oh-reh-hah deh-reh-chah)

I need to put this medication into each eye; left eye; right eye.
Necesito poner este medicamento en cada ojo; ojo izquierdo; ojo derecho.
(Neh-seh-see-toh poh-nehr ehs-teh meh-dee-kah-mehn-toh ehn kah-dah oh-hoh; oh-hoh
   ees-kee-ehr-doh; oh-hoh deh-reh-choh)

PREPARING FOR DISCHARGE

The generic name for this medication is _____.
El nombre genérico (sin marca) de este medicamento es _____.
(Ehl nohn-breh heh-neh-ree-koh [seen mahr-kah] deh ehs-teh meh-dee-kah-mehn-toh ehs)

The trade name for this medication is _____.
El nombre comercial de este medicamento es _____.
(Ehs nohm-breh koh-mehr-see-ahl deh ehs-teh meh-dee-kah-mehn-toh ehs)

Take the medication exactly as prescribed.
Tome el medicamento exactamente como se receta.
(Toh-meh ehl meh-dee-kah-mehn-toh ehx-ahk-tah-mehn-teh koh-moh seh reh-seh-tah)

You can safely break a scored tablet in half.
Puede partir por la mitad la tableta que tiene una muesca (marca).
(Poo-eh-deh pahr-teer pohr lah mee-tahd lah tah-bleh-tah keh tee-eh-neh oo-nah
   moo-ehs-kah [mahr-kah])

Do not crush or chew enteric-coated, extended-release, or sustained-release tablets
or capsules.
No aplaste (triture) o mastique una tableta con capa entérica, de acción prolongada o de
mantenimiento.
(Noh ah-plahs-teh [tree-too-reh] oh mahs-tee-keh oo-nah tah-bleh-tah kohn-kah-pah
ehn-teh-ree-kah, deh ahk-see-ohn proh-lohn-gah-dah oh deh mahn-teh-nee-mee-ehn-toh)

If you miss a dose:
Si pierde una dosis:
(See pee-ehr-deh oo-nah doh-sees:)

—take it as soon as you remember it.
tómela tan pronto se acuerde.
(toh-meh-lah tahn prohn-toh seh ah-koo-ehr-deh)

—wait until the next dose.
espere hasta la siguiente dosis.
(ehs-peh-reh ahs-tah lah see-ghee-ehn-teh doh-sees)

—do not double the next dose.
No doble la siguiente dosis.
(noh doh-bleh lah see-ghee-ehn-teh doh-sees)

—contact your physician.
llame a su médico.
(yah-meh ah soo meh-dee-koh)

Do not stop taking your medication without first speaking with your physician.
No deje de tomar su medicamento sin hablar primero con su médico.
(Noh deh-heh deh toh-mahr soo meh-dee-kah-ehn-toh seen ah-blahr pree-meh-roh kohn
soo meh-dee-koh)

Do not drink alcohol while taking this medication.
No tome alcohol cuando tome este medicamento.
(Noh toh-meh ahl-kohl koo-ahn-doh toh-meh ehs-teh meh-dee-kah-mehn-toh)

Do not drive or operate machinery while taking this medication.
No maneje o use maquinaria cuando toma este medicamento.
(Noh mah-neh-heh oh oo-seh mah-kee-nah-ree-ah koo-ahn-doh toh-mah ehs-teh
meh-dee-kah-mehn-toh)

Notify your physician right away if you experience a dangerous side effect.
Llame a su médico inmediatamente si tiene efectos secundarios peligrosos.
(Llah-meh ah soo meh-dee-koh een-meh-dee-ah-tah-mehn-teh see tee-eh-neh
eh-fehk-tohs seh-koon-dah-ree-ohs peh-lee-groh-sohs)

Check with your physician before taking any over-the-counter medications.
Cheque con su médico antes de tomar medicamentos sin receta.
(Cheh-keh kohn soo meh-dee-koh ahn-tehs deh toh-mahr meh-dee-kah-mehn-tohs seen reh-seh-tah)

Notify your physician if you are pregnant or are planning to become pregnant while taking this medication.
Dígale a su médico si está embarazada o planea el embarazo cuando toma este medicamento.
(Dee-gah-leh ah soo meh-dee-koh see ehs-tah ehm-bah-rah-sah-dah oh plah-neh-ah ehl ehm-bah-rah-soh koo-ahn-doh toh-mah ehs-teh meh-dee-kah-mehn-toh)

Notify your physician if you are breastfeeding while taking this medication.
Dígale a su médico si está amamantando (dando de pecho) cuando toma este medicamento.
(Dee-gah-leh ah soo meh-dee-koh see ehs-tah ah-mah-mahn-tahn-doh [dahn-doh deh peh-choh] koo-ahn-doh toh-mah ehs-teh meh-dee-kah-mehn-toh)

Refill your prescription right away, unless you don't need it anymore.
Rellene su receta inmediatamente, a menos que no la necesite.
(Reh-yeh-neh soo reh-seh-tah een-meh-dee-ah-tah-mehn-teh, ah meh-nohs keh noh lah neh-seh-see-teh)

PROPER MEDICATION STORAGE

Discard expired medications because they may become dangerous or ineffective.
Tire los medicamentos con fecha vencida (caducados) porque pueden ser peligrosos o inefectivos.
(Tee-reh lohs meh-dee-kah-mehn-tohs kohn feh-chah behn-see-dah [kah-doo-kah-dohs] pohr-keh poo-eh-dehn sehr peh-lee-groh-sohs oh een-eh-fehk-tee-bohs)

Keep all medications out of the reach of children at all times.
Guarde todos los medicamentos fuera del alcance de los niños todo el tiempo.
(Goo-ahr-deh toh-dohs lohs meh-dee-kah-mehn-tohs foo-eh-rah dehl ahl-kahn-seh deh lohs nee-nyohs toh-doh ehl tee-ehm-poh)

Store the medication:
Almacene (guarde) el medicamento:
(Ahl-mah-seh-neh [goo-ahr-deh] ehl meh-dee-kah-mehn-toh:)

—in its original container.
en su empaque original.
(ehn-soo ehm-pah-keh oh-ree-hee-nahl)

—in a cool, dry place.
en un lugar fresco y seco.
(ehn oon loo-gahr frehs-koh ee seh-koh)

—away from heat.
lejos del calor.
(leh-hohs dehl kah-lohr)

—at room temperature.
a temperatura ambiente
(ah tehm-peh-rah-too-rah ahm-bee-ehn-teh)

—out of direct sunlight.
fuera de la luz directa del sol.
(foo-eh-rah deh lah loos dee-rehk-tah dehl sohl)

—in the refrigerator.
en el refrigerador.
(ehn ehl reh-free-heh-rah-dohr)

English	Spanish	Pronunciation
Selected Drug Classes	**Clasificación de Drogas Selectas (Medicamentos Selectos)**	**(Klah see-fee-kah-see-ohn deh droh-gahs seh-lehk-tahs [Meh-dee-kah-mehn-tohs Seh-lehk-tohs])**
Analgesic (narcotic, non-narcotic)	Analgésico (narcótico, no narcótico)	(Ah-nahl-heh-see-koh [nahr-koh-tee-koh, noh nahr-koh-tee-koh])
Antacid	Antiácido	(Ahn-tee-ah-see-doh)
Antianginal	Antianginoso	(Ahn-tee-ahn-hee-noh-soh)
Antianxiety	Ansiolítico	(Ahn-see-oh-lee-tee-koh)
Antiarrhythmic	Antiarrítmico	(Ahn-tee-ah-reet-mee-koh)
Antibiotic	Antibiótico	(Ahn-tee-bee-oh-tee-koh)
Anticoagulant	Anticoagulante	(Ahn-tee-koh-ah-goo-lahn-teh)
Anticonvulsant	Anticonvulsivo	(Ahn-tee-kohn-bool-see-boh)
Antidepressant	Antidepresivo	(Ahn-tee-deh-preh-see-boh)
Antidiarrheal	Antidiarréicos	(Ahn-tee-dee-ah-reh-ee-kohs)
Antifungal	Antimicótico	(Ahn-tee-mee-koh-tee-koh)
Antihistamine	Antihistamínico	(Ahn-tee-ees-tah-mee-nee-koh)
Antihyperlipemic	Antihiperlipémico	(Ahn-tee-ee-pehr-lee-peh-mee-koh)
Antihypertensive	Antihipertensivo	(Ahn-tee-ee-pehr-tehn-see-boh)
Anti-inflammatory	Anti-inflamatorio; Contra la inflamación	(Ahn-tee-een-flah-mah-toh-ree-oh; kohn-trah lah een-flah- mah-see-ohn)
Antimigraine	Antimigrañoso	(Ahn-tee-mee-grah-nyoh-soh)
Antiparkinsonian	Contra el Parkinson	(Kohn-trah ehl Pahr-keen-sohn)
Antipsychotic	Medicamentos sicóticos	(Meh-dee-kah-mehn-tohs see-koh-tee-kohs)
Antipyretic	Antitérmicos	(Ahn-tee-tehr-mee-kohs)
Antiseptic	Antiséptico	(Ahn-tee-sehp-tee-koh)
Antispasmodic	Antiespasmódico	(Ahn-tee-ehs-pahs-moh-dee-koh)

Continued

English	Spanish	Pronunciation
Antithyroid	Antitiroideos	(Ahn-tee-tee-roh-ee-deh-ohs)
Antituberculosis	Antifímicos	(Ahn-tee-fee-mee-kohs)
Antitussive	Antitusígenos	(Ahn-tee-too-see-heh- nohs)
Antiviral	Antivirales	(Ahn-tee-bee-rah-lehs)
Appetite suppressant	Antisupresivos del apetito	(Ahn-tee-soo-preh-see-bohs dehl ah-peh-tee-toh)
Appetite stimulant	Estimulantes del apetito	(Ehs-tee-moo-lahn-tehs dehl ah-peh-tee-toh)
Bronchodilator	Bronquoliticos	(Brohn-kee-oh-lee-tee-kohs)
Cancer chemotherapy	Quimioterapia de Cancer	(Kee-mee-oh teh-rah-pee-ah deh kahn-sehr)
Decongestant	Anticongestivo	(Ahn-tee-kohn-hehs-tee-boh)
Digestant	Digestible	(Dee-hehs-tee-bleh)
Diuretic	Diurético	(Dee-oo-reh-tee-koh)
Emetic	Emético	(Eh-meh-tee-koh)
Fertility	Inductor de la Ovulación	(Een-doohk-tohr deh lah Oh-boo-lah-see-ohn)
Herbal	Medicamentos Naturales	(Meh-dee-kah-mehn-tohs Nah-too-rah-lehs, Ee-ehr-bhas Meh-dee- see-nah-lehs)
Hypnotic	Hipnótico	(Eep-noh-tee-koh)
Insulin	Insulina	(Een-soo-lee-nah)
Laxative	Laxante	(Lahx-ahn-teh)
Mineral	Mineral	(Mee-neh-rahl)
Muscle relaxant	Relajante Muscular	(Reh-lah-hahn-teh Moos-koo-lahr)
Oral contraceptive	Anticonceptivos Orales	(Ahn-tee-kohn-sehp-tee-bohs Oh-rah-lehs)
Oral hypoglycemic	Hipoglicémico Oral	(Ee-poh-glee-seh-mee-koh Oh-rahl)
Sedative	Sedantes	(She-dahn-tehs)
Steroid	Esteroide	(Ehs-teh-roh-ee-deh)
Thyroid Hormone	iroideos, Hormona Tiroide	(Tee-roh-ee-deh-ohs, Ohr-moh-nah Tee-roh-ee-deh)
Vaccine	Vacuna	(Bah-koo-nah)

Continued

Administration Routes	Modo de Uso	(Moh-doh deh Oo-soh)
By mouth	Oral	(Oh-rahl)
Intradermal	Intradérmica	(Een-trah-dehr-mee-kah)
Intramuscular	Intramuscular	(Een-trah-moos-koo-lahr)
Intravenous	Intravenosa	(Een-trah-beh-noh-sah)
Nasal	Nasal	(Nah-sahl)
Oral	Oral	(Oh-rahl)
Otic	Ótica	(Oh-tee-kah)
Patch	Parche	(Pahr-cheh)
Rectal	Rectal	(Rehk-tahl)
Subcutaneous	Subcutanea	(Soob-koo-tah-neh-ah)
Sublingual	Sublingual	(Soob-leen-goo-ahl)
Topical	Topical, Local	(Toh-pee-kahl, Loh-kahl)
Vaginal	Vaginal	(Bah-hee-nahl)
Drug Preparations	Presentación del Medicamento	(Preh-sehn-tah-see-ohn dehl Meh-dee-kah-mehn-toh)
Capsule	Cápsula	(Kahp-soo-lah)
Cream	Crema	(Kreh-mah)
Drops	Gotas	(Goh-tahs)
Elixir	Elixir, Jarabe	(Eh-leex-eer, Hah-rah-beh)
Fluid	Liquido	(Lee-kee-doh)
Gel	Gel, Jalea	(Hehl, Hah-leh-ah)
Inhaler	Inhalador*	(Een-ah-lah-dohr)
Injection	Inyección	(Een-yehk-see-ohn)
Liquid	Liquido	(Lee-kee-doh)
Lotion	Loción	(Loh-see-ohn)
Lozenge	Trocisco, pastilla	(Troh-sees-koh, Pahs-tee-yah)

English	Spanish	Pronunciation
Ointment	Ungüento	(Oon-goo-ehn-toh)
Pill	Píldora, Pastilla	(Peel-doh-rah, Pahs-tee-yah)
Powder	Polvo	(Pohl-boh)
Spray	Spray	(Sp-rah-ee)
Suppository	Supositorio	(Soo-poh-see-toh-ree-oh)
Syrup	Jarabe	(Hah-rah-beh)
Tablet	Tableta	(Tah-bleh-tah)
Administration Frequency	**Frecuencia de la Administración**	**(Freh-koo-ehn-see-ah deh lah Ahd-mee-nees-trah-see-ohn)**
Once a day	Una vez por día; diariamente	(Oo-nah behs pohr dee-ah; dee-ah-ree-ah-mehn-teh)
Twice a day	Dos veces por día	(Dohs beh-sehs pohr dee-ah)
Three times a day	Tres veces por día	(Trehs beh-sehs pohr dee-ah)
Four times a day	Cuatro veces por día	(Koo-ah-troh beh-sehs pohr dee-ah)
Every other day	Cada tercer día	(Kah-dah tehr-sehr dee-ah)
Once a week	Una vez por semana	(Oo-nah behs pohr seh-mah-nah)
Every 4 h	Cada cuatro horas	(Kah-dah koo-ah-troh oh-rahs)
Every 6 h	Cada seis horas	(Kah-dah she-ees oh-rahs)
Every 8 h	Cada ocho horas	(Kah-dah oh-choh oh-rahs)
Every 12 h	Cada doce horas	(Kah-dah doh-seh oh-rahs)
In the morning	En la mañana	(Ehn lah mah-nyah-nah)
In the afternoon	En la tarde	(Ehn lah tahr-deh)
In the evening	En la noche	(Ehn lah noh-cheh)
Before bedtime	Antes de acostarse	(Ahn-tehs deh ah-kohs-tahr-seh)
Before meals	Antes de la comida; Antes del alimento	(Ahn-tehs deh lah koh-mee-dah; Ahn-tehs dehl ah-lee-mehn-toh)
With meals	Con los alimentos; con la comida	(Kohn lohs ah-lee-mehn-tohs; Kohn lah koh-mee-dah)

After meals	Después de los alimentos, Después de la comida	(Dehs-poo-ehs deh lohs ah-lee-mehn-tohs; Dehs-poo-ehs deh lah koh-mee-dah)
Only when you need it	Solo cuando la necesite	(Soh-loh koo-ahn-doh lah neh-seh-see-teh)
When you have (pain)	Cuando tiene (dolor)	(Koo-ahn-doh tee-eh-neh) (doh-lohr)
50 Common Side Effects	**Cincuenta Efectos Secundarios Comúnes**	**(Seen-koo-ehn-tah Eh-fehk-tohs Seh-koon-dah-ree-ohs Koh-moo-nehs)**
Abdominal cramps	Retorción abdominal	(Reh-tohr-see-hohn ahb-doh-mee-nahl)
Abdominal pain	Dolor abdominal	(Doh-lohr ahb-doh-mee-nahl)
Abdominal swelling	Inflamación abdominal	(Een-flah-mah-see-ohn ahb-doh-mee-nahl)
Anxiety	Ansiedad	(Ahn-see-eh-dahd)
Blood in the stool	Sangre en el excremento	(Sahn-greh ehn ehl ehx-kreh-mehn-toh)
Blood in the urine	Sangre en la orina	(Sahn-greh ehn la oh-ree-nah)
Bone pain	Dolor de hueso*	(Doh-lohr deh oo-eh-soh)
Chest pain	Dolor de pecho	(Doh-lohr deh peh-choh)
Chest pounding	Palpitación; latidos fuertes o en el pecho	(Pahl-pee-tah-see-ohn; lah- tee-dohs foo-ehr-tehs ehnehl peh-choh)
Chills	Escalofrío	(Ehs-kah-loh-free-oh)
Confusion	Confusión	(Kohn-foo-see-ohn)
Constipation	Constipación, estreñimiento	(Kohns-tee-pah-see-ohn, ehs-treh-nyee-mee-ehn-toh)
Cough	Tos	(Tohs)
Mental depression	Depresión mental	(Deh-preh-see-ohn mehn-tahl)
Diarrhea	Diarrea	(Dee-ah-reh-ah)
Difficult urination	Dificultad al orinar	(Dee-fee-kool-tahd ahl oh-ree-nahr)
Difficulty breathing	Dificultad al respirar	(Dee-fee-kool-tahd ahl rehs-pee-rahr)

Continued

English	Spanish	Pronunciation
Difficulty sleeping	Dificultad al dormir	(Dee-fee-kool-tahd ahl dohr-meer)
Dizziness	Mareos; vahídos	(Mah-reh-ohs; bah-ee-dohs)
Dry mouth	Boca seca	(Boh-kah seh-kah)
Easy bruising	Fragilidad capilar; le salen moretones con facilidad	(Frah-hee-lee-dahd kah-pee-lahr; leh sah-lehn moh-reh-toh-nehs kohn fah-see-lee-dahd)
Faintness	Desvanecimiento; sintió un vahído	(Dehs-bah-neh-see-mee-ehn-toh; seen-tee-oh oon bah-ee-doh)
Fatigue	Fatiga, cansancio	(Fah-tee-gah, kahn-sahn-see-oh)
Fever	Fiebre	(Fee-eh-breh)
Frequent urination	Orina frecuente	(Oh-ree-nah freh-koo-ehn-teh)
Headache	Dolor de cabeza	(Doh-lohr deh kah-beh-sah)
Impotence	Impotencia	(Eem-poh-tehn-see-ah)
Increased appetite	Aumento en el apetito	(Ah-oo-mehn-toh ehn ehl ah-peh-tee-toh)
Increased gas	Flatulencia	(Flah-too-lehn-see-ah)
Increased perspiration	Aumento en el sudor	(Ah-oo-mehn-toh ehn ehl soo-dohr)
Indigestion	Indigestión	(Een-dee-hehs-tee-ohn)
Itching	Comezón	(Koh-meh-sohn)
Loss of appetite	Pérdida en el apetito	(Pehr-dee-dah ehn ehl ah-peh-tee-toh)
Menstrual changes	Cambios en la menstruación; cambio en el ciclo menstrual	(Kahm-bee-ohs ehn la mehns-truh-ah-see-ohn; Kahm-bee-oh ehn ehl see-kloh mehns-truh-ahl)
Mood changes	Cambio en el humor; cambio en la disposición	(Kahm-bee-oh ehn ehl oo-mohr, Kahm-bee-oh ehn lah dees-poh-see-see-ohn)
Muscle pain	Dolores musculares	(Doh-loh-rehs moos-koo-lah-rehs)
Muscle aches	Achaques musculares	(Ah-chah-kehs moos-koo-lah-rehs)
Muscle cramps	Calambre muscular	(Kah-lahm-breh moos-koo-lahr)
Nasal congestion	Congestión nasal	(Kohn-hehs-tee-ohn nah-ahl)

English	Spanish	Pronunciation
Nausea	Nausea	(Nah-oo-seh-ah)
Ringing in the ears	Zumbido en los oidos	(Soom-bee-doh ehn lohs oh-ee-dohs)
Skin rash	Erupción en la piel	(Eh-roop-see-ohn ehn lah pee-ehl)
Swelling of the hands, legs, or feet	Hinchazón en las manos, piernas, o pies	(Een-chah-sohn ehn lahs mah-nohs, pee-ehr-nahs, oh pee-ehs)
Vaginal bleeding	Sangrado vaginal	(Sahn-grah-doh bah-hee-nahl)
Vision changes	Cambios en la visión; cambios en la vista	(Kahm-bee-ohs ehn lah bee-see-ohn; cahm-bee-ohs ehn lah bees-tah)
Vomiting	Vomitando	(Boh-mee-tahn-doh)
Weakness	Debilidad	(Deh-bee-lee-dahd)
Weight gain	Aumento de peso	(Ah-oo-mehn-toh deh peh-soh)
Weight loss	Pérdida de peso	(Pehr-dee-day deh peh-soh)
Wheezing	Resollar; respiración sibilante	(Reh-soh-yahr; rehs-pee-rah-see-ohn see-bee-lahn-teh)

From *Mosby's 2006 Drug Consult for Nurses.* St. Louis, 2006, Mosby.

APPENDIX C
FDA PREGNANCY CATEGORIES

Medications should be used during pregnancy only if clearly needed.

A: Adequate and well-controlled studies have failed to show a risk to the fetus in the first trimester of pregnancy (also, no evidence of risk has been seen in later trimesters). Possibility of fetal harm appears remote.

B: Animal reproduction studies have failed to show a risk to the fetus, no adequate and well-controlled studies have been done in pregnant women.

C: Animal reproduction studies have shown an adverse effect on the fetus, and no adequate and well-controlled studies in have been done in humans. However, the benefits may warrant use of the drug in pregnant women despite potential risks.

D: Positive evidence has been found of human fetal risk based on data from investigational or marketing experience or from studies in humans, but the potential benefits may warrant use of the drug despite potential risks (e.g., use in life-threatening situations in which other medications cannot be used or are ineffective).

X: Animal or human studies have shown fetal abnormalities, and/or there is evidence of human fetal risk based on adverse reaction data from investigational or marketing experience where the risks in using the medication clearly outweigh potential benefits.

From *2009 Saunders Nursing Drug Handbook*, St. Louis, 2009, Saunders.

APPENDIX D

Normal Laboratory Values

HEMATOLOGY/COAGULATION

Test	Specimen	Normal Range
Activated partial thromboplastin time (aPTT)	Whole blood	25-35 s
Erythrocyte count (RBC count)	Whole blood	M: 4.3-5.7 million cells/mm³ F: 3.8-5.1 million cells/mm³
Hematocrit (HCT, Hct)	Whole blood	M: 39%-49%, F: 35%-45%
Hemoglobin (Hb, Hgb)	Whole blood	M: 13.5-17.5 g/dL, F: 12.0-16.0 g/dL
Leukocyte count	Whole blood	4.5-11.0 thousand cells/mm³
(WBC count)		
Leukocyte differential count	**Whole blood**	
Basophils		0%-0.75%
Eosinophils		1%-3%
Lymphocytes		23%-33%
Monocytes		3%-7%
Neutrophils—bands		3%-5%
Neutrophils—segmented		54%-62%
Mean corpuscular hemoglobin (MCH)	Whole blood	26-34 pg/cell
Mean corpuscular hemoglobin concentration (MCHC)	Whole blood	31%-37% Hb/cell
Mean corpuscular volume (MCV)	Whole blood	80-100 fL
Partial thromboplastin time (PTT)	Whole blood	60-85 sec
Platelet count (thrombocyte count)	Whole blood	150-450 thousand/mm³
Prothrombin time (PT)	Whole blood	11-13.5 s
RBC count (see Erythrocyte count)		

CLINICAL CHEMISTRY (SERUM PLASMA/URINE)

Test	Specimen	Normal Range
Alanine aminotransferase (ALT, SGPT)	Serum	0-55 units/L
Albumin	Serum	3.5-5 g/dL
Alkaline phosphatase	Serum	M: 53-128 units/L, F: 42-98 units/L
Anion gap	Plasma or serum	5-14 mEq/L
Aspartate aminotransferase (AST, SGOT)	Serum	0-50 units/L
Bilirubin (conjugated direct)	Serum	0-0.4 mg/dL
Bilirubin (total)	Serum	0.2-1.2 mg/dL
Calcium (total)	Serum	8.4-10.2 mg/dL
Carbon dioxide (CO_2) total	Plasma or serum	20-34 mEq/L
Chloride	Plasma or serum	96-112 mEq/L
Cholesterol (total)	Plasma or serum	Less than 200 mg/dl
C-reactive protein	Serum	68-8200 ng/mL
Creatine kinase (CK)	Serum	M: 38-174 units/L, F: 26-140 units/L
Creatine kinase isoenzymes	Serum	Fraction of total: Less than 0.04-0.06
Creatinine	Plasma or serum	M: 0.7-1.3 mg/dl, F: 0.6-1.1 mg/dL
Creatinine clearance	Plasma or serum and urine	M: 90-139 mL/min/1.73 m^2 F: 80-125 mL/min/1.73 m^2
Free thyroxine index (FTI)	Serum	Adults: 70-105 mg/dL
Glucose	Serum	Older than 60 yr: 80-115 mg/dL
Hemoglobin A$_{1c}$	Whole blood	5.6%-7.5% of total Hgb
Homovanillic acid (HVA)	Urine, 24 h	1.4-8.8 mg/day

17-Hydroxycorticosteroids (17-OHCS)	Urine, 24 h	M: 3-10 mg/day, F: 2-8 mg/day
Iron	Serum	M: 65-175 mcg/dL
		F: 50-170 mcg/dL
Iron-binding capacity, total (TIBC)	Serum	250-450 mcg/dL
Lactate dehydrogenase (LDH)	Serum	0-250 units/L
Magnesium	Serum	1.3-2.3 mg/dL
Oxygen (PO₂)	Whole blood, arterial	83-100 mm Hg
Oxygen saturation	Whole blood, arterial	95%-98%
pH	Whole blood, arterial	7.35-7.45
Phosphorus, inorganic	Serum	2.7-4.5 mg/dL
Potassium	Serum	3.5-5.1 mEq/L
Protein (total)	Serum	6-8.5 g/dL
Sodium	Plasma or serum	136-146 mEq/L
Specific gravity	Urine	1.002-1.030
Thyrotropin (hTSH)	Plasma or serum	2-10 mU/mL
Thyroxine (T₄) total	Serum	5-12 mcg/dL
Triglycerides (TG)	Serum, after 12-h fast	20-190 mg/dL
Tri-iodothyronine resin uptake test (TxRU)	Serum	22%-37%
Urea nitrogen	Plasma or serum	7-25 mg/dL
Urea nitrogen/creatinine ratio	Serum	12/1-20/L
Uric acid	Serum	M: 3.5-7.2 mg/dL
		F: 2.6-6 mg/dL
Vanillylmandelic acid (VMA)	Urine, 24 h	2-7 mg/day

From *2009 Saunders Nursing Drug Handbook*, St. Louis, 2009, Saunders.

APPENDIX E
ERROR-PRONE DRUG NAME ABBREVIATIONS

Drug Name Abbreviations	Intended Meaning	Misinterpretation	Correction
ARA A	Vidarabine	Mistaken as cytarabine (ARA C)	Use complete drug name
AZT	Zidovudine (Retrovir)	Mistaken as azathioprine or aztreonam	Use complete drug name
CPZ	Compazine (prochlorperazine)	Mistaken as chlorpromazine	Use complete drug name
DPT	Demerol-Phenergan-Thorazine	Mistaken as diphtheria-pertussis-tetanus (vaccine)	Use complete drug name
DTO	Diluted tincture of opium or deodorized tincture of opium (Paregoric)	Mistaken as tincture of opium	Use complete drug name
HCl	Hydrochloric acid or hydrochloride	Mistaken as potassium chloride ("H" is misinterpreted as "K")	Use complete drug name unless expressed as salt of a drug
HCT	Hydrocortisone	Mistaken as hydrochlorothiazide	Use complete drug name
HCTZ	Hydrochlorothiazide	Mistaken as hydrocortisone (seen as HCT250 mg)	Use complete drug name
$MgSO_4$,**	Magnesium sulfate	Mistaken as morphine sulfate	Use complete drug name
MS, MSO_4,**	Morphine sulfate	Mistaken as magnesium sulfate	Use complete drug name
MTX	Methotrexate	Mistaken as mixtoxantrone	Use complete drug name
PCA	Procainamide	Mistaken as patient-controlled analgesia	Use complete drug name
PTU	Propylthiouracil	Mistaken as mercaptopurine	Use complete drug name
T3	Tylenol with codeine no. 3	Mistaken as liothyronine	Use complete drug name
TAC	Triamcinolone	Mistaken as tetracaine, Adrenalin, cocaine	Use complete drug name
TNK	TNKase	Mistaken as "TPA"	Use complete drug name
$ZnSO_4$	Zinc sulfate	Mistaken as morphine sulfate	Use complete drug name

Official "Do Not Use" List1 May 2005

Do Not Use	Potential Problem	Use Instead
U (unit)	Mistaken for "0" (zero), the number "4" (four) or "cc"	Write "unit"
IU (International Unit)	Mistaken for IV (intravenous) or the number 10 (ten)	Write "International Unit"
Q.D., QD, q.d., qd (daily)	Mistaken for each other	Write "daily"
Q.O.D., QOD, q.o.d, qod (every other day)	Period after the Q mistaken for "I" and the "O" mistaken for "I"	Write "every other day"
Trailing zero (X.0 mg)*	Decimal point is missed	Write X mg
Lack of leading zero (.X mg)		Write 0.X mg
MS	Can mean morphine sulfate or magnesium sulfate	Write "morphine sulfate"
MSO₄ and MgSO₄	Confused for one another	Write "magnesium sulfate"

^{1} Applies to all orders and all medication-related documentation that is handwritten (including free-text computer entry) or on pre-printed forms.

*Exception: A "trailing zero" may be used only where required to demonstrate the level of precision of the value being reported, such as for laboratory results, imaging studies that report size of lesions, or catheter/tube sizes. It may not be used in medication orders or other medication-related documentation.

Copyright © The Joint Commission, 2009. Reprinted with permission.

Additional Abbreviations, Acronyms and Symbols
(For possible future inclusion in the Official "Do Not Use" List)

Do Not Use	Potential Problem	Use Instead
> (greater than)	Misinterpreted as the number "7" (seven) or the letter "L"	Write "greater than"
< (less than)	Confused for one another	Write "less than"
Abbreviations for drug names	Misinterpreted due to similar abbreviations for multiple drugs	Write drug names in full
Apothecary units	Unfamiliar to many practitioners	Use metric units
	Confused with metric units	
@	Mistaken for the number "2" (two)	Write "at"
cc	Mistaken for U (units) when poorly written	Write "mL" or "milliliters"
μg	Mistaken for mg (milligrams) resulting in one thousand-fold overdose	Write "mcg" or "micrograms"

Copyright © The Joint Commission, 2009. Reprinted with permission.

GLOSSARY

Abortifacient Any treatment or substance that facilitates loss (abortion) of a fetus

Absorption The passage of nutrients and medicines across the barriers that separate the body from the environment

Accommodation The changes that occur in the ocular lens to allow it to focus to various distances

ACE Angiotensin-converting enzyme; facilitates the transformation of angiotensin I to angiogensin II, a potent vascoconstrictor, in the lungs

Acidification The conversion to an acid environment

Acidosis Elevated acid content of the blood resulting from the accumulation of acid (H^+) or loss of bicarbonate ($HCO3^-$); the pH of blood is lowered

Acoustic nerve The eighth cranial nerve; carries sensory information about hearing and equilibrium to the various parts of the brain

Acquired immunity Immunity resulting from exposure to an antigen or infectious agent

Acute A symptom or condition that appears suddenly

Adaptogen A substance with a nonspecific action that casues improved resistance to physical and mental stress

Addison disease Condition resulting in a decrease in the adrenocortical hormones, mineralocorticoids and glucocorticoids, that causes symptoms, including muscle weakness and weight loss

Adenoma An abnormal growth of glandular epithelial tissue

Adjuvant A substance added to a drug to enhance its action

Adrenalin The hormone that binds to adrenergic receptors and causes the fight or flight response; also known in the United States as *epinephrine*

Adrenergic Relating to a class of drugs that affects the sympathetic nervous system

Adverse effect Unintended, undesirable effect of a drug

Aerobic Organisms that need oxygen to survive; vs. anaerobic

Afferent Neuronal impulses that travel from the body toward the central nervous system (CNS)

Agonist A substance that activates a membrane receptor

AIDS Acquired immunodeficiency syndrome; a condition of a gradually weakened immune system that results from a viral infection

Alcoholic extract Solid fraction of plant material obtained after extraction with ethanol

Alkaloid Organic compound containing nitrogen as part of a herterocyclic ring; often highly active as a drug

Alkalosis The decrease of acidity of the blood resulting from the accumulation of alkali or reduction of acid content; the pH of blood is raised

Allergen A substance that triggers an allergic reaction

Alligation A method of determining the needed amounts of two different concentrations to prepare a needed concentration

Allopathy A medical system that uses substances to cause an effect different or counter to those caused by the condition under treatment

Alopecia Loss of hair

Amenorrhea Absence or suppression of menses

Amino acid Macromolecule that forms the building blocks of proteins

Anabolism To build up; the constructive phase of metabolism

Anaerobic Organisms that live in the absence of oxygen; vs. aerobic

Analeptic A substance that stimulates the central nervous system

Analgesic A drug that reduces the perception of pain

Anaphylactic shock A severe allergic reaction that causes airway obstruction; bronchoconstriction and circulatory collapse that will cause death if not treated immediately

Androgen Male sex hormone originating from the cholesterol family

Anemia A deficiency of circulating red blood cells; a symptom of disease, not a disease

Anesthetic A substance that causes localized or general loss of sensation

Angina pectoris Chest pain related to coronary heart diease

Antacid An agent that counteracts acidity in the stomach

Antagonist Agent that binds at a receptor site and prevents or lessens the effect of other agents that would bind there

Anthelmintic A substance that kills or expels intestinal worms

Antiarrhythmic Agents that restore normal rhythm and conduction of the heart

Antibiotic Chemical agent used to stop microorganism growth or replication; generally refers to agents used to treat infections caused by bacteria and parasites

Antibiotic spectrum The variety of microbes a particular antibiotic can treat. Broad-spectrum agents can treat many organisms, whereas narrow-spectrum agents treat only a few

Antibody Protein that neutralizes or destroys antigens; also known as *immunoglobulin*

Anticoagulant A substance that prevents or delays blood from clotting

Anticonvulsant Agent that prevents or controls seizures

Antidepressant Agent that counters a clinical state of depression

Antidote A substance that counteracts toxic effects of a poison

Antiemetic An agent that prevents or relieves nausea and vomiting

Antigen The marker on cell surfaces that stimulates the production of antibodies

Antihistamine A substance that blocks the action of histamine and relieves allergic symptoms

Antihypertensive A substance that reduces blood pressure

Anti-inflammatory A substance that reduces swelling, redness, and pain

Antimicrobial Chemical agent that prevent the growth of or that kill microorganisms

Antimycotic Antifungal agent

Antineoplastic An agent used to prevent the development, proliferation, or growth of neoplastic cells; a medication used in treatment of abnormal cells

Antioxidant A substance that is able to protect cells or counteract the damage caused by oxidation and oxygen-free radicals

Antipruritic A drug that relieves, or prevents, itching

Antipsychotic Drug that manages a variety of psychiatric conditions, including schizophrenia, delirium/dementia, agitation, paranoia, and mania

Antipyretic A substance that reduces fever

Antiseptic A substance that slows or stops and the growth of microorganisms on skin and mucous membranes

Antispasmodic A substance that reduces smooth muscle spasms

Antitussive A drug that relieves or suppresses cough

Anuria The inability to urinate

Anxiety Feelings of apprehension, dread, and fear unrelated to any danger or threat

APAP *N*-acetyl-para-amino-phenol; also known generically as *acetaminophen* or *paracetamol*

Aperitif A drink that stimulates the appetite

Apnea Absence of breathing

Apothecary Latin term for *pharmacist*

Appendicitis Inflammation of the appendix

Aqueous extract Soluble fraction of plant material obtained after extraction with water

Aqueous humor Lymph-type fluid that is found in the eye

Aromatherapy The medicinal use of aroma substances

Arrhythmia Variation from the normal rate, regularity, or conduction of the heart's rhythm

Arteriosclerosis Conditions that cause arterial walls to thicken and lose elasticity

Artery A vessel that carries oxygenated blood from the heart to the tissues of the body

Arthritis Inflammation of joints

Aseptic technique Procedures used to maintain sterility

Asthenia Diminishing strength and energy

Asthma A condition in which narrowing of the airways impairs breathing

Astringent Substance (often a tannin) that shrinks or constricts body tissues

Ataxia Loss of muscle coordination

Atherosclerosis Thickened, irregular inner arterial walls related to plaque build-up

Attenuated An altered or weakened live vaccine made from the disease organism that the vaccine protects against

Auditory canal The passage from the opening of the external ear to the eardrum

Auditory ossicles Three small bony structures in the ear: malleus, incus, and stapes

Autoimmune disease A condition in which a person's tissues are attacked by his or her immune system; abnormal antigen-antibody reaction

Autonomic Literally, self-controlling or involuntary

Autonomic nervous system (ANS) Division of the nervous system that controls the involuntary body functions; includes the sympathetic and parasympathetic divisions

Auxiliary label A label attached to a container with information related to the medication inside

Avitaminosis Vitamin deficiency

Axon The part of a nerve cell that conducts impulses away from the cell body

Ayurveda A lifestyle-based holistic medical system originating in India 5000 years ago

Bacteria Unicellular organisms that live on a host

Bactericidal Agents that kill bacteria

Bacteriostatic Agents that prevent the growth of bacteria but do not kill them

Benign A nonmalignant growth of tumor cells; not recurrent

Benign prostatic hypertrophy Nonmalignant enlargement of the prostate gland; properly called *benign prostatic hyperplasia*

Beta-carotene An orange plant pigment that is converted in the body to vitamin A

Binary fission The method by which a single cell divides into two separate cells

Biology The study of life

Biopsy A procedure in which a piece of tissue is removed from a patient for examination and diagnosis; to take a sample of the whole

Bipolar disorder Mood disorder in which a patient alternates between excessive phases of manic and depressive episodes

Blister pack Container usually made of plastic that holds a single-dose tablet or capsule

Blood-brain barrier A barrier formed by special characteristics of capillaries in the brain to prevent certain chemicals from moving into the brain

Blood urea nitrogen (BUN) A laboratory test that measures the nitrogen waste in blood in the form of urea

Bradycardia Slow beating of the heart; in adults, <60 beats/min

Bradykinin A peptide in the inflammatory pathway that is a potent vasodilator and causes pain, contraction, and inflammatory reactions in tissues

Brand name/tradename Trademark of a drug or device registered by the originating manufacturing company

Bronchitis Inflammation of the mucous membranes of the bronchi

Bronchodilator A substance that reduces bronchial muscle spasm

Bulk compounding A larger quantity of medication

Bulk forming Fiber used as a stimulant to the intestines or to cause a feeling of fullness to decrease appetite

Cachexia Weight loss caused by chronic illness or prolonged emotional stress

Calibration Determination of the accuracy of an instrument or measuring device against a standard

Cancer Malignant and abnormally invasive growth of cells, known as *neoplasms*

Candidiasis Infection with the fungus *Candida albicans* or related species, also called *a yeast infection*

Capillary Minute blood vessel that connects the ends of the arterioles to the venules, where exchanges of nutrients and wastes, O_2, and CO_2 occurs

Carbohydrates Chemical substances that include sugars, glycogen, starches, and cellulose; composed of carbon, hydrogen, and oxygen molecules

Carcinogen A substance or chemical that can increase the risk of developing cancer

Carcinoma Malignant growth of epithelial cells

Carminative A substance that reduces flatulence, or intestinal gas

Catabolism To break down; the destructive phase of metabolism

Catalyst A molecule that allows chemical reactions to take place rapidly but is not altered in the reaction

Cataract Loss of transparency of the lens of the eye

Cell body The main part of a neuron from which axons and dendrites extend

Cerebrospinal fluid (CSF) Fluid that fills the ventricles of the brain, the spaces of the brain and spinal cord, and the arachnoid layer of the meninges

Cervical The region from the base of the skull to the upper chest or thorax

Chemotherapy The treatment of a disease with toxic chemical substances to slow the disease process or to kill cells

Chiropractic A therapy system that uses manual manipulation of the joints and muscles to relieve organ and muscle dysfunction

Chloasma Hyperpigmentation of skin, limited or confined to a certain area

Chronic obstructive pulmonary disease (COPD) A disease process where the lungs have decreased ability for gas exchange; types include emphysema and chronic bronchitis

Chyme Food of a soupy acidic consistency as it passes from mixing with stomach enzymes into the small intestine

Clinical pharmacist Pharmacist who directly monitors patient medications and health in inpatient, ambulatory, and some community settings

Clinical trial The research phases of new drug development

CNS Central nervous system; composed of the brain and spinal cord

Coagulate To solidify or change from a fluid state to a more solid state

Code blue A coded message to indicate an emergency in a hospital situation, usually cardiopulmonary arrest

Coenzyme A compound that activates an enzyme

Cofactor Usually a vitamin, mineral, or molecule that must be present for other factors to be active in a chemical reaction

Colic Abdominal pains caused by smooth muscle contraction of an abdominal organ, usually accompanied by nausea, vomiting, and perspiration

Commission E Recommendations of a group of German experts in the 1990s regarding the usefulness and efficacy of plant drugs

Communication The ability to express oneself in such a way that one is readily and clearly understood

Competency The capability or proficiency to perform a function

Compounding The act of mixing, reconstituting, and packaging a drug

Condyloma Warts of the genital-anal region, usually caused by a virus of the Papilloma group

Cone Photoreceptor that perceives color (daylight vision) in the retina of the eye

Confidentiality To keep privileged information from being disclosed without the patient's consent

Congestive heart failure (CHF) Accumulation of blood in the lungs and circulatory system resulting from the inability of the heart to pump all of the blood that is delivered to it

Conjunctiva The mucous membranes of the eyes and eyelids

Constipation Decreased frequency of bowel movements leading to difficulty with elimination and dry hard feces/stools

Continuing Education (CE) Professional education beyond the basic technical level, usually required for license maintenance and renewal

Cornea The transparent tissue covering the anterior portion of the eye

Corpus luteum A group of cells in the ovary that secrete estrogen and progesterone and have released an egg

Cough reflex An automated response caused by stimulation of sensory nerves in the respiratory system that clears air passages of foreign substances and mucus by a forceful expiration

Cream A hydrophilic base

Cretinism Condition in which the development of the brain and body is inhibited by a congenital lack of thyroid hormones

Crohn disease Chronic inflammation of the intestinal tract

Cushing disease Syndrome in which an increase in secretions of the adrenal cortex create symptoms such as a moon face and deposits of fat on the upper back (buffalo hump)

Cyclooxygenase Enzymes that catalyze prostaglandin and other inflammation chemical biosynthesis inhibited by COX inhibitors, aspirin, and similar agents

Cycloplegia Paralysis of the ciliary muscle in the eye

Cystic fibrosis An inherited disorder that causes the production of very thick mucus in the respiratory tract as a result of impaired chloride ion flow; affects the pancreas and sweat glands

Cystitis Inflammation of the urinary bladder, possibly caused by a bacterial infection

Cytotoxic A substance that is toxic to cells

Debride To remove dead or damaged tissue

Decoction Watery extract obtained by boiling, used in making plant medicines

Decongestants Drugs that reduce swelling of the mucous membranes by constricting dilated nasal blood vessels, reducing nasal congestion and opening air passages

Dementia Loss of individually acquired mental skills; Alzheimer disease is a severe form

Dendrite The part of a neuron that receives impulses

Deoxyribonucleic acid (DNA) The complex nucleic acids that are base for genetic continuance

Depot An area of the body where a substance can be stored for later distribution

Depression A mental state characterized by sadness; changes in sleep, appetite, and sex drive; feelings of loss and grief, hopelessness. May include suicidal thoughts; associated with low concentrations of dopamine, noradrenaline, or serotonin

Dermatitis Inflammation of the skin associated with itching and burning

Desquamation A normal process of shedding the top layer of the skin, also known as *exfoliation*

Diabetes mellitus Chronic abnormally high blood sugar levels caused by inadequate production or use of insulin

Diagnosis The assessment of the cause of a condition

Dialysis The passage of a solute through a semipermeable membrane to remove toxic materials and to maintain fluid, electrolyte, and pH of the body system; often used to describe treatment when the kidneys no longer function in end-stage renal disease (ESRD)

Diaphoretic A substance that increases sweating

Diarrhea Watery, loose stools, abnormal to the patient's usual frequency

Dietary supplement A substance that is marketed and sold as a nonfood, nondrug item but not as a therapeutic agent; often includes vitamins, minerals, herbs, and medicines from nonallopathic medical systems

Digestion The mechanical, chemical, and enzymatic action of breaking food into molecules that can be absorbed and then used in metabolism

Diuresis The secretion and passage of large amounts of urine from the body

Diuretic An agent that increases urine output

DNA Deoxyribonucleic acid; the biomolecules in the cells of most living things that store genetic information

Dogma A code of beliefs based on tradition rather than fact

Dromotropic An agent that alters the conduction velocity of a nerve cell

Dropsy Outdated term for hydrops

Drug Enforcement Agency (DEA) Federal agency within the Department of Justice that regulates the use of controlled substances

Dysentery Inflammation of the colon; often caused by bacteria or viruses, accompanied by pain and severe diarrhea

Dysmenorrhea Painful menstruation

Dyspepsia Indigestion

Dystonia Symptoms that include twisting, repeated jerking movements, and/or abnormal posture

Dysuria Painful urination

Eczema Inflammation of the skin with redness, itching, and oozing vesicular lesions

Edema A local or generalized condition in which body tissues retain an excessive amount of tissue fluid outside of the blood vessels

Efferent The conduction of electrical impulses away from the central nervous system toward the body

Electrolytes Charged elements

Elixir A base solution that is a mixture, emulsion, or suspension of alcohol and water

Emesis Vomiting

Endometriosis Condition where tissue resembling endometrium is found outside the uterine cavity, usually in the pelvic area

Endometrium The mucus membrane lining of the uterus, where a fertilized egg implants

Endorphins Peptides made by the body with actions similar to morphine

Enteritis Inflammation of the intestines

Enzyme A protein that speeds up a chemical reaction by reducing the amount of energy required to initiate a reaction; also called a *biological catalyst*

Epilepsy A chronic brain condition characterized by seizures and loss of consciousness

Erythema Redness of the skin resulting from capillary dilation

Essential oil Mixture of volatile terpenoids responsible for the taste and smell of many plants, especially spices, the basic ingredients used in aromatherapy

Estrogen A family of related compounds serving as female sex hormones

Ethics The values and morals that are used within a profession

Eustachian tube A passage that connects the middle ear to the nasopharynx (throat)

Euthyroid Normal functioning thyroid gland

Excretion Elimination of waste products through stools, urine, sweat, and breath

Exophthalmos Abnormal protrusion or prominence of the eyeball, usually as a result of increased thyroid hormone, also called *proptosis*

Expectorant Chemical that loosens and thins bronchial secretions for ease of removal through coughing

Extract A concentrated preparation in semiliquid, solid, or dry powder of the soluble fraction of plant material

Extrapyramidal Side effects of antipsychotic medications that include parkinsonism, dystonia, and tremors

Euthyroid Normal functioning thyroid gland

Facts and Comparisons Reference book found in most pharmacies containing detailed information on all medications

Facultative anaerobe A microorganism that can live with or without oxygen

Fallopian tubes Narrow passage tube connecting an ovary with the uterus

Fat-soluble Drugs that are absorbed into the body's fat layer

Fat-soluble vitamin Vitamin that is soluble in fat and therefore is stored in body fat; vitamins A, D, E, and K are fat soluble

FDA Food and Drug Administration

Fertilization The process by which the sperm unites with the ovum to create a new life

Floor stock Supplies kept on hand in different units of a hospital

Food and Drug Administration (FDA) Federal agency that regulates the manufacture and safeguarding of medications

Formulary A list of preferred drugs to be stocked by the pharmacy; also a list of drugs covered by an insurance company

Fungicide An agent that kills fungus

Gamete Sex cell of reproduction: ovum and sperm

Gastritis Inflammation of the stomach lining

Gauge The size of the needle opening; smaller-gauge numbers indicate larger openings

Generic name Name assigned to a medication by the FDA; nonproprietary name of a drug

Globulin A protein that is insoluble in water; immune globulins protect against diseases

Glucose Simple six-carbon sugar; one of the basic building blocks of energy used by the body

Goiter Condition in which the thyroid is enlarged, commonly from a lack of iodine known as *simple goiter,* or because of a tumor, known as *toxic goiter*

Government insurance Includes Medicaid and Medicare

Gram The basic unit of mass (weight) of the metric system, equal to the weight of a cubic centimeter (cc) or a milliliter (mL) of water

Gram-negative bacteria Bacteria that are unable to keep crystal violet stain when washed in acid alcohol because of a phospholipid outer membrane that prevents staining

Gram-positive bacteria Bacteria that are able to keep crystal violet stain when washed in acid alcohol as the result of a thick peptidoglycan that holds stain

Graves disease Hyperplasia or hypersecretion of the thyroid, causing exophthalmos, diffuse goiter, and skin changes; usually autoimmune in origin

Hallucinogen A substance that induces the perception of objects that are not actually present

Health Insurance Portability and Accountability Act of 1996 (HIPAA) Federal act designed to protect patients' privacy

Heartburn Uncomfortable burning sensation in the chest, rising toward the throat, because of the return of stomach acid into the esophagus

Helminth Multicellular worm

Hematuria Blood in the urine

Hemoglobin The iron-containing molecule that carries oxygen to and carbon dioxide from body tissues

Hemolysis Breakdown of red blood cells

Hemorrhage Profuse bleeding

Hemorrhoid Known commonly as *piles*; painful and swollen anal vein

Hemostatic A substance or procedure that reduces or stops bleeding

Hepatitis Inflammation of the liver

Hepatotoxic Toxic to the liver

Herb A plant that is used for its medicinal properties

Herpes simplex Localized infection on the lips or genitalia, caused by the herpes virus

Histamine A chemical produced by mast cells and released during inflammation reactions; it interacts with tissues to produce itching, vasodilation, and decreased blood pressure as part of an allergic reaction

HIV Human immunodeficiency virus; associated with AIDS

HMO Health Maintenance Organization

Hodgkin disease A cancer of lymph cells (lymphoma) that originates in one lymph node and later spreads to other organs

Homeopathy A holistic therapy based on the belief that medicinal remedies causing specific symptoms can be used to treat an illness that manifests the same symptoms

Homeostasis The equilibrium pertaining to the internal balance of body functions

Horizontal flow hood Environment for the preparation of sterile products

Hormone Chemical substances produced and secreted into the bloodstream by an endocrine gland, resulting in physiologic responses at target tissues elsewhere in the body

Household system A system of measurement commonly used for weight, volume, and length in the United States

HPLC High-performance liquid chromatography; a technique used to analyze chemical compounds and extracts

Hydrophilic Any substance that easily dissolves into water

Hydrophobic Any substance that does not go into or mix in water

Hyperalimentation Parenteral nutrition for patients who are unable to eat solids or liquids

Hypercalcemia Unusually high concentration of calcium in the blood

Hyperemia Abnormal blood accumulation in a localized part of the body

Hyperglycemia Abnormally high glucose concentration in the bloodstream

Hyperlipidemia High lipid values in the blood, triglycerides >160 mg/dL, and cholesterol >200 mg/dL

Hyperplasia Abnormal increase in the growth of an organ attributable to cells dividing and increasing in number

Hypertension High blood pressure, >140/90 mm Hg

Hypertonic solution Fluid having a higher osmotic pressure than blood or another body fluid

Hypertrophy Abnormal increase in the size of an organ, with cell numbers remaining constant

Hypervitaminosis A disorder caused by the accumulation of too many vitamins in the body; more common with fat-soluble vitamins

Hypnotic A substance that induces sleep

Hypocalcemia Low concentration of calcium in the blood

Hypoglycemia Abnormally low glucose concentration in the bloodstream

Hypoplasia Incomplete or underdevelopment of an organ or tissue

Hypotension Abnormally low blood pressure

Hypothermia Low body temperature

Icterus Jaundice, yellowish discoloration of body organs such as skin and eyes resulting from bile pigments from the liver not being metabolized properly

Immunity Protection of the body through resistance to infection via factors in the immune system, the immune response of the body, or agents such as vaccinations

In utero In the uterus, before birth

In vitro In the laboratory or test tube

In vivo In a living animal or human

Inert ingredient An ingredient that has little or no effect on body functions

Inflammation Localized swelling, redness, pain, and heat, usually as a result of an infection or injury

Influenza An acute and highly contagious respiratory tract infection caused by one of many influenza viruses

Infusion Introduction of a fluid into the body through a vein

Ingestion The act of taking in food or liquid

Inhibit To stop or hold back; to keep a reaction from taking place

Inotropic A substance that affects the force or energy of contraction of muscles

Inpatient A hospitalized patient

Inpatient pharmacy A pharmacy in a hospital or institutional setting

Insomnia Difficulty falling or staying asleep

Insulin A hormone of the pancreas that controls the level of glucose in the blood

Intrinsic factor A naturally produced protein that is necessary for the absorption of vitamin B_{12}

Invasive The tendency for a tumor or mass to move into tissues or organs in close proximity

Ion channel Membrane proteins that can form water-containing pores so that mineral ions can enter or leave cells

Jaundice Yellowish discoloration of body organs such as skin and eyes, caused by bile pigments not being metabolized properly

Kcal Kilocalorie; a measurement of energy or heat expended or used up in a chemical activity; the amount of heat needed to change the temperature of 1 kg of water 1° Celsius

Keratolytic A drug that causes shedding of the outer layer of the skin

Labyrinth A system of cavities or canals; in the inner ear, the bony maze composed of the vestibular utricle, saccule, cochlea, and three semicircular canals

Lactation Production and secretion of milk by female mammary glands

Laminar flow hood Environment for the preparation of sterile products

Laxative A substance that loosens stool forming in the bowels

Legend drug Drug that requires a prescription for dispensing

Leukopenia Low white blood cell count

Leukemia A progressive disease marked by malignancy of the blood-forming cells found in the hemopoietic tissues, organs, and bloodstream, causing the circulation of abnormal blood cells

Leukorrhea Vaginal discharge of white or yellowish fluid

Ligand A substance that binds to a receptor

Liniment Ointment for topical application

Lipid Fat and fatty acid; substance soluble in nonpolar solvents and insoluble in water

Lipid-lowering A substance that lowers triglyceride or cholesterol levels in blood

Lipophilic A substance soluble in oil or a nonpolar solvent

Lumbar The region of the back that includes the area between the ribs and the pelvis

Lymphoma A term used to describe a malignant disorder of lymphoid tissue

Maceration A preparation that is made by adding cold water to the required amount of drug or plant material, which is allowed to soak at room temperature for 6-8 h before it is strained

Macro Large

Malaria A parasitic disease caused by *Plasmodium* parasites; transmitted to humans by mosquitoes

Malignant An invasive and destructive pattern of rapid, abnormal cell growth; often fatal

Mania A form of psychosis characterized by uncontrolled and excessive excitement, elevated mood, and exalted feelings

MAO The enzyme monoamine oxidase, catalyses the removal of amine groups from dopamine and norepinephrine

MAO inhibitor Inhibitor of monoamine oxidase that degrades the neurotransmitters epinephrine, norepinephrine, dopamine, and serotonin

MAR Medication administration record

Mastitis Inflammation of the breast

Mastodynia Pain in swollen female breasts

Materia medica Listing of the various materials from plants, animals, or minerals that are used in medical and healing systems

Melanoma A malignant tumor or neoplasm of the pigment-producing cells of skin and mucosa; may metastasize to other organs

Menopause Permanent cessation of menstruation resulting from decreased production of female sex hormones; a natural phenomenon around age 50 in which the woman completes her reproductive phase of her life

Menorrhagia Abnormally severe menstruation

Metabolism The physical and chemical changes that take place within an organism to maintain life

Metastasis The movement or spread of cancerous cells through the body to organs in distant areas

Meter Basic measurement of length in the metric system

Metered dose inhaler (MDI) A dispenser for supplying medications to the lungs through inhalation

Micro Small

Microbial Refers to minute living organisms visible with a microscope, fungi, protozoa, and bacteria

Microbiology The study of microscopic organisms

Microgram One one-thousandth of a milligram; metric unit of measure; 10^{-6} g

Microtubules Linear tubular structure of cells essential for cell division and transport process in the cell

Micturition Urination

Migraine Recurrent condition of severe pain in the head often accompanied by symptoms such as nausea and visual disturbances

Milligram One one-thousandth of a gram; metric unit of measure; 10^{-3} grams

Mineralocorticoid The steroid of the adrenal cortex, primarily aldosterone, which regulates salt metabolism

Miosis Contraction of the pupil resulting in less light going into the eye

Mitochondrion Important compartment of eukaryotic cells; site of the Krebs cycle and respiration chain, production of ATP

Mitosis Cellular reproduction that creates two identical daughter cells from the parent cell's DNA

Molecular biosynthesis The making of chemical compounds within a living organism

Monoamine oxidase (MAO) An enzyme (includes MAO-A and MAO-B) found in the nerve terminals, the neurons, and liver cells; inactivates chemicals such as tyramine, catecholamines, serotonin, and certain medications

Monograph Medication information sheet that includes side effects, dosage forms, indications, and other important information; must be provided by the manufacturer to FDA

Morals Ethics; honorable beliefs

Morphology Appearance, including shape, size, structure, and stain characteristics of organisms; study of organisms without studying the function

Mortar and pestle A bowl and rounded knob used to grind substances into fine powder

Mucilage A solution of viscous or slimy substances, usually polysaccharides, that form a protective layer over inflamed mucosal tissues

Mucolytic Substance that dissolves mucus, such as in the bronchus

Mucosa Mucous tissue layer on the inside of the respiratory, gastrointestinal tract

Mucus Clear, viscous secretion formed by mucous membranes

Multiple sclerosis Disorder of the central nervous system caused by a destruction of the myelin around axons in the brain and spinal cord, leading to various neurologic symptoms

Mutagenic A substance that induces genetic mutations

Muscarinic Relating to acetylcholine receptor type and cholinergic function of the parasympathetic nervous systems, including decrease in heart rate, dilation of arterioles, increase in gut motility, and stimulation of glands

Mutation An unexpected change in the molecular structure within the DNA, sometimes causing a permanent change in the expression of proteins in cells

Myalgia Nonlocalized muscle pain

Mycosis Fungal disease

Mydriasis Dilation of the pupil

Myopia Nearsightedness

Myxedema Condition associated with the a decrease in overall thyroid function in adults; also known as *hypothyroidism*

Narcotic A controlled substance that acts on the central nervous system to relieve pain

National Association of Boards of Pharmacy (NABP) National organization for members of state boards of pharmacy

Naturopathy A holistic system of healing that emphasizes the body's inherent power of regaining balance and harmony

Necrosis Death of cells or tissue

Negative feedback A self-regulating mechanism in which the output of a system has input or control on the process; a factor within a system that causes a corrective action to return the system to normal range

Neoplasm An abnormal tissue growth

Nephritis Kidney inflammation

Nerve terminal The end portion of the neuron where nerve impulses cause chemical to be released; these neurochemicals cross a small space, the synaptic cleft, to carry the impulse to another neuron

Neuralgia Severe pain along nerve ends

Neuron The functional unit of the nervous system

Neurosis Mental illness arising from stress or anxiety in the patient's environment without loss of contact with reality; phobias can be listed in this category; vs. psychosis

Neurotransmitter Chemicals in synapses of neurons that relay signals; important neurotransmitters are acetylcholine, epinephrine, norepinephrine, dopamine, serotonin, histamine, glycine, GABA, glutamate, endorphins, and peptides

Nicotinic Relating to acetylcholine receptor subtype and cholinergic function the autonomic nervous system, especially at the ganglion and neuromuscular junction, causing skeletal muscle changes and widespread organ regulation

NKDA No known drug allergy

NKFA No known food allergy

Nocturia Nightly urge to urinate

Nonproductive cough Cough that does not produce mucous secretions from the respiratory tract

Normal flora Microorganisms that reside harmlessly in the body and do not cause disease but may aid the host organism

Nosocomial infection An infection acquired while hospitalized

NSAID Nonsteroidal anti-inflammatory drug

Nucleic acid The molecule bases contained within deoxyribonucleic acid (DNA)

Nutritional supplement A preparation that supplies additional nutrients or active compounds to the body that may not be obtained by the normal diet

Ointment A semisolid hydrophobic medicinal preparation used topically

On-call A medication to be administered when directed, usually for preanesthesia

Oncogene A previously normal gene that may be adversely affected by infection, such as a retrovirus, which causes a mutation and may produce cancer

Oocyte or ovum The female reproductive germ cell

Ophthalmic Pertaining to the eye

Orbit The bone casing of the eye

*Organic Term used for products grown and processed without use of artificial chemicals, such as hormones, pesticides, or plastic derivatives; wild-harvested materials usually qualify

Osteoporosis Condition associated with the decrease of bone mass and the softening of the bones, increasing the possibility of bone fractures

OTC Over-the-counter; a drug sold without prescription in the United States, nonlegend medications

Otic Pertaining to the ear

Otitis Inflammation of the ear

Outpatient pharmacy Pharmacies that serve patients in their communities; pharmacies that are not in inpatient facilities

Oxytocic Speeding up of parturition, or birth

Oxytocin A pituitary gland hormone that stimulates lactation, induces uterine contractions and labor

Paget disease Condition affecting older adults in which the density of the bones decreases

Palliative Brings relief but does not cure

PAR Periodic automatic replacement

Parasite Organism that uses a host for nourishment and reproduction without benefiting the host

Parasympathetic nervous system Division of the autonomic nervous system that functions during restful situations; slows the heart rate, increases intestinal smooth muscle and gland activity, and relaxes sphincter muscles

Parenteral Medication administered by routes outside the gut or enteric system; common routes include subcutaneous, intravenous, and intramuscular injection

Parkinson disease A progressive neurologic disease caused by degeneration of the substantia nigra and a reduction in dopamine concentrations, marked by lack of muscular coordination and mental deterioration, manifesting in unnaturally slow or rigid movements

Passive immunity Resistance to infection acquired through a transfer of antibodies from outside the body, from mother to child, from animal contact, or from vaccinations; vs. active immunity

Pathogen A microorganism that can cause disease

Peptic ulcer An ulcerative condition of the lower esophagus, stomach, or duodenum, often resulting from the bacterium *Helicobacter pylori*

Peptidoglycan The substance that comprises bacterial cell walls, thicker in gram-positive than in gram-negative microbes

Periodontitis Inflammation of the area around a tooth

Peripheral nervous system (PNS) The division of the nervous system outside the brain and spinal cord

Peripheral parenteral Injection of a medication into the veins located on the periphery of the body system, in arms or legs, instead of a central vein or artery

Peristalsis Waves of involuntary contraction of the smooth muscles of the digestive system

Pharmacist Person who dispenses drugs and counsels patients about drugs

Pharmacodynamics The study of how medicinal substances work in the body

Pharmacognosy The study of herbal drugs and their identification, properties, and uses

Pharmacokinetics The study of how medicinal substances are absorbed, moved, distributed, metabolized, and excreted

Pharmacology The study of the nature, properties, and uses of drugs and their effects on the body

Pharmacopoeia An official publication listing all the various drugs that may be used

Phlegm Catarrhal secretion or sputum

Phosphodiesterase Important enzyme of signal transduction; inactivates cAMP or cGMP

Phospholipids Phosphorylated lipids that are the building blocks of cell membranes

Photosensitization Increased sensitivity to sunlight

Physician's Desk Reference **(PDR)** Reference book of medications

Phytotherapy Application of plant drugs or products derived from plants to cure diseases or to relieve symptoms

Placebo Drug preparation without active ingredient that cannot be distinguished from the original drug

Placebo effect An improvement of a health condition that cannot be ascribed to the treatment used

PMS Premenstrual syndrome, now called *premenstrual dysphoric disorder,* PMDD; usually occurs a few days before menstruation with symptoms of fear, irritability, changing mood, insomnia, headache, swollen breasts, abdominal pain, edema, decreased libido; thought to result from changing sex hormone levels causing hypoglycemia and endogenous opioid release

POS Point of sale

Poultice A semisolid mass of plant materials in oil or water applied to the skin

PPO Preferred Provider Organization

Pre-op A drug ordered to be given before surgery, or preoperatively

PRN *Pro re nata* (Latin); take as needed

Prodrug A substance that is converted to its active form within the body

Productive cough Cough that expectorates mucous secretions from the respiratory tract

Professionalism Conforming to the principles of conduct (work ethics) as accepted by others in the profession

Prophylaxis Treatment given before an event to prevent the event from happening

Prostaglandins Physiologically active substances in the cell membrane of tissues that cause stimulation of muscles and numerous other metabolic effects; released during cell damage. Promote the inflammatory process, including pain, swelling, heat

Prostate A gland at the base of the male bladder that secretes a fluid that forms a part of semen, stimulating sperm motility

Protectant A substance that acts as a barrier between the skin and an irritant

Protocol A set of standards and guidelines within which a facility works

Proton A subatomic particle of an atom that holds a positive charge; the hydrogen ion, H^+

Protozoa Kingdom Protista; unicellular organisms that are usually parasites

Pruritus Itching

Psoriasis Skin condition caused by an enhanced growth of dermal cells, resulting in the production of excess skin, or dandruff

Psychosis A mental illness characterized by loss of contact with reality; vs. necrosis

Psychotherapeutic Relating to classes of drugs or agents that affect the mind and brain; categories include tricyclic antidepressants, SSRIs, and phenothiazines

Psychotropic A substance that affects the mind or mood

Pyretic A substance that induces fever

Recall When a drug or device must be returned to the manufacturer because of a failure to meet FDA standards

Receptor Protein, often attached to a cell membrane, that has a binding site for another molecule called a *ligand*, important for signal transduction in cells

Reconstitution To mix a liquid and a powder to form a suspension or solution

Remission The span of time during which a disease, such as cancer, is not spreading

Resorption Uptake of a substance through the skin or a mucous membrane

Rheumatism General term referring to painful joints

Rhinitis Inflammation of the mucosal lining of the nose; runny nose

ROA Route of administration

Rods Photoreceptors that respond to dim light and are responsible for black and white color (night vision)

RTS Return to stock

Rx Latin for *recipe*, commonly used to mean *prescription*, legend drug, prescription drug

Sarcoma A malignant, neoplastic growth arising from connective tissue

Saturated fat Fat with fatty acids saturated with hydrogen, therefore without double bonds, such as animal fats, coconut oil; more easily taken up by the body and therefore unfavorable; vs. unsaturated fat

Schizophrenia A group of mental disorders characterized by inappropriate emotions and unrealistic thinking

Script A prescription

Sedative-hypnotic Central nervous system depressants used to induce sleep; tranquilizer

Semen The fluid released from penis during orgasm that contains sperm

Shaman Medicine person who holds a high place of honor in a tribe and emphasizes spiritual connection

Sig Medication directions written in pharmacy terms on a prescription

Sitz-bath An immersion bath used for medicinal purposes

Solute The ingredient that is dissolved into a solution

Solution A water base in which the ingredients dissolve completely

Solvent The greater part of a solution; what the ingredient is dissolved into

Somatic The motor neurons that control voluntary actions of the skeletal muscles

Soporific A substance that induces or promotes sleep

Spasm Involuntary contraction of muscles

Species Latin origin meaning *kind* or *type*; used to differentiate one biologic item from another

Spondylitis Inflammation of vertebrae

Sputum Fluid coughed up from the lungs and bronchial tissues

STAT order A medication order that must be filled as soon as possible, usually within 5-15 min

Steroid Messenger chemical produced by the body; helps to fight inflammation and pain

Sunscreen A substance that protects the skin from ultraviolet light, which causes sunburns

Suspension A solution is which the powder does not dissolve into the base and must be shaken before using

Symbiotic A close relationship between two species, in which both can benefit

Sympathetic nervous system Division of the autonomic nervous system that functions during stressful situations; accelerates the heart rate, constricts blood vessels, and raises blood pressure; mediated by α- and β-adrenergic receptors

Sympathomimetic Resembling the adrenergic effects of the sympathetic nervous system

Synapse The space between which neurons are connected with each other or with target tissues via neurotransmitters as a way of converting electrical into chemical signals

Synergistic The phenomenon that the combined effect of two or more substances is greater than the sum of their individual effects

Synthesis The formation of components within a body system

Synthetic Medication made in a laboratory or factory

Syrup A sugar-based liquid solution intended to ease oral administration of a drug

Systemic Affecting the entire body rather than individual body parts

Tachycardia Fast beating of the heart; in adults, more than 100 beats/min

Tardive dyskinesia Unwanted side effects of taking dopamine blockers that include slow, rhythmical involuntary movements that are either generalized or specific to one muscle group

Taxonomy The science of classification and nomenclature of organisms

TCM Traditional Chinese Medicine; one of the oldest therapeutic systems of mankind still in use

Tea An infusion made by pouring boiling water over a measured quantity of dried plant material and leaving it for a while to steep; vs. maceration

Teratogenic A substance that causes abnormal growth in an embryo

Testosterone The male sex hormone

Therapeutic Curative treatment that is effective

Thoracic Related to the chest or thorax

Thrombin An enzyme that is converted in coagulating blood from prothrombin, which reacts with fibrinogen, converting it into fibrin, which is essential in the formation of blood clots; tested by performing a prothrombin time (PT) or partial thromboplastin time (PTT) blood test

Thrombolytic Medication used to break up a thrombus or blood clot

Thrush A fungal infection of mucous membranes marked by white patches, caused by *Candida* spp.

Thyroxine Known as T_4; contains four ions of iodine

Tincture A base solution of alcohol

Tinnitus Ringing noise in the ear

Tisane An herbal tea often made from flowers that is not as strong as an infusion

Tonic A substance that maintains or restores health and vigor, usually taken over a lengthy period

Topical application External application on the skin

Total parenteral nutrition (TPN) Large-volume IV nutrition administered through the central vein (subclavian vein), allowing for a higher concentration of solutions

Tourette syndrome A neurologic disorder characterized by multiple motor tics, lack of muscle coordination, and involuntary movements that are often accompanied by grunts and barks

Toxicology Science that studies toxins and their effects in humans or animals

Toxoid A toxin that has been rendered harmless but still invokes an antigenic response

Trace elements Chemical elements that are needed by the body in very small amounts

Tradename Brand name drug; the company that first applies for a patent on the chemical structure of a medication or generic name is allowed to name the product with a patented name

Transporter A membrane protein that catalyzes the transport of a molecule from one side of a biomembrane to the other side

Tri-iodothyronine Known as T_3; contains three ions of iodine

Tuberculosis A bacterial disease caused by *Mycobacterium tuberculosis* that affects the lungs and later other organs, often chronic and fatal if not treated

Tumor An abnormal growth of tissue, can be benign or malignant

Tympanic membrane A membrane that separates the external ear from the middle ear

Ulcer A lesion on the skin or a mucous membrane; a lesion on the mucosal lining of the stomach or intestines that causes burning pain, bleeding, and maldigestion

Unit dose A single dose of a drug delivered in one time period

Universal Precautions A set of standards that lowers the possibility of infection

Unsaturated fat Fat with fatty acids with double bonds between the carbon atoms instead of hydrogens, such as olive oil and canola oil

Urinary calculus Concrete formation of salts, usually stone, in the ureters

Urticaria A skin eruption of itching wheals

Vaccine Toxoids or attenuated viral components that are given to create a response from the body that results in immunity

Varicose veins Abnormally distended veins

Vasoconstrictor A substance that causes narrowing of the blood vessels

Vasodilation Widening of the blood vessels that allows for increased blood flow

Vector A carrier, especially one who transfers an infective agent from one host to another without getting the disease; for example, a mosquito bite transfers malaria from the mosquito's saliva without the mosquito having the disease

Vein A vessel that carries deoxygenated blood toward the heart

Vertical flow hood Environment for the preparation of chemotherapy treatments

Vertigo Sensation of instability

Villus A projection from the surface of a mucous membrane; in the gastric tract, these projections increase the surface area for the absorption of nutrients and liquids in the small intestines

Virology The study of viruses

Virus Infectious complex of macromolecules that contain their genetic information either as DNA or RNA; replicates by using the host's cell parts to form new viral particles

Viscosity The thickness of a solution or fluid

Vitamin An organic substance that occurs in many foods and is necessary in trace amounts for the normal metabolic functioning of the human body

Volatile oil Various terpenoids that evaporate easily; usually add taste and smell to plants

Volume The amount of substance enclosed within a container

Vomit The expulsion of matter from the stomach via the mouth

Wild-crafting The collection of medicinal material from natural plant populations in a sustainable way

Workers' compensation A government-required and enforced coverage for workers injured on the job

Yeast Simple eukaryotic cells belonging to the fungus kingdom; *Candida* spp. commonly infect vulnerable human mucous membranes

*Some definitions from Hopper T: *Mosby's Pharmacy Technician, Principles and Practice.* St. Louis, 2004, Saunders.

INDEX

A

A200 Lice, 1244–1246
abacavir, 1–2
abarelix, 2–4
Abbocillin VK [AUS], 1228–1230
abciximab, 4–6
Abelcet, 100–103
Abenol [CAN], 12–14
Abilify, 123–125
Abraxane, 1187–1188
Abreva, 503–504
absorbable gelatin sponge, 6–7
Absorbine Jr. Antifungal, 1550–1551
acamprosate, 7–8
acarbose, 8–9
Accolate, 1634–1635
AccuNeb, 34–36
Accupril, 1366–1368
Accutane, 853–854
acebutolol, 10–12
Acenorm [AUS], 250–252
Aceon, 1243–1244
Acetadote, 18–19
acetaminophen, 12–14
Acetasol, 16–17
acetazolamide, 14–16
acetic acid, 16–17
Acetoxyl [CAN], 177–178
acetylcysteine, 18–19
acetylsalicylic acid, 130–133
Aciclovir-BC IV [AUS], 21–24
Acid Jelly, 16–17
Acidic Vaginal Jelly, 16–17
Acihexal [AUS], 21–24
Aci-Jel, 16–17
Aciphex, 1372–1373
acitretin, 19–21
Aclin [AUS], 1472–1473
Aclovate, 36–37
Acova, 122–123
Actacode [AUS], 379–381
Act-3 [AUS], 788–790
Acticin, 1244–1246
Actidose with Sorbitol, 314–315
Actidose-Aqua, 314–315
Actigall, 1590–1591
Actilyse, 58–60
Actimmune, 832–833
Actiq, 638–643
Activase [AUS], 58–60
Activase Cathflo, 58–60
Actonel, 1398–1399
Actos, 1284–1285
Actrapid [AUS], 813–815
Acular, 868–871

Acular LS, 868–871
Acular PF, 868–871
acyclovir, 21–24
Acyclo-V [AUS], 21–24
Aczone, 415–416
Adalat 5 [AUS], 1113–1115
Adalat 10 [AUS], 1113–1115
Adalat 20 [AUS], 1113–1115
Adalat CC, 1113–1115
Adalat Oros [AUS], 1113–1115
adalimumab, 24–26
adapalene, 26–27
Adderall, 98–100
Adderall XR, 98–100
adefovir dipivoxil, 27–28
Adenocard, 28–30
Adenocor [AUS], 28–30
Adenoscan, 28–30
adenosine, 28–30
Adipex-P, 1256–1257
Adipost, 1249–1250
AD-Nephrin, 1259–1262, 1266–1268
Adoxa, 523–526
Adrenalin, 562–566
Adrenaline Injection [AUS], 562–566
Adriamycin, 521–522
Adrucil, 668–669
Advate, 115–116
Advil, 788–790
Aerius, 435–437
AeroBid, 662–664
Aerobin [GERMANY], 1513–1515
Aerodil [AUS], 596–600
Aerodyne Retard [AUSTRIA], 1513–1515
Aerospan HFA, 662–664
Aerosporin, 1296–1298
A-Fil, 114–115
Afonilum Forte [GERMANY],
    1513–1515
Afonilum Mite [GERMANY], 1513–1515
Afonilum Retard, 1513–1515
Afrin, 1179–1180
Afrin Children's Strength Nose Drops,
    1179–1180
Afrin 12-Hour, 1179–1180
Af-Taf [ISRAEL], 1259–1262, 1263–1266
Aftate Antifungal, 1550–1551
agalsidase-ß, 30–31
Aggrastat, 1539–1540
Agrylin, 109–110
AHF. *See* antihemophilic factor
A-HydroCort, 769–773
Airomir [AUS], 34–36
Akamin [AUS], 1037–1038
AK-Con, 1087–1088

AK-Dilate, 1259–1262, 1263–1266, 1266–1268
AK-Fluor, 665–667
Akne-Mycin, 585–589
AK-Pred, 1314–1316
AK-Sulf, 1466–1467
AK-Tate [CAN], 1314–1316
AK-Tob, 1541–1544
Alamast, 1215–1216
Ala-Quin, 359–360
Alavert, 922–923
Albalon Liquifilm [AUS], 1087–1088
Albalon Relief [NEW ZEALAND], 1259–1262, 1263–1266
albendazole, 31–33
Albenza, 31–33
Albert [CAN], 1240–1241
Albumex [AUS], 33–34
albumin, human, 33–34
Albuminar, 33–34
Albutein, 33–34
albuterol, 34–36
alclometasone, 36–37
Alcomicin [CAN], 719–723
Aldactone, 1454–1456
Aldara, 800–801
Aldazine [AUS], 1519–1520
Aldecin [AUS], 165–167
Aldecin Hayfever Aqueous Nasal Spray [AUS], 165–167
aldesleukin, 37–40, 833–835
Aldomet, 1003–1004
alefacept, 40–42
alemtuzumab, 42–43
alendronate, 44–45
Alepam [AUS], 1170–1172
Alertec [CAN], 1047–1048
Aleve, 1088–1091
Alferon N, 825–826
alfuzosin, 45–46
Alimta, 1213–1215
Alinia, 1119–1120
aliskiren, 46–47
alitretinoin, 47–48
Alka-Seltzer Gas Relief, 1436–1437
Allegra, 646–647
Allegron [AUS], 1138–1140
Aller-Chlor, 325–327
Allerdryl [CAN], 491–495
Allermax Aqueous [AUS], 1052–1053
Allfen, 743–744
Alli [OTC], 1160–1161
Allohexal [AUS], 49–51
allopurinol, 49–51
Allosig [AUS], 49–51

Almarion [THAILAND], 1513–1515
almotriptan, 51–52
Alocril, 1096–1097
Alodox, 523–526
Alomide, 916–917
Alophen, 192–193
Aloprim, 49–51
Alora, 596–600
alosetron, 52–54
Aloxi, 1189–1190
Alphacin [AUS], 103–106
Alphagan P, 208–209
Alphamax [AUS], 94–96
Alphanate, 115–116
AlphaNine SD, 625–626
Alphapress [AUS], 760–762
Alphapril [AUS], 550–553
Alphaquin HP, 777–778
Alphatrex, 181–183
alprazolam, 54–56
alprostadil, 56–58
Altace, 1375–1377
Altaryl, 491–495
alteplase, 58–60
Alternagel, 62–63
Alti-Azathioprine [CAN], 149–150
Alti-Clobetasol [CAN], 360–361
Altinac, 1571–1573
Alti-Sulfasalazine [CAN], 1467–1469
Altoprev, 928–929
aluminum acetate/acetic acid, 63–66
aluminum chloride hexahydrate, 60–61
aluminum hydroxide, 62–63
aluminum hydroxide/magnesium carbonate, 63–66
aluminum hydroxide/magnesium hydroxide, 63–66
aluminum hydroxide/magnesium hydroxide simethicone, 63–66
aluminum hydroxide/magnesium trisilicate, 63–66
aluminum hydroxide/magnesium trisilicate/simethicone, 63–66
aluminum salts, 63–66
aluminum sulfate/calcium acetate, 63–66
Alupent, 974–976
Alustra, 777–778
Alu-Tab, 62–63
Alvesco, 337–338
amantadine hydrochloride, 66–68
Amaryl, 724–725
Amatine, 1030–1031
ambenonium, 68–69
Ambien, 1645
AmBisome, 100–103

ambrisentan, 69–70
amcinonide, 71–72
Amerge, 1091–1092
Americaine Anesthetic Lubricant, 174–175
Americaine Otic, 174–175
A-Methapred, 1008–1011
Ametop [CAN], 1505–1508
Amevive, 40–42
Amicar, 77–79
Amidate, 1647
amifostine, 72–73
amikacin, 73–75
Amikin, 73–75
amiloride hydrochloride, 76–77
aminocaproic acid, 77–79
aminophylline, 79–81
aminosalicylic acid, 81–82
5-Aminosalicylic acid, 973–974
Aminoxin, 1359–1361
amiodarone, 82–85
amitriptyline, 85–87
Amlactin, 89–90
amlexanox, 87–88
amlodipine, 88–89
ammonium lactate, 89–90
Amnesteem, 853–854
amobarbital, 90–92
Amohexal [AUS], 94–96
amoxapine, 92–94
amoxicillin, 94–96, 1223–1225
amoxicillin/clavulanate, 96–98
amoxicillin/clavulanate potassium, 1223–1225
Amoxil, 94–96
amphetamine, 98–100
Amphocin, 100–103
Amphojel [CAN], 62–63
Amphotec, 100–103
amphotericin B, 100–103
amphotericin B cholesteryl, 100–103
amphotericin B lipid complex, 100–103
ampicillin, 1223–1225
ampicillin sodium, 104–106
ampicillin/sulbactam, 106–108
ampicillin/sulbactam sodium, 1223–1225
Amprace [AUS], 550–553
amyl nitrite, 108–109
Amyl Nitrite, 108–109
Amytal sodium, 90–92
Anadrol, 1180–1182
Anafranil, 364–366
anagrelide, 109–110
anakinra, 110–111
Analpram-HC, 1309–1310

Anamorph [AUS], 1057–1061
Anandron [CAN], 1115–1116
Anapolon [CAN], 1180–1182
Anaprox, 1088–1091
Anaprox DS, 1088–1091
Anaspaz, 784–786
anastrozole, 111–113
Anatensol [AUS], 673–674
Anbesol, 174–175
Anbesol Baby Gel, 174–175
Anbesol Maximum Strength, 174–175
Ancef, 276–278
Ancobon, 657–659
Andriol [CAN], 1502–1505
Androderm, 1502–1505
AndroGel, 1502–1505
Android, 1011–1012
Android-10, 1011–1012
Android-25, 1011–1012
Andropository [CAN], 1502–1505
Androxy, 671–673
Anesthetics, general, 1647
Anexate [CAN], 660–662
Anexsia, 764–767
Ange 28 [JAPAN], 898–900
Anginine [AUS], 1123–1126
Angiomax, 197–198
Angiscein, 665–667
anidulafungin, 113–114
Anpec [AUS], 1609–1612
Ansaid, 679–680
Antabuse, 500–501
Antara, 634–636
Antenex [AUS], 457–461
Anthra-Derm, 114–115
Anthra-forte [CAN], 114–115
anthralin, 114–115
Anthranol [CAN], 114–115
Anthrascalp [CAN], 114–115
antihemophilic factor, 115–116
Antilirium, 1275–1276
Antiminth, 1355–1356
Antispas, 167–169
Antispasmodic, 167–169
Antivert, 950–951
Antizol, 687–689
Anturane, 1469–1470
Anusol, 1309–1310
Anusol-HC, 769–773
Anzatax [AUS], 1187–1188
Anzemet, 507–508
Apexicon, 471–472
Aphrodyne, 1632–1633
Aphthasol, 87–88
Apidra, 815–817

Apo-Acetaminophen [CAN], 12–14
Apo-Acetazolamide [CAN], 14–16
Apo-Allopurinol [CAN], 49–51
Apo-Alpraz [CAN], 54–56
Apo-Amitriptyline [CAN], 85–87
Apo-Amoxi [CAN], 94–96
Apo-Ampi [CAN], 104–106
Apo-Atenol [CAN], 135–137
Apo-Baclofen [CAN], 159–160
Apo-Benztropine [CAN], 178–180
Apo-Bisacodyl [CAN], 192–193
Apo-Bromocriptine [CAN], 210–212
Apo-C [CAN], 126–128
Apo-Cal [CAN], 241–244
Apo-Carbamazepine [CAN], 254–256
Apo-Cefaclor [CAN], 272–274
Apo-Cephalex [CAN], 308–310
Apo-Chlordiazepoxide [CAN], 318–320
Apo-Chlorpropamide [CAN], 329–331
Apo-Chlorthalidone [CAN], 331–332
Apo-Cimetidine [CAN], 343–345
Apo-Clomipramine [CAN], 364–366
Apo-Clonazepam [CAN], 366–368
Apo-Cromolyn [CAN], 389–391
Apo-Desipramine [CAN], 433–435
Apo-Diazepam [CAN], 457–461
Apo-Diflunisal [CAN], 472–474
Apo-Diltiaz [CAN], 482–486
Apo-Dipyridamole [CAN], 496–498
Apo-Docusate [CAN], 504–505
Apo-Doxy [CAN], 523–526
Apo-Enalapril [CAN], 550–553
Apo-Erythro Base [CAN], 585–589
Apo-Etodolac [CAN], 615–617
Apo-Fenofibrate [CAN], 634–636
Apo-Ferrous Gluconate [CAN], 644–645
Apo-Ferrous Sulfate [CAN], 644–645
Apo-Fluconazole [CAN], 654–657
Apo-Fluphenazine [CAN], 674–676
Apo-Flurazepam [CAN], 678–679
Apo-Folic [CAN], 686–687
Apo-Furosemide [CAN], 702–704
Apo-Gain [CAN], 1039–1041
Apo-Gemfibrozil [CAN], 714–716
Apo-Haloperidol [CAN], 750–752
Apo-Hydro [CAN], 762–764
Apo-Hydroxyquine [CAN], 779–781
Apo-Hydroxyzine [CAN], 782–784
Apo-Ibuprofen, 788–790
Apo-Imipramine [CAN], 798–800
Apo-Indomethacin [CAN], 808–811
Apo-Ipravent [CAN], 836–838
Apo-ISDN [CAN], 851–853
Apo-K [CAN], 1303–1306
Apo-Keto [CAN], 866–868

Apo-Ketoconazole [CAN], 864–866
Apokyn, 116–118
Apo-Lactulose [CAN], 874–876
Apo-Lamotrigine [CAN], 878–880
Apo-Levocarb [CAN], 257–259
Apo-Lisinopril [CAN], 912–914
Apo-Loperamide [CAN], 918–919
Apo-Lorazepam [CAN], 923–926
Apo-Loxapine [CAN], 929–930
Apo-Mefenamic [CAN], 955–957
Apo-Megestrol [CAN], 959–960
Apo-Methazolamide [CAN], 987–988
Apo-Methotrexate [CAN], 992–994
Apo-Methyldopa [CAN], 1003–1004
Apo-Metoclop [CAN], 1013–1015
Apo-Metoprolol [CAN], 1017–1020
Apo-Metronidazole [CAN], 1020–1023
Apo-Midazolam [CAN], 1028–1030
apomorphine, 116–118
Apo-Nabumetone, 1069–1070
Apo-Nadol [CAN], 1071–1072
Apo-Naprosyn [CAN], 1088–1091
Apo-Nifed [CAN], 1113–1115
Apo-Nitrofurantoin [CAN], 1120–1122
Apo-Norflox [CAN], 1135–1136
Apo-Oflox [CAN], 1144–1146
Apo-Oxazepam [CAN], 1170–1172
Apo-Pentoxifylline SR [CAN], 1240–1241
Apo-Pen-VK [CAN], 1228–1230
Apo-Pindol [CAN], 1282–1283
Apo-Piroxicam [CAN], 1289–1290
Apo-Prednisone [CAN], 1316–1318
Apo-Primidone [CAN], 1320–1321
Apo-Propranolol [CAN], 1345–1348
Apo-Quin-G [CAN], 1368–1370
Apo-Quinidine [CAN], 1368–1370
Apo-Ramipril [CAN], 1375–1377
Apo-Ranitidine [CAN], 1377–1379
Apo-Selegiline [CAN], 1424–1425
Apo-Sertraline [CAN], 1428–1430
Apo-Simvastatin [CAN], 1437–1438
Apo-Sotalol [CAN], 1451–1452
Apo-Sucralfate [CAN], 1463–1464
Apo-Sulfatrim [CAN], 376–378
Apo-Sulfinpyrazone [CAN], 1469–1470
Apo-Sulin [CAN], 1472–1473
Apo-Tamox [CAN], 1482–1484
Apo-Temazepam [CAN], 1489–1490
Apo-Terazosin [CAN], 1496–1497
Apo-Terbinafine [CAN], 1497–1499
Apo-Tetra [CAN], 1508–1509
Apo-Thioridazine [CAN], 1519–1520
Apo-Ticlopidine [CAN], 1528–1529
Apo-Timol [CAN], 1530–1532
Apo-Timop [CAN], 1530–1532

Apo-Tobramycin [CAN], 1541–1544
Apo-Tolbutamide [CAN], 1546–1547
Apo-Trazodone [CAN], 1568–1569
Apo-Tremethoprim [CAN], 1581–1582
Apo-Triazo [CAN], 1575–1576
Apo-Trihex [CAN], 1578–1579
Apo-Trimip [CAN], 1583–1584
Apo-Verap [CAN], 1609–1612
Apo-Warfarin [CAN], 1627–1629
Apo-Zidovudine [CAN], 1639–1640
apraclonidine hydrochloride, 118–119
aprepitant, 119–120
Apresoline, 760–762
Apriso, 973–974
Aproven [AUS], 836–838
Aqua Gem E, 1622–1623
Aqua Mephyton, 1277–1278
Aquachloral Supprettes, 315–317
Aquaear [AUS], 16–17
Aquasol A, 1618–1620
Aquasol E, 1622–1623
Aquatensen, 1000–1001
Aqueous Charcodote [CAN], 314–315
Ara-C, 403–404
Aralen [CAN], 321–323
Aralen hydrochloride, 321–323
Aralen phosphate, 321–323
Aramine, 976–977
Aranesp, 419–421
Aratac [AUS], 82–85
Arava, 883–884
Aredia, 1191–1192
Arestin, 1037–1038
arformoterol tartrate, 120–122
argatroban, 122–123
Aricept, 509–510
Arimidex, 111–113
aripiprazole, 123–125
Aristocort, 1316–1318
Aristospan, 1316–1318
Arixtra, 690–691
Armophylline [FRANCE], 1513–1515
Armour Thyroid, 1522–1523
Aromasin, 622–623
arsenic trioxide, 125–126
Artane, 1578–1579
Arthexin [AUS], 808–811
Asacol, 973–974
Ascendin, 92–94
ascorbic acid, 126–128
Ascriptin, 130–133
Asig [AUS], 1366–1368
Asmanex Twisthaler, 1052–1053
Asmasalon [PHILIPPINES], 1513–1515
Asmol CFC-Free [AUS], 34–36

asparaginase, 128–130
Asperal-T [BELGIUM], 1513–1515
aspirin, 130–133
Aspro [AUS], 130–133
Astelin, 152–153
AsthmaNephrin, 562–566
Astramorph, 1057–1061
Atacand, 245–247
Atarax, 782–784
Atasol [CAN], 12–14
atazanavir sulfate, 133–135
AteHexal [AUS], 135–137
atenolol, 135–137
Atgam, 931–932
Ativan, 923–926
atomoxetine, 137–139
atorvastatin, 139–140
atovaquone, 140–141
atropine, 141–143
atropine sulfate, 141–143
Atropt [AUS], 141–143
Atrovent, 836–838
Atrovent Aerosol [AUS], 836–838
Atrovent Nasal [AUS], 836–838
Attenta [AUS], 1006–1008
Augmentin, 96–98
Augmentin ES 600, 96–98
Augmentin XR, 96–98
auranofin, 143–145
Auro Ear Drops, 256–257
aurothioglucose, 145–147
Auscap [AUS], 669–671
Auscard [AUS], 482–486
Ausclav Duo 400 [AUS], 96–98
Ausclav Duo Forte [AUS], 96–98
Ausclav [AUS], 96–98
Ausgem [AUS], 714–716
Auspril [AUS], 550–553
Ausran [AUS], 1377–1379
Austyn [KOREA], 1513–1515
Avage, 1485–1486
Avandia, 1409–1410
Avanza [AUS], 1041–1042
Avapro, 838–839
Avastin, 186–188
Avelox, 1061–1062
Avelox IV, 1061–1062
Aventyl, 1138–1140
Avinza, 1057–1061
Avirax [CAN], 21–24
Avita, 1571–1573
Avodart, 533–534
Avonex, 827–828, 828–830
Axert, 51–52
Axid, 1129–1130

Axid AR, 1129–1130
Aygestin, 1132–1134
azacitidine, 147–148
Azactam, 155–157
Azasan, 149–150
azathioprine, 149–150
Azdone, 764–767
azelaic acid, 151
azelastine, 152–153
Azelex, 151
azithromycin, 153–155
Azo-Gesic, 1248–1249
Azopt, 209–210
Azo-Standard, 1248–1249
AZT, 1639–1640
aztreonam, 155–157
Azulfidine, 1467–1469
Azulfidine EN-tabs, 1467–1469

B

Babee Cof Syrup, 455–457
Babee Teething, 174–175
bacampicillin, 1223–1225
Baciguent, 158–159
Baci-IM, 158–159
bacitracin, 158–159
Bacitracin, 158–159
Backache Relief, 942–943
Baclo [AUS], 159–160
baclofen, 159–160
Bactrim, 376–378
Bactrim DS, 376–378
Bactroban, 1063–1064
BAL in Oil, 487–489
Balmex, 1641
Balminil [CAN], 743–744
Balminil Decongestant [CAN],
    1352–1354
balsalazide, 161
Bancap HC, 764–767
Banophen, 491–495
Barbidonna, 167–169
Barophen, 167–169
Basaljel [CAN], 62–63
basiliximab, 161–163
Bausch & Lomb Computer Eye Drops,
    731–733
Bayer, 130–133
Baygam [CAN], 801–803
Bayhep B, 756–757
BCG, intravesical, 163–164
Bebulin VH, 625–626
becaplermin, 164–165
Beclodisk [CAN], 165–167
Becloforte Inhaler [CAN], 165–167

beclomethasone dipropionate, 165–167
Beconase AQ, 165–167
Becotide [AUS], 165–167
Bedoz [CAN], 392–394
Beesix, 1359–1361
belladonna alkaloids, 167–169
belladonna and opium, 169–171
Bellalphen, 167–169
Bellatal, 167–169
Benadryl, 491–495
benazepril, 171–173
BeneFix, 625–626
Benicar, 1149–1150
Benicar HCT, 1149–1150
Benoquin, 1053–1054
Benoxyl [CAN], 177–178
Ben-Tann, 491–495
bentoquatam, 173
Bentrop [AUS], 178–180
Bentyl, 465–467
Bentylol [CAN], 465–467
Benuryl [CAN], 1321–1323
Benylin E [CAN], 743–744
Benzac, 177–178
Benzac AC, 177–178
Benzac AC Wash, 177–178
Benzac W, 177–178
Benzac W Wash, 177–178
Benzagel, 177–178
Benzagel Wash, 177–178
Benzashave, 177–178
benzocaine, 174–175
Benzodent, 174–175
benzonatate, 176
Benzoxyl [CAN], 177–178
benzoyl peroxide, 177–178
benztropine, 178–180
beractant, 180–181
Betaderm [CAN], 181–183
Betaferon, 828–830, 830–832
Betaloc [CAN], 1017–1020
betamethasone, 181–183
Betapace, 1451–1452
Betapace AF, 1451–1452
Betaseron, 828–830
Beta-Sol [AUS], 1517–1518
Betatrex, 181–183
Beta-Val, 181–183
Betaxin [CAN], 1517–1518
betaxolol, 183–185
Betnesol [CAN], 181–183
Betoptic-S, 183–185
Betoquin [AUS], 183–185

bevacizumab, 186–188
Bex [AUS], 130–133
bexarotene, 188–190
Bexxar, 1560–1562
Biaxin, 353–355
Biaxin XL, 353–355
bicalutamide, 190–191
Bicillin LA, 1225–1227
BiCNU, 264–265
Biltricide, 1312–1313
bimatoprost, 191–192
Biocef, 308–310
BioContact Cold 12 Hour Relief Non
    Drowsy [CAN], 1352–1354
BioQuin Durules [CAN], 1368–1370
Biquinate [AUS], 1368–1370
bisacodyl, 192–193
Bisalax [AUS], 192–193
Bismed [CAN], 193–195
bismuth subsalicylate, 193–195
bisoprolol, 195–196
bivalirudin, 197–198
Blenamax [AUS], 198–200
Blenoxane, 198–200
bleomycin sulfate, 198–200
Bleph-10, 1466–1467
Blocadren, 1530–1532
Bluboro, 63–66
B&O Supprettes 15-A, 169–171
B&O Supprettes 16-A, 169–171
Bonamine [CAN], 950–951
Bonine, 950–951
Boniva, 787–788
Bontril PDM, 1249–1250
Bontril Slow-Release, 1249–1250
Borofair, 16–17
bortezomib, 200–201
bosentan, 202–203
Botox, 203–205
botulinum toxin type A, 203–205
botulinum toxin type B, 205–206
Bretylate [CAN], 207–208
bretylium, 207–208
Bretylium Tosylate-Dextrose, 207–208
Brevibloc, 590–593
Brevital, 1647
Brevoxyl, 177–178
Brevoxyl Cleansing, 177–178
Brevoxyl Wash, 177–178
Bricanyl [CAN], 1499–1400
brimonidine, 208–209
brinzolamide, 209–210
bromocriptine, 210–212
Bromohexal [AUS], 210–212

brompheniramine, 212–214
Bronchoretard [GERMANY], 1513–1515
Bronsolvan [INDONESIA], 1513–1515
Brovana, 121–122
BroveX, 212–214
BroveX CT, 212–214
Brufen [AUS], 788–790
Buckley's DM Cough, 455–457
Buckley's Mixture, 455–457
budesonide, 214–216
Bufferin, 130–133, 942–944
bumetanide, 216–218
Bumex, 216–218
Buminate, 33–34
bupivacaine, 218–222
Buprenex, 222–223
buprenorphine, 222–223
bupropion, 223–225
Burinex [CAN], 216–218
Buscopan [CAN], 784–786
BuSpar, 225–226
Buspirex [CAN], 225–226
buspirone, 225–226
Bustab [CAN], 225–226
busulfan, 226–228
Busulfex, 226–228
butabarbital sodium, 228–229
butenafine, 229–230
Butisol, 228–229
butoconazole, 230–231
butorphanol, 231–233

C
cabergoline, 234–235
Cafcit, 235–236
Cafergot [CAN], 579–581
caffeine citrate, 235–236
Calan, 1609–1612
Calan SR, 1609–1612
Calcibind, 307–308
Calciferol, 1620–1621
Calciject, 241–244
Calcijex, 240–241
Calcimar, 238–239
Calcione, 241–244
calcipotriene, 237–238
Calciquid, 241–244
calcitonin, 238–239
Calcitrate, 241–244
calcitriol, 240–241
Calcium Disodium Versenate, 538–540
calcium EDTA, 538–540
Calcium Leucovorin [AUS], 887–889
calcium salts, 241–244
Caldesene Powder, 1589

calfactant, 244–245
Calsan [CAN], 241–244
Calsup [AUS], 241–244
Caltine [CAN], 238–239
Caltrate, 241–244
Camilla, 1132–1134
Campath, 42–43
Campral, 7–8
Camptosar, 839–841
Cancidas, 269–271
candesartan, 245–247
Candyl-D [AUS], 1289–1290
Canesten [CAN], 373–374
Capastat [AUS], 248–249
Capastat Sulfate, 248–249
capecitabine, 247–248
Capex, 664–665
Capoten, 250–252
capreomycin, 248–249
capsaicin, 249–250
Captohexal [AUS], 250–252
captopril, 250–252
Capurate [AUS], 49–51
Carac, 668–669
Carafate, 1463–1464
carbachol, 253
Carbacot, 991–992
carbamazepine, 254–256
carbamide peroxide, 256–257
Carbatrol, 254–256
carbenicillin, 1223–1225
carbidopa/levodopa, 257–259
carboplatin, 259–261
carboprost, 261–263
Cardcal [AUS], 482–486
Cardene, 1108–1111
Cardene IV, 1108–1111
Cardene SR, 1108–1111
Cardizem, 482–486
Cardizem CD, 482–486
Cardizem LA, 482–486
Cardol [AUS], 1451–1452
Carimune, 801–803
carisoprodol, 263–264
carmustine, 264–265
Caroptic, 253
carteolol, 265–267
Cartia XT, 482–486
carvedilol, 267–269
Casodex, 190–191
caspofungin acetate, 269–271
castor oil, 271–272
Cataflam, 461–464
Catapres, 368–370
Catapres TTS, 368–370

Cathflo Activase, 58–60
Caverject, 56–58
Caverject Impulse, 56–58
c7E3, 4–6
Ceclor, 272–274
Ceclor CD, 272–274
Cecon, 126–128
Cedax, 297–298
Cedocard [CAN], 851–853
cefaclor, 272–274
cefadroxil, 274–275
cefazolin, 276–278
cefdinir, 278–280
cefditoren, 280–281
cefepime, 281–283
cefixime, 283–285
Cefizox, 298–300
Cefkor [AUS], 272–274
Cefkor CD [AUS], 272–274
Cefotan, 287–289
cefotaxime, 285–287
cefotetan, 287–289
cefoxitin, 289–291
cefpodoxime, 291–293
cefprozil, 293–294
ceftazidime, 294–296
ceftibuten, 297–298
Ceftin, 303–305
ceftizoxime, 298–300
ceftriaxone, 300–302
cefuroxime, 303–305
Cefzil, 293–294
Celebrex, 305–306
celecoxib, 305–306
Celestone, 181–183
Celexa, 351–353
CellCept, 1066–1068
cellulose sodium phosphate, 307–308
Celontin, 998–1000
Cenestin, 600–602
Cenolate, 126–128
Cepacol, 174–175
cephalexin, 308–310
Ceporex [AUS], 308–310
Ceptaz, 294–296
Cerebyx, 699–700
Cerezyme, 795–796
Cerubidine, 424–427
Cervidil, 489–491
C.E.S. [CAN], 600–602
Cetacaine, 174–175
Ceta-Plus, 764–767
cetirizine, 310–311
cetuximab, 311–313
cevimeline, 313–314

C-Flox [AUS], 347–350
Chantix, 1604–1605
CharcoAid-G, 314–315
charcoal, activated, 314–315
Charcoal Plus DS, 314–315
Charcocaps, 314–315
Chardonna-2, 167–169
Chemet, 1462–1463
Chiggerex, 174–175
Chiggertox, 174–175
chloral hydrate, 315–317
chloramphenicol, 317–318
Chlorate, 325–327
chlordiazepoxide, 318–320
chlorhexidine gluconate, 320–321
Chlorhexidine Mouthwash [AUS], 320–321
Chlorhexidine Obstetric Lotion [AUS], 320–321
Chlorohex Gel [AUS], 320–321
Chlorohex Gel Forte [AUS], 320–321
Chlorohex Mouth Rinse [AUS], 320–321
Chloromycetin, 317–318
chloroquine, 321–323
chloroquine phosphate, 321–323
chlorothiazide, 323–325
Chlorphen, 325–327
chlorpheniramine, 325–327
Chlorpromanyl [CAN], 327–329
chlorpromazine, 327–329
chlorpropamide, 329–331
Chlorsig [AUS], 317–318
chlorthalidone, 331–332
Chlor-Trimeton, 325–327
Chlor-Trimeton Allergy, 325–327
Chlor-Trimeton Allergy 8 Hour, 325–327
Chlor-Trimeton Allergy 12 Hour, 325–327
Chlor-Tripolon [CAN], 325–327
chlorzoxazone, 332–333
Cholac, 874–876
cholecalciferol, 1620–1621
cholestyramine resin, 333–335
choline magnesium trisalicylate, 335–336
Chronovera [CAN], 1609–1612
Cialis, 1480–1481
Cibalith-S, 914–916
ciclesonide, 337–338
ciclopirox, 339–340
cidofovir, 340–342
Cidomycin [CAN], 719–723
Cilamox [AUS], 94–96
Cilicaine VK [AUS], 1228–1230
Ciloquin [AUS], 347–350
cilostazol, 342–343
Ciloxan, 347–350
Cimehexal [AUS], 343–345

cimetidine, 343–345
cinacalcet, 346–347
Cipramil [AUS], 351–353
Cipro, 347–350
ciprofloxacin, 347–350
Ciproxin [AUS], 347–350
cisplatin, 350–351
citalopram, 351–353
Citracal, 241–244
Citrate of Magnesia, 938–942
Citro-Mag [CAN], 938–942
citrovorum factor, 887–889
Citrucel, 1002–1003
Claforan, 285–287
Clamoxyl [AUS], 94–96, 96–98
Clamoxyl Duo 400 [AUS], 96–98
Clamoxyl Duo Forte [AUS], 96–98
Claravis, 853–854
Clarinex, 435–437
Clarinex Redi-Tabs, 435–437
Claripel, 777–778
clarithromycin, 353–355
Claritin, 922–923
Claritin RediTab, 922–923
Clavulin [CAN], 96–98
Clavulin Duo Forte [AUS], 96–98
Clear Eyes [AUS], 1087–1088
Clearplex, 177–178
clemastine, 355–356
Cleocin, 356–358
Cleocin-T, 356–358
Climara, 596–600
Clinac BPO, 177–178
Clindamax, 356–358
clindamycin, 356–358
Clindesse, 356–358
Clinoril, 1472–1473
clioquinol, 359–360
clobetasol, 360–361
clocortolone, 361–362
Cloderm, 361–362
Cloderm [CAN], 361–362
clofarabine, 362–363
Clofen [AUS], 159–160
Clolar, 362–363
Clomhexal [AUS], 363–364
Clomid, 363–364
Clomid [CAN], 363–364
clomiphene, 363–364
clomipramine, 364–366
Clonapam [CAN], 366–368
clonazepam, 366–368
clonidine, 368–370
clopidogrel, 370–371
Clopine [AUS], 374–376

Clopram [AUS], 364–366
clorazepate, 371–373
Closina [AUS], 397–398
Clotrimaderm [CAN], 373–374
clotrimazole, 373–374
cloxacillin, 1223–1225
clozapine, 374–376
Clozaril, 374–376
CO Ramipril [CAN], 1375–1377
codeine, 379–381
Codeine Linctus [AUS], 379–381
Codeine Phosphate Injection, 379–381
Codiclear DH, 764–767
Codimal A, 212–214
Codral Period Pain [AUS], 788–790
Cogentin, 178–180
Co-Gesic, 764–767
Cognex, 1476–1477
Colace, 504–505
Colax-C [CAN], 504–505
Colazal, 161
colchicine, 381–382
Colchicine, 381–382
Coldcough, 764–767
colesevelam, 382–383
Colestid, 383–385
Colestid [CAN], 383–385
colestipol, 383–385
Colgout [AUS], 381–382
Colhist, 212–214
Colo-Fresh, 193–195
Cologel, 1002–1003
Coloxyl [AUS], 504–505
CoLyte, 1295–1296
Combantrin [CAN], 1355–1356
Commit, 1111–1113
Compazine, 1329–1332
Compound W, 1413–1415
Compound W One Step Wart Remover,
    1413–1415
Comtan, 557–559
Concerta, 1006–1008
Condyline [CAN], 1290–1291
Condyline Paint [AUS], 1290–1291
Condylox, 1290–1291
Congest [CAN], 600–602
conivaptan, 385–386
Constilac, 874–876
Constulose, 874–876
Contin [CAN], 379–381
Copaxone, 723–724
Copegus, 1387–1389
Coras [AUS], 482–486
Cordarone, 82–85
Cordarone X [AUS], 82–85

Cordilox SR [AUS], 1609–1612
Cordran, 676–677
Cordran SP, 676–677
Coreg, 267–269
Coreg CR Dilatrend [AUS], 267–269
Corgard, 1071–1072
Cormax, 360–361
Correctol, 504–505
Cortaid, 769–773
Cortate [AUS], 386–387
Cortef cream [AUS], 769–773
Cortic cream [AUS], 769–773
Cortic DS [AUS], 769–773
Cortifoam [AUS], 769–773
cortisone, 386–387
Cortizone-5, 769–773
Cortizone-10, 769–773
Cortone [CAN], 386–387
Cortrosyn, 388–389
Corvert, 790–792
Cosig Forte [AUS], 376–378
Cosudex [AUS], 190–191
cosyntropin, 388–389
Cotazym-S [AUS], 1193–1195
Cotazym-S Forte [AUS], 1193–1195
co-trimoxazole, 376–378
Coumadin, 1627–1629
Covera-HS, 1609–1612
Cozaar, 926–927
Creomulsion Cough, 455–457
Creomulsion for Children, 455–457
Creon, 1193–1195
Creo-Terpin, 455–457
Crestor, 1411–1412
Crinone, 1333–1335
Crixivan, 806–808
Crolom, 389–391
cromolyn, 389–391
Cronasma [GERMANY], 1513–1515
crotamiton, 391–392
Cruex Aerosol, 1589
Cruex Cream, 1589
Cruex Powder, 1589
Crysanal [AUS], 1088–1091
Cubicin, 416–419
Cuprimine, 1221–1223
Curosurf, 1299–1300
Cutivate, 681–683
cyanocobalamin, 392–394
Cyanokit, 778–779
cyclobenzaprine, 394–395
Cycloblastin [AUS], 395–397
Cyclocort, 71–72
Cyclomen [CAN], 410–412
cyclophosphamide, 395–397

cycloserine, 397–398
cyclosporine, 398–401
Cylert, 1216–1218
Cylex, 174–175
Cymbalta, 532–533
Cymevene [AUS], 708–712
cyproheptadine, 401–403
Cysporin [AUS], 398–401
Cystospaz, 784–786
Cystospaz-M, 784–786
Cytamen [AUS], 392–394
cytarabine, 403–404
Cytomel, 910–912
Cytosar [CAN], 403–404
Cytosar-U, 403–404
Cytotec, 1042–1043
Cytovene, 708–712
Cytoxan, 395–397

D

dacarbazine, 405–406
daclizumab, 407–408
Dacogen, 427–428
Dalacin [CAN], 356–358
Dalmane, 678–679
dalteparin, 408–410
danazol, 410–412
Dandruff, 1413–1415
Dantrium, 412–415
dantrolene, 412–415
Daonil [CAN], 729–731
Dapa-tabs [AUS], 804–806
dapsone, 415–416
Dapsone, 415–416
daptomycin, 416–419
Daraprim, 1361–1362
darbepoetin alfa, 419–421
darifenacin hydrobromide, 421–423
Darvon, 1343–1345
Darvon-N [CAN], 1343–1345
dasatinib, 423–424
daunorubicin, 424–427
DaunoXome, 424–427
Dayhist Allergy, 355–356
Daypro, 1169–1170
DDAVP, 437–439
ddI, 467–469
Debrox, 256–257
Decadron, 441–445
Deca-Durabolin, 1085–1086
decitabine, 427–428
Declomycin, 432–433
Decofed, 1352–1354
deferoxamine, 429–430
Dehydral [CAN], 988–989

Dek-Quin, 359–360
Del Aqua, 177–178
Delatestryl, 1502–1505
delavirdine, 430–432
Delestrogen, 596–600
Delsym 12-Hour, 455–457
Deltasone, 1316–1318
Demadex, 1558–1560
demeclocycline, 432–433
Demerol, 965–967
Demser, 1023–1024
Denavir, 1220–1221
Deo-Q Syrup [KOREA], 1513–1515
Depacon, 1595–1597
Depakene, 1595–1597
Depakene syrup, 1595–1597
Depakote, 1595–1597
Depakote ER, 1595–1597
Depakote Sprinkle, 1595–1597
Depen, 1221–1223
DepoDur, 1057–1061
Depo-Estradiol, 596–600
Depo-Medrol, 1008–1011
Depo-Nisolone [AUS], 1008–1011
Depo-Provera, 954–955
Depo-Provera Contraceptive, 954–955
Depotest [CAN], 1502–1505
Depo-Testosterone, 1502–1505
Deptran [AUS], 517–519
Deralin [AUS], 1345–1348
Derm-Aid cream [AUS], 769–773
Dermaid soft cream [AUS], 769–773
Dermaid [AUS], 769–773
Derma-Smooth/FS, 664–665
Dermoplast, 174–175
Dermovate [CAN], 360–361
Desenex Powder, 1589
Desenex Soap, 1589
Desferal [CAN], 429–430
Desferal Mesylate, 429–430
desipramine, 433–435
desloratadine, 435–437
desmopressin, 437–439
Desocort [CAN], 439–440
Desonate, 439–440
desonide, 439–440
DesOwen, 439–440
desoximetasone, 440–441
Desoxyn, 985–986
Despec-SF, 1259–1262, 1263–1266
Desquam-E, 177–178
Desquam-X, 177–178
Desyrel, 1568–1569
Detaine, 174–175

Detrol, 1551–1552
Detrol LA, 1551–1552
Detussin, 764–767
Devrom, 193–195
dexamethasone, 441–445
Dexamphetamine [AUS], 453–455
Dexasone [CAN], 441–445
dexchlorpheniramine, 446–447
Dexedrine, 453–455
Dexedrine Spansule, 453–455
Dexferrum, 841–843
Dexiron [CAN], 841–843
dexmedetomidine hydrochloride, 447–449
Dexmethsone [AUS], 441–445
dexmethylphenidate, 450–451
dextran, 451–453
dextroamphetamine, 98–100, 453–455
dextromethorphan, 455–457
Dextrostat, 453–455
D.H.E. 45, 480–482
DHS Sal, 1413–1415
DiaBeta, 729–731
Diabetic Tussin, 743–744
Diabetic Tussin Allergy Relief, 325–327
Diabinese, 329–331
Diamox, 14–16
Diamox Sequels, 14–16
Diastat, 457–461
Diazemuls [CAN], 457–461
diazepam, 457–461
Diazepam Intensol, 457–461
Dibenzyline, 1254–1256
Dicarbosil, 241–244
Dichlotride [AUS], 762–764
diclofenac, 461–464
Diclohexal [AUS], 461–464
Diclotek [CAN], 461–464
dicloxacillin, 464–465, 1223–1225
dicyclomine, 465–467
didanosine, 467–469
Didronel, 614–615
diethylpropion, 470–471
Differin, 26–27
diflorasone, 471–472
Diflucan, 654–657
diflunisal, 472–474
Digibind, 478–480
DigiFab, 478–480
Digitek, 474–478
digoxin, 474–478
digoxin immune Fab, 478–480
Dihydergot [AUS], 480–482
dihydroergotamine, 480–482
Dilacor XR, 482–486
Dilantin, 1268–1272

Dilantin-125, 1268–1272
Dilantin Infatab, 1268–1272
Dilantin Kapseals, 1268–1272
Dilatrate, 851–853
Dilaudid, 773–776
Dilaudid HP, 773–776
Diltahexal [AUS], 482–486
Diltia XT, 482–486
Diltiamax [AUS], 482–486
diltiazem, 482–486
Dilzem [AUS], 482–486
dimenhydrinate, 486–487
dimercaprol, 487–489
Dimetane, 212–214
Dimetane Extentabs, 212–214
Dimetapp, 212–214, 922–923
Dimetapp 12 Hour Non Drowsy
    Extentabs, 1352–1354
Dimetapp Decongestant, 1352–1354
Dimetapp Sinus Liquid Caps [AUS],
    1352–1354
dinoprostone, 489–491
Diocto, 504–505
Diodex [CAN], 441–445
Diodoquin [CAN], 835–836
Diofluor [CAN], 665–667
Diosulf [CAN], 1466–1467
Diovan, 1599–1600
Diovol [CAN], 63–66
Diovol EX [CAN], 63–66
Diovol Plus [CAN], 63–66
Dipentum, 1151–1152
Diphedryl, 491–495
Diphenhist, 491–495
diphenhydramine, 491–495
diphenoxylate/atropine, 495–496
Diprivan, 1647
Diprivan Recofol [AUS], 1340–1343
Diprolene, 181–183
dipyridamole, 496–498
disopyramide, 498–500
DisperDose, 305–306
DisperMox, 94–96
Disprin [AUS], 130–133
disulfiram, 500–501
Ditenaten [GERMANY], 1513–1515
Dithiazide [AUS], 762–764
Dithrocream [AUS], 114–115
Drithocreme, 114–115
Ditropan, 1175–1176
Ditropan XL, 1175–1176
Diuril, 323–325
divalproex sodium, 1595–1597
Divigel, 596–600
Dixarit [CAN], 368–370

Doan's Extra Strength, 942–943
dobutamine, 501–503
docosanol, 503–504
docusate, 504–505
Docusoft-S, 504–505
dofetilide, 505–507
DOK, 504–505
dolasetron, 507–508
Dolobid, 472–474
Dolophine, 983–985
Doloxene [AUS], 1343–1345
Domeboro, 63–66
DOM-Ursodiol C [CAN], 1590–1591
donepezil, 509–510
Donnapine, 167–169
Donnatal, 167–169
Donnatal Extentabs, 167–169
dopamine, 510–513
Dopamine Injection [AUS], 510–513
Dopar, 894–895
Dopram, 514–516
Doral, 1363–1364
dornase alfa, 513–514
Doryx, 523–526
D.O.S., 504–505
Dostinex, 234–235
Dovonex, 237–238
doxapram, 514–516
doxepin, 517–519
doxercalciferol, 519–521
Doxil, 521–522
Doxine, 1359–1361
doxorubicin, 521–522
Doxsig [AUS], 523–526
Doxy-100, 523–526
Doxycin [CAN], 523–526
doxycycline, 523–526
Doxyhexal [AUS], 523–526
Doxylin [AUS], 523–526
Dr. Scholl's Callus Remover, 1413–1415
Dr. Scholl's Clear Away, 1413–1415
Dramamine, 486–487
Drisdol, 1620–1621
Dritho-Scalp, 114–115
dronabinol, 526–527
droperidol, 528–530
Drosin [INDIA], 1259–1262, 1263–1266
drotrecogin alfa, 530–531
Droxine [AUS], 902–904
Drysol, 60–61
d4T, 1457–1459
D-Tal, 167–169
DTIC [CAN], 405–406
DTIC-Dome, 405–406
Ducene [AUS], 457–461

Dulcolax, 192–193, 504–505
duloxetine, 532–533
Duofem [GERMANY], 898–900
DuoFilm, 1413–1415
DuoPlant, 1413–1415
Duphalac [CAN], 874–876
Durabolin [CAN], 1085–1086
Duraclon, 368–370
Duragesic, 638–643
Duralith [CAN], 914–916
Duramorph, 1057–1061
Duricef, 274–275
Duride [AUS], 851–853
dutasteride, 533–534
Duvoid [CAN], 185–186
Dylix, 535–536
Dymadon [AUS], 12–14
Dynacin, 1037–1038
DynaCirc, 855–856
DynaCirc CR, 855–856
dyphylline, 535–536
Dyrenium, 1573–1575
Dysport [AUS], 203–205
Dytan, 491–495

E

ECEEZ [INDIA], 898–900
EC-Naprosyn, 1088–1091
econazole, 537
Ecostatin [CAN], 537
Ecotrin, 130–133, 942–944
edetate calcium disodium, 538–540
edetate disodium, 540–541
Edex, 56–58
EES, 585–589
efalizumab, 541–542
efavirenz, 543–545
Effer K, 1303–1306
Effexor, 1607–1609
Effexor XR, 1607–1609
eflornithine, 545–546
Efrin-10 [ISRAEL], 1259–1262, 1263–1266
Efrisel [INDONESIA], 1259–1262, 1263–1266
Efudex, 668–669
Efudix [AUS], 668–669
E-Gems, 1622–1623
Egocort cream [AUS], 769–773
Elavil, 85–87
Eldepryl, 1424–1425
Eldopaque, 777–778
Eldopaque Forte, 777–778
Eldoquin, 777–778
Elestat, 561–562
Elestrin, 596–600

eletriptan, 546–547
Elidel, 1279–1280
Eligard, 889–891
Elimite, 1244–1246
Elixofilina [MEXICO, PERU], 1513–1515
Elixophyllin, 1513–1515
ElixSure, 491–495
ElixSure Cough, 455–457
Elmiron, 1237–1238
Elocon Cream [AUS], 1052–1053
Elocon Ointment [AUS], 1052–1053
Elon Dual Defense Anti-Fungal Formula
    Solution, 1589
Eloxatin, 1165–1167
Elspar, 128–130
Eltroxin [CAN], 902–904
Emadine, 547–548
Emcin, 585–589
Emcort, 769–773
emedastine, 547–548
Emend, 119–120
Emetrol, 1274–1275
Emgel, 585–589
Emsam, 1424–1425
emtricitabine, 548–550
Emtriva, 548–550
Emulsoil, 271–272
Enablex, 421–423
enalapril, 550–553
Enbrel, 608–610
Endantadine [CAN], 66–68
Endep [AUS], 85–87
Endone [AUS], 1176–1178
Endoxan Asta [AUS], 395–397
Endoxon Asta [AUS], 395–397
Enduron, 1000–1001
enfuvirtide, 553–555
English-Spanish drug phrases translator,
    1648–1665
Enjuvia, 600–602
enoxaparin, 555–557
entacapone, 557–559
Entocort EC, 214–216
Entrophen [CAN], 130–133
Enulose, 874–876, 1002–1003
Enzone, 1309–1310
Epaq Inhaler [AUS], 34–36
ephedrine, 559–561
Epifoam, 1309–1310
epinastine, 561–562
epinephrine, 562–566
EpiPen, 562–566
EpiQuin Micro, 777–778
Epitol, 254–256
Epivir, 876–877

Epivir-HBV, 876–877
eplerenone, 566–567
epoetin alfa, 568–571
Epogen, 568–571
epoprostenol, 571–573
Eprex [CAN], 568–571
eprosartan, 573–574
eptifibatide, 574–576
Eraxis, 113–114
Erbitux, 311–313
ergocalciferol, 1620–1621
Ergodryl Mono [AUS], 579–581
ergoloid mesylates, 576–577
Ergomar, 579–581
Ergomar [CAN], 480–482
ergonovine, 577–579
Ergostat, 579–581
ergotamine, 579–581
Ergotrate, 577–579
erlotinib, 581–582
ERO Ear, 256–257
Errin, 1132–1134
Error-prone drug name abbreviations,
    1670–1672
Ertaczo, 1427–1428
ertapenem, 582–585
Ery, 585–589
Eryacne [AUS], 585–589
Erybid [CAN], 585–589
Eryc LD [AUS], 585–589
EryDerm, 585–589
Erygel, 585–589
EryPed, 585–589
Ery-Tab, 585–589
Erythrocin, 585–589
Erythromid [CAN], 585–589
erythromycin, 585–589
erythropoietin, 568–571
escitalopram, 589–590
Esidrix, 762–764
Eskalith, 914–916
esmolol, 590–593
esomeprazole, 593–595
Esoterica Regular, 777–778
estazolam, 595–596
Estrace, 596–600
Estraderm, 596–600
Estraderm MX [AUS], 596–600
estradiol, 596–600
Estradot [CAN], 596–600
Estrasorb, 596–600
Estring, 596–600
EstroGel, 596–600
estrogens, conjugated, 600–602
estrogens, esterified, 602–604

estropipate, 605–606
eszopiclone, 607–608
etanercept, 608–610
ethambutol, 610–611
ethionamide, 611–612
Ethmozine, 1056–1057
ethosuximide, 612–614
Ethyol, 72–73
Etibi [CAN], 610–611
etidronate, 614–615
etodolac, 615–617
etomidate, 1647
Etopophos, 617–621
etoposide, 617–621
Euflex [CAN], 680–681
Euflexxa, 759–760
Euglucon [CAN], 729–731
Eulexin, 680–681
Euphylong [ISRAEL, HONG KONG],
    1513–1515
Euphylong Retardkaps [GERMANY],
    1513–1515
Euphylong SR [PHILIPPINES], 1513–1515
Eurax, 391–392
Eutroxsig [AUS], 902–904
Evamist, 596–600
Everone [CAN], 1502–1505
Evista, 1373–1375
Evoxac, 313–314
Exact Acne Medication, 177–178
exemestane, 622–623
Ex-lax, 1426–1427
Extendryl, 764–767
EZ-Char, 314–315
ezetimibe, 623–624

F
Fab, 4–6
Fabrazyme, 30–31
Factive, 716–717
factor IX complex, 625–626
factor IX concentrates, 625–626
factor viii. *See* antihemophilic factor
Factrel, 736–737
famciclovir, 626–628
famotidine, 628–631
Famvir, 626–628
Fareston, 1556–1557
Faslodex, 701–702
Fastin, 1256–1257
Faverin [AUS], 685–686
FazaClo, 374–376
FDA pregnancy categories, 1666
felbamate, 631–633
Felbatol, 631–633

Feldene, 1289–1290
felodipine, 633–634
Fem pH, 16–17
Femara, 886–887
Femilax, 192–193
Femiron, 644–645
Femizol-M, 1026–1027
Femring, 596–600
Femstat One [CAN], 230–231
Femtrace, 596–600
Fenac [AUS], 461–464
Fenesin, 743–744
fenofibrate, 634–636
Fenoglide, 634–636
fenoprofen, 636–638
fentanyl, 638–643
Fentora, 638–643
Feostat, 644–645
Fer-Gen-Sol, 644–645
Fergon, 644–645
Fer-In-Sol, 644–645
Fer-Iron, 644–645
Ferretts, 644–645
Ferrlecit, 1443–1445
Ferro-Gradumet [AUS], 644–645
Ferro-Sequels, 644–645
ferrous salts, 644–645
Feverall, 12–14
Fexicam [CAN], 1289–1290
fexofenadine, 646–647
Fiberall, 1354–1355
Fibercon, 1294–1295
Fibersol, 1294–1295
Fibsol [AUS], 912–914
filgrastim, 647–650
Finacea, 151
finasteride, 650–651
Finevin, 151
Fisamox [AUS], 94–96
Fiv-Canasa, 973–974
Flagyl, 1020–1023
Flagyl ER, 1020–1023
Flamazine [CAN], 1434–1436
flavocoxid, 651–652
flavoxate, 652–653
Flebogamma, 801–803
flecainide, 653–654
Flector, 461–464
Fleet Babylax, 731–733
Fleet Enema, 1272–1274
Fleet Glycerin Suppositories for Adults,
    731–733
Fleet Glycerin Suppositories for Children,
    731–733
Fleet Liquid Glycerin Suppositories for
    Adults and Children, 731–733

Fleet Maximum-Strength Glycerin Suppositories, 731–733
Fleet Phospho Soda, 1272–1274
Flexeril, 394–395
Flexitec [CAN], 394–395
Flixotide Disks [AUS], 681–683
Flixotide Inhaler [AUS], 681–683
Flolan, 571–573
Flomax, 1484–1485
Flonase, 681–683
Florinef, 659–660
Florone [CAN], 471–472
Flovent, 681–683
Flovent Diskus, 681–683
Flovent HFA, 681–683
Floxin, 1144–1146
Floxin Otic, 1144–1146
flucloxacillin, 1223–1225
fluconazole, 654–657
flucytosine, 657–659
fludrocortisone, 659–660
Flugerel [AUS], 680–681
Flumadine, 1397–1398
flumazenil, 660–662
flunisolide, 662–664
fluocinolone acetonide, 664–665
Fluoderm [CAN], 664–665
Fluohexal [AUS], 669–671
Fluor-A-Day, 667
fluorescein, 665–666
Fluorescite, 665–667
Fluorets, 665–667
fluoride, sodium, 667
Fluorigard, 667
Fluor-I-Strip, 665–667
Fluor-I-Strip-AT, 665–667
Fluoroplex, 668–669
fluorouracil, 668–669
Fluotic [CAN], 667
fluoxetine, 669–671
fluoxymesterone, 671–673
fluphenazine, 673–674
fluphenazine decanoate, 674–676
fluphenazine enanthate, 674–676
fluphenazine hydrochloride, 674–676
Flura-Drops, 667
flurandrenolide, 676–677
flurazepam, 678–679
flurbiprofen, 679–680
flutamide, 680–681
Flutamin [AUS], 680–681
fluticasone, 681–683
fluvastatin, 684–685
fluvoxamine, 685–686
Focalin, 450–451

Focalin XR, 450–451
Foille, 174–175
Foille Medicated First Aid, 174–175
Foille Plus, 174–175
folic acid, 686–687
folinic acid, 887–889
Folvite, 686–687
Folvite-parenteral, 686–687
fomepizole, 687–689
fomivirsen, 689–690
fondaparinux, 690–691
Foradil Aerolizer, 691–693
Foradile [AUS], 691–693
formoterol, 691–693
Formulex [CAN], 465–467
Fortamet, 978–981
Fortaz, 294–296
Forteo, 1501–1502
Fortum [AUS], 294–296
Fosamax, 44–45
fosamprenavir, 693–694
foscarnet, 694–696
Foscavir, 694–696
fosfomycin, 696–697
fosinopril, 697–699
fosphenytoin, 699–700
Fosrenol, 882–883
Fostex 10% BPO, 177–178
4-Way Decongestant Moisturizing Relief, 1630–1631
Fragmin, 408–410
Freezone, 1413–1415
Froben [CAN], 679–680
Frovan, 700–701
frovatriptan, 700–701
Frusehexal [AUS], 702–704
Frusid [AUS], 702–704
5FU, 668–669
Fugerel [AUS], 680–681
Ful-Glo, 665–667
fulvestrant, 701–702
Fungi-Guard, 1550–1551
Fungizone, 100–103
Fung-O, 1413–1415
Fungoid AF Solution, 1589
Furacin, 1122–1123
Furadantin, 1120–1122
furosemide, 702–704
Fuzeon, 553–555

G

gabapentin, 705–706
Gabitril, 1523–1524
galantamine, 706–708
Gamimune N, 801–803

gamma benzene hexachloride, 907–908
Gammagard S/D, 801–803
Gammar-P-IV, 801–803
Gamunex, 801–803
ganciclovir, 708–712
Ganidin, 743–744
Gantin [AUS], 705–706
Gantrisin, 1470–1471
Garamycin, 719–723
Gastrocrom, 389–391
Gastro-Stop [AUS], 918–919
Gas-X, 1436–1437
gatifloxacin, 712–713
Gaviscon, 63–66
Gaviscon Extra Strength, 63–66
Gaviscon Liquid, 63–66
gefitinib, 713–714
Gelfoam, 6–7
Gelusil [CAN], 63–66
Gelusil Extra Strength [CAN], 63–66
Gemfibromax [AUS], 714–716
gemfibrozil, 714–716
gemifloxacin, 716–717
gemtuzumab ozogamicin, 717–719
Genahist, 491–495
Genaphed, 1352–1354
Genasym, 1436–1437
Gen-Clobetasol [CAN], 360–361
General anesthetics, 1647
Generlac, 874–876
Gengraf, 398–401
Genlac [AUS], 874–876
Genoptic, 719–723
Genoral [AUS], 605–606
Genox [AUS], 1482–1484
Gentacidin, 719–723
Gentak, 719–723
gentamicin, 719–723
Gen-Timolol [CAN], 1530–1532
Gentlax, 192–193
Gentran, 451–453
Gen-Warfarin [CAN], 1627–1629
Geodon, 1641–1642
Gestrol LA, 781–782
glatiramer, 723–724
Glauctabs, 987–988
Gleevec, 793–795
Gliadel, 264–265
Glimel [AUS], 729–731
glimepiride, 724–725
glipizide, 726–727
Glivec [AUS], 793–795
GlucaGen, 727–729
Glucagen [AUS], 727–729
GlucaGen Diagnostic Kit, 727–729

Glucagon, 727–729
Glucagon Diagnostic Kit, 727–729
Glucagon Emergency Kit, 727–729
glucagon hydrochloride, 727–729
Glucobay [AUS], 8–9
GlucoNorm [CAN], 1379–1381
Glucophage, 978–981
Glucophage XL, 978–981
Glucotrol, 726–727
Glucotrol XL, 726–727
glyburide, 729–731
glycerin, 731–733
Glycon [CAN], 978–981
glycopyrrolate, 733–735
Glynase, 729–731
GlyOxide, 256–257
Glyquin, 777–778
Glyrol, 731–733
Glyset, 1033–1034
Godafilin [SPAIN], 1513–1515
Godochom Solution, 1589
gold sodium thiomalate, 145–147, 735–736
Gold-50 [AUS], 145–147
GoLYTELY, 1295–1296
gonadorelin acetate, 736–737
gonadorelin hydrochloride, 736–737
Gopten [AUS], 1564–1565
Gordofilm, 1413–1415
goserelin, 738–739
granisetron, 739–742
granulocyte macrophage colony-stimulating factor, 1419–1421
Grifulvin V, 742–743
griseofulvin, 742–743
Grisovin [AUS], 742–743
Gris-PEG, 742–743
guaifenesin, 743–744
guanabenz, 744–746
guanfacine, 746–747
Guiatuss, 743–744
Gynazole-1, 230–231
Gynecure [CAN], 1535–1536
Gyne-Lotrimin, 373–374
Gynodiol, 596–600

H

Habitrol [CAN], 1111–1113
halcinonide, 748
Halcion, 1575–1576
Haldol, 750–752
Haldol Decanoate, 750–752
Halfprin, 130–133
halobetasol, 749
Halog, 748

Halog-E, 748
haloperidol, 750–752
Halotestin, 671–673
Halotestin [CAN], 671–673
Haponal, 167–169
H-B-Vax II [AUS], 756–757
HDA Toothache, 174–175
Hectorol, 519–521
Helixate FS, 115–116
Hemabate, 261–263
Hemocyte, 644–645
Hemofil M, 115–116
Hepalean [CAN], 753–756
heparin, 753–756
Heparin injection B.P. [AUS], 753–756
Heparin Leo, 753–756
hepatitis B immune globulin (human),
    756–757
Hepsera, 27–28
Heptovir [CAN], 876–877
Herceptin, 1567–1568
Hespan, 757–759
hetastarch, 757–759
Hexadrol [CAN], 441–446
Hexit [CAN], 907–908
Hextend, 757–759
Hiprex, 988–989
Hip-Rex [CAN], 988–989
Histussin D, 764–767
Humalog, 813–815
Humalog Mix 75/25, 813–815
human leukocyte interferon (antiviral),
    825–826
Humanate P, 115–116
Humatin, 1201–1202
Humegon, 963–965
Humibid LA, 743–744
Humira, 24–26
Humulin 70/30, 813–815
Humulin 50/50 NPH Lispro mixture,
    813–815
Humulin L, 813–815
Humulin N, 813–815
Humulin R, 813–815
Hurricane, 174–175
Hyalgan, 759–760
hyaluronan, 759–760
Hyate C, 115–116
Hycamtin, 1554–1556
Hycet, 764–767
Hycodan, 764–767
Hycodan [CAN], 768–769
Hycomine Compound, 764–767
Hycor [AUS], 769–773
Hycor eye ointment [AUS], 769–773

Hycosin, 764–767
Hycotuss, 764–767
Hydergine [CAN], 576–577
Hydopa [AUS], 1003–1004
hydralazine, 760–762
Hydramine Nytol [CAN], 491–495
Hydrisalic, 1413–1415
Hydrocet, 764–767
hydrochlorothiazide, 762–764
Hydrocil, 1354–1355
hydrocodone, 764–767
hydrocodone bitartrate, 768–769
hydrocodone/acetaminophen, 764–767
hydrocodone/aspirin, 764–767
hydrocodone/chlorpheniramine,
    764–767
hydrocodone/chlorpheniramine/
    phenylephrine/acetaminophen/caffeine,
    764–767
hydrocodone/guaifenesin, 764–767
hydrocodone/homatropine, 764–767
hydrocodone/ibuprofen, 764–767
hydrocodone/pseudoephedrine,
    764–767
hydrocortisone, 359–360, 769–773
Hydrogesic, 764–767
Hydromet, 764–767
Hydromorph Contin [CAN], 773–776
hydromorphone, 773–776
Hydropane, 764–767
hydroquinone, 777–778
hydroxocobalamin, 778–779
hydroxychloroquine, 779–781
hydroxyprogesterone, 781–782
hydroxyzine, 782–784
Hygroton [AUS], 331–332
hyoscyamine, 784–786
Hyosine, 784–786
HyperRHO S/D Full Dose, 1385–1387
HyperRHO S/D Mini Dose,
    1385–1387
Hypnovel [AUS], 1028–1030
Hysone [AUS], 769–773
Hytone, 769–773

I
ibandronate, 787–788
Ibilex [AUS], 308–310
ibuprofen, 788–790
ibutilide, 790–792
IL-2, 37–40, 833–835, 1158–1160
IL-11, 1158–1160
iloprost, 792–793
imatinib, 793–795
Imdur, 851–853

imiglucerase, 795–796
Imigran [AUS], 1473–1475
imipenem-cilastatin, 796–798
imipramine, 798–800
imiquimod, 800–801
Imitrex, 1473–1475
immune globulin IV, 801–803
Imodium [AUS], 918–919
Imodium A-D, 918–919
Imtrate [AUS], 851–853
Imukin [AUS], 832–833
Imuran, 149–150
Inamrinone, 803–804
inamrinone lactate, 803–804
Inapsine, 528–530
Indahexal [AUS], 804–806
indapamide, 804–806
Inderal, 1345–1348
Inderal LA, 1345–1348
indinavir, 806–808
Indocid [CAN], 808–811
Indocin, 808–811
Indocin IV, 808–811
Indocin-SR, 808–811
indomethacin, 808–811
Infant Mylicon, 1436–1437
Infasurf, 244–245
Infed, 841–843
Infergen, 826–827
Inflamase Forte, 1314–1316
Inflamase Mild, 1314–1316
infliximab, 811–813
Infufer [CAN], 841–843
Infumorph, 1057–1061
INH, 847–849
Innohep, 1534–1535
InnoPran XL, 1345–1348
Insensye [AUS], 1135–1136
Insig [AUS], 804–806
Insomn-Eze [AUS], 1335–1338
Inspra, 566–567
insulin, 813–815
Insulin Aspart, 813–815
Insulin Glargine, 813–815
insulin Glulisine, 815–817
Insulin Lente, 813–815
Insulin Lispro, 813–815
Intal, 389–391
Integrilin, 574–576
interferon alfa-2a, 817–819
interferon alfa-2a/2b, 819–822
interferon alfa-2b, 822–825
interferon alfacon-1, 826–827
interferon alfa-n3, 825–826
interferon beta-1a, 827–828

interferon beta-1a/b, 828–830
interferon beta-1b, 830–832
interferon gamma-1b, 832–833
Interleukin-2, 37–40, 833–835
interleukin-11, 1158–1160
Intron-A, 819–822, 822–825
Invanz, 582–585
Inversine, 949–950
Invirase, 1417–1419
Inza [AUS], 1088–1091
iodoquinol, 835–836
Ionamin, 1256–1257
Ionil, 1413–1415
Ionil Plus, 1413–1415
Ionsys, 638–643
Iopidine, 118–119
Iosopan Plus, 937–938
ipratropium, 836–838
Iquix, 896–898
irbesartan, 838–839
Iressa, 713–714
irinotecan, 839–841
iron dextran, 841–843
iron sucrose, 843–844
Iscover [AUS], 370–371
ISMO, 851–853
isocarboxazid, 844–846
isoetharine hydrochloride, 846–847
isoetharine mesylate, 846–847
Isogen [AUS], 851–853
isoniazid, 847–849
isoproterenol, 849–851
Isoptin SR, 1609–1612
Isopto Carbachol, 253
Isopto Cetamide, 1466–1467
Isopto Frin [AUS], 1266–1268
Isopto Frin [BELGIUM, CZECH REPUBLIC,
     ECUADOR, MALAYSIA], 1259–1262,
     1263–1266
Isopto Hyoscine, 1421–1422
IsoptoCarpin, 1278–1279
IsoptoFrin, 1259–1262
Isordil, 851–853
isosorbide dinitrate, 851–853
isosorbide mononitrate, 851–853
Isotamine [CAN], 847–849
isotretinoin, 853–854
Isotrex [CAN], 853–854
isradipine, 855–856
Istadol, 1530–1532
Istubol, 1482–1484
Isuprel, 849–851
I-tositumomab, 1560–1562
itraconazole, 856–859
Iveegam EN, 801–803

Ivermectin (systemic), 859–860
IvyBlock, 173

J

Jantoven, 1627–1629
Jezil [AUS], 714–716
Jolivette, 1132–1134

K

Kadian, 1057–1061
Kaletra, 919–922
Kalma [AUS], 54–56
Kaluril [AUS], 76–77
kanamycin sulfate, 861–862
Kantrex, 861–862
Kaochlor, 1303–1306
Kaon, 1303–1306
Kaon-Cl, 1303–1306
Kaopectate, 193–195
Kapanol [AUS], 1057–1061
Karvea [AUS], 838–839
Kayexalate, 1446–1447
K-Dur, 1303–1306
Keflex, 308–310
Keflor [AUS], 272–274
Keftab, 308–310
Kefurox, 303–305
Kefzol, 276–278
Kemadrin, 1332–1333
Kenalog, 1316–1318
Kepivance, 1188–1189
Keppra, 892–893
Keppra XR, 892–893
Keralyt, 1413–1415
Kerlone, 183–185
Kerr Insta-Char, 314–315
Ketalar, 862–864, 1647
ketamine, 1647
ketamine hydrochloride, 862–864
Ketek, 1486–1487
ketoconazole, 864–866
ketoprofen, 866–868
ketorolac tromethamine, 868–871
Key-E, 1622–1623
Key-E Kaps, 1622–1623
Kidrolase [CAN], 128–130
Kineret, 110–111
Kinidin Durules [AUS], 1368–1370
Kinson [AUS], 257–259
Kionex, 1446–1447
Klacid [AUS], 353–355
Klean-Prep [CAN], 1295–1296
Klexane [CAN], 555–557
Kliovance [AUS], 596–600
Klonopin, 366–368

K-Lor, 1303–1306
Klor-Con EF, 1303–1306
K-Lor-Con M 15, 1303–1306
K-Lyte, 1303–1306
K-Lyte DS, 1303–1306
Koate DVI, 115–116
Kogenate FS, 115–116
Konsyl, 1354–1355
K-Phos ME, 1272–1274
K-Phos Neutral, 1272–1274
Kripton [AUS], 210–212
KSR-600 [AUS], 1303–1306
KSR [AUS], 1303–1306
Ku-Zyme, 1193–1195
Kwelcof, 764–767
Kwellada-P [CAN], 1244–1246
Kytril, 739–742

L

labetalol hydrochloride, 872–874
Laboratory values, normal,
      1667–1669
Lac-Hydrin, 89–90
Lac-Hydrin Five, 89–90
LAClotion, 89–90
lactulose, 874–876
Lamictal, 878–880
Lamictal cD, 878–880
Lamisil, 1497–1499
Lamisil AT, 1497–1499
lamivudine, 876–877
lamotrigine, 878–880
Lanacane, 174–175
Lanoxin, 474–478
lansoprazole, 880–882
lanthanum carbonate, 882–883
Lantus, 813–815
Largactil [CAN], 327–329
Lariam, 957–958
Larodopa, 894–895
Lasix, 702–704
Lasma [ISRAEL, ENGLAND],
      1513–1515
Latisse, 191–192
Latycin [AUS], 1508–1509
Ledermycin [AUS], 432–433
Ledertrexate [AUS], 992–994
leflunomide, 883–884
Lente Iletin II, 813–815
lepirudin, 884–885
Lescol, 684–685
Lescol XL, 684–685
Letairis, 69–70
letrozole, 886–887
leucovorin calcium, 887–889

Leukine, 1419–1421
Leunase [AUS], 128–130
leuprolide acetate, 889–891
levalbuterol, 891–892
Levaquin, 896–898
Levate [CAN], 85–87
Levatol, 1218–1219
Levbid, 784–786
levetiracetam, 892–893
Levitra, 1603–1604
levodopa, 894–895
Levo-Dromoran, 900–902
levofloxacin, 896–898
Levonelle [NEW ZEALAND], 898–900
levonorgestrel, 898–900
Levophed, 1130–1132
levorphanol, 900–902
Levothroid, 902–904
levothyroxine, 902–904
Levoxyl, 902–904
Levsin, 784–786
Levsinex, 784–786
Levsin/SL, 784–786
Lexapro, 589–590
Lexiva, 693–694
Librium, 318–320
lidocaine hydrochloride, 904–907
Lidoderm, 904–907
Lignocaine Gel [AUS], 904–907
Limbrel, 651–652
lindane, 907–908
Lindane, 907–908
linezolid, 908–910
Lioresal, 159–160
Liotec [CAN], 159–160
liothyronine T$_3$, 910–912
Lipazil [AUS], 714–716
Lipex [AUS], 1437–1438
Lipitor, 139–140
Lipofen, 634–636
liposomal amphotericin B, 100–103
Liqui-Char, 314–315
Lisodur [AUS], 912–914
lisinopril, 912–914
Lithicarb [AUS], 914–916
lithium carbonate, 914–916
lithium citrate, 914–916
Lithobid, 914–916
Locoid, 769–773
lodoxamide tromethamine, 916–917
Lodrane 12 Hour, 212–214
Lofenoxal [AUS], 495–496
Lofibra, 634–636
LoKara, 439–440
Lomine [CAN], 465–467

Lomotil, 495–496
Lonavar [AUS], 1167–1168
Loniten, 1039–1041
Lonox, 495–496
Loperacap [CAN], 918–919
loperamide, 918–919
Lopid, 714–716
lopinavir/ritonavir, 919–922
Lopresor [AUS], 1017–1020
Lopressor, 1017–1020
Loprox, 339–340
loratadine, 922–923
lorazepam, 923–926
Lorazepam Intensol, 923–926
Lorcet 10/650, 764–767
Lorcet Plus, 764–767
Lorcet-HD, 764–767
Loroxide, 177–178
Lortab, 764–767
losartan, 926–927
Losec [CAN], 1154–1156
Lotensin, 171–173
Lotrel, 928–929
Lotrimin, 373–374
Lotrimin Ultra, 229–230
Lotronex, 52–54
Lovan [AUS], 669–671
lovastatin, 928–929
Lovenox, 555–557
Lovir [AUS], 21–24
Lowsium Plus, 937–938
Loxapac [CAN], 929–930
loxapine, 929–930
Loxitane, 929–930
Lozide [CAN], 804–806
Lozol, 804–806
L.P.V. [AUS], 1228–1230
Lucrin [AUS], 889–891
Lucrin Depot Inj [AUS], 889–891
Ludiomil, 946–948
Lufyllin, 535–536
Lumigan, 191–192
Luminal, 1252–1254
Lunesta, 607–608
LupiCare, 1413–1415
LupiCare Psoriasis, 1413–1415
LupiCare II Psoriasis, 1413–1415
Lupron, 889–891
Lupron Depot, 889–891
Lupron Depot Ped, 889–891
Luride, 667–668
Lustra, 777–778
Lustra-AF, 777–778
Lutrepulse, 736–737
Luvox, 685–686

Luxiq, 181–183
Luvox CR, 685–686
lymphocyte immune globulin N, 931–932
lyrica, 933–935
Lyrica, 933–935
Lysodren, 1044–1045

M

Maalox, 63–66
Maalox Max, 63–66
Maalox Fast Release Liquid, 63–66
Maalox TC, 63–66
Mabthera [AUS], 1404–1405
Macrobid, 1120–1122
Macrodantin, 1120–1122
mafenide, 936–937
magaldrate, 937–938
Mag-Delay SR, 938–942
Magicul [AUS], 343–345
magnesium, 938–942
magnesium salicylate, 942–943
Mag-Ox 400, 938–942
Malocide [FRANCE], 1361–1362
Malsalate, 942–943
mannitol, 944–946
maprotiline, 946–948
Marcaine, 218–222
Marcaine Spinal, 218–222
Marevan [AUS], 1627–1629
Margesic H, 764–767
Marinol, 526–527
Marplan, 844–846
Matulane, 1328–1329
Mavik, 1564–1565
Maxair, 1287–1288
Maxair Autohaler, 1287–1288
Maxalt, 1406–1407
Maxalt-MLT, 1406–1407
Maxidex, 441–445
Maxidone, 764–767
Maxipime, 281–283
Maxivate, 181–183
Maxolon [AUS], 1013–1015
Maxor [AUS], 1154–1156
Mebaral, 967–969
mebendazole, 948–949
mecamylamine, 949–950
meclizine hydrochloride, 950–951
meclofenamate sodium, 952–953
Meclomen [CAN], 952–953
Mectizan [CAN], 859–860
Mediplast, 1413–1415
Medrol, 1008–1011
medroxyprogesterone acetate, 954–955
mefenamic acid, 955–957

mefloquine, 957–958
Mefoxin, 289–291
Megace, 959–960
Megacillin [CAN], 1227–1228
Megafol [AUS], 686–687
megestrol acetate, 959–960
Megostat [AUS], 959–960
Melanex, 777–778
Melfiat, 1249–1250
Melipramine [AUS], 798–800
Melizide [AUS], 726–727
Mellaril, 1519–1520
Melleril [AUS], 1519–1520
meloxicam, 960–961
Melpaque HP, 777–778
Melquin-3, 777–778
Melquin HP, 777–778
memantine hydrochloride, 961–962
Menest, 602–604
Menopur, 963–965
Menostar, 596–600
menotropins, 963–965
Mentax, 229–230
meperidine hydrochloride, 965–967
mephobarbital, 967–969
Mephyton, 1277–1278
meprobamate, 969–971
Mepron, 140–141
Merbentyl [AUS], 465–467
Mericaine, 1326–1328
Meridia, 1431–1432
Meropenem, 971–972
Merrem IV, 971–972
mesalamine, 973–974
Mesasal [CAN], 973–974
M-Eslon, 1057–1061
Mestinon, 1357–1359
Mestinon SR [CAN], 1357–1359
Mestinon Timespan, 1357–1359
Metadate CD, 1006–1008
Metadate ER, 1006–1008
Metadol [CAN], 983–985
Metalyse [AUS], 1492–1493
Metamucil, 1354–1355
Metaoxedrin [DEN, NOR, SWE], 1259–1262, 1263–1266
Metaoxedrin [DENMARK, NORWAY, SWEDEN], 1259–1263
metaproterenol sulfate, 974–976
metaraminol, 976–977
metaxalone, 977–978
metformin hydrochloride, 978–981
methacholine, 981–982
methadone hydrochloride, 983–985
Methadone Intensol, 983–985

Methadose, 983–985
methamphetamine, 985–986
methazolamide, 987–988
methenamine, 988–989
Methergine, 1004–1006
methicillin, 1223–1225
methimazole, 989–991
Methoblastin [AUS], 992–994
methocarbamol, 991–992
methohexital, 1647
methotrexate sodium, 992–994
methoxsalen, 995–997
methscopolamine bromide, 997–998
methsuximide, 998–1000
methyclothiazide, 1000–1001
methylcellulose, 1002–1003
methyldopa, 1003–1004
methylergonovine, 1004–1006
Methylin, 1006–1008
Methylin ER, 1006–1008
methylphenidate hydrochloride, 1006–1008
methylprednisolone, 1008–1011
methyltestosterone, 1011–1012
metipranolol hydrochloride, 1012–1013
metoclopramide, 1013–1015
Metohexal [AUS], 1017–1020
metolazone, 1015–1017
Metolol [AUS], 1017–1020
metoprolol tartrate, 1017–1020
MetroCream, 1020–1023
MetroGel, 1020–1023
Metrogyl [AUS], 1020–1023
MetroLotion, 1020–1023
metronidazole hydrochloride, 1020–1023
Metronidazole IV [AUS], 1020–1023
Metronide [AUS], 1020–1023
metyrosine, 1023–1024
Mevacor, 928–929
mexiletine hydrochloride, 1024–1025
Mexitil, 1024–1025
mezlocillin, 1223–1225
MG217 Sal-Acid, 1413–1415
Miacalcin, 238–239
Micanol, 114–115
Micardis, 1488–1489
Micatin, 1026–1027
miconazole, 1026–1027
Micozole [CAN], 1026–1027
MICRhogam, 1385–1387
Micro-K, 1303–1306
Microlut [COLOMBIA], 898–900
Micronase, 729–731
microNephrin, 562–566
Micronor, 1132–1134
Microval [COLOMBIA], 898–900

Microzide, 762–764
Midamor, 76–77
midazolam, 1647
midazolam hydrochloride, 1028–1030
midodrine, 1030–1031
Mifeprex, 1031–1033
mifepristone, 1031–1033
miglitol, 1033–1034
miglustat, 1034–1035
Migranal, 480–482
Milnox [CAN], 1039–1041
Milophene, 363–364
Milophene [CAN], 363–364
milrinone lactate, 1035–1036
Miltown, 969–971
Minax [AUS], 1017–1020
Minidiab [AUS], 726–727
Minims Phenylephrine HCL 10%
    [SOUTH AFRICA], 1259–1262,
    1263–1266
Minims Phenylephrine Hydrochloride
    [ENG], 1259–1262, 1263–1266
Minims-Prednisolone [CAN], 1314–1316
Minipress, 1313–1314
Minirin, 437–439
Minirin [AUS], 437–439
Minitran, 1123–1126
Minocin, 1037–1038
minocycline hydrochloride, 1037–1038
Minomycin [AUS], 1037–1038
minoxidil, 1039–1041
Mintezol, 1516–1517
Miostat, 253
MiraLax [OTC], 1295–1296
Mirapex, 1307–1309
Mirena [CHINA, COLOMBIA, GERMANY,
    HONG KONG, ISRAEL, KOREA, PHILIPPINES,
    SOUTH AFRICA, THAILAND], 898–900
Mireze [CAN], 1096–1097
mirtazapine, 1041–1042
misoprostol, 1042–1043
mitotane, 1044–1045
mitoxantrone, 1045–1047
Moban, 1050–1052
Mobic, 960–961
Mobilis [AUS], 1289–1290
modafinil, 1047–1048
Modane, 192–193
Modecate [AUS], 673–674, 674–676
Moditen [CAN], 673–674, 674–676
moexipril hydrochloride, 1048–1050
molindone, 1050–1051
Mollifene Ear Wax Removing,
    256–257
mometasone furoate monohydrate,
    1052–1053

Monarc M, 115–116
Monistat [CAN], 1026–1027
Monistat-1, 1535–1536
Monistat-3, 1026–1027
Monistat-7, 1026–1027
Monistat-Derm, 1026–1027
Monitan [CAN], 10–12
monobenzone, 1053–1054
Monoclate-P, 115–116
Monodox, 523–526
Monodur Durules [AUS], 851–853
Monoket, 851–853
Mononine, 625–626
Monopril, 697–699
Monotard [AUS], 813–815
montelukast, 1054–1056
Monurol, 696–697
8-MOP, 995–997
moricizine hydrochloride, 1056–1057
morphine, 1057–1061
Morphine Mixtures [AUS], 1057–1061
Mosco Corn and Callus Remover,
   1413–1415
Motrin, 788–790
Moxacin [AUS], 94–96
Moxamox [AUS], 94–96
Moxatag, 94–96
moxifloxacin hydrochloride, 1061–1063
MS Contin, 1057–1061
MS Mono [AUS], 1057–1061
MSIR, 1057–1061
Mucinex, 743–744
Mucomyst, 18–19
mupirocin, 1063–1064
Murelax [AUS], 1170–1172
Murine Ear Drops, 256–257
Muro 128, 1442–1443
muromonab-CD3, 1064–1066
Muse, 56–58
Myambutol, 610–611
Mycelex, 373–374
Mycelex-3 2%, 230–231
Mycelex OTC, 373–374
Myciguent, 1100–1102
Mycinettes, 174–175
Mycobutin, 1390–1391
mycophenolate mofetil, 1066–1068
Mycostatin, 1140–1141
Mydfrin, 1259–1262, 1263–1266,
   1266–1268
My-E, 585–589
Mykrox, 1015–1017
Mylanta [CAN], 63–66
Mylanta Double Strength [CAN], 63–66
Mylanta Extra Strength Liquid, 63–66

Mylanta Extra Strength [CAN], 63–66
Mylanta Gas, 1436–1437
Mylanta Liquid, 63–66
Mylanta Regular Strength [CAN], 63–66
Myleran, 226–228
Mylotarg, 717–719
Myobloc, 205–206
Myochrysine, 145–147, 735–736
Myocrisin [AUS], 145–147, 735–736
Myoquin [AUS], 1368–1370
Myotonachol [CAN], 185–186
Myrac, 1037–1038
Mysoline, 1320–1321
Mysteclin [AUS], 1508–1509
Mytelase, 68–69

N

Nabi-HB, 756–757
nabumetone, 1069–1070
nadolol, 1071–1072
nafarelin, 1073–1074
Nafcil, 1074–1075
nafcillin, 1223–1225
nafcillin sodium, 1074–1075
naftifine, 1076
Naftin, 1076
nalbuphine hydrochloride, 1077–1079
Nalfon, 636–638
Nallpen, 1074–1075
nalmefene hydrochloride, 1079–1080
naloxone hydrochloride, 1081–1082
naltrexone hydrochloride, 1083–1084
Namenda, 961–962
nandrolone decanoate, 1085–1086
naphazoline, 1087–1088
Naphcon, 1087–1088
Naprelan, 1088–1091
Naprogesic [AUS], 1088–1091
Naprosyn, 1088–1091
naproxen, 1088–1091
naproxen sodium, 1088–1091
Naramig [AUS], 1091–1092
naratriptan, 1091–1092
Narcan, 1081–1082
Nardil, 1250–1252
Nasahist B, 212–214
Nasal Mist, 1442–1443
Nasal Moist, 1442–1443
Nasalcrom, 389–391
Nasalide, 662–664
Nasarel, 662–664
Nasonex, 1052–1053
Nasonex Nasal Spray [AUS], 1052–1053
Natacyn, 1094
natalizumab, 1092–1094

natamycin, 1094
nateglinide, 1095–1096
Natrecor, 1104–1105
Natrilix [AUS], 804–806
Natrilix-SR [AUS], 804–806
Natulan [CAN], 1328–1329
Nature-Thyroid NT, 1522–1523
Navane, 1520–1521
Navelbine, 1616–1618
ND Stat, 212–214
Nebcin, 1541–1544
NebuPent, 1230–1232
nedocromil sodium, 1096–1097
nefazodone hydrochloride, 1097–1099
Nefoben [ARGENTINA], 1513–1515
Nefrin-Ofteno [COSTA RICA, DOMINICAN
    REPUBLIC, EL SALVADOR, GUATEMALA,
    HONDURAS, NICARAGUA, PANAMA],
    1259–1262, 1263–1266
nelfinavir, 1099–1100
Nemasol [CAN], 81–82
Nembutal, 1234–1237
Neobiphyllin [CHINA], 1513–1515
NeoCeuticals Acne Spot Treatment,
    1413–1415
Neo-Estrone [CAN], 602–604
NeoFradin, 1100–1102
Neofrin, 1259–1262, 1263–1266
neomycin sulfate, 1100–1102
Neoprofen, 788–790
Neoral, 398–401
Neosar, 395–397
neostigmine, 1102–1104
NeoStrata AHA, 777–778
Neostrata HQ, 777–778
Neosulf [AUS], 1100–1102
Neo-Synephrine, 1259–1262,
    1266–1268
Neosynephrine 10% Chibret [FRA],
    1259–1262, 1263–1266
Neosynephrine Faure 10% [FRA],
    1259–1262, 1263–1266
Neo-Synephrine Ophthalmic, 1259–1262,
    1263–1266
Neo-Synephrine Ophthalmic Viscous 10%
    [AUS], 1259–1262, 1263–1266
Neosynephrine [BELGIUM, SWE],
    1259–1262, 1263–1266
Neosynephrin-POS [KOR], 1259–1262,
    1263–1266
Nephro-Fer, 644–645
Neptazane, 987–988
nesiritide, 1104–1105
Nestrex, 1359–1361
Neulasta, 1207–1208

Neulin SA [SOUTH AFRICA],
    1513–1515
Neulin-SR [TAIWAN], 1513–1515
Neumega, 1158–1160
Neupogen, 647–650
Neur-Amyl [AUS], 90–92
Neurontin, 705–706
Neutra-Phos, 1272–1274
NeutroGard, 667
Neutrogena Acne Mask, 177–178
Neutrogena Acne Wash, 1413–1415
Neutrogena Body Clear, 1413–1415
Neutrogena Clear Pore, 1413–1415
Neutrogena Clear Pore Shine Control,
    1413–1415
Neutrogena Healthy Scalp, 1413–1415
Neutrogena Maximum Strength T/Sal,
    1413–1415
Neutrogena On The Spot Acne Patch,
    1413–1415
Neutrogena On The Spot Acne Treatment,
    177–178
nevirapine, 1105–1107
Nexium, 593–595
niacin, 1107–1108
Niacor, 1107–1108
Niaspan, 1107–1108
nicardipine hydrochloride, 1108–1111
NicoDerm [CAN], 1111–1113
NicoDerm CQ, 1111–1113
Nicorette, 1111–1113
Nicorette Plus [CAN], 1111–1113
nicotine, 1111–1113
Nicotinex, 1107–1108
nicotinic acid, 1107–1108
Nicotrol, 1111–1113
Nicotrol NS, 1111–1113
Nicotrol Patch [CAN], 1111–1113
NidaGel [CAN], 1020–1023
Nifecard [AUS], 1113–1115
Nifedicol XL, 1113–1115
nifedipine, 1113–1115
Nifehexal [AUS], 1113–1115
Nilandron, 1115–1116
Nilstat [CAN], 1140–1141
nilutamide, 1115–1116
nimodipine, 1116–1117
Nimotop, 1116–1117
Nipent, 1238–1240
Nipride [CAN], 1126–1129
nisoldipine, 1118–1119
nitazoxanide, 1119–1120
Nitradisc [AUS], 1123–1126
Nitrek, 1123–1126
Nitro-Bid, 1123–1126

Nitro-Dur, 1123–1126
nitrofurantoin, 1120–1122
nitrofurazone, 1122–1123
Nitrogard, 1123–1126
nitroglycerin, 1123–1126
Nitroject [CAN], 1123–1126
Nitrolingual, 1123–1126
Nitrong-SR, 1123–1126
Nitropress, 1126–1129
nitroprusside, 1126–1129
NitroQuick, 1123–1126
Nitrostat, 1123–1126
Nitro-Tab, 1123–1126
Nix, 1244–1246
nizatidine, 1129–1130
Nizoral, 864–866
Nizoral AD, 864–866
Nolvadex, 1482–1484
Nolvadex-D [CAN], 1481–1483
Nora-BE, 1132–1134
Norco, 764–767
norepinephrine bitartrate, 1130–1132
norethindrone, 1132–1134
Norflex, 1161–1162
norfloxacin, 1135–1136
Norfloxacine [CAN], 1135–1136
norgestrel, 1136–1138
Noritate, 1020–1023
Norlevo [FRANCE, SOUTH AFRICA],
    898–900
Norlutate [CAN], 1132–1134
Normal laboratory values, 1667–1669
Normodyne, 872–874
Noroxin, 1135–1136
Norpace, 498–500
Norpace CR, 498–500
Norplant System, 898–900
Norplant 36 [ISRAEL], 898–900
Norpramin, 433–435
Nor-QD, 1132–1134
nortriptyline hydrochloride, 1138–1140
Norvasc, 88–89
Norventyl, 1138–1140
Norvir, 1402–1404
Norvisec [CAN], 1402–1404
Noten [AUS], 135–137
Novamoxin [CAN], 94–96
Novantrone, 1045–1047
Novasen [CAN], 130–133
Novasal, 942–943
Novasone Cream [AUS], 1052–1053
Novasone Lotion [AUS], 1052–1053
Novasone Ointment [AUS], 1052–1053
Novo Minocycline [CAN], 1037–1038
Novo Sundac [CAN], 1472–1473

Novo-Acebutolol [CAN], 10–12
Novo-Alprazol [CAN], 54–56
Novo-Ampicillin [CAN], 104–106
Novo-AZT [CAN], 1639–1640
Novocain, 1326–1328
Novo-Captoril [CAN], 250–252
Novo-Cholamine [CAN], 333–335
Novocimetine [CAN], 343–345
Novo-Clobetasol [CAN], 360–361
Novo-Clopamine [CAN], 364–366
Novoclopate [CAN], 371–373
Novo-Cycloprine [CAN], 394–395
Novo-Desipramine [CAN], 433–435
Novo-Difenac [CAN], 461–464
Novo-Diflunisal [CAN], 472–474
Novo-Diltiazem [CAN], 482–486
Novodipiradol [CAN], 496–498
Novo-Doxepin [CAN], 517–519
Novo-Ducosate [CAN], 504–505
Novo-Famotidine [CAN], 628–631
Novo-Fluoxetine [CAN], 669–671
Novo-Flutamide [CAN], 680–681
Novo-Furan [CAN], 1120–1122
Novo-Gemfibrozil [CAN], 714–716
Novohydroxyzin [CAN], 782–784
Novohylazin [CAN], 760–762
Novo-Ipramide [CAN], 836–838
Novo-Keto-EC, 866–868
Novolexin [CAN], 308–310
Novolin 70/30, 813–815
Novolin L, 813–815
Novolin N, 813–815
Novolin R, 813–815
NovoLog, 813–815
NovoLog Mix 70/30 Long Acting,
    813–815
Novo-Loperamide [CAN], 918–919
Novolorazepam [CAN], 923–926
Novomedopa [CAN], 1003–1004
Novo-Medrone [CAN], 954–955
Novo-Mepro [CAN], 969–971
Novo-Metformin [CAN], 978–981
Novomethacin [CAN], 808–811
Novo-Mucilax [CAN], 1354–1355
Novo-Nadolol [CAN], 1071–1072
Novo-Naprox [CAN], 1088–1091
Novonidazol [CAN], 1020–1023
Novo-Nifedin [CAN], 1113–1115
Novo-Norfloxacin [CAN], 1135–1136
Novopen-G [CAN], 1227–1228
Novo-Pen-VK [CAN], 1228–1230
Novoperidol [CAN], 750–752
Novopirocam [CAN], 1289–1290
Novopoxide [CAN], 318–320
Novo-Prednisolone [CAN], 1314–1316

Novoprofen [CAN], 788–790
Novo-Rabeprazole EC [CAN], 1372–1373
Novo-Ramipril [CAN], 1375–1377
Novo-Ranitidine [CAN], 1377–1379
Novorapid [AUS], 813–815
Novosalmol [CAN], 34–36
Novo-Selegiline [CAN], 1424–1425
Novo-Sertraline [CAN], 1428–1430
Novo-Sotalol [CAN], 1451–1452
Novo-Soxazole [CAN], 1470–1471
Novospiroton [CAN], 1454–1456
Novo-Sucralfate [CAN], 1463–1464
Novo-Tamoxifen [CAN], 1482–1484
Novo-Temazepam [CAN], 1489–1490
Novo-Terazosin [CAN], 1496–1497
Novo-Terbinafine [CAN], 1497–1499
Novotetra [CAN], 1508–1509
Novothyrox [CAN], 902–904
Novo-Tolmetin [CAN], 1549–1550
Novo-Trazodone [CAN], 1568–1569
Novotrimel [CAN], 376–378
Novo-Tripramine [CAN], 1583–1584
Novo-Triptyn [CAN], 85–87
Novo-Veramil SR [CAN], 1609–1612
Novo-Veramil [CAN], 1609–1612
Novo-Warfarin [CAN], 1627–1629
Noxafil, 1300–1301
NPH, 813–815
Nu-Ampi [CAN], 104–106
Nubain, 1077–1079
Nudopa [AUS], 1003–1004
Nuelin [PUERTO RICO, COSTA RICA, DENMARK,
    DOMINICAN REPUBLIC, EL SALVADOR,
    FINLAND, HONDURAS, MALAYSIA, NORWAY,
    PANAMA, PHILIPPINES], 1513–1515
Nuelin SA [SOUTH AFRICA, ISRAEL, COSTA
    RICA, DOMINICAN REPUBLIC, EL SALVADOR,
    GUATEMALA, HONDURAS, PANAMA],
    1513–1515
Nuelin SR [ISRAEL, AUSTRALIA, HONG KONG,
    MALAYSIA, THAILAND], 1513–1515
Nu-Ipratropium [CAN], 836–838
NuLev, 784–786
NuLytely, 1295–1296
Nu-Mefenamic [CAN], 955–957
Nu-Metop [CAN], 1017–1020
Numorphan, 1182–1184
Nu-Naprox [CAN], 1088–1091
Nupercainal Hydrocortisone Cream,
    769–773
Nu-Propranolol [CAN], 1345–1348
Nuquin HP, 777–778
Nurofen [AUS], 788–790
Nu-Sulfinpyrazone [CAN], 1469–1470
Nu-Tetra [CAN], 1508–1509

Nu-Trimipramine [CAN], 1583–1584
Nyaderm, 1140–1141
Nydrazid, 847–849
Nyefax [AUS], 1113–1115
nystatin, 1140–1141
Nystop, 1140–1141
Nytol, 491–495

O
Obezine, 1249–1250
Oby-Cap, 1256–1257
Occlusal [CAN], 1413–1415
Occlusal-HP, 1413–1415
Ocean, 1442–1443
Octagam, 801–803
Octostim [CAN], 437–439
octreotide, 1142–1143
octreotide acetate, 1142–1143
Ocuclear, 1179–1180
Ocufen, 679–680
Ocuflox, 1144–1146
Ocu-Phrin, 1259–1262, 1263–1266
Ocupress, 265–267
Ocusert, 1278–1279
Ocusert Pilo-40, 1278–1279
Odrik [AUS], 1564–1565
Oesclim [CAN], 596–600
ofloxacin, 1144–1146
Oftan-Metaoksedrin [FIN], 1259–1262,
    1263–1266
Ogen, 605–606
OKT3, 1064–1065
olanzapine, 1146–1148
olmesartan medoxomil, 1149–1150
olopatadine, 1150–1151
olsalazine sodium, 1151–1152
Olux, 360–361
omalizumab, 1152–1154
Omedia, 174–175
omeprazole, 1154–1156
Omnaris, 337–338
Omnicef, 278–280
Oncaspar, 1205–1206
Oncovin, 1615–1616
Oncovin [AUS], 1613–1614
ondansetron hydrochloride, 1156–1158
Onkotrone [AUS], 1045–1047
Onxol, 1187–1188
Opana, 1182–1184
Opana ER, 1182–1184
Ophthacet, 1466–1467
oprelvekin, 1158–1160
Opticrom, 389–391
Optimal [AUS], 1530–1532
OptiPranolol, 1012–1013

Optistin [ITL], 1259–1262, 1263–1266
Optivar, 152–153
Orabase-B, 174–175
Orajel, 174–175
Orajel Baby, 174–175
Orajel Baby Nighttime, 174–175
Orajel Maximum Strength, 174–175
Orajel Perioseptic, 256–257
Oramorph SR, 1057–1061
Orap, 1280–1282
Orapred, 1314–1316
Orasol, 174–175
Oraxyl, 523–526
Orazinc, 1641
Oretic, 762–764
Oreton Methyl, 1011–1012
Organidin, 743–744
Orinase, 1546–1547
Orinase Diagnostic, 1545–1546
orlistat, 1160–1161
Oroxine [AUS], 902–904
Orphenace [CAN], 1161–1162
orphenadrine, 1161–1162
Orthoclone, 1064–1065
Ortho-Est, 605–606
Orthovisc, 759–760
Orudis [AUS], 866–868
Orudis KT [CAN], 866–868
Orudis SR [AUS], 866–868
Oruvail, 866–868
Oruvail SR [AUS], 866–868
OsCal, 241–244
oseltamivir, 1162–1164
Osmitrol, 944–946
Osmoglyn, 731–733
Ostoforet [CAN], 1620–1621
Otic Domeboro, 63–66
Otocain, 174–175
Otricaine, 174–175
Otrivin Nasal Drops, 1630–1631
Otrivin Nasal Spray, 1630–1631
Otrivin Nasal Spray with Eucalyptol
    [CAN], 1630–1631
Otrivin Nasal Spray with Moisturizers
    [CAN], 1630–1631
Otrivin Pediatric Nasal Drops, 1630–1631
Otrivin Pediatric Nasal Spray, 1630–1631
Otrivin With M-D Pump [CAN], 1630–
    1631
Otrivin With Measured-Dose Pump [CAN],
    1630–1631
Otrivin with Moisturizers Measured Dose
    Pump [CAN], 1630–1631
Ovol [CAN], 1436–1437
Ovrette, 1136–1138

oxacillin, 1164–1164, 1223–1225
oxaliplatin, 1165–1167
Oxandrin, 1167–1168
oxandrolone, 1167–1168
oxaprozin, 1169–1170
oxazepam, 1170–1172
oxcarbazepine, 1172–1174
oxiconazole, 1174–1175
Oxis [AUS], 691–693
Oxistat, 1174–1175
Oxizole [CAN], 1174–1175
Oxsoralen, 995–997
Oxsoralen-Ultra, 995–997
Oxy 10 Balance Spot Treatment, 177–178
Oxy 10 Balanced Medicated Face Wash,
    177–178
Oxy Balance, 1413–1415
Oxy Balance Deep Pore, 1413–1415
Oxy [AUS], 177–178
oxybutynin, 1175–1176
oxycodone, 1176–1178
OxyContin, 1176–1178
Oxyderm [CAN], 177–178
Oxydose, 1176–1178
OxyFast, 1176–1178
OxyIR, 1176–1178
oxymetazoline, 1179–1180
oxymetholone, 1180–1182
oxymorphone hydrochloride, 1182–1184
Oxynorm [AUS], 1176–1178
oxytocin, 1185–1186
Oxytrol, 1175–1176

P

Pacerone, 82–85
paclitaxel, 1187–1188
Palafer [CAN], 644–645
palifermin, 1188–1189
Palladone, 773–776
Palmer's Skin Success Acne, 177–178
Palmer's Skin Success Acne Cleanser,
    1413–1415
Palmer's Skin Success Fade Cream,
    777–778
Palmitate A, 1618–1620
palonosetron, 1189–1190
Pamelor, 1138–1140
pamidronate disodium, 1191–1192
Pamine, 997–998
Pamine Forte, 997–998
Pamprin, 1088–1091
Panadol [AUS], 12–14
Panafcort [AUS], 1316–1318
Panamax [AUS], 12–14
Pancof, 764–767

Pancrease [CAN], 1193–1195
Pancrease MT, 1193–1195
Pancreatin, 1193–1195
pancrelipase, 1193–1195
Panglobulin, 801–803
panitumumab, 1195–1196
Panixine, 305–306
PanOxyl, 177–178
PanOxyl Aqua Gel, 177–178
PanOxyl-AQ, 177–178
PanOxylBar, 177–178
Panretin, 47–48
Pantoloc, 1196–1197
pantoprazole, 1196–1197
Parafon Forte DSC, 332–333
Paralgin [AUS], 12–14
Paraplatin, 259–261
paregoric, 1198–1199
paricalcitol, 1199–1201
Pariet [CAN], 1372–1373
Parlodel, 210–212
Parnate, 1565–1567
paromomycin, 1201–1202
paroxetine hydrochloride, 1202–1205
Parvolex [CAN], 18–19
Paser, 81–82
Pataday, 1150–1151
Patanase, 1150–1151
Patanol, 1150–1151
Paxam [AUS], 366–368
Paxeva, 1202–1205
Paxil, 1202–1205
Paxil CR, 1202–1205
PCE, 585–589
PediaCare Long-Acting Cough, 455–457
Pediacare Nighttime, 491–495
Pediaflor, 667
Pediapred, 1314–1316
Pedi-Boro, 63–66
Pedisilk, 1413–1415
pegaspargase, 1205–1206
Pegasys, 1208–1210
pegfilgrastim, 1207–1208
peginterferon alfa-2a, 1208–1210
peginterferon alfa-2b, 1210–1212
PEG-Intron, 1210–1212
Peglyte [CAN], 1295–1296
pegvisomant, 1212–1213
PemADD, 1216–1218
PemADD CT, 1216–1218
pemetrexed, 1213–1215
pemirolast potassium, 1215–1216
pemoline, 1216–1218
penbutolol, 1218–1219
penciclovir triphosphate, 1220–1221

penicillamine, 1221–1223
penicillin, 1223–1225
penicillin G benzathine, 1223–1225, 1225–1227
penicillin G potassium, 1223–1225, 1227–1228
penicillin V potassium, 1223–1225, 1228–1230
Penlac, 339–340
Pentacarinat [CAN], 1230–1232
Pentam-300, 1230–1232
pentamidine isethionate, 1230–1232
Pentasa, 973–974
pentazocine hydrochloride, 1232–1234
pentobarbital, 1234–1237
pentosan polysulfate, 1237–1238
pentostatin, 1238–1240
Pentothal, 1647
pentoxifylline, 1240–1241
Pentoxifylline [CAN], 1240–1241
Pentoxyl, 1240–1241
Pepcid, 628–631
Pepcid AC, 628–631
Pepto-Bismol, 193–195
Peptol [CAN], 343–345
Perdiem, 1354–1355
Perforomist, 691–693
pergolide mesylate, 1242–1243
Pergonal, 963–965
Periactin, 401–403
Peridex, 320–321
Peridol [CAN], 750–752
perindopril, 1243–1244
PerioChip, 320–321
PerioGard, 320–321
Periostat, 523–526
Perisol, 320–321
Permapen, 1225–1227
Permax, 1242–1243
permethrin, 1244–1246
Permitil, 673–674, 674–676
perphenazine, 1246–1247
Persantin [AUS], 496–498
Persantin 100 [AUS], 496–498
Persantin SR [AUS], 496–498
Persantine, 496–498
Pertofran [AUS], 433–435
Pethidine Injection [AUS], 965–967
Pfizerpen, 1227–1228
PGE$_2$. See dinoprostone
Phanasin, 743–744
Pharphylline [NETHERLANDS], 1513–1515
Phazyme, 1436–1437
Phenadoz, 1335–1338
Phenazo [CAN], 1248–1249

phenazopyridine hydrochloride, 1248–1249
Phendiet, 1249–1250
Phendiet-105, 1249–1250
phendimetrazine, 1249–1250
phenelzine sulfate, 1250–1252
Phenergan, 1335–1338
phenobarbital, 1252–1254
Phenobarbitone [AUS], 1234–1237, 1252–1254
Phenoptic, 1259–1262, 1263–1266
phenoxybenzamine, 1254–1256
Phentercot, 1256–1257
phentermine, 1256–1257
phentolamine, 1257–1259
Phenylephrine [NETHERLANDS], 1259–1262, 1263–1266
phenylephrine (systemic), 1259–1262
phenylephrine (topical), 1263–1266
phenylephrine hydrochloride, 1266–1268
phenytoin, 1268–1272
Phenytoin sodium, 1268–1272
Phillips', 504–505
Phillips Milk of Magnesia, 938–942
PHL-Ursodiol C [CAN], 1590–1591
PhosLo, 241–244
phosphorated carbohydrate solution, 1274–1275
Phyllocontin, 79–81
Phylobid [SOUTH AFRICA, INDIA], 1513–1515
Physeptone [AUS], 983–985
physostigmine, 1275–1276
phytonadione, 1277–1278
Pilo-20, 1278–1279
pilocarpine hydrochloride, 1278–1279
Pilopt Eyedrops, 1278–1279
Pima, 1302–1303
pimecrolimus, 1279–1280
pimozide, 1280–1282
pindolol, 1282–1283
Pin-Rid, 1355–1356
Pin-X, 1355–1356
pioglitazone, 1284–1285
piperacillin, 1223–1225, 1285–1287
piperacillin/tazobactam, 1223–1225, 1285–1287
pirbuterol, 1287–1288
Pirohexal-D [AUS], 1289–1290
piroxicam, 1289–1290
Pitocin, 1185–1186
Pitressin, 1605–1607
Pitrex [CAN], 1550–1551
pivampicillin, 1223–1225
pivmecillinam, 1223–1225

Placil [AUS], 364–366
Plan B, 898–900
Plaquenil, 779–781
Plasbumin, 33–34
Platinol-AQ, 350–351
Plavix, 370–371
Plegine, 1249–1250
Plenaxis, 2–4
Plendil, 633–634
Pletal, 342–343
PMS-Amantadine [CAN], 66–68
PMS-Chloral Hydrate [CAN], 315–317
PMS-Ducosate [CAN], 504–505
PMS-Ipratropium [CAN], 836–838
PMS-Isoniazid [CAN], 847–849
PMS-Lactulose [CAN], 874–876
PMS-Lindane [CAN], 907–908
PMS-Mefenamic Acid [CAN], 955–957
PMS-Methylphenidate [CAN], 1006–1008
PMS-Metoprolol [CAN], 1017–1020
PMS-Norfloxacin [CAN], 1135–1136
PMS-Opium & Belladonna [CAN], 169–171
PMS-Pseudoephedrine [CAN], 1352–1354
PMS-Sertraline [CAN], 1428–1430
PMS-Sodium Polystyrene Sulfonate [CAN], 1446–1447
PMS-Sotalol [CAN], 1451–1452
PMS-Temazepam [CAN], 1489–1490
PMS-Timolol [CAN], 1530–1532
PMS-Tobramycin, 1541–1544
PMS-Trazodone [CAN], 1568–1569
PMS-Ursodiol C [CAN], 1590–1591
Pneumotussin, 764–767
Podocon-25, 1292–1293
Pododerm, 1292–1293
podofilox, 1290–1291
podophyllum resin, 1292–1293
polycarbophil, 1294–1295
polyethylene glycol-electrolyte solution, 1295–1296
Polygam S/D, 801–803
poly-L-lactic acid, 1294–1295
Polymox, 94–96
polymyxin B, 1296–1298
polymyxin B sulfate, 1298–1299
Polytrim, 1298–1299
Ponstan [CAN], 955–957
Ponstel, 955–957
Pontocaine, 1505–1508
Pontocaine Niphanoid, 1505–1508
poractant alfa, 1299–1300
Pork, 813–815
posaconazole, 1300–1301

Postinor-2 [ISRAEL, NEW ZEALAND, SINGAPORE], 898–900
potassium acetate, 1303–1306
potassium bicarbonate-citrate, 1303–1306
potassium chloride, 1303–1306
potassium gluconate, 1303–1306
potassium iodide, 1302–1303
potassium phosphates, 1272–1274
potassium salts, 1303–1306
pralidoxime, 1306–1307
Pramin [AUS], 1013–1015
pramipexole, 1307–1309
Pramosome, 1309–1310
Pramox HC [CAN], 1309–1310
pramoxine, 1309–1310
Prandase [CAN], 8–9
Prandin, 1379–1381
Prasig [AUS], 1313–1314
Prasone [TAIWAN], 1309–1310
Pratisol [AUS], 1313–1314
Pravachol, 1310–1311
pravastatin, 1310–1311
Prax, 1309–1310
praziquantel, 1312–1313
prazosin hydrochloride, 1313–1314
Precedex, 447–449
Precose, 8–9
Pred Forte, 1314–1316
Pred Mild, 1314–1316
prednisolone, 1314–1316
prednisone, 1316–1318
Prednisone Intensol, 1316–1318
Prefrin, 1259–1262, 1266–1268
Prefrin [AUSTRIA, ECUADOR, GREECE, HONG KONG, INDONESIA, NEW ZEALAND, SOUTH AFRICA, THAILAND], 1259–1263, 1263–1266
pregabalin, 933–935
Pregnancy categories, FDA, 1666
Prelone, 1314–1316
Prelu-2, 1249–1250
Premarin, 600–602
Premarin Crème [AUS], 600–602
Preparation H Hydrocortisone, 769–773
Prepidil Gel, 489–491
Presolol [AUS], 872–874
Pressin [AUS], 1313–1314
Pressyn [CAN], 1605–1607
Pretz-D, 559–561
Prevacid, 880–882
Prevacid IV, 880–882
Prevacid Solu-Tab, 880–882
Prevalite, 333–335
Prialt, 1638–1639

Priftin, 1394–1395
Prilosec, 1154–1156
Prilosec OTC, 1154–1156
Primacin [AUS], 1319–1320
Primacor, 1035–1036
primaquine, 1319–1320
Primatene Mist, 562–566
Primaxin, 796–798
Primaxin IM, 796–798
primidone, 1320–1321
Primsol, 1581–1582
Principen, 104–106
Prinivil, 912–914
Pritor [AUS], 1488–1489
Privigen, 801–803
Privine, 1087–1088
ProAmatine, 1030–1031
Pro-Banthine, 1339–1340
probenecid, 1321–1323
Probitor [AUS], 1154–1156
procainamide hydrochloride, 1323–1325
procaine, 1326–1328
procarbazine hydrochloride, 1328–1329
Procardia, 1113–1115
Procardia XL, 1113–1115
Pro-C [AUS], 126–128
Prochieve, 1333–1335
prochlorperazine, 1329–1332
Pro-cid [AUS], 1321–1323
Procrit, 568–571
Proctocream, 1309–1310
Proctofoam [US, ENG, GERMANY], 1309–1310
procyclidine, 1332–1333
Procytox [CAN], 395–397
Prodium, 1248–1249
Pro-Fast HS, 1256–1257
Pro-Fast SA, 1256–1257
Pro-Fast SR, 1256–1257
Profilnine, 625–626
progesterone, 1333–1335
Progout [AUS], 49–51
Prograf, 1477–1480
Pro-Lax [CAN], 1295–1296
Proleukin, 37–40, 833–835
Prolixin, 673–674, 674–676
Prolixin Decanoate, 673–674
Proloprim, 1581–1582
promethazine hydrochloride, 1335–1338
Prometrium, 1333–1335
Pronestyl, 1323–1325
Propa pH, 1413–1415
propafenone hydrochloride, 1338–1339
propantheline, 1339–1340
Propanthl [CAN], 1339–1340

Propecia, 650–651
propofol, 1340–1343, 1646
propoxyphene hydrochloride, 1343–1345
propoxyphene napsylate, 1343–1345
propranolol hydrochloride, 1345–1348
Propranolol Intensol, 1345–1348
propylthiouracil, 1348–1349
Propylthiouracil, 1348–1349
Propyl-Thyracil [CAN], 1348–1349
Proscar, 650–651
prostacyclin, 571–573
Prostigmin, 1102–1104
Prostin E2, 489–491
Prostin VR Pediatric, 56–58
protamine sulfate, 1349–1350
Protamine Sulfate, 1349–1350
Protamine [CAN], 1349–1350
Protheo [CHINA], 1513–1515
Protocort, 769–773
Protonix, 1196–1197
Protopam Chloride, 1306–1307
Protopic, 1477–1480
protriptyline, 1351–1352
Protropin, 1449
Proventil, 34–36
Proventil Repetabs, 34–36
Provera, 954–955
Provigil, 1047–1048
Provocholine, 981–982
Proxigel, 256–257
Prozac, 669–671
Prozac Weekly, 669–671
Prudoxin, 517–519
Pryi, 1359–1361
pseudoephedrine, 1352–1354
Psoralen, 995–997
Psorcon-e, 471–472
Psoriatec, 114–115
psyllium, 1354–1355
Pulmicort Flexhaler, 214–216
Pulmicort Respules, 214–216
Pulmicort Turbuhaler, 214–216
Pulmidur [AUSTRIA, GERMANY], 1513–1515
Pulmozyme, 513–514
Pupiletto Forte [INDIA], 1259–1262, 1263–1266
Purge, 271–272
Purinol [CAN], 49–51
P.V. Carpine Liquifilm Ophthalmic Solution [AUS], 1278–1279
P-V Tussin, 764–767
Pyralin EN [AUS], 1467–1469
pyrantel pamoate, 1355–1356
pyrazinamide, 1356–1357

Pyrazinamide, 1356–1357
Pyridium, 1248–1249
pyridostigmine bromide, 1357–1359
pyridoxine hydrochloride, 1359–1361
pyrimethamine, 1361–1362
Pyroxin [AUS], 1359–1361

Q

Q-Dryl, 491–495
Qualaquin, 1371
quazepam, 1363–1364
Quenalin, 491–495
Questran [CAN], 333–335
Questran Lite [AUS], 333–335
quetiapine, 1364–1366
Quibron-T, 1513–1515
Quibron-T SR [US, CANADA, INDONESIA], 1513–1515
Quilonum SR [AUS], 914–916
Quinaglute Dura-Tabs, 1368–1370
quinapril, 1366–1368
Quinate [CAN], 1368–1370
Quinbisu [AUS], 1368–1370
Quinidex Extentabs, 1368–1370
quinidine, 1368–1370
quinine, 1370–1371
Quinoctal [AUS], 1368–1370
Quinsul [AUS], 1368–1370
Quixin, 896–898
Qvar, 165–167

R

rabeprazole, 1372–1373
Rafen [AUS], 788–790
Ralodantin [AUS], 1120–1122
Ralovera [AUS], 954–955
raloxifene, 1373–1375
ramipril, 1375–1377
Rani-2 [AUS], 1377–1379
Ranihexal [AUS], 1377–1379
ranitidine, 1377–1379
Ran-Rabeprazole [CAN], 1372–1373
Rapamune, 1438–1439
Raphon, 562–566
Rapilysin [AUS], 1383–1385
Raptiva, 541–542
Rastinon [AUS], 1546–1547
RatioLactulose [CAN], 874–876
ratio-Ramipril [CAN], 1375–1377
Razadyne, 706–708
Reactine [CAN], 310–311
Rebetol, 1387–1389
Rebif, 827–828, 828–830
Recombinate, 115–116
Rectasol, 1259–1262, 1263–1266

Rectocort, 1309–1310
Rectogesic [AUS], 1123–1126
Redoxon [CAN], 126–128
Reese's Pinworm Caplets, 1355–1356
Reese's Pinworm Medicine, 1355–1356
ReFacto, 115–116
Refenesen, 743–744
Refludan, 884–885
Regaine [AUS], 1039–1041
Regitine, 1257–1259
Reglan, 1013–1015
Regranex, 164–165
Regular Iletin II, 813–815
Regulex [CAN], 504–505
Relafen, 1069–1070
Relagard, 16–17
Relenza, 1636–1637
Relpax, 546–547
Remeron, 1041–1042
Remeron Soltab, 1041–1042
Remicade, 811–813
Remodulin, 1570–1571
Remular, 332–333
Remular-S, 332–333
Renagel, 1430
Renedil [CAN], 633–634
Renitec [AUS], 550–553
Renova, 1571–1573
ReoPro, 4–6
repaglinide, 1379–1381
Replens [CAN], 1294–1295
Reprexain, 764–767
Repronex, 963–965
Requip, 1407–1409
Rescriptor, 430–432
reserpine, 1381–1382
Respax [AUS], 34–36
RespiGam, 1382–1383
respiratory syncytial immune globulin,
    1382–1383
Resprim [AUS], 376–378
Resprim Forte [AUS], 376–378
Restasis, 398–401
Restoril, 1489–1490
Retavase, 1383–1385
reteplase, 1383–1385
Retin-A, 1571–1573
Retin-A Micro, 1571–1573
Retre-Gel, 174–175
Retrovir, 1639–1640
Revatio, 1432–1433
Revex, 1079–1080
ReVia, 1083–1084
Reyataz, 133–135
Rheomacrodex, 451–453

Rheumatrex, 992–994
Rhinalar [CAN], 662–664
Rhinocort Aqua, 214–216
Rhinocort Aqueous [AUS], 214–216
Rhinocort Hayfever [AUS], 214–216
rho (D) immune globulin, 1385–1387
Rhodis [CAN], 866–868
RhoGAM, 1385–1387
Rhophylac, 1385–1387
Rhotral [CAN], 10–12
Rhotrimine [CAN], 1583–1584
Rhoxal-orphenadrine [CAN],
    1161–1162
RibaPak, 1387–1389
Ribasphere, 1387–1389
ribavirin, 1387–1389
RID Spray, 1244–1246
Ridaura, 143–145
rifabutin, 1390–1391
Rifadin, 1391–1393
rifampin, 1391–1393
rifapentine, 1394–1395
rifaximin, 1395–1396
Rilutek, 1396–1397
riluzole, 1396–1397
Rimactane, 1391–1393
rimantadine, 1397–1398
Rimycin [AUS], 1391–1393
Riomet, 978–981
Riopan Plus, 937–938
Riphenidate [CAN], 1006–1008
risedronate, 1398–1399
Risperdal, 1399–1402
Risperdal Consta, 1399–1402
Risperdal M-Tabs, 1399–1402
risperidone, 1399–1402
Ritalin, 1006–1008
Ritalin LA, 1006–1008
Ritalin SR, 1006–1008
ritonavir, 1402–1404
Rituxan, 1404–1405
rituximab, 1404–1405
Rivotril [CAN], 366–368
rizatriptan, 1406–1407
RMS, 1057–1061
Robafen, 455–457
Robaxin, 991–992
Robidone [CAN], 768–769
Robidrine [CAN], 1352–1354
Robinul, 733–735
Robinul Forte, 733–735
Robinul Injection [AUS], 733–735
Robitussin, 743–744
Robitussin CoughGels, 455–457
Robitussin Honey Cough, 455–457

Robitussin Maximum Strength Cough, 455–457
Robitussin Pediatric Cough, 455–457
Robitussion [AUS], 455–457
Rocaltrol Vectical, 240–241
Rocephin, 300–302
Rodex, 1359–1361
Rofact [CAN], 1391–1393
Roferon-A, 817–819, 819–822
Rogaine, 1039–1041
Rogaine Extra Strength, 1039–1041
Romazicon, 660–662
ropinirole, 1407–1409
Rosig [AUS], 1289–1290
Rosig-D [AUS], 1289–1290
rosiglitazone, 1409–1410
rosuvastatin, 1411–1412
Rowasa, 973–974
Roxanol, 1057–1061
Roxicodone, 1176–1178
Roxicodone Intensol, 1176–1178
Roxin [AUS], 1135–1136
Rozex [AUS], 1020–1023
Rynacrom [AUS], 389–391
Rythmodan [CAN], 498–500
Rythmol, 1338–1339
Rythmol SR, 1338–1339

S
S2, 562–566
SalAc, 1413–1415
Salac, 1413–1415
Sal-Acid, 1413–1415
Salactic, 1413–1415
Salagen, 1278–1279
Salazopyrin [CAN], 1467–1469
Salazopyrin EN [AUS], 1467–1469
Salazopyrin EN-Tabs [CAN], 1467–1469
salicylic acid, 1413–1415
SalineX, 1442–1443
salmeterol, 1416–1417
Salofalk [CAN], 973–974
Sal-Plant, 1413–1415
Sanctura, 1587–1588
Sandimmune, 398–401
Sandimmune Neoral [AUS], 398–401
Sandoglobulin [AUS], 801–803
Sandostatin, 1142–1143
Sandostatin LAR, 1142–1143
Sandoz-Ramipril [CAN], 1375–1377
Sandrena Gel [AUS], 596–600
Sani-Supp, 731–733
saquinavir, 1417–1419
Sarafem, 669–671
sargramostim, 1419–1421

Scheinpharm Desonide [CAN], 439–440
Sclerosal, 1481–1482
Scopace, 1421–1422
scopolamine, 1421–1422
Scot-tussin, 743–744
Scot-Tussin Diabetes CF, 455–457
SeaMist, 1442–1443
Seba-Gel, 177–178
Sebizole [AUS], 864–866
secobarbital, 1422–1423
Seconal, 1422–1423
Sectral, 10–12
Selax [CAN], 504–505
selegiline, 1424–1425
Selgene [AUS], 1424–1425
Semi-Daonil [AUS], 729–731
Semi-Euglucon [AUS], 729–731
Senexon, 1426–1427
senna, 1426–1427
Senna-Glen, 1426–1427
Sennatural, 1426–1427
Senokot, 1426–1427
Sensipar, 346–347
Sensorcaine, 218–222
Sensorcaine-MPF, 218–222
Septra, 376–378
Septra DS, 376–378
Septrin [AUS], 376–378
Septrin Forte [AUS], 376–378
Serax, 1170–1172
Serenace [AUS], 750–752
Serepax [AUS], 1170–1172
Serevent Diskus, 1416–1417
Serevent Inhaler and Disks [AUS], 1416–1417
Seromycin, 397–398
Serophene, 363–364
Serophene [CAN], 363–364
Seroquel, 1364–1366
Seroquel XR, 1364–1366
Serpasil [CAN, INDONESIA], 1381–1382
Serpasol [SPAIN], 1381–1382
sertaconazole, 1427–1428
sertraline, 1428–1430
Serzone, 1097–1099
Setamol [AUS], 12–14
sevelamer, 1430
sibutramine, 1431–1432
Sigmaxin [AUS], 474–478
Sigmetadine [AUS], 343–345
Silace, 504–505
Siladryl, 491–495
sildenafil, 1432–1433
Silphen, 491–495
Silphen DM, 455–457

Siltussin, 743–744
Silvadene, 1434–1436
silver nitrate, 1433–1434
silver sulfadiazine, 1434–1436
simethicone, 1436–1437
Simulect, 161–163
simvastatin, 1437–1438
Sinemet, 257–259
Sinemet CR, 257–259
Sinex 12-Hour Long-Acting, 1179–1180
Singulair, 1054–1056
Siquent Hycor [AUS], 769–773
sirolimus, 1438–1439
Skelaxin, 977–978
Skelid, 1529–1530
Slo-Bid Gyrocaps, 1513–1515
Slo-Niacin, 1107–1108
Slo-Salt, 1442–1443
Slo-Theo [HONG KONG], 1513–1515
Slow-Fe, 644–645
Slow-K [AUS], 1303–1306
Slow-Mag, 938–942
sodium bicarbonate, 1439–1442
sodium chloride, 1442–1443
sodium ferric gluconate complex,
    1443–1445
sodium oxybate, 1445–1446
sodium polystyrene sulfonate, 1446–1447
Sodium Sulamyd, 1466–1467
Soflax [CAN], 504–505
Solaquin, 777–778
Solaquin Forte, 777–778
Solaraze, 461–464
Solarcaine, 174–175
Solavert [AUS], 1451–1452
Solganal, 145–147
solifenacin, 1448–1449
Solone [AUS], 1314–1316
Solosin [GERMANY], 1513–1515
Solprin [AUS], 130–133
Solu-Cortef, 769–773
Solugel [CAN], 177–178
Solu-Medrol, 1008–1011
Soma, 263–264
Somac [AUS], 1196–1197
somatrem, 1449
Somavert, 1212–1213
Sominex, 491–495
Somnote, 315–317
Somofillina [ITALY], 1513–1515
Sonata, 1635–1636
Sone [AUS], 1316–1318
Sorbidin [AUS], 851–853
sorbitol, 1450
Soriatane, 19–21

Sorine, 1451–1452
Sotab [AUS], 1451–1452
Sotacor [AUS], 1451–1452
Sotahexal [AUS], 1451–1452
sotalol, 1451–1452
Sotret, 853–854
Spacol, 167–169, 784–786
Spacol T/S, 784–786
Spanish-English drug phrases translator,
    1648–1665
Span-K [AUS], 1303–1306
Spasmolin, 167–169
Spasquid, 167–169
Spectazole, 537
Spectinomycin, 1453
Spectracef, 280–281
Spiractin [AUS], 1454–1456
Spiriva, 1537–1538
spironolactone, 1454–1456
Sporanox, 856–859
Spren [AUS], 130–133
Sprycel, 423–424
SPS, 1446–1447
Squibb HC [AUS], 769–773
SSD, 1434–1436
SSD AF, 1434–1436
SSKI, 1302–1303
Stadol, 231–233
Stadol NS, 231–233
Stagesic, 764–767
Stamoc [CAN], 1635–1636
stanozolol, 1456–1457
Starlix, 1095–1096
Statex [CAN], 1057–1061
stavudine, 1457–1459
Stavzor, 1595–1597
Stelax [AUS], 159–160
Stemetil [CAN], 1329–1332
Stemzine, 1329–1332
Sterapred, 1316–1318
Sterapred DS, 1316–1318
Stilnox [AUS], 1645
Stimate, 437–439
Stocrin [AUS], 543–545
Strattera, 137–139
Strepfen [AUS], 679–680
Streptase, 1459–1461
streptokinase, 1459–1461
streptomycin, 1461–1462
Striant, 1502–1505
Stri-dex, 1413–1415
Stri-dex Body Focus, 1413–1415
Stri-dex Facewipes To Go, 1413–1415
Stri-dex Maximum Strength, 1413–1415
Stromectol, 859–860

Sublimaze, 638–643
Subutex, 222–223
succimer, 1462–1463
sucralfate, 1463–1464
Sudafed, 1352–1354
Sudafed 12 Hour, 1352–1354
Sudafed 24 Hour, 1352–1354
Sudafed 12hr [AUS], 1352–1354
Sular, 1118–1119
sulfabenzamide/sulfacetamide/
    sulfathiazole, 1465
sulfacetamide, 1465, 1466–1467
Sulfair, 1466–1467
sulfamethoxazole/trimethoprim, 376–378
Sulfamylon, 936–937
sulfasalazine, 1467–1469
Sulfatrim Pediatric, 376–378
sulfinpyrazone, 1469–1470
sulfisoxazole, 1470–1471
Sulfizole [CAN], 1470–1471
Sulfolax, 504–505
sulindac, 1472–1473
sumatriptan, 1473–1475
Sumycin, 1508–1509
Sunspot Cream [AUS], 1413–1415
Supartz, 759–760
Suprax, 283–285
Surmontil, 1583–1584
Survanta, 180–181
Sustiva, 543–545
Suvalan [AUS], 1473–1475
Symax SL, 784–786
Symax SR, 784–786
Symmetrel, 66–68
SymTan, 764–767
Synalar, 664–665
Synarel, 1073–1074
Synthroid, 902–904
Syntocinon INJ [AUS], 1185–1186
Synvisc Injection, 759–760
Syprine, 1576–1577

T
tacrine, 1476–1477
tacrolimus, 1477–1480
tadalafil, 1480–1481
Tagamet, 343–345
Tagamet HB, 343–345
Talacen, 1232–1234
talc powder, sterile, 1481–1482
Talwin, 1232–1234
Talwin Compound, 1232–1234
Talwin NX, 1232–1234
Tambocor, 653–654
Tamiflu, 1162–1164

Tamofen [CAN], 1482–1484
Tamosin [AUS], 1482–1484
tamoxifen, 1482–1484
tamsulosin, 1484–1485
Tapazole, 989–991
Tarceva, 581–582
Targretin, 188–190
Taro-Desoximetason [CAN], 440–441
Taro-Warfarin [CAN], 1627–1629
Tasmar, 1547–1549
Tavist Allergy, 355–356
Tavist ND, 922–923
Taxol, 1187–1188
Tazac [AUS], 1129–1130
tazarotene, 1485–1486
Tazicef, 294–296
Tazidime, 294–296
Tazocin [CAN], 1285–1287
Tazorac, 1485–1486
Taztia XT, 482–486
T-Diet, 1256–1257
Tebrazid [CAN], 1356–1357
Tegretol, 254–256
Tegretol CR [AUS], 254–256
Tegretol XR, 254–256
Tekturna, 46–47
Telfast [AUS], 646–647
telithromycin, 1486–1487
telmisartan, 1488–1489
temazepam, 1489–1490
Temgesic [CAN], 222–223
Temodal [AUS], 1490–1492
Temodar, 1490–1492
Temovate, 360–361
temozolomide, 1490–1492
Tempra, 12–14
tenecteplase, 1492–1493
Tenex, 746–747
teniposide, 1493–1495
tenofovir, 1495–1496
Tenolin [CAN], 135–137
Tenopt [AUS], 1530–1532
Tenormin, 135–137
Tensig [AUS], 135–137
Teobid [COLOMBIA], 1513–1515
Teoclear [KOREA], 1513–1515
Teoclear LA [ARGENTINA], 1513–1515
Teofilina Retard [COLOMBIA],
    1513–1515
Teolixir [SPAIN], 1513–1515
Teolong [MEXICO], 1513–1515
Teosona [ARGENTINA], 1513–1515
Teramine, 1256–1257
Terazol [CAN], 1500–1501
Terazol 3, 1500–1501

Terazol 7, 1500–1501
terazosin, 1496–1497
terbinafine, 1497–1499
terbutaline, 1499–1500
terconazole, 1500–1501
Teril [AUS], 254–256
teriparatide, 1501–1502
Tertroxin [AUS], 910–912
Tessalon Perles, 176
Testim, 1502–1505
Testoderm, 1502–1505
Testoprel, 1502–1505
testosterone, 1502–1505
Testred, 1011–1012
tetracaine, 1505–1508
tetracycline, 1508–1509
tetrahydrozoline hydrochloride,
    1510–1511
Tetrex [AUS], 1508–1509
Teveten, 573–574
thalidomide, 1511–1512
Thalitone, 331–332
Thalomid, 1511–1512
Theo PA [INDIA], 1513–1515
Theo von CT [GERMANY], 1513–1515
Theo-2 [BELGIUM], 1513–1515
Theo-24, 1513–1515
Theo-Bros [GREECE], 1513–1515
Theochron, 1513–1515
Theo-Dur, 1513–1515
Theolair, 1513–1515
Theolair S [PERU], 1513–1515
Theolair SR, 1513–1515
Theolan [KOREA, TAIWAN], 1513–1515
Theolin [SINGAPORE], 1513–1515
Theolin SR [SINGAPORE], 1513–1515
Theolong [JAPAN], 1513–1515
Theomax [SPAIN], 1513–1515
Theon [SWITZERLAND], 1513–1515
theophylline, 1513–1515
Theoplus Retard [AUSTRIA, GREECE],
    1513–1515
Theoplus [BULGARIA, SINGAPORE, SPAIN],
    1513–1515
Theospirex Retard [AUSTRIA, SWITZERLAND],
    1513–1515
Theostat LP [FRANCE], 1513–1515
Theotard [ISRAEL], 1513–1515
Theo-Time, 1513–1515
Theotrim [ISRAEL], 1513–1515
Theovent LA [HONG KONG], 1513–1515
TheraCys, 163–164
thiabendazole, 1516–1517
Thiamilate, 1517–1518
thiamine, 1517–1518

Thiola, 1536–1537
Thiopental, 1647
Thioprine [AUS], 149–150
thioridazine, 1519–1520
Thioridazine Intensol, 1519–1520
thiothixene, 1520–1521
Thorazine, 327–329
3TC, 876–877
Thyro-Block [CAN], 1302–1303
thyroid, 1522–1523
tiagabine, 1523–1524
Tiazac, 482–486
Ticar, 1524–1526
ticarcillin, 1223–1225, 1524–1526
*ticarcillin disodium/clavulanate
    potassium,* 1526–1528
ticarcillin/clavulanate, 1223–1225
Tice BCG, 163–164
Ticlid, 1528–1529
ticlopidine, 1528–1529
Tigan, 1580–1581
Tikosyn, 505–507
Tilodene [AUS], 1529–1530
tiludronate, 1528–1529
Timentin, 1526–1528
timolol, 1530–1532
Timoptic, 1530–1532
Timoptic OccuDose, 1530–1532
Timoptic XE, 1530–1532
Timoptol XE [AUS], 1530–1532
Timoptol [AUS], 1530–1532
Tinactin Antifungal, 1550–1551
Tinactin Antifungal Jock Itch, 1550–1551
Tinaderm, 1550–1551
Tinamed, 1413–1415
Tindamax, 1532–1534
Ting, 1550–1551
tinidazole, 1532–1534
tinzaparin, 1534–1535
tioconazole, 1535–1536
Tiodilax [ARGENTINA], 1513–1515
tiopronin, 1536–1537
tiotropium, 1537–1538
tirofiban, 1539–1540
Tiseb, 1413–1415
Titralac, 241–244
tizanidine, 1540–1541
TNKase, 1492–1493
TOBI, 1541–1544
tobramycin sulfate, 1541–1544
Tobrex, 1541–1544
Tofranil, 798–800
Tofranil-PM, 798–800
tolazamide, 1544–1545
tolbutamide, 1546–1547

tolcapone, 1547–1549
Tolectin, 1549–1550
Tolectin DS, 1549–1550
Tolinase, 1544–1545
tolmetin, 1549–1550
tolnaftate, 1550–1551
Tol-Tab, 1546–1547
tolterodine, 1551–1552
Topace [AUS], 250–252
Topamax, 1553–1554
Topicaine [AUS], 174–175
Topicort, 440–441
Topicort-LP, 440–441
topiramate, 1553–1554
Toposar, 617–621
topotecan, 1554–1556
Toprol XL, 1017–1020
Toradol, 868–871
toremifene, 1556–1557
torsemide, 1558–1560
tositumomab/iodine 131, 1560–1562
T-Phyl, 1513–1515
Tracleer, 202–203
tramadol, 1562–1564
Tramal [AUS], 1562–1564
Tramal SR [AUS], 1562–1564
Trandate, 872–874
trandolapril, 1564–1565
Trans-Derm Scop, 1421–1422
Transderm-V [CAN], 1421–1422
Transiderm Nitro [AUS], 1123–1126
Trans-Ver-Sal, 1413–1415
Tranxene, 371–373
Tranxene SD, 371–373
Tranxene SD Half-Strength, 371–373
tranylcypromine, 1565–1567
trastuzumab, 1567–1568
trazodone, 1568–1569
Trecator, 611–612
Trelstar Depot, 1586–1587
Trelstar LA, 1586–1587
Trental, 1240–1241
treprostinil, 1570–1571
tretinoin, 1571–1573
Trexall, 992–994
Triaminic Long-Acting Cough, 455–457
triamterene, 1573–1575
Triaz, 177–178
Triaz Cleanser, 177–178
triazolam, 1575–1576
Tricor, 634–636
Tricosal, 335–336
trientine, 1576–1577
trifluridine, 1577–1578
Triglide, 634–636

trihexyphenidyl, 1578–1579
Trilafon, 1246–1247
Trileptal, 1172–1174
Trilisate, 335–336
Tri-Luma, 664–665
TriLyte, 1295–1296
trimethobenzamide, 1580–1581
trimethoprim, 376–378, 1581–1582
trimethoprim sulfate, 1298–1299
trimipramine, 1583–1584
Trimox, 94–96
Trinipatch [CAN], 1123–1126
Triostat, 910–912
trioxsalen, 1585–1586
Triptil [CAN], 1351–1352
triptorelin pamoate, 1586–1587
Trisenox, 125–126
Trisilate, 942–943
Trisoralen, 1585–1586
Trivagizole 3, 373–374
Trocaine, 174–175
Tronolane, 1309–1310
trospium, 1587–1588
Trosyd [CAN], 1535–1536
Truxazole, 1470–1471
Truxophyllin, 1513–1515
Tryptanol [AUS], 85–87
T-Tab, 371–373
Tums, 241–244
Tussigon, 764–767
Tussin, 743–744
Tussionex, 764–767
Twinject, 562–566
Tylenol, 12–14
Tylenol Children's Simply Cough,
    455–457
Tyrex [PERU], 1513–1515
Tysabri, 1092–1094
Tyzine, 1510–1511
Tyzine Pediatric, 1510–1511

U
Ulcidine [CAN], 628–631
Ulcyte [AUS], 1463–1464
Ultradol [CAN], 615–617
Ultram, 1562–1564
Ultramop [CAN], 995–997
Ultrase, 1193–1195
Ultravate, 749
Unasyn, 106–108
undecylenic acid, 1589
Unicontin-400 Continus [INDIA],
    1513–1515
Uni-Dur, 1513–1515
Unifyl Retard [SWITZERLAND], 1513–1515

Uniparin [AUS], 753–756
Unipen, 1074–1075
Uniphyl, 1513–1515
Uniphyl CR [KOREA], 1513–1515
Uniphyllin [TAIWAN], 1513–1515
UniphyllinContinus [SOUTH AFRICA], 1513–1515
Unisom Sleepgels [AUS], 491–495
Unithroid, 902–904
Univasc, 1048–1050
Univol [CAN], 63–66
Urasal [CAN], 988–989
Urecholine, 185–186
Uremide [AUS], 702–704
Urex, 988–989
Urex-M [AUS], 702–704
Urispas, 652–653
Uristat, 1248–1249
Urocarb [AUS], 185–186
Uro-KP-Neutral [CAN], 1272–1274
Uro-Mag, 938–942
Uroxatral, 45–46
Urso, 1590–1591
Urso [CAN], 1590–1591
ursodiol, 1590–1591
Uvadex, 995–997

V
Vagifem, 596–600
Vagistat, 1535–1536
VaHaxan [CAN], 1598–1599
valacyclovir, 1592–1593
Valcyte, 1593–1595
valganciclovir, 1593–1595
Valium, 457–461
Valpam [AUS], 457–461
valproate sodium, 1595–1597
valproic acid, 1595–1597
valrubicin, 1598–1599
valsartan, 1599–1600
Valstar, 1598–1599
Valtrex, 1592–1593
Vancocin, 1601–1603
Vancocin CP [AUS], 1601–1603
Vancocin HCL Pulvules [AUS], 1601–1603
vancomycin, 1601–1603
Vaniqa, 545–546
Vantin, 291–293
Vaprisol, 385–386
vardenafil, 1603–1604
varenicline, 1604–1605
Vasocardal CD [AUS], 482–486
Vasocon, 1087–1088
vasopressin, 1605–1607

Vasotate, 16–17
Vasotec, 550–553
Vastin [AUS], 684–685
V-Cillin-K, 1228–1230
Vectavir [SOUTH AFRICA, COSTA RICA, DOMINICAN REPUBLIC, EL SALVADOR, GERMANY, GUATEMALA, HONDURAS, ISRAEL, NICARAGUA, PANAMA], 1220–1221
Vectibix, 1195–1196
Veetids, 1228–1230
Velban, 1613–1614
Velbe [AUS], 1613–1614
Velcade, 200–201
venlafaxine, 1607–1609
Venofer, 843–844
Ventavis, 792–793
Ventolin, 34–36
Ventolin CFC-Free [AUS], 34–36
Veracaps SR [AUS], 1609–1612
Veracolate, 192–193
Verahexal [AUS], 1609–1612
verapamil, 1609–1612
Verdeso, 439–440
Verelan, 1609–1612
Verelan PM, 1609–1612
Vermox, 948–949
Versed, 1028–1030, 1647
verteporfin, 1612–1613
Vesanoid, 1571–1573
VESIcare, 1448–1449
Vfend, 1623–1625
Viadur, 889–891
Viagra, 1432–1433
Vibramycin, 523–526
Vibra-Tabs, 523–526
Vicks 44 Cough Relief, 455–457
Vicodin Tuss, 764–767
Vicodin, 764–767
Vicodin ES, 764–767
Vicodin HP, 764–767
Vicoprin, 764–767
Vicoprofen, 764–767
Vidaza, 147–148
Videx, 467–469
Videx-EC, 467–469
Vigamox, 1061–1062
Vikela [FRANCE], 898–900
vinblastine sulfate, 1613–1614
Vincasar PFS, 1615–1616
vincristine sulfate, 1615–1616
vinorelbine, 1616–1618
Vioform-Hydrocortisone Cream, 359–360
Vioform-Hydrocortisone Mild Cream, 359–360

Vioform-Hydrocortisone Mild Ointment, 359–360
Vioform-Hydrocortisone Ointment, 359–360
Viokase, 1193–1195
Viracept, 1099–1100
Viramune, 1105–1107
Virazole, 1387–1389
Viread, 1495–1496
Virilon, 1011–1012
Virilon IM [CAN], 1502–1505
Viroptic, 1577–1578
Visine, 1510–1511
Visken, 1282–1283
Vistafrin [SPA], 1259–1262, 1263–1266
Vistaril, 782–784
Vistide, 340–342
Vistosan [GER], 1259–1262, 1263–1266
Visudyne, 1612–1613
Vitabee 6, 1359–1361
vitamin A, 1618–1620
vitamin B_1, 1517–1518
vitamin B_3, 1107–1108
vitamin B_6, 1359–1361
vitamin B_{12}, 392–394, 778–779. See cyanocobalamin
vitamin C. See ascorbic acid
vitamin D, 1620–1621
vitamin D_2, 1620–1621
vitamin D_3, 1620–1621
vitamin E, 1622–1623
Vitrasert, 708–712
Vitravene, 689–690
Vitussin, 764–767
Vivactil, 1351–1352
Vivelle Dot, 596–600
Vivitrol, 1083–1084
Vivol [CAN], 457–461
Volmax, 34–36
Voltaren Emulgel [AUS], 461–464
Voltaren Ophthalmic, 461–464
Voltaren Rapid [AUS], 461–464
Voltaren XR, 461–464
voriconazole, 1623–1625
vorinostat, 1625–1626
Vosol, 16–17
VoSpire ER, 34–36
VP-16, 617–621
Vumon, 1493–1495
V.V.S., 1465

W

warfarin sodium, 1627–1629
Wart-Off Maximum Strength, 1413–1415
Welchol, 382–383

Wellbutrin, 223–225
Wellbutrin SR, 223–225
Wellbutrin XL, 223–225
Wellcovorin, 887–889
Wellvone [AUS], 140–141
WestCort, 769–773
Westhroid, 1522–1523
Winpred [CAN], 1316–1318
WinRho SDF, 1385–1387
Winstrol, 1456–1457
Wymox, 94–96
Wytensin, 744–746

X

Xanax, 54–56
Xanax XR, 54–56
Xanthium [SINGAPORE], 1513–1515
Xantivent [SWITZERLAND], 1513–1515
Xeloda, 247–248
Xenical, 1160–1161
Xerac AC, 60–61
Xifaxan, 1395–1396
Xigris, 530–531
Xolair, 1152–1154
Xopenex, 891–892
XPECT, 743–744
Xpect, 764–767
X-Prep, 1426–1427
Xylocaine, 904–907
Xylocaine Aerosol [AUS], 904–907
Xylocaine Ointment [AUS], 904–907
Xylocaine Viscous Topical Solution [AUS], 904–907
Xylocard [CAN], 904–907
xylometazoline, 1630–1631
Xyntha, 115–116
Xyrem, 1445–1446

Y

Yocon, 1632–1633
Yodoxin, 835–836
Yohimbe, 1632–1633
yohimbine, 1632–1633

Z

Zactin [AUS], 669–671
zafirlukast, 1634–1635
zaleplon, 1635–1636
Zanaflex, 1540–1541
zanamivir, 1636–1637
Zantac, 1377–1379
Zantac-75, 1377–1379
Zantac-EFFERdose, 1377–1379
Zantryl, 1256–1257
Zapzyt, 177–178

Zapzyt Acne Wash, 1413–1415
Zapzyt Pore Treatment, 1413–1415
Zaroxolyn, 1015–1017
Zavesca, 1034–1035
Zazole, 1500–1501
Zeasorb AF, 1026–1027
Zebeta, 195–196
Zeffix [AUS], 876–877
Zelapar, 1424–1425
Zemplar, 1199–1201
Zenapax, 407–408
Zerit, 1457–1459
Zestril, 912–914
Zetia, 623–624
Ziagen, 1–2
Zicam Cool Mist Spray, 455–457
ziconotide, 1638–1639
zidovudine, 1639–1640
Zilactin, 174–175
Zilactin Baby, 174–175
Zilactin-L [CAN], 904–907
zileuton, 1640–1641
Zinacef, 303–305
Zinamide [AUS], 1356–1357
zinc oxide, 1641
zinc sulfate, 1641
Zincaps [AUS], 1641
Zinnat [AUS], 303–305
ziprasidone, 1641–1642
Zithromax, 153–155
Zithromax TRI-PAK, 153–155
Zithromax Z-PAK, 153–155
Zocor, 1437–1438
Zofran, 1156–1158
Zofran ODT, 1156–1158

Zoladex, 738–739
Zoladex Implant [AUS], 738–739
Zoladex LA, 738–739
zoledronic acid, 1642–1643
Zolinza, 1625–1626
zolmitriptan, 1644–1645
Zoloft, 1428–1430
zolpidem tartrate, 1645
Zometa, 1642–1643
Zomig, 1642–1643
Zomig Rapimelt [CAN], 1642–1643
Zomig-ZMT, 1642–1643
Zonalon, 517–519
Zone-A, 1309–1310
Zonegran, 1646
zonisamide, 1646
Zostrix, 249–250
Zosyn, 1285–1287
Zoton [AUS], 880–882
Zovirax, 21–24
Zumenon [AUS], 596–600
Zyban, 223–225
Zyban sustained release [AUS], 223–225
Zyclir [AUS], 21–24
Zydol [AUS], 1562–1564
Zydone, 764–767
Zyflo, 1640–1641
Zyloprim, 49–51
Zymar, 712–713
Zyprexa, 1146–1148
Zyprexa Intramuscular, 1146–1148
Zyprexa Zydis, 1146–1148
Zyrtec, 310–311
Zyvox, 908–910
Zyvoxam, 908–910